THE HEART AND CARDIOVASCULAR SYSTEM

Scientific Foundations

THE HEART AND CARDIOVASCULAR SYSTEM

Scientific Foundations

Volume 2

Editors

Harry A. Fozzard, M.D.
The Otho S. A. Sprague Professor of Medical Sciences
The University of Chicago
Chicago, Illinois

Edgar Haber, M.D.
Higgins Professor of Medicine
Harvard Medical School
Chief, Cardiac Unit
Massachusetts General Hospital
Boston, Massachusetts

Robert B. Jennings, M.D.
Professor and Chairman
Department of Pathology
Duke University Medical Center
Durham, North Carolina

Arnold M. Katz, M.D.
Professor of Medicine
Head, Division of Cardiology
The University of Connecticut
School of Medicine
Farmington, Connecticut

Howard E. Morgan, M.D.
Evan Pugh Professor of Physiology
Chairman, Department of Physiology
The Milton S. Hershey Medical Center
Hershey, Pennsylvania

Raven Press 🐦 New York

Raven Press, 1140 Avenue of the Americas, New York, New York 10036

Made in the United States of America

Library of Congress Cataloging-in-Publication Data

The Heart and cardiovascular system.

Includes index.
1. Cardiovascular system.   2. Heart.
3. Cardiology.   I. Fozzard, Harry A. (Harry Allen),
1931–   . [DNLM. 1. Cardiovascular System—
physiology.   2. Heart—physiology.   3. Heart
Diseases. WG 202 H436]
QP102.H397   1986   612.1   86-24775
ISBN 0-88167-126-6

9   8   7   6   5   4   3   2   1

Preface

Cardiovascular medicine today is a rich and powerful tool. Physicians can intervene effectively because of sophisticated and accurate diagnostic methods, specific drugs, reconstructive surgery that requires suspension of cardiovascular function for hours, and knowledge to prevent disease. How did all of this happen?

The first half of this century witnessed an explosion of knowledge in physics, chemistry, and physiology. Such landmark achievements as those of Alexis Carrel in blood vessels, Einthoven with the electrocardiogram, Courand, Richards, and Forssman with the cardiac catheter, all recognized by receiving Nobel prizes, laid the groundwork for this spectacular change in cardiovascular medicine. The mark that they and their physiologist colleagues have made on medical practice surrounds us, because we have translated this science into practical applications in individual lives.

Where will we find the future of cardiovascular medicine? An equivalent explosion of knowledge in biology and biochemistry has followed that in the more physical sciences. We have discovered that cardiovascular science has no definable boundaries, because progress in nerve conduction, carbohydrate metabolism, antibody production, protein structure, and every other area of biological science is of direct importance to progress in cardiovascular medicine. Our opportunities extend even further, embracing engineering, statistics, and psychology. Donald Fredrickson, former Director of the National Institutes of Health, clearly stated the challenge to us when he called upon us to bring this great body of knowledge to medical usefulness in the next half-century.

If there are no boundaries to the sciences important to cardiovascular medicine, how can we cope with our need to know? Here rests the mission of this book. We, the Editors, selected some talented authors to present their views of the problems facing this area of science, the tools we have to study them, and the possible solutions we may achieve. We have made every effort to ignore classical disciplinary boundaries, because we feel they are not relevant to our mission. In this book you will find biochemistry, pathology, molecular biology, physiology, computer science, physics, and anything else that we feel deserves its place in cardiovascular science.

This book will be of value to medical students and graduate students in the biological sciences who want to identify problems in cardiovascular science. We expect trainees in medical specialties and postdoctoral science trainees to draw from the technical discussion the tools they may use in their research. We hope more senior investigators will use it as a source of ideas. For the Editors it has been an exercise in expanding scientific horizons, and we hope it may be as valuable for you.

Inevitably, some areas are treated briefly. We decreased attention to certain areas that we felt were adequately considered by other texts. And we sought to keep the book within bounds of readability by heavy use of reference lists, to guide you to the best sources for more intensive study.

The first part of the book provides background and general information that may be of greater value for the student or the scientist entering a new area. A large section is organized according to methods that are common to broad areas of cardiovascular research, discussed by experts and innovators in these areas. These methods range from recombinant DNA to quantitative angiographic imaging. The second part is a balanced discussion of some central basic research areas and their problems and opportunities. The third part contains consideration of disease states and interventions.

We, the Editors, have a vision of spectacular progress in cardiovascular medicine, based on the rich resources of biological science. We offer this book as a step toward that goal.

Contents

Section II. Cellular Aspects of Cardiac Function

Sarcolemmal Membrane Transport

Excitability

Section III. Pathophysiology and Pharmacology

Hypertrophy and Hypertension

Pharmacologic Intervention

Contributors

Morton F. Arnsdorf *Section of Cardiology, The University of Chicago Hospitals and Clinics, 950 East 59th Street, Chicago, Illinois 60637*

Evelyn L. Ball *The Cellular and Molecular Research Laboratory, Jackson 13, Massachusetts General Hospital, Boston, Massachusetts 02114*

Martha Barlai-Kovach *Radiology Research, Research 5, Massachusetts General Hospital, Boston, Massachusetts 02114*

Dr. Clive M. Baumgarten *Department of Physiology and Biophysics, Medical College of Virginia, Richmond, Virginia 23298*

Dr. J. Thomas Bigger *Departments of Medicine and Pharmacology, Columbia University College of Physicians and Surgeons, 630 West 168th Street, New York, New York 10032*

Dr. Mordecai P. Blaustein *Department of Physiology, University of Maryland School of Medicine, 655 West Baltimore Street, Baltimore, Maryland 21201*

Dr. John R. Blinks *Department of Pharmacology, Mayo Foundation, Rochester, Minnesota 55905*

Charles A. Boucher *Cardiac Unit, Bullfinch 1, Massachusetts General Hospital, Boston, Massachusetts 02114*

Robert C. Bourge *Division of Cardiovascular Disease, Department of Medicine, University of Alabama, Birmingham, Alabama 35294*

Richard W. Briggs *The Milton S. Hershey Medical Center, The Pennsylvania State University, Hershey, Pennsylvania 17933*

Arthur M. Brown *Department of Physiology and Biophysics, University of Texas Medical Branch, Galveston, Texas 77550*

Lawrence Bugaisky *Department of Medicine, The University of Chicago, 950 East 59th Street, Chicago, Illinois 60637*

William J. Bugni *Suncoast Chapter Cardiovascular Research Laboratory, Department of Internal Medicine, University of South Florida, Tampa, Florida 33612*

Robert C. Canby *Cardiac NMR Laboratory, Division of Cardiovascular Disease, Department of Medicine, University of Alabama, Birmingham, Alabama 35294*

O. A. Carretero *Hypertension Research Division, Henry Ford Hospital, 2799 W. Grand Boulevard, Detroit, Michigan 48202*

Balvin H. L. Chua *Department of Physiology, Pennsylvania State University, 500 University Drive, Hershey, Pennsylvania 17033*

I. S. Cohen *Department of Physiology and Biophysics, Health Sciences Center, State University of New York, Stony Brook, New York 11794-8661*

Jay N. Cohn *Cardiovascular Division, Department of Medicine, University of Minnesota Medical School, Minneapolis, Minnesota 55455*

Jackie D. Corbin *Howard Hughes Medical Institute, Vanderbilt University Medical Center, 702 Light Hall, Nashville, Tennessee 37232*

Peter B. Corr *Cardiovascular Division, Washington University School of Medicine, 660 South Euclid Avenue, St. Louis, Missouri 63110*

Robert K. Crane *Department of Physiology and Biophysics, University of Medicine and Dentistry, Rutgers Medical School, P.O. Box 101, Piscataway, New Jersey 08854*

N. B. Datyner *Department of Physiology and Biophysics, Health Sciences Center, State University of New York, Stony Brook, New York 11794-8661*

Harold T. Dodge *Professor of Medicine, Division of Cardiology, University of Washington School of Medicine, Seattle, Washington 98195*

George Dubyak *Assistant Professor, Physiology and Biophysics, Case Western Reserve University School of Medicine, Cleveland, Ohio 44106*

Victor J. Dzau *Division of Vascular Medicine and Atherosclerosis, Brigham and Women's Hospital, Department of Medicine, Harvard Medical School, 75 Francis Street, Boston, MA 02115*

David A. Eisner *Department of Physiology, University College London, Gower Street, London WC1E 6BT, England*

William T. Evanochko *Cardiac NMR Laboratory, Division of Cardiovascular Disease, Department of Medicine, University of Alabama, Birmingham, Alabama 35294*

John T. Fallon *Department of Pathology, Shirners Burn Institute 2, Massachusetts General Hospital, 55 Fruit Street, Boston, Massachusetts 02114*

Barbara B. Farmer *Departments of Medicine and Pharmacology, Krannert Institute of Cardiology, Indiana School of Medicine, Indianapolis, Indiana 42223*

John W. Fleming *Department of Pharmacology and Toxicology, Department of Medicine, Krannert Institute of Cardiology, Indiana University School of Medicine, Indianapolis, Indiana 46223*

Harry A. Fozzard *The Otho S. A. Sprague Professor of Medical Sciences, The University of Chicago, 950 East 59th Street, Chicago, Illinois 60637*

Alan M. Fujii *Department of Pediatrics, Harvard Medical School, Pediatric Cardiology, Children's Hospital, Joint Program in Neonatology, Brigham & Women's Hospital, Boston, Massachusetts 02115*

Leonard S. Gettes *Division of Cardiology, School of Medicine, The University of North Carolina, 349 Clinical Sciences Building, Chapel Hill, North Carolina 27514*

W. R. Gibbons *Department of Physiology and Biophysics, University of Vermont College of Medicine, Burlington, Vermont 05405*

Linda D. Gillam *Assistant Professor of Cardiology, Newington Veterans Administration Center, Newington, Connecticut 06111*

Robert F. Gilmour, Jr. *Associate Professor of Pharmacology and Medicine, Indiana University School of Medicine, 1100 West Michigan Street, Indianapolis, Indiana 46223*

G. A. Gintant *Department of Physiology and Biophysics, Health Sciences Center, State University of New York, Stony Brook, New York 11794-8661*

Herman K. Gold *Cardiac Unit, Massachusetts General Hospital, 55 Fruit Street, Boston, Massachusetts 02114*

Stanley M. Goldin   *Associate Professor and Director, Pharmacological Sciences Training Program, Department of Pharmacology, Harvard Medical School, Boston, Massachusetts 02115*

Ellen E. Gordon   *Department of Internal Medicine, University of Iowa Hospitals & Clinics, Iowa City, Iowa 52442*

Robert M. Graham   *Cellular and Molecular Research Laboratory, Cardiac Unit, Massachusetts General Hospital, Harvard Medical School, Boston, Massachusetts 02114*

Frank J. Green   *Department of Medicine, Department of Pharmacology, Krannert Institute of Cardiology, Indiana University School of Medicine, Indianapolis, Indiana 46223*

Robert B. Gunn   *Department of Physiology, Emory University School of Medicine, Atlanta, Georgia 30322*

Edgar Haber   *Higgins Professor of Medicine, Harvard Medical School, Chief, Cardiac Unit, Massachusetts General Hospital, Boston, Massachusetts 02114*

Burt B. Hamrell   *Department of Physiology and Biophysics, College of Medicine, University of Vermont, Burlington, Vermont 05405*

Leo G. Herbette   *Department of Medicine, University of Connecticut Health Center, Farmington, Connecticut 06032*

Edward W. Holmes   *Professor of Medicine, Assistant Professor of Biochemistry, Duke University Medical Center, Durham, North Carolina 27710*

Charles J. Homcy   *Massachusetts General Hospital, New England Regional Primate Research, 1 Pine Hill Drive, Southborough, Massachusetts 01772*

Jose Icardo   *Department of Anatomy, University of Santander, Santander, Spain*

Smilja Jakovcic   *Department of Medicine, The University of Chicago, 950 E. 59th Street, Chicago, Illinois 60637*

Joseph S. Janicki   *Division of Cardiology, Michael Reese Hospital, University of Chicago, Chicago, Illinois 60616*

Michael J. Janse   *Department of Cardiology and Experimental Cardiology, University of Amsterdam, Academisch Medisch Centrum Interuniversity Cardiology Institute, Amsterdam, The Netherlands*

Robert B. Jennings   *Department of Pathology, Duke University Medical Center, Durham, North Carolina 27710*

Larry R. Jones   *Krannert Institute of Cardiology, Departments of Medicine and Pharmacology, Indiana University School of Medicine, Indianapolis, Indiana 46202*

Arnold M. Katz   *Cardiology Division, Department of Medicine, University of Connecticut, Farmington, Connecticut 06032*

Ban An Khaw   *Cellular and Molecular Research Laboratory, Cardiac Unit, Massachusetts General Hospital, Harvard Medical School, Boston, Massachusetts 02114*

R. P. Kline   *Department of Pharmacology, Columbia College of Physicians and Surgeons, 630 W. 168th Street, New York, New York 10032*

Edward G. Lakatta   *Cardiovascular Section, Clinical Physiology Branch, Gerontology Research Center, National Institute on Aging, National Institutes of Health, Baltimore, Maryland 21224*

Stephen M. Lanier   *Cellular and Molecular Research Laboratory, Cardiac Unit, Massachusetts General Hospital, Harvard Medical School, Boston, Massachusetts 02114*

Robert C. Leinbach   *Cardiac Unit, Massachusetts General Hospital, Boston, Massachusetts 02114*

Robert A. Levine   *Cardiac Ultrasound, Massachusetts General Hospital, Boston, Massachusetts 02114*

Peter J. Longabaugh   *Cellular and Molecular Research Laboratory, Massachusetts General Hospital, Boston, Massachusetts 02114*

Francis J. Manasek   *Department of Anatomy, Department of Pediatrics, The Committee on Developmental Biology, The University of Chicago, Chicago, Illinois 60637*

Chellakere K. Manjunath   *Department of Medicine, The University of Chicago, 5841 South Maryland Avenue, Chicago, Illinois 60637*

Eduardo Marban   *Division of Cardiology, Department of Medicine, The Johns Hopkins Hospital, Baltimore, Maryland 21205*

Gary R. Matsueda   *The Cellular and Molecular Research Laboratory, Massachusetts General Hospital, Boston, Massachusetts 02114*

Jacques Merab   *Department of Medicine, Columbia University College of Physicians and Surgeons, Presbyterian Hospital, 630 W. 168th Street, New York, New York 10032*

Howard E. Morgan   *Department of Physiology, Pennsylvania State University, 500 University Drive, Hershey, Pennsylvania 17033*

Meredith Mudgett-Hunter   *Cellular and Molecular Research Laboratory, Massachusetts General Hospital, Boston, Massachusetts 02114*

Atsuyo Najamura   *Department of Anatomy, University of Chicago, Chicago, Illinois 60637*

A. Nasjletti   *Department of Pharmacology, University of Tennessee, 874 Union Avenue, Memphis, Tennessee 38163*

Eva J. Neer   *Department of Medicine, Brigham and Women's Hospital, Harvard Medical School, Boston, Massachusetts 02114*

Jiří Novotný   *Massachusetts General Hospital, 55 Fruit Street, Boston, Massachusetts 02114*

Robert Okada   *Cardiology of Tulsa Incorporated, 6585 South Yale, 800 William Medical Building, Tulsa, Oklahoma 74136*

R. A. Olsson   *Suncoast Chapter Cardiovascular Research Laboratory, Department of Internal Medicine, University of South Florida, Tampa, Florida 33612*

Ernest Page   *Department of Medicine, University of Chicago, 5841 South Maryland Avenue, Chicago, Illinois 60637*

Gerald M. Pohost   *Cardiac NMR Laboratory, Division of Cardiovascular Disease, Department of Medicine, University of Alabama, Birmingham, Alabama 35294*

James D. Potter   *Department of Pharmacology, P.O. Box 016189, University of Miami School of Medicine, Miami, Florida 33101*

S. F. Rabito   *Hypertension Research Division, Henry Ford Hospital, 2799 W. Grand Boulevard, Detroit, Michigan 48202*

Keith A. Reimer *Department of Pathology, Box 3712, Duke University Medical Center, Durham, North Carolina 27710*

R. J. Ridge *Creative Biomolecules, 35 South Street, Hopkinton, Massachusetts 01748*

Alison M. Robinson-Steiner *Howard Hughes Medical Institute, Vanderbilt University, Nashville, Tennessee 37232*

Linda M. Rolnitzky *Department of Medicine, Division of Cardiology, Columbia College of Physicians and Surgeons, 630 W. 168th Street, New York, New York 10032*

Michael R. Rosen *Professor of Pharmacology, Professor of Pediatrics, Columbia College of Physicians and Surgeons, 630 W. 168th Street, New York, New York 10032*

Louise Russo *Department of Physiology, The Pennsylvania State University, Hershey, Pennsylvania 17033*

Antonio Scarpa *Professor and Chairman, Department of Physiology and Biophysics, Case Western Reserve University School of Medicine, Cleveland, Ohio 44106*

Kurt Schwarz *Bleerstr. 57, 4019 Monheim, Federal Republic of Germany*

A. G. Scicli *Hypertension Research Division, Henry Ford Hospital, 2799 W. Grand Boulevard, Detroit, Michigan 48202*

Nisar A. Shaikh *Department of Medicine and Clinical Biochemistry, Clinical Science Division, Medical Science Building, University of Toronto, Toronto, Ontario M5S 1A8, Canada*

Florence H. Sheehan *Department of Medicine, Division of Cardiology, University of Washington School of Medicine, Seattle, Washington 98195*

John T. Shepherd *Department of Physiology and Biophysics, Mayo Medical School, Rochester, Minnesota 55905*

Shey-Shing Sheu *Departments of Pharmacology and Physiology, University of Rochester School of Medicine and Dentistry, 601 Elmwood Avenue, Rochester, New York 14642*

Sanjeev G. Shroff *Division of Cardiology, Michael Reese Hospital, University of Chicago, Chicago, Illinois 60616*

Vivienne-Elizabeth Smith *Cardiology Division, Department of Medicine, University of Connecticut, Farmington, Connecticut 06032*

Andrew P. Somlyo *Pennsylvania Muscle Institute, University of Pennsylvania, School of Medicine, B42 Anatomy-Chemistry, Philadelphia, Pennsylvania 19104*

Avril Somlyo *Pennsylvania Muscle Institute, University of Pennsylvania, School of Medicine, B42 Anatomy-Chemistry, Philadelphia, Pennsylvania 19104*

Joachim R. Sommer *Duke University and Veterans Administration Medical Center, 2500 Erwin Road, Durham, North Carolina 27710*

Edmund H. Sonnenblick *Department of Medicine, Albert Einstein College of Medicine, 1300 Morris Park Avenue, Bronx, New York 10461*

C. Frank Starmer *Departments of Medicine and Computer Science, Duke University Medical Center, Durham, North Carolina 27710*

H. William Strauss *Department of Radiology, Massachusetts General Hospital, Boston, Massachusetts 02114*

John E. Strobeck *Cardiac Care, Valley Hospital, Ridgewood, New Jersey 07451*

Judith L. Swain *Assistant Professor, Medicine and Physiology, Duke University Medical Center, Durham, North Carolina 27710*

Lauren Sweeney *Department of Anatomy, Department of Pediatrics, The University of Chicago, Chicago, Illinois 60637*

Hitoshi Takenaka *Department of Hygiene, Miyazaki Medical College, Miyazaki 889-16, Japan*

Edwin W. Taylor *Department of Molecular Genetics, The University of Chicago, Chicago, Illinois 60637*

Patrick K. Umeda *Department of Medicine, The University of Chicago, 950 E. 59th Street, Chicago, Illinois 60637*

Dorothy E. Vatner *New England Regional Primate Research Center, 1 Pine Hill Drive, Southborough, Massachusetts 01772*

Stephen F. Vatner *New England Regional Primate Center, 1 Pine Hill Drive, Southborough, Massachusetts 01772*

John L. Walker *Department of Physiology, University of Utah, Salt Lake City, Utah 84132*

K. D. Warber *Department of Pharmacology, University of Miami School of Medicine, P.O. Box 016189, Miami, Florida 33101*

August M. Watanbe *Departments of Medicine and Pharmacology, The Krannert Institute of Cardiology, Indiana University School of Medicine, Indianapolis, Indiana 46223*

James Watras *Cardiology Division, Department of Medicine, University of Connecticut, Farmington, Connecticut 06032*

Peter A. Watson *Department of Physiology, The Pennsylvania State University, Hershey, Pennsylvania 17033*

Karl T. Weber *Division of Cardiology, Michael Reese Hospital, University of Chicago, Chicago, Illinois 60616*

Myron L. Weisfeldt *Professor of Medicine, Cardiology Division, Johns Hopkins University Hospital, Blalock 536, Baltimore, Maryland 21205*

Arthur E. Weyman *Associate Professor of Medicine, Director, Non-Invasive Cardiac Laboratory, Massachusetts General Hospital, Boston, Massachusetts 02114*

Lewis T. Williams *Howard Hughes Medical Institute, The University of California, 3rd and Parnassus, San Francisco, California 94143*

Saul Winegrad *Department of Physiology, University of Pennsylvania, Philadelphia, Pennsylvania 19104*

A. L. Wit *Department of Pharmacology and Pediatrics, Columbia College of Physicians and Surgeons, 630 W. 168th Street, New York, New York 10032*

Francis X. Witkowski *Cardiovascular Division, Washington University School of Medicine, 660 South Euclid Avenue, St. Louis, Missouri 63110*

Kathryn A. Yamada *Cardiovascular Division, Washington University School of Medicine, 660 South Euclid Avenue, St. Louis, Missouri 63110*

Tsunehiro Yasuda *Radiology, Massachusetts General Hospital, Boston, Massachusetts 02114*

Atsuko Yatani   *Department of Physiology and Biophysics, University of Texas Medical Branch, Galveston, Texas 77550*

Radovan Zak   *Department of Medicine, Department of Pharmacology and Physiological Sciences, The University of Chicago, Chicago, Illinois 60637*

Douglas P. Zipes   *Professor of Medicine, Indiana University School of Medicine, Krannert Institute of Cardiology, 1100 West Michigan Street, Indianapolis, Indiana 46223*

Randall M. Zusman   *Cardiac Unit, Hypertension Division, Massachusetts General Hospital, Harvard Medical School, Boston, Massachusetts 02114*

THE HEART AND CARDIOVASCULAR SYSTEM

Scientific Foundations

The Heart and Cardiovascular System,
edited by H. A. Fozzard et al.
Raven Press, New York © 1986.

CHAPTER 37

Contractile Proteins and Phosphorylation

Kimbrough D. Warber and James D. Potter

The composition of the contractile units of striated cardiac muscle are virtually identical to that of the more extensively studied voluntary skeletal muscle. Parallel arrays of thick and thin filaments are interdigitated so as to allow energy-coupled "sliding" motions along or between the filaments during contraction and relaxation. A primary focus of research into muscle contraction has been to understand the various molecular events governing the interrelationships between these filaments.

The asymmetric myosin proteins compose the bipolar thick filaments. A single myosin molecule consists of two heavy chains associated as an α-helical coiled-coil "tail," each of which terminates at one end in a globular domain or "head." The two heads occur at the same end of the essentially dimeric myosin molecule. In a given thick filament, each of several dimeric myosin molecules is oriented in such a manner that the myosin tails of each half of the filament all point toward the middle of the filament, thereby orienting the protruding myosin heads in the opposite directions along the filament. The midregion of the filament is bare of the protruding heads. The insolubility of the tail or rod portion of myosin in solutions of ionic strength less than 0.3 (physiologic ionic strength ≈ 0.15) drives the self-assembled aggregation of myosins to form the bipolar thick filaments. Tryptic or chymotryptic digestion of the dimeric myosin yields myosin heavy chain (light meromyosin; LMM) and heavy meromyosin (HMM) (24). The HMM consists of the globular heads (subfragment 1; S1) and a flexible hinge region of the myosin rod (subfragment 2; S2). Either S1 or S2 can be obtained by further digestion of HMM with papain or chymotrypsin, respectively (24). The S1 portion of HMM contains the

myosin ATPase (EC 3.6.1.3) activity, which when activated by actin interaction and with Mg^{2+} as a cofactor, provides the chemical energy for contraction from hydrolysis of ATP to ADP and P_i. This hydrolysis is followed by a coordinated sequential release of P_i and ADP. The mechanism and kinetics of the coupling of energy release and contraction likely involve several intermediate complexes of actin, myosin, ADP, and P_i and are currently subjects of extensive scrutiny and debate (see *Chapter* 38). Also associated with each S1 region of HMM is a pair of complementary light-chain species, LC1 and LC2. The LC2 species is phosphorylatable (46) and is generally referred to as P light chain or P-LC (35,39,43).

C protein is also an integral part of the thick filament of skeletal and cardiac myofibrils (26). This protein is located in the middle one-third of each half of the A band in striated muscle filaments (27). In various muscle types, C proteins have been shown to have differing molecular weights and immunologic properties, but C protein interactions with myosin, actin, and actomyosin appear identical regardless of isoform examined. *In vitro,* C protein can bind to the rod portion of myosin aggregates and to the S2 region of HMM, but not to the S1 portion. This thick-filament protein can also bind to filamentous actin and to myofibrillar thin filaments. In association with myosin aggregates, C protein can inhibit or slightly activate the actin-activated ATPase of the myosin, depending on whether the ionic-strength conditions are very low or near physiologic, respectively (26,45). The binding pattern and the influence of C protein on myosin ATPase are currently used to assay for C-protein function in various preparations of this component. Whereas C protein may primarily contribute to the structural arrangement of the thick filament, its effect on myosin ATPase activity suggests a modulating role as well (14,45).

The thin filament is composed of filamentous actin, tropomyosin, and troponin. Filamentous actin (F actin) is a self-assembled double-stranded helical array of actin monomers (G actin). The precise structure and orientation of G actin in the polymeric state are unknown and are subjects of continuing investigations (e.g., X-ray diffraction, site-specific chemical cross-linking, electron microscopy). Tropomyosin, a coiled-coil helical dimer approximately 40 nm long, is thought to be specifically associated with the actin polymer along the helical grooves of the actin double strand. However, recent preliminary electron microscopic studies of frozen-hydrated preparations suggest that such helical grooves may be nonexistent (11), so that the exact way in which tropomyosin associates with actin remains unresolved. Troponin is a complex of three protein subunits, each of which contributes a distinct property to the functional complex. The nature of the subunits and their interactions will be discussed later. The three thin-filament proteins (actin, tropomyosin, troponin) are associated in a molar ratio of 7:1:1 and together are considered the principal regulatory unit that initiates striated muscle contraction (for review, see ref. 10).

Although the composition of the functional muscle unit (sarcomere) is well established, the biochemical and intermolecular and intramolecular interactions that allow heart muscle cells to adjust their contractile activities to varying hemodynamic demands and hormonal stimuli are not yet well understood. The identification of protein phosphorylation as a control process in myofibrils (for review, see ref. 28) suggests a physiologic means of regulation of the protein interactions in cardiac muscle. Several of the myofibrillar proteins in heart muscle have been shown to exist in a phosphorylated state. These include two subunits of troponin (TnT, TnI, as discussed later), certain of the myosin light chains, tropomyosin, and C protein, all of which can be phosphorylated *in vivo* (1). Monomeric G actin from some skeletal and smooth muscles has recently been found able to be phosphorylated *in vitro* (4) and may exist phosphorylated *in vivo*. The significance of G-actin phosphorylation for F-actin formation and function (and whether or not this can occur in cardiac actin) remains to be elucidated. An intriguing question that has fostered much research is the role, if any, played by any one or any combination of the phosphorylations in altering cardiac muscle function. Equally intriguing is how phosphorylation functions in normal cardiac muscle contraction.

TROPONIN

As mentioned earlier, cardiac troponin (CTn) is a complex of three proteins: TnC, TnI, and TnT. This complex confers Ca^{2+} sensitivity to myofibrillar activation. Calcium is bound by the cardiac TnC subunit (CTnC; MW 18,459), which somehow conveys the "calcium-bound" signal to or through cardiac TnT (CTnT; MW ~ 38,000) and cardiac TnI (CTnI; MW 23,550) (for review, see ref. 33). Cardiac TnT is the tropomyosin-binding subunit through which the CTn complex is strongly associated with thin-filament tropomyosin. Gel-exclusion chromatography indicates that CTnT is a highly asymmetric molecule. In the absence of CTn-bound Ca^{2+} or of the CTnC-CTnT complex, the CTnI subunit inhibits actin activation of myosin ATPase activity; hence, CTnI is termed the inhibitory subunit.

Troponin, which can be obtained by high-salt (1 M KCl) extraction of detergent-treated, ethanol-dehydrated ether powder of cardiac muscle (31), is fractionated to its component subunits by sequential isoelectric and salt precipitations, followed by ion-exchange chromatography. Integrity and purity of the isolated subunits can be determined by sodium dodecyl sulfate polyacrylamide-gel electrophoresis (SDS-PAGE). Whereas whole troponin is soluble at physiologic ionic strength ($\mu \approx 0.15$), in the absence of CTnC the isolated CTnI and CTnT subunits are essentially insoluble except at high ionic strength ($\mu = 0.3$ and 0.5, respectively).

The interactions of the individual subunits of CTn are of prime interest, because Ca^{2+} binding and/or phosphorylation are but single events in an interwoven cascade of changes in the myofibrillar protein interactions that result in contraction. Reconstitution experiments have shown that CTnT interacts primarily with cardiac tropomyosin (CTm); viscosity and sedimentation methods indicate that these proteins associate with a molar stoichiometry of 1:1. Nuclear magnetic resonance (NMR) studies of fragments of cardiac Tm and TnT, along with pH titration of a histidine residue on TnT, suggest a specific interaction between the N-terminal regions of the two proteins in which the intact portion of Tm including residues 1 to 11 is particularly important (5). These data seem to provide a direct measure of a strongly site-specific CTm-CTnT interaction already suggested by the consistent molar stoichiometry of association. CTnT also interacts with the CTnI subunit, but only when two sulfhydryls on CTnI are reduced, also with a 1:1 stoichiometry. The characteristic stoichiometry of the CTnT-CTnI interaction, as determined by gel-exclusion chromatography, suggests that the associations are specific and probably critical in the functional myofibril. It must be noted, however, that these determinations are made at relatively high nonphysiologic ionic strengths because of the insolubility of CTnT and CTnI in the absence of CTnC. Interaction between CTnT and CTnC is weak *in vitro* and quite probably nonspecific, occurring only in the presence of Ca^{2+} and at low ionic strength (32). Indeed, even at saturating ratios of CTnC-CTnT, less than 0.5 mole CTnC per mole CTnT is bound. Extrapolation of these *in vitro* results to the *in vivo* system must be done cautiously, because the summary interactions of the several proteins in the intact myofibril system *in vivo* may involve a specific CTnC-CTnT interaction that only appears weak and nonspecific in the simpler binary complexes of CTnC and CTnT *in vitro*.

On the other hand, CTnC forms a stable stoichiometric 1:1 complex with CTnI, regardless of free Ca^{2+} levels. Studies of interactions using isolated peptide fragments of CTnC (22,41) and studies of chemical reactivity of lysine residues in CTnC during subunit interactions (15) suggest that CTnC contains two identifiable sites that interact specifically with CTnI. Because CTnI likewise contains two sites that interact specifically with CTnC (33), it appears that CTnC and CTnI each contain two sites that direct a specific interaction between the two subunits. Finally, CTnI will bind to cardiac actin or actin-CTm, but not to CTm alone. The actin-specific binding of CTnI in myofibrils inhibits actomyosin ATPase.

Thus, it appears that whole troponin functions as a specifically ordered interaction of CTnT-CTnI-CTnC, depicted schematically in Fig. 1. However, interaction between CTnT and CTnC cannot be ruled out absolutely in the functioning filament. In terms of initiation of contraction events in response to transient increases in free calcium in the myofibril, the interaction between the CTnI-CTnC and actin-CTm complexes is pivotal, as this is likely the single Ca^{2+}-affected interaction leading to activation (disinhibition) of actomyosin ATPase activity.

Because the identifications of specific sequences involved in the interactions between CTnC and CTnI and between CTm and CTnT are based largely on methods of chemical modification or fragmentation of the proteins involved, the results do not necessarily reflect the interactions between these proteins in their native states in the intact muscle. These and similar investigations should be interpreted conservatively. Methods involving minimal or no protein modifications are required for identifying interactive regions or residues to confirm the importance of putatively identified sequences involved in supposed specific interactions between any of the several myofibrillar proteins. For example, monospecific antibodies can be used to localize specific structures (determinants) contained in a particular protein such as actin (36) or egg-white lysozyme (37). By identifying the target structure for which the antibody is specific, it should be possible to probe the interactions involving the target structure or whole protein containing the structure. This has been done in cell receptors for nerve growth factor (7) and among phosphorylase kinase subunits (17) in studies in which the structures being investigated were not directly modified and so presumably interacted in a native fashion, albeit *in vitro*.

In cardiac muscle, TnC has three sites that bind calcium. Two sites that have a high affinity for Ca^{2+}

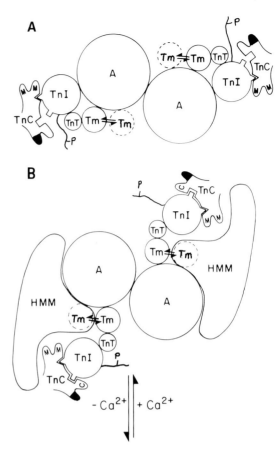

FIG. 1. Model for troponin regulation of cardiac muscle contraction by cardiac troponin. A = actin; Tm = tropomyosin; HMM = heavy meromyosin portion of thick-filament myosin (containing ATPase activity); TnT = tropomyosin-binding subunit of troponin (Tn); TnI = actomyosin-ATPase-inhibitory subunit of Tn; TnC = calcium-binding subunit of Tn; M = Mg^{2+}; C = Ca^{2+}. The darkened area shown in cardiac TnC represents a region structurally analogous to one of two Ca^{2+}-specific sites in skeletal TnC but that does not bind Ca^{2+} in the cardiac subunit (32). Note association of TnT with Tm and TnI throughout. **A:** In the absence of Ca^{2+}, only the Ca^{2+}-Mg^{2+} sites of CTnC contain metal ion (Mg^{2+}), with no metal in the single Ca^{2+}-specific site. TnI is shown to be associated with actin, inhibiting force generation by inhibiting actomyosin ATPase. **B:** With increasing free-Ca^{2+} concentration, contraction is initiated, depending on "dissociation" of CTnI from actin and showing Tm as pivotal for the overall vicinity of CTn and actin in regulatory interplay. The disinhibition results from occupation of the Ca^{2+}-specific site by Ca^{2+}, movement of Tm away from its "blocking" position on actin, and HMM association with actin. Not shown is the less likely interaction of CTnC and CTnT. Displacement of Mg^{2+} by Ca^{2+} at the Ca^{2+}-Mg^{2+} sites during pCa-contraction coupling may occur, but not to a significant extent during the time course of normal contraction. The TnI subunit is shown as phosphorylated in the model, though normal contraction events may or may not involve phosphorylation at all times.

($K_{Ca^{2+}} = 1.4 \times 10^7\ M^{-1}$) and also bind Mg^{2+} competitively are termed the Ca^{2+}-Mg^{2+} sites. The third site, called the Ca^{2+}-specific site, binds Ca^{2+} exclusively, but at a lower affinity ($K_{Ca^{2+}} = 2.5 \times 10^5\ M^{-1}$). The values (listed in Table 1) have been measured by indirect

TABLE 1. *Comparison of the Ca^{2+}-binding properties of cardiac muscle TnC, TnC-TnI complex, and Tn*

Protein[a]	MgCl$_2$ concentration (M)	n_1[b] (mol/mol)	K_1[c] (M^{-1})	n_2[d] (mol/mol)	K_2[c,e] (M^{-1})
CTnC	—	2	1.4×10^7	1	2.5×10^5
	4×10^{-3}	2	3.6×10^6	1	2.5×10^5
CTnC-CTnI	—	2	3.2×10^8	1	1×10^6
	4×10^{-3}	2	3.2×10^7	1	1×10^6
CTn	—	2	3.7×10^8	1	2.5×10^6
	4×10^{-3}	2	2.4×10^7	1	2.4×10^6

[a] Cardiac (C) calcium-binding (TnC) and actomyosin-inhibitory (TnI) subunits, and whole troponin (Tn).
[b] For the Ca^{2+}-Mg^{2+} sites.
[c] Values determined by direct binding measurements.
[d] For the Ca^{2+}-specific sites.
[e] Values corroborated by indirect fluoresence-change measurements, using fluorescently labeled CTnC subunit.
Adapted from Potter et al. (32).

(fluorescence-probe changes) and direct (isotope-equilibrium dialysis) binding assays. The Ca^{2+}-specific site is believed to be the Ca^{2+}-binding site that regulates myocardial contraction, because activation of cardiac myofibrillar ATPase occurs over the same range of free-calcium concentrations as does binding to that site. Furthermore, the rapid time course of the activation-contraction-relaxation-activation cycle requires a similarly rapid association-dissociation of Ca^{2+}, which can be met only by the Ca^{2+}-specific site (for review, see ref. 32). Note, too, the effect of complex formation of CTnC with CTnI or in whole CTn on the apparent binding affinities of both classes of sites (Table 1). In both complexes, binding affinity is increased by an order of magnitude.

PHOSPHORYLATION

Phosphorylation of the cardiac contractile proteins is routinely detected, located, and quantified by ^{32}P incorporation under various experimental conditions. Although techniques of radiolabeling are quite sensitive and easily quantified, several considerations must be kept in mind in designing the use of the radiolabel. When radiolabeling is done *in vivo* or in an isolated organ system *in vitro* to be followed by extraction and analysis of the substrate, phosphatase activity must be minimized during extraction, as this enzyme can catalyze nonspecific dephosphorylation that results in loss of labeled substrate. This can be achieved by rapid freezing using liquid nitrogen and/or homogenization in ice-cold trichloroacetic acid (3,43). Conversely, attention must be given to minimize the possibility of phosphorylation by nonspecific activation of protein kinases during preparative manipulations. Here, too, freeze-clamping and tissue processing on ice are effective in minimizing such

artifacts. Protein extractions must eliminate nucleic acids and phospholipids that probably also will be radiolabeled and might contaminate preparations of the target protein. Nucleic acids can be removed by diethylaminoethyl (DEAE)-cellulose chromatography or by digestions of protein extracts with RNase and DNase (21). Either method minimizes loss of labile phosphoprotein components. Acid chloroform-methanol extraction works well to remove phospholipids (2,21), but may incur loss of acid-labile phosphoproteins. Urea/SDS-PAGE has been reported to successfully separate phospholipid contaminants from protein, as well (2). Of course, the most direct evidence of a *bona fide* protein phosphorylation comes with the isolation and identification of the phosphate-bound amino acid residue. Some phosphoryl amino acids are quite labile under conditions of classic chemical (acid) hydrolysis (2). Proteolytic digestion, on the other hand, proceeds under milder conditions favorable to the retention of added phosphoryl groups. Properly done, enzymatic proteolysis can also provide sequencing data at the same time (8,9). It is to be expected that in any system, other than *in vitro* constructs of highly purified and well-characterized component proteins, the proteins are likely already partially phosphorylated before labeling. This inevitably means even the sensitive radiolabel approach will underestimate actual protein phosphorylation. Analytical phosphate assays must therefore be used in conjunction with the radiolabel method whenever practicable. Sensitivities in the micromolar and nanomolar range are available in certain colorimetric assays (16,40).

TROPONIN SUBUNITS

Of the troponin subunits, only CTnI and CTnT have been identified in the phosphorylated form. Comparison of the amino acid sequence of CTnI with that of skeletal TnI shows that the former contains an additional 26 residues at the N terminal not present in STnI. At position 20 of this additional sequence is a serine residue that contains the protein hydroxyl group that accepts phosphate to form phosphoserine during phosphorylation. At physiologic pH, phosphoserine is ionized; hence, the effect of phosphorylation-dephosphorylation of protein serine residues is a change in the net charge of the target protein. The milieu surrounding the serine-20 of CTnI is dominated by basic amino acid residues that provide the cationic environ usually required for phosphorylations by 3':5'-cyclic-adenosine-monophosphate-dependent protein kinase (cAMPdPK) (44). In fact, this serine residue is rapidly converted to phosphoserine by this enzyme *in vitro*. *In situ* in beating rabbit hearts, catecholamine-induced phosphorylation of CTnI occurs exclusively and also quite rapidly at serine-20.

It is important that *in vitro* and *in vivo* phosphorylations be carefully distinguished. Most phosphoproteins were initially described in results of *in vitro* studies of the suitability of the proteins as substrates for various phosphorylation enzyme systems. Often the particular phosphorylation is then sought *in vivo*. For example, *in vitro*, phosphorylase b kinase catalyzes the phosphorylation of cardiac muscle TnI at a serine residue at position 72 and, to a markedly lesser extent, threonine-138, threonine-162, and serine-20 (25). However, extraction of CTnI from whole heart shows only serine-20 to be phosphorylated. Indeed, the serine-20 was significantly phosphorylated before *in vitro* incubation of the subunit with phosphorylase b kinase, indicating that the other sites reported are phosphorylated only by virtue of their exposure in the isolated *in vitro* situation. Even simply complexing CTnI with CTnC *in vitro* significantly blocked the phosphorylase-b-kinase-catalyzed phosphorylation of the other residues listed. The cAMPdPK, which is considered to function physiologically to phosphorylate CTnI, will phosphorylate serine-20 and another serine at position 146, both significantly. Again, however, in the presence of CTnC or as whole CTn, only the serine-20 is actually phosphorylated. Hence, simply because a residue can be phosphorylated *in vitro* does not mean that the residue is phosphorylated, or even accessible to phosphorylation, *in vivo*.

Three principal sites of phosphorylation have been identified in rabbit skeletal TnT. The first site is the N-terminal serine. Phosphorylation of this residue is substantial in STnT from *in vivo* ^{32}P-labeled muscle. Phosphorylation *in vitro* is considerably decreased in the presence of added STnC, as is phosphorylation of the other sites at serine-149(150) and serine-156(157). The difference in extent of phosphorylation indicates that associated STnC does not block STnT serine-1 *in vivo*, though it appears to do so *in vitro*. Involvement of any of the phosphorylations of STnT in skeletal muscle

regulatory interactions is yet to be established. Much less is known about the phosphorylation of CTnT. Still, by strength of analogy and functional homology between CTnT and STnT, phosphorylation similar to that seen in STnT might be expected in CTnT as well. Although part of the phosphate detected in intact cardiac troponin has been putatively associated with the CTnT subunit, no definite results have been forthcoming (1).

MYOSIN LIGHT CHAINS

Research into the location, mechanism, and influence of phosphorylation of the phosphorylatable light chains (P-LC) of myosin has been quite extensive in the past decade. *In vitro* phosphorylation of myosin light chains (MW $\approx$ 18,000–20,000) has been reported in all three muscle types: skeletal, smooth, and cardiac (39). In heart, a specific protein kinase called myosin light-chain kinase (MLCK) is responsible for the phosphorylation of the P-LC. The MLCK is indirectly Ca^{2+}-dependent, as it is activated by Ca^{2+}-calmodulin complex formed when calmodulin binds Ca^{2+} (39,46). Whereas it seems clear that calmodulin, which contains four Ca^{2+}-binding sites, must bind a minimum of three Ca^{2+} per mole in order to activate the calmodulin-sensitive kinase, it is unclear how cooperative that binding might be. Characterization of how the binding of Ca^{2+} to calmodulin results in modulation of enzyme function is currently enjoying extensive attention (6,12,18,20).

The cardiac P-LC appear to be phosphorylated at a serine residue in the N-terminal region of the protein sequence that, similar to the serine-20 region of CTnI, contains the basic amino acid residues that provide the necessary cationic environment for protein kinase activity. It is generally accepted that the P-LC are phosphorylated *in vivo*, but no correlation between the extent of phosphorylation and altered myocardial function has been established. It is difficult to "freeze" a functioning heart in a particular clearly defined state of contraction or relaxation when the heartbeat is rapid (35); even normal heart rates are generally too rapid for manual freezing. The use of hearts from poikilotherms, which can be slowed to 5 to 8 beats per minute while in the cold, has been introduced recently (35). Such a model should permit the heart to be frozen in a discrete contraction state, with the time-course effects of administration of agonists and antagonists more readily controlled. In first reports, a measurable clear difference in the levels of light-chain phosphorylation in systole versus diastole was observed.

Experimentally, another hindrance to definition of a relation between P-LC phosphorylation and myocardial function was suggested by the observation that skeletal muscle myosin became unresponsive to phosphorylation after storage at 0°C for 5 days. Fresh preparations stored on ice no longer than 5 days showed increases in Mg^{2+}-ATPase activity correlated with increases in the phosphate content of P-LC. Myosin stored 7 days had a higher ATPase activity in the absence of P-LC phosphorylation compared with fresher myosin, and the activity did not increase significantly with increasing phosphate content of the myosin P-LC (30). For the cardiac system, sensitivity to preparation and storage may be a critical factor in experimental approaches to modification and functional studies. Such "artificial" influences must be accounted for and avoided, if possible, to gain a truer system for *in vitro* study.

TROPOMYOSIN

Of the α- and β-tropomyosin subunits of skeletal tropomyosin, only α-tropomyosin is found to be phosphorylated *in vivo* (23). The amino acid sequence in the vicinity of the serine-283 residue, which is the phosphorylation site, is unique among the myofibrillar proteins. Indeed, the uniqueness may be why neither phosphorylase b kinase nor cAMPdPK is able to phosphorylate α-tropomyosin *in vitro*. The reason for the selective phosphorylation of α-tropomyosin *in vivo*, while β-tropomyosin is not phosphorylated, despite the high degree of sequence homology between the two, is unknown. The minor sequence differences that have been described imply a remarkably subtle degree of fine specificity of substrate recognition. The enzyme responsible for the α-component-specific phosphorylation is certainly a fascinating problem in itself, its possible relation to myocardial function notwithstanding. Though the preceding description is based on studies of frog skeletal muscle, similar phosphoryl amino acid assays have identified an identical phosphorylated peptide from the cardiac tropomyosin in rabbits (1).

C PROTEIN

Little is known of the primary structure or phosphorylation site(s) of cardiac C protein, partly because of the fact that this protein was originally identified as a contaminant of myosin preparations (26). It is known, however, that C protein is phosphorylated *in situ* in isolated perfused heart, particularly in response to norepinephrine. Conversely, administration of acetylcholine leads to dephosphorylation of phosphoryl cardiac C protein (14). As mentioned earlier, the considerable heterogeneity of the various isoforms of C protein in different muscles is in contrast with the strong similarity of binding properties and effects on ATPase activity so far described among the isoforms of the protein. Definition of the relation between structure and function for each of the isoforms is certainly necessary for further clarification of the role of C protein in cardiac contractility.

FUNCTIONAL SIGNIFICANCE OF PHOSPHORYLATION

Myosin Light-Chain Phosphorylation

Whereas a strong correlation has been reported for skeletal (3,30) or smooth muscle (13) light-chain phosphorylation and contraction, reflecting perhaps a mechanism of increasing actin-myosin interaction, no such relation has been unequivocally demonstrated for heart muscle. The significance of P-LC phosphorylation in heart muscle remains obscure, particularly for mammalian heart. In turtle heart, a high "basal" level of phosphorylation of light chains is observed in the resting (diastolic) heart. From this level, a moderate increase in P-LC phosphorylation was seen during systole, indicating that increased phosphorylation, when detectable, accompanies myocardial contraction. The significance of the high basal level of phosphorylation in diastole is unknown. The observations that light-chain phosphorylation appears to decrease actomyosin ATPase activity *in vivo* and that slowly beating hearts have low actomyosin ATPase activity suggest that increased phosphorylation of the light chains during systole might predispose the heart muscle to subsequent relaxation (35). The lower level of phosphorylation in diastole implies a dephosphorylation process, presumably by a phosphatase, though no such process has been directly identified. Dephosphorylation, like phosphorylation, must also play an important role in regulation.

Another indication that phosphorylation of the P-LC of myosin may play a role in cardiac muscle regulation is the positive inotropic effect of catecholamines, which increase cellular cAMP levels. Because agents that increase cAMP also increase Ca^{2+} influx into the cell, the resulting increase in intracellular free Ca^{2+} increases Ca^{2+} binding to calmodulin, which modulates MLCK activity in both smooth and cardiac muscle, although by significantly different mechanisms (1,46). In the cardiac cell, the Ca^{2+}-calmodulin complex increases the phosphorylation of myosin P light chain. Recent evidence suggests that this increase in phosphoryl light chain is due to a Ca^{2+}-calmodulin-dependent increase in the affinity of the MLCK for its substrate, the P-LC (LC-2) of (bovine) cardiac myosin (46). Nonetheless, it is not yet clear if phosphorylation of cardiac myosin light chain modifies myocardial contractility, or even if the phosphate content of the light chains is physiologically significant.

Troponin Phosphorylation

Under steady-state conditions, CTn in myofibrils binds Ca^{2+} significantly at concentrations of free Ca^{2+} that are not associated with ATPase activation in myofibrillar preparations. At pCa ($-$log molar free-Ca^{2+} concentration) values greater than 7.5, no myofibrillar ATPase is measured, although the free Ca^{2+} is within the range of the $K_{Ca^{2+}}$ for binding to the Ca^{2+}-Mg^{2+} sites (Fig. 2). Only above pCa 7.0 do free-Ca^{2+} levels result in myofibrillar ATPase activity. These observations indicate titration of the high-affinity Ca^{2+}-Mg^{2+} sites at nonactivating free-Ca^{2+} levels, followed then by Ca^{2+} binding to the single lower-affinity Ca^{2+}-specific site. The "second phase" of Ca^{2+} binding activates actomyosin ATPase.

Alteration of Ca^{2+} binding by cardiac troponin that results from CTnI phosphorylation is apparently confined to the Ca^{2+}-specific site. Indirect binding experiments, designed to label CTn fluorescently at the TnC subunit, have shown changes in the fluorescence of the probe *in situ* that provide a sensitive indication of the extent of binding of Ca^{2+}. Binding of Ca^{2+} is essentially the same at pCa above 7.5 for either CTn containing phosphoryl-CTnI or CTn containing nonphosphorylated CTnI. Binding of the cation occurs at lower pCa for either CTn, but the second phase of the binding curve is shifted slightly to the right (approximately 0.5 pCa unit) (Fig. 2) for CTn containing phosphoryl-CTnI. It does not matter experimentally if the CTnI is phosphorylated by cAMPdPK before complexation into whole CTn or *in situ* in the complex. Only the fluorescence change occurring within the range of free Ca^{2+} at which the Ca^{2+}-specific site binds the cation is affected by CTnI phosphorylation. This hints at the singular importance of Ca^{2+} binding at the Ca^{2+}-specific site and provides evidence of a critical effect of subunit phosphorylation on troponin-mediated sensitivity to free Ca^{2+} in the myofibril (38). That critical effect is an apparent decrease in the relative affinity of whole CTn for Ca^{2+} at the Ca^{2+}-specific site.

Evidence is accumulating that different levels of free Mg^{2+} will also alter myofibrillar ATPase activity and the relation between free-Ca^{2+} levels and tension devel-

opment (see Table 1). The on/off rates for Ca^{2+} at the Ca^{2+}-Mg^{2+} sites are probably not fast enough for Ca^{2+} binding to have an effect on myofibril activity, via those sites, as immediate as the contractile response to transient changes in free-Ca^{2+} levels would seem to require. Rather, it is the association-dissociation of Ca^{2+} at the Ca^{2+}-specific site that is generally associated with changing contractility as free-Ca^{2+} transients occur. There is as yet no evidence to discount the possibility that changing fractional saturation of the Ca^{2+}-Mg^{2+} sites of CTnC by Ca^{2+} (none, one, or both sites occupied by Ca^{2+}), reflecting recent Ca^{2+} transient (and hence contraction) history for the myofibril, might work in concert with other relatively instantaneous changes to modulate myocardial activity. Thus, the putative roles of Mg^{2+} and of the Ca^{2+}-Mg^{2+} sites in maintaining structural integrity of the CTnC subunit (47) may be more critical than current data would indicate. Compelling as such suggestions may seem, definition of the influence of the Ca^{2+}-specific and the Ca^{2+}-Mg^{2+} sites in myocardial function and how phosphorylation of one subunit (CTnI) works to modify the function of another subunit (CTnC) or of whole cardiac troponin remains open to investigation.

Computer modeling of the time course of Ca^{2+} binding to various cell receptors has been developed (34) using an exponential expression to estimate qualitatively the free-Ca^{2+} transients believed to occur in sarcoplasm during a muscle contraction. Others (32,38) have constructed a model based on this useful approach to predict the effect of phosphorylation of CTnI on Ca^{2+} binding during an *in vivo* heart muscle beat. Calculations made on the basis of measured rate constants for Ca^{2+} dissociation and the pCa of half-saturation measured directly in phosphorylated and nonphosphorylated CTn using fluorescence probes resulted in the Ca^{2+}-binding-response model depicted in Fig. 3 for two different free-Ca^{2+} transients. Calculation of the pCa transients involved the following equation:

$$pCa_{(t)} = pCa_{(relax)} - A(e^{t/f} - e^{-t/r})$$

where $pCa_{(relax)}$ is assumed to be 8.0, the steady-state resting level; A is the amplitude factor; r and f are the rising and falling time constants, respectively. The two transients depicted involve a minimum pCa of 5.7 (Fig. 3A; $A = 3.301$; $r = 10$ msec; $f = 120$ msec) and a minimum pCa of 5.4 (Fig. 3B; $A = 3.73$). With these (or similar) transient parameters to drive the model, computer solution of the following equations can be used:

$$Ca_{(t)} = 10^{(-pCa_{(t)})}$$

$$dCaX_{(t)}/dt = k_{on} \cdot Ca_{(t)} \cdot (100 - CaX_{(t)}) - k_{off} \cdot CaX_{(t)}$$

Here, X represents the Ca^{2+}-specific site of CTnC in CTn. The expression $CaX_{(t)}$ is the percentage of saturation of this site; k_{on} and k_{off} are rate constants for Ca^{2+}

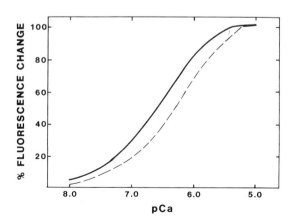

FIG. 2. Relationship between pCa and percentage change in fluorescence of labeled CTn [with 2-(4'-iodoacetamidoanilino)naphthalene-6-sulfonic acid; IAANS] reconstituted with nonphosphorylated (*solid curve*) or phosphorylated (*broken curve*) CTnI. (Adapted from ref. 38.)

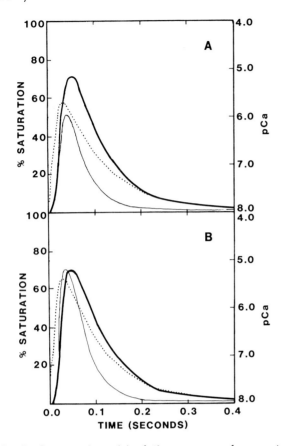

FIG. 3. Computed model of time course of percentage saturation of Ca^{2+}-specific sites with Ca^{2+} in nonphosphorylated (*bold curve*) and phosphorylated (*light curve*) CTnI, in response to a transient increase in free Ca^{2+} (*dot curve*). **A:** pCa of free-Ca^{2+} peak = 5.7; **B:** pCa of free-Ca^{2+} peak = 5.35. (From ref. 38, with permission.)

association and dissociation, respectively. Initial values of CaX are assumed to be the steady-state value (8.0) at pCa = pCa$_{(relax)}$. Calcium-binding titration of fluorescence-labeled CTn (labeled via the CTnC subunit) (Fig. 2) supports an assumption that phosphorylation of the TnI subunit shifts the pCa range for binding at the Ca^{2+}-specific site lower by 0.5 unit in whole CTn. Calculation of the saturation of the Ca^{2+}-specific site based on the modeling parameters generates the predictions shown in Fig. 3. In both Fig. 3A and 3B, phosphorylation of CTn is reflected in a reduced peak saturation of the Ca^{2+}-specific binding site. At the same time, the phosphorylation also increases the off rate of Ca^{2+} binding.

Keeping in mind that the depictions are a modeling system, if it is assumed that tension would develop roughly parallel to saturation of the Ca^{2+}-specific site with Ca^{2+}, the model indicates that CTnI phosphorylation in cardiac myofibrils could, at least in part, figure significantly in the well-known increased rate of relaxation and shortened contraction-relaxation cycle times that occur during positive inotropy. This is especially

significant in terms of adjusting the transient amplitude to simulate the changes in Ca^{2+} flux out of and into the sarcoplasmic reticulum (SR) that likewise occur in response to β-adrenergic stimulation and phosphorylation of the SR (see *Chapter* 35). The adjustment leads to the same prediction of the Ca^{2+}-binding transient in the model.

Interestingly, then, two separate phosphorylations appear to modulate cardiac myofibril troponin function in producing the inotropic perturbation seen in the presence of catecholamines. An increase in intracellular cAMP as a second messenger after catecholamine binding to the β-receptors leads to an increase in cAMPdPK activity that results in phosphorylation of both the SR and the CTnI. It is the SR phosphorylation that increases the rates of flux of sarcoplasmic calcium into and out of the sarcomere. Concomitant with the increased calcium flow, CTnI phosphorylation decreases the affinity of CTn in the myofibril for Ca^{2+} at the regulatory Ca^{2+}-specific site. If contractions occur even roughly in tandem with transients of CTn-bound Ca^{2+}, then the decreased affinity for Ca^{2+} seen in CTn containing phosphoryl-CTnI could account for the accelerated rates of relaxation (lusitropic effect) and subsequently shortened contraction cycles (chronotropic effect) widely reported in hearts responding to β-adrenergic agonists. Confirmation of a direct coupling of these two phosphoryl-dependent responses (increased Ca^{2+} flux rates and decreased CTn affinity for Ca^{2+}) in cardiac myofibrils requires further investigation. Critically, the rates of these processes modeled for CTn phosphorylation are compatible with the timing of the altered response of the working heart to β-adrenergic stimulation both *in vivo* and *in vitro*.

Recently, a kinetic model has been presented that, also using computer simulation, describes a relationship between myosin light-chain phosphorylation and isometric tension (19). The model is composed of three features related to smooth-muscle contraction: Ca^{2+}-calmodulin-dependent MLCK activation, P-LC phosphorylation-dephosphorylation in myosin, and conversion of the myosin light-chain phosphorylation to isometric tension. Similar contraction-related events have been suggested for cardiac muscle as well (35,39,46). A key assumption of the model, which successfully simulates many experimentally obtained results, is a cooperativity of phosphorylation of the P-LC of the two "heads" of the dimeric myosin molecule (29). That is, phosphorylation of the P-LC in one pair of myosin-associated light chains promotes the subsequent phosphorylation of the P-LC in the remaining pair of light chains associated with the other myosin head.

For continued elucidation of the details of the interwoven events of contractile regulation, the importance of modeling, which simulates known results and which predicts as-yet-unknown phenomena that can be examined in the laboratory, is patently obvious.

C-Protein Phosphorylation

With so little known about the basic role of the association of C protein with cardiac myofibrillar thick filaments, it is difficult to speculate on the functional significance of the phosphorylation-dephosphorylation of this protein. Norepinephrine is well known to increase the relaxation rate of cardiac muscle, likely because of increased pumping of Ca^{2+} by the SR and increased rates of Ca^{2+} dissociation from troponin leading to an effective decrease in the sensitivity of the contractile machinery to the cation. Phosphorylation of C protein in perfused, isolated hearts has been shown to increase measurably on addition of norepinephrine (14). However, an unequivocal correlation between C-protein phosphorylation and changes in myocardial contractility has not been established. In the absence of a direct correlation, it has been suggested that C-protein modification may affect heart by somehow setting limits governing cardiac relaxation that would be regulated directly by some other process (e.g., changes in intracellular Ca^{2+}, or changes in myofibrillar sensitivity to Ca^{2+}). Those limits would change as the phosphorylation of C protein changed. It has been suggested that phosphorylation of C protein could promote or hinder C-protein-actin interactions, terminating a contraction or prolonging it, respectively. These hypotheses, as well as the basic nature of C-protein structure and function, remain central issues in the characterization of this poorly understood myofibrillar component. Fundamental questions of structure, criteria of purity, functional assays, and association will require much investigation.

SUMMARY

The events and functional components involved in contraction of cardiac muscle are quite similar to those identified in skeletal muscle. Evidence continues to accumulate that all of the principal protein components of the contractile array are phosphorylated *in situ* under a variety of conditions. The troponin C subunit is a notable exception. This is true for cardiac as well as for skeletal muscle. What remains in question is the functional and/or structural influence of phosphorylation-dephosphorylation. Just as significant uncertainty remains with regard to what, if any, correlation exists between phosphorylations and myofibrillar events, how possible correlations might be effected is even less clearly understood. Indeed, it seems few phosphorylations can be directly correlated with changes in cardiac contractility. Although this may in part reflect experimental limitations, it is much more likely that phosphorylations of the myofibrillar proteins in heart do not exert their effect(s) directly. This appears particularly to be the case involving reduced affinity of CTnC for calcium upon CTnI phosphorylation. It is reasonable, then, to postulate that the protein phosphorylations in cardiac muscle exert modulating influences on discrete other, more direct regulations. There is no discounting the possibility that the major consequence of any (or all) of the phosphorylations is more simply structural, however. Much work remains to be done, both in identifying sites of phosphorylation for several myofibrillar proteins and in defining the consequences and mechanics of the effects of the phosphorylations that do occur. For example, finer resolution of the time course of perturbations versus phosphorylations or of phosphorylations versus subsequent contractility changes would enhance definition of myocardial phosphorylations as cause or effect or both.

REFERENCES

1. Bárány, M., and Bárány, K. (1980): Phosphorylation of the myofibrillar proteins. *Annu. Rev. Physiol.*, 42:275–292.
2. Bárány, M., Bárány, K., Gaetjens, E., and Steinschneider, A. (1977): Isolation of phosphorylated acid chloroform/methanol-soluble proteins from live frog muscle. *Biochim. Biophys. Acta*, 491:387–397.
3. Bárány, K., Ledvora, R. F., Vander Meulen, D. L., and Bárány, M. (1983): Myosin light chain phosphorylation during contraction of chicken fast and slow skeletal muscles. *Arch. Biochem. Biophys.*, 225:692–703.
4. Brauer, M., and Sykes, B. D. (1984): Phosphorylated G-actin in smooth and skeletal muscle—a P-31 NMR study. *Biophys. J.*, 45:239a.
5. Brisson, J.-P., Sykes, B. D., Golosinska, K., and Smillie, L. B. (1984): Nuclear magnetic resonance study of muscle regulation: Tropomyosin-troponin complex. *Biophys. J.*, 45:239a.
6. Burger, D., Cox, J. A., Comte, M., and Stein, E. A. (1984): Sequential conformational changes in calmodulin upon binding of calcium. *Biochemistry*, 23:1966–1971.
7. Chandler, C. E., Parsons, L. M., Hosang, M., and Shouter, E. M. (1984): A monoclonal antibody modulates the interaction of nerve growth factor with PC12 cells. *J. Biol. Chem.*, 259:6882–6889.
8. Collins, J. H., and Elzinga, M. (1975): The primary structure of actin from rabbit skeletal muscle. Three cyanogen bromide peptides that are insoluble at neutral pH. *J. Biol. Chem.*, 250:5906–5911.
9. Collins, J. H., Greaser, M. L., Potter, J. D., and Horn, M. J. (1977): Determination of the amino acid sequence of troponin C from rabbit skeletal muscle. *J. Biol. Chem.*, 252:6356–6362.
10. Ebashi, S. (1980): Regulation of muscle contraction. *Proc. R. Soc. London [Biol.]*, 207:259–286.
11. Egelman, E. H. (1985): The structure of F-actin. *J. Muscle Res. Cell Motil.*, 6:129–151.
12. Harper, J. F. (1983): Antigenic structure of calmodulin: Production and characterization of antisera specific for plant calmodulins of Ca^{2+}-replete *vs.* Ca^{2+}-free calmodulins. *J. Cyclic Nucleotide Protein Phosphorylation Res.*, 9:3–17.
13. Hartshorne, D. J., and Siemankowski, R. F. (1981): Regulation of smooth muscle actomyosin. *Annu. Rev. Physiol.*, 43:519–530.
14. Hartzell, H. C. (1984): Phosphorylation of C-protein in intact amphibian cardiac muscle. Correlation between ^{32}P-incorporation and twitch relaxation. *J. Gen. Physiol.*, 83:563–588.
15. Hitchcock, S. E. (1981): Study of the structure of troponin-C by measuring the relative reactivities of lysines with acetic anhydride. *J. Mol. Biol.*, 147:153–173.
16. Itaya, K., and Ui, M. (1966): A new micromethod for the colorimetric determination of inorganic phosphate. *Clin. Chim. Acta*, 14:361–366.
17. Jennisen, H. P., Peterson-Von Gehr, J. K. H., and Botzet, G. (1985): Activation and inhibition of phosphorylase kinase by monospecific antibodies against preparatively isolated alpha, beta, and gamma subunits. *Eur. J. Biochem.*, 147:619–630.

18. Johnson, J. D., Holroyde, M. J., Crouch, T. H., Solaro, R. J., and Potter, J. D. (1981): Fluorescence studies of the interaction of calmodulin with myosin light chain kinase. *J. Biol. Chem.*, 256: 12194–12198.

19. Kato, S., Osa, T., and Ogasawara, T. (1984): Kinetic model for isometric contraction in smooth muscle on the basis of myosin phosphorylation hypothesis. *Biophys. J.*, 46:35–44.

20. Klee, C. B., Crouch, T. H., and Richman, P. G. (1980): Calmodulin. *Annu. Rev. Biochem.*, 49:489–515.

21. Kleinsmith, L. J., Allfrey, V. G., and Mirsky, A. E. (1966): Phosphoprotein metabolism in isolated lymphocyte nuclei. *Proc. Natl. Acad. Sci. USA*, 55:1182–1189.

22. Leavis, P. C., Rosenfeld, S. S., Gergely, J., Grabarek, Z., and Drabikowski, W. (1978): Proteolytic fragments of troponin C. *J. Biol. Chem.*, 253:5452–5459.

23. Mak, A., Smillie, L. B., and Bárány, M. (1978): Specific phosphorylation at serine-283 of α-tropomyosin from frog skeletal and rabbit skeletal and cardiac muscle. *Proc. Natl. Acad. Sci. USA*, 75: 3588–3592.

24. Margossian, S. S., and Lowey, S. (1982): Preparation of myosin and its subfragments from rabbit skeletal muscle. In: *Methods in Enzymology, Vol. 85*, edited by D. W. Frederiksen and L. W. Cunningham, pp. 55–71. Academic Press, New York.

25. Moir, A. J. G., and Perry, S. V. (1980): Phosphorylation of rabbit cardiac-muscle troponin I by phosphorylase kinase. The effect of adrenalin. *Biochem. J.*, 191:547–554.

26. Offer, G., Moos, C., and Starr, R. (1973): A new protein of the thick filaments of vertebrate skeletal myofibrils. *J. Mol. Biol.*, 74: 653–676.

27. Pepe, F. A., and Drucker, B. (1975): The myosin filament. III. C-protein. *J. Mol. Biol.*, 99:609–617.

28. Perry, S. V. (1979): The regulation of contractile activity in muscle. *Biochem. Soc. Trans.*, 7:593–617.

29. Persechini, A., and Hartshorne, D. J. (1981): Phosphorylation of smooth muscle myosin: Evidence for cooperativity between the myosin heads. *Science*, 213:1383–1385.

30. Persechini, A., and Stull, J. T. (1984): Phosphorylation kinetics of skeletal muscle myosin and the effect of phosphorylation on actomyosin adenosine triphosphatase activity. *Biochemistry*, 23: 4144–4150.

31. Potter, J. D. (1982): Preparation of troponin and its subunits from rabbit skeletal and bovine cardiac muscle. In: *Methods in Enzymology, Vol. 85*, edited by D. W. Frederiksen and L. W. Cunningham, pp. 241–263. Academic Press, New York.

32. Potter, J. D., Holroyde, M. J., Robertson, S. P., Solaro, R. J., Kranias, E. G., and Johnson, J. D. (1982): The regulation of cardiac muscle contraction by troponin. In: *Cell and Muscle Motility, Vol. 2*, edited by R. M. Dowben and J. W. Shay, pp. 245–255. Plenum, New York.

33. Potter, J. D., and Johnson, J. D. (1982): Troponin. In: *Calcium and Cell Function, Vol. II*, edited by W. Cheung, pp. 145–173. Academic Press, New York.

34. Robertson, S. P., Johnson, J. D., and Potter, J. D. (1981): The time course of Ca^{++} exchange with calmodulin, troponin, parvalbumin, and myosin in response to tansient increases in Ca^{++} *Biophys. J.*, 34:559–569.

35. Sayers, S. T., and Bárány, K. (1983): Myosin light chain phosphorylation during contraction of turtle heart. *FEBS Lett.*, 154: 305–310.

36. Simpson, P. A., Spudich, J. A., and Parham, P. (1984): Monoclonal antibodies prepared against *Dictyostelium* actin: Chartacterization and interactions with actin. *J. Cell. Biol.*, 99:287–295.

37. Smith-Gill, S. J., Lavoie, T. B., and Mainhart, C. R. (1984): Antigenic regions defined by monoclonal antibodies correspond to structural domains of avian lysozyme. *J. Immunol.*, 133:384–393.

38. Solaro, R. J., Robertson, S. P., Johnson, J. D., Holroyde, M. J., and Potter, J. D. (1981): Troponin-I phosphorylation: A unique regulator of the amount of calcium required to activate cardiac myofibrils. In: *Cold Spring Harbor Conferences on Cell Proliferation. Vol. 8B: Protein Phosphorylation*, edited by O. M. Rosen and E. G. Krebs, pp. 901–911. Cold Spring Harbor Laboratory, Cold Spring Harbor, New York.

39. Stull, J. T., Blumenthal, D. K., Manning, D. R., and High, C. W. (1980): Regulation of myosin phosphorylation in different types of muscles. In: *Calcium-Binding Proteins: Structure and Function*, edited by F. L. Siegel, E. Carafoli, R. H. Kretsinger, D. H. MacLennan, and R. H. Wasserman, pp. 263–270. Elsevier/North Holland, New York.

40. Stull, J. T., and Buss, J. E. (1977): Phosphorylation of cardiac troponin by cyclic adenosine 3′:5′-monophosphate-dependent protein kinase. *J. Biol. Chem.*, 252:851–857.

41. Weeks, R. A., and Perry, S. V. (1978): Characterization of a region of the primary sequence of troponin C involved in calcium ion-dependent interaction with troponin I. *Biochem. J.*, 173:449–457.

42. Westwood, S. A., Hudlicka, O., and Perry, S. V. (1984): Phosphorylation *in vivo* of the P light chain of myosin in rabbit fast and slow skeletal muscles. *Biochem. J.*, 218:841–847.

43. Westwood, S. A., and Perry, S. V. (1981): The effect of adrenaline on the phosphorylation of the P light chain of myosin and troponin I in the perfused rabbit heart. *Biochem. J.*, 197:185–193.

44. Williams, R. E. (1976): Phosphorylated sites in substrates of intracellular protein kinases: A common feature in amino acid sequences. *Science*, 192:473–474.

45. Yamamoto, K., and Moos, C. (1983): The C-proteins of rabbit red, white, and cardiac muscles. *J. Biol. Chem.*, 258:8395–8401.

46. Zimmer, M., Göbel, C., and Hofmann, F. (1984): Calmodulin activates bovine-cardiac myosin light-chain kinase by increasing the affinity for myosin light-chain 2. *Eur. J. Biochem.*, 139:295–301.

47. Zot, H. G., and Potter, J. D. (1982): A structural role for the Ca^{2+}-Mg^{2+} sites on troponin C in the regulation of muscle contraction. Preparation and properties of troponin C depleted myofibrils. *J. Biol. Chem.*, 257:7678–7683.

The Heart and Cardiovascular System,
edited by H. A. Fozzard et al.
Raven Press, New York © 1986.

CHAPTER **38**

Mechanism and Energetics of Actomyosin ATPase

Edwin W. Taylor

WHAT CAN BE LEARNED FROM THE MECHANISM AND ENERGETICS OF THE ACTOMYOSIN ATPase ENZYME

In one sense the mechanism of muscle contraction is well understood. There is general agreement that contraction is brought about by a cyclic interaction of myosin cross-bridges with the thin filaments which causes the development of force. This cycle is coupled to the hydrolysis of ATP. Mechanical models of the cycle have been proposed (35) which relate a structural change in the actomyosin complex to the production of a force by stretching a spring attached to the cross-bridge. Hill and Eisenberg (15,16,30) have described a general formalism which relates the mechanical force exerted by the spring to changes in the rate and equilibrium constants of the enzyme mechanism. By making plausible assumptions, the physiological properties of muscle can be calculated from the mechano-chemical model.

The purpose of kinetic studies is to determine the set of intermediates which make up the enzyme cycle and measure the rate constants of the transitions between pairs of intermediate states. The kinetic mechanism is the basis for construction of the mechano-chemical

model. Since the equilibrium constants for each step give the changes in free energy, the kinetic scheme provides the information for a calculation of the energetics of the contraction cycle.

The current status of the biochemical mechanism and its relation to structural and mechanical properties of muscle is the subject of this review. Emphasis is placed on clarifying the assumptions which underlie the kinetic analysis and the assignment of intermediates to cross-bridge states.

A SIMPLE BIOCHEMICAL MODEL

The essential features of the mechano-chemical model can be understood in terms of a simple biochemical scheme and the corresponding mechanical cycle. The mechanical model is based on the observations that the cross-bridges behave like independent passive springs for very fast stretches or releases of the muscle (19,35). The cross-bridge cycle can be described by four states as illustrated by the version of a familiar diagram shown in Fig. 1. Only one head of the myosin molecule is shown. In state 1 the bridge has completed a cycle and is exerting a force represented by a stretched spring. The

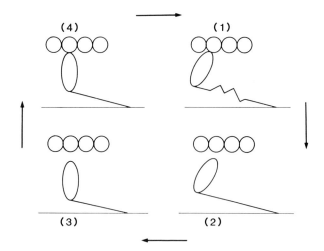

FIG. 1. A simple contraction model (isometric cycle). A single head of myosin is shown in the illustration. In state 1 the bridge has completed a cycle and is developing a force symbolized by the stretched spring in the S-2 region. The bridge detaches to give state 2 and undergoes a structural change to yield state 3. The detached bridges are probably in almost free rotation about the S-1,S-2 junction, and the different orientation shown for state 3 is meant to indicate a change in state. The cross-bridge reattaches in state 4 at an orientation shown as 90°, but the actual angle is not known. The transition to state 1 rotates the bridge and a force is developed by stretching the spring in S-2. The diagram is simplified by selecting a bridge whose position relative to the nearest actin site is such that attachment in state 4 occurs without distortion of the spring in S-2. In general, both attached states will exert a force in the positive or negative direction.

cross-bridge detaches to give state 2. It undergoes a change in state to give state 3 which reattaches to the thin filament in a different orientation (state 4). The orientation of the detached bridge in states 2 and 3 is probably the same since the bridge is free to rotate about a swivel at the base, but states 2 and 3 are drawn at a different orientation to indicate that the states are different in a manner which has to be specified in the model. The orientation in state 4 is not known and it is drawn as 90° for illustration. The transition to state 1 rotates the bridge to 45° and stretches the spring. The length of the myosin head may be as much as 15 nm, thus the rotation could displace the thin filament or stretch the spring by 10 nm per cycle. A range for the spring of 8 to 12 nm is inferred from rapid release experiments (19). In isometric contraction the cycle continues to turn and the fraction of bridges in state 1 exert a force. In an isotonic contraction the thin filament moves relative to the myosin and the energy stored in the spring is converted to external work.

The diagram is simplified to describe a bridge which matches an actin site and binds without stretching or compressing the spring in state 3. In general, all attached states may exert a force in the positive or negative

direction depending on the relative position of the actin site and the preferred orientation of the state (45° or 90°).

The simplest biochemical model will have four states which correspond to the four states of the mechanical cycle. The complex of a myosin head with an actin unit of the thin filament is denoted AM; and T, D, and P_i refer to ATP, ADP, and phosphate, respectively. The binding of T to AM produces very rapid dissociation of the protein complex which occurs an order of magnitude faster than the hydrolysis step. Thus, state 1 should correspond to AM and state 2 to $M \cdot T$. The remaining states are specified by assuming that the change in structure to form state 3 is coupled to the hydrolysis step and the biochemical state $AM \cdot D \cdot P_i$ binds to actin in a different orientation. The biochemical scheme is

$$\begin{array}{ccc} AM \cdot D \cdot P_i & \longrightarrow & AM + D + P_i \\ +A \uparrow & +T \downarrow & -A \\ M \cdot D \cdot P_i & \longleftarrow & M \cdot T \cdot \end{array}$$

This simple scheme is supported by various pieces of biochemical evidence. The rate of dissociation of the reaction products from myosin is slow (0.05 sec^{-1}) while the rate constant of the hydrolysis step is 100 sec^{-1}. Myosin gives a "phosphate burst" when mixed with ATP (38) since after the first ATP is hydrolyzed, the reaction is rate-limited by the slow dissociation of products from the enzyme site. Actin activates myosin ATPase by a factor of 500 or more with little change in the rate of the actual hydrolysis step. Activation must be caused primarily by the increase in the rate of dissociation of the $AM \cdot D \cdot P_i$ state. There is a relatively large free energy change for the transition of $AM \cdot D \cdot P_i$ to $Am + D + P_i$ which could provide the energy to stretch the spring. At this stage the discussion is not intended to be quantitative but the coupling of ATP hydrolysis to mechanical work is expected to occur at the product release step rather than the actual hydrolysis step.

The simple model is introduced to illustrate the concept that transitions in a biochemical scheme can be correlated with steps in a mechanical cycle. It also shows that particular properties of actomyosin ATPase, the rapid dissociation by ATP, the phosphate burst, the activation by increase in the rate of product release, appear to be related in a simple way to the requirements of the mechanical cycle. However there are serious problems with the simple model. It is drawn as a one-way cycle which must be an approximation to the actual reaction in which all the steps are reversible. In fact, the product of the equilibrium constants taken around the cycle is equal to the equilibrium constant of ATP hydrolysis. The reversal of each step must be included to obtain the equilibrium constants which are necessary to determine the energetics of the mechanism. The hydrolysis step is shown only for myosin which allows the pathway to be represented by a single cycle (39). Although dissociation is much faster than hydrolysis, reversal of the dissociation step gives the state $AM \cdot T$ which could hydrolyze ATP to give $AM \cdot D \cdot P_i$ directly, which would appear to rotate the cross-bridge in the wrong direction. Finally, the model assumes that the preferred orientation for reattachment is determined by a change in state of myosin which is coupled to the hydrolysis step. This is an assumption of the model and other assumptions could be made. An important question is the correlation of biochemical states with cross-bridge orientation. The modification of the simple model to take account of recent biochemical evidence will be considered in a later section.

METHODS OF KINETIC ANALYSIS

The objective of kinetic studies is to obtain as complete a description as possible of the steps in the enzyme cycle and to determine the rate and equilibrium constants of each step. To illustrate the procedure we consider a simple reaction, the binding of ADP to myosin. The reversal of this reaction is presumed to be part of the pathway of product dissociation in the enzyme cycle. The reaction occurs in at least two steps, an initial step in which the ADP forms a collision complex at the binding site followed by a change in conformation of the enzyme (and possibly the ADP as well) in which the nucleotide becomes more strongly bound. The change in structure of the protein may be confined to the immediate vicinity of the binding site, but in some cases the change in structure could be transmitted to other regions of the protein. The kinetic scheme is $M + D \overset{K_0}{\rightleftharpoons} M(D) \overset{k_1}{\underset{k_{-1}}{\rightleftharpoons}} M_1 \cdot D$ where (D) indicates a collision intermediate and subscript 1 denotes a new structural state of the protein. The formation of the M(D) intermediate is not expected to alter the structure of the protein.

The change in structure can be detected by a change in the environment of a fluorescent group, either intrinsic to the protein (tryptophan) or extrinsic (a fluorophore attached to a particular amino acid residue). A fluorescent substrate analog could also be used, such as etheno-ATP. Other signals are a change in absorbance or a change in the ionization of protein side-chains. The release or uptake of hydrogen ions can be converted to a change in absorption by including a pH indicator dye in the solution. All of these methods have been used to measure the binding of ADP to myosin.

The kinetic equations are easily obtained for this example. The collision complex M(D) is essentially in equilibrium with D during the binding reaction. If D is in excess the reaction is a first order process, $M_1 \cdot D / M_t = a[1 - \exp(-\lambda t)]$ where $\lambda = K_0 D/(K_0 D + 1)$ $(k_1 +$

$k_{-1})$ and M_t is the total concentration of M. λ is the apparent first order rate constant. The time course is fitted by a single exponential term which gives the value of λ. The variation of λ with the concentration of ADP fits a hyperbola from which the value of K_0 can be determined. The maximum rate at infinite ligand concentration is $(k_1 + k_{-1})$. At equilibrium $M_1 \cdot D/M_t = a$, thus $a = K_0 K_1 D/[1 + K_0(1 + K_1)D]$ where $K_1 = k_1/k_{-1}$.

The quantity obtained by an equilibrium binding measurement is $K = K_0(1 + K_1)$. In general the value of K_1 will be much larger than unity, thus $K = K_0 K_1$ and $a = KD/(1 + KD)$.

Thus the parameters which define the model can be obtained from measurements of the apparent rate constant as a function of ligand concentration and a measurement of the equilibrium constant. Actual data for ADP binding fits the simple model approximately with values of $K_0 = 10^4 M^{-1}$, $k_1 = 100$ sec^{-1}, and $k_{-1} = 1$ sec^{-1} at 20°.

The hydrolysis cycle of ATP involves several states and the difficulty in determining the kinetic parameters increases markedly with the number of states. If there are two first-order transitions in our example the mechanism is

$$M_0 + D \overset{K_0}{\rightleftharpoons} M(D) \overset{k_1}{\underset{k_{-1}}{\rightleftharpoons}} M_1 \cdot D \overset{k_2}{\underset{k_{-2}}{\rightleftharpoons}} M_2 \cdot D.$$

This mechanism is probably a better representation of the ADP reaction (8). If states 1 and 2 give different amplitudes for the signal that is measured, the two steps will contribute to the signal with different rate constants and the time course is $1 + b \exp(-\lambda_1 t) + c \exp(-\lambda_2 t)$. Determination of the two apparent rate constants requires a fit to five parameters, λ_1, λ_2, b, c, and the total signal amplitude. It is evident that a mechanism with more than two first-order transitions can not be analyzed using a single signal. Ideally, a separate signal should be found for each intermediate state in a complex mechanism. In practice, the fluorescence generally receives contributions from more than one intermediate and the only other signal, in the case of ATP hydrolysis, is the measurement of the formation of phosphate in the hydrolysis step. This is done by stopping the reaction with acid at various short intervals after mixing with substrate, and this method, although valuable in determining the mechanism, is subject to larger errors than the optical methods.

Most of the evidence on the kinetic mechanism has been obtained by the stop-flow and quench-flow techniques, but valuable data can be collected by perturbation of the steady state by means of a temperature or pressure jump. In particular cases nuclear magnetic resonance (NMR) can provide evidence on transitions between intermediates at equilibrium (48). Important results have been obtained by the study of oxygen isotope exchange (reviewed by Sleep and Smith in ref. 50). Since reversal of the hydrolysis step can lead to exchange of oxygen between water and reaction intermediates, the rate constant for this step can be determined.

Application of all of the available techniques still leaves some ambiguity in the more complex schemes discussed in the next section. However, any scheme, no matter how complex, must satisfy certain thermodynamic relations. A cycle starting with myosin plus ATP and ending with myosin plus ADP and phosphate

$$M + T \overset{K_0}{\rightleftharpoons} M(T) \overset{K_1}{\rightleftharpoons} M_1T \rightleftharpoons \cdots \overset{K_{n-1}}{\rightleftharpoons} M + D + P_i$$

satisfies the condition that the product of the n equilibrium constants taken around the cycle, $K_0 K_1 K_2 \cdots K_{n-1} = K_{ATP}$, the equilibrium constant of ATP hydrolysis (approximately 10^5 M at pH 7).

A partial cycle, for example, the association of different myosin states with actin,

$$
\begin{array}{ccc}
AM(T) & \overset{K_b}{\longrightarrow} & AM_1 \cdot T \\
K_a \big\uparrow & & \big\downarrow K_c \\
M(T) & \underset{K_d}{\longrightarrow} & M_1 \cdot T
\end{array}
$$

satisfies the relation $K_a K_b K_c K_d = 1$ for the equilibrium constants taken in the same sense around the loop. In the discussion of kinetic schemes it is more convenient to use association constants for the binding of myosin states to actin and to take the forward direction of the transitions in the direction of the hydrolysis reaction. The relation becomes $K_a K_b = K_c K_d$ where K_a and K_c are association constants and K_b and K_d are equilibrium constants for the formation of state 1. Dissociation of actomyosin by ATP occurs because K_c is reduced by a factor of 10^4 compared to K_a and therefore K_b must be reduced by the same factor compared to K_d.

CURRENT BIOCHEMICAL MODELS

The scheme that was used in a previous section to introduce the idea of a mechanochemical cycle has to be expanded to include collision intermediates, the reversal of all of the reactions and the presence of a direct hydrolysis step. An AM·D and an M·D state are included on the assumption that these states are intermediates that occur on the reaction pathway although this point has not been clearly established. The mechanism is

$$
\begin{array}{ccccccccccccc}
AM + T & \overset{K_0'}{\longrightarrow} & AM(T) & \overset{K_1'}{\longrightarrow} & AM \cdot T & \overset{K_2'}{\longrightarrow} & AM \cdot D \cdot P_i & \overset{K_3'}{\longrightarrow} & AM \cdot D & \overset{K_4'}{\longrightarrow} & AM(D) & \overset{(K_0')^{-1}}{\longrightarrow} & AM + D \\
10^8 \updownarrow & & 10^8 \updownarrow & & 10^4 \updownarrow & & 10^4 \updownarrow & & 10^6 \updownarrow & & 10^8 \updownarrow & & 10^8 \updownarrow \\
M + T & \underset{K_0}{\longrightarrow} & M(T) & \underset{K_1}{\longrightarrow} & M \cdot T & \underset{K_2}{\longrightarrow} & M \cdot D \cdot P_i & \underset{K_3}{\longrightarrow} & M \cdot D & \underset{K_4}{\longrightarrow} & M(D) & \underset{(K_0)^{-1}}{\longrightarrow} & M + D
\end{array}
$$

(Scheme 1)

The equilibrium constants are taken in the direction of the hydrolysis reaction. The product of the equilibrium constants is 3×10^5 M. The values shown beside the vertical arrows are the association constants of the myosin states. The set of rate and equilibrium constants is given in Table 1. The values of the constants are in some cases an order of magnitude estimate to illustrate the general properties of the system. The association constants to actin are very dependent on ionic strength. The values correspond to a very low ionic strength (20–30 mM).

The steps on the myosin line are based on the following observations. The binding of ATP and ADP are two-step reactions involving the formation of a collision intermediate ($K_0 = 10^3$–10^4 M^{-1}) and the values of K_0 are similar for both ligands. The rate constant for the transition to M·T(k_1) is 500 sec^{-1} or larger based on the formation of a strongly bound complex with nucleotide and a small enhancement of tryptophan fluorescence. The corresponding step for ADP has a rate-constant (k_{-4}) of 100 sec^{-1} obtained from enhancement of fluorescence (59). The equilibrium constant K_1 is 10^8 for ATP (24,40) and the corresponding step for

ADP has a value of 10^3 $(K_4)^{-1}$. The hydrolysis step has a rate constant (k_2) of 50 to 100 sec^{-1} depending on the ionic strength, and the equilibrium constant is small ($K_2 = 1$ to 10 for a range of pH, ionic strength, and temperatures) (9,58). The value of K_2 is obtained from the size of the initial rapid hydrolysis step and from the rate of oxygen exchange (50). K_3, which includes phosphate dissociation, has not been directly measured and is estimated from reversal of hydrolysis and the equilibrium constant of ATP hydrolysis (24,40). The value is 1 to 10 M.

The steady state rate is 0.05 to 0.1 sec^{-1} and since the steps up to M·D·P$_i$ are all fast (k ≥ 100 sec^{-1}) either step 3 or step 4 must be slow. Phosphate is weakly bound to M and more weakly to M·D (10^2–10^3 M^{-1}), thus reversal of step 3 can be ignored (1). The steady state rate is thus given by $[K_3/(K_3 + 1)] k_3 k_4/(k_3 + k_4)$. At low temperature there is evidence for accumulation of an intermediate after M·D·P$_i$, hence k_3 and k_4 are comparable in magnitude, but at 20° only one step is detected (20). Therefore $k_4 > k_3$ and $k_3 \cong 0.1$ sec^{-1}. The rate constant of ADP dissociation measured for the

TABLE 1. *Rate and equilibrium constants of scheme 1*

Step	M states		AM states		Actin association constants (M^{-1})
	Equilibrium constants	Rate constants (sec^{-1})	Equilibrium constants	Rate constants (sec^{-1})	
0 ATP binding	$10^3 \, M^{-1}$	Rapid equilibrium	$10^3 \, M^{-1}$	Rapid equilibrium	M(T) 10^8
1 Isomerization of ATP state	10^8	$500\text{--}1000/10^{-5}$	10^4	1000/1	$M \cdot T \; 10^4$
2 Hydrolysis	3–10	50–100/10	1–3	30/10	$M \cdot D \cdot P_i \; 10^4$
3 P_i dissociation	1	0.1/–	1–10	20–80/–	$M \cdot D \; 10^6$
4 Isomerization of ADP states	$10^{-3}\text{--}10^{-2}$	1/100	1–10	500/–	M(D) 10^8
5 ADP dissociation	$(10^3\text{--}10^4 \, M^{-1})^{-1}$	Rapid equilibrium	$(10^2\text{--}10^3 \, M^{-1})^{-1}$ (?)	Rapid equilibrium	M 10^8

Values of equilibrium constants are order of magnitude estimates for steps 3 and 4; only K_3K_4 or $K'_3K'_4$ are measured (24,40). Association constants of myosin states are very dependent on ionic strength and values refer to about 30 mM ionic strength. $M \cdot D$. and $AM \cdot D$ are assumed to be on the hydrolysis pathway and the ADP binding constants are used to determine equilibrium constants of the pathway (3, 26). Temperature approximately 20°.

$M \cdot D$ complex is approximately $1 \; sec^{-1}$ (1). Therefore the rate-limiting step is the slow dissociation of phosphate from the $M \cdot D \cdot P_i$ state.

The reaction of AM with ATP also involves the formation of a collision intermediate ($K_0 \simeq 10^3 \, M^{-1}$). The corresponding step for ADP binding is assumed to have the same association constant. The AM(T) state undergoes a very fast conformation change to form $AM \cdot T$ ($k'_1 \geq 1,000 \; sec^{-1}$). This state dissociates at a rate of $1,000 \; sec^{-1}$ or larger and the degree of association indicates a binding constant of approximately $10^4 \, M^{-1}$. Dissociation is rate-limited by the transition of $AM \cdot T$ because a maximum rate is observed for actomyosins of slower muscles (42). The dissociation step is reversible since the combination of an association constant of $10^4 \, M^{-1}$ and a rate constant of dissociation of $1,000 \; sec^{-1}$ or larger gives a rate constant for association of $10^7 \, M^{-1} \, sec^{-1}$. Thus, the dissociation-reassociation step is essentially in equilibrium on the time scale of the ATPase cycle.

The rate and equilibrium constants of the hydrolysis step can not be measured directly by transient kinetics because other steps in completing the cycle make a significant contribution to the amplitude and apparent rate constant of this transition. Calculations based on plausible models of the complete cycle give rate and equilibrium constants for the $AM \cdot T$ hydrolysis step which are comparable to the values for the $M \cdot T$ hydrolysis step (46,52). At most there is a three- to fourfold decrease in the rate-constant k'_2 compared to k_2 and a three- or fourfold decrease in the equilibrium constant.

ADP binding gives only a small decrease in association of AM and the binding constant is 10^3 to $10^4 \, M^{-1}$ compared to $10^6 \, M^{-1}$ for the binding of ADP to myosin (3,26). The association constant of $M \cdot D$ is obtained from the other three equilibrium constants of a partial cycle and is approximately $10^6 \, M^{-1}$. The binding of phosphate to AM is weak but values are not available.

The equilibrium constant for the transition of $AM \cdot D \cdot P_i$ to $AM \cdot D + P_i$ is calculated from the other equilibrium constants ($K'_3 \simeq 10 \, M$). Thus the transitions in the direction of dissociation of products are much more favorable for AM than for M. The rate constant for ADP dissociation from $AM \cdot D$ is $\geq 500 \; sec^{-1}$ (62), thus this step is not rate-limiting for fast muscle actomyosin since the maximum rate of the cycle is 10 to $20 \; sec^{-1}$. The rate-limiting step is either hydrolysis or phosphate dissociation. Since neither step has been directly measured the rate constants are calculated from a model of the cycle. If the rate of the hydrolysis step is essentially the same for AM and M, then phosphate dissociation is rate-limiting and k'_3 is 20 to $30 \; sec^{-1}$ at 20° and low ionic strength (52,53). If the hydrolysis step is three or four times smaller for AM it could be rate-limiting and k'_3 is approximately $80 \; sec^{-1}$ (46). In either case actin activation is explained by a large increase in the rate of phosphate dissociation from $0.1 \; sec^{-1}$ for the $M \cdot D \cdot P_i$ state to 20 to $80 \; sec^{-1}$ for the $AM \cdot D \cdot P_i$ state.

The scheme is consistent with most of the kinetic studies from several laboratories but there are discrepancies which will be considered in the next section. It is a useful model because the rate constants are known for most steps within a factor of two and at worst some equilibrium constants could be in error by a factor of ten. The model is sufficiently complex to serve as the basis for a mechanochemical model. It has to be stressed that some of the constants are calculated from the model and if a more complex scheme is adopted the constants will have to be altered. The scheme differs from the simple Lymn-Taylor model discussed in a previous section primarily by including the direct hydrolysis step explicitly. The extra states $AM \cdot D$ and $M \cdot D$. were introduced by assumption as being on the main pathway in order to be able to use the data on ADP reactions to complete the specification of all the constants. Both states would be present in small amounts in the steady state cycle and they have very little effect on the kinetic behavior.

A number of assumptions have been made in formulating the scheme and before interpreting kinetic schemes as contraction models we wish to make these assumptions explicit. The scheme contains several first-order steps (isomerizations) which have been referred to as conformational changes. Although any isomerization could be called a conformational change we wish to distinguish between local structural changes in the vicinity of the active site and large scale changes in structure which alter the binding of myosin to actin and/or the orientation of the cross-bridge. These transitions are referred to as nonlocalized or global changes. The nucleotide and actin binding sites are separated by 5 nm or more (4,13). Thus the transition to the $M \cdot T$ state must be a global transition since it alters the binding site for actin. Important problems are to determine which of the set of transitions of the kinetic scheme are local changes, which alter the global structure of myosin, and how many structural transitions occur.

An important assumption of the scheme is that the transitions occur in a linear order, such as $M \cdot D \rightarrow M(D) \rightarrow M + D$. The simplicity of the model allowed the intermediates to be specified by the ligands which are bound, i.e., T, D, $D \cdot P_i$ but $M \cdot D$ in the example is a different structural state than M with a different affinity for actin. If the state is labeled by a subscript to denote a possible conformation of myosin then it is evident that the reaction could branch. The scheme becomes

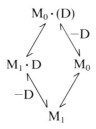

where M_0 and M_1 are two states of myosin, and from the principle of reversibility the state M_1 can exist in the absence of ligand. Thus, some assumption has been introduced to simplify the scheme. Since only the upper branch is included in the scheme it is assumed that the direct dissociation of D from state $M_1 \cdot D$ is much slower than the isomerization to $M_0 \cdot (D)$ followed by rapid dissociation of the collision complex. This rule is followed for ATP and ADP states but not for P_i states since $AM \cdot D \cdot P_i$ dissociates into $AM \cdot D + P_i$. Thus it is assumed that a conformational change occurs which essentially traps the nucleotide in the active site and the change must be reversed before nucleotide is released but phosphate is able to leave the site without a structural change. Additional evidence is needed to support this assumption and for more complex schemes the problem of branching is a serious limitation on the testibility of models.

A kinetic criterion can be applied to distinguish local versus global transitions. A change in rate or equilibrium constants for corresponding transitions of AM versus M implies the transmission of an interaction between the nucleotide and actin binding sites. This criterion is clearly satisfied for the transitions to the $M \cdot T$ and $M \cdot D$ states and since they have different affinity for actin they could correspond to different structural states of myosin. A difficulty with arriving at a consistent interpretation of the model is that several nucleotides and pyrophosphate dissociate AM and the nucleotide and pyrophosphate complexes have different affinities for actin. It is unlikely that each complex corresponds to a different structural state of myosin. The difficulty may be that the model is too simple and a self-consistent scheme could be obtained by introducing an additional nucleotide state.

The hydrolysis step shows only a small interaction with actin. The hydrolysis step may be a local transition, but a small change in the actin binding region or in a region of myosin that does not interact with the actin binding site can not be ruled out.

The interpretation of structural changes induced by nucleotide binding is strengthened by studies on chemical modification and energy transfer. The binding of nucleotides alters the region of myosin containing the two reactive sulphydryl groups SH-1 and SH-2 (6). Conversely, modification of SH-1 alters the rate constants of several steps in the scheme (51). The SH-1 group is 2.5 to 3.9 nm distant from the active site (57,60). Nucleotide binding reduces the distance between the sulphydryl groups by 0.6 to 0.7 nm (12). The two sulphydryl groups can be cross-linked in a myosin nucleotide complex to form a disulphide bond and the nucleotide or pyrophosphate is trapped at the active site (61). The disulphide bridged state (pPDM-myosin) is very weakly bound to actin, comparable to the binding of $M \cdot T$ or $M \cdot D \cdot P_i$ (7). The half-life of the trapped nucleotide is the order of 10 to 20 hr which is similar to the $M \cdot D \cdot V_i$ complex, and in both cases the nucleotide is released rapidly on formation of a complex with actin (23). The evidence suggests a structural interaction between the nucleotide site and the SH-1, SH-2 region which is transmitted to the actin binding region (4).

Progress in identifying the actin binding regions has been made by cross-linking studies and by renaturation of possible myosin domains. S-1 is cleaved by trypsin and a variety of proteolytic enzymes into three large peptides of 25, 50, and 20 kDa.

$$N \overline{\quad^{25}\quad | \quad^{50}\quad | \quad^{20}\quad} C$$

The active site has been assigned to the 25 KDa fragment (56) with a part of the 50 kDa fragment participating in the binding site (26). The SH-1 and SH-2 groups are ten residues apart approximately in the center of the 20 kDa piece. The C-terminal end is connected to the S-2 segment.

S-1 can be cross-linked to actin by a carbodiimide which introduces a peptide bond between a basic side chain of S-1 and a carboxyl side-chain of actin (43). Although there is some disagreement, S-1 appears to be cross-linked to a single actin (8,27,43,55) either to the 20 kDa or to the 50 kDa peptides, but not both. The sites have been localized to the 18 to 20 region of the 20 kDa piece and the 27 to 35 region of the 50 kDa piece numbering from the C-terminal end of S-1 (8).

The renatured 20 kDa piece binds very strongly to actin (44) which suggests that the binding site that is affected by nucleotide is in the 20 kDa domain. The SH groups are some distance from the cross-linked region as measured along the backbone chain and may be 2 nm distant from the actin contact (63). Thus, the structural change may be transmitted through the SH group region to the actin binding site which is consistent with distances obtained from energy transfer (4).

The renatured 50 kDa fragment also binds to actin although not as strongly as the 20 kDa piece (45). Cleavage at the 50–20 boundary reduces the affinity of S-1 for actin in the presence of ATP but V_M of the ATPase is unchanged. It is probable that there is a second actin binding site in the 50 kDa peptide which has a smaller binding constant. The cross-links to actin in both the 50 kDa and 20 kDa regions of S-1 are made to the same region of actin close to the N-terminal end (54). A cross-link is also formed between the C-terminal end of actin (CYS 374) and a light chain of S-1 (54). A hypothetical diagram of actin-myosin contacts is presented in Fig. 2.

The chemical evidence also provides some support for the assumption of a linear sequence of steps in the kinetic scheme. Nucleotide or pyrophosphate is trapped in the active site by forming the disulphide bridge. The stability of the complex is comparable to the $M \cdot ADP \cdot V_i$ or the $M \cdot T$ complex (22). Phosphate is slowly released from the $ADP \cdot P_i$ complex, but ADP release appears to require a conformation change and the rate is greatly accelerated by binding of actin. Complexes of etheno-ADP and etheno-ATP with S-1 are resistant to fluorescence-quenching by a small molecule such as acrylamide (47). Thus, the evidence supports the trapping of substrate in a pocket by a structural change induced by substrate interactions and stabilized by formation of a disulphide bond between the two reactive SH groups.

A More Complex Model

The kinetic scheme may be oversimplified because various studies of nucleotide binding (47,48,59), acto-

myosin dissociation (2,59), and the distribution of substrate and product intermediates in the steady state cycle (52,62) are not completely accounted for by the set of intermediates in the model. Stein et al. (52,53) have postulated an additional transition between $AM \cdot D \cdot P_i$ states.

$$\begin{array}{ccc}
AM \cdot D \cdot P_{iI} \overset{K}{\underset{}{\rightleftharpoons}} AM \cdot DP_{iII} & \overset{500\ S^{-1}}{\longleftarrow} & AM \cdot D \\
\downarrow \qquad \qquad K \downarrow & & \downarrow \\
M \cdot D \cdot P_{iI} \overset{}{\underset{}{\rightleftharpoons}} M \cdot D \cdot P_{iII} & \overset{slow}{\longleftarrow} & M \cdot D
\end{array}$$

K is approximately 1/6 for both transitions but the rate constants are three times smaller for the transition between AM states compared to M states. This transition from state I, formerly called the refractory state, to state II is the rate-limiting step at high actin concentrations such that the system is largely associated. The extra step accounts for the ratio of product to substrate states and for the larger apparent association constant obtained from the actin concentration dependence of the ATPase relative to the actual binding constant. There are some disagreements on the interpretation of this type of evidence (46,47). In this model there is no difference in association constants of the two product states and a small change in rate constants for the corresponding M and AM states, thus the transition does not appear to involve an important structural change. This is a small variation on the scheme we have discussed which may remove some discrepancies, but it is not likely to be significantly different as the basis for a mechanochemical model.

An extra step has also been proposed based on the studies of nucleotide binding (47,48,59). Two first-order transitions are observed and since both appear to reduce the affinity for actin both may involve structural changes.

$$M_0 + L \overset{K_0}{\rightleftharpoons} M_0(L) \overset{k_1}{\rightleftharpoons} M_1 \cdot L \overset{k_2}{\rightleftharpoons} M_2 \cdot L$$

where L is ATP or ADP, etheno-ATP or etheno-ADP, and AMPPNP. Subscripts are used to distinguish possible structural states. The rate constants are similar to di- and triphosphates which suggests that the same states are formed. In the case of etheno-ATP, the hydrolysis step is an order of magnitude slower than step 2 and therefore there are three isomerizations in the mechanism. However, with ATP step 2 and the hydrolysis step occur at similar rates and it is not clear that they are separate steps.

Shriver and Sykes (48) have also proposed a mechanism with two transitions between nucleotide states. A scheme which includes all of the suggestions is

$$\begin{array}{ccccccccccccc}
AM_0 & \!\!-\!\! & AM_0(T) & \overset{(1)}{\!-\!} & AM_1 \cdot T & \overset{(2)}{\!-\!} & AM_2 \cdot T & \overset{(3)}{\!-\!} & AM_2 \cdot D \cdot P_i & \overset{(4)}{\!-\!} & AM_1 \cdot D(P_i) & \overset{(5)}{\!-\!} & AM_1 \cdot D & \overset{(6)}{\!-\!} & AM_0 D \\
\updownarrow & & \updownarrow & & \updownarrow & & \updownarrow & & \updownarrow & & \updownarrow & & \updownarrow & & \updownarrow \\
M_0 & \!\!-\!\! & M_0(T) & \!-\! & M_1 \cdot T & \!-\! & M_2 \cdot T & \!-\! & M_2 \cdot D \cdot P_i & \!-\! & M_1 \cdot D \cdot (P_i) & \!-\! & M_1 \cdot D & \!-\! & M_0 D
\end{array}$$

(Scheme 2)

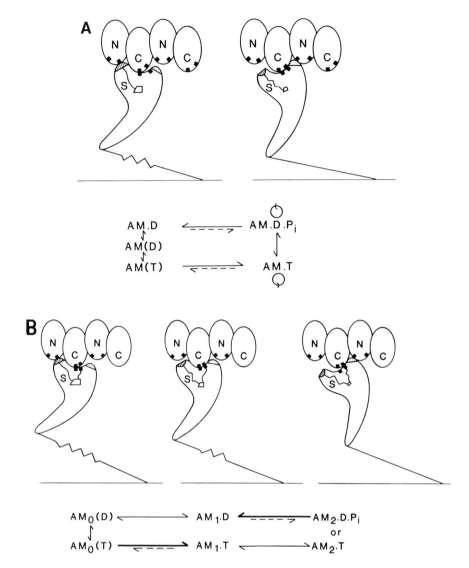

FIG. 2. Hypothetical contraction models. S indicates the SH-1,SH-2 region; substrate binding site is shown by the polygon; internal springs indicate interactions propagated between substrate and actin binding sites. Three myosin-actin binding regions are shown as *shaded, stippled,* and *filled areas* of the myosin. Actin monomer units labeled N and C are on the two long pitch helices of F-actin, but the helical twist is not shown. N and C could refer to N- and C-terminal regions of the elongated actin monomer units. *Heavy arrows* connecting biochemical states indicate energetically favorable transitions (equilibrium constant much larger than ten). *Circle with arrow* denotes states which are in rapid equilibrium for detachment-reattachment. These states will be distributed over the set of nearest neighbor actin sites to minimize the strain energy in the external spring in S-2.

The major cycle is counter-clockwise. **A:** One-step model: There is a single structural transition of myosin. The transition to AM·T weakens actin binding and permits rotation of the bridge in a single step as proposed by Eisenberg and Greene (52). The hydrolysis step is a local transition with no structural change. Detachment and reattachment of M·T and M·D·P_i states will occur in the major pathway as indicated by the *circular arrows*. Rotation to the "90°" state is represented by a detachment of the strong binding site in the 20 kDa domain (*shaded*) by interaction with the substrate-induced transition (internal spring) together with the formation of a new contact (*stippled*) possibly in the 50 kDa domain. Both domains can be covalently cross-linked to the same N-terminal region of two different actin monomer units. Cleavage of the ATP reduces the interaction between the substrate and actin binding sites and rebinding of the 20 kDa domain returns the bridge to the original orientation and "opens" the active site pocket with release of P_i. Rotations of actin monomer units may facilitate the transitions between myosin states. **B:** Two-step model: There are two structural transitions of myosin to give states 1 and 2. In the simpler case AM_1·T and AM_1·D have the same orientation as AM_0, but the strong contact is broken or weakened by interaction with the nucleotide site. Rotation occurs in the transition to state 2 with the formation of a new actin contact. This transition could be coupled to the hydrolysis step (modified Lymn-Taylor model) or to a second structural change induced by interaction with the nucleotide (AM_2·T) and the hydrolysis step is a local transition. The remaining steps are the same as in model **A.** State 1 could have an intermediate orientation (as drawn) in order to accommodate models which require a two-step rotation of the cross-bridge in the power stroke. In either case the AM_1·D and AM_1·T states are distinguished by the stronger binding and slower rate of dissociation of the former. In the diagram the stretched configuration of the spring should be associated with the AM_1· D state.

The relation between the two transitions in substrate binding and the two or three transitions in product release is not clear. In the scheme of Stein et al. (52) the $AM_1 \cdot D(P_i)$ state is formed slowly and decays very rapidly, consequently this intermediate is always present in very small amounts. The nature of the bound phosphate is not known and it is shown as (P_i) since it could be a collision complex, although Stein et al. regard the two product states as similar. Since phosphate release is very rapid the scheme could be condensed to $AM_2 \cdot D \cdot P_i \leftrightharpoons AM_1 \cdot D + P_i$ with little effect on the kinetic properties. Omission of the corresponding myosin state $M_1 \cdot D \cdot (P_i)$ gives the symmetric scheme of Rosenfeld and Taylor (13,46). In this scheme there are two structural changes induced by substate binding which are reversed in product release and the hydrolysis step is a local transition. Although $AM_1 \cdot D(P_i)$ may be present in small amounts in the ATPase cycle if phosphate dissociation is very fast, the state can be formed in the presence of high concentrations of phosphate. Oxygen exchange studies of reversal of the reaction in the presence of phosphate indicate the presence of two product intermediate states and a value for K_4 of about ten (49).

At present, there is insufficient evidence to properly test scheme 2, and different rate-constants and equilibrium constants have been assigned to the steps in product release by various authors in fitting the models to the steady-state cycle. The rate-limiting step for actomyosin could be a transition which follows hydrolysis (step 4) as proposed by Stein et al., or a transition before hydrolysis (step 2), or the hydrolysis step itself (step 3). It is clear that some actomyosin transition is slower or less favorable than the corresponding myosin transition. A further problem is whether a self-consistent scheme can be formulated in the sense that the intermediates can be labeled with a set of subscripts which refer to configurational states of myosin (29,48,58). In this case the association constants to actin are properties of the states, thus $M_1 \cdot T$ and $M_1 \cdot D$ should have the same association constants. This is a very strong restriction and it has not been satisfied by any of the schemes.

It is not appropriate to select any one model at this time as the best description of the mechanism. However, the general features of the mechanism are reasonably clear and the simpler model (scheme 1) is useful as a basis for an approximate description of mechano-chemical coupling.

Energetics and Models of Contraction

The energetics of the cycle has been discussed by several authors (15,16,25,42,50). The question is what fraction of the free energy of ATP hydrolysis is potentially available to do mechanical work. The first step in answering the question is to obtain a set of basic free-energy levels for the hydrolysis of ATP in solution. Scheme 1 will be used because a set of equilibrium constants is available for the transitions. The steps involving the binding of ATP and dissociation of products are second-order reactions and the free-energy change depends on the concentrations of the ligands. The remaining steps are first-order reactions (isomerizations) and the basic free-energy levels are defined by $-\Delta G_b = RT \ln K$ where K is the equilibrium constant of the transition. The second order reactions, such as ATP binding, can be expressed in the form $K_0[T] = [AM(T)]/[AM]$ and the quantity $K_0[T]$ is an effective first-order equilibrium constant. The basic free-energy change $-\Delta G_b = RT \ln (K_0[T])$ is therefore the change in free energy for the transition from AM to AM(T) at the concentration of ATP present in the system. The sum $\Sigma \Delta G_b$ for all the steps in the cycle is equal to the free energy of ATP hydrolysis at the concentrations of ATP, ADP, and P_i present in the system, $\Delta G(\text{hydrolysis}) = \Delta G^0 + RT \ln [ADP] [P_i]/[ATP]$. In muscle the concentrations are roughly 10^{-3} M, 10^{-5} M, and 10^{-3} M, respectively.

In scheme 1 we had

$$AM \xrightleftharpoons[10^3]{} AM(T) \xrightleftharpoons[10^4]{} AM \cdot T \xrightleftharpoons[3]{} AM \cdot D \cdot P_i \xrightleftharpoons[10]{} AM \cdot D \xrightleftharpoons[1]{} AM(D) \xrightleftharpoons[(10^3)^{-1}]{} AM$$

and the product of the equilibrium constants is 3×10^5 M which is a standard free-energy change for ATP hydrolysis of 7.3 kcal per mole. In terms of effective first-order

equilibrium constants and basic free energy changes for the ligand concentrations given above

$$AM \xrightleftharpoons{} AM(T) \xrightleftharpoons{} AM \cdot T \xrightleftharpoons{} AM \cdot D \cdot P_i \xrightleftharpoons{} AM \cdot D \xrightleftharpoons{} AM(D) \xrightleftharpoons{} AM$$

	K	1		10^4	3		10^4	1		$10^2 = 3 \times 10^{10}$
	$-\Delta G$	0		5.36	0.6		5.36	0		2.68 = 14 kcal

Note that addition of free energies is equivalent to multiplication of first-order equilibrium constants and the product of the constants is 3×10^{10} and RT ln(Kproduct) equals 14 kcal. The product of the Ks is K_{hyd} [ATP]/[ADP] [P_i]. Thus, the relationship could be

expressed in terms of equilibrium constants without introducing free energies.

The values of some of the Ks could be in error by a factor of 10. It is also assumed that the main pathway is the dissociation of phosphate in step 3 which is the primary contribution to the free-energy decrease in this step. The basic free-energy levels are the appropriate quantities for a discussion of the maximum efficiency of the mechanochemical reaction (for a full treatment of this question see Simmonds and Hill, refs. 32,32). In terms of a simple spring model (Fig. 1 or 2) all attached states that are displaced from their equilibrium positions will exert a force. The displacement will occur primarily by rotation of the cross-bridge at some transition in the cycle and step 3 is the most probable transition. Approximately 40% of the free-energy change is available in this step. If states AM(D) and AM also contribute to the force, the efficiency could be 60%. The maximum energy conversion efficiency in muscle is about 50% (37), thus the biochemical mechanism is feasible. This statement of the problem of efficiency is clearly very approximate since we have essentially stated that about half the free-energy change occurs after hydrolysis and a large free-energy drop or a large equilibrium constant is necessary in the force-producing step. It is surprising that the step which leads to detachment of the bridge (step 2) has such a large equilibrium constant since a value of 10^2 would be sufficient to drive this step in the direction of dissociation.

To proceed further with the problem, a detailed model is required. Eisenberg et al. (16) have studied the properties of plausible, if somewhat oversimplified, models which are helpful in understanding how the system might work. The properties of the system are easier to understand if the myosin head is visualized as a rigid body attached to an extensible and compressible spring, as in the figures, but these are not necessary properties of the system. The connection between biochemical transitions and mechanochemical transitions can be understood by assuming that each biochemical state binds to actin in a particular orientation such as 45° or 90°. A transition from the 90° state to the 45° state will rotate the tip of the cross-bridge a distance L. If the relative positions of the actin site and the myosin origin in the thick filament are such that the attachment in the 90° state occurred without stretching the spring, then the rotation stretches the spring a distance L and energy $1/2(aL^2)$ is stored in the spring. This energy is a free energy since we could envisage a process in which the energy could be converted to external work. An equilibrium constant could be assigned to the spring, $\Delta G_{sp} = -RT \ln K_{sp}$ where ΔG_{sp} is the energy stored in the spring. Since it is a positive number, K_{sp} is less than one. If we assume that the transition $AM \cdot D \cdot P_i$ to $AM \cdot D$ with equilibrium constant K_3 rotates the bridge, the mechanochemically coupled transition has equilibrium constant $K_3 K_{sp}$ and the free-energy change is reduced by the energy stored in the spring. This procedure could be applied to all of the transitions between attached states to obtain a new set of equilibrium constants and

a set of association constants for binding to actin. Each attached state exerts a force positive or negative depending on the stretch of the spring in that state. The force will, in general, be different for all bridges, since the periodicities of the myosin in the thick filaments and the actin sites in the thin filaments are different. An average over the range of extension of the springs has to be made to calculate macroscopic properties. The Hill-Eisenberg formulation allows the biochemical model to be converted to a mechanical model. Two assumptions are required. First, it is necessary to obtain the rate constants since only the equilibrium constant is specified by including the factor K_{sp}. The simplest assumption is to multiply the forward rate constant by the factor $\sqrt{K_{sp}}$ and divide the reverse rate constant by the same factor. Second, the association constants of the myosin states in the kinetic scheme are second-order constants and to obtain the binding constants in the lattice an effective myosin concentration has to be assumed. Applications of this procedure to kinetic schemes are presented in detail in a number of papers by Eisenberg and Hill (15,16,30).

The first step in formulating a model is to assign cross-bridge orientations to the biochemical states. The question is whether the properties of the biochemical scheme indicate how the orientation states should be chosen. Scheme 1 has one major conformation change induced by substrate binding which is reversed in the product release steps. The large free-energy change for the $AM \cdot D \cdot P_i$ to $AM \cdot D$ step suggests that this step corresponds to cross-bridge rotation. If $AM \cdot D \cdot P_i$ is assigned to a 90° state, the remaining choice to make is the orientation of the $AM \cdot T$ state. The simplest assumption is that there is only one structural change in the cycle, and the transition which weakens actin binding also alters the orientation of the bridge; thus, the $AM \cdot T$ state corresponds to a 90° orientation. This is the model proposed by Greene and Eisenberg (14). The authors suggest that orientation should be correlated with the strength of binding and the weakly bound states, $AM \cdot T$ and $AM \cdot D \cdot P_i$, are 90° states while the strongly bound states, AM and $AM \cdot D$, are 45° states. A pictorial representation is shown in Fig. 2. The transition induced by substrate detaches the binding site in the 20 kDa domain and the head rotates to make a new contact with a different actin unit. Bond cleavage reduces the interaction with the 20 kDa domain, and interaction with actin leads to rebinding of this region and release of reaction products. An obvious problem with the model is that the transition to the $AM \cdot T$ state has an equilibrium constant in solution of 10^4 and the transition will be favorable for most bridges in the lattice because the spring energy is probably of the order of 5 or 6 kcal per mole ($K_{sp} = 10^{-4}$–10^{-5}). Therefore, the majority of the attached bridges would rotate in the wrong direction at this step. The problem is not too serious because the

AM·T state is weakly bound and dissociates very rapidly. The bridge is expected to reattach to a different actin. Both the AM·T and AM·D·P$_i$ bridges will distribute among actin sites exerting positive and negative forces which sum to nearly zero. The force in the isometric state is developed by the AM·D state which must be sufficiently strongly bound that force is not dissipated by detachment-reattachment. In this model, as in most models, an additional assumption is needed because in solution the AM·D state has a very short lifetime and is converted back to AM·T by dissociation of ADP and rebinding of ATP. Assumptions such as having the release of ADP occur only at the end of the rotation or suggesting that the rotation does not quite go to completion (14) are arbitrary postulates that cover up a serious problem.

A second interpretation of the kinetic scheme is that there are two structural transitions, a detachment of one actin binding site in the transition to AM·T and a further transition at the hydrolysis step because there is a small interaction at this step detected by a slower rate constant and an increase in the degree of dissociation. The AM·T state is then a weakly bound 45° state and AM·D·P$_i$ is a 90° state. The remaining steps are interpreted in the same manner as in the first model. The hypothetical steps are illustrated in Fig. 2. The most probable cross-bridge trajectory has to be determined by a reasonable choice of the parameters as it was in the first model. Since the first transition does not alter the orientation of the bridge, it is independent of the force and rapid detachment and reattachment occurs. The second step could occur by detachment, hydrolysis and reattachment, or by direct hydrolysis and rotation of the cross-bridge in the wrong direction. Because the direct hydrolysis step is slower and has a small equilibrium constant, this pathway will be unfavorable except for those bridges which start with a fairly large positive stretch. The ratio of fluxes for the direct and the dissociation pathways depends on the AM·T association constant. An approximate calculation shows that if the probability of attachment of AM·T is 0.9 for an unstrained bridge the direct pathway will contribute 10% of the flux. The dissociation pathway predominates at the expense of slowing the reaction because hydrolysis occurs primarily on the detached bridges.

The second interpretation is the pathway proposed originally by Lymn and Taylor (39), but it is introduced here for a different reason. The earlier attempts to relate the kinetic scheme to the cross-bridge cycle assumed that the major pathway in solution would determine the major pathway in the muscle. It is evident from the discussion that the pathway is partly determined by the constraints imposed by the forces generated in the lattice. It is unlikely that the two interpretations can be distinguished by the biochemical evidence. In view of the structural evidence to be considered in the next section, there is a question whether any such distinction is meaningful.

The kinetic scheme on which this discussion is based is probably oversimplified. Scheme 2 allows for two structural changes in substrate binding and product release and it could be accommodated to models which require two-step rotation of cross-bridges. An example of such a model is also given in Fig. 2, but the difficulty in establishing a correlation of biochemical states with cross-bridge orientations even in the simpler model indicates that it is not profitable to pursue more complex explanations at present.

Biochemical Models and Cross-Bridge Dynamics

Attempts to understand the mechanism from the biochemical standpoint reach a limit set by the need to incorporate the dynamic behavior of the cross-bridge into the model. A direct approach to this problem has been initiated by Trentham and Goldman by generating ATP photochemically in muscle fibers. The kinetic behavior can be studied under conditions in which the forces can influence the biochemical processes. The initial results show a gratifying agreement between rate processes measured in the muscle and the corresponding reactions in solution (20,21). Cross-bridge detachment by ATP is a very fast process and, although the maximum rate has not yet been measured, the apparent second-order rate constant is similar to the value in solution (5×10^5 M^{-1} sec^{-1}). A phosphate burst with similar rate constant and amplitude to solution values was also obtained (18). An effect of force on rate constants has not been clearly shown in the studies so far reported but this method promises to be the most important approach to the problem.

An important question is whether the mechanochemical models presented in the last section are in accord with the available evidence on cross-bridge dynamics. The assumption made in the discussion was that a particular orientation could be assigned to each biochemical state so that an unstrained bridge has a minimum free energy when bound in a 45° or 90° orientation. A bridge in a strained state maintains the same orientation and the strain is taken up in a spring attached to the base of the bridge. This is essentially the model introduced by Huxley and Simmonds (35). We expect the interaction between two proteins to cover a moderately large contact area which would not permit a large rotation without breaking the bond. The attached bridges would be expected to have a narrow angular distribution about their stable attachment angles. A different interpretation has been proposed by Eisenberg and Hill (16) who consider that rotation occurs only when the thick and thin filament lattices undergo relative movement, consequently the attached bridges will have a large angular distribution. Both descriptions are useful in formulating simple models and need not correspond to the actual system.

The efforts to determine the distribution of bridges and the dynamics of attached bridges have led to apparently conflicting results. The X-ray diffraction evidence indicates that most of the cross-bridges are attached in the active state, but the myosin periodicity in the thick filaments of 14.3 nm is maintained (36). The intensity of the 14.3 nm reflection is not very different in rest and in the active state which shows that the rotational and axial disorder of the bridges is comparable in both states. Quick stretches or releases cause a transient decrease in intensity, but it is not clear whether the fall in intensity is caused by a rotation or an increase in axial disorder. The simplest interpretation is that bridges can rotate about the S1-S2 junction, and in the active state the bridges find the nearest actin primarily by rotating rather than stretching a spring in S2. The bridges in the active state would then be distributed about a fairly wide range of angles with a small axial disorder but this disorder is increased in quick stretches and releases (36).

Measurements of orientation by fluorescence polarization, dichroism, and electron spin resonance give different results. Fluorescence polarization of etheno-ATP bound to myosin heads gave essentially the same orientation in rigor and active states (64). Dichroism measurements of a label attached to the SH-1 sulphydryl group fitted a single orientation in the active state (5), although the angle was different than the rigor angle. A spin label attached to SH-1 showed that 20% of the heads are immobilized and have the same orientation as the rigor state, and the remainder are in rapid rotation and indistinguishable from detached heads in the relaxed state (10). No evidence was obtained for two populations of attached bridges distributed about two orientation angles such as 45° and 90° (11). The results are difficult to interpret since there is a disagreement, but it may be significant that none of the measurements give the results that might have been expected of either two populations of bridges at definite angles or a wide distribution of angles in the active state versus a narrow distribution in rigor.

Huxley and Kress (34) have proposed as a solution to these difficulties that in active muscle only 20% of the bridges are in a force generating state corresponding to the population detected by the spin-label. Consequently, the spring has a larger force constant and tension is generated by a smaller rotation. A displacement of 4 nm would correspond to a rotation of 15° which might be consistent with the narrow distribution of angles for the strongly bound bridges observed in the electron spin resonance (ESR) measurements. The remaining bridges are weakly attached over a wide range of angles and could account for the apparent range of 12 nm for the spring which seems to be required by force redevelopment in quick releases (19).

How do these results affect the interpretation of the biochemical models? The biochemical evidence also indicates that there are two populations of attached bridges, weakly bound $AM \cdot T$ and $AM \cdot D \cdot P_i$ states which are in rapid equilibrium for attachment and detachment and strongly bound states [$AM \cdot D$, AM(D), AM] as emphasized by Greene and Eisenberg (14). The relative amounts of the two populations will depend on the assumptions made in deriving a model, but models could be adjusted to give 20% of strongly bound states. The weakly attached states which may be bound to a single actin domain are expected to show rotational and also axial disorder from interchange between actin binding sites. Recent evidence indicates that the monomer units in F-actin have some freedom of rotation (17). The actin filament is flexible and the internal motions are enhanced by interaction with myosin in the presence of ATP (65). Thus, a fairly large rotation of bound heads may be permitted for the weakly attached states without a large distortion of the actin-myosin contacts. However, the ESR results appear to require a fast rotation over a 90° angular range which is a larger disorder than expected from these considerations. If this interpretation is correct, the question of whether $AM \cdot T$ is a weakly bound 45° or 90° state is not meaningful.

The requirement of a small rotation at the force-generating step but a larger angular distribution for the whole population of attached states may be met by assigning more than two orientations to the biochemical intermediates. $M \cdot D$ has a different affinity for actin than $M \cdot T$, and M and could have its most stable orientation at an angle which is between the values assigned to the product state and rigor state. This suggestion has been made for the state generated by AMPPNP binding (41). The transition to $AM \cdot D$ has a large free-energy change but the steps to AM(D) and AM give much smaller changes. The evidence could be interpreted as a two-step rotation as proposed by Huxley and Simmons (35). The second step could be unfavorable in the isometric state because of the large activation energy from an increase in the stretch of the spring, but the transition would be completed in a quick release and contribute to the apparent range of the spring. The reinterpretation of the cycle (34) may have much in common with the Huxley and Simmonds model. The two-step mechanism does not appear to be in agreement with the ESR results, but the spin-probe reports the orientation of its environment and not the orientation of the entire bridge unless the bridge is rigid. As discussed by A. F. Huxley, the elastic elements can be in the cross-bridge head as well as in S-2, and force can be developed without a rotation of the cross-bridge as a whole (33).

The simple spring models are useful in formulating models of the biochemical cycle but the dynamic behavior of the cross-bridge is more complex than expressed in the diagrams and as yet it is poorly understood.

REFERENCES

1. Bagshaw, C. R., and Trentham, D. R. (1974): The characterization of myosin-product complexes and of product-release steps during the magnesium ion-dependent adenosine triphosphatase reaction. *Biochem. J.,* 141:331–349.
2. Biosca, J. A., Barman, T. E., and Travers, F. (1984): Transient kinetics of the binding of ATP to acto S1. *Biochemistry,* 23:2428–2436.
3. Biosca, J. A., Greene, L. E., and Eisenberg, E. (1985): Binding of PPi and AMP-PNP to crosslinked and non-crosslinked Acto-S-1. *Biophys. J.,* 47:308a.
4. Botts, J., Takoshi, R., Torgerson, P., Hozumi, T., Muhlrad, A., Mornet, D., and Morales, M. (1984): On the mechanism of energy transduction in myosin subfragment 1. *Proc. Natl. Acad. Sci. U.S.A.,* 81:2060–2064.
5. Burghardt, T. P., Ando, T., and Borejdo, J. (1983): Evidence for cross bridge order in contraction of glycerinated skeletal muscle. *Proc. Natl. Acad. Sci. U.S.A.,* 80:7515–7519.
6. Burke, M., and Riesler, E. (1977): Effect of nucleotide binding on the proximity of essential sulfhydryl groups of myosin. Chemical probing of movement of residues during conformational transitions. *Biochemistry,* 16:5559–5563.
7. Chalovich, J. M., Greene, L. E., and Eisenberg, E. (1983): Cross-linked myosin subfragment 1: A stable analogue of the subfragment-1 ATP. *Proc. Natl. Acad. Sci. U.S.A.,* 80:4909–4913.
8. Chen, T., Applegate, D., and Reisler, E. (1985): Crosslinking of actin to myosin subfragment 1: Course of reaction and stoichiometry of products. *Biochemistry,* 24:137–144.
9. Chock, S. P., Chock, P. B., and Eisenberg, E. (1979): The mechanism of the skeletal muscle myosin ATPase. II. Relationship between the fluorescence enhancement induced by ATP and the initial Pi burst. *J. Biol. Chem.,* 254:3236–3243.
10. Cook, R., Crowder, M. S., and Thomas, D. D. (1982): Orientation of spin labels attached to cross-bridges in contracting muscle fibers. *Nature (Lond.),* 300:776–778.
11. Cooke, R., Crowder, M. S., Wendt, C. H., Barnett, V. A., and Thomas, D. D. (1984): Muscle Cross-bridges: Do They Rotate? In: *Contractile Mechanisms in Muscle,* edited by G. H. Pollack and H. Sugi, pp. 413–423. Plenum Press, New York.
12. Dalbey, R. E., Weiel, J., and Yount, R. G. (1983): Förster energy transfer measurements of thiol 1 to thiol 2 distances in myosin subfragment 1. *Biochemistry,* 22:4696–4706.
13. Dos Remedios, C. G., and Cooke, R. (1984): Fluorescence energy transfer between probes on actin and probes on myosin. *Acta Biochim. Biophys.,* 788:193–205.
14. Eisenberg, E., and Greene, L. E. (1980): The relation of muscle biochemistry to muscle physiology. *Ann. Rev. Physiol.,* 42:293–309.
15. Eisenberg, E., and Hill, T. L. (1978): A cross-bridge model of muscle contraction. *Prog. Biophys. Mol. Biol.,* 33:55–82.
16. Eisenberg, E., Hill, T. L., and Chen, Y. (1980): Cross-bridge model of muscle contraction. *Biophys. J.,* 29:195–227.
17. Engelman, E. H., Francis, N., and DeRosier, D. J. (1983): Helical disorder and the filament structure of F-actin are elucidated by the angle-layered aggregate. *J. Mol. Biol.,* 166:605–629.
18. Ferenczi, M. A., Homsher, E., and Trentham, D. R. (1984): The kinetics of magnesium adenosine triphosphate cleavage in skinned muscle fibers of the rabbit. *J. Physiol.,* 352:575–599.
19. Ford, L. E., Huxley, A. F., and Simmonds, R. M. (1977): Tension responses to sudden length change in stimulated frog muscle fibers near slack length. *J. Physiol.,* 269:441–515.
20. Goldman, Y. E., Hibberd, M. G., and Trentham, D. R. (1984): Relaxation of rabbit psoas muscle fibers from rigor by photochemical generation of adenosine-5'-triphosphate. *J. Physiol.,* 354:577–604.
21. Goldman, Y. E., Hibberd, M. G., and Trentham, D. R. (1984): Initiation of active contraction by photogeneration of ATP in rabbit psoas muscle fibers. *J. Physiol.,* 354:605–624.
22. Goodno, C. C. (1979): Inhibition of myosin ATPase by vanadate ion. *Proc. Natl. Acad. Sci. U.S.A.,* 76:2620–2624.
23. Goodno, C. C., and Taylor, E. W. (1982): Inhibition of actomyosin ATPase by vanadate. *Proc. Natl. Acad. Sci. U.S.A.,* 79:21–25.
24. Goody, R. S., Hofmann, W., and Mannherz, H. G. (1977): The binding constant of ATP to myosin S1 fragment. *Eur. J. Biochem.,* 78:317–324.
25. Goody, R. S., and Holmes, K. C. (1983): Cross-bridges and the mechanism of muscle contraction. *Acta Biochim. Biophys.,* 726:13–39.
26. Grammer, J. C., Czarnecki, J. J., and Yount, R. G. (1985): Photoaffinity labelling of myosin subfragment-1 by 2-azido-ADP. *Biophys. J.,* 47:306a.
27. Greene, L. E. (1984): Stoichiometry of actin-S-1 crosslinked complex. *J. Biol. Chem.,* 259:7363–7366.
28. Greene, L. E., and Eisenberg, E. (1980): Dissociation of the actin-subfragment 1 complex by adenylyl-5'-yl imidodiphosphate, ADP, and PPi. *J. Biol. Chem.,* 255:543–547.
29. Greeves, M. A., Goody, R. S., and Gutfreund, H. (1984): Kinetics of acto-S1 interaction. *J. Muscle Res. Cell Motil.,* 5:351–361.
30. Hill, T. L. (1974): Theoretical formalism for the sliding filament model of contraction of striated muscle. *Prog. Biophys. Mol. Biol.,* 28:267–340.
31. Hill, T. L., and Simmonds, R. L. (1976): Free energy levels and entropy production associated with biochemical kinetic diagrams. *Proc. Natl. Acad. Sci. U.S.A.,* 73:95–99.
32. Hill, T. L., and Simmonds, R. L. (1976): Free energy levels and entropy production in muscle contraction and in related solution systems. *Proc. Natl. Acad. Sci. U.S.A.,* 73:336–340.
33. Huxley, A. F. (1974): Muscular contraction. *J. Physiol.,* 243:1–43.
34. Huxley, H. E., and Kress, M. (1985): Crossbridge Behavior during muscle contraction. *J. Muscle Res. Cell Motil.* 6:153–161.
35. Huxley, A. F., and Simmonds, R. M. (1971): Proposed mechanism of force generation in striated muscle. *Nature,* 233:533–538.
36. Huxley, H. E., Simmonds, R. M., Faruqi, A. R., Kress, M., Bordas, J., and Koch, M. H. J. (1983): Changes in X-ray reflections from contracting muscle during rapid mechanical transients. *J. Mol. Biol.,* 169:469–506.
37. Kushmerick, M. J., and Davies, R. E. (1969): The chemical energetics of muscle contraction. II. The chemistry, efficiency and power of maximally working sartorius muscles. *Proc. Roy. Soc. B,* 174:315–353.
38. Lymn, R. W., and Taylor, E. W. (1970): Myosin-product complex and its effect on the steady-state rate of nucleoside triphosphate hydrolysis. *Biochemistry,* 9:2975–2983.
39. Lymn, R. W., and Taylor, E. W. (1971): Mechanism of adenosine triphosphate hydrolysis by actomyosin. *Biochemistry,* 10:4617–4624.
40. Mannherz, H. G., Schenk, H., and Goody, R. S. (1974): Synthesis of ATP from ADP and inorganic phosphate at the myosin-subfragment 1 active site. *Eur. J. Biochem.,* 48:287–295.
41. Marston, S. B., Rodger, C. D., and Tregear, R. T. (1976): Changes in muscle crossbridges when β,γ-imido-ATP binds to myosin. *J. Mol. Biol.,* 104:263–276.
42. Marston, S. B., and Taylor, E. W. (1980): Comparison of the myosin and actomyosin ATPase mechanisms of the four types of vertebrate muscles. *J. Mol. Biol.,* 139:573–600.
43. Mornet, D., Bertrand, R., Pantel, P., Audemard, E., and Kassab, R. (1981): Structure of the actin-myosin interface. *Nature (Lond.),* 292:301–306.
44. Muhlrad, A., and Morales, M. (1984): Isolation and partial renaturation of proteolytic fragments of the myosin head. *Proc. Natl. Acad. Sci. U.S.A.,* 81:1003–1007.
45. Muhlrad, A., Ue, K., and Kaspzrak, A. (1985): Structural characterization and actin interaction of isolated renatured fragments of myosin S-1. *Biophys. J.,* 47:347a.
46. Rosenfeld, S. S., and Taylor, E. W. (1984): The ATPase mechanism of skeletal and smooth muscle acto-subfragment 1. *J. Biol. Chem.,* 259:11908–11919.
47. Rosenfeld, S. S., and Taylor, E. W. (1984): Reactions of 1-N[6]-

ethenoadenosine nucleotides with myosin subfragment 1 and acto-subfragment 1 of skeletal and smooth muscle. *J. Biol. Chem.*, 259: 11920–11929.

48. Schriver, J. W., and Sykes, B. D. (1981): Phosphorus-31 nuclear magnetic resonance evidence for two conformations of myosin subfragment-1-nucleotide complexes. *Biochemistry*, 20:2004–2012.

49. Sleep, J. A., and Hutton, R. L. (1980): Exchange between inorganic phosphate and adenosine 5'-triphosphate in the medium by acto-myosin subfragment 1. *Biochemistry*, 19:1276–1283.

50. Sleep, J. A., and Smith, S. J. (1981): Actomyosin ATPase and muscle contraction. *Curr. Top. Bioenerg.*, 11:239–286.

51. Sleep, J. A., Trybus, K. M., Johnson, K. A., and Taylor, E. W. (1981): Kinetic studies of normal and modified heavy meromyosin and subfragment-1. *J. Muscle Res. Cell Motil.*, 2:373–399.

52. Stein, L. A., Chock, P. B., and Eisenberg, E. (1984): The rate-limiting step in the actomyosin adenosinetriphosphatase cycle. *Biochemistry*, 23:1555–1563.

53. Stein, L. A., Schwartz, R. P., Chock, P. B., and Eisenberg, E. (1979): Mechanism of actomyosin adenosine triphosphatase. Evidence that adenosine 5'-triphosphate hydrolysis can occur without dissociation of the actomyosin complex. *Biochemistry*, 18:3895–3909.

54. Sutoh, K. (1982): Identification of myosin-binding sites on the actin sequence. *Biochemistry*, 21:3654–3661.

55. Sutoh, K. (1983): Mapping of actin-binding sites on the heavy chain of myosin subfragment-1. *Biochemistry*, 22:1579–1585.

56. Szilagyi, L., Balint, M., Sreter, F. A., and Gergely, J. (1979): Photoaffinity labelling with an ATP analog of the N-terminal peptide of myosin. *Biochem. Biophys. Res. Comm.*, 87:936–945.

57. Tao, T., and Lamkin, M. (1981): Excitation energy transfer studies on the proximity between SH$_1$ and the adenosinetriphosphatase site in myosine subfragment 1. *Biochemistry*, 20:5051–5055.

58. Taylor, E. W. (1977): Transient phase of adenosine triphosphate hydrolysis by myosin, heavy meromyosin, and subfragment 1. *Biochemistry*, 16:732–740.

59. Trybus, K. M., and Taylor, E. W. (1982): Transient kinetics of adenosine 5'-diphosphate and adenosine 5'-(β,γ-Imidotriphosphate) binding to subfragment 1 and actosubfragment 1. *Biochemistry*, 21:1284–1294.

60. Weiel, J., Perkins, W. J., and Yount, R. G. (1982): Use of phase-modulation fluorescence lifetime analyses to determine spatial relationships in myosin subfragment one by energy transfer. *Biophys. J.*, 37:265a.

61. Wells, J. A., and Yount, R. G. (1979): Active site trapping of nucleotides by crosslinking two sulfhydryls. *Proc. Natl. Acad. Sci. U.S.A.*, 76:4966–4970.

62. White, H. D. (1977): Energetics and mechanism of actomyosin adenosine triphosphatase. *Biophys. J.*, 17:40a.

63. Yamamoto, K., Sekine, T., and Sutoh, K. (1984): Spatial relationship between SH$_1$ and the actin binding site on myosin subfragment-1 surface. *FEBS Lett.*, 176:75–78.

64. Yanigida, T. (1981): Angles of nucleotides bound to cross-bridges in glycinerated muscle fiber at various concentrations of ϵ-ATP, ϵ-ADP and ϵ-AMPPNP detected by polarized fluorescence. *J. Mol. Biol.*, 146:539–560.

65. Yanagida, T., Nakase, M., Nishiyama, K., and Oosawa, F. (1984): Direct observation of motion of single F-actin filaments in the presence of myosin. *Nature (Lond.)*, 307:58–60.

The Heart and Cardiovascular System,
edited by H. A. Fozzard et al.
Raven Press, New York © 1986.

CHAPTER 39

Relaxation and Diastolic Properties of the Heart

Vivienne-Elizabeth Smith, Myron L. Weisfeldt, and Arnold M. Katz

The ability of the left ventricle to pump blood depends both on the interaction of the heart with the circulation and on the properties of the myocardium itself. (This chapter will consider the properties of the left ventricle as representative of those of the entire myocardium.) The importance of the circulation in regulating cardiac function is manifest in the role of venous return (preload), which delivers the blood to be pumped by the ventricle, in determining end-diastolic volume. In addition, the resistance to flow through the arterial system (afterload), which defines the load against which the venous return must be pumped out of the ventricle, plays a major role in determining the work of the ventricle.

The performance of the left ventricle is also influenced by the properties of the myocardial cells, which must both shorten to eject blood from the ventricle and lengthen so as to allow the ventricle to fill. Although attention has traditionally focused on the contractile or systolic performance of the heart, the ability of the heart to pump blood also reflects its relaxation or diastolic properties. Finally, the pumping characteristics of the left ventricle, like those of any pump, are defined by the frequency at which the pump cycles (heart rate).

The volume of blood ejected by the left ventricle during each stroke of the pump is, of course, the stroke volume, which is the difference between the volume of blood in the ventricle at the beginning of its stroke (end-diastolic volume, EDV) and that contained in the ventricle at the end of systole (end-systolic volume, ESV). In considering the left ventricle as a pump, the dependence of stroke volume on both EDV and ESV means that stroke volume can be modified by two independent, though interrelated, properties of the myocardium. These are the ability of the ventricle to empty during systole, which encompasses the contractile or inotropic properties of the heart, and the ability of the ventricle to fill during diastole, which involves the relaxation or lusitropic properties of the ventricle.

This chapter describes the relaxation properties of the heart, that is, the recovery of the heart following contraction after each beat. Relaxation can be defined as the process whereby the ventricular myocardium returns to its resting state following contraction, so that if there is no event that initiates contraction, there will be no relaxation to be studied. According to this definition, relaxation ends when the myocardium is returned to the state that existed before initiation of contraction. Thus, we do not consider relaxation to include steady-state diastolic tone or steady-state diastolic contractile-element activity. Although steady-state diastolic activity is of great importance as one of the determinants of passive left ventricular filling, it is not encompassed by this definition nor the concept of contraction–relaxation cycles.

SIGNIFICANCE OF RELAXATION IN PHYSIOLOGICAL ADAPTATION AND DISEASE

Rapid physiological regulation of the speed of relaxation is essential to allow the heart to adapt to increased loads or stress. One can consider the portion of relaxation that can be measured *in vivo* to encompass the interval from maximum shortening (end-systole) to the time that residual interaction of contractile elements no longer contributes to ventricular filling (the end of the rapid-filling phase). At a heart rate of 60 beats/min, with each cardiac cycle lasting 1,000 msec, the interval described will last approximately 150 msec. Thus, at that low heart rate, relaxation would not be inordinately long, because it would occupy 15% of the cardiac-cycle duration. If, with exercise, the heart rate increased threefold to 180 beats/min, and if the duration of relaxation per cycle remained fixed at 150 msec, then for each 1,000-msec period relaxation would encompass 450 msec or nearly half of the entire time available. The remaining 550 msec would be the only time available for the threefold increase in the amount of blood ejected and for filling of the ventricle to occur. Clearly, such a circumstance might not allow adequate time for filling because of incomplete relaxation between beats.

Fortunately, the normal physiological adaptation, especially in young individuals in whom heart rate can reach 180 beats/min during vigorous exercise, is readily accomplished by activation of mechanisms that shorten systole and speed the rate of relaxation. The most important of these mechanisms is an enhancement of relaxation that is caused indirectly by an increase in sympathetic tone and directly as a result of adjustment within the myocardium to the increase in heart rate itself. Relaxation has been shown to be enhanced by increased heart rate (1,2), but this shortening of the duration of relaxation is only modest. By far the most profound effect on the time course of relaxation and the most important physiological adaptation is that related to the increase in sympathetic tone (3). As a result of the greater speed of relaxation, the period of relaxation is shortened in proportion to rate. In our example, at a rate of 180/min, the duration of relaxation would shorten to approximately 50 msec per cycle, meaning that as a function of total cycle time, relaxation would continue to occupy 15% of total cycle time.

With endurance conditioning (4) there is evidence of additional physiological enhancement of relaxation. As will be discussed later, an essential adaptation to exercise conditioning takes the form of an increased rate of Ca^{2+} removal by the sarcoplasmic reticulum. Aging, on the other hand, results in prolongation of relaxation, in part based on age-associated decreases in Ca^{2+} transport by the sarcoplasmic reticulum. Fortunately, the relaxing effects of sympathetic stimulation are maintained with

age, so that with the lower heart-rate response to exercise that occurs in older individuals there is adequate shortening of relaxation to allow filling to proceed normally. In chronic disease states characterized by increases in sympathetic activity and heart rate there is some enhancement of relaxation. It remains unclear whether the enhancement of the rate of relaxation that accompanies hyperthyroidism is based solely on increased sensitivity to catecholamines or whether there is some change within the relaxing system as well.

It is now clear that relaxation abnormalities play major roles in the pathogenesis of a number of forms of cardiac disease, including heart failure, and that relaxation is more readily impaired by ischemia and pressure overload than is contraction (5–10). These findings can be explained by the greater effect of a deficit in chemical energy to slow the Ca^{2+} fluxes that occur during relaxation than during contraction and by a greater reserve capacity for the Ca^{2+} fluxes involved in systole than in diastole (*vide infra*).

Although beat-to-beat changes in relaxation are related in large part to changes in the rates of Ca^{2+} movement within the cardiac cell, rates of relaxation may also be influenced by changes in contractile protein composition. In muscle from hyperthyroid rats, for example, isomyosin composition is changed from the normal of 12% V_1 and 88% V_3 to 90% V_1 and 10% V_3 isomyosin. Relaxation is more rapid in hyperthyroid muscle, although this acceleration of relaxation is not nearly as striking as the shortening of contraction. With pressure-overload hypertrophy, in which both contraction and relaxation are slowed and the V_3 isoform becomes the predominant myosin heavy chain, contraction is slowed more than relaxation is slowed. In these experimental models, changes in myosin isoform (11) may complement changes (as yet poorly understood) in Ca^{2+} uptake by the sarcoplasmic reticulum (*vide infra*).

ENERGY DEPENDENCE OF Ca^{2+} FLUXES RESPONSIBLE FOR RELAXATION

The greater sensitivity of the Ca^{2+} fluxes involved in relaxation to an energy deficit can thus be attributed in part to the fact that the delivery of activator Ca^{2+} to the contractile proteins is a passive process, whereas relaxation requires that Ca^{2+} be actively transported against a concentration gradient (12,13). Thus, activation is initiated when Ca^{2+} diffuses through membrane channels from the extracellular space and sarcoplasmic reticulum, where Ca^{2+} concentration is in the millimolar range, into the cytosol, where Ca^{2+} concentration is approximately 0.1 μM. These downhill fluxes of activator Ca^{2+} are much more rapid than the active processes responsible for the Ca^{2+} fluxes that effect relaxation. For example, Ca^{2+} entry via a single sarcolemmal Ca^{2+} channel has been estimated to be approximately

TABLE 1. *Balances between Ca^{2+} fluxes during activation and relaxation in the myocardium*

A. Surface areas of membranes in the myocardium (16) ($\mu m^2/\mu m^3$)	
Sarcolemma + t tubules (SL)	~0.3
Sarcoplasmic reticulum (SR)	~1.2
B. Densities of Ca^{2+} channels and Ca^{2+}-pump sites (sites/μm^2)	
Ca^{2+} channels in the cardiac SL (17,18)	1–5
Ca^{2+}-pump proteins in cardiac SR (11,19)	6,000
C. Number of sites/μm^3 [A × B]	
Sarcolemma + t tubules	~1
Sarcoplasmic reticulum	~7,000
D. Rates of Ca^{2+} fluxes involved in activation and relaxation (ions/sec)	
Activation (flux through a Ca^{2+} channel) (14)	~3,000,000
Relaxation (flux by a Ca^{2+}-pump site) (15)	~30
E. "Ca^{2+} flux reserve capacity" (ions/sec · μm^3) [C × D]	
Activation	~3,000,000
Relaxation	~210,000

3,000,000 ions per second (14), whereas the ATP-dependent flux of Ca^{2+} through a single Ca^{2+}-pump site of the sarcoplasmic reticulum, which relaxes the heart, is much slower, approximately 30 ions per second (15), or 1/100,000 the rate of Ca^{2+} entry through a Ca^{2+} channel. This intrinsic slowness of the Ca^{2+} fluxes responsible for relaxation is partially overcome by a very high density of Ca^{2+}-pump proteins in the membranes of the sarcoplasmic reticulum (Table 1), but the myocardium remains susceptible to an imbalance between the rates of Ca^{2+} entry and removal from the cytosol.

The greater sensitivity of relaxation than of contraction to an imbalance between energy production and energy utilization probably reflects both the smaller "reserve" capacity for Ca^{2+} removal from the myocardial cytosol (Table 1) and the fact that a deficit in myocardial ATP supply slows the Ca^{2+} pump of the sarcoplasmic reticulum and thereby impairs Ca^{2+} transport out of the cytosol. The ability of a small decrease in ATP supply to impair relaxation may reflect an important allosteric effect of ATP to stimulate the Ca^{2+} pump, whereas a more profound fall in ATP concentration, to levels at which this nucleotide serves as the energy donor for active transport of Ca^{2+}, would lead to contracture (12,13,20,21) (see *Chapter 35*). It is mainly for this reason that relaxation (lusitropic) abnormalities have been found to be more prominent than contraction (inotropic) abnormalities in both ischemic and hypertrophied hearts, in which energy demand tends to outstrip energy supply.

CLINICAL MEASUREMENTS OF CARDIAC FUNCTION

Our present view of the pumping action of the heart can be traced back to the original description of the Frank-Starling relationship almost a century ago. The monumental studies of these early physiologists led to the traditional view that the pumping action of the heart reflects mainly the ability of the ventricles to eject blood and that the major importance of increases in diastolic pressure and volume was their ability to increase cardiac work according to Starling's law of the heart. Until the introduction of cardiac catheterization in the 1940s, traditional measurements of cardiac function involved only estimates of pressures and flow rather than indices related to the myocardium itself. During the 1960s, largely because of application of the concepts of muscle mechanics into cardiology, efforts were made to separate the effects of altered properties of the myocardium from those arising from hemodynamic abnormalities due to valvular and other structural abnormalities involving the heart. Knowledge derived from muscle mechanics, along with early input from biochemical approaches to myocardial function, led efforts to understand the pumping of the heart in failure to focus on "myocardial contractility." Because cardiology at that time was undergoing a major shift in emphasis as a result of the development of cardiac catheterization, it was logical that myocardial function came to be defined by the technology then available, notably pressure measurements obtained during cardiac catheterization. Measurements of the rates of pressure rise in the ventricles ($+dP/dt$) were followed by application of a variety of velocity indices (V_{max}, V_{CF}, etc.) that, while initially based on pressure measurements, attempted to express the contractile process in terms of muscle shortening so as to quantify myocardial contractility.

Those measurements provided insights regarding moment-to-moment changes in the contractile state of cardiac muscle when repeated measurements of the same index were made in the same individual or experimental animal. However, severe limitations in this approach were found when attempts were made to compare individuals, particularly those with normal, mildly abnormal, and severely abnormal ventricles. As has already been pointed out, myocardial contractility describes only one aspect of overall left ventricular function. Thus, to characterize overall left ventricular pump function, it is also necessary to consider its relaxation properties.

The heart can utilize a number of adaptive mechanisms in order to compensate for a reduction in myocardial contractility. In addition to changes in intrinsic contractile properties, compensation can be improved by cavity enlargement, hypertrophy, and adaptations such as changes in fiber angle and muscle bundle direction. These morphological adaptive mechanisms can be called into play during chronic conditions in which there is an increase in the hemodynamic load on the ventricle, such as in hypertension, aortic stenosis, or valvular regurgitation. The specific adaptations to each of these increases in load include shape and conformational adaptations as well as changes in myocardial contractility. With such adaptations, pump function can be markedly improved even though contractility may not be modified. Thus, over the last several years there

has been a redirection of studies of clinical hemodynamics to include characterization of pump function from an engineering viewpoint. The approaches of Suga and Sagawa (22) and others (see *Chapter* 42) now form the basis of important approaches to study of left ventricular function.

This engineering approach uses pressure–volume or pressure–dimension loops in assessing overall contractility. Regression lines relating end-systolic pressure to end-systolic dimension with varying afterload form the basis of assessments of chamber contractile function that facilitate our understanding of the processes of relaxation and filling. As shown in Fig. 1A, the isovolumic period of relaxation is followed by the period of rapid filling. If relaxation is prolonged, then the time course of rapid filling is slowed and delayed, as shown in this figure. Finally, if relaxation is prolonged sufficiently or heart rate is sufficiently rapid, then even at end-diastole there may not be sufficient time for relaxation to be completed. This phenomenon, termed incomplete relaxation, is characterized by incomplete filling of the left ventricle and an elevated left ventricular end-diastolic pressure, as shown in Fig. 1B. These relaxation

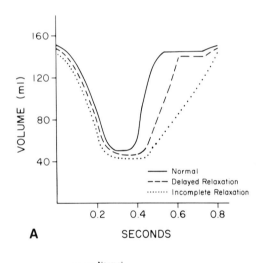

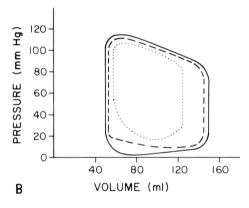

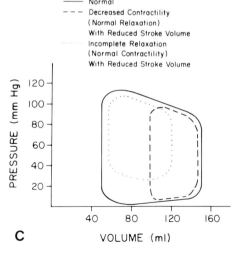

FIG. 1. A: Time–volume curves for a normal beat, a beat with prolonged relaxation, and a beat with relaxation sufficiently prolonged to result in incomplete relaxation with reduced stroke volume. **B:** Pressure–volume loops for the beats shown in A. **C:** Pressure–volume loops for a normal beat, one with decreased contractility with reduced stroke volume, and one with incomplete relaxation with reduced stroke volume.

abnormalities, in turn, can lead to all of the consequences of inadequate cardiac filling that one ordinarily associates with decreased pump function of the ventricle due to systolic abnormalities. In this context, it is equally detrimental when a decreased stroke volume is caused by too prolonged relaxation and inadequate filling, as it is when similar decreases in pump function and inadequate stroke volume are caused by decreased contractile activity. These circumstances are illustrated in Fig. 1C, which shows examples in which stroke volumes are equally decreased as a result of incomplete relaxation and as a result of decreased contractile function.

A number of investigators have utilized analysis of the fall in intraventricular pressure during isovolumic relaxation in an effort to obtain an index of myocardial relaxation (vide infra). More recently, clinical studies of relaxation have come to rely on newer noninvasive methods such as imaging and Doppler echocardiography and radionuclide ventriculography. With these techniques, patterns of ventricular wall motion and chamber filling, rather than direct measurements of pressure, are used to evaluate left ventricular function. Furthermore, these noninvasive methods allow serial studies of the heart in which it is possible to quantify aspects of contraction, relaxation, and filling.

Although measurements of the time course of left ventricular pressure fall are more difficult to obtain clinically than are those that define the filling of the ventricles, the decrease in left ventricular pressure more directly reflects properties of left ventricular relaxation than do indices derived from volume measurements. It should be clearly understood that during the normal cardiac cycle it is primarily the phase of rapid filling (between the time the mitral valve opens and the nadir of left ventricular pressure) during which ventricular relaxation determines the time course of filling in diastole (Fig. 1A). At the end of rapid filling, or the onset of diastasis, the time course and the extent of left ventricular filling are determined largely by the passive diastolic properties of the ventricle, the amplitude of left atrial contraction, and various other factors (vide infra) not related to relaxation per se.

The effect of prolonged relaxation is demonstrated in the middle curve of Fig. 1A, where the rapid-filling phase is protracted. In this example, the time course of diastolic filling is determined by the time course of ventricular relaxation throughout approximately 50% of diastolic filling, that is, from the end-systolic volume of approximately 50 ml to a mid-diastolic volume of 120 ml. In contrast, where ventricular relaxation is incomplete, as shown in the bottom curve of the same figure, the time course and extent of ventricular relaxation affect the rate of ventricular filling throughout diastole.

With incomplete relaxation, the passive diastolic properties of the ventricle will not determine the extent of diastolic filling, because relaxation will not proceed to completeness at any time during filling. The stiffness of the fully relaxed ventricle bears no constant relationship to the time course or extent of rapid filling (vide infra). Left atrial pressure also will not be a major determinant of the extent of diastolic filling when the left ventricular cavity volume is limited entirely by the time course or extent of ventricular cardiac muscle relaxation. During diastole, when relaxation is complete, left atrial pressure becomes a more important determinant of filling.

In contrast to the volume changes that occur during the ventricular filling period (some of which relate to "active" relaxation, and some to pressure differences between the ventricle and left atrium), the time course of left ventricular pressure fall reflects uniformly the relaxation properties of the ventricle. There are, however, several limitations to this approach based on pressure measurements. These include difficulties in measuring rapid changes in left ventricular pressure accurately, making it necessary to use catheter-tip micromanometers for accurate assessment of the time course of left ventricular pressure fall. With aortic valvular regurgitation, the period of isovolumic relaxation may be short or nonexistent. Under these circumstances, left ventricular relaxation properties cannot be assessed from measurements of the time course of pressure fall. Although isovolumic relaxation begins (in the absence of aortic regurgitation) at the time of maximum rate of pressure fall (maximum negative dP/dt), the time of mitral valve opening is not clearly evident unless echocardiographic measurements are made simultaneously. Thus, some variability in measurements based on analysis of pressure fall may result from inclusion of periods during which the ventricle is still relaxing but already beginning to fill. Finally, it should be recognized that the time course of pressure fall reflects the net characteristics of all regions of the ventricle. Thus, it is not clear whether or not the time course of left ventricular pressure fall is useful or valid in assessing left ventricular relaxation under circumstances in which there is ventricular inhomogeneity, such as in ischemic heart disease. If a significant portion of the left ventricle is relaxing at a rate different from that for the rest of the ventricle, these differently behaving regions will influence the time course of overall ventricular pressure fall in a complex manner. Such complexity almost certainly has resulted in deviation from simple models for assessing left ventricular relaxation (23). The validity of these approaches and such models as indices of left ventricular relaxation remains an open question. Specific approaches to analysis of pressure fall will be presented later.

DIASTOLIC PROPERTIES OF THE MYOCARDIUM

Cardiac muscle is characterized by a high level of resting tension and low diastolic compliance. For detailed review of this subject, refer to Gaasch et al. (23a). Because cardiac muscle has a relatively lower resting compliance than, for example, skeletal muscle, the heart has a very steep resting length–tension curve. The terms that can be used to describe the passive properties of the myocardium (24) include the following:

Stress: Force per unit of cross-sectional area, e.g., dynes/cm².

Strain: A fractional, or percentage, change in dimension caused by application of stress.

Compliance or distensibility: The change in volume that accompanies a change in pressure, i.e., dV/dP, or $(dP/dV) - 1$. *Specific compliance* is the change in volume per unit of total volume (dV/V) that accompanies a change in pressure, i.e., $dV/V\,dP$.

Elastic stiffness (or tangent modulus) is the slope of a stress–strain curve, that is, the amount of stress needed to cause a given strain. This is referred to in this chapter in a nonphysical way simply as *stiffness,* that is, the tendency of the myocardium to resist stretching (a strain) in response to an increase in tension (a stress).

Elasticity: The property of a material to return from a stressed state to its original conformation when the stresses are removed.

The mechanism responsible for the high diastolic stiffness of cardiac muscle is not clearly understood. Some of the high resistance to stretch can probably be attributed to structures that lie outside the myocardial cells (25), for example, collagen (26). Intracellular structures, including the cytoskeletal protein *desmin* (27), or *connectin,* an elastic protein found in both the myofibrils and muscle cell membranes (28), also appear to contribute to the high diastolic stiffness of the myocardium.

Another quite different mechanism for the low compliance of the myocardium is suggested by the finding of spontaneous oscillations in sarcomere length in unstimulated myocardial cells (29). These oscillations, which can generate significant levels of diastolic tension, are due to low levels of contractile interactions between the thick and thin filaments initiated by cyclic release of Ca^{2+} from the sarcoplasmic reticulum. Even though the contractile responses to this spontaneous Ca^{2+} release are not induced by an action potential, this cause for diastolic stiffness represents a manifestation of the processes of excitation-contraction coupling that are discussed in other chapters. These tension oscillations, which are similar to aftercontractions, may be of considerable importance in the pathogenesis of filling abnormalities in the heart.

EVALUATION OF DIASTOLIC PROPERTIES OF THE HEART

Diastolic function can be evaluated clinically by such simple methods as auscultation of a third or fourth heart sound that implies that the ventricle has become more stiff and unable to fill normally. These simple clinical tools, though of some use in patient evaluation and screening, are nonspecific and thus of little use in quantitative research. Thus, optimal evaluation of diastolic function requires measurements of the time course of changes in either ventricular pressure or volume during the cardiac cycle. Diastolic time intervals derived from apex and phonoechocardiography may be of use in certain instances in which loading conditions are relatively normal (*vide infra*).

Evaluation of Diastolic Function Using Pressure Data

Initial attempts to use the time course of fall of left ventricular pressure to index relaxation concentrated on the maximum rate of left ventricular pressure fall (maximum negative dP/dt). Although maximum negative dP/dt is determined by the time course of left ventricular relaxation, it is also extremely load-dependent (30). This dependence is marked for systolic pressure in that the higher the level of pressure at peak systole and at the onset of isovolumic relaxation (the time of maximum negative dP/dt), the greater the value of maximum negative dP/dt.

A number of early studies in isolated muscle showed that the time course of tension fall in both cardiac and skeletal muscle could be approximated by an exponential process. There is some evidence that the fundamental relaxing process involving calcium uptake by the sarcoplasmic reticulum may well be exponential. Data from a number of laboratories have shown that the time course of left ventricular pressure fall, when measured carefully in normal left ventricles, approximates an exponential function to a remarkable degree of certainty (31–33) and that attempts to fit pressure-fall data to a higher or lower order of functions are less successful than attempts to fit the time course of left ventricular pressure fall during isovolumic relaxation to a single exponential function.

If the close approximation of isovolumic pressure fall to an exponential function reflects a fundamental aspect of the process of relaxation, some of the relationships between load and the time constant for the exponential fall in pressure become clear. Increasing the level from which the ventricular pressure begins its exponential fall during relaxation would likely have little effect on the time course of this process of relaxation. Hence, the time constant would be unaffected by the magnitude of peak left ventricular pressure and uninfluenced by the level of pressure at the onset of the exponential phase of pressure fall. At higher levels of pressure from which the exponential fall in pressure begins, there would be a greater absolute rate of left ventricular pressure fall, so that maximum negative dP/dt would increase, but there would be no change in the time constant.

The relationship between load and the decline in tension in isolated muscle has important implications for the determinants of the rate at which pressure falls in the ventricle. When mammalian cardiac muscle is allowed to shorten isometrically during a single contraction, sudden unloading causes a significant acceleration of the decay of tension decline (34). This important influence has been characterized extensively by Brutsaert and colleagues (35,36), who have shown that the relaxation properties of cardiac muscle are influenced by a complex interplay between load-dependent and time-dependent properties of the mechanisms responsible for the decay of tension in the muscle within a single contraction. Loads which are applied early in the cardiac cycle will effectively delay relaxation, whereas those applied later in systole will prompt premature, more rapid relaxation (35,36). Recently, Gaasch et al. have demonstrated this phenomenon in the working canine left ventricle. In both "ejecting" and "isovolumic" beats, quick stretch was produced by addition of 6 ml volume in 15 msec either shortly after aortic valve opening or near aortic valve closure. In the former, relaxation was delayed, whereas in the latter it occured earlier and more rapidly (23a).

Experiments in a number of laboratories have attempted to determine if the time constant for the exponential pressure fall in the intact ventricle is independent of load or if it depends to some extent on loading conditions. The initial studies of Weiss, Frederiksen, and Weisfeldt (31) showed a clear load dependence of the time constant of pressure fall at values of load that approached isovolumic tension. That is, there was a shortening of the time constant (or an acceleration of the process of relaxation) when the heart was allowed to shorten, as compared with isovolumic conditions. This observation is analogous to similar observations made in skeletal muscle, in which it was shown that the duration of relaxation was rather markedly abbreviated on going from an isometric contraction to an isotonic contraction. However, increasing the extent of muscle shortening caused little further acceleration of relaxation, so that skeletal muscle relaxation exhibits little load dependence except during changes from isometric contraction to totally unloaded contraction. In cardiac muscle that is contracting in an isometric fashion, many investigators have shown that rapid stretches, releases, or sinusoidal forcing functions decrease force development and accelerate relaxation. A series of studies performed by Wiegner and Bing (37) showed that in isolated cardiac muscle, much greater load dependence exists than was apparent in those initial studies in vivo; however, the studies of Wiegner and Bing were performed at lower than physiological temperature. When similar studies were carried out at more physiological temperatures in the same apparatus, which allowed a physiological loading sequence, with tension falling before muscle lengthening (as occurs in vivo), much less load dependence and an exponential tension fall were seen (38–40).

Investigators in a number of laboratories have shown greater evidence of load dependence in intact hearts than did the initial studies of Weisfeldt and associates. Because the time constant has been shown by all laboratories to be shortened by catecholamines, which are known to enhance ventricular myocardial relaxation (3), great care must be taken in the performance of such studies to eliminate neurogenic influences that might enhance or decrease sympathetic tone and thereby modify relaxation. If, for example, the aorta is cross-clamped to increase proximal aortic pressure during contraction and peak arterial pressure rises, baroreceptor stimulation would be expected to decrease sympathetic tone and thereby lead to prolongation of the time constant. This prolongation of the time constant might not be evidence of load dependence, but instead would reflect withdrawal of sympathetic nervous tone that, as already described, would prolong relaxation in cardiac muscle. In the majority of the studies demonstrating load dependence, there was a somewhat greater tendency toward load dependence at high loads than at low loads. Despite this load dependence, this index remains the most direct measurement of the relaxation properties of the left ventricle.

In studies in which the measured pressure was the transmural pressure, that is, where the extracavitary left ventricular pressure was atmospheric pressure, as is the case in most isolated heart preparations, the exponential phase of pressure pumping can be described as

$$P = P_0 e^{-t/T} \quad [1]$$

T is the negative inverse slope of the line relating $\ln P$ and t, which is commonly obtained by plotting P versus t on a semilog scale and obtaining the slope of the linear least-squares regression analysis of the data. However, in cases in which there is a base-line shift in the pressure record or in which there is an extracavitary pressure present (such as low pleural pressure, pericardial pressure, right ventricular pressure) that is, different from zero, a different formula must be used (41). If that P_B is this external pressure that is constant throughout the cardiac cycle, then the record pressure is described by the following equation:

$$P = P_0 e^{-t/T} + P_B \quad [2]$$

In this case, T can no longer be obtained simply by plotting P versus t on a semilog scale and performing a linear least-squares fit, because $\ln P$ is no longer a linear function of t; instead, it is $\ln(P - P_B)$ that is a linear function of t. Thus, the difficulty can be circumvented by plotting the logarithm of the difference between P and P_B, rather than P versus t.

However, if one does not know or cannot measure the value of P_B (again assumed to be constant), as would be the case for a closed-chest animal in which the outside pressure is not recorded, one can still obtain T easily by using an alternative approach. If equation (2) is differentiated with respect to time, one obtains the following equation:

$$dP/dt = -P_0e^{-t/T}/T \qquad [3]$$

Substituting equation (2) back into equation (3), one obtains

$$dP/dt = -\ln(P - P_B)/T \qquad [4]$$

If one now plots dP/dt versus P and performs a linear least-squares regression, the slope of the line obtained is independent of P_B, and only the intercept of the line is influenced by P_B. Attempts to examine the load dependence of the time constant determined from the slope of the relationship between dP/dt and P have resulted in a similar picture of relatively little load dependence of this index. Again, P determined by this approach is remarkably sensitive to the enhancement of relaxation produced by catecholamines and relatively insensitive to inotropic agents that do not enhance relaxation.

Evaluation of Diastolic Function Using Echocardiographic Data and Diastolic Time Intervals

Both two-dimensional echocardiography and M-mode echocardiography can be used to evaluate left ventricular relaxation and left ventricular filling. The periods of interest in the functioning heart include isovolumic relaxation, rapid filling, slow filling (diastasis), and atrial augmentation of filling (Fig. 2). In general, quantitative echocardiographic data are more simply obtained in the M-mode, because this method provides a continuous recording of time-dependent changes in the positions of the walls of the ventricle. Time intervals can be referred to components of the simultaneously recorded electrocardiogram or phonocardiogram. A number of measurements can be made by this method (42–44). Isovolumic relaxation time has been represented in several ways: by the interval from either the aortic closure sound, A_2, or the echographic aortic closure point to mitral valve opening (MVO), or by the interval from end-systole (the minimal end-systolic dimension, i.e., where the first derivative of the left ventricular dimension curve goes to zero, see Fig. 3) to MVO. Shaver and Rahko (44) have shown that A_2 corresponds to the incisura of the high-fidelity aortic pressure curve and that MVO falls within ±10 msec of the crossover between left atrial and left ventricular pressure. Methods that consider aortic valve closure as the onset of isovolumic relaxation will yield slightly shorter isovolumic relaxation times than those which consider the onset of relaxation to begin with increasing cavity dimension. The ability of these intervals to represent actual myocardial relaxation time will depend on preload and afterload. For example, if systemic arterial pressure is elevated, A_2 will occur sooner, thereby lengthening the A_2-to-MVO interval. The O point of the apex cardiogram corresponds approximately with the nadir of the left ventricular pressure curve; its timing can be influenced by a number of factors, particularly ventricular geometry.

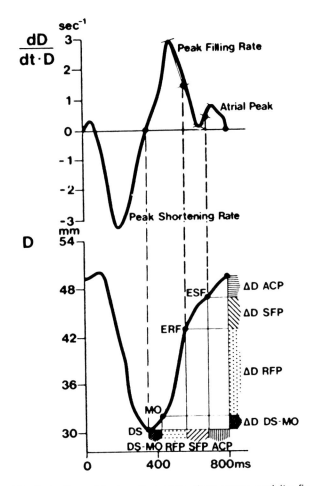

FIG. 2. Left ventricular dimension–time curve and its first derivative as obtained by echocardiographic analysis of left ventricular wall motion showing different phases of left ventricular filling and emptying. Abbreviations: ACP, filling due to atrial systole; D, dimension; DS, end-systolic dimension; ERF, end of phase of rapid filling; ESF, end of phase of slow filling; MO, mitral valve opening; RFP, rapid-filling phase; SFP, slow-filling phase; t, time. (From ref. 42, with permission.)

The echocardiogram also allows measurements of left ventricular cavity dimensions throughout the cardiac cycle. When these dimensions are expressed in relation to time, derivative functions can be analyzed that also characterize ventricular relaxation and filling (Fig. 2). The rapid-filling period has attracted much recent interest because, as previously stated, it is the portion of the ventricular filling period most governed by active muscle relaxation. By M-mode echocardiography, the rapid-filling period begins after MVO and is considered to end where the normalized rate of lengthening has fallen to 50% of its peak value (43). Rapid-filling time can be expressed as a percentage of the total filling time, as expressed by Hanrath et al. (42), as can the periods of slow filling and atrial augmentation. Similarly, the percentages of total left ventricular diameter increase during rapid filling, slow filling, and atrial augmentation can also be calculated from the data in Fig. 2 (42).

Further information with regard to the relationship of left ventricular relaxation and the time course of left ventricular filling has recently emanated from the use of focused Doppler techniques with anatomic localization of the beam by echocardiography. Such measurements have already been utilized to demonstrate an age-related decrease in the maximum velocity of early filling that is almost certainly a consequence of age-related prolongation of left ventricular relaxation (45).

Unfortunately, neither direct measurements of pressure nor diastolic time intervals can specify precisely the termination of cardiac muscle relaxation, because the chamber may be continuing to dissipate tension and pressure even as it fills. It is probable, although still somewhat uncertain, that the end of relaxation corresponds to the end of the rapid-filling interval in normal hearts.

Evaluation of Diastolic Function Using Radionuclide Ventriculography

When the peripheral blood pool is labeled with a radiopharmaceutical, it is possible to generate dynamic images of the left ventricular cavity (46). Such images are of the moving ventricular blood pool rather than of the ventricular walls themselves (in contrast to echocardiography). The EKG can be used to "gate" or control an acquisition sequence of images from which a representative composite cardiac cycle is created by superimposing information from 200 to 400 individual cycles. An operator-selected region of interest can be then defined. When the region of interest is defined as the left ventricular cavity, the multiple-frame images of one or many cardiac cycles can be reconstructed by computer into time–activity or time–volume curves for the left ventricle. Because radionuclide ventricular volume curves are derived directly from images, and simply represent the change in (radioactive) counts with respect to time, no assumptions are made about the geometry of the chamber, an advantage particularly when studying disease states in which ventricular geometry may be abnormal, or ventricular shape changes during the cardiac cycle.

Volume curves can be derived from both imaging and nonimaging counting devices. When the conventional gamma camera is used, the region of interest is visualized. If a nonimaging nuclear probe is used, the region of interest is selected by a positioning algorithm that relies on the cyclic change in radioactivity over the left ventricle (48). The gamma camera tends to provide more reliable data when hearts with markedly heterogeneous wall motion, markedly increased or decreased contractile performance, or unusual geometry are studied. The nuclear probe, however, can provide high-resolution curves with lower doses of isotope and shorter imaging times, an advantage when serial studies are contemplated. In addition, the probe allows analysis of cardiac function on a beat-to-beat basis; this is not feasible with conventional gamma-camera imaging because of poor count statistics of individual cycles with the latter.

A number of different methods have been applied to analyze quantitatively both the ejection and filling phases of the ventricular volume curve. Prior to curve analysis, the raw data must be processed so as to reduce variability and errors due to "noise" (radioactive scatter from structures outside the region of interest). One method that has been applied in recent clinical studies is based on fitting the raw-count data to a high-order polynomial function. Subsequently, curves of the first-derivative functions are generated in order to locate and assign values to the peak rates of ejection and filling. Curve fitting has the advantage of greatly reducing data variability due to noisy curves, but may require somewhat complex mathematical modeling in order to accurately express "native" ventricular performance. It is possible that a given model may not be valid across a wide range of abnormal ventricular function; moreover, one mathematical model may fit a particular set of data from a subject but not another set of data from the same subject. With an alternative method of analysis for volume curves, the noise is first reduced by temporal smoothing; then time-related functions of the smoothed "native" volume curve are analyzed. With the latter method, fewer mathematical assumptions regarding ventricular performance are made. The volume curve is therefore more likely to reveal subtle changes; however, the results are more observer-dependent, and the effect of noise may be greater than with curve fitting.

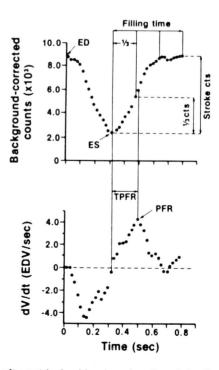

FIG. 3. Left ventricular blood-pool radioactivity–time curve and its first derivative as obtained by a nuclear-camera analysis of left ventricular wall motion showing different phases of left ventricular filling and emptying. Abbreviations: cts, radionuclide counts; ED, end-diastole; ES, end-systole; $\frac{1}{3}$, the first third of diastole; PFR, peak filling rate; TPFR, time to peak filling rate. (From ref. 47, with permission.)

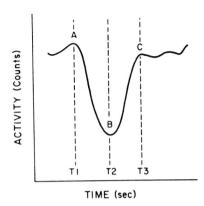

FIG. 4. Schematic left ventricular time–activity curve: A = end-diastolic counts measured at time T1; B = end-systolic counts measured at time T2; C = rapid-filling counts measured at time T3. Dashed vertical lines define the ejection period (T2 − T1) and rapid-filling period (T3 − T2). (From ref. 10, with permission.)

The first-third (of diastole) filling fraction is calculated as the percentage of end-diastolic counts achieved during the first third of the diastolic interval (Fig. 3). This parameter represents the initial filling behavior of the left ventricle and theoretically reflects left ventricular relaxation more closely than do those parameters that include a larger fraction of the filling interval. The peak filling rate and the time to achieve the peak filling rate are calculated from the first-derivative function of the left ventricular time–activity (volume) curve (Fig. 3) and have been utilized in numerous clinical studies of ventricular performance. The average rapid-filling rate (Fig. 4) results from simple division of rapid-filling volume (point C minus point B) by rapid-filling interval (time T3 minus time T2), with normalization for the end-diastolic volume (point A). The average rapid-filling rate is generally calculated from the unfitted curve, because it requires identification of the end of rapid filling. The average rapid-filling rate will, by definition, reflect abnormalities in the extent of relaxation that result in reduced rapid-filling volume, a phenomenon that is not quantified by either the first-third filling fraction or the peak filling rate.

The effect of heart rate on the rapid-filling phase has not been satisfactorily studied. Hence, the results of studies in which the effect of heart rate on filling parameters has not been considered should be interpreted with caution. A number of physiological influences can alter cycle length, so that the practice of simply "correcting" filling-rate data for variations in heart rate may not be justified when a changing physiological variable such as sympathetic tone could affect both the cycle length and the relaxation rate independently. At increased heart rates, ventricular diastasis may be sufficiently shortened to result in superimposition of atrial stroke volume on rapid-filling volume. This phenomenon is particularly likely to occur when the rapid-filling time

is prolonged. In this instance, neither the peak nor the average filling rate reliably reflects either the time course or the extent of rapid left ventricular filling. Finally, information about ventricular filling derived from the global volume curve may not represent the relaxation behavior of different regions of the ventricle, a limitation that should be considered when the effects of interventions on ventricular filling behavior are being studied.

SIGNIFICANCE OF RELAXATION MEASUREMENTS

The mechanisms that are responsible for the fall in pressure during isovolumic relaxation ($-dP/dt$) are fundamentally different from those responsible for filling ($+dV/dt$) (Table 2). Although the biochemical and biophysical bases for the dissipation of both tension [indexed by the time constant of pressure fall (T)] and filling ($+dV/dt$) of the ventricle are still incompletely understood, it is likely that T reflects mainly the rates at which Ca^{2+} is removed from the contractile proteins and at which the active bonds linking actin and myosin are dissipated. Early filling can similarly be viewed as an index of Ca^{2+} removal rate; however, when there is delayed relaxation, the filling occurring later in diastole more closely reflects passive properties and left atrial pressure. When relaxation changes occur in conditions such as hypertrophy and hyperthyroidism, these changes reflect altered myosin isoenzyme profiles as well. A

TABLE 2. *Possible mechanisms for impaired diastolic function*

Impaired isovolumic relaxation ($-dP/dt$)
  Prolongation of the active state of muscle
    Increased Ca^{2+} affinity of troponin
    Decreased rate of dissociation of actin-myosin interactions
    Decreased rate of Ca^{2+} transport by sarcoplasmic reticulum
  Decreased elastic recoil of myocardium
  Lack of true isometricity
    Localized wall-motion abnormalities
    Aortic regurgitation
Impaired filling ($+dV/dt$ or EDV → ESV)
  Impaired ejection (increased ESV)
  Incomplete removal of activator Ca^{2+} from troponin
    Increased Ca^{2+} affinity of troponin
    Decreased Ca^{2+} sensitivity of sarcoplasmic reticulum
  Persistence of actin-myosin interactions (rigor bonds)
  Aftercontractions
  Fibrosis or infiltrative disease of myocardium
  Hypertrophy, increased wall thickness
  Hypoplasia, decreased chamber size
  Mechanical factors
    Pericardial constriction or tamponade
    Mitral stenosis
  Interactions between right and left ventricles
  Inadequate filling time, tachycardia

Adapted from ref. 7.

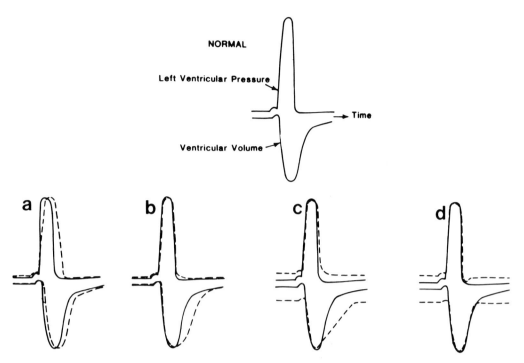

FIG. 5. Schematic diagram illustrating possible relaxation abnormalities. **Top:** Representation of normal left ventricular pressure and volume curves. **Bottom:** Theoretical illustrations of four types of relaxation abnormalities: **a:** slowing of isovolumic relaxation ($-dP/dt$) that delays filling without slowing filling rate ($+dV/dt$) or reducing the extent of filling (ESV $\rightarrow$ EDV); **b:** slowing of filling rate ($+dV/dt$) that occurs without reducing $-dP/dt$ or the extent of filling (ESV $\rightarrow$ EDV); **c:** slowing of filling rate ($+dV/dt$) that is accompanied by a decrease in the extent of filling (ESV $\rightarrow$ EDV) but no change in $-dP/dt$; **d:** impaired filling (ESV $\rightarrow$ EDV) that occurs without changes in either $-dP/dt$ or filling rate ($+dV/dt$). (From ref. 9, with permission.)

schematic diagram showing some theoretical relaxation abnormalities is shown in Fig. 5.

Abnormalities in Isovolumic Relaxation

Abnormalities in isovolumic relaxation, which are manifest as a decreased rate of pressure fall and a prolonged time constant (T) during the interval between aortic valve closure and mitral valve opening, can result from a variety of mechanisms. Some of these mechanisms are intrinsic to the myocardium, and others arise from influences acting on the heart itself (Table 2). Relaxation is related to the breaking of the bonds linking actin and myosin that are responsible for contraction. These two proteins begin to dissociate shortly after removal of activator Ca^{2+} from its binding sites on troponin, a process that is effected by uphill transport of Ca^{2+} by the ATP-dependent Ca^{2+} pump of the sarcoplasmic reticulum. From a theoretical point of view, therefore, slowing of isovolumic relaxation will be expected to occur when the rate of Ca^{2+} transport into the sarcoplasmic reticulum is reduced, or when Ca^{2+} fails to dissociate normally from the Ca^{2+}-binding sites on troponin. The latter situation can arise when the Ca^{2+} affinity of troponin is increased. In other words, T can be lengthened when the "inactivation" of excitation-contraction coupling is abnormally slow. The rate at

which pressure falls during isovolumic relaxation will also be slowed by an impairment of the dissociation of actin from myosin after Ca^{2+} is removed from troponin. Because the elastic recoil in the walls of the heart also contributes to relaxation, a loss of this elasticity will slow this phase of isovolumic relaxation. Finally, a lack of true isometricity during isovolumic relaxation, as is seen in aortic insufficiency or when there is an expansile ventricular aneurysm, will also reduce $-dP/dt$ and likewise prolong T or make pressure fall nonexponential.

Abnormalities of Filling

Impaired filling may be manifest as a reduced rate ($+dV/dt$) or extent of ventricular filling (ESV $\rightarrow$ EDV, the difference between end-diastolic and end-systolic volumes). The abnormalities that slow the dissipation of pressure within the ventricle ($-dP/dt$) may be quite different from those that impair filling, particularly as diastole progresses (Table 2). It should be noted, however, that a delay in dissipation of tension by the walls of the left ventricle can reduce the rate of ventricular filling or the extent of filling (Fig. 1A).

The major link between abnormalities of contraction and of relaxation resides in the fact that incomplete emptying (an inotropic abnormality) increases end-systolic volume. This increased residual volume in the ventricle, in turn, reduces the volume of blood that can enter the ventricle during the subsequent diastole (Table 2), so that a contraction abnormality will indirectly impair the ability of the ventricle to fill. Sudden decreases in left atrial pressure, as well as changes in the ventricular passive diastolic stiffness or restriction of left ventricular filling by virtue of pericardial restraint, also influence ventricular filling. The factor that is dominant in overall filling will change from one situation to another. The pericardium, myocardial diastolic tone, passive properties, left atrial pressure, and the characteristics of ventricular relaxation, either alone or in combination, may be the controlling factor that modifies ventricular filling.

Filling of the ventricle can also be reduced by any mechanism that inhibits removal of activator Ca^{2+} from the cytosol at the end of systole. Slowing of the rate of this Ca^{2+} removal will be expected to both prolong T and slow $+dV/dt$, whereas incomplete removal of cytosolic Ca^{2+} will decrease ESV → EDV. Most important of the mechanisms that remove Ca^{2+} from the cytosol at the end of systole is the Ca^{2+} pump of the sarcoplasmic reticulum, but both sodium/calcium exchange and a sarcolemmal Ca^{2+} pump also lower the cytosolic Ca^{2+} concentration to levels that will cause this cation to be completely dissociated from troponin.

An important and recently described mechanism that can impair filling is persistence of oscillatory Ca^{2+} release from the sarcoplasmic reticulum during diastole (29) (*vide supra*). This mechanism is also responsible for generation of aftercontractions, which represent spontaneous redevelopment of tension in cardiac muscle in the absence of an observed action potential. Aftercontractions are seen after intense inotropic stimulation, when the sarcoplasmic reticulum spontaneously releases Ca^{2+} in early diastole. Persistence of rigor bonds linking the myosin cross-bridge to the thin filament, even in the absence of troponin-bound Ca^{2+}, provides another theoretical explanation for impaired filling.

Ventricular filling can also be impaired by changes in the ventricular wall that do not involve the contractile system, notably fibrosis or infiltrative disease of the heart. Hypertrophy, by increasing wall thickness, may impair filling because of the greater mass of tissue to be stretched and because of uneven distribution of stress across the wall of the ventricle. Other abnormalities of chamber geometry, notably hypoplasia, also can impair filling. Increased intramyocardial tension, such as occurs as a result of lymphatic obstruction or the edema caused by myocardial injury, or when increased coronary artery pressure causes engorgement of the coronary circulation, can also reduce ventricular filling. Changes in the geometry of the interventricular septum caused by an abnormality of one ventricle can alter the filling of the other, as exemplified by the impaired right ventricular filling caused by septal hypertrophy in patients suffering from concentric hypertrophy of the left ventricle.

Finally, filling of the ventricle can also be reduced by such mechanical factors as mitral stenosis, pericardial tamponade, and constrictive pericarditis. In conditions in which one ventricle suddenly becomes dilated, as occurs where there is an acute depression of regional or global function or a sudden increase in preload or afterload, the normal pericardium becomes restricting and limits filling of the opposite ventricle. Acute right ventricular infarction or massive pulmonary emboli, for example, can cause marked pericardial restriction to left ventricular filling.

HEMODYNAMIC EFFECTS OF RELAXATION ABNORMALITIES

Some of the hemodynamic consequences of the relaxation abnormalities discussed earlier are shown schematically in Figs. 1 and 5 (41). The patterns drawn in Fig. 5 are based largely on theoretical considerations, but may resemble those for data obtained by analyses of ventricular volume data now becoming available from both noninvasive and invasive clinical studies.

One clear and graphic example of the importance of incomplete left ventricular relaxation in overall hemodynamics is illustrated by hypotensive ventricular tachycardia in subjects with relatively normal ventricular systolic function (49). As stated earlier, one circumstance in which left ventricular relaxation compromises overall ventricular function through restricting ventricular filling occurs when heart rate is very rapid, and it is well recognized that there is a greater likelihood of hypotension and syncope as the rate of a ventricular tachycardia increases. It had been assumed that the mechanism of hypotension during such episodes of ventricular tachycardia was relative myocardial ischemia due to the increasing oxygen demands of very rapid ventricular rates, along with increased sympathetic tone, and interference with contraction of the ventricle due to the asynchronous activation and prolonged activation of the ventricle due to the arrhythmia itself. Recently, simultaneous echocardiographic and pressure measurements have been performed in patients who had had episodes of symptomatic ventricular arrhythmia during induced ventricular tachycardia. Figure 6 (left) shows the pressure–dimension loops for normal sinus rhythm and for ventricular tachycardia in 2 patients. For the first patient, the loops during sinus rhythm are compared only with a single loop during ventricular tachycardia. These loops are very similar in appearance to the example of incomplete relaxation shown in Fig. 1B. Stroke volume is profoundly reduced, and the end-systolic pressure–dimension point during the ventricular tachycardia appears to fall on an end-systolic pressure–volume line that would be typical for a normal ventricle. Thus, systolic function during hypotensive ventricular tachycardia is not greatly altered, but stroke volume and therefore systolic pressure are markedly reduced as a result of incomplete relaxation. This is shown in more rigorous

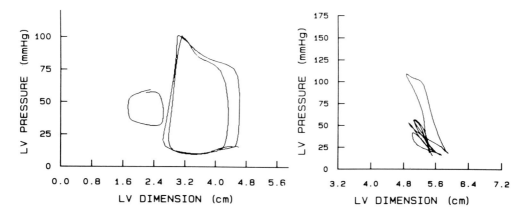

FIG. 6. Left: Pressure–dimension loops in sinus rhythm (*large*) and during ventricular tachycardia (*small*) from a patient with near-normal ventricular function. Displacement of the ventricular tachycardia loop to the left and upward in relation to the loop in sinus rhythm indicates marked reduction in cavity size with a high end-diastolic pressure due to incomplete relaxation. **Right:** The pressure–dimension loops for the last three beats of ventricular tachycardia (*small loops*) and the first sinus beat after conversion to sinus rhythm are plotted together with two preventricular tachycardia beats. As ventricular tachycardia ends, left ventricular pressure falls immediately to join the diastolic pressure–dimension line of the two control sinus beats. (From ref. 49, with permission.)

fashion in Fig. 6 in the more complex loop on the right. In a different patient, two beats of a sinus rhythm and the last three beats of ventricular tachycardia and the

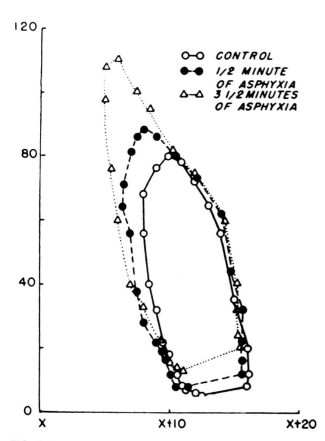

FIG. 7. Pressure–volume loops constructed from representative beats during each of three periods of progressive asphyxia in an anesthetized, open-chest dog. The abscissa is left ventricular volume (in cc), expressed as the increment over an arbitrary volume *x*, and the ordinate is left ventricular pressure (in mm Hg). (From ref. 53, with permission of the American Heart Association.)

first postventricular tachycardia beat are shown. Here it is clear that the moment that the ventricular tachycardia is interrupted, left ventricular pressure falls and dimension increases to normal values for this heart. When the ventricle contracts with its first beat after the tachycardia, contractility is, if anything, higher than the level of contractility prior to the episode of ventricular tachycardia. Again, during the last three beats of ventricular tachycardia, the decreases in left ventricular stroke volume and left ventricular pressure are entirely related to the decrease in left ventricular filling due to incomplete left ventricular relaxation.

It has already been pointed out that relaxation abnormalities often play major roles in the pathogenesis of heart failure. Further, relaxation is more readily impaired by ischemia and pressure overload than is contraction. For example, increased left ventricular diastolic stiffness occurs during attacks of angina and following myocardial infarction (50–52), a phenomenon that was observed many years ago in experimental animals (53) (Fig. 7). The resulting decrease in ventricular distensibility probably contributes to the increased left ventricular filling pressure and congestive symptoms observed during spontaneous and pacing-induced angina. This phenomenon has important clinical diagnostic and therapeutic implications. Ventricular hypertrophy caused by hypertrophic cardiomyopathy (54) and chronic hemodynamic overloading of the left ventricle is also associated with abnormalities in diastolic function (6–10,55,56), and there is evidence that these abnormalities may be among the earliest signs of impaired left ventricular function (10). Of interest is the finding that, unlike the pathological hypertrophy caused by chronic pressure overload, the hypertrophy associated with intermittent strenuous exercise in otherwise healthy individuals is not accompanied by detectable abnormalities in left ventricular systolic or diastolic function (57–59).

REFERENCES

1. Frederickson, J. W., Weiss, J. L., and Weisfeldt, M. L. (1978): Time constant of isovolumic pressure fall: Determinants in the working left ventricle. *Am. J. Physiol.*, 235:H701–H706.
2. Raff, G. L., and Glantz, S. A. (1981): Volume loading shows left ventricular isovolumic relaxation rate: Evidence of load-dependent relaxation in the intact dog heart. *Circ. Res.*, 48:813–824.
3. Katz, A. M. (1983): Cyclic adenosine monophosphate effects on the myocardium: A man who blows hot and cold with one breath. *J. Am. Coll. Cardiol.*, 2:143–149.
4. Schaible, T. F., and Scheuer, J. (1979): Cardiac function in hypertrophied hearts from chronically exercised female rats. *J. Appl. Physiol. (Respirat. Environ. Exercise Physiol.)*, 46:854–860.
5. Brutsaert, D. L., and Meijler, F. L. (1980): Introduction: Relaxation and diastole. II. Proceedings of the Fifth Workshop on Contractile Behavior of the Heart. *Eur. Heart J. [Suppl. A]*, 1:1.
6. Grossman, W., and Barry, W. H. (1980): Diastolic pressure–volume relations in the diseased heart. *Fed. Proc.*, 39:148–155.
7. Rankin, J. S., and Olson, C. O. (1980): The diastolic filling of the left ventricle. *Eur. Heart J. [Suppl. A]*, 1:95–105.
8. Bonow, R. O., Bacharach, S. L., Green, M. V., Kent, K. M., Rosing, D. R., Lipson, L. C., Leon, M. B., and Epstein, S. E. (1981): Impaired left ventricular filling in patients with coronary artery disease: Assessment with radionuclide angiography. *Circulation*, 64:315–323.
9. Smith, V. E., and Katz, A. M. (1983): Inotropic and lusitropic abnormalities in the genesis of heart failure. *Eur. Heart J. [Suppl. A]*, 4:7–17.
10. Smith, V. E., Schulman, P., Karimeddini, M. K., White, W. B., Meeran, M. K., and Katz, A. M. (1985): Rapid filling in left ventricular hypertrophy. II. Pathological hypertrophy. *J. Am. Coll. Cardiol.* 5:869–874.
11. Alpert, N. R., Mulieri, L. A., and Litten, R. Z. (1982): Isoenzyme contribution to economy of contraction and relaxation in normal and hypertrophied hearts. In: *International Erwin Riesch Symposium*, Tubingen, pp. 103–157.
12. Tada, M., Yamamoto, T., and Tonomura, Y. (1978): Molecular mechanisms of active calcium transport by sarcoplasmic reticulum. *Physiol. Rev.*, 58:1–79.
13. Katz, A. M. (1984): Calcium fluxes across the sarcoplasmic reticulum. *Persp. Cardiovasc. Res.* 9:53–66.
14. Tsien, R. W. (1983): Calcium channels in excitable cell membranes. *Annu. Rev. Physiol.*, 45:341–358.
15. Shigekawa, M., Finegan, J.-A. M., and Katz, A. M. (1976): Calcium transport ATPase of canine cardiac sarcoplasmic reticulum. A comparison with that of rabbit fast skeletal muscle sarcoplasmic reticulum. *J. Biol. Chem.*, 251:6894–6900.
16. Anversa, P., Olivetti, G., Melissari, M., and Loud, A. V. (1980): Stereological measurement of cellular and subcellular hypertrophy and hyperplasia in the papillary muscle of adult rat. *J. Mol. Cell. Cardiol.*, 12:781–795.
17. Colvin, R. A., Ashavaid, T. F., and Herbette, L. (1985): Structure-function studies of canine cardiac sarcolemmal membranes. I. Estimation of receptor site densities. *Biochim. Biophys. Acta*, 812:601–608.
18. Herbette, L., MacAlister, T., Ashavaid, T. F., and Colvin, R. A. (1985): Structure-function studies of canine cardiac sarcolemmal membranes. II. Structural organization of the sarcolemmal membrane as determined by electron microscopy and lamellar x-ray diffraction. *Biochim. Biophys. Acta*, 812:609–623.
19. Napolitano, C. A., Cooke, P., Segalman, K., and Herbette, L. (1983): Organization of calcium pump protein dimers in the isolated sarcoplasmic reticulum membrane. *Biophys J.*, 42:119–125.
20. Shigekawa, M., Dougherty, J. P., and Katz, A. M. (1978): Reaction mechanism of Ca^{2+}-dependent ATP hydrolysis by skeletal muscle sarcoplasmic reticulum in the absence of added alkali metal salts. I. Characterization of steady state ATP hydrolysis and comparison with that in the presence of KCl. *J. Biol. Chem.*, 253:1442–1450.
21. Nakamura, Y., and Tonomura, Y. (1982): The binding of ATP to the catalytic and the regulatory site of Ca^{2+},Mg^{2+}-dependent ATPase of the sarcoplasmic reticulum. *J. Bioeng. Biomed.*, 14:307–318.
22. Suga, H., Sagawa, K., and Shoukas, A. A. (1973): Load independence of the instantaneous pressure–volume ratio of the canine left ventricle and effects of epinephrine and heart rate on the ratio. *Circ. Res.*, 32:314–322.
23. Rousseau, M. F., Veriter, C., Detry, J. M. R., Brasseur, L., and Pouleur, H. (1980): Impaired early left ventricular relaxation in coronary artery disease: Effects of intracoronary nifedipine. *Circulation*, 62:764–772.
23a. Gaasch, W. H., Apstein, C. S., and Levine, H. J. (1985): Diastolic properties of the left ventricle. In: *The Ventricle: Basic and Clinical Aspects*, edited by H. J. Levine and W. H. Gaasch. Martinus Nijhoff, Boston, pp. 143–170.
24. Mirsky, I., and Parmley, W. W. (1973): Assessment of passive elastic stiffness for isolated heart muscle and the intact heart. *Circ. Res.*, 33:233–243.
25. Tarr, M., Trank, J. W., Leiffer, P., and Shepherd, N. (1979): Sarcomere length-resting relation in single frog atrial cardiac cells. *Circ. Res.*, 45:554–559.
26. Borg, T. K., and Caulfield, J. B. (1981): The collagen matrix of the heart. *Fed. Proc.*, 40:2037–2041.
27. Price, M. G. (1984): Molecular analysis of intermediate filament cytoskeleton—a putative load-bearing structure. *Am. J. Physiol.*, 246:H556–H572.
28. Maruyama, K., Matsubara, S., Natori, R., Nonomura, Y., Kimura, S., Ohashi, K., Murakami, F., Handa, S., and Eguchi, G. (1977): Connectin, an elastic protein of muscle. Characterization and function. *J. Biochem. (Tokyo)*, 82:317–337.
29. Lakatta, E. G., Capogrossi, M. C., Kort, A. A., and Stern, M. D. (1985): Spontaneous myocardial Ca oscillations: An overview with emphasis on ryanodine and caffeine. *Fed. Proc. (in press)*.
30. Weisfeldt, M. L., Scully, H. E., Frederiksen, J., Rubinstein, J. J., Phost, G. M., Beierholm, E., Bello, A. G., and Daggett, W. M. (1974): Hemodynamic determinants of maximum negative *dP/dt* and periods of diastole. *Am. J. Physiol.*, 227:613–621.
31. Weiss, J. L., Frederiksen, J. W., and Weisfeldt, M. L. (1976): Hemodynamic determinants of the time-course of fall in canine left ventricular pressure. *J. Clin. Invest.*, 58:751–760.
32. Karliner, J. S., LeWinter, M. M., Mahler, F., Engler, R., and O'Rourke, R. A. (1977): Pharmacologic and hemodynamic influences on the rate of isovolumic left ventricular relaxation in the normal conscious dog. *J. Clin. Invest.*, 60:511–521.
33. Gaasch, W. H., Blaustein, A. S., and Adam, D. (1980): Myocardial relaxation. IV. Mechanical determinants of the time course of left ventricular pressure decline during isovolumic relaxation. *Eur. Heart J. [Suppl. A]*, 1:111–117.
34. Brady, A. J. (1965): Time and displacement dependence of cardiac contractility: Problems in defining the active state and force-velocity relations. *Fed Proc.*, 24:1410–1420.
35. Brutsaert, D. L., DeClerck, N. M., Goethals, M. A., and Housmans, P. R. (1978): Relaxation of ventricular cardiac muscle. *J. Physiol. (Lond.)*, 283:469–480.
36. Goethals, M. A., Housmans, P. R., and Brutsaert, D. L. (1980): Load-dependence of physiologically relaxing cardiac muscle. *Eur. Heart J. [Suppl. A]*, 1:81–87.
37. Wiegner, A. W., and Bing, O. H. L. (1974): Isometric relaxation of rat myocardium at end-systolic length. *Circ. Res.*, 43:865–869.
38. Wiegner, A. W., and Bing, O. H. L. (1982): Mechanics of myocardial relaxation: Application of a model to isometric and isotonic relaxation of rat myocardium. *J. Biomechanics*, 15:831–840.
39. Nakamura, Y., Wiegner, A. W., and Bing, O. H. L. (1981): Does load alter the time constant of isometric relaxation? *Circulation*, 64:177 (abstract).
40. Elzinga, G., and Westerhof, N. (1980): Reply to comments on "How to quantify pump function in the heart." *Circ. Res.*, 46:303–304.
41. Weisfeldt, M. L., Weiss, J. L., Frederiksen, J. T., and Yin, F. C. P. (1980): Quantification of incomplete left ventricular relaxation: Relationship to the time constant for isovolumic pressure fall. *Eur. J. Cardiol.*, 1:119–129.
42. Hanrath, P., Mathey, D. G., Siegert, R., and Bleifeld, W. (1980): Left ventricular relaxation and filling patterns in different forms of left ventricular hypertrophy: An echocardiographic study. *Am. J. Cardiol.*, 45:15–23.

43. Decoodt, P. R., Mathey, D. G., Swan, H. J. C. (1976): Automated analysis of the left ventricular diameter time curve from echocardiographic recordings. *Comput. Biomed. Res.,* 9:549–558.

44. Shaver, J. A., and Rahko, P. S. (1986): The use of diastolic time intervals in clinical cardiology. *Prog. Cardiovasc. Dis. (in press).*

45. Miyatake, K., Okamoto, M., Kinoshita, N., Owa, M., Nakasone, I., Sakakibara, H., and Nimura, Y. (1984): Augmentation of atrial contribution to left ventricular inflow with aging as assessed by intracardiac Doppler flowmetry. *Am. J. Cardiol.,* 53:586–589.

46. Wagner, H. N., Jr., Wake, R., Nickoloff, E., and Natarajan, T. K. (1976): The nuclear stethoscope: A simple device for generation of left ventricular volume curves. *Am. J. Cardiol.,* 38:747–750.

47. Inouye, I., Massie, B., Loge, D., Topic, N., Silverstein, D., Simpson, P., and Tubau, J. (1984): Abnormal left ventricular filling: An early finding in mild to moderate systemic hypertension. *Am. J. Cardiol.,* 53:120–126.

48. Berger, H. J., Davies, R. A., Batsford, W. P., Hoffer, P. B., Gottschalk, A., and Zaret, B. L. (1981): Beat-to-beat left ventricular performance assessed from the equilibrium cardiac blood pool using a computerized nuclear probe. *Circulation,* 63:133–142.

49. Lima, J. A. C., Weiss, J. L., Guzman, P. A., Weisfeldt, M. L., Reid, P. R., and Traill, T. A. (1983): Incomplete filling and incoordinate contraction as mechanisms of hypotension during ventricular tachycardia in man. *Circulation,* 68:928–938.

50. Gaasch, W. H., Levine, H. J., Quinones, M. A., and Alexander, J. F. (1976): Left ventricular compliance mechanisms and clinical implications. *Am. J. Cardiol.,* 38:645–653.

51. Barry, W. H., Porovoker, J. K., Alderman, E. L., and Harrison, D. C. (1974): Changes in diastolic stiffness and tone to the left ventricle during angina pectoris. *Circulation,* 49:255–263.

52. Papietro, S. E., Cogheau, H. C., Fisserman, D., Russell, R. O., Rackley, C. E., and Rogers, W. J. (1979): Impaired maximal rate of left ventricular relaxation in patients with coronary artery disease and left ventricular dysfunction. *Circulation,* 59:984–990.

53. Katz, A. M., Katz, L. N., and Williams, F. L. (1955): Registration of left ventricular volume curves in the dog with the systemic circulation intact. *Circ. Res.,* 6:588–593.

54. Lipson, L. C., Maron, B. J., Leon, M. B., and Epstein, S. E. (1981): Effects of verapamil on left ventricular systolic function and diastolic filling in patients with hypertrophic cardiomyopathy. *Circulation,* 64:787–796.

55. Grossman, W., McLaurin, L. P., Moss, S. P., Stefadouros, M., and Young, D. T. (1974): Wall thickness and diastolic properties of the left ventricle. *Circulation,* 49:129–135.

56. Grossman, W., McLaurin, L. P., and Stefadouros, M. (1974): Left ventricular stiffness associated with chronic pressure and volume overload in man. *Circ. Res.,* 35:793–800.

57. Schaible, T. F., and Scheuer, J. (1981): Cardiac function in hypertrophied hearts from chronically exercised female rats. *J. Appl. Physiol.,* 50:1140–1145.

58. Carew, T. E., and Covell, J. W. (1978): Left ventricular function in exercise-induced hypertrophy in dogs. *Am. J. Cardiol.,* 42:82–88.

59. Granger, C. B., Karimeddini, M. K., Smith, V. E. E., Shapiro, H. R., Katz, A. M., and Riba, A. L. (1985): Rapid filling in left ventricular hypertrophy. I. Physiological hypertrophy. *J. Am. Coll. Cardiol.,* 5:862–868.

The Heart and Cardiovascular System,
edited by H. A. Fozzard et al.
Raven Press, New York © 1986.

CHAPTER 40

Length Modulation of Muscle Performance: Frank-Starling Law of the Heart

Edward G. Lakatta

For at least 150 years biomedical scientists have appreciated the effect of stretch to enhance myocardial performance. The most convincing or perhaps the most popular demonstrations of this effect came around the turn of the century in the isolated heart experiments of Frank and Starling (36), which showed that an increase in diastolic volume caused increases in systolic performance. Although subsequent studies have shown that the stretch effect persists across a range of myocardial contractile states, other physiologists have maintained that it plays only a minor role augmenting ventricular function in normal man during high myocardial contractile states, e.g., during exercise (36). The main reason for this ambiguity regarding whether or not Starling's law of the heart has physiological relevance in human healthy subjects is that reflex mechanisms, i.e., catecholamine modulation of myocardial performance, heart rate, vascular impedance, and coronary flow, interact with length modulation of myocardial performance and, when effective, can overshadow the effect of fiber stretch or even prevent an increase in end-diastolic volume during stress. Another reason for ambiguity regarding the role of the Frank-Starling mechanism during exercise has been the difficulty in measuring cardiac volume during exercise.

Recent advances in noninvasive ultrasound technology and radionuclide imaging of the heart have made possible a reinvestigation of the role of the Frank-Starling mechanism in the augmentation of stroke volume during upright exercise in healthy human subjects (Fig. 1). These studies have demonstrated that both end-diastolic and stroke volume increase and contribute to the increase in cardiac output during exercise, particularly in elderly subjects, in whom the increase in end-diastolic volume and stroke volume occurs without a substantial decrease in the end-systolic volume. This is the Frank-Starling mechanism, and the composite data in Fig. 1 clearly demonstrate that it is indeed utilized to augment stroke volume to meet the need for increased cardiac output during exercise, and that, in particular, increased reliance on this mechanism occurs with advancing age, when the effectiveness of catecholamine modulation of myocardial performance and stroke volume is diminished (61,63). Although an increase in end-diastolic volume may affect several factors that determine the heart's pumping capacity, its effect to stretch the myocardial fibers and the resultant change in muscle performance is the focus of the present chapter.

LENGTH MODULATION OF CONTRACTILE FORCE IN CARDIAC MUSCLE: PERSPECTIVES FROM MEASUREMENTS OF MUSCLE LENGTH AND FORCE

In cardiac muscle isolated from the heart and studied *in vitro* a change in resting length over a relatively

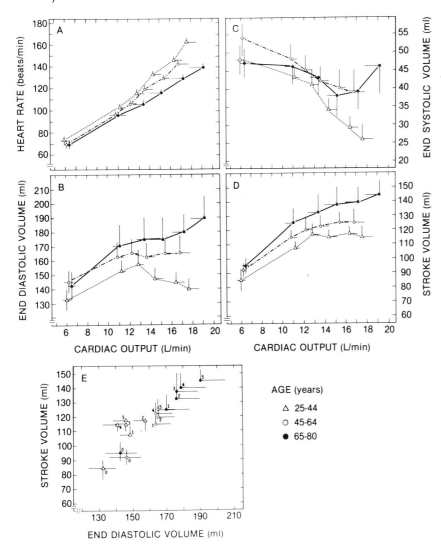

FIG. 1. Relationship of heart rate (**A**), end-diastolic volume (**B**), end-systolic volume (**C**), and stroke volume (**D**) to cardiac output at rest (*left most points*) and during graded upright bicycle exercise in human subjects of three age groups who have been screened rigorously to exclude the presence of both clinical and occult cardiovascular disease. The relationship between stroke and end-diastolic volumes is depicted in **E** (at rest, 0; during progressive exercise, 1–5). The major point of the figure is that a *unique* mechanism for augmentation of cardiac output during exercise does not exist in all subjects. (Adapted from ref. 81.)

narrow range (approximately 15%) can produce large changes in the extent of shortening and force developed during the contraction in response to an external stimulation (Fig. 2). The mechanisms of this effect of fiber length to modulate muscle performance have been and continue to be the focus of considerable study, and our concepts regarding these mechanisms have evolved both with improvements in existing technology and with application of innovative technology to these studies.

Pioneering studies of cardiac muscle followed the rationale of studies performed earlier in skeletal muscle: Mechanical properties (force and displacement) were measured as a function of length prior to excitation and of time and length following excitation (1,10,84). The results of these studies and their interpretation, to a first approximation, concurred with those in skeletal muscle: The viscoelastic properties of cardiac muscle exhibited a transient change following excitation, which was manifest as a twitch or contraction, construed as a turning on of an "active state" which then waned with time. By

making length changes at different times prior to or during the contraction, and measuring the resulting instantaneous change in force or displacement and the secondary slower changes in these variables, the mechanical properties of the muscle could be further categorized into "active" and "passive"; it was fashionable to interpret these in the context of analog models with an "active" force generator ("contractile element"), arranged in various series and/or parallel schemes with inert or "passive" viscous and elastic elements. Subsequent studies in both skeletal and cardiac muscle, however, have shown that critical assumptions made in conceptualizing such models, i.e., that the properties of the passive elastic elements do not vary with time and that the passive and active properties could be truly independently measured, were not correct (83); hence, the popularity of this modeling approach in studies of muscle has dwindled. Nonetheless, these studies were critical in laying the groundwork for our understanding of cardiac muscle function.

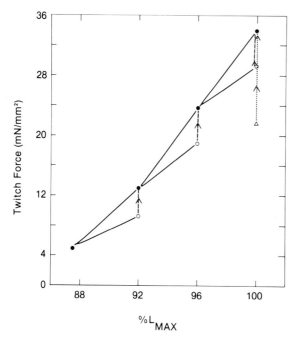

FIG. 2. Effect of a change in resting muscle length on the force development in a subsequent contraction (twitch) in isolated cat right ventricular papillary muscle. An increase of muscle length of about 15%, i.e., from 0.85% L_{max} to L_{max}, that length at which twitch force following excitation is maximal, causes an eightfold increase in twitch force. Note that the relation between twitch force and length is not unique but varies with time following a stretch, i.e., a secondary slow increase in twitch force can occur, the magnitude of which varies with the magnitude of stretch and previous history of the muscle. The steady state length-twitch force relationship is indicated by *solid circles*. The *open circles* indicate the initial twitch force with a stretch from prior equilibration at 87% L_{max} to 92%, 96%, or to 100% L_{max}. The secondary slow increase is indicated by the *dashed line*. The effect of a stretch of greater magnitude, i.e., from equilibration at 87% to 100% L_{max} is indicated by the *triangle* and the secondary slow increase by the *dotted line*. Note in particular that the magnitude of the secondary change in force with this greater stretch from 87% L_{max} to L_{max} is approximately equal to the *sum* of the time-dependent secondary changes in force following the three smaller stretches, and approximate 40% of the steady state force development at L_{max}. (Adapted from ref. 66, with permission.)

Another line of investigation in cardiac muscle was concerned less with the description of the mechanical properties of muscle but more with investigation of the processes that governed excitation and contractile activation which accounted for the change in force following excitation (6). The results of these studies are not usually interpreted in the context of mechanical engineering models but rather in excitation-activation-contraction schemes (99) that are analogous to models of a cardiac cell and to a first approximation represent the "contractile element" in the engineering models of muscle. A general schematic of a model of this sort is depicted in Fig. 3,

the essential feature of which is that following excitation, activation of the myofilaments occurs due to an increase in myoplasmic [Ca], Ca_i, producing myofilament displacement and force production. The level of myofilament activation following a given excitation varies with the extent of the Ca^{2+}-myofilament interaction and can be altered by changes in the Ca_i transient or by changes in the affinity of the myofilaments for Ca^{2+}. Thus, changes in myofilament displacement and force performance at a *given* resting muscle length can be considered to occur via changes in the effectiveness of excitation-activation-contraction coupling. It was evident early on that this could be varied by changes in the rate and pattern of stimulation, i.e., the Bowditch phenomenon or rate treppe, by changes in the $[Ca^{2+}]$ in the solution bathing the muscle, and by many additional physical and pharmacologic influences as well (51). These factors were referred to as "inotropic" interventions and the resultant changes in muscle performance were referred to as changes in "contractility" or "inotropic state." Is it possible that the resting length of the fiber could also modulate muscle performance by altering the extent of myofilament activation following excitation?

One simple experimental approach to this question would be to determine whether the response to inotropic influences, i.e., the Bowditch phenomenon or a change in $[Ca^{2+}]$ in the fluid bathing the muscle, proceeded more efficiently when induced at longer than at shorter resting muscle lengths. It has indeed been shown (Fig. 4A) that the kinetics of the force staircase on stimulation from quiescence in cat papillary muscles are more rapid in muscles at longer than at a shorter resting lengths, i.e., less time (or number of excitations) is required to complete the transient (or any given portion of it) at the longer versus the shorter length. In addition, if the bathing fluid $[Ca^{2+}]$ is abruptly increased at a constant stimulation rate (Fig. 4B) the resulting force staircase to the new steady state level at the higher Ca^{2+} is more rapid when the muscle has been equilibrated at the longer than the shorter muscle length. Experiments of this type indicate that factor(s) that govern the effectiveness of the excitation-activation-contraction cycle (Fig. 3) are length-dependent, i.e., this coupling is more effective at longer than at shorter muscle lengths.

If factor(s) that govern contractile activation are less effective at shorter muscle lengths, the length-developed tension relations (as depicted in Fig. 2) at different "contractile" or "inotropic" states should not be superimposable. Rather, the relative decline in tension with a given reduction in muscle length should be less at a higher inotropic state than at a lower one when, by definition, contractile activation at any given muscle length is diminished. Simple measurements of twitch force across a range of muscle lengths at different contractile states would determine if this were the case,

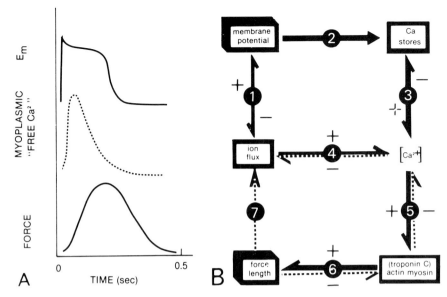

FIG. 3. A: Schematic illustration of the approximate time course of excitation-activation-contraction coupling. From *top* to *bottom,* the transients are of cell membrane potential, myoplasmic [Ca^{2+}] as measured by the photoprotein aequorin, and force. **B:** Schematic diagram of some interactions between membrane potential and contraction in the heart. The sequence in excitation-activation-contraction coupling may be followed via the *heavy black arrows* (mainly clockwise). Ion fluxes across the sarcolemma [1+] determine the membrane potential, which itself can provide a driving force for ion movements [1−]. The changes in membrane potential are a function of the ionic equilibrium potentials and conductances. The depolarization [2] causes a rise in myoplasmic [Ca^{2+}] derived from intracellular stores [3+]. This results directly from the depolarization or possibly from Ca^{2+}-induced Ca^{2+} release. The Ca^{2+} within the myoplasm combines with troponin-C [5+] allow an actin-myosin interaction requiring ATP and resulting in force development [6+]. As, or probably before, the membrane repolarizes, the sarcoplasmic reticulum sequesters Ca^{2+} [5−; 3−] permitting relaxation to occur [6−]. Ca^{2+} can also leave the myoplasm by a metabolically dependent Ca^{2+} pump or by Na$^+$, Ca^{2+}-exchange [4−]. Force and length changes could influence membrane events (contraction-activation-excitation feedback) by processes depicted by the *dotted lines.* For example, these mechanical alterations could change ionic fluxes across the sarcolemma by affecting permeability or diffusion gradients directly [7]. Indirectly [6−; 5−], force and length changes could influence the membrane by altering myoplasmic [Ca^{2+}]. This may influence ionic flux [4−], and, hence, membrane potential [1+] by modulation of the electrochemical gradient for Ca^{2+} and, thus, modulation of the slow Ca^{2+} channel, outward potassium currents, "leak" currents, the electrogenic Na/Ca exchange, or the nonspecific cation conductance referred to as the oscillatory or transient inward (TI) current. (Adapted from ref. 59, with permission.)

and, indeed, when the inotropic state is altered by changing the rate and pattern of stimulation (Fig. 5A), a given reduction in muscle length causes a greater relative decline in contractile force at a lower than at a higher inotropic state (Fig. 5C). Figs. 5B and 5D show that this not only applies for peak twitch force but also for the *maximum rate* of force development. Although thus far we have not been concerned with experiments designed to ask what particular factor(s) that modulate excitation-activation-contraction coupling (as depicted in Fig. 3) are length-dependent, Figs. 5B and 5D provide some very useful information in this regard. They clearly indicate that the length-dependence is manifest rather early following excitation, since dT/dt_{max} occurs early (at about 30% of the time to peak force) with respect to the time course of contraction. Similar shifts in the relative developed tension-length curve are observed in cat papillary muscle when the length-tension relation is measured in different bathing [Ca^{2+}], either acutely following changes in length (3) or in the steady state as in Fig. 4B. The results of studies in Figs. 4 and 5

demonstrate that simple measurements of force and resting length permit strong inference that resting length modulates the effectiveness of excitation-activation-contraction coupling (44). An important corollary of the results of studies of this sort is that inotropic perturbations have a greater *relative* effect to alter the twitch force at lower than at higher resting muscle lengths.

SARCOMERE AS THE FORCE-PRODUCING UNIT

As theories of the anatomical basis of muscle contraction emerged, the sarcomere (Fig. 6A) was emphasized as the functional unit or "contractile element" of the muscle, and it was found that a change in resting muscle length over a certain range was paralleled by a proportional change in average sarcomere length. The advent of technology to monitor and control the sarcomere length in contracting muscle permitted a new approach toward investigation of the role of sarcomere length in governing force production in muscle.

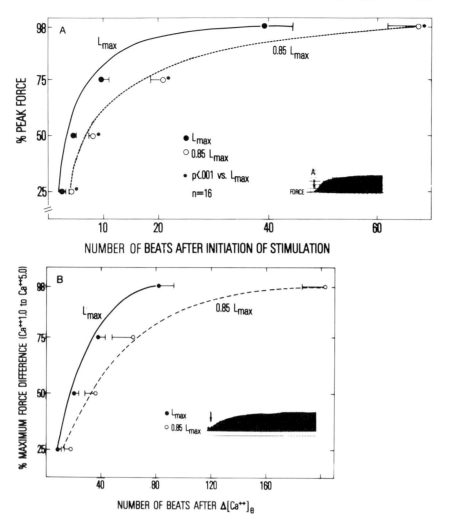

FIG. 4. A (inset): Stimulation of quiescent papillary muscle at a rate of 24 min^{-1} (arrow) results in a progressive increase in twitch force in each subsequent beat until a new steady state is achieved (force staircase). When muscles ($N = 16$) are pre-equilibrated at the shorter muscle length (0.85 L_{max}), the number of beats to complete 98% of the staircase, or any portion of it, is about twice that required when the muscles had been pre-equilibrated at the longer length (L_{max}). The computed function (continuous or dashed line) was derived by normalizing the mean exponential equation $DF = DF_{max}[1 - (\alpha_1 e^{b}1^x + \alpha_2 e^{b}2^x)]$ to DF_{max} at that length. DF is developed twitch force in a given beat, DF_{max} is 98% of maximum DF achieved in the transient, and x is the beat number of the staircase at each length. Both b_1 and b_2 were greater (50% and 75%, respectively) at L_{max} than at 0.85 L_{max} ($p < 0.001$). The solid circles (L_{max}) and open circles (0.85 L_{max}) represent the mean number of beats to reach a given level of relative force as measured directly at each length, and fit the computed function at $r = 0.95 \pm 0.009$. The number of beats required to reach each of the given levels of relative force (25%, 50%, 75%, or 98%) is significantly greater at the shorter length than at L_{max}, $p < 0.001$. Steady state twitch force was 4.49 ± 0.46 g/mm^2 L_{max} and 1.67 ± 0.20 g/mm^2 at 0.85 L_{max}. Resting force was $17 \pm 0.04\%$ and $28 \pm 0.02\%$ of total force at 0.85 L_{max} and L_{max}, respectively. Cross-sectional area was 0.61 ± 0.06 mm^2. B (inset): An increase in [Ca^{2+}] in the fluid [Ca]$_e$ bathing cat papillary muscles stimulated regularly at 24 min^{-1} (arrow) results in a progressive increment in force in each beat (staircase) until a new steady state is achieved. The curves represent the mean Ca^{2+} staircase in six muscles, constructed from the mean exponential function $\dfrac{\text{force difference}}{\text{max force difference}} = 1 - \alpha e^{bx}$ at each length. The solid circles (L_{max}) and (open circles) (0.85 L_{max}) are the measured number of beats to reach a given level of the staircase in each muscle and averaging the number for six muscles at each length. The difference in the function described by the four points at L_{max} versus that at 0.85 L_{max} is significant ($p < 0.005$). Mean peak DF in g/mm^{-2} in [Ca^{2+}]$_o$ of 5.0 mM was 5.60 ± 1.0 at L_{max} and 3.33 ± 0.92 at 0.85 L_{max}. Mean DF in [Ca^{2+}]$_e$ of 1.0 mM was 3.52 ± 0.99 at L_{max} and 1.05 ± 0.34 at 0.85 L_{max}. The mean difference in DF in [Ca^{2+}]$_e$ of 5.0 and 1.0 mM (the Ca^{2+} staircase) was 2.08 ± 0.24 at L_{max} and 2.29 ± 0.58 g/mm^{-2} at 0.85 L_{max}. Cross-sectional area was 0.54 ± 0.14 mm^2. (From ref. 68.)

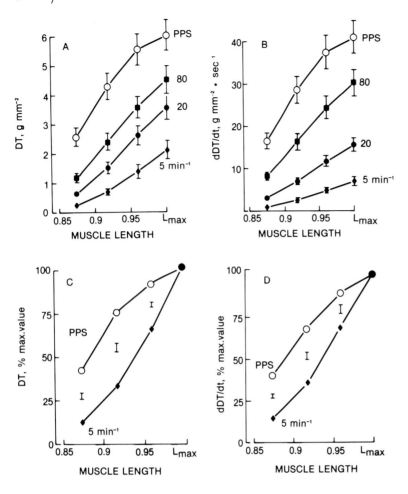

FIG. 5. Length-tension curves in isolated cat papillary muscles ($N = 10$) for peak developed tension (**A**: DT, g/mm^{-2}) and for the maximum rate of tension development (**B**: dDT/dt) under steady state conditions during regular stimulation at a low inotropic state, i.e., regular stimulation at 5 min^{-1} and at a higher inotropic state, i.e., at stimulation rates of 20 and 80 min^{-1} or paired pulse stimulation (PPS) at 20 pairs min^{-1}. Data are expressed mean ± SEM. $L_{max} = 4.84 \pm 0.39$ mm; cross-section area = 0.47 ± 0.05 mm^2; $[Ca]_e = 2.25$ mM. Resting tension at L_{max} was $15.4 \pm 2.0\%$ of the total tension. **C** and **D**: Data for paired pulse stimulation and 5 min^{-1} in **A** and **B**, respectively, have been normalized to the value at L_{max} in each muscle. *Vertical bars* are the standard error of the mean difference at each length. The measurements in this study were made in the steady state at both lengths. It is noteworthy that the ratio of dT/dt in the potentiated beat following a single interpolated early stimulus to that during regular stimulated beat does not vary with length (5). (From ref. 66, with permission.)

Skeletal Muscle Fibers

Evidence from light microscopic studies in skeletal muscle indicated that during the contraction the actin or thin filaments were drawn over the myosin or thick filaments; furthermore, this "sliding" of the filaments was hypothesized to occur by attachments between the filaments ("cross-bridges") that could be observed by X-ray diffraction and that seemed to project from certain areas of the thick filament at regularly spaced intervals (Fig. 6A). In the evolution of theory regarding the mechanism of force production by muscle, it was hypothesized that the *number* of attached cross-bridges between thick and thin filaments determined the force that could be generated by the fiber (32). In order to substantiate this hypothesis, the experimental strategy was to maintain *both* the level of myofilament activation and the sarcomere length constant during the contraction; i.e., it was necessary that the preparations be "activation-clamped" at the maximum level and "sarcomere length-clamped" at varying sarcomere lengths, and thus at varying cross-bridge numbers. Activation clamping at the maximum level was thought to be achieved in these intact skeletal muscle fibers by tetanizing the preparation (i.e., fusing the individual twitch contractions by rapid

stimulation) at low temperatures. Length clamping was accomplished by monitoring markers placed on the surface of the muscle; should the distance between two markers begin to decline during the tetanus, a stretch was applied to the end of the muscle to return the markers to their original position. This feedback monitoring of intermarker distance was performed continuously throughout the tetanus (32). It was also important that not just mean sarcomere length be held constant, but that all the sarcomeres in the fiber be at constant length to avoid the "creep" phenomenon (32). Variation in the number of cross-bridges could be accomplished by the changing resting length of the preparation, since the attachment of the side projections had a fixed distribution along the myosin filaments. In other words, over a certain range of sarcomere lengths, the number of cross-bridges varied directly with sarcomere length, and the range of sarcomere lengths over which this occurs is from 2.2 μm, where the number of cross-bridge attachments is at a maximum, to 3.6 μm at which no bridges are attached (Fig. 6A). The results of the experiment (Fig. 6B) did indeed demonstrate a linear decrease in force as sarcomere length was increased (and cross-bridge numbers decreased) over that range of lengths (Fig. 6B); furthermore, force declined to naught

A

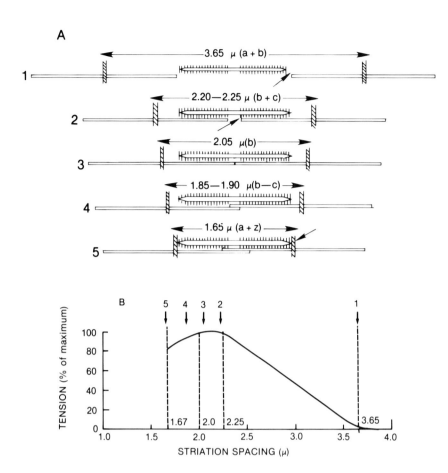

FIG. 6. A: Schematic diagram of the thick (myosin) and thin (actin) filaments, and of the spacing of the lateral projections from myosin that attach to actin to form cross-bridges. Sarcomere length is the distance between "Z lines," which are dense areas resulting from the overlap of actin fibers of sarcomeres in series. Note that when the sarcomere length is 3.65 μm, no cross-bridge attachment between thick and thin filaments can occur; when sarcomere length is 2.20–2.25 μm, the maximum number of bridges is formed. Reduction of sarcomere length from 2.20 to 2.05 μm does not decrease the number of cross-bridges because the central part of myosin (C band) has no projections. It is particularly important to note that reduction of sarcomere length from 2.05 to 1.85–1.64 μm does not reduce the number of cross-bridges from the maximum number but does result in double actin overlap. **B:** Force measured during a tetanic activation at 0°C as a function of sarcomere length (as in 1–5 in A) in tetanized skeletal muscle. Note that force is zero at zero myofilament overlap, i.e., at sarcomere length of 3.6 μm at which no cross-bridges exist between myosin and actin. Maximum force occurs when the number of cross-bridges is maximum and no double overlap of actin occurs (2.0–2.25). Force decreases 20% when sarcomere length is reduced from 2.0 to 1.65, a length range where the *number* of cross-bridges does not change. (From ref. 32, with permission.)

at 3.6 μm (32). Thus, the sarcomere defined anatomically, was now also construed as the functional unit in muscle and the sliding filament/cross-bridge hypothesis as the mechanism of force development seemed substantiated. Also, more recently, this experiment has been repeated with similar results in fibers in which the sarcolemma had been removed and in which Ca^{2+} activation of myofilaments was controlled directly by buffered solutions (47). However, there is still substantial debate as to whether or not the cross-bridge model as currently expounded provides a satisfactory explanation for force development in muscle, since with constant filament activation under other experimental conditions a unique relation between sarcomere length and force development from sarcomere lengths 2.2 to 3.6 is not always observed (28,91).

Intact Cardiac Muscle

An analogous approach to relate sarcomere length to force production might be considered to explain the length modulation of force in the myocardium. However, restoring forces, inhomogeneity of contractile segment

lengths within isolated cardiac muscle, changes in sarcomere length during contraction, and the appropriate modeling of "resting force" pose problems. Additionally, a nonuniformity of thin filament length has also been reported in cardiac muscle (80).

When ventricular myocardium or muscle is stretched to that length (L_{max}) at which maximum twitch force (or maximum rate of force development) occurs, the *average* resting sarcomere length is about 2.3 μm. However, in isolated cardiac ventricular muscle (or in the intact left ventricle) it is not possible (as it is in skeletal muscle) to stretch the resting sarcomeres to lengths greater than this (44,88,100). Rather, beyond this length, the cells seem to resist further stretch, and continued application of stretch at the ends of isolated muscle produces excessive passive force and results in damage to the ends of the preparation. Similarly, chronic ventricular dilatation in the heart is associated with intersarcomere misalignment or slippage between adjacent parallel sarcomeres (100). [It is noteworthy that in atrial muscle (75) or in isolated single cells of frog atria or ventricle (28,90) and dog ventricle (28), sarcomere length can be increased to well over 3 μm when the cell is stretched.]

Restoring Forces

A reduction in filling volume in the intact heart or of the resting length in isolated muscle from the L_{max} results in a more or less parallel reduction in average sarcomere length until slack length [usually about 1.85–1.9 μm but as low as 1.6 in one study (48)] is reached. Slack length is that length to which the myocardial sarcomeres lengthen following a stimulated contraction in the absence of an externally applied stretch, or, stated in other words, that length to which the myocardial sarcomere can be *passively* shortened without evidence of a "restoring force" manifest visually as myofilament filament buckling (44). Passive reductions in the preparation length to those below slack length in *muscle* or in the ventricle are not paralleled by proportional changes in length of all sarcomeres. Thus, the range of *resting* sarcomere lengths we must be concerned with in explaining the Frank-Starling mechanism in cardiac muscle is 2.3 to 2.4 to about 1.8 μm. Since slack length in isolated cardiac myocytes (28) is the same as that in intact muscle, the origin of this restoring force must be intracellular. These forces, which are possibly related to double overlap of actin, are of functional significance if sarcomere length is *actively* shortened to lengths below slack length during contraction (Fig. 6A). In addition, *inter*cellular restoring forces, i.e., due to cell branching and extracellular collagen (97), are present at all lengths and could theoretically impede active shortening and might reduce twitch force as measured at the ends of the preparation. Thus, both types of restoring forces as well as average sarcomere length, per se, must be considered when attempting to determine the mechanisms of the steepness of the resting length-developed force relation in cardiac muscle as depicted in Fig. 2. It has already been argued, however, that in order to account for the shift in the relative length-developed tension curve with inotropic state (Fig. 5), the restoring forces themselves would have to vary with inotropic state; this seems unlikely if they are considered to be passive in origin (44). Thus, restoring forces, per se, cannot entirely account for the steep length-tension curve in cardiac muscle as depicted in Fig. 2.

Average Sarcomere Length Changes
During Contraction

In isolated cardiac muscle contracting in the apparently isometric mode (i.e., *ends* of muscle not permitted to shorten during contraction) as in Figs. 2, 4, and 5, considerable (up to 17%) sarcomere shortening can occur in the center of the muscle at the expense of stretching the cells near the mounted ends (20,57). This artifactual compliance at the ends of the preparation has been attributed both to localized damage due to mounting of the preparation (20,57) and to uncoiling collagen within the tendinous end in the case of papillary

muscles (98), and the contribution of each factor probably depends on the method used to mount the preparation. These nonuniformities of length among contractile segments within isolated cardiac muscle can be demonstrated by monitoring muscle segment or sarcomere lengths in various regions of the muscle (33,43,48,49,92) (examples are shown in Figs. 7 and 8). In Fig. 7 note that during a contraction in which the muscle ends are held constant, the segment at the end of the preparation lengthens, that in the middle shortens, and that in an intermediate area between the two shortens, but to a different extent and with a different time course than that of the central segment. Because of this inhomogeneity, force measured at the ends of the muscle peaks while shortening in the central segments is still occurring and the end segments are already lengthening.

Sarcomere length during contraction can be measured either from photomicrographs, which has been accomplished both in rat and rabbit preparations (48,49), and from measurements of the laser diffraction pattern, which, in intact preparations, has been accomplished successfully only in thin, right ventricular papillary or trabecular muscles from the rat. Figure 7B illustrates the effect of a change in resting muscle length on the average sarcomere length measured via laser diffraction in a given muscle segment both at rest and at the time of peak force during contractions in isometric (really auxotonic) rat papillary muscles. Note (lower panel) that (a) changes in the average resting sarcomere length parallel changes in resting muscle length from L_{max} to 83% L_{max} where twitch force production is about 25% of that at L_{max}; (b) the average sarcomere length decreases during contraction. (Shortening of the myocardium *in situ* occurs during the cardiac systole so that in some ways the "internal" shortening in these preparations does indeed mimic the intact heart.) This internal shortening of sarcomeres or muscle segments during a contraction can be prevented by applying a stretch to the ends of the muscle (see below).

In attempting to define a relation of twitch force production and sarcomere length, the sarcomere length at peak force in the contraction might be more important than the resting sarcomere length. Studies of the sort depicted in Fig. 5 have been repeated and the data related to average sarcomere length *at the peak of the contraction* rather than to resting sarcomere or muscle length (Fig. 8). Note that the length–tension relation derived in this way is still very steep and when the muscle is more highly activated, i.e., when twitch force is potentiated by changes in the pattern of stimulation, the reduction in force with decreasing sarcomere length is substantially less than during regular stimulation. Thus, a comparison of Figs. 5C and 8 indicates that regardless of whether contractile force is related to the average sarcomere length or muscle length measured at

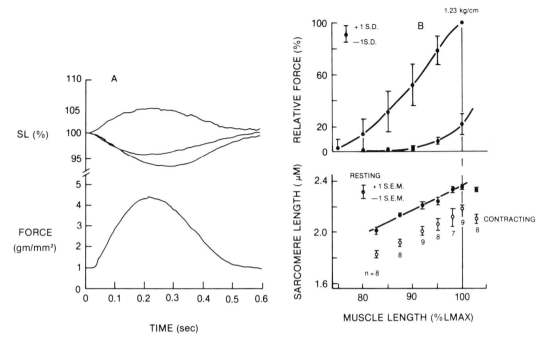

FIG. 7. A: Segment length (SL) changes as percent of resting level from (*top to bottom*) end, intermediate, and central segments of a ferret papillary muscle, together with a simultaneous force trace during an "isometric" contraction at L_{max}. The area within a segment can be assessed via a magnetic induction technique because intact muscle exhibits constant volume, and when a change in segment length occurs, it causes a change in the cross-sectional area that produces a change in the magnetic field sensed by a coil placed around the segment. Photomicrographic tracking of opaque spheres within capillaries of the preparation corroborated the validity of this technique for measuring segment length. The segment length method confirms the results of studies that utilized the laser diffraction method to monitor sarcomere length during contraction, i.e., substantial inhomogeneity in sarcomere lengths occurs within the preparation. (From ref. 43.) B: Effect of variation of muscle length on force and average sarcomere length measured by laser diffraction of isolated rat papillary muscles. Muscle length is expressed as a fraction of L_{max}, the length at which maximum active force is produced. *Top* = length-tension relations. The peak active (caused by an excitation) tensions (*top panel, upper points*) averaged 1.23 ± 0.53 SD kg/cm^2 at optimal length. The ratio of active to resting force (*top panel, lower points*) at optimal length averaged 5:1. *Bottom* = average sarcomere length in resting muscle (*solid circle*) and at time of peak contractile force (*open circle*). A moderately consistent amount of sarcomere shortening occurred during the contraction at all lengths; n = the number of data points in each group. Note the relatively narrow range of average sarcomere lengths that encompass the length-tension diagram. (From ref. 57.)

rest, or to sarcomere length at the time of peak contraction, the relative reduction in force at high inotropic states is less than at lower inotropic states.

Resting Force

Figures 7B and 8 illustrate that resting force increases in cardiac muscle as the resting or initial sarcomere length is increased. This has been found in all studies of cardiac muscle and uncertainty regarding its origin poses yet another problem in interpreting the load or force on the sarcomeres during contraction, and thus relating contractile force to sarcomere length. Resting force been modeled in various ways, and whether or not to subtract the resting force present at the beginning of the contraction from the total force at the time of peak of contraction depends on the model chosen. In one model the internal sarcomere shortening is construed as causing the passive load to shift to the sarcomeres; thus, in this model, no subtraction of passive force is

required. In an alternative modeling scheme, other elements within the muscle are construed as bearing this passive force, and subtraction of it from total force during contraction is required. This problem has been elegantly addressed in a recent review (44).

Inhomogeneity of Sarcomere Length

Whereas it has been in vogue to reference cardiac muscle performance to average sarcomere length within a muscle segment, as in Figs. 7B and 8 (see Fig. 21 also), inhomogeneities of sarcomere length *within a segment* (Fig. 9), as evidenced from sarcomere diffraction patterns themselves (33,57,92) and from intensity fluctuations in the optical field of the scattered laser beam (57,67), can pose a formidable obstacle to a strict quantitative description of the dependence of muscle mechanical properties on sarcomere length, as has been accomplished in skeletal muscle (Fig. 6). This sarcomere length inhomogeneity is not sensed by measures of

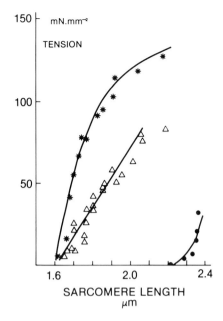

FIG. 8. Relation between the passive (*circle*), the active tension during regular stimulation at 12 min⁻¹ (*triangle*), and that due to post rest frequency potentiation (*asterisk*), and average sarcomere length measured via laser diffraction in a segment of isolated rat papillary muscles at the peak of the isometric contraction. Note the similarities of these curves with those in Fig. 5C, i.e., with a reduction in length twitch force (active tension) falls more steeply in less potentiated muscles. It is important to note that the species studied here is rat whereas in Fig. 5 cat muscle was studied. To date it has not been possible to monitor sarcomere length during contraction via the laser diffraction pattern in species other than rat probably due to the geometry of the tissue, as only thin and relative flat muscles will suffice. (From ref. 92, with permission.)

segment length by external markers on the muscle surface, or by other methods of monitoring segment length (Fig. 7A). In addition to factors that may be purely mechanical in origin, spontaneous sarcomere oscillations due to spontaneous Ca²⁺ oscillations (15,52–56,64,67,69,79,89,96) can be an important cause of the observed sarcomere length inhomogeneity, particularly in rat cardiac muscle. These Ca²⁺ oscillations occur asynchronously within and among cells causing there inhomogeneity of sarcomere length due to asynchronous myofilament activation. This results in a broadening of

the first-order diffraction peak and causes intensity fluctuations in laser light scattered by the muscle (Fig. 10). Asynchronous oscillations among parallel cells within the muscle implies asynchronous oscillatory parallel sarcomere loading and complicates the modeling of "resting" force obtained in experiments in which such oscillations occur.

In the absence of intentional experimental Ca²⁺ overload, these Ca²⁺ oscillations cannot be sensed by chemiluminescent Ca²⁺ indicators, such as aequorin or Ca²⁺ electrodes, but can have been sensed by aequorin when they become exaggerated as cell Ca²⁺ loading is enhanced (79,56,96). Estimates of the localized increase in [Ca²⁺] due to the spontaneous oscillatory release range from 4 to 40 μM (79,96). In rat ventricular muscle, the tissue most often utilized to study the effects of sarcomere lengths on muscle performance, these oscillations are present in the apparently quiescent state even when bathing [Ca]ₒ is 2 mM (54) and have been attributed to spontaneous release of Ca²⁺ from the sarcoplasmic reticulum (24,54,89,64), which has been shown to occur in all mammalian cardiac tissues once a threshold level of cell Ca²⁺ loading is achieved (54).

The period of spontaneous oscillations ranges from less than 0.1 to 0.2 Hz under normal Ca²⁺ loading of the intact rat ventricular muscle preparation, and can reach levels up to about 4 to 7 Hz (53) as cellular Ca²⁺ loading increases (64). Stimulation of the preparation at frequencies greater than the spontaneous oscillation frequency can suppress the oscillations (14,16). At very high Ca²⁺ loads, produced either by catecholamines or cardiac glycosides, reductions in the bathing [Na⁺], or elevations in the bathing [Ca²⁺], the time for their appearance following the prior excitation is reduced and the oscillations are present in the diastole interval (55). In single adult rat or rabbit isolated cardiac cells contracting in a high inotropic state with catecholamines, spontaneous oscillations can be detected in the interstimulus period even when the interstimulus interval is as low as 80 msec (14). The summation of these asynchronous myofilament oscillations results in a Ca²⁺-dependent diastolic tone (54,56,67,89), which itself interferes with analog modeling of resting force as purely passive (Fig. 10). During regular stimulation, oscillations appear after

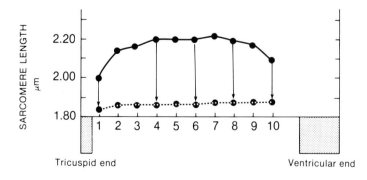

FIG. 9. Average sarcomere length measured at rest (**top curve**) and at the peak of the isometric contraction (**lower curve**) in different regions (numbered 1–10 on the abscissa) of an isotonic rat papillary muscle. Note the inhomogeneity of sarcomere length both at rest and during contraction and the inhomogeneity in the sarcomere length change (magnitude of *arrow*) during the contraction. (From ref. 92, with permission.)

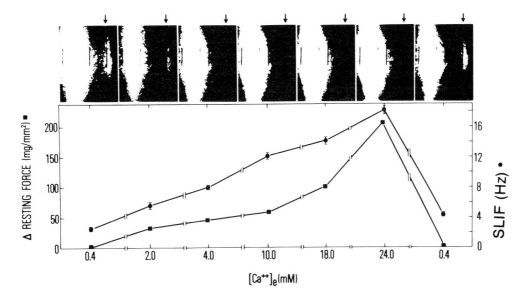

FIG. 10. Effect of superfusate $[Ca^{2+}]$, Ca_e, on sarcomere diffraction pattern (**top**), resting force, and scattered light intensity fluctuations (SLIF) of a laser beam illuminating a rat papillary muscle in the unstimulated state. Note that as Ca_e is increased the first order diffraction band (*arrows*) blurs and then fades completely; this is accompanied by an increase in resting force and SLIF frequency. Both the increased SLIF and resting force are reversed and the first order diffraction band returns when Ca_e is decreased back to control (0.4 mM) level. (From ref. 67.) When rat preparations such as this are illuminated with incoherent light and monitored in a phase contrast microscope at high magnification, sarcomere oscillations due to waves of contraction originating in cells and propagating for various distances are observed (89); these oscillations are asynchronous within and among cells. Increasing the Ca_e increases the frequency of these spontaneous myofilament oscillations and causes greater sarcomere length inhomogeneity. The resultant asynchronous myofilament displacement within the preparation summates (89) to produce a Ca^{2+}-dependent component of resting force (which is very small compared to the total resting force). While the sarcomere motion that causes SLIF is due to periodic spontaneous Ca^{2+} oscillations (53,89), the SLIF frequency (in Hz) is determined not only by the frequency of the mechanical oscillations but also by their amplitude relative to the wavelength of the laser beam (600 nm), and therefore does not indicate the true oscillation frequency (54).

a finite time following a prior excitation, and their appearance coincides with a gradual increase in resting force from a nader (hyperrelaxation), which either then reaches the pre-excitation level monotonically or passes through a transient maximum, sometimes referred to as an aftercontraction (29,55). That the oscillations vary with stretch (see below) further complicates studies to relate Starling's law of the heart to the sarcomere length.

Ryanodine or moderately high concentrations of caffeine (54,64,89), each of which interferes with sarcoplasmic reticulum Ca^{2+}-uptake release, can abolish these oscillations. Additionally, when Ba^{2+} or Sr^{3+} is substituted for Ca^{2+} in the bathing fluid, the oscillations also cease (52), as it appears these ions are not taken up and spontaneously released by the sarcoplasmic reticulum as easily as Ca^{2+}. Frog myocardium does not exhibit these oscillations even under situations of high Ca^{2+} loading, and this can be attributed to a paucity of sarcoplasmic reticulum, or to a high threshold for frog sarcoplasmic reticulum to oscillate; this is consistent with the current hypothesis that transsarcolemmal Ca influx, rather than sarcoplasmic reticulum Ca^{2+} release, seems to be the primary mechanism of excitation-activation-contraction coupling in the frog myocardium (25).

Thus, these observations indicate that referencing

twitch force production measured across a range of muscle lengths in the intact cardiac muscle to sarcomere length, as has been done in skeletal muscle, has proven difficult due to (a) the presence of resting force, (b) the possible influence of restoring forces that are encountered over the range of average sarcomere lengths pertinent to the Frank-Starling mechanisms, (c) the observation that sarcomere lengths at rest are not homogeneous either among or within muscle segments, and (d) changes in both the average sarcomere length and the extent of sarcomere length during contraction in conventionally mounted isolated cardiac muscle. In addition to the difficulty in achieving uniform sarcomere length, since cardiac muscle cannot be tetanized, activation cannot be kept constant at a given muscle or sarcomere length, i.e., activation cannot be clamped at the maximum level as in intact skeletal muscle. Thus, if the length-dependence of contractile force in cardiac muscle is to be compared to that of skeletal muscle (85,86), it must compared to the skeletal muscle *twitch*, not the tetanus. In the skeletal muscle *twitch*, unlike the tetanus, there is no unique relationship of twitch force to sarcomere length (18,74), and the simple interpretation that a change in twitch force is due to the change in the cross-bridge number or sarcomere geometry cannot be entertained. Rather, a length-dependence of contractile activation becomes a viable mechanism to explain the length-dependence of twitch force in skeletal muscle (18,74).

Single Myocardial Cells

Studies in single cardiac cells under conditions in which sarcomere inhomogeneities are minimal would seem to be the simplest preparation with an intact sarcolemma in which to relate the mechanical performance to the sarcomere length. The effect of sarcomere and cell length on the sarcomere velocity and force produced in intact single frog atrial cells (90) has recently been determined. These cells are quite long and their ends can be wrapped about cantilevered rods so that length can be varied and force measured. In addition, since these cells are only 1 to 2 myofibrils wide, sarcomere performance is assumed to be uniform across the width of the cell, i.e., total force is distributed equally between the parallel fibers (90) so that guessing which analog model to choose to interpret the result is not required. The experiment in Fig. 11 depicts such a cell contracting auxotonically from two different sarcomere lengths. Note that the shortening velocity (rate of change of sarcomere length) over a range of sarcomere lengths during the development of force was greater when the preparation contracted from the longer *initial* sarcomere length, even though the absolute force was greater than at the shorter length. Note also that the sarcomere length at peak force was the same in the two contractions. Thus, it appears that initial stretch rather than final sarcomere length reached, at least in this type of cell, is the determinant of the force produced. Similar findings were also observed in cells stretched to higher sarcomere lengths in which resting force is present, as well as in relatively isotonic contractions (90). Earlier studies in intact frog atrial strands also indicated that over the sarcomere length range above 2.2 μm, a longer initial sarcomere length was capable of supporting greater loads during contraction than shorter initial sarcomere lengths (75). These results in frog tissue, which indicate the importance of initial sarcomere length on the subsequent force and velocity achieved during contraction, are not consistent with the concept that the force-velocity relation depends on the instantaneous sarcomere or tissue length (i.e., independent of initial length or time) as has been suggested in mammalian cardiac muscle (11,37). However, the situation in the mammalian cell is somewhat more complex due to the apparent greater participation of the sarcoplasmic reticulum in the contraction. Further studies in mammalian myocytes are required to determine the extent to which this observation made in frog cardiac cells holds for mammalian cells as well.

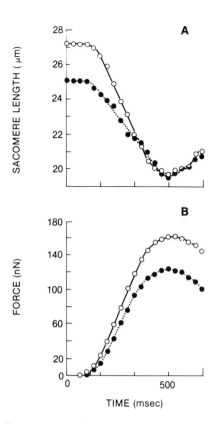

FIG. 11. Time course of sarcomere shortening and force development (change from resting force) during auxotonic twitch contractions beginning from two different initial sarcomere lengths in an isolated single frog atrial cell. The performance of the same groups of 10 sarcomeres was analyzed in both contractions. Force beam compliance was 0.21 μM/mN. (It is noteworthy that slack length is about 2.4 μM in frog atrial cells.) (From ref. 90, with permission.)

TIME-DEPENDENT CHANGES IN CARDIAC MUSCLE PERFORMANCE FOLLOWING CHANGES IN RESTING LENGTH

Although studies over a range of muscle or sarcomere lengths in the steady state strongly suggest an interaction of initial (resting) length and excitation-activation coupling in determining the strength of the cardiac contraction, an additional experimental strategy in cardiac muscle, i.e., to monitor the preparation over time following a length change, indicates this interaction even more directly. When cardiac muscle is stretched an initial increase in twitch force occurs, and this is followed by a slow secondary increase in isometric force or in the extent of isotonic shortening (Fig. 12A). (These time-dependent changes in twitch force following a change in muscle length are the cause for the difference in the acute versus steady-state length-twitch tension curves in Fig. 2.) The time course and magnitude of this secondary change varies with the magnitude of stretch (see Fig. 2), with the inotropic state at which the muscle was equilibrated prior to the stretch (66), and the milieu in which the muscle contracts following the

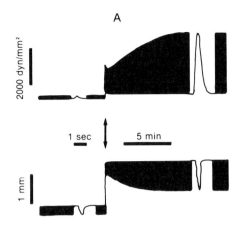
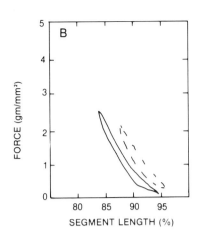

FIG. 12. **A:** Effect of a stretch (*arrow*) on isometric force (**top**) and the extent of shortening in isotonic contractions (**bottom**) in cat papillary muscle stimulated at 12 min^{-1} at 30°C in bathing fluid [Ca^{2+}] of 2.2 mM. Note that following the initial increase in force or shortening, a slow secondary increase in both parameters occurred. (From ref. 35, with permission.) **B:** Relationship between central segment length and force during an auxotonic contraction shortly after a reduction in length when the muscle had been pre-equilibrated at L_{max} (*solid loop*) and following a stretch to the same length when the muscle had been pre-equilibrated at 80% L_{max} (*dotted loops*). The presence of a loop and its counterclockwise rotation is due to the inhomogeneity of segment shortening across the muscle (see Fig. 7A). The difference between the two loops, i.e., greater shortening and greater force production at the same length following pre-equilibration at L_{max} then pre-equilibration at 0.80 L_{max} is the equivalent of the slow change in force and shortening that occurs following a stretch in A. This is a typical behavior also obtained in cat and monkey muscles. (From ref. 43, with permission.)

stretch. When considering these slow changes in muscle performance that follow a stretch, it is important to bear in mind the *marked* species differences in the relative level of activation in a given experimental milieu. For example, in rat cardiac muscle equilibrated in [Ca]$_o$ of 2.5 mM, the effectiveness excitation-activation coupling at low frequencies of stimulation appears saturated even at low lengths and no, or a very minor, secondary time-dependent increase in force occurs following a stretch. In lower [Ca]$_e$ in the rat muscle, these secondary changes do indeed occur (4) and ought to be considered in the experimental design (33,92). In the experiment in Fig. 12A, experimental conditions were such that prior to the length increase, excitation-activation-contraction coupling was far from the maximum level that could be achieved.

Because of the inhomogeneities within segments of the muscle noted in Figs. 7 and 9, in particular those caused by the damaged ends, it might be hypothesized that artifactual adaptations within these end regions might occur with time following a stretch, and that the change in contractile performance with time measured across the whole preparation as in Fig. 12A might not be due to a genuine augmentation of excitation-activation-contraction coupling within the central or undamaged portions of the muscle (43). However, experiments undertaken to address this issue, and which utilized the segment length monitoring technique as above (Fig. 7), do indeed indicate that a time-dependent change in the contractile performance occurs within the central muscle segments with time following a length change. This is illustrated in Fig. 12B which depicts a substantial difference in the force-segment length relation measured during contraction with a change in length depending on whether the preparation had been pre-equilibrated at a longer or a shorter length.

In the intact heart, a sudden and constant increase in aortic and ventricular pressure causes initial increase in ventricular volume; this is followed by a secondary slow increase in myocardial performance that results in enhanced pump performance during the maintenance of the higher afterload, thus allowing the ventricle to decrease toward its original size. This has sometimes been referred to as the Anrep effect, or "homeometric autoregulation," in contrast to "heterometric autoregulation" or the Frank-Starling effect that pertains to situations in which ventricular size remains increased (82). This secondary increase in myocardial performance could be attributable to the secondary increase in force and shortening within the myocardium as demonstrated in the muscle preparations following a stretch in Fig. 12 (albeit that in the muscle experiment the ends of the muscle remain fixed at the long length, whereas in studies in the intact heart the ventricle is permitted to undergo a reduction in size). Thus, explanations for the Anrep effect in the intact heart need not invoke transient regional ischemia with stretch followed by a redistribution of coronary flow (78), although a concomitant redistribution of flow may also occur. In fact, on the basis of the experiments in Figs. 2, 4, 5, 8, 11, and 12 from which a length-dependence excitation-activation coupling of cardiac muscle can be inferred, *both* "homeometric" and "heterometric" autoregulation (82) can be construed as resulting from an effect of stretch to enhance contractile activation, and, thus, can be considered as two facets of the same phenomenon.

MECHANISMS OF THE LENGTH-DEPENDENCE OF EXCITATION-ACTIVATION-CONTRACTION COUPLING

The factors that determine myofilament activation, and thus the force of contraction, fall into three general categories: those that modulate the transient increase in myoplasmic $[Ca^{2+}]$ that occurs subsequent to excitation; those that modulate the extent of Ca^{2+} myofilament interaction at a given myoplasmic $[Ca^{2+}]$; and those that determine the extent of synchronization among the individual contractile units (54,64), though this has not usually been emphasized previously in models of excitation-activation-contraction coupling. Studies of the effects of length on each of these factors require experimental strategies that go beyond measurements of force and shortening relative to sarcomere cell or muscle length.

Length Effects on Ca^{2+} Release into the Myoplasm Following Excitation

The strategy here has been to measure the effect of length on the transient change in myoplasmic $[Ca^{2+}]$ that results from excitation. This can be estimated utilizing the chemiluminescent protein, aequorin. At lengths and conditions corresponding roughly to those of the *steady state* length-tension curve depicted in Fig. 2, the increase in contractile force at longer muscle lengths is associated with an increase in the peak of the myoplasmic $[Ca^{2+}]$ transient, as well as alterations in the shape of this transient (Fig. 13). This result has been interpreted to indicate that more Ca^{2+} is released into the myoplasm subsequent to excitation in cardiac muscle contracting in the steady state at longer lengths than in the steady state at shorter lengths (4). The enhancement of the peak aequorin luminescence does not occur immediately on the length increase, however, but develops slowly with time following a stretch and parallels the slow changes in force that occur following the length change; thus, it may be the immediate cause for the slow change in contractile force that follows a length change. It is important, here, to remember that the peak aequorin luminescence samples the free $[Ca^{2+}]$ in the myoplasm. In order to achieve the 1 μM to 10 μM increase in the concentration of free myoplasmic Ca^{2+} following excitation, as estimated by the aequorin luminescence, roughly two orders of magnitude greater

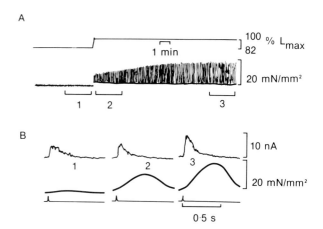

FIG. 13. Effect of an increase in muscle length from 0.82 L_{max} to L_{max} on (**A**) twitch force, and on (**B**) aequorin luminescence (**top**) and twitch (**lower**) in a cat papillary muscle. The aequorin luminescence and force in **B** are the averaged levels in time periods 1, 2, and 3 in **A**. Note that in the steady state at the longer length (period 3) the enhanced twitch force is preceded by an increase in peak aequorin luminescence. Also note that immediately following stretch, twitch force had increased, but peak aequorin luminescence did not increase from the level at the shorter length. (Adapted from ref. 4, with permission.)

Ca^{2+} must be released, due to binding to cellular proteins, e.g., calmodulim, the sarcoplasmic reticulum itself, and the myofilaments (25). A change in the binding of Ca^{2+} by these structures cannot be directly sensed in the peak aequorin luminescence. In this regard, with an increase in muscle length, the apparent affinity of the myofilaments for Ca^{2+} is enhanced (see below). Thus, it is possible that an enhanced release of Ca^{2+} into the myoplasm occurs immediately with stretch, and is offset by enhanced myofilament binding, with no appreciable change in peak aequorin luminescence.

Other experimental strategies have been utilized to determine whether length may alter the Ca^{2+} release following excitation. A length-dependence of Ca^{2+} release might occur either via a length-dependence of the trigger for Ca^{2+} release or from a net change in Ca^{2+} loading of the intracellular release sites (Fig. 3). In considering the length effect on mechanisms of Ca^{2+} release it is important to emphasize that a change in the geometry of membranes and organelles, as well as a change in myofilament geometry, occurs when a cell or muscle is stretched. Thus, one possible mechanism of either a "masked" time-independent, or of the observed time-dependent increase in aequorin luminescence, and presumably in $[Ca]_i$, following a stretch (Fig. 13), might be an effect of stretch on the physical properties of the membraneous structures.

Transversely oriented folds as well as vesicular invaginations called caveoli are present in sarcolemma and can amplify surface membrane area. Quantitative morphologic studies utilizing freeze-fracture techniques in skeletal and cardiac muscle have indicated that passive stretch may alter the contribution of these folds to total plasmalemal surface area (21,71). In skeletal muscle fibers, estimates of the surface area contained within the folds and caveoli at muscle lengths that correspond to an average sarcomere length 2.4 μm are about 40% (21). A substantial change in surface area could occur as the sarcolemma unfolds or caveoli open with stretching. In rabbit cardiac muscle, plasmalemmal folds were observed over resting muscle lengths corresponding to sarcomere lengths 1.60 to 2.3 μm, i.e., that range of interest in the Frank-Starling law of the heart. The contribution of these folds to effective surface membrane area can be estimated from Fig. 14 that depicts the effect of stretch on the percent of apparent plasmalemmal area occupied by t-tubular openings. Note that the surface density of t-tubular openings exhibits an approximate linear decrease with increasing length. This has been interpreted to be due to an unfolding of plasmalemmal folds with increasing muscle length (71). This plasmalemmal unfolding with stretch may alter the functional states of channels, pumps, carriers, or receptors contained within them or caveoli, and this could provide a mechanism which could mediate a length effect on transsarcolemmal ion flux. In this regard it is noteworthy that stretch has been observed to cause a change in Ca^{2+} flux in resting skeletal muscle (31) and of Na^+ flux in cardiac muscle (39). Further experimentation with Ca^{2+} and Na^+ ion-selective electrodes might provide useful additional information on this issue.

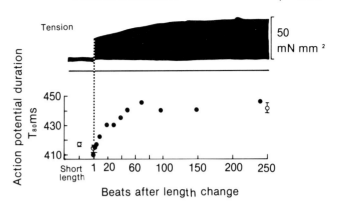

FIG. 15. Changes in tension and action potential duration (time to 80% repolarization on stretching the muscle from 80% L_{max} to L_{max}. Both panels are on the same time scale. *Open circles* indicate the average durations measured from selected beats on the above record. *Open symbols with bars* are mean $\pm$ 1 SE for control beat, first beat at L_{max}, and steady state beat at L_{max} obtained by repeating the above procedure six times on the same muscle. (From ref. 2, with permission.)

Stretch-related changes in sarcolemmal geometry may or may not be manifest in concomitant changes of cell membrane potential. Studies of the effect of a length change on transmembrane potential in a given cell are difficult to implement because in the vast majority of cases the electrode becomes dislodged following a length change. However, in some studies which have successfully made such measurements, the effect of an abrupt stretch on resting membrane potential in isolated cardiac muscle seems to vary with the extent of the stretch, the species, and the experimental conditions employed, particularly with regard to Ca^{2+} loading of this tissue; some studies show no effect (59). Whereas the effect of stretch on the action transmembrane action potential has also provided varied results (59), in an experiment made under nearly identical conditions to that in Fig. 13, a stretch initially caused a modest transient decrease in action potential duration that was followed by a secondary increase which paralleled the major portion of the secondary increase in force (Fig. 15). Although this change in action potential duration appears to relate to the increase in twitch force, it need not be implied that the change in the twitch force is directly caused by the change in action potential duration. Several Ca^{2+}-dependent ionic channels, both inward and outward going, or electrogenic ionic carrier mechanisms, or pumps, modulate the action potential duration. For example, an increase in Ca^{2+} influx via slow inward current (Fig. 3) could explain the observation in Fig. 15; this could be modulated by the increase in Ca_i as manifest in the increase in peak aequorin luminescence during the secondary transient, as in Fig. 13 (76). Similarly, other studies have demonstrated that verapamil has retarded the time course of the slow increase in force (66). Alternatively, a reduction in K^+ outward currents would tend to prolong the

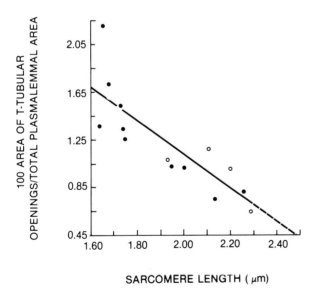

SARCOMERE LENGTH (μm)

FIG. 14. Percent of apparent plasmalemmal fracture face area occupied by t-tubular openings as a function of cell and sarcomere length in rabbit ventricular papillary muscle. Data have been fitted by the method of least squares to the $y = (1.41\%/\mu M) \times \pm 3.97$ ($r = 0.81$). *Solid circles* = experiments with normal (1.4 mM) Ca^{2+}; *open circles* = experiments in which Ca^{2+} was omitted. (From ref. 71, with permission.)

transmembrane action potential. The evidence for enhanced [Ca]ᵢ release in Fig. 13 with time following the stretch (Fig. 13) might enhance, rather than retard outwardly directed current via K⁺ channels subject to Ca modulation. Also, in the new steady state following the stretch, the increase in Ca²⁺ released into the myoplasm (Fig. 13) could prolong the transmembrane action potential by its effect on the electrogenic Na⁺, Ca²⁺-exchange or on the conductance of the recently described (19) Ca²⁺-dependent nonspecific cation channel (TI). Because of the multiplicity of possible mechanisms involved to explain a stretch-induced change in the action potential and because of the interaction (feedback) among these mechanisms (Fig. 3), the effect of length on each must be studied individually in voltage clamp and ion flux studies in future studies.

Enhanced Ca²⁺ release from an intracellular store (Fig. 3), all else equal, would serve to enhance the aequorin luminescence such as that in Fig. 13. Experiments in cardiac cells in which the sarcolemma has been mechanically removed have been interpreted to indicate the sarcoplasmic Ca²⁺-release mechanisms are length-dependent (26,67). Contractions caused by Ca²⁺-induced Ca²⁺ release from the sarcoplasmic reticulum within these preparations exhibit a steep dependence on length (Fig. 16). When the experiment is repeated utilizing caffeine to trigger Ca²⁺ release (caffeine is considered to be a more effective trigger than Ca²⁺ for Ca²⁺ release) the decline in contraction strength with decreasing stretch of the preparation and decreasing sarcomere length is markedly reduced. In fact, over a wide range of lengths, the phasic contractions induced by caffeine did not differ from the tonic level of force measured at each

length in the presence of steady maximally activating pCa (discussed later). This result can be interpreted to indicate that Ca²⁺ loading of sarcoplasmic reticulum, the source of Ca²⁺ during both the Ca²⁺- and caffeine-induced phasic contractions in these experiments, did not vary with length but that the Ca²⁺-induced release of Ca²⁺ was affected by length or the degree of stretch. More recent experiments in which the myosin was extracted from this skinned-cell preparation by a brief prior period of exposure to a bathing solution of high ionic strength, directly demonstrates the effect of stretch on Ca²⁺-induced Ca²⁺ release as measured by the Ca²⁺ indicator, Arsenazo III (23). The implication of these results is that the effectiveness of Ca²⁺ as a trigger, perhaps via a length-induced change in its diffusion pathway causing a change in the rate (24) at which its concentration changes at the surface of the sarcoplasmic reticulum, is altered by the stretch of the preparation.

Scattered light intensity fluctuations (SLIF) due to spontaneous sarcoplasmic reticulum Ca²⁺ release in intact rat isolated cardiac muscle and measured by laser spectroscopy (as discussed in conjunction with Fig. 10) also exhibit a steep length-dependence (Fig. 17). Note that SLIF measured at each muscle length in the steady state 5 min following the cessation of stimulation, increase with muscle length. Since SLIF frequency varies with conditions that vary cell Ca²⁺ loading (15,52–55,64, 67,89,95,96), this result might be interpreted to indicate that length influences cell Ca²⁺ loading. This would also explain the length-dependent increase of the peak aequorin luminescence with time following a length increase (Fig. 13). However, the result in Fig. 17 could also be interpreted as an effect of stretch to enhance

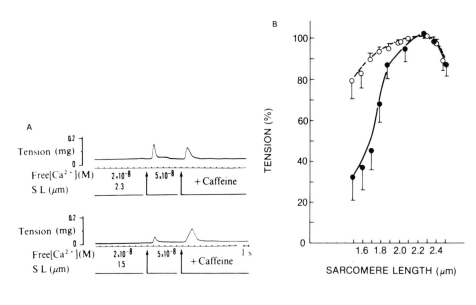

FIG. 16. A: The experimental protocol at sarcomere lengths of 2.3 and 1.5 μm. Note that Ca²⁺ release, indicated by a force transient, does not occur when the cell is bathed in 2 × 10⁻⁸ M Ca²⁺; but when free Ca²⁺ is increased to 5 × 10⁻⁸ M a force transient occurs and is smaller in magnitude at the lower length. In contrast, force transients elicited by caffeine are similar at both lengths. B: The effect of stretch on force produced by Ca²⁺-induced release of Ca²⁺ (solid circle) or by caffeine-induced Ca²⁺ release (open circle) from the sarcoplasmic reticulum in rat cardiac cells in which the sarcolemma had been mechanically dissected. Each point on the curves is the mean ± SE of 12–15 cells. Sarcomere length reported is that during a contraction. Force in each preparation has been normalized to the maximum measured for that type of contraction. (From ref. 26, with permission.)

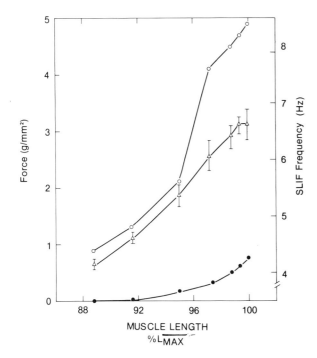

FIG. 17. Resting force (*solid circles*); scattered light intensity fluctuations (SLIF) (*triangles*) measured as in Fig. 10 in the steady state at varying resting muscle lengths (mean ±of 5 determinations) and force in a test twitch (*open circles*) measured at each length in a cat papillary muscle. (Adapted from ref. 67.)

myofilament Ca^{2+} binding (see below) through mechanisms that could be independent of cell or sarcoplasmic reticulum Ca^{2+} loading.

It has long been appreciated that resting heat and O_2 consumption increase with stretch, e.g., the Feng effect as described in skeletal muscle (30). Whereas one interpretation of this has suggested that anoxia in the core of the muscle reduces O_2 consumption at shorter lengths, it has been demonstrated recently, quite conclusively, that core hypoxia at short lengths can explain only a very small part of the increase in O_2 consumption with stretch in cardiac muscle (72). The "cardiac Feng effect," however, may relate to the length-dependence of the Ca^{2+} oscillations as in Fig. 17. That spontaneous Ca^{2+} oscillations may affect resting heat and O_2 consumption is supported by the observation that both resting heat and the frequency of oscillations decrease with time following the mounting the muscle *in vivo* (54,73), and that steady levels of resting heat in rat myocardium in which oscillations are prominent compared to other species, is twofold that in species in which the oscillations, do not occur in physiological Ca_o (54,73). This oscillatory Ca^{2+} cycling between the sarcoplasmic reticulum and myofilaments requires ATP utilization both for myofilament shortening and Ca^{2+} pumping at the sarcoplasmic reticulum and sarcolemma, and thus, as might be expected, increases O_2 consumption and heat production above those levels measured during experiments in

which such oscillations are not present. A related observation is that low concentrations of caffeine, which cause an increase in the frequency of the spontaneous Ca^{2+} oscillations in the heart (13,16,55), can cause *de novo* spontaneous oscillations to occur in frog skeletal muscle (58) and also potentiate the Feng effect (17). Although the substantial increase in resting force with an increase in resting length (Fig. 8) is largely passive in origin, a component of Ca^{2+}-dependent resting tone due to the average effect of the spontaneous asynchronous Ca^{2+} oscillations (Fig. 10) might also be expected to increase with resting length, as the oscillations change their characteristics with a change in length. Note that in Fig. 17, a fairly good correlation between resting force and SLIF occurs over the range of lengths up to L_{max} and that the slope of this relationship is much less than between SLIF and twitch force (i.e., milligrams for resting force and grams for twitch force). Further increases in length beyond L_{max} markedly increase resting force, but suppress and abolish oscillations (not shown for this muscle, but see ref. 67). This has been attributed, in part, to the effect of a large passive force to retard or prevent oscillatory myofilament shortening in response to the Ca^{2+} oscillations (67). The graded and asynchronous electromechanical behavior in response to stimulation that has been observed to occur following stretch in rat cardiac muscle, but not in that from other species that do not exhibit the spontaneous Ca^{2+} oscillations under similar conditions (87), may be related to the effect of stretch on spontaneous Ca^{2+} oscillations as observed in Fig. 17. Additionally, stretching of rat cardiac muscle throughout the contraction in order to prevent "internal shortening" (92) or following a large stretch from a lower length (8) causes or enhances "aftercontractions" that can be modeled by partial synchronization of these spontaneous cell Ca^{2+} oscillations (64,89). Length-dependent spontaneous mechanical oscillations also have been observed during stimulated contractions in mammalian (cat) but not frog ventricular muscle under conditions when the sarcoplasmic reticulum buffering capacity is reduced and the action potential is prolonged by substituting Sr^+ for Ca^{2+} in the bathing fluid (38).

Length Effect on the Ca^{2+}-Myofilament Interaction

Results in Figures 5, 8, 13, 16, and 17 suggest a length-dependence of myofilament activation during a contraction and predict that if it were possible to maintain constant myofilament activation (i.e., to maintain steady rather than phasic activation during a contraction), the level of Ca^{2+} activation at which the preparations were "clamped" would be a major determinant of the magnitude of force-length relation. Experiments of this sort can be made either by soaking small bundles of isolated muscle in a detergent, e.g., Triton-X, to "chemically skin" the membranes within the preparation, or by mechanically removing the sarcolemma (as in Fig. 16). Application of solutions with graded constant pCa to such a preparation results in graded steady levels of force (Fig. 18A). These studies, in which no electrical excitation is needed for activation, have provided information regarding the range of $[Ca^{2+}]$ to which the myofilaments respond following excitation. Figure 18B shows that when sarcomere length is reduced from L_{max}, when pCa is clamped at a low, an intermediate, and at a level required for maximum myofilament activation in small bundles of rat papillary muscles, the drop in force is highly dependent on the level at which activation is clamped. Stated in other words, for a given change in

sarcomere overlap, the change in force was greater when Ca^{2+} activation of the myofilaments was clamped at a lower level. Thus, there is no unique function relating the change in force with a change in average sarcomere length. This indicates that sarcomere length is not an *independent* modulator of force production in cardiac muscle and suggests that the length-tension curves in muscles with intact membranes as depicted in Figs. 2 and 8 cannot be attributed in large measure to changes in sarcomere length that accompany changes in muscle length.

The question now arises as to whether in muscle with the sarcolemma intact, a change in the level of myofil-

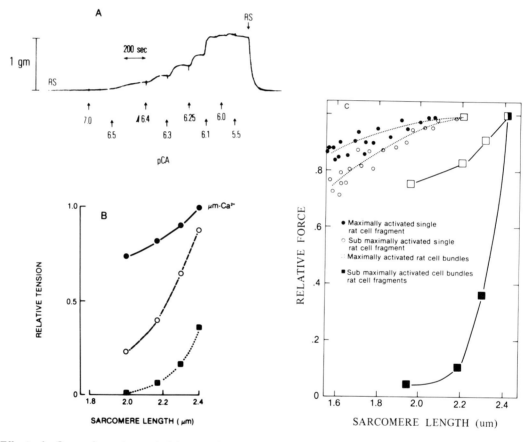

FIG. 18. A: Effect of pCa on force in a rat right ventricular preparation which had previously been made hyperpermeable to Ca^{2+} and EGTA by "chemical skinning" of the muscle for 30 min in 1% Triton-X. The pCa of the relaxing solution, RS, is >8. It is important to note that the steepness of this relation and the pCa required for maximal activation varies among the many published papers in which it was determined. These differences are likely due to differing methods used to "skin" and mount the preparation and different constants used to calculate the free pCa in the buffer used. (From ref. 93.) **B:** Length-force curves for maximal and submaximal steady contractions of chemically skinned ventricular muscle bundle of the rat. All forces are expressed as a fraction of the force produced by activating the preparation with $[Ca^{2+}]$ 100 μmoles/liter at a sarcomere length of 2.4 μm. The **top curve** shows the variation of force production with changed sarcomere length in maximal $[Ca^{2+}]$ (100 μmoles/liter), in the **middle** for 5 μmoles/liter, and the **lower** for $[Ca^{2+}]$ of 2.5 μmoles/liter. (From ref. 40.) **C:** Effect of the level of myofilament Ca^{2+} activation on the reduction of force as sarcomere length is reduced over that range that is applicable to the Frank-Starling law of the heart. The force in multicellular rat preparations (*squares*) from B at the maximal (*open symbols*) and at submaximal (*solid symbols*) Ca^{2+} activation have been normalized to their respective absolute level at sarcomere lengths 2.4 μm; the single cell preparation (*circles*) was mechanically skinned as in **Fig. 16** and maximally activated (pCa 5, *solid symbol*) or submaximally activated (pCa 6, *open symbol*). Note that in the multicellular preparations a marked decline (>90%) of force occurred with a reduction in length during submaximal activation; in contrast during maximum Ca^{2+} activation only a 25% reduction in force occurred in the multicellular preparation, and only a 5% reduction occurred in the maximally activated single cell preparation. (From refs. 23, 26, 40, 67, with permission; and A. Fabiato, *private communication*.)

ament Ca^{2+} activation is the only determinant of the length-tension relationship, e.g., that relationship depicted in Figs. 2 and 8. If this were the case, force should not decrease from the maximum level when sarcomere length is reduced in experimental preparations in which activation is maintained constant at the maximum level. That the absolute force in *maximally* Ca^{2+}-activated multicellular rat preparations (Fig. 18C) declined 25% with a change in length from 2.4 to 2.0 suggests that some other factor(s) in addition to activation might be operative when length is changed over this range. Intracellular restoring forces would not be expected to be encountered during contraction over this range of sarcomere lengths, since it is above slack length. However, in experiments, such as in Fig. 18C, sarcomere lengths have been measured prior to, rather than during Ca^{2+} activation. As indicated previously, during activation, sarcomeres shorten in cardiac muscle and the inhomogeneity observed at rest increases. This makes precise measurement of sarcomere length during Ca^{2+} activation difficult in the "skinned" multicellular preparation, particularly at the lower resting length (40,46). Thus, during Ca^{2+} activation *some* of the sarcomeres within the preparation might reach lengths less than slack length, and the issue of a contribution of restoring forces might be raised to account for this decline. In addition, cellular branching and intercellular connective tissue might act as "restoring force" with a reduction in length (97). Thus, the influence of restoring forces is a plausible mechanism for the 25% decline noted in the maximally activated multicellular preparation in Fig. 18C. Maximally activated mechanically skinned *single* cardiac cells exhibit only a 5% decline of force of sarcomere length (measured *during* contraction) over an equivalent length range (Fig. 18C) and a 10 to 12% decrease when sarcomere length is reduced to 1.6 μm. As in multicellular preparations, the curve is steeper when the myofilaments are submaximally activated. The conclusion drawn from the maximally activated curves in Fig. 18C is that only 12 to 25% of the force change with a change in length can be attributed to nonmyofilament activation mechanisms. The difference between the single and multicellular preparations may in part be explained by *intercellular* restoring forces (45).

A factor that has been raised in the interpretation of the results in skinned fibers (Fig. 18) is that in skinned preparations myofilament lattice swells at any length, and constant myofilament lattice volume is not maintained when length is changed, as it is in preparations in which the sarcolemma is intact (i.e., Fig. 8). Thus, at short lengths the separations among the myofilaments might be greater than at long lengths, and this may reduce force production. However, this is not seen to be the case since agents added to vary the osmolarity and swelling do not affect the shape of the maximally activated length-tension curve over the range of lengths

in Fig. 18, and at lower lengths actually enhance force (27).

Regardless of the mechanism for the force decline with a decrease in length in the maximally activated cardiac preparations in Fig. 18, it must be considered that its magnitude is relatively small. Thus, the major portion of the decrease in force with a reduction in intact muscle, i.e., Figs. 2 and 8, must be attributed to a decline in the extent of myofilament activation with decreasing length.

That contractile force changes immediately following a length change, without a detectible change in the $[Ca]_i$ transient (Fig. 13), may indicate that some mechanism other than a change in $[Ca]_i$ following excitation is required to explain the immediate change in contractile force. Stated in other words, all of the difference in steady state force at low and high resting lengths might not be attributable to a length-dependence of Ca^{2+} release (Fig. 16) as manifest in the Ca^{2+} transient following excitation (Fig. 13). Another experimental approach in bundles of cardiac fibers in which the sarcolemma and membraneous organelles had been "chemically skinned" (Fig. 18) has examined whether the myofilament-Ca^{2+} interaction is length-dependent. At lower lengths, a lower pCa (higher $[Ca^{2+}]$) was required to produce a given *relative* level of force (Fig. 19A). A length-dependent shift of the force-pCa curves in experiments of this sort has been interpreted to indicate a change in sensitivity of the myofilaments for Ca^{2+}. In this particular study, the magnitude of the force shift was such that at the pCa required for 50% contractile activation at the long length, the force at the low length was reduced by a factor of 1.6. The Ca^{2+} affinity for myofilaments also varies at lengths longer than 2.2 μm (Fig. 19B). In atrial muscle, long sarcomeres are observed (75) and a shift in the myofilament force-pCa relation may indeed have a role in the stretch response of this tissue. Thus, in cardiac muscle there is evidence that the myofilament Ca^{2+} affinity is altered over the entire range of sarcomere lengths depicted for skeletal muscle in Fig. 6. This cannot be attributed simply to a change in cross-bridge numbers since that number decreases with increasing lengths over the range employed in Fig. 19B, and does not change over the length range in Fig. 19A. In intact cardiac fibers in which contractile activation at maximum levels can neither be achieved nor clamped constant (i.e., Figs. 2 and 8), the altered myofilament Ca^{2+} sensitivity precludes the demonstration of a plateau in the length-tension relation similar to that found in maximally activated skeletal muscle (Fig. 6B). Additional studies that directly measure the effect of stretch on Ca^{2+} binding by myofilaments are required to determine whether the shifts in the curves in Fig. 19 are, in fact, due to altered myofilament Ca^{2+} sensitivity or some other factors that would produce a similar result. The observation in tetanized skeletal muscle that

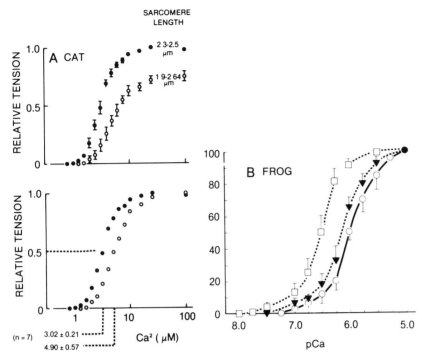

FIG. 19. A: $[Ca^{2+}]$-force curves for chemically-skinned cat ventricular muscle bundles at long and short sarcomere lengths. Each point shows pooled data for seven preparations in which the force production at a given $[Ca^{2+}]$ was measured at resting sarcomere lengths of 2.3–2.5 μm and 1.9–2.04 μm. The *bars* on the points show $\pm$ 1 SE of the mean where this exceeds the diameter of the plotted point. In the **top panel** all forces are expressed as a fraction of the maximum force produced at the longer sarcomere length. The **bottom panel** shows the data from top panel after normalization so that the forces produced at each sarcomere length are expressed as a fraction of the maximum absolute force at that sarcomere length. (From ref. 40, with permission.) **B:** Effect of varying the mean sarcomere length on the relation between pCa and relative tension in 3- to 7-μm wide completely or partially skinned cells from the frog ventricle. *Open circles* correspond to an active (measured during activation) sarcomere length of 2.20–2.30 μm, *solid triangles* to an active sarcomere length of 2.60–2.70 μm, and *open squares* to an active sarcomere length of 3.00–3.10 μm. The tension developed by a given cell at a given pCa and sarcomere length was expressed as a percentage of the tension developed by the same cell at that same sarcomere length and at pCa 5.0, i.e., at maximum activation. Each point corresponds to the mean and each vertical bar to 1 SD. (From ref. 28.)

stretch causes an increase in force with a decrease in peak aequorin luminescence has also been interpreted to result from a shift in the myofilament affinity for Ca^{2+} (7). If this is indeed the case, then the observation that in cardiac muscle force increases acutely with stretch, with no corresponding decrease in peak aequorin luminescence (Fig. 13), might substantiate the hypothesis that Ca^{2+} release from the sarcoplasmic reticulum at a given Ca^{2+}-loading level is acutely increased by an increase in cell length (Fig. 16).

Myofilament "Deactivation Due to Shortening"

Several studies have indicated that muscle fiber shortening during a contraction causes a decreased duration of force-generating capacity in both skeletal (22,41,46) and cardiac muscle (9,11), and that the extent of this decrease depends on the speed and duration of the shortening (70). Since the myofilament Ca^{2+} affinity is length-dependent, as noted above, does a decrease in length during the muscle shortening that occurs during a contraction reduce myofilament Ca^{2+} affinity and thus "deactivate" the myofilaments?

Studies (4,34,42,60) utilizing aequorin to measure myoplasmic $[Ca^{2+}]$ have observed that when a muscle is allowed to shorten following stimulation, the decay of the Ca^{2+} transient is retarded compared to that accompanying an isometric transient. This "extra" light associated with shortening in some instances appears as a secondary "hump" in the declining phase of the

aequorin light (Fig. 20A). An hypothesis to explain the "extra" light has been extrapolated from an earlier suggestion that the Ca^{2+} affinity of troponin C is enhanced when rigor links rather than cycling cross-bridges are formed between the thick and thin filaments (94). According to the sliding filament cross-bridge theory of muscle contraction, sliding of the thin filaments over the thick filaments occurs via continuous deattachment and reattachment when Ca^{2+} is maintained above threshold for activation following excitation. If the observations when rigor attachments connect the myofilaments can be extrapolated to be the case when Ca^{2+}-activated cross-bridges connect the myofilaments (40,46), then any situation that results in more cross-bridge cycling (or fewer cross-bridges per unit time) would result in less Ca^{2+} binding. It would be expected that shortening during an isotonic (or auxotonic) contraction (as opposed to the purely isometric contraction) produces a situation in which the average time of cross-bridge unattachment increases, since detachment occurs following each power stroke. However, this hypothesis regarding the role of the cross-bridge in myofilament binding is weakened by the observation that Ca^{2+} affinity of the myofilaments increases with length over that range of muscle lengths where the number of cross-bridges actually decreases (Fig. 19). Regardless of the mechanism for altered myofilament Ca^{2+} affinity with a reduction in length, less Ca^{2+} would be bound at shorter lengths leaving more in the myoplasm as reflected in the declining phase of the aequorin transient (Fig. 20A).

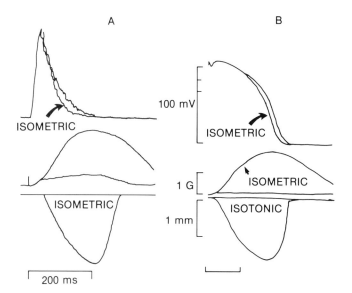

FIG. 20. **A:** Effect of shortening during a contraction on the transient on aequorin luminescence (**top**), force (**middle**), and length (**lower**) trace of a ferret papillary muscle. Note that the duration of force production decreases when shortening is permitted to occur during a contraction and that this is associated with a prolongation of the relaxation phase of aequorin. **B:** Transmembrane action potential (**top**), twitch force (**middle**), and length trace (**bottom**) in cat papillary muscle when contracting isometrically (ends of preparation fixed) and when allowed to shorten (end of preparation allowed to move, i.e., an isotonic contraction. (From ref. 60, with permission.)

That the myofilaments become a less effective Ca^{2+} sink at the shorter sarcomere lengths that are encountered near the end of the shortening period could explain previous observations that active shortening during a contraction is associated with decreased duration and intensity of force-generating capacity in muscle. The enhanced myoplasmic $[Ca^{2+}]$ that results from this shortening might also be expected to modulate Ca^{2+}-dependent transsarcolemmal currents or carrier mechanisms (Fig. 3), and thus alter the transsarcolemmal action potential (59). Prolongation of the action potential has indeed been observed when muscle shortens during contraction (ref. 59; Fig. 20B) and could result from Ca^{2+} activation of some of the electrogenic processes described above. Moreover, higher myoplasmic $[Ca^{2+}]$ at a *critical* time in the cardiac cycle, i.e., when the sarcoplasmic reticulum has resequestered sufficient Ca^{2+}, and when the myoplasmic $[Ca^{2+}]$ still constitutes an effective trigger for Ca^{2+} release (24), might be expected to trigger a second release of Ca^{2+} from the sarcoplasmic reticulum (Figs. 16 and 17), which might be expected to have a further impact on membrane potential. Indeed, shortening "deactivation" caused late in the cardiac cycle by releasing the end of the muscle under conditions when buffering capacity of sarcoplasmic reticulum is reduced (38), does indeed cause mechanical oscillations;

and the Ca_i oscillations that drive these mechanical oscillations are the possible modulators of the concomitantly observed voltage oscillations (50,77).

Considering that the apparent Ca^{2+} affinity of the myofilaments increases at longer *resting* lengths (Fig. 19), it might be hypothesized that an increase in resting length might counteract shortening deactivation, i.e., following the same extent of shortening in a fiber that begins to shorten from a long length versus that from a shorter length, the longer fiber would have more Ca^{2+} remaining bound at the end of shortening period. This should delay the dissipation of contractile force in the presence of a decrease in the late phase aequorin light; indeed, that prolonged relaxation time at long versus short muscle length accompanied by an earlier decay in aequorin luminescence is compatible with the notion that more Ca^{2+} remains bound to the myofilament later in the contraction at longer versus shorter muscle lengths (4). Moreover, one would predict from the greater apparent Ca^{2+} binding at longer resting lengths (Fig. 19) that a muscle that begins to contract from a longer resting sarcomere length than from a shorter one, would, at the *same* sarcomere length during contraction, exhibit greater contractile function, i.e., velocity- as well as force-developing capacity. This is indeed the case in the single frog atrial cell as illustrated in Fig. 11. In fact it might be speculated that the effect of initial sarcomere length to enhance contractile activation in Fig. 11 is indeed observed because virtually no "shortening deactivation" occurs in frog myocardium (12).

In the "isometric" contraction in isolated cardiac muscle, even though the overall muscle length is fixed (as in Figs. 2 and 8), substantial (5–17%) shortening of central sarcomeres (Figs. 7 and 8) occurs due to stray compliance at the ends of the preparation (20,33,43,48,49,57,92,98). In addition to causing a shift to shorter sarcomere lengths during contraction, this shortening might, per se, also be expected to deactivate the myofilaments. Could "shortening deactivation" during contraction (as in Fig. 20) be more pronounced in a muscle when contraction is initiated from shorter versus longer resting muscle lengths (as in Fig. 2)? Could this be yet another mechanism for the Frank-Starling law of the heart? This issue has been addressed by monitoring the extent of internal shortening during contractions that originate from different resting lengths, by monitoring the spacing between markers applied to the external surface of the center of the muscle (49), or by monitoring average sarcomere length in a central segment either microscopically (48) or by laser diffraction (33,57,92). The general result obtained has been that the extent of internal shortening is greater at intermediate muscle lengths than at L_{max} or at very short lengths (20,33,43,48,49,57,92,98). Thus, the extent of "internal" shortening, does not exhibit a clear monotonic dependence on the resting length (Fig. 7B).

Another approach to determine whether shortening "deactivation" accounts for the steep length-tension relations in Figs. 2 and 8 is to offset the shortening that occurs during the contraction by a stretch applied to the end of the muscle (49,92). At a *given* resting length this results, as expected from the interpretation of the experiments regarding shortening deactivation, in a greater force development and rate of rise of force in the contraction (Fig. 21A inset). When segment length during contraction is controlled, it is observed that the *relative* length-tension curves in the presence and absence of internal shortening are superimposable (Fig. 21A). Also, the shapes of length-tension curve in contractions in which internal sarcomere shortening occurs and in which it is prevented by a counterstretch at the muscle end do not differ (Fig. 21B). In the curves in Fig. 21, it is noteworthy that the sarcomere lengths at the peak of contraction when internal shortening occurred, i.e., muscle isometric, are shorter than at rest, whereas in

the other curve, i.e., sarcomere isometric, sarcomere length at rest and contraction do not differ. Thus, both resting sarcomere length and the final sarcomere length achieved at peak force are important determinants of the *absolute* force-length relation. The resting sarcomere length is important in that it reflects the stretch on the cell, which may determine the effectiveness of Ca^{2+} loading and release (Figs. 11, 13, 14, and 16) and Ca^{2+} bound to the myofilaments at the onset of contraction (Fig. 19); the final sarcomere length is important because it reflects the extent of shortening during the contraction, and thus the degree of shortening deactivation (Fig. 20). Yet except for a scaling factor for the difference in the absolute force at any given length due to shortening deactivation, the two curves in either Fig. 21A or 21B do not differ substantially in steepness. Thus, the *shape* of either the absolute (Fig. 21B) or relative length-tension relation (Fig. 21A) cannot depend on the final sarcomere length achieved during contraction, but rather

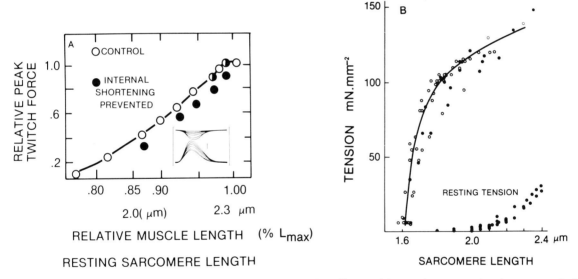

FIG. 21. A *(inset)*: Sequence of length and force records showing the effects of increasing amounts of servo control applied to a rabbit papillary muscle at a given resting sarcomere length. The **upper** series of traces are length signals from a photoelectronic spot follower. These indicate changes in separation of markers on the muscle surface, where length decreases as indicated by a downward deflection. A corresponding series of twitches is shown **below**. The smallest twitch is associated with the largest deflection in the length signal records. Between each twitch, the gain of the servo system was increased. This caused the end of the muscle attached to the servo motor to be driven so as to diminish progressively the amount of change in marker separation during a twitch. Finally, servo gain was increased to the point at which, during a twitch, there was a just perceptible deflection in the length signal trace. The largest twitch amplitude corresponds to a tension of about 8 g/mm⁻². The data points in the figure indicate peak twitch force for contractions in rabbit papillary muscles in which internal shortening was allowed to occur *(open symbols)* and for those in which this shortening was prevented by applying a stretch necessary to maintain the spacing between markers in the center of the muscle constant throughout the contraction *(solid symbols)*. Twitch force is normalized to that value obtained at L_{max} (2.3 μm) in each condition. The stretch applied to the end of the muscle to maintain segment length in the center of the muscle constant during contraction results in a sufficient force applied to the muscle, i.e., the "resting" force usually present prior to onset of a contraction and which usually decreases during the contraction in this experimental mode is maintained throughout the contraction; whether to subtract this force from the total force developed by the muscle at the peak of the contraction requires a choice of an analog model (44). The approach used here was to subtract passive force from both curves. (From ref. 49.) **B:** Relations between *active* tension and length from contractions in thin rat papillary muscles (Ca_e = 2.5 mM) in which sarcomere length during contraction was held constant *(solid circles)* does not differ from the sarcomere length-total tension (isometric twitch tension plus "passive" tension) relation derived from isometric contractions in *(open circles)* during which 8–14% internal shortening occurred. This approach is model-dependent (see A and the text in conjunction with Fig. 8). (From ref. 92, with permission.)

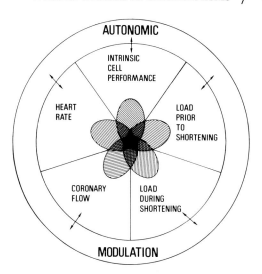

only on resting length since the sets of curves depicted in either Fig. 21A or 21B are similar in shape but had in common resting length, but not final sarcomere length. The same conclusion was reached in other studies in which a similar relative tension-sarcomere length curves were observed in muscles that exhibited markedly different extents of internal shortening (98).

SUMMARY

The results of studies of the last decade clearly indicate that resting muscle length modulates the extent of myofilament contractile activation (45). Thus, the resting fiber length (or preload) and "contractile" or "inotropic" state of the myocardium can no longer be theoretically considered as independent determinants of myocardial performance, as was formerly thought to be the case, and as is still expounded in some current textbooks of cardiology and medicine. Similarly, since the fiber length during a contraction also determines the extent of myofilament Ca^{2+} activation, and since this length is determined by the load encountered during shortening (afterload), neither can afterload be considered independent of contractile state. Rather, the level of excitation-activation-contraction coupling is length-dependent, and myofilament activation varies with length at the onset of the cardiac contraction and continues to vary as length changes during the contraction, as the fiber shortens.

The modulation of stroke volume and cardiac output in the intact organism must be considered to occur from the interdependency of several factors (Fig. 22) the relative contribution of which can vary, depending on the particular moment of observation. In experimental studies conditions can be altered such that the expression of one or more of these factors becomes dominant; this, however, does not imply dominance of that individual factor in the intact circulation. Rather, the scheme in Fig. 22 portrays all factors *interacting* in a feedback manner such that in a steady state the performance of the system could be modulated within a narrow range. The example in Fig. 1 offers a particularly clear illustration of this: During exercise, a greater autonomic modulation of excitation-activation-contraction coupling and heart rate occurred in the younger than in the older subjects, as suggested by the greater increase in heart rate and reduction in end-systolic volume in the younger versus older subjects. Thus, the role of an augmentation of filling volume in increasing cardiac output is minimized in younger subjects. In the elderly subjects, however, a substantial reduction in end-systolic volume did not occur and the increase in heart rate was less than in the younger subjects, suggesting a diminished autonomic modulation and possibly an increased afterload compared to the younger subjects. However, cardiac output was maintained at the same level as the younger

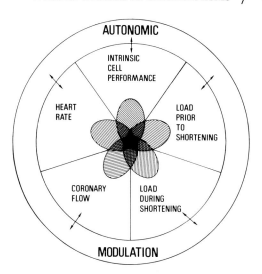

FIG. 22. Multiple interdependent factors modulate cardiac function. The importance of the contribution of each factor as a determinant of cardiac function in the intact organism varies with the status of the organism (see text for details). (From ref. 62.)

subjects via ventricular dilatation and enhanced stroke volume, i.e., via the Frank-Starling mechanism. Likewise, disease states and pharmacologic therapeutic interventions, depending on their impact on each of the factors in Fig. 22, alter the relative contribution of that factor in determining cardiac output. For example, the often observed, but heretofore unexplained, flattening of the "Starling curve" in patients with congestive heart failure may be explained, in part, by a reduced contribution of length-dependent contractile activation due to an abnormality in the excitation-activation-contraction coupling that results from the pathophysiology of a particular disease state. However, even under conditions when the effect of length or preload is altered, each of the other factors must also be considered as determinants of performance, because the summation of these effects, in fact, determines the myocardial fiber length or preload at which the myocardium operates.

REFERENCES

1. Abbott, B. C., and Mommaerts, W. F. H. M. (1959): A study of inotropic mechanisms in the papillary muscle preparation. *J. Gen. Physiol.*, 42:533–551.
2. Allen, D. G. (1977): On the relationship between action potential duration and tension in cat papillary muscle. *Cardiovasc. Res.*, 11:210–218.
3. Allen, D. G., Jewell, B. R., and Murray, J. W. (1974): The contribution of activation processes to the length-tension relation of cardiac muscle. *Nature*, 248:606–607.
4. Allen, D. G., and Kurihara, S. (1982): The effects of muscle length on intracellular calcium transients in mammalian cardiac muscle. *J. Physiol.*, 327:79–94.
5. Anderson, P. A. W., Manring, A., and Johnson, E. A. (1973): Force-frequency relationship: A basis for a new index of cardiac contractility. *Circ. Res.*, 33:665–671.
6. Blinks, J. R., and Koch-Weser, J. (1963): Physical factors in the

analysis of the actions of drugs on myocardial contractility. *Pharmacol. Rev.*, 15:531–599.

7. Blinks, J. R., Rudel, R., and Taylor, S. R. (1978): Calcium transients in isolated amphibian skeletal muscle fibers: Detection with aequorin. *J. Physiol.*, 277:291–323.

8. Bozler, E., and Delahayes, J. F. (1973): Mechanical and electrical oscillations in cardiac muscle of the turtle. *J. Gen. Physiol.*, 62:523–534.

9. Brady, A. J. (1967): Onset of contractility in cardiac muscle. *J. Physiol.*, 184:560–580.

10. Brady, A. J. (1967): Mechanics of isolated papillary muscle. In: *Factors Influencing Myocardial Contractility*, edited by R. D. Tanz, F. Kavaler, and J. Roberts, pp. 53–64. Academic Press, New York.

11. Brutsaert, D. L., and Sonnenblick, E. H. (1969): Force-velocity-length-time relations of the contractile elements in heart muscle of the cat. *Circ. Res.*, 24:137–149.

12. Brutsaert, D. L., DeClerck, N. M., Goethal, M. A., and Housmans, P. R. (1978): Relaxation of ventricular muscle. *J. Physiol.*, 283:469–480.

13. Capogrossi, M. C., Fraticelli, A., and Lakatta, E. G. (1984): Ca^{++} release from the sarcoplasmic reticulum: different effects of ryanodine and caffeine (abstract). *Fed. Proc.*, 43:820.

14. Capogrossi, M. C., Fraticelli, A., Spurgeon, H. A., and Lakatta, E. G. (1984): Electrical suppression of spontaneous Ca^{2+} oscillations in adult cardiac cells (Abstr.). *Clin. Res.*, 32:472A.

15. Capogrossi, M. C., Kort, A. A., Spurgeon, H. A., and Suarez-Isla, B. A., and Lakatta, E. G. (1984): Spontaneous contractile waves and stimulated contractions exhibit the same Ca^{++} and species dependence in isolated cardiac myocytes and papillary muscles (abstract). *Biophys. J.*, 45:94a.

16. Capogrossi, M. C., and Lakatta, E. G. (1985): Frequency modulation of synchronization of spontaneous oscillations in cardiac cells. *Am. J. Physiol.*, 248:H412–H418.

17. Clinch, N. F. (1968): On the increase in rate of heat production caused by stretch in frog's skeletal muscle. *J. Physiol.*, 196:397–414.

18. Close, R. I. (1972): The relations between sarcomere length and characteristics of isometric twitch contractions of frog sartorius muscle. *J. Physiol.*, 220:745–762.

19. Colquhoun, D., Neher, E., Reuter, H., and Stevens, C. F. (1981): Inward current channels activated by intracellular Ca in cultured cardiac cells. *Nature*, 294:752–754.

20. Donald, T. C., Reeves, D. N. S., Reeves, R. C., Walker, A. A., and Hefner, L. L. (1980): Effect of damaged ends in papillary muscle preparations. *Am. J. Physiol.*, 238:H14–H23.

21. Dulhunty, A. F., and Franzini-Armstrong, C. (1975): The relative contributions of the folds and caveolae to the surface membrane of frog skeletal muscle fibers at different sarcomere lengths. *J. Physiol.*, 250:513–539.

22. Edman, K. A. P. (1975): Mechanical deactivation induced by active shortening in isolated muscle fibres of the frog. *J. Physiol.*, 246:255–275.

23. Fabiato, A. (1980): Sarcomere length dependence of calcium release from the sarcoplasmic reticulum of skinned cardiac cells demonstrated by differential microspectrophotometry with Arsenzo III (abstract). *J. Gen. Physiol.*, 76:15a.

24. Fabiato, A. (1981): Myoplasmic free calcium concentration reached during the twitch of an intact isolated cardiac cell and during calcium-induced release of calcium from the sarcoplasmic reticulum of a skinned cardiac cell from the adult rat or rabbit ventricle. *J. Gen. Physiol.*, 78:457–497.

25. Fabiato, A. (1983): Calcium-induced release of calcium from the cardiac sarcoplasmic reticulum. *Am. J. Physiol.*, 245(14):C1–C14.

26. Fabiato, A., and Fabiato, F. (1975): Dependence of the contractile activation of skinned cardiac cells on the sarcomere length. *Nature*, 256:54–56.

27. Fabiato, A., and Fabiato, F. (1976): Dependence of calcium release, tension generation and restoring forces on sarcomere length in skinned cardiac cells. *Eur. J. Cardiol.*, 4(Suppl.):13–27.

28. Fabiato, A., and Fabiato, F. (1978): Myofilament-generated tension oscillations during partial calcium activation and activation dependence of the sarcomere length-tension relation of skinned cardiac cells. *J. Gen. Physiol.*, 72:667–699.

29. Feigl, E. O. (1967): Effects of stimulation frequency on myocardial extensibility. *Circ. Res.*, 20:447–458.

30. Feng, T. P. (1932): The effect of length on the resting metabolism of muscle. *J. Physiol.*, 74:441–454.

31. Frank, J. S., and Winegrad, S. (1976): Effect of muscle length on ^{45}Ca efflux in resting and contracting skeletal muscle. *Am. J. Physiol.*, 231:555–559.

32. Gordon, A. M., Huxley, A. F., and Julian, F. J. (1966): The variation in isometric tension with sarcomere length in vertebrate muscle fibers. *J. Physiol.*, 184:170–192.

33. Gordon, A. M., and Pollack, G. H. (1980): Effects of calcium on the sarcomere length-tension relation in rat cardiac muscle. *Circ. Res.*, 47:610–619.

34. Gordon, A. M., and Ridgway, E. B. (1978): Calcium transients and relaxation in single muscle fibers. *Eur. J. Cardiol.*, 7(Suppl.):27–34.

35. Gulch, R. W., and Jacob, R. (1975): The effect of sudden stretches on length-tension- and force-velocity relations of mammalian cardiac muscle. *Pfluegers Arch.*, 357:335–347.

36. Guz, A. (1974): Chairman's introduction. In: *The Physiological Basis of Starling's Law of the Heart*, edited by R. Porter and D. W. Fitzsimons, pp. 1–6. Associated Scientific, Amsterdam.

37. Henderson, A. H., and Brutsaert, D. L. (1974): Force-velocity-length relationship in heart muscle: Lack of time-independence during twitch contractions of frog ventricle strips with caffeine. *Pfluegers Arch.*, 348:59–64.

38. Henderson, A. H., and Cattell, M. R. (1976): Length-induced changes in activation during contraction. A study of mechanical oscillations in strontium-mediated contractions of cat and frog heart muscle. *Circ. Res.*, 38:289–296.

39. Hercus, V. M., McDowall, R. J. S., and Mendel, D. (1955): Sodium exchanges in cardiac muscle. *J. Physiol.*, 129:177–183.

40. Hibberd, M. G., and Jewell, B. R. (1982): Calcium-and length-dependent force production in rat ventricular muscle. *J. Physiol.*, 329:527–540.

41. Hill, A. V. (1964): The effect of tension in prolonging the active state in a twitch. *Proc. R. Soc. Lond. (Biol.)*, 159:589–595.

42. Housman, P., Lee, N. K. M., and Blinks, J. R. (1983): Active shortening retards the decline of the intracellular calcium transient in mammalian heart muscle. *Science*, 221:159–161.

43. Huntsman, L. L., Joseph, D. S., Oiye, M. Y., and Nichols, G. L. (1979): Auxotonic contractions in cardiac muscle segments. *Am. J. Physiol.*, 237:H131–H138.

44. Jewell, B. R. (1977): A re-examination of the influence of muscle length on myocardial performance. *Circ. Res.*, 40:321–330.

45. Jewell, B. R. (1982): Activation of contraction in cardiac muscle. *Mayo Clin. Proc.*, 57(Suppl.):6–13.

46. Jewell, B. R., and Wilkie, D. R. (1960): The mechanical properties of relaxing muscle. *J. Physiol.*, 152:30–47.

47. Julian, F. J., and Moss, R. L. (1980): Sarcomere length-tension relations of frog skinned muscle fibres at lengths above the optimum. *J. Physiol.*, 304:529–539.

48. Julian, F. J., and Sollins, M. R. (1975): Sarcomere length-tension relation in living rat papillary muscle. *Circ. Res.*, 37:299–308.

49. Julian, F. J., Sollins, M. R., and Moss, R. L. (1976): Absence of a plateau in length-tension relationship of rabbit papillary muscle when internal shortening is prevented. *Nature*, 260:340–342.

50. Kass, R. S., Tsien, R. W., and Weingart, R. (1978): Ionic basis of transient inward current induced by strophanthidin in cardiac Purkinje fibres. *J. Physiol.*, 281:209–226.

51. Koch-Weser, J., and Blinks, J. R. (1963): The influence of the interval between beats on myocardial contractility. *Pharmacol. Res.*, 15:601–652.

52. Kort, A. A., and Lakatta, E. G. (1983): Rest potentiation in cardiac muscle is associated with cell Ca^{2+} oscillations (abstract). *Circulation*, 68(Part II):III-72.

53. Kort, A. A., and Lakatta, E. G. (1984): Propagation velocity and frequency of spontaneous microscopic waves in intact rat papillary muscles are Ca^{2+}-dependent (abstract). *Biophys. J.*, 45:94a.

54. Kort, A. A., and Lakatta, E. G. (1984): Calcium-dependent mechanical oscillations occur spontaneously in unstimulated mammalian cardiac tissues. *Circ. Res.*, 54:396–404.

55. Kort, A. A., and Lakatta, E. G. (1985): Ca^{2+}-dependent oscillations in rat cardiac muscle: Transient state measurements following regular electrical depolarization. *Biophys. J.*, 47:280a.

56. Kort, A. A., Lakatta, E. G., Marban, E., Stern, M. D., and Wier, W. G. (1985): Fluctuations in intracellular calcium concentration and their effect on tonic tension in canine cardiac Purkinje fibres. *J. Physiol.,* 367:291–308.

57. Krueger, J. W., and Pollack, G. H. (1975): Myocardial sarcomere dynamics during isometric contraction. *J. Physiol.,* 251:627–643.

58. Kumbarachi, N. M., and Nastuk, W. L. (1982): Action of caffeine in excitation-contraction coupling of frog skeletal muscle fibres. *J. Physiol.,* 325:295.

59. Lab, M. J. (1982): Contraction-excitation feedback in myocardium. Physiological basis and clinical relevance. *Circ. Res.,* 50:757–766.

60. Lab, M. J., Allen, D. G., and Orchard, O. H. (1984): The effects of shortening on intracellular calcium and on the action potential in mammalian ventricular muscle. *Circ. Res.,* 55:825–829.

61. Lakatta, E. G. (1980): Age-related alterations in the cardiovascular response to adrenergic mediated stress. *Fed. Proc.,* 39:3173–3177.

62. Lakatta, E. G. (1983): Determinants of cardiovascular performance: modification due to aging. *J. Chronic Dis.,* 36:15–30.

63. Lakatta, E. G. (1985): Altered autonomic modulation of cardiovascular function with adult aging: perspectives from studies ranging from man to cell. In: *Pathobiology of Cardiovascular Injury,* edited by H. L. Stone and W. B. Weglicki, pp. 441–460, Martinus Nijhoff, Boston.

64. Lakatta, E. G., Capogrossi, M. C., Kort, A. A., and Stern, M. D. (1985): Spontaneous myocardial Ca oscillations: an overview with emphasis on ryanodine and caffeine. *Fed. Proc.* 44:2977–2983.

65. Lakatta, E. G., and Henderson, A. H. (1977): Starling's law reactivated. *J. Mol. Cell. Cardiol.,* 9:347–351.

66. Lakatta, E. G., and Jewell, B. R. (1977): Length-dependent activation; its effect on the length-tension relation in cat ventricular muscle. *Circ. Res.,* 40:251–257.

67. Lakatta, E. G., and Lappe, D. L. (1981): Diastolic scattered light fluctuation, resting force and twitch force in mammalian cardiac muscle. *J. Physiol.,* 315:369–394.

68. Lakatta, E. G., and Spurgeon, H. A. (1980): Force staircase kinetics in mammalian cardiac muscle: modulation by muscle length. *J. Physiol.,* 299:337–352.

69. Lappe, D. L., and Lakatta, E. G. (1980): Intensity fluctuation spectroscopy monitors contractile activation in 'resting' cardiac muscle. *Science,* 207:1369–1371.

70. Leach, J. K., Brady, A. J., Skipper, B. J., and Millis, D. L. (1980): Effects of active shortening on tension development of rabbit papillary muscle. *Am. J. Physiol.,* 238(7):H8–H13.

71. Levin, K. R., and Page, E. (1980): Quantitative studies on plasmalemmal folds and caveolae of rabbit ventricular myocardial cells. *Circ. Res.,* 46:244–255.

72. Loiselle, D. S. (1982): Stretch-induced increase in resting metabolism of isolated papillary muscle. *Biophys. J.,* 38:185–194.

73. Loiselle, D. S., and Gibbs, C. L. (1979): Species differences in cardiac energetics. *Am. J. Physiol.,* 237:H90–H98.

74. Lopez, J. R., Wanek, L. A., and Taylor, S. R. (1981): Skeletal muscle: length-dependent effects of potentiating agents. *Science,* 214:79–82.

75. Manring, A., Nassar, R., and Johnson, E. A. (1977): Light diffraction of cardiac muscle: An analysis of sarcomere shortening and muscle tension. *J. Mol. Cell. Cardiol.,* 9:441–459.

76. Marban, E., and Tsien, R. W. (1982): Enhancement of calcium current during digitalis inotropy in mammalian heart: positive feedback regulation by intracellular calcium. *J. Physiol.,* 329:589–614.

77. Matsuda, H., Noma, A., Kurachi, Y., and Irisawa, H. (1982): Transient depolarization and spontaneous voltage fluctuations in isolated single cells from guinea pig ventricles. Calcium-mediated membrane potential fluctuations. *Circ. Res.,* 51:142–151.

78. Monroe, R. G., Gamble, W. J., Lafarge, C. G., and Vatner, S. F. (1974): Homeometric autoregulation. In: *The Physiological Basis of Starling's Law of the Heart,* edited by R. Porter and D. W. Fitzsimons, pp. 257–277. Associated Scientific, Amsterdam.

79. Orchard, C. H., Eisner, D. A., and Allen, D. G. (1983): Oscillations of intracellular Ca^{2+} in mammalian cardiac muscle. *Nature,* 304:735–738.

80. Robinson, T. F., and Winegard, S. (1979): The measurement and dynamic implications of thin filament lengths in heart muscle. *J. Physiol.,* 286:607–619.

81. Rodeheffer, R. J., Gerstenblith, G., Becker, L. C., Fleg, J. L., Weisfeldt, M. L., and Lakatta, E. G. (1984): Exercise cardiac output is maintained with advancing age in healthy human subjects: cardiac dilatation and increased stroke volume compensate for a diminished heart rate. *Circulation,* 69:203–213.

82. Sarnoff, S. J., Mitchell, J. H., Gilmore, J. P., and Remensnyder, J. P. (1960): Homeometric autoregulation in the heart. *Circ. Res.,* 8:1077–1091.

83. Simmons, R. M., and Jewell, B. R. (1974): Mechanics and medols of muscular contraction. *Recent Adv. Physiol.,* 9:87–147.

84. Sonnenblick, E. H. (1962): Force-velocity relations in mammalian heart muscle. *Am. J. Physiol.,* 202:931–939.

85. Sonnenblick, E. H. (1968): Correlation of myocardial ultrastructure and function. *Circulation,* 38:29–44.

86. Sonnenblick, E. H., and Skelton, C. L. (1974): Reconsideration of the ultrastructural basis of cardiac length-tension relations. *Circ. Res.,* 35:517–526.

87. Spear, J. F., and Moore, E. N. (1972): Stretch-induced excitation and conduction disturbances in the isolated rat myocardium. *J. Electrocardiol.,* 5:15–24.

88. Spotnitz, H. M., Sonnenblick, E. H., and Spiro, D. (1966): Relationship of ultrastructure to function in the intact heart; sarcomere structure relative to pressure-volume curves of intact left ventricles of dog and cat. *Circ. Res.,* 18:49–66.

89. Stern, M. D., Kort, A. A., Bhatnagar, B. M., and Lakatta, E. G. (1983): Scattered-light intensity fluctuations in diastolic rat cardiac muscle caused by spontaneous Ca^{++}-dependent cellular mechanical oscillations. *J. Gen. Physiol.,* 82:119–153.

90. Tarr, M., Trank, J. W., Goertz, K. K., and Leiffer, P. (1981): Effect of initial sarcomere length on sarcomere kinetics and force development in single frog atrial cardiac cells. *Circ. Res.,* 49:767–774.

91. Ter Keurs, H. E. D. J., Iwazumi, T., and Pollack, G. H. (1978): The sarcomere length-tension relation in skeletal muscle. *J. Gen. Physiol.,* 72:565–592.

92. Ter Keurs, H. E. D. J., Rijnsburger, W. H., Henuingen, R. V., and Nagelsmit, M. J. (1980): Tension development and sarcomere length in rat cardiac trabeculae. Evidence of length-dependent activation. *Circ. Res.,* 46:703–714.

93. Walford, G. D., Gerstenblith, G., and Lakatta, E. G. (1984): Effect of sodium on calcium-dependent force in unstimulated rat cardiac muscle. *Am. J. Physiol.,* 246(15):H222–H231.

94. Weber, A., and Murray, J. M. (1973): Molecular control mechanisms in muscle contraction. *Physiol. Rev.,* 53:612–673.

95. Weiss, R., and Morad, M. (1981): Intrinsic birefringence signal preceding the onset of contraction in heart muscle. *Science,* 213:663–666.

96. Wier, W. G., Kort, A. A., Stern, M. D., Lakatta, E. G., and Marban, E. (1983): Cellular calcium fluctuations in mammalian heart: Direct evidence from noise analysis of aequorin signals in Purkinje fibers. *Proc. Natl. Acad. Sci. USA,* 80:7367–7371.

97. Winegrad, S. (1980): The importance of passive elements in the contraction of the heart. In: *Cardiac Dynamics,* edited by J. Baan, A. C. Arntzenius, and E. L. Yellin, pp. 11–23. Martinus Nijhoff, The Hague.

98. Wohlfart, B., Grimm, A. F., and Edman, K. A. P. (1977): Relationship between sarcomere length and active force in rabbit papillary muscle. *Acta Physiol. Scand.,* 101:155–164.

99. Wood, E. G., Heppner, R. L., and Weidmann, S. (1969): Inotropic effects of electric currents. I. Positive and negative effects of constant electric currents of current pulses applied during cardiac action potential. II. Hypothesis; calcium, excitation-contraction coupling and inotropic effects. *Circ. Res.,* 24:409–445.

100. Yoran, C., Covell, J. W., and Ross, J., Jr. (1973): Structural basis for the ascending limb of left ventricular function. *Circ. Res.,* 32:297–303.

The Heart and Cardiovascular System,
edited by H. A. Fozzard et al.
Raven Press, New York © 1986.

CHAPTER 41

Smooth Muscle Structure and Function

Andrew P. Somlyo and Avril V. Somlyo

The diversity of the many, vascular and visceral, smooth muscles, is expressed by their different sensitivities to drugs and neurotransmitters, as well as by differences in their electrophysiological properties, shape, size, and detailed ultrastructure. The purpose of this chapter, however, is to provide not a detailed catalogue of the numerous species and organ-related properties of smooth muscle, but an introduction and overview for the nonspecialist. Nevertheless, this generalized survey should not mislead the reader to a stereotyped view of "smooth muscle," because only an awareness of the great diversity of smooth muscles will permit the development of drugs having selective effects on different vascular beds, and the identification of the cellular processes that, if altered, change physiological diversity to cellular pathology.

GENERAL STRUCTURE

Smooth muscle cells are fusiform or branched cells approximately 100 to 500 μm long and 2 to 6 μm diameter, with a very large surface area/volume ratio (2.5 μm^{-1}, including surface vesicles). The surface vesicles, or caveolae, increase the surface membrane area by about 75%. The cells are embedded in connective tissue, and the extracellular space can be from 12 to 40% of the tissue volume. Arterial and uterine smooth muscle cells synthesize collagen, elastin, glycoproteins, and proteoglycans. These connective tissue elements contribute to the distribution of forces developed by smooth muscle, and are dramatically illustrated in the freeze-fractured, deep-etched preparation shown in Fig. 1, where the attachment of the glycosaminoglycans of the basement membrane to the smooth muscle cell membrane, as well as to the collagen and elastin fibrils in the extracellular space, can be readily visualized.

Cell-to-Cell Conduction

Electrical and metabolic coupling between smooth muscle cells occurs through regions of close apposition between the outer leaflets of the plasma membranes of neighboring cells. A regular lattice of particles is found within these regions, called gap junctions, of the plasma membrane. There is a spectrum of sizes and numbers of gap junctions among different smooth muscles: "single unit" smooth muscles that are characterized by relatively extensive conducted electrical activity, contain a greater number of gap junctions. This is consistent with the junctions acting as low resistance pathways for the rapid spread of the electrical signal throughout the tissue. In the rat uterus, gap junctions have been reported to appear at the time of parturition, and could therefore be involved in the coordination of muscle contraction during labor. Gap junctions are dynamic structures, and the coupling resistance can change with ionic changes,

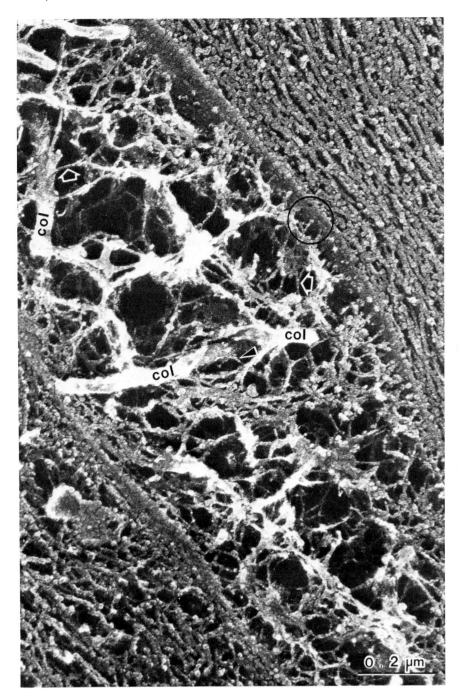

FIG. 1. Extracellular matrix between two smooth muscle cells of the rabbit portal vein showing a dense network of fibrils (*open white arrows*) attached to collagen (COL) fibers or to basement membrane fibrils that frequently terminate with a granule on the outer leaflet of the plasma membrane (*encircled region*). Occasionally fibrils appear to terminate with finger-like processes grasping the collagen fiber (*large arrowhead*). Note the granular material of varying size attached to the fibrillar network. Prefixed, cryoprotected with 30% methanol, frozen, deep-etched, and rotary shadowed. [From Somlyo, A. V. and Franzini-Armstrong, C. (1985): *Experientia,* 41:841–856.]

Ca^{2+}, and pH. These structures may also be involved in metabolic coupling, as small molecules, such as amino acids, sugars, phosphorylated sugars, and nucleotides can cross through the junctions.

CONTRACTILE APPARATUS

Filamentous Proteins

Smooth muscle cells contain three types of filaments (Figs. 2 and 3): thick (myosin), thin (actin), and intermediate.

Myosin

The *thick* (myosin) *filaments* are significantly longer (2.2 μm) in smooth than in vertebrate striated muscle (1.5 μm). In mature smooth muscle, though not necessarily in cultured cells, myosin is in the filamentous form, regardless of whether the muscle is contracted or relaxed or of the extent of myosin phosphorylation. The filaments have tapered ends, but it is not known whether these filaments are bipolar, with a central bare zone, as in striated muscles. The *in situ* myosin filaments have cross-bridges with a periodicity (14.3 nm) similar to

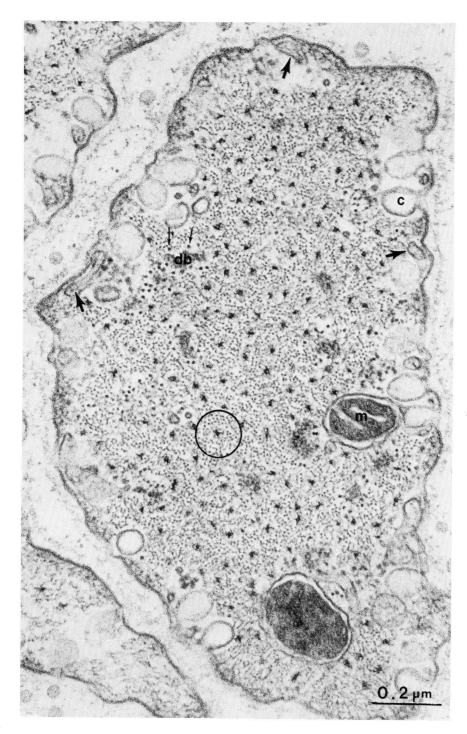

FIG. 2. Transverse section of a cell from the rabbit *vas deferens* showing transversely sectioned thick (myosin) filaments surrounded by actin filaments (*encircled region*) as well as dense bodies (db) that are the equivalent of the Z bands of striated muscles, and associated 10 nm filaments (*small arrows*). Surface couplings, where the sarcoplasmic reticulum is apposed to the plasma membrane, are also present (*large arrows*). Invaginations of the surface membrane called caveolae (c) and mitochondria (m) are also indicated.

that of striated muscle myosin filaments. Although immunologically distinct from skeletal and cardiac myosin, smooth muscle myosin molecules (MW 470,000 daltons) are ultrastructurally indistinguishable from these other myosins, having two globular heads joined to a 150-nm-long tail. Two light chains (20,000 and 17,000 daltons) are associated with each head. The 20,000-dalton light chains are involved in smooth muscle regulation (see Contractile Regulation section, below).

Unlike skeletal muscle myosin, the shape of isolated smooth muscle myosin molecules is sensitive to the state of phosphorylation of the 20,000-dalton light chain and to the ionic strength and Mg^{2+} content of the suspending solutions. By altering these parameters, the *isolated* molecules can assume an extended (6 S) or folded (10 S) configuration that is accompanied by differences in their respective sedimentation velocities in the ultracentrifuge. Such large-scale folding of molecules

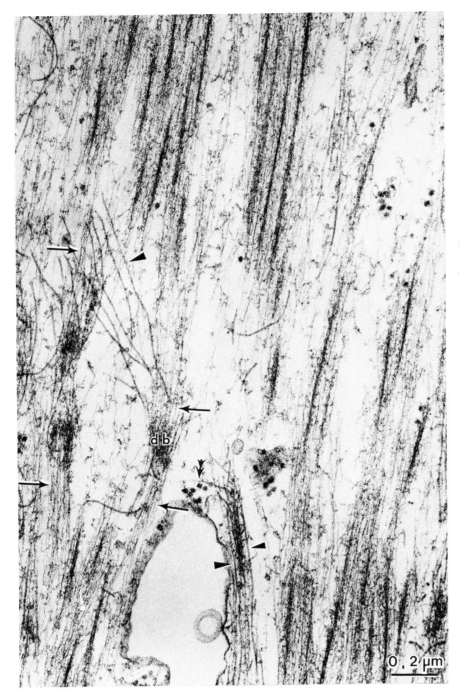

FIG. 3. Longitudinal section of a saponin-skinned portal vein smooth muscle cell. The filaments are spread out, revealing the relationship of the dense bodies with associated actin to the neighboring myosin filaments. Thin filaments (*arrows*) that emerge from cytoplasmic dense bodies (db) can be traced to where they are adjacent to (overlap) the myosin filaments. The 10-nm filaments (*arrowheads*) do not run parallel to the sarcomere-like units, but appear to interconnect dense bodies (*double arrowhead*) (From Bond, M., and Somlyo, A. V. (1982): *J. Cell Biol.*, 95:403–413.)

cannot occur in the filaments *in situ,* but small conformational changes in the head region due to the same process could play a role in contractile regulation.

Actin

Actin, in smooth as well as in striated muscle, is the main constituent of the thin *filaments.* Filamentous actin is a two-stranded helix made up of actin monomers of MW 42,500, and is found in all muscle cells, as well as in many other cell types. Smooth muscle F-actin can activate skeletal muscle myosin ATPase and, like other actins, binds tropomyosin that lies in the groove on either side of the actin filament. Except for a few amino acids at the N-terminus, the sequence is similar to that of other actins. The stoichiometry of tropomyosin to actin in smooth muscle is similar to that in striated muscles, and smooth muscle tropomyosin still retains the troponin-binding site, although troponin is absent in smooth muscles. Filamin, a high molecular weight, actin-binding protein is present in high concentrations in smooth muscle, and is thought to be associated with thin filaments. Its function is not known.

One of the striking features of smooth muscle is the relative content of contractile proteins. The *weight* ratio of actin:myosin in smooth muscle, 1.5 to 3:1, is the reverse of that (1:3) in rabbit skeletal muscle. The number of myosin filaments and the amount of myosin in smooth muscle is approximately five times less than in skeletal muscle. These differences are obvious from inspection of electron micrographs (i.e., Fig. 2): The ratio of actin to myosin filaments is approximately 13:1, compared with 2:1 in vertebrate striated muscle. The length of the actin filaments has not been directly measured, but estimates from counts of actin:myosin filaments and mass ratios suggest a value of 1 to 2 μm. The actin:myosin ratio is somewhat higher in (at least some) arterial than in venous smooth muscles.

Intermediate Filaments

Intermediate filaments (10 nm) are not directly involved in the contractile process, and are found in a variety of other cell types. In normal vascular smooth muscle, intermediate filaments form a "cytoskeleton" linking the dense bodies throughout the cell (Fig. 3). In transversely sectioned smooth muscle cells, their round profiles surround the dense bodies (Fig. 2). These and similar filaments (neurofilaments, glial filaments, epidermal keratin filaments) are found in a great variety of cells (fibroblasts, endothelial cells, cardiac muscle, developing skeletal muscle, etc.) and are polymers of small "families" of proteins. The intermediate filaments of smooth muscles are composed of two proteins, desmin or vimentin, which may occur alone or both within the same cell. There is a massive increase in 10 nm filaments in hypertrophied vascular smooth muscle, in cultured cells, and in some pathological states.

Dense Bodies

Dense bodies are scattered throughout the cytoplasm of smooth muscle cells, and also occur as patches on the inner aspect of the plasma membrane. They are the equivalent of the Z bands of striated muscles and contain α-actinin, a protein also found in the Z bands. α-Actinin causes gelation and cross-links actin filaments *in vitro* and, therefore, probably plays a role in anchoring the thin filaments to the dense bodies. In addition to α-actinin, the plasma membrane-bound dense bodies contain another identified protein, vinculin, that is also present in other cell types (e.g., cardiac muscle). Actin filaments insert both on the "free floating" dense bodies in the cytoplasm and on the plasma membrane-bound dense bodies. When the actin filaments are labeled with the S-1 subfragment of myosin (Fig. 3), the arrowheads formed by the label point away from the (membrane-bound or cytoplasmic) dense body on which the thin

filaments insert. This polarity of actin filaments at dense bodies is analogous to that observed at the Z lines or skeletal muscle. There is some alignment of the myosin filaments into small groups of three to five, and the association of such groups with actin filaments and dense bodies on either side forms a small contractile unit (Fig. 3).

MECHANICS AND ENERGETICS

The orientation and proportion of smooth muscle, as well as the content and distribution of extracellular matrix proteins (Fig. 1) (e.g., collagen, elastic, glycoproteins, and proteoglycans) vary considerably among blood vessels and hollow viscera containing smooth muscle. These factors, in addition to the contractile and passive elastic properties of smooth muscle cells, determine the mechanical properties (e.g., the length-tension curve, the force-velocity relationship) of smooth muscle bundles and blood vessels. The passive length-tension curve of arterial smooth muscles shows significant passive tension at the optimal tissue length for maximal force development, in contrast to striated muscles that develop maximal force at a length where passive tension is absent. The length-tension curves of other smooth muscles resemble that of striated muscle, in showing a maximum active force at near-zero passive tension, but their active force-length curve is still broader than that of skeletal muscle.

Source of Energy

Smooth muscles derive a large proportion (more than 30%) of their energy requirements from aerobic glycolysis, and the balance from oxidative phosphorylation. In some smooth muscles most of the energy requirements of the membrane Na-pump are met by glycolysis.

Force

Smooth muscle, in spite of its much lower myosin content, can develop as much force/cell cross-section as skeletal muscles. As the amount of force developed is proportional to the number of cross-bridges acting in parallel, the 46% greater length of the smooth muscle myosin filaments could account for some of the extra force developed by smooth, compared to striated, muscle myosin. In addition, the actomyosin ATPase activity that reflects the cross-bridge cycling rate is much lower in smooth than in skeletal muscle. The lower rate of cross-bridge cycling would favor a larger number of cross-bridges being in the attached state at any one time during contraction. The high actin/myosin ratio of smooth muscles would also increase the probability of the attached state for a given cross-bridge. Single smooth muscle cells develop comparable force/area as bundles, suggesting that the vectorial addition of forces developed by the many individual smooth muscle cells, displaced relative to each other, is not required for the large total force/unit area.

Speed of Contraction

The maximum speed of contraction of smooth muscle, even in isolated single cells, is very slow (e.g., 10 sec to peak tension). The shortening speed is proportional to the myosin ATPase activity, which is lower in slow muscles.

Energy Usage During Force Development and Tension Maintenance

The average rate of energy usage is higher during force development than during maintenance (e.g., in the rabbit taenia coli it is about four times greater). The energy usage and force developed by, respectively, the frog sartorius at 0°C and the rabbit taenia coli at 18°C are compared in Fig. 4. The frog, even at lower T°, develops tension 50 times faster and uses 50 times as much energy. The calculated cross-bridge cycle time in smooth muscle is much slower (e.g., for Fig. 4, it is about 150 times slower when corrected for same T°). Measurements of actomyosin ATPase rates (20–30 times slower) are consistent with these calculations.

Economy of Energy Usage During Tension Maintenance

The term economy is defined as the force/cross-sectional area divided by the rate of energy utilization. Many smooth muscles must maintain contractions over long periods of time without fatiguing, e.g., the vascular wall during various modes of regulation of the circulation.

A general characteristic of smooth muscle is that it has a much greater economy of tension maintenance than skeletal muscle, e.g., the taenia has 100-fold higher economy than frog sartorius (at the same T°). A *catch-like state* occurs under some conditions in mammalian smooth muscle: This is characterized by tension maintenance without active tension development upon quick release (absence of "active state").

ELECTROPHYSIOLOGY AND ION DISTRIBUTION

Resting Membrane Potential and Na, K, and Cl Distribution

The resting membrane potential (RMP) of smooth muscle ranges between approximately −40 to −60 mV. Smooth muscles showing spontaneous, rhythmic electrical activity (e.g., portal vein, intestinal smooth muscle) generally have a less negative membrane potential. The surface membrane of smooth muscle, as of many other cells, behaves as an (imperfect) K electrode, and the RMP is largely, but not exclusively, determined by the ratio between the intracellular and extracellular K concentrations. The intracellular K^+:Na^+:Cl^- concentration ratios and the respective relative membrane permeabilities (P_K, P_{Na}, P_{Cl}) vary in different smooth muscles. The contribution of E_{Na} and E_{Cl} $\left(Na^+ \text{ and } Cl^- \text{ equilibrium potentials, e.g., } E_{Na} = \dfrac{RT}{zF} \ln \dfrac{Na_o}{Na_i}\right)$ to the RMP probably accounts for its departure from E_K. The intracellular Cl^- in smooth muscle is high, much higher than expected on the basis of passive distribution, and probably reflects operation of a large active, but electrically silent, inward Cl^- transport mechanism. The electrogenic Na^+ pump can also make a small (3–10 mV) contribution to the magnitude of the RMP, and it has been suggested

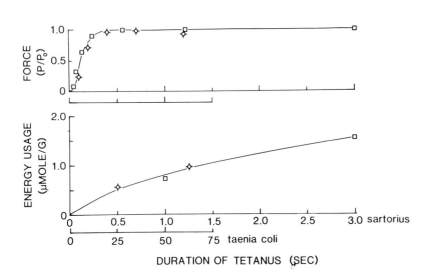

FIG. 4. Comparison of the relative rates of force development and associated energy usage under isometric conditions in the frog sartorius at 0°C and rabbit taenia coli at 18°C. Note the 50-fold difference in time scales for the two muscles: the frog develops tension 50 times faster and its rate of chemical usage is 50 times greater. *Square:* data for frog sartorius; *circle:* data for taenia coli. (From Butler, T. M., and Siegman, M. J. (1982): *Fed. Proc.*, 41:204–208.)

that this contribution is somewhat increased in vascular smooth muscle of hypertensive (SHR) rats, although the resting membrane potential is not changed.

Excitatory drugs and neurotransmitters depolarize smooth muscle, while *some* inhibitory (relaxant) drugs cause hyperpolarization. However, it is important to realize that the effects of drugs and transmitters on smooth muscle contraction and relaxation are not dependent *solely* on their effects on the RMP and/or action potential (see below). The depolarizing effect of drugs is largely due to their increasing P_{Na} and P_{Cl}. Under normal conditions the increase in membrane Ca permeability (P_{Ca}) and associated Ca current makes only a small contribution to the total depolarizing current. Excitatory drugs generally also increase the P_K directly, or through a Ca-induced increase in K-permeability. This effect causes hyperpolarization, because the RMP of most smooth muscles is less negative than the K-equilibrium potential (E_K), and so can oppose the depolarizing action of increased P_{Na} and P_{Cl}. Some of the variability in the depolarizing action of excitatory drugs in different smooth muscles is probably due to these varying, and sometimes opposing effects on P_{Na}, P_{Cl}, and P_K and to variations in intracellular Na, K, and Cl (i.e., E_{Na}, E_K, E_{Cl}) at any one time. A given neurotransmitter or drug can increase different ion permeabilities in different smooth muscles and, in some smooth muscles, drug-induced depolarization can also be caused by a *decrease* in P_K.

Smooth muscles have been classified into two general types, depending on whether they (normally) do or do not generate action potentials: (a) *Spike generating, phasic smooth muscles* (e.g., intestinal and uterine) that generate action potentials spontaneously or in response to depolarizing, excitatory stimuli; and (b) *gradedly responsive, tonic smooth muscles* (e.g., rabbit main pulmonary artery, aorta, trachealis) with a nonregenerative electrical response, similar to the end-plate potential, to excitatory agents. As implied by the above nomenclature, K-contractures of gradely responsive smooth muscles tend to be more sustained (tonic), while those of spike-generating smooth muscles tend to be more phasic. However, the rate of relaxation of K-contractures is rather sensitive to changes in extracellular Ca^{2+} and temperature, and, like all classifications, the distinction between the two types of smooth muscles is not always a sharp one.

Action Potentials

Some, though not all, smooth muscles generate action potentials spontaneously or in response to stimulation. The rate of depolarization of these action potentials ranges from 2 to 12 V/sec, and their duration is variable: In guinea pig taenia coli, the duration at half maximum

amplitude is approximately 10 to 20 msec. The action potential current may be carried by Na^+ or Ca^{2+}, in varying proportion, depending on the type of smooth muscle. For example, Na^+ seems to be the major current carrier in uterine, but Ca^{2+} in taenia coli smooth muscle. Action potentials in smooth muscle, even those for which Na^+ is the major current carrier, are resistant to tetrodotoxin. Action potentials can also be induced in smooth muscles that normally do not generate them, by agents [e.g., tetraethylammonium (TEA) or barium] that reduce P_K. The current carrier is generally Ca^{2+}, as shown by the inhibition of such action potentials by Ca^{2+}-free solutions and by Ca^{2+}-entry blocking agents.

EXCITATION-CONTRACTION COUPLING

The two major forms of excitation-contraction (E-C) coupling in smooth muscle are *electromechanical coupling and pharmacomechanical coupling*. It is important to recognize that these two mechanisms *can operate simultaneously,* and contraction stimulated by a single excitatory agent may be mediated by exclusively electromechanical (e.g., twitch evoked by an action potential), solely pharmacomechanical (e.g., drug-induced contraction of completely depolarized muscle), or by combined electromechanical and pharmacomechanical coupling (probably many drug and transmitter-induced contractions of normally polarized smooth muscles). The *primary* trigger of contraction by either mechanism of E-C coupling is a rise in cytoplasmic free Ca^{2+}, although it is probable that as our understanding of the details of smooth muscle regulation is refined, secondary mechanisms of E-C coupling, independent of Ca^{2+}, will be recognized (see Contractile Regulation section, below).

Electromechanical Coupling

Electromechanical coupling is the mechanism that influences contraction through changes in membrane potential. Depolarization and/or action potentials cause an increase in cytoplasmic free Ca^{2+} and, therefore, contraction, whereas hyperpolarization of the surface membrane (e.g., by β-adrenergic stimulation) causes relaxation through the reverse process.

The relative contributions of, respectively, extracellular and intracellular sources of activator Ca to E-C coupling, under physiological conditions, have yet to be quantitated. They probably vary with both the type of smooth muscle and the stimulus. Electromechanical coupling may utilize both sources. The Ca^{2+} current flowing through an action potential is *insufficient* to account for the amount of total activator Ca^{2+} required to cause contraction. Because of this and the persistence of spontaneous contractions in the absence of extracellular Ca^{2+} in *some* smooth muscles, it is likely that electromechanical coupling of *action potentials* involves the release of Ca from the sarcoplasmic reticulum. Large Ca influxes have been measured during prolonged depolarization with high K and/or excitatory drugs such as norepinephrine. The tonic components of some smooth muscles are also more sensitive to Ca-entry blockers and to the removal of extracellular Ca^{2+}, than are the initial "fast" components of drug-induced contractions. Therefore, it is often thought that electromechanical coupling by graded depolarization is mediated largely by the influx of extracellular Ca^{2+} through Ca channels opened by depolarization. However, the removal of extracellular Ca could also uncouple contractions by interfering with intracellular release or could simply cause an abnormal loss of intracellular Ca. Similarly, Ca-entry blockers, like all drugs, have multiple effects and some are known to enter smooth muscle. Therefore, a decisive statement regarding the extent to which, respectively, the influx of extracellular or the release of intracellular Ca^{2+} causes contraction induced by graded depolarization will have to await more detailed and quantitative studies.

Pharmacomechanical Coupling

Pharmacomechanical coupling has been defined as the stimulation of contraction or relaxation by mechanism(s) independent of changes in membrane potential. The drug-induced contractions of smooth muscles that are completely depolarized in high K solutions and, hence, cannot have their membrane potential altered by drugs, represent "pure" pharmacomechanical coupling. Drug-induced contractions without any *detectable* depolarization have sometimes been observed in normally polarized smooth muscle, and are presented as examples of exclusively pharmacomechanical coupling. Technically, this is difficult to prove conclusively, as contraction without any depolarization of smooth muscle bundles containing large groups of cells is always subject to the question whether the cells from which electrical activity is recorded are identical to the contracting ones. Theoretically, such a mechanism is certainly feasible: For example, the hyperpolarizing effect of a drug due to increased P_K could cancel out the depolarizing action of increased P_{Na} and/or P_{Cl}, without preventing pharmacomechanical Ca release or Ca influx.

The physiologically most relevant form of pharmacomechanical coupling occurs together with depolarization, when normal, polarized smooth muscles are stimulated by neurotransmitters. The relatively small (few mV) depolarizing action of the excitatory drugs under these conditions is usually insufficient to account for the magnitude of the accompanying contractions, which are much larger than contractions caused by comparable depolarization with high K or electrical current. It is

likely that, during submaximal activation, electromechanical and pharmacomechanical coupling operate simultaneously, at least in gradedly responsive smooth muscles.

The contributions of, respectively, extracellular influx or intracellular [from the sarcoplasmic reticulum (SR)] release of Ca to pharmacomechanical coupling remain to be quantitated. Because drugs can cause maximal contractions in *depolarized smooth muscles in the absence of extracellular Ca^{2+}*, it is now clear that pharmacomechanical coupling can operate through the release of Ca from the SR. The evidence supporting the contribution of Ca influx to pharmacomechanical coupling, as in the case of electromechanical coupling, is based largely on measurements of ^{45}Ca influx in drug-stimulated depolarized smooth muscle, and on the inhibitory effects of Ca^{2+}-free solutions and Ca-entry blockers.

Very recent evidence suggests that inositol 1,4,5-trisphosphate (InsP$_3$) mediates Ca release during pharmacomechanical coupling. In view of the persistence of pharmacomechanical coupling in the absence of extracellular Ca, the influx of extracellular Ca^{2+} is *not* required for the release of intracellular Ca (Ca-induced Ca release). Excitatory transmitters stimulate phosphatidylinositol turnover in the membranes of a variety of cells, and InsP$_3$, one of the metabolites produced as the result of phosphatidylinositol breakdown, is probably a second messenger that releases Ca from the endoplasmic reticulum, the intracellular Ca store of non-muscle cells. Even more recently, it has been shown with ^{45}Ca flux and Ca-selective electrode studies that InsP$_3$ also releases Ca from the sarcoplasmic reticulum of saponin-permeabilized smooth muscle (Fig. 5) (preparations in which the membranes are hyperpermeable to large molecules, such as enzymes and ATP). Furthermore, sustained contractions can be evoked in saponin-permeabilized main pulmonary artery smooth muscle (Fig. 6), and this contraction can be graded by graded concentrations of InsP$_3$. The amount of Ca released, like the amount released by norepinephrine in main pulmonary artery, appears to be sufficient to evoke a maximal contraction. In addition, stimulation of phosphatidylinositol breakdown by excitatory agents (carbamylcholine on trachealis smooth muscle) persists in smooth muscles depolarized with high K, which is consistent with the mechanism of pharmacomechanical coupling. Therefore, the evidence is highly suggestive that at least part of pharmacomechanical coupling is mediated by stimulation of phosphatidylinositol breakdown followed by InsP$_3$-induced Ca release. There is, however, no information yet about the role, if any, of InsP$_3$ on the effect of excitatory drugs on membrane permeability (i.e., Ca-influx) or on electromechanical coupling. Furthermore, in a broader sense, pharmacomechanical modulation of contraction may also occur independently of not only the membrane potential, but also of cytoplasmic free Ca^{2+}, as for

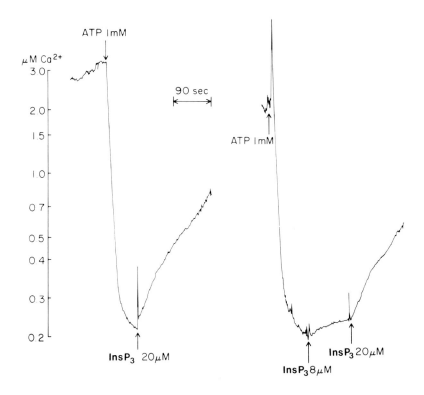

FIG. 5. Changes in free Ca^{2+} measured by a Ca^{2+}-selective electrode in a cuvet (0.5 ml volume) containing no EGTA and no added calcium solution and digitonin (0.005%, 10 min)-permeabilized strips of rabbit main pulmonary artery. Mitochondrial calcium uptake was blocked by 2 mM KCN and 0.5 nmoles oligomyocin/mg tissue. The addition of ATP produced a time-dependent decrease of $[Ca^{2+}]$ in the bathing solution. This accumulation into cellular sites was reversed by addition of $InsP_3$ which increased the $[Ca^{2+}]$ in the bathing solution. [From Somlyo, A. V., Bond, M., Somlyo, A. P., and Scarpa, A. (1985): *Proc. Natl. Acad. Sci.*, 82:5231–5235.]

example, through phosphorylation of myosin light chain kinase by the cyclic AMP-dependent protein kinase (Fig. 7) (see Contractile Regulation section, below).

Calcium Efflux

The major active Ca efflux system is via the ATP-dependent active Ca transport of the plasma membrane, mediated by a Ca^{2+}-ATPase regulated by calmodulin. Na^+-Ca^{2+} exchange that derives energy from the (inward-directed) transmembrane Na gradient may also contribute, but the magnitude of its contribution is not well defined and appears to be small under physiological conditions. The operation of an active Ca transport system is essential for the maintenance of steady-state Ca levels, given the influx of Ca under the influence of normal stimuli.

SARCOPLASMIC RETICULUM AND MITOCHONDRIA

Sarcoplasmic Reticulum

The SR is an intracellular membrane system of tubules and, in some species, flattened cisternae. It is *not* in direct communication with the extracellular space, as indicated by its exclusion of extracellular markers and its K, Na, and Cl content. The SR occupies from 1.5 to 7.5% of the cell volume in smooth muscle, compared to about 3.5% in rat and 0.5% in frog heart, and 10 to

13%, in frog skeletal muscle. The largest volumes of the SR occur in the smooth muscle of large elastic arteries (e.g., rabbit main pulmonary artery, Fig. 8) that also show the greatest persistence of contraction in the absence of extracellular calcium. The taenia coli and rabbit portal mesenteric vein, both phasic muscles, contain relatively small volumes (1.5–2.5%) of SR and lose their responsiveness more readily in Ca-free solutions. However, even this small 2% volume of SR can store sufficient calcium for activating a near maximal contraction when released. The norepinephrine-induced release of calcium from the (junctional and central) SR in vascular smooth muscle has been directly measured with electron probe X-ray microanalysis.

Regions where the tubules of SR approach the surface membrane are called surface couplings (Fig. 9). These are functionally important specializations between the SR and the plasma membrane, where a 12- to 18-nm space between the cytoplasmic leaflets of the two membrane systems is spanned by quasi-periodic bridging structures. These resemble the surface couplings of cardiac muscle and the triads in skeletal muscles. In smooth muscle, these are probably the sites where depolarization, action potentials, drugs, and transmitters release calcium stored in the junctional SR.

As in striated muscles, stored calcium has also been directly localized in the SR of smooth muscle. In smooth muscle cells in which the membranes are made hyperpermeable and exposed to 10^{-6} M calcium, the SR accumulates calcium. This calcium concentration of 10^{-6} M is in the range (probably 3×11^{-7}–5×10^{-6})

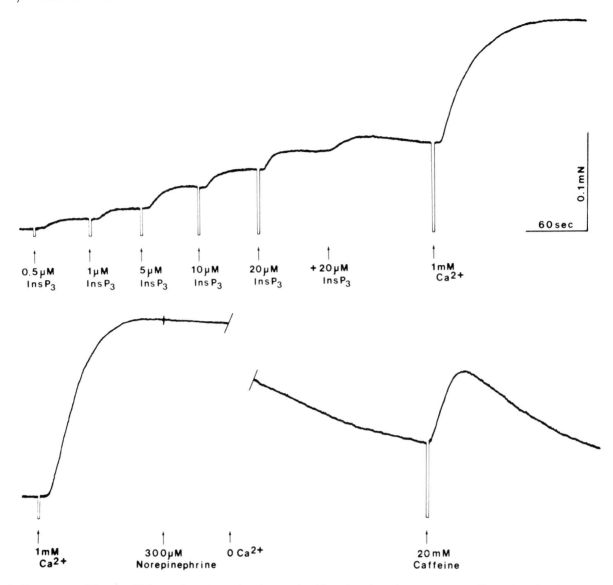

FIG. 6. Force record from a 180-μm diameter strip of saponin-skinned main pulmonary artery illustrating the dependence of force development on $InsP_3$ concentration, the maximal Ca^{2+}-dependent produced force and the size of the caffeine-releasable Ca store. The last $InsP_3$ stimulus was added topically, resulting in a much higher transient local concentration of $InsP_3$. Maximal skinning is indicated by the absence of a norepinephrine-induced contraction in the presence of 1 mM Ca^{2+}. The downward deflections represent exchanges of the bathing solution. The 0 EGTA bathing solution contains 3 μM Ca^{2+}. [From Somlyo, A. V., Bond, M., Somlyo, A. P., and Scarpa, A. (1985): *Proc. Natl. Acad. Sci.*, 82:5231–5235.]

where force is developed in smooth muscle and, therefore, the affinity of the SR for Ca is high enough to sequester Ca and so cause relaxation. Microsomal SR preparations showing energy-dependent Ca uptake have been isolated from smooth muscle, and Ca electrode studies of saponin-permeabilized smooth muscle (Fig. 5) show the operation of an ATP-dependent (non-mitochondrial) Ca-pump that is blocked by vanadate.

The release of ^{45}Ca from pre-loaded smooth muscle provides additional evidence of an intracellular store involved in activating contraction and assists in localizing this store to the SR because: (a) the amount of ^{45}Ca released and the magnitudes of contractions evoked by various stimulators are proportional; (b) neurotransmit-

ters and caffeine, an agent known to affect the SR, release Ca from the same store; (c) the effect of caffeine persists in smooth muscles in which the surface membrane is partially destroyed by saponin, but the SR is intact.

Mitochondria

The evidence is now overwhelming that the SR plays the major physiological role as the calcium storage site, and that the mitochondria accumulate Ca only when cytoplasmic Ca^{2+} is *abnormally* high. The apparent K_m of mitochondria for Ca uptake (approximately 17 μM) is higher than that of the SR, and suggests that the

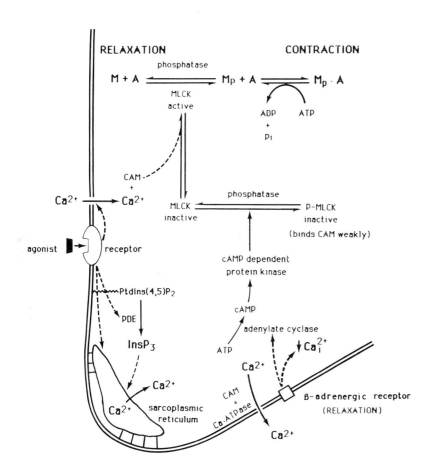

FIG. 7. Schematic representation showing the generation of intracellular signals that regulate smooth muscle contraction. Agonists stimulate a rise in intracellular Ca^{2+} through calcium release from the sarcoplasmic reticulum possibly by inositol trisphosphate ($InsP_3$), a product of agonist-stimulated hydrolysis of phosphatidylinositol 4,5 P_2 (PtdIns), by a phosphodiesertase, and by other unknown mechanisms, or by stimulated Ca^{2+} influx. Ca^{2+} binds to calmodulin that permits the binding of calmodulin to myosin light chain kinase. The active calmodulin-myosin kinase complex phosphorylates the 20,000 dalton light chain of myosin, resulting in cross-bridge cycling and contraction (M_pA). Dephosphorylation of myosin by a phosphatase promotes relaxation. β-adrenergic agents bring about relaxation by stimulating adenylate cyclase resulting in an increase intracellular cyclic AMP causing hyperpolarization, decreasing cytoplasmic calcium, and activating protein kinase by liberating a catalytic subunit that can phosphorylate myosin kinase. The phosphorylated kinase binds calmodulin much more weakly than the unphosphorylated kinase. The net effect of this sequence is to inhibit phosphorylation of myosin, thus favoring relaxation. Abbreviations: M = myosin; M_p = phosphorylated (LC_{20}) myosin; A = actin; MLCK = myosin light chain kinase; CAM = calmodulin; $InsP_3$ = inositol 1,4,5-trisphosphate.

mitochondria *cannot* efficiently accumulate Ca^{2+} in the physiological range, but become effective buffers of cell Ca when cell death is threatened by massive Ca^{2+} influx. Mitochondria do not accumulate detectable amounts of Ca even when smooth muscles are maximally contracted for 30 min. The high endogenous mitochondrial Ca content of mitochondria isolated from atherosclerotic blood vessels may reflect the effects of vascular smooth muscle damage, and such cells containing Ca-loaded mitochondria may become initial sites of vascular calcification. Smooth muscle mitochondria contain an active, bidirectional Mg-transport system.

CONTRACTILE REGULATION

The regulation of contractile proteins in smooth muscle is distinctly different from that in skeletal and cardiac muscle. Skeletal muscle actomyosin (with or without tropomyosin) has a high Mg^{2+}-ATPase activity which, in the absence of troponin, is insensitive to calcium. The addition of the regulatory protein, troponin, inhibits the Mg^{2+}-ATPase activity. Calcium acts as a de-repressor and removes the inhibitory effect of troponin. In smooth muscle, in contrast, Ca acts as a true activator of the inherently low actomyosin ATPase activity. Smooth muscle does contain tropomyosin, in the same stoichiometry to actin as in striated muscle, but does not

contain troponin. Nevertheless, activation of smooth muscle myosin Mg^{2+}-ATPase by actin (normally) requires calcium, at a concentration similar to that required to initiate contraction.

It is now generally accepted that the activation of smooth muscle actomyosin is initiated by the phosphorylation of the 20,000-dalton light chains of the myosin molecule (Fig. 7). This phosphorylation is mediated by a myosin light chain kinase (MLCK), and makes myosin activatable by actin. The activation of actomyosin ATPase activity as a result of myosin phosphorylation is not unique to smooth muscle, and occurs in several non-muscle systems, such as platelets and lymphocytes. The active MLCK is composed of two distinct proteins, the smaller of these subunits (MW 17,000) is calmodulin, has four Ca-binding sites, and is the Ca receptor of the MLCK. When cytoplasmic free Ca^{2+} rises (to about 5×10^{-7}–5×10^{-6}) and Ca is bound to three or four of the binding sites, the Ca-calmodulin complex interacts with the larger subunit to form the active MLCK. As long as cytoplasmic Ca^{2+} remains high, the phosphorylated myosin undergoes repeated cycles of actin-mediated ATP hydrolysis, as the cross-bridges cycle. When Ca^{2+} falls below threshold, the concentration of the calcium-calmodulin complex falls, and the active form of MLCK decreases. A second enzyme, a myosin light chain

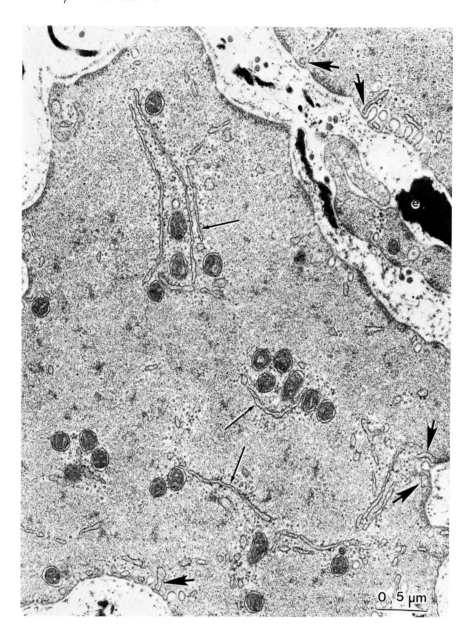

FIG. 8. Transversely sectioned smooth muscle from the rabbit main pulmonary artery, showing the centrally located sarcoplasmic reticulum (*small arrows*) as well as regions where the reticulum approaches the cell membrane and forms surface couplings (*large arrows*). Darkly stained elastin (e) is seen in the extracellular space. (From Somlyo, A. V. (1980): In: *The Handbook of Physiology: The Cardiovascular System: Vol. II. Vascular Smooth Muscle,* edited by D. F. Bohr, A. P. Somlyo, and H. V. Sparks, pp. 33–67. American Physiological Society, Bethesda.)

FIG. 9. Transverse section from rabbit portal vein showing a surface coupling of sarcoplasmic reticulum (SR) with the cell membrane. Dense periodic structures (*arrows*) are present across the 15–20 nm junctional gap between SR and the plasma membrane. (From Somlyo, A. V. 1980: In: *The Handbook of Physiology: The Cardiovascular System: Vol. II. Vascular Smooth Muscle,* edited by D. F. Bohr, A. P. Somlyo, and H. V. Sparks, pp. 33–67. American Physiological Society, Bethesda.)

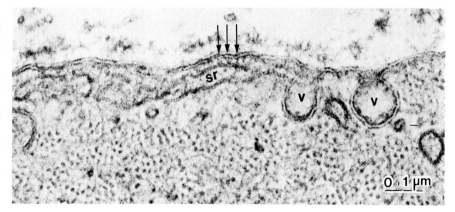

phosphatase, dephosphorylates the light chains, and the myosin returns to its inactive state and the muscle relaxes.

The following is some of the evidence supporting the above scheme of activation in smooth muscle: (a) In intact muscle, the phosphorylation of the light chains precedes and is proportional to the magnitude of activation of contraction, and a similar correlation is found between phosphorylation and ATPase activity in isolated actomyosin preparations and in intact smooth muscle (however, this correlation may not be linear); (b) phosphorylation of myosin light chains by an artificially produced, Ca-insensitive MLCK can produce contraction in the absence of Ca^{2+} in skinned smooth muscles; and (c) dephosphorylation of the myosin light chains in skinned smooth muscle by phosphatase causes relaxation.

The existence of other contractile regulatory mechanisms, in addition to myosin light chain phosphorylation, is indicated by the fact that the latter stages of (tonic) contraction of smooth muscle can be regulated by Ca, independently of light chain phosphorylation. Indeed, in some smooth muscles the proportion of phosphorylated light chains may decline to resting levels, while tension is still maintained. Proteins other than MLCK have been isolated from smooth muscle with regulatory properties, at least *in vitro*. The best characterized of these is caldesmon, a 120,000- to 150,000-dalton actin-binding protein that is released from actin by Ca-calmodulin.

Myosin light chain kinase itself has two sites that can be phosphorylated by the cyclic AMP-dependent protein kinase. The activity of MLCK declines when *both* sites are phosphorylated, and it has been suggested that phosphorylation of MLCK by the cyclic AMP-dependent protein kinase may play a role in β-adrenergic relaxation of smooth muscle (Fig. 7). Inasmuch as the cyclic AMP-dependent protein kinase can not phosphorylate the large (catalytic) subunit of MLCK when Ca-calmodulin is bound to it, it is unlikely that this mechanism plays a major role in relaxing maximally contracted smooth muscles in which the catalytic subunit is fully saturated with Ca-calmodulin. The mechanism of β-adrenergic relaxation is complex, and may include hyperpolarization of the surface membrane and stimulation of Ca-pumps.

ACKNOWLEDGMENTS

The authors research has been supported by HL15835 to the Pennsylvania Muscle Institute, and work reported from their laboratory includes studies conducted with postdoctoral associates supported by Cardiovascular Training Grant HL07499. We thank Mrs. M. Ridgell for preparation of the manuscript.

BIBLIOGRAPHY

This bibliography is intended to reflect the evolution of research on smooth muscle during the last 15 years, with an emphasis on the most recent developments, rather than providing a comprehensive bibliography. The authors regret the necessity of excluding numerous very informative publications from this list.

General

Bohr, D. F., Somlyo, A. P., and Sparks, H. V. (1980): *The Handbook of Physiology: The Cardiovascular System: Vascular Smooth Muscle, Vol. II.* American Physiology Society, Bethesda.
Bulbring, E., Brading, A. F., Jones, A. W., and Tomita, T. (1980): *Smooth Muscle: An Assessment of Current Knowledge.* Edward Arnold Press, Oxford.
Stephens, N. W. (1984): *Smooth Muscle Contraction.* Dekker, New York.

Structure

Ashton, F. T., Somlyo, A. V., and Somlyo, A. P. (1975): The contractile apparatus of vascular smooth muscle: Intermediate high voltage stereo electron microscopy. *J. Mol. Biol.,* 98:17–29.
Berner, P. F., Franck, E., Holtzer, H., and Somlyo, A. P. (1981): The intermediate filament proteins of rabbit vascular smooth muscle: Immunofluorescent studies of desmin and vimentin. *J. Muscle Res. Cell Motility,* 2:439–452.
Berner, P. F., Somlyo, A. V., and Somlyo, A. P. (1981): Hypertrophy-induced increase of intermediate filaments in vascular smooth muscle. *J. Cell Biol.,* 88:96–101.
Bond, M., and Somlyo, A. V. (1982): Dense bodies and actin polarity in vertebrate smooth muscle. *J. Cell. Biol.,* 95:403–413.
Burnstock, G. (1975): Innervation of vascular smooth muscle: histochemistry and electron microscopy. *Clin. Exp. Pharmacol. Physiol.,* 2:7–20.
Chandra, T. S., Nath, N., Suzuki, H., and Seidel, J. C. (1985): Modification of thiols of gizzard myosin alters ATPase activity, stability of myosin filaments, and the 6-10 S conformational transition. *J. Biol. Chem.,* 260:202–207.
Craig, R., and Megerman, J. (1977): Assembly of smooth muscle myosin into side-polar filaments. *J. Cell. Biol.,* 75:990–996.
Craig, R., Smith, R., and Kendrick-Jones, J. (1983): Light chain phosphorylation controls the conformation of vertebrate non-muscle and smooth muscle myosin molecules. *Nature,* 302:436–439.
Devine, C. E. (1978): Morphology and ultrastructure. In: *Microcirculation,* edited by G. Kaley, B. M. Altura, and B. W. Zweifach, pp. 3–39. University Park Press, Baltimore.
Devine, C. E., and Rayns, D. G. (1975): Freeze-fracture studies of membrane systems in vertebrate muscle. II. Smooth Muscle. *J. Ultrastruct. Res.,* 51:293–306.
Forbes, M. S. (1982): Ultrastructure of vascular smooth muscle cells in mammalian heart. In: *The Coronary Artery,* edited by S. Kalsner, pp. 3–58. Oxford University Press, New York.
Forbes, M. S., and Sperelakis, N. (1982): Bridging junctional processes in couplings of skeletal, cardiac, and smooth muscle. *Muscle and Nerve,* 5:674–681.
Gabella, G. (1979): Smooth muscle cell junctions and structural aspects of contraction. *Br. Med. Bull.,* 35:213–218.
Gabella, G. (1981): Structure of smooth muscles. In: *Smooth Muscle: An Assessment of Current Knowledge,* edited by E. Bulbring, A. F. Brading, A. W. Jones, and T. Tomita, pp. 1–46. Edward Arnold Press, Oxford.
Gabella, G. (1983): An introduction to the structural variety of smooth muscles. In: *Vascular Neuroeffector Mechanisms, 4th International Symposium,* edited by J. A. Bevan et al., pp. 13–35. Raven Press, New York.
Gabella, G. (1984): Structural apparatus for force transmission in smooth muscles. *Physiol. Rev.,* 64:455–477.
Garfield, R. E., and Somlyo, A. P. (1985): Structure of smooth muscle. In: *Calcium and Smooth Muscle Contractility,* edited by A. K. Grover and E. E. Daniel, pp. 1–36. Humana Press, Clifton, New Jersey.
Geiger, B., Dutton, A. H., Tokuyasu, T., and Singer, S. J. (1981): Immunoelectron microscope studies of membrane-microfilament inter-action: Distribution of alpha-actinin, tropomyosin, and vin-

culin in intestinal epithelial brush border and chicken gizzard smooth muscle cells. *J. Cell Biol.*, 91:614–618.

Heumann, H-G. (1976): The subcellular localization of calcium in vertebrate smooth muscle: Calcium-containing and calcium-accumulating structures in muscle cells of mouse intestine. *Cell Tissue Res.*, 169:221–231.

Ikebe, M., Barsotti, R. J., Hinkins, S., and Hartshorne, D. J. (1984): Effects of magnesium chloride on smooth muscle actomyosin adenosine-5'-triphosphatase activity, myosin conformation, and tension development in glycerinated smooth muscle fibers. *Biochemistry*, 23:5062–5068.

Komuro, T., and Burnstock, G. (1980): The fine structure of smooth muscle cells and their relationship to connective tissue in the rabbit portal vein. *Cell Tissue Res.*, 210:257–267.

Lee, R. M. K. W., Forrest, J. B., Garfield, R. E., and Daniel, E. E. (1983): Ultrastructural changes in mesenteric arteries from spontaneously hypertensive rats. *Blood Vessels*, 20:72–91.

Litwin, J. A. (1980): Cell membrane features of rabbit arterial smooth muscle. A freeze-fracture study. *Cell Tissue Res.*, 212:341–350.

Matsumura, F., and Lin, J. J.-C. (1982): Visualization of monoclonal antibody binding to tropomyosin on native smooth muscle thin filaments by electron microscopy. *J. Mol. Biol.*, 157:163–171.

Prescott, L., and Brightman, M. W. (1976): The sarcolemma of *Aplysia* smooth muscle in freeze-fracture preparations. *Tissue Cell*, 8:241–258.

Schollmeyer, J. E., Furcht, L. T., Goll, J. E., Robson, R. M., and Stromer, M. H. (1976): Localization of contractile proteins in smooth muscle cells and in normal and transformed fibroblasts. In: *Cell Motility, Vol. 3-A*, edited by R. Goldman, T. Pollard, and J. Rosenbaum, pp. 361–388. Cold Spring Harbor Laboratories, Cold Spring Harbor, New York.

Small, J. V. (1985): Geometry of actin-membrane attachments in the smooth muscle cell: the localizations of vinculin and alpha-actinin. *EMBO J.*, 4:45–50.

Small, J. V., and Sobieszek, A. (1980): The contractile apparatus of smooth muscle. *Int. Rev. Cytol.*, 64:241–306.

Somlyo, A. P., and Somlyo, A. V. (1975): Ultrastructure of smooth muscle. In: *Methods in Pharmacology, Vol. 3*, edited by E. E. Daniel and D. M. Paton, pp. 3–45. Plenum Press, New York.

Somlyo, A. P., Devine, C. E., Somlyo, A. V., and Rice, R. V. (1973): Filament organization in vertebrate smooth muscle. *Philos. Trans. R. Soc., Lond. (Biol.)*, 265:223–229.

Somlyo, A. P., Garfield, R. E., Chacko, S., and Somlyo, A. V. (1975): Golgi organelle response to the antibiotic X537A. *J. Cell Biol.*, 66:425–443.

Somlyo, A. P., Somlyo, A. V., Devine, C. E., and Rice, R. V. (1971): Aggregation of thick filaments into ribbons in mammalian smooth muscle. *Nature*, 231:243–246.

Somlyo, A. P., Somlyo, A. V., Shuman, H., Sloane, B., and Scarpa, A. (1978): Electron probe analysis of calcium compartments in cryo sections of smooth and striated muscles. *Ann. NY Acad. Sci.*, 307:523–544.

Somlyo, A. V. (1979): Bridging structures spanning the junctional gap at the triad of skeletal muscle. *J. Cell Biol.*, 80:743–750.

Somlyo, A. V. (1980): Ultrastructure of vascular smooth muscle. In: *The Handbook of Physiology: The Cardiovascular System: Vascular Muscle*, edited by D. F. Bohr, A. P. Somlyo, and H. V. Sparks, pp. 33–67. American Physiological Society, Bethesda.

Somlyo, A. V., Butler, T. M., Bond, M., and Somlyo, A. P. (1981): Myosin filaments have phosphorylated light chains in relaxed smooth muscle. *Nature*, 294:567–570.

Somlyo, A. V., and Franzini-Armstrong, C. (1985): New views of smooth muscle structure using freezing, deep-etching and rotary shadowing. *Experientia*, 41:841–856.

Somlyo, A. V., and Somlyo, A. P. (1971): Strontium accumulation by sarcoplasmic reticulum and mitochondria vascular smooth muscle. *Science*, 174:955–958.

Suzuki, H., Onishi, H., Takahashi, K., and Watanabe, S. (1978): Structure and function of chicken gizzard myosin. *J. Biochem. (Tokyo)*, 84:1529–1542.

Trybus, K. M., and Lowey, S. (1984): Conformational states of smooth muscle myosin. *J. Biol. Chem.*, 259:8564–8571.

Trybus, K. M., Huiatt, T. W., and Lowey, S. (1982): A bent monomeric conformation of myosin from smooth muscle. *Proc. Natl. Acad. Sci. USA*, 158:6151–6155.

Tsukita, S., Tsukita, S., Usukura, J., and Ishikawa, H. (1982): Myosin filaments in smooth muscle cells of the guinea pig taenia coli: a freeze-substitution study. *Eur. J. Cell Biol.*, 28:195–201.

Mechanics and Energetics

Arner, A. (1982): Energy turnover and mechanical properties of smooth muscle with observations on vascular smooth muscle structure and function in the hypertensive rat. *Acta Physiol. Scand.*, 505:1–62.

Arner, A. (1983): Force-velocity relation in chemically skinned rat portal vein. Effects of Ca^{2+} and Mg^{2+}. *Pfluegers Arch.*, 397:6–12.

Arner, A., and Hellstrand, P. (1983): Activation of contraction and ATPase activity in intact and chemically skinned smooth muscle of rat portal vein. Dependence on Ca^{++} and muscle length. *Circ. Res.*, 53:695–702.

Butler, T. M., and Davies, R. E. (1980): High-energy phosphates in smooth muscle. In: *The Handbook of Physiology: The Cardiovascular System: Vascular Smooth Muscle, Vol. II*, edited by D. F. Bohr, A. P. Somlyo, and H. V. Sparks, pp. 237–252. American Physiological Society, Bethesda.

Butler, T. M., and Siegman, M. J. (1983): Chemical energy usage and myosin light chain phosphorylation in mammalian smooth muscle. *Fed. Proc.*, 42:57–61.

Butler, T. M., Siegman, M. J., and Mooers, S. U. (1983): Chemical energy usage during shortening and work production in mammalian smooth muscle. *Am. J. Physiol.*, 244:C234–C242.

Butler, T. M., Siegman, M. J., and Mooers, S. U. (1984): Chemical energy usage during stimulation and stretch of mammalian smooth muscle. *Pfluegers Arch.*, 401:391–395.

Chapman, J. B., Gibbs, C. L., and Loiselle, D. S. (1982): Myothermic, polarographic, and fluorometric data from mammalian muscles. Correlations and an approach to a biochemical synthesis. *Fed. Proc.*, 41:176–184.

Cox, R. H. (1979): Contribution of smooth muscle to arterial wall mechanics. *Basic Res. Cardiol.*, 74:1–9.

Davey, D. F., Gibbs, C. L., and McKirdy, H. C. (1975): Structural, mechanical and myothermic properties of rabbit rectococcygeus muscle. *J. Physiol. (Lond.)*, 248:207–230.

Dobrin, P. B. (1978): Mechanical properties of arteries. *Physiol. Rev.*, 58:397–460.

Driska, S. P., Damon, D. N., and Murphy, R. A. (1978): Estimates of cellular mechanics in an arterial smooth muscle. *Biophys. J.*, 24:525–540.

Gabella, G. (1976): The force generated by a visceral smooth muscle. *J. Physiol. (Lond.)*, 263:199–213.

Gibbs, C. L., and Loiselle, D. S. (1980): Effect of temperature on mechanical and myothermic properties of rabbit smooth muscle. *Am. J. Physiol.*, 238:C49–C55.

Greven, K., Rudolph, K. H., and Hohorst, B. (1976): Creep after loading in the relaxed and contracted smooth muscle (*Taenia coli* of the guinea pig) under various osmotic conditions. *Pfluegers Arch.*, 362:255–260.

Halpern, W., Mulvany, M. J., and Warshaw, D. M. (1978): Mechanical properties of smooth muscle cells in the walls of arterial resistance vessels. *J. Physiol. (Lond.)*, 275:85–101.

Hellstrand, P., and Paul, R. J. (1983): Phosphagen content, breakdown during contraction, and O_2 consumption in rat portal vein. *Am. J. Physiol.*, 244:C250–C258.

Herlihy, J. T., and Murphy, R. A. (1973): Length-tension relationship of smooth muscle of the hog carotid artery. *Circ. Res.*, 33:275–283.

Iyengar, M. R., Fluellen, C. E., and Iyengar, C. L. (1982): Creatine kinase from the bovine myometrium: purification and characterization. *J. Muscle Res. Cell Motility*, 3:231–244.

Krisanda, J. M., and Paul, R. J. (1984): Energetics of isometric contraction in porcine carotid artery. *Am. J. Physiol.*, 246:C510–C519.

Meiss, R. A. (1982): Transient responses and continuous behavior of active smooth muscle during controlled stretches. *Am. J. Physiol.*, 242:C146–C158.

Meiss, R. A. (1984): Nonlinear force response of active smooth muscle subjected to small stretches. *Am. J. Physiol.*, 246:C114–C124.

Mooers, S. U., Butler, T. M., Davies, R. E., and Siegman, M. J. (1980): Chemical energetics of force development, force mainte-nance, and relaxation in mammalian smooth muscle. *J. Gen. Physiol.,* 76:609–629.

Mulvany, M. J., and Halpern, W. (1977): Contractile properties of small arterial resistance vessels in spontaneously hypertensive and normotensive rats. *Circ. Res.,* 41:19–26.

Mulvany, M. J., and Warshaw, D. M. (1979): The active tension-length curve of vascular smooth muscle related to its cellular components. *J. Gen. Physiol.,* 74:85–104.

Murphy, R. A. (1976): Contractile system function in mammalian smooth muscle. *Blood Vessels,* 13:1–23.

Paul, R. J. (1981): Smooth muscle: Mechanochemical energy conversion relations between metabolism and contractility. In: *Physiology of the Gastrointestinal Tracts,* edited by L. R. Johnson, pp. 269–288. Raven Press, New York.

Paul, R. J., Doerman, G., Zeugner, C., and Ruegg, J. C. (1983): The dependence of unloaded shortening velocity on Ca^{++}, calmodulin, and duration of contraction in "chemically skinned" smooth muscle. *Circ. Res.,* 53:342–351.

Peterson, J. W. (1982): Effect of histamine on the energy metabolism of K^+-depolarized hog carotid artery. *Circ. Res.,* 50:848–855.

Peterson, J. W., and Gluck, E. (1982): Energy cost of membrane depolarization in hog carotid artery. *Circ. Res.,* 50:839–847.

Pfitzer, G., Peterson, J. W., and Ruegg, J. C. (1982): Length dependence of calcium activated isometric force and immediate stiffness in living and glycerol extracted vascular smooth muscle. *Pfluegers Arch.,* 394:174–181.

Rosenfeld, S. S., and Taylor, E. W. (1984): The ATPase mechanism of skeletal and smooth muscle acto-subfragment. *J. Biol. Chem.,* 259:11908–11919.

Ruegg, J. C. (1971): Smooth muscle tone. *Physiol. Rev.,* 51:201–248.

Speden, R. N. (1984): Active reactions of the rabbit ear artery to distension. *J. Physiol. (Lond.),* 351:631–643.

Siegman, M. J. (1983): Chemical energy usage during shortening and work production in mammalian smooth muscle. *Am. J. Physiol.,* 244:C234–C242.

Siegman, M. J., Butler, T. M., Mooers, S. U., and Davies, R. E. (1976): Calcium-dependent resistance to stretch and stress relaxation in resting smooth muscles. *Am. J. Physiol.,* 231:1501–1508.

Siegman, M. J., Butler, T. M., Mooers, S. U., and Michalek, A. (1984): Ca^{2+} can affect V_{max} without changes in myosin light chain phosphorylation in smooth muscle. *Pfluegers Arch.,* 401:385–390.

Somlyo, A. V., and Somlyo, A. P. (1967): Active state and catch-like state in rabbit main pulmonary artery. *J. Gen. Physiol.,* 50:168–169.

Stephens, N. L., Cardinal, R., and Simmons, B. (1977): Mechanical properties of tracheal smooth muscle: effects of temperature. *Am. J. Physiol.,* 233:C92–C98.

Uvelius, B. (1976): Isometric and isotonic length-tension relations and variations in cell length in longitudinal smooth muscle from rabbit urinary bladder. *Acta Physiol. Scand.,* 97:1–12.

Vermue, N. A., and Nicolay, K. (1983): Energetics of smooth muscle taenia caecum of guinea-pig: a ^{31}P-NMR study. *FEBS Lett.,* 156:293–297.

Warshaw, D. M., and Fay, F. S. (1983): Cross-bridge elasticity in single smooth muscle cells. *J. Gen. Physiol.,* 82:157–199.

Warshaw, D. M., and Fay, F. S. (1983): Tension transients in single isolated smooth muscle cells. *Science,* 219:1438–1441.

Electrophysiology and Ion Distribution

Aaronson, P., and van Breemen, C. (1981): Effects of sodium gradient manipulation upon cellular calcium, ^{45}Ca fluxes and cellular sodium in the guinea-pig taenia coli. *J. Physiol. (Lond.),* 319:443–461.

Aickin, C. C., and Brading, A. F. (1983): Towards an estimate of chloride permeability in the smooth muscle of guinea-pig vas deferens. *J. Physiol. (Lond.),* 336:179–197.

Aickin, C. C., Brading, A. F., and Burdyga, Th. V. (1984): Evidence for sodium-calcium exchange in the guinea-pig ureter. *J. Physiol. (Lond.),* 347:411–430.

Anderson, N. C., Ramon, F., and Snyder, A. (1971): Studies on

calcium and sodium in uterine smooth muscle excitation under current-clamp and voltage-clamp conditions. *J. Gen. Physiol.,* 58:322–339.

Benham, C. D., and Bolton, T. B. (1983): Patch-clamp studies of slow potential-sensitive potassium channels in longitudinal smooth muscle cells of rabbit jejunum. *J. Physiol. (Lond.),* 340:469–486.

Brading, A. F. (1975): Sodium/sodium exchange in the smooth muscle of the guinea-pig taenia coli. *J. Physiol. (Lond.),* 251:79–105.

Casteels, R. (1971): The distribution of chloride ions in the smooth muscle cells of the guinea-pig's taenia coli. *J. Physiol. (Lond.),* 214:225–243.

Casteels, R., Droogmans, G., and Hendrickx, H. (1971): Membrane potential of smooth muscle cells in K-free solution. *J. Physiol. (Lond.),* 217:281–295.

Casteels, R., and Suzuki, H. (1980): The effect of histamine on the smooth muscle cells of the ear artery of the rabbit. *Pfluegers Arch.,* 387:17–25.

Cole, W. C., Garfield, R. E., and Kirkaldy, J. S. (1985): Gap junctions and direct intercellular communication between rat uterine smooth muscle cells. *Am. J. Physiol.,* 249:C20–C31.

Daniel, E. E., and Sarna, S. (1978): The generation and conduction of activity in smooth muscle. *Annu. Rev. Pharmacol. Toxicol.,* 18:145–166.

Den Hertog, A. (1981): Calcium and the α-action of catecholamines on guinea-pig taenia caeci. *J. Physiol. (Lond.),* 316:109–125.

Farley, J. M., and Miles, P. R. (1977): Role of depolarization in acetylcholine-induced contractions of dog trachealis muscle. *J. Pharmacol. Exp. Ther.,* 201:199–205.

Ferrero, J. D., and Frischknecht, R. (1983): Different effector mecha-nisms for ATP and adenosine hyperpolarization in the guinea-pig taenia coli. *Eur. J. Pharmacol.,* 87:151–154.

Golenhofen, K., and Hermstein, N. (1975): Differentiation of calcium activation mechanisms in vascular smooth muscle by selective suppression with verapamil and D 600. *Blood Vessels,* 12:21–37.

Haeusler, G. (1983): Contraction, membrane potential, and calcium fluxes in rabbit pulmonary arterial muscle. *Fed. Proc.* 42:263–268.

Haeusler, G., and Thorens, S. (1980): Effects of tetraethylammonium chloride on contractile, membrane and cable properties of rabbit artery muscle. *J. Physiol. (Lond.),* 303:203–224.

Hamon, G., and Worcel, M. (1979): Electrophysiological study of the action of angiotensin II on the rat myometrium. *Circ. Res.,* 45:234–243.

Harder, D. R. (1980): Comparison of electrical properties of middle cerebral and mesenteric artery in cat. *Am. J. Physiol.,* 239:C23–C26.

Harder, D. R. (1980): Membrane electrical effects of histamine on vascular smooth muscle of canine coronary artery. *Circ. Res.,* 46:372–277.

Hermsmeyer, K. (1976): Electrogenesis of increased norepinephrine sensitivity of arterial vascular muscle in hypertension. *Circ. Res.,* 38:362–367.

Hermsmeyer, K. (1981): Membrane potential mechanisms in experi-mental hypertension. In: *New Trends in Arterial Hypertension, INSERM Symposium No. 17,* edited by M. Worcel et al., pp. 175–187. Elsevier/North-Holland, Amsterdam.

Hirst, G. D. S. (1977): Neuromuscular transmission in arterioles of guinea-pig submucosa. *J. Physiol. (Lond.),* 273:263–275.

Hirst, G. D. S., and Neild, T. O. (1980): Some properties of spontaneous excitatory junction potentials recorded from arterioles of guinea-pigs. *J. Physiol. (Lond.),* 303:43–60.

Hirst, G. D. S., and van Helden, D. F. (1982): Ionic basis of the resting potential of submucosal arterioles in the ileum of the guinea-pig. *J. Physiol. (Lond.),* 333:53–67.

Johansson, B. (1971): Electromechanical and mechanoelectrical coupling in vascular smooth muscle. *Angiologica,* 8:129–143.

Jones, A. W. (1980): Content and fluxes of electrolytes. In: *The Handbook of Physiology, The Cardiovascular System. Vol. II: Vascular Smooth Muscle,* edited by D. F. Bohr, A. P. Somlyo, and H. V. Sparks, pp. 253–300. American Physiological Society, Bethesda.

Jones, A. W., and Miller, L. A. (1978): Ion transport in tonic and phasic vascular smooth muscle and changes during deoxycortico-sterone hypertension. *Blood Vessels,* 15:83–92.

Kajiwara, M., and Casteels, R. (1983): Effects of Ca-antagonists on neuromuscular transmission in the rabbit ear artery. *Pfluegers Arch.*, 396:1–7.

Kao, C. Y., and McCullough, J. R. (1975): Ionic currents in the uterine smooth muscle. *J. Physiol. (Lond.)*, 246:1–36.

Kitamura, K., and Kuriyama, H. (1979): Effects of acetylcholine on the smooth muscle cell of isolated main coronary artery of the guinea-pig. *J. Physiol. (Lond.)*, 293:119–133.

Kuriyama, H., and Suzuki, H. (1978): Electrical property and chemical sensitivity of vascular smooth muscles in normotensive and spontaneously hypertensive rats. *J. Physiol. (Lond.)*, 285:409–424.

Kuriyama, H., Ito, Y., Suzuki, H., Kitamura, K., and Itoh, T. (1982): Factors modifying contraction-relaxation cycle in vascular smooth muscles. *Am. J. Physiol.*, 243:H641–662.

Ljung, B., Isaksson, O., and Johansson, B. (1975): Levels of cyclic AMP and electrical events during inhibition of contractile activity in vascular smooth muscle. *Acta Physiol. Scand.*, 94:154–166.

Lombard, J. H., Willems, W. J., and Stekiel, W. J. (1984): Role of vascular smooth muscle transmembrane potential in control of the microcirculation. *Microcirc. Endothel. Lymphat.*, 1:25–55.

Marshall, J. M. (1977): Modulation of smooth muscle activity by catecholamines. *Fed. Proc.*, 36:2450–2455.

Mironneau, J. (1976): Effects of oxytocin on ionic currents underlying rhythmic activity and contraction in uterine smooth muscle. *Pfluegers Arch.*, 363:113–118.

Mironneau, J., and Savineau, J.-P. (1980): Effects of calcium ions on outward membrane currents in rat uterine smooth muscle. *J. Physiol. (Lond.)*, 302:411–425.

Morgan, K. G. (1983): Comparison of membrane electrical activity of cat gastric submucosal arterioles and venules. *J. Physiol. (Lond.)*, 345:135–147.

Morgan, K. G. (1983): Electrophysiological differentiation of α-receptors on arteriolar smooth muscle. *Am. J. Physiol.*, 244:H540–H545.

Mulvany, M. J., Nilsson, H., and Flatman, J. A. (1982): Role of membrane potential in the response of rat small mesenteric arteries to exogenous noradrenaline stimulation. *J. Physiol. (Lond.)*, 332:363–373.

Osa, T., and Ogasawara, T. (1979): Influence of magnesium on the β-inhibition of catecholamines in the uterine circular muscle of estrogen-treated rats. *Jpn. J. Physiol.*, 29:339–352.

Prehn, J. L., and Bevan, J. A. (1983): Facial vein of the rabbit. Intracellularly recorded hyperpolarization of smooth muscle cells induced by β-adrenergic receptor stimulation. *Circ. Res.*, 52:465–470.

Prosser, C. L., and Mangel, A. W. (1982): Mechanisms of spike and slow wave pacemaker activity in smooth muscle cells. In: *Cellular Pacemakers. Mechanisms of Pacemaker Generation, Vol. 1*, edited by D. O. Carpenter, pp. 273–301. Wiley, New York.

Purves, R. D. (1974): Muscarinic excitation: A microelectrophoretic study on cultured smooth muscle cells. *Br. J. Pharmacol.*, 52:77–86.

Shuba, M. F. (1980): Smooth muscle of the ureter: the nature of excitation and the mechanisms of action of catecholamines and histamine. In: *Smooth Muscle: An Assessment of Current Knowledge*, edited by E. Bulbring, A. F. Brading, A. W. Jones, and T. Tomita, pp. 377–384. Edward Arnold Press, Oxford.

Shuba, M. F., and Vladimirova, I. A. (1980): Action of apamin on nerve-muscle transmission and the effects of ATP and noradrenaline in smooth muscles. In: *Advances in the Physiological Sciences Molecular and Cellular Aspects of Muscle Function, Vol. 5*, edited by E. Varga, A. Kover, T. Kovacs, and L. Kovacs, pp. 111–126. Pergamon Press, New York.

Sims, S. M., Daniel, E. E., and Garfield, R. E. (1982): Improved electrical coupling in uterine smooth muscle is associated with increased numbers of gap junctions at parturition. *J. Gen. Physiol.*, 80:353–375.

Sperelakis, N. (1982): Electrophysiology of vascular smooth muscle of coronary artery. In: *The Coronary Artery*, edited by S. Kalsner, pp. 118–167. Oxford University Press, New York.

Suzuki, H. (1981): Effects of endogenous and exogenous noradrenaline on the smooth muscle of guinea-pig mesenteric vein. *J. Physiol. (Lond.)*, 321:495–512.

Suzuki, H., and Twarog, B. M. (1982): Membrane properties of smooth muscle cells in pulmonary arteries of the rat. *Am. J. Physiol.*, 242: H900–H906.

Trapani, A., Matsuki, N., Abel, P. W., and Hermsmeyer, K. (1981):

Norepinephrine produces tension through electromechanical coupling in rabbit ear artery. *Eur. J. Pharmacol.*, 72:87–91.

Walsh, J. V., and Singer, J. J. (1981): Voltage clamp of single freshly dissociated smooth muscle cells: Current-voltage relationships for three currents. *Pfluegers Arch.*, 390:207–210.

Excitation-Contraction Coupling: Electrophysiology and Structural Aspects

Aalkjaer, C., and Mulvany, M. J. (1983): Sodium metabolism in rat resistance vessels. *J. Physiol. (Lond.)*, 343:105–116.

Aaronson, P., and van Breemen, C. (1981): Effects of sodium gradient manipulation upon cellular calcium, ^{45}Ca fluxes and cellular sodium in the guinea-pig taenia coli. *J. Physiol. (Lond.)*, 319:443–461.

Aickin, C. C., Brading, A. F., and Burdyga, T. V. (1984): Evidence for sodium-calcium exchange in the guinea-pig ureter. *J. Physiol. (Lond.)*, 347:411–430.

Baron, C. B., Cunningham, M., Strauss, J. F., and Coburn, R. F. (1984): Pharmacomechanical coupling in smooth muscle may involve phosphatidylinositol metabolism. *Proc. Natl. Acad. Sci. USA*, 81:6899–6903.

Berridge, M. J., and Irvine, R. F. (1984): Inositol trisphosphate, a novel second messenger in cellular signal transduction. *Nature*, 312:315–321.

Blaustein, M. P. (1977): Sodium ions, calcium ions, blood pressure regulation, and hypertension: a reassessment and a hypothesis. *Am. J. Physiol.*, 232:C165–C173.

Bolton, T. B. (1979): Mechanisms of action of transmitters and other substances on smooth muscle. *Physiol. Rev.*, 59:607–718.

Bond, M., Kitazawa, T., Somlyo, A. P., and Somlyo, A. V. (1984): Release and recycling of calcium by the sarcoplasmic reticulum in guinea pig portal vein smooth muscle. *J. Physiol. (Lond.)*, 355: 677–695.

Brading, A. (1981): Ionic distribution and mechanisms of transmembran ion movements in smooth muscle. In: *Smooth Muscle: An Assessment of Current Knowledge*, edited by E. Bulbring, A. F. Brading, A. W. Jones, and T. Tomita, pp. 93–104. University of Texas Press, Austin.

Brading, A. F., Burnett, M., and Sneddon, P. (1980): The effect of sodium removal on the contractile responses of the guinea-pig taenia coli to carbachol. *J. Physiol. (Lond.)*, 306:411–429.

Bulbring, E. (1955): Correlation between membrane potential, spike discharge and tension in smooth muscle. *J. Physiol. (Lond.)*, 128: 200–221.

Bulbring, E., and Szurszewski, J. H. (1974): The stimulant action of noradrenaline (α-action) on guinea-pig myometrium compared with that of acetylcholine. *Proc. R. Soc. Lond. (Biol.)*, 185:225–262.

Casteels, R. (1980): Electro- and pharmacomechanical coupling in vascular smooth muscle. *Chest*, 78:150–156.

Casteels, R., and Droogmans, G. (1981): Exchange characteristics of the noradrenaline-sensitive calcium store in vascular smooth muscle cells of rabbit ear artery. *J. Physiol. (Lond.)*, 317:263–279.

Casteels, R., and Raeymaekers, L. (1979): The action of acetylcholine and catecholamines on an intracellular calcium store in the smooth muscle cells of the guinea-pig taenia coli. *J. Physiol.*, 294: 51–68.

Coburn, R. (1977): The airway smooth muscle cell. *Fed. Proc.*, 36: 2692–2697.

Deth, R., and Casteels, R. (1977): A study of releasable Ca fractions in smooth muscle cells of the rabbit aorta. *J. Gen. Physiol.*, 69: 401–416.

Deth, R. C., and Lynch, C. J. (1981): Mobilization of a common source of smooth muscle Ca^{2+} by norepinephrine and methylxanthines. *Am. J. Physiol.*, 240:C239–C247.

Deth, R., and van Breemen, C. (1974): Relative contributions of Ca^{2+} influx and cellular Ca^{2+} release during drug induced activation of the rabbit aorta. *Pfluegers Arch.*, 348:13–22.

Deth, R., and van Breemen, C. (1977): Agonist induced release of intracellular Ca^{2+} in the rabbit aorta. *J. Membrane Biol.*, 30:363–380.

Devine, C. E., Somlyo, A. V., and Somlyo, A. P. (1972): Sarcoplasmic reticulum and excitation-contraction coupling in mammalian smooth muscle. *J. Cell Biol.*, 52:690–718.

Droogmans, G., Raeymaekers, L., and Casteels, R. (1977): Electro- and pharmacomechanical coupling in the smooth muscle cells of the rabbit ear artery. *J. Gen. Physiol.*, 70:129–148.

Endo, M., Yagi, S., and Iino, M. (1982): Tension-pCa relation and sarcoplasmic reticulum responses in chemically skinned smooth muscle fibers. *Fed. Proc.*, 41:2245–2250.

Evans, D. H. L., Schild, H. O., and Thesleff, S. (1958): Effects of drugs on depolarized plain muscle. *J. Physiol. (Lond.)*, 143:474–485.

Fay, F. S., Shlevin, H. H., Granger, W. C., and Taylor, S. R. (1979): Aequorin luminescence during activation of single isolated smooth muscle cells. *Nature*, 280:506–508.

Fleckenstein, A. (1983): *Calcium Antagonism in Heart and Smooth Muscle. Experimental Facts and Therapeutic Prospects.* Wiley, New York.

Forbes, M. S., Rnnels, M. L., and Nelson, E. (1979): Caveolar systems and sarcoplasmic reticulum in coronary smooth muscle cells of the mouse. *J. Ultrastruct. Res.*, 67:325–339.

Haeusler, G. (1972): Differential effect of verapamil on excitation-contraction coupling in smooth muscle and on excitation-secretion coupling in adrenergic nerve terminals. *J. Pharmacol. Exp. Ther.*, 180:672–682.

Hellstrand, P., and Arner, A. (1980): Contraction of the rat portal vein in hypertonic and isotonic medium: mechanical properties and effects of Mg^{2+}. *Acta Physiol. Scand.*, 110:59–67.

Hermsmeyer, K., Trapani, A., and Abel, P. W. (1981): Membrane potential-dependent tension in vascular smooth muscle. In: *Vasodilatation*, edited by P. M. Vanhoutte and I. Leusen, pp. 273–284. Raven Press, New York.

Ito, Y., Kitamura, K., and Kuriyama, H. (1979): Effects of acetylcholine and catecholamines on the smooth muscle cells of the procine coronary artery. *J. Physiol.*, 294:595–611.

Itoh, T., Kajiwara, M., Kitamura, K., and Kuriyama, H. (1982): Roles of stored calcium on the mechanical response evoked in smooth muscle cells of the porcine coronary artery. *J. Physiol. (Lond.)*, 322:107–125.

Itoh, T., Kuriyama, H., and Suzuki, H. (1983): Differences and similarities in the noradrenaline- and caffeine-induced mechanical responses in the rabbit mesenteric artery. *J. Physiol. (Lond.)*, 337:609–629.

Johansson, B. (1981): Vascular smooth muscle reactivity. *Annu. Rev. Physiol.*, 43:359–370.

Johansson, B., and Somlyo, A. P. (1980): Electrophysiology and excitation-contraction coupling. In: *The Handbook of Physiology. The Cardiovascular System, Vascular Smooth Muscle, Vol. II*, edited by D. F. Bohr, A. P. Somlyo, and H. V. Sparks, pp. 301–324. American Physiological Society, Bethesda.

Jones, A. (1980): Content and fluxes of electrolytes. In: *The Handbook of Physiology. Cardiovascular System, Vascular Smooth Muscle, Vol. II*, edited by D. F. Bohr, A. P. Somlyo, and H. V. Sparks, pp. 301–324. American Physiological Society, Bethesda.

Jones, A. W., and Miller, L. A. (1978): Ion transport in tonic and phasic vascular smooth muscle and changes during deoxycorticosterone hypertension. *Blood Vessels*, 15:83–92.

Jones, A. W., Somlyo, A. P., and Somlyo, A. V. (1973): Potassium accumulation in smooth muscle and associated ultrastructural changes. *J. Physiol. (Lond.)*, 232:247–273.

Kao, C. W., and Nishiyama, A. (1969): Ion concentrations and membrane potentials of myometrium during recovery from cold. *Am. J. Physiol.*, 217:525–531.

Kowarski, D., Shuman, H., Somlyo, A. P., and Somlyo, A. V. (1985): Calcium release by norepinephrine from central sarcoplasmic reticulum in rabbit main pulmonary artery smooth muscle. *J. Physiol. (Lond.)*, 366.

Kuriyama, H. (1981): Excitation-contraction coupling in various visceral smooth muscles. In: *Smooth Muscle: An Assessment of Current Knowledge*, edited by E. Bulbring, A. F. Brading, A. W. Jones, and T. Tomita, pp. 171–198. University of Texas Press, Austin.

Kyozuka, M. (1983): Contraction of rat uterine smooth muscle in Ca-free high K solution. *Biomed. Res.*, 4:523–532.

Leijten, P. A. A., and van Breemen, C. (1984): The effects of caffeine on the noradrenaline-sensitive calcium store in rabbit aorta. *J. Physiol.*, 357:327–339.

Mangel, A. W., Nelson, D. O., Rabovsky, J. L., Prosser, C. L., and

Connor, J. A. (1982): Depolarization-induced contractile activity of smooth muscle in calcium-free solution. *Am. J. Physiol.*, 242:C36–C40.

Morgan, J. P., and Morgan, K. G. (1984): Stimulus-specific patterns of intracellular calcium levels in smooth muscle of ferret portal vein. *J. Physiol.*, 351:155–167.

Mulvany, M. J., Aalkjaer, C., and Petersen, T. T. (1984): Intracellular sodium, membrane potential, and contractility of rat mesenteric small arteries. *Circ. Res.*, 54:740–749.

Popescu, L. M., and Diculescu, I. (1975): Calcium in smooth muscle sarcoplasmic reticulum in situ: Conventional and X-ray analytical electron microscopy. *J. Cell Biol.*, 67:911–918.

Sinback, C. N., and Shain, W. (1980): Chemosensitivity of single smooth muscle cells to acetylcholine, noradrenaline, and histamine in vitro. *J. Cell. Physiol.*, 102:99–112.

Sitrin, M. D., and Bohr, D. F. (1971): Ca and Na interaction in vascular smooth muscle contraction. *Am. J. Physiol.*, 220:1124–1128.

Somlyo, A. P. (1984): Cellular site of calcium regulation. *Nature*, 309:516–517.

Somlyo, A. P. (1985): Excitation-contraction coupling and the ultra-structure of smooth muscle. *Circ. Res.*, 57:497–507.

Somlyo, A. P., and Somlyo, A. V. (1970): Vascular smooth muscle: II. Pharmacology of normal and hypertensive vessels. *Pharmacol. Rev.*, 22:249–353.

Somlyo, A. P., and Somlyo, A. V. (1971): Electrophysiological correlates of the inequality of maximal vascular smooth muscle contraction elicited by drugs. In: *Vascular Neuroeffector Systems*, edited by J. A. Bevan, R. F. Furchgott, and A. P. Somlyo, pp. 216–226. Karger, Basel.

Somlyo, A. P., and Somlyo, A. V. (1981): Effects and subcellular distribution of magnesium in smooth and striated muscle. *Fed. Proc.*, 40:2667–2671.

Somlyo, A. P., Devine, C. E., Somlyo, A. V., and North, S. R. (1971): Sarcoplasmic reticulum and the temperature-dependent contraction in vitro. *J. Cell. Physiol.*, 102:99–112.

Somlyo, A. P., Somlyo, A. V., and Shuman, H. (1979): Electron probe analysis of vascular smooth muscle: Composition of mitochondria, nuclei and cytoplasm. *J. Cell Biol.*, 81:316–335.

Somlyo, A. P., Somlyo, A. V., and Smiesko, V. (1972): Cyclic AMP and vascular smooth muscle. In: *Advances in Cyclic Nucleotide Research: Vol. 1*, edited by R. Paoletti, and G. A. Robinson, pp. 175–194. Raven Press, New York.

Somlyo, A. P., Somlyo, A. V., Shuman, H., and Endo, M. (1982): Calcium and monovalent ions in smooth muscle. *Fed. Proc.*, 41:2883–2890.

Somlyo, A. V., and Somlyo, A. P. (1968): Electromechanical and pharmacomechanical coupling in vascular smooth muscle. *J. Pharmacol. Exp. Ther.*, 159:129–145.

Somlyo, A. V., Bond, M., Somlyo, A. P., and Scarpa, A. (1985): Inositol-trisphosphate (InsP3) induced calcium release and contraction in vascular smooth muscle. *Proc. Natl. Acad. Sci. USA* 82:5231–5235.

Somlyo, A. V., Haeusler, G., and Somlyo, A. P. (1970): Cyclic adenosine-monophosphate: Potassium-dependent action on vascular smooth muscle membrane potential. *Science*, 169:490–491.

Somlyo, A. V., Shuman, H., and Somlyo, A. P. (1977): Elemental distributions in striated muscle and effects of hypertonicity: Electron probe analysis of cryo sections. *J. Cell Biol.*, 74:828–857.

Somlyo, A. V., Vinall, P., and Somlyo, A. P. (1969): Excitation-contraction coupling and electrical events in two types of vascular smooth muscle. *Microvasc. Res.*, 1:354–373.

Suematsu, E., Hirata, M., Hashimoto, T., and Kuriyama, H. (1984): Inositol 1,4,5-trisphosphate releases Ca^{2+} from intracellular store sites in skinned single cells of porcine coronary artery. *Biochem. Biophys. Res. Commun.*, 120:481–485.

Surprenant, A., Neild, T. O., and Holman, M. E. (1983): Effects of nifedipine on nerve-evoked action potentials and consequent contractions in rat tail artery. *Pfluegers Arch.*, 396:342–349.

Trapani, A., Matsuki, N., Abel, P. W., and Hermsmeyer, K. (1981): Norepinephrine produces tension through electromechanical coupling in rabbit ear artery. *Eur. J. Pharmacol.*, 72:87–91.

van Breemen, C., Aaronson, P., and Loutzenhiser, R. (1979): Sodium-calcium interactions in mammalian smooth muscle. *Pharmacol. Rev.*, 30:167–208.

Van Eldere, J., Raeymaekers, L., and Casteels, R. (1982): Effect of isoprenaline on intracellular Ca uptake and on Ca influx in arterial smooth muscle. *Pfluegers Arch.*, 395:81–83.

Isolated Membranes and Organelles

Akerman, K. E. O., and Wikstrom, M. K. F. (1979): (Ca^{2+} + Mg^{2+})-stimulated ATPase activity of rabbit myometrium plasma membrane is blocked by oxytocin. *FEBS Lett.*, 97:283–285.

De Schutter, G., Wuytack, F., Verbist, J., and Casteels, R. (1984): Tissue levels and purification by affinity chromatography of the calmodulin-stimulated Ca^{2+}-transport ATPase in pig antrum smooth muscle. *Biochim. Biophys. Acta*, 773:1–10.

Chiesi, M., Gasser, J., and Carafoli, E. (1984): Properties of the Ca-pumping ATPase of sarcoplasmic reticulum from vascular smooth muscle. *Biochem. Biophys. Res. Commun.*, 124:797–806.

Grover, A. K., Kwan, C.-Y., Luchowski, E., Daniel, E. E., and Triggle, D. J. (1984): Subcellular distribution of [^{3}H]Nitrendipine binding in smooth muscle. *J. Biol. Chem.*, 259:2223–2226.

Moore, L., Hurwitz, L., Davenport, G. R., and Landon, E. J. (1975): Energy-dependent calcium uptake activity of microsomes from the aorta of normal and hypertensive rats. *Biochim. Biophys. Acta*, 413:432–443.

Morel, N., Wibo, M., and Godfraind, T. (1981): A calmodulin-stimulated Ca^{2+} pump in rat aorta plasma membranes. *Biochim. Biophys. Acta*, 644:82–88.

Piascik, M. T., Babich, M., and Rush, M. E. (1983): Calmodulin stimulation and calcium regulation of smooth muscle adenylate cyclase activity. *J. Biol. Chem.*, 258:10913–10918.

Popescu, L. M., and Ignat, P. (1983): Calmodulin-dependent Ca^{2+}-pump ATPase of human smooth muscle sarcolemma. *Cell Calcium*, 4:219–235.

Raeymaekers, L., and Hasselbach, W. (1981): Ca^{2+} uptake, Ca^{2+}-ATPase activity, phosphoprotein formation and phosphate turnover in a microsomal fraction of smooth muscle. *Eur. J. Biochem.*, 116:373–378.

Raeymaekers, L., Casteels, R., Wuytack, F., and Deschutter, G. (1982): Demonstration of the phosphorylated intermediates of the Ca^{2+}-transport ATPase in a microsomal fraction and in a Ca^{2+} + Mg^{2+}-ATPase purified from smooth muscle by means of calmodulin affinity chromatography. *Biochim. Biophys. Acta*, 693:45–52.

Raeymaekers, L., Wuytack, F., Eggermont, J., De Schutter, G., and Casteels, R. (1983): Isolation of a plasma-membrane fraction from gastric smooth muscle. *Biochem. J.*, 210:315–322.

Scarpa, A., Vallieres, J., Sloane, B. F., and Somlyo, A. P. (1979): Smooth muscle mitochondria. *Methods Enzymol.*, 55:6065.

Sloane, B. F. (1980): Isolated membranes and organelles from vascular smooth muscle. In: *The Handbook of Physiology. The Cardiovascular System, Vascular Smooth Muscle, Vol. II*, edited by D. F. Bohr, A. P. Somlyo, and H. V. Sparks, pp. 121–132. American Physiological Society, Bethesda.

Sloane, B. F., Scarpa, A., and Somlyo, A. P. (1978): Vascular smooth muscle mitochondria: Magnesium content and transport. *Arch. Biochem. Biophys.*, 189:409–416.

Suematsu, E., Hirata, M., and Kuriyama, H. (1984): Effects of cAMP-dependent protein kinases, and calmodulin on Ca^{2+} uptake by highly purified sarcolemmal vesicles of vascular smooth muscle. *Biochim. Biophys. Acta*, 773:83–90.

Thorens, S. (1982): Ca^{2+}-dependent phosphorylation and Ca^{2+} uptake in membrane fractions of the mesenteric artery. *J. Muscle Res. Cell Motility*, 3:419–436.

Vallieres, J., Fortier, M., Somlyo, A. V., and Somlyo, A. P. (1978): Isolation of plasma membranes from rabbit myometrium. *Int. J. Biochem.*, 9:487–498.

Vallieres, J., Scarpa, A., and Somlyo, A. P. (1975): Subcellular fractions of smooth muscle: Isolation, substrate utilization and Ca^{++} transport by main pulmonary and artery and mesenteric vein mitochondria. *Arch. Biochem. Biophys.*, 170:659–669.

Verbist, J., Wuytack, F., De Schutter, G., Raeymaekers, L., and Casteels, R. (1984): Reconstitution of the purified calmodulin-dependent (Ca^{2+} + Mg^{2+})-ATPase from smooth muscle. *Cell Calcium*, 5:253–263.

Wikstrom, M., Ahonen, P., and Luukkaine, T. (1975): The role of mitochondria in uterine contraction. *FEBS Lett.*, 56:120–123.

Wuytack, F., and Casteels, R. (1980): Demonstration of a (Ca^{2+} + Mg^{2+})-ATPase activity probably related to Ca^{2+} transport in the microsomal fraction of porcine coronary artery smooth muscle. *Biochim. Biophys. Acta*, 595:257–263.

Wuytack, F., De Schutter, G., and Casteels, R. (1980): The effect of calmodulin on the active calcium-ion transport and (Ca^{2+} + Mg^{2+})-dependent ATPase in microsomal fractions of smooth muscle compared with that in erythrocytes and cardiac muscle. *Biochem. J.*, 190:827–831.

Wuytack, F., Raeymaekers, L., De Schutter, G., and Casteels, R. (1982): Demonstration of the phosphorylated intermediates of the Ca^{2+}-transport ATPase in a microsomal fraction and in a (Ca^{2+} + Mg^{2+})-ATPase purified from smooth muscle by means of calmodulin affinity chromatography. *Biochim. Biophys. Acta*, 693:45–52.

Wuytack, F., Raeymaekers, L., Verbist, J., De Smedt, H., and Casteels, R. (1984): Evidence for the presence in smooth muscle of two types of Ca^{2+} transport ATPase. *Biochem. J.*, 224:445–451.

Contractile Regulation

Adelstein, R. S., and Eisenberg, E. (1980): Regulation and kinetics of the actin-myosin-ATP interaction. *Annu. Rev. Biochem.*, 49:921–956.

Aksoy, M. O., Mras, S., Kamm, K. E., and Murphy, R. A. (1983): Ca^{2+}, cAMP, and changes in myosin phosphorylation during contraction of smooth muscle. *Am. J. Physiol.*, 245:C255–C270.

Bailin, G. (1984): Structure and function of a calmodulin-dependent smooth muscle myosin light chain kinase. *Experientia*, 40:1155–1188.

Barron, J. T., Barany, M., Barany, K., and Storti, R. V. (1980): Reversible phosphorylation and dephosphorylation of the 20,000-dalton light chain of myosin during the contraction-relaxation-contraction cycle of arterial smooth muscle. *J. Biol. Chem.*, 255:6238–6244.

Bond, M., Shuman, H., Somlyo, A. P., and Somlyo, A. V. (1984): Total cytoplasmic calcium in relaxed and maximally contracted rabbit portal vein smooth muscle. *J. Physiol. (Lond.)*, 357:185–201.

Butler, T. M., and Siegman, M. J. (1982): Chemical energics of contraction in mammalian smooth muscle. *Fed. Proc.* 41:204–208.

Cavadore, J.-C., Molla, A., Harricane, M.-C., Gabrion, J., Benyamin, Y., and Demaille, J. G. (1982): Subcellular localization of myosin light chain kinase in skeletal, cardiac, and smooth muscles. *Proc. Natl. Acad. Sci. USA*, 79:3475–3479.

Chacko, S. (1981): Effects of phosphorylation, calcium ion, and tropomyosin on actin-activated adenosine 5′-triphosphatase activity of mammalian smooth muscle myosin. *Biochemistry*, 20:702–707.

Chacko, S., and Rosenfeld, A. (1982): Regulation of actin-activated ATP hydrolysis by arterial myosin. *Proc. Natl. Acad. Sci. USA*, 79:292–296.

Chatterjee, M., and Murphy, R. A. (1983): Calcium-dependent stress maintenance without myosin phosphorylation in skinned smooth muscle. *Science*, 221:464–466.

Conti, M. A., and Adelstein, R. S. (1981): The relationship between calmodulin binding and phosphorylation of smooth muscle myosin kinase by the catalytic subunit of 3′:5′ cAMP-dependent protein kinase. *J. Biol. Chem.*, 256:3178–3181.

de Lanerolle, P., Nishikawa, M., Yost, D. A., and Adelstein, R. S. (1984): Increased phosphorylation of myosin light chain kinase after an increase in cyclic AMP in intact smooth muscle. *Science*, 223:1415–1417.

DiSalvo, J., and Gifford, D. (1983): An aortic spontaneously active phosphatase dephosphorylates myosin and inhibits actin-myosin interaction. *Biochem. Biophys. Res. Commun.*, 111:906–911.

DiSalvo, J., and Gifford, D. (1983): Spontaneously active and ATP Mg-dependent protein phosphatase activity in vascular smooth muscle. *Biochem. Biophys. Res. Commun.*, 111:912–918.

DiSalvo, J., and Jiang, M. J. (1982): The ATP Mg-dependent phosphatase is present in mammalian vascular smooth muscle. *Biochem. Biophys. Res. Commun.*, 108:534–540.

Di Salvo, J., Gifford, D., and Jiang, M. J. (1983): Properties and function of phosphatases from vascular smooth muscle. *Fed. Proc.*, 42:67–71.

Driska, S. P., Aksoy, M. O., and Murphy, R. A. (1981): Myosin light chain phosphorylation associated with contraction in arterial smooth muscle. *Am. J. Physiol.*, 240:C222–C233.

Ebisawa, K. (1983): Ca^{2+} regulation not associated with phosphorylation of myosin light chain in aortic intima smooth muscle. *J. Biochem.*, 93:935–937.

Endo, M., Kitazawa, T., Yagi, S., Iino, M., and Kakuta, T. (1977): Some properties of chemically skinned smooth muscle fibers. In: *Excitation-Contraction in Smooth Muscle*, edited by R. Casteels, T. Godfraind, and J. C. Ruegg, pp. 199–210. Elsevier/North-Holland, Amsterdam.

Filo, R. S., Bohr, D. F., and Ruegg, J. C. (1963): Glycerinated skeletal and smooth muscle: Calcium and magnesium dependence. *Science*, 147:1581–1583.

Gagelmann, M., Ruegg, J. C., and DiSalvo, J. (1984): Phosphorylation of the myosin light chains and satellite proteins in detergent-skinned arterial smooth muscle. *Biochem. Biophys. Res. Commun.*, 120:933–938.

Gallis, B., Edelman, A. M., Casnellie, J. E., and Krebs, E. G. (1983): Epidermal growth factor stimulates tyrosine phosphorylation of the myosin regulatory light chain from smooth muscle. *J. Biol. Chem.*, 258:13089–13093.

Gorecka, A., Aksoy, M. O., and Hartshorne, D. J. (1976): The effect of phosphorylation of gizzard myosin on actin activation. *Biochem. Biophys. Res. Commun.*, 71:325–331.

Guth, K., and Junge, J. (1982): Low Ca^{2+} impedes cross-bridge detachment in chemically skinned taenia coli. *Nature*, 300:775–776.

Hartshorne, D. J., and Gorecka, A. (1980): Biochemistry of the contractile proteins of smooth muscle. In: *The Handbook of Physiology. The Cardiovascular System, Vascular Smooth Muscle, Vol. II*, edited by D. F. Bohr, A. P. Somlyo, and H. V. Sparks, pp. 93–120. American Physiological Society, Bethesda.

Hartshorne, D. J., and Mrwa, U. (1982): Regulation of smooth muscle actomyosin. *Blood Vessels*, 19:1–18.

Hartshorne, D. J., and Siemankowski, R. F. (1981): Regulation of smooth muscle actomyosin. *Annu. Rev. Physiol.*, 43:519–530.

Ikebe, M., Barsotti, R. J., Hinkins, S., and Hartshorne, D. J. (1984): Effects of magnesium chloride on smooth muscle actomyosin adenosine-5'-triphosphatase activity, myosin conformation, and tension development in glycerinated smooth muscle fibers. *Biochemistry*, 23:5062–5068.

Janis, R. A., Barany, K., Barany, M., and Sarmiento, J. G. (1981): Association between myosin light chain phosphorylation and contraction of rat uterine smooth muscle. *FEBS Lett.*, 154:3–11.

Kakiuchi, R., Inui, M., Morimoto, K., Kanda, K., Sobue, K., and Kakiuchi, S. (1983): Caldesmon, a calmodulin-binding, F actin-interacting protein, is present in aorta, uterus and plates. *FEBS Lett.*, 154:351–356.

Kaminski, E. A., and Chacko, S. (1984): Effects of Ca^{2+} and Mg^{2+} on the actin-activated ATP hydrolysis by phosphorylated heavy meromyosin from arterial smooth muscle. *J. Biol. Chem.*, 259:9104–9108.

Kendrick-Jones, J., Cande, W. Z., Tooth, P. J., Smith, R. C., Scholey, J. M. (1983): Studies on the effect of phosphorylation of the 20,000 M_r light chain of vertebrate smooth muscle myosin. *J. Mol. Biol.*, 165:139–162.

Klee, C. B., and Vanaman, T. C. (1982): Calmodulin. In: *Advances in Protein Chemistry, Vol. 35*, edited by C. B. Anfinsen, J. T. Edsall, and F. M. Richards, pp. 213–321. Academic Press, New York.

Kreye, V. A. W., Ruegg, J. C., and Hofmann, F. (1983): Effect of calcium-antagonist and calmodulin-antagonist drugs on calmodulin-dependent contractions of chemically skinned vascular smooth muscle from rabbit renal arteries. *Naunyn-Schmiedebergs Arch. Pharmacol.*, 323:85–89.

Litten, R. Z., Solaro, R. J., and Ford, G. D. (1979): Nature of the calcium regulatory system of bovine arterial actomyosin. *Blood Vessels*, 16:26–34.

Maelncik, D. A., Anderson, S. R., Bohnert, J. L., and Shalitin, Y. (1982): Functional interactions between smooth muscle myosin light chain kinase and calmodulin. *Biochemistry*, 21:4031–4039.

Marston, S. B. (1982): The regulation of smooth muscle contractile proteins. *Prog. Biophys. Mol. Biol.*, 41:1–41.

Mikawa, T., Nonomura, Y., Hirata, M., Ebashi, S., and Kakiuchi, S. (1978): Involvement of an acidic protein in regulation of smooth muscle contraction by the tropomyosin-leiotonin system. *J. Biochem.*, 84:1633–1636.

Moreland, R. S., and Ford, G. D. (1982): The influence of Mg^{2+} on the phosphorylation and dephosphorylation of myosin by an actomyosin preparation from vascular smooth muscle. *Biochem. Biophys. Res. Commun.*, 106:652–659.

Nag, S., and Seidel, J. C. (1983): Dependence on Ca^{2+} and tropomyosin of the actin-activated ATPase activity of phosphorylated gizzard myosin in the presence of low concentrations of Mg^{2+}. *J. Biol. Chem.*, 258:6444–6449.

Nag, S., Nath, N., Carlos, A., and Seidel, J. C. (1984): Requirement of Ca^{2+} and tropomyosin (TM) for actin-activated ATPase activity of phosphorylated forms of pulmonary and gizzard myosin with gizzard or skeletal muscle actin. *Biophys. J.*, 45:44a.

Ngai, P. K., Carruthers, C. A., and Walsh, M. P. (1984): Isolation of the native form of chicken gizzard myosin light-chain kinase. *Biochem. J.*, 218:863–870.

Nishikawa, M., de Lanerolle, P., Lincoln, T. M., and Adelstein, R. S. (1984): Phosphorylation of mammalian myosin light chain kinases by the catalytic subunit of cyclic AMP-dependent protein kinase and by cyclic GMP-dependent protein kinase. *J. Biol. Chem.*, 259:8429–8436.

Nonomura, Y., and Ebashi, S. (1980): Calcium regulatory mechanism in vertebrate smooth muscle. *Biomed. Res.*, 1:1–14.

Ochiai, K., Umazume, Y., and Maruyama, M. (1981): Augmentation by calmodulin of Ca^{2+}-induced tension development in saponin-treated (chemically skinned) rat uterine smooth muscle fibers. *Biomed. Res.*, 2:714–717.

Onishi, H., Iijima, S., Anzai, H., and Watanabe, S. (1979): Possible role of myosin light chain phosphatase in the relaxation of chicken gizzard muscle. *J. Biochem.*, 86:1283–1290.

Onishi, H., Umeda, J., Uchiwa, H., and Watanabe, S. (1982): Purification of gizzard myosin light-chain phosphatase, and reversible changes in the ATPase and superprecipitation activities of actomyosin in the presence of purified preparations of myosin light-chain phosphatae and kinase. *J. Biochem.*, 91:265–271.

Pato, M. D., and Adelstein, R. S. (1983): Purification and characterization of a multisubunit phosphatase from turkey gizzard smooth muscle. *J. Biol. Chem.*, 258:7047–7054.

Pato, M. D., and Adelstein, R. S. (1983): Characterization of a Mg^{2+}-dependent phosphatase from turkey gizzard smooth muscle. *J. Biol. Chem.*, 258:7055–7058.

Persechini, A., and Hartshorne, D. J. (1983): Ordered phosphorylation of the two 20,000 molecular weight light chains of smooth muscle myosin. *Biochemistry*, 22:470–476.

Ruegg, J. C., DiSalvo, J., and Paul, R. J. (1982): Soluble relaxation factor from vascular smooth muscle: A myosin light chain phosphatase. *Biochem. Biophys. Res. Commun.*, 106:1126–1133.

Ruegg, J. C., Pfitzer, G., Zimmer, M., and Hofmann, F. (1984): The calmodulin fraction responsible for contraction in an intestinal smooth muscle. *FEBS Lett.*, 170:383–386.

Ruegg, J. C., Sparrow, M. P., and Mrwa, U. (1981): Cyclic-AMP mediated relaxation of chemically skinned fibres of smooth muscle. *Pfluegers Arch.*, 390:198–201.

Schneider, M., Sparrow, M., and Ruegg, J. C. (1981): Inorganic phosphate promotes relaxation of chemically skinned smooth muscle of guinea-pig taenia coli. *Experientia*, 37:980–982.

Sellers, J. R., and Pato, M. D. (1984): The binding of smooth muscle myosin light chain kinase and phosphatases to actin and myosin. *J. Biol. Chem.*, 259:7740–7746.

Sellers, J. R., Eisenberg, E., and Adelstein, R. S. (1982): The binding of smooth muscle heavy meromyosin to actin in the presence of ATP. *J. Biol. Chem.*, 257:13880–13883.

Sheetz, M. P., Chasan, R., and Spudich, J. A. (1984): ATP-dependent movement of myosin *in vitro*: Characterization of a quantitative assay. *J. Cell Biol.*, 99:1867–1871.

Siegman, M. J., Butler, T. M., Mooers, S. U., and Michalek, A. (1984): Ca^{2+} can affect V_{max} without changes in myosin light chain phosphorylation in smooth muscle. *Pfluegers Arch.*, 401:385–390.

Silver, P. J., and DiSalvo, J. (1979): Adenosine 3':5'-monophosphate-mediated inhibition of myosin light chain phosphorylation in bovine aortic actomyosin. *J. Biol. Chem.*, 254:9951–9954.

Silver, P. J., and Stull, J. T. (1982): Regulation of myosin light chain and phosphorylase phosphorylation in tracheal smooth muscle. *J. Biol. Chem.*, 257:6145–6150.

Silver, P. J., and Stull, J. T. (1984): Phosphorylation of myosin light chain and phosphorylase in tracheal smooth muscle in response to KCl and carbachol. *Mol. Pharmacol.*, 25:267–274.

Silver, P. J., Dachiw, J., and Ambrose, J. M. (1984): Effects of calcium antagonists and vasodilators on arterial myosin phosphorylation and actin-myosin interactions. *J. Pharmacol. Exp. Ther.*, 230:141–148.

Small, J. V., and Sobieszek, A. (1977): Ca-regulation of mammalian smooth muscle actomyosin *via* a kinase-phosphatase-dependent phosphorylation and dephosphorylation of the 20,000-M_r light chain of myosin. *Eur. J. Biochem.*, 76:521–530.

Sobue, K., Morimoto, K., Inui, M., Kanda, K., and Kakiuchi, S. (1982): Control of actin-myosin interaction of gizzard smooth muscle by calmodulin- and caldesmon-linked flip-flop mechanism. *Biomed. Res.*, 3:188–196.

Sobue, K., Muramoto, Y., Fujita, M., and Kakiuchi, S. (1981): Calmodulin-binding protein from chicken gizzard that interacts with F-actin. *Biochem. Int.*, 2:469–476.

Sobue, K., Muramoto, Y., Fujita, M., and Kakiuchi, S. (1981): Purification of a calmodulin-binding protein from chicken gizzard that interacts with F-actin. *Proc. Natl. Acad. Sci. USA*, 78:5652–5655.

Sparrow, M. P., Pfitzer, G., Gagelmann, M., and Ruegg, J. C. (1984): Effect of calmodulin, Ca^{2+}, and cAMP protein kinase on skinned tracheal smooth muscle. *Am. J. Physiol.*, 246:C308–C314.

Strzelecka-Golaszewska, H., and Sobieszek, A. (1981): Activation of smooth muscle myosin by smooth and skeletal muscle actins. *FEBS Lett.* 134:197–202.

Strzelecka-Golaszewska, H., Hinssen, H., and Sobieszek, A. (1984): Influence of an actin-modulating protein from smooth muscle on actin-myosin interaction. *FEBS Lett.*, 177:209–216.

Stull, J. T., and Blumenthal, D. K. (1980): Regulation of contraction by myosin phosphorylation. A comparison between smooth and skeletal muscles. *Biochem. Pharmacol.*, 29:2537–2543.

Walsh, M. P., Bridenbaugh, R., Kerrick, W. G. L., and Hartshorne, D. J. (1983): Gizzard Ca^{2+}-independent myosin light chain kinase: evidence in favor of the phosphorylation theory. *Fed. Proc.*, 42:45–50.

Walsh, M. P., Dabtowska, R., Hinkins, S., and Hartshorne, D. J. (1982): Calcium-independent myosin light chain kinase of smooth muscle. Preparation by limited chymotryptic digestion of the calcium ion dependent enzyme, purification, and characterization. *Biochemistry*, 21:1919–1925.

Walsh, M. P., Hinkins, S. Muguruma, M., and Hartshorne, D. J. (1983): Identification of two forms of myosin light chain kinase in turkey gizzard. *FEBS Lett.*, 153:156–160.

Walsh, M. P., Persechini, A., Hinkins, S., and Hartshorne, D. J. (1981): Is smooth muscle myosin a substrate for the cAMP-dependent protein kinase? *FEBS Lett.*, 126:107–110.

Werth, D. K., Haeberle, J. E., and Hathaway, D. R. (1982): Purification of a myosin phosphatase from bovine aortic smooth muscle. *J. Biol. Chem.*, 257:7306–7309.

Yamaguchi, M., Ver, A., Carlos, A., and Seidel, J. C. (1984): Modulation of the actin-activated adenosinetriphosphatase activity of myosin by tropomyosin from vascular and gizzard smooth muscles. *Biochemistry*, 23:774–779.

Zimmer, M., and Hofmann, F. (1984): Calmodulin antagonists inhibit activity of myosin light-chain kinase independent of calmodulin. *Eur. J. Biochem.*, 142:393–397.

The Heart and Cardiovascular System,
edited by H. A. Fozzard et al.
Raven Press, New York © 1986.

CHAPTER **42**

Measurement of Ventricular Function in the Experimental Laboratory

Karl T. Weber, Joseph S. Janicki, and Sanjeev G. Shroff

The heart is an integral part of the body's gas transport system that links the metabolizing tissues and their need for O_2 to the atmosphere. At the same time that O_2 is used to sustain oxidative metabolism, CO_2 is being produced. CO_2 needs to be expelled into the atmosphere if a life-threatening acidosis is to be avoided. The heart and lungs, together with hemoglobin, permit the body's internal respiration (O_2 uptake and CO_2 production) to be accommodated on a moment-to-moment basis as metabolic requirements dictate.

The movement of air and blood into and out of the thorax is a highly integrated process that is performed by the cardiopulmonary unit. The left heart is responsible for the delivery of O_2 to the tissues while the right heart delivers blood poor in O_2, but rich in CO_2, to the lungs. The function of the right and left heart has to be balanced with respect to the tissues as well as with one another. Numerous circulatory, neurohumoral, and metabolic factors are known to influence and control cardiac performance. These extrinsic stimuli, together with the intrinsic behavior of the myocardium, regulate ventricular function.

Since the discovery by William Harvey that the heart plays the central role in the circulation of blood, the study of cardiac performance has attracted an enormous interest. The study of ventricular function has been central to this scientific inquiry. The approach to the measurement of ventricular function in the laboratory, however, has been varied. Broadly speaking, several fundamental lines of investigation have emerged: (a) The heart has been studied in isolation devoid of circulatory control and humoral stimuli. With this approach it has been possible to examine the intrinsic behavior of the myocardium. (b) The heart has been studied coupled to the circulation, but where the metabolic requirements of the tissues are relatively constant because the experimental animal is anesthetized. Here the heart functions independently of the tissues. From this vantage point it is possible to examine the coupled behavior of the two mechanical systems, the heart and circulation. (c) The heart has been studied in the intact, awake, and metabolically active animal, where exercise can be used as a physiologic stress on the cardiopulmonary unit. Here the heart and its integrative behavior and control, with respect to the remainder of the organism and the lungs, can be examined.

A detailed discussion of each of these areas is beyond the scope of this chapter. We have arbitrarily elected to review the first two of these areas. We also recognize at the outset that it will not be possible to provide an exhaustive review of these areas and therefore wish to direct the interested reader to several excellent publications on the subject (1,12,13,15). Our approach in the space available is to focus more narrowly and to rely heavily on our own experience with the measurement of ventricular function.

METHOD I: THE HEART IN ISOLATION

In isolating the heart from the remainder of the body and circulation it is possible to examine ventricular function in a setting where the heart is devoid of external stimuli that normally influence its behavior. On a conceptual basis, ventricular function can be examined from two vantage points. The first view is to consider the ventricles to represent *mechanical pumps.* The relevant parameters in the analysis are ventricular pressure, volume, and flow. Historically, this has been the approach that emerged from the laboratories of Otto Frank and Ernest Starling at the turn of the century, where ventricular function was expressed in terms of the heart's displacement of blood (stroke volume) and the work (stroke work) it performed.

A second approach is to analyze ventricular performance based on the recognition that the ventricles are *muscular pumps* composed of muscle fibers tethered and supported within a connective tissue network. Accordingly, the description of ventricular function is given in terms that describe the behavior of cardiac muscle. This is a more recent approach whose primary motivation was to distinguish disturbances in ventricular function that are related to alterations in the myocardium, per se, from those that affect the ventricular chamber. The relevant parameters here are instantaneous muscle force (or stress) and length, and the indices of ventricular function become the extent and velocity of fiber shortening. It should be noted that with today's technology it is not possible to directly measure force and length of individual muscle fibers in the intact heart. Instead, these variables are computed from the measurements of ventricular pressure, volume, flow, and muscle mass, and certain assumptions about chamber geometry.

Experimental Approach

The removal of a heart from any properly anesthetized experimental animal and its subsequent perfusion on the bench can be accomplished with relative ease, provided proper attention is paid to anatomic detail. What is more important to the subsequent performance of the isolated heart is the ischemic period between the heart's isolation and its subsequent perfusion. This interval must be kept to a minimum. The choice of perfusate is also important. Various crystalloid perfusates that are aerated with O_2 and CO_2 have been chosen for this purpose. In our experience the heart performs best when

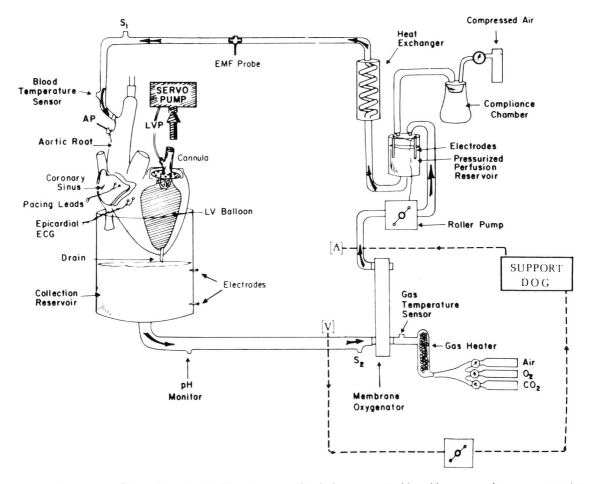

FIG. 1. Schematic representation of our isolated heart preparation being supported by either a membrane oxygenator system or a support dog. The *dashed line* indicates the support equipment that is bypassed when a support dog is used. Venous (V) blood is returned to either support system and reoxygenated. Arterial (A) blood is pumped to the perfusion reservoir. S_1 and S_2 represent arterial and venous blood sampling ports, respectively; AP represents the aortic perfusion pressure catheter, and LVP a left ventricular (LV) pressure (p) gauge. (From ref. 6, with permission.)

the perfusate carries O_2 directly bound to hemoglobin rather than its being dissolved in solution. Thus, we prefer to perfuse the isolated heart with blood. In the case of smaller laboratory animals (e.g., rabbit and rat), however, this may not be practical because of the large quantity of blood required to prime the perfusion apparatus. Hemoglobin or washed erythrocyte solutions may be preferable here. In our isolated canine heart studies we perfuse the heart in cross-circulation with another dog (6) and thus eliminate the need for mechanical oxygenation and a large reservoir of blood. A diagrammatic representation of this preparation is given in Fig. 1.

The study of ventricular function in the isolated heart requires the monitoring of ventricular volume and pressure. Current day pressure transducers, which are inexpensive and easy to use, provide high fidelity tracings. On the other hand, monitoring ventricular volume is more difficult. Our approach to the measurement of volume is to insert a very distensible balloon into the ventricular chamber via the left atrium. Since the coronary arteries are perfused via the aorta (the aortic valve is closed), the left ventricle is essentially devoid of blood except for that draining from the Thebesian veins. This small quantity of blood, representing 5% or less of total coronary flow, can be vented through a tube inserted at the apex of the ventricle. The balloon can be attached to a calibrated syringe so that the volume of fluid added to the balloon, and hence the volume of the ventricle, can be measured directly. To obtain absolute volume, the volume of the balloon material itself must be determined and added to the volume of fluid in the balloon.

Care must be taken to insure that the balloon does not herniate through the mitral or aortic valves during ventricular contraction. Finally, the proper seating of the balloon in the ventricle can be ensured by severing the chordal attachments of each papillary muscle, and by attaching silk suture to the tip of the balloon which can be brought through the sump tube that was inserted at the apex of the left ventricle.

Once instrumented, the mechanical behavior of the ventricle can now be examined. The simplest approach is to have the ventricle contract isovolumetrically around the balloon. In this setting the ventricle does not displace a volume from the balloon. Instead, it simply contracts around the balloon raising balloon pressure; hence the term *isovolumetric* contraction. To create an *ejecting* preparation requires a more involved system. We have developed a mechanical servo system for this purpose the details of which are presented elsewhere (6). In brief (see Fig. 2), the balloon is connected to this system so that its interior is a continuum with the hydraulic unit that is composed of a piston-cylinder arrangement and electronics. Potentiometer output from the servo piston provides a continuous record of intraventricular volume. Intraventricular pressure measured inside the balloon is used as the input signal for the servo logic, which is designed to maintain left ventricular end-diastolic and ejection pressures at predetermined or preset levels. An isovolumetric contraction can also be obtained by locking the piston in its end-diastolic position.

Other features of our isolated heart preparation include the following: (a) Coronary perfusion pressure is maintained at preset levels by having a pressurized reservoir

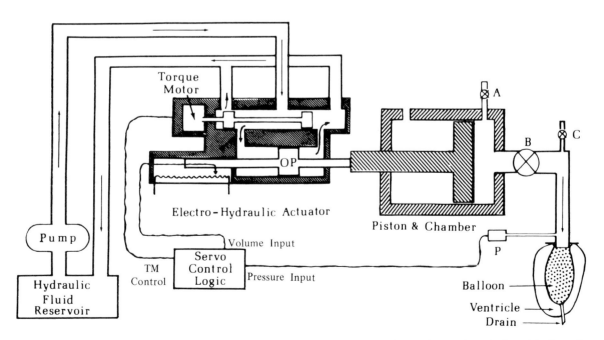

FIG. 2. Schematic representation of the servo pump system used to continuously monitor and control ventricular volume and pressure. A, B, and C represent manual valves; P, intraventricular pressure; OP, the output piston; and TM, the torque motor. The actuator alters the position of the piston, which in turn displaces fluid either into or out of the balloon. (From ref. 6, with permission.)

that receives blood from the dog in cross-circulation. This makes coronary perfusion independent of the support dog's circulation. (b) Heart rate is maintained at preset levels by atrial pacing. (c) Coronary blood flow is continuously monitored by the insertion of a cannulating electromagnetic flow probe into the perfusion line. (d) Coronary sinus effluent is sampled via a cannulating catheter. (e) The arteriovenous O_2 difference across the heart is continuously monitored by having the aortic perfusate and coronary sinus effluent directed to an O_2 difference analyzer (3). (f) Venous effluent is returned to the support dog by roller pump.

Mechanics of the Muscular Pump

The dynamics of either ventricle may be expressed in terms of the force that its muscle fibers generate and the rate and extent of their shortening. The sequence of events that occur within the myocardium during the cardiac cycle may be described as follows. During ventricular filling, the myocardium is stretched; at the end of the diastolic filling period, a force distends the muscular wall stretching its muscle fibers to a given length. This distending force has been termed the *preload* and is a function of chamber size and shape, and distensibility of the muscular wall (*vide infra*). From its diastolic length, muscle fibers are depolarized and mechanical contraction follows.

The contraction of these muscle fibers generates a force within the myocardium, which causes the development of pressure inside the ventricular chamber. Once chamber pressure exceeds that of the aorta or pulmonary artery, or the preset ejection pressure in the case of the servo system, ejection begins. Fiber shortening now displaces a given volume from the ventricle. The shortening of the muscle fibers occurs against a force, or shortening load, termed the *afterload*. Like preload, afterload is dependent on both chamber pressure and chamber size and shape. Because chamber configuration and pressure are changing throughout the ejection period, afterload has a time-varying value. In the normal heart, afterload peaks shortly after ejection begins and then declines throughout the remainder of ejection. The heart is therefore able to partially unload itself; it does not contract isotonically.

Concepts of Force, Stress, Tension, and Fiber Length

Direct measurements of force and length for a particular muscle fiber in the intact myocardium cannot be performed with current technology. However, a global description of muscle dynamics can be developed for the myocardium. According to this view, the summated contraction of all fibers determines wall shortening and, hence, chamber volume displacement. For this purpose, we have chosen a simplified derivation of wall force and fiber length, which are described below.

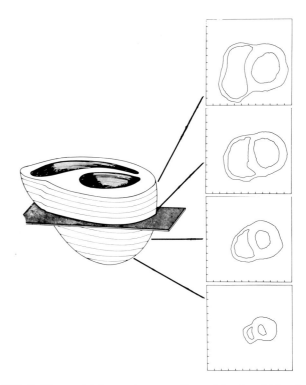

FIG. 3. The ventricles and myocardium of the heart bisected by an imaginary horizontal plane. For either ventricle, net wall force is a function of the pressure inside the ventricle and the cross-sectional area of its chambers included in the plane. See text for discussion. (From ref. 32, with permission.)

If we envision the ventricular chamber, containing blood under pressure, and its surrounding myocardium as being divided by an imaginary plane, as represented in Fig. 3, then a force is created on either side of the plane that tends to pull the myocardium apart. The magnitude of this force is a function of chamber pressure and the area of the chamber included in the plane. Under the condition of static equilibrium, this force must be counterbalanced by an equal and opposite force (i.e., wall force) that exists within the rim of the subtended myocardium and holds the two halves of the myocardium together. This computed force is a net result of the summation of the forces generated by individual muscle fibers. Thus, the net wall force may be calculated as the product of chamber pressure and the cross-sectional area of the chamber included in any given plane. Hefner et al. (4) have validated this concept by measuring the force recorded from a strain gauge that held together two edges of a slit made in the myocardium.

The distribution of wall force (*g*) across a cross-sectional area of myocardium (cm^2) represents wall *stress* (g/cm^2). Stress is the force borne by an unit area of myocardium.

The growth of muscle is thought to be a function of muscle *tension*. Tension (g/cm) describes the force that exists along a unit length of muscle. Because the myocardium is thick-walled, the application of the tension

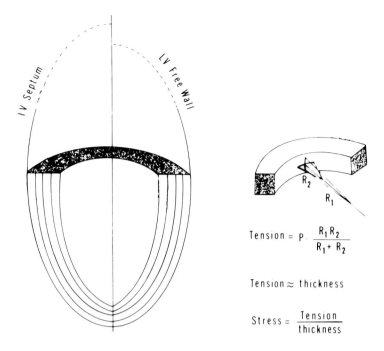

$$\text{Tension} = p \cdot \frac{R_1 R_2}{R_1 + R_2}$$

$$\text{Tension} \approx \text{thickness}$$

$$\text{Stress} = \frac{\text{Tension}}{\text{thickness}}$$

FIG. 4. The concept of tension is best applied to thin-walled structures. If the left ventricle is viewed as consisting of a series of nested shells of finite thickness then the tension existing at any point along the surface of one of these shells is related to the product of chamber pressure and the two principal radii of curvature (R_1 and R_2). Because the radius of curvature is larger for the septum than the free wall or apex of the left ventricle, septal tension and thickness must be greater than the other regions of the ventricle. Stress expresses tension per unit wall thickness. (From ref. 23, with permission.)

concept can be facilitated by considering the myocardium and its muscle fibers to be represented by a set of nested, concentric shells of finite thickness as shown in Fig. 4. The tension that exists at a point along the surface of any given shell, can then be related to the pressure and the principal radii of curvature (R_1 and R_2) at that point (23). Hence, for any given pressure, the tension developed by a muscle fiber is a function of chamber geometry. The complex shape of the ventricle dictates that there will be differences in regional tension. Variations that exist in myocardial wall thickness suggest that systolic wall stress, or systolic tension per unit thickness, is uniform despite the complex shape of the ventricle. Such a homogeneous distribution of stress favors an ordered process of ventricular contraction. If stress were not uniformly distributed, the performance of the muscular pump would be compromised by a distortion in shape and wall motion at regions of higher stress.

Finally, a midwall circumferential muscle *length* is chosen to represent the average length over the entire thickness of the myocardium (see Fig. 5). The change in circumferential length from end-diastole to end-systole is considered the *extent* to which these fibers have shortened, whereas the rate of change of length with respect to time in systole represents the *velocity* of shortening.

Isovolumetric Force-Length Relation

Over the years we have always assumed a spherical geometry for the left ventricle. As a result, only one force-length relation is required to describe the contractile behavior of the heart as a muscular pump (24–28). The maximum force that the myocardium will develop for any chamber volume can be found in the isovolumetrically beating heart. If the ventricle is progressively

FIG. 5. A circumferential length for the mid-wall of the myocardium is chosen to represent muscle fiber length. Ro = outside radius, Ri = internal radius, and Rm = mid-wall radius. (From ref. 33, with permission.)

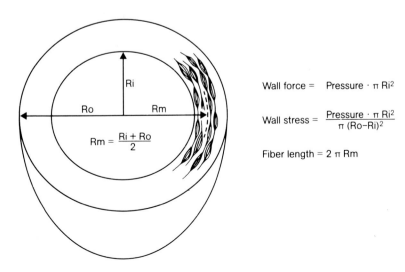

$$Rm = \frac{Ri + Ro}{2}$$

$$\text{Wall force} = \text{Pressure} \cdot \pi\, Ri^2$$

$$\text{Wall stress} = \frac{\text{Pressure} \cdot \pi\, Ri^2}{\pi\, (Ro - Ri)^2}$$

$$\text{Fiber length} = 2\, \pi\, Rm$$

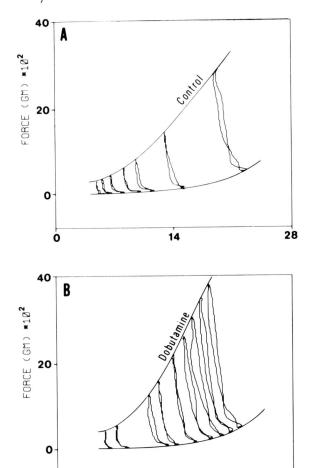

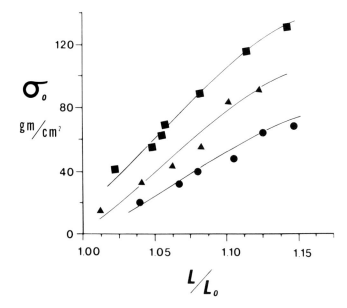

FIG. 7. Manipulations of contractile state and the maximal isovolumetric stress-length (normalized by L_o, length at zero end-diastolic pressure) relation is shown for two different infusion rates of norepinephrine. Note that the extent of this manipulation is a function of the norepinephrine infusion rate. *solid circles,* basal; *solid triangles,* norepinephrine 0.69 μg/min; *solid squares,* norepinephrine 1.36 μg/min. (From ref. 25, with permission.)

FIG. 6. The maximal force-diameter relation obtained from the isovolumetrically beating left ventricle of the isolated canine heart. Chamber diameter was measured along the minor axis of the ventricle between the lateral free wall and interventricular septum using piezoelectric crystals implanted on the endocardium and the sonomicrometry technique. **A:** Control data; **B:** following dobutamine (6 μg/min). (From ref. 28, with permission.)

stretched by sequentially increasing its filling volume, we would find an increase in both the end-diastolic and systolic forces that the ventricle will generate from any given level of filling volume. In Fig. 6 (panel A), the relation between ventricular force and chamber diameter (a quantity proportional to muscle length) is given over the physiological range of filling pressure (i.e., 1–25 mm Hg). This relation depicts a fundamental property of cardiac muscle, namely, the dependence of developed force on fiber length. This has also been termed the Frank-Starling relation.

Within the physiologic range of filling volumes, the peak isovolumetric force-length relation of the intact myocardium does not exhibit a maximum. In addition, with the exception of the lower range of filling volumes, this relation can be considered linear. With the assumption of linearity, the slope of this relation accurately

reflects the contractile state of the heart (*vide infra*). This is unlike isolated cardiac muscle where developed isometric force peaks and then subsequently declines as muscle is progressively stretched.

Pharmacological or intrinsic alterations in the contractile state of the myocardium result in nonparallel shifts in the developed force-length relation. Positive or negative inotropic interventions, for example, raise or reduce the slope of this relation, respectively. This response is depicted in Fig. 6 (panel B) where dobutamine, a synthetic catecholamine, is seen to raise the force developed for any particular end diastolic dimension. The degree of augmentation in the maximum force-length relation is a function of the rate of the catecholamine infusion (25) as illustrated in Fig. 7. In the failing heart, on the other hand, this relation is shifted to the right with a reduced slope.

Under physiologic conditions, the slope of the peak isovolumetric force-length relation is proportional to the contractile state of the myocardium. Therefore, parallel shifts in the force-length relation of a given ventricle, do not connote an alteration in myocardial contractile state. For example, a parallel upward shift is observed when the end-diastolic volume of the contralateral ventricle is raised (29).

Limit to Fiber Shortening

The isovolumetric developed force-length relation establishes a limit to which the fibers of the ejecting ventricle will shorten or, equivalently, to which the ventricle is able to reduce its volume during ejection (26). The force that exists in the wall at end-ejection is equal to the maximum developed or peak isovolumetric force that the muscle length at end-ejection can sustain. To illustrate this point further, several force-length loops obtained in the ejecting isolated heart are presented in Fig. 8 along with the corresponding isovolumetric force-length relations (dashed lines). In panel A, four force-length loops are given for four different afterloads. From an initial end-diastolic length (point *a*) the ventricle generates force until the onset of ejection (point *b*). Force peaks shortly after the onset of ejection and then declines during the remainder of ejection. As soon as a force is achieved that is maximum for the given systolic length, the muscle fiber no longer shortens (point *c*). The ventricle has reached its isovolumetric condition (broken line). Another contraction, which had a higher afterload represented by *def*, also ceases to shorten when the maximum force-length relation is attained. In panel B, the afterload has been varied from the same onset ejection force and end-diastolic length to create three different end-systolic lengths. In each case, however, shortening ceases when the isovolumetric force-length relation is attained (broken line).

From these findings it should be apparent that end-systolic length is independent of end-diastolic length and the ejection force that exists at the onset of ejection. These latter conditions merely serve to determine the starting points of each contraction. End-systolic length is solely a function of end-systolic force and is insensitive to the force-length trajectory preceeding the attainment of this end-systolic force. The equivalence of the peak isovolumetric and end-systolic force-length relations also have been verified during variations in myocardial contractile state (panel C of Fig. 8) as well. Therefore, the ejecting ventricle contracts within the confines of the diastolic and peak isovolumetric force-length relations.

The end-systolic force-length relation provides an estimate of the peak isovolumetric force-length curve. Hence, in deriving this relation, the contractile state of the myocardium can be quantitated in the ejecting ventricle. In order to adequately describe the slope of the relation, at least three and preferably more force-length points must be obtained without altering contractility.

Determinants of Fiber Shortening

The limit to myocardial shortening has been identified as the maximal isovolumetric or end-systolic force-length relation. Moreover, shortening is independent of those conditions of length and load that exist at the onset of contraction (or end-diastole). Instead, the fibers comprising the heart's muscular wall are responsive to the shortening load that is present at each instant of ejection (25,27). The influence of *instantaneous shortening load* on the extent and rate of shortening has been studied in the isolated heart (10–12). Four different afterloaded contractions are shown in Fig. 9 along with the rate and extent of midwall circumferential fiber shortening. Each contraction begins from the same preload. In panel A, the contractions are shown in the force-length domain together with the isovolumetric force-length relation (broken line). For each contraction, the extent of fiber shortening is determined by instantaneous force, or afterload, opposing shortening. Shortening is greatest in beat *a*, having the least shortening load. The responsiveness of the velocity of shortening to instantaneous shortening load is depicted in panel B of Fig. 9. It can be seen that for a given muscle length, the instantaneous velocity is greatest for the contraction

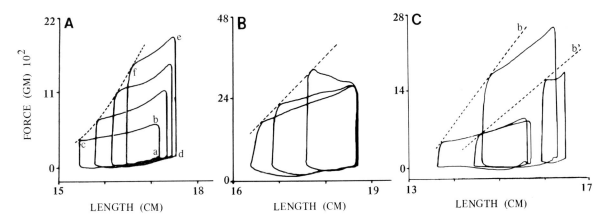

FIG. 8. The close interrelationship between the isovolumetric maximal force-length relation (*dashed line*) and the end-systolic force-length relation of ejecting contractions from three isolated hearts. **A:** Four counterclockwise force-length loops are given for an ejecting ventricle. End-diastole, onset, and end-ejection are denoted by *a, b, c,* and *d, e, f,* respectively, in the widest and tallest loops. **B:** Three contractions in which end-diastolic length and initial shortening load were identical. However, because the trajectory of instantaneous shortening load was varied, three different end-systolic lengths were obtained. **C:** The equivalence of the isovolumetric and end-ejection force-length relations is preserved following the pharmacological depression in contractile state (propranolol, 0.1 mg/min; line *b'*). Line *b* represents the control state. (From ref. 25, with permission.)

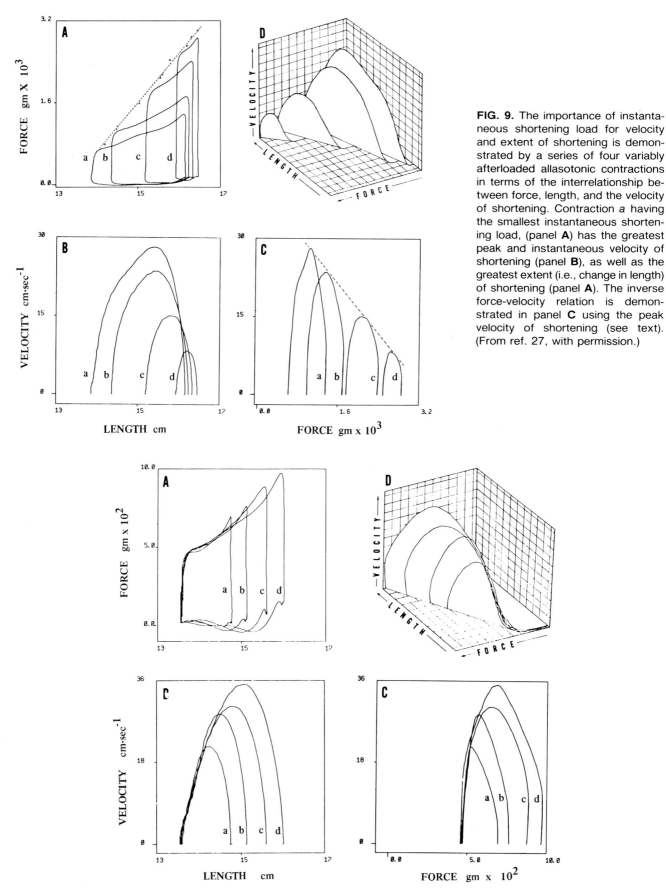

FIG. 9. The importance of instantaneous shortening load for velocity and extent of shortening is demonstrated by a series of four variably afterloaded allasotonic contractions in terms of the interrelationship between force, length, and the velocity of shortening. Contraction *a* having the smallest instantaneous shortening load, (panel **A**) has the greatest peak and instantaneous velocity of shortening (panel **B**), as well as the greatest extent (i.e., change in length) of shortening (panel **A**). The inverse force-velocity relation is demonstrated in panel **C** using the peak velocity of shortening (see text). (From ref. 27, with permission.)

FIG. 10. The importance of instantaneous shortening length for the velocity and extent of shortening is demonstrated by a series of contractions, each of which traverses an essentially identical trajectory of instantaneous shortening load. As end-diastolic fiber length is progressively raised from beats *a* to *d*, the instantaneous shortening length becomes greater (panel **A**). Thus, for the same shortening load, the peak and instantaneous velocity of shortening and the extent of shortening are greatest for beat *d* (panel **B** and see text). (From ref. 27, with permission.)

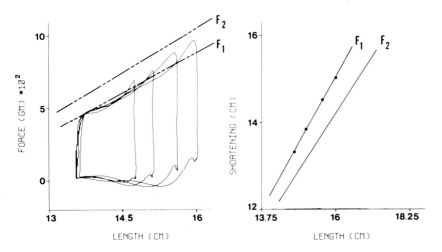

FIG. 11. The ventricular function curve may be derived from the shortening-length relation of the muscular pump. In the **left hand panel**, the common instantaneous length-load trajectory has been simplified and represented by the *broken line* labeled F_1. Because instantaneous shortening length has been progressively increased in these contractions having the same shortening load, the extent of shortening will increase. This is demonstrated by the linear relation between the extent of shortening and end diastolic length relation shown in the **right hand panel**. For a greater shortening load trajectory, F_2, the slope of the linear shortening-length relation would be reduced; hence, there is less shortening for any equivalent initial length. (From ref. 23, with permission.)

having the smallest shortening load (i.e., beat *a*). In addition, peak velocity is inversely proportional to shortening load. This inverse force-velocity relation is depicted in panel C and represents a fundamental property of the muscle. Finally, panel D summarizes, in three dimensions, the interrelationship between shortening velocity, fiber length, and shortening load for the four contractions.

The second determinant of wall shortening is the *instantaneous shortening length.* In Fig. 10, instantaneous shortening length has been raised by increasing the initial or onset contraction length while instantaneous shortening load has been held constant. Consequently, each beat traverses the common trajectory within the shortening load-length domain and thus the same end-systolic force-length point is reached (panel A). The rate and extent of each contraction's shortening are quite different, and a function of instantaneous shortening length. Contraction *d,* which has the greatest instantaneous shortening length, shortens with the greatest peak and instantaneous shortening velocity (panel B) and to the greatest extent (panel A). Moreover, it is apparent that instantaneous shortening velocity is not a function of contraction duration since each beat reaches the common velocity-length trajectory (panel B) at a different time during ejection. Panel C indicates that once the common load or force is reached, the force-velocity trajectories of all four contractions superimpose, even though the instantaneous lengths are different. Finally, in panel D, the interrelationships among shortening load, length, and velocity are depicted in three dimensions.

The traditional estimate of pump function, the ventricular function curve, defined as the relation between stroke volume and the filling volume of the ventricle, may be derived from shortening load-length relationships. For each constant shortening load trajectory shown in Figs. 11 and 12 and labeled (F_1, $F_2 \cdots F_n$), the extent of fiber shortening increases in linear fashion as the initial (i.e., end-diastolic) length is progressively raised. As the shortening load becomes greater (e.g., $F_2 > F_1$) the amount of shortening is less for any equivalent length. The ventricular function curve can be derived by examining the response of stroke volume (or shortening) to increments in end-diastolic volume (or length). In an intact circulation, the shortening load progressively increases with increments in end-diastolic volume or length. Therefore, the ventricular function curve (broken line in Fig. 12) is simply the shortening-length relationship obtained at progressively increasing values of shortening load.

The third major determinant of fiber shortening is the *contractile state* of the myocardium. The decline in fiber shortening seen during a pharmacological depression

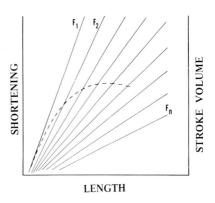

FIG. 12. A series of shortening-length relations could be constructed for a range of ever increasing shortening load trajectories, F_1, F_2, . . . , F_n. In the intact animal, the derivation of the ventricular function curve during volume loading is associated with increased intracardiac and intravascular volumes, and hence increasing shortening loads. The resultant stroke volume to diastolic volume (fiber length) relation, therefore, traverses those shortening-length relations as indicated by the *dashed line.* (Modified from ref. 23, with permission.)

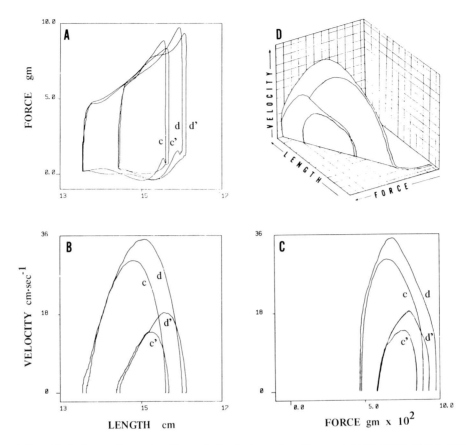

FIG. 13. The interrelationship between force, length, and shortening when the contractile state of the myocardium has been pharmacologically reduced by propranolol (0.07 mg/min). Following β-blockade, the rate and extent of shortening of contractions c' and d' are reduced from the control beats c and d despite the similar conditions of initial length, instantaneous length, and shortening load (see text). (From ref. 27, with permission.)

of contractile state with the β-adrenergic receptor antagonist, propranolol, is illustrated in Fig. 13. The control state of contractility (beats c and d) are given for comparable conditions of instantaneous shortening load and length. Following propranolol, the isovolumetric force-length relation (not shown) and the end-systolic force-length relation are each shifted downward or to the right (panel C, Fig. 8). Thus, the instantaneous velocity and extent of shortening are both reduced (beats c' and d'). On the other hand, a positive shift in contractile state with a catecholamine, for example, would increase the rate and extent of shortening above that observed for the control state. By utilizing the trajectories of instantaneous force, length, and shortening velocity, a three-dimensional representation of their interrelationship can be constructed as shown in panel D of Fig. 13. Intrinsic or pharmacological shifts in contractile state either increase or decrease the dimensions of this three-dimensional surface.

Mechanics of the Mechanical Pump

In addition to the concepts of cardiac muscle and the muscular pump, ventricular function may be described

in terms of its properties as a mechanical pump. The mechanical properties of the ventricular chamber, first in diastole as the ventricle is filled, and then in systole as blood is ejected, play a key role in determining ventricular function.

At this point, it would be appropriate to distinguish between the mechanical properties of the ventricular chamber from those of the myocardium described in the foregoing discussion. The *chamber* mechanical properties are generally computed from the pressure-volume relation of the ventricle. On the other hand, the *myocardial* mechanical properties are computed from its stress-strain relation. The primary goal of assessing the stress-strain relation is to obtain a measure of the intrinsic mechanical properties of the myocardium that are independent of shape and size of the ventricle and also of the external forces, such as pericardial and intrathoracic pressures.

Elastic and Viscous Properties

A purely elastic system will deform and completely recover from its deformation independently of the rate with which the deforming stress is applied. The *elastic* behavior of the ventricular chamber and the myocardium can be quantitated by the pressure-volume and stress-strain (or tension-length) relations, respectively. Like most biological tissue, however, the myocardium does not demonstrate purely elastic behavior. The heart also exhibits a *viscous* property which dictates that the mechanical behavior of the heart is also dependent on flow or strain rate. The elastic and viscous properties together determine the extent and the rate of shortening in response to a given transmural pressure or stress (30). Viscous properties are often ignored, especially at end-diastole and end-systole, where rate-dependent processes are usually quite small. However, during the rapid filling phase of diastole or the ejection period of systole, the computation of elasticity based solely on a purely elastic model will be in substantial error.

Mechanical Properties in Diastole

The diastolic portion of the cardiac cycle begins when the ejection of blood from the ventricle has ceased, or just prior to aortic valve closure; it terminates when the myocardium is depolarized. The diastolic period is broken down into five phases as shown in Fig. 14: proto-

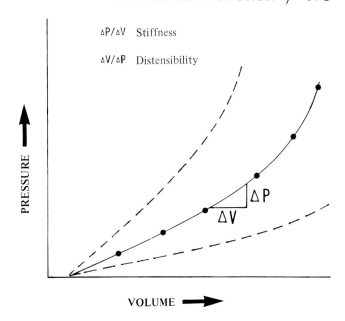

FIG. 15. A diagrammatic representation of the end-diastolic pressure-volume (*P-V*) relation for the left ventricle. Chamber stiffness is approximated from the slope ($\Delta P/\Delta V$) of this relation by using a monoexponential curve fitting routine. An increase or decrease in chamber stiffness is depicted by the relations (*dashed lines*) shown above or below normal curve (*solid line*). (From ref. 35, with permission.)

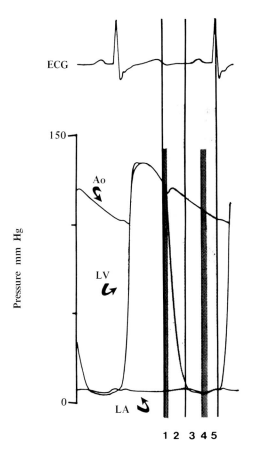

FIG. 14. The five phases of diastole are depicted from the pressure tracings of the left ventricle, aorta, and left atrium. (See text for discussion.) (From ref. 35, with permission.)

diastole, isovolumetric relaxation, rapid filling, diastasis, and atrial contraction, labeled 1 to 5 in Fig. 14. After the contraction of the atria there is a point in time when atrial and ventricular pressures are essentially equal. This connotes the hemodynamic endpoint of diastole. Ventricular filling at end-diastole is complete and, consequently, the viscous effects (i.e., proportional to flow or strain rate) are minimal. Thus, at end-diastole the pressure-volume relation primarily reflects the elastic behavior of the myocardium. In contrast, the pressure-volume relation obtained throughout the filling period (i.e., from the onset of rapid filling period to end-diastole) is influenced by both the elastic and viscous properties of the system. In the following section we focus our attention only on the mechanical properties at end-diastole and not on the instantaneous pressure-volume or stress-strain relations throughout diastole.

The end-diastolic pressure-volume relation is typically nonlinear for filling pressures greater than 5 mm Hg. The slope of this relation ($\Delta P/\Delta V$) is a measure of the static *chamber stiffness*. The inverse of chamber stiffness, termed *compliance* or *distensibility,* is $\Delta V/\Delta P$. Due to the nonlinear nature of the pressure-volume relation (see Fig. 15), chamber stiffness varies with filling or end-diastolic pressure. In using a monoexponential curve fitting routine to analyze the end-diastolic pressure-volume data (usually for end-diastolic pressure greater than 5 mm Hg), the slope or chamber stiffness can be linearly related to chamber pressure (2). The slope of this linear relation is termed the *chamber stiffness con-*

stant. An increase in the steepness of the pressure-volume relation will result in an increase in the chamber stiffness while a rightward parallel shift in the pressure-volume relation will not affect chamber stiffness.

Factors Influencing Mechanical Properties in Diastole

In order to induce changes in *myocardial mechanical properties,* the composition of the myocardium has to change. Cardiac disease may induce a change in myocardial stiffness through a variety of mechanisms (e.g., ischemia, increased collagen concentration). These intrinsic alterations of the myocardium must be distinguished from the extrinsic factors (e.g., pericardium or the interplay between the ventricles) that will only alter *chamber* stiffness and the pressure-volume relation (8). In the latter case, the myocardium is not diseased, only chamber stiffness is altered. Such a situation frequently presents itself for the left ventricle when the right heart is enlarged. As we discuss more fully later in the chapter, the left ventricle as a chamber may appear stiffer under these circumstances because the position of the interventricular septum is altered, thereby altering the geometry of the left ventricle.

Extramyocardial factors primarily influence the *ventricular pressure-volume relationship* or *chamber stiffness* (8). These include heart rate, the level of left ventricular ejection pressure, coronary blood volume, and the pericardium.

Increases in *heart rate* shorten diastole and, as a result, systole occupies a greater percentage of the cardiac cycle. Below 170 beats/min, the diastolic pressure-volume relation is insensitive to this reduction in diastolic interval. Above 170 beats/min relaxation is incomplete which causes an elevated ventricular pressure for any given end-diastolic volume. Consequently, the end-diastolic pressure-volume relation is shifted to the left. In circumstances where the mitral or tricuspid valve is diseased and its orifice for ventricular filling is narrowed, elevations in heart rate above 100 to 120 beats/min may prohibit the adequate filling of the ventricle while leading to acute atrial distension.

Studies in our laboratory (7) have indicated that the end-diastolic pressure-volume relation of the left ventricle is also altered by the level of its *ejection pressure.* From a constant filling volume, an increase in ejection pressure results in a decline in end-diastolic pressure. The magnitude of the change in filling pressure is dependent on the absolute increment in ejection pressure and the ventricular chamber volume before the perturbation in pressure. The fact that end-diastolic pressure falls following an elevation in ejection pressure indicates that the pressure-volume relation is shifted to the right. These observations leave little doubt that alterations in diastolic distensibility occur with increments in arterial pressure and serve to explain similar observations noted with interventions that are unavoidably accompanied by increments in arterial pressure (e.g., catecholamines and paired pacing).

Another factor that will alter the diastolic properties of the chamber is the *coronary blood volume.* A modest increment in the end-diastolic pressure-volume relation is observed with an elevation in coronary perfusion pressure and a greater distention of the coronary circulation. This swelling of the myocardium, termed the "erectile" response, accounts for a decline in chamber distensibility.

To this point, the physiologic factors that we have reviewed have a minor effect on diastolic chamber stiffness. Other factors, such as the pericardium and the mechanical interplay between ventricles play a more important role (8,29). Each of these factors are considered in more detail elsewhere in this chapter. In brief, however, the parietal *pericardium,* which forms a discrete sac surrounding the ventricles and atria, will significantly influence the pressure-volume relation of each chamber. The effect of the pericardium is demonstrated in Fig. 16 where the diastolic pressure-volume relation for each ventricle is presented before and after pericardiectomy. In order to minimize the effects of right and left ventricular interaction (*vide infra*), these data have been presented when the filling pressure in the contralateral ventricle was zero. Removal of the pericardium resulted in a significant decrease in chamber stiffness. The de-

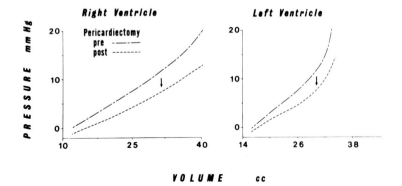

FIG. 16. The parietal pericardium, which is contiguous with both ventricles, will significantly influence the diastolic pressure-volume relation of each ventricle. Removal of the pericardium results in a downward, nonparallel shift of the end diastolic pressure-volume curves. (From ref. 8, with permission.)

crease in chamber stiffness following pericardiectomy is a function of the ventricle's filling volume; the greatest reduction is noted at higher filling volumes. With the pericardium intact, each ventricular chamber appears to be stiffer. Thus, the pericardium can be viewed as restraining the acute distension of the ventricles and the atria. More gradual increments in heart size, as occur with growth from infancy to adulthood or in the failing heart, are not constrained by the pericardium; in fact, the pericardial space is increased and the pericardial pressure-volume relation shifts to the right.

Mechanical Properties in Systole

In the following section, we present the methods for quantitating the mechanical properties of the ventricular chamber during systole.

Instantaneous ventricular systolic pressure is primarily a function of several factors, including the time during systole, chamber volume, flow, and contractile state. Chamber *elastance* (mm Hg/ml) describes the relationship between chamber pressure and volume. In a manner analogous to an elastic bag, the higher the volume in the chamber, the greater the pressure inside the chamber. However, unlike a passive elastic bag, chamber elastance during systole is not constant; instead, it increases with time in systole. This is evident from the observation that chamber pressure increases with time even for a fixed chamber volume (i.e., an isovolumetric contraction). Thus, ventricular pressure-volume relations during systole can be described in terms of a time-varying elastance. Chamber *resistance,* (mm Hg·sec/ml) on the other hand, describes the property of the chamber that is flow-dependent. Conceptually, the role of resistance can be viewed as subtracting from the pressure that would have existed for either a purely elastic system or a condition with zero flow. In the case of an isovolumetric contraction, where there is no ejection, ventricular pressure first increases and then declines. Figure 17 (panel A) illustrates pressure-volume relations for an isovolumetric contraction at various times in systole. The slope of each pressure-volume line represents ventricular elastance at a given instant in systole. An ejecting beat is superimposed on these isovolumetric pressure-volume relations and is represented by the pressure-volume loop in Fig. 17 (panel B). During the isovolumetric period of systole, when there is no flow, ventricular pressure is governed by the elastic behavior and therefore the ejecting beat pressure-volume points during the period fall on the isovolumetric pressure-volume relations. During the ejection period, however, ventricular pressure falls below that predicted by pure elastic behavior. The difference (ΔP) in predicted (based on pure elastic behavior) and actual pressure is due to the resistive behavior of the ventricle. Ventricular resistance, for a

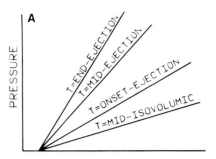

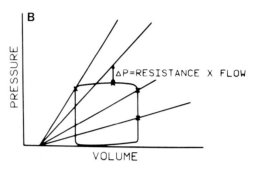

FIG. 17. The elastance of the pump may be described by its pressure-volume relation. If there was no flow from the ventricle, the four pressure-volume relations shown in panel **A** would pertain. During ejection, however **(B)**, when flow occurs, ventricular resistance results in a reduction in pressure (ΔP) that is generated, and hence the pressure-volume loop does not reach the elastic relation during this period. (From ref. 31, with permission.)

given time and volume in systole, is defined as this pressure difference divided by the flow.

Experimental evidence (16,19,21) indicates that ventricular pressure-volume-time relations during systole can be adequately quantitated by a time-varying elastance. Furthermore, the elastance function is independent of the external loading conditions, i.e., end-diastolic volume and ejection pressure. This is depicted in Fig. 18 where the solid curves represent ventricular elastance as a function of time for various combinations of end-diastolic volume and ejection pressure. On the other hand, when the contractile state is raised by a catecholamine, such as dobutamine, elastance (broken curve in Fig. 18) is significantly altered such that it reaches a higher maximum in a shorter period of time. Ventricular elastance (especially its peak value) can be used to represent the intrinsic force-generating capability of the heart because of its insensitivity to external loading conditions and its behaving in a predictable manner with variations in contractile state.

Similar to elastance, ventricular resistance is not constant during systole; instead it varies throughout systole (5,19). However, ventricular resistance for a given combination of systolic time, volume, and contractile state is uniquely related to the corresponding isovolumetric pressure (i.e., for the same time, volume, and contractile

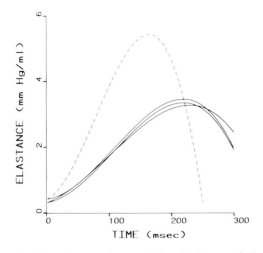

FIG. 18. The time-varying systolic elastance of the left ventricle is not influenced by the variations in loading conditions [i.e., end-diastolic volume and ejection pressure (*solid lines*)]. Changes in contractility alter elastance. For example, dobutamine, a synthetic catecholamine, will raise elastance (*dashed curve*). (From ref. 35, with permission.)

state but with zero flow) (5,18). As shown in Fig. 19, this relationship between resistance and isovolumetric pressure is linear and independent of changes in end-diastolic volume, ejection pressure, and contractile state (18,19).

It should be emphasized that ventricular systolic elastance and resistance are strictly phenomenologic descriptions of chamber mechanical properties. Elastance describes the volume- and time-dependence of pressure, while resistance describes flow-dependence. At present, one can only speculate as to the physical basis of these global properties. For example, elastance and resistance may be a manifestation of the force-length and force-velocity relations of the constituent muscle fibers, respectively. However, factors other than the properties of

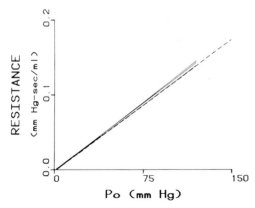

FIG. 19. Left ventricular systolic resistance is a linear function of ventricular isovolumetric pressure (Po) (see text). This linear relationship is not affected by alterations in loading condition [i.e., end-diastolic volume and ejection pressure (*solid lines*) or contractility (*dashed lines*)]. (From ref. 35, with permission.)

the individual muscle fibers (e.g., collagen concentration, geometry, muscle mass) may also contribute to the measured values of elastance and resistance.

In a manner similar to diastolic chamber stiffness, ventricular systolic elastance and resistance represent chamber properties and not myocardial properties. In order to derive the myocardial properties so as to facilitate comparisons among hearts with varying sizes and shapes, one has to appropriately normalize pressure, volume, and flow. For this purpose, one can transform pressure, volume, and flow to stress, strain, and strain rate, respectively. However, since stress and strain have multiple components and an additional variable (i.e., strain rate) is present, this process will result in a relatively large number of relations and, therefore, may have limited practical utility. Another approach to normalization is to concentrate on specific aspects of the elastance and resistance functions (e.g., peak elastance and the slope of resistance-pressure relationship) and derive empirical normalization factors based on simultaneous experiments performed on the intact ventricle and isolated papillary muscle from the same ventricle. These experiments have not yet been performed and it is clear that much work needs to be done in this area.

Factors Influencing the Mechanical Properties in Systole

Since an explicit description of myocardial mechanical properties is not currently available, the following discussion primarily focuses on those factors which influence the chamber mechanical properties.

The effects of various factors on ventricular elastance has generally been studied for the left ventricle in terms of quantities that are derived from the entire elastance function: peak elastance (E_{max}) and the volume axis intercept of the peak elastance (V_d). As noted earlier, variations in arterial load or end-diastolic volume do not affect E_{max} or V_d (10,19) whereas increases in contractile state with catecholamines (e.g., dobutamine) significantly increases E_{max} without altering the intercept (19,21). Finally, an increase in right ventricular systolic pressure and end-diastolic volume result in a decrease in V_d without any change in E_{max} (29). These observations suggest that an increase or decrease in E_{max} can be interpreted to represent an augmentation or depression of contractile state, respectively. However, a change in V_d alone is difficult to interpret.

Factors influencing ventricular resistance have not been studied. However, based on our preliminary studies (18), we believe that the rate-limiting process of the contractile apparatus is one of the major determinants of chamber ventricular resistance. In addition, it is possible that the extracellular components (e.g., collagen), shearing forces between myocardial fibers, and geometric deformation during systole may contribute to chamber resistance. The relative contributions of each of these components needs further evaluation.

Factors Influencing Ventricular Systolic Performance

In the following discussion we briefly discuss the three major factors (i.e., ejection pressure, end-diastolic volume, and contractile state) that influence ventricular performance in terms of stroke volume and stroke work. This analysis is based on the mean values of measurements such as pressure and volume and should be contrasted with that presented earlier, where instantaneous muscle force-length-velocity variables were used. This pressure-volume analysis will be useful in describing the coupling of the heart to the circulation, as described in the subsequent section.

The hemodynamic performance of the pump may be considered by using the mean values of ejection pressure and flow and the stroke volume. Figure 20 depicts the inverse relationships that exist between stroke volume

and mean ejection rate with mean ejection pressure (24,25). For any given end-diastolic volume, as the level of *ejection pressure* increases, the stroke volume and ejection rate fall. Eventually, ejection pressure reaches a level such that there is no ejection. This is an isovolumetric contraction, where there is no flow or volume ejected; it is represented by the points which intersect the abscissa. From the inverse slope of the systolic flow to ejection pressure relation, the flow-dependent or resistance properties of the pump may be derived. The elastic properties of the pump, on the other hand, are reflected in the slope of the relation between stroke volume and ejection pressure. As the contractile state of the pump is compromised (see right panel, Fig. 20), systolic elastance will fall. Of equal importance is the fact that when elastance falls (e.g., the failing heart), the slope of this relation is increased so that the ventricle is influenced to a greater extent by changes in ejection pressure. Hence, the failing heart has become more sensitive to its arterial load.

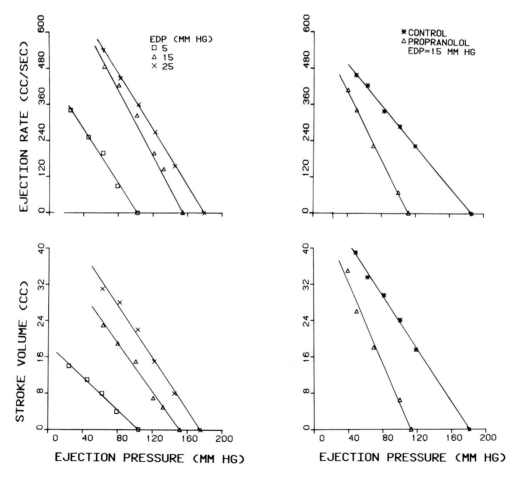

FIG. 20. The behavior of the heart as a pump may be described by its mean flow and stroke volume to ejection pressure relations. For any given filling pressure [end-diastolic pressure (EDP) in **left panels**], the greater the ejection pressure the less the stroke volume and rate of ejection. As filling pressure is raised, the flow and volume displaced from the chamber increases for any given ejection pressure. Compared to the normal heart, the failing heart (**right panels;** propranolol) generates less flow and displaces less volume from its chamber for any given ejection pressure. In addition, it becomes more sensitive to ejection pressure (small increments in ejection pressure will significantly reduce the stroke volume). (From ref. 31, with permission.)

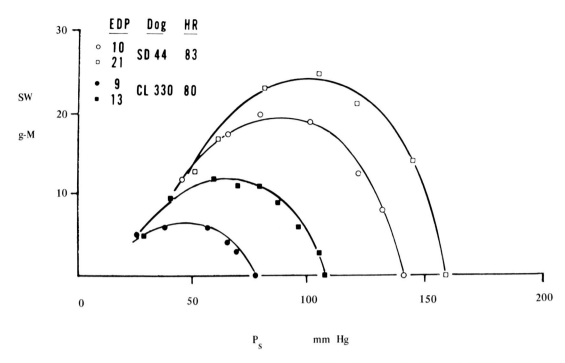

FIG. 21. Influence of end-diastolic pressure (EDP) on the parabolic relation between stroke work (SW) and ejection pressure (P$_s$) is given for two different dog hearts. HR is heart rate in beats/min (see text). (From ref. 24, with permission.)

For any given ejection pressure, the larger the *end-diastolic volume* the greater the stroke volume and the rate of ejection. This volume-dependent property of the pump has been termed the Frank-Starling mechanism. If one considers the interrelationship between ejection pressure and the volume ejected we have a representation of systolic work, where stroke work equals the force exerted over a unit distance (24). For a given diastolic volume, stroke work normally rises and falls over the physiologic range of ejection pressure. Peak work generally occurs at the expected normal range of arterial pressures (e.g., 80–140 mm Hg). Beyond this point, stroke volume falls and work declines (see Fig. 21). Thus, the normal ventricle operates at the peak of its work-load curve. In order for it to perform at its peak during increments of ejection pressure, there must be a corresponding increase in diastolic volume.

Finally, the *contractile state* of the pump will determine the volume and rate of ejection for any given filling volume and ejection pressure. Contractility, or contractile state, are terms used to describe this property of the pump which is independent of its filling volume and arterial load, but sensitive to neurohumoral influences (e.g., plasma norepinephrine) and dependent on the intrinsic constituents (e.g., myosin isoform composition) of its myocardium.

Interplay and Interdependence of the Right and Left Ventricles

To ensure proper O$_2$ and CO$_2$ transport and a steady state of fluid balance and nutrient exchange across the lungs and circulation, pulmonary and systemic blood flow must be balanced relative to one another. The equilibrium that normally exists between the right and left hearts is promoted by their anatomic arrangement which, conceptually speaking, may be represented as two muscular pumps aligned in series via their mechanical coupling by the lungs. Several anatomical and physiologic factors also provide for the interplay between ventricles (34). These include the muscle fibers that interconnect the ventricular free walls and intraventricular septum, the mobile interventricular septum itself, the pericardium, and intrapleural pressure. Collectively, these factors create and foster an interdependence between the ventricles.

Muscle Fibers

For many years it was thought that the myocardium was composed of discrete muscle bundles. Each ventricle was thought to have a distinct composition of several of these muscles. More recent evidence, however, indicates that these muscle bundles probably do not exist. Instead, the myocardium should be considered as a continuum of wound muscle fibers (20). Irrespective of one's viewpoint, the alignment of muscle fibers within the interventricular septum and ventricular free walls will determine, in part, the interaction of the ventricles.

In the interventricular septum, muscle fiber alignment resembles that of the left ventricle, so that the left ventricular side of the septum has an orientation of fibers similar to that of the left ventricular subendocardium, while the right ventricular side of the septum and its fibers resemble the epicardial fibers of the left ventricular free wall (14). Morphologically, therefore, the septum resembles the left ventricle. The concentric reduction of the left ventricular chamber during systole would also support the view, from a functional standpoint, that the septum and left ventricle behave as a unit. The alignment of fibers within the right ventricular free wall and its attachments to the septum and left ventricle remain undefined. Nevertheless, these attachments would promote the interdependence between ventricles by creating a radial force that draws the right ventricular free wall into the septum, thereby aiding in right ventricular emptying.

Interventricular Septum

The septum is a deformable structure that separates the two ventricles. Its position and curvature relative to the ventricles is determined by the distribution of forces across its surface. Radial and axial forces are present on both its right and left ventricular surfaces. A radial force is created by the tethering or pulling of the muscle fibers in the septum toward the free wall of each ventricle. From the information presented earlier on the alignment of muscle fibers within the septum, this radial force will dominate in the direction of the left ventricular free wall. The axial force is related to ventricular pressure

and septal surface area. Normally, the difference in pressure between the ventricles creates an axial force that bows the septum toward the right ventricle.

Acute variations in right ventricular volume or pressure alter the distribution of this axial force and, thereby, septal position and motion. When this occurs, the geometry of the left ventricle is distorted and the distensibility of its chamber is reduced. The left ventricle now appears to be stiffer.

Pericardium

The pericardium surrounds the heart. The viscoelastic properties of the pericardium determine intrapericardial pressure for any given intrapericardial volume. Both the atria and ventricles are subjected to intrapericardial pressure. For normal ventricular volumes the pericardium imposes little, if any, physical constraint and, therefore, intrapericardial and intrapleural pressures are equivalent. During diastole, the interplay between the ventricles is modestly enhanced by the pericardium. In systole, as cardiac volume declines, the pericardium imposes no constraint on the behavior of the ventricles.

During an acute increase in heart size, the viscoelastic limits of the pericardium are brought into play. Here, intrapericardial pressure rises to produce a positive external pressure on the external surfaces of both ven-

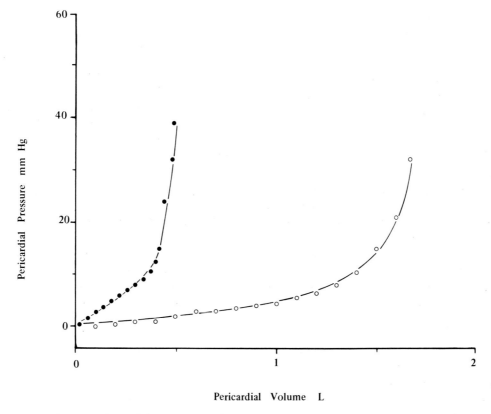

FIG. 22. The pressure-volume relation of the canine. Volume represents only the amount of blood added to the pericardial space and does not include the volume of cardiac muscle and cardiac chambers. The curve on the left (*solid circles*) was obtained in the normal pericardium. The curve on the right (*open circles*) was obtained in an animal with a large and chronic pericardial effusion. (From ref. 35, with permission.)

tricles. This serves to lower the transmural pressure of the ventricles and thereby ventricular filling. A pericardial effusion may also create a positive extracardiac pressure. The more severe the effusion or the more rapid its onset, the greater its propensity to compromise cardiac filling as the viscoelastic properties of the pericardium are once again introduced (see Fig. 22). An intrapericardial pressure of 12 mm Hg or more represents the point at which the pressure in each cardiac chamber will be equalized (9). It is at this point that ventricular filling is severely compromised. As a result, cardiac output falls and systemic hypotension appears.

METHOD II: THE HEART COUPLED TO THE CIRCULATION

The heart and the circulation represent two individual mechanical systems that are coupled to each other. Under the conditions of coupled equilibrium, the pressure, volume, and flow variables measured at any point in the cardiovascular system are determined by the mechanical properties of each system and their mutual interactions. In this respect, the terms *cardiac output* and *arterial pressure*, which are actually determined by the joint interaction of heart and circulation, could be misconstrued. On the surface, one might suppose that the cardiac output was solely determined by the heart and not the vasculature. Similarly, the term arterial pressure suggests that only the vasculature determines it. In reality, both these variables are determined by the mutual interaction of heart and circulation. Finally, the analysis of coupling is based on variables such as pressure, volume, and flow. Therefore, chamber mechanical properties (e.g., elastance and resistance), and not the myocardial properties, are useful in such an endeavor.

Experimental Approach

The open chest preparation has been used extensively to study ventricular function with the heart coupled to the circulation. Because the animal is anesthetized, the numerous circulatory, neurohumoral, and metabolic factors that are known to influence and control cardiac performance are relatively constant making it possible to evaluate the interaction between the heart and circulation. In addition, the animal could be pharmacologically blocked to further insure against reflexive adjustments of the contractile state of the heart and tonicity of the vasculature.

The choice of anesthesia is critical and should take into account its duration and effects on the cardiovascular system. All anesthetic agents will depress cardiac function, some more so than others. Pentobarbital is one of the more commonly used agents because it is inexpensive, easy to use, fast-acting and long-lasting. However, associated with its use is a tachycardia and a decreased

stroke volume. Less hemodynamic alterations are seen with halothane. Its use, however, requires special equipment and careful attention to the rate of administration throughout the experiment. There is no ideal anesthesia, each has its advantages and disadvantages, and one should be evermindful of its effects on the cardiovascular system.

A median sternotomy provides maximum exposure of the heart and its major vessels. In order to assess cardiac function and cardiovascular coupling, one needs to measure ventricular and vascular pressures, ventricular outflow, and ventricular volume. For pressure measurements, the solid state, catheter tip mounted pressure transducers are preferable because of their high fidelity and insensitivity to catheter motion or catheter whip. To measure ventricular pressure, the catheter is either inserted through the wall of the ventricle or via one of the cardiac valves. The arterial pressure catheter is positioned in close proximity to the flow probe. Flow is commonly measured using an electromagnetic flow device (3). The flow probe, which consists of a magnetic coil for generating a magnetic field and electrodes for measuring the voltage induced by the ionic blood flowing through the magnetic field, is placed around the vessel at the site of interest. For the systemic circulation this is usually the ascending aorta; and for the pulmonary circulation, it is the root of the pulmonary artery. A major disadvantage of this preparation compared to the isolated heart is the inability to measure directly the ventricular volume. Instead, indirect techniques, such as the measurements of several ventricular dimensions with sonomicrometry crystals, one- or two-dimensional echocardiography, or angiography are used. In the remainder of the chapter it will become evident how this preparation together with the measurements of vascular pressure and ventricular volume (indirect), pressure and flow can be used to assess *in vivo* cardiac performance and cardiovascular coupling.

Coupling to the Arterial Circulation

The following discussion is limited to the coupling of the left ventricle to the systemic arterial circulation. Conceptually, one can analyze the coupling of the right ventricle to the pulmonary arterial circulation in a similar manner. The intrinsic chamber mechanical properties of the left ventricle are its elastance and resistance, as we have described earlier in the chapter. Similarly, the mechanical properties of the systemic arterial circulation can be represented by its input impedance spectrum, a detailed description of which can be found elsewhere (11). Briefly, the arterial circulation does not act as a pure resistance; instead, the load imposed on the left ventricle is frequency-dependent. In addition, the pressure and flow events are not exactly in phase, and the phase difference is also a function of frequency. Impedance is a more complete definition of the mechanical properties of the arterial circulation. The input impedance spectrum is often approximated by a three-element modified Windkessel (36) consisting of: (a) systemic vascular resistance (Rp); (b) the collective compliance of the arterial circulation (C); and (c) characteristic impedance of the arteries (Rc). Rp is primarily determined by the resistance of small vessels and arterioles, C represents the overall static compliance ($\Delta V / \Delta P$) of the arterial circulation; and Rc is primarily a property of major arteries. If one has a knowledge of ventricular elastance and resistance throughout systole and parameters, Rp, C, and Rc, one can predict the entire time-course of pressure and flow that would result when these two systems are coupled to each other. These results cannot be presented as explicit analytical equations; instead, one derives the results from numerical solution of a set of coupled differential equations. On the other hand, if one is only interested in predicting the average values of the resultant variables (e.g., average arterial pressure, stroke volume, or cardiac output), and not in the exact time-course, then one can simplify the analysis considerably. The simplified analysis results in explicit analytical expressions for pressures and flows and can also be represented graphically. One such example is discussed below.

The left ventricle and its arterial load are characterized in terms of average pressure-flow relations in Fig. 23. For the arterial load, this relationship is represented by the line demonstrating the proportional increase in mean arterial pressure as the flow through the arteries is increased. The inverse of the slope of this relation represents systemic vascular resistance. In other words, when systemic vascular resistance is reduced, the slope becomes steeper. Similarly, the left ventricle is represented by a relationship between mean flow (i.e., cardiac output) and mean ejection pressure (similar to those in Fig. 20) for a given end-diastolic volume and contractile state. An increase in the end-diastolic volume shifts this relationship to the right in a parallel fashion, whereas an augmentation of the contractile state shifts this relationship such that the extrapolated flow axis intercept (i.e., cardiac output for zero ejection pressure) is invariant while the ejection pressure axis intercept (i.e., ejection pressure for zero cardiac output) is increased. In order to couple these two relationships and establish the point of equilibrium (i.e., the intersection point), one needs to have a common variable represented by the pressure axis. We have observed that there exists a linear relation between mean ejection pressure and mean arterial pressure (i.e., mean arterial pressure = $k \cdot$ mean ejection pressure). The proportionality coefficient (k) is dependent on the arterial load parameters, Rp and C and heart rate. However, the ratio of k within the physiologic range of arterial load and heart rate is small. In addition, the conceptual discussion of the coupling analysis presented here is not affected by the variations of k with arterial load. Having converted the mean arterial pressure to mean ejection pressure, one can now calculate the equilibrium point as the intersection of the arterial and ventricular relations (see Fig. 23). At this equilibrium point, the capability of the cardiac pump to generate pressure at a given flow balances the pressure required to force the same flow through the arterial load.

In the above example we have purposely simplified the actual conditions and focused, in effect, on average values of pressure and flow. The pulsatile nature of cardiac contraction, however, introduces many complexities. For example, in addition to the systemic vascular resistance, the arterial compliance (C) also affects the cardiac output such that the cardiac output declines as C is reduced. Sunagawa et al. (22) have incorporated the effects of heart rate, Rp, C in their analysis of left ventricular-arterial coupling and have derived an analytical expression for predicting the equilibrium stroke volume from the intrinsic properties of the two mechanical systems: the left ventricle and the arterial load. Finally, it should be noted that the aortic

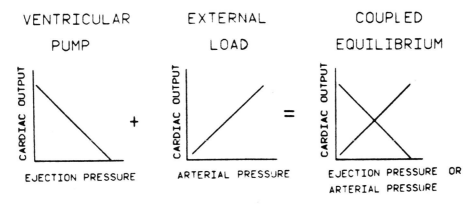

FIG. 23. The functional coupling of the heart to the systemic arterial circulation may be represented according to the scheme which relates the flow and pressure variables of each system (**left and middle panels**). When coupled, cardiac output, ejection pressure, and arterial pressure are uniquely determined by the intersection of the two curves (coupled equilibrium in **right panel**). (From Ref. 31, with permission.)

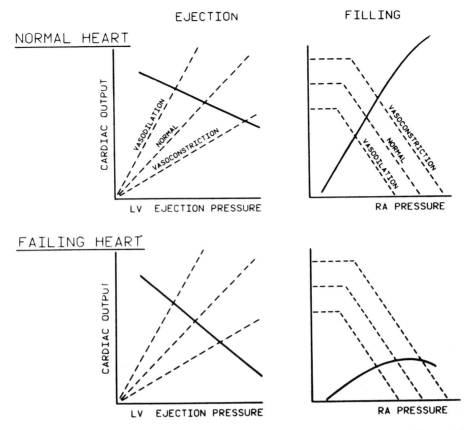

FIG. 24. The coupling of the pump to the arterial (ejection) and venous (filling) circulations. The relation for the heart is represented as the *heavy line,* while the vasculature is given as the *dashed lines.* The normal heart is primarily regulated by the venous return; arterial resistance has little effect. In the failing heart, however, arterial resistance becomes dominant (see text). (From ref. 31, with permission.)

input impedance spectrum, which is a complete description of arterial load, was simplified in terms of the three elements, Rp, C, and Rc. In doing so, one effectively ignores the reflected pressure and flow waves that are known to exist in the arterial system (11). These reflections may affect cardiac output independent of the absolute magnitude of the load (i.e., values of Rp, C, and Rc). The relative importance of reflected waves in determining left ventricular-arterial coupling is unknown at present.

The degree to which the left ventricle and arterial circulation interact to contribute to the generation of the equilibrium pressure and flow is determined in part by the functional state of the left ventricle itself. In other words, the amount of change in the equilibrium cardiac output for a given change in arterial load is dependent on the properties (e.g., the cardiac output-ejection pressure relation) of the left ventricular pump. For example, the cardiac output-ejection pressure relation for a normal ventricle is relatively more horizontal (i.e., cardiac output is less sensitive to changes in ejection pressure) than that of a failing ventricle (see left panel, Fig. 24). Accordingly, the interaction between the left ventricle and the arterial load is relatively modest for a normal left ventricle, whereas the failing left ventricle is quite

sensitive to changes in arterial load (see left panels, Fig. 24).

Coupling to the Venous Circulation

In addition to the coupling that exists between the left ventricle and arterial circulation, a similar coupling is present between the right ventricle and venous circulation. The classic analysis of this venous coupling by Guyton (3) follows the logic outlined earlier for the arteries. The right heart is a flow generator; the venous circulation its filling reservoir. Each can be described by its own unique pressure-flow relation shown in Fig. 25 and which have traditionally been termed the ventricular function curve for the right ventricle and the venous return curve for the venous circulation, respectively. The cardiac output or, more specifically, pulmonary blood flow, and right atrial pressure form this coupling and equilibrium point. At equilibrium, the capacity of the venous system to return flow to the right heart against a given filling pressure is balanced by the ability of the heart to generate flow when it is distended by the given filling pressure.

Sarnoff (17) has popularized the term *ventricular function curve* to describe the relationship between the

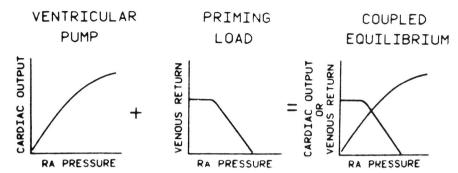

FIG. 25. The functional coupling of the heart to the systemic venous circulation may be represented according to the scheme that relates the flow and pressure variables of each system (**left and middle panel**). When coupled, cardiac output, venous return, and right atrial pressure are uniquely determined by the intersection of the two curves (coupled equilibrium in **right panel**). (From ref. 31, with permission.)

mechanical work of the ventricle and its filling volume and emphasized the fact that alterations in the functional state of the ventricle are best described by a "family" of such curves. In man or in the intact animals, the ventricular function curve is usually obtained during intravascular volume expansion, where arterial load is increased. As a result, pump output is measured under conditions of varying arterial pressure. Ideally, the ventricular function curve would best be determined for a given level of ejection pressure, as shown in the right panels of Fig. 24. The heavy, superimposed curve depicts the Frank-Starling relation and the fact that the ventricle can eject more when it is filled with a larger diastolic volume. In addition, various other factors influence the function curve, including the diastolic properties of the chamber. For example, the more the ventricle is dis-

tended, the stiffer it becomes, and increments in filling pressure are consequently less effective in increasing diastolic volume. Increments in arterial loading diminish pump output for any given filling volume and, therefore, also affect the relation. These two factors are the primary reasons for the curvature which exists in the ventricular function curve. Additional factors that may contribute to this response include the interaction between the atria and ventricles in diastole, atrial contraction, and the pericardium.

The Heart Coupled to the Arterial and Venous Circulations

The coupling between either ventricle and its respective circulation obviously occurs in similar fashion. Altera-

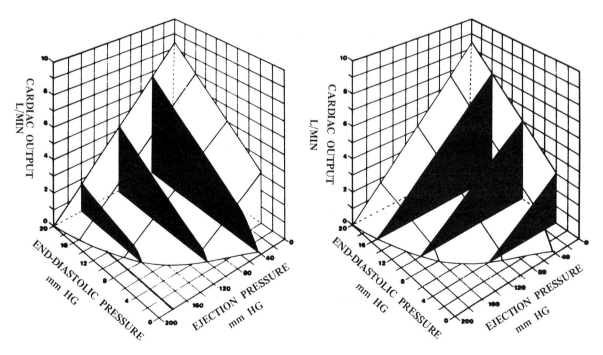

FIG. 26. The three-dimensional surface depicting the interrelationship between cardiac output, left ventricular filling pressure, and ejection pressure. On the **left,** three ventricular function curves are given. On the **right,** the cardiac output-ejection pressure relations are represented for three filling pressures (see text). (From ref. 19, with permission.)

tions in the coupling between either system will affect the other. To visualize this joint coupling and its influence on the heart, it is useful to consider the two pressure-flow relations within a three-dimensional surface (31). Figure 26 depicts the two representations of ventricular function in the plane of venous coupling on the left and the plane of arterial coupling on the right. Together, they can be integrated into one overall surface. This three-dimensional surface reflects the fact that with increases in filling pressure from 4 to 10 and to 16 mm Hg, and thereby diastolic volume, the corresponding ejection pressure to cardiac output relation is shifted upward in a parallel manner. Thus, a greater stroke volume can be generated by a more distended ventricle (i.e., the Frank-Starling relation) for any systolic pressure. Contrariwise, increasing systolic pressure (e.g., from 40 to 100 to 160 mm Hg as shown on the left) will depress the ventricular function curve such that at any filling pressure, cardiac output is reduced.

REFERENCES

1. Braunwald, E., Ross, J., and Sonnenblick, E. H. (1976): *Mechanisms of Contraction of the Normal and Failing Heart.* Little, Brown, Boston.
2. Gaasch, W. H., Bing, O. H., and Mirsky, I. (1982): Chamber compliance and myocardial stiffness in left ventricular hypertrophy. *Eur. Heart J.,* 3:139–145.
3. Guyton, A. C., Farish, C. A., and Williams, J. W. (1957): An improved arterio-venous oxygen difference recorder. *J. Appl. Physiol.,* 10:145–147.
4. Hefner, L. L., Sheffield, L. T., Cobbs, G. C., and Klip, W. (1962): Relation between mural force and pressure in the left ventricle of the dog. *Circ. Res.,* 11:654–663.
5. Hunter, W. C., Janicki, J. S., Weber, K. T., and Noordergraaf, A. (1983): Systolic mechanical properties of the left ventricle: effects of volume and contractile state. *Circ. Res.,* 52:319–327.
6. Janicki, J. S., Reeves, R. C., Weber, K. T., Donald, T. C., and Walker, A. A. (1974): The application of a pressure-servo system developed to study ventricular dynamics. *J. Appl. Physiol.,* 37: 736–741.
7. Janicki, J. S., and Weber, K. T. (1977): Ejection pressure and the diastolic left ventricular pressure-volume relation. *Am. J. Physiol.,* 232:H545–552.
8. Janicki, J. S., and Weber, K. T. (1980): Factors influencing the diastolic pressure-volume relation of the cardiac ventricles. *Fed. Proc.,* 139:133–140.
9. Janicki, J. S., Shroff, S. G., and Weber, K. T. (1986): Influence of extracardiac forces on the cardiopulmonary unit. *Cardiac/Vascular Coupling,* edited by F. C-P. Vir, pp. 371–413. Springer-Verlag, New York.
10. Maughan, W. L., and Sunagawa, K. (1984): Factors affecting the end-systolic pressure-volume relationship. *Fed. Proc.,* 43:2408–2410.
11. Milnor, W. R. (1982): *Hemodynamics.* Williams & Wilkins, Baltimore.
12. Mirsky, I., Ghista, D. N., and Sandler, H. (1974): Cardiac Mechanics. *Physiological, Clinical and Mathematical Considerations.* Wiley, New York.
13. Noble, M. I. M. (1979): *The Cardiac Cycle.* Blackwell, Oxford.
14. Pearlman, E. S., Weber, K. T., Janicki, J. S., Pietra, G. G., and Fishman, A. P. (1982): Muscle fiber orientation and connective tissue content in the hypertrophied human heart. *Lab. Invest.,* 46: 158–164.
15. Rushmer, R. F. (1976): *Cardiovascular Dynamics.* Saunders, Philadelphia.
16. Sagawa, K., Suga, H., Shoukas, A. A., and Bakalar, K. M. (1977): End-systolic pressure/volume ratio: a new index of ventricular contractility. *Am. J. Cardiol.,* 40:748–753.
17. Sarnoff, S. J., and Berglund, E. (1954): Ventricular function. I. Starling's law of the heart studied by means of simultaneous right and left ventricular function curves in the dog. *Circulation,* 9:706–718.
18. Shroff, S. G., Janicki, J. S., and Weber, K. T. (1985): Evidence and quantitation of left ventricular systolic resistance. *Am. J. Physiol.,* 249:H358–H370.
19. Shroff, S. G., Janicki, J. S., and Weber, K. T. (1983): Left ventricular systolic dynamics in terms of its chamber mechanical properties. *Am. J. Physiol.,* 245:H110–H124.
20. Streeter, D. D., Jr., Sponitz, H. W., Patel, D. J., Ross, J., Jr., and Sonnenblick, E. H. (1969): Fiber orientation in canine left ventricle during diastole and systole. *Circ. Res.,* 24:339–347.
21. Suga, H., Sagawa, K., and Shoukas, A. A. (1973): Load independence of instantaneous pressure-volume ratio of the canine left ventricle and effects and epinephrine and heart rate on the ratio. *Circ. Res.,* 32:314–322.
22. Sunagawa, K., Sagawa, K., and Maughan, W. L. (1984): Ventricular interaction with the loading system. *Ann. Biomed. Eng.,* 12:163–189.
23. Weber, K. T., Reichek, N., Janicki, J. S., and Shroff, S. (1981): The pressure overloaded heart. Physiological and clinical correlates. *The Heart in Hypertension,* edited by B. Strauer, pp. 287–306. Springer-Verlag, Berlin.
24. Weber, K. T., Janicki, J. S., Reeves, R. C., and Hefner, L. L. (1974): Determinants of stroke volume in isolated canine heart. *J. Appl. Physiol.,* 37:742–747.
25. Weber, K. T., Janicki, J. S., Reeves, R. C., and Hefner, L. L. (1976): Factors influencing left ventricular shortening in isolated canine heart. *Am. J. Physiol.,* 230:419–426.
26. Weber, K. T., Janicki, J. S., and Hefner, L. L. (1976): Left ventricular force-length relations of isovolumic and ejecting contractions. *Am. J. Physiol.,* 231:337–343.
27. Weber, K. T., and Janicki, J. S. (1977): Instantaneous force-velocity-length relations in isolated dog heart. *Am. J. Physiol.,* 232:H241–H249.
28. Weber, K. T., and Janicki, J. S. (1980): The dynamics of ventricular contraction: Force, length and shortening. *Fed. Proc.,* 39:188–195.
29. Weber, K. T., Janicki, J. S., Shroff, S. G., and Fishman, A. P. (1981): Contractile mechanics and interaction of the right and left ventricles. *Am. J. Cardiol.,* 47:686–695.
30. Weber, K. T., and Hawthorne, E. W. (1981): Descriptors and determinants of cardiac shape. *Fed. Proc.,* 40:2005–2010.
31. Weber, K. T., Janicki, J. S., Hunter, W. C., Shroff, S. G., Pearlman, E. S., and Fishman, A. P. (1982): The contractile behavior of the heart and its functional coupling to the circulation. *Prog. Cardiovasc. Dis.,* 24:375–400.
32. Weber, K. T., Janicki, J. S., and Shroff, S. (1983): Mechanical and structural aspects of the hypertrophied human myocardium. In: *Cardiac Hypertrophy in Hypertension,* edited by R. C. Tarazi and J. B. Dunbar, p. 201–210. Raven Press, New York.
33. Weber, K. T., Janicki, J. S., Likoff, M. J., Shroff, S. G., and Andrews, V. (1983): Chronic cardiac failure: Pathophysiologic and therapeutic considerations. *Triangle,* 22:1–9.
34. Weber, K. T., Janicki, J. S., Shroff, S. G., and Likoff, M. J. (1983): The cardio-pulmonary unit. The body's gas transport system. *Clin. Chest Med.,* 4:101–110.
35. Weber, K. T., and Janicki, J. S. (1986): *CardioPulmonary Exercise Testing—Physiologic Principles and Clinical Applications.* Saunders, Philadelphia.
36. Westerhof, N., Elzinga, G., and Sipkema, P. (1971): Artificial arterial system for pumping hearts. *J. Appl. Physiol.,* 228:776–781.

The Heart and Cardiovascular System,
edited by H. A. Fozzard et al.
Raven Press, New York © 1986.

CHAPTER **43**

Protein Phosphorylation in the Heart

Alison M. Robinson-Steiner and Jackie D. Corbin

There is increasing evidence that protein phosphorylation is intimately involved in the regulation of heart contraction and metabolism. A number of the proteins phosphorylated in heart have been identified, but in many cases the precise way in which phosphorylation controls their behavior is not certain. Historically, cyclic AMP-dependent protein kinase reactions in heart received much attention after elucidation of the control mechanism for glycogen metabolism in liver and skeletal muscle. However, now there is interest in kinases activated by agents other than cyclic AMP, such as cyclic GMP, Ca²⁺-calmodulin, and phospholipids, as well as by unknown factors; and various hormones and neurotransmittors have been considered as their primary regulators. Protein phosphatases, which have been less well studied than the kinases, may also prove to play a significant role in heart regulatory mechanisms. This chapter outlines the nature of the phosphorylated heart proteins, the respective kinases and phosphatases involved, and their possible relevance in control of cardiac function.

METHODOLOGY

Measurement of Protein Phosphorylation

For an excellent discussion of the quantitative analysis of protein phosphorylation the reader is referred to Manning et al. (146). Protein phosphorylation can be determined chemically or by the incorporation of radioactive inorganic phosphate ($^{32}P_i$). Many proteins will incorporate radioactivity when heart tissue is incubated or perfused with $^{32}P_i$, as can be seen by gel electrophoresis of the tissue extract, followed by autoradiography to locate radioactive protein bands. Some phosphorylated proteins can be identified and isolated, in many cases, rapidly, with a high degree of purity using specific antibody precipitation; and the extent of ^{32}P incorporation estimated in terms of moles of phosphate if the specific radioactivity of the $[\gamma\text{-}^{32}P]ATP$ formed in the tissue is determined (30,79,150). To measure phosphorylation *in vitro* of a purified protein substrate, a known amount is incubated with a purified kinase, $[\gamma\text{-}^{32}P]ATP$

and any other required co-factors, and the protein precipitated to measure ^{32}P incorporation. Likewise, in the assay commonly used for measuring protein kinase activity, histone or a synthetic peptide substrate is adsorbed on phosphocellulose paper using phosphoric acid (186). Most commonly, protocols for investigation of ^{32}P incorporation into heart proteins involve sodium dodecyl sulphate (SDS) polyacrylamide gel electrophoresis of a whole extract, a general protein precipitate of an extract, or an antibody precipitate. Radioactivity in protein bands can be estimated qualitatively by the intensity of bands in the autoradiograph or measured quantitatively by counting the radioactivity in an antibody precipitate or a gel slice containing the band. It should be mentioned that ^{32}P incorporation may be an imperfect method to determine the role of cyclic AMP or other agents in protein phosphorylation since identification of protein bands is difficult. (See the list of pitfalls in ref. 132.)

When measuring protein-bound phosphate by a chemical method, it is essential to have a pure protein. Although sensitive assays have been developed, larger amounts of protein than are needed for the determination of ^{32}P incorporation may often be required to obtain sufficient protein-bound phosphate for the chemical assay, and thus chemical methods are not often used for measuring phosphate of protein bands in gel slices. Chemical methods generally involve washing of the protein and removal of nonphosphoester-bound phosphate before hydrolysis in 0.1 N NaOH to release protein-bound phosphate for assay (146). Direct chemical measurements of phosphate are more accurate than ^{32}P incorporation and have advantages in some situations since they detect the presence of endogenous protein-bound phosphate which may turn over slowly, as well as the extra ^{32}P incorporated in an experiment.

Intact Heart

Heart protein phosphorylation can be studied in intact animals using injection of ^{32}P$_i$ or chemical measurement of protein-bound phosphate, but more frequently a perfused heart preparation is used. The heart is removed from the animal and perfused in either the normal *in vivo* direction (working heart) (157,207), or in the reverse direction by the Langendorff procedure (155). A pressure transducer can be attached to the system and pressure development and frequency recorded. To measure phosphorylation, ^{32}P$_i$ can be included in the perfusion buffer but even a preperfusion period of 60 min may not be sufficient for complete equilibration of ^{32}P$_i$ with cellular ATP (150). The perfused heart system lends itself particularly well to studies of hormone effects since a hormone can be added to the perfusion buffer and its effects on heart rate and contractile force recorded before removal of heart tissue for further analysis. Usually the

heart tissue is freeze-clamped with tongs cooled in liquid nitrogen and ground to a fine powder before suspension in buffer appropriate for the protein(s) being investigated. It is important to include agents such as sodium fluoride (NaF), ethyldiaminetetraacetate (EDTA), SDS, phosphate, and specific inhibitors of kinase and phosphatase activities to prevent changes in phosphorylation state from occurring in the extract.

In Vitro Studies

Phosphorylation has been studied in cultured neonatal heart cells (80,116) as well as in myocytes prepared from adult hearts (methods reviewed in ref. 55). Hormones can be added to the incubation medium but changes in rate and strength are technically more difficult to measure than in the perfused heart. Action potentials in isolated heart cells have been recorded using microelectrodes (15,166). Alteration of the permeability properties of heart cells has been useful for probing regulators of phosphorylation (148,229). Protein phosphorylation has also been studied using sarcolemma or sarcoplasmic reticulum membrane preparations which are believed to be pure and not contaminated by each other (13,98,215,216). [γ-^{32}P]ATP, and not ^{32}P$_i$, is used with subcellular fractions or isolated heart proteins, and agents such as NaF can be added to prevent excessive endogenous ATPase activities (215). Endogenous phosphorylation may be measured in subcellular fractions, or purified substrate proteins or protein kinases may be added to subcellular fractions to investigate phosphorylation by endogenous protein kinases or of endogenous substrates, respectively.

PROTEINS PHOSPHORYLATED IN HEART

General Spectrum Studies

In studies with perfused heart (6,121,128,135,196), rat ventricular slices (46), rat myocytes (164), and cultured heart cells (80,117) incubated with ^{32}P$_i$, as many as thirty phosphoproteins are resolved by electrophoresis on SDS-polyacrylamide gels. Some of the phosphorylated bands have been identified, although often tentatively, as myosin light chain (M_r 20,000), phosphorylase (M_r 94,000), myosin light chain phosphatase (M_r 70,000), troponin T (M_r 37,000), troponin I (M_r 28,000), and phospholamban. Isoproterenol and catecholamines cause marked changes in the extent of phosphorylation of five or more of the bands (46,121,128,135,164,196). In most cases there is increased ^{32}P incorporation into protein bands including those believed to be C-protein (M_r 150,000–155,000), phosphorylase, troponin I, myosin light chain, and phospholamban, but in at least one case (protein band of M_r 30,000) decreased ^{32}P incorporation occurs (46). In studies with subcellular fractions, cyclic AMP-dependent and Ca^{2+}-calmodulin-dependent protein kinases are found in both sarcoplasmic reticulum and sarcolemmal fractions as well as in the cytosol (13,57,98,120,215). Walsh et al. (220) detected two phosphoproteins (identified as A and B) in a purified sarcolemmal fraction from rat heart. The A protein (M_r 36,000) is phosphorylated by both cyclic AMP-independent and cyclic AMP-dependent protein kinases, whereas the B protein (M_r 27,000) is phosphorylated by cyclic AMP-dependent protein kinase (cAK) and in response to epinephrine. The B protein might have a role in modulation of Ca^{2+} transport and is possibly the same as a phosphorylatable protein of M_r 24,000 which interconverts to a form of M_r 9,000 (126). Two proteins of M_r 6,000 to 8,000 and M_r 21,000 to 24,000 (probably phospholamban) are rapidly phosphorylated in dog cardiac sarcoplasmic reticulum when cyclic AMP and cAK or Ca^{2+} and calmodulin are present, but endogenous phosphorylation is much slower (13). Phosphorylase and Ca^{2+}-Mg^{2+}-ATPase are also phosphorylated in the sarcoplasmic reticulum (13,98). There still remains much confusion regarding the nature of peptides phosphorylated in different membrane fractions, and whether or not the peptides correspond between different studies (215).

Table 1 is a list of proteins identified as being phosphorylated in heart. (Other phosphorylatable proteins are listed in refs. 59, 122.) Phosphorylation is of particular interest if it is associated with altered behavior, since this may indicate possible regulatory function (see refs. 122 and 151 for a set of criteria for establishing that phosphorylation of an enzyme may be physiologically significant).

Phosphorylation of Proteins Involved in the Contractile Process

Myosin P-light chain or myosin light chain 2 (M_r 20,000) is phosphorylated in heart, whereas myosin heavy chain (M_r 200,000) and myosin light chain 1 (M_r 26,000) are not (6,46,97,116,165). P-light chain isolated from perfused rat heart contains 0.5 to 0.6 moles phosphate/mole, and this is not affected by epinephrine or change in perfusate Ca^{2+} concentrations (97). Phosphorylation of P-light chain is not obligatory for the interaction of actin and myosin in heart (97) and it is not clear what regulatory role myosin light chain phosphorylation may have in heart muscle where control of contraction is effected primarily via troponin. Recent reviews (18,26,165) discuss possible effects of cardiac myosin phosphorylation and compare heart with skeletal and smooth muscle.

Myosin light chain kinase (MLCK) is believed to be responsible for phosphorylation of P-light chain (26).

TABLE 1. *Phosphorylation of cardiac proteins*

Protein phosphorylated	Kinases shown to cause phorphorylation	Effect of phosphorylation
Myosin P-light chain	MLCK	?
Myosin light chain kinase	cAK, MLCK	Decreases activity
Troponin I	cAK, Phos. kinase	Increases Ca^{2+} removal from troponin; promotes relaxation
Troponin T	cAK, Phos. kinase	?
Phospholamban	cAK, Phos. kinase Calmodulin-dependent PK	Promotes relaxation; stimulates Ca^{2+} pump of SR
Ca^{2+}-ATPase of sarcolemma (or associated protein)	cAK, Phos. kinase	Activates to extrude Ca^{2+}
Phosphorylase	Phos. kinase	Increases activity
Phos. kinase	cAK, Phos. kinase	Increases activity
Glycogen synthase	cAK, Phos. kinase cAMP-independent PK	Decreases activity
cAMP-dependent PK		
Type I	cGK	Promotes activation
Type II	cAK	Promotes activation by cAMP
C subunit	cAK	?
cGMP-dependent PK	cGK	Promotes activation by cGMP
Pyruvate dehydrogenase	PDH kinase	Decreases activity

Abbreviations: MLCK = myosin light chain kinase; Phos. kinase = phosphorylase kinase; cAK = cAMP-dependent protein kinase; cGK = cGMP-dependent protein kinase; PK = protein kinase; SR = sarcoplasmic reticulum; PDH = pyruvate dehydrogenase.

The Ca^{2+}-dependent enzyme purified from beef heart is dimeric with subunits of M_r 85,000 to 94,000 (221,233). Binding of Ca^{2+} and calmodulin to purified MLCK causes activation. The heart enzyme is phosphorylated by catalytic subunit of cAK (C subunit), Ca^{2+}-calmodulin-dependent autophosphorylation, or both, resulting in the incorporation of 1 mole phosphate/mole MLCK (233). The slow rate of the C subunit-catalyzed phosphorylation of heart MLCK casts doubt on its physiological significance (233). In addition, for the smooth muscle enzyme, calmodulin appears to inhibit phosphorylation by C subunit (34). Phosphorylation is believed to decrease MLCK activity, but this has not been fully investigated in heart (18,59).

Both troponin I and troponin T (but not troponin C) are phosphorylated in heart, and phosphorylation of troponin I is believed to regulate Ca^{2+} interactions with cardiac myofibrils (18,229). Troponin I is phosphorylated preferentially at serine 20 by cAK, and at serine 72 and threonines 138 and 162 by phosphorylase kinase (154). Phosphate bound at serine 20 is likely to be important in control of contraction since changes in phosphorylation of this site, but not the others, occur when rabbit heart is perfused with epinephrine (154). Phosphorylase kinase probably does not phosphorylate troponin I *in vivo* since troponin I phosphorylation occurs as expected in hearts from phosphorylase kinase-deficient (I-strain) mice (52), and the sites phosphorylated by phosphorylase kinase are not accessible in the presence of troponin C (154). In rat heart perfused with increasing concentrations of epinephrine there is a good correlation under most, but not all, conditions between increased phosphorylation of troponin I and increasing force of contraction (50,51). In the process of muscle contraction troponin I is responsible for inhibition of actomyosin Mg^{2+}-ATPase in the absence of Ca^{2+}, and binding of Ca^{2+} to troponin C results in a reversal of this inhibitory effect of troponin I, thereby allowing contraction to occur. Phosphorylation of troponin I may decrease the sensitivity of the actomyosin Mg^{2+}-ATPase to Ca^{2+} and help stabilize the contractile response of the myocardium to β-adrenergic agonists and speed up relaxation (18,154,229). In the bovine cardiac troponin complex, phosphorylation of troponin I by cAK decreases the concentration of Ca^{2+} required to achieve 50% binding to troponin C, and increases the rate of removal of Ca^{2+} from the troponin complex (180). Since phosphorylation increases the sensitivity of troponin I to proteolysis by a cardiac Ca^{2+}-activated neutral protease, phosphorylation by cAK could control troponin destruction in a situation such as myocardial infarction when cyclic AMP levels and intramuscular protease activities increase (212).

Despite numerous studies much is still unknown regarding the nature of phospholamban and its regulatory role in contraction. It is uncertain whether phospholamban is confined to the sarcoplasmic reticulum or whether it, or a very similar proteolipid named calciductin by Demaille et al. (18), is also bound to the sarcolemma (18,57,98,215). Phospholamban is a proteolipid of M_r 22,000, but its ability to dissociate into smaller forms has added confusion to its identification in phosphorylation studies. Louis et al. (139) reported that canine cardiac phospholamban reversibly dissociates into fragments of M_r 11,000, 15,000, and 20,000 when sarcoplasmic reticulum is solubilized in 1% SDS and heated at 71°C for 2 min in 1 mM $MgCl_2$, and they proposed that phospholamban is a trimer of subunits of M_r 11,000, 8,000, and 4,000. On the other hand, Kirchberger and Antonetz (113) found that phospholamban in dog heart microsomes dissociates into forms of M_r 11,000 and 5,500 upon boiling the SDS-treated form of M_r 22,000. Triton X-100 also causes the formation of a form of M_r 11,000 (113). Phospholamban purified from dog cardiac sarcoplasmic reticulum is phosphorylated by cAK to a level of 0.15 moles phosphate/mole protein (12), and its properties alter to become resistant to trypsin digestion or deoxycholate solubilization (13). Early studies had shown increased Ca^{2+} uptake in association with phosphorylation of phospholamban by cAK in cardiac microsomes from dog, cat, rabbit, and guinea pig (114). Phospholamban is also phosphorylated by exogenous phosphorylase kinase and by an endogenous membrane-bound, calmodulin-dependent protein kinase (18,129,206). Different phosphorylation sites are involved, with ^{32}P incorporation and the increases in Ca^{2+} uptake and Ca^{2+}-dependent ATPase activity being additive with cyclic AMP- or calmodulin-dependent phosphorylation (26,129,206). From studies in perfused rat heart using fluphenazine to inhibit Ca^{2+}- plus calmodulin-dependent phosphorylation of phospholamban, or propanolol to inhibit isoproterenol-stimulated cyclic AMP-dependent phosphorylation (128), it is believed that Ca^{2+}-dependent phospholamban kinase may be a permanent Ca^{2+} sensor which activates the Ca^{2+} pump when free Ca^{2+} increases during systole, thereby helping to induce relaxation. β-Adrenergic agonists which increase cyclic AMP and activate cAK can increase relaxation by hyperactivation of the Ca^{2+} pump due to the additional cyclic AMP-dependent phosphorylation of phospholamban (18,26,128,129). Although several steps in the Ca^{2+}-ATPase reaction sequence are stimulated by sarcoplasmic reticulum phosphorylation (119) and the Ca^{2+}-Mg^{2+}-ATPase has been isolated (12), the exact mechanism by which phospholamban phosphorylation can stimulate the Ca^{2+} pump is not clear. Ca^{2+}-transport activity in rat cardiac sarcoplasmic reticulum also increases following phosphorylation by a Ca^{2+}-activated, phospholipid-dependent protein kinase (130). Phosphorylation by cAK of cardiac sarcoplasmic reticulum affects the external Ca^{2+}-binding sites but the proteins involved are not known (145).

The sarcolemmal Ca^{2+}-ATPase responsible for transport of Ca^{2+} out of myocardial cells also appears to be activated by phosphorylation (18). The turnover rate of Ca^{2+}-ATPase in dog heart sarcolemmal vesicles increases with phosphorylation apparently by cAK and decreases upon dephosphorylation by phosphorylase phosphatase (20). The Ca^{2+}-pump affinity for Ca^{2+} also increases upon cyclic AMP-dependent phosphorylation in dog heart sarcolemma (126), but stimulation of Ca^{2+} transport in pig heart sarcolemmal membranes is small unless both C subunit and calmodulin are present together (217). However, the purified sarcolemmal Ca^{2+}-ATPase is not itself phosphorylated by ATP and cAK suggesting that it is not the target of the regulatory phosphorylation (21). A possible candidate is the dog heart sarcolemmal protein of M_r 9,000 which is phosphorylated by both Ca^{2+}- plus calmodulin- and cyclic AMP-dependent protein kinases (126). Neither cyclic AMP- nor calmodulin-dependent phosphorylation of bovine cardiac sarcolemmal membranes affects potassium-stimulated Ca^{2+} uptake by the Na^+-Ca^{2+} exchanger (57), the other means of transporting Ca^{2+} out of the cell (18).

Phosphorylation of Enzymes Involved in Glycogen Metabolism

Much of the previous work on glycogen metabolism used skeletal muscle and liver systems, but many features apply also to heart. Numerous reviews describe the properties and regulation of muscle and liver phosphorylase, phosphorylase kinase, and glycogen synthase (19,31,59,122,159,199) and this section focuses on the more recent studies of the heart enzymes. Phosphorylation of phosphorylase (M_r 94,000) has been demonstrated in intact cells and sarcoplasmic reticulum, and is increased by treatment with isoproterenol, epinephrine, and norepinephrine (46,164) which activate cAK and phosphorylase kinase. Phosphorylase kinase is itself phosphorylated and activated by cAK, cyclic GMP-dependent protein kinase (cGK), and autophosphorylation (Ca^{2+}-dependent), as well as being activated by a Ca^{2+}-dependent proteolytic enzyme (19,31,59,122,159, 199). Phosphorylase kinase from beef heart, which differs from the skeletal muscle enzyme in its smaller α subunit (denoted α') (151), has a molecular weight (MW) of about 1.3×10^6, and is composed of four subunits: α' (M_r 134,000), β (M_r 125,000), and γ (M_r 48,000), with stoichiometry $\alpha'_1\beta_{1.01}\gamma_{1.35}$ together with small amounts of δ (M_r 20,000) which is believed to be calmodulin (35). In the presence of C subunit and $[\gamma-^{32}P]$ATP, both α' and β subunits are phosphorylated and the increased activity correlates with phosphate incorporation into both α' and β subunits (35,36). α'-Subunit phosphorylation starts at a slower rate than β-subunit phosphorylation, but reaches a higher maximum level of incorporation. Once β-subunit phosphorylation is maximal at

1 mole phosphate/mole phosphorylase kinase (4 moles β subunits), cyclic AMP-dependent phosphorylation of the α' subunit continues to activate the bovine heart enzyme (36). The α' subunit is also phosphorylated by a cyclic AMP-independent reaction, probably representing autocatalysis (205). A close relationship between ^{32}P incorporation into the immunoprecipitated enzyme and activation of phosphorylase kinase by epinephrine is found in perfused rat hearts (151).

Phosphorylation and inactivation of glycogen synthase involves multisite phosphorylation catalyzed by a number of different kinases. When bovine heart glycogen synthase which is 95% in the dephosphorylated I form (independent of glucose 6-phosphate) is incubated with bovine heart C subunit and a low concentration of ATP, 1 mole phosphate/mole subunit is incorporated, and the I form decreases to 50% (153). With a higher ATP concentration 2 moles phosphate/mole subunit is incorporated and there is almost total conversion to the D form that is dependent on glucose 6-phosphate for activity. The extent of phosphorylation up to 2 moles phosphate/mole subunit correlates linearly with conversion of glycogen synthase to the D form, using either or both of cAK and a cyclic AMP-independent protein kinase from beef heart (153,174). Cleavage by cyanogen bromide to separate phosphorylated sites reveals that predominantly one peptide is phosphorylated by cAK at low ATP concentrations, compared with two peptides at higher concentrations (153). Likewise, glycogen synthase is phosphorylated at multiple sites in perfused rat heart (150), and these sites are similar to those phosphorylated in the rabbit skeletal muscle enzyme (150,197). Presumably, heart glycogen synthase, as well as phosphorylase kinase, will be shown to be phosphorylated by protein kinases other than cAK, such as a Ca^{2+}-calmodulin-dependent protein kinase (168). Only under certain conditions, such as depleted cardiac glycogen levels, is epinephrine found to increase phosphorylation and decrease glycogen synthase activity (150,174).

Phosphorylation of Other Proteins

Phosphorylation of the cyclic AMP-dependent and cyclic GMP-dependent protein kinases are discussed in later sections.

The link between pyruvate formation and the citric acid cycle is the formation of acetyl CoA. This occurs in the matrix space of mitochondria, catalyzed by the pyruvate dehydrogenase complex. The complex includes a minimum of three enzymes, the dehydrogenase, a lipoyl transacetylase, and a dihydrolipoyl dehydrogenase. The dehydrogenase, which contains two α and two β chains, is the enzyme which is phosphorylated.

The activity of pyruvate dehydrogenase (PDH) in heart can be regulated by a cyclic AMP-independent kinase and a phosphatase intrinsic to its mitochondrial complex (199). Incorporation of about 0.5 mole phosphate/mole α subunit occurs rapidly and almost exclusively at site 1, resulting in nearly complete inactivation of PDH (236). Partial phosphorylation at sites 2 and 3 occurs slowly up to a maximum of 1.5 moles phosphate/mole α subunit corresponding to 3 serine residues phosphorylated/mole $\alpha_2\beta_2$ complex (110,236). Phosphorylation of site 1 correlates with loss of activity, while phosphorylation at the other two sites inhibits reactivation by the phosphatase (110). PDH in perfused rat heart is activated by epinephrine and isoproterenol (83,149), but it is not known whether this involves kinase regulation or Ca^{2+} activation of the specific phosphatase which is loosely associated with the complex (110,199).

Liver phosphofructokinase has recently been shown to be regulated by fructose-2,6-bisphosphate (62,171,214) which is formed from fructose 6-phosphate in a reaction catalyzed by 6-phosphofructo 2-kinase/fructose-2,6-bisphosphatase (170). Phosphorylation of liver 6-phosphofructo 2-kinase/fructose-2,6-bisphosphatase by cAK inactivates the kinase activity and activates the phosphatase activity (172), but it remains to be seen whether this regulates cardiac phosphofructokinase. Fructose-2,6-bisphosphate concentrations in heart decrease in ischemia, but are not changed by epinephrine perfusion (88,89). Although phosphofructokinase may be phosphorylated in skeletal muscle and liver (122), there is no suggestion of this in heart. In perfused rat heart phosphofructokinase is activated by epinephrine in an α-adrenergic, cyclic AMP-independent mechanism and is not reactivated by phosphatases (167).

CYCLIC AMP-DEPENDENT PROTEIN KINASE

Identification of Heart Cyclic AMP-Dependent Protein Kinase

A section is devoted to cAK since it plays such a significant role in regulation of contractility. cAK is a tetramer consisting of 2 regulatory (R) subunits and 2 catalytic (C) subunits. (Reviews of the properties of cAK are found in refs. 19,59,122,159.) Activation occurs upon cyclic AMP binding to R subunit thereby releasing C subunit which is catalytically active in the absence of the inhibitory R subunit. Once cyclic AMP concentrations decrease, C subunits reassociate with R subunits to reform the inhibited holoenzyme.

$$R_2C_2 + 4\,cAMP \rightleftharpoons R_2cAMP_4 + 2C$$

Two major classes of cAK, recognized by their elution at different salt concentrations from a diethylaminoethyl (DEAE)-cellulose column, differ in their R subunit which exists in at least two isozyme forms. This is based on DEAE-cellulose elution, immunological tests, amino acid composition data, peptide mapping, reassociation experiments, and gel electrophoresis (19,39,75). Differences between the type I and type II holoenzymes in their susceptibility to dissociation by salt or histone is important when measuring protein kinase activity, since the composition of the extraction buffer can change the extent of dissociation. cAK activity is usually determined as an activity ratio, i.e., activity in the absence of added cyclic AMP divided by activity in the presence of sufficient cyclic AMP to achieve maximum activity. By SDS gel electrophoresis, free R^I and R^{II} have M_rs of 49,000 and 56,000, respectively, while the M_r of C subunit is 41,000 (19).

R subunits can be identified in crude extracts of heart by labeling with 8-azido[^{32}P]cAMP, which is then covalently attached by photolysis before separation of radioactive bands by SDS-polyacrylamide gel electrophoresis (16,98,175,187,223). Specificity of 8-azido-cAMP binding is confirmed by its ability to be competitively inhibited by cyclic AMP, and the amount and proportions of R^I and R^{II} are estimated using appropriate controls to ensure full saturation. This method has located cAK in the sarcolemma (98) and sarcoplasmic reticulum (121) of heart as well as in the soluble fraction. A concentration of KCl greater than 150 mM in extraction buffers prevents nonspecific adsorption of free C subunit to particulate material (106). The remaining membrane-bound cAK is almost entirely type II, indistinguishable from the soluble type II isozyme (41,98), and represents approximately 20 to 30% of the total cAK in beef or rat heart (38,41) and 50% in rabbit heart (16,41). The proportions of the two isozymes in the cytosol also vary in hearts of different species. Beef heart cytosol contains predominantly the type II isozyme, and is thus chosen for isolation of the enzyme for extensive characterization (38,41,59,175,184). Indeed, many original studies of cAK used the bovine heart enzyme, and its properties seem to be very similar in other tissues. Rat and mouse hearts contain more than 80% of the type I form; whereas guinea pig heart contains greater than 90% type II; and human, dog, and rabbit hearts contain approximately equal amounts of the two isozymes (38,183).

Protein Kinase Inhibitor

Another protein besides R subunit which binds tightly to C subunit to inhibit its activity is the low-MW, acid- and heat-stable protein kinase inhibitor protein. This inhibitor can possibly control C subunit *in vivo* since enough of it is present in rabbit skeletal muscle to inhibit basal protein kinase activity (8). Although there have been few studies of its physiological role, protein kinase inhibitor is frequently used to test for cAK-catalyzed phosphorylations. Protein kinase inhibitor exhibits a variety of forms differing in charge and size (227). Three distinct charge isomers are separable by

DEAE-cellulose chromatography of the bovine heart form, and each exists as two molecular size species, I and I'. After purification from rabbit skeletal muscle, the probable physiological I form has a MW of 22,000 by gel exclusion chromatography, 10,000 to 11,000 by SDS gel electrophoresis, and 8,300 to 8,700 by amino acid analysis (227). Protein kinase inhibitor is believed to inhibit C subunit by interaction with the C subunit Mg^{2+}-ATP complex, and in its mode of interaction shares many similarities with R (228).

Physical Properties of R and C Subunits

The amino acid sequences for both R^{II} (208) and C (192,193) subunits of the bovine heart enzyme have recently been completed. This complements earlier work on R subunit which by proteolytic cleavage localized domains of the protein responsible for various functions such as cyclic AMP binding, phosphorylation, and interaction with C subunit (59,210), and led to schematic models of the domains in R^{II} (60) and R^{I} (178). The primary structure of bovine heart R^{II} indicates considerable homology between two regions of the polypeptide chain: residues 135 to 256 and 257 to 400 (208). These two sequences could represent the two cyclic AMP binding sites known to be present in each subunit, and presumably result from internal gene duplication (see later section). On each side of the autophosphorylation site at serine-95 there are two extremely acidic regions (residues 73–83 and 104–111), one or both of which may be involved in interaction with C subunit (208). Surprisingly the MW of R^{II} calculated from sequence data of the 400 amino acids is 45,084 which is considerably lower than the M_r of 56,000 determined by SDS-polyacrylamide gel electrophoresis. X-ray crystallographic studies are currently in progress to provide a three-dimensional model of R^{II}.

Bovine heart C subunit contains 350 residues with its MW calculated to be 40,580 (192,193). It has an N-terminal blocking group of n-tetradecanoic acid which is amide-linked to glycine (23,192). C subunit can catalyze autophosphorylation and when isolated contains more than 1 mole phosphate/mole protein (9). There are two phosphorylation sites, threonine-196 and serine-337, which are relatively close to the two cysteine residues of 198 and 342 (192,193). (Studies of active site-directed reagents and kinetics with both normal substrates and analogs to investigate the nature of the active site, its reactive cysteine residue, and the reaction mechanism of C subunit are reviewed in refs. 19,59,210.) The synthetic peptide often called kemptide, Leu-Arg-Arg-Ala-Ser-Leu-Gly (43,84,110), contains a sequence of amino acids similar to that frequently found at sites in proteins phosphorylated by C subunit (19,31,70,159). It has been suggested that this particularly good substrate should be used in comparisons of protein kinase activities

in various tissues (44). A synthetic peptide derived from a second frequently found phosphorylation site sequence, that of the β subunit of phosphorylase kinase, may also be useful since fluorescence changes as peptide phosphorylation proceeds can be monitored continuously (142). Studies with this other site sequence suggest that the tertiary structure as well as the primary structure play a role in substrate specificity of C subunit (237). A three-dimensional model for the arrangement of substrates at the active site has been constructed from kinetic studies and using electron spin resonance and nuclear magnetic resonance techniques (72). The active complex is an enzyme-ATP-metal bridge, and inhibition of C subunit activity in the holoenzyme is achieved by R subunit blocking the binding site of the protein substrate. Recent kinetic studies which attempt to explain apparent inconsistencies of previous data concluded that with kemptide as substrate, C subunit follows a steady state ordered B_i-B_i kinetic mechanism with nucleotide binding first (226,228).

Regulation by Cyclic AMP

It was found that the beef heart R subunit binds 2 moles of cyclic AMP on each subunit (42). That these two sites differ from one another (59) is indicated by the biphasic curve of dissociation of [³H]cAMP bound to R^{I} or R^{II} upon the addition of excess unlabeled cyclic AMP (48,178) and the biphasic quenching of the fluorescence of $1,N^6$-etheno-cAMP as it binds to R (127). [³H]cAMP dissociates more rapidly from site 2 than from site 1 which has a higher affinity for cyclic AMP (178). The inclusion of certain analogs of cyclic AMP during the binding of [³H]cAMP to either R^{I} or R^{II} can prevent [³H]cAMP binding at one of the two sites (178). Thus 8-bromo-cAMP enhances the fast component of the [³H]cAMP dissociation curve suggesting that 8-bromo-cAMP binds at site 1 (the slower dissociating site) preferentially to cyclic AMP (178). Analogs of cyclic AMP with modifications at the 8-position generally prefer site 1, and those with modifications at the 6-position prefer site 2 (40,178). With the holoenzyme, but not free R subunit, an analog specific for one site is able to stimulate binding of another analog at the other site (179). Thus, 8-bromo-cAMP which selects site 1 stimulates the binding of [³H]cyclic inosine monophosphate (cIMP) to site 2 (40,179). Studies with [³H]cAMP and 8-azido[³²P]cAMP indicated that in like manner an analog selective for site 2 stimulates binding of an analog selective for site 1 and as with [³H]cIMP the order of potency differs for the type I and type II holoenzymes (40,182). This difference is a potential way of distinguishing between the two isozymes. In crude heart extracts from rat (181), dog, guinea pig, and rabbit (183) the stimulation pattern of [³H]cIMP-binding by analogs is consistent with the relative proportions of the two isozymes. Mg^{2+}-ATP is necessary for maximum stimulation of binding of one analog by another with the type I, but not the type II purified holoenzyme (40,181); and Mg^{2+}-ATP concentrations are already high enough in fresh heart extracts (181,183). Mg^{2+}-ATP prevents dissociation of the type I holoenzyme (19) and magnifies the difference between binding rates in the presence or absence of a stimulatory analog by slowing both rates to be linear when binding is measured (181).

The ability of an analog bound at one site to stimulate cyclic nucleotide binding at the other suggests that such cooperativity can occur *in vivo*, with the binding of cyclic AMP at one site stimulating binding at the other. Kinetic studies of cyclic AMP binding to bovine heart free R^{II} subunit indicate that binding of cyclic AMP at site 2 affects the rates of cyclic AMP association to and dissociation from site 1, and that site 2 can interact with cyclic AMP only after site 1 is occupied (161,162). Consistent with this, only site 1 of bovine heart type II holoenzyme contains bound cyclic AMP at very low subsaturating cyclic AMP concentrations (179). Rates of [^{3}H]cIMP binding in extracts from rat heart perfused in the absence and presence of epinephrine and 3-isobutyl-1-methylxanthine can test such intersite interactions *in vivo* (181). If the increased intracellular cyclic AMP binds only at site 1, the rate of [^{3}H]cIMP binding is expected to increase since site-2 binding sites will not decrease and site-1 binding would stimulate site-2 binding. The rate of [^{3}H]cIMP binding actually decreases suggesting that both sites become occupied upon elevation of tissue cyclic AMP leaving fewer unoccupied sites to which [^{3}H]cIMP can bind (181). This is consistent with binding of endogenous cyclic AMP at site 1 promoting rapid binding of a second cyclic AMP molecule at site 2. It is not known if such apparent site interaction occurs between two sites on the same or different R subunits of the holoenzyme.

The nature of the site(s) responsible for kinase activation could potentially be determined convincingly if analogs could be found which are so highly selective for each site that they do not bind significantly at the other. Studies with analogs of less than ideal selectivity disagree as to which site is responsible for activation. The site-2 selective analog, cIMP, is more efficient at activating bovine heart type II protein kinase than cyclic AMP (179), whereas site-1 binding appears to be responsible for activation in studies correlating activation with binding of 8-azido-cAMP to type II (111) and a series of analogs to type I (45). However, neither study considers the possible involvement of site 2 and considerable 8-azido-cAMP binding can occur at site 2 (162). Furthermore, comparison of analog binding to free R^I with activation of the holoenzyme (45) does not seem valid since the binding characteristics of R alter upon association with C subunit (161,179). The potency of over 80 different analogs as activators of rabbit skeletal muscle type-I protein kinase correlates with the mean affinity for sites 1 and 2 rather than with the affinity for only one site (163). This, together with the finding that a combination of two analogs, one site-1 selective and the other site-2 selective, activates protein kinase synergistically suggests that both sites 1 and 2 are involved in the process of activation (163,182). It does not necessarily eliminate the possibility that binding at one particular site actually triggers the activation, but binding at the other may be required to get sufficient binding at the site ultimately responsible for activation (182). The degree of synergism between two analogs in activating protein kinase correlates with their selectivity (163). The order of potency of analogs in their synergistic effect with an analog selective for the other site is very similar to their order of effectiveness to stimulate analog binding (182). Cooperativity in cyclic nucleotide binding is apparent in the activation curves with cyclic AMP for both the type I and type II holoenzymes from rat heart (182). Kinetic and analog activation studies generally agree that cyclic AMP binds to the holoenzyme to form a ternary complex before dissociation of the ternary complex into R_2cAMP_4 and C (59,72). Measurements of fluorescence and circular dichroic changes suggest that cyclic AMP binding to free R^I induces a conformational or structural change, and activation of type-I holoenzyme by cyclic AMP appears to require the binding of four molecules of cyclic AMP before release of C subunit (198). Cyclic AMP dissociation is cooperative when titrating the R^I dimer containing bound $1,N^6$-etheno-cAMP, with C subunit (198). However, the nature of the inter- and intra-chain interactions between binding sites during activation are not yet resolved. Analog selectivity can be used to map the steric conformation of the cyclic AMP binding sites of cAK, and cyclic AMP is believed to bind in a *syn* conformation at both sites (40,49). Analogs have been used to probe the activation of cAK in intact adipose tissue cells (10), and similar techniques may prove to be useful in heart.

Compartmentalization

A number of observations of the behavior of cAK suggest that the enzyme may be compartmentalized within the heart cell. Whereas activation of protein kinase generally correlates with tissue cyclic AMP concentrations, the protein kinase activity ratio or bound cyclic AMP sometimes increases to a greater extent than would be expected from the increase in cyclic AMP concentration, and occasionally the activity ratio changes without a detectable change in tissue cyclic AMP concentrations (182). A possible explanation in some cases could be the cooperativity of cyclic AMP binding and protein kinase activation (182). However, this cannot explain the findings in perfused rat and rabbit hearts and incubated rabbit cardiomyocytes where isoproterenol or prostaglandin E_1 each increase cyclic AMP concentrations and protein kinase activity ratios, but only isoproterenol activates phosphorylase, inhibits glycogen synthase, and increases phosphorylation of troponin I (16,17,81,103). Compartmentalization of cAK into bound and soluble forms offers an explanation since cyclic AMP concentrations increase and cAK activity decreases in the particulate fraction with isoproterenol but not prostaglandin E_1, although both increase soluble cAK activity (16,17). Measurement of unoccupied cyclic AMP binding sites in perfused rabbit hearts by 8-azido[^{32}P]cAMP binding also indicates that isoproterenol increases bound cyclic AMP in both soluble and particulate fractions whereas prostaglandin E_1 increases soluble bound cyclic AMP only (16). Perfusion of rat heart with epinephrine or 3-isobutyl-1-methylxanthine increases cyclic AMP binding in both particulate and cytosolic fractions, with release of C subunit into the soluble fraction when cyclic AMP binds to particulate R subunits (106). Membrane-bound cAK offers the potential for specificity of hormone action with hormone receptor, adenylate cyclase, cAK, and phosphorylatable protein organized in a localized area of the cell (16,17,41,164). Such postulated compartmentalization together with cooperative effects of cyclic AMP on cAK would allow activation without large increases in heart cyclic AMP, but more investigation is required and specific antibodies may prove particularly useful. For example, R^I, R^{II}, and C subunits have been immunocytochemically located in the area of the sarcoplasmic reticulum and periodic cross-bands of rat skeletal muscle (117), and specific fluorescent antibodies have located R^I and R^{II} in the nucleus of MCF-7 human breast cancer cells before redistribution of R^{II} to the cytoplasm and plasma membrane region upon progression of growth (99). Measurements of the absolute levels using monospecific antibodies (137) and of the activation state (136) of each isozyme in heart fractions may be potentially useful for investigating the functions of R^I and R^{II}. The suggestion that protein kinase subunits can undergo translocation from cytosol to nucleus has remained controversial and most of the evidence has been obtained in tissues other than heart. It has been suggested that the ability of bovine heart R^{II} to form a specific complex with chromatin constituents may provide a basis for R^{II}-specific translocation to the nucleus, thereby causing isozyme-type selectivity (225).

Phosphorylation of R

A marked difference between the type I and type II holoenzymes is that type II undergoes autophosphorylation, whereas type I does not (19,59,60,65,85,184). A phosphoprotein phosphatase isolated from bovine cardiac muscle catalyzes dephosphorylation of the phosphorylated free R^{II} subunit as well as phosphorylase, histone,

and casein (28). The phosphatase is inhibited by P_i and ATP and activated by manganese, but is inactive with the holoenzyme form of cAK in the absence of cyclic AMP (28). It has also been reported recently that protein phosphatase-2B (see later) purified from bovine heart readily dephosphorylates the autophosphorylation site of R^{II} in a calmodulin-dependent reaction that is inhibited by C subunit (14). In rat heart cytosol there is a phosphoprotein phosphatase activity which dephosphorylates R^{II} and is stimulated by cyclic AMP, presumably by interaction of cyclic AMP with the substrate (213). Despite differences in the parameter investigated, phosphorylation generally promotes the rate of dissociation of R and C subunits by cyclic AMP, thus increasing catalytically active enzyme (53,72,85). Dephosphorylated R^{II} subunits reassociate with C subunits to form holoenzyme to a 10-fold higher concentration of cyclic AMP than would phosphorylated R^{II} (176,177). However, there is no good evidence for a physiological role of phosphorylation in control of type II protein kinase activity (184). Phosphorylated R^{II} accounts for 82% of the total cardiac R^{II} in intact rats injected with $^{32}P_i$ (213) and purified bovine heart R^{II} generally contains between 1 and 3 moles phosphate/mole subunit (60,188). Sites in addition to the autophosphorylation site (serine-95) may be phosphorylated, possibly by kinases other than C subunit, without changes in enzyme properties (60,82,188). With high added C subunit concentrations, approximately 2 moles phosphate/mole subunit is incorporated into bovine heart R^{II}, whether dephosphorylated or containing 2 moles endogenous phosphate/mole subunit (188). In a preparation of bovine heart R^{II} containing 1.3 moles phosphate/mole subunit, most of the phosphate is associated with a peptide containing serines-74 and -76, which are phosphorylated preferentially by glycogen synthase kinase-5 *in vitro* (82). Less than 0.1 mole phosphate/mole subunit is associated with the autophosphorylation site together with serines-46 and -47, which are preferentially phosphorylated by glycogen synthase kinase-3 (82). Preferential phosphorylation of serine-95 by C subunit (82) may be primarily responsible for the altered behavior of R^{II} and its decreased mobility on SDS-polyacrylamide gel electrophoresis using a Tris-glycine buffer system (85,175). However, recent studies in our laboratory suggest that heart R^{II} from all species may not behave similarly (183) (see later).

Although phosphorylation of R^I has not been investigated in heart, phosphorylated forms of R^I are detectable in rat and bovine skeletal muscles by isoelectric focusing (66), and R^I from bovine skeletal muscle is phosphorylated up to 2 moles phosphate/mole subunit by high concentrations of beef lung cGK (65). This phosphorylation is promoted by cyclic AMP, suggesting that R^I containing bound cyclic AMP is probably the substrate. C subunit does not phosphorylate free R^I (65). However, cGK is unlikely to phosphorylate R^I *in vivo* since the reaction occurs very slowly *in vitro,* and R^I phosphorylated *in vivo* does not lose inhibitory activity towards C subunit nor half of its cyclic AMP binding sites as occurs upon R^I phosphorylation *in vitro* by cGK (64). One site phosphorylated by cGK in R^I is a serine residue in a sequence which shows many similarities to that surrounding serine-95 in R^{II} (77). Nucleotide-free R^I is a competitive inhibitor of phosphorylation reactions of cGK suggesting that R^I has an inhibitory domain for cGK as well as for C subunit consistent with the postulated close relationship between the cyclic AMP- and cyclic GMP-dependent protein kinases (see later).

Microheterogeneity

The first indication that more than one form of R^{II} exists was the finding that the peak of rat adipose tissue type II protein kinase activity eluted from DEAE-cellulose columns at a lower NaCl concentration than did rat heart type II, and the two could be separated when a mixture of the peak fractions was rechromatographed (39). More recently, specific antibodies distinguished a class of R^{II} present only in neural tissues which differs markedly from heart R^{II} (54,187). Whereas the two R^{II} classes are indistinguishable by SDS-polyacrylamide gel electrophoresis, elution from a DEAE-cellulose column or Sepharose-6B column, sucrose density gradient centrifugation, and isoelectric focusing of 8-azido[^{32}P]cAMP-labeled R^{II} subunits (54,187), there are differences in the two-dimensional tryptic peptide maps and in the main phosphorylated peptide (75). In addition, upon auto-phosphorylation with [γ-^{32}P]ATP, ^{32}P is incorporated into two immunoprecipitable bands of M_r 55,000 and 57,000 with the bovine brain holoenzyme, whereas only the slower migrating, higher M_r band of the bovine heart enzyme is labeled with ^{32}P (187). The ^{32}P incorporated into bovine brain R^{II} of M_r 55,000 could represent phosphorylation either at sites different to those phosphorylated in the more slowly migrating M_r 57,000 form or of another M_r 55,000 form of brain R^{II}, which upon phosphorylation does not change its mobility (187). Studies in our laboratory indicate differences in R^{II} from hearts of various species in their electrophoretic mobility on a standard Tris-glycine SDS-polyacrylamide gel system (183). At least four forms have been detected according to M_r and the effect of phosphorylation on electrophoretic mobility (Table 2). Those forms which shift to a more slowly migrating band on SDS gel electrophoresis after phosphorylation are designated type IIA, and those which do not shift are termed type IIB. No difference in R^I from these heart species has thus far been detected by SDS-gel electrophoresis. In view of the differences in electrophoretic mobility of R^{II} together with the finding that type I in some tissues does not elute where expected on DEAE-cellulose chromatography (143), immunoreactivity with antibodies against specific subclasses of R^I and R^{II} may be required ultimately for isozyme type classification. Although photolabeling with 8-azido[^{32}P]cAMP followed by determination of M_r of radioactive bands upon gel electrophoresis is useful for screening tissue extracts, not all R reacting immunologically as R^{II} or R^I migrates at M_r 54,000 to 56,000 and M_r 48,000 to 49,000, respectively (225). Such an immunological technique would also eliminate other cyclic AMP binding proteins which are not R subunit (48,204), as well as being able to quantitate R^I and R^{II} in heterologous systems (225). Weber et al. (225) summa-

TABLE 2. *Distribution of subclasses of type II R subunit*

	Apparent M_r by SDS gels	Shifts detectably to lower mobility form on standard SDS gels after phosphorylation	Tissue
Type IIA (ungulates, carnivores)	56,000	Yes	Bovine heart Porcine heart
	54,000	Yes	Canine heart Equine heart
Type IIB (rodents, lagomorphs, primates, ungulates)	52,000	No	Rabbit heart Guinea pig heart Bovine brain
	56,000	No	Rat heart Rabbit skeletal muscle Rat liver
	51,000	No	Rat brain Rat adipose tissue Monkey (*E. patas*) heart
	Equal mixture of 52,000 and 56,000	52,000 No 56,000 Yes	Bovine lung

rizes some of the immunoreactive R^I and R^{II} variants already found in mammalian tissues. Some variants may prove to be proteolytic breakdown products of R^I and R^{II}, and endogenous proteolysis of R may possibly serve some function *in vivo*. Although there are small interspecies differences such as two amino acids in 27 residues in the sequence surrounding lysine-72 in the ATP-binding site of C subunit from bovine and porcine hearts (192), C subunit from various tissues of the same species appears to have identical M_r, amino acid compositions, isoelectric points, and two-dimensional maps of tryptic peptides (59,75). However, two active forms of C subunit with different isoelectric points are found in rabbit skeletal muscle (9), and an inactive "mute" C subunit which can be activated by protein kinase inhibitor is detectable in rat muscle (63).

CYCLIC AMP-INDEPENDENT PROTEIN KINASES

Phosphorylase Kinase

Cardiac phosphorylase kinase is activated by Ca^{2+} ions and by phosphorylation by a number of kinases, but it is not certain which kinase(s) are important *in vivo* (see previous section). Although the α subunit differs, cardiac and skeletal muscle phosphorylase kinase have similar MWs, subunit stoichiometry, Ca^{2+} sensitivity, and increased activity in response to elevated cyclic AMP concentrations (35). Activity changes correlate well with β-subunit phosphorylation in skeletal muscle phosphorylase kinase (59,199), but the situation is less clear for the cardiac enzyme. Thus, while β-subunit phosphorylation accompanied by very little change in α'-subunit phosphorylation activates the cardiac enzyme, phosphorylation of the α' subunit also causes activation (205). It is uncertain whether prior phosphorylation of β subunit is obligatory for cyclic AMP-dependent phosphorylation of α' subunit since cyclic AMP-dependent phosphorylation of α' subunit is not known to occur without β-subunit phosphorylation which precedes that of the α' subunit in time course studies (205). On the other hand, autophosphorylation of the α' subunit occurs without β subunit phosphorylation, and probably involves sites different to those phosphorylated by cAK (205). The sites phosphorylated by cAK on heart phosphorylase kinase will presumably resemble those on skeletal muscle α and β subunits (31,159,199). Although the physiological role of autophosphorylation is unknown, cyclic AMP-dependent activation of phosphorylase kinase is likely to be a physiologically important reaction. The major substrate for phosphorylase kinase *in vivo* is probably phosphorylase, but the purified enzyme also phosphorylates itself, troponin I, tropinin T, glycogen synthase, cardiac sarcolemma, and phospholamban. Some of these substrates are not competitive

inhibitors of phosphorylase, suggesting that two catalytic sites exist (59,199). One catalytic site may be on the γ subunit and the other possibly on the β subunit, although in its ability to be phosphorylated the β subunit seems likely to have a regulatory function (59,199). Further investigation of the catalytic site(s) is necessary and may help to determine whether phosphorylation of other substrates besides phosphorylase is physiologically significant.

Myosin Light Chain Kinase

This calmodulin-sensitive, Ca^{2+}-regulated protein kinase is likely to be specific for P-light chain in the heart since its activity *in vitro* is very low with substrates such as casein, phosphorylase b, histone IIA, and phosvitin (221). Regulation of catalytic activity in smooth muscle MLCK involves removal of an inhibitory domain by calmodulin, and phosphorylation makes the inhibitory domain harder to remove (59). The inhibitory domain may block binding of myosin P-light chain in a manner thus analogous to the ability of R to prevent binding of peptide substrate to C subunit. Presumably, control of cardiac MLCK will be similar, although myosin phosphorylation effects different regulation in smooth muscle and nonmuscle tissues where it is a prerequisite for activation of Mg^{2+}-ATPase activity by actin (59) (see previous section). The relative contributions of MLCK and cAK to myosin P-light chain phosphorylation in intact heart is not known. The Ca^{2+} sensitivity of MLCK makes it a prime candidate for regulation of the contractile process.

Glycogen Synthase Kinases

Phosphorylation of cardiac glycogen synthase is catalyzed by at least three types of protein kinase including cAK, Ca^{2+}-dependent protein kinases, and cyclic nucleotide- and Ca^{2+}-independent protein kinases (153, 174,197). In skeletal muscle some specific glycogen synthase kinases have been identified which are selective for one or more of the six or more phosphorylation sites in glycogen synthase (200). However, no cardiac cyclic nucleotide-independent glycogen synthase phosphorylating activity has yet been given the name glycogen synthase kinase, mainly because it is difficult to establish the occurrence *in vivo* of a particular phosphorylation reaction. Inhibition by the protein kinase inhibitor protein, and effects of Ca^{2+} and EGTA have been used to assess the proportions of different glycogen synthase kinase activities in skeletal muscle (199), but such studies have not been performed in heart.

Phospholipid-Sensitive, Ca^{2+}-Dependent Protein Kinase

A phospholipid-sensitive, Ca^{2+}-dependent protein kinase (protein kinase C) purified from bovine heart has a M_r of 83,500 and a sedimentation coefficient of 5.6S (232). Both phosphatidylserine and Ca^{2+} are essential for activity, and calmodulin cannot substitute for phospholipids. Phosphatidylserine is the most effective of a number of phospholipids tested, and the kinase also requires magnesium (232). The substrate specificity of the phospholipid-sensitive, Ca^{2+}-dependent protein kinase is very different from that of cyclic nucleotide-dependent protein kinases and the calmodulin-sensitive, Ca^{2+}-dependent protein kinases (230). Histone H1 and myelin basic protein are good substrates for the purified bovine heart enzyme, although histone H2B, pyruvate kinase, phosphorylase kinase, myosin light chain, protamine, phosvitin, and peptides containing the phosphorylation sites of histone H2B and pyruvate kinase are poorly phosphorylated (230). The phospholipid-sensitive protein kinase does, however, share a property in common with the calmodulin-sensitive protein kinases in that both are inhibited by trifluoperazine and N-(6-aminohexyl)-5-chloro-1-naphthalenesulfonamide (230,231). There may be a common mechanism of enzyme activation for the calmodulin- and phospholipid-sensitive, Ca^{2+}-dependent protein kinases requiring hydrophobic interactions between the enzymes and their co-factors (231). It is not clear what role the phospholipid-sensitive, Ca^{2+}-dependent protein kinase may play in the heart. Both the enzyme and endogenous substrates in rat and guinea pig heart appear to be distributed in the cytosol and particulate fractions (230,232), and phosphorylation by a cytosolic Ca^{2+}-activated, phospholipid-dependent protein kinase increases Ca^{2+}-transport ATPase activity in cardiac sarcoplasmic reticulum (130).

Cyclic GMP-Dependent Protein Kinase

The function of cGK in most tissues is still unclear; despite a large number of *in vitro* substrates there are no well established physiological substrates. (For review of the properties of cGK see refs. 59,70,132.) cGK purified from bovine heart is similar to the more studied enzyme from bovine lung (58). cGK is composed of two identical subunits of M_r 74,000 to 82,000 which may be linked in part by disulfide bridges (58,133). Despite being composed of a single type of subunit, cGK shows many similarities with cAK (see later section). The enzyme is activated by binding cyclic GMP to a regulatory domain at the N-terminal region of the molecule which is separable by proteolysis from a catalytic domain at the C-terminal end (59,132,133). Like R subunit, each monomer of cGK has two cyclic nucleotide binding sites, but one site (site 2) is of low affinity allowing very rapid dissociation of cGMP (37,132,141). These sites exhibit differences in cGMP analog specificity (37,132,141). cGK undergoes autophosphorylation, but there is disagreement as to whether or not cGK can be phosphorylated by C subunit (86,133).

cGMP has been reported to stimulate (86,141), have no effect on (61), or inhibit (133) autophosphorylation, but it is agreed that in the presence of cGMP, 1 mole of phosphate is incorporated per mole of subunit monomer. Cyclic AMP stimulates autophosphorylation of cAK, resulting in similar (61) or greater (86) incorporation than with cyclic GMP (2 moles phosphate/mole subunit). Autophosphorylation renders cGK more susceptible to activation by cyclic GMP (61). cGK can be activated by trypsin cleavage at a hinge region close to the autophosphorylation site (133). The amino acid sequence immediately adjacent to the autophosphorylated threonine residue is quite different from the autophosphorylation site in R^{II} and the site in R^I phosphorylated by cGK (209). The ATP-binding site of bovine lung cGK exhibits homology with that of C subunit (78,192) but the catalytic mechanism has not been studied (59).

Many substrates which are phosphorylated by cAK *in vitro* are also phosphorylated by cGK *in vitro*, although generally at considerably lower rates (59,61,132,133). cGK does, however, exhibit some specificity when compared with cAK. One of two serine residues (32 and 36) in histone H2B and one of two corresponding serine residues in synthetic peptide analogs is phosphorylated preferentially by each kinase (59,70). Rabbit skeletal muscle R^I is phosphorylated by cGK in the presence of cyclic AMP, but not by C subunit (65). A cytosolic brain protein of M_r 23,000 called G-protein is phosphorylated more effectively by cGK than cAK (2). Smooth muscle has also been reported to contain cGK-specific substrates (24,132). A protein in rat heart cytosol of M_r 70,000 is phosphorylated in response to cyclic GMP preferentially to cyclic AMP (235).

Changes in cyclic GMP concentrations accompany changes in cardiac function raising the possibility of a regulatory role for cyclic GMP-dependent phosphorylation (165). Acetylcholine produces a dose-dependent increase in both cyclic GMP and cGK in perfused rat heart (134). Cyclic GMP may be compartmentalized in heart since sodium nitroprusside which increases cardiac cyclic GMP concentrations does not increase cGK activity or decrease contractile force as does acetylcholine (134). The decreased heart contractility is probably not mediated by the increased cyclic GMP concentration since it can occur with low acetylcholine concentrations and no accompanying increase in tissue cyclic GMP concentrations (152,165). Cyclic GMP concentrations can be increased by an α-adrenergic mechanism (104), but data are conflicting as to whether cyclic GMP can counteract β-adrenergic effects mediated by cyclic AMP (132,165). In the frog ventricle, cyclic GMP has been postulated to counteract effects of cyclic AMP on contractility as well as regulating cyclic AMP levels (195). The concentration of Ca^{2+} required for half the maximum tension decreases and phosphate incorporation into several protein bands increases upon the addition of cyclic GMP and cGK to chemically skinned porcine cardiac muscle fibers (169). However, this effect may not occur *in vivo* since proteins such as troponin I which are phosphorylated in the *in vitro* system may not be accessible to cGK in the intact cell (169). There has been a report recently that cyclic GMP can decrease ventricular Ca^{2+} efflux by effects on the sarcolemmal Ca^{2+} pump (29). Rat heart cyclic GMP concentrations increase with cardiac hypertrophy as in other situations of cell growth (158). Other techniques available to investigate the role of cGK in heart include the use of antiserum inhibition of cGK-catalyzed phosphorylation (222), 8-azido[^{32}P]cIMP labeling of cGK (25), and immunocytochemical techniques to locate cGK and cyclic GMP (201). cGK is more difficult to study than cAK since it is present at low levels in most tissues, and it is present together with proteins of unknown function which also bind cyclic GMP specifically and with high affinity (59,132).

Pyruvate Dehydrogenase Kinase

PDH kinase (MW approximately 50,000) is tightly bound to the mitochondrial PDH complex and is highly specific for the α subunit of pyruvate carboxylase, although it slowly phosphorylates added casein (59,199). The amino acid sequences surrounding the three phosphorylated serine residues (199,236) are clearly distinct from the phosphorylation site sequences in glycogen synthase or phosphorylase kinase. PDH kinase is stimulated by acetyl CoA and NADH and inhibited by pyruvate, coenzyme A, and NAD^+, but the specific nature of its interaction with these substrates and products of the PDH reaction is not known (59). One problem in studying PDH kinase is its presence in only small amounts compared with the other polypeptide chains of the large PDH complex (199).

Other Kinases

Two protein kinases which are not stimulated by either cyclic AMP or calmodulin have recently been purified from bovine heart mitochondrial membranes, but their substrates and function are not known (115). Protein kinases different from those already described are known and some of these, or kinases like them, may subsequently be shown to exist in heart. Of much recent interest are protein kinases which specifically phosphorylate tyrosine, rather than serine or threonine residues (59,90). For example, cyclic nucleotide-independent phosphorylation of tyrosine residues on the epidermal growth factor receptor occurs upon binding of epidermal growth factor to cell membranes of A-431 human epidermoid carcinoma cells (22). The epidermal growth factor receptor-kinase complex prepared from A-431 cells (MW 170,000) phosphorylates itself as well as other proteins (32). The receptor, kinase, and substrate domains appear to be linked, possibly covalently (32). This may represent a prototype for some hormonally activated protein kinases since a similar tyrosine-specific protein kinase activity is associated with other growth receptors such as the purified insulin receptor in human placenta and 3T3-L1 adipocytes (100,202), and may prove to be widespread in most insulin-sensitive cells. Insulin-dependent phosphorylation of its receptor generates an activated insulin-independent receptor protein kinase (185) (see ref. 59 for other protein kinases which have been described in noncardiac tissues). There are doubtless many unidentified protein kinases responsible for endogenous phosphorylation of cardiac proteins.

Evolutionary Relationships Among Protein Kinases

Because of similarities in several key properties of cyclic AMP- and cyclic GMP-dependent protein kinases, it was suggested in 1977 (68,131) that these enzymes are related in evolution. More direct evidence are the amino acid sequence homologies in both the regulatory and catalytic components of both major isozymes of cAK and cGK (78,192). Based on studies of the domains of cyclic nucleotide binding and catalytic activity (42,59,133), it is proposed that these kinases are structurally related as shown in Fig. 1. All three kinases possess two cyclic nucleotide-binding sites on a regulatory component and a single catalytic site on a catalytic component. Intrachain cyclic nucleotide binding for each is positively cooperative, and there are also possibly interchain-binding interactions. The cyclic nucleotide-binding component inhibits the catalytic component, at least in part, by competition with protein substrates, and the inhibition is relieved by cyclic nucleotide binding

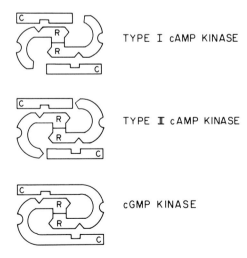

FIG. 1. Hypothesis for structural similarities between cyclic nucleotide-dependent protein kinases. The two different cyclic nucleotide binding sites on each regulatory component (R) are indicated by a *triangle* and *semicircle*. The catalytic site on the catalytic component (C) is denoted by a *rectangle*.

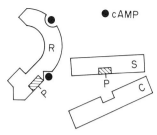

FIG. 2. Competition between regulatory component and substrate for catalytic component of cAMP-dependent protein kinase. The regulatory component (R) has two cAMP-binding sites denoted by a *semicircle* and *triangle* and the substrate (S) and R each have a site (P) which can be phosphorylated by interaction with the catalytic site (*rectangle*) on the catalytic component (C).

(see previous sections). This mechanism is illustrated in Fig. 2. It is likely that cGK, like cAK (208), possesses internal amino acid sequence homology corresponding to the two intrachain cyclic nucleotide-binding sites which presumably evolved through contiguous gene duplication, i.e., duplication within the start and stop signals of the gene. On the other hand, the three kinase homologous groups shown in Fig. 1 probably evolved through discrete gene duplication. Because each has two apparently highly conserved intrachain cyclic nucleotide-binding sites, contiguous gene duplication may have occurred early in evolution, at least before the discrete gene duplication that led to separate cyclic AMP- and cyclic GMP-dependent protein kinases. From the dis-

cussion below, it also seems probable that the existence of the catalytic component of cGK on the same protein chain as the regulatory component is the result of gene fusion.

The evolutionary relationships among protein kinases undoubtedly extend beyond the cyclic nucleotide-dependent protein kinases, since many kinases have physical and kinetic properties in common. As amino acid and gene sequencing data become available, many familiar protein kinases will probably be shown to possess homologies. The recent finding that the amino acid sequence (deduced from the corresponding nucleotide sequence) of viral *src* gene products, which are protein kinases catalyzing phosphorylation of tyrosine residues (see previous section), is homologous with that of the C subunit of mammalian cAK suggests that these proteins are distantly related (7). Although unexpected because of both evolutionary distance and the different amino acid residues phosphorylated in protein substrates, it thus appears that the catalytic components of many protein kinases may be derived from a common ancestral protein kinase. The regulatory components of cyclic nucleotide-dependent protein kinases are certainly closely related, but for other protein kinases one can only speculate that some may also have inhibitory regulatory components not necessarily related to R subunit which are competitive with protein substrates, the competition derived at least in part from the presence of an auto-phosphorylation site, or pseudo-autophosphorylation site, on the regulatory component. A cyclic AMP-binding

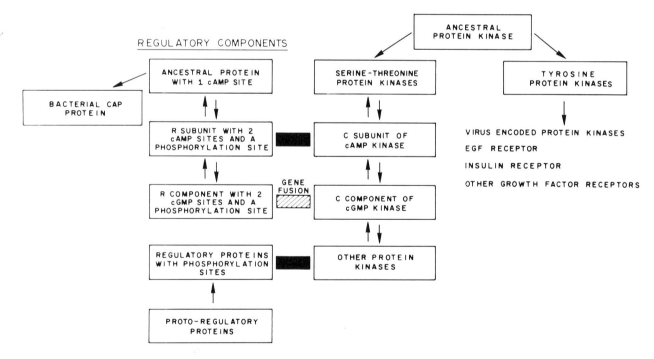

FIG. 3. Possible evolutionary relationships among protein kinases. Regulatory and catalytic components of protein kinases may remain separate or become part of one peptide chain by gene fusion as in cGK.

protein of bacteria, also known as the CAP (catabolic activator protein) or CRP protein (cyclic AMP receptor protein), is devoid of a protein kinase component, but is, nevertheless, quite homologous with R subunit of mammalian cAK (224). It seems logical that a possible mechanism during evolution for developing high affinity between a protein kinase catalytic protein and a potential regulatory protein would be through the existence of a phosphorylation site(s) on the regulatory protein, which might develop into a good competitive inhibitor of other protein substrate(s) of the kinase in a manner similar to cAK and cGK (Fig. 2). It is probably not fortuitous that regulatory components of several protein kinases contain one or more phosphorylation sites. A scheme depicting the postulated independent evolution of the regulatory and catalytic components of protein kinases is shown in Fig. 3. In the practice of studying protein kinases, consideration of their ancestral relationships, which extrapolate information from one protein kinase to another, should prove fruitful, although the differences between the enzymes determine their separate physiological functions.

PROTEIN PHOSPHATASES

The identification of protein phosphatases responsible *in vivo* for dephosphorylation of specific proteins has proved to be difficult because of the small amounts present in tissues; and conversion into forms of different molecular weights during purification make it difficult to interrelate different preparations. Cohen et al. recently clarified the situation by designating that protein phosphatase activities involved in regulating the major pathways of intermediary metabolism can be represented by four enzymes grouped into two different classes (94). The classification is based on whether the phosphatase is sensitive (type 1) or not (type 2) to inhibition by heat stable inhibitor-1 and inhibitor-2, and whether it is specific for the β (type 1) or α (type 2) subunit of phosphorylase kinase (94). Subclasses of type 2, designated A, B, and C, differ in substrate specificity and regulators (94). Protein phosphatase-1, which may exist in at least three forms, has broad substrate specificity and is regulated by inhibitor-1 and inhibitor-2. Protein phosphatases-2A and -2C also have broad substrate specificities, but type 2C has very low phosphorylase and histone phosphatase activities and is regulated by magnesium. Protein phosphatase-2A has no known regulators and can exist in three forms (95). Protein phosphatase-2B, originally called calcineurin (203), is regulated by Ca^{2+} and calmodulin and can be distinguished by specific inhibition by trifluoperazine. Type 2B is the most specific of the four phosphatases, catalyzing dephosphorylation at a significant rate of only α subunit,

inhibitor-1, myosin light chains (94), and the autophosphorylation site of R^{II} (14). Examination of the amino acid sequence around at least 20 phosphorylated serine and threonine residues in protein substrates, and the relative lack of specificity for several phosphorylated synthetic peptide analogs (211) suggest that the primary sequence around the phosphorylation site is not important in conferring protein phosphatase specificity. Although most protein phosphatases fit the above classification, there are other protein phosphatases such as PDH phosphatase and the phosphatases responsible for dephosphorylation of tyrosine residues on proteins, including the phosphorylated insulin and epidermal growth factor receptors (94).

In extracts of rabbit heart, protein phosphatase-2A accounts for the majority of the phosphatase activity, while protein phosphatase-1 exhibits approximately one-third of the activity found for type 2A (96). Protein phosphatases-2B and -2C each show less than 10% of the activity found for type 2A (96). The role of each of the four protein phosphatases in dephosphorylating particular proteins has been assessed in rabbit skeletal muscle, but not in heart muscle (96). Three of four previously described histone phosphatases from dog heart appear to represent the three forms of protein phosphatase-2A, while the fourth histone phosphatase activity can be further separated into two activities corresponding to protein phosphatases-1 and -2C (95). Phosphoprotein phosphatases which dephosphorylate myosin light chain (97), phospholamban (129), and R^{II} (28,213) have been reported in heart, and a phosphoseryl protein phosphatase which also dephosphorylates tyrosine residues has been prepared from bovine heart (27). However, classification requires investigation of the effect of inhibitor-1 and inhibitor-2 and the subunit specificity with phosphorylase kinase.

Regulation of the activity of protein phosphatases in heart may simply reflect the classification scheme. Thus, activation of protein phosphatase-2B by Ca^{2+} and calmodulin may prove to be important in heart during each cycle of contraction and relaxation. Protein phosphatase-1 is sensitive to inhibition by inhibitors-1 and -2 which are postulated to regulate phosphatase activity *in vivo* (95,96). Inhibitor-1 inhibits protein phosphatase-1 activity only after phosphorylation by cAK, and phosphorylation of inhibitor-1 in skeletal muscle *in vivo* increases in response to epinephrine but decreases with insulin (96,159). On the other hand, phosphorylation of inhibitor-2 by glycogen synthase kinase-3 and Mg^{2+}-ATP causes it to dissociate from protein phosphatase-1 (95,96). It is not known which protein phosphatase is responsible for dephosphorylation of inhibitor-1 and inhibitor-2. It should be mentioned, however, that some workers regard regulation by the inhibitors to be an artifact of *in vitro* preparations (112,125).

CONTROL OF HEART FUNCTION BY PROTEIN PHOSPHORYLATION

Current opinion favors both protein phosphorylation and Ca^{2+} to be intimately involved in the mechanism of muscle contraction. Moreover, they are tightly interrelated since Ca^{2+} activates some protein kinases, and protein phosphorylation may regulate Ca^{2+} concentrations by controlling Ca^{2+}-binding protein affinity and/or Ca^{2+} pumps (18,174). The efficiency of such regulation also ensures sufficient energy production by the metabolic pathways for use in contraction. Thus, Ca^{2+} bound to calmodulin is an integral part of phosphorylase kinase and MLCK, and cAK regulates phosphorylase kinase activity and phosphorylates troponin I (see previous section). The extent of protein phosphorylation must also be controlled by protein phosphatase activity, but this is not well understood.

Agents Which Affect Heart Contractile Force and Metabolism

Both Ca^{2+} concentrations and cAK activity can be controlled by hormonal and neural stimulation of cardiac cells. Little work has been done on neural control of cardiac protein phosphorylation, per se, since in most studies in perfused systems the heart is denervated. Perfusion studies with norepinephrine, epinephrine, and acetylcholine together with α- or β-antagonists, or with α- and β-agonists are used to delineate molecular events involved in regulation of heart rate and contractility. This may indeed mimic neural control since in bullfrog heart perfused *in situ,* stimulation of the left vagosympathetic trunk (in the presence of atropine to inhibit parasympathetic effects) is associated with increased ventricular contractility, increased cyclic AMP concentrations, cAK activity, and phosphorylase activity (56). This response is blocked by propanolol suggesting that a β-adrenergic mechanism is involved. Likewise, in rat, guinea pig, or rabbit hearts perfused with epinephrine, norepinephrine, or isoproterenol (β-agonist), contractile force, cyclic AMP concentrations, cAK activity, and phosphorylase activity all increase, and glycogen synthase activity decreases (81,106,108,174,218). The rate of relaxation is also increased by these agents (218). Epinephrine activation of cAK occurs principally via a β-adrenergic mechanism, although some α-adrenergic activation is also apparent (104). cAK activation also correlates well with increased contractile force in perfused guinea pig heart treated with a nonadrenergic agent, histamine (107). Increased phosphorylation of a number of cardiac proteins occurs in response to epinephrine or isoproterenol (see previous section), and many of the effects of catecholamines and histamine can be explained, at least in part, by phosphorylation of heart proteins which is probably cyclic AMP- or Ca^{2+}-dependent.

Adenosine, which increases in the heart in response to decreased oxygen supply or increased oxygen demand attenuates catecholamine responses by reducing β-adrenergic activation of adenylate cyclase (47). Acetylcholine antagonizes the β-adrenergic effects of epinephrine in perfused rat heart and when the α-blocker, phentolamine, is present the antagonistic action of acetylcholine on phosphorylase activation can be accounted for by the decreased cAK activity (92,108). Methacholine inhibits the cyclic AMP-induced phosphorylation of troponin I in hyperpermeable rat ventricle (229). Speculative explanations for the antagonistic effect of acetylcholine include inhibition of receptor interaction with adenylate cyclase, activation of phosphatase(s), or activation of cyclic AMP phosphodiesterase (229). Although cyclic GMP concentrations may increase with acetylcholine (see previous section), cyclic GMP does not mediate an antiadrenergic action (132).

Role of Cyclic AMP-Dependent Phosphorylation

There has been debate in the past as to whether changes in cyclic AMP concentration can explain all the inotropic, chronotropic, and relaxant effects attributed to β-adrenergic stimulation (18,102,165). The present belief is that cyclic AMP-dependent protein phosphorylation can increase both contractile force and rate of relaxation by controlling Ca^{2+} movements across the sarcolemmal membrane and Ca^{2+} sensitivity of the contractile machinery (Fig. 4) (18,102,165). Activated cAK phosphorylates troponin I and phospholamban resulting in release of Ca^{2+} from the troponin complex and increased Ca^{2+} uptake by the sarcoplasmic reticulum and sarcolemma, thereby promoting relaxation (see previous section). Contractile force is enhanced by more available Ca^{2+}, and cyclic AMP-dependent phosphorylation of some component of the Ca^{2+} channel may enhance this by increasing the upstroke velocity of the slow action potentials due to an increased number of slow Ca^{2+} channels (4,15,18,165,219). Injection of cyclic AMP, injection of C subunit, or incubation with epinephrine all increase the slow inward current carried by Ca^{2+} in isolated guinea pig ventricular myocytes, and the amplitude of isotonic contraction increases while relaxation occurs faster (15,166). It has been suggested, however, that β-adrenergic stimulation may activate Ca^{2+} channels directly without detectable changes in heart cyclic AMP concentrations (92). Although Fig. 4 applies principally to a contractile cell, some aspects also apply to pacemaker cells and Purkinje fiber cells. Thus, the β-adrenergic-mediated increase in heart rate is believed to be due to an increased slow inward current carried mainly by Ca^{2+}, but also by Na^+, which creates a steeper pacemaker potential and an increased rate of rise and height of the action potential (87). Conduction through the Purkinje fiber system is also facilitated by

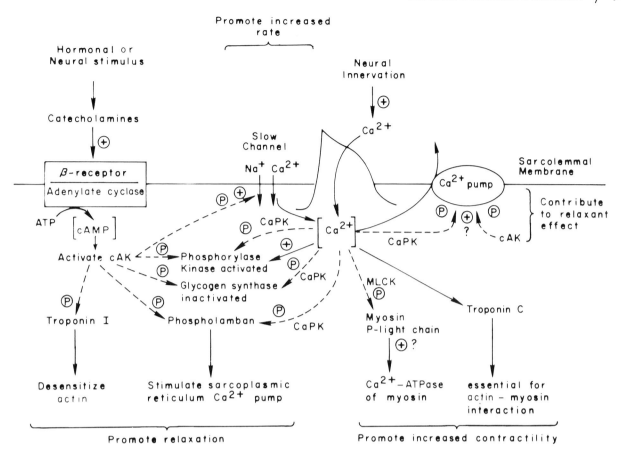

FIG. 4. Control by Ca^{2+} and cAMP of protein phosphorylation involved in cardiac contractile events. Abbreviations: CaPK = Ca^{2+}-calmodulin-dependent protein kinase; MLCK = myosin light chain kinase; cAK = cAMP-dependent protein kinase; *encircled P* = phosphorylation; *encircled cross* = stimulatory effect; ? = effect on or nature of protein phosphorylated uncertain. (Scheme derived from refs. 102 and 165.)

the faster-rising action potentials (87). As is indicated in Fig. 4, cAK-dependent phosphorylation of some membrane component probably controls the number of functional Ca^{2+} channels, but data in pacemaker and conducting cells are scarce.

While there do appear to be relationships between cyclic AMP and changes in heart function, the exact nature and role of the proteins which are phosphorylated as part of the molecular mechanism causing these changes in heart function is not well understood. Although cAK is believed to phosphorylate phosphorylase kinase (151), glycogen synthase (150), troponin I (50,51) and a M_r 27,000 sarcolemmal protein (220) in response to epinephrine in perfused rat heart, the phosphorylation of each follows a slightly different time course suggesting that other factors can regulate cyclic AMP-dependent phosphorylation (151). Possibly these include the phosphorylation state of additional sites on the substrate, or compartmentalization of the substrate and cAK. It may be difficult to distinguish between Ca^{2+}- and cyclic AMP-dependent protein phosphorylation *in vivo*, particularly since Ca^{2+} has multiple roles in cardiac cells including that of a possible third messenger for cyclic

AMP (165), and cyclic AMP-dependent phosphorylation regulates Ca^{2+} binding and transport across membranes of the cardiac cell (18). Raising perfusate Ca^{2+} concentrations increases contractile force and phosphorylase activity without any increase in tissue cyclic AMP concentrations or cAK activity (104), but it is not known if changes in protein phosphorylation also occur.

Role of Cyclic AMP-Independent Phosphorylation

Hormones or agonists used experimentally or therapeutically which interact with β-adrenergic receptors activate adenylate cyclase thereby generating cyclic AMP, whereas those interacting with α-adrenergic receptors exert their effects via Ca^{2+} as indicated in Fig. 4 (174). There are, however, other less well understood mechanisms of control of cardiac protein phosphorylation. Cyclic GMP seems likely to regulate protein phosphorylation, but although cyclic GMP causes a direct negative inotropic effect in cardiac muscle, neither a role for cGK in this effect nor substrate proteins for cGK have been established (132). Insulin activates glycogen synthase presumably via modification of its phosphorylation state by a process that is independent of cyclic AMP and Ca^{2+} (174). The mechanism by which insulin alters phosphorylation of this and possibly other proteins in heart is not clear. Insulin could control protein phosphatase activity by regulation of inhibitor-1 phosphorylation (see previous section). Insulin activation of cyclic AMP-dependent phosphorylation which inactivates plasma membrane low K_m cyclic AMP phosphodiesterase may explain the ability of insulin to counteract the effect of agents which increase cyclic AMP in adipose tissue and liver (138,147). However, insulin does not reverse the increased cyclic AMP concentrations and cAK activity caused by glucagon in perfused rat heart (105). Insulin activation of PDH in adipocyte mitochondria involves a chemical mediator, which activates PDH phosphatase (173). This action of insulin may also apply to heart PDH (83), but whereas epinephrine activates PDH in perfused rat heart it inhibits the adipose tissue enzyme (149). The insulin receptor itself is autophosphorylated in the presence of insulin in various cell types, but it is not known whether this controls intracellular events in heart (see previous section).

Long-Term Control of Cardiac Protein Phosphorylation

Protein phosphorylation patterns in heart are altered by disease or chronic changes in hormonal status of the animal. In starved or diabetic rats, cardiac PDH is in a less activated, more phosphorylated state due to increased PDH kinase activity (91). Diabetes also appears to decrease the ability of the heart to accumulate cyclic AMP (93). In hypothyroid rats the type II isozyme of cardiac cAK increases relative to the type I isozyme and the level of the protein kinase inhibitor decreases (74). Although the proportions of the two isozymes do not change, total and soluble cAK activity decrease as do membrane phosphorylation and Ca^{2+} uptake by the sarcoplasmic reticulum in hypertrophied hearts of spontaneously hypertensive rats (11). Total protein kinase activity and the proportions of the isozymes of cAK in mouse heart also change during growth from fetus to adult (144). Ischemia in rat heart caused by coronary ligation results in a change in the ventricular fibrillation threshold which is related to the resulting increased cyclic AMP concentrations (140). Protein phosphorylation state may be important in changes in heart function in development and in disease states, and this is potentially an interesting but rather neglected area.

Regulation of Coronary Blood Flow by Protein Phosphorylation

Protein phosphorylation occurring in the smooth muscle of the coronary vessels is predicted to regulate coronary blood flow because cyclic AMP and cyclic GMP promote relaxation of bovine coronary arterial

smooth muscle apparently by activation of the respective protein kinases (132,156), and calcium-dependent MLCK phosphorylates myosin light chains (1,76,132). MLCK is presumably regulated by changes in intracellular free Ca^{2+} brought about by various agents, but whether or not MLCK itself is a physiological substrate for the cyclic nucleotide-dependent protein kinases thereby linking the Ca^{2+} and cyclic nucleotide systems, is controversial.

Although agents that elevate cyclic AMP cause coronary artery relaxation (5,33,124,191,194), the increased coronary flow induced by sympathetic stimulation (87) can be explained only partly by direct effects of β-adrenergic cyclic AMP production in coronary vessels. Sympathetic stimulation of cardiac contractile activity and the associated increase in metabolic activity causes accumulation of vasodilator metabolites such as adenosine, an agent which causes relaxation by elevating cyclic AMP (67,234), thus promoting phosphorylation of a specific protein(s) linked to the contractile mechanism. The adenosine receptors mediating this effect are termed "Ra receptors" because analogs which mimic adenosine require an intact *ribose* moiety and are linked to adenylate cyclase in an *activating* manner (234).

Cyclic GMP may also be a "second messenger" in relaxing coronary vessels. In fact, the best evidence for a physiological role of cyclic GMP in any system has come from studies of vascular smooth muscle (132): (a) Nitrate vasodilators cause elevations in cyclic GMP that correlate with vascular smooth muscle relaxation (3,73,123,190); (b) high concentrations of cyclic GMP and cGK are present in vascular smooth muscle (132); (c) nitrate vasodilators activate cGK (132); (d) substrates for cGK are present in smooth muscle tissues (24); (e) phosphodiesterase inhibitors selective for inhibition of cyclic GMP hydrolysis relax coronary smooth muscle (118,123); (f) exogenous 8-bromo-cGMP causes relaxation of several smooth muscle preparations (156,189). Although the evidence is suggestive, it is not known if cyclic GMP and cGK mediate effects of hormones, neurotransmittors, and other agents on vascular smooth muscle relaxation. The ability of 8-bromo-cGMP to block the α-adrenergic effect of norepinephrine on contraction (71,101,132) suggests that the cyclic GMP elevation caused by acetylcholine might be a negative feedback to dampen the increased contraction. A general role of cyclic GMP, as well as of cyclic AMP, could be to decrease intracellular free Ca^{2+}. Thus, cyclic nucleotide-dependent protein phosphorylation could underlie the mechanism for lowering Ca^{2+}, thereby leading to muscle relaxation.

ACKNOWLEDGMENTS

We thank Diane Smithson for typing this manuscript. The work performed in our laboratory was supported in part by research grant AM 15988 from the National Institutes of Health. A. Robinson-Steiner is a recipient of a Juvenile Diabetes Foundation Fellowship.

REFERENCES

1. Adelstein, R. S., Conti, M. A., and Pato, M. D. (1980): Regulation of myosin light chain kinase by reversible phosphorylation and calcium-calmodulin. *Ann. NY Acad. Sci.*, 356:142.

2. Aswad, D. W., and Greengard, P. (1981): A specific substrate from rabbit cerebellum for guanosine 3':5'-monophosphate-dependent protein kinase I. Purification and characterization. *J. Biol. Chem.*, 256:3487–3493.

3. Axellson, K. L., Wikberg, J. E. S., and Andersson, R. G. G. (1979): Relationship between nitroglycerine, cyclic GMP, and relaxation of vascular smooth muscle. *Life Sci.*, 24:1779–1786.

4. Azuma, J., Sawamura, A., Harada, H., Tanimoto, T., Ishiyama, T., Morita, Y., Yamamura, Y., and Sperelakis, N. (1981): Cyclic adenosine monophosphate modulation of contractility via slow Ca^{2+} channels in chick heart. *J. Mol. Cell. Cardiol.*, 13:577–587.

5. Bär, H. (1974): Cyclic nucleotides and smooth muscle. *Adv. Cyclic Nucleotide Res.*, 4:195–237.

6. Bárány, K., Bárány, M., Hager, S. R., and Sayers, S. T. (1983): Myosin light chain and membrane protein phosphorylation in various muscles. *Fed. Proc.*, 42:27–32.

7. Barker, W. C., and Dayhoff, M. O. (1982): Viral *src* gene products are related to the catalytic chain of mammalian cAMP-dependent protein kinase. *Proc. Natl. Acad. Sci. USA*, 79:2836–2839.

8. Beavo, J. A., Bechtel, P. J., and Krebs, E. G. (1974): Activation of protein kinase by physiological concentrations of cyclic AMP. *Proc. Natl. Acad. Sci. USA*, 71:3580–3583.

9. Bechtel, P. J., Beavo, J. A., and Krebs, E. G. (1977): Purification and characterization of catalytic subunit of skeletal muscle adenosine 3':5'-monophosphate-dependent protein kinase. *J. Biol. Chem.*, 252:2691–2697.

10. Beebe, S., and Corbin, J. D. (1983): Stimulation of protein kinase and lipolysis in adipocytes by cAMP analogs and epinephrine. *Fed. Proc.*, 42:2256.

11. Bhalla, R. C., Gupta, R. C., and Sharma, R. V. (1982): Distribution and properties of cAMP-dependent protein kinase isozymes in the myocardium of spontaneously hypertensive rat. *J. Mol. Cell. Cardiol.*, 14:33–39.

12. Bidlack, J. M., Ambudkar, I. S., and Shamoo, A. E. (1982): Purification of phospholamban, a 22,000-dalton protein from cardiac sarcoplasmic reticulum that is specifically phosphorylated by cyclic AMP-dependent protein kinase. *J. Biol. Chem.*, 257:4501–4506.

13. Bidlack, J. M., and Shamoo, A. E. (1980): Adenosine 3',5'-monophosphate-dependent phosphorylation of a 6,000 and a 22,000 dalton protein from cardiac sarcoplasmic reticulum. *Biochim. Biophys. Acta*, 632:310–325.

14. Blumenthal, D. K., and Krebs, E. G. (1983): Dephosphorylation of cAMP-dependent protein kinase regulatory subunit (type II) by calcineurin (protein phosphatase 2B). *Biophys. J.*, 41:409a.

15. Brum, G., Flockerzi, V., Hofmann, F., Osterrieder, W., and Trautwein, W. (1983): Injection of catalytic subunit of cAMP-dependent protein kinase into isolated myocytes. *Pfluegers Arch.*, 398:147–154.

16. Brunton, L. L., Hayes, J. S., and Mayer, S. E. (1981): Compartments of cyclic AMP and protein kinase in heart: data supporting their existence and speculations on their subcellular basis. *Cold Spring Harbor Symp.*, 8:227–235.

17. Buxton, I. L. O., and Brunton, L. L. (1983): Compartments of cyclic AMP and protein kinase in mammalian cardiomyocytes. *J. Biol. Chem.*, 258:10233–10239.

18. Capony, J.-P., Cavadore, J.-C., Demaille, J. G., Derancourt, J., Ferraz, C., Haiech, J., Kilhoffer, M.-C., LePeuch, C. J., LePeuch, D. A. M., Martin, F., Molla, A., and Rinaldi, M. (1983): The control of contractility by protein phosphorylation. *Adv. Cyclic Nucleotide Res.*, 15:337–371.

19. Carlson, G. M., Bechtel, P. J., and Graves, D. J. (1979): Chemical and regulatory properties of phosphorylase kinase and cyclic AMP-dependent protein kinase. *Adv. Enzymol.*, 50:41–115.

20. Caroni, P., and Carafoli, E. (1981): Regulation of Ca^{2+}-pumping ATPase of heart sarcolemma by a phosphorylation-dephosphorylation process. *J. Biol. Chem.*, 256:9371–9373.

21. Caroni, P., Zurini, M., Clark, A., and Carafoli, E. (1983): Further characterization and reconstitution of the purified Ca^{2+}-pumping ATPase of heart sarcolemma. *J. Biol. Chem.*, 258:7305–7310.

22. Carpenter, G., King, L., and Cohen, S. (1979): Rapid enhancement of protein phosphorylation in A-431 cell membrane preparations by epidermal growth factor. *J. Biol. Chem.*, 254:4884–4891.

23. Carr, S. A., Biemann, K., Shoji, S., Parmelee, D. C., and Titani, K. (1982): n-Tetradecanoyl is the NH$_2$-terminal blocking group of the catalytic subunit of cyclic AMP-dependent protein kinase from bovine cardiac muscle. *Proc. Natl. Acad. Sci. USA*, 79:6128–6131.

24. Casnellie, J. E., and Greengard, P. (1974): Guanosine 3':5'-cyclic monophosphate-dependent phosphorylation of endogenous substrate proteins in membranes of mammalian smooth muscle. *Proc. Natl. Acad. Sci. USA*, 71:1891–1895.

25. Casnellie, J. E., Ives, H. E., Jamieson, J. D., and Greengard, P. (1980): Cyclic GMP-dependent protein phosphorylation in intact medial tissue and isolated cells from vascular smooth muscle. *J. Biol. Chem.*, 255:3770–3776.

26. Cavadore, J.-C., LePeuch, C. J., Walsh, M. P., Vallet, B., Molla, A., and Demaille, J. G. (1981): Calcium-calmodulin-dependent phosphorylations in the control of muscular contraction. *Biochimie*, 63:301–306.

27. Chernoff, J., Li, H.-C., Cheng, Y.-S. E., and Chen, L. B. (1983): Characterization of a phosphotyrosyl protein phosphatase activity associated with a phosphoseryl protein phosphatase of Mr = 95,000 from bovine heart. *J. Biol. Chem.*, 258:7852–7857.

28. Chou, C.-K., Alfano, J., and Rosen, O. M. (1977): Purification of phosphoprotein phosphatase from bovine cardiac muscle that catalyzes dephosphorylation of cyclic AMP-binding protein component of protein kinase. *J. Biol. Chem.*, 252:2855–2859.

29. Church, J. G., and Sen, A. K. (1983): Regulation of canine heart sarcolemmal Ca^{2+}-pumping ATPase by cyclic GMP. *Biochim. Biophys. Acta*, 728:191–200.

30. Cogoli, J. M., and Dobson, J. G. (1981): An easy and rapid method for the measurement of [γ-^{32}P]ATP specific radioactivity in tissue extracts obtained from *in vitro* rat heart preparations labeled with ^{32}Pi. *Anal. Biochem.*, 110:331–337.

31. Cohen, P. (1978): The role of cyclic-AMP-dependent protein kinase in the regulation of glycogen metabolism in mammalian skeletal muscle. *Curr. Top. Cell. Regul.*, 14:117–196.

32. Cohen, S., Ushiro, H., Stoscheck, C., and Chinkers, M. (1982): A native 170,000 epidermal growth factor receptor-kinase complex from shed plasma membrane vesicles. *J. Biol. Chem.*, 257:1523–1531.

33. Collins, G. A., and Sutter, M. C. (1975): Quantitative aspects of cyclic AMP and relaxation in the rabbit anterior mesenteric-portal view. *Can. J. Physiol. Pharmacol.*, 53:989–997.

34. Conti, M. A., and Adelstein, R. S. (1981): The relationship between calmodulin binding and phosphorylation of smooth muscle myosin kinase by the catalytic subunit of 3':5' cAMP-dependent protein kinase. *J. Biol. Chem.*, 256:3178–3222.

35. Cooper, R. H., Sul, H. S., McCullough, T. E., and Walsh, D. A. (1980): Purification and properties of the cardiac isoenzyme of phosphorylase kinase. *J. Biol. Chem.*, 255:11794–11801.

36. Cooper, R. H., Sul, H. S., and Walsh, D. A. (1981): Phosphorylation and activation of the cardiac isoenzyme of phosphorylase kinase by the cAMP-dependent protein kinase. *J. Biol. Chem.*, 256:8030–8038.

37. Corbin, J. D., and Døskeland, S. O. (1983): Studies of two different intrachain cGMP-binding sites of cGMP-dependent protein kinase. *J. Biol. Chem.*, 258:11391–11397.

38. Corbin, J. D., and Keely, S. L. (1977): Characterization and regulation of heart adenosine 3':5'-monophosphate-dependent protein kinase isozymes. *J. Biol. Chem.*, 252:910–918.

39. Corbin, J. D., Keely, S. L., and Park, C. R. (1975): The distribution and dissociation of cyclic adenosine 3':5'-monophosphate-dependent protein kinases in adipose, cardiac, and other tissues. *J. Biol. Chem.*, 250:218–225.

40. Corbin, J. D., Rannels, S. R., Flockhart, D. A., Robinson-Steiner, A. M., Tigani, M. C., Døskeland, S. O., Suva, R., and Miller,

J. P. (1982): Effect of cyclic nucleotide analogs on intrachain site 1 of protein kinase isozymes. *Eur. J. Biochem.*, 125:259–266.

41. Corbin, J. D., Sugden, P. H., Lincoln, T. M., and Keely, S. L. (1977): Compartmentalization of adenosine 3':5'-monophosphate and adenosine 3':5'-monophosphate-dependent protein kinase in heart tissue. *J. Biol. Chem.*, 252:3854–3861.

42. Corbin, J. D., Sugden, P. H., West, L., Flockhart, D. A., Lincoln, T. M., and McCarthy, D. (1978): Studies on the properties and mode of action of the purified regulatory subunit of bovine heart adenosine 3':5'-monophosphate-dependent protein kinase. *J. Biol. Chem.*, 253:3997–4003.

43. Daile, P., Carnegie, P. R., and Young, J. D. (1975): Synthetic substrate for cyclic AMP-dependent protein kinase. *Nature*, 257:416–418.

44. De La Houssaye, B. A., and Masaracchia, R. A. (1983): Standardization of the assay for the catalytic subunit of cyclic AMP-dependent protein kinase using a synthetic peptide substrate. *Anal. Biochem.*, 128:54–59.

45. de Wit, R. J. W., Hoppe, J., Stec, W. J., Baraniak, J., and Jastorff, B. (1982): Interaction of cAMP derivatives with the "stable" cAMP-binding site in the cAMP-dependent protein kinase type I. *Eur. J. Biochem.*, 122:95–99.

46. Dobson, J. G. (1981): Catecholamine-induced phosphorylation of cardiac muscle proteins. *Biochim. Biophys. Acta*, 675:123–131.

47. Dobson, J. G. (1983): Mechanism of adenosine inhibition of catecholamine-induced responses in heart. *Circ. Res.*, 52:151–160.

48. Døskeland, S. O., and Øgreid, D. (1981): Binding proteins for cyclic AMP in mammalian tissues. *Int. J. Biochem.*, 13:1–19.

49. Døskeland, S. O., Øgreid, D., Ekanger, R., Sturm, P. A., Miller, J. P., and Suva, R. H. (1983): Mapping of the two intrachain cyclic nucleotide binding sites of adenosine cyclic 3',5'-phosphate dependent protein kinase I. *Biochemistry USA*, 22:1094–1101.

50. England, P. J. (1975): Correlation between contraction and phosphorylation of the inhibitory subunit of troponin in perfused rat heart. *FEBS Lett.*, 50:57–60.

51. England, P. J. (1976): Studies on the phosphorylation of the inhibitory subunit of troponin during modification of contraction in perfused rat heart. *Biochem. J.*, 160:295–304.

52. England, P. J. (1977): Phosphorylation of the inhibitory subunit of troponin in perfused hearts of mice deficient in phosphorylase kinase. Evidence for the phosphorylation of troponin by adenosine 3':5'-phosphate-dependent protein kinase *in vivo*. *Biochem. J.*, 168:307–310.

53. Erlichman, J., Rosenfeld, R., and Rosen, O. M. (1974): Phosphorylation of a cyclic adenosine 3':5'-monophosphate-dependent protein kinase from bovine cardiac muscle. *J. Biol. Chem.*, 249:5000–5003.

54. Erlichman, J., Sarkar, D., Fleischer, N., and Rubin, C. S. (1980): Identification of two subclasses of type II cAMP-dependent protein kinases. Neural-specific and non-neural protein kinases. *J. Biol. Chem.*, 255:8179–8184.

55. Farmer, B. B., Mancini, M., Williams, E. S., and Watanabe, A. M. (1983): Isolation of calcium tolerant myocytes from adult rat hearts: review of the literature and description of a method. *Life Sci.*, 33:1–18.

56. Fiscus, R. R., and Mayer, S. E. (1982): Neural regulation of cyclic AMP, cyclic AMP-dependent protein kinase, and phosphorylase in bullfrog ventricular myocardium. *Circ. Res.*, 51:551–559.

57. Flockerzi, V., Mewes, R., Ruth, P., and Hofmann, F. (1983): Phosphorylation of purified bovine cardiac sarcolemma and potassium-stimulated calcium uptake. *Eur. J. Biochem.*, 135:131–142.

58. Flockerzi, V., Speichermann, N., and Hofmann, F. (1978): A guanosine 3':5'-monophosphate-dependent protein kinase from bovine heart muscle. Purification and phosphorylation of histone I and IIb. *J. Biol. Chem.*, 253:3395–3399.

59. Flockhart, D. A., and Corbin, J. D. (1982): Regulatory mechanisms in the control of protein kinases. *CRC Crit. Rev. Biochem.*, 12:133–186.

60. Flockhart, D. A., Watterson, D. M., and Corbin, J. D. (1980): Studies on functional domains of the regulatory subunit of bovine

61. Foster, J. L., Guttmann, J., and Rosen, O. M. (1981): Autophosphorylation of cGMP-dependent protein kinase. *J. Biol. Chem.*, 256:5029–5036.

62. Furuya, E., and Uyeda, K. (1980): An activation factor of liver phosphofructokinase. *Proc. Natl. Acad. Sci. USA*, 77:5861–5864.

63. Gagelmann, M., Reed, J., Kübler, D., Pyerin, W., and Kinzel, V. (1980): Evidence for a "mute" catalytic subunit of cyclic AMP-dependent protein kinase from rat muscle and its mode of activation. *Proc. Natl. Acad. Sci. USA*, 77:2492–2496.

64. Geahlen, R. L., Allen, S. M., and Krebs, E. G. (1981): Effect of phosphorylation on the regulatory subunit of the type I cAMP-dependent protein kinase. *J. Biol. Chem.*, 256:4536–4540.

65. Geahlen, R. L., and Krebs, E. G. (1980): Regulatory subunit of the type I cAMP-dependent protein kinase as an inhibitor and substrate of the cGMP-dependent protein kinase. *J. Biol. Chem.*, 255:1164–1169.

66. Geahlen, R. L., and Krebs, E. G. (1980): Studies on the phosphorylation of the type I cAMP-dependent protein kinase. *J. Biol. Chem.*, 255:9375–9379.

67. Gerlach, E., Schrader, J., and Nees, S. (1979): Sites and mode of action of adenosine in the heart. I. Coronary System. In: *Physiological and Regulatory Functions of Adenosine and Adenine Nucleotides*, edited by H. P. Baer and G. I. Drummond, pp. 127–136. Raven Press, New York.

68. Gill, G. N. (1977): A hypothesis concerning the structure of cAMP- and cGMP-dependent protein kinase. *J. Cyclic Nucleotide Res.*, 3:153–162.

69. Glass, D. B., and Krebs, E. G. (1980): Protein phosphorylation catalyzed by cyclic AMP-dependent and cyclic GMP-dependent protein kinases. *Annu. Rev. Pharmacol. Toxicol.*, 20:363–388.

70. Glass, D. B., and Krebs, E. G. (1982): Phosphorylation by guanosine 3':5'-monophosphate-dependent protein kinase of synthetic peptide analogs of a site phosphorylated in histone H2B. *J. Biol. Chem.*, 257:1196–1200.

71. Goldberg, N. D., O'Dea, R. F., and Haddox, M. K. (1973): Cyclic GMP. *Adv. Cyclic Nucleotide Res.*, 3:155–223.

72. Granot, J., Mildvan, A. S., and Kaiser, E. T. (1980): Studies of the mechanism of action and regulation of cAMP-dependent protein kinase. *Arch. Biochem. Biophys.*, 205:1–17.

73. Gruetter, C. A., Barry, B. K., McNamara, D. B., Gruetter, D. Y., Kadowitz, P. J., and Ignarro, L. J. (1979): Relaxation of bovine coronary artery and activation of coronary arterial guanylate cyclase by nitric oxide, nitroprusside, and a carcinogenic nitrosamine. *J. Cyclic Nucleotide Res.*, 5:211–224.

74. Hagino, Y., and Tachibana, M. (1981): Effect of hypothyroid status on adenosine 3',5'-monophosphate-dependent protein kinase of skeletal, heart and diaphragm muscle of rats. *Jpn. J. Pharmacol.*, 31:1005–1012.

75. Hartl, F. T., and Roskoski, R. (1983): Cyclic adenosine 3':5'-monophosphate-dependent protein kinase. Comparison of type II enzymes from bovine brain, skeletal muscle, and cardiac muscle. *J. Biol. Chem.*, 258:3950–3955.

76. Hartshorne, D. J., and Pereschini, A. J. (1980): Phosphorylation of myosin as a regulatory component in smooth muscle. *Ann. NY Acad. Sci.*, 356:130.

77. Hashimoto, E., Takio, K., and Krebs, E. G. (1981): Studies on the site in the regulatory subunit of type I cAMP-dependent protein kinase phosphorylated by cGMP-dependent protein kinase. *J. Biol. Chem.*, 256:5604–5607.

78. Hashimoto, E., Takio, K., and Krebs, E. G. (1982): Amino acid sequence at the ATP-binding site of cGMP-dependent protein kinase. *J. Biol. Chem.*, 257:727–733.

79. Hawkins, P. T., Michell, R. H., and Kirk, C. J. (1983): A simple assay method for determination of the specific radioactivity of the γ-phosphate group of ^{32}P-labeled ATP. *Biochem. J.*, 210:717–720.

80. Hayes, J. S., Bowling, N., King, K. L., and Boder, G. B. (1982): Evidence for selective regulation of the phosphorylation of myocyte proteins by isoproterenol and prostaglandin E$_1$. *Biochim. Biophys. Acta*, 714:136–142.

81. Hayes, J. S., Brunton, L. L., and Meyer, S. E. (1980): Selective activation of particulate cAMP-dependent protein kinase by

isoproterenol and prostaglandin E₁. *J. Biol. Chem.*, 255:5113–5119.

82. Hemmings, B. A., Aitken, A., Cohen, P., Rymond, M., and Hofmann, F. (1982): Phosphorylation of the type-II regulatory subunit of cyclic-AMP-dependent protein kinase by glycogen synthase kinase 3 and glycogen synthase kinase 5. *Eur. J. Biochem.*, 127:473–481.

83. Hiraoka, T., DeBuysere, M., and Olson, M. S. (1980): Studies of the effects of β-adrenergic agonists on the regulation of pyruvate dehydrogenase in the perfused rat heart. *J. Biol. Chem.*, 255:7604–7609.

84. Hjelmquist, G., Andersson, J., Edlund, B., and Engström, L. (1974): Amino acid sequence of a (^{32}P)phosphopeptide from pig liver pyruvate kinase phosphorylated by cyclic 3′,5′-AMP-stimulated protein kinase and γ-(^{32}P)ATP. *Biochem. Biophys. Res. Commun.*, 61:509–513.

85. Hofmann, F., Beavo, J. A., Bechtel, P. J., and Krebs, E. G. (1975): Comparison of adenosine 3′:5′-monophosphate-dependent protein kinases from rabbit skeletal and bovine heart muscle. *J. Biol. Chem.*, 250:7795–7801.

86. Hofmann, F., and Gensheimer, H.-P. (1983): Cyclic AMP-dependent protein kinase does not phosphorylate cyclic GMP-dependent protein kinase *in vitro*. *FEBS Lett.*, 151:71–75.

87. Honig, C. R. (1981): *Modern Cardiovascular Physiology*. Little, Brown, Boston.

88. Hue, L. (1982): Role of fructose 2,6-bisphosphate in the stimulation of glycolysis by anoxia in isolated hepatocytes. *Biochem. J.*, 206:359–365.

89. Hue, L., Blackmore, P. F., Shikama, H., Robinson-Steiner, A., and Exton, J. (1982): Regulation of fructose 2,6-bisphosphate content in rat hepatocytes, perfused hearts and perfused hindlimbs. *J. Biol. Chem.*, 257:4308–4313.

90. Hunter, T., and Sefton, B. M. (1980): Transforming gene product of Rous sarcoma virus phosphorylates tyrosine. *Proc. Natl. Acad. Sci. USA*, 77:1311–1315.

91. Hutson, N. J., and Randle, P. J. (1978): Enhanced activity of pyruvate dehydrogenase kinase in rat heart mitochondria in alloxan-diabetes or starvation. *FEBS Lett.*, 92:73–76.

92. Ingebretsen, C. G. (1980): Interaction between alpha and beta adrenergic receptors and cholinergic receptors in isolated perfused rat heart: effects on cAMP-protein kinase and phosphorylase. *J. Cyclic Nucleotide Res.*, 6:121–132.

93. Ingebretsen, W. R., Peralta, C., Monsher, M., Wagner, L. K., and Ingebretsen, C. G. (1981): Diabetes alters the myocardial cAMP-protein kinase cascade system. *Am. J. Physiol.*, 240:H375–H382.

94. Ingebritsen, T. S., and Cohen, P. (1983): The protein phosphatases involved in cellular regulation. I. Classification and substrate specificities. *Eur. J. Biochem.*, 132:255–261.

95. Ingebritsen, T. S., Foulkes, J. G., and Cohen, P. (1983): The protein phosphatases involved in cellular regulation. 2. Glycogen metabolism. *Eur. J. Biochem.*, 132:263–274.

96. Ingebritsen, T. S., Stewart, A. A., and Cohen, P. (1983): The protein phosphatases involved in cellular regulation. 6. Measurement of type-1 and type-2 protein phosphatases in extracts of mammalian tissues; an assessment of their physiological roles. *Eur. J. Biochem.*, 132:297–307.

97. Jeacocke, S. A., and England, P. J. (1980): Phosphorylation of myosin light chains in perfused rat heart. Effect of adrenaline and increased cytoplasmic calcium ions. *Biochem. J.*, 188:763–768.

98. Jones, L. R., Maddock, S. W., and Hathaway, D. R. (1981): Membrane localization of myocardial type II cyclic AMP-dependent protein kinase activity. *Biochim. Biophys. Acta*, 641:242–253.

99. Kapoor, C. L., and Cho-Chung, Y. S. (1983): Compartmentalization of regulatory subunits of cyclic adenosine 3′:5′-monophosphate-dependent protein kinases in MCF-7 human breast cancer cells. *Cancer Res.*, 43:295–302.

100. Kasuga, M., Fujita-Yamaguchi, Y., Blithe, D. L., and Kahn, C. R. (1983): Tyrosine-specific protein kinase activity is associated with the purified insulin receptor. *Proc. Natl. Acad. Sci. USA*, 80:2137–2141.

101. Katsuki, S., and Murad, F. (1977): Regulation of adenosine cyclic 3′,5′-monophosphate and guanosine cyclic 3′,5′-monophosphate levels and contractility in bovine tracheal smooth muscle. *Mol. Pharmacol.*, 13:330–341.

102. Katz, A. (1979): Role of the contractile proteins and sarcoplasmic reticulum in the response of the heart to catecholamines: An historical review. *Adv. Cyclic Nucleotide Res.*, 11:303–343.

103. Keely, S. L. (1979): Prostaglandin E₁ activation of heart cAMP-dependent protein kinase: apparent dissociation of protein kinase activation from increases in phosphorylase activity and contractile force. *Mol. Pharmacol.*, 15:235–245.

104. Keely, S. L., Corbin, J. D., and Lincoln, T. (1977): *Alpha* adrenergic involvement in heart metabolism: effects on adenosine cyclic 3′,5′-monophosphate, adenosine cyclic 3′,5′-monophosphate-dependent protein kinase, guanosine cyclic 3′,5′-monophosphate, and glucose transport. *Mol. Pharmacol.*, 13:965–975.

105. Keely, S. L., Corbin, J. D., and Park, C. R. (1975): Regulation of adenosine 3′:5′-monophosphate-dependent protein kinase. Regulation of the heart enzyme by epinephrine, glucagon, insulin and 1-methyl-3-isobutylxanthine. *J. Biol. Chem.*, 250:4832–4840.

106. Keely, S. L., Corbin, J. D., and Park, C. R. (1975): On the question of translocation of heart cAMP-dependent protein kinase. *Proc. Natl. Acad. Sci. USA*, 72:1501–1504.

107. Keely, S. L., and Eiring, A. (1979): Involvement of cAMP-dependent protein kinase in the regulation of heart contractile force II. *Am. J. Physiol.*, 236:H84–H91.

108. Keely, S. L., Lincoln, T. M., and Corbin, J. D. (1978): Interaction of acetylcholine and epinephrine on heart cyclic AMP-dependent protein kinase. *Am. J. Physiol.*, 234:H432–H438.

109. Kemp, B. E., Graves, D. J., Benjamini, E., and Krebs, E. G. (1977): Role of multiple basic residues in determining the substrate specificity of cyclic AMP-dependent protein kinase. *J. Biol. Chem.*, 252:4888–4894.

110. Kerbey, A. L., and Randle, P. J. (1979): Role of multisite phosphorylation in regulation of pig heart pyruvate dehydrogenase phosphatase. *FEBS Lett.*, 108:485–488.

111. Kerlavage, A. R., and Taylor, S. S. (1982): Site-specific cyclic nucleotide binding and dissociation of the holoenzyme of cAMP-dependent protein kinase. *J. Biol. Chem.*, 257:1749–1754.

112. Khatra, B. S., and Soderling, T. R. (1983): Rabbit muscle glycogen x̄ bound phosphoprotein phosphatases: substrate specificities and effects of inhibitor-1. *Arch. Biochem. Biophys.*, 227:39–51.

113. Kirchberger, M. A., and Antonetz, T. (1982): Phospholamban: dissociation of the 22,000 molecular weight protein of cardiac sarcoplasmic reticulum into 11,000 and 5,500 molecular weight forms. *Biochem. Biophys. Res. Commun.*, 105:152–156.

114. Kirchberger, M. A., and Tada, M. (1976): Effects of adenosine 3′,5′-monophosphate-dependent protein kinase on sarcoplasmic reticulum isolated from cardiac and slow and fast contracting skeletal muscles. *J. Biol. Chem.*, 251:725–729.

115. Kitagawa, Y., and Racker, E. (1982): Purification and characterization of two protein kinases from bovine heart mitochondrial membrane. *J. Biol. Chem.*, 257:4547–4551.

116. Klein, I., Levey, J. S., and Gondek, M. (1982): Characterization of the phosphoprotein profile in spontaneously beating cultured rat heart cells. *Proc. Soc. Exp. Biol. Med.*, 170:19–24.

117. Koide, Y., Beavo, J. A., Kapoor, C. L., Spruill, W. A., Huang, H.-L., Levine, S. N., Ong, S.-L., Bechtel, P. J., Yount, W. J., and Steiner, A. L. (1981): Hormonal effects of the immunocytochemical location of 3′,5′-cyclic adenosine monophosphate-dependent protein kinase in rat tissues. *Endocrinology*, 109:2226–2238.

118. Kramer, G. L., and Wells, J. N. (1979): Effects of phosphodiesterase inhibitors on cyclic nucleotide levels and relaxation of pig coronary arteries. *Mol. Pharmacol.*, 16:813–822.

119. Kranias, E. G., Mandel, F., Wang, T., and Schwartz, A. (1980): Mechanism of the stimulation of calcium ion dependent adenosine triphosphatase of cardiac sarcoplasmic reticulum by adenosine 3′,5′-monophosphate dependent protein kinase. *Biochemistry USA*, 19:5434–5439.

120. Kranias, E. G., Schwartz, A., and Jungmann, R. A. (1982): Characterization of cyclic 3′:5′-AMP-dependent protein kinase in sarcoplasmic reticulum and cytosol of canine myocardium. *Biochim. Biophys. Acta*, 709:28–37.

121. Kranias, E. G., and Solaro, R. J. (1983): Coordination of cardiac

sarcoplasmic reticulum and myofibrillar function by protein phosphorylation. *Fed. Proc.*, 42:33–38.

122. Krebs, E. G., and Beavo, J. A. (1979): Phosphorylation-dephosphorylation of enzymes. *Annu. Rev. Biochem.,* 48:923–959.

123. Kukovetz, W. R., Holzmann, S., Wurm, A., and Pöch, G. (1979): Evidence for cyclic GMP mediated relaxant effects of nitro-compounds in coronary smooth muscle. *Naunyn-Schmiedebergs Arch. Pharmacol.*, 310:129–138.

124. Kukovetz, W. P., Pöch, G., Holzmann, S., Wurm, A., and Rinner, J. (1978): Role of cyclic nucleotides in adenosine-mediated regulation of coronary flow. *Adv. Cyclic Nucleotide Res.,* 9:397–409.

125. Laloux, M., and Hers, H. G. (1979): Native and latent forms of skeletal muscle phosphorylase phosphatase. *FEBS Lett.,* 105:239–243.

126. Lamers, J. M. J., Stinis, H. T., and DeJonge, H. R. (1981): On the role of cyclic AMP and Ca^{2+}-calmodulin-dependent phosphorylation in the control of $(Ca^{2+} + Mg^{2+})$-ATPase of cardiac sarcolemma. *FEBS Lett.,* 127:139–143.

127. LaPorte, D. C., Builder, S. E., and Storm, D. R. (1980): Spectroscopic studies of the cAMP binding sites of the regulatory subunits of types I and II protein kinase. *J. Biol. Chem.,* 255:2343–2349.

128. LePeuch, C. J., Guilleux, J.-C., and Demaille, J. G. (1980): Phospholamban phosphorylation in the perfused rat heart is not solely dependent on β-adrenergic stimulation. *FEBS Lett.,* 114:165–168.

129. LePeuch, C. J., Haiech, J., and Demaille, J. G. (1979): Concerted regulation of cardiac sarcoplasmic reticulum calcium transport by cyclic adenosine monophosphate dependent and calcium-calmodulin-dependent phosphorylations. *Biochemistry USA,* 18:5150–5157.

130. Limas, C. J. (1980): Phosphorylation of cardiac sarcoplasmic reticulum by a calcium-activated, phospholipid-dependent protein kinase. *Biochem. Biophys. Res. Commun.,* 96:1378–1383.

131. Lincoln, T. M., and Corbin, J. D. (1977): Adenosine 3′:5′-cyclic monophosphate- and guanosine 3′:5′-cyclic monophosphate-dependent protein kinases: Possible homologous proteins. *Proc. Natl. Acad. Sci. USA,* 74:3239–3243.

132. Lincoln, T. M., and Corbin, J. D. (1983): Characterization and biological role of the cGMP-dependent protein kinase. *Adv. Cyclic Nucleotide Res.,* 15:139–192.

133. Lincoln, T. M., Flockhart, D. A., and Corbin, J. D. (1978): Studies on the structure and mechanism of activation of the guanosine 3′:5′-monophosphate-dependent protein kinase. *J. Biol. Chem.,* 253:6002–6009.

134. Lincoln, T. M., and Keely, S. L. (1981): Regulation of cardiac cyclic GMP-dependent protein kinase. *Biochim. Biophys. Acta,* 676:230–244.

135. Lindemann, J. P., Jones, L. R., Hathaway, D. R., Henry, B. G., and Watanabe, A. M. (1983): β-Adrenergic stimulation of phospholamban phosphorylation and Ca^{2+}-ATPase activity in guinea pig ventricles. *J. Biol. Chem.,* 258:464–471.

136. Livesey, S. A., Kemp, B. E., Re, C. A., Partridge, N. C., and Martin, T. J. (1982): Selective hormonal activation of cyclic AMP-dependent protein kinase isoenzymes in normal and malignant osteoblasts. *J. Biol. Chem.,* 257:14983–14987.

137. Lohmann, S. M., Schwoch, G., Reiser, G., Port, R., and Walter, U. (1983): Dibutyryl cAMP treatment of neuroblastoma-glioma hybrid cells results in selective increase in cAMP-receptor protein (R-I) as measured by monospecific antibodies. *EMBO J.,* 2:153–159.

138. Loten, E. G., and Sneyd, J. G. T. (1970): An effect of insulin on adipose-tissue adenosine 3′:5′-cyclic monophosphate phosphodiesterase. *Biochem. J.,* 120:187–193.

139. Louis, C. F., Maffitt, M., and Jarvis, B. (1982): Factors that modify the molecular size of phospholamban, the 23,000 dalton cardiac sarcoplasmic reticulum phosphoprotein. *J. Biol. Chem.,* 257:15182–15186.

140. Lubbe, W. F., Nguyen, T., and West, E. J. (1983): Modulation of myocardial cyclic AMP and vulnerability to fibrillation in the rat heart. *Fed. Proc.,* 42:2460–2464.

141. Mackenzie, C. W. (1982): Bovine lung cyclic GMP-dependent protein kinase exhibits two types of cyclic GMP-binding sites. *J. Biol. Chem.,* 257:5589–5593.

142. Malencik, D. A., and Anderson, S. R. (1983): Characterization of a fluorescent substrate for the adenosine 3′,5′-cyclic monophosphate-dependent protein kinase. *Anal. Biochem.,* 132:34–40.

143. Malkinson, A. M., Beer, D. S., Wehner, J. M., and Sheppard, J. R. (1983): Elution of the regulatory subunit of cAMP-dependent protein kinase type I isozyme derived from epididymal fat within the type II isozyme chromatographic peak. *Biochem. Biophys. Res. Commun.,* 112:214–220.

144. Malkinson, A. M., Hogy, L., Gharrett, A. J., and Gunderson, T. J. (1978): Ontogenetic studies of cyclic AMP-dependent protein kinase enzymes from mouse heart and other tissues. *J. Exp. Zool.,* 205:423–431.

145. Mandel, F., Kranias, E. G., and Schwartz, A. (1983): The effect of cAMP-dependent protein-kinase phosphorylation on the external Ca^{2+}-binding-sites of cardiac sarcoplasmic reticulum. *J. Bioenerg. Biomembr.,* 15:179–194.

146. Manning, D. R., DiSalvo, J., and Stull, J. T. (1980): Protein phosphorylation: quantitative analysis *in vivo* and in intact cell systems. *Mol. Cell. Endocrinol.,* 19:1–19.

147. Marchmont, R. J., and Houslay, M. D. (1981): Characterization of the phosphorylated form of the insulin-stimulated cyclic AMP phosphodiesterase from rat liver plasma membranes. *Biochem. J.,* 195:653–660.

148. McClellan, G. B., and Winegrad, S. (1980): Cyclic nucleotide regulation of the contractile proteins in mammalian cardiac muscle. *J. Gen. Physiol.,* 75:283–295.

149. McCormack, J. G., and Denton, R. M. (1981): The activation of pyrurate dehydrogenase in the perfused rat heart by adrenaline and other inotropic agents. *Biochem. J.,* 194:639–643.

150. McCullough, T. E., and Walsh, D. A. (1979): Phosphorylation of glycogen synthase in the perfused rat heart. *J. Biol. Chem.,* 254:7336–7344.

151. McCullough, T. E., and Walsh, D. A. (1979): Phosphorylation and dephosphorylation of phosphorylase kinase in the perfused rat heart. *J. Biol. Chem.,* 254:7345–7352.

152. Metsä-Ketelä, T., Kuosa, R., and Vapaatalo, H. (1980): Temporal dissociation between the negative inotropism and the increase in cyclic GMP level induced by choline esters in spontaneously beating rat atria preparations. *Acta Physiol. Scand.,* 110:83–87.

153. Mitchell, J. W., Mellgren, R. L., and Thomas, J. A. (1980): Phosphorylation of heart glycogen synthase by cAMP-dependent protein kinase. Regulatory effects of ATP. *J. Biol. Chem.,* 255:10368–10374.

154. Moir, A. J. G., and Perry, S. V. (1980): Phosphorylation of rabbit cardiac muscle troponin I by phosphorylase kinase. The effect of adrenaline. *Biochem. J.,* 191:547–554.

155. Morgan, H. E., Henderson, M. J., Regen, D. M., and Park, C. R. (1961): Regulation of glucose uptake in muscle. I. The effects of insulin and anoxia on glucose transport and phosphorylation in the isolated, perfused heart of normal rats. *J. Biol. Chem.,* 236:253–261.

156. Napoli, S. A., Gruetter, C. A., Ignarro, L. J., and Kadowitz, P. J. (1980): Relaxation of bovine coronary arterial smooth muscle by cyclic GMP, cyclic AMP and analogs. *J. Pharmacol. Exp. Ther.,* 212:469–473.

157. Neely, J. R., Liebermeister, H., Battersby, E. J., and Morgan, H. E. (1967): Effect of pressure development on oxygen consumption by isolated rat heart. *Am. J. Physiol.,* 212:804–814.

158. Nichols, J. R., and Gonzalez, N. C. (1982): Increase in myocardial cell cGMP concentration in pressure-induced myocardial hypertrophy. *J. Mol. Cell. Cardiol.,* 14:181–183.

159. Nimmo, H. G., and Cohen, P. (1977): Hormonal control of protein phosphorylation. *Adv. Cyclic Nucleotide Res.,* 8:145–266.

160. Øgreid, D., and Døskeland, S. O. (1981): The kinetics of the interaction between cyclic AMP and the regulatory moiety of protein kinase II. Evidence for interaction between the binding sites for cyclic AMP. *FEBS Lett.,* 129:282–286.

161. Øgreid, D., and Døskeland, S. O. (1981): The kinetics of association of cyclic AMP to the two types of binding sites associated with protein kinase II from bovine myocardium. *FEBS Lett.,* 129:287–292.

162. Øgreid, D., and Døskeland, S. O. (1982): Activation of protein kinase isoenzymes under near physiological conditions. Evidence that both types (A and B) of cAMP binding sites are involved in

the activation of protein kinase by cAMP and 8-N₃-cAMP. *FEBS Lett.*, 150:161–166.

163. Øgreid, D., Døskeland, S. O., and Miller, J. P. (1983): Evidence that cyclic nucleotides activating rabbit muscle protein kinase I interact with both types of cAMP binding sites associated with the enzyme. *J. Biol. Chem.*, 258:1041–1049.

164. Onorato, J. J., and Rudolph, S. A. (1981): Regulation of protein phosphorylation by inotropic agents in isolated rat myocardial cells. *J. Biol. Chem.*, 256:10697–10703.

165. Opie, L. H. (1982): Role of cyclic nucleotides in heart metabolism. *Cardiovasc. Res.*, 16:483–507.

166. Osterrieder, W., Brum, G., Hescheler, J., and Trautwein, W. (1982): Injection of subunits of cyclic AMP-dependent protein kinase into cardiac myocytes modulates Ca²⁺ current. *Nature*, 298:576–578.

167. Patten, G. S., Filsell, O. H., and Clark, M. G. (1982): Epinephrine regulation of phosphofructokinase in perfused rat heart. A calcium ion-dependent mechanism mediated via α-receptors. *J. Biol. Chem.*, 257:9480–9486.

168. Payne, E., and Soderling, T. R. (1980): Calmodulin-dependent glycogen synthase kinase. *J. Biol. Chem.*, 255:8054–8056.

169. Pfitzer, G., Rüegg, J. C., Flockerzi, V., and Hofmann, F. (1982): cGMP-dependent protein kinase decreases calcium sensitivity of skinned cardiac fibers. *FEBS Lett.*, 149:171–175.

170. Pilkis, S. J., El-Maghrabi, M., McGrane, M., Pilkis, J., Fox, E., and Claus, T. H. (1982): Fructose 2,6-bisphosphate: a mediator of hormone action at the fructose 6-phosphate/fructose 1,6-bisphosphate substrate cycle. *Mol. Cell. Endocrinol.*, 25:245–266.

171. Pilkis, S. J., El-Maghrabi, M. R., Pilkis, J., Claus, T. H., and Cumming, D. A. (1981): Fructose 2,6-bisphosphate. A new activator of phosphofructokinase. *J. Biol. Chem.*, 256:3171–3174.

172. Pilkis, S. J., Walderhaug, M., Murray, K., Beth, A., Venkataramu, S. D., Pilkis, J., and El-Maghrabi, M. R. (1983): 6-Phosphofructo-2-kinase/fructose 2,6-bisphosphatase from rat liver. Isolation and identification of a phosphorylated intermediate. *J. Biol. Chem.*, 258:6135–6141.

173. Popp, D. A., Kiechle, F. L., Kotagal, N., and Jarett, L. (1980): Insulin stimulation of pyruvate dehydrogenase in an isolated plasma membrane-mitochondrial mixture occurs by activation of pyruvate dehydrogenase phosphatase. *J. Biol. Chem.*, 255:7540–7543.

174. Ramachandran, C., Angelos, K. L., Sivaramakrishnan, S., and Walsh, D. A. (1983): Regulation of cardiac glycogen synthase. *Fed. Proc.*, 42:9–13.

175. Rangel-Aldao, R., Kupiec, J. W., and Rosen, O. M. (1979): Resolution of the phosphorylated and dephosphorylated cAMP-binding proteins of bovine cardiac muscle by affinity labeling and two-dimensional electrophoresis. *J. Biol. Chem.*, 254:2499–2508.

176. Rangel-Aldao, R., and Rosen, O. M. (1976): Dissociation and reassociation of the phosphorylated and nonphosphorylated forms of adenosine 3′:5′-monophosphate-dependent protein kinase from bovine cardiac muscle. *J. Biol. Chem.*, 251:3375–3380.

177. Rangel-Aldao, R., and Rosen, O. M. (1977): Effect of cAMP and ATP on the reassociation of phosphorylated and nonphosphorylated subunits of the cAMP-dependent protein kinase from bovine cardiac muscle. *J. Biol. Chem.*, 252:7140–7145.

178. Rannels, S. R., and Corbin, J. D. (1980): Two different intrachain cAMP binding sites of cAMP-dependent protein kinases. *J. Biol. Chem.*, 255:7085–7088.

179. Rannels, S. R., and Corbin, J. D. (1981): Studies on the function of the two intrachain cAMP binding sites of protein kinase. *J. Biol. Chem.*, 256:7871–7876.

180. Robertson, S. P., Johnson, J. D., Holroyde, M. J., Kranias, E. G., Potter, J. D., and Solaro, R. J. (1982): The effect of troponin I phosphorylation on the Ca²⁺-binding properties of the Ca²⁺-regulatory site of bovine cardiac troponin. *J. Biol. Chem.*, 257:260–263.

181. Robinson-Steiner, A. M., and Corbin, J. D. (1982): Stimulation of [³H]cIMP binding by cAMP analogs in extracts of perfused rat hearts. *J. Biol. Chem.*, 257:5482–5489.

182. Robinson-Steiner, A. M., and Corbin, J. D. (1983): Probable involvement of both intrachain cAMP binding sites in activation of protein kinase. *J. Biol. Chem.*, 258:1032–1040.

183. Robinson-Steiner, A. M., Beebe, S., Rannels, S. R., and Corbin,

J. D. (1984): Microheterogeneity of type II cAMP-dependent protein kinase in various mammalian species and tissues. *J. Biol. Chem.*, 259:10576–10605.

184. Rosen, O. M., and Erlichman, J. (1975): Reversible autophosphorylation of a cyclic 3′:5′-AMP-dependent protein kinase from bovine cardiac muscle. *J. Biol. Chem.*, 250:7788–7794.

185. Rosen, O. M., Herrera, R., Olowe, Y., Petruzzelli, L. M., and Cobb, M. H. (1983): Phosphorylation activates the insulin receptor tyrosine protein kinase. *Proc. Natl. Acad. Sci. USA*, 80:3237–3240.

186. Roskoski, R. (1983): Assays of protein kinase. *Methods Enzymol.*, 99:3–6.

187. Rubin, C. S., Fleischer, N., Sarkar, D., and Erlichman, J. (1981): Neural-specific and nonneural protein kinases: subclasses of type-II protein kinases. *Cold Spring Harbor Symp.*, 8:1333–1346.

188. Rymond, M., and Hofmann, F. (1982): Characterization of phosphorylated and dephosphorylated regulatory subunit of cAMP-dependent protein kinase II. *Eur. J. Biochem.*, 125:395–400.

189. Schultz, K. D., Bohme, E., Kreye, V. A. W., and Schultz, G. (1979): Relaxation of hormonally stimulated smooth muscular tissues by the 8-bromo derivative of cyclic GMP. *Naunyn-Schmiedebergs Arch. Pharmacol.*, 306:1–9.

190. Schultz, K. D., Schultz, K., and Schultz, G. (1977): Sodium nitroprusside and other smooth muscle-relaxants increase cyclic GMP levels in rat ductus deferens. *Nature*, 265:750–751.

191. Seidel, C. L., Schnarr, R. L., and Sparks, H. V. (1975): Coronary artery cyclic AMP content during adrenergic receptor stimulation. *Am. J. Physiol.*, 229:265–274.

192. Shoji, S., Ericsson, L. H., Walsh, K. A., Fischer, E. H., and Titani, K. (1983): Amino acid sequence of the catalytic subunit of bovine type II adenosine cyclic 3′,5′-phosphate dependent protein kinase. *Biochemistry USA*, 22:3702–3709.

193. Shoji, S., Parmelee, D. C., Wade, R. D., Kumar, S., Ericsson, L. H., Walsh, K. A., Neurath, H., Long, G. L., Demaille, J. G., Fischer, E. H., and Titani, K. (1981): Complete amino acid sequence of the catalytic subunit of bovine cardiac muscle cyclic AMP-dependent protein kinase. *Proc. Natl. Acad. Sci. USA*, 78:848–851.

194. Silver, P. J., Schmidt-Silver, C., and DiSalvo, J. (1982): β-Adrenergic relaxation and cAMP kinase activation in coronary arterial smooth muscle. *Am. J. Physiol.*, 242:H177–H184.

195. Singh, J., and Flitney, F. W. (1981): Inotropic responses of the frog ventricle to dibutyryl cyclic AMP and 8-bromo cyclic GMP and related changes in endogenous cyclic nucleotide levels. *Biochem. Pharmacol.*, 30:1475–1481.

196. Sistare, F. D., Lichtenberg, L., Sugg, R. G., McFarland, S. A., and Villar-Palasi, C. (1981): Effects of isoproterenol treatment of isolated perfused rat hearts on myofibrillar phosphorylation and ATPase activity. *J. Cyclic Nucleotide Res.*, 7:85–93.

197. Sivaramakrishnan, S., High, C. W., and Walsh, D. A. (1982): Regulation of cardiac glycogen synthase by phosphorylation: catalysis of inactivation by cAMP-dependent and cAMP-independent protein kinases and comparison with the phosphorylation of the skeletal muscle enzyme. *Arch. Biochem. Biophys.*, 214:311–325.

198. Smith, S., White, H. D., Siegel, J. B., and Krebs, E. G. (1981): Cyclic AMP-dependent protein kinase I: Cyclic nucleotide binding, structural changes, and release of the catalytic subunits. *Proc. Natl. Acad. Sci. USA*, 78:1591–1595.

199. Soderling, T. R. (1979): Regulatory functions of protein multisite phosphorylations. *Mol. Cell. Endocrinol.*, 16:157–179.

200. Soderling, T. R., and Khatra, B. S. (1982): Regulation of glycogen synthase by multiple protein kinases. In: *Calcium and Cell Function, Vol. III*, edited by W. Y. Cheung, pp. 189–221. Academic Press, New York.

201. Spruill, W. A., Koide, Y., Huang, H.-L., Levine, S. N., Ong, S.-H., Steiner, A. L., and Beavo, J. A. (1981): Immunocytochemical localization of cyclic guanosine monophosphate-dependent protein kinase in endocrine tissues. *Endocrinology*, 109:2239–2248.

202. Stadtmauer, L. A., and Rosen, O. M. (1983): Phosphorylation of exogenous substrates by the insulin receptor-associated protein kinase. *J. Biol. Chem.*, 258:6682–6685.

203. Stewart, A. A., Ingebritsen, T. S., and Cohen, P. (1983): The protein phosphatases involved in cellular regulation. 5. Purification

and properties of a Ca²⁺/calmodulin-dependent protein phosphatase (2B) from rabbit skeletal muscle. *Eur. J. Biochem.*, 132:289–295.

204. Sugden, P. H., and Corbin, J. D. (1976): Adenosine 3′:5′-cyclic monophosphate-binding proteins in bovine and rat tissues. *Biochem. J.*, 159:423–437.

205. Sul, H. S., Cooper, R. H., Whitehouse, S., and Walsh, D. A. (1982): Cardiac phosphorylase kinase. Modulation of the activity by cAMP-dependent and cAMP-independent phosphorylation of the α′ subunit. *J. Biol. Chem.*, 257:3484–3490.

206. Tada, M., Inui, M., Yamada, M., Kadoma, M., Kuzuya, T., Abe, H., and Kakiuchi, S. (1983): Effects of phospholamban phosphorylation catalyzed by adenosine 3′:5′-monophosphate- and calmodulin-dependent protein kinases on calcium transport ATPase of cardiac sarcoplasmic reticulum. *J. Mol. Cell. Cardiol.*, 15:335–346.

207. Taegtmeyer, H., Hems, R., and Krebs, H. A. (1980): Utilization of energy-providing substrates in the isolated working rat heart. *Biochem. J.*, 186:701–711.

208. Takio, K., Smith, S. B., Krebs, E. G., Walsh, K. A., and Titani, K. (1982): Primary structure of the regulatory subunit of type II cAMP-dependent protein kinase from bovine cardiac muscle. *Proc. Natl. Acad. Sci. USA*, 79:2544–2548.

209. Takio, K., Smith, S. B., Walsh, K. A., Krebs, E. G., and Titani, K. (1983): Amino acid sequence around a "hinge" region and its "autophosphorylation" site in bovine lung cGMP-dependent protein kinase. *J. Biol. Chem.*, 258:5531–5536.

210. Taylor, S. S., Kerlavage, A. R., Zoller, M. J., Nelson, N. C., and Potter, R. L. (1981): Nucleotide-binding sites and structural domains of cAMP-dependent protein kinases. *Cold Spring Harbor Symp.*, 8:3–18.

211. Titanji, V. P. K., Ragnarsson, U., Humble, E., and Zetterqvist, O. (1980): Phosphopeptide substrates of a phosphoprotein phosphatase from rat liver. *J. Biol. Chem.*, 255:11339–11343.

212. Toyo-oka, T. (1982): Phosphorylation with cyclic adenosine 3′:5′ monophosphate-dependent protein kinase renders bovine cardiac troponin sensitive to degradation by calcium-activated neutral protease. *Biochem. Biophys. Res. Commun.*, 107:44–50.

213. Uno, I. (1980): Phosphorylation and dephosphorylation of the regulatory subunit of cyclic 3′:5′-monophosphate-dependent protein kinase (type II) *in vivo* and *in vitro*. *Biochim. Biophys. Acta*, 631:59–69.

214. Van Schaftingen, E., Hue, L., and Hers, H. G. (1980): Control of the fructose 6-phosphate/fructose 1,6-bisphosphate cycle in isolated hepatocytes by glucose and glucagon. *Biochem. J.*, 192:887–895.

215. Veleema, J., Noordam, P. C., and Zaagsma, J. (1983): Comparison of cyclic AMP-dependent phosphorylation of sarcolemma and sarcoplasmic reticulum from rat cardiac ventricle muscle. *Int. J. Biochem.*, 15:675–684.

216. Veleema, J., and Zaagsma, J. (1981): Purification and characterization of cardiac sarcolemma and sarcoplasmic reticulum from rat ventricle muscle. *Arch. Biochem. Biophys.*, 212:678–688.

217. Vetter, R., Haase, H., and Will, H. (1982): Potentiating effect of calmodulin and catalytic subunit of cyclic AMP-dependent protein kinase on ATP-dependent Ca²⁺-transport by cardiac sarcolemma. *FEBS Lett.*, 148:326–330.

218. Vittone, L., Grassi, A., Chiappe, L., Argel, M., and Cingolani, H. E. (1981): Relaxing effect of pharmacologic interventions increasing cAMP in rat heart. *Am. J. Physiol.*, 240:H441–H447.

219. Vogel, S., and Sperelakis, N. (1981): Induction of slow action potentials by microiontophoresis of cyclic AMP into heart cells. *J. Mol. Cell. Cardiol.*, 13:51–64.

220. Walsh, D. A., Clippinger, M. S., Sivaramakrishnan, S., and McCullough, T. E. (1979): Cyclic adenosine monophosphate

221. Walsh, M. P., Vallet, B., Autric, F., and Demaille, J. G. (1979): Purification and characterization of bovine cardiac calmodulin-dependent myosin light chain kinase. *J. Biol. Chem.*, 254:12136–12144.

222. Walter, U., Miller, P., Wilson, F., Menkes, D., and Greengard, P. (1980): Immunological distinction between guanosine 3′:5′-monophosphate-dependent and adenosine 3′:5′-monophosphate-dependent protein kinases. *J. Biol. Chem.*, 255:3757–3762.

223. Walter, U., Uno, I., Liu, A. Y.-C., and Greengard, P. (1977): Identification, characterization and quantitative measurement of cyclic AMP receptor proteins in cytosol of various tissues using a photoaffinity ligand. *J. Biol. Chem.*, 252:6494–6500.

224. Weber, I. T., Takio, K., Titani, K., and Steitz, T. A. (1982): The cAMP binding domains of the regulatory subunit of cAMP-dependent protein kinase and the catabolite gene activator protein are homologous. *Proc. Natl. Acad. Sci. USA*, 79:7679–7683.

225. Weber, W., Schwoch, G., Schröder, H., and Hilz, H. (1981): Analysis of cAMP-dependent protein kinases by immunotitration: multiple forms-multiple functions? *Cold Spring Harbor Symp.*, 8:125–140.

226. Whitehouse, S., Feramisco, J. R., Casnellie, J. E., Krebs, E. G., and Walsh, D. A. (1983): Studies on the kinetic mechanism of the catalytic subunit of the cAMP-dependent protein kinase. *J. Biol. Chem.*, 258:3693–3701.

227. Whitehouse, S., and Walsh, D. A. (1982): Purification of a physiological form of the inhibitor protein of the cAMP-dependent protein kinase. *J. Biol. Chem.*, 257:6028–6032.

228. Whitehouse, S., and Walsh, D. A. (1983): Mg-ATP²⁻-dependent interaction of the inhibitor protein of the cAMP-dependent protein kinase with the catalytic subunit. *J. Biol. Chem.*, 258:3682–3692.

229. Winegrad, S., McClellan, G., Horowits, R., Tucker, M., Lin, L.-E., and Weisberg, A. (1983): Regulation of cardiac contractile proteins by phosphorylation. *Fed. Proc.*, 42:39–44.

230. Wise, B. G., Glass, D. B., Chou, C.-H. J., Raynor, R. L., Katoh, N., Schatzman, R. C., Turner, R. S., Kibler, R. F., and Kuo, J. F. (1982): Phospholipid-sensitive Ca²⁺-dependent protein kinase from heart. II. Substrate specificity and inhibition by various agents. *J. Biol. Chem.*, 257:8489–8495.

231. Wise, B. C., and Kuo, J. F. (1983): Modes of inhibition by acylcarnitines, adriamycin and trifluoperazine of cardiac phospholipid-sensitive calcium-dependent protein kinase. *Biochem. Pharmacol.*, 32:1259–1265.

232. Wise, B. C., Raynor, R. L., and Kuo, J. F. (1982): Phospholipid-sensitive Ca²⁺-dependent protein kinase from heart. I. Purification and general properties. *J. Biol. Chem.*, 257:8481–8488.

233. Wolf, H., and Hofmann, F. (1980): Purification of myosin light chain kinase from bovine cardiac muscle. *Proc. Natl. Acad. Sci. USA*, 77:5852–5855.

234. Wolff, J., Londos, C., and Cooper, D. M. F. (1981): Adenosine receptors and the regulation of adenylate cyclase. *Adv. Cyclic Nucleotide Res.*, 14:199–214.

235. Wrenn, R. W., and Kuo, J. F. (1981): Cyclic GMP-dependent phosphorylation of an endogenous protein from rat heart. *Biochem. Biophys. Res. Commun.*, 101:1274–1280.

236. Yeaman, S. J., Hutcheson, E. F., Roche, T. E., Pettit, F. H., Brown, J. R., Reed, L. J., Watson, D. C., and Dixon, G. H. (1978): Sites of phosphorylation on pyruvate dehydrogenase from bovine kidney and heart. *Biochemistry USA*, 17:2364–2370.

237. Zetterqvist, Ö., and Ragnarrson, U. (1982): The structural requirements of substrates of cyclic AMP-dependent protein kinase. *FEBS Lett.*, 139:287–290.

dependent and independent phosphorylation of sarcolemma membrane proteins in perfused rat heart. *Biochemistry USA*, 18:871–877.

The Heart and Cardiovascular System,
edited by H. A. Fozzard et al.
Raven Press, New York © 1986.

CHAPTER 44

Nucleotide Metabolism in Cardiac Muscle

Judith L. Swain and Edward W. Holmes

Purine, pyrimidine, and pyridine nucleotides, nucleosides, and bases play important roles in cardiac metabolism. This chapter describes analytical methods for quantitating nucleotide, nucleoside, and base pools, as well as methods for determining rates of nucleotide synthesis and degradation. The pathways involved in nucleotide synthesis and degradation are reviewed, and the changes produced with ischemia and hypertrophy are delineated. The relationship of nucleotide metabolism to myocardial function and viability is discussed, followed by strategies for increasing purine nucleotide synthesis.

STRUCTURE OF PURINE, PYRIMIDINE, AND PYRIDINE COMPOUNDS

Purines are heterocyclic compounds containing carbon and nitrogen atoms, while pyrimidines contain a single six-membered ring composed of carbon and nitrogen. The structures of the purine bases (adenine, hypoxanthine, xanthine, guanine) and the pyrimidine bases (uracil, cytosine) are illustrated in Fig. 1. Nucleosides consist of a purine or pyrimidine base with the addition of ribose. The nucleosides adenosine, guanosine, inosine, cytidine, and uridine consist of the corresponding base (adenine, guanine, hypoxanthine, cytosine, or uracil)

with a ribose at the 9 position of the purine ring or at the 1 position of the pyrimidine ring. As an example of this class of compounds the structure of the nucleoside inosine is illustrated in Fig. 2. Nucleotides are phosphoric acid esters of the nucleosides, and exist as either 5'-mono-, di-, or triphosphates. For illustration, the structure of adenosine-5'-triphosphate is shown in Fig. 3. The pyridine nucleotides contain a molecule of adenosine-5'-diphosphate and nicotinamide mononucleotide. The structure of nicotinamide adenine dinucleotide (NAD^+) is shown in Fig. 4. NADH is formed by the reduction of NAD^+ through the addition of a H^+ and two electrons on carbon atom 4 of the quinoid ring. In nicotinamide adenine dinucleotide phosphate ($NADP^+$) the 2'-hydroxyl of ADP is esterified with phosphoric acid. $NADP^+$ is reduced to NADPH in an analogous fashion to that described above for NAD^+.

ANALYTICAL METHODS

Preparation of Tissue for Analysis of Nucleotides, Nucleosides, and Bases

Since creatine phosphate and nucleotides are chemically labile and they are quickly catabolized when the

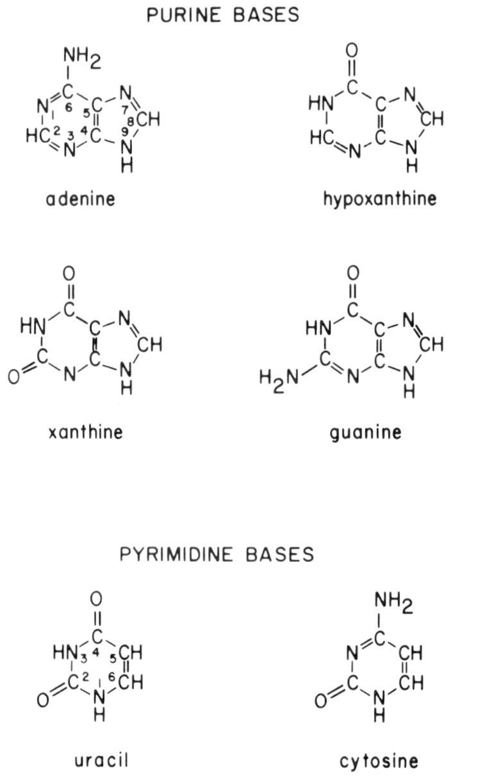

PURINE BASES

adenine

hypoxanthine

xanthine

guanine

PYRIMIDINE BASES

uracil

cytosine

FIG. 1. Structure of purine and pyrimidine bases.

blood supply to the heart is interrupted, the tissue to be analyzed must be rapidly frozen *in situ* to arrest all further metabolism (2). Cardiac tissue can be frozen *in situ* using Wollenberger tongs precooled in liquid nitrogen or isopentane, a technique referred to as "freeze-clamping." If repetitive samples are needed, the myocardial tissue samples can be removed by a rotary drill apparatus equipped with a hollow drill bit (63), or with a biopsy needle (64), and the tissue immediately frozen in liquid nitrogen or isopentane. The latter coolant is preferred by some investigators because of its more rapid diffusion into the tissue and resultant speeding of the freeze-clamping process. More sophisticated devices are available consisting of a drill bit attached to a vacuum system, where the sample is frozen in less than

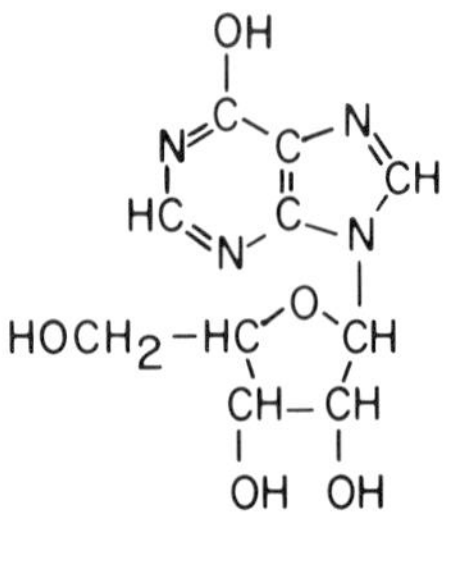

FIG. 2. Structure of inosine.

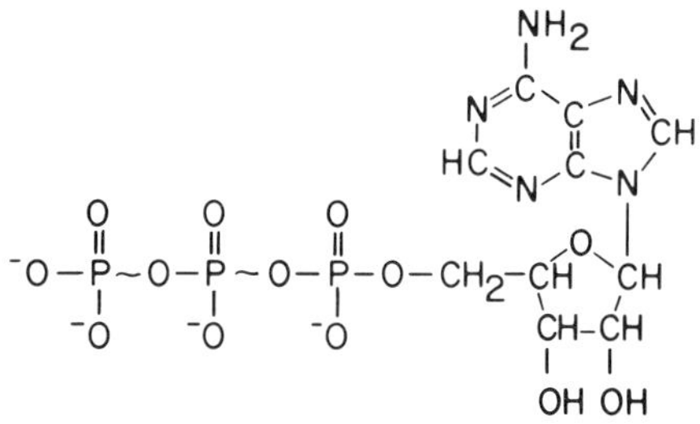

FIG. 3. Structure of adenosine triphosphate (ATP).

1 sec after removal from the myocardium (1,24,72). Tissue obtained by any of the methods can be stored for days under liquid nitrogen until processed, without change in content of most nucleotides, nucleosides, or bases.

Nucleotides, nucleosides, bases, and creatine phosphate are usually extracted from the tissue with acid solutions (73), except when quantitating the reduced forms of the pyridine nucleotides (35). (NADH and NADPH are acid labile and are usually extracted under alkaline conditions.) The frozen tissue is added directly to dilute trichloroacetic or perchloric acid and the tissue homogenized in an ice bath for several minutes. The homogenate is centrifuged to remove the insoluble material (protein, DNA, etc.) and the supernatant containing the nucleotides, nucleosides, and bases neutralized by either removing the trichloroacetic acid with a mixture of freon and tri-*N*-octylamine or ether, or by precipitating the perchlorate anion by the addition of potassium hydroxide. The solutions containing the neutralized nucleotides, nucleosides, or bases can then be stored for many months at $-70°C$ until analyzed. Various combinations of the above extraction, neutralization, and storage procedures have been successfully employed, but it is important to document that recovery of nucleotide, nucleoside, and base standards is adequate in the experimenter's own hands with whatever procedure is selected.

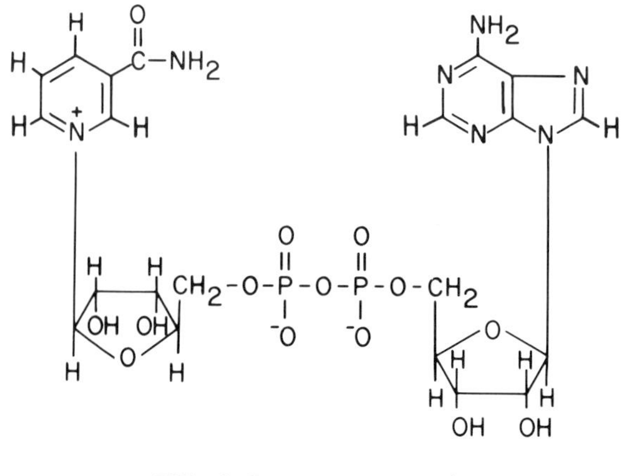

FIG. 4. Structure of NAD+.

Analysis of Tissue for Nucleotides, Nucleosides, and Bases

Nucleotides and their derivatives and creatine phosphate can be quantitated by enzymatic methods or by high performance liquid chromatography. Enzymatic analysis relies on the specificity of an enzyme to generate a product or consume a substrate in a reaction which is dependent on the content of nucleotide, nucleoside, or base in the extract. The measured change in content of the substrate or product is then used to quantitate the amount of the nucleotide in the extract. Spectrophotometric, fluorimetric, or radiochemical techniques can be used for these quantitations.

The enzymatic assay of ATP illustrates the principles involved (6). When the extract of tissue containing ATP is added to a cuvette containing luciferase isolated from the luminous organ of the firefly, light is produced:

$$\text{ATP} + \text{luciferin} \underset{\text{luciferase}}{\overset{\text{Mg}^{2+}, \text{O}_2}{\rightleftharpoons}}$$

$$\text{adenyl-oxyluciferin} + \text{H}_2\text{O} + \text{light}$$

The product, light, is quantitated with a photometer, and the amount of light produced is proportional to the amount of ATP in the extract. The ATP content of a tissue extract can also be quantitated using the phosphoglycerate kinase reaction coupled to the NADH-dependent glyceraldehyde-3-phosphate dehydrogenase reaction. The two reactions are:

$$\text{3-phosphoglycerate} + \text{ATP} \underset{\text{Mg}^{2+}}{\overset{\text{phosphoglycerate kinase}}{\rightleftharpoons}}$$

$$\text{1,3-diphosphoglycerate} + \text{ADP}$$

$$\text{1,3-diphosphoglycerate} + \text{NADH} + \overset{\text{G-3-P dehydrogenase}}{\text{H}^+} \rightarrow$$

$$\text{glyceraldehyde-3-phosphate} + \text{NAD}^+ + \text{phosphate}$$

The reduction in optical density at 340 nm, a measure of NADH consumption, is quantitated spectrophotometrically; the amount of NADH consumed is proportional to the amount of 1,3-diphosphoglycerate generated in the ATP-dependent phosphoglycerate kinase reaction.

Similar linked assays are available for other nucleotides, nucleosides, and bases. Creatine phosphate can be determined by coupling the ATP produced in the creatine kinase reaction to one of the above assays, or it can be determined directly by incubating tissue extract with ^{14}C-ADP and creatine phosphokinase (63). The ^{14}C-ATP produced in this reaction is separated from radiolabeled ADP by thin-layer chromatography and quantitated in a scintillation spectrophotometer.

When many nucleotides or derivatives are to be quantitated in a single sample, rather than perform multiple enzymatic analyses, it is preferable to analyze the sample by high performance liquid chromatography. In this technique individual compounds are identified by the time required for elution from a chromatographic column, and by the relative absorbance at different UV wavelengths. Quantification is achieved by comparison of peak heights or areas under the peaks to known concentrations of standard compounds applied to the column under the same conditions. Various chromatographic separations have been used for nucleotide analyses of cardiac tissue. For determination of adenine nucleotides alone, either anion exchange, paired ion exchange, or reverse phase chromatography (20,36,73) appears to be adequate. If other purine, pyrimidine, and pyridine nucleotides are to be quantitated in the same extract, anion exchange chromatography may be preferable (57). In anion exchange chromatography, the phosphate groups of the nucleotides are ionized when the mobile phase is at an appropriate pH (2.4–4.5). The more negatively charged nucleoside triphosphates are retained longer than the diphosphates, and the diphosphates longer than the monophosphates. The retention of the compounds on the column is also influenced by the ionic strength of the buffer. Separation of individual purine or pyrimidine compounds within these classes of nucleoside phosphates is determined by constituents of the ring and by groups substituted on the ring. Because of these considerations, one cannot rely on retention time alone for identification of compounds. "Enzyme shift," i.e., transfer of a peak from one elution position to another by a specific enzyme reaction, is a definitive method of identification of a compound detected in a high performance liquid chromatogram (HPLC). In the chromatograph illustrated in Fig. 5, purine, pyrimidine, and pyridine nucleotides are separated on an anion exchange column by varying both the pH and ionic strength of the buffer system during the elution. A gradient elution such as this usually enhances the resolution, but it also increases the time required when compared to isocratic separations. Thus, another consideration in choosing a separation system is the degree of resolution needed versus the time required to achieve this resolution.

When quantitating nucleosides, bases, and creatine phosphate, reverse phase or paired anion exchange chromatography (26,39,58) provides good resolution of these compounds. The polarity of the mobile phase is varied to separate individual nucleosides and bases, and gradient elutions and isocratic separations are available. Choice of a system depends on the resolution required.

Other methods are also available for quantitation of nucleotide pools. Isotachophoresis has been used to measure nucleotide concentration in extracts from heart and skeletal muscle (49,52). Nuclear magnetic resonance (NMR) spectroscopy is a noninvasive procedure that

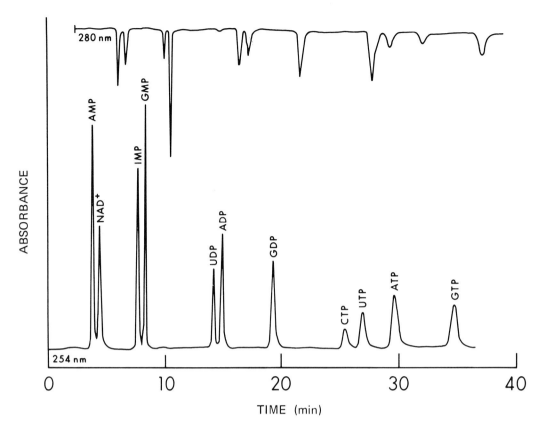

FIG. 5. Separation of purine, pyrimidine, and pyridine nucleotides by HPLC using an anion exchange column. The conditions are: 100% buffer A (5 mM $NH_4H_2PO_4$, pH 2.8) to 100% buffer B (750 mM $NH_4H_2PO_4$, pH 3.8) in a 40-min linear gradient at 2.0 ml/min.

can be used to obtain a relative estimate of ATP, creatine phosphate, and inorganic phosphate concentrations in tissue extracts, in isolated organs, and *in vivo*. This technique is discussed in *Chapter 13*.

PATHWAYS OF PURINE NUCLEOTIDE SYNTHESIS AND CATABOLISM

There are two pathways for purine nucleotide synthesis in the heart (18): formation of the purines through the *de novo* pathway, and reutilization of purine nucleosides and bases through the salvage pathways.

Purine Nucleotide Synthesis *De Novo*

The pathway of purine biosynthesis *de novo* consists of 10 reactions which culminate in formation of the parent purine nucleotide, inosine 5′-monophosphate (IMP). The reactions of this pathway are indicated in Fig. 6. An associated reaction, which strictly speaking is not a component of this pathway, leads to the synthesis of phosphoribosylpyrophosphate (PP-ribose-P) via the phosphorylation of ribose-5-phosphate by ATP:

$$\text{ribose-5-phosphate} + \text{ATP} \xrightarrow{\text{Mg}^{2+}, \text{P}_i} \text{PP-ribose-P} + \text{AMP}$$

This reaction is catalyzed by the enzyme PP-ribose-P synthetase.

The first unique reaction in purine biosynthesis is the formation of phosphoribosylamine (PRA). The amide nitrogen of glutamine (or NH_3) displaces PP_i from carbon 1 of PP-ribose-P in this reaction:

$$\text{PP-ribose-P} + \text{glutamine} + H_2O \xrightarrow{\text{Mg}^{2+}}$$

$$\text{PRA} + \text{glutamic acid} + PP_i \qquad [1]$$

This reaction is catalyzed by the enzyme glutamine phosphoribosylpyrophosphate amidotransferase, and the activity of this enzyme is one of the principle determinants of the rate of purine biosynthesis (29). When ammonia is the substrate, the enzyme functions as an aminotransferase. There are data to suggest that the amidotransferase and aminotransferase activities are enzymatic functions of the same protein in mammalian cells.

Glycine is added to the nascent purine ring in the next reaction in this pathway:

$$\text{PRA} + \text{glycine} + \text{ATP} \rightarrow$$

$$\text{glycinamide ribonucleotide} + \text{ADP} + \text{P}_i \qquad [2]$$

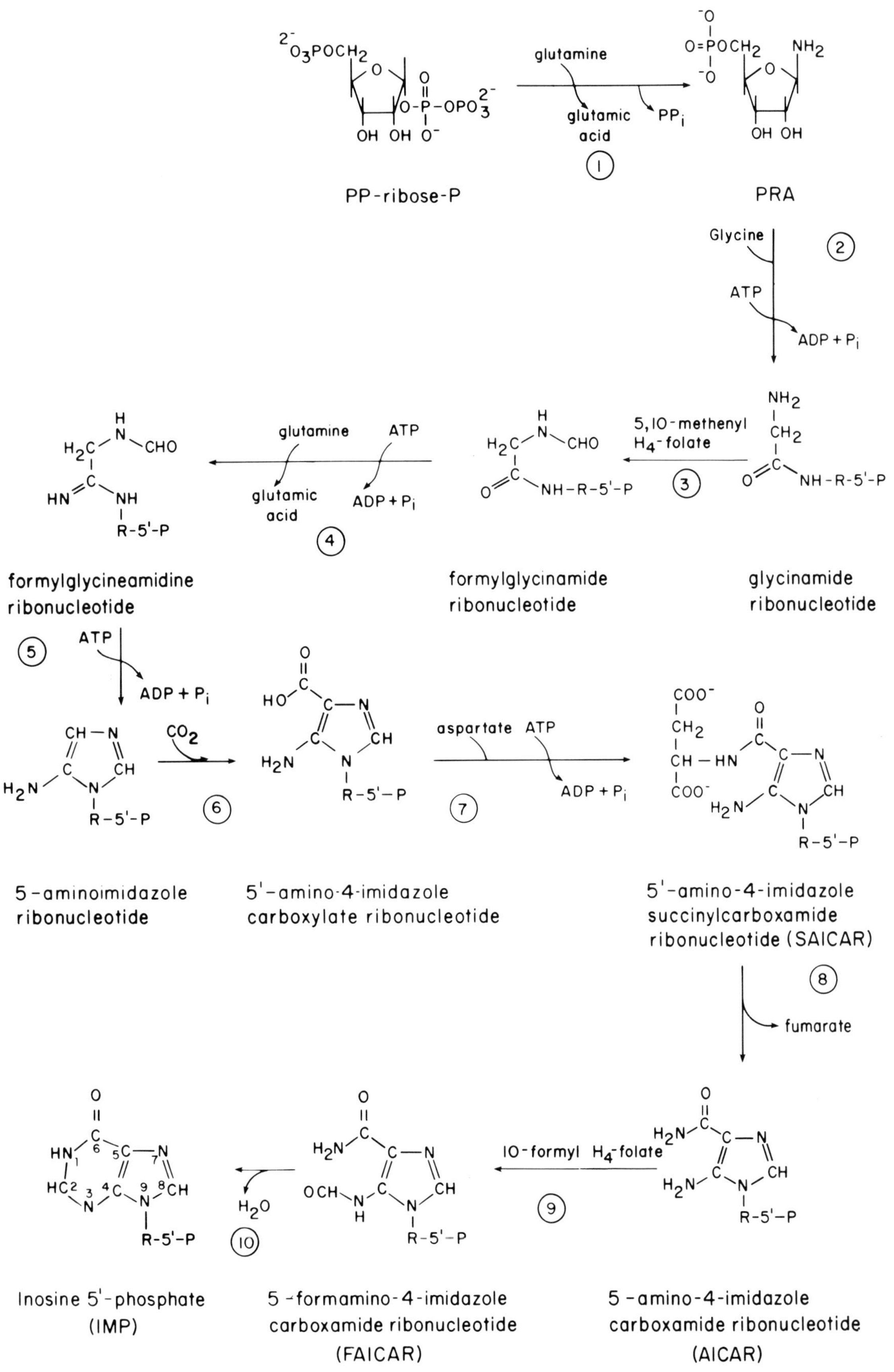

FIG. 6. Pathway of purine synthesis *de novo*.

The addition of a formyl group donated by a tetrahydrofolic acid (THFA) derivative and the addition of an amide group from glutamine in two separate reactions results in the formation of an amadine compound:

glycinamide ribonucleotide

$$+ 5,10\text{-methenyl } H_4\text{-folate} + H_2O \rightarrow \qquad [3]$$

formylglycineamide ribonucleotide

$$+ \text{ THFA} + H^+$$

formylglycineamide ribonucleotide

$$+ \text{ glutamine} + \text{ATP} + H_2O \xrightarrow{Mg^{2+}} \qquad [4]$$

formylglycineamidine ribonucleotide

$$+ \text{ glutamic acid} + \text{ADP} + P_i$$

Ring closure then occurs resulting in the formation of a 5-membered imidazole ring:

formylglycineamidine ribonucleotide + ATP $\xrightarrow{Mg^{2+},K^+}$ [5]

5-aminoimidazole ribonucleotide + ADP + P_i

A carbonyl group is added by fixation of CO_2:

5-aminoimidazole ribonucleotide + CO_2 ⇄ [6]

5-amino-4-imidazole carboxylate ribonucleotide

and aspartic acid condenses with the newly added carbonyl group:

5-amino-4-imidazole carboxylate ribonucleotide

$$+ \text{ aspartate} + \text{ATP} \xrightarrow{Mg^{2+}} 5\text{-amino-4-imidazole}$$

succinylcarboxamide ribonucleotide [7]

$$\text{(SAICAR)} + \text{ADP} + P_i$$

The SIACAR thus formed is cleaved by a bifunctional lyase enzyme:

SAICAR ⇄ fumarate + 5-amino-4-

imidazolecarboxamide ribonucleotide (AICAR) [8]

This same lyase enzyme catalyzes a similar reaction in the interconversion pathway leading from IMP to AMP, hence the term, bifunctional. AICAR receives a formyl group from another folic acid derivative, formyl-THFA:

AICAR + 10-formyl H_4-folate $\overset{K^+}{\rightleftarrows}$

5'-formamino-4-imidazolecarboxamide [9]

ribonucleotide (FAICAR) + THFA

and ring closure results in the formation of the parent purine nucleotide inosine 5'-monophosphate (IMP):

$$\text{FAICAR} \rightleftarrows \text{IMP} + H_2O \qquad [10]$$

Four moles of ATP are consumed in synthesizing one mole of IMP via the *de novo* pathway (one additional mole of ATP is needed for the formation of PP-ribose-P). The carbon atoms of the resulting purine ring are supplied by glycine (positions 4 and 5), formate (positions 2 and 8), and CO_2 (position 6). The nitrogen atoms are supplied by glycine (position 7), glutamine or NH_3 (positions 3 and 9), and aspartic acid (position 1).

Salvage Synthesis of Purine Nucleotides

Purine nucleotides are also synthesized by reutilizing or salvaging the purine ring in nucleosides and bases (Fig. 7). The purine ring in adenosine can reenter the nucleotide pool by two different routes. Adenosine can be directly phosphorylated to AMP through a reaction catalyzed by adenosine kinase:

$$\text{adenosine} + \text{ATP} \rightarrow \text{AMP} + \text{ADP} \qquad [12]$$

Alternatively, adenosine can be deaminated by adenosine deaminase to the nucleoside inosine, and inosine can undergo phosphorolysis by purine nucleoside phosphorylase to form the base hypoxanthine. Hypoxanthine can be salvaged through phosphoribosylation in a reaction catalyzed by hypoxanthine-guanine phosphoribosyltransferase:

$$\text{adenosine} + H_2O \rightarrow \text{inosine} + NH_3 \qquad [13]$$

$$\text{inosine} + P_i \rightleftarrows \text{hypoxanthine} + \text{ribose-1-P} \qquad [14]$$

$$\text{hypoxanthine} + \text{PP-ribose-P} \rightarrow \text{IMP} + PP_i \qquad [15]$$

Inosine is not directly reutilized for nucleotide synthesis since mammalian cells do not contain appreciable inosine kinase activity (4).

The purine base adenine can be used for nucleotide synthesis in a manner analogous to hypoxanthine:

$$\text{Adenine} + \text{PP-ribose-P} \rightarrow \text{AMP} + PP_i \qquad [16]$$

with the reaction catalyzed by the enzyme adenine phosphoribosyltransferase. While most mammalian tis-

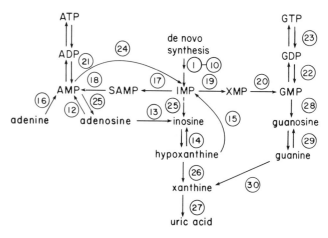

FIG. 7. Salvage synthesis, interconversion, and catabolism of purine nucleotides.

TABLE 1. *Concentrations of nucleosides and bases in human and canine plasma*

Nucleosides and bases	Plasma concentration (μM)	
	Human	Dog
Adenosine	<0.10	<0.10
Inosine	0.40	0.39
Hypoxanthine	2.63	0.51
Xanthine	0.93	—
Adenine	ND	ND

ND = not determined.

sues, including heart, are rich in both phosphoribosyl-transferase activities (41), little, if any, nucleotide is formed from adenine because mammalian tissues lack appreciable adenosine phosphorylase activity (60). Consequently, little adenine is produced and plasma adenine concentrations are too low to detect. In contrast, hypoxanthine is readily available in plasma in most mammals, and it is the major source of salvageable purine. Table 1 lists the plasma concentrations reported for the various purine nucleosides and bases in humans and dogs (9,19,74). Once hypoxanthine is oxidized to xanthine, a reaction which occurs primarily in the liver and intestine in man, the purine base is lost, since neither xanthine nor urate (the oxidation product of xanthine) can be salvaged in mammalian cells.

Synthesis of Adenine and Guanine Nucleotides from IMP

IMP formed from either *de novo* or salvage synthesis is located at an important branchpoint in the purine biosynthetic pathway since it can be used to synthesize AMP or GMP. The synthesis of AMP occurs in a two-step reaction catalyzed sequentially by adenylosuccinate (SAMP) synthetase and SAMP lyase (Fig. 7):

$$IMP + aspartate + GTP \rightarrow SAMP + GDP + P_i \quad [17]$$

$$SAMP \rightarrow AMP + fumarate \quad [18]$$

As pointed out earlier, SAMP lyase is a bifunctional enzyme which also catalyzes the cleavage of SAICAR in the *de novo* pathway. The formation of GMP occurs in a two-step reaction utilizing NAD^+ and glutamine:

$$IMP + NAD^+ + H_2O \xrightarrow{K^+}$$
$$xanthosine\text{-}5'\text{-}monophosphate\ (XMP) \quad [19]$$
$$+ NADH + H^+$$

$$XMP + glutamine + ATP \xrightarrow{Mg^{2+}}$$
$$GMP + glutamic\ acid + AMP + PP_i \quad [20]$$

The nucleoside diphosphates ADP and GDP are synthe-

sized from the monophosphates through the action of nucleoside monophosphate kinases which are specific for the adenosine (reaction 21) or guanosine nucleotides (reaction 22) (Fig. 7). GDP is phosphorylated to GTP by a general nucleoside diphosphate kinase (reaction 23), which is not base specific, and ATP is the phosphate donor in this reaction. ADP is phosphorylated to ATP by either substrate level phosphorylation in the glycolytic pathway or by oxidative phosphorylation in mitochondria. In many mammalian cells the adenine and guanine nucleotides can be interconverted by deamination of AMP and GMP to the common intermediate IMP. However, in adult myocardium both AMP deaminase and GMP reductase activities are low and little IMP is formed via these pathways (30,66).

Purine Nucleotide Catabolism

ATP is the major energy source in the cell and this nucleoside triphosphate is hydrolyzed by various ATPases, as well as serving as the phosphate donor in multiple kinase reactions. ADP produced in these reactions is either rephosphorylated, or is a substrate for the adenylate kinase reaction (Fig. 7).

$$2\ ADP \rightleftarrows ATP + AMP$$

The AMP thus formed can be deaminated to IMP by adenylate deaminase (reaction 24) or dephosphorylated to adenosine by a specific cytosol 5'-nucleotidase (reaction 25) (Fig. 7). In the heart the predominant pathway for AMP catabolism is hydrolysis to adenosine since cytosol 5'-nucleotidase activity is greater than adenylate deaminase activity in cardiac tissue (59). The adenosine formed from AMP is further metabolized to inosine by adenosine deaminase (reaction 13) and inosine then undergoes phosphorolysis to hypoxanthine (reaction 14) (Fig. 7). Hypoxanthine is oxidized to xanthine and ultimately uric acid (reactions 26 and 27) (Fig. 7). These two reactions are catalyzed by xanthine oxidase and are essentially irreversible. GDP enters the catabolic pathway by reversal of the guanylate kinase reaction and the resultant GMP is hydrolyzed to guanosine (reaction 28). Guanosine undergoes phosphorolysis to guanine (reaction 29) (Fig. 7). Both of the latter reactions are catalyzed by the same nucleotidase and phosphorylase as described in AMP and inosine catabolism. Guanine is deaminated by a specific deaminase (reaction 30) (Fig. 7) and the resultant xanthine oxidized to urate by xanthine oxidase.

Control of Purine Nucleotide Synthesis and Catabolism

The rate-limiting step in the pathway of purine biosynthesis is the production of PRA, a reaction catalyzed by the enzyme PP-ribose-P amidotransferase. The substrate PP-ribose-P is an allosteric activator of PP-ribose-

P amidotransferase, and, consequently, this metabolite is an important regulator of the rate at which purines are synthesized by the *de novo* pathway (29). PP-ribose-P is also required for nucleotide synthesis via the salvage pathway. PP-ribose-P production is determined by the activity of the enzyme PP-ribose-P synthetase (5). The enzyme exists in multiple forms, varying in size from 60,000 daltons to as large as 1,900,000 daltons. The larger forms appear to be the most catalytically active. The activity of this enzyme is controlled in a complex manner by not only substrate concentration but also by the nucleotide end products of the purine, pyrimidine, and pyridine pathways. The product of the reaction, PP-ribose-P, does not appear to be an important inhibitor under physiologic conditions. A large number of purine, pyrimidine, and pyridine nucleotides have been shown to individually inhibit PP-ribose-P synthetase activity, and the degree of inhibition appears to depend on the total nucleotide concentration rather than individual nucleotide concentrations. Some studies have suggested that the energy charge in the cell, which determines the ratio of mono- to di- to triphosphates, may also play a role in controlling the activity of PP-ribose-P synthetase. However, there may be a special role for purine nucleoside diphosphates, such as ADP, in the control of this enzyme, since patients have been described in whom PP-ribose-P activity is increased in association with a decrease in sensitivity of this enzyme to inhibition by ADP and GDP. In addition to nucleotide effectors, there are several other intracellular metabolites which affect the activity of PP-ribose-P synthetase. The enzyme has an obligatory requirement for inorganic phosphate, and orthophosphate is a potent allosteric activator of this enzyme. Under some conditions, orthophosphate concentrations may play a role in controlling the activity of this enzyme in the cell. 2,3'-Diphosphoglycerate is another potential effector of the activity of PP-ribose-P synthetase.

The activity of PP-ribose-P synthetase in heart has not been well characterized but may be limiting under certain conditions. Under normoxic conditions prior to and following an ischemic period, both *de novo* and salvage nucleotide synthesis take place at less than maximal rates. Since both pathways require PP-ribose-P as substrate, it has been postulated that the PP-ribose-P concentration is not saturating for either pathway under these conditions. However, it should be pointed out that PP-ribose-P concentrations have not been measured directly in any myocyte preparation. PP-ribose-P is labile and special precautions are required in determining tissue content of this metabolite. Indirect measures of PP-ribose-P content, sometimes referred to as PP-ribose-P availability, have been reported for myocardium by determining the amount of radiolabeled adenine [the adenine phosphoribosyl transferase (APRT) reaction is PP-ribose-P dependent] which is incorporated into

purine nucleotides under various conditions (76). These types of experiments have been used to support the hypothesis that PP-ribose-P concentrations are limiting for *de novo* (and possibly salvage) nucleotide synthesis in control and normoxic postischemic myocardium. Thus PP-ribose-P synthetase activity may be an important determinant of the rate of nucleotide synthesis in the heart through its control of PP-ribose-P concentration, and as discussed below this may be a reasonable step at which to intervene in attempts to increase nucleotide production in postischemic myocardium.

The first unique and rate-limiting step in the pathway of *de novo* synthesis is the formation of PRA, a reaction catalyzed by PP-ribose-P amidotransferase (29). PP-ribose-P is an obligatory substrate for the enzyme, and either glutamine or ammonia can be used as the nitrogen donor. In most mammalian cells amidotransferase activity is controlled in part by the PP-ribose-P concentration, since this substrate is not present in saturating concentrations. The glutamine concentrations are probably saturating in most cells and affect the activity of this enzyme to a lesser extent. The activity of the enzyme is also controlled by the concentration of purine nucleotides in the cell. This enzyme is inhibited by nucleoside monophosphates to a greater extent than diphosphates, and by diphosphates to a greater extent than by triphosphates. Inhibitory and catalytic sites of the enzyme are distinct and interact allosterically. The feedback inhibition produced by nucleotides can be overcome by increasing the PP-ribose-P concentration.

These opposing actions of PP-ribose-P and purine nucleotides are explained at the molecular level by the finding that the enzyme exists in two forms in mammalian cells, a large, inactive form (270,000 daltons), and a small, active form (133,000) (28). In the presence of nucleotides, the enzyme is converted to the large inactive form, but with increasing concentrations of PP-ribose-P the enzyme shifts back to the small active form. PP-ribose-P amidotransferase activity is present in the heart, and total activity in cardiac extracts has been estimated to be 21.4 nmoles/hr/g (61). The distribution of this enzyme between the active versus inactive forms in various physiological conditions in the heart is unknown. The rate of *de novo* purine synthesis in the heart is slow and has been estimated to be between 5 and 8 nmoles/hr/g in the rat heart (77). Only a twofold increase in the rate of *de novo* synthesis occurs in the postischemic period. These values for *de novo* synthetic rate in heart approach those for total amidotransferase activity and suggest that limitation of amidotransferase activity as well as substrate (PP-ribose-P) availability may be important determinants of the rate of *de novo* synthesis in myocardium. This conclusion has potential implications for interventions aimed at increasing purine nucleotide pools through increasing PP-ribose-P concentrations.

The rate of purine nucleotide synthesis via salvage

pathways has been measured at 6 to 20 nmoles/hr/g in isolated rat hearts utilizing adenine, adenosine, inosine, and hypoxanthine as precursors (46,54). The rate of nucleotide synthesis via these pathways is apparently dependent on the concentration of nucleoside or base in the perfusate, since the total activities of adenosine kinase (11.6 μmoles/hr/g) (3), adenine phosphoribosyl-transferase (96 μmoles/hr/g) and hypoxanthine phos-phoribosyltransferase (14–16 μmoles/hr/g) (41) in tissue extracts greatly exceed the measured rates of nucleotide synthesis by the salvage pathways in myocardium. These results suggest that the concentrations of nucleosides and bases in the plasma play a significant role in determining the rate of nucleotide synthesis via the salvage pathways in the heart. Other factors, such as intracellular concentrations of co-substrates for these salvage reactions, like PP-ribose-P and ATP, may also be important determinants of rate of nucleotide synthesis via the salvage pathways in pathological conditions such as ischemic and postischemic myocardium. Unfortu-nately, few of the *in vitro* studies have been performed at physiological concentrations of nucleosides or bases, so it is not possible to predict how important the salvage pathways are quantitatively in repleting nucleotide pools in postischemic myocardium.

The branchpoint in the purine pathway leading from IMP to either AMP or GMP synthesis is also tightly regulated in mammalian cells and control of this branchpoint determines the relative rates of ATP and GTP synthesis. The activity of the first enzyme in the pathway leading to AMP formation, i.e., SAMP synthe-tase, is controlled by substrate availability (IMP and GTP concentrations) and by the concentration of the end product of this branch of the pathway, i.e., AMP (25). IMP dehydrogenase activity, the first reaction leading to GMP synthesis, is controlled by substrate availability (IMP) and the concentration of the end product of this branch of the pathway, i.e., GMP (25). The regulation of these two enzymes at the IMP branch-point assures a balanced synthesis of adenine and guanine nucleotides in the cell, and it prevents unneeded metab-olism of IMP to adenine and guanine nucleotides when these pools are replete in the cell. However, when a pool like the ATP and/or GTP pool is reduced during ischemia, the regulation at this branchpoint operates to effectively shunt any newly formed IMP from the *de novo* or salvage pathways into the adenine and/or guanine nucleotide pools during the postischemic period (62). Similarly, if these pools are at control levels already, it is unlikely that attempts to increase ATP and GTP pools to supra-normal levels by increasing IMP will be successful. Thus, it is not reasonable to attempt to expand ATP and GTP pools to greater than physiological levels as a protective mechanism prior to ischemic insult to the myocardium (57).

Catabolism of purine nucleotides to nucleosides and

bases is another control point at which regulatory mech-anisms are operative in myocardial, as well as other cell types. Hydrolysis of nucleotides to nucleosides is cata-lyzed by a class of enzymes referred to as 5'-nucleotidases. In myocardium there are at least two distinct types of 5'-nucleotidase, i.e., a soluble form found in the sarco-plasm and a membrane form located on the outside of the plasma membrane, hence the term ecto-5'-nucleoti-dase. The latter ecto enzyme is not thought to be important in purine nucleotide catabolism in most cell types because of its location on the outer surface of the cell membrane. The cytoplasmic enzyme is quite active in myocardium, 319 μmoles/hr/g (10), and it is probably responsible for hydrolysis of most of the AMP, as well as IMP and GMP, formed from ATP and GTP catab-olism during ischemia. The cytosolic 5'-nucleotidase has regulatory properties that are distinct from those of the ecto enzyme (10). The cytosolic enzyme is an allosteric protein, and ATP is a potent activator of this enzyme. Thus, under control conditions when ATP pools are normal, any purine monophosphate formed via the *de novo* or salvage pathways will likely be hydrolyzed since the cytosolic enzyme is activated by ATP. During isch-emia when ATP levels are reduced, the activity of cytosolic 5'-nucleotidase is reduced, and this will tend to slow the rate of nucleotide hydrolysis and preserve the nucleotide pools in the cell. These regulatory prop-erties of cytosol 5'-nucleotidase are important to keep in mind when devising strategies aimed at preserving nucleotide pools during myocardial ischemia. A phar-macologic agent that specifically inhibited cytosolic 5'-nucleotidase would potentially be useful in preserving nucleotide pools if it were given prior to the ischemic insult. This type of agent might be useful during coronary artery bypass grafting when myocardial blood flow is compromised.

Measurement of Rates of Nucleotide Synthesis and Degradation

Static measurements of nucleotide pools only reflect the balance between the rate of nucleotide synthesis and the rate of degradation. Methods employing radiolabeled compounds are available to directly measure synthetic rates, and these methods have been employed with fetal hearts, isolated perfused hearts, and *in vivo* in rodents (37,46,54,66,68,76,77). Studies of nucleotide synthesis in larger animals, such as dogs, have been limited because of the quantity of radiolabeled compound re-quired.

Adenine nucleotides can be synthesized by the *de novo* pathway, or by the salvage pathway. In the second reaction in the *de novo* pathway, a glycine molecule is incorporated into the imidazole portion of the nascent purine ring (Fig. 6). The rate of *de novo* synthesis can be determined by quantitating the amount of radioactivity incorporated into purine nucleotide pools and by measuring the specific activity of the radiolabeled glycine in the cell or tissue at various times following the administration of [^{14}C] or [H^3]-labeled glycine. This technique requires the isolation of glycine from the cell or tissue to determine its specific activity, as well as the isolation of a given purine nucleotide pool. The former requires an amino acid analyzer and the latter can be performed by HPLC or by ion exchange chromatography columns. Radiolabeled glycine can be administered for a sufficient period of time to attain a constant intracellular specific activity before obtaining samples for determination of radioactivity in the nucleotide pools, or the specific activity of glycine can be experimentally determined at each time point a sample is taken for nucleotide analysis. The rate of *de novo* synthesis may be overestimated in the intact animal if labeled nucleotides in the heart or other organs, such as the liver, are catabolized to nucleosides and bases that then circulate back to the heart and enter the nucleotide pool through the salvage pathway. If the radiolabel in glycine is randomized into other compounds that can also be incorporated into the purine ring, this will also lead to overestimation of the rate of *de novo* synthesis. Other labeled compounds, such as [^{15}N]-glutamine, [^{14}C]-formate (incorporated into folate pools), and [^{14}C]-CO$_2$, have also been used to determine the rate of *de novo* synthesis in various noncardiac tissues. Estimates of rates of *de novo* purine synthesis in myocardium have varied with the animal model and specific isotope used. No incorporation of glycine into the adenine nucleotide pool could be detected in cultured fetal mouse heart (37). Using [^{14}C] glycine, the rate of *de novo* adenine nucleotide synthesis has been estimated to be 1.3 nmoles/g/hr in the isolated perfused rat heart and 8.4 nmoles/g/hr *in situ* (75–77), assuming no uptake of circulating purine from other organs or glycine conversion to other intermediates.

Nucleotide synthesis via salvage pathways can also be estimated using radiolabeled precursors. ^{14}C-Labeled adenosine, inosine, hypoxanthine, and adenine have been administered to isolated perfused hearts and rates of incorporation into nucleotide pools measured (46,54,66). The rate of incorporation of these four compounds is similar, and has been measured to be 6 to 30 nmoles/g/hr. None of these measurements have been corrected for intracellular isotope specific activity, but this may be less of a problem than mentioned above with regard to glycine utilization because of the small size of the intracellular pool of purine nucleosides and bases compared to that of glycine.

Nucleotide catabolism can be estimated with the "pulse-chase" method. After the nucleotide pool of interest has been labeled by a short "pulse" with the appropriate radioactive precursor, a "chase" of unlabeled isotope is administered to dilute the radiolabeled compound and prevent further radiolabel from entering the nucleotide pool. At various intervals following the chase, the nucleotide pool is isolated and the amount of residual radioactivity determined. Intact cells are relatively impermeable to phosphorylated compounds such as nucleotides, and consequently radiolabeled nucleotides will be retained in the cell. In isolated organs or cultured cells, the effluent or media can be sampled over time for the appearance of radiolabeled nucleosides and bases. A more detailed description of the methods used for assessing the rates of synthesis and degradation of intracellular compounds can be found in *Chapter* 9.

Turnover of a very active metabolite such as ATP cannot be quantitated by the technique described above for measuring the rate of adenine nucleotide catabolism because ADP is rapidly rephosphorylated in oxygenated, substrate-replete myocardium. However, with the advent of newer NMR techniques, it is now possible to directly assess *in vivo* the turnover rate of ATP (and creatine phosphate) pools in myocardium using different energy pulses to saturate selective pools of phosphorous containing compounds (7) (see *Chapter* 13).

PYRIMIDINE NUCLEOTIDE SYNTHESIS AND CATABOLISM

Pyrimidine Synthesis *De Novo*

Both *de novo* and salvage pathways exist for the synthesis of pyrimidine nucleotides. One difference between purine and pyrimidine nucleotide synthesis via the respective *de novo* pathways is that in the latter class of nucleotides the pyrimidine ring is completed before the addition of ribose-5-phosphate (Fig. 8).

The first unique reaction in pyrimidine synthesis *de novo* is the formation of carbamyl phosphate:

$$2 \text{ ATP} + \text{glutamine (or NH}_3\text{)} + \text{HCO}_3^-$$
$$+ \text{ H}_2\text{O} \xrightarrow{\text{Mg}^{2+}, \text{K}^+} \text{carbamyl phosphate} \qquad [1]$$
$$+ 2 \text{ ADP} + \text{P}_i + \text{glutamate}$$

This reaction is catalyzed by carbamyl phosphate synthetase. Two distinct isozymes of this protein are found in mammalian cells: The first, found in liver mitochondria, is used to synthesize carbamyl phosphate for the urea cycle and NH$_3$ is the nitrogen donor in this reaction; the second, present in the cytoplasm of most cells, is used to synthesize carbamyl phosphate for use in pyrimidine synthesis, and glutamine is the nitrogen donor in this reaction. In certain urea cycle defects carbamyl phosphate can diffuse out of the mitochondria and enter the pyrimidine biosynthetic pathway, indicating that these two pathways are not totally separate.

The next step in pyrimidine synthesis is the formation of carbamyl aspartate, a reaction catalyzed by the cytosolic enzyme aspartate transcarbamylase:

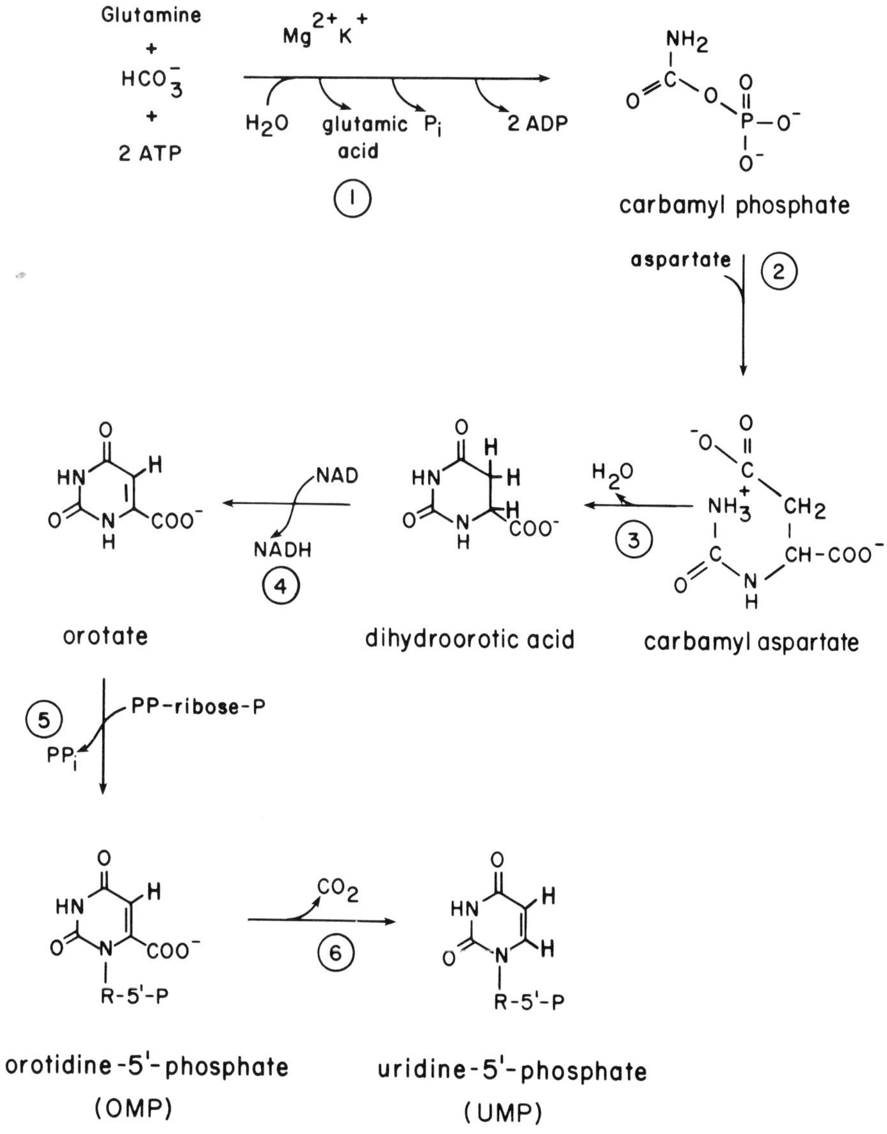

FIG. 8. Pathway of pyrimidine synthesis *de novo.*

carbamyl-phosphate + L-aspartate →

$$\text{carbamyl-aspartate} \quad [2]$$

Ring closure is catalyzed by dihydroorotase:

$$\text{carbamyl aspartate} \rightarrow \text{dihydroorotic acid} \quad [3]$$

The oxidation of dihydroorotic acid to orotate:

dihydroorotic acid + NAD + O_2 →

$$\text{orotate} + H_2O_2 + \text{NADH} \quad [4]$$

is catalyzed by dihydroorotic acid dehydrogenase, an enzyme that is located in the mitochondria. This is the only reaction in the pyrimidine pathway that is not located in the cytoplasm.

The next two reactions in *de novo* synthesis are catalyzed by a single protein containing both the orotate phosphoribosyltransferase and orotidine-5'-phosphate decarboxylase activities. The first step is the formation of orotidine-5'-phosphate:

orotate + PP-ribose-P $\xrightarrow{\text{Mg}^{2+}}$

$$\text{orotidine 5'-phosphate (OMP)} + \text{PP}_i \quad [5]$$

followed by decarboxylation of the OMP:

$$\text{OMP} \rightarrow \text{uridine 5'-phosphate (UMP)} + CO_2 \quad [6]$$

Salvage Synthesis of Pyrimidine Nucleotides

Similar to the purine pathways, pyrimidine nucleotides can be formed from either pyrimidine nucleosides or bases. Unlike orotate, there is no phosphoribosyltransferase in mammalian cells that accepts the pyrimidine base uracil as a substrate. Instead uracil is first ribosylated to the nucleoside uridine by uridine phosphorylase:

$$\text{uracil} + \text{ribose-1-phosphate} \leftrightarrow \text{uridine} + P_i$$

Uridine is then phosphorylated to UMP by uridine kinase:

$$uridine + ATP \rightarrow UMP + ADP$$

UMP is phosphorylated to UDP and then to UTP with ATP donating the high energy phosphate bond in each step. These two reactions are catalyzed by the specific pyrimidine nucleoside monophosphate kinase and non-specific nucleoside disphosphate kinase, respectively. Cytidine triphosphate (CTP) can be formed directly from UTP via the following reaction:

$$UTP + glutamine + ATP \xrightarrow{Mg^{2+}} CTP + ADP$$
$$+ P_i + H_2O + glutamic\ acid$$

CTP can also be synthesized via a reutilization pathway similar to that for uridine nucleotides: cytidine is phosphorylated to CMP in a reaction catalyzed by uridine kinase and CMP is metabolized to CTP by phosphate transfers from ATP in reactions catalyzed by the specific pyrimidine nucleoside monophosphate kinase and the nonspecific nucleoside diphosphate kinase, respectively.

Catabolism of Pyrimidine Nucleotides

Pyrimidine triphosphates can be dephosphorylated by the reversible nucleoside diphosphate kinase reaction, and the diphosphates converted to the nucleoside 5′-monophosphates CMP and UMP by specific kinases. A 5′-nucleotidase specific for pyrimidine monophosphates hydrolyzes CMP and UMP to the nucleosides, cytidine and uridine. Cytidine deaminase deaminates cytidine to uridine, and phosphorolysis of uridine by pyrimidine nucleoside phosphorylase results in the formation of the base uracil. Uracil is subsequently oxidized by dihydrouracil dehydrogenase, and dihydrouracil is hydrolyzed by dihydropyrimidinase:

$$uracil + NADP^+ \rightarrow dihydrouracil + NADPH + H^+$$

$$dihydrouracil \rightarrow carbamyl\ propionate$$

Deamination and hydrolysis to β-alanine is the final step in pyrimidine degradation:

$$carbamyl\ propionate + H_2O \rightarrow$$
$$NH_3 + CO_2 + \beta\text{-}alanine$$

Control of Pyrimidine Nucleotide Synthesis

The enzymatic activities that catalyze the six reactions that comprise the *de novo* pathway of pyrimidine nucleotide synthesis (Fig. 8) require only three proteins, since two of these proteins are multifunctional enzymes. The first three reactions (carbamyl phosphate to dihydroorotate) are catalyzed by a trifunctional protein that has been termed complex A (38). The carbamyl phosphate synthetase activity of complex A, like the first unique reaction in the purine biosynthetic pathway, appears to be the rate-limiting step in pyrimidine bio-synthesis. ATP and PP-ribose-P allosterically activate the enzyme, while the end product of the pathway, UTP, feedback inhibits this reaction. Channeling of the substrates and products for the three enzyme activities contained in complex A has been demonstrated *in vitro,* and this is postulated to be a mechanism of preventing significant accumulation of these intermediates in the cell.

Following the oxidation of dihydroorotate by dihydroorotate oxidase in the mitochondria, the final two steps in pyrimidine biosynthesis (orotate → OMP → UMP) are catalyzed by the cytosolic bifunctional protein which has been termed UMP synthase (38). The activity of the first enzyme in this complex, orotate phosphoribosyltransferase, may be rate limiting for pyrimidine nucleotide biosynthesis under some conditions, i.e., high ATP and reduced pyrimidine nucleotide and PP-ribose-P concentrations. Under these conditions carbamyl phosphate synthetase activity is stimulated leading to enhanced orotate production, and phosphoribosyltransferase activity becomes dependent on PP-ribose-P availability. These conditions may obtain in cells or organs exposed to purine substrates in the absence of exogenous pyrimidines. The OMP formed in the first reaction of the enzyme complex remains bound to the protein where it becomes the substrate for the second reaction, i.e., the orotidine 5′-phosphate decarboxylase activity. This bifunctional enzyme provides yet another example of substrate channeling in the pyrimidine biosynthetic pathway.

INTERRELATIONSHIP BETWEEN PURINE AND PYRIMIDINE METABOLISM

Reutilization of both purine and pyrimidine bases for nucleoside monophosphate synthesis requires PP-ribose-P. Likewise, the activity of the rate-limiting steps of the *de novo* pathways leading to both purine and pyrimidine nucleotide synthesis are controlled by the PP-ribose-P concentration in the cell. Thus, rates of *de novo* and salvage synthesis of both purine and pyrimidine nucleotides are dependent on the availability of PP-ribose-P in the cell, and this key intermediate may coordinate the production of these two classes of ribonucleotides. It follows that depletion of PP-ribose-P may lead to a decrease in the rate of both purine and pyrimidine synthesis in the cell. If myocardial ischemia were to result in a decrease in PP-ribose-P content, this substrate might become rate limiting for purine and pyrimidine nucleotide synthesis during the post ischemic period. As discussed later, interventions designed to increase the rate of PP-ribose-P synthesis, i.e., ribose administration, have been employed to increase the rate of repletion of both purine and pyrimidine nucleotide pools in the myocardium.

PYRIDINE NUCLEOTIDE METABOLISM

NAD^+ and $NADP^+$ are obligatory co-factors and serve as electron acceptors for numerous oxidation reactions that are important for energy generation in the myocardium. NAD^+ is essential for mitochondrial oxidative phosphorylation and glycolysis; under certain circumstances NAD^+ and NADH availability may become limiting factors for energy generation.

NAD^+ can be synthesized *de novo* from tryptophan, or it can be synthesized from nicotinamide by two separate pathways (Fig. 9). *De novo* synthesis of NAD^+ requires the oxidation of tryptophan to kynurenine, followed by hydroxylation to 3-hydroxykynureninic acid. Further metabolism leads to the formation of α-amino-β-carboxymuconic δ-semialdehyde and quinolinic acid. Quinolinic acid undergoes decarboxylation and phosphoribosylation to form nicotinic acid mononucleotide. (Although nicotinic acid mononucleotide can be synthesized as described above in most mammals, the amount that is produced by this pathway is variable and nicotinic acid is usually considered to be an essential nutrient in

most species.) The AMP portion of ATP is added to nicotinic acid mononucleotide in the next reaction in this pathway to produce nicotinic acid adenine dinucleotide, and amidation of this intermediate leads to formation of NAD^+.

NAD^+ can also be synthesized from nicotinamide obtained from dietary sources. Nicotinamide is deaminated to nicotinic acid; nicotinic acid mononucleotide, nicotinic acid adenine dinucleotide, and NAD^+ are produced as described above. NAD^+ can be formed from nicotinamide by a second series of reactions: nicotinamide is first phosphoribosylated and ADP is then added to form NAD^+. $NADP^+$ is synthesized by phosphorylation of the 2'-hydroxyl group of the ADP moiety of NAD^+.

CHANGES IN PURINE AND PYRIMIDINE METABOLISM WITH CARDIAC HYPERTROPHY

Myocardial hypertrophy secondary to a sustained increase in cardiac workload is associated with an increase

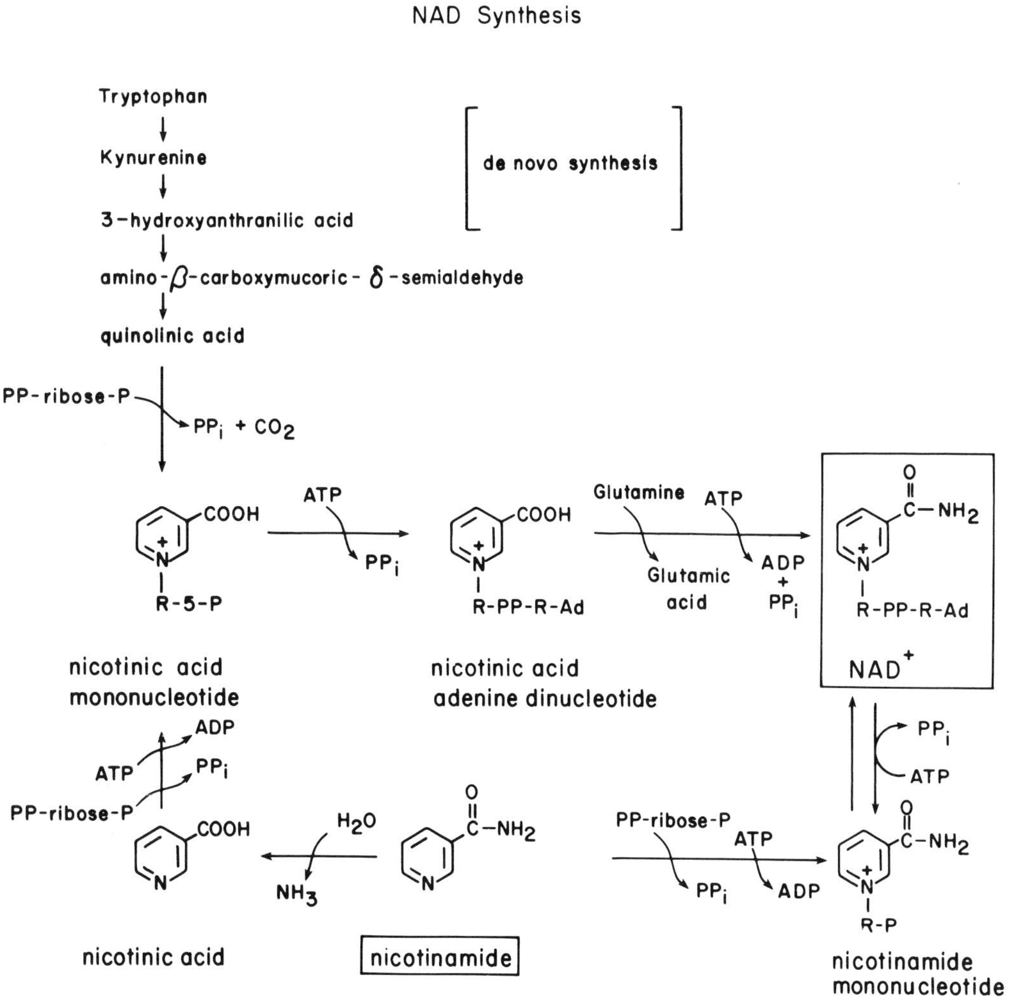

NAD Synthesis

FIG. 9. Pathways of NAD^+ synthesis.

in the synthesis of purine and pyrimidine ribonucleotides, RNA, and protein (56,78). The increase in purine and pyrimidine ribonucleotide production is required to supply the precursors needed for increased RNA synthesis. Pools of purine and pyrimidine ribonucleotides have been reported to be increased, decreased, or unchanged depending on the model of hypertrophy and the time following the hypertrophic stimulus at which the pool sizes were assessed. However, in all situations in which the rate of purine or pyrimidine nucleotide synthesis has been determined, production of these nucleotides is increased.

The biochemical mechanism(s) linking the mechanical stimulus, i.e., pressure overload, to the observed changes in myocardial metabolism is unknown. Several mechanisms have been proposed, and some investigators have suggested that changes in either the pool size or rate of turnover of adenine nucleotides may be the signal that initiates the increase in protein synthesis observed during hypertrophy (44). This is a potentially attractive hypothesis since ATP consumption is the most immediate and direct biochemical consequence of increased muscle contractility. However, several laboratories have reported no correlation between adenine nucleotide pool sizes and the development of cardiac hypertrophy in intact animals (78). It remains to be determined whether changes in turnover of adenine nucleotide pools and increased production of purine nucleotide catabolites, such as adenosine, inosine, and hypoxanthine, may act as biochemical signals leading to cardiac hypertrophy.

EFFECTS OF ISCHEMIA AND REPERFUSION ON NUCLEOTIDE CONTENT

Effects of Ischemia and Reperfusion on Purine Catabolism and Synthesis

When oxygen becomes limiting in the myocardium (i.e., during hypoxia) and oxygen plus other substrates become limiting during ischemia, the rate of catabolism of nucleoside triophosphates exceeds the rate of synthesis, resulting in a decrease in the cellular content of these compounds (31,32,37,45,54,63,67). The decrease in ATP content of myocardium is, in part, accounted for by an increase in ADP and AMP content during ischemia and hypoxia. With ischemia, AMP is degraded to adenosine, inosine, and hypoxanthine resulting in an increase in the tissue concentrations of these nucleosides and base. During hypoxia when oxygen is limiting but flow is normal, the nucleosides and bases accumulate to a lesser extent because these metabolites diffuse out of the cell, and they are taken up by the perfusate leaving the heart (7). During ischemia, when both oxygenation and perfusion are reduced, the "washout" of catabolites is decreased. In both animal models and patients the

appearance of purine nucleosides and bases have been demonstrated in coronary sinus effluent during episodes of ischemia (16,42). During reperfusion of the myocardium following ischemia, the purine nucleotide, nucleoside, and base content of the heart remain depressed as a result of the "washout" that occurred during ischemia.

Because the myocardial content of pyrimidine nucleotides is normally 30- to 60-fold less than the purine nucleotide content, pyrimidine di- and mononucleotides are less easily quantitated. Pyrimidine nucleoside triphosphate pools have been measured during ischemia, and a decrease in myocardial content of these compounds demonstrated. For the technical reasons stated above no increases in pyrimidine mono- or diphosphates, nor nucleosides or bases have been reported during ischemia. The degree of pyrimidine nucleotide depletion observed during ischemia and the subsequent rate of repletion during myocardial reperfusion parallel the changes seen in the purine nucleotide pools with ischemia and reperfusion (63).

Similar changes occur in the myocardial content of pyridine nucleotides with ischemia. During myocardial ischemia NAD^+ is initially reduced to NADH, and subsequently both NAD^+ and NADH are catabolized to nicotinamide and nicotinic acid. The latter two compounds can be lost from the cell during reperfusion. Most investigators have not quantitated both NAD^+ and NADH in myocardium since acid extraction which degrades NADH has usually been employed to remove the nucleotides from the tissue. As a result, limited data are available on the time course of changes in NADH during ischemia and reperfusion. However, it is known that NAD^+ + NADH content decreases during ischemia and remains below control levels for some time during reperfusion (63). The rate of repletion of pyridine nucleotide pools during reperfusion after an ischemic event is unknown.

Myocardial content of nucleotides, as well as the magnitude of the changes produced by ischemia and the duration of these changes following reperfusion, vary with assay method and experimental model. As an example of the types of changes observed, the results of nucleotide analyses obtained from a study performed in the authors' laboratory are shown in Fig. 10. In this study, open chest dogs underwent occlusion of the left anterior descending coronary artery for 12 min followed by coronary reperfusion for 60 min. Serial samples were taken from the nonischemic, ischemic, and reperfused regions. Nucleotide and creatine phosphate pools decreased during ischemia. During reperfusion, creatine phosphate content was restored rapidly while nucleotide pools remained depleted. Other studies indicate that under some experimental conditions purine nucleotide pools may remain depleted for many days following an ischemic event (14,55,62,63).

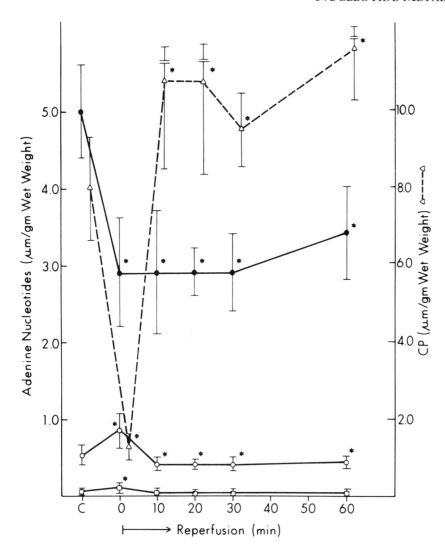

FIG. 10. ATP (*solid circle*), ADP (*open circle*), AMP (*square*) and creatine phosphate (CP) (*triangle*) content of tissue samples taken from ischemic regon during control conditions (C), during coronary occlusion (O), and at various times during reperfusion. Results are expressed as μmoles/g wet wt $\pm$ 1 SD. *Asterisk* indicates $p < 0.05$ compared with control.

The rapid increase in creatine phosphate content has been interpreted to indicate that energy production by the mitochondria is not limiting in postischemic myocardium. Thus, prolonged depletion of purine and pyrimidine nucleotide pools does not appear to be secondary to a defect in energy generation, but rather it is secondary to nucleotide catabolism during ischemia and loss of nucleosides and bases during reperfusion. Repletion of nucleotide pools is limited by the availability of purine and pyrimidine substrates.

RELATIONSHIP OF NUCLEOTIDE METABOLISM TO MYOCARDIAL FUNCTION AND VIABILITY

Until recently it was held that when coronary perfusion was restored after a brief period of ischemia (less than 15 min) myocardial function returned to normal rapidly. A number of studies utilizing various models indicate that myocyte function does not immediately return to

control with reperfusion or reoxygenation, but rather improves slowly over time (12,27,40,43,71). The time course of improvement in function is biphasic, with a rapid and substantial improvement initially followed by a period of gradual return of function to control levels. The time required for complete recovery of function has been shown to vary from 24 hr to 7 days.

Several studies have documented a temporal relationship between the slow repletion of nucleotide pools following an ischemic episode and the slow return of normal myocardial function (11,22,23,48,50,53,70). This temporal relationship forms the basis for the hypothesis that repletion of nucleotide pools is at least one determinant of myocardial function in the postischemic state. In other studies, improvement in function after an ischemic (or hypoxic) episode is not correlated with repletion of ATP pools (13,34,45,47,67,69). No studies have conclusively demonstrated a cause and effect relationship between repletion of nucleotide pools and return of myocardial function in the postischemic state. One method for testing this relationship is to selectively alter the rate of repletion of nucleotide pools and then determine whether this produces a change in myocardial function. Myocardial dysfunction and nucleotide depletion can be produced by the infusion of isoproterenol. If animals are pretreated with ribose, an agent designed to increase adenine nucleotide synthesis, the fall in nucleotide pools is prevented and myocardial function is preserved (79). This observation would suggest a link between adenine nucleotide metabolism and myocardial function, but no studies of this type have as yet been reported in postischemic myocardium.

Myocardial nucleotide content has also been hypothesized to be a determinant of cell viability (32,33,67). The basis for this hypothesis is the correlation between the decrease in nucleotide content below a certain level and the onset of irreversible changes in the myocardium during ischemia or during the incubation of myocardial tissue samples under hypoxic conditions *in vitro*. As with the postulated relationship between nucleotide metabolism and myocardial function, studies have not yet documented a cause and effect relationship between nucleotide pool size and cell viability.

INTERVENTIONS TO INCREASE PURINE NUCLEOTIDE SYNTHESIS

A variety of compounds have been administered in an attempt to increase purine synthesis in the myocardium. ATP and creatine phosphate have been added to the solutions of blood perfusing the heart, but rapid catabolism of these compounds in blood or tissues and slow transport of these phosphorylated compounds across cell membranes has limited the usefulness of this approach. Consequently, repletion of purine nucleotide pools has focused on supplying purine substrates or cofactors for either the *de novo* or salvage pathways. The most useful compounds are those that penetrate cell membranes rapidly and specifically affect the pathways leading to nucleotide synthesis.

Three approaches to increasng purine nucleotide synthesis *in vivo* have received the most attention experimentally. One approach has been to enhance *de novo* synthesis. The optimal compound for this approach should enter the pathway distal to the rate-limiting step (the reaction catalyzed by PP-ribose-P amidotransferase) and not require co-substrates that might be present in limiting concentrations in the myocardium (i.e., PP-ribose-P). One agent that fulfills these criteria and has been successfully used to increase nucleotide synthesis is 5-amino-4-imidazole carboxamide ribonucleoside (AICAriboside) (57,62,65). This compound is rapidly taken up by cardiac myocytes and phosphorylated to the ribotide AICAR, an intermediate that enters the *de novo* pathway distal to the PP-ribose-P amidotransferase

step. Nucleotide pools have been successfully restored in postischemic myocardium using this compound (62). However, the compound has a biphasic effect on nucleotide synthesis. At low concentrations it enhances nucleotide synthesis, whereas at high concentrations nucleotide synthesis is inhibited (57). Other interventions specifically designed to increase *de novo* synthesis have not been evaluated.

Another approach has been to selectively enhance synthesis of purine nucleotides through the salvage pathways. A number of agents have been used for this purpose. The nucleoside adenosine has received the most attention. Adenosine enters cells rapidly and it is phosphorylated to AMP in a reaction catalyzed by adenosine kinase. Incorporation of this nucleoside into the nucleotide pool can be further facilitated by administering an adenosine deaminase inhibitor such as erythro-9-(2-hydroxy-3-nonyl)adenine hydrochloride (EHNA). Adenosine together with EHNA has been shown to effectively replete nucleotide pools after aortic cross-clamping in open-chest dogs on cardiopulmonary bypass (15). Another nucleoside, inosine, has also been shown to preserve nucleotide pools (17,21). When inosine is administered prior to myocardial ischemia in isolated hearts, adenine nucleotide content is maintained at higher levels than in untreated hearts (17). As discussed earlier, inosine cannot be used directly for nucleotide synthesis, but it undergoes phosphorolysis to hypoxanthine and the latter compound is used in the hypoxanthine phosphoribosyl transferase (HPRT) reaction for IMP synthesis. When inosine undergoes phosphorolysis, ribose-1-phosphate is generated which may provide substrate for PP-ribose-P synthesis and thus facilitate the reutilization to hypoxanthine. The bases hypoxanthine and adenine are also incorporated into nucleotide pools through reactions which require PP-ribose-P as a co-substrate. The successful use of these agents to replete nucleotide pools in the postischemic state has not been reported.

A third approach to increasing purine nucleotide synthesis is to increase myocardial content of PP-ribose-P, a potentially limiting substrate for both the *de novo* and salvage pathways in normal tissues. It has been postulated that PP-ribose-P content is reduced even further in ischemic and postischemic hearts. This has prompted several groups of investigators to attempt to increase PP-ribose-P availability in myocardium by administering ribose to the intact animal or isolated perfused heart (51,77). Ribose is postulated to enter the cell and be phosphorylated to ribose-5-phosphate, thereby enhancing PP-ribose-P production. Studies with intact rodents and isolated perfused hearts have documented that ribose administration leads to an increase in the rate of purine nucleotide synthesis via the *de novo* pathway. Experiments have not been performed to assess the effect of ribose on nucleotide synthesis via the salvage pathways. These same studies have shown that depletion of myocardial nucleotide pools induced by isoproteronol administration to rats can be prevented by pretreatment of the animal with ribose. The rate of nucleotide repletion in isolated perfused hearts previously subjected to ischemia can also be enhanced by administration of ribose (51).

In conclusion, a number of different approaches have been shown to have potential for enhancing purine nucleotide synthesis in myocardial cells. However, comparative studies have not yet been performed during the postischemia period in intact animals or even in the same *in vitro* model, and thus no single approach has been judged to be superior. Myocardial function has not been measured *in vivo* in association with the application of these interventions designed to accelerate the rate of repletion of nucleotide pools in the postischemic period. Consequently, it has not been established whether these interventions can improve myocardial function. As pointed out earlier, these studies are essential in order to test the hypothesis that nucleotide depletion contributes to myocardial dysfunction in the postischemic state.

ACKNOWLEDGMENTS

This work was supported in part by the Howard Hughes Medical Institute (EWH) and by National Institutes of Health grants R01AM12413 and R01HL26831. Dr. Swain is an Established Investigator of the American Heart Association.

We wish to thank Carolyn S. Mills for expert secretarial assistance.

REFERENCES

1. Allard, J. R., Conhaim, R. L., Vlahakes, G. J., O'Neill, M. J., and Hoffman, I. E. (1981): Rapid-freezing transmural cardiac biopsy drill. *Am. J. Physiol.*, 240:H126–H132.
2. Allison, T. B., Ramey, C. A., and Holsinger, J. W., Jr. (1978): Effects on labile metabolites of temporal delay in freezing biopsy samples of dog myocardium in liquid nitrogen. *Cardiovasc. Res.*, 12:162–166.
3. Arch, J. R. S., and Newsholme, E. A. (1978): Activities and some properties of 5'-nucleotidase, adenosine kinase and adenosine deaminase in tissues from vertebrates and invertebrates in relation to the control of the concentration and the physiological role of adenosine. *Biochem. J.*, 174:965–977.
4. Becker, M. (1976): Regulation of purine nucleotide synthesis: Effects of inosine on normal and HGPRT-deficient fibroblasts. *Biochim. Biophys. Acta*, 435:132–144.
5. Becker, M. A. (1978): Abnormalities of PRPP metabolism leading to an overproduction of uric acid. *Handbook Exp. Pharmacol.*, 51:155–178.
6. Bergmeyer, H. V. (1965): *Methods of Enzymatic Analysis.* Academic Press, New York.
7. Berne, R. M. (1983): Cardiac nucleotides in hypoxia: Possible role in regulation of coronary blood flow. *Am. J. Physiol.*, 204:317–322.
8. Bittl, J. A., and Ingwall, J. S. (1983): Direct investigation of creatine kinase kinetics and ATP synthesis in the isolated rat heart: A 31P-NMR study. *Circulation*, 68:III-E.
9. Boulieu, R., Bory, C., Baltassat, P., and Gonnet, C. (1983): Hypoxanthine and xanthine levels determined by high-performance liquid chromatography in plasma, erythrocyte, and urine samples from healthy subjects: the problem of hypoxanthine level evolution as a function of time. *Anal. Biochem.*, 129:398–404.
10. Bounous, C. G., Sabina, R. L., Hettleman, B. D., Swain, J. L., and Holmes, E. W. (1981): Basis for accumulation of IMP in fast-twitch muscle following ATP degradation. *Clin. Res.*, 29:428A.
11. Braunwald, E., and Kloner, R. A. (1982): The stunned myocardium: Prolonged post-ischemic ventricular dysfunction. *Circulation*, 66:1146–1149.
12. Bush, L. R., Buja, L. M., Samowitz, W., Rude, R. W., Wathen, M., Tilton, G. D., and Willerson, J. T. (1983): Recovery of left ventricular segmental function after long-term reperfusion following temporary coronary occlusion in conscious dogs. Comparison of 2- and 4-hour occlusions. *Circ. Res.*, 53:248–263.
13. Chiong, M. A., Berezny, G. M., and Winton, T. L. (1978): Metabolism of the isolated perused rabbit heart. I. Responses to anoxia and reoxygenation. II. Energy stores. *Can. J. Physiol. Pharmacol.*, 56:844–856.
14. DeBoer, L. W. V., Ingwall, J. S., Kloner, R. A., and Braunwald, E. (1980): Prolonged derangements of canine myocardial purine metabolism after a brief coronary artery occlusion not associated with anatomic evidence of necrosis. *Proc. Natl. Acad. Sci. USA*, 77:5471–5475.
15. Foker, J. E., Einzig, S., and Wang, T. (1980): Adenosine metabolism and myocardial preservation: Consequences of adenosine catabolism on myocardial high-energy compounds and tissue blood flow. *J. Thorac. Cardiovasc. Surg.*, 80:506–516.
16. Fox, A. C., Reed, G. E., Meilman, H., and Silk, B. B. (1979): Release of nucleosides from canine and human hearts as an index of prior ischemia. *Am. J. Cardiol.*, 43:52–58.
17. Goldhaber, S. Z., Pohost, G. M., Kloner, R. A., Andrews, E., Newell, J. B., and Ingwall, J. B. (1982): Inosine: A protective agent in an organ culture model of myocardial ischemia. *Circ. Res.*, 51:181–188.
18. Goldthwait, D. A. (1957): Mechanisms of synthesis of purine nucleotides in heart muscle extracts. *J. Clin. Invest.*, 36:1572–1578.
19. Harmsen, E., DeJong, J. W., and Serruys, P. W. (1981): Hypoxanthine production by ischemic heart demonstrated by high pressure liquid chromatography of blood purine nucleosides and oxypurines. *Clin. Chim. Acta*, 115:73–84.
20. Harmsen, E., DeTombe, P. P., and Dejong, J. W. (1982): Simultaneous determination of myocardial adenine nucleotides and creatine phosphate by high-performance liquid chromatography. *J. Chromatogr.*, 230:131–136.
21. Harmsen, E., DeTombe, P. P., DeJong, J. W., and Achterberg, P. W. (1984): Enhanced ATP and GTP synthesis from hypoxanthine or inosine after myocardial ischemia. *Am. J. Physiol.*, 246:H37–H43.
22. Hearse, D. J., and Chain, E. B. (1972): The role of glucose in the survival and recovery of the anoxic isolated perfused rat heart. *Biochem. J.*, 128:1125–1133.
23. Hearse, D. J., Stewart, D. A., and Chain, E. B. (1974): Recovery from cardiac bypass and elective cardiac arrest: The metabolic consequences of various cardioplegic procedures in the isolated rat heart. *Circ. Res.*, 35:448–457.
24. Hearse, D. J., Yellon, D. M., Chappell, D. A., Wyse, R. K. H., and Ball, G. R. (1981): A high velocity impact device for obtaining multiple, contiguous, myocardial biopsies. *J. Mol. Cell. Cardiol.*, 13:197–206.
25. Henderson, J. F. (1978): Purine nucleotide interconversions. *Handbook Exp. Pharmacol.*, 51:75–88.
26. Henderson, R. J., Jr., and Griffin, C. A. (1981): Analysis of adenosine, inosine and hypoxanthine in suspensions of cardiac myocytes by high-performance liquid chromatography. *J. Chromatogr.*, 226:202–207.
27. Heyndrickx, G. R., Millard, R. W., McRitchie, R. J., Maroko, P. R., and Vatner, S. F. (1975): Regional myocardial functional

and electrophysiological alterations after brief coronary artery occlusion in conscious dogs. *J. Clin. Invest.,* 56:978–985.

28. Holmes, E. W., Wyngaarden, J. B., and Kelley, W. N. (1973): Human glutamine PP-ribose-P amidotransferase: Two molecular forms interconvertible by purine ribonucleotides and PP-ribose-P. *J. Biol. Chem.,* 248:6035–6040.

29. Holmes, E. W. (1978): Regulation of biosynthesis *de novo.* In: *Uric Acid,* edited by W. N. Kelley, I. M. Weiner, pp. 21–42. Springer-Verlag, New York.

30. Imai, S., Riley, A. L., and Berne, R. M. (1964): Effect of ischemia on adenine nucleotides in cardiac and skeletal muscle. *Circ. Res.,* 15:443–449.

31. Isselhard, W., Lauterjung, K. L., Witte, J., Ban, T., Hubner, G., Giersberg, O., Heugel, E., and Hirt, H. J. (1975): Metabolic and structural recovery of left ventricular canine myocardium from regional complete ischemia. *Eur. Surg. Res.,* 7:136–155.

32. Jennings, R. B., Hawkins, H. K., Lowe, J. E., Hill, M. L., Klotman, S., and Reimer, K. A. (1978): Relation between high energy phosphate and lethal injury in myocardial ischemia in the dog. *Am. J. Pathol.,* 92:187–214.

33. Jennings, R. B., and Reimer, K. A. (1981): Lethal myocardial ischemic injury. *Am. J. Pathol.,* 102:241–255.

34. Jolly, S. R., Menahan, L. A., and Gross, G. J. (1981): Diltiazem in myocardial recovery from global ischemia and reperfusion. *J. Mol. Cell. Cardiol.,* 13:359–372.

35. Jones, D. P. (1981): Determination of pyridine dinucleotides in cell extracts by high-performance liquid chromatography. *J. Chromatogr.,* 225:446–449.

36. Juengling, E., and Kammermeier, H. (1980): Rapid assay of adenine nucleotides or creatine compounds in extracts of cardiac tissue by paired-ion reverse-phase high-performance liquid chromatography. *Anal. Biochem.,* 102:358–361.

37. Kaufman, I. A., Hall, N. F., DeLuca, M. A., Ingwall, J. S., and Mayer, S. E. (1977): Metabolism of adenine nucleotides in the cultured fetal mouse heart. *Am. J. Physiol.,* 233:H282–H288.

38. Keppler, D., and Holstege, A. (1982): Pyrimidine nucleotide metabolism and its compartmentation. In: *Metabolic Compartmentation,* edited by H. Sies, pp. 147–203. Academic Press, Orlando, Florida.

39. Klabunde, R. E., Winser, C. L., Ito, C. S., and Mayer, S. E. (1979): Measurement of adenosine and inosine in heart samples by high pressure liquid chromatography. *J. Mol. Cell. Cardiol.,* 11:707–715.

40. Kloner, R. A., DeBoer, L. W. V., Darsee, J. R., Ingwall, J. S., and Braunwald, E. (1981): Recovery from prolonged abnormalities of canine myocardium salvaged from ischemic necrosis by coronary reperfusion. *Proc. Natl. Acad. Sci. USA,* 78:7152–7156.

41. Krenitsky, T. (1969): Tissue distribution of purine ribosyl- and phosphoribosyltransferases in the Rhesus monkey. *Biochim. Biophys. Acta,* 179:506–509.

42. Kugler, G. (1979): The effect of pindolol on myocardial release of inosine, hypoxanthine and lactate during pacing-induced angina. *J. Pharmacol. Exp. Ther.,* 209:185–189.

43. Lavallee, M., Cox, D., Patrick, T. A., and Vatner, S. F. (1983): Salvage of myocardial function by coronary artery reperfusion 1, 2, and 3 hours after occlusion in conscious dogs. *Circ. Res.,* 53:235–247.

44. Meerson, F. Z., and Pomoinitsky, V. D. (1972): The role of high-energy phosphate compounds in the development of cardiac hypertrophy. *J. Mol. Cell. Cardiol.,* 4:571–597.

45. Mochizuki, S., and Neely, J. R. (1980): Energy metabolism during reperfusion following ischemia. *J. Physiol. (Paris),* 76:805–812.

46. Namm, D. H. (1973): Myocardial nucleotide synthesis from purine bases and nucleosides. *Circ. Res.,* 33:686–695.

47. Neely, J. R., Rovetto, M. J., Whitmer, J. T., and Morgan, H. E. (1973): Effects of ischemia on function and metabolism of the isolated working rat heart. *Am. J. Physiol.,* 225:651–658.

48. Nishioka, K., and Jarmakani, J. M. (1982): Effect of ischemia on mechanical function and high-energy phosphates in rabbit myocardium. *Am. J. Physiol.,* 242:H1077–H1083.

49. Oerlemans, F., van Bennekom, C., and DeBruyn, C. (1981): Metabolite profiling of human muscle extracts by isotachophoresis. *J. Inherited Metab. Dis.,* 4:109–110.

50. Ohhara, H., Kanaide, H., Yoshimura, R., Okada, M., and Nakamura, M. (1981): A protective effect of coenzyme Q_{10} on ischemia and reperfusion of the isolated perfused rat heart. *J. Mol. Cell. Cardiol.,* 13:65–74.

51. Pasque, M. K., Spray, T. L., Pellom, G. L., Van Trigt, P., Peyton, R. B., and Currie, W. B. (1982): Ribose-enhanced myocardial recovery following ischemia in the isolated working rat heart. *J. Thorac. Cardiovasc. Surg.,* 83:390–398.

52. Perez, J. A., Mateo, F., and Melendez-Hevia, E. (1982): Nucleotide isotachophoretic assay: Method and application for determination of ATP/ADP ratio in several rat tissues. *Electrophoresis,* 3:102–106.

53. Reibel, D. K., and Rovetto, M. J. (1978): Myocardial ATP synthesis and mechanical function following oxygen deficiency. *Am. J. Physiol.,* 234:H620–H624.

54. Reibel, D. K., and Rovetto, M. J. (1979): Myocardial adenosine salvage rates and restoration of ATP content following ischemia. *Am. J. Physiol.,* 237:H247–H252.

55. Reimer, K. A., Hill, M. L., and Jennings, R. B. (1981): Prolonged depletion of ATP and of the adenine nucleotide pool due to delayed resynthesis of adenine nucleotides following reversible myocardial ischemic injury in dogs. *J. Mol. Cell. Cardiol.,* 13:229–239.

56. Rossi, A., Olivares, J., and Ray, A. (1981): Changes in myocardial pyrimidine nucleotide levels following repeated injections of iso-proterenol in rats. *Pfluegers Arch.,* 390:5–9.

57. Sabina, R. L., Kernstine, K. H., Boyd, R. L., and Holmes, E. W. (1982): Metabolism of 5-amino-4-imidazolecarboxamide riboside cardiac and skeletal muscle. *J. Biol. Chem.,* 257:10178–10183.

58. Sabina, R. L., Swain, J. L., Hines, J. J., and Holmes, E. W. (1983): A comparison of methods for quantitation of metabolites in skeletal muscle. *J. Appl. Physiol.,* 55:624–627.

59. Saleen, Y., Niveditha, T., and Sadasivudu, B. (1982): AMP deaminase, 5'-nucleotidase and adenosine deaminase in rat myocardial tissue in myocardial infarction and hypothermia. *Experientia,* 38:776–777.

60. Snyder, F. F., and Henderson, J. R. (1973): Alternative pathways of deoxyadenosine and adenosine metabolism. *J. Biol. Chem.,* 248:5899–5904.

61. Swain, J. L., and Holmes, E. W. (1980): *De novo* adenine nucleotide synthesis in myocardium. *Fed. Proc.,* 39:1089.

62. Swain, J. L., Hines, J. J., Sabina, R. L., and Holmes, E. W. (1982): Accelerated repletion of ATP and GTP pools in postischemic canine myocardium using a precursor of purine de novo synthesis. *Circ. Res.,* 51:102–105.

63. Swain, J. L., Sabina, R. L., McHale, P. A., Greenfield, J. C., Jr., and Holmes, E. W. (1982): Prolonged myocardial nucleotide depletion after brief ischemia in the open-chest dog. *Am. J. Physiol.,* 242:H818–H826.

64. Swain, J. L., Sabina, R. L., Peyton, R. B., Jones, R. N., Wechsler, A. S., and Holmes, E. W. (1982): Derangements in myocardial purine and pyrimidine nucleotide metabolism in patients with coronary artery disease and left ventricular hypertrophy. *Proc. Natl. Acad. Sci. USA,* 79:655–659.

65. Thomas, C. B., Meade, J. C., and Holmes, E. W. (1981): Aminoimidazole carboxamide ribonucleoside toxicity: A model for study of pyrimidine starvation. *J. Cell. Physiol.,* 107:335–344.

66. Tsuboi, K. K., and Buckley, N. M. (1965): Metabolism of perfused C-14-labeled nucleosides and bases by the isolated heart. *Circ. Res.,* 16:343–352.

67. Vary, T. C., Angelakos, E. T., and Schaffer, S. W. (1979): Relationship between adenine nucleotide metabolism and irreversible ischemic tissue damage in isolated perfused rat heart. *Circ. Res.,* 45:218–225.

68. Verdys, M., Aussedat, J., Olivares, J., Ray, A., and Rossi, A. (1983): A method for measuring free-nucleotide pool sizes and incorporation of labeled precursors: its application in studying myocardial pyrimidine nucleotides. *Anal. Biochem.,* 132:137–141.

69. Vial, C., Crozatier, B., Goldschmidt, D., and Font, B. (1982): Adenine nucleotide content and regional function during ischemia and reperfusion in canine ventricular myocardium. *Basic Res. Cardiol.,* 77:645–655.

70. Watts, J. A., Koch, C. D., and LaNove, K. F. (1980): Effects of

Ca^{2+} antagonism on energy metabolism: Ca^{2+} and heart function after ischemia. *Am. J. Physiol.,* 238:H909–H919.

71. Weiner, J. M., Apstein, C. S., Arthur, J. H., Pirzada, F. A., and Hood, W. B., Jr. (1976): Persistence of myocardial injury following brief periods of coronary occlusion. *Cardiovasc. Res.,* 10:678–686.

72. Wikman-Coffelt, J., and Coffelt, R. J. (1982): A stimulator-regulated rapid-freeze clamp for terminating metabolic processes of the heart during normal physiological working conditions. *IEEE Trans. Biomed. Eng.,* BME-29:448–453.

73. Zakaria, M., and Brown, P. R. (1981): High-performance liquid column chromatography of nucleotides, nucleosides and bases. *J. Chromatogr.,* 226:267–290.

74. Zakaria, M., Brown, P. R., Farnes, M. P., and Barker, B. E. (1982): HPLC analysis of aromatic amino acids, nucleosides, and bases in plasma of acute lymphocytic leukemics on chemotherapy. *Clin. Chim. Acta,* 126:69–80.

75. Zimmer, H.-G., Trandelenburg, C., Kammermeier, H., and Gerlach, E. (1973): *De novo* synthesis of myocardial adenine nucleotides in the rat. *Circ. Res.,* 32:635–640.

76. Zimmer, H-G., and Gerlach, E. (1977): Studies on the regulation of the biosynthesis of myocardial adenine nucleotides. In: *Purine Metabolism in Man. II: Regulation of Pathways and Enzyme Defects,* edited by M. M. Muller, E. Kaiser, and J. E. Seegmiller, pp. 40–49. Plenum Press, New York.

77. Zimmer, H-G. (1980): Restitution of myocardial adenine nucleotides: Acceleration by administration of ribose. *J. Physiol. (Paris),* 76:769–775.

78. Zimmer, H-G., Steinkopff, G., Ibel, H., and Koschine, H. (1980): Is the ATP decline a signal for stimulating protein synthesis in isoproterenol-induced cardiac hypertrophy? *J. Mol. Cell. Cardiol.,* 12:421–426.

79. Zimmer, H.-G. (1983): Normalization of depressed heart function in rats by ribose. *Science,* 220:81–82.

The Heart and Cardiovascular System,
edited by H. A. Fozzard et al.
Raven Press, New York © 1986.

CHAPTER 45

Protein Synthesis and Degradation

Howard E. Morgan, Balvin H. L. Chua, Peter A. Watson, and Louise Russo

Studies of protein synthesis and degradation are important because of the continuous turnover of cardiac proteins and the central role of these processes in physiologic and pathologic growth of the heart. Research in this field is strongly dependent on related investigations in systems from prokaryotes, simple eukaryotes, cultured cell lines, and mammalian cells and tissue. The large majority of findings that delineate the pathways of protein synthesis and degradation and the mechanisms of control have arisen from noncardiac systems. The extent to which studies of macromolecular turnover depend on fundamental research is steadily increasing with the application of molecular and cell biological techniques to studies of contractile proteins, cell membranes, receptors, and other cellular organelles. As a result, research in these areas requires a broad base of knowledge well beyond topics usually considered to be the province of cardiac biochemistry, physiology, and pharmacology.

Development of knowledge of the pathways of protein synthesis and degradation has involved usual procedures of cell fractionation, protein purification, development of assays for partial reactions of peptide-chain initiation, elongation and termination, and reconstitution of these purified components (86). In regard to protein synthesis, these approaches have led to detailed knowledge of reactions involved in initiation and elongation of peptide chains, but additional catalytic factors may remain to be discovered, because the activity of reconstituted systems is far below the rates observed in intact cells

(93,116). Inability to reconstitute rates of peptide-chain initiation as rapid as those observed in intact cells represents an important weakness in studies of control mechanisms, because this group of reactions constitutes an important site of regulation by hormones, substrates, and mechanical activity of heart.

Although substantial progress has been made in defining the pathway of protein synthesis, the sequence of reactions in protein degradation remains uncertain (79). Proteolysis is thought to involve cytoplasmic as well as lysosomal proteases. In regard to studies of regulation of proteolysis in heart, lack of identification of flux-generating step(s) has resulted in studies that describe factors controlling protein degradation and correlate the rate of proteolysis with activities of proteolytic enzymes and with morphology, density, and fragility of lysosomes. The energy dependence of protein degradation provides the incentive to search for ATP-dependent proteases and to define the molecular mechanisms by which energy is used to control protein breakdown, such as direct effects of ATP on proteases and the need for ATP to conjugate ubiquitin to proteins and thus to commit them to hydrolysis (51,52,123,124). Similarly, the presence of calcium-dependent proteases in the nonlysosomal compartment of the cell has led to studies of the role of cytosolic Ca^{2+} concentration in control of proteolysis (61,89).

In this chapter, an approach to studies of protein synthesis and degradation is described. Principles that are important to these studies are stressed. Data are presented when needed to illustrate the principle at hand.

REGULATION OF PROTEIN SYNTHESIS

Measurement of Rate

The most common problem in measurement of rates of protein synthesis is determination of the specific radioactivity of the precursor pool of amino acid used for peptide-chain initiation and elongation. Calculation of rates of protein synthesis using specific radioactivities of extracellular or intracellular phenylalanine gives rates that vary with perfusate phenylalanine concentration (Fig. 1). When the specific radioactivity of tRNA-bound phenylalanine is used, the rate of protein synthesis is constant; histidine incorporation also is unchanged over this range of phenylalanine concentrations. These results are consistent with two models of amino acid compartmentation (Figs. 2 and 3). The compartmentation problem has been solved by use of the specific radioactivity of phenylalanine bound to tRNA and elevation of perfusate phenylalanine to 0.4 mM, a concentration at which the specific activities of extracellular, intracellular, and tRNA-bound amino acids are the same (75,84). *In vivo*, a similar principle has been adopted: injection of a large dose of free amino acid that tends to equalize these same specific activities (29,41,47). When the specific radioactivity of the precursor pool is rigorously determined (29), absolute rates of protein synthesis can be calculated (nanomoles amino acid incorporated per gram

of tissue per hour). Attention must be given to selection of the radioactive amino acid used to monitor the rates. Ideally, the amino acid should be transported rapidly and not metabolized by the heart. Phenylalanine and tyrosine have these properties and are used most frequently for measurements of this rate. *In vivo* measurements commonly employ leucine or phenylalanine because of their greater solubility.

Even if the precursor specific activity is not rigorously measured, relative rates of synthesis of specific proteins can be determined (28,111). In this approach, incorporation of radioactivity into a specific protein is compared with incorporation of radioactivity into whole-heart protein. The specific protein must be highly purified by conventional fractionation procedures or by immunological methods.

Whether absolute or relative rates of protein synthesis are measured, cellular heterogeneity complicates assessment of the rate. The assumption that is implicit in these measurements is that the specific radioactivity of the indicator amino acid is the same in both muscle and nonmuscle cells. If the rate is modified by an experimental variable, cardiac muscle cells can be prepared to be certain that these cells share in the effect (139).

Finally, the properties of the isolated tissue preparation used for studies of protein synthesis and degradation are crucial (36,81). Cells of the preparation must be intact and supplied saturating quantities of oxygen and oxidative substrate. Under these conditions, tissue contents of ATP and creatine phosphate are stable for periods of several hours. Rates of protein synthesis should equal

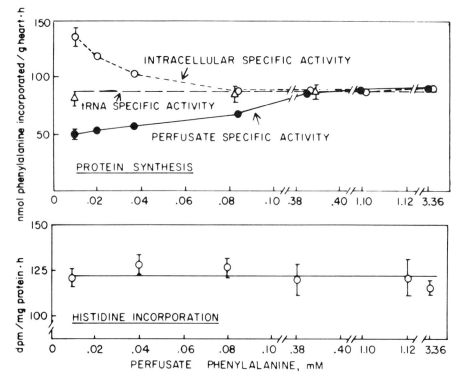

FIG. 1. Effect of perfusate phenylalanine concentration on rates of protein synthesis and histidine incorporation into heart protein. A preliminary perfusion of rat hearts for 10 min with buffer containing phenylalanine at the concentrations indicated, 15 mM glucose, and normal plasma concentrations of other amino acids is followed by recirculation of the same buffer containing [^{14}C]phenylalanine for either 90 min (phenylalanyl-tRNA specific activity) or 180 min (specific activity of perfusate and intracellular phenylalanine). Intracellular specific activity is calculated as described previously (75), as is the specific activity of phenylalanyl-tRNA. Each value represents the mean ± SE. In the phenylalanyl-tRNA experiments, six hearts were pooled for each determination. (From ref. 84, with permission.)

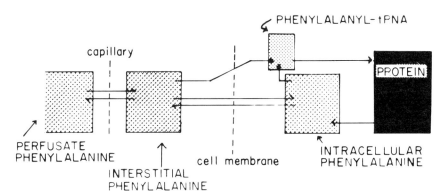

FIG. 2. Model of amino acid compartmentation involving acylation of phenylalanine from both intracellular and extracellular pools. The solution of this model by compartmental analysis and the derived rate constants and equations have been presented elsewhere (75). (From ref. 84, with permission.)

rates of proteolysis and be equal to rates that occur *in vivo*. Isolated rat hearts perfused either as working preparations or Langendorff preparations meet these criteria. In these preparations, rates of synthesis in specific areas of heart can be assessed, following a period of perfusion, by dissection of right and left ventricular free walls, septum, and atria (97). Rates of synthesis in atria are substantially higher than in ventricles. This finding stresses the importance of avoiding contamination of one tissue with the other. Other heart preparations that are useful for measurements of rates of synthesis and degradation are cultured fetal heart cells (18,39,119), freshly isolated and rapidly attached muscle cells from adult rats (96), and fetal mouse hearts in organ culture (138). Cultured fetal heart cells are suitable for these studies if care is taken to avoid contamination of the culture with other cell types or with dead cells. Muscle cells isolated by enzymatic digestion of adult hearts contain round as well as rod-shaped cells. This situation complicates measurements of rates of protein synthesis by addition of radioactive amino acids to isolated cells because of heterogeneity of the preparation. Fetal mouse hearts in organ culture offer an opportunity for experiments of longer duration, but heart size must be 2 mm or less to prevent diffusion limitations to supplies of oxygen and substrates. The small size of the fetal mouse heart restricts its usefulness for many biochemical studies. Furthermore, these hearts are in negative nitrogen balance. Heart slices and homogenates are not suitable for studies of control of protein synthesis.

Identification of Important Rate-Controlling Steps

Control of the rate of protein synthesis is investigated by measuring the overall rate and tissue content of intermediates in the pathway (Fig. 4). Methods for rigorous estimates of the rate were discussed earlier. Intermediates in the pathway that can be measured in a quantitative or semiquantitative manner in heart muscle are amino acid content, content of amino acids bound to tRNA, and percentage of RNA in ribosomal subunits. Only qualitative estimates of polysome content are possible; entrapment of polysomes in the pellet of contractile protein prevents more precise measurements.

The size of the free amino acid pool reflects the balance between rates of inward amino acid transport and protein degradation that supply this pool and protein synthesis and amino acid efflux and metabolism that deplete the pool. Amino acid availability does not appear to restrict the rate of protein synthesis in rat heart under the experimental conditions that have been studied thus far (86). For example, insulin accelerates amino acid transport and the rate of protein synthesis, but reduces tissue content of several amino acids (101). These findings indicate that the hormone accelerates utilization of intracellular free amino acids for protein synthesis to a greater extent than it increases their supply. Restraint of proteolysis by insulin also contributes to the decline in free amino acid content. Similarly, inhibition of protein synthesis observed in anoxic hearts is not due to decreased amino acid availability (63).

FIG. 3. Model of amino acid compartmentation involving two intracellular pools. The solution of this model by compartmental analysis and the derived rate constants and equations have been presented elsewhere (75). (From ref. 84, with permission.)

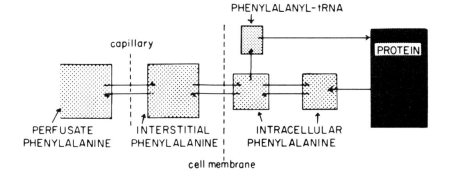

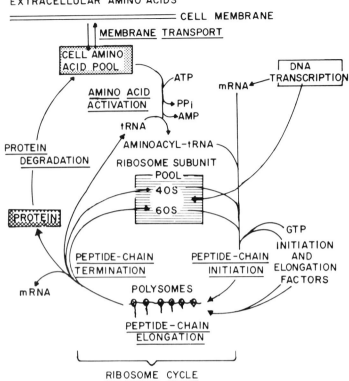

EXTRACELLULAR AMINO ACIDS

FIG. 4. Pathway of protein turnover. Amino acids are supplied to the intracellular pool by either membrane transport or protein degradation. Intracellular amino acids are activated to form aminoacyl derivatives by combination with tRNA. Polymerization of activated amino acids into protein is catalyzed by a series of ribosome-dependent reactions that make up the ribosome cycle. These reactions include initiation of peptide chains on the ribosomes and elongation and termination of chains. Peptide-chain initiation refers to binding of messenger RNA (mRNA) and initiator-tRNA (methionyl-tRNA$_f$) to the small ribosomal subunit (40S), followed by the binding of the large subunit (60S). Both steps require GTP and initiation factors. Peptide-chain elongation refers to successive addition of activated amino acids as determined by the code contained within mRNA. This process is dependent on elongation factors. When the protein is complete, the peptide chain and ribosomal subunits are released into the cytoplasm. Protein degradation refers to reactions catalyzed by proteases and results in the release of free amino acids into the intracellular pool (From ref. 86, with permission of the American Physiological Society.)

The content of amino acids bound to tRNA has not been rigorously measured in heart muscle. Leucyl-tRNA is found to be unchanged in hearts supplied 1 mM as compared with 0.2 mM leucine, indicating that stimulation of protein synthesis by leucine is not due to greater availability of this substrate of protein synthesis (80). Interpretation of the tissue content of tRNA-bound amino acids is complicated by the fact that there are multiple species of tRNA for most amino acids. As a result, a change in content of a minor species of aminoacyl-tRNA complementary to a particular nucleotide triplet might not be detected if the total of that amino acid bound to tRNA is measured. In liver, the content of tRNA-bound amino acid did not change over a wide range of amino acid concentrations in the extracellular fluid (37). Most tRNA appears to be charged with amino acids at a given time, but difficulties in measurement of the charged compared with uncharged species of a given tRNA leave the problem unresolved.

Evidence cited earlier suggests that amino acid supply, either of the free or tRNA-bound form, does not restrict protein synthesis and that ribosome-catalyzed reactions include the flux-generating step. Faster rates of peptide bond formation result from either greater efficiency or capacity for protein synthesis or both. Efficiency is defined as the quantity of protein synthesized per amount of RNA per time, whereas capacity represents the total amount of protein synthetic machinery that is present, including ribosomes, mRNA, initiation factors, and elongation factors. Capacity is assessed by measuring

the content of total RNA or rRNA per gram of tissue. Ribosomal RNA amounts to 85% of total RNA in most tissues, including heart (142). However, as will be discussed later, measurements of total RNA and rRNA give an accurate reflection of the capacity for synthesis only if sufficient mRNA is present to allow most ribosomal subunits to be present as polysomes.

The efficiency of protein synthesis in heart is found to be more commonly controlled by rates of peptide-chain initiation than elongation (86). *In vivo,* the availability of substrates and hormones and the operation of mechanical factors, such as aortic pressure, result in rates of peptide-chain initiation in rat heart that are fast enough to leave only about 12% of total RNA in ribosomal subunits (117,139). Perfusion of rat hearts *in vitro* with only glucose as oxidative substrate results in development of a block in peptide-chain initiation, as indicated by a fall in the rate of protein synthesis and an increase in the amount of total RNA in ribosomal subunits to about 20% (67). This block is not due to an acute deficiency of mRNA, because addition of fatty acids in the presence of actinomycin D rapidly restores subunit content to *in vivo* levels (100). These findings indicate that there is sufficient mRNA in rat heart to allow most subunits to be present as polysomes and to be active in protein synthesis.

Faster protein synthesis in rat hearts induced to hypertrophy by aortic banding or injection of pharmacological doses of thyroxine is dependent on the presence of more ribosomes and mRNA. Synthesis of only more total mRNA results in only a small increase in synthesis, because 90% of subunits are already active in making new protein (87,117). However, an increase in relative abundance of a particular mRNA has a large effect on synthesis of that protein; for example, synthesis of the α heavy chain of myosin increases markedly within 24 hr after thyroxine injection because of higher tissue content of its mRNA (30). Greater abundance of the skeletal muscle form of actin mRNA also increases early in the course of thyrotoxic cardiac hypertrophy (114). It is not known if sufficient total mRNA is present in hearts of species other than rat to prevent limitation of peptide-chain initiation by mRNA availability. Whether or not the availability of mRNA, as compared with ribosomes, limits protein synthesis in human hearts is unknown.

Limitations of present methods for identification of rate-controlling steps in protein synthesis include lack of methods for measurement of many intermediates in the pathway and availability of only semiquantitative methods for others. For example, native 40S subunits can be measured in liver by extraction in low-ionic-strength buffer, fixation, and separation on cesium chloride density gradients (50,56). In muscle, these measurements are more difficult because of entrapment of subunits in the resulting actomyosin gel that forms in low-ionic-strength buffer (65). As a result, formation of the preinitiation 40S complex has not been assessed as a rate-controlling step in heart muscle. Recovery of ribosomal subunits free of initiation factors by extraction in high-ionic-strength buffer is only semiquantitative. When hearts are perfused with buffer containing puromycin, about 63% of total RNA is recovered in ribosomal subunits (83). If recovery had been quantitative, 85% of total RNA should have been recovered. Thus, the presence of only 12% of total RNA in ribosomal subunits is indicative of the presence of sufficient mRNA to saturate peptide-chain initiation, but a more quantitative estimate is desirable. In cell suspensions, rates of peptide-chain elongation are estimated by measurements of transit times. These measurements depend on the rapidity of appearance of particle-bound radioactive amino acid, representing peptidyl-tRNA on ribosomes, followed by transfer of radioactivity to soluble protein (33,55). These measurements indicate that the time required to make an average protein once a peptide chain is initiated is about 2 min. Attempts were made to carry out such experiments in groups of perfused rat hearts to determine if anoxia inhibited peptide-chain elongation. The attempt was unsuccessful because of the variability introduced by the use of separate hearts for each time point, as compared with aliquots from a cell suspension. In regard to enzyme isolation, the difficulty of recovering polysomes from hearts homogenized in low-ionic-strength buffer impedes purification of initiation factors. In liver, an important purification step is the isolation of poly-somes to which initiation factors are bound, followed by release of these factors by exposure to high-salt buffer (93). If the ionic strength of heart homogenates is increased to improve polysome recovery, initiation factors are released and must be purified from the bulk of soluble proteins. Despite these limitations, control of protein synthesis by substrates, hormones, and mechanical activity has been described. However, the limitations listed earlier have restricted studies of the molecular mechanisms by which these regulatory events are achieved.

FACTORS CONTROLLING THE RATE OF SYNTHESIS

Control of Efficiency with Which Ribosomes Synthesize Protein

Discoveries of factors that control the efficiency of protein synthesis in heart have depended to a large extent on *in vitro* experiments using perfused rat hearts. In this experimental model, many factors that affect peptide-chain initiation *in vivo* are removed by provision of only glucose or pyruvate as oxidative substrate and by exposure to a low aortic pressure (67,86). Despite the lack of hormones and substrates that are present *in vivo*, energy availability is well maintained, as assessed by contents of ATP and creatine-P and the creatine-P/creatine ratio. After about 1 hr of *in vitro* perfusion of Langendorff preparations at an aortic pressure of 60 mm Hg with buffer containing glucose, a block in peptide-chain initiation develops, as indicated by a decrease of about 40% in the rate of protein synthesis and an increase in the percentage of total RNA in ribosomal subunits from 10% to 20%. Assessment of the effectiveness of factors controlling the efficiency of synthesis is best carried out by measuring the rate of synthesis and the contents of intermediates in the pathway of synthesis during the second or third hour of perfusion. The regulatory factors prevent the development of initiation block or reverse it once it has occurred (83,100).

Hormonal Control

Hormones that affect the efficiency of synthesis by maintaining *in vivo* rates of peptide-chain initiation are insulin and epinephrine and other catecholamines (86). In regard to insulin, the questions that have been asked are whether or not physiological concentrations of the hormone are effective, whether or not the insulin effect is dependent on accelerated rates of glycolysis or increased tissue content of glycolytic intermediates, and whether or not an increase in energy availability is responsible for the effect (36). The outcome of the experiments is that the maximal hormone effect is achieved with insulin concentrations in the range found in plasma, that insulin is effective in hearts supplied pyruvate rather than glucose and in which the contents of glucose-6-P are low and unchanged, and that the hormone does not affect energy availability in hearts oxidizing pyruvate but continues to increase rates of protein synthesis. Although some possible mechanisms of the insulin effect have been ruled out, the biochemical mechanism remains undefined. As noted earlier, amino acid availability also was excluded as a mechanism of the insulin effect (101).

Epinephrine accelerates protein synthesis in the perfused rat heart (16). In this case, interpretation of the effect as a direct β-receptor-mediated phenomenon is complicated by increased contractility and heart rate and decreased ATP content that follow addition of the catecholamine. Effects of catecholamines on protein synthesis under circumstances in which changes in mechanical activity are inhibited by agents such as tetrodotoxin have not been sought.

Substrate Control

Substrate availability modifies the rates of protein synthesis in heart by affecting the efficiency of synthesis (67,100). In hearts supplied either pyruvate or glucose, a block in peptide-chain initiation develops after approximately 1 hr of perfusion. In the case of pyruvate, the content of ATP is well maintained, and creatine-P and the creatine-P/creatine ratio are substantially elevated. These findings indicate that development of the initiation block is not due to impaired energy availability. However, addition of free fatty acid or a variety of other noncarbohydrate substrates prevents the development of block or reverses it once it has developed. The range of compounds that are effective includes palmitate, oleate, octanoate, β-hydroxybutyrate, acetoacetate, and acetate. As in the case of insulin, the effect of palmitate addition is not inhibited by perfusion in the presence of actinomycin D. Although changes in energy availability do not appear to account for the effects of noncarbohydrate substrates on peptide-chain initiation, the biochemical mechanism(s) of the effect is unknown. A major reason for lack of progress on this point is the absence of an *in vitro* protein-synthesizing system derived from heart muscle that would initiate peptide chains in an efficient manner. Intermediates in the metabolism of noncarbohydrate substrates could modify rates of peptide chain through covalent modification or allosteric regulation of initiation factors. In skeletal muscle supplied with glucose, a block in peptide-chain initiation develops in mixed skeletal muscle but not in soleus (35). The tissue specificity of the effects of starvation, diabetes, and noncarbohydrate substrates on protein synthesis is similar to the specificity of these effects on glycolysis

(91). Inhibition of phosphofructokinase by an elevated tissue content of citrate accounts for glycolytic inhibition following fatty acid addition. There appears to be a physiological advantage during starvation to sparing heart from development of a block in peptide-chain initiation in that white skeletal muscle can be in severe negative nitrogen balance and the resulting free amino acids used for gluconeogenesis and maintenance of blood glucose without such severe effects on heart.

Leucine appears to be another regulator of protein synthesis that ameliorates the effects of starvation (6,14,15,82,100). Plasma concentrations of branched-chain amino acids, leucine, isoleucine, and valine increase in severely diabetic animals, as well as during starvation. Addition of leucine, but not isoleucine and valine, in concentrations of 0.5 mM or greater accelerates peptide-chain initiation in hearts with a block at this step. This effect is shared by the keto acids of all three branched-chain amino acids, as well as several other metabolites in the degradative pathway of these compounds. A question that has been asked in regard to the mechanisms of these effects is whether they are due to a greater availability of leucyl-tRNA, of leucine itself, or of the content of a leucine metabolite, or are due to improved energy availability. As noted earlier, the tissue content of leucyl-tRNA does not increase as the perfusate leucine is raised (80), and reduced energy levels do not account for development of the initiation block. Whether leucine itself or a metabolite accounts for reversal of the block is unknown. In skeletal muscle, leucine, but not its keto acid, α-ketoisocaproate, is effective in accelerating protein synthesis (7). Tunicamycin, an inhibitor of protein glycosylation, blocks the stimulatory effect of leucine on protein synthesis in skeletal muscle, but has not been tested in heart (99).

Control by Mechanical Factors

The mechanical activity of the heart affects the efficiency of protein synthesis by accelerating both peptide-chain initiation and elongation. Initial studies of this phenomenon were carried out by Schreiber et al. (113) in baby guinea pig hearts and by Hjalmarson and Isaksson (58) in rat heart. Increased pressure work as compared with volume work was linked to faster rates of synthesis. Studies from this laboratory (63) and studies by Schreiber et al. (112) demonstrated that inhibition of contraction by tetrodotoxin or elevated perfusate potassium levels had no effect on the rate of protein synthesis in Langendorff preparations supplied an aortic pressure of 60 mm Hg or less. Takala (122) and Kira et al. (66) observed that the rate of protein synthesis was increased by elevation of perfusion pressure of Langendorff preparations from 60 to 120 mm Hg and that this effect was still present in hearts that were arrested and had a drain in the ventricle. In arrested-drained hearts, elevation of aortic perfusion pressure does not increase oxygen consumption as it does in control-beating or beating-drained hearts. When considered in terms of the mechanical parameter most closely linked to acceleration of protein synthesis, beating, contractility, and intraventricular-pressure development are excluded. Increased aortic pressure results in greater intravascular volume and sarcomere length and in stretch of the ventricular wall (88,98,132). Stretch of isolated papillary muscles, skeletal muscle, and cultured myotubes also increases the rate of protein synthesis (5,95,121,130).

Biochemical mechanisms that link stretch of muscle to faster rates of protein synthesis have been reported to be related to increased availability of Ca^{2+} and accelerated production of prostaglandins (27,94,105). In skeletal muscle, addition of the Ca^{2+} ionophore A23187 accelerates protein synthesis, whereas the effects of stretch are blocked by Ca^{2+} removal and addition of EDTA. Direct measurements of cytosolic free Ca^{2+} were not carried out in these experiments. The stimulatory effect of stretch on protein synthesis in skeletal muscle is blocked by the cyclooxygenase inhibitor indomethacin and is mimicked by addition of $PGF_{2\alpha}$ and PGE_2. Similar studies recently have been carried out in the perfused rat heart (48,49). An increase in aortic pressure from 60 to 120 mm Hg accelerates protein synthesis in arrested-drained hearts over a range of perfusate Ca^{2+} concentrations from 0.6 to 5.1 mM, in the presence of 0.1 mM EDTA. In these preparations, energy availability is well maintained. In control beating hearts, an increase in perfusate Ca^{2+} from 0.6 to 5.1 mM increases heart rate and oxygen consumption and decreases energy availability but has no effect on the rate of protein synthesis. These studies provide no support for a role for Ca^{2+} availability as an important controlling factor in cardiac protein synthesis. Whether or not lower concentrations of extracellular Ca^{2+} would inhibit protein synthesis and prevent the stimulatory effect of increased aortic pressure cannot be explored because of the instability of Langendorff preparations, as manifested by loss of proteins and nucleotides from the preparation at lower perfusate Ca^{2+} concentrations. In regard to prostaglandins, addition of meclofenamate reduces the rate of appearance of a prostacyclin metabolite, 6-keto-$PGF_{2\alpha}$, and PGE_2 in the perfusion medium, but has no effect on the rate of protein synthesis either at 60 or 120 mm Hg aortic pressure. These studies provide no support for the proposal that accelerated prostaglandin production is linked to the effects of stretch on protein synthesis. At the present time, the intracellular mediator that links stretch of the ventricular wall to faster rates of protein syntheses in heart is unknown.

Control by Energy Availability

Impairment of oxygen delivery in anoxic and ischemic hearts results in inhibition of protein synthesis (63,86).

Both peptide-chain initiation and elongation are energy-requiring processes, and analysis of ribosomal-subunit content indicates that the balance between rates of peptide-chain initiation and elongation is unchanged in energy-deficient hearts as compared with control hearts. These findings indicate that both initiation and elongation of chains are inhibited. Inhibition of synthesis is not due to impairment of contractile activity, because the rate does not fall in hearts exposed to tetrodotoxin. The rate of synthesis is restored if oxygen is resupplied before irreversible damage occurs.

Significance of Control of Peptide-Chain Initiation

In rat heart, sufficient mRNA is present to result in only 12% of total RNA in ribosomal subunits, and a variety of factors operate to accelerate peptide-chain initiation. For example, the content of ribosomal subunits does not change in hearts of diabetic rats despite severe insulin deficiency, because plasma concentrations of fatty acids and ketone bodies rise and maintain rates of peptide-chain initiation (100). In short, the rat heart is protected in the intact animal from a fall in efficiency of protein synthesis by hormones, substrates, and mechanical activity. Only under drastic conditions such as anoxia or ischemia does the efficiency of synthesis fall markedly. In such a well-protected setting, can efficiency of synthesis increase *in vivo* in response to a demand such as pressure overload and represent an important factor in the genesis of cardiac hypertrophy? Overall protein synthesis does increase in rat hearts supplied saturating concentrations of insulin when aortic pressure is raised from 60 to 120 mm Hg, suggesting that the answer may be positive (66). The difficulty in answering this question is that small increments in rates of protein synthesis, if maintained for days or weeks, result in marked cardiac hypertrophy, if the rate of protein degradation is unchanged. These small changes (<5%) are not detectable because of the variability that is encountered when groups of 6 to 12 hearts are used to estimate the rate of synthesis.

Thus far, the efficiency of synthesis has been discussed in terms of synthesis of whole-heart protein. An equally important or perhaps more important question is whether or not insulin, noncarbohydrate substrates, or increased aortic pressures favor initiation of translation of one mRNA species as compared with another and result in faster synthesis of a specific protein. If so, translational control, in addition to transcriptional control, of protein synthesis will be important (102,116). Examples of preferential translation of endogenous compared with viral mRNA have been observed in cultured cells (44). This phenomenon is due to differing affinities for mRNA binding to initiation factors. If increased aortic pressure results in accelerated translation of messages for RNA polymerases and ribosomal proteins in heart, translational control will be an important factor in cardiac hypertrophy. Early studies attempted to assess whether or not addition of insulin results in synthesis of specific proteins, using one-dimensional polyacrylamide gels (141). The hormone accelerates synthesis of all proteins, but the analytical method is too crude for rigorous examination of the specificity of synthesis. The question whether or not translational control is important in heart needs further study using two-dimensional gels, high specific radioactivity of precursor amino acid, and imposition of the factors that accelerate peptide-chain initiation.

Extrapolation of results obtained with hearts of adult rats to other species and ages of animals may not be justified. If peptide-chain initiation is significantly restricted by the availability of mRNA in hearts of other animals and man, mRNA synthesis will be important not only for the rate of synthesis of a specific protein but also for total heart protein. Investigation of the control of synthesis in hearts of other animals is needed to assess how broadly results in rat heart can be applied.

Control of Capacity for Synthesis

Growth of a wide variety of cells and tissues is associated with greater content of ribosomes per tissue mass (92). In *Escherichia coli,* not only are the numbers of ribosomes higher but also the activities of initiation and elongation factors are increased during rapid growth (59). The same situation is probably true in mammalian tissues, including heart. During hypertrophy that follows aortic banding in rats, faster synthesis of rRNA, tRNA, and mRNA occurs (34,68,129). In thyrotoxic hypertrophy, mRNA and rRNA contents of rat heart increase 59 and 29%, respectively (143). The larger increase in mRNA content has been suggested to account for the rapid growth, because it corrects a deficit in mRNA availability. As discussed earlier, we do not believe that mRNA availability is deficient in control rat hearts, but rather that greater tissue contents of ribosomes and mRNA are essential for growth. Rates of synthesis of ribosomal proteins have been measured during thyrotoxic hypertrophy (117), and measurements of rates of synthesis of mRNA and rRNA are in progress in this laboratory.

An increased tissue content of ribosomes depends on the balance between rates of formation and degradation of mature cytoplasmic ribosomes. Rates of ribosome formation depend on synthesis of preribosomal RNA (pre-rRNA), a 45S molecule that is processed to yield 28S, 18S, and 5S RNA. The efficiency of processing is unknown in heart but is reported to vary widely in other cells (19,21,54,103,104). During processing, rRNA is methylated on about 2% of ribose moieties to yield the 2-*O*-methyl derivatives; all of these methylated nucleotides are preserved in mature rRNA (73,135). In the

case of ribosomal proteins (r-protein), the situation is even more complex. Approximately 70 r-proteins are involved, the genes for which are widely dispersed in multiple copies in the genome (25,26,78). In some cases, all but one copy are pseudogenes that lack introns. The mRNAS for r-proteins are translated on cytoplasmic ribosomes, and newly formed proteins are transported into the nucleus, where they bind to the newly made rRNA. Faster synthesis of r-proteins is associated with either unchanged or increased contents of r-protein mRNA, depending on the cell or tissue involved, indicating that either translational or transcriptional control of r-protein formation can occur (32,40,43,109). Contents of r-protein mRNAs have not been measured in heart. If rRNA synthesis is inhibited, r-proteins have no binding sites available. In these circumstances, the half-life of r-proteins is 0.5 hr to 2 hr instead of the several days for r-proteins in mature ribosomes (136). The details of binding of specific r-proteins to newly made rRNA are unknown. Similarly, events in final ribosome assembly and transport from the nucleus have not been defined. In studies of the rate of formation of ribosomes in thyrotoxic hearts that we reported earlier (117), r-proteins were labeled with [^{3}H]phenylalanine, and the appearance of radioactivity in ribosomal subunits was measured. The time between addition of radioactivity and appearance of radioactive subunits was 10 to 12 min. However, these hearts were homogenized using a Polytron that caused breakage of some nuclei, as indicated by release of DNA into the cytosol. As a result, our earlier studies probably assessed the rapidity of synthesis of r-proteins and their binding to rRNA in the nucleus. More recently, hearts are homogenized with a Dounce homogenizer, and release of DNA into the cytosol is not observed. In these circumstances, the lag between addition of [^{3}H]phenylalanine and the appearance of radioactive ribosomal subunits is approximately 30 min. The additional 20 min that are needed for appearance of these radioactive particles presumably represent the time required for ribosome assembly and transport across the nuclear membrane into the cytosol (127). Degradation of mature cytoplasmic ribosomes appears to occur as a unit and is suggested to involve lysosomes (128).

Measurements of rates of rRNA and mRNA synthesis involve the same principles described for protein synthesis, but are more complex, because nonmetabolized precursors are not available, and RNA synthesis occurs in the nucleus, whose pool of nucleotides may not have the same specific radioactivity as nucleotides in the cytosol. *De novo* synthesis of purine and pyrimidine bases occurs at slow rates in heart (2,74). As a result, nucleosides are the only available precursor for rigorous estimates of RNA synthesis. These compounds enter the nucleotide pool via salvage pathways. Uridine is used for studies of RNA synthesis because the tissue content of UTP is low relative to ATP (42) and because UTP and UDPG can be resolved readily from other compounds by high-pressure liquid chromatography (17). The UTP pool is pulse-labeled by exposure to [³H]uridine, and the nucleoside is washed from the heart. The specific radioactivity of tissue UTP remains unchanged over the next 2 hr of perfusion. Incorporation of radioactivity into pre-rRNA, 18S rRNA, and mRNA over the 2-hr perfusion period is used to calculate rates of synthesis of these RNA species based on specific radioactivity of tissue UTP and specific radioactivity of UMP in a specific segment of 45S pre-rRNA that contains a portion of the 18S sequence. The 45S pre-rRNA is recovered by hybridization to a complementary RNA probe, and unhybridized portions of the molecule are removed by ribonuclease digestion. The UMP content and sequence of this portion of 18S rRNA are known (8). The specific radioactivity of UMP in pre-rRNA is calculated from the amount of [³H] radioactivity incorporated into the segment that hybridizes with the RNA probe, and the amount of pre-rRNA from specific radioactivity of the ³²P-labeled probe. If the specific radioactivity of UMP in pre-rRNA is the same as that of tissue UTP, UTP specific radioactivities will be used routinely for calculation of rates of rRNA synthesis. If the specific radioactivity of UMP in pre-rRNA differs from the specific radioactivity of tissue UTP, the UMP specific activity will be used as a monitor of the specific radioactivity of nuclear UTP. The major problem in the use of uridine as a precursor for studies of RNA synthesis is its rapid hydrolysis by uridine phosphorylase to uracil and ribose-1-P. Uridine phosphorylase activity is high in endothelial cells of capillaries, and the enzyme degrades uridine before it can reach muscle cells (107). This problem has been solved by addition of a competitive inhibitor of the enzyme to the perfusate used to pulse-label the UTP pool. This approach provides a rigorous method for measurements of synthesis of pre-rRNA, rRNA, and mRNA and allows the effects of hormones and mechanical performance to be examined.

Hormonal Control

The tissue content of RNA (mg/g) is elevated in hearts induced to hypertrophy by injection of pharmacological doses of thyroxine (117) and is decreased in hearts of hypophysectomized, starved, or diabetic rats (67,86,139). Because approximately 85% of total RNA is rRNA, measurements of RNA content reflect changes in the rRNA pool. Parallel changes in total RNA and rRNA content occur in hearts of thyroxine-injected rats. RNA and protein are present in approximately equal amounts in mature ribosomes. Thus far, rates of ribosome formation have been monitored by incorporation of newly made ribosomal proteins into cytoplasmic ribosomes. After 3 days of thyroxine injections, rat

hearts hypertrophy approximately 15 to 20%, and RNA content increases 30% (117). In order to achieve this increase in RNA content, larger effects on rates of ribosome formation are required. Four to eight hours after the first thyroxine injection, rates of ribosome formation are 30% higher, and 24 to 36 hr after instituting thyroxine treatment, the rate of ribosome formation is twice as fast. Whether faster r-protein synthesis depends on more efficient translation of preexisting r-protein mRNAs or higher tissue contents of these mRNAs has not been determined. Rates of pre-rRNA and rRNA synthesis have not been investigated.

Insulin accelerates r-protein synthesis in chick embryo fibroblasts to a much greater extent than it increases overall protein synthesis (24,60). These findings have been interpreted to indicate that the hormone results in preferential translation of r-protein mRNA. In perfused rat hearts, rates of r-protein incorporation into ribosomes and rates of whole-heart protein synthesis increase to similar extents in the 2 hr following hormone addition (117). These findings do not provide evidence for preferential translation of r-protein mRNA in rat heart.

Hearts from diabetic rats have lower RNA contents (139). To our surprise, the rate of incorporation of newly made r-proteins into cytoplasmic ribosomes is increased in severely insulin-deficient hearts (L. Russo, *unpublished observations*). Three days after insulin withdrawal, rates of cytoplasmic ribosome formation are twice as fast as in control hearts. Tissue contents of r-protein mRNAs have not been measured. Rates of whole-heart protein synthesis decreased approximately 20% at this time. Faster rates of ribosome formation, together with decreased RNA content in diabetic heart, indicate that degradation of mature cytoplasmic ribosomes is accelerated to a greater extent than ribosome synthesis. Overall protein degradation increases approximately twofold at this time in this model of diabetes, and lysosomal latency and density are decreased (13). These findings indicate that r-protein synthesis is protected in hearts of diabetic rats from effects of insulin deficiency. The factors that account for this protection are unknown.

Increased tissue content of mRNA for the α heavy chain of myosin follows treatment of hormone-deficient animals with thyroxine (30). This topic is dealt with in detail in *Chapter 46*. The time course of this effect is similar to that of the effects of thyroxine injection on rates of r-protein synthesis.

Control by Mechanical Factors

Initial studies of control of RNA synthesis in heart involved a pressure-overload model of cardiac hypertrophy that was induced by aortic banding (68). These studies indicated that all classes of RNA were synthesized at more rapid rates, but absolute rates could not be calculated because the specific radioactivity of the precursor nucleotide pool was not known. In these studies, the activity of RNA polymerase was found to increase in nuclei from hypertrophying hearts (90). Interpretation of changes in RNA polymerase activity in terms of the mechanism of muscle cell hypertrophy was uncertain because the majority of nuclei were derived from non-muscle cells; this problem was solved by separation of muscle and nonmuscle cells (20). In addition, imposition of an acute pressure overload resulted in depletion of ATP and focal areas of necrosis in the ventricular wall (3,118). Rates of protein synthesis increase in hearts from rats subjected to aortic banding; RNA content is elevated to a similar extent. This model of hypertrophy has not been used for a detailed examination of ribosome synthesis because of the deficiencies outlined earlier. It is doubtful that such studies would be worthwhile. More suitable models include rapid cardiac growth that is induced (a) by replacement doses of thyroid hormone administered to hypothyroid animals (57) or (b) by swimming exercise of female rats (53), as well as the rapid growth that occurs normally in the left ventricular free wall of animals in the period immediately after birth.

In vitro effects of cardiac work and increased aortic pressure on rates of incorporation of r-proteins into cytoplasmic ribosomes have not been thoroughly studied (117). Whether or not stretch of the ventricular wall induced by higher aortic pressure has a preferential effect to accelerate synthesis of r-protein or rRNA under more physiological conditions remains to be investigated.

Significance of Control of Capacity for Protein Synthesis

Increased ribosome and mRNA contents clearly are important factors leading to cardiac hypertrophy in rats. Without these changes, rates of protein synthesis could not increase to a significant extent, because existing ribosomal subunits are already engaged in synthesizing protein at an optimal rate. An understanding of the mechanisms that control synthesis of pre-rRNA, rRNA, and mRNA may reveal the nature of the intracellular mediator that links the effects of thyrotoxicosis and increased work of the heart to faster synthesis of these compounds.

REGULATION OF PROTEIN DEGRADATION

Measurement of Rate

Rates of protein degradation are measured more easily in isolated muscle preparations than *in vivo.* In perfused rat hearts or isolated atria, proteolysis is measured in two ways. First, net release of an amino acid that is incorporated into protein but not otherwise metabolized is estimated, along with the rate of protein synthesis employing the same compound or another amino acid with the same properties (101). Net release plus the rate of protein synthesis equals the rate of degradation. This method has the advantage that it does not require the use of inhibitors of protein synthesis, but the disadvantage that the rate of proteolysis is derived from two measurements, each of which has a level of error. The second method is to delete the indicator amino acid from the perfusion or incubation medium, to add an inhibitor of protein synthesis, such as cycloheximide, and to measure release of an amino acid such as phenylalanine into the incubation medium (10,14). This method has the advantage of greater sensitivity, but the disadvantage that inhibitors of protein synthesis restrain protein degradation in other tissues, such as liver. In heart, both methods of measuring protein degradation give the same value within experimental errors of the methods. In both methods, amino acid release is best measured using a tRNA-binding assay (9,106). This assay measures amounts in the range of 50 to 500 pmol, is specific, and can be carried out readily in large numbers of samples. In liver and cultured cells, a third method of measurement involving release of radioactivity from prelabeled protein is commonly employed (140). When radioactive amino acids are injected into whole animals, most of the radioactivity is incorporated into liver, and relatively little into heart. The specific radioactivity of protein that is achieved in heart following *in vivo* injection is too low to allow this method to be used conveniently for estimates of proteolysis.

In vivo rates of protein degradation are calculated from rates of protein synthesis and net changes in weight of the heart (4,69). These estimates suffer from problems of measuring the rate of protein synthesis *in vivo* and the need to measure changes in tissue weight over periods of days, whereas protein synthesis usually is determined at only a single time during this interval. If no growth occurs, the rate of proteolysis equals the rate of protein synthesis. Earlier attempts to estimate rates of protein degradation *in vivo* involved injection of a pulse of radioactive amino acid followed by measurements of the rate of disappearance of radioactivity from muscle protein (45,76). These measurements are compromised by reutilization of radioactive amino acids produced by proteolysis for protein synthesis. Finally, release of 3-methylhistidine that cannot be reincorporated into protein is employed as an index of degradation of muscle proteins (77,137). This and other methylated amino acids are produced by posttranslational modification of contractile proteins; in the case of actin, 3-methylhistidine is produced. Excretion of 3-methyl-histidine in the urine of animals and humans is used to monitor muscle proteolysis; these estimates are compromised by release of 3-methylhistidine from nonmuscle sources, including intestine. Release of methylated amino acids has not been used to estimate rates of cardiac proteolysis either *in vivo* or *in vitro*. Turnover of contractile proteins with half-lives of 6 to 10 days yields too little of the amino acid derivative for convenient estimates of the rate in isolated heart preparations. *In vivo*, the contribution of heart to appearance of 3-methylhistidine in urine is minor in comparison with the remainder of the body.

Degradation of specific proteins is estimated by measurements of changes in enzyme activity or immunologically reactive protein after an inducing agent is removed or synthesis of protein is inhibited (9). Measurements of enzyme protein with specific antibodies is preferred, because these estimates do not depend on development of optimal conditions for assay of enzyme activity (115). If degradation of a specific protein is to be assessed in *in vitro* experiments, the protein must have a half-life in the range of minutes or hours. The most common choices for these measurements are the enzymes involved in polyamine synthesis, including ornithine decarboxylase and *S*-adenosylmethionine decarboxylase.

Identification of the Pathway

Proteases are present in cytosol and in lysosomes of cardiac muscle cells (79). A major unresolved question is the contributions of these groups of proteases to overall protein degradation and to hydrolysis of specific proteins. Is there a unique flux-generating step in protein degradation that commits a protein molecule to destruction? If the initial proteolytic event occurs in cytosol, can hydrolysis to free amino acids also be accomplished in this compartment, or must the peptide fragments be transported into lysosomes for complete hydrolysis?

Hydrolysis by these groups of proteases is distinguished by the use of lysosomotropic reagents, of specific protease inhibitors, and of correlation between rates of proteolysis and latency, density, or morphology of lysosomes (70,79). None of these approaches gives unambiguous answers. Lysosomes take up basic compounds because of a large pH gradient across the lysosomal membrane or accumulate free amino acids as a result of intralysosomal hydrolysis of amino acid esters that readily penetrate lysosomal membranes (71). As a result of accumulation of these compounds, intralysosomal pH increases, but there is no assurance that lysosomal proteolysis falls to zero. If protein degradation is inhibited 50% by exposure of tissue to a lysosomotropic agent, the result cannot be interpreted to mean that 50% of proteolysis is cytosolic and 50% lysosomal. The specificity of protease inhibitors is based on binding or reaction with specific amino acids at or near the active site (70,105). As a result, groups of proteases, such as those with sulfhydryl groups,

react with a given protease inhibitor. These proteases may be in either cytosol or lysosomes. Lack of penetration of some protease inhibitors into the cell also impairs their value in tissue preparations. For example, pepstatin, a small peptide that is a potent inhibitor of cathepsin D, does not block proteolysis in heart because of its low membrane permeability (133). Finally, changes in the latency of lysosomal enzymes or the density or morphology of these organelles, together with a reduced rate of proteolysis, have been interpreted to indicate that insulin restrains protein breakdown by affecting this organelle (72). This conclusion is qualitative, not quantitative. Whether the hormone affects lysosomes directly or indirectly by restraining the activity of a flux-generating step in the cytosol is unknown.

As discussed earlier in regard to protein synthesis, identification of the pathway of protein degradation has been hindered by inability to reconstitute a cell-free protein-degradation system in which lysosomes take up and degrade protein. Protein that is already sequestered is degraded by isolated lysosomes, but additional protein is not taken up (134). Energy is needed for sequestration of protein and for maintenance of a pH gradient across the lysosomal membrane (1,110), but addition of ATP and an energy-generating system has not allowed isolated lysosomes to sequester protein. Heart presents an additional difficulty in isolation of lysosomes (13). As compared with liver, lysosome content in heart is low, and the large quantity of contractile protein entraps lysosomes in heart homogenates. Furthermore, greater force is required to homogenize heart than liver. As a result, more lysosomes are broken. These problems have been partially overcome by digestion of heart with Nagase, a bacterial protease, and by use of high salt concentrations to solubilize contractile proteins (13). Nevertheless, lysosomes have not been obtained from heart without extensive contamination with mitochondria or other cellular membranes. Yields of even partially purified lysosomes are low. Success has been achieved in the purification of lysosomal, Ca^{2+}-activated, and ATP-dependent proteases from muscle, but these purified enzymes do not completely degrade protein to free amino acids.

FACTORS CONTROLLING THE RATE OF PROTEIN DEGRADATION

Control of proteolysis is studied more easily in isolated heart preparations, but the physiological significance of control mechanisms that are identified may be difficult to deduce. Differences in the control of protein breakdown in heart as compared with skeletal muscle also have been reported. For example, the rate of proteolysis is Ca^{2+}-dependent in skeletal muscle, but not in heart (27,49,105). Whether differences in mechanisms of control are real or artifacts of the tissue preparations that are used is uncertain. Isolated perfused hearts and isolated atria have intact cells that are well supplied with oxygen and substrates. Rates of protein degradation and protein synthesis can be brought into balance if *in vivo* levels of aortic pressure, hormones, and oxidizable substrates are provided (81). Isolated skeletal muscle preparations that are most commonly used for studies of protein degradation are the isolated rat diaphragm, extensor digitorum longus, or soleus (38,105). None of these preparations is perfused, so that access of oxygen and substrates to the center of the preparation is dependent on their thickness. In the case of the diaphragm, all of the muscle cells are cut, and often the preparation is further divided into quarters. Cut muscles are heterogeneous in that they contain areas near the cut border where intracellular contents readily exchange with extracellular constituents. The isolated skeletal muscle preparations are in severe negative nitrogen balance, with rates of proteolysis three to five times the rates of protein synthesis. Sufficient care has not been taken in many experiments to document that energy availability is maintained, that lactate/pyruvate ratios are in a physiological range, and that the muscles are maintained at rest length. In the case of control of proteolysis by Ca^{2+} availability, Ca^{2+} has been omitted from the incubation medium, and a Ca^{2+} chelator added (64). It is not clear whether the lower rate of proteolysis that is observed under these conditions is due to loss of membrane integrity secondary to Ca^{2+} removal or to depletion of ATP and creatine-P. Control of proteolysis in skeletal muscle needs to be reinvestigated using preparations in which the muscles are at rest length, the cells are well supplied with oxygen and substrates via the capillary bed, nitrogen balance can be achieved, and energy availability is maintained. The perfused rat hind limb or hemicorpus would be a suitable preparation for identification of factors that regulate proteolysis in skeletal muscle and for studies of mechanisms of regulation (62,108). Only when these conditions are met can differences in regulation between heart and skeletal muscle be concluded to be real, and not artifacts of a defective skeletal muscle preparation.

Hormonal Control

Protein degradation in heart is restrained by addition of insulin, β-adrenergic agonists, and glucagon to isolated hearts (16,72,101). Rates of proteolysis are accelerated in hearts from diabetic animals (13). The concentration of insulin needed to inhibit proteolysis is in the physiological range, but larger effects can be obtained with pharmacological concentrations of the hormone (11). The effect of insulin on the rate of proteolysis is detected within 30 min, whereas the latency of lysosomes increases

within 15 min after addition of insulin (101). In hearts perfused in the absence of insulin, autophagic vacuoles appear, and the content of dense lysosomes decreases (72). These changes are prevented or reversed by addition of insulin. These findings indicate that insulin is an important regulator of protein degradation and that the hormone modifies the property of cardiac lysosomes.

Isoproterenol, epinephrine, and phenylephrine inhibit protein degradation, but the concentration of isoproterenol (10^{-8} M) that is required is two orders of magnitude lower than the concentrations of epinephrine and phenylephrine (*unpublished observations*). The inhibitory effect of isoproterenol is blocked by the β-adrenergic antagonist propranolol. When cardiac contraction is inhibited by tetrodotoxin, a blocker of fast sodium channels, isoproterenol does not inhibit proteolysis, although it increases cyclic AMP (*unpublished observations*). These findings indicate that the isoproterenol effect may be secondary to effects of the catecholamine on contraction of heart.

Glucagon in concentrations greater than 10^{-8} M increases the cyclic AMP content of isolated hearts and reduces the rate of protein degradation (16). Glucagon has no effect on energy availability, as monitored by contents of ATP and creatine-P (*unpublished observations*). Heart rate and contractile force are increased by glucagon, but the magnitudes of these effects are not as great as with isoproterenol. It is not known whether or not tetrodotoxin will inhibit the effect of glucagon on proteolysis. The physiological significance of the effect of glucagon on protein degradation is unknown.

When the hormonal status of rats is modified *in vivo* by hypophysectomy, cardiac size decreases by 25% over a period of 8 days (57). Removal of these hearts from the animals and perfusion under simulated *in vivo* conditions results in the same rates of protein degradation in control and hormone-deficient animals. In contrast, administration of pharmacological doses of thyroxine results in 15% greater cardiac mass after 3 days (117). Rates of protein degradation are unchanged in hearts from thyrotoxic rats as compared with control rats. These studies suggest that variations in rates of proteolysis are not important factors in growth and atrophy of the heart induced by deficiency or excess of thyroid hormone.

Control by Substrate Availability

When hearts are removed from overnight-fasted rats and perfused *in vitro* with buffer that contains either glucose or pyruvate as sole exogenous substrate, the rate of proteolysis is approximately three times the rate of protein synthesis (48,49). Rates of protein degradation in hearts supplied glucose are reduced by provision of 1.5 mM palmitate (85) and by a mixture of 1.5 mM palmitate and 10 mM DL-β-hydroxybutyrate (81). The mixture of palmitate and β-hydroxybutyrate is effective in both Langendorff and working preparations. Acetate and propionate also inhibit protein degradation (14). These findings indicate that the availability of noncarbohydrate substrates improves nitrogen balance by both accelerating protein synthesis and inhibiting protein degradation.

Branched-chain amino acids inhibit proteolysis, and this effect is due to leucine (6,7,14). Additions of isoleucine and valine in concentrations of 1 or 2 mM to the perfusion medium of hearts supplied glucose have no effect on protein breakdown (14). However, intermediates in the pathway of oxidation of all three amino acids inhibit proteolysis. These findings raise the question whether leucine or a metabolic product inhibits protein degradation. When oxidative decarboxylation of leucine is inhibited by provision of pyruvate as oxidative substrate, leucine still blocks the rate of proteolysis, suggesting that either leucine itself or its transamination product, α-ketoisocaproate, is responsible for the effect (12). However, a positive correlation between the inhibition of protein degradation and intracellular concentrations of α-ketoisocaproate is not apparent. Leucine analogs have no effect on proteolysis, except for leucinol, an amino alcohol that behaves as a lysosomotropic agent.

Control by Mechanical Factors

Protein degradation and protein synthesis are controlled by the same mechanical factors in heart muscle (49,66). Cardiac work reduces the rates of proteolysis in working hearts supplied glucose as substrate, when compared with Langendorff preparations perfused at an aortic pressure of 60 mm Hg (81). An inhibitory effect of cardiac work cannot be demonstrated in the presence of more physiological substrate mixtures, such as glucose, fatty acid, and ketone bodies or glucose, lactate, and insulin. The mechanical factor most closely linked to inhibition of protein degradation is explored in the same manner as for protein synthesis in control-beating, beating-drained, and arrested-drained Langendorff hearts by elevation of aortic pressure from 60 to 120 mm Hg (49). In each case, proteolysis is inhibited during the second hour of perfusion, when aortic pressure is raised. As is the case of protein synthesis, these findings indicate that stretch of the ventricular wall is the mechanical event most closely linked to inhibition of protein breakdown.

These findings in heart muscle agree with studies of the acute effects of stretch in skeletal muscle or cultured myotubes, in which greater muscle length inhibits the rate of proteolysis (5,69,131). After longer periods of continuous stretch *in vivo,* skeletal muscle growth is associated with faster rates of protein breakdown, but

an even larger acceleration of protein synthesis (46). Accelerated proteolysis is observed in hearts removed from rats subjected to aortic banding 3 days earlier when they are perfused *in vitro* as working preparations (118). The significance of this finding for the mechanism of hypertrophy is uncertain, because focal necrosis of the ventricular wall occurs in this model of acute pressure overload (3). Faster proteolysis may be associated with healing of these necrotic areas of myocardium. These findings stress the importance of using models of cardiac growth that do not involve tissue necrosis or depletion of adenine nucleotide pools for evaluation of the role of protein degradation in cardiac hypertrophy.

Control by Energy Availability

Both degradation and synthesis of protein are inhibited in hypoxic, anoxic, and ischemic hearts (10). Reduced rates of proteolysis also occur in a variety of cells and tissues as ATP stores are reduced (79). The energy requirement for protein breakdown may involve the need for ATP to couple ubiquitin to proteins destined for hydrolysis (51), for an ATP-dependent protease (22,23,123,124), for maintenance of an acidic intralysosomal pH (22,110), for sequestering protein into lysosomes, and for formation of autophagic vacuoles (1). In perfused rat hearts, ischemia is a more potent inhibitor of proteolysis than anoxia, and rates of protein synthesis and degradation are more nearly in balance in ischemic hearts than in anoxic hearts (10). Anoxia and ischemia appear to affect initial steps in the degradative pathway, because they block the decrease in activity of S-adenosylmethionine decarboxylase, as well as the appearance of perfusate phenylalanine in hearts exposed to cycloheximide (10). A further mechanism for restraint of proteolysis in energy-poor hearts is accumulation of metabolic products, such as lactate and hydrogen ions. These metabolites accumulate to much higher concentrations in ischemic hearts than in anoxic hearts, and this accumulation appears to account for the more marked inhibition of proteolysis in ischemic muscle than in anoxic muscle (10). Both perfusate lactate and decreased extracellular pH reduce rates of protein breakdown in aerobic and anoxic rat hearts.

Mechanisms of Control of Proteolysis

A unifying control mechanism has been sought to explain the inhibitory effects of insulin, fatty substrates, leucine, α-ketoisocaproate, stretch, and energy depletion on proteolysis. The intracellular mediators that are suggested to be involved in control of protein breakdown in skeletal muscle are the redox state (11,31,125,126), availability of Ca^{2+}, and prostaglandin production

(27,94,105,121). In regard to insulin, the hormone effect is not accounted for by decreased energy availability or by the oxidation-reduction state of the cells (11); the effects of calcium availability or cyclooxygenase inhibitors in restraint of proteolysis by insulin have not been studied. Possible mechanisms for inhibition of proteolysis by fatty substrates have not been investigated. Leucine and/or α-ketoisocaproate do not block protein breakdown as a result of their oxidation or a change in redox state (11,12). The effects of calcium availability and synthesis of prostaglandins on inhibition of proteolysis by leucine have not been examined. The effects of stretch on proteolysis are not modified by calcium availability or the presence of cyclooxygenase inhibitors (49). Stretch secondary to increased aortic pressure is not the result of decreased energy availability (49). Inhibition of proteolysis in anoxic and ischemic hearts have defined biochemical mechanisms, as discussed earlier, but a unifying mechanism for the control of proteolysis by insulin, leucine, and stretch has not emerged.

CONCLUSIONS

Future studies of the control of protein synthesis and degradation in heart must focus on the molecular mechanisms of regulation. Cell-free systems are needed for studies of peptide-chain initiation and protein breakdown. In each case, these systems should be reconstituted from purified components. Studies of this type have proved difficult in heart because of the presence of large amounts of contractile proteins that entrap ribosomes and lysosomes. In intact hearts or isolated cells, synthesis of specific tissue components that can account for faster growth requires study. These components include total mRNA, mRNAs for specific proteins, and ribosomes. Rigorous measurements of synthesis rates for RNA and protein must be employed. Continued attention must be given to the suitability of tissue preparations as experimental models. Future work should not focus, however, on descriptive studies of factors that modify synthesis and degradation in cells or tissues. Mechanisms of regulation should be the focus of future work.

REFERENCES

1. Ahlberg, J., Henell, F., and Gluamann, H. (1982): Proteolysis in isolated autophagic vacuoles from rat liver. *Exp. Cell Res.*, 142: 373–383.
2. Aussedat, J., Ray, A., and Rossi, A. (1984): Uridine incorporation in normal and ischemic perfused rat heart. *Mol. Physiol.*, 6:247–256.
3. Bishop, S. P., and Melsen, L. R. (1976): Myocardial necrosis, fibrosis, and DNA synthesis in experimental cardiac hypertrophy induced by sudden pressure overload. *Circ. Res.*, 39:238–245.
4. Bonnin, C. M., Sparrow, M. P., and Taylor, R. R. (1983): Increased protein synthesis and degradation in the dog heart during thyroxine administration. *J. Mol. Cell. Cardiol.*, 15:245–250.
5. Booth, F. W., Nicholson, W. F., and Watson, P. A. (1982): Influence of muscle use on protein synthesis and degradation. In: *Exercise and Sport Sciences Review,* edited by R. L. Terjung, pp. 27–48. Franklin Institute Press, New York.
6. Buse, M. G., and Reid, S. S. (1975): Leucine: A possible regulator of protein turnover in muscle. *J. Clin. Invest.*, 56:1250–1261.
7. Buse, M. G., and Weigand, D. A. (1977): Studies concerning the specificity of the effect of leucine on the turnover of proteins in muscles of control and diabetic rats. *Biochim. Biophys. Acta,* 475:81–89.
8. Chan, Y. L., Gutell, R., Noller, H. F., and Wool, I. G. (1984): The nucleotide sequence of a rat 18S ribosomal ribonucleic acid gene and a proposal for the secondary structure of 18S ribosomal ribonucleic acid. *J. Biol. Chem.*, 259:224–230.
9. Chua, B. L., Kao, R. L., Rannels, D. E., and Morgan, H. E. (1978): Hormonal and metabolic control of proteolysis. *Biochem. Soc. Symp.*, 43:1–15.
10. Chua, B. L., Kao, R. L., Rannels, D. E., and Morgan, H. E. (1979): Inhibition of protein degradation by anoxia and ischemia in perfused rat hearts. *J. Biol. Chem.*, 254:6617–6623.
11. Chua, B. H. L., and Kleinhans, B. J. (1985): Effect of redox potential on protein degradation in perfused rat heart. *Am. J. Physiol.*, 248:E726–731.
12. Chua, B. H. L., Kleinhans, B. J., and Lautensack-Belser, N. (1985): Is leucine effect on protein degradation mediated by α-ketoisocaproate in rat heart? *Fed. Proc.*, 44:1091.
13. Chua, B. H. L., Long, W. M., Latuensack, N., Lins, J. A., and Morgan, H. (1983): Effects of diabetes on cardiac lysosomes and protein degradation. *Am. J. Physiol. (Cell Physiol.,* 4), 245:C91–C100.
14. Chua, B. H. L., Siehl, D. L., and Morgan, H. E. (1979): Effect of leucine and metabolites of branched chain amino acids on protein turnover in heart. *J. Biol. Chem.*, 254:8358–8369.
15. Chua, B. H. L., Siehl, D. L., and Morgan, H. E. (1980): A role for leucine in regulation of protein turnover in working rat hearts. *Am. J. Physiol. (Endocrinol. Metab.,* 2), 239:E510–E514.
16. Chua, B. L., Watkins, C. A., Siehl, D. L., and Morgan, H. E. (1978): Effect of epinephrine and glucagon on protein turnover in perfused rat heart. *Fed. Proc.*, 37:1332.
17. Chua, B. H. L., Watson, P., Kleinhans, B., and Morgan, H. E. (1985): Effect of 5-benzyloxybenzylacylouridine on the labeling of UTP and RNA in perfused rat heart. *Fed. Proc.*, 44:1773.
18. Clark, W. A., and Zak, R. (1981): Assessment of fractional rates of protein synthesis in cardiac muscle cultures after equilibrium labeling. *J. Biol. Chem.*, 256:4863–4870.
19. Cooper, H. L., and Gibson, E. M. (1971): Control of synthesis and wastage of ribosomal ribonucleic acid in lymphocytes. II. The role of protein synthesis. *J. Biol. Chem.*, 246:5059–5066.
20. Cutilletta, A. F. (1981): Muscle and nonmuscle cell RNA polymerase activities in early myocardial hypertrophy. *Am. J. Physiol. (Heart Circ. Physiol.,* 9), 240:H901–H907.
21. Dabeva, M. D., and Dudov, K. P. (1982): Transcriptional control of ribosome production in regenerating rat liver. *Biochem. J.,* 208:101–108.
22. DeMartino, G. N. (1983): Identification of a high molecular weight alkaline protease in rat heart. *J. Mol. Cell. Cardiol.*, 15: 17–29.
23. DeMartino, G. N., and Goldberg, A. L. (1979): Identification and partial purification of an ATP-stimulated alkaline protease in rat liver. *J. Biol. Chem.*, 254:3712–3715.
24. DePhilip, R. M., Rudert, W. A., and Lieberman, I. (1980): Preferential stimulation of ribosomal protein synthesis by insulin and in the absence of ribosomal and messenger ribonucleic acid formation. *Biochemistry*, 19:1662–1669.
25. D'Eustachio, P., Meyuhas, O., Ruddle, F., and Perry, R. P. (1981): Chromosomal distribution of ribosomal protein genes in the mouse. *Cell*, 24:307–312.
26. Dudov, K. P., and Perry, R. P. (1984): The gene family encoding the mouse ribosomal protein L32 contains a uniquely expressed intron-containing gene and an unmutated processed gene. *Cell*, 37:457–468.
27. Etlinger, J. D., Kameyama, T., Toner, K., Van der Westhuyzen, D., and Matsumoto, K. (1980): Calcium and stretch-dependent regulation of protein turnover and myofibrillar assembly in

muscle. In: *Plasticity of Muscle,* edited by D. Pette, pp. 541–557. W. deGruyter & Co., Berlin.

28. Evans, C. D., Schreiber, S. S., Oratz, M., and Rothschild, M. A. (1981): Relative synthesis of cardiac contractile proteins. Evidence for synthesis from the same precursor pool. *Biochem. J.,* 194: 673–678.

29. Everett, A. W., Prior, G., and Zak, R. (1981): Equilibration of leucine between the plasma compartment and leucyl-tRNA in the heart, and turnover of cardiac myosin heavy chain. *Biochem. J.,* 194:365–368.

30. Everett, A. W., Sinha, A. N., Umeda, P. K., Jakovcic, S., Rabinowitz, M., and Zak, R. (1984): Regulation of myosin synthesis by thyroid hormone: Relative change in the α- and β-myosin heavy chain mRNA levels in rabbit hearts. *Biochemistry,* 23:1596–1599.

31. Fagan, J. M., and Goldberg, A. L. (1985): The rate of protein degradation in isolated skeletal muscle does not correlate with reduction-oxidation status. *Biochem. J.,* 227:689–694.

32. Faliks, D., and Meyuhas, O. (1982): Coordinate regulation of ribosomal protein mRNA level in regenerating rat liver. Study with corresponding mouse cloned cDNAs. *Nucleic Acids Res.,* 10:789–801.

33. Fan, H., and Penman, S. (1970): Regulation of protein synthesis in mammalian cells. II. Inhibition of protein synthesis at the level of initiation during mitosis. *J. Mol. Biol.,* 50:655–670.

34. Fanburg, B. L., and Posner, B. I. (1968): RNA synthesis in experimental cardiac hypertrophy in rats. I. Characterization and kinetics of labeling. *Circ. Res.,* 23:123–135.

35. Flaim, K. E., Copenhaver, M. E., and Jefferson, L. S. (1980): Effects of diabetes on protein synthesis in fast- and slow-twitch rat skeletal muscle. *Am. J. Physiol. (Endocrinol. Metab.,* 2), 239: E88–E95.

36. Flaim, K. E., Kochel, P. J., Kira, Y., Kobayashi, K., Fossell, E. T., Jefferson, L. S., and Morgan, H. E. (1983): Insulin effects on protein synthesis are independent of glucose and energy metabolism. *Am. J. Physiol. (Cell Physiol.,* 14), 245:C133–C143.

37. Flaim, K. E., Peavy, D. E., Everson, W. V., and Jefferson, L. S. (1982): The role of amino acids in the regulation of protein synthesis in perfused rat liver. *J. Biol. Chem.,* 257:2932–2938.

38. Frayn, K. N., and Maycock, P. F. (1979): Regulation of protein metabolism by a physiological concentration of insulin in mouse soleus and extensor digitorum longus muscles: Effects of starvation and scald injury. *Biochem. J.,* 184:323–330.

39. Frelin, C. (1980): The regulation of protein turnover in newborn rat heart cell cultures. *J. Biol. Chem.,* 255:11149–11155.

40. Gantt, J. S., and Key, J. L. (1985): Coordinate expression of ribosomal protein mRNAs following auxin treatment of soybean hypocotyls. *J. Biol. Chem.,* 260:6175–6181.

41. Garlick, P. J., McNurlan, M. A., and Preedy, V. R. (1980): A rapid and convenient technique for measuring the rate of protein synthesis in tissues by injection of [³H]phenylalanine. *Biochem. J.,* 192:719–723.

42. Gertz, B. J., Haugaard, E. S., and Haugaard, N. (1980): Effects of thyroid hormone on UTP content and uridine kinase activity of rat heart and skeletal muscle. *Am. J. Physiol. (Endocrinol. Metab.,* 1), 238:E443–E449.

43. Geyer, P. K., Meyuhas, O., Perry, R. P., and Johnson, L. F. (1982): Regulation of ribosomal protein mRNA content and translation in growth-stimulated mouse fibroblasts. *Mol. Cell. Biol.,* 2:685–693.

44. Godefroy-Colburn, T., and Thach, R. E. (1981): The role of mRNA competition in regulating translation. IV. Kinetic model. *J. Biol. Chem.,* 256:11762–11773.

45. Goldberg, A. L. (1969): Protein turnover in skeletal muscle. *J. Biol. Chem.,* 244:3217–3222.

46. Goldspink, D. F. (1978): The influence of passive stretch on the growth and protein turnover of the denervated extensor digitorum longus muscle. *Biochem. J.,* 174:595–602.

47. Goldspink, D. F., and Kelly, F. J. (1984): Protein turnover and growth in the whole body, liver and kidney of the rat from the foetus to senility. *Biochem. J.,* 217:507–516.

48. Gordon, E. E., Kira, Y., and Morgan, H. E. (1985): Dependence of protein synthesis on aortic pressure and calcium availability. In: *Advances in Myocardiology,* edited by P. Harris and P. A. Poole-Wilson, pp. 145–156. Plenum, New York.

49. Gordon, E. E., Kira, Y., Demers, L. M., and Morgan, H. E. (1986): Aortic pressure as a determinant of cardiac protein degradation. *Am. J. Physiol., (in press).*

50. Henshaw, E. C., Guiney, D. G., and Hirsch, C. A. (1973): The ribosome cycle in mammalian protein synthesis. I. The place of monomeric ribosomes and ribosomal subunits in the cycle. *J. Biol. Chem.,* 248:4367–4376.

51. Hershko, A., and Ciechanover, A. (1982): Mechanisms of intracellular protein breakdown. *Annu. Rev. Biochem.,* 51:335–365.

52. Hershko, A., Heller, H., Ganoth, D., and Ciechanover, A. (1978): Mode of degradation of abnormal globin chains in rabbit reticulocytes. In: *Protein Turnover and Lysosome Function,* edited by H. L. Segal and D. J. Doyle, pp. 149–169. Academic Press, New York.

53. Hickson, R. C., Hammons, G. T., and Holloszy, J. O. (1979): Development and regression of exercise-induced cardiac hypertrophy in rats. *Am. J. Physiol. (Heart Circ. Physiol.,* 5), 236: H268–H272.

54. Hill, J. M. (1975): Ribosomal RNA metabolism during renal hypertrophy. Evidence of decreased degradation of newly synthesized ribosomal RNA. *J. Cell. Biol.,* 64:260–265.

55. Hille, M. B., and Albers, A. A. (1979): Efficiency of protein synthesis after fertilization of sea urchin eggs. *Nature,* 278:469–471.

56. Hirsch, C. A., Cox, M. A., Van Venrooij, W. J. W., and Henshaw, E. C. (1973): The ribosome cycle in mammalian protein synthesis. II. Association of the native smaller ribosomal subunit with protein factors. *J. Biol. Chem.,* 248:4377–4385.

57. Hjalmarson, A. C., Rannels, D. E., Kao, R., and Morgan, H. E. (1975): Effects of hypophysectomy, growth hormone, and thyroxine on protein turnover in heart. *J. Biol. Chem.,* 250:4556–4561.

58. Hjalmarson, A., and Isaksson, O. (1972): *In vitro* work load and rat heart metabolism. I. Effect on protein synthesis. *Acta Physiol. Scand.,* 86:126–144.

59. Howe, J. G., and Hershey, J. W. B. (1983): Initiation factor and ribosome levels are coordinately controlled in *Escherichia coli* growing at different rates. *J. Biol. Chem.,* 258:1954–1959.

60. Ignotz, G. G., Hokari, S., DePhilip, R. M., Tsukada, K., and Lieberman, I. (1981): Lodish model and regulation of ribosomal protein synthesis by insulin-deficient chick embryo fibroblasts. *Biochemistry,* 20:2550–2558.

61. Imahori, K. (1982): Calcium-dependent neutral protease: Its characterization and regulation. In: *Calcium and Cell Function, Vol. III,* edited by W. Y. Cheung, pp. 473–485. Academic Press, New York.

62. Jefferson, L. S., Koehler, J. O., and Morgan, H. E. (1972): Effect of insulin on protein synthesis in skeletal muscle of an isolated perfused rat hemicorpus preparation. *Proc. Natl. Acad. Sci. USA,* 69:816–820.

63. Jefferson, L. S., Wolpert, E. B., Giger, K. E., and Morgan, H. E. (1971): Regulation of protein synthesis in heart muscle. III. Effect of anoxia on protein synthesis. *J. Biol. Chem.,* 246:2171–2178.

64. Kameyama, T., and Etlinger, J. D. (1979): Calcium-dependent regulation of protein synthesis and degradation in muscle. *Nature,* 279:344–346.

65. Kelly, F. J., and Jefferson, L. S. (1985): Control of peptide-chain initiation in rat skeletal muscle. *J. Biol. Chem.,* 260:6677–6683.

66. Kira, Y., Kochel, P. J., Gordon, E. E., and Morgan, H. E. (1984): Aortic perfusion pressure as a determinant of cardiac protein synthesis. *Am. J. Physiol. (Cell Physiol.,* 15), 246:C247–C258.

67. Kochel, P. J., Kira, Y., Gordon, E. E., and Morgan, H. E. (1984): Effects of noncarbohydrate substrates on protein synthesis in hearts from fed and fasted rats. *J. Mol. Cell. Cardiol.,* 16:371–383.

68. Koide, T., and Rabinowitz, M. (1969): Biochemical correlates of cardiac hypertrophy. II. Increased rate of RNA synthesis in experimental cardiac hypertrophy in the rat. *Circ. Res.,* 24:9–18.

69. Laurent, G. J., Sparrow, M. P., and Millward, D. J. (1978): Turnover of muscle protein in the fowl. Changes in rates of protein synthesis and breakdown during hypertrophy of the anterior and posterior latissimus dorsi muscles. *Biochem. J.,* 176: 407–417.

70. Libby, P., and Goldberg, A. L. (1980): The control and mechanism of protein breakdown in striated muscle: Studies with selective inhibitors. In: *Degradative Processes in Heart and Skeletal Muscle,*

edited by K. Wildenthal, pp. 201–222. Elsevier/North-Holland, Amsterdam.

71. Long, W. M., Chua, B. H. L., Lautensack, N., and Morgan, H. E. (1983): Effects of amino acid methylesters on cardiac lysosomes and protein degradation. *Am. J. Physiol.*, 245:C101–C112.

72. Long, W. M., Chua, B. H. L., Munger, B. L., and Morgan, H. E. (1984): Effects of insulin on cardiac lysosomes and protein degradation. *Fed. Proc.*, 43:1295–1300.

73. Maden, B. E. H., and Salim, M. (1974): The methylated nucleotide sequences in HeLa cell ribosomal RNA and its precursors. *J. Mol. Biol.*, 88:133–164.

74. Matsushita, S., and Fanburg, B. L. (1970): Pyrimidine nucleotide synthesis in the normal and hypertrophying rat heart. *Circ. Res.*, 27:415–428.

75. McKee, E. E., Cheung, J. Y., Rannels, D. E., and Morgan, H. E. (1978): Measurement of the rate of protein synthesis and compartmentation of heart phenylalanine. *J. Biol. Chem.*, 253:1030–1040.

76. Millward, D. J. (1980): Protein turnover in skeletal and cardiac muscle during normal growth and hypertrophy. In: *Degradative Processes in Heart and Skeletal Muscle*, edited by K. Wildenthal, pp. 161–196. Elsevier/North-Holland, Amsterdam.

77. Millward, D. J., Bates, P. C., Grimble, G. K., Brown, J. G., Natlan, M., and Rennie, M. J. (1980): Quantitative importance of nonskeletal muscle sources of $N\gamma$-methylhistidine in urine. *Biochem. J.*, 190:225–228.

78. Monk, R. J., Meyuhas, O., and Perry, R. P. (1981): Mammals have multiple genes for individual ribosomal proteins. *Cell*, 24:301–306.

79. Morgan, H. E., Chua, B., and Beinlich, C. J. (1980): Regulation of protein degradation in heart. In: *Degradative Processes in Heart and Skeletal Muscle*, edited by K. Wildenthal, pp. 87–112. Elsevier/North-Holland, Amsterdam.

80. Morgan, H. E., Chua, B. H., Boyd, T. A., and Jefferson, L. S. (1981): Branched-chain amino acids and the regulation of protein turnover in heart and skeletal muscle. In: *Metabolism and Clinical Implications of Branched Chain Amino and Ketoacids*, edited by M. Walser and J. R. Williamson, pp. 217–226. Elsevier/North-Holland, New York.

81. Morgan, H. E., Chua, B. H. L., Fuller, E. O., and Siehl, D. L. (1980): Regulation of protein synthesis and degradation during *in vitro* cardiac work. *Am. J. Physiol. (Endocrinol. Metab., 1)*, 238:E431–E442.

82. Morgan, H. E., Earl, D. C. N., Boradus, A., Wolpert, E. B., Giger, K., and Jefferson, L. S. (1971): Regulation of protein synthesis in heart muscle. I. Effect of amino acid levels on protein synthesis. *J. Biol. Chem.*, 246:2152–2162.

83. Morgan, H. E., Jefferson, L. S., Wolpert, E. B., and Rannels, D. E. (1971): Regulation of protein synthesis in heart muscle. II. Effect of amino acid levels and insulin on ribosomal aggregation. *J. Biol. Chem.*, 246:2163–2170.

84. Morgan, H. E., McKee, E. E., and Cheung, J. Y. (1978): Effect of compartmentation of heart phenylalanine on measurements of protein synthesis and amino acid transport. In: *Microenvironments and Metabolic Compartmentation*, edited by P. A. Srere and R. W. Estabrook, pp. 97–107. Academic Press, New York.

85. Morgan, H. E., and Rannels, D. E. (1975): The control of protein degradation in the isolated perfused rat heart. In: *Alcohol and Abnormal Protein Biosynthesis, Biochemical Clinical*, edited by M. Oratz and S. S. Schreiber, pp. 233–246. Pergamon Press, New York.

86. Morgan, H. E., Rannels, D. E., and McKee, E. E. (1979): Protein metabolism of the heart. In: *Handbook of Physiology: The Cardiovascular System, Vol. I*, edited by R. M. Berne and N. Sperelakis, pp. 845–871. American Physiological Society, Bethesda.

87. Morgan, H. E., Siehl, D., Chua, B. H. L., and Lautensack-Belser, N. (1985): Faster protein and ribosome synthesis in hypertrophying heart. *Basic Res. Cardiol.*, 80(Suppl. 2):115–118.

88. Morgenstern, C., Höljes, U., Arnold, G., and Lochner, W. (1973): The influence of coronary perfusion pressure and coronary flow on intracoronary blood volume and geometry of the left ventricle. *Pfluegers Arch.*, 340:101–111.

89. Murachi, T. (1983): Intracellular Ca^{2+} protease and its inhibitor protein: Calpain and calpastatin. In: *Calcium and Cell Function*,

Vol. IV, edited by W. Y. Cheung, pp. 377–410. Academic Press, New York.

90. Nair, K. G., Cutilletta, A. F., Zak, R., Koide, T., and Rabinowitz, M. (1968): Biochemical correlates of cardiac hypertrophy. I. Experimental model, changes in heart weight, RNA content, and nuclear RNA polymerase activity. *Circ. Res.*, 23:451–462.

91. Neely, J. R., and Morgan, H. E. (1974): Relationship between carbohydrate and lipid metabolism and energy balance of heart muscle. *Annu. Rev. Physiol.*, 36:413–459.

92. Nomura, M., Gourse, R., and Baughman, G. (1984): Regulation of the synthesis of ribosomes and ribosomal components. *Annu. Rev. Biochem.*, 53:75–117.

93. Ochoa, S. (1983): Regulation of protein synthesis initiation in eukaryotes. *Arch. Biochem. Biophys.*, 223:325–349.

94. Palmer, R. M., Reeds, P. J., Atkinson, T., and Smith, R. H. (1983): The influences of changes in tension on protein synthesis and prostaglandin release in isolated rabbit muscles. *Biochem. J.*, 214:1011–1014.

95. Peterson, M. B., and Lesch, M. (1972): Protein synthesis and amino acid transport in the isolated rabbit right ventricular papillary muscle. Effect of isometric tension development. *Circ. Res.*, 31:317–327.

96. Piper, H. M., Probst, I., Schwartz, P. Hütter, J. F., and Spieckermann, P. G. (1982): Culturing of calcium stable adult cardiac myocytes. *J. Mol. Cell. Cardiol.*, 14:397–412.

97. Preedy, V. R., Smith, D. M., Kearney, N. F., and Sugden, P. H. (1985): Regional variation and differential sensitivity of rat heart protein synthesis *in vivo* and *in vitro*. *Biochem. J.*, 225:487–492.

98. Poche, R., Arnold, G., and Gahlen, D. (1971): The influence of coronary perfusion pressure on metabolism and ultrastructure of the arrested aerobically perfused isolated guinea pig heart. *Virchows Arch. B*, 8:252–266.

99. Pryor, J. C., and Buse, M. G. (1984): Tunicamycin prevents stimulation of protein synthesis by branched chain amino acids in isolated rat muscles. *Biochem. Biophys. Res. Commun.*, 125:149–156.

100. Rannels, D. E., Hjalmarson, A. C., and Morgan, H. E. (1974): Effects of noncarbohydrate substrates on protein synthesis in heart muscle. *Am. J. Physiol.*, 226:528–539.

101. Rannels, D. E., Kao, R., and Morgan, H. E. (1975): Effect of insulin on protein turnover in heart muscle. *J. Biol. Chem.*, 250:1694–1701.

102. Ray, B. K., Lawson, G., Kramer, J. C., Cladaras, M. H., Grifo, J. A., Abramson, R. D., Merrick, W. C., and Thach, R. E. (1985): ATP-dependent unwinding of messenger RNA structure by eukaryotic initiation factors. *J. Biol. Chem.*, 260:7651–7658.

103. Raikow, R. B., and Vaughan, M. H. (1980): Synthesis of proteins and RNA of the 60S ribosomal subunit in HeLa cells recovering from valine deprivation. *J. Cell. Physiol.*, 102:81–89.

104. Rizzo, A. J., and Webb, T. E. (1972): Regulation of ribosome formation in regenerating rat liver. *Eur. J. Biochem.*, 27:136–144.

105. Rodemann, H. P., Waxman, L., and Goldberg, A. L. (1982): The stimulation of protein degradation in muscle by Ca^{2+} is mediated by prostaglandin E_2 and does not require the calcium-activated protease. *J. Biol. Chem.*, 257:8716–8723.

106. Rubin, I. B., and Goldstein, G. (1970): An ultrasensitive isotope dilution method for the determination of L-amino acids. *Anal. Biochem.*, 33:244–254.

107. Rubio, R., and Berne, R. M. (1980): Localization of purine and pyrimidine nucleoside phosphorylases in heart, kidney and liver. *Am. J. Physiol. (Heart Circ. Physiol., 8)*, 239:H721–730.

108. Ruderman, N. B., and Berger, M. (1974): The formation of glutamine and alanine in skeletal muscle. *J. Biol. Chem.*, 249:5500–5506.

109. Schmidt, T., Chen, P. S., and Pellegrini, M. (1985): The induction of ribosome biosynthesis in a nonmitotic secretory tissue. *J. Biol. Chem.*, 260:7645–7650.

110. Schneider, D. J. (1981): ATP-dependent acidification of intact and disrupted lysosomes. *J. Biol. Chem.*, 256:3858–3864.

111. Schreiber, S. S., Evans, C. D., Oratz, M., and Rothschild, M. A. (1982): Problems in evaluating cardiac protein synthesis. *J. Mol. Cell. Cardiol.*, 14:307–312.

112. Schreiber, S. S., Hearse, D. J., and Rothschild, M. (1977): Protein

synthesis in prolonged cardiac arrest. *J. Mol. Cell. Cardiol.,* 9: 87–100.

113. Schreiber, S. S., Oratz, M., and Rothschild, M. A. (1966): Protein synthesis in the overloaded mammalian heart. *Am. J. Physiol.,* 211:314–318.

114. Schwartz, K., Moalic, J. M., de la Bastie, D., Wisnewsky, C., Bouveret, P., Bercovici, J., and Swynghedauw, B. (1985): Messenger RNA complexity and expression of skeletal and cardiac actin genes during rat cardiac hypertrophy. *J. Muscle Res.,* 6:61.

115. Seely, J. E., and Pegg, A. E. (1983): Changes in mouse kidney ornithine decarboxylase activity are brought about by changes in the amount of enzyme protein as measured by radioimmunoassay. *J. Biol. Chem.,* 258:2496–2500.

116. Shatkin, A. J. (1985): mRNA cap binding proteins: Essential factors for initiating translation. *Cell,* 40:223–224.

117. Siehl, D., Chua, B. H. L., Lautensack-Belser, N., and Morgan, H. E. (1985): Faster protein and ribosome synthesis in thyroxine-induced hypertrophy of rat heart. *Am. J. Physiol. (Cell Physiol.,* 17), 248:C309–C319.

118. Siehl, D. L., Gordon, E. E., Kira, Y., Chua, B. H. L., and Morgan, H. E. (1985): Protein degradation in the hypertrophic heart. In: *Lysosomes: Their Role in Protein Breakdown,* edited by H. Glaumann and F. J. Ballard, (in press).

119. Simpson, P. (1985): Stimulation of hypertrophy of cultured neonatal rat heart cells through a α_1-adrenergic receptor and induction of beating through an α_1- and β_1-adrenergic receptor interaction. Evidence for independent regulation of growth and beating. *Circ. Res.,* 56:884–894.

120. Smith, R. H., Palmer, R. M., and Reeds, P. J. (1983): Protein synthesis in isolated rabbit forelimb muscles. The possible role of metabolites of arachidonic acid in the response to intermittent stretching. *Biochem. J.,* 214:153–161.

121. Smith, D. M., and Sugden, P. H. (1983): Stimulation of left-atrial protein synthesis rates by increased left-atrial filling pressures in the perfused working rat heart *in vitro. Biochem. J.,* 216:537–542.

122. Takala, T. (1981): Protein synthesis in the isolated perfused rat heart. Effects of mechanical work load, diastolic ventricular pressure, and coronary flow on amino acid incorporation and its transmural distribution into left ventricular protein. *Basic Res. Cardiol.,* 76:44–61.

123. Tanaka, K., Waxman, L., and Goldberg, A. L. (1983): ATP serves two distinct roles in protein degradation in reticulocytes, one requiring and one independent of ubiquitin. *J. Cell Biol.,* 96:1580–1585.

124. Tanaka, K., Waxman, L., and Goldberg, A. L. (1984): Vanadate inhibits the ATP-dependent degradation of proteins in reticulocytes without affecting ubiquitin conjugation. *J. Biol. Chem.,* 259: 2803–2809.

125. Tischler, M. E. (1980): Is regulation of proteolysis associated with redox state changes in rat skeletal muscle? *Biochem. J.,* 192:963–966.

126. Tischler, M. E., and Fagan, J. M. (1982): Relationship of the reduction oxidation state to protein degradation in skeletal and atrial muscle. *Arch. Biochem. Biophys.,* 217:191–201.

127. Tsurugi, K., Morita, T., and Ogata, K. (1972): Studies on the metabolism of ribosomal structural proteins of regenerating rat liver. *Eur. J. Biochem.,* 25:117–128.

128. Tsurugi, K., Morita, T., and Ogata, K. (1974): Mode of degradation of ribosomes in regenerating rat liver *in vivo. Eur. J. Biochem.,* 45:119–126.

129. Turto, H. (1972): Experimental cardiac hypertrophy and the synthesis of poly(A) containing RNA and of myocardial proteins in the rat: The effect of digitoxin treatment. *Acta Physiol. Scand.,* 101:144–154.

130. Vandenburgh, H. H. (1983): Cell shape and growth regulation in skeletal muscle: Exogenous versus endogenous factors. *J. Cell Physiol.,* 116:363–371.

131. Vandenburgh, H., and Kaufman, S. (1980): Protein degradation in embryonic skeletal muscle. Effect of medium, cell type, inhibitors and passive stretch. *J. Biol. Chem.,* 255:5826–5833.

132. Vogel, W. M., Apstein, C. S., Briggs, L. L., Gaasch, W. H., and Ahn, J. (1982): Acute alterations in left ventricular diastolic chamber stiffness. Role of the "erectile" effects of coronary arterial pressure and flow in normal and damaged hearts. *Circ. Res.,* 51:465–478.

133. Ward, W. F., Chua, B. L., Li, J. B., Morgan, H. E., and Mortimore, G. E. (1979): Inhibition of basal and deprivation-induced proteolysis by leupeptin and pepstatin in perfused rat liver and heart. *Biochem. Biophys. Res. Commun.,* 87:92–98.

134. Ward, W. F., and Mortimore, G. E. (1978): Compartmentation of intracellular amino acids in rat liver. *J. Biol. Chem.,* 253: 3581–3587.

135. Warner, J. R. (1974): The assembly of ribosomes in eukaryotes. In: *Ribosomes,* edited by H. Nomura, A. Tissieres, and P. Lengel, pp. 461–468. Cold Spring Harbor Laboratory, Cold Spring Harbor, N.Y.

136. Warner, J. R. (1977): In the absence of ribosomal RNA synthesis, the ribosomal proteins of HeLa cells are synthesized normally and degraded rapidly. *J. Mol. Biol.,* 115:315–333.

137. Wassner, S. J., and Li, J. B. (1982): N^τ-methylhistidine release: Contributions of rat skeletal muscle, GI tract, and skin. *Am. J. Physiol.,* 243:E293–E297.

138. Wildenthal, K. (1971): Long-term maintenance of spontaneously beating mouse hearts in organ culture. *J. Appl. Physiol.,* 30:153–157.

139. Williams, I. H., Chua, B. H. L., Sahms, R. H., Siehl, D., and Morgan, H. E. (1980): Effects of diabetes on protein turnover in cardiac muscle. *Am. J. Physiol. (Endocrinol. Metab.,* 2), 239: E178–E185.

140. Woodside, K. H., and Mortimore, G. E. (1972): Suppression of protein turnover by aminoacids in the perfused rat liver. *J. Biol. Chem.,* 247:6474–6481.

141. Wool, I. G., Stirewalt, W. S., Kurihara, K., Low, R. B., Bailey, P., and Oyer, D. (1968): Mode of action of insulin in the regulation of protein biosynthesis in muscle. *Recent Prog. Hormone Res.,* 24:139–208.

142. Young, V. R. (1970): The role of skeletal and cardiac muscle in the regulation of protein metabolism. In: *Mammalian Protein Metabolism, Vol. 4,* edited by H. N. Munro and J. B. Allison, pp. 585–662. Academic, New York.

143. Zähringer, J., and Klaubert, A. (1982): The effect of triiodothyronine on the cardiac mRNA. *J. Mol. Cell. Cardiol.,* 14:559–571.

The Heart and Cardiovascular System,
edited by H. A. Fozzard et al.
Raven Press, New York © 1986.

CHAPTER 46

RNA Transcription in Heart Muscle

Patrick K. Umeda, Smilja Jakovcic, and Radovan Zak

It is generally recognized that the protein synthesis of a cell closely corresponds to its RNA content. Thus, the amount of RNA in protein-exporting tissues, such as the liver and pancreas, is higher than that in nonsecreting organs, such as skeletal and cardiac muscles. Nevertheless, the normal myocardium has considerable capacity for protein synthesis because of the rapid turnover of its constituent proteins. For example, myosin, which contributes close to a quarter of total cardiac proteins, has a half-life of about 6 days. When the myocardium enlarges during compensatory hypertrophy, increased synthesis of RNA is the most striking and consistent change that has been reported in the literature. During the early phase of hypertrophy there is a direct correlation between the degree of cardiac enlargement and the amount of RNA per unit mass of tissue. Analysis of newly synthesized RNA by sucrose-gradient centrifugation has revealed that all classes of RNA are being synthesized at approximately equal rates.

The accumulation of RNA during myocardial growth results from increases in the activities of DNA-dependent RNA polymerases I, II, and III (which synthesize ribosomal, messenger, and transfer RNAs, respectively). However, during the early stages, these increases in activity lag behind the change in RNA synthesis detected by *in vivo* incorporation of labeled precursors. Therefore, the initial rise in RNA synthesis apparently results from an increase in the template available for transcription.

Early studies of RNA synthesis in heart muscle clearly demonstrated that there are dramatic changes in gene transcription or expression during myocardial growth. Analysis of total RNA, however, has serious limitations, because the growth response of the heart involves not only overall cardiac enlargement but also a change in the composition of its constituent proteins. Thus, to obtain a true growth response, it is necessary to follow the transcription of individual genes rather than overall RNA synthesis. In recent years, analysis of the molecular changes in cardiac muscle has progressed quite rapidly. The following review will describe some general aspects of regulation of gene expression in eukaryotes and discuss recent advances in understanding the molecular basis for cardiac muscle growth.

CONTROL OF GENE EXPRESSION IN EUKARYOTES: AN OVERVIEW

During the past decade, most of the reaction steps involving translation of genetic information encoded in the nucleotide sequence of the DNA molecule into the amino acid sequence of the polypeptide chain have been elucidated. With the development of new biochemical techniques that permit isolation and modification of genes of known function, it is now possible to study the controlling regions in eukaryotic genes and to identify the molecules within cells that are involved in turning individual genes on and off during differentiation and development.

Gene expression in eukaryotes is influenced basically by two mechanisms: first, by alterations in structure of the genes, such as loss, amplification, rearrangement, and modification of their DNA sequences; second, by direct modulation of gene transcription, posttranscriptional processing, and mRNA translation. It is primarily the latter type of regulation that will be addressed in this review.

Sequence Organization of Eukaryotic DNA and Chromosome Structure

In eukaryotes, the amount of DNA per haploid genome vastly exceeds the DNA required to specify the respective polypeptides. For example, only 1% of the mammalian genome is thought to correspond to single-copy genes encoding most protein and gene-specific controlling sequences. Although part of the remaining 99% of the DNA is likely to be involved in forming a higher-order structure of eukaryotic chromosomes, most of it may be functionally neutral for insertions and deletions and may be derived by a continuous flux of such events.

The excess DNA that contributes to the complexity of eukaryotic genome is due, in part, to segments of repeated nucleotide sequences of various lengths (1,2). These sequences belong to several classes, based on their copy number per haploid genome. The most highly repetitive ones are approximately 300 bp in length and are present at about 10^6 copies. They are usually clustered in the heterochromatin and are not transcribed, and their function remains unknown. Segments of DNA that have less regular repeats and are represented at about 10^3 copies belong to the class of moderate repetitive sequences, which are interspersed throughout the genomic DNA, and could be found even within structural genes. They may be relatively short (<1 kb) or long (1–10 kb), and their tendency to reassociate intramolecularly because of palindromic sequences may result in the secondary structures found in the nuclear transcripts. The precise pattern of interspersion varies even in a given species. The scattered locations of these sequences, however, could reflect their capacity to transpose during evolution, thus resulting in rearrangements of chromosome structure.

In primates, there is one class of moderately repetitive sequences that are distinguished by their susceptibility to cleavage with the restriction endonuclease, AluI. This family of sequences, commonly referred to as the Alu family, consists of 150 to 300 nucleotide regions that are widely dispersed in the genome. Similar Alu-like families of interspersed repeats have been found in other mammals, and the ubiquity of these sequences has prompted many suggestions as to their function (3,4). They have been implicated as organizers of chromatin structure, origins of DNA replication, recognition sites

for tissue-specific transcription, and interruptions in homologous genes that block gene conversion. Their true role, however, remains to be established.

Besides the repetitive DNAs, another characteristic of the eukaryotic genome that contributes to the observed excess of DNA is the reiteration of genes themselves. Most notable are the genes coding for ribosomal RNA and histones, which are organized in tandemly repeated clusters (5). Most reiterated genes are separated by spacer segments of DNA that are not transcribed. However, some gene families (e.g., actin) may be widely dispersed in the genome. In addition, eukaryotes are unique in that the protein-coding regions of nearly all of their genes are interrupted. The expressed nucleotide sequences (exons) of a single gene are interdispersed by silent noncoding intervening sequences (introns) (6) that further add to the size of the genome. Finally, the eukaryotic genome may contain nonfunctional genes, or pseudogenes. Although homologous to expressed genes, pseudogenes contain altered sequences that prevent them from expressing a functional biological molecule. Members of one class have a molecular structure of exons and introns very similar to that of their related expressed genes, but contain mutations that render them inactive. These pseudogenes most likely arise by duplication and mutation of expressed genes and are usually closely linked to the parental gene (7). Another group of pseudogenes, called processed genes (8), are highly homologous DNA copies of the mRNA coded by their parental genes. They do not contain introns and are located at chromosomal sites remote from that of the expressed gene. Processed pseudogenes are probably generated by reverse transcription of a mature mRNA and subsequent integration of the cDNA intermediate into the genome of the organism.

The complexity of gene regulation in eukaryotes is also reflected by the structure of the chromosome. In the nucleus, genomic DNA is associated with two classes of proteins, the highly basic histones and a variety of nonhistone chromosomal proteins, to form the nucleoprotein material referred to as chromatin. Within chromatin, the DNA and protein are organized into repeating units called nucleosomes. Each nucleosome contains several hundred supercoiled base pairs of DNA wound around an octamere of histones. The nucleosomes are held together by a segment of the same DNA molecule called a linker DNA. Thus, the resulting chromatin fiber is a flexible chain of an uninterrupted and unbranched DNA molecule with beads of nucleosomes formed along its length. The packing of nucleosomes into helical arrays results in the higher-order solenoid structures found in chromosomes. It has been suggested that histone H1 is essential for the stability of this higher-order chromatin form. The association of nonhistone proteins with chromatin is less clear; it is believed that they do not function as building blocks but may play a role in gene expression and in the condensation of nucleosome cores.

At present, the significance of the complex organization of the eukaryotic genome is not completely understood. Undoubtedly, however, it is related to the needs for processing large amounts of DNA-encoded information.

Transcriptional Control

Although the information available about the regulation of gene expression in eukaryotes is still fragmentary, the regulatory mechanisms are likely to be much more complex than in prokaryotes. The vast diversity of cells in the animal body, all containing virtually identical genomes, indicates that an individual cell expresses only a small part of its full genetic potential. Consequently, at any given time only a small portion of total DNA serves as a template for the synthesis of mRNA.

The actual mechanisms responsible for activating genes and rendering them accessible for transcription by RNA polymerase remain largely obscure. From our current knowledge of gene organization, one can postulate the interplay of three factors: (a) the conformation of chromatin, (b) the regulatory nucleotide sequences of the gene, and (c) the activity and/or amount of RNA polymerase.

Chromatin Conformation

Because of the compact structure of the chromosome, the potential for expression or transcription of a gene is primarily determined by the chromatin conformation. For example, staining with basic dyes distinguishes two types of chromatin structures. Regions of the chromosomes that do not stain (euchromatin) correspond primarily to coding sequences, whereas the staining heterochromatin contains nontranscribed sequences. Moreover, active genes have an altered nucleosome structure that results in a chromosomal domain that shows increased sensitivity to nucleases. Within this altered domain, sites that are hypersensitive to DNAse digestion can also be identified. The latter sites are usually localized in the flanking regions of active genes and probably reflect a relaxed configuration of the DNA in these regions (9).

Although the mechanism that generates this "open" conformation is not known, active chromatin is distinguished by the presence of variant or modified histones. DNAse-sensitive regions are generally depleted of histone H1. This is consistent with the hypothesis that histones act as blocking agents, thereby inhibiting RNA synthesis on the DNA template. Active genes also contain hyperacetylated histones; however, the role of this modification in the activation of transcription is not known. Another characteristic of active nucleosomes is the presence of specific histone-like proteins such as those of the high-mobility group (HMG), which bind at the junction of internucleosomal DNA. Recently, positive regulatory control by nonhistone proteins with sequence-specific DNA binding properties has been described (10). These include several transcription factors (11,12) and the glucocorticoid hormone receptor complex (10).

Another mechanism that may contribute to altering the structure of nucleosomes is DNA modification. In general, the degree of methylation of DNA, primarily at cytosine residues, is inversely related to gene activation (13). The correlation between gene activation and hypomethylation appears to be further strengthened by the observation that inhibition of methylation with the cytidine analogue 5-azacytidine results in reactivation of fetal globin genes in adult reticulocytes. Irrespective of the differences between active and nonactive chromatin, it is generally believed that the first step in gene activation may be the unfolding of a tightly packed chromatin fiber. Thus, the role of topoisomerase enzymes and the formation of the left-handed Z-form DNA are also being examined as possible primary events in the activation process (14).

Regulatory DNA Sequences

Considerable progress has been made recently in elucidating the role of DNA sequences in the regulation of transcription. The current view of the structural organization of a protein gene is shown in Fig. 1.

The structures of ribosomal RNA, tRNA, and 5S RNA genes are slightly different and will not be considered here. The gene consists of a series of exons and introns that are bound on either side by noncoding regions that contain controlling sequences for initiation and termination of transcription by RNA polymerase. The intron-exon junctions in higher eukaryotes have highly conserved consensus sequences, suggesting a common splicing mechanism (15). On either side, adjacent to the genes are flanking regions that contain various regulatory sequences and the domains containing DNAse hypersensitive sites. Within the 5' flanking region there are at least three elements that are required to promote efficient initiation of transcription by RNA polymerase II: the initiation or cap site (16), and the TATA (17) and CAAT (17) boxes localized at −25 to −31 and −81 bp upstream, respectively. The TATA box, which is present in almost all the genes reported so far, is believed to be involved in recognition of the precise location of the transcription initiation site, whereas CAAT sequences appear to be necessary for efficient binding of polymerase II.

The promoter region also contains additional sequences generally located >100 bp from the cap site (18) that either enhance transcription of a gene or are implicated in the regulation of transcription in response to effector molecules, or both. Enhancer elements have a remarkable ability to function in either orientation,

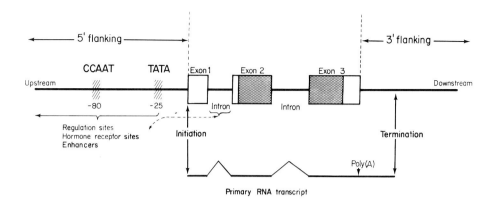

FIG. 1. General features of a eukaryotic gene. Exons are indicated by boxes, with the *shaded regions* corresponding to the protein coding sequences. The *unshaded portions* at the 5' and 3' ends designate the nontranslated mRNA sequences. Although regulatory sequences are generally found in the 5' flanking regions, hormone-receptor-binding sites and enhancers have also been identified in the first intron in growth-hormone and immunoglobulin heavy-chain genes, respectively.

whether they are in front of, within, or downstream from the gene. Although very few eukaryotic enhancers have been characterized so far (19,20), they are believed to act as bidirectional entry sites for RNA polymerase II, and as such are responsible for the increased efficiency of transcription. Recently, enhancer elements have been found to induce an altered chromatin structure resulting in a nucleosome-free region (21). Short enhancer-like repeated elements have also been identified with consensus sequences in the various locations of the 5' flanking regions, sometimes forming a palindromic structure that may be of regulatory significance. Unlike the TATA box, these sequences are unique to a specific set of genes and may convey tissue-specific gene expression (22,23).

Thus, the eukaryotic promoter extends over a large region composed of different functional elements. The conservation of nucleotide sequences among functionally related regulatory elements suggests that they serve as binding sites for protein factors, such as a hormone receptor. The molecular events involved in regulation of transcription following such protein-DNA interaction are not yet clear. It is possible that such interactions could lead to a change in the conformation of the double helix, a signal that can be transmitted over some distance and lead to local melting at the TATA box, the site for binding of RNA polymerase and initiation factors to DNA.

RNA Polymerase II

In addition to changes occurring in the nucleosome structure, control of transcription could also involve modulating the activity of RNA polymerase (24). There are three types of polymerases (I, II, and III) with distinct physical and functional properties in eukaryotic nuclei. Types I and III transcribe the genes coding for ribosomal, transfer, and 5S RNAs, whereas RNA polymerase II catalyzes the synthesis of mRNA. Thus, it is the selectivity of polymerase II that determines to a large extent which protein-coding genes will be expressed in a given cell.

RNA polymerase II is a large molecule composed of at least 11 subunits ranging from 10,000 to 220,000 daltons molecular mass. Transcription of the DNA template by RNA polymerase II (Pol II) is a complex reaction that requires, in addition to four ribonucleotides, divalent ions (Mg^{2+} and Mn^{2+}) and several protein factors that participate in the initiation, elongation, and termination of the polynucleotide chain. The isolated enzyme is incapable of selective initiation of transcription at mRNA promoters on naked DNA. However, addition either of soluble whole-cell extracts or of recently purified specificity factors results in accurate transcriptional initiation at various mRNA promoters (25). The transcriptional factors identified thus far direct specific initiation of sets of genes and also of individual genes *in vitro* (25). The presence of gene-specific transcription factors suggests a mechanism of control in which subsets of cellular genes are regulated by an array of specificity factors that direct initiation by Pol II at the respective DNA-binding sites.

Although the initiation of transcription is probably the major controlling step in gene expression, differential termination of transcription may also be an important factor (26). The generation of different mRNAs by alternate RNA splicing of the 3' terminal exons of a gene may well depend on the use of different sites for either termination or polyadenylation or both. Lately, the concept of transcriptional control dependent on DNA rearrangement has gained more support, because such a mechanism has been described in several systems, including the formation of immunoglobulin genes.

The primary result of transcription is a direct copy of the genome sequences from the initiation to the termination site. The transcript is generally larger than its mature cytoplasmic counterpart, because it still contains all the intervening sequences. Compared with ribosomal RNA or tRNA transcripts, primary mRNA transcripts have a broad size distribution of 0.1 to 100 kb and hence are referred to as heterogeneous nuclear RNA (hnRNA). These rather long RNA chains are quite unstable and are found associated with sets of proteins, resulting in ribonucleoprotein complexes (27,28). There is considerable evidence to suggest sequence-specific RNA-protein interactions that result in different sensitivities to nuclease digestion (29). Because only one-fourth of the hnRNA is processed to cytoplasmic RNA, most of the hnRNA turns over entirely within the nucleus, and the function of the unstable sequences is not known (26).

Posttranscriptional Control

The second level of gene control reflects (a) the sequence of events that convert a primary RNA transcript to a mature mRNA, commonly referred to as RNA processing (26), and (b) the transport of mRNA from the nucleus to the cytoplasm.

RNA Processing

The processing of hnRNA begins very rapidly after the start of transcription and prior to its completion (26). First, enzymatically catalyzed modifications occur at both ends of the pre-mRNA chain. Most of the 5′ ends become methylated by the addition of 7-methyl-guanosine, a process referred to as capping. Strong evidence indicates that the 5′ cap structure is crucial for mRNA stability and serves to enhance the ribosome binding. At the 3′ end, after cleavage of the mRNA, a stretch of about 200 adenylic residues is added to almost all cellular mRNAs by the action of a specific enzyme, poly(A)polymerase. There are some data to suggest that polyadenylation helps mediate subsequent RNA processing and the export of the mature mRNA from the nucleus and may also be important for cytoplasmic stabilization of the mRNA. However, the significance of polyadenylation remains unclear, because some mRNAs, notably those for histones and heat-shock proteins, are not polyadenylated. Finally, internal methylation of adenosine residues of mRNA precursors may occur, but very little is known about its mechanism or its function during subsequent mRNA maturation.

In order to convert the RNA transcript into a mRNA molecule that codes for a complete protein, intervening sequences that are present in the primary transcript must be removed. Identification of the components of the enzymatic machinery that are involved in the splicing process is only just beginning. The specificity of splicing may be directed by small nuclear RNAs that contain sequences complementary to consensus splice junctions (30). In the simple type of processing, the primary transcript is converted into only one mature mRNA by cleavage and joining at the intron-exon junctions, possibly by the concerted actions of endonuclease and ligase. In more complex splicing schemes, the primary transcript may give rise to several functionally different

mRNAs by the splicing of alternate exon sequences. In the process of splicing, most of the mass of the primary RNA transcripts is removed and degraded, and only about 5% of the total RNA mass transcribed is exported to the cytoplasm. The selection of which completed mRNAs in the cell nucleus are exported to the cytoplasm may depend on specific molecular export signals that have not yet been defined. Thus, the complexity of mRNA processing infers several possibilities for control of gene expression at this level.

Nucleocytoplasmic Transport

Very little is known about nucleocytoplasmic transport of RNA through the numerous pores that exist in nuclear membranes. Proteins that interact with RNA in the nucleus, forming ribonucleoprotein particles (RNP), could play an important role in the passage from the nucleus to the cytoplasm and as such contribute to a final possible step of posttranscriptional control (29).

Translational Control

There are several processes that affect the translation of mRNA molecules after they reach the cytoplasm. These include (a) mRNA turnover, (b) storage or masking of mRNA, and (c) formation of mRNA-ribosome complexes.

mRNA Turnover

Messenger RNA stability resulting from differential turnover is an important aspect of translational control. Most eukaryotic mRNAs turn over with a half-life of 5 to 15 hr. However, the turnover of specific mRNAs may be modulated during transitions from one synthetic program to another. Following terminal differentiation of skeletal muscle, mRNAs encoding contractile proteins have longer half-lives than other cellular mRNAs. Likewise, during mammalian erythroblast differentiation (31), and during development of the slime mold *Dictyostelium discoideum* (32), specific mRNAs are selectively retained, while a large fraction of total cellular mRNA is degraded. In some instances, these effects can be demonstrated for individual mRNA species. For example, casein (33) and vitellogenin (34) mRNAs are selectively stabilized following hormonal stimulation by prolactin and estrogens, respectively. Thus, even though the synthesis of individual mRNAs is transcriptionally regulated, the cytoplasmic mRNA levels (and hence expression of the gene) may also be modulated through differential degradation of mRNAs.

Storage of mRNA

Another mechanism that could contribute to the rate at which mRNA is translated involves the masking or storage of mRNA in an inactive form. This occurs in the sea urchin oocyte, where maternal histone mRNAs are specifically sequestered into RNP particles and not translated until the egg is fertilized (35). Similarly, while normal protein synthesis is shut down during heat shock, the mRNAs for these proteins remain intact in the cytoplasm (36). Thus, the formation of mRNP complexes reflects a mechanism to prevent degradation of mRNAs that are not being translated.

Formation of mRNA-Ribosome Complexes

Finally, the formation of mRNA-ribosome complex represents yet another possible level of regulation. The molecular events that underlie protein synthesis are very complex. Three main classes of RNAs, mRNA, tRNA, and rRNA, are involved in the process, with rRNA playing a part in the crucial ribosome mRNA-tRNA recognition event. Initiation, elongation, and termination reactions require a complex catalytic machinery to guide the events of protein synthesis on the ribosome. Specifically, aminoacyl-tRNA synthetase, peptidyl transferase, and the availability of high-energy phosphates are necessary for reactions to occur. Phosphorylation of the initiation factor responsible for placing the methionyl-transfer RNA on the ribosome, of aminoacyl-tRNA synthetase, and of a protein that is a component of the smaller ribosomal subunit (37), as well as changes in the conformation of ribosomes, may add to the complex interplay of factors involved in protein synthesis and its regulation.

Posttranslational Control

Protein Modification

Several types of posttranslational control could account for the final concentration of a particular protein in a given cell. Most polypeptides undergo covalent modification after being released from the ribosome. Phosphorylation, adenylation, and methylation, as well as formation of disulfide cross-linkage, are examples of some common reversible modifications that occur in the cytosol and regulate the biological activity of the protein. Likewise, permanent attachment of prosthetic groups is required for enzymatic or biochemical function, as are the modifications of proteins that leave the cytosol, such as glycosylation of secretory proteins. In addition, proteolytic cleavage of a primary translation product can result in peptides with different biological activities (38).

Protein Turnover

All proteins in the cell undergo continued degradation and resynthesis, resulting in a constant turnover of

protein. Therefore, the amount of any protein in a given cell depends not only on the rate of its synthesis, which is largely controlled by the synthesis of its mRNA in the nucleus, but also on the rate at which it is degraded. Because different proteins have different inherent susceptibilities to the degradation process, they turn over at markedly different rates. Thus, differential protein turnover is one of the possible means by which a particular cell may regulate expression of a gene. Although little is known about the mechanisms of intracellular proteolysis, altering the rate of protein degradation may be one response to regulatory signals, along with the metabolic demand in some tissues (39,40).

Summary

Although all of the steps in the pathway leading from DNA to protein may participate in controlling gene expression in eukaryotes, the primary level of regulation probably occurs during synthesis of the mRNA transcript in the cell nucleus. The molecular events that influence the transcription of a gene are still largely unknown. However, delineations of genomic sequences that are involved in turning on cellular genes and analyses of transcription initiation of individual genes now permit characterization of the effector molecules involved in regulating mRNA synthesis. It is likely that these effectors correspond to proteins specifying transcriptional specificity factors, enhancer recognition proteins, or enzymes directly involved in altering chromatin conformation or structure. DNA-protein interactions and enhancer sequences are likely to play important roles, because they probably change the structure of the chromosome in the vicinity of the respective gene, allowing the RNA polymerase to bind and transcribe the gene. The types of regulatory proteins that operate during differentiation and distinguish one cell type from another remain to be elucidated.

RNA TRANSCRIPTION AND PROCESSING IN HEART MUSCLE

Both qualitative and quantitative changes in the patterns of myofibrillar protein synthesis and gene expression occur during cardiac muscle growth. The changes reflect the responses of the heart to a variety of physiologic and environmental stimuli. With the development of recombinant DNA technology, it is now possible to identify and delineate the expression of individual contractile protein genes and to directly analyze the molecular mechanisms that differentially regulate and orchestrate the expression of these genes.

Markers of Specific Genes: Polymorphism of Contractile Proteins

Multiple molecular forms of contractile, regulatory, and sarcoplasmic proteins have been identified in both muscle and nonmuscle tissues. We are only now beginning to appreciate the large repertoire of different isoforms, their developmental and tissue-specific expressions, the complex splicing mechanisms that lead to some of this diversity, and their relevance to muscle function (41).

Myosin

Myosin is a key structural enzymatic protein of muscle. It is composed of two 200,000-dalton heavy chains and two sets of light chains between 15,000 and 27,000 daltons. The heavy chains form the major structural features of the molecule, which consists of an α-helical rod and two globular heads containing the ATPase activity and the actin-binding sites. The myosin ATPase activity appears to be a major determinant of muscle function, because it is directly correlated with contractile velocity (42). Differences in ATPase activity, in turn, depend primarily on the heavy chains, as indicated by measurements of the enzymatic activity of heavy chains isolated under nondenaturing conditions (43) and of myosin in which the light chains have been exchanged (44).

Multiple molecular forms of myosin heavy chains have been identified in fast, slow, and cardiac muscle by partial amino acid sequencing (45), peptide mapping (46,47), and immunological techniques (48–52). Furthermore, within each muscle type, additional forms of myosin heavy chains have been identified. Thus, fast (53–56), slow (57–59), and cardiac (60–63) tissues all contain at least two different forms of myosin heavy chains. Genomic blot analysis (64,65) suggests the existence of six to eight separate genes. However, the diversity of heavy-chain forms in skeletal muscle may be quite extensive, because developmentally distinct embryonic, neonatal, and adult myosin heavy chains (66) are also expressed in multiple forms (67).

In mammalian ventricular muscle there are at least two forms of myosin heavy chains, α and β, specifying myosins of relatively high and low ATPase activities, respectively (47). The expression of these forms follows a defined developmental pattern (68,69) and can be markedly altered by thyroid hormones (47), by insulin (70), by androgens (71), and by the imposition of a pressure work overload (60). Additional heavy chains have been identified in avian Purkinje fibers (63) and in rat (72), rabbit (73), and bovine (74) myocardium. However, it is unclear whether the variant cardiac isoforms represent allelic variants of the α and β cardiac myosin heavy chains or correspond to unique isoforms with distinct structural and enzymatic properties. In contrast, atrial muscles contain predominantly the α myosin heavy chain, whereas in avian ventricles only the β isoform is expressed (75). In the latter tissues, the expression of the respective heavy-chain isoforms does not change with thyroid hormone administration. Thus,

regulation of cardiac myosin heavy-chain expression also varies in different species and in atrial heart muscle.

Distinct myosin heavy-chain isoforms are also expressed in early muscle development. Immunologic analyses have indicated that fast, slow, and cardiac myosins are co-expressed in early embryonic skeletal and cardiac muscle (76). Recent investigations, however, revealed that prior to differentiation, chick somitic myoblasts expressed cardiac-like myosin at the time when no skeletal fast or slow isoforms could be detected (77). Whether this primordial cardiac-like isoform represents either an adult cardiac myosin or an additional isoform that is expressed in the somite is unclear.

The myosin light chains also occur in multiple polymorphic forms. They are integral parts of the globular myosin heads, but their functional role is still unclear. The two major types of light chains are the alkali light chains, LC_1 (19,000–22,000 daltons) and LC_3 (16,000 daltons) in skeletal muscle, and the phosphorylatable or regulatory light chains, LC_2 (17,000–20,000 daltons) (41). Distinct alkali and regulatory LCs are expressed in fast, slow, and atrial muscles. In ventricular muscle, however, LC_2 is identical with the isoform expressed in slow skeletal muscle (78,79), and the same may be true for LC_1 (78,80). A variant of LC_2 has also been reported in the latter tissues (81). In addition, a distinct developmentally expressed isoform of LC_1 has been identified in all embryonic mammalian striated muscle tissues, including atria (78,82,83). Interestingly, the embryonic LC_1 appears to be reexpressed during cardiac hypertrophy (84). Although the alkali and regulatory LCs have different primary structures and are encoded by separate genes (85–87), some of the variants within each class may be similar to the skeletal alkali LC_1 and LC_3 in that they are generated by alternate RNA splicing from a single gene.

Actin

The actins represent a family of highly conserved proteins found in abundance in all eukaryotes. They are major components of the cytoskeleton (88) in nonmuscle cells and of the myofibrillar arrays in muscle cells (89). Functionally they are involved in as diverse roles as cell motility, mitosis, and muscle contraction. Protein sequencing has identified six actin isoforms (90) in birds and mammals. Distinct muscle-specific or α actins are found in skeletal, cardiac, vascular smooth, and enteric smooth muscles. The α actins are highly homologous to one another, even from such diverse organisms as yeast and mammals (91). The β and γ variants are part of the cytoskeletal (cytoplasmic) actins and differ only in 25 of 375 amino acids from the α isoforms. Each actin isozyme contains a unique 18-residue N-terminal sequence that is responsible for the isoelectric-point differences between the isoproteins. Moreover, all six isoforms are encoded by at least one gene, and in the case of β

actin, there may be as many as 20 copies of the gene in mammals (92,93).

Tropomyosin

Tropomyosins are a family of related proteins that are widely distributed in nature. In muscle, tropomyosin occurs bound to actin in the thin filament and serves to mediate the effect of calcium on the actomyosin interaction. By two-dimensional peptide mapping, two isoforms, α and β, are known to exist in skeletal fast and slow muscle fibers as homodimers (94). However, recently, in rabbit, γ and δ variants were resolved in slow muscle by two-dimensional gel analyses (95,96). Additional α variants are present in the heart (97) and in smooth muscle, and still another type is found in nonmuscle tissues (98,99). The high degree of homology between different tropomyosin isoforms suggests that there are separate genes that evolved from a common ancestral gene. Alternatively, recent characterizations of tropomyosin genes show that the strong sequence conservation between these isoforms results from alternate RNA splicing of a single gene (100,101).

Troponin

Troponin is the component of the thin filament that confers calcium sensitivity on actomyosin in the presence of tropomyosin. It is composed of three subunits: a calcium-binding subunit, Tn-C, an inhibitory subunit, Tn-I, and a tropomyosin-binding subunit, Tn-T. As with other myofibrillar proteins, each of the subunits occurs in multiple polymorphic forms that are expressed in a tissue-specific fashion. By protein sequencing, distinct Tn-I and Tn-T subunits have been characterized in fast, slow, and cardiac muscles (102), whereas Tn-C subunits in cardiac and slow skeletal muscles are identical (103) and differ from that in fast muscle (104). Structural analysis reveals that the various Tn-T isoforms have identical sequences except for isoform-specific regions at the N terminus and a small segment near the C terminus (105). In similarity to the skeletal alkali LCs (85,86), isolation and characterization of the Tn-T gene (106) indicates that different Tn-T isoforms arise from alternate splicing of exons encoding the conserved and divergent regions. A similar mechanism may possibly give rise to the Tn-C isoforms. Thus, the expression of different troponin isoforms is primarily regulated at the level of RNA processing.

Analysis of α and β Myosin Heavy-Chain mRNA Expression in Cardiac Muscle

As indicated earlier, the expression of α and β cardiac myosin heavy chains has been studied most extensively in two model systems, during development and after thyroid hormone administration. Because a detailed review of myosin heavy-chain expression in cardiac muscle is provided in chapter 63 of this volume, we shall focus primarily on molecular genetic analysis of heavy-chain expression.

Isolation and Characterization of cDNA Probes for α and β Myosin Heavy-Chain mRNAs

So far, complementary DNA clones have been constructed for the α and β myosin heavy chains of rat (72) and rabbit (107,108) ventricles. By restriction endonuclease mapping and DNA sequencing, the clones correspond to about 3.5 kb of the 3' portion of the 6–7-kb mRNA including the 3' nontranslated region. The cloned regions include the carboxy-terminal portion of the globular head or subfragment 1 (107), the entire subfragment-2 region, and 90% of the remaining rod portion of the molecule (72,108). Complementary DNA clones specifying residues at the N terminus have not been constructed, and clones encoding additional cardiac heavy-chain isoforms have not been isolated. However, a variant rat α myosin heavy-chain mRNA having a distinct 3' nontranslated sequence has been identified by molecular cloning (72,109), and a rabbit β myosin heavy-chain mRNA variant has been detected by S1 nuclease mapping (110). At the present time, it is unclear if the latter variants represent genetic polymorphism, arise from alternate splicing, or correspond to additional myosin heavy-chain genes.

Sequence analysis of cardiac cDNA clones has revealed that the α and β myosin heavy chains are highly homologous, but are distinct proteins. There is at least 95% homology in the overlapping amino acid sequences, as well as a high degree of similarity to heavy chains from rabbit fast skeletal muscle (87%) and from distant species, such as the nematode (50%). The slight differences in homology between cardiac and skeletal heavy chains are consistent with generation of the two cardiac isoforms after the divergence of cardiac and skeletal myosin genes. In contrast, the evolutionary constraints on noncoding sequences are apparently less than on protein-coding sequences, and the 3' nontranslated regions of the α and β cardiac mRNAs show marked sequence divergence (72). Relatively high sequence divergences in the nontranslated regions are generally observed in other gene families (111), though notably not with the cardiac and skeletal actins (112).

Although the conservation of coding sequences makes it difficult to distinguish the α and β heavy-chain mRNAs using conventional hybridization techniques, it is possible to measure their relative abundances using a powerful method that maps sequence divergence in the two mRNAs with S1 nuclease (113). As shown in Fig. 2, an end-labeled cDNA probe spanning an area of

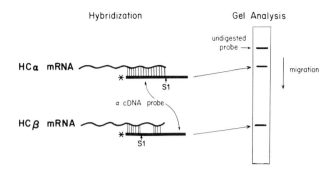

Hybridization   Gel Analysis

HCα mRNA

HCβ mRNA

FIG. 2. Principle of S1 nuclease mapping analysis. In this example, the α cDNA probe is labeled at the 3′ terminus (asterisk) and is complementary to the 3′ end of the mRNA.

divergence between the α and β mRNAs is hybridized to the mRNAs, and the hybrids are treated with single-strand-specific S1 nuclease. Because of the homology between the cardiac myosin heavy-chain mRNAs, the probe hybridizes to both mRNAs. However, only hybridization to the homologous mRNA protects the cDNA sequences from digestion with the nuclease, whereas hybridization to the heterologous mRNA results in cleavage of the probe at sites of sequence divergence. Following fractionation by gel electrophoresis, hybridization of the probe to each mRNA is indicated by labeled fragments of different lengths. Thus, the method allows detection of specific mRNAs based on small sequence differences alone, and because only a single probe is used, it also provides information on the relative amount of each mRNA species by the radioactivity associated with each band.

Myosin Heavy-Chain Expression During Development

The changes in expression of the ventricular α and β myosin heavy chains during development are well documented. Using labeled cDNA probes in an S1 nuclease mapping procedure, the roles of transcriptional or translational mechanisms in regulating the expression of the proteins have been evaluated in rabbit (114) and rat (109) ventricles. During fetal and adult life there is a direct correlation between the relative ratios of the mRNAs and the relative amounts of the α and β myosin heavy chains. The results indicate that the cardiac heavy chains are translated in the same proportion as the respective mRNAs, and therefore the differential expression of the cardiac myosin heavy-chain genes during development occurs primarily at the pretranslational level, i.e., at the level of either transcriptional initiation or posttranscriptional processing.

In contrast to the ventricle, atrial muscle appears to express only the α form of the protein throughout development. Analysis of the mRNA sequences in atrial muscle of rabbit (108) and rat (109) hearts by S1

nuclease mapping reveals only the presence of a mRNA that is indistinguishable from ventricular heavy-chain α mRNA in the 3′ nontranslated region and in a number of coding regions extending to the N terminus of the protein (109,115). Thus, regulation of myosin heavy-chain expression in atrial muscle also occurs at the pretranslational level. Moreover, the apparent identity of the atrial and ventricular α myosin heavy-chain mRNAs indicates that the same gene is differentially regulated in both tissues. Thus, understanding the factors involved in this differential regulation of cardiac heavy-chain genes in atria and ventricles would also provide insight into the molecular mechanisms involved in cellular differentiation.

Myosin Heavy-Chain Expression in Different Thyroid States

Thyroid hormones have a dramatic effect on the expression of the ventricular α and β myosin heavy chains (116). Along with conversion to synthesis of the α form of the protein, there is a corresponding increase in the relative amount of α myosin heavy-chain mRNA (109,110). In fact, changes in the relative synthesis rates of the α and β heavy chains after thyroid hormone administration correlate directly with the relative abundances of the two mRNAs (110). Thus, in similarity to the changes in expression during development, modulation of α and β myosin heavy-chain expression by thyroid hormone is also regulated at the pretranslational level.

Direct evidence for transcriptional regulation of myosin heavy-chain expression has been obtained from recent studies on the transcription of α and β heavy-chain genes in isolated nuclei (117). In these experiments, heart nuclei from hypothyroid rabbits before and after their treatment with 3,5,3′-triiodothyronine (T_3) were incubated *in vitro* with radioactive nucleotide triphosphates to label nuclear transcripts. Hybridization of the labeled RNA to sequence-specific probes for the α and β myosin heavy-chain genes (117) indicated that T_3 treatment resulted in approximately a 10-fold increase in the relative transcription of the heavy-chain α gene and a decrease in the specific transcription of the heavy-chain β gene. The large change in transcription clearly demonstrates that the effect of thyroid hormone on myosin heavy-chain expression is primarily regulated at the level of transcriptional initiation.

Whether or not thyroid hormone directly participates in transcriptional activation of the α heavy-chain genes and whether or not there are secondary effects of the hormone on mRNA turnover and stability are not known. However, because effects of thyroid hormone on other response genes such as growth-hormone gene (118) have been postulated to be mediated through chromatin binding of a nuclear thyroid hormone receptor, it is possible that a similar mechanism regulates cardiac myosin heavy-chain gene expression.

Thus, the use of molecular cloning techniques to obtain cDNA clones for cardiac myosin heavy chains has rapidly provided a detailed picture of the structures of heavy-chain isoforms in cardiac muscle and their developmental and tissue-specific patterns of expression. This approach has permitted analysis of mRNA expression in heart muscle and has provided further insights into the mechanisms regulating one family of myofibrillar proteins. It has also provided a path to a more detailed understanding of the molecular mechanisms regulating the expression of myofibrillar proteins through isolation of the respective genes.

Characterization of Myosin Heavy-Chain Genes in Cardiac Muscle

Molecular analysis of the myosin heavy-chain gene family is still in its early stages. Genomic clones encoding nematode (119), *Drosophila* (120,121), chicken (64), rat (65,122,123), rabbit (124), and human (125,126) myosin heavy chains have been isolated, but only the nematode genes, the rat embryonic skeletal genes, and the rabbit and rat cardiac genes have been characterized in great detail.

At least three myosin heavy-chain genes for the body-wall musculature in the nematode, *Caenorhabditis elegans* (119), have been completely sequenced. The genes are approximately 8.0 kbp long and contain up to eight short introns. In these genes, the locations of the introns do not correlate with the proteolytic subfragments of the heavy chain (i.e., S1, S2, and LMM), and they also vary between the genes. Thus, in the nematode there is little correlation between exons and either major structural or functional domains of the protein. Because the gene is three times smaller than mammalian myosin genes (*vide infra*), the apparent random locations of introns may reflect the reduction of noncoding or inter-

vening sequences from a larger ancestral gene during evolution of this invertebrate.

In contrast, the cardiac myosin heavy-chain genes of both rabbit (124) and rat (123) ventricular muscles encompass approximately 25 kbp of genomic DNA. The genes have a complex structure of coding and intervening sequences specifying mRNAs of 6 to 6.5 kb. As shown in Fig. 3, an entire rabbit α heavy-chain gene, reconstructed in two overlapping genomic clones, is divided into at least 37 exons ranging in size from 30 to 300 bp. The 5′ terminal exon contains the transcriptional initiation site and 15 nucleotides of the 5′ non-translated mRNA sequences, whereas the 3′ terminal exon of the gene encodes 7 amino acids at the C terminus and all of the 3′ nontranslated region of the mRNA. The 5′ half of the β heavy-chain gene, encoding the entire S1 and 275 amino acids of the S2 portion of the protein, has a similar organization. Corresponding exons of both genes are similar in size, but are interrupted by introns that differ markedly in both length and nucleotide sequence. Because the coding regions are highly homologous, the intron differences are a major distinguishing feature of the cardiac myosin genes. The two genes are also tandemly linked in the genome (123). In the rat, the α and β myosin heavy-chain genes have been reconstructed from overlapping genomic clones spanning over 50 kbp of genomic DNA. Within this region, the β heavy-chain gene is located approximately 4 kbp upstream from the α heavy-chain gene. Because the β heavy-chain gene is primarily expressed in the embryo, and the α heavy-chain gene in adult rats, the 5′-to-3′ orientation of the fetal and adult genes is similar to the arrangement of the β-globin gene family (127). The linkage of the two genes and the similarity in the positions of the introns indicate that the α and β genes arose by gene duplication.

Partial characterization of at least six other mammalian myosin heavy-chain genes indicates that they are structurally similar to the cardiac genes in both size and

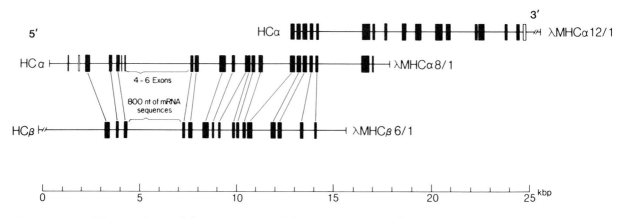

FIG. 3. Structures of the rabbit α and β ventricular myosin heavy-chain genes. *Shaded boxes* designate protein-coding exons; *open boxes* represent the 5′ and 3′ nontranslated mRNA sequences.

complex organization of coding and intervening sequences. Sequence analyses of limited portions of these genes indicate that intron positions in the coding regions of the rabbit cardiac genes are conserved in two rat sarcomeric myosin heavy chain genes (123,128) and in a human myosin heavy chain gene (H. P. Vosberg, unpublished data). In contrast to the situation for the nematode, conservation of a complex gene structure in mammals suggests an evolutionary advantage in generating diversity in the protein either at the genomic level or through alternate RNA splicing. An example of the latter has been documented in *Drosophila* (120,121), in which a single myosin heavy-chain gene gives rise to three distinct transcripts that are differentially expressed during development.

The structures of the 5′ terminus and promoter regions of the cardiac myosin heavy-chain genes have recently been characterized in detail (Fig. 4). In the rabbit α heavy-chain gene, the transcriptional initiation starts approximately 900 nucleotides (nt) from the N-terminal coding exon. The flanking region of the gene contains consensus TATA and CAAAT promoter sequences located 26 and 59 nt upstream of the cap site, respectively. The sequence organization of the 5′ end of the gene is unique among eukaryotes in that the first two exons encode only 5′ nontranslated sequences, and this suggests some functional role for sequences in the nontranslated exons or sequences in the 5′ introns in regulating transcription and expression of the α heavy-chain mRNA. There is very little sequence homology with the 5′ portion of the β heavy-chain gene, which is consistent with the differential expressions of the two heavy chains.

The α heavy-chain gene also contains a number of interesting sequence elements that may be of regulatory significance. Sequence comparison with the rat α heavy-chain gene identifies a 400-bp region immediately upstream of the cap site that is conserved not only in its nucleotide sequence (>80% homology) but also in its location relative to the translational initiation site. Downstream, the sequences are divergent, with only short regions of homology, none of which correspond to the nontranslated exons. The sequence homology in the 400-bp region is comparable to that observed in the protein-coding sequences (115) and strongly suggests that this region contains additional sequence elements (such as enhancers) that are important in regulating the expression of the α heavy-chain gene. In addition, Fig. 4 also shows regions of the α myosin heavy-chain gene that are highly homologous to regions in the rat growth-hormone gene (129). The sequence GTGTGGTTTG is exactly conserved, and the sequence CTCCTGTC-TCCTGTCTCTCT is identical in 20 of 21 nt. The former has similarities to a core enhancer sequence (130), and the latter is repeated imperfectly in the α heavy-chain gene. Both conserved sequences are located in the first introns of the respective genes. Because growth-hormone gene expression is regulated by thyroid hormone, the sequence homology suggests additional regions that may be important in thyroid hormone regulation of α myosin heavy-chain gene expression.

PERSPECTIVE

In the latter half of this review we have focused mainly on the myosin heavy chains of cardiac muscle

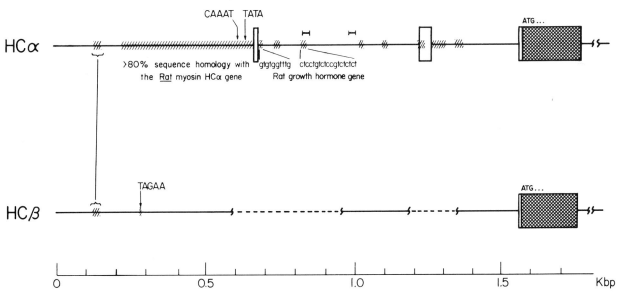

FIG. 4. The 5′ flanking regions of the rabbit α and β myosin heavy-chain genes. Protein-coding regions are indicated by *shaded boxes,* and 5′ nontranslated regions are *unshaded.* Regions of homology between the rabbit and rat α myosin heavy-chain genes are indicated by *hatched areas.* The portions of the β myosin heavy-chain gene that have not been sequenced are indicated by *broken lines.*

because of their importance in both the structure and contractile function of the heart. Over the last few years, the molecular approach to study these proteins has rapidly increased our understanding of heavy-chain polymorphism, its correlation to contractile function, and the mechanisms involved in regulating their expression. With the current characterizations of the cardiac genes, we are in a position to delineate the molecular components (i.e., regulatory gene sequences and putative protein factors) that control expression of these genes during development and in response to environmental stimuli. Elucidating the mechanisms that regulate expression of these genes will be an important step in understanding the process by which the effects of external stimuli are transmitted to the changes in gene expression that modulate cardiac muscle growth and function.

Myosin heavy chain, however, is only one of many protein constituents of cardiac muscle. It is quite clear that other proteins are modulated both qualitatively and quantitatively through mechanisms that may be different from that for the heavy chain. The future challenge for molecular biology will be to decipher the patterns of expression and regulation of other protein components and to identify the networks that integrate expression of these proteins and regulate cardiac muscle physiology.

ACKNOWLEDGMENTS

This investigation was supported in part by USPHS grants HL09172, HL20592, and HL16637 from the National Institutes of Health, by grants from the Muscular Dystrophy Association, by an Established Investigatorship of the American Heart Association (P.K.U.), and by funds contributed in part by the Chicago Heart Association.

REFERENCES

1. Davidson, E. H., and Posakony, J. W. (1982): Repetitive sequence transcripts in development. *Nature,* 297:633–635.
2. Jelinek, W. R., and Schmid, C. W. (1982): Repetitive sequences in eukarotic DNA and their expression. *Annu. Rev. Biochem.,* 51:813–844.
3. Sun, L., Paulson, K. E., Schmid, C. W., Kadyk, L., and Leinwand, L. (1984): Non-Alu family interspersed repeats in human DNA and their transcriptional activity. *Nucleic Acids Res.,* 12:2669–2690.
4. Spence, S. E., Young, R. M., Garner, K. J., and Lingrel, J. B. (1985): Localization and characterization of members of a family of repetitive sequences in the goat β-globin locus. *Nucleic Acids Res.,* 13:2171–2186.
5. Brown, D. D. (1981): Gene expression in eukaryotes. *Science* 211:667–674.
6. Berget, S. M., Moore, C., and Sharp, P. A. (1977): Spliced segments at the 5′ terminus of adenovirus 2 late mRNA. *Proc. Natl. Acad. Sci. USA,* 74:3171–3175.
7. Little, P. F. R. (1982): Globin pseudogenes. *Cell,* 28:683–684.
8. Sharp, P. A. (1983): Conversion of RNA to DNA in mammals: Alu-like elements and pseudogenes. *Nature* 301:471–472.
9. Weisbrod, S. (1982): Active chromatin. *Nature,* 297:289–295.
10. Groner, B., Kennedy, N., Skroch, P., Hynes, N. E., and Ponta, H. (1984): DNA sequences involved in the regulation of gene expression by glucocorticoid hormones. *Biochim. Biophys. Acta,* 781:1–6.
11. Emerson, B. M., and Felsenfeld, G. (1984): Specific factor conferring nuclease hypersensitivity at the 5′ end of the chicken adult β-globin gene. *Proc. Natl. Acad. Sci. USA,* 81:95–99.
12. Wu, C. (1984): Two protein-binding sites in chromatin implicated in the activation of heat-shock genes. *Nature* 309:229–234.
13. Doerfler, W. (1983): DNA methylation and gene activity. *Annu. Rev. Biochem.,* 52:93–124.
14. Nordheim, A., and Rich, A. (1983): Negatively supercoiled Simian Virus 40 contains Z-DNA segments with transcriptional enhancer sequences. *Nature,* 303:674–679.
15. Breathnach, R., Benoist, C., O'Hare, K., Gannon, F., and Chambon, P. (1978): Ovalbumin gene: Evidence for a leader sequence in mRNA and DNA sequences at exon-intron boundaries. *Proc. Natl. Acad. Sci. USA,* 75:4853–4857.
16. Venkatesan, S., and Moss, B. (1980): Donor and receptor specificities of HeLa cell mRNA guanylyltransferase. *J. Biol. Chem.,* 255:2835–2842.
17. Breathnach, R., and Chambon, P. (1981): Organization and expression of eukaryotic split genes coding for protein. *Annu. Rev. Biochem.,* 50:349–383.
18. Khoury, G., and Gruss, P. (1983): Enhancer elements. *Cell,* 33: 313–314.
19. Boss, A. M. (1983): Enhancer elements in immunoglobulin genes. *Nature,* 303:281–282.
20. Walker, M. D., Edlund, T., Boulet, A. M., and Rutter, W. J. (1983): Cell-specific expression controlled by the 5′ flanking region of insulin and chymotrypsin genes. *Nature,* 306:557–561.
21. Jongstra, J., Reudelhuber, T. L., Oudet, P., Benoist, C., Chae, C. B., Jeltsch, J. M., Mathis, D. J., and Chambon, P. (1984): Induction of altered chromatin structures by simian virus 40 enhancer and promoter elements. *Nature,* 307:708–714.
22. McKnight, S. T., and Kingsbury, R. (1982): Transcriptional control signals of a eukaryotic protein-coding gene. *Science,* 217: 316–324.
23. Dierks, P., Van Ooyen, A., Cochran, M. D., Dobkin, C., Reiser, J., and Weissmann, C. (1983): Three regions upstream from the cap site are required for efficient and accurate transcription of the rabbit β-globin gene in mice BT6 cells. *Cell,* 32:695–706.
24. Lewis, M. K., and Burgess, R. R. (1982): Eukaryotic RNA polymerase. In: *The Enzymes,* ed. 3, *Vol. 15B,* edited by P. D. Boyer, pp. 109–153. Academic Press, New York.
25. Dynan, W. S., and Tjian, R. (1983): Isolation of transcription factors that discriminate between different promoters recognized by RNA polymerase II. *Cell,* 32:669–680.
26. Darnell, E. J. (1982): Variety in the level of gene control in eukaryotic cells. *Nature,* 297:365–371.
27. Kinniburgh, A. J., and Martin, T. E. (1976): Detection of mRNA sequences in nuclear 30S ribonucleoprotein subcomplexes. *Proc. Natl. Acad. Sci. USA,* 73:2725–2729.
28. Stevienin, J., Gattoni, R., Gallinaro-Matringe, H., and Jacob, M. (1978): Nuclear ribonucleoprotein particles contain specific proteins and unspecific non-histone nuclear protein. *Eur. J. Biochem.,* 84:541–549.
29. Flint, S. J. (1984): Processing of mRNA precursors in eukaryotic cells. In: *RNA Processing,* edited by D. Aperion, pp. 151–179.
30. Lerner, M. R., Boyle, J. A., Mount, S. M., Wolin, S. L., and Steitz, J. A. (1980): Are snRNPs involved in splicing? *Nature,* 283:220–224.
31. Aviv, H., Voloch, Z., Bastos, R., and Levy, S. (1976): Biosynthesis and stability of globin mRNA in cultured erythroleukemic Friend cells. *Cell,* 8:495–503.
32. Chung, S., Landfear, S. M., Blumberg, D. D., Cohen, N. S., and Lodish, H. F. (1981): Synthesis and stability of developmentally regulated *Dictyostelium* mRNAs are affected by cell-cell contact and cAMP. *Cell,* 24:785–797.
33. Guyette, W. A., Matusik, R. J., and Rosen, J. M. (1979): Prolactin-mediated transcriptional and posttranscriptional control of casein gene expression. *Cell,* 17:1013–1023.
34. Brock, M. L., and Shapiro, D. J. (1983): Estrogen stabilizes vitellogenin mRNA against cytoplasmic degradation. *Cell,* 34: 207–214.
35. Showman, R. M., Wells, D. E., Anstrom, J., Hursh. D. A, and

Raff, R. (1982): Message specific sequestration of maternal histone mRNA in the sea urchin egg. *Proc. Natl. Acad. Sci. USA,* 79: 5944–5947.

36. DiDomenico, B.-J., Bugaisky, G. E., and Lindquist, S. (1982): Heat shock and recovery are mediated by different translational mechanisms. *Proc. Natl. Acad. Sci. USA,* 79:6181–6185.

37. Clemens, M. (1983): Protein phosphorylation and translation of messenger RNAs. *Nature,* 302:110.

38. Roberts, J. L., and Herbert, E. (1977): Characterization of a common precursor to corticotropin and β-lipotropin: Cell free synthesis of the precursor and identification of corticotropin peptides in the molecule. *Proc. Natl. Acad. Sci. USA,* 74:4826–4830.

39. Conde, R. D., and Scornik, O. A. (1976): Role of protein degradation in the growth of livers after a nutritional shift. *Biochem. J.,* 158:385–390.

40. Albin, R., Dowell, R. T., Zak, R., and Rabinowitz, M. (1973): Synthesis and degradation of mitochondrial components in hypertrophied rat heart. *Biochem. J.,* 136:629–637.

41. Buckingham, M. E., and Minty, A. J. (1983): Contractile protein genes. In: *Eukaryotic Genes: Their Structure, Activity, and Regulation,* edited by R. A. Flavell, S. P. Gregory, and N. MacLean, pp. 365–395. Butterworth, London.

42. Barany, M. (1967): ATPase activity of myosin correlated with speed of muscle shortening. *J. Gen. Physiol.,* 50:197–218.

43. Sivaramakrishnan, M., and Burke, M. (1982): The free heavy chain of vertebrate skeletal myosin subfragment I shows full enzymatic activity. *J. Biol. Chem.,* 257:1102–1105.

44. Wagner, P. D. (1981): Formation and characterization of myosin hybrids containing essential light chains and heavy chains from different muscle myosins. *J. Biol. Chem.,* 256:2493–2498.

45. Huszar, G. (1972): Developmental changes of the primary structure and histidine methylation in rabbit skeletal muscle myosin. *Nature [New Biol.],* 240:260–264.

46. Brevet, A., and Whalen, R. G. (1978): Comparative structural analysis of myosin after limited tryptic hydrolysis by use of two dimensional gel electrophoresis. *Biochimie,* 60:459–466.

47. Flink, I. L., Rader, J. H., and Morkin, E. (1979): Thyroid hormone stimulates synthesis of a cardiac isozyme. *J. Biol. Chem.,* 254:3105–3110.

48. Masaki, T. (1974): Immunochemical comparison of myosins from chicken cardiac, fast white, slow red, and smooth muscle. *J. Biochem. (Tokyo),* 76:441–449.

49. Arndt, I., and Pepe, F. A. (1975): Antigenic specificity of red and white muscle myosin. *J. Histochem.,* 23:159–168.

50. Gauthier, G. F., and Lowey, S. (1977): Polymorphism of myosin among skeletal muscle fiber types. *J. Cell Biol.,* 74:760–779.

51. Gauthier, G. F., and Lowey, S. (1979): Distribution of myosin isoenzymes among skeletal muscle fiber types. *J. Cell Biol.,* 81: 10–25.

52. Pierobon-Bormioli, S., Sartore, S., Dalla Libera, L., Vitadello, M., and Schiaffino, S. (1981): "Fast" isomyosins and fiber types in mammalian skeletal muscle. *J. Histochem. Cytochem.,* 29: 1179–1188.

53. Starr, R., and Offer, G. (1973): Polarity of the myosin molecule. *J. Mol. Biol.,* 81:17–31.

54. Elzinga, M., Behar, K., and Walton, G. (1980): Sequences and proposed structure of a 17,000 dalton CNBr fragment from C-terminus of myosin. *Fed. Proc.,* 39:2169 (abstract).

55. Dalla Libera, L., Sartore, S., Pierobon-Bormioli, S., and Schiaffino, S. (1980): Fast-white and fast-red isomyosins in guinea pig muscles. *Biochem. Biophys. Res. Commun.,* 96:1662–1670.

56. Zweig, S. E. (1981): The muscle specificity and structure of two closely related fast-twitch white muscle myosin heavy chain isozymes. *J. Biol. Chem.,* 256:11847–11853.

57. Rushbrook, J. I., and Stracher, A. (1979): Comparison of adult, embryonic and dystrophic myosin heavy chains from chicken muscle by sodium dodecyl sulfate/polyacrylamide gel electrophoresis and peptide mapping. *Proc. Natl. Acad. Sci USA,* 76:4331–4334.

58. Hoh, J. F. Y. (1978): Light chain distribution of chicken skeletal muscle myosin isoenzymes. *FEBS Lett.,* 90:297–300.

59. Umeda, P. K., Zak, R., and Rabinowitz, M. (1980): Purification of messenger ribonucleic acids for fast and slow myosin heavy chains by indirect immunoprecipitation of polysomes from embryonic chick skeletal muscle. *Biochemistry,* 19:1955–1965.

60. Lompre, A. M., Schwartz, K., d'Albis, A., Lacombe, G., Thiem, N. V., and Swynghedauw, B. (1979): Myosin isoenzyme redistribution in chronic heart overload. *Nature,* 282:105–107.

61. Hoh, J. F. Y., Yeoh, G. P. S., Thomas, M. A. W., and Higginbottom, L. (1979): Structural differences in the heavy chains of rat ventricular myosin isozymes. *FEBS Lett.,* 97:330–334.

62. Chizzonite, R. A., Everett, A. W., Clark, W. A., Jakovcic, S., Rabinowitz, M., and Zak, R. (1982): Isolation and characterization of two molecular variants of myosin heavy chain from rabbit ventricle. *J. Biol. Chem.,* 257:2056–2065.

63. Sartore, S., Gorza, L., Pierobon-Bormioli, S., and Schiaffino, S. (1978): Immunohistochemical evidence for myosin polymorphism in the chicken heart. *Nature,* 274:82–83.

64. Robbins, J., Freyer, G. A., Chisholm, D., and Gilliam, T. C. (1982): Isolation of multiple genomic sequences coding for chicken myosin heavy chain protein. *J. Biol. Chem.,* 257:549–556.

65. Wydro, R. M., Nguyen, H. T., Gubits, R. M., and Nadal-Ginard, B. (1983): Characterization of sarcomeric myosin heavy chain genes. *J. Biol. Chem.,* 258:670–678.

66. Whalen, R. G., Schwartz, K., Bouveret, P., Sell, S., and Gros, F. (1979): Contractile protein isozymes in muscle development: Identification of an embryonic form of myosin heavy chain. *Proc. Natl. Acad. Sci. USA,* 76:5197–5201.

67. Umeda, P. K., Kavinsky, C. J., Sinha, A. M., Hsu, H.-J., Jakovcic, S., and Rabinowitz, M. (1983): Cloned mRNA sequences for two types of embryonic myosin heavy chains from chick skeletal muscle. II. Expression during development using S1 nuclease mapping. *J. Biol. Chem.,* 258:5206–5214.

68. Hoh, J. F. Y., McGrath, P. A., and Hale, P. T. (1977): Electrophoretic analysis of multiple forms of rat cardiac myosin: Effect of hypophysectomy and thyroxine replacement. *J. Mol. Cell. Cardiol.,* 10:1053–1076.

69. Pope, B., Hoh, J. F. Y., and Weeds, A. (1980): The ATPase activities of rat cardiac myosin isoenzymes. *FEBS Lett.,* 118: 205–208.

70. Dillman, W. (1980): Diabetes mellitus induces changes in cardiac myosin of the rat. *Diabetes,* 29:579–582.

71. Malhotra, A., Schaible, T. F., Karell, M., and Scheuer, J. (1983): Effects of gonadectomy and testosterone replacement on cardiac myosin in male rats. *Circulation,* 68:III-7.

72. Mahdavi, V., Periasamy, M., and Nadal-Ginard, B. (1982): Molecular characterization of two myosin heavy chain genes expressed in the adult heart. *Nature,* 297:659–664.

73. Everett, A. W., Sinha, A. M., Umeda, P. K., Jakovcic, S., Rabinowitz, M., and Zak, R. (1984): Regulation of myosin synthesis by thyroid hormone: Relative change in the α- and β-myosin heavy chain mRNA levels in rabbit heart. *Biochemistry,* 23:1596–1599.

74. Flink, I. L., and Morkin, E. (1983): Evidence for two distinct β-heavy chains in bovine cardiac myosin. *Circulation,* 68:III-7.

75. Clark, W. A., Chizzonite, R. A., Everett, A. W., Rabinowitz, M., and Zak, R. (1982): Species correlations between cardiac isomyosins. A comparison of electrophoretic and immunological properties. *J. Biol. Chem.,* 257:5449–5454.

76. Masaki, T., and Yoshizaki, C. (1974): Differentiation of myosin in chick embryos. *J. Biochem. (Tokyo),* 76:123–131.

77. Sweeney, L. J., Clark, W. A., Umeda, P. K., Zak, R., and Manasek, F. J. (1984): Immunofluorescence analysis of the primordial myosin detectable in embryonic striated muscle. *Proc. Natl. Acad. Sci. USA,* 81:797–800.

78. Whalen, R. G., Butler-Browne, G. S., and Gros, F. (1978): Identification of a novel form of myosin light chain present in embryonic muscle tissue and cultured muscle cells. *J. Mol. Biol.,* 126:415–431.

79. Weeds, A. G. (1976): Light chains from slow-twitch muscle myosin. *Eur. J. Biochem.,* 66:157–173.

80. Frank, G., and Weeds, A. G. (1974): The amino acid sequence of the alkali light chains of rabbit skeletal muscle myosin. *Eur. J. Biochem.,* 44:317–334.

81. Westwood, S. A., and Perry, S. V. (1982): Two forms of the P light chain of myosin in rabbit and bovine hearts. *FEBS Lett.,* 142:31–34.

82. Wikman-Coffelt, J., and Srivastava, S. (1979): Differences in atrial and ventricular myosin light chain LC₁. *FEBS Lett.*, 106: 207–212.

83. Matsuda, G., Maita, T., Kato, Y., Chen, J. I., and Unegane, T. (1981): Amino acid sequences of the cardiac L-2A and gizzard 17,000 M_r light chains of chicken muscle myosin. *FEBS Lett.*, 135:232–236.

84. Cummins, P. (1982): Transitions in human atrial and ventricular myosin light chain isoenzymes in response to cardiac-pressure-overload-induced hypertrophy. *Biochem. J.*, 205:195–204.

85. Nabeshima, Y. I., Fujii-Kuriyama, Y., Muramatsu, M., and Ogata, K. (1984): Alternative transcription and two modes of splicing result in two myosin light chains from one gene. *Nature*, 308:333–338.

86. Periasamy, M., Strehler, E. E., Garfinkel, L. I., Gubits, R. M., Ruiz-Opazo, N., and Nadal-Ginard, B. (1984): Fast skeletal muscle myosin light chain 1 and 3 are produced from a single gene by a combined process of differential RNA transcription and splicing. *J. Biol. Chem.*, 259:13595–13604.

87. Winter, B., Klapthor, H., Wiebauer, K., Delius, H., and Arnold, H. H. (1985): Isolation and characterization of the chicken cardiac myosin light chain (L-2A) gene. *J. Biol. Chem.*, 260: 4478–4483.

88. Korn, E. D. (1978): Biochemistry of actomyosin-dependent cell motility (a review). *Proc. Natl. Acad. Sci. USA*, 75:588–599.

89. Potter, J. D. (1974): Content of troponin, tropomyosin, actin and myosin in rabbit-skeletal muscle myofibrils. *Arch. Biochem. Biophys.*, 162:436–441.

90. Vandekerckhove, J., and Weber, K. (1978): At least six different actins are expressed in a higher mammal: Analysis based on the amino-acid sequence of the amino-terminal tryptic peptide. *J. Mol. Biol.*, 126:783–802.

91. Ng, R., and Abelson, J. (1980): Isolation and sequence of the gene for actin in *Saccharomyces cerevisiae. Proc. Natl. Acad. Sci. USA*, 77:3912–3916.

92. Humphries, S. E., Whittall, R., Minty, A., Buckingham, M., and Williamson, R. (1981): There are approximately 20 actin genes in the human genome. *Nucleic Acids Res.*, 9:4895–4908.

93. Leavitt, J., Gunning, P., Porreca, P., Ng, S. Y., Lin, C. S., and Kedes, L. (1984): Molecular cloning and characterization of mutant and wild-type human β-actin genes. *Mol. Cell. Biol.*, 4: 1961–1969.

94. Billeter, R., Heizmann, C. W., Reist, U., Howald, H., and Jenny, E. (1981): α- and β-tropomyosin in typed single fibers of human skeletal muscle. *FEBS Lett.*, 132:133–136.

95. Heeley, D. H., Dhott, G. K., Frearson, N., Perry, S. V., and Vrbova, G. (1983): The effect of cross-innervation on the tropomyosin composition of rabbit skeletal muscle. *FEBS Lett.*, 152: 282–286.

96. Heeley, D. H., Dhoot, G. K., and Perry, S. V. (1985): Factors determining the subunit composition of tropomyosin in mammalian skeletal muscle. *Biochem. J.*, 226:461–468.

97. Mak, A. S., Lewis, W. G., and Smillie, L. B. (1979): Amino acid sequences of rabbit skeletal β and cardiac tropomyosins. *FEBS Lett.*, 105:232–234.

98. Fine, R. E., and Blitz, A. L. (1975): A chemical comparison of tropomyosins from muscle and non-muscle tissues. *J. Mol. Biol.*, 95:447–454.

99. Cummins, P., and Perry, S. V. (1974): Chemical and immunochemical characterization of tropomyosins from striated and smooth muscle. *Biochem. J.*, 141:43–49.

100. Bautch, V. L., and Storti, R. V. (1983): Identification of a cytoplasmic tropomyosin gene linked to two muscle tropomyosin genes in *Drosophila. Proc. Natl. Acad. Sci. USA*, 80:7123–7127.

101. Ruiz-Opazo, N., Weinberger, J., and Nadal-Ginard, B. (1985): Comparison of α-tropomyosin sequences from smooth and striated muscle. *Nature*, 315:67–70.

102. Syska, H., Perry, S. V., and Trayer, I. P. (1974): A new method of preparation of troponin I (inhibitory protein) using affinity chromatography: Evidence for three different forms of troponin I in striated muscle. *FEBS Lett.*, 40:253–257.

103. Wilkinson, J. M. (1980): Troponin from rabbit slow skeletal and cardiac muscles is the product of a single gene. *Eur. J. Biochem.*, 103:179–188.

104. Dhoot, G. K., Frearson, N., and Perry, S. V. (1979): Polymorphic forms of troponin T and troponin C and their localization in striated muscle cell types. *Exp. Cell. Res.*, 122:339–350.

105. Medford, R. M., Nguyen, H. T., Destree, A. T., Summers, E., and Nadal-Ginard, B. (1984): A novel mechanism of alternative RNA splicing for the developmentally regulated generation of troponin-T isoforms from a single gene. *Cell* 38:409–421.

106. Breitbart, R. E., Nguyen, H. T., Medford, R. M., Destree, A. T., Mahdavi, V., and Nadal-Ginard, B. (1985): Intricate combinatorial patterns of exon splicing generate multiple regulated troponin-T isoforms from a single gene. *Cell*, 41:67–82.

107. Sinha, A. M., Umeda, P. K., Kavinsky, C. J., Rajamanickam, C., Hsu, H.-J., Jakovcic, S., and Rabinowitz, M. (1982): Molecular cloning of mRNA sequences for cardiac α and β myosin heavy chains; expression in ventricles of normal, hypothyroid and thyrotoxic rabbits. *Proc. Natl. Acad. Sci. USA*, 79:5847–5851.

108. Sinha, A. M., Friedman, D. J., Nigro, J. M., Jakovcic, S., Rabinowitz, M., and Umeda, P. K. (1984): Expression of rabbit ventricular α-myosin heavy chain messenger RNA sequences in atrial muscle. *J. Biol. Chem.*, 259:6674–6680.

109. Lompre, A.-M., Nadal-Ginard, B., and Mahdavi, V. (1984): Expression of the cardiac ventricular α- and β-myosin heavy chain genes is developmentally and hormonally regulated. *J. Biol. Chem.*, 259:6437–6446.

110. Everett, A. W., Sinha, A. M., Umeda, P. K., Jakovcic, S., Rabinowitz, M., and Zak, R. (1984): Regulation of myosin synthesis by thyroid hormone: Relative change in the α- and β-myosin heavy chain mRNA levels in rabbit heart. *Biochemistry*, 23:1596–1599.

111. Konkel, D. A., Maizel, J. V., and Leder, P. (1979): The evolution and sequence comparison of two recently diverged mouse chromosomal β-globin gene. *Cell*, 18:865–873.

112. Mayer, Y., Czosnek, H., Zeelon, P. E., Yaffe, D., and Nudel, U. (1984): Expression of the genes coding for the skeletal muscle and cardiac actins in the heart. *Nucleic Acids Res.*, 12:1087–1100.

113. Orkin, S. H., and Goff, S. C. (1981): The duplicated human α-globin genes: Their relative expression as measured by RNA analysis. *Cell*, 24:245–345.

114. Sinha, A. M., Everett, A. W., Umeda, P. K., Zak, R., Jakovcic, S., and Rabinowitz, M. (1982): Developmental expression of mRNAs for α and β rabbit ventricular myosin heavy chains using cloned cDNA probes. *Circ.* 66:II-259.

115. Kavinsky, C. J., Umeda, P. K., Levin, J. E., Sinha, A. M., Nigro, J. M., Jakovcic, S., and Rabinowitz, M. (1984): Analysis of cloned mRNA sequences encoding subfragment 2 and part of subfragment 1 of α- and β-myosin heavy chains of rabbit heart. *J. Biol. Chem.*, 259:2775–2781.

116. Hoh, J. F. Y., and Egerton, L. J. (1979): Action of triiodothyronine on the synthesis of rat ventricular myosin isoenzymes. *FEBS Lett.*, 101:143–148.

117. Umeda, P. K., Levin, J. E., Sinha, A. M., Cribbs, L. L., Darling, D. S., Ende, D. J., Hsu, H.-J., Dizon, E., and Jakovcic, S. (1986): Molecular anatomy of cardiac myosin heavy chain genes. In: *Molecular Biology of Muscle Development 1985*, edited by C. Emerson, D. Fischman, B. Nadal-Ginard, and M. A. Q. Siddiqui. Alan R. Liss, Inc., New York.

118. Spindler, S. R., Mellon, S. H., and Baxter, J. D. (1982): Growth hormone gene transcription is regulated by thyroid and glucocorticoid hormones in cultured rat pituitary tumor cells. *J. Biol. Chem.*, 257:11627–11632.

119. Karn, J., Brenner, S., and Barnett, L. (1983): Protein structural domains in the *Caenorhabditis elegans* unc-54 myosin heavy chain gene are not separated by introns. *Proc. Natl. Acad. Sci. USA*, 80:4253–4257.

120. Bernstein, S. I., Mogami, K., Donady, J. J., and Emerson, C. P., Jr. (1983): *Drosophila* muscle myosin heavy chain encoded by a single gene in a cluster of muscle mutations. *Nature*, 302:393–397.

121. Rozek, C. E., and Davidson, N. (1983): *Drosophila* has one myosin heavy-chain gene with three developmentally regulated transcripts. *Cell*, 32:23–34.

122. Nudel, U., Katcoff, D., Carmon, Y., Zevin-Sonkin, D., Levi, Z., Shaul, Y., Shani, M., and Yaffe, D. (1980): Identification of

recombinant phages containing sequences from different rat myosin heavy chain genes. *Nucleic Acids Res.,* 8:2133–2146.

123. Mahdavi, V., Chambers, A. P., and Nadal-Ginard, B. (1984): Cardiac α- and β-myosin heavy chain genes are organized in tandem. *Proc. Natl. Acad. Sci. USA,* 81:2626–2630.

124. Friedman, D. J., Umeda, P. K., Sinha, A. M., Hsu, H.-J., Jakovcic, S., and Rabinowitz, M. (1984): Characterization of genomic clones specifying rabbit α- and β-ventricular myosin heavy chains. *Proc. Natl. Acad. Sci. USA,* 81:3044–3048.

125. Appelhans, H., and Vosberg, H. P. (1983): Characterization of a human genomic DNA fragment coding for a myosin heavy chain. *Hum. Genet.,* 65:198–203.

126. Leinwand, L. A., Saez, L., McNally, E., and Nadal-Ginard, B. (1983): Isolation and characterization of human myosin heavy chain genes. *Proc. Natl. Acad. Sci. USA,* 80:3716–3720.

127. Efstratiadis, A., Posakony, J. W., Maniatis, T., Lawn, R. M., O'Connell, C., Spritz, R. A., DeRiel, J. K., Forget, B. G., Weisman, S. M., Slightom, J. L., Blechl, A. E., Smithies, O., Baralle, F. E., Shoulders, C. C., and Proudfoot, N. J. (1980): The structure and evolution of the human β-globin gene family. *Cell,* 21:653–668.

128. Strehler, E. E., Mahdavi, V., Periasamy, M., and Nadal-Ginard, B. (1985): Intron positions are conserved in the 5′ end region of myosin heavy-chain genes. *J. Biol. Chem.,* 260:468–471.

129. Barta, A., Richards, R. I., Baxter, J. D., and Shine, J. (1981): Primary structure and evolution of rat growth hormone gene. *Proc. Natl. Acad. Sci. USA,* 78:4867–4871.

130. Weiher, H., Konig, M., and Gruss, P. (1983): Multiple point mutations affecting the simian virus 40 enhancer. *Science,* 219: 626–631.

The Heart and Cardiovascular System,
edited by H. A. Fozzard et al.
Raven Press, New York © 1986.

CHAPTER **47**

Cardiogenesis: Developmental Mechanisms and Embryology

Francis J. Manasek, Jose Icardo, Atsuyo Nakamura, and Lauren Sweeney

Cardiac morphogenesis has been studied extensively using a variety of anatomical techniques, and many of the major events of developmental anatomy have been described, at least to the level of the light microscope. Although there is still much descriptive morphological work that can be done, especially at the ultrastructural level, major advances in understanding developmental mechanisms probably will not result solely from morphological studies. Indeed, the level of understanding of shape that can be derived solely from studying shape is very limited. It is our firm belief that shape, and the development of shape, can be understood only in mechanistic terms and that the regulators of shape generation are ultimately to be found at the level of gene expression. Consequently, we need to understand the control of gene expression as well as the assembly of gene products into larger units. In essence, we argue that there is a biochemical basis for anatomic shape and that the biochemistry underlying even relatively complex morphogenic events can be discerned. We do not imply that there is simple causality. Rather, it is recognized that anatomic shape is the product of an integration of lower-order events. Clearly, there must be a series of links between biological shape and cell activity functions, and we are confident that it will be possible to discern these links.

Much of the present chapter will attempt to present cardiogenesis as a dynamic sequence of events, and we shall attempt to emphasize mechanisms wherever possible. In writing this chapter we have the optimistic feeling that we are tantalizingly close to understanding some of the basic mechanisms regulating major events of early heart development but that we are, in most cases, still far from understanding the connection between the genome and much of the shape of the heart. We simply do not know which genes have possible morphoregulatory functions and how their products might interact to produce a reproducible biological shape. We believe that a major conceptual block has been the virtual absence of falsifiable mechanistic hypotheses. We still do not know what questions to ask for many events of heart development. We have tried to keep this in mind while writing this chapter, and we have tried to place, as much as possible, anatomic events in a dynamic and mechanistic perspective.

EARLY EMBRYOLOGY OF HEART CELLS

The development of the embryonic heart begins long before any evidence of cardiac tissue can be recognized morphologically. The presence of cells with heart-forming capacity can be demonstrated throughout the blastula and gastrula stages by different methods. With the formation of the primitive streak and the beginning of gastrulation, prospective heart cells cluster progressively and become localized in a bilaterally paired area of the lateral mesoderm. By the stage of 3 to 4 somites, mesodermal cells group in the midregion of the cephalic portion of the splanchnic mesoderm, forming a crescent of cardiogenic material, the precardiac mesoderm (117,118,121,122). These precardiac mesodermal cells are cardiac myocyte precursors. Some cells sort out of the splanchnic mesoderm and form a loose cellular network between the endoderm and the precardiac mesoderm. This loose network organizes later into tubes, giving rise to the endocardium. Thus, when the heart anlage is first morphologically recognizable, it is a paired structure formed of premyocardial cells, preendocardial cells, and associated extracellular material. The subsequent fate of the heart primordium is linked inextricably to foregut formation. The precardiac areas are brought progressively toward the embryonic midline concomitant with the formation of the endodermal foregut. Once formed, the precardiac mesoderm migrates as a coherent sheet of cells that stretches and bends, but with the cells retaining their position relative to each other (138). However, preendocardial cells appear to migrate relatively free from each other in the endomesodermal space. They later organize into tubes that are connected cranially with the primitive aortic roots and caudally with the veins entering the heart.

Little is known of the mechanisms that regulate the migration of the pre-heart cells and their progressive localization within the cardiogenic crescent. It was suggested that the endodermal basal surface might provide directional information for the migration of precardiac mesoderm (27). The basal surface of the endoderm is very rich in fibronectin (56), and the precardiac mesoderm could be using this fibronectin to migrate on the endoderm. However, evidence to confirm this suggestion has not been attained to date (70). The migration of the preendocardial cells could also be oriented by the glycoprotein content of the endodermal basal surface (56), but, again, no direct experimental proof is yet available. Another possible explanation of the progressive clustering of the pre-heart cells is that these cells may undergo changes in cell surface properties that make them aggregate, sort out, and differentiate histotypically. Embryonic chick heart cells in vitro show changes in intercellular adhesion characteristics with age (3). However, the possibility of a similar phenomenon occurring during the formation of the cardiogenic crescent in vivo remains

speculative. The continued migration toward the embryonic midline brings the paired primordia together; they contact each other and fuse. The fusion of the paired anlage takes place along the longitudinal embryonic axis and results in the formation of a single tubular structure that is the beginning of the tubular heart (113).

In chicks, the premyocytes are histologically undifferentiated prior to formation of the tubular heart. After the heart tube forms, beating begins and cardiac function is established. In rodents and possibly other mammals, differentiation and tube formation are not separate events. The beginning of beating is related structurally to the first appearance of myofibrils in the myocyte cytoplasm. Myofibrils, initially consisting of only a few sarcomeres, are at first scattered. As the embryo grows and beating becomes well established, myocytes become progressively filled with myofibrils (77), indicating a rapid increase in accumulation of contractile proteins. Although early fibrils may appear to be aligned randomly when examined by the electron microscope, recent work (106) has shown that they form a regular pattern with respect to the tubular heart. The arrangement of myofibrils may be very important in later morphogenesis. Moreover, myofibrillogenesis seems to be necessary for normal morphogenesis. Recent work has focused on the expression of contractile proteins in embryonic striated muscle, particularly in later heart development. This problem, as related to myosin expression during early heart development, is explored in the next section.

Acquisition of Cardiac Muscle Phenotype as Determined by Expression of Contractile Protein Isoforms

An integral component of cardiac differentiation is the development of myocardial contractility. This requires the coordinated expression of the muscle-specific contractile proteins and their organization into myofibrils. The developing heart expresses muscle-specific contractile proteins in organized myofibrils from early stages of cardiac looping (77). The myocardium at these stages is morphologically homogeneous (75), but already has different intrinsic rates of contraction in the future ventricular, atrial, and sinus venosus regions (153a). As these regions of the heart become differentiated morphologically, they undergo changes in function. The biochemical status of the myocardium in response to these functional changes is largely unknown.

Very little investigation has been done on the contractile protein phenotype of the embryonic heart during these very early stages of organogenesis. Because different forms of contractile proteins are associated in the adult with different functional capabilities (5,15), transitions in genetic expression of these isoforms in the embryonic heart could provide an important biochemical basis for cardiac development.

Contractile Protein Phenotype of the Adult Heart

The myocardium of the adult vertebrate atrium and that in the ventricle have different contractile characteristics that are associated with the expression of different contractile protein isoforms, principally those of myosin (26,160). Furthermore, the myosin phenotype is altered in abnormal physiologic and hormonal states (19,25, 49,167). The other contractile proteins (actin, tropomyosin, and troponin T, I, and C) have been shown to have cardiac- and skeletal-muscle-specific forms, but no differences have been found between the forms expressed in the atria and ventricles (24,31,36,161,162).

With respect to myosin, variations in isomyosin composition can occur at all levels of myocardial organization. Individual myocytes can express more than one myosin simultaneously (125,127). Myocytes singly or in groups can have a myosin composition that differs from the surrounding myocardium (49,126). In some cases these differences may represent distinctions between specialized conduction tissue and surrounding myocardium (40,146). There can also be gradients in myosin expression from endocardial to epicardial surfaces of the ventricle (33,126), as well as differences in myosin expression between left and right ventricles and atria (40,143).

Isomyosins differ in both their heavy-chain (HC) and light-chain (LC) subunit compositions. The expression of different myosin IIC subunits is correlated with biochemical differences in the enzymatic Ca^{2+}-activated ATPase activity of myosins (19), while the presence of different LC subunits does not seem to alter these properties (20). Recent evidence suggests that the two HC subunits that are expressed in ventricular myosins, designated HC_α and HC_β (49,50), are similar to, if not identical with, the HCs expressed in atrial myosins (20,25,40,133). The HC_α has a twofold to threefold greater level of ATPase activity than the more efficient HC_β (166). This difference, in turn, helps determine functional differences (speed of contraction) and electrophysiologic differences (shape of the action potential) between cardiac isomyosins (15,128,130,160). Unlike myosin HC expression, however, the LCs expressed in cardiac isomyosins are specific to either atria or ventricles (116).

A slower isoform, containing exclusively HC_β, is the predominant myosin expressed in the ventricles of most species (V_3) (72), while a faster isoform, containing exclusively HC_α, predominates in the atria (A_1, Table 1). This is true for man and for frequently used experimental animals such as the chicken (22). Other animals (in particular, smaller mammals with high metabolic

TABLE 1. *Cardiac contractile proteins*

Myosin: cardiac HC and LC subunits
  Ventricle
    $V_1 = (HC_\alpha)_2 (LC_{1V})_2 (LC_{2V})_2$
    $V_2 = (HC_\alpha HC_\beta) (LC_{1V})_2 (LC_{2V})_2$
    *$V_3 = (HC_\beta)_2^* (LC_{1V})_2 (LC_{2V})_2$
  Atrium
    *$A_1 = (HC_\alpha)_2 (LC_{1A})_2^* (LC_{2A})_2$
    $A_2 = (HC_\beta)_2 (LC_{1A})_2^* (LC_{2A})_2$
Actin
  *α cardiac
Tropomyosin
  *α = cardiac, fast skeletal
Troponin T, I, C subunits
  *T cardiac
  +I cardiac
  *C cardiac

Note: Asterisk indicates cardiac isoforms expressed in embryonic skeletal muscle; plus sign indicates skeletal isoform expressed in embryonic cardiac muscle

rates, such as the rat, mouse, and rabbit) express the V_3 isoform in the ventricle of the embryo and in old age, but express a faster form, V_1, containing exclusively HC_α, as well as an intermediate V_2 form ($HC_\alpha HC_\beta$) in the ventricle of the neonate and young adult (22,49, 50,72). Experimental work has shown that species whose intrinsic genetic program includes expression of more than one myosin in the ventricle are often converted to expression of a different isomyosin under a number of altered physiologic conditions. For example, hyperthyroidism induces a shift to V_1, while hypertrophy and pressure overload induce a shift to V_3 (19,25,134,167). Atrial myosin expression, on the other hand, seems to be less responsive to functional challenges in all animals studied (20). The one interesting exception to this may well be the human atrium, which shifts toward expression of A_2 myosin (containing exclusively HC_β) in atrial hypertrophy induced by mitral valve obstruction (129).

Myosin Phenotype of the Embryonic Heart

All evidence suggests that the embryonic ventricle expresses the slower, V_3, isoform of myosin regardless of the type expressed later in the adult ventricle (72). The exact stage at which transitions to neonatal or adult forms is made is not yet clear, nor has the full range of myosin types expressed in most species during embryonic development been investigated.

Embryonic skeletal muscle expresses myosin subunits unique to the embryonic state (37,74,150,159). However, there is no evidence that cardiac muscle expresses any unique embryonic myosin subunits. The myosin HCs expressed initially in the embryonic chick atrium include the adult atrial myosin (HC_α) (39), but we have found that they also appear to include ventricular myosin HC$_\beta$ (142).

A myosin heavy chain with the same immunological properties as cardiac ventricular heavy chain is the earliest HC form detectable in the chick. It is expressed at the initial stages of muscle-specific myosin expression in all forms of striated muscle, thus making the ventricular isoform a "primordial" muscle myosin (141).

Expression of HC$_\beta$ gradually ceases in the atrium. By the time the mature four-chambered configuration is acquired, atrial expression of this myosin HC has stopped. Further, a myosin HC with the same immunological properties as this ventricular myosin is also expressed in the earliest somite stages of skeletal muscle development in the chick and is present through a long period of embryonic development (141). Evidence has also shown that both cultured and regenerating skeletal muscles express a myosin with cardiac immunological properties (14,41) as part of a reversion to the embryonic contractile protein phenotype (4).

This evidence has led to a revision of earlier concepts of myosin expression in developing muscle, which suggested that all muscle initially expressed all myosin types and became restricted to expression of "appropriate" myosins only with development (98). It appears that differentiation may trigger the expression of cardiac ventricular (V$_3$) myosin HC in all striated muscle, which later becomes repressed in skeletal muscle and the atrium. Work is now under way to characterize this primordial myosin fully and to determine the timing of its expression in different muscle types as a possible clue to understanding the normal factors involved in its expression. Further, analysis of the expression of primordial myosin in the cardiac chambers of species such as the mouse and rat, which express several myosins in the ventricle, will determine how widespread this pattern is. When this evidence is combined with recent studies on embryonic myosin LC, actin, and troponin expression, it appears that cardiac forms of all these contractile proteins are expressed in skeletal muscle during its embryonic development (Table 1) (13,112,148,158). This suggests that the initial muscle-specific genetic program includes the expression of the cardiac muscle phenotype.

Techniques of Contractile Protein Analysis

A number of technical approaches have been used to provide the analyses of contractile protein expression described earlier. Biochemical and immunochemical techniques have been invaluable in determining the identity of myosin from bulk tissue. The biochemical methods employed include determination of the molecular weight (MW) and charge of the whole molecule by means of its electrophoretic mobility on acrylamide gels (native gel electrophoresis), analysis of the MW of separated subunits under denaturing conditions on SDS-polyacrylamide gels, and analysis of peptide fragments produced by proteolytic cleavage of myosin in one-dimensional or two-dimensional gel electrophoresis (19,22,49,74,159).

Amino acid sequences can be determined for the smaller contractile protein forms such as myosin LC subunits and actin, and for selected regions of the larger molecules such as myosin HC subunits. Techniques include determining the extent of sequence homology between mRNAs and cDNA probes from known myosins by S$_1$ nuclease mapping (112,133,150,162).

The enzymatic activity of the myosin molecule, and specifically its HC subunits, can be determined by measuring its calcium- or actin-activated ATPase activity (40,128,143,146).

Immunofluorescence localization with well-characterized antibodies to specific contractile protein isoforms has become a powerful tool in assessing the regional and cellular distributions of isomyosins (37,41,141,148). It is also a particularly sensitive technique for detecting minor myosin species that can go undetected with some biochemical techniques. Moreover, immunofluorescence techniques are invaluable in detecting patterns of contractile protein expression in embryonic tissues. Not only do the minute volumes of embryonic heart tissue make carrying out a number of biochemical procedures virtually impossible, but extraction of purified myosin from embryonic muscle is often much more difficult than from adult material. Immunochemical techniques utilizing antibodies include competitive radioimmunoassay (RIA), which determines the relative affinity of a test myosin for the antibody in comparison with the affinity of a known myosin for the same antibody (19,21). Immunoblot analysis allows determination of the peptide fragments of myosin that stain with peroxidase-labeled myosin antibody.

In addition to all of these tools used to characterize the myosin content of the normal myocardium, experimental techniques have been developed to subject the heart *in vivo* to different hormonal, pressure, and electrophysiologic conditions. Culture techniques have been employed to test the effect of alterations of some of these same parameters *in vitro*. These techniques have only recently been applied to the embryonic heart to study the changes in myosin isoforms they may induce.

Future Challenges

The work done in recent years on myosin expression has generated as many questions as it has answered concerning the nature of the intrinsic genetic program for myosin expression and the degree to which it is affected at all stages of development by extrinsic phenomena. In embryonic skeletal muscle, for example, there is a whole series of myosin isoform changes that occur prior to any demonstrable functional changes.

Embryonic cardiac ventricular muscle, which undergoes continuous functional changes during its development, expresses only one myosin in many species.

Further, it appears from our work on the chick that the atrium shows a greater variability in myosin expression during development than does the ventricle, which is in contrast to the known greater flexibility of response of the adult ventricle to extrinsic stimuli. Clearly, the biologic reason for the expression of many different myosins may be related to factors other than simple changes in overt muscle function, and many more questions can be raised. Why do adult cardiac myocytes, which are functionally (electrogenically) coupled, express different myosin isoforms in individual adjacent cells, or in gradients across the myocardial wall? What function is served by the expression of several different isoforms simultaneously within the same myocyte? Why are some regions of the adult and neonatal heart (ventricles) more able to alter their myosin composition than others (atria)?

CARDIAC EXTRACELLULAR MATRIX

Cells produce and excrete a number of products that are incorporated into their surroundings and create their immediate environment. In addition to water and ions, the structural constituents of connective tissues are generally grouped into four types: collagen, glycosaminoglycans, noncollagenous glycoproteins, and elastin.

While the nature and the properties of connective tissues depend primarily on the molecular properties, composition, and organization of their components, the type of connective tissue depends on the cell types that produce it. Thus, the properties and the influences of connective tissues on cells change temporally and spatially with alterations in cellular physiology and biochemistry. Such changes in the interactions between the cells and their environment are essential for embryonic development of multicellular organisms.

In addition to becoming overt, functional cardiac muscle, the embryonic myocardium has at least one other major function; it produces the bulk of the early heart's extracellular matrix (76,79,80). Indeed, evidence suggests that myocardial cells *in vitro* can respond to the matrix molecules they synthesize (89).

Embryonic Cardiac Connective Tissue

The cardiac jelly is the extracellular matrix of the early embryonic vertebrate heart and makes up the bulk of space located between the developing myocardium and endocardium. It is produced largely by the myocardium (81). The cardiac jelly layer undergoes extensive modifications as the heart transforms into a four-chambered organ. In this process, most of the cardiac jelly layer becomes part of the subendocardial connective

tissue of the adult heart. However, the subepicardial connective tissue, the true connective tissue of the myocardium, and vascular adventitia (77,78) are formed separately as mesenchymal cells invade the heart.

Components of the Cardiac Jelly

It has been recognized that most of the major components of connective tissues are present in the cardiac jelly and that they are possibly different both qualitatively and quantitatively from those found in adult connective tissue.

Matrix composition has been determined primarily by ultrastructural, autoradiographic, or histochemical studies, or by limited synthetic analysis of components. Although it is possible to distinguish in the cardiac jelly the major classes of connective tissue components, relatively little is known about their molecular heterogeneity. The main reason for this difficulty is the minute size of the developing heart, which does not provide enough material to readily allow detailed chemical or structural analysis. This is extremely unfortunate, because such structural diversity may be related specifically to the various developmental processes.

Collagen

There are at least five, and possibly more, genetically distinct collagen types (12,71,132). They are designated types I to V and type I trimer, and they have different alpha polypeptide chains. Types I, II, and III usually appear as interstitial fibrillar forms and are called "interstitial collagen." Type IV is localized in basal laminae and is a collageneous protein with a different amino acid composition and slightly larger than the interstitial collagens (60). Type IV collagen does not have a fibrillar form and is believed to be arranged in a three-dimensional network (147). Type V has an amino acid composition similar to type IV and is often localized in basal lamina of certain types of cells (97,119), but also can have a fibrillar form (47,155,156). These different types of collagens have more or less distinct distributions among animal tissues and organs.

In the past few years, immunohistochemical and immunocytochemical techniques became available to identify and detect even very small amounts of collagen *in situ*. The major limitations here are the specificity of antibody and the preservation and the availability of antigenic sites after sample preparation. Purified polyclonal antibodies and monoclonal antibodies appear to overcome those limitations well when they are used in conjunction with enzymatic unmasking of antigenic sites. The greatest advantages of these techniques are not only visualization of collagens in association with other histologic structures *in situ* but also the possibility of following the temporal and spatial changes in the distribution of the different collagen types that occur associated with cardiac developmental events.

In the chick embryo heart, the earliest (day 2 of development) type of collagen detected biochemically is type I (59). It is not clear when type IV collagen begins to appear, but by the third day of development the rate of type IV collagen synthesis already reaches its peak and gradually decreases thereafter, suggesting the presence of considerable amounts of this type of collagen (144). In contrast to the biochemical studies, an indirect immunofluorescence study revealed that type IV collagen is the earliest collagen to appear in the mouse embryo heart (68). This collagen lines the basal surfaces of endocardium and myocardium by the eighth day, which is equivalent to about stage 9 to 10 in the chick embryo. The discrepancy between the cardiac biochemical work and the immunofluorescence studies could be due to species differences, but is equally likely the result of different techniques used. The appearance of type IV is followed within a day by the appearance of types I and III, with a distribution pattern similar to that of type IV.

In these early developing tubular hearts, types I, III, and IV collagens all appear within basal lamina of myocardium and endocardium. This is unusual, because type I and type III are interstitial collagens and appear as fibrillar forms in older embryos or in adults. The localization of types I and III collagens in the basal lamina of young embryonic hearts may suggest that types I, III, and IV may be real structural components of early basal laminae. This possibility seems to be substantiated by an ultrastructural study showing that collagenous microfibrils began to appear within or associated with electron-dense basal lamina material (59,73).

As the heart develops further and the myocardium is invaded by mesenchymal cells, types I and III collagens become the major collagens of the heart. This was shown both by biochemical extraction methods (7,34,100,144) and by immunohistochemical studies (11,154). Although the presence of type V was confirmed by immunohistochemical techniques (47,154), alpha-1 (I) trimer has not been localized so far. Morris and McClain (102) found alpha chains very similar to those of type II in bovine heart valves; however, Hendrix (47) was unable to find type II collagen with immunohistochemical technique in the 12-day chick embryo heart and in the 16-week human embryo heart. This discrepancy may again indicate species differences, or perhaps that type II collagen appears in valves much later in development.

In the postnatal rat heart, collagen changes quantitatively, but not qualitatively. Types III and I are the predominant types in myocardial endomysium and perimysium, with the same distribution (11). Similar results were also obtained with human hearts (154). Anti-type-IV antibody stains the surfaces of myocytes (presumably

their basal laminae), and type V is localized primarily around the blood vessels (11).

Thus, all types of collagens seem to appear in the normal heart during its morphogenic development. Types I and IV collagens appear very early, but types I and III collagen eventually become the major types in later embryonic and adult heart. These changes may be significant for heart morphogenesis, but their exact roles in development are not understood at the present time. The anatomic distribution of collagen fibrils, together with other components of connective tissue, undergoes significant changes with age. They form a complex interconnected system suspected to have important physiological functions.

At later stages of embryonic life, each myocyte becomes invested by a basal lamina and is associated with some collagen fibrils. However, a well-developed fiber system does not appear to be present. After birth, the rat heart gradually develops a complex matrix fiber network that reaches maturity in its complexity at about 15 days post partum (10). Collagen fibrils appear to organize into several distinct structures. Fine bundles of collagen fibrils, "struts," bridge the lateral surfaces of cells. The struts course from myocyte to myocyte or from myocyte to capillary endothelial cells. A "weave" pattern of collagen fibers also develops, separating myocytes into groups and anchoring myocytes through a number of struts. Larger, longer, tendonlike collagen fiber bundles binding neighboring collagen weaves complete the interconnecting system of the entire myocardium. The postnatal organization of the collagen fiber network is thought to be somehow related to the functional changes that the heart undergoes during postnatal development.

During this period the systemic blood pressure rises dramatically, and the cardiac output also increases significantly (51). Consequently, the heart wall needs to be modified so that such physiological changes can be accommodated. The intermyocytic struts and the basal-lamina-associated fine microfibrils appear to prevent "slippage" between myocytes within a weave and participate in the transmission of tension generated by myocytes even when intercalated discs are experimentally disassociated (16,163). Intermyocytic struts are in a relaxed state during systole, but the struts between myocytes and capillaries appear to be in tension. The reverse is true during diastole. It was suggested that the myocyte-capillary struts maintain the capillaries open during systole to ensure uninterrupted blood flow against high wall pressure during contraction (16). The development of collagen weave is believed to provide the myocardium with the required rigidity for maintenance of shape and integrity of the heart wall under increased luminal pressure. In the presence of the lathyritic agent beta-aminopropionitrile (BAPN), which inhibits cross-linking of collagen molecules, collagen weave fails to form, and the heart develops aneurysms and eventually ruptures (9). In addition, this weave pattern of collagen fibers is thought to provide viscoelastic properties even though the collagen fiber itself is not viscoelastic (16).

Glycosaminoglycans

Glycosaminoglycans (GAGs) are a major component of extracellular matrices and are distributed throughout animal connective tissues. GAGs are long linear molecules with the repeating disaccharide unit (hexuronic acid–hexosamine). They are classified according to the kind of hexuronic acid (glucuronic acid or iduronic acid), hexosamine (N-acetyl glucosamine or N-acetyl galactosamine), position and degree of sulfation within the repeating unit, the mode of linkages between hexose units, and the size of molecules. GAGs are hyaluronic acid (HA), chondroitin-4-sulfate (CH4-S), chondroitin-6-sulfate (CH6-S), dermatan sulfate (DS), keratan sulfate (KS), heparan sulfate (HS)/heparin (H). All of these, except HA, appear in vivo as proteoglycans in which more than one GAG molecule is attached noncovalently to a common core protein. A number of these proteoglycan monomers attach noncovalently to HA, with the attachment site on one end of the core protein. This noncovalent bond is stabilized by two link proteins (62,63). This HA-proteoglycan complex forms an extremely large three-dimensional aggregate.

Each disaccharide unit of GAGs contains one or more carboxyl or sulfate groups and is ionized at physiological conditions. Therefore, the proteoglycan complex is not only a large three-dimensional network but also a highly negatively charged one. These negatively charged groups repulse each other, so that the complex tends to have a huge extended molecular configuration and domain. The negatively charged groups also attract and concentrate cations as counter-ions, which creates an osmotic pressure to hydrate. These physicochemical properties of proteoglycans may exert tremendous physical influences on the cellular components of tissues and organs, especially in embryos (23).

The presence of acid mucopolysaccharides (acidic proteoglycans) in the cardiac jelly of early developing hearts has been demonstrated by histochemical, autoradiographic, and biochemical analysis. These studies have revealed that the GAG content of the cardiac jelly changes both quantitatively and qualitatively during heart development.

The cardiac jelly of early tubular hearts (H.H. stages 9–11) is rich in hyaluronate, chondroitin, and undersulfated chondroitin sulfate. However, by H.H. stage 11$^+$, fully sulfated chondroitin sulfate begins to appear and eventually becomes a major component (90). Histochemical techniques have also suggested the presence of minute amounts of strongly anionic sulfated GAGs (probably heparin, dermatan, or keratan sulfate) along

the basal surface of the myocardium at stage 11 (53). Similarly, the presence of a heparin-like proteoglycan was detected just prior to cushion tissue development (38).

Similar developmental changes occur in the cushion tissue, where cardiac jelly continues to enlarge even after it decreases rapidly in other parts of the heart. The major GAGs in the cushion are hyaluronate and chondroitin sulfate. However, the invading endocardial cushion cells appear to modify the ground substance from principally hyaluronate to primarily chondroitin sulfate as the cells migrate through (92). The sulfated GAGs are initially chondroitin sulfate A and C, but dermatan sulfate (chondroitin sulfate B) begins to appear later and becomes prominent as the embryo develops further (91). This trend appears to continue even after birth. Bulk compositional analysis of heart valves from young and old animals indicates that the relative amount of dermatan sulfate gradually increases with age (101). Thus, the cardiac GAGs appear to undergo a transition from primarily nonsulfated or low-sulfated GAGs (hyaluronate, chondroitin) to highly sulfated, strong anionic GAGs throughout life.

Although GAGs are basically simple repeating polymers of disaccharide units, they can form considerably diverse proteoglycan aggregates. Recent results suggest the presence of such diverse proteoglycans from different sources (32,42,58). Because we do not know the heterogeneity of heart proteoglycans, it is erroneous to dismiss such proteoglycan heterogeneities as developmentally insignificant. In fact, embryonic myocytes in vitro are capable of responding rapidly to environmental GAG concentration changes (89). Such changes could be effected by the production of closely related but different GAG aggregates. So far, no attempts have been made to determine possible heterogeneity. It may be possible to use immunological techniques for this, but extreme care should be exercised in the interpretation of immunological data for proteoglycans (61).

Glycoproteins

Glycoproteins are proteins with one or more covalently attached short sugar chains. Glycoproteins apparently appear very early in the developing heart (82). Biochemical characterization of early embryonic heart glycoproteins has been difficult, and isolation and characterization of individual glycoproteins have not been done. To date, only fibronectin has been identified unequivocally in the developing heart.

There are at least two types of fibronectin: plasma fibronectin and cell surface fibronectin (cellular fibronectin). They are antigenically and functionally very similar to each other; yet they are definitely different. For example, plasma fibronectin cannot functionally fully substitute cellular fibronectin. Both types of fibronectin appear to be products of two separate genes (1,164,165).

Fibronectin has two similar subunit polypeptide chains (A and B) that are covalently bound by disulfide bridges at or near the carboxylic terminals. Each subunit has several well-defined functional domains that bind to different ligands such as cells, heparin, and collagen. All of the observed biological functions of fibronectin are due to these discrete functional domains that make the molecule functionally divalent.

In the heart, the distribution of fibronectin seems to be associated with cellular movements or rearrangements prior to expression of their final phenotypic characteristics (56,57). It might be interesting to see if fibronectin is expressed when adult myocardium is damaged and fibroblastic reorganization takes place to form scar.

In chick embryo hearts, ^{3}H-fucose is rapidly incorporated into glycoproteins (45,82). Newly synthesized glycoproteins become progressively larger as the heart develops. These glycoproteins appear to be associated covalently or noncovalently with other structural components of the cardiac jelly to form extremely large aggregates, which are retained even by a large-pore filter (3–0.8 μm pore size) (83).

It is interesting to note that large proportions of the fucosylated glycoproteins of the early developing heart form large aggregates that are sensitive to testicular hyaluronidase (82,83). Some of this fucosylated glycoprotein could be similar to the one that is reported to be a specific hyaluronic-acid-binding glycoprotein (30).

Elastin

Late in embryonic development, elastic fibers become ultrastructurally identifiable in the heart. However, little is known about their time of production, source, and chemistry.

Anatomic Organization of Cardiac Jelly

Cardiac jelly is not a homogeneous gel. Rather, it contains a number of structural inclusions, such as fibrillar collagen, amorphous masses of electron-dense anionic material, and noncollagenous filaments. The distribution and orientation of such inclusions would be expected to influence profoundly the mechanical properties of the cardiac jelly, hence probably the shape of the heart.

In the tubular heart, a well-organized and readily demonstrable system of radially oriented filaments (extending from endocardium to myocardium) has been demonstrated by conventional histology and by transmission, as well as scanning electron microscopy (53,108,114). This matrical filamentous system is present and organized radically long before cushions form. The composition of these filaments is unclear; they are

sensitive to general proteases, but not to purified collagenase or hyaluronidase (105). Most likely their alignment is dependent on both the physical-chemical properties of the matrix and the geometry of the system.

The dorsal mesocardium region appears to be particularly rich in material that extends from the ventral floor of the foregut to the endocardium (54,59). This material, probably mostly glycoproteins, forms part of a complex longitudinal argyrophylic fiber system that extends along the length of the heart (Nakamura, *unpublished observation*), forming yet a second organized structural system within the cardiac matrix.

The myocardial basal lamina is initially incomplete. Its formation occurs first in the dorsal mesocardium region and only later extends to the rest of the myocardium (75).

Fibrillar collagen distribution and orientation have not been examined thoroughly for most stages. Early in tubular heart formation there is only a small amount of fibrillar collagen detectable, and it does not appear to have any particular regional distribution or orientation (76,77).

Cushion Tissue Formation

During development, cardiac jelly accumulates in specific regions such as the atrioventricular canal and the bulbus cordis, forming distinct structures that protrude into the cardiac lumen. These structures, the endocardial cushions, are the forerunners of septal and valvular structures (69,120). Many commonly observed congenital heart defects are related to abnormal development of cushion tissue (153).

Although the anatomical changes in the distribution of the cardiac jelly matrix are quite apparent, no clear explanation of these changes has been provided to date. The classic flow molding theories (6,18) suggested displacement of the cardiac jelly from zones of high hemodynamic stress to zones of low hemodynamic stress. Endocardial cushions would then develop in these low-pressure zones. These theories seem to be overly simplistic, and they do not account for the resistance that the viscous cardiac jelly would present to such a displacement.

Two important events occur during early cushion development: (a) regional thickening of acellular cardiac jelly and (b) invasion of these masses by mesenchyme derived from the endocardium. Little experimental work has been done on the mechanisms of regional matrix hypertrophy (see the later section on hemodynamics). Endocardium overlying these masses becomes "activated," and mesenchymatous progeny invade the matrix (94). These cells probably use the radially oriented matrix filaments as directional cues in their centrifugal migration (114). As they populate the cushion matrix, they apparently change the GAG composition (92), reducing the amount of hyaluronate and increasing the amount of chondroitin sulfate. Experimental studies *in vitro* suggest that hyaluronate and some proteinaceous components of the matrix stimulate mesenchyme to invade three-dimensional collagen gels (8,123). However, it appears that some developmental maturation of the endocardium is also necessary (124).

There is at this point little doubt that the cushion tissue (CT) cells interact closely with the matrical components of the cardiac jelly (35). It appears clear that the CT cells, like any other migrating mesenchymal cell, can modify the composition and organization of the external milieu through which they move. However, the precise role played by the cardiac jelly matrix in cushion development is still under investigation.

A distinctive feature of embryonic cell movements is their extraordinary directionality (149). It is clear that the environment through which cells move must exert some kind of influence on the migratory processes. However, we do not know yet how extracellular matrices provide directional information for cell migration. Contact guidance and chemotaxis (93,95) have been factors implicated in the control of directionality of CT cell migration. However, the demonstration *in vivo* of the existence of these controlling mechanisms has been, at least, ambiguous. Contrary to the reports that suggest a directing role for the cardiac jelly in CT cell migration, recent *in vitro* (Kinsella and Fitzharris, 1982) and *in vivo* (57) evidence supports the view that the CT cells may be able to control their own migratory behavior. Protraction and retraction of migratory appendages, combined with responses to other cells and to the substratum, may effectively direct the migration of the CT cells toward the myocardium (57). Thus, the cardiac jelly would play only a secondary role during the formation of endocardial cushion tissue. A full understanding of the complex interactions that occur between the migrating CT cells and the cardiac jelly matrix awaits further investigation.

Up to this point we have concerned ourselves largely with early developmental processes at the cell and tissue level, and with the development of the extracellular matrix. These events must, in our opinion, be linked, temporally and functionally, and be integrated in such a manner as to produce and regulate the overall anatomy of the heart. In other words, heart shape is a high-order integrated expression of these processes. This is difficult to prove, and the gaps between the reductionist data and the shape of the organ are enormous. In the ensuing sections we shall try to juxtapose ideas in such a way as to suggest possible links between cells, cell activities, and shape.

The morphogenic mechanisms that mold and shape the embryonic heart appear to be different in different periods of development. The initial events (establishment of the tubular heart) seem to be linked to the migration

of sheets of cells over an underlying matrix and their subsequent deformation, whereas much of later development involves migration of individual cells and subsequent remodeling of tissue masses (84).

During the formation of the heart rudiment, premyocardial splanchnic mesoderm moves bilaterally toward the embryonic midline as a continuous sheet of epithelial cells. Although it may be possible that there is some directional information in the underlying matrix that provides cues or signals that are read by the migrating sheet of cells, such directional signals may not be necessary.

MORPHOGENESIS OF THE HEART TUBE

To date there is no experimentally verified mechanism that has been shown to regulate any of the dramatic changes in shape that characterize the tubular heart during the processes of looping. Intuitively obvious mechanisms, such as differential cell division, do not appear to be of significance in tube morphogenesis (81,82,135,137), and others, such as "differential cell adhesion," are sufficiently vague and nonspecific to be experimentally meaningless. In the past several years our laboratory has been concerned with looping as a general type of embryonic deformation. By recognizing the fact that early heart tube morphogenesis is a true physical deformation (84), we were able to construct a model that not only incorporates the descriptive and experimental data but also makes predictions and is, most importantly, falsifiable. In this section we shall explore this biomechanical model of heart looping and attempt to show how it provides the theoretical framework for linking the biochemistry of the component cells and matrix to the rapidly changing gross anatomy of the heart tube.

EPITHELIAL NATURE OF THE HEART

At the early stages of cardiogenesis, vertebrate embryos are histologically (although certainly not functionally) relatively simple organisms, consisting largely of sheets of epithelia with relatively little mesenchymatous tissue. The heart is organized similarly, and the myocardium is a true epithelium. Early embryonic epithelia are separated from each other by rather broad expanses of extracellular matrix (ECM), which consists principally of GAGs (79,80,136) and is synthesized by the embryonic epithelia. An important point we wish to emphasize is that such an anatomic arrangement (sheets of cells enclosing a matrix) can create, by itself, alterations of shape.

Early stages of development have components that are similar, in many ways, to the inflation of a balloon, with the biological epithelia analogous to the distensible balloon and the matrix elaborated by them analogous to the inflating gas. If the system is not to change, then an equilibrium must be reached, with the wall of the balloon (or the epithelium) being sufficiently strong to resist deformation by any outward pressure of the contents. The shape and the change of shape of an epithelial system that contains a matrix are thus dependent on several factors, each of which can, in principle, be analyzed separately.

Mechanical deformation: An increase or expansion of the underlying ECM will deform the epithelium only if the force exerted by the expanding ECM exceeds the elastic modulus of the overlying epithelium. This is the simplest mechanism and represents a simple deformation involving, so far, no information transfer or control of the deformation.

Control of deformation: Regulation of deformational epithelial shape change can be effected at several anatomic and biochemical levels. Obviously, the force of the deformation can be controlled by controlling the ECM. Such control can take the form of regulation of the total amount of matrix synthesized, the rate at which it is secreted by the cells, and both the temporal and geographic distributions of secretory activity. Control could also be effected by regulating the volume of ECM in an indirect manner. Such control could result from regulation of matrix hydration by the overlying epithelium. This could occur if the epithelium had a transport function. Obviously, such a physiological activity, if present, should be detectable in embryonic epithelia, and its detection would lend support to this mechanism. Force generation is apparently related to the composition of the cardiac matrix and its physical chemical properties. Proteoglycans are polyanionic molecules with an extremely large molecular domain that tend to attract cationic counter-ions, trap water, and exclude other molecules (131). These molecular properties can be translated into mechanical forces or work (96,99, 107,151). A proteoglycan gel, in which proteoglycan molecules are stabilized by binding to a structural fibrillar system, can exert work by changing its volume by hydration or dehydration. Because the molecules have a huge hydrated molecular domain, a relatively small number of molecules can occupy a rather large volume. Thus, if newly synthesized proteoglycan molecules are excreted in a dehydrated form and hydrate as soon as they are in the matrix, the result will be a disproportionate increase in the gel space. Furthermore, proteoglycan molecules exclude other soluble materials from their molecular domain and reduce the space available to other molecules. This increases the practical concentrations of other molecules and sets up an osmotic pressure to hydrate and consequently to swell more. The polyanionic nature of proteoglycans attracts counter ions, and this also creates an osmotic pressure.

Finally, we must consider the physical properties of the epithelia. If they are too strong, then the matrix will be unable to expand and deform them. Clearly, to achieve shape change, epithelial compliance must be such as to permit deformations (strain) when the epithelia are subjected to the stress imposed by the matrix. Regulation of epithelial compliance would regulate the possible deformation that the epithelium can undergo. More compliant areas would tend to expand more than less compliant areas. There is some compelling evidence that the early embryonic myocardium demonstrates regionally different compliances. Some of the pioneering particle-marking experiments done by Stalsberg and DeHaan (139) showed that strains on the myocardial surface during looping were different in different regions. This observation was repeated in a series of experiments by Manasek and associates, and the observed strains were analyzed quantitatively (66,86). Briefly, these studies showed that the ventral surface of the myocardium expanded more rapidly than some other areas, such as the region near the dorsal mesocardium or the conotruncal region. Recent studies utilizing a servo-null instrument to measure matrix pressure in the looping heart failed to demonstrate regional pressure differences that could explain these different strains. Pressures were uniform throughout the matrix. This implies that the myocardium itself must have regionally different compliances. It was shown (88) that as the tubular heart develops, individual myocytes within the wall appear to become more flattened and also to lose their wrinkled appearance. These surface characteristics are different in different regions of the developing myocardium, and it was possible to correlate them with regions exhibiting different strains. It may be proposed that the wrinkles, or microplicae, on the myocyte surfaces represent excess membrane. Those cells with a large excess of membrane could flatten out more rapidly and acquire a greater surface/volume ratio, whereas those cells with less "excess membrane" could not flatten out as much and consequently would be prevented from changing their surface/ volume ratio appreciably. Cells would, in effect, become less compliant as they "used up" their microplicae. Lower compliance, in turn, means that these areas are "stiffer" and less able to be deformed. This model was tested using a rubber balloon (88). When the dorsal mesocardium region was stiffened (e.g., compliance lowered) and the balloon inflated slightly, the balloon bent, mimicking the bending component of the looping process.

The heart does not simply swell uniformly in all dimensions; rather, it demonstrates a significant degree of asymmetry. This suggests that in addition to having gross regional variations in compliance, the myocardium must also be anisotropic. Anisotropy within the myocardial wall would be sufficient to cause the developmental asymmetries that are seen during looping, including the dextral rotation that is such a prominent and necessary part of looping.

BIOLOGICAL FIBER SKELETONS

Control of bending by means of wall anisotropy is rather common in hydrostatically supported organisms. A hydrostatically supported organism is one that has an internal pressure that is relatively higher than that outside the organism. The high internal pressure provides support for the organism, essentially by providing turgor. Many hydrostatically supported organisms do not have skeleton systems that bear compressive forces; rather, their skeletons are such that they bear tensile forces. These skeletons are in the form of fibers, generally collagenous in nature. Typically, fiber skeletons have unique winding patterns, and the deformation that the organism can undergo is a function of the pattern into which these fibers are wound. For example, a simple helical winding can bend very readily, but a double winding consisting of two helices of opposite sense does not bend well; for more detailed summaries of fiber systems, see Wainwright et al. (157) and Manasek et al. (88). Because the tubular embryonic heart has all the characteristics of a hydrostatically supported structure (85), it is interesting to consider the possibility that its bending and rotation are regulated by a wound fiber system within the wall (Fig. 1). We can envision a fiber system with a geometry that could permit differential bending and also act to prevent unlimited bending, two requirements if the system is to both deform and stop deforming (106). The fiber system would not need to be static, because the system is developing, and different parts of it could appear at different times during the maturation of the tubular heart. By analogy to lower organisms, we would expect such a system to be extracellular. However, careful examination of the extracellular compartment during this period failed to reveal any evidence for the existence of an extracellular wound fiber system (see the foregoing matrix section of this chapter).

MYOCARDIAL INTRACELLULAR FIBER SYSTEM

A clue to the possible intracellular location of a fiber system came from experiments showing that the myocardium had to undergo normal cytodifferentiation in order for the heart tube to undergo normal morphogenesis. Briefly, if myocardial cytodifferentiation or myofibrillar assembly was inhibited experimentally, the heart tube did not bulge normally and did not rotate (81,87). Clearly there is a link between cardiac myocyte phenotypic expression and overall organ morphogenesis, and it appears that gene expression alone is not sufficient, but that there has to be assembly of gene products into myofibrils.

More recent studies have demonstrated the existence of a very complex fiber system in the myocardium of the tubular heart. The myocardial fiber system can be demonstrated by mild detergent extraction of intact myocardia, with subsequent examination by means of scanning electron microscopy (88). These studies demonstrate the presence of a complex system of intracellular fibers within the myocardium. To date it is not possible to identify precisely which ones are myofibrils and which ones are components of the nonmyofibrillar cytoskeleton, and the complexity of the system makes quantitative morphogenic analysis difficult. However, some general conclusions can be drawn. There are regional differences in both orientation and density of the fibers, and the fiber pattern changes with developmental age. In an approximate sense, the general fiber orientation is such that it appears consistent with the hypothesis that the fibers are involved in regulating myocardial anisotropy, hence act as regulators of the deforming pressure derived from the matrix.

In summary, this model relates the biosynthetic activities of the myocardium (matrix synthesis as well as intracellular fiber synthesis) to the regulation of changing heart shape. It departs from more conventional ways of viewing embryonic development in that it does not concentrate solely on biochemically mediated developmental interactions between, for example, matrix and cells, nor does it even invoke such putative interactions, but rather asks a question somewhat more fundamental to morphogenesis: What are the morphological consequences of materials with these physical properties,

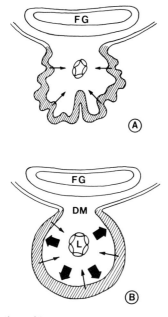

FIG. 1. Generation of hydrostatic pressure within the cardiac jelly. A: Flaccid myocardium (shaded) elaborates GAG and inward pressure (arrows) that results in turgor. B: Additional synthesis or hydration (thin arrows) creates increased outward pressure (bold arrows) that is translated into rotation and bending by myocardial anisotropy. FG, foregut; L, lumen; DM, dorsal mesocardium.

arranged in such an anatomic fashion? Obviously we cannot develop such models in the absence of adequate biochemical and cytological data, but these data taken in isolation do not provide adequate models for morphogenesis.

THE HEART AT POST-LOOPING STAGES: MODIFICATIONS OF EXTERNAL FORM

Whereas looping is related to mechanical deformation and can be modeled in a semiquantitative fashion, later stages of heart development are much more complex. In post-loop stages, heart shape is modified by a number of mechanisms such as differential growth, cell migration, and possibly cell death and hemodynamic factors. There are no unifying comprehensive models that can be applied to these later stages, and different events, such as trabeculation, valve remodeling, and septal closure, are the results of different mechanisms.

The external changes undergone by the heart at post-looping stages are illustrated in Fig. 2. These changes have been recently reviewed (55), and only a brief account will follow here. The bulbus cordis increases in length, especially in the area of the truncus, and bends around a transverse axis. The point of maximal bending marks the separation between conus and truncus. As a whole, the bulbus cordis changes its position lateral to the primitive atrium to a medial and ventral position between the right and left developing atria. At the same time, the trunco-conal junction is displaced progressively toward the ventricle by both the greater lengthening of the truncus and the progressive incorporation of the conus into the ventricular region. It has to be stressed that these changes in position and relation of the trunco-conal region are not the result of active displacements, but rather of asymmetric reorganization and differential growth of the different parts of the heart. The mechanisms controlling these changes are unknown. The spatial relationship of the bulbus cordis to the embryonic axis remains constant throughout this period of rapid changes (140).

The primitive ventricle loses progressively its saccular aspect and becomes trapezoidal. The sharp demarcation between the conus and the ventricular region flattens progressively as the ventral wall of the conus is invaded by myocardial trabeculae. The interventricular sulcus appears in the ventral surface of the ventricular region marking the zone where the interventricular septum will develop. From these early stages the apex of the ventricle is already occupied by the left ventricle.

The primitive atrium undergoes a process of rapid expansion, at first mainly toward the left side. Thus, the left side of the atrium is, for a brief period of time, larger than the right side. The appearance of the inter-atrial sulcus marks the zone where the interatrial septum (septum primum) will develop. In the meantime, the

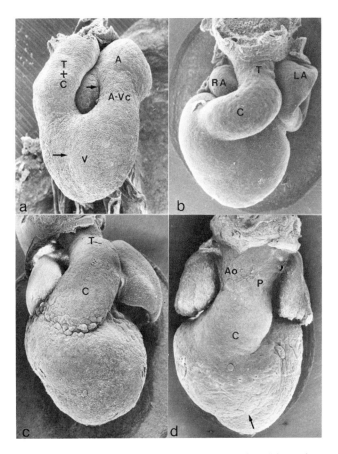

FIG. 2. Scanning electron micrographs of chick embryo hearts showing the shape changes undergone by the heart at post-looping stages (ventral views). A, atrium; Ao, aorta; A-Vc, atrioventricular canal; C, conus; LA, left atrium; P, pulmonary artery; RA, right atrium; T, truncus; V, ventricle. **(a):** Third day of incubation. At this stage the bulbus cordis (T + C) cannot be separated into its two components. Arrows indicate the interatrial and interventricular sulci. **(b):** Fourth day of incubation. The bulbus increases in length and bends around a transverse axis. The point of maximal bending marks the separation between conus and truncus. The left atrium is larger than the right one. **(c):** Fifth day of incubation. The right atrium is expanding rapidly now. **(d):** Sixth day of incubation. The proximal segments of the aorta and the pulmonary artery are already formed, but there is not external separation yet. Arrow indicates interventricular sulcus. The apex of the heart is already formed by the left ventricle.

atrioventricular sulcus becomes a narrow, distinct region, the atrioventricular canal.

The sinus venosus is situated on the dorsal aspect of the heart, and its subsequent development presents some special characteristics. Part of the sinus venosus and its venous affluents are progressively incorporated into the dorsal wall of the right atrium. The division of the internal aspect of the mature right atrium into trabeculated and smooth parts has its origin in this embryologic characteristic. The fate of the portion of the sinus venosus that is not incorporated into the atrial wall varies along the phylogenetic ladder. Whereas in birds that part of the sinus venosus remains as a distinct structure, in mammals it is transformed into the coronary sinus.

INTERNAL CHANGES

Trabeculation

The rapid growth of the primitive ventricle is accompanied internally by a process of diverticulation that changes dramatically the structural appearance of the ventricular wall. At the final stages of loop formation, large intercellular spaces develop in the myocardial layer. As a result, the previously compact myocardium is divided into two layers: a compact or external layer and a spongy or internal layer (64). At the same time, the endocardium forms outpocketings that grow into the cardiac jelly, directed toward the myocardium. When these outpocketings contact the myocardium, the smooth inner myocardial surface is disrupted at the site of all junctions, and the endocardium expands into the myo-

cardial wall (77), forming primitive trabeculae. These primitive trabeculae are soon isolated from the wall of the ventricle and are transformed into slender cords of myocardial tissue invested by endocardium (Fig. 3). It is interesting to point out that the first isolated cords, observed in the heart apex, are oriented parallel to each other and run in a dorsoventral direction. As the ventricular chambers expand centrifugally, the trabeculae adopt a definite radial orientation, presumably in the direction of the ventricular growth.

The development of the trabecular network has several important advantages. In the absence of trabeculation the ventricular wall would become too heavy and compact for the heart to fulfill its contractile functions adequately. Trabeculation permits the easy access of blood to the thickened ventricular wall. Also, coalescence of the first trabeculae in the ventricular apex forms the primordium of the muscular interventricular septum.

The fate of the embryonic trabeculae varies. At later stages of development the ventricular wall again undergoes a process of compaction, and most of the trabeculae

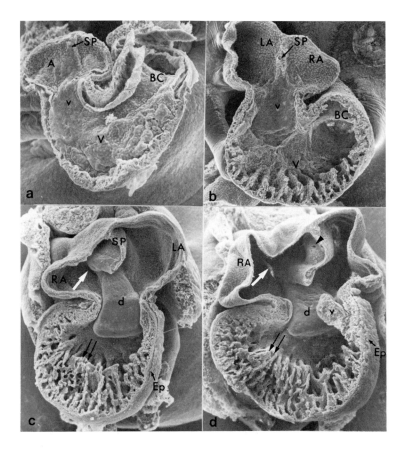

FIG. 3. Scanning electron micrographs of chick embryo hearts showing several aspects of internal remodeling. The hearts have been dissected frontally. **Top:** Ventral half of the specimens. **Bottom:** dorsal half. A, primitive atrium; BC, bulbus cordis; d, dorsal endocardial cushion; Ep, epicardium; LA, left atrium; RA, right atrium; SP, septum primum; v, ventral endocardial cushion; V, ventricle. **(a):** Third day of incubation. The primitive atrium appears separated from the ventricle by the atrioventricular canal. The septum primum and the ventral endocardial cushion are beginning to form. The bulbus cordis has been also opened. **(b):** At the end of the third day of incubation the septum primum and the ventral endocardial cushion are more marked. The left atrium appears larger than the right one. **(c):** Four and a half days of incubation. The left atrium is still larger than the right one. The septum primum is prominent, and it is reaching the cranial aspect of the dorsal endocardial cushion. The opening of the sinus venosus (*white arrow*) appears as a slitlike opening in the dorsal aspect of the right atrium. **(d):** Fifth day of incubation. The two atria are similar in size. The septum primum has reached the dorsal endocardial cushion. Some foraminae (*arrowhead*) appear in the septum primum. The opening of the sinus venosus is indicated (*white arrow*). The broken line of the epicardium appears in (c) and (d). Note in (b)–(d) the progressive changes in shape and structure of the ventricular region. The ventricular trabeculae appear well marked at the end of the third day of incubation (b) and are oriented ventrodorsally. Later (c, d) the trabeculae acquire a more radial disposition. The anlage of the interventricular septum (*double arrow*) appears to form by coalescence of some of the primitive trabeculae (c, d).

are incorporated into the ventricular wall. Others coalesce to form the papillary muscles, and some others atrophy and develop into the chordae tendineae.

Virtually nothing is known about the mechanisms that trigger the beginning of the trabeculation process, nor about the interactions that are likely to occur between endocardium and myocardium. Staining for fibronectin increases with the beginning of trabeculation (56), decreasing progressively as the embryo matures. However, the significance of the changes in the pattern of fibronectin staining remains obscure. The mechanisms of endocardial invasion of the myocardium are also unclear. Hyaluronidase activity increases at trabeculation stages (104,110), and it may disrupt the structural organization of the existing cardiac jelly, facilitating the progression of the endocardial outgrowths. Also at these stages, plasminogen activator activity can be detected by casein overlays (Manasek, *unpublished observations*). However, it is still unknown if the proteolytic activity is confined to the endocardium or to the myocardium, or if both tissue layers produce the plasminogen activator. On the other hand, proteolytic activity is also present in every other part of the heart tested, suggesting that the activity detected represents a generalized phenomenon during processes of rapid remodeling and shaping.

Heart Partitioning

The formation of the heart septa begins independently in the atrioventricular canal, atrium, bulbus cordis, and ventricle. All these septa become united later in development to make two independent circulatory channels. There are two basic mechanisms by which a hollow structure, like the heart, is divided into separate compartments (152). One involves the active growing of two opposite masses of tissue that eventually meet each other and fuse. Septa formed this way are at first large and bulky, and only secondarily are transformed into thin septa. The second mechanism is a more passive process. A segment of the heart increases in diameter very slowly while the immediate segments on each side expand rapidly. The division formed in this way is at first incomplete, and an opening is always left. This opening is located normally in an eccentric position, and it is eventually closed by tissue derived from nearby structures (67,152). The division of the atrioventricular canal and the septation of the bulbus cordis are examples of the first, active, mechanism. The interatrial and interventricular septa are examples of the second, more passive, mechanism.

Interatrial Septum

The interatrial septum develops as a thin myocardial partitioning that originates in the dorsocephalic wall of the atrium. This partitioning, the septum primum, grows

with a concave free border toward the atrioventricular canal (Fig. 3). The orifice situated between the free border of the septum primum and the atrioventricular endocardial cushions is called the foramen primum. With continued growth the free border of the septum primum reaches the superior aspect of the dorsal and ventral endocardial cushions and merges with them.

Under these conditions, because no pulmonary circulation has developed, and because the opening of the sinus venosus has shifted in the meantime to the right atrium, the closure of the foramen primum should exclude the left atrium from the embryonic circulation. To assure the blood supply for the left side of the heart, a new communication, the foramen secundum, opens in the dorsal aspect of the septum primum. In birds the foramen secundum is represented by a series of small perforations, the foramina secunda, formed of thin strands of myocardium covered by endocardium. Invasive behavior of the endocardium that dislodges the continuous myocardial layer, and programmed cell death, appear to be basic mechanisms involved in the formation of the foramina secunda in the chick, as reviewed by Morse et al. (103). The suggestion that focal ruptures of the septum primum could be provoked by increased right atrial pressure (17) appears to be incorrect, because the foramina form in the absence of blood flow (48), indicating that hemodynamics are not involved in this process.

ROLE OF HEMODYNAMICS IN CARDIAC DEVELOPMENT

Many shape changes during cardiac development have been classically attributed to maintenance of normal flow patterns. Indeed, hemodynamic alterations appear superficially to be common mechanisms by which many teratogens exert an effect on the heart. A wide variety of indirect, as well as direct, experimental manipulations of the volume and path of blood flow have repeatedly been demonstrated to result in the generation of congenital heart defects. The emphasis that has been placed on studying the specifics of hemodynamically-induced defects has to some extent distracted researchers from the basic developmental questions. It was long thought sufficient to merely consider the effect of flow volume on the heart as "molding" the heart, but it is clear that this is a nonexplanation, because it proposes no mechanisms for the molding. Even worse, this concept has obstructed research in the entire area of functional-structural interaction in heart development, because it has come to connote for many biologists the outmoded idea of a passive biologic structure being shaped by the dynamic of flow, when in fact the questions should be posed in terms of the dynamic interactions between the flow volume and the living tissue responding to the flow (21). If normal flow patterns are required for cardiogenesis both during organ formation and throughout its subsequent growth, what is the exact mechanism of that effect? In other words, how do cells respond to flow, how do they recognize changes, and how is this translated to organ shape?

For example, it seems reasonable to postulate that the endocardium should respond to flow, because it represents the cellular interface between the bloodstream and the rest of the heart. Some modifications of endocardial cell morphology have been shown after experimental modifications of blood flow (115). However, the relation existing between those findings and the morphology of the endocardium under normal flow conditions is difficult to evaluate. In high-shear-stress areas, such as the ventricular face of the semilunar valves (52) and the part of the atrial wall that funnels into the atrioventricular canal, endocardial cells appear oriented to the direction of the blood flow. In recent experiments, the left vitelline vein was severed at 2.5 days of incubation, and the embryos were reincubated until the fifth day of development. This procedure causes redistribution of the blood flow through the right vitelline vein and the right atrium. When the inner surface of the right atrium of the experimental embryo was observed, endocardial cells situated to the right of the opening of the sinus venosus appeared arranged in a predominantly lateral direction. This kind of orientation was not observed in control embryos.

Although this experiment demonstrates that flow alterations can alter endocardial cell polarity, it does not provide a cellular mechanism for the response. Furthermore, the mechanism by which such a response may be translated into a regulator of heart shape is still, at best, speculative.

HEART PARTITIONING

Division of the atrioventricular canal is brought about by formation of two masses of cushion tissue (Fig. 3). One of these masses develops in the dorsal wall of the atrioventricular canal, and the other develops in the ventral wall. The dorsal and ventral endocardial cushions grow toward each other, meet in the central part of the canal, and fuse. The fusion of the dorsal and ventral endocardial cushions results in the formation of a single structure, the cushion septum, that separates the primitive lumen into right and left atrioventricular apertures. At about the same time two small masses of cushion tissue, the lateral endocardial cushions, develop in the lateral margins of the primitive canal. When the septum cushion has been formed, the right and left atrioventricular orifices are totally circled by cushion tissue. These masses of cushion tissue will contribute to formation of the membranous portion of the interventricular septum and to formation of the atrioventricular valves.

The mechanisms regulating the fusion of the endo-

cardial cushions are still poorly understood. Elsewhere in the embryo, fusion processes usually occur in association with programmed cell death. Fusion of the palatine shelves (46) and fusion of the primitive endocardial tubes (109) are clear examples of morphogenic processes in which cell death is involved. However, during endocardial cushion fusion, images of cell death are seldom observed.

As the cushions come together, endocardial cells from opposite sides extend fingerlike projections into the lumen, become adherent, and form occasional tight and gap junctions (44). No clear evidence of cell fusion between opposite endocardial cells has been presented. As the merging of the cushions begins, endocardial cells behind the edge of fusion lose their typical epithelial characteristics, develop pseudopodia and filopodia, and become indistinguishable from the rest of the CT cells (43). The mesenchymal transformation of the endocardial cells at these stages probably is similar to the phenomenon that takes place during the earlier formation of the endocardial cushions.

Formation of the interventricular septum appears to be related intimately to the process of myocardial trabeculation (Fig. 3). The primitive trabeculae seem to coalesce at the ventricular apex forming the primordium of the interventricular septum. The septum grows with its concave free border toward the atrioventricular canal. The orifice situated between the free border of the septum and the atrioventricular canal is called the primary interventricular foramen. As the septum grows higher, its posterior horn reaches the right border of the septum cushion and fuses with it. A second orifice, the secondary interventricular foramen, is then formed between the septum cushion, the free border of the interventricular septum, and the anterior wall of the ventricle. Thus, at this stage of development, the primitive ventricle has been divided into right and left chambers. The two ventricles communicate through the secondary interventricular foramen. Because the aperture of the bulbus cordis lies to the right of the interventricular septum, the only possible communication between the left ventricle and the bulbus cordis is through the secondary interventricular foramen. We now see the importance of the right-side deviation of the interventricular septum. Should the septum grow straight and merge with the center of the septum cushion, the left ventricle could never communicate with the bulbus cordis, and both great vessels would originate from the right ventricle. The secondary interventricular foramen never closes and is used in connecting the aorta with the left ventricle.

The septation of the bulbus cordis is carried out in the same basic manner as the division of the atrioventricular canal. Two sets of endocardial cushions, the truncal and conal ridges, develop in the truncoconal portion of the heart. The truncal ridges are located in the dextrodorsal and sinistroventral walls of the truncus.

They are the dextrodorsal and sinistroventral truncal ridges. Similar structures, the dextrodorsal and sinistroventral conal ridges, appear in the conus. Conal and truncal ridges develop following a spiraling course, and they merge with each other in the following manner: The sinistroventral conal ridge becomes continuous with the dextrodorsal truncal ridge, and the dextrodorsal conal ridge becomes continuous with the sinistroventral truncal ridge. The two systems cross each other at the truncoconal junction (Fig. 4). Thus, along the entire length of the conotruncus, two systems of spiraling ridges project into the lumen, establishing, at this time, an incomplete division.

While this is occurring, the portion of the heart that connects the conotruncus with the aortic arches becomes a distinct region, the truncoaortic sac. Division of the truncoaortic sac is achieved by formation of a spur of mesenchymal tissue called the aortopulmonary septum. The aortopulmonary septum, which presents a horseshoe-shaped form, originates between the fourth and sixth aortic arches and grows downward toward the truncus until it meets the truncal ridges. It follows a spiraling

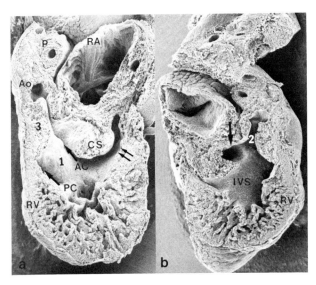

FIG. 4. Scanning electron micrographs of a 6-day chick embryo heart. The heart has been sectioned longitudinally and both halves are presented. Ao, aorta; CS, cushion septum; IVS, interventricular septum; P, pulmonary artery; RA, right atrium; RV, right ventricle; 1, dextrodorsal conal ridge; 2, sinistroventral conal ridge; 3, sinistroventral truncal ridge. (a): Right segment of the specimen (seen from the left). The dextrodorsal conal ridge is continuous with the right side of the cushion septum. The spiraling fusion of the truncoconal ridges has established at this time an incomplete division of the truncoconus. The pulmonic conus (PC) and aortic conus (AC) can be seen in this picture. Double arrow indicates the right atrioventricular canal. (b): Left segment of the specimen (seen from the right). The secondary interventricular foramen (*arrow*) appears as a tunnellike communication between the ventricles. The sinistrodorsal conal ridge is continuous with the anterior margin of the interventricular septum.

course that is continued downward by the truncoconal ridges. The spiraling trajectory of the aorta and pulmonary artery is due in part to the course followed by the aortopulmonary septum.

After the aortopulmonary septum meets the truncal ridges, the ridges meet each other and fuse. Following fusion of the truncal ridges, the conal ridges also meet each other and fuse, and the septum of the conus becomes continuous with the septum of the truncus.

Perhaps one of the most controversial aspects of heart development is the way in which the septation of the bulbus cordis is described by different workers. The controversy arises not only from the different terminology used by different authors (65) but also from the radically different ways of approaching the morphogenesis of this region. Explanations different than the one presented here can be found, for example, in Thompson et al. (145), Anderson et al. (2), and Orts Llorca et al. (111).

FORMATION OF THE AORTIC VESTIBULUM

Formation of the truncal septum has divided the truncus into aortic and pulmonic channels. They will form later the initial portions of the aorta and pulmonary artery. The conus septum is dividing the conus into a posteromedial (aortic) portion and an anterolateral (pulmonic) portion. These channels are about to form the outflow tract portions of the left and right ventricles, respectively (Fig. 5).

The enlargement of the right ventricle and the displacement to the right of the atrioventricular canal bring the aortic division of the conus above the interventricular foramen. The dextrodorsal conus ridge blends with the right lateral cushion and with the right side of the cushion septum. Then the conus septum blends with the ventral part of the interventricular septum, and the left ventricle becomes continuous with the aortic channel. A small communication, the tertiary interventricular foramen, persists between the right ventricle and the aortic vestibulum. The tertiary interventricular foramen is bordered dorsally by the cushion septum, caudally by the interventricular septum, and ventrally by the conus septum. The three structures grow toward each other and close the foramen, forming the origin of the membranous portion of the adult interventricular septum (55,152).

It is not surprising that one of the most, if not the most, frequent heart malformations is the presence of an interventricular communication. The complexity of the successive steps that result in separation of the aortic and pulmonic circulations makes it very susceptible to the influence of diverse teratogens. Although most of the experimental studies have been centered on analysis of gross morphologic changes, we cannot forget that this septation process is basically that of a growing mesenchymal tissue. Perhaps study of cell-matrix interactions,

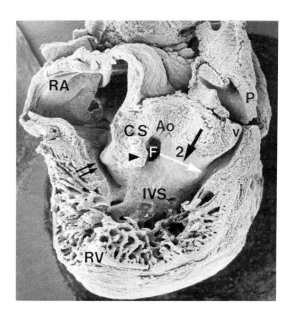

FIG. 5. Scanning electron micrograph of a chick embryo heart at the middle of the sixth day of incubation. The heart has been dissected through the right atrium (RA), the right atrioventricular aperture (*double arrow*), and the right ventricle (RV). In front of the interventricular foramen (F) the fusion of the conal ridges is taking place, but the inferior part of the sinistroventral conal ridge (2) is still unfused. The dextro-dorsal conal ridge (left out of the dissection) blends with the cushion septum (CS). The line of fracture passes through the zone of blending (*arrowhead*). The continued fusion of the conal ridges in a downward direction (*black arrow*) together with the growing of the right side of the cushion septum along the top of the interventricular foramen (direction of growth marked by arrowhead) isolate the ventricular foramen from the right ventricle. Then the interventricular foramen becomes part of the aortic vestibulum, and in this sense the aorta is transferred to the left ventricle. Ao indicates the position of the aortic outflow tract (most of it has been removed). The future position of the tertiary interventricular foramen is indicated by the white arrow. P, pulmonary artery; v, semilunar valve cusp.

and their experimental modifications, that occur during heart septation will be a better way to approach the problem of the development of congenital heart malformations.

CONCLUSION

It is perhaps a truism to state that heart shape is dependent ultimately on the genome. Even those events having, as we are beginning to show, an immediate dependence on the geometry of the developing organ and the physical properties of various of its components depend on the proper sequence of gene expression to produce the gene products that create the physical properties that control the deformation. Later events of cardiogenesis that involve even more complex activities have a more tortuous route leading from the genome to

the shape of the organ. This chapter has attempted to show, by summarizing some of the salient points of cardiogenesis viewed at different levels of organization, the current state of work on these problems. Gene expression and synthesis of gene products are problems that are clearly amenable to investigation, and much current research is focused on these areas. Anatomic development of the heart may have been described more or less to an adequate degree. The most glaring gaps appear to be in the area between these two levels of biologic organization. Except for the restricted case of looping, we have no mechanistic models that provide us with testable predictions. Emphasis should be placed on developing hypotheses that are falsifiable. Moreover, it appears that an entirely biochemical view of developmental regulation may not suffice. It is becoming more apparent that biomechanical factors are important in the shaping of anatomic form. These are probably not simplistic or intuitive processes such as have been proposed in several instances in the past, but rather are more akin to engineering problems. They can be modeled, analyzed, and developed experimentally, and the interaction of the geometry of nascent organs and the biochemical processes occurring within them must be understood. We should consider that biochemistry influences anatomy, and anatomy influences biochemistry.

ACKNOWLEDGMENTS

Original work presented here was supported by USPHS grant HL-13831 to F.J.M. L.S. is a Fellow of the Chicago Heart Association. This work was begun when J.M.I. was a recipient of a Fullbright-MEC grant. We thank Ms. Joan Hives for her support during the many international versions of the manuscript.

REFERENCES

1. Akiyama, S. K., Yamada, K. M., and Hayashi, M. (1981): The structure of fibronectin and its role in cellular adhesion. *J. Supramol. Struct. Cell Biochem.,* 16:345–358.
2. Anderson, R. H., Wilkinson, J. L., Arnold, R., and Lubkiewicz, K. (1974): Morphogenesis of bulboventricular malformations. I. Considerations of embryogenesis in the normal heart. *Br. Heart J.,* 36:242–255.
3. Atherton, B. T., and DeHaan, R. L. (1978). Developmental changes in the adhesion of embryonic chick heart cells. *J. Cell Biol.,* 79:54a.
4. Bandman, E., Matsuda, R., Micou-Eastwood, J., and Strohman, R. (1981): In vitro translation of RNA from embryonic and from adult chicken pectoralis muscle produces different myosin heavy chains. *FEBS Lett.,* 136:301–305.
5. Barany, M. (1967): ATPase activity of myosin correlated with speed of muscle shortening. *J. Gen. Physiol.,* 50:197–216.
6. Barthel, H. (1960): *Missbildungen des menschieblen Herzens.* Theime, Stuttgart.
7. Bashey, R. I., Bashey, H. M., and Jimenez, S. A. (1978): Characterization of pepsin-solubilized bovine heart valve collagen. *Biochem. J.,* 173:885–894.
8. Bernanke, D. H., and Markwald, R. R. (1979): Effects of hyaluronic acid on cardiac cushion tissue cells in collagen matrix culture. *Tex. Rep. Biol. Med.,* 39:271–285.

9. Borg, T. K., and Caufield, J. B. (1979): Collagen in the heart. *Tex. Rep. Biol. Med.,* 39:321–333.

10. Borg, T. K., and Caufield, J. B. (1981): The collagen matrix of the heart. *Fed. Proc.,* 40:2037–2041.

11. Borg, T. K., Gay, R. E., and Johnson, L. D. (1982): Changes in the distribution of fibronectin and collagen during development of the neonatal rat heart. *Collagen Rel. Res.,* 2:211–218.

12. Bornstein, P., and Sage, H. (1980): Structurally distinct collagen types. *Annu. Rev. Biochem.,* 49:957–1003.

13. Buckingham, M. E., Carvatti, M., Minty, A., Robert, B., Alonso, S., Cohen, A., Daubas, P., and Weydert, A. (1982): Skeletal muscle myogenesis: The expression of actin and myosin in mRNAs. *Adv. Exp. Med. Biol.,* 158:331–347.

14. Cantini, M., Sartore, S., and Schiaffino, S. (1980): Myosin types in cultured muscle cells. *J. Cell Biol.,* 85:903–909.

15. Carey, R. A., Bove, A. A., Coulson, R. L., Packman, D. L., and Spann, J. F. (1979): Correlation between cardiac muscle myosin ATPase activity and velocity of muscle shortening. *Biochem. Med.,* 21:235–245.

16. Caufield, J. B., and Borg, T. K. (1979): The collagen network of the heart. *Lab. Invest.,* 40:364–372.

17. Chang, C. (1931): The formation of the interatrial septum in chick embryos. *Anat. Rec.,* 50:9–22.

18. Chang, C. (1932): On the reaction of the endocardium to the blood stream in the embryonic heart with special reference to the endocardial thickenings in the atrioventricular canal and bulbus cordis. *Anat. Rec.,* 51:253–265.

19. Chizzonite, R. A., Everett, A. W., Clark, W. A., Jakovcic, S., Rabinowitz, M., and Zak, R. (1982): Isolation and characterization of two molecular variants of myosin heavy chains from rabbit ventricle: Change in their content during normal growth and after treatment with thyroid hormone. *J. Biol. Chem.,* 257:2056–2065.

20. Chizzonite, R., Everett, A. W., Prior, G., and Zak, R. (1985): Identical α-myosin heavy chains in atria and ventricles from hypothyroid, euthyroid and hyperthyroid rabbit hearts. *J. Biol. Chem.,* 260:5445–5451.

21. Clark, E. B. (1984): Functional aspects of cardiac development. In: *Growth of the Heart in Health and Disease,* edited by R. Zak, pp. 81–104. Raven Press, New York.

22. Clark, W. A., Chizzonite, R. A., Everett, A. W., Rabinowitz, M., and Zak, R. (1982): Species correlations between cardiac isomyosins. A comparison of electrophoretic and immunological properties. *J. Biol. Chem.,* 257:5449–5454.

23. Comper, W. D., and Laurent, T. C. (1978): Physiological function of connective tissue polysaccharides. *Physiol. Rev.,* 58:255–315.

24. Cummins, P., and Perry, S. V. (1974): Chemical and immuno-chemical characteristics of tropomyosins from striated and smooth muscle. *Biochem. J.,* 141:43.

25. Dalla Libera, L., and Sartore, S. (1981): Immunological and biochemical evidence for atrial-like isomyosin in thyrotoxic rabbit ventricle. *Biochim. Biophys. Acta,* 669:84–92.

26. Dalla Libera, L., Sartore, S., and Schiaffino, S. (1979): Comparative analysis of chicken atrial and ventricular myosins. *Biochim. Biophys. Acta,* 581:283–294.

27. DeHaan, R. L. (1964): Cell interactions and oriented movements during development. *J. Exp. Zool.,* 157:127–138.

28. DeHaan, R. L. (1965): Morphogenesis of the vertebrate heart. In *Organogenesis,* edited by R. L. DeHaan and H. Ursprung, pp. 377–419. Holt, Rinehart and Winston, New York.

29. DeHaan, R. L. (1968): Emergence of form and function in the embryonic heart. *Dev. Biol. [Suppl.],* 2:208–250.

30. Delpech, A., and Delpech, B. (1984): Expression of hyaluronic acid-binding glycoprotein, hyaluronectin (HN), in the developing rat embryo. *Dev. Biol.,* 101:391–400.

31. Dhoot, G. K., Fearson, N., and Perry, S. V. (1979): Polymorphic forms of troponin-T and troponin-C and their localization in striated muscle cell type. *Exp. Cell Res.,* 122–339.

32. Dietrich, C. P., Nader, H. B., and Straus, A. H. (1983): Structural differences of heparan sulfates according to the tissue and species of origin. *Biochem. Biophys. Res. Commun.,* 111:865–871.

33. Eisenberg, B. R., Edwards, J. A., and Zak, R. (1983): Isomyosin antibody and Ca^{2+}-activated ATPase redistribution in rabbit ventricle during development. *J. Cell Biol.,* 97:50a.

34. Epstein, E. H., and Munderloh, N. H. (1975): Isolation and characterization of CNBr peptides of human 1(III)$_3$ collagen and tissue distribution of 1(I)$_2$ and 1(III)$_3$ collagens. *J. Biol. Chem.,* 250:9304–9312.

35. Fitzharris, T. P., and Markwald, R. R. (1982): Cellular migration through the cardiac jelly matrix: A stereoanalysis by high-voltage electron microscopy. *Dev. Biol.,* 92:315–329.

36. Garrels, J. I., and Gibson, W. (1976): Identification and characterization of multiple forms of actin. *Cell,* 9:793–805.

37. Gauthier, G. F., Lowey, S., Benfield, P. A., and Hobbs, A. W. (1982): Distribution and properties of myosin isozymes in developing avian and mammalian skeletal muscle fibers. *J. Cell Biol.,* 92:471–484.

38. Gessner, I. H., Lorincz, A. E., and Bostrom, H. (1965): Acid mucopolysaccharide content of the cardiac jelly of the chick embryo. *J. Exp. Zool.,* 160:291–298.

39. Gonzalez-Sanchez, A., and Bader, D. (1984): Immunochemical analysis of myosin heavy chains in the developing chicken heart. *Dev. Biol.,* 103:151–158.

40. Gorza, L., Sartore, S., and Schiaffino, S. (1982): Myosin types and fiber types in cardiac muscle. 2. Atrial myocardium. *J. Cell Biol.,* 95:838–845.

41. Gorza, L., Sartore, S., Triban, C., and Schiaffino, S. (1983): Embryonic-like myosin heavy chains in regenerating chicken muscle. *Exp. Cell Res.,* 143:395–403.

42. Hascall, V. C., and Hascall, G. K. (1981): Protoeoglycans. In: *Cell Biology of Extracellular Matrix,* edited by E. D. Hay, pp. 39–63. Plenum Press, New York.

43. Hay, D. A. (1978): Development and fusion of the endocardial cushions. In: *Morphogenesis and Malformations of the Cardiovascular System,* edited by G. C. Rosenquist and D. Bergsma, pp. 69–90. Alan R. Liss, New York.

44. Hay, D. A., and Low, F. N. (1972): The fusion of dorsal and ventral endocardial cushions in the embryonic chick heart: A study in fine structure. *Am. J. Anat.,* 133:1–24.

45. Hay, D. A., and Markwald, R. R. (1981): Localization of fucose-containing substances in developing atrioventricular cushion tissue. In: *Perspectives in Cardiovascular Research. 5. Mechanisms of Cardiac Morphogenesis and Teratogenesis,* edited by T. Pexieder, pp. 197–211. Raven Press, New York.

46. Hayward, A. F. (1969): Ultrastructural changes in the epithelium during fusion of the palatal processes in rats. *Arch. Oral Biol.,* 14:661–678.

47. Hendrix, M. J. C. (1981): Localization of collagen types in the embryonic heart and aorta using immunohistochemistry. In: *Perspectives in Cardiovascular Research 5,* edited by T. Pexieder, pp. 213–225. Raven Press, New York.

48. Hendrix, M. J. C., Brailey, J. L., Brown, B. J., and Sorrentino, J. M. (1983): The development of the atrial septum in the absence of hemodynamic pressure. *Anat. Rec.,* 205:80a.

49. Hoh, J. F. Y., McGrath, P. A., and Hale, P. T. (1978): Electrophoretic analysis of multiple forms of rat cardiac myosin: Effect of hypophysectomy and thyroxine replacement. *J. Mol. Cell Cardiol.,* 10:1053–1076.

50. Hoh, J. F. Y., Yeoh, G. P. S., Thomas, M. A. W., and Higginbottom, L. (1979): Structural differences in the heavy chains of rat ventricular myosin isoenzymes. *FEBS Lett.,* 97:330–334.

51. Hopkins, F., McCutcheon, E. P., and Wekstein, D. R. (1973): Postnatal changes in rat ventricular function. *Circ. Res.,* 32:685–691.

52. Hurle, J. M., and Colvee, E. (1983): Changes in the endothelial morphology of the developing semilunar heart valves. A TEM and SEM study in the chick. *Anat. Embryol.,* 167:67–83.

53. Hurle, J. M., Icardo, J. M., and Ojeda, J. L. (1980): Compositional and structural heterogeneity of the cardiac jelly of the chick embryo tubular heart: A TEM, SEM and histochemical study. *J. Embryol. Exp. Morphol.,* 56:211–223.

54. Hurle, J. M., and Ojeda, J. L. (1977): Cardiac jelly arrangement during the formation of the tubular heart of the chick embryo. *Acta Anat.,* 98:444–455.

55. Icardo, J. M. (1984): The growing heart: An anatomical perspective. In: *Growth of the Heart in Health and Disease,* edited by R. Zak, pp. 41–80. Raven Press, New York.

56. Icardo, J. M., and Manasek, F. J. (1983): Fibronectin distribution

during early chick embryo heart development. *Dev. Biol.*, 95:19–30.

57. Icardo, J. M., and Manasek, F. J. (1984): An indirect immunofluorescence study of the distribution of fibronectin during the formation of the cushion tissue mesenchyme in the embryonic heart. *Dev. Biol.*, 101:336–345.

58. Inoue, S., and Iwasaki, M. (1976): Dermatan sulphate–chondroitin sulphate copolymers from umbilical cord. Isolation and characterization. *J. Biochem. (Tokyo)*, 80:513–524.

59. Johnson, R. C., Manasek, F. J., Vinson, W., and Seyer, J. (1974): The biochemical and ultrastructural demonstration of collagen during early heart development. *Dev. Biol.*, 36:252–271.

60. Kefalides, N. A. (1973): Structure and biosynthesis of basement membranes. *Int. Rev. Connect. Tissue Res.*, 6:63–104.

61. Keiser, H. D. (1982): The immunology of proteoglycans. *Connect. Tissue Res.*, 10:101–108.

62. Kimura, J. H., Hardingham, T. E., Hascall, V. C., and Solursh, M. (1979): Biosynthesis of proteoglycans and their assembly into aggregates in cultures of chondrocytes from the swarm rat chondrosarcoma. *J. Biol. Chem.*, 254:2600–2609.

63. Kimura, J. H., Hardingham, T. E., and Hascall, V. C. (1980): Assembly of newly synthesized proteoglycan and link protein into aggregates in cultures of chondrosarcoma chondrocytes. *J. Biol. Chem.*, 255:7134–7143.

63.aKinsella, M. G. and Fitzharris, T. P. (1982): Control of cell migration in atrioventricular pads during chick early heat development: Analysis of cushion tissue migration *in vitro*. *Develop. Biol.*, 91:1–10.

64. Kurkiewicz, T. O. (1909): O histogenezie miesnia sarcowego zwierzat kregowych. *Bull. Acad. Sci. Cracovie*, pp. 148–191.

65. Laane, H. M. (1974): The nomenclature of the arterial pole of the embryonic heart. IV. Discussion and conclusion. *Acta Morphol. Neerl.-Scand.*, 12:195–210.

66. Lacktis, J. W., and Manasek, F. J. (1978): An analysis of deformation during a normal morphogenic event. In: *Morphogenesis and Malformation of the Cardiovascular System*, edited by G. C. Rosenquist and D. Bergsma, pp. 205–227. Alan R. Liss, New York.

67. Langman, J., and Van Mierop, L. H. S. (1968): Development of the cardiovascular system. In: *Heart Disease in Infants, Children and Adolescents*, edited by A. J. Moss and F. H. Adams, pp. 3–25. Williams & Wilkins, Baltimore.

68. Leivo, I., Vaheri, A., Timpl, R., and Wartiovaara, J. (1980): Appearance and distribution of collagens and laminin in the early mouse embryo. *Dev. Biol.*, 76:100–114.

69. Lillie, F. R. (1908): *The Development of the Chick* (3rd ed., 1965, revised by H. L. Hamilton). Holt, Rinehart and Winston, New York.

70. Linask, K. K., and Lash, J. W. (1983): Directional cell migration of precardiac mesoderm cells in the early chick embryo. *J. Cell Biol.*, 97:319a.

71. Linsenmayer, T. F. (1981): Collagen. In: *Cell Biology of Extracellular Matrix*, edited by E. D. Hay, pp. 5–37. Plenum Press, New York.

72. Lompre, A. M., Mercadier, J. J., Wisnewsky, C., Bouveret, P., Pantaloni, C., d'Albis, A., and Schwartz, K. (1981): Species and age dependent change in the relative amounts of cardiac myosin isoenzymes in mammals. *Dev. Biol.*, 84:286–290.

73. Low, F. N. (1968): Extracellular connective tissue fibrils in the chick embryo. *Anat. Rec.*, 160:93–108.

74. Lowey, S., Benfield, P. A., LeBlanc, D. D., and Waller, G. S. (1983): Myosin isozymes in avian skeletal muscles. I. Sequential expression of myosin isozymes in developing chicken pectoralis muscles. *J. Muscle Res. Cell Motil.*, 4:695–716.

75. Manasek, F. J. (1968): Embryonic development of the heart. I. A light and electron microscopic study of myocardial development in the early chick embryo. *J. Morphol.*, 125:329–366.

76. Manasek, F. J. (1970): Sulfated extracellular matrix production in the embryonic heart and adjacent tissues. *J. Exp. Zool.*, 174:415–440.

77. Manasek, F. J. (1970): Histogenesis of the embryonic myocardium. *Am. J. Cardiol.*, 25:149–168.

78. Manasek, F. J. (1971): The ultrastructure of embryonic myocardial blood vessels. *Dev. Biol.*, 26:42–54.

79. Manasek, F. J. (1975): The extracellular matrix of the early embryonic heart. In: *Developmental and Physiological Correlates of Cardiac Muscle*, edited by M. Lieberman and E. T. Sano, pp. 1–20. Raven Press, New York.

80. Manasek, F. J. (1975): The extracellular matrix: A dynamic component of the developing embryo. In: *Current Topics in Developmental Biology*, edited by A. A. Moscona and A. Monroy, pp. 35–102. Academic Press, New York.

81. Manasek, F. J. (1976): Heart development: Interactions involved in cardiac morphogenesis. In: *The Cell Surface in Animal Embryogenesis and Development*, edited by G. Poste and G. Nicholson, pp. 545–598. Elsevier/North Holland, Amsterdam.

82. Manasek, F. J. (1976): Glycoprotein synthesis and tissue interactions during establishment of the functional embryonic chick heart. *J. Mol. Cell. Cardiol.*, 8:389–402.

83. Manasek, F. J. (1977): Structural glycoproteins of the embryonic cardiac extracellular matrix. *J. Mol. Cell. Cardiol.*, 9:425–439.

84. Manasek, F. J. (1981): Determinants of heart shape in early embryos. *Fed. Proc.*, 40:2011–2016.

85. Manasek, F. J. (1983): Control of early embryonic heart morphogenesis: A hypothesis. In: *Development of the Cardiovascular System*, Ciba Foundation Symposium 100, pp. 4–19. Pitman, London.

86. Manasek, F. J., Burnside, M. B., and Waterman, R. E. (1972): Myocardial cell shape change as a mechanism of embryonic heart looping. *Dev. Biol.*, 29:349–371.

87. Manasek, F. J., Kulikowski, R. R., and Fitzpatrick, L. (1978): Cytodifferentiation: A causal antecedent of looping? In: *Morphogenesis and Malformation of the Cardiovascular System*, edited by G. C. Rosenquist and D. Bergsma, pp. 161–178. Alan R. Liss, New York.

88. Manasek, F. J., Kulikowski, R. R., Nakamura, A., Nguyenphuc, Q., and Lacktis, J. W. (1984): Early heart development: A new model of cardiac morphogenesis. In: *Growth of the Heart in Health and Disease*, edited by R. Zak, pp. 105–130. Raven Press, New York.

89. Manasek, F. J., Lacktis, J. W., Aiton, J., and Lieberman, M. (1981): Synthesis and distribution of glycopeptides and glycosaminoglycans in cultures of embryonic heart cells. In: *Perspectives in Cardiovascular Research 5*, edited by T. Pexieder, pp. 181–195. Raven Press, New York.

90. Manasek, F. J., Reid, M., Vinson, W., Seyer, J., and Johnson, R. (1973): Glycosaminoglycan synthesis by the early embryonic chick heart. *Dev. Biol.*, 35:332–348.

91. Markwald, R. R., and Adams Smith, W. N. (1972): Distribution of mucosubstances in the developing rat heart. *J. Histochem. Cytochem.*, 20:896–907.

92. Markwald, R. R., Fitzharris, T. P., Bank, H., and Bernanke, D. H. (1978): Structural analysis on the matrical organization of glycosaminoglycans in developing endocardial cushions. *Dev. Biol.*, 62:292–316.

93. Markwald, R. R., Fitzharris, T. P., Bolender, D. L., and Bernanke, D. H. (1979): Structural analysis of cell: Matrix interaction during morphogenesis of atrioventricular cushion tissue. *Dev. Biol.*, 69:634–654.

94. Markwald, R. R., Fitzharris, T. P., and Manasek, F. J. (1977): Structural development of endocardial cushions. *Am. J. Anat.*, 148:85–120.

95. Markwald, R. R., Funderberg, F. M., and Bernanke, D. H. (1979): Glycosaminoglycans: Potential determinants in cardiac morphogenesis. *Tex. Rep. Biol. Med.*, 39:253–270.

96. Maroudas, A., and Bannon, C. (1981): Measurement of swelling pressure in cartilage and comparison with osmotic pressure of constituent proteoglycans. *Biorheology*, 18:619–632.

97. Martinez-Hernandez, A., Gay, S., and Miller, E. J. (1982): Ultrastructural localization of type V collagen in rat kidney. *J. Cell Biol.*, 92:343–349.

98. Masaki, T., and Yoshizaki, C. (1974): Differentiation of myosin in chick embryos. *J. Biochem. (Tokyo)*, 76:123–131.

99. Mayer, F. (1983): Macromolecular basis of globular protein exclusion and of swelling pressure in loose connective tissue (umbilical cord). *Biochim. Biophys. Acta*. 755:388–399.

100. McClain, P. E. (1974): Characterization of cardiac muscle collagen. *J. Biol. Chem.*, 249:2303–2311.

101. Moretti, A., and Whitehouse, M. W. (1963): Changes in the mucopolysaccharide composition of bovine heart valves with age. *Biochem. J.,* 87:396–402.

102. Morris, S. C., and McClain, P. E. (1972): Heterogeneity in the CNBr peptides from striated muscle and heart valve collagen. *Biochem. Biophys. Res. Commun.,* 47:27–43.

103. Morse, D. E., Rogers, C. S., and McCaan, P. S. (1984): Atrial septation in the chick and rat-A review. *J. Submicrosc. Cytol.,* 16:259–272.

104. Nakamura, A. (1980): Cardiac hyaluronidase activity of chick embryos at the time of endocardial cushion formation. *J. Mol. Cell. Cardiol.,* 12:1239–1248.

105. Nakamura, A., and Manasek, F. J. (1981): An experimental study of the relation of cardiac jelly to the shape of the early chick embryonic heart. *J. Embryol. Exp. Morphol.,* 65:235–256.

106. Nakamura, A., Kulikowski, R. R., Lacktis, J. W., and Manasek, F. J. (1980): Heart looping: A regulated response to deforming forces. In: *Etiology and Morphogenesis of Congenital Heart Disease,* edited by R. Van Praagh and A. Takao, pp. 81–98. Future, New York.

107. Nakamura, A., and Manasek, F. J. (1978): Experimental studies of the shape and structure of isolated cardiac jelly. *J. Embryol. Exp. Morphol.,* 43:167–183.

108. Nakamura, A., and Manasek, F. J. (1978): Cardiac jelly fibrils: Their distribution and organization. In: *Morphogenesis and Malformation of the Cardiovascular System,* edited by G. C. Rosenquist and D. Bergsma, pp. 229–250. Alan R. Liss, New York.

109. Ojeda, J. L., and Hurle, J. M. (1975): Cell death during the formation of the tubular heart of the chick embryo. *J. Embryol. Exp. Morphol.,* 33:523–534.

110. Orkin, R. W., and Toole, B. P. (1978): Hyaluronidase activity and hyaluronate content of the developing chick embryo heart. *Dev. Biol.,* 66:308–320.

111. Orts Llorca, F., Puerta Fonolla, J., and Sabrado Perez, J. (1981): Morphogenesis of the ventricular flow pathways in man (bulbus cordis and truncus arteriosus). In: *Mechanisms of Cardiac Morphogenesis and Teratogenesis,* edited by T. Pexieder, pp. 17–30. Raven Press, New York.

112. Paterson, B. M., and Eldridge, J. D. (1984): Cardiac actin is the major sarcomeric isoform expressed in embryonic avian skeletal muscle. *Science,* 224:1436–1438.

113. Patten, B. M. (1968): The development of the heart. In: *Pathology of the Heart and Blood Vessels,* ed. 3, edited by S. E. Gould, pp. 20–90. Charles C Thomas, Springfield, Ill.

114. Patten, B. M., Kramer, T. C., and Barry, A. (1948): Valvular action in the embryonic heart by localized apposition of endocardial masses. *Anat. Rec.,* 102:299–311.

115. Pexieder, T. (1976): Effects de l'hemodynamique sur la morphologie de l'endocarde embryonnaire. *Bull. Assoc. Anat.,* 60:163–170.

116. Price, K. M., Littler, W. A., and Cummins, P. (1980): Human atrial and ventricular myosin light chain subunits in the adult and during development. *Biochem. J.,* 191:571–580.

117. Rawles, M. E. (1936): A study in the localization of organ-forming areas of the chick blastoderm of the head process stage. *J. Exp. Zool.,* 72:271–315.

118. Rawles, M. E. (1943): The head-forming areas of the early chick blastoderm. *Physiol. Zool.,* 16:22–47.

119. Roll, F. J., Madri, J. A., Albert, J., and Furthmayr, H. (1980): Codistribution of collagen type IV and AB2 in basement membranes and mesangium of the kidney. *J. Cell Biol.,* 85:597–616.

120. Romanoff, A. L. (1960): *The Avian Embryo.* Macmillan, New York.

121. Rosenquist, G. C. (1960): A radiographic study of labeled grafts in the chick blastoderm. Development from primitive streak to stage 12. *Contrib. Embryol.,* 263:71–110.

122. Rudnick, D. (1944): Early history and mechanics of the chick blastoderm. *Q. Rev. Biol.,* 19:187–212.

123. Runyan, R. B., Kitten, G. T., and Markwald, R. R. (1982): Proteins of the embryonic extracellular matrix: Regional and temporal correlation with tissue interaction in the heart. In: *Extracellular Matrix,* edited by S. Hawkes and J. L. Wang, pp. 153–157. Academic Press, New York.

124. Runyan, R. B., and Markwald, R. R. (1983): Invasion of mes-

enchyme into three-dimensional collagen gels: A regional temporal analysis of interaction in embryonic heart tissue. *Dev. Biol.,* 95:108–114.

125. Samuel, J. L., Rappaport, L., Mercadier, J. J., Lompre, A. M., Sartore, S., Triban, C., Schiaffino, S., and Schwartz, K. (1983): Distribution of myosin isozymes within single cardiac cells: An immunohistochemical study. *Circ. Res.,* 52:200–209.

126. Sartore, S., Gorza, L., Bormioli, S. P., Libera, L. D., and Schiaffino, S. (1981): Myosin types and fiber types in cardiac muscle. I. Ventricular myocardium. *J. Cell Biol.,* 88:226–233.

127. Sartore, S., Pierobon-Bormioli, S., and Schiaffino, S. (1978): Immunohistochemical evidence for myosin polymorphism in the chicken heart. *Nature (Lond.),* 274:82–83.

128. Scheuer, J., and Bahn, A. K. (1979): Cardiac contractile proteins. Adenosine triphosphatase activity and physiological function. *Circ. Res.,* 45:1–12.

129. Schiaffino, S., Gorza, L., Sartore, S., and Thornell, L. E. (1985): Developmental and adaptive changes of atrial isomyosins. In: *The Development of the Cardiovascular System,* edited by M. J. Legato, (in press). Martinus Nijhoff, The Hague.

130. Schwartz, K., LeCarpentier, Y., Martin, J. L., Lompre, A. M., Mercadier, J. J., and Swynghedauw, B. (1981): Myosin isoenzymic distribution correlates with speed of myocardial contraction. *J. Mol. Cell. Cardiol.,* 13:1074–1075.

131. Shubert, M., and Hamerman, D. (1968): *A Primer on Connective Tissue Biochemistry.* Lea & Febiger, Philadelphia.

132. Shupp-Byrne, D. E., and Church, R. L. (1982): "Embryonic" collagen (type 1 trimer) a1-chains are genetically distinct from type I collagen a1-chains. *Collagen Rel. Res.,* 2:481–494.

133. Sinha, A. M., Friedman, D. J., Nigro, J. M., Jakovcic, S., Rabinowitz, M., and Umeda, P. K. (1984): Expression of rabbit ventricular β-myosin heavy chain messenger RNA sequences in atrial muscle. *Proc. Natl. Acad. Sci. U.S.A.,* 259:6674–6680.

134. Sinha, A. M., Umeda, P. K., Kavinsky, C. J., Rajamanickam, C., Hsu, H.-J., Jakovcic, S., and Rabinowitz, M. (1982): Molecular cloning of mRNA sequences for cardiac α- and β-form myosin heavy chains: Expression in ventricles of normal, hypothyroid, and thyrotoxic rabbits. *Proc. Natl. Acad. Sci. U.S.A.,* 79:5847–5851.

135. Sissman, N. J. (1966): Cell multiplication rates during development of the primitive cardiac tube in the chick embryo. *Nature (Lond.),* 210:504.

136. Solursh, M., Fisher, M., and Singley, C. T. (1979): The synthesis of hyaluronic acid by ectoderm during early organogenesis in the chick embryo. *Differentiation,* 14:77–85.

137. Stalsberg, H. (1970): The mechanism of dextral looping of the embryonic heart. *Am. J. Cardiol.,* 215:265.

138. Stalsberg, H., and DeHaan, R. L. (1968): Endodermal movements during foregut formation in the chick embryo. *Dev. Biol.,* 18:198–215.

139. Stalsberg, H., and DeHaan, R. L. (1969): The precardiac areas and the formation of the tubular heart in the chick embryo. *Dev. Biol.,* 19:128.

140. Steding, G., and Seidl, E. (1980): Contribution to the development of the heart. I. Normal development. *J. Thorac. Cardiovasc. Surg.,* 28:386–409.

141. Sweeney, L. J., Clark, W. A., Umeda, P. K., Zak, R., and Manasek, F. J. (1984): Immunofluorescence analysis of the primordial myosin detectable in embryonic striated muscle. *Proc. Natl. Acad. Sci. U.S.A.,* 81:797–800.

142. Sweeney, L. J., Zak, R., and Manasek, F. J. (1984): Changes in atrial myosin heavy chain expression during differentiation of the embryonic chick heart. *Circulation,* 70(Suppl II): 196.

143. Syrovy, I., Delcayre, C., and Swynghedauw, B. (1979): Comparison of ATPase activity and light subunits in myosins from left and right ventricles and atria in seven mammalian species. *J. Mol. Cell. Cardiol.,* 11:1129–1135.

144. Thompson, R. P., Fitzharris, T. P., Denslow, S., and Carwile, E. (1979): Collagen synthesis in the developing chick heart. *Tex. Rep. Biol. Med.,* 39:305–319.

145. Thompson, R. P., Wong, Y.-M. M., and Fitzharris, T. P. (1983): A computer graphic study of cardiac truncal septation. *Anat. Rec.,* 206:207–214.

146. Thornell, L. E., and Forsgren, S. (1982): Myocardial cell hetero-

geneity in the human heart with respect to myosin ATPase activity. *Histochem. J.,* 14:479–490.

147. Timple, R., Oberbaumer, I., Furthmayr, H., and Kuhn, K. (1982): Macromolecular organization of type IV collagen. In: *New Trends in Basement Membrane Research,* edited by K. Kuhn, Schoene, and R. Timpl, pp. 57–67. Raven Press, New York.

148. Toyota, N., and Shimada, Y. (1981): Differentiation of troponin in cardiac and skeletal muscles in chicken embryos as studied by immunofluorescence microscopy. *J. Cell Biol.,* 91:497–504.

149. Trinkaus, J. P. (1980): Formation of protrusions of the cell surface during tissue cell movement. In: *Tumor Cell Surfaces and Malignancy,* edited by R. O. Hynes and C. F. Fox, pp. 887–906. Alan R. Liss, New York.

150. Umeda, P. K., Kavinsky, C. J., Sinha, A. M., Hsu, H. J., Jakovcic, S., and Rabinowitz, M. (1983): Cloned mRNA sequences for two types of embryonic myosin heavy chains from chick skeletal muscle. II. Expression during development using S1 nuclease mapping. *J. Biol. Chem.,* 258:5206–5214.

151. Urban, J. P. G., Maroudas, A., Bayliss, M. T., and Dillon, J. (1979): Swelling pressures of proteoglycans at the concentrations found in cartilaginous tissues. *Biorheology,* 16:447–464.

152. Van Mierop, L. H. S. (1979): Morphological development of the heart. In: *Handbook of Physiology,* Sect. 2, Vol. 1, *The Heart,* pp. 1–27. American Physiological Society, Bethesda.

153. Van Mierop, L. H. S., Alley, R. D., Kanssel, J. W., and Stranahan, A. (1963): The anatomy and embryology of endocardial cushion defects. *J. Thorac. Cardiovasc. Surg.,* 43:71–96.

153.a Van Mierop, L. H. S. and Bertuch, C. J. (1967): Development of arterial blood pressure in the chick embryo. *Am. J. Physiol.,* 212:43–48.

154. von der Mark, K. (1981): Localization of collagen types in tissues. *Int. Rev. Connect. Tissue Res.,* 9:265–324.

155. von der Mark, K., and Ocalan, M. (1982): Immunofluorescent localization of type V collagen in the chick embryo with monoclonal antibodies. *Collagen Rel. Res.,* 2:541–555.

156. von der Mark, K., Sasse, J., von der Mark, H., and Kuhn, U. (1982): Changes in the distribution of collagen types during embryonic development. *Connect. Tissue Res.,* 10:37–42.

157. Wainwright, S. A., Biggs, W. D., Currey, J. D., and Gosline, J. M. (1976): *Mechanical Design in Organisms.* Wiley, New York.

158. Whalen, R. G., and Sell, S. M. (1980): Myosin from fetal hearts contains the skeletal muscle embryonic light chain. *Nature (Lond.),* 286:731–733.

159. Whalen, R. G., Sell, S. M., Eriksson, A., and Thornell, L. E. (1982): Myosin subunit types in skeletal and cardiac tissues and their developmental distribution. *Dev. Biol.,* 91:485–490.

160. Wikman-Coffelt, J., Refsum, H., Hollosi, G., Rouleau, L., Chuck, L., and Parmley, W. W. (1982): Comparative force-velocity relation and analysis of myosin of dog atria and ventricles. *Am. J. Physiol.,* 243:H391–H397.

161. Wilkinson, J. M. (1980): Troponin C from rabbit slow skeletal and cardiac muscles is the product of a single gene. *Eur. J. Biochem.,* 103:179.

162. Wilkinson, J. M., and Grand, R. J. A. (1978): Comparison of amino acid sequence of troponin I from different striated muscles. *Nature (Lond.),* 271:31.

163. Winegrad, S., and Robinson, T. F. (1978): Force generation among cells in the relaxing heart. *Eur. J. Cardiol. [Suppl.],* 7:63–70.

164. Yamada, K. M. (1983): Cell surface interactions with extracellular materials. *Annu. Rev. Biochem.,* 52:761–799.

165. Yamada, K. M., and Kennedy, D. W. (1979): Fibroblast cellular and plasma fibronectins are similar but not identical. *J. Cell Biol.,* 80:492–498.

166. Yazaki, Y., Ueda, S., Nagai, R., and Shimada, K. (1979): Cardiac atrial myosin adenosine triphosphatase of animals and humans. Distinctive enzymatic properties compared with cardiac ventricular myosin. *Circ. Res.,* 45:522–527.

167. Zak, R., Chizzonite, R. A., Everett, A. W., and Clark, W. A. (1982): Study of ventricular isomyosins during normal and thyroid hormone induced cardiac growth. *J. Mol. Cell. Cardiol. [Suppl. 3],* 14:111–117.

The Heart and Cardiovascular System,
edited by H. A. Fozzard et al.
Raven Press, New York © 1986.

CHAPTER **48**

Coronary Circulation

R. A. Olsson and William J. Bugni

Raffiniert ist der Herr Gott, aber boshaft ist er nicht.
                                        A. Einstein

. . . the esential characteristics of science are: (1) It is guided by natural law; (2) It has to be explanatory by reference to natural law; (3) It is testable against the empirical world; (4) Its conclusions are tentative, i.e., are not necessarily the final word; and (5) It is falsifiable. . . .
                                        W. R. Overton (280)

This chapter deals with four questions that we feel will provide the central themes for future research in coronary physiology: How do the chemical and physical determinants of coronary flow interact during particular physiological responses? What metabolites control coronary flow? How does regulation of coronary flow differ from one cardiac chamber to another? How do events in discrete elements of the cardiac microcirculation determine the overall behavior of the coronary circulation? Accordingly, this chapter will not be a comprehensive review of coronary physiology. At best, such an effort would only duplicate several recent major reviews (42,117,235) as well as incisive reviews that have provided different interpretations or have dealt with

more specialized topics (19,21,37,38,170,187,269,282, 356,390,399). Rather, we shall begin with a brief synopsis of the several determinants of coronary flow in order to orient the reader, and then consider several selected topics in detail. The discussion of each topic usually centers on one or more articles that illustrate the kinds of experiments that have been used to attack problems in coronary physiology. We have chosen these topics because they emphasize the need for additional research and also because they emphasize the interactions of the various determinants of coronary flow. At times these interactions can be quite subtle, and experimental separation and quantitation of the individual contributions to an overall response can prove exceedingly difficult. We shall conclude with a survey of some recent experiments that appear to have opened up new areas for future research.

DETERMINANTS OF MYOCARDIAL PERFUSION

Physical as well as chemical factors determine myocardial perfusion. Two of the five determinants of coronary blood flow are purely physical: coronary perfusion pressure and intramural myocardial pressure. A third (myogenic vascular tone) is in essence a chemical response (myocyte relaxation) to a physical stimulus (stretch). Two determinants are, ultimately, chemical in nature: the local responses to endogenous or blood-borne metabolites and the influences of both major divisions of the autonomic nervous system. The physical determinants of coronary flow vary phasically from moment to moment throughout the cardiac cycle. The phasic coronary flow waveform is an expression of the dynamic interplay of these factors. Myogenic, metabolic, and neural mechanisms operate over a longer time base, exerting a tonic influence on coronary resistance, or, if they change myocardial perfusion, changing it at a rate that requires several to many heartbeats to achieve full expression.

Coronary driving pressure is the *primum mobile* for myocardial perfusion. It is identical with aortic root pressure unless there is coronary obstruction, in which case the pressure distal to the obstruction becomes the effective inflow pressure for the system.

Cardiac contraction generates a tissue pressure that opposes coronary driving pressure. This intramyocardial pressure consists of two components: compression of the contents of the cardiac interstitial space by myofiber shortening, augmented by pressure transmitted from the cavity of the cardiac chamber.

Myogenic tone reflects the innate propensity of all kinds of smooth muscle to contract in response to stretch. Coronary vascular smooth muscle is no exception, generating tension in response to the transmural pressure differential. Indeed, much of the high basal resistance characteristic of the coronary circulation appears to be myogenic in origin.

Locally produced metabolites seem to be important determinants of coronary vascular resistance. The metabolic hypothesis of coronary blood flow regulation posits that myocytes release vasodilatory metabolites in proportion to their work rate, thus, in effect, regulating their own supply of substrates. The metabolic hypothesis takes two forms, depending on the stimulus to the production of vasodilator. One view holds that cardiac contraction generates a momentary imbalance between oxygen supply and demand and that this "micro-hypoxia" is the stimulus to metabolite release. An alternative view is that vasodilator release is a metabolic concomitant of cardiac contraction and that micro-hypoxia is unnecessary. The list of candidate vasoregulators includes oxygen, carbon dioxide, potassium, glycolytic intermediates such as acetate, purines such as adenosine or its phosphates, and prostacyclin. All are vasodilators that presumably act by opposing the mechanisms that generate basal tone. Experimental evidence to be reviewed later does not support the ascendancy of any one metabolite over the others, and, indeed, several may act

in concert to affect metabolic control. Emerging evidence that endothelial cells elaborate vasoactive metabolites indicates that metabolic events within the blood vessels themselves may contribute to local flow control.

The nearly simultaneous developments of selective autonomic agonists and antagonists, as well as the development of instrumented models using conscious dogs, have greatly enhanced our understanding of neural control of the coronary circulation. All elements of the vegetative nervous system, α-adrenergic vasoconstrictor influences as well as cholinergic and β-adrenergic vasodilatory influences, participate to variable degrees in the control of myocardial perfusion. In addition to being important tonic determinants of coronary resistance, autonomic reflexes may contribute prominently to dynamic flow responses such as that to exercise.

INSTANTANEOUS FLOW IN CORONARY ARTERIES AND VEINS

A recording of instantaneous coronary flow rate reflects the interplay of all the determinants, both tonic and dynamic, of myocardial perfusion. Estimates of mean flow rate, such as those obtained by one of the indicator dilution methods or by electronic processing of a flow meter signal, are quite appropriate for studying a tonic influence such as that of cardiac metabolism and certainly have contributed a great deal to what is known today about the regulation of myocardial perfusion. However, a phasic flow curve contains valuable additional information, particularly about the physical determinants of coronary flow. The technical means for obtaining phasic flow curves have been available for some time, but exploitation is hampered by a rather primitive understanding of what a change in instantaneous flow rate means.

A goal of coronary physiology should be to understand the actions and interactions of the several determinants of coronary flow to a degree that will permit prediction of instantaneous coronary flow rate, at any moment in the cardiac cycle and under any set of physiological circumstances. The following summary of the present state of knowledge about phasic coronary flow patterns is an attempt to stimulate further research toward a fuller understanding of their meaning.

Owing to its size, temperament, and husbandry, the dog has provided most of what is known about phasic coronary flow patterns. Information from other species, although more limited in scope, suggests that coronary flow patterns in the dog probably represent those of mammals generally.

Left Ventricular Epicardial Arteries

Figure 1A is a tracing of aortic root pressure and blood flow rate in the left anterior descending and

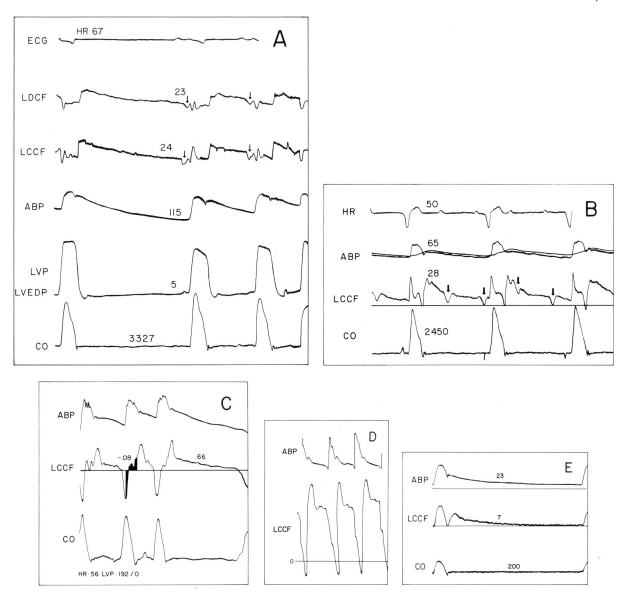

FIG. 1. Examples of phasic flow patterns in left coronary branches of awake dogs. **A:** Normal pattern in a dog resting quietly some weeks after thoracotomy for instrumentation. From above downward, curves are electrocardiograms (ECG), flow in the anterior descending (LDCF) and circumflex (LCCF) branches of the left coronary artery, aortic root (ABP) and left ventricular cavitary (LVP) pressures, and cardiac output (CO). Numbers indicate mean heart rate (HR), blood flow rates (ml/min), and pressures (mm Hg). Note the similarity of the flow patterns in the coronary branches, the atrial coves (*arrows*) in the coronary flow curves, and the pronounced sinus arrhythmia typical of this experimental preparation. **B:** From a dog with experimental heart block during ventricular pacing at 50/min, showing how atrial coves follow the P wave of the electrocardiogram. (From ref. 297, with permission.) **C:** From a dog with congenital subaortic stenosis. In the second beat, systolic flow is shaded to illustrate how early systolic backflow may result in net negative forward flow during this phase of the cardiac cycle. Numbers refer to stroke systolic and diastolic flow volumes, and the horizontal line through the coronary flow curve is the zero-flow reference. (From ref. 298, with permission of the American Heart Association, Inc.) **D:** Coronary flow response to left stellate ganglion stimulation in a conscious dog, illustrating how the positive inotropic effect of this intervention produces late systolic backflow. (From ref. 148, with permission.) **E:** In the late stages of cardiovascular decompensation following hemorrhage, showing how systolic coronary flow constitutes a large fraction of stroke coronary flow. (From ref. 147, with permission.)

circumflex coronary arteries of a conscious, resting dog. The singular attribute of left coronary flow is that it is predominantly diastolic. Unlike other vascular beds, wherein flow is mainly systolic, 60 to 85% of left coronary inflow occurs in diastole (156). Such a low fraction of systolic flow reflects, first of all, the shorter

duration of this phase of the cardiac cycle and, more important, the indirect effects, resistive as well as capacitative, of compressive forces exerted by myocardium surrounding the intramural coronary arteries.

During myocardial relaxation at the end of systole, the coronary flow rate rises rapidly to a zenith early in diastole and then falls as diastolic runoff from the root of the aorta lowers coronary perfusion pressure. One would expect that retarded myocardial relaxation, such as that brought about by ischemia, would reduce early diastolic acceleration of blood into the coronary arteries. Our casual observations suggest that this may be so, but systematic studies addressing this question apparently have never been performed. In some dogs, particularly those with low heart rates, early diastolic coronary flow undergoes one or more rather marked oscillations that damp out by late diastole and that do not seem to be related to corresponding oscillations of aortic pressure (see, for example, Fig. 12). Their genesis is unknown.

In dogs in sinus rhythm, left coronary inflow falls transiently by as much as a third late in diastole, the so-called atrial cove (158). Several pieces of evidence show that atrial systole generates this flow transient. First, it coincides with small vibrations in the aortic pressure curve that are due to atrial systole (293). Second, similar coronary flow transients accompany each atrial systole in dogs with surgical heart block (297) (Fig. 1B). Because the circumflex branch of the left coronary artery supplies atrium as well as ventricle, the atrial cove could reflect systolic compression of atrial intramural branches. However, the cove persists after ligation of the major atrial branches of this artery (34) and, moreover, is present in recordings of flow in the left anterior descending branch, which lacks an atrial distribution (Fig. 1A). In sum, this evidence shows that the atrial curve is due to compression of ventricular intramural branches during the rise in ventricular cavitary pressure due to atrial systole.

Coronary flow falls precipitously at the onset of ventricular systole. A normal flow curve may actually show a momentary reversal of flow at this time. The flow rate remains low throughout systole, tending to rise somewhat during midsystole and fall again at the end of this portion of the cardiac cycle. The systolic flow waveform varies substantially from dog to dog and, in some instances, from day to day in a given dog. It now appears that the systolic waveform in an epicardial coronary artery is the resultant of antegrade systolic flow impelled by coronary flow pressure, opposed by retrograde flow of blood expressed from intramural vessels by the action of systolic intramyocardial pressure (348). Coronary flow tracings obtained from dogs with idiopathic hypertrophic subaortic stenosis (IHSS), from dogs during stellate ganglion stimulation, and from dogs in hemorrhagic shock support this interpretation. When intramyocardial pressure is enhanced by outflow tract obstruction or β-adrenergic stimulation, the coronary flow tracing exhibits prominent early systolic backflow (Figs. 1C and 1D). By contrast, the systolic component of flow to the hypodynamic ventricle of an animal in hemorrhagic shock constitutes a substantial fraction of total stroke flow (Fig. 1E).

Right Ventricular Epicardial Arteries

Phasic flow in the right coronary artery differs from that in a left coronary branch primarily in the magnitude of the systolic flow rate, which is approximately as high as that in diastole (Fig. 2). This difference owes to the lower systolic compressive forces in the right ventricle, which are apparently too small to effectively oppose antegrade flow (153). A right coronary flow tracing, like that of a left coronary branch, may contain an atrial cove (224).

Comparisons of right coronary flow patterns in 5 dogs with congenital valvular pulmonic stenosis (Figs. 2B and 2C) show that the systolic component of flow decreases as an inverse function of systolic right ventricular pressure. When stenosis is severe, the right coronary flow pattern resembles that of a left coronary branch, and, when extreme, there may even be systolic backflow. By contrast with the left coronary flow pattern of dogs with left ventricular outflow tract obstruction, the retrograde systolic right coronary flow of extreme pulmonic stenosis occurs late in systole. Whether or not this finding in one dog is generalizable and, if so, the reason for the difference between the two conditions should be investigated further. Little is known about how reactive hyperemia affects phasic right coronary flow, other than that both systolic flow and diastolic flow increase. There is very little information on the phasic right coronary flow responses to interventions such as nerve stimulation or hemorrhage, which seem fertile areas for future research.

Septal and Left Ventricular Intramural Arteries

The anterior septal artery of the dog arises from the abepicardial surface of the left coronary artery or near the origin of its anterior descending branch (94,154,391) and penetrates directly into the septal myocardium. Several anatomic features of this artery make it of special interest to physiologists. Owing to the short extramural course of this artery, usually only 1 or 2 mm, its phasic flow pattern should be relatively free of the inertial, resistive, and capacitative effects that doubtless modify the phasic flow profiles of epicardial coronary arteries. For part of its course, the septal artery runs immediately under the endocardium of the right ventricle, and so the extravascular compression exerted on it is intermediate between that of an epicardial and a deep intramural coronary artery. Varying the degree of extramural systolic compression on the septal artery is a feasible experimental intervention; one need only raise the right ventricular systolic pressure, for example, by pulmonary artery obstruction. The venous drainage of the septal artery differs from that of other left coronary branches in that it is by way of thebesian channels that empty directly into the right ventricle rather than by

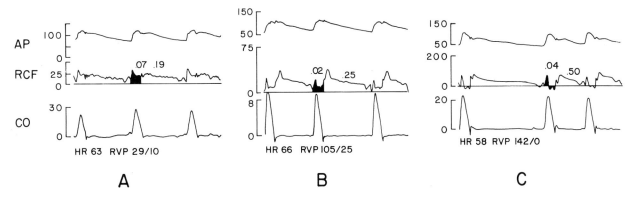

FIG. 2. Phasic right coronary flow patterns. From top to bottom, curves are aortic root pressure (AP, mm Hg), right coronary flow rate (RCF, ml/min), and cardiac output (CO, liters/min). **A:** Normal dog, showing the high flow rate in systole typical of this coronary branch. In the second beat, systolic stroke flow is shaded to illustrate that in the right coronary artery, systolic flow makes a larger contribution to total stroke flow, 27% in this example, than in left coronary branches. **B** and **C:** From dogs with congenital pulmonic stenosis, showing how chronic right ventricular systolic overload decreases the systolic contribution to total right coronary flow. HR, heart rate; RVP, right ventricular cavitary pressure. (From ref. 224, with permission.)

way of the coronary sinus (244,296). In principle, at least, one should be able to manipulate the septal venous drainage by altering right ventricular cavitary pressure. Finally, the anatomical location of this artery makes registration of its phasic flow profile a technically formidable undertaking; indeed, we can find only two reports that describe phasic flow rate and one that describes phasic flow velocity profiles in this artery.

Eckstein and his colleagues described measurements of septal flow made by means of an orifice meter (104). Although flow rate is not directly proportional to pressure differential in this method of measurement, such curves nonetheless yield accurate information about flow rate and its phasic variations, and it is possible to reconstruct true flow profiles by recourse to calibration curves. These authors found (Fig. 3A) that septal flow is antegrade throughout diastole. Isovolumic systole causes retrograde flow, but flow then reverts to antegrade by midsystole and remains so for the rest of this phase of the cardiac cycle. Raising pulmonary artery systolic pressure to a level approximating that in the aorta abolishes the transeptal systolic pressure gradient and, in a functional sense, renders the septal artery less superficial. This maneuver exaggerates both early systolic backflow and early diastolic forward flow, while reducing midsystolic flow to nearly zero (Fig. 3B). These authors also described a separate set of experiments aimed at measuring septal intramyocardial pressure. The septal artery was isolated by cannulation, and right ventricular systolic pressure was raised to levels near those in the aorta by pulmonary artery obstruction. Septal artery flow in midsystole was then measured as coronary perfusion pressure was lowered. The intramyocardial pressure, i.e., the perfusion pressure at which midsystolic flow ceased, was approximately twofold higher than aortic pressure.

Eckstein and his colleagues ascribed early systolic backflow in the septal arteries solely to events on the arterial side of the circulation, because coronary venous flow is systolic: ". . . at some location there is a reversal of direction from which point forward flow continues distally and backward flow occurs centrally, at least, during the early phase of ventricular systole." Further, these authors attributed the exaggerated early diastolic forward flow during pulmonary artery constriction to filling of the main septal trunk, a capacitative effect, rather than to actual capillary flow.

A similar experiment by Carew and Covell (66) employed an electromagnetic flow meter and plastic snare for a zero-flow reference on the septal artery. A second

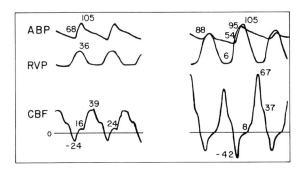

FIG. 3. Septal artery flow profiles obtained in an open-chest dog by means of an orifice meter. Curves are, from top downward, aortic pressure (ABP, mm Hg), right ventricular cavitary pressure (RVP, mm Hg), and coronary flow (CBF, ml/min). Note that the output of an orifice meter is not a linear function of flow rate. **Left:** At a normal right ventricular pressure. **Right:** During pulmonary artery constriction that raised right ventricular systolic pressure above aortic pressure. Note that early systolic flow is retrograde and that acute right ventricular pressure overload accentuates this backflow. (From ref. 104, with permission.)

flow meter and snare on the left circumflex branch permitted comparisons of the timing of flow oscillations in the two arteries. The oscillations in septal artery flow were directionally similar to those that Eckstein measured with the orifice meter, a notable exception being that early systolic backflow was either absent or negligible. One cannot tell whether this difference owes to some shortcoming of the orifice meter or to the possibility that the snare used for septal artery occlusion, which must have been very close to the electromagnetic flow meter, might have altered the contact between the flow meter and vessel and thus systematically shifted the zero reference. These authors also estimated intramyocardial systolic pressure by raising right ventricular pressure. Flow ceased when the pressures in the two ventricles were equal, indicating that intramyocardial pressure is no higher than intracavitary pressure. Whether this estimate or Eckstein's is correct depends crucially on which investigator established the zero-flow reference accurately. If Carew's estimate is too low or if Eckstein's is too high, the two studies will be in agreement.

Comparisons of septal and circumflex branch flow curves showed that the decrease in flow at the onset of systole began approximately 25 msec earlier in the septal artery than in the left circumflex branch. Electrically pacing the left ventricle from the free wall either reduced this time differential or reversed it, indicating that the earlier onset of systole in the septal artery flow tracing reflects the earlier activation of the interventricular septum.

Chilian and Marcus (70) placed miniature Doppler sensors on the septal artery and, for comparison, on the left anterior descending branch, as well as on one of its small branches just proximal to the point at which it penetrated into the myocardium. Owing to phasic variations in coronary artery diameter throughout the cardiac cycle (366,370), variations in flow velocity (units are LT^{-1}) do not correspond exactly to flow rate (units are L^3T^{-1}). However, these phasic variations in arterial caliber are only a few percent, small enough that a velocity profile approximates the flow profile reasonably well and certainly reflects the direction of flow accurately. Turning off the current that activates the piezoelectric crystal of a Doppler sensor generates a signal that coincides with that registered during mechanical occlusion of the vessel. Accordingly, the use of a Doppler sensor obviates the need for mechanical zero and circumvents the possibility of artifact in the flow zero due to movement of the flow meter during aterial occlusion.

Septal and perforating epicardial flow velocity profiles are similar to each other, but certainly not similar to flow velocity in the anterior descending branch (Fig. 4). Early systolic retrograde flow in the intramural coronary branches is the most prominent difference and is a result that confirms Eckstein's observation. Vasodilation produced by dipyridamole, nitroglycerin, or 20-sec occlusion of the left coronary artery enhanced both forward early systolic flow in the anterior descending branch and retrograde flow in the septal branch.

Left Ventricular Veins

Flow in the epicardial veins in the left ventricle varies phasically during the cardiac cycle, but unlike the predominantly diastolic flow on the arterial side of the

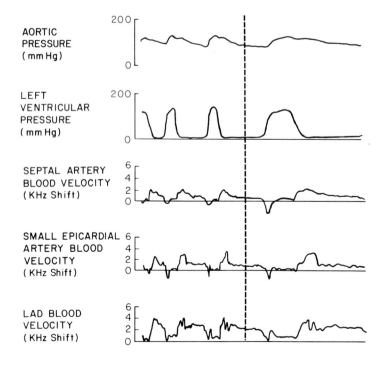

FIG. 4. Septal artery blood flow velocity profiles obtained by means of Doppler velocity meters in an open-chest dog. Note the early systolic backflow in the septal and small epicardial artery curves that is not present in the left anterior descending (LAD) curve. The *vertical dashed line* indicates a change in recording speed. (Redrawn from Fig. 2 of ref. 70, with permission.)

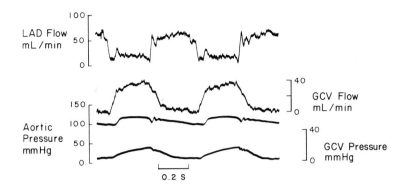

FIG. 5. Phasic flow and pressure curves from the left anterior descending (LAD) coronary artery and great cardiac vein (GCV) of an open-chest dog. Note that whereas arterial inflow is predominantly diastolic, venous outflow is almost exclusively systolic. (From unpublished experiments by Dr. Nobuyuki Yamada in the authors' laboratory.)

circulation, venous outflow is confined almost exclusively to systole (Fig. 5). Such an out-of-phase relationship between coronary inflow and outflow, particularly the negligible venous outflow during diastole, the time of greatest arterial inflow, is undeniable evidence that myocardial intramural blood volume oscillates throughout the cardiac cycle. Indeed, a mass balance approach, which includes measurements of both phasic arterial inflow and venous outflow, seems particularly appropriate for studies of coronary capacitance.

Probably because of their small size, there have been no studies of phasic flow profiles in the anterior cardiac veins. Such observations would be of great interest in view of the important differences between phasic right and left coronary inflow patterns, differences that suggest that the determinants of perfusion in the right and left ventricles differ at least quantitatively.

Although technical means to measure flow in the thebesian channels draining the interventricular septum are not now available and may never be, such observations would be of exceedingly great interest. These veins have an entirely intramural course and, by analogy with flow in the septal artery, will be freer of capacitance effects than will flow in an epicardial vein. The septal thebesian veins drain into the right ventricle, a chamber whose systolic pressure is substantially higher than that of the right atrium, the terminus of the coronary sinus and anterior cardiac veins. Accordingly, there is no reason to believe that flow in these veins is exclusively systolic, or even predominantly so.

MYOGENIC CORONARY TONE

Myogenic tone, as the term implies, is the intrinsic property of all types of smooth muscle to contract in response to stretch. In vascular smooth muscle the transmural pressure differential is the stimulus to the development of myogenic tone. Electrophysiological studies of cat cerebral arteries show that myocyte membrane potential and vessel caliber vary inversely, and the frequency of "pacemaker-like" action potentials varies directly with transmural pressure differential between 0 and 140 mm Hg. Still higher pressures will

lower the membrane potential to such an extent that pacemaker activity is suppressed. Increasing the extracellular $[Ca^{2+}]$ or blocking nerve excitation by tetrodotoxin (Na^+ channel blocker) or phentolamine (α-adrenergic receptor antagonist) increases the pressure dependence of the membrane potential, whereas lowering extracellular $[Ca^{2+}]$ or blocking Ca^{2+} entry with verapamil decreases it (165). Observations such as these suggest that voltage-dependent Ca^{2+} channels may mediate myogenic tone, but how gating is coupled to membrane stretch remains a mystery. In the coronary circulation the capacity to autoregulate and the singularly high basal tone characteristic of this vascular bed appear to be myogenic in origin.

Autoregulation

Investigations in organs other than the heart have shown that changes in vascular transmural pressure differential, either increases or decreases, evoke dynamic resistance changes that are very strongly dependent on the rate of pressure change (149–151,184). A mathematical model based on measurements of the mechanical properties of blood vessels and only a minimum number of assumptions predicts the dynamics of myogenic vascular responses quite well (50). The coronary circulation exhibits the same dynamic responses to step increases and decreases in perfusion pressure, i.e., transmural pressure differential, as other vascular beds (Fig. 6A). Whether or not such coronary responses show the same rate dependence as in other vascular beds is unknown.

Autoregulation, the capacity of a vascular bed to adjust its resistance so as to maintain blood flow constant in the face of changes in perfusion pressure, is a static manifestation of myogenic tone. The points on the pressure-flow curve demonstrating autoregulation (Fig. 6B) represent the steady-state flow rates reached at the end of dynamic responses such as those shown in Fig. 6A. If perfusion pressure is changed very slowly so as to avoid dynamic responses, the resulting pressure-flow curve resembles Fig. 6B very closely. The coronary circulation exhibits a substantial capacity for autoregulation, maintaining flow very nearly constant over a

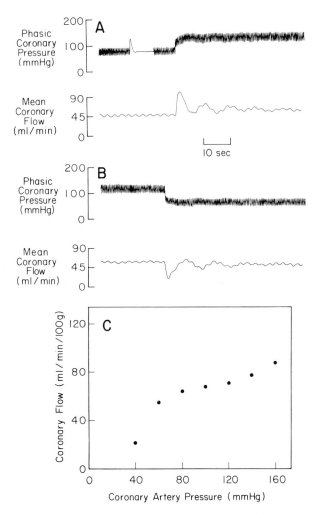

FIG. 6. Dynamic and static coronary autoregulatory flow responses to a step increase **(A)** and a step decrease **(B)** in coronary perfusion pressure of 50 mm Hg. Note that the dynamic flow responses consist of a series of damped oscillations that ultimately reach a new steady-state level only slightly different from that prior to the change in perfusion pressure. **C:** Steady-state coronary flow rate is relatively independent of perfusion pressure over the autoregulatory range, which in this example extends between roughly 60 and 120 mm Hg. (Redrawn from original records kindly furnished by Dr. William P. Dole, University of Iowa.)

range of mean perfusion pressures whose bounds are, roughly, 60 to 70 mm Hg and 120 to 140 mm Hg. However, the capacity to autoregulate is not unlimited; owing to limits on the ability of the coronary vascular smooth muscle to further contract or relax, the coronary flow rate is pressure-dependent above or below the "autoregulatory range."

Basal Coronary Tone

Considered in light of the high and continuous rate of cardiac oxygen consumption (6–10 ml/min/100 g), basal coronary resistance is remarkably high. By contrast,

the brain and the kidney consume oxygen at rates as high as or higher than that for the heart (on a per weight basis). However, the ratios of cerebral and renal vascular resistances to oxygen consumption rates for these organs are approximately two and five times lower, respectively, than that for the heart. Presumably a high coronary resistance confers some sort of biological advantage, perhaps an evolutionary one, but what this advantage might be is unknown.

Myogenic coronary constriction seems the likeliest explanation for the bulk of basal coronary tone. Regrettably, there is not much direct evidence to support this inference, which instead rests to an uncomfortably large degree on exclusion of other tonic vasoconstrictor influences. Foremost among the alternative mechanisms is α-adrenergic vasoconstriction, which clearly is present during exercise, for example, and appears to modulate coronary flow responses to exercise (308,356). However, experimental ablation of adrenergic vasoconstriction shows that this influence is quantitatively not sufficient to account for basal coronary tone. Coronary resistance in conscious dogs after convalescence from total cardiac denervation is approximately twice as high (not lower) as that in dogs with intact cardiac innervation (157). The $M\dot{V}O_2$ for such denervated hearts is approximately half that in control dogs, suggesting that the change in resistance may reflect a reduction in metabolic vasodilation, perhaps β_1-adrenergically mediated. "Chemical sympathectomy" achieved by intracoronary administration of 6-hydroxydopamine, a neurotoxic catecholamine analog, is said to reduce regional coronary vascular resistance (177). However, destruction of cardiac sympathetics by painting the epicardium with phenol does not change basal coronary resistance (69). Because the two experimental approaches produce similar degrees of tissue catecholamine depletion and insensitivity to pharmacological agents that release catecholamines, it is difficult to reconcile these discordant results. Finally, selective α_1-adrenergic blockade with drugs such as prazosin has a relatively small effect on coronary resistance. In sum, these lines of evidence suggest that there is probably an α_1-adrenergic component of basal coronary tone, but it is rather modest.

There is now evidence that different cellular mechanisms mediate the myogenic and adrenergic components of basal coronary tone. Pharmacological doses of adenosine are often used to abolish coronary autoregulatory tone in order to examine, for example, the interaction of the resistive and capacitative properties of this vascular bed (see pages 1002–1005). Even when autoregulation is abolished by supramaximal doses of adenosine, it is possible to raise coronary conductance further by unselective α-adrenergic blockade with phentolamine (373). Whether the heart or coronary blood vessels produce metabolites that are coronary vasoconstrictors is uncertain (see pages 995–997).

If myogenic tone is responsible for the singularly high basal resistance of the coronary circulation, what is the stimulus that generates it? The coronary circulation differs from that of other vascular beds in the magnitude of the changes in vascular transmural pressure that occur within each cardiac cycle as a consequence of the large fluctuations in intramyocardial pressure. Despite the limitations of intramyocardial pressure measurements, there seems little doubt that the difference between systolic and diastolic cardiac intramural pressures is larger than that in other organs, wherein "tissue pressure" is presumably relatively constant and the change in vascular transmural pressure is simply the difference between the systolic and diastolic perfusion pressures. However, the magnitude of the cyclical transmural pressure differential does not tell the entire story, for available evidence suggests that this differential is smaller in the subepicardium than in the subendocardium, exactly the opposite of the apparent autoregulatory capacities of these regions (see pages 1012–1013). Future work must determine how both the magnitude and the rate of change of coronary vascular smooth muscle stretch might influence myogenic tone. Because the available information about myogenic tone comes from experiments in which stretch was aperiodic, future studies should also search for force- and frequency-dependent effects and for interactions between the two.

In hearts under constant-pressure perfusion from a reservoir, a fall in coronary resistance on cessation of the heartbeat is clear evidence of the importance of cardiac systole as a determinant of stroke coronary resistance (316). One wonders whether or not the loss of a potential stimulus to myogenic tone, i.e., the oscillation in coronary transmural pressure, also contributes to such a resistance change and, if so, to what extent. Indeed, studying the effects of cyclical changes in coronary perfusion pressure during prolonged asystoles may yield insights into the characteristics of myogenic responses generally and of their contribution to regulation of coronary flow.

METABOLIC REGULATION OF CORONARY FLOW

The apparent dependence of left coronary flow on $M\dot{V}O_2$ is the foundation for the hypothesis that the heart regulates its own blood supply by elaborating coronary vasodilators in proportion to its rate of energy expenditure. The high degree of covariance between coronary flow and $M\dot{V}O_2$ shown in Fig. 7 is typical of the results of many such experiments in a number of laboratories. Depending on how one interprets the correlation between coronary flow and $M\dot{V}O_2$, it is possible to construct two general models for metabolic regulation of coronary flow. Both models postulate the release of

a vasodilatory metabolite, but they differ fundamentally with regard to the stimulus for its production and, accordingly, the relationships among cardiac energy expenditure, $M\dot{V}O_2$, the rate of metabolite production, and coronary resistance. One interpretation is that $M\dot{V}O_2$ and coronary flow are causally related, rather than merely covariant, i.e., that metabolite production is oxygen-dependent (Fig. 8A). An alternative interpretation is that the covariance of coronary flow and $M\dot{V}O_2$ is coincidental (Fig. 8B). The model that derives from this interpretation envisions that some concomitant of cardiac activity, for example, the action potential, serves as the stimulus to metabolite production and considers $M\dot{V}O_2$ as only an indirect index of metabolite production. Henceforth we shall refer to these as the oxygen-dependent and oxygen-independent models.

The oxygen-dependent model has served as a useful guide to research that has now revealed weaknesses in this model that are sufficient to force its rejection. On the other hand, the oxygen-independent model offered as a substitute is gravely weakened by its imprecision. The major strength of the oxygen-dependent model was that it provided precise experimentally testable predictions about the quantitative relationships among $M\dot{V}O_2$, metabolite production, and coronary resistance. Implicit in that model was the concept of a small imbalance between oxygen supply and demand that led to hypoxia, the actual stimulus to metabolite production. Experimental proof of the generalizability of the model depended on demonstrating that coronary resistance was uniquely related to $M\dot{V}O_2$, which clearly was not the case. Because heart muscle can meet its oxygen needs by altering oxygen extraction, such as during exercise (197,308), as well as by altering coronary flow, coronary flow cannot be uniquely related to $M\dot{V}O_2$. Additionally, the micro-hypoxia postulated to be the signal that drives metabolite production has not yet been demonstrated experimentally.

The oxygen-independent model successfully skirts the problem of oxygen extraction as the determinant of $M\dot{V}O_2$, as well as the need to postulate micro-hypoxia. However, this model will remain of dubious usefulness unless metabolite production can be linked to something more concrete than "cardiac activity." In its present form, this model is difficult to test experimentally.

Direct quantitative proof of either model becomes immensely more complicated if, as is quite possible, more than one metabolite controls coronary resistance (105). Future work may well force us to reject altogether the notion of a unitary hypothesis for metabolic regulation of coronary flow. Just as the discovery of quantum dynamics, with its ultimate indeterminacy, forced abandonment of classical physics with its philosophical deterministic foundation, so may metabolic control of coronary flow turn out to be less deterministic than the covariance of coronary flow and $M\dot{V}O_2$ would imply.

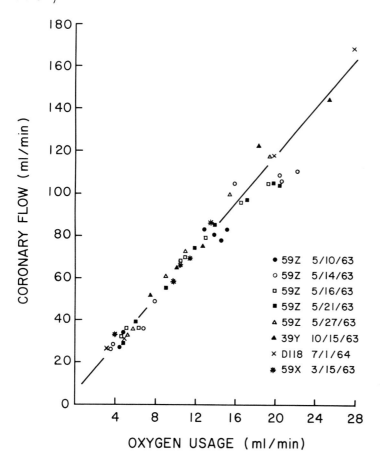

FIG. 7. Relationship of coronary flow and MV̇O₂ in conscious dogs, each of which is represented by a separate symbol. (From ref. 197, with permission.)

- ● 59Z 5/10/63
- ○ 59Z 5/14/63
- □ 59Z 5/16/63
- ■ 59Z 5/21/63
- △ 59Z 5/27/63
- ▲ 39Y 10/15/63
- × DII8 7/1/64
- ＊ 59X 3/15/63

Irrespective of the type and degree of linkage between coronary flow and metabolism, endogenous metabolites do appear to influence coronary resistance. Berne (40) has proposed criteria for establishing that adenosine is a coronary vasoregulatory metabolite: (a) the substance must be a potent dilator of the coronary resistance vessels; (b) there must be an endogenous source of the mediator; (c) the substance should have access to the arterioles and be present under basal physiological conditions; (d) the concentration reached in the interstitial fluid (ISF) must be capable of eliciting vasodilation, and there should be a close relationship between the ISF

concentration and coronary flow rate (dose-response relationship); (e) the time course of oxygen deficit (either decreased oxygen supply or increased oxygen demand) should parallel the increment in coronary flow rate; (f) the physiological effect, at different concentrations of the endogenous mediator, should be mimicked by exogenous administration of the substance; (g) agents that potentiate or attenuate the action of administered mediator should elicit a similar effect on endogenously liberated mediator; and (h) a direct cause-and-effect relationship should be established under all physiological and pathophysiological conditions among change and

FIG. 8. Diagrammatic representations of the oxygen-dependent (A) and oxygen-independent (B) models of metabolic control of coronary flow. See text for discussion.

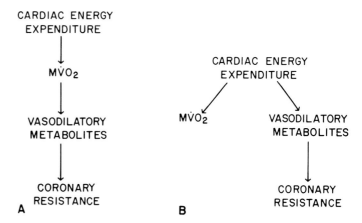

coronary blood flow and adenosine release. An additional criterion is that the receptor or the chemical process that initiates coronary relaxation be known (279). With the exception of criteria (e) and (h), which apply only to oxygen-dependent models, these criteria apply to any metabolite and thus are applicable as we now consider the candidacies of the various metabolites proposed as coronary regulators. It is fair to say at the outset that none of the candidate vasodilators meets all of these criteria.

Oxygen

The hypothesis that oxygen acts directly on coronary vascular smooth muscle posits that as $M\dot{V}O_2$ rises, PO_2 in the vicinity of the coronary resistance vessels falls, thereby initiating relaxation. In a sense, the depletion of a metabolite rather than its production qualifies this as a metabolic hypothesis. The support for this hypothesis is generally ambiguous. Studies of the coronary microcirculation that demonstrate the intermittent perfusion of individual vascular units (354,365) admit the possibility of a hypoxic stimulus to smooth muscle relaxation and complements evidence that hyperoxia elicits coronary vasoconstriction (309,345). Recent evidence suggests that hypoxic coronary vasodilation is endothelium-dependent (65) and is probably mediated by prostaglandins (64). Whether or not PO_2 in the endothelium of resistance vessels falls to levels that would elicit this type of vasodilation is uncertain.

A necessary consequence of the PO_2 hypothesis is that in order for the coronary circulation to protect the heart from hypoxia, the precapillary sphincters must be more sensitive to hypoxia than the parenchymal cardiocytes (269). The only available evidence (measurement by means of a cartesian diver) shows that the basal oxygen consumption rate in isolated noncoronary microvessels is 0.5 to 0.6 nmole/min per gram dry weight (178), a rate more than 10-fold lower than $M\dot{V}O_2$ under conditions of basal cardiac activity. However, this evidence from relatively large microvessels does not rule out the possibility that the muscle of precapillary sphincters has a much higher rate of oxygen usage. Whether or not PO_2 in the walls of the resistance vessels, which carry arterial blood, ever falls low enough to cause myocyte relaxation is unknown. Larger microvessels maintain tone until PO_2 is equal to or less than 5 mm Hg, a level well below the PO_2 of coronary venous blood (132). Again, the lack of oxygen sensitivity of these larger vessels may not represent the situation in the resistance vessels, but there is as yet no experimental support for this possibility.

Cytochrome aa_3 is a logical candidate for a vascular oxygen receptor, but poisoning this enzyme with cyanide causes less relaxation of vascular smooth muscle than does hypoxia (72). There is no support for an alternative oxygen receptor, nor is there a mechanism known whereby oxygen depletion could otherwise initiate relaxation.

An experiment by Gellai et al. (132) suggested that although oxygen by itself may not regulate coronary flow, it could act in concert with other metabolites to do so. Isolated coronary microvessels that were insensitive to hypoxia were "conditioned" by addition of adenosine to the organ bath and thereupon exhibited PO_2-dependent relaxation.

Carbon Dioxide/H^+

The preponderantly aerobic metabolism of cardiac muscle generates carbon dioxide continuously and in a proportion to $M\dot{V}O_2$ that is determined by the respiratory quotient. Being highly diffusible, carbon dioxide has no difficulty reaching the coronary resistance vessels. Indeed, the diffusibility of this gas suggests a feedback model of coronary flow regulation in which the stimulus to coronary vasodilation, carbon dioxide accumulation, is modulated by enhanced washout of this metabolite. Essentially all the support for the hypothesis that PCO_2 controls coronary flow comes from studies in which arterial PCO_2 was the independent variable. Many such studies have shown that hypercapnia increases and hypocapnia decreases coronary flow; Feigl (117) has critically reviewed this extensive literature. Although this experimental approach is a good first step and the unanimity of the observations is impressive, evidence of this sort is not particularly persuasive, because it begs the central issue: What is the relationship between the coronary flow rate and the concentration of *endogenous* carbon dioxide? We can find no evidence on this crucial point. Further, the mechanism by which carbon dioxide might alter the contractile state of vascular smooth muscle is unknown.

Potassium

Several observations have suggested that potassium could link coronary flow to cardiac effort. Potassium efflux is a concomitant of cardiac systole, net efflux from the heart changing concordantly with heart rate, contractile force (202,361,362), or state of oxygenation (201). Further, intracoronary administration of potassium causes coronary vasodilation in the beating heart (59,337).

The experiment that probably best defined the role of potassium in coronary regulation was a comparison by Murray et al. (252) of the time courses of changes in coronary resistance and coronary plasma $[K^+]$ following a step increase in heart rate. This experiment entailed measuring coronary perfusion pressure and coronary

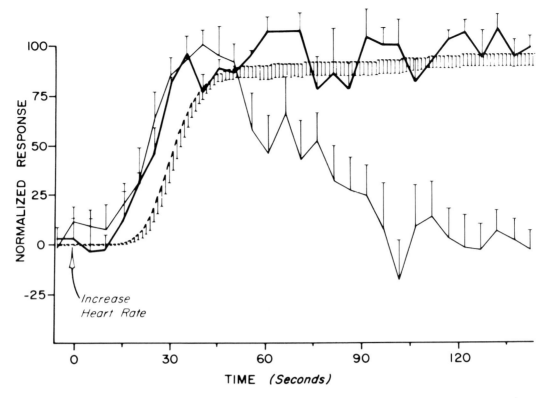

FIG. 9. Time courses of changes in coronary vascular resistance (*dash line*) and coronary venous plasma K$^+$ (*thick solid line,* 6 dogs; *thin solid line,* 3 dogs) in response to a step increase in heart rate at time zero. An upward deflection in the curve depicting coronary resistance indicates vasodilation. (From ref. 252, with permission.)

sinus oxygen content and [K$^+$] in open-chest dogs during constant-rate perfusion of the left coronary artery. As expected, electrical pacing at a rate 75 beats per minute above control caused a sustained increase in MV̇O$_2$ and, as shown in Fig. 9, a sustained decrease in coronary resistance. Coronary venous [K$^+$] initially rose in inverse proportion to coronary resistance, reaching a peak level ~ 0.5 mEq/liter higher than control. In 6 of 9 dogs, [K$^+$] then declined to control levels even though resistance remained unchanged. For reasons that were not identified, 3 dogs exhibited sustained increases in coronary sinus [K$^+$]. By reference to earlier studies of coronary vasoactivity and the permeability × surface area product for K$^+$ (253), these authors concluded that interstitial [K$^+$] reached levels that could account for about half of the change in coronary resistance and that other mechanisms, perhaps metabolic, accounted for the rest of the initial resistance response. In the 6 dogs in which venous [K$^+$] rose and then fell, other mechanisms must have been responsible for the entirety of the sustained response. In other words, potassium may have facilitated the development, but not the maintenance, of active hyperemia.

Acetate

Among the many intermediates of glycolytic metabolism, only acetate is a coronary vasodilator in dogs (221,245). The acetate concentrations needed to cause coronary vasodilation are in the millimolar range; whether or not such concentrations ever obtain in the cardiac interstitium is unknown. Likewise, the mechanism by which acetate causes coronary relaxation is unknown; that there would be a vascular receptor requiring millimolar concentrations of ligand for activation seems unlikely. Accordingly, the possibility that acetate contributes significantly to the regulation of coronary blood flow seems remote.

Prostaglandins

In contrast to the evidence linking prostaglandins to flow regulation in organs such as the kidney, the evidence for coronary flow control by prostaglandins is at best indirect. Coronary microvessels have the capacity to synthesize prostaglandins (137). Prostacyclin is an extremely powerful coronary relaxant *in vitro* (260).

Strong arguments oppose a prostaglandin hypothesis. There is, at present, no model that explains how prostaglandin synthesis might be coupled to cardiac effort. More compelling evidence, such as correlation of tissue prostaglandin levels with coronary resistance, does not exist. Prostaglandin synthesis inhibitors have little or no effect on coronary vasomotion (172).

Adenosine

Following experiments by Drury and Szent-Gyorgyi demonstrating the coronary vasoactivity of adenosine (102), Lindner and Rigler (222) crystallized this nucleoside from cardiac muscle extracts (where it probably arose from postmortem degradation of adenine nucleotides) and proposed the hypothesis that adenosine is a physiological regulator of coronary flow. For 30 years this idea received little attention, but in 1963, Berne (39) and Gerlach et al. (136) simultaneously began reinvestigations of this hypothesis. Augmented by the work of their students and others, this inquiry continues today. The recognition that adenosine may have a regulatory role in other organs, especially in brain, has stimulated research that has contributed significant insights into the possible role of adenosine in coronary regulation. Recent reviews summarize evidence for the regulatory role of adenosine (21,40,41,61,62,78,122).

Heart muscle contains a substrate, adenosine monophosphate (AMP), and the phosphohydrolases capable of generating adenosine, but as yet the site(s) and mechanism(s) of its production are uncertain. An account of the research toward an understanding of how adenosine is formed in heart muscle chronicles how significantly knowledge (or ignorance) of the compartmentalization of enzymes and substrates has influenced the direction of this research.

A series of electron micrographic histochemical studies that demonstrated 5'-nucleotidase activity in the cardiac sarcolemma (48,49,146,310,313) served as the basis for the earliest model of cardiac adenosine production. The discovery that ADP and ATP inhibit the catalytic activity of partially purified cardiac 5'-nucleotidase (22,106,360) provided a convenient explanation for the observation that only a very minor fraction of the enzyme activity in heart muscle, which totals approximately 0.5 μmole/min per gram in dogs, could account for measured rates of adenosine production, approximately 5 to 10 nmoles/min per gram (267). As is the case in most eukaryotic cells, this cardiac 5'-nucleotidase is an ectoenzyme; i.e., its catalytic site is on the external surface of the plasmalemma (85,86,124). Whereas this fact could account for the release of adenosine directly into the cardiac interstitium, it posed a serious problem: Given the consensus that plasma membranes are impermeable to nucleoside phosphates, how could AMP cross the sarcolemma to reach the putative site of adenosine production? Experiments suggesting that the ecto 5'-nucleotidase of heart muscle either contains or is functionally associated with an AMP permease (47,125) have been challenged (321). More recent experiments have shown that inhibitors, such as concanavalin A, adenosine-5'-α,β-methylene diphosphonate, or antibodies against the enzyme can suppress the hydrolysis of AMP nearly completely but have no influence on adenosine produc-

tion by heart muscle (333) or blood leukocytes (107,394). Such results mean that the ecto 5'-nucleotidase of heart muscle probably plays no role in the control of coronary flow.

The tentative identification within the last several years of not just one but two hitherto unsuspected cardiac 5'-nucleotidases, one cytosolic, the other mitochondrial, is an embarrassment of riches. A model of cardiac adenosine production based on either enzyme circumvents the problems of the ecto 5'-nucleotidase model very nicely, but in the case of the cytosolic enzyme, the substitute model encounters new difficulties in the form of substrate compartmentalization.

Schutz and his associates have provided evidence (333) that approximately 20% of the AMP phosphohydrolase activity of guinea pig heart muscle meets one operational criterion of a "soluble" enzyme; i.e., it is not sedimented by centrifugation for 2 hr at 200,000 $\times$ g. Rat heart homogenates contain a similar amount of unsedimentable AMP phosphohydrolase activity (R. A. Olson, *unpublished observations*). This cytoplasmic nucleotidase appears to be the pyrimidine-selective 5'-nucleotidase found in a number of tissues (107,181,230), although information about regulation of the cardiac enzyme by, for example, metal ions and nucleoside diphosphates and triphosphates is not available. The CMP-selective 5'-nucleotidase of human placenta appears to be Mg^{2+}-dependent and is competitively inhibited by ADP and ATP (K_i = 15 μM and 90 μM, respectively) and noncompetitively inhibited by inorganic phosphate (P_i) (K_i = 22 mM) (230). Owing to this sort of regulation by ADP and ATP and the compartmentalization of AMP, the role of the cytosolic 5'-nucleotidase in cardiac adenosine metabolism is uncertain. It now appears that mitochondria contain well over 90% of the cardiac AMP pool (60,346); accordingly, the cytosolic enzyme probably operates at a substrate concentration of 1 μM or at most only a few micromolar, whereas its catalytic activity is antagonized by ADP and ATP concentrations in the millimolar range.

Recognizing that mitochondria contain most of the AMP in cardiac cells and that coronary flow appears to correlate with the cardiac muscle ratio [ATP/(ADP + P_i)] (265), Bukoski et al. (56,57) are now examining the hypothesis that mitochondria are the seat of cardiac adenosine production. Initial *in vitro* studies showed that rat heart mitochondria release adenosine during incubation at 30°C. Substrates such as the combination of pyruvate plus malate stimulated adenosine release, whereas ADP, the ATPase inhibitor oligomycin, and the nucleotide translocase inhibitor atractyloside all inhibited adenosine release. Neither PO_2 nor [Ca^{2+}] influenced adenosine release. These workers have subsequently reported finding a 5'-nucleotidase activity in mitochondrial suspensions that cannot be accounted for by contamination with sarcolemmal 5'-nucleotidase (57).

These studies have not as yet characterized the catalytic or the regulatory properties of the mitochondrial enzyme. However, these interesting preliminary communications rekindle the hope that, at last, the site of cardiac adenosine formation may be identified. Because mitochondria contain cytochrome aa_3, the physiological "oxygen sensor," ultimately it may be possible to link adenosine production to $M\dot{V}O_2$.

The adenosine hypothesis predicts that there will be a quantitatively unique dependence of coronary resistance on the concentration of this nucleoside in the vicinity of the coronary resistance vessels, i.e., in the cardiac interstitial space. This is an exceedingly stringent criterion that, because of limitations in the methods for assaying adenosine and compartmentalization of this nucleoside within the heart, has resisted experimental proof. The earliest studies of the concentration of adenosine in heart muscle employed a spectrophotometric assay (268) in which heart extracts were treated sequentially with xanthine oxidase, nucleoside phosphorylase, and adenosine deaminase. The increases in uric acid concentrations that followed the addition of each enzyme measured, respectively, the concentrations of hypoxanthine, inosine, and adenosine in the muscle extract. Contamination of nucleoside phosphorylase by adenosine deaminase was recognized, but this was thought to introduce a systematic underestimate of adenosine of less than 30%. This analytical method yielded an estimate of adenosine concentration in cardiac muscle of 0.2 to 0.3 nmoles/g wet weight (268,312). Because the adenosine deaminase and adenosine kinase activities of cardiac muscle are high and these enzymes were thought to be exclusively intracellular, it was reasoned that in order for the cardiac adenosine pool to exist at all, it must be situated in the interstitial space. Given the drawbacks of the assay method, the estimated interstitial adenosine concentration of approximately 1 μM agreed reasonably well with the coronary vasoactivity of exogenous adenosine.

By the mid-1970s, improved assay methods showed that the original estimates of the amount of adenosine in heart muscle were too low by nearly an order of magnitude. The new estimates showed that under basal conditions, heart muscle adenosine content was between 1 and 2 nmoles/g wet weight (327). If distributed only in the cardiac interstitium, this much adenosine would have a concentration between 5 and 10 μM, more than enough to cause maximum coronary vasodilation. Because the normal state of the coronary circulation is certainly not one of maximum vasodilation, the model of an exclusively extracellular adenosine compartment had to be wrong.

The discovery that S-adenosylhomocysteine hydrolase (SAH) is an intracellular adenosine-binding protein (167) and that this enzyme accounts for an intracellular adenosine compartment in many organs, including the heart (317), resolved the discrepancy between cardiac muscle adenosine content and coronary resistance. As its name implies, one function of SAH is to catalyze the hydrolysis of S-adenosylhomocysteine, a product of S-adenosylmethionine-dependent methylations (367). This activity is important because it prevents product inhibition of the enzymes that catalyze, for example, several steps in catecholamine metabolism and also phospholipid synthesis. However, the poise of the equilibrium mediated by SAH strongly favors synthesis. In the absence of homocysteine, a low-affinity substrate, SAH exhibits high-affinity reversible binding of adenosine (367).

Although it is now clear that adenosine bound to SAH accounts for the bulk of the intracardiac adenosine pool (276,330), the physiological significance of this intracellular adenosine compartment is uncertain. In order to demonstrate hydrolysis of S-adenosylhomocysteine by SAH, it is necessary to remove adenosine as fast as it is formed, e.g., by deamination (79). The net result of this stratagem is not production of adenosine, but rather formation of one of its metabolites. In vitro experiments have shown that the [^{3}H]adenosine-SAH complex dissociates very slowly, the half-time being 2.5 hr when dissociation is driven by an excess of unlabeled ligand and over 6 hr when the complex is incubated with adenosine deaminase (276). To the extent that such in vitro experiments pertain to adenosine metabolism in the beating heart, it is difficult to visualize how adenosine in the intracellular compartment might participate in coronary vasoregulation.

The existence of a major intracellular compartment in the cardiac adenosine pool greatly complicates tests of the adenosine hypothesis that rely on correlations of coronary resistance with the adenosine concentration in the interstitial space. Unless future work establishes that the sizes of the interstitial and intracellular compartments change concordantly during physiological responses—and there is no reason to assume a priori that they should—studies that correlate cardiac muscle adenosine content with coronary flow rate (227,228,277,318) must be considered uninterpretable.

There is at present no consensus as to how to measure adenosine concentration in the cardiac interstitium. Release of adenosine into coronary venous blood is probably driven by diffusion down a concentration gradient. However, the release rate does not seem to be a simple function of the permeability × surface area product for adenosine (231). Rather, uptake by endothelial cells (and, under certain circumstances, perhaps even release from these cells) (262,263,286,287) doubtless obscures the true interstitial concentration. Adenosine accumulates in pericardial superfusates (242,312), but owing to uptake by the parietal pericardium (163), superfusate concentrations will be lower by an uncertain amount than those in the interstitial space. Epicardial diffusion wells (163) constitute, together with the cardiac interstitium, a closed two-compartment system. In principle, the concentration of adenosine in such a well should at equilibrium equal that in the interstitial space. This method yields estimates of interstitial adenosine concentration in hearts under basal conditions that are surprisingly high: 0.5 μM (163), a level that is well within the range at which exogenous adenosine is vasoactive (274,328). A subsequent preliminary communication (162) has described diffusion well adenosine concentrations that are somewhat lower, approximately 0.3 μM, in dogs whose coronary circulations retained the capacity to autoregulate. The adenosine concentration in cardiac lymph collected proximal to a node (229) is another approach to estimating interstitial concentration. Further work will be necessary to gauge the extent to which metabolism of adenosine by lymphatic endothelium alters lymph adenosine concentrations during transit to the collecting site.

To date, most tests of the adenosine hypothesis have compared some index of cardiac interstitial adenosine concentration with either $M\dot{V}O_2$ or some index of cardiac performance. Almost invariably such comparisons were made under steady-state conditions. There is now evidence that cardiac adenosine levels oscillate during the cardiac cycle, rising during systole and returning to a basal level during the succeeding diastole (363). Improved quick-freezing devices (388,389) have the potential to precisely define the time course of these dynamic changes so that they can be compared, for example, under various levels of cardiac work load. Such an experimental approach could be the means to discriminate between oxygen-dependent and oxygen-independent models of adenosine production.

The proof of the adenosine hypothesis must include an explanation of how interstitial adenosine levels are controlled during physiological responses. A mass balance approach recognizes that the concentration of adenosine will be the resultant of the rate of adenosine release into the interstitial space, minus losses from it, either through washout into coronary venous blood or through uptake by the cells that constitute its boundaries. At this time, there is no way to directly measure adenosine release. Measurement of the rate of washout, which is possible, plus measurements of the rate of cellular uptake would, under steady-state conditions, provide indirect estimates of adenosine production rate. Past studies of the uptake of exogenous radiolabeled adenosine by beating hearts (208,271,278) have been justly criticized for not accounting for endothelial uptake of adenosine (261–263). Unless this problem can be circumvented, a quantitative explanation of the control of interstitial adenosine concentration will remain elusive.

Studies in a variety of mammalian and nonmammalian cells have shown that nucleoside inward transport is a nearly universal phenomenon. Studies employing chick embryo cardiocytes (257) and isolated perfused rat hearts (259) have shown that heart cells are no exception to this general rule. These cells take up adenosine by a combination of simple and carrier-mediated diffusion. The carriers that mediate this transport are nonconcentrative; i.e., they catalyze transport down a concentration gradient, and they are inhibited enantio-selectively by certain adenosine analogs (271), by a number of 6-(benzylthio)purine nucleosides (282), and by drugs as chemically diverse as dipyridamole (293), diltazem (282), and benzodiazepines (71). Although transport inhibitors are potentially useful tools for quantitative studies of adenosine release rate, this potential is yet to be fully exploited.

Understanding the mechanism by which adenosine initiates coronary relaxation is a third major element in the proof of the adenosine hypothesis. A specific receptor on the surface of the coronary myocyte mediates the vasoactivity of adenosine (270,329); vascular relaxation is not endothelium-dependent (128). The attributes of the coronary receptor are identical with those of the low-affinity stimulatory (R_a or A2) adenosine receptor of adenylate cyclase (Table 1). Moreover, adenosine and A2-receptor-selective analogs stimulate the release of cyclic AMP by cultured vascular smooth muscle cells (4,139,145). Such a similarity suggests that coronary relaxation by adenosine may share a final common

TABLE 1. *Comparison of adenylate cyclase A2 (R_a) with coronary adenosine receptor*

Characteristic	A2	Coronary	Refs.
Cell surface	Yes	Yes	269,328
Stimulate adenylate cyclase	Yes	Yes	212,242
Forskolin potentiation	Yes	Yes	214
Theophylline inhibition	Yes	Yes	1,2,59,324
GTP dependence	Yes	Yes	242
Adenosine potency	Micromolar	Micromolar	273,327
Selective adenosine analog potency	NECA > R-PIA[a]	MPR NECA 150 MPR R-PIA 4.5	216

NECA = N-ethyladenosine-5'-uronamide; R-PIA = N[6]-R-1-phenyl-2-propyladenosine; MPR = molar potency ratio vs. adenosine.

pathway with the receptors of other vasodilatory agonists that act through adenylate cyclase, such as the β-adrenergic receptor. Accordingly, the results of experiments employing agonists other than adenosine could provide useful insights to guide future research on the mechanism of adenosine relaxation.

Events in the coronary myocyte subsequent to adenosine receptor occupancy are unclear. Electrophysiological studies have shown that adenosine reduces the slow inward current of the action potential of the coronary myocyte (166), but whether this reflects inhibition of the inward movement of Ca^{2+} (32) or inhibition of the outward movement of K^+ (182) is uncertain. Such evidence does not necessarily mean that the adenosine receptor is part of a so-called receptor-operated ion channel. Research in several laboratories appears to be converging on the idea that cyclic AMP-dependent protein phosphorylation plays a central role in the smooth muscle relaxation initiated by those agonists, including adenosine, that operate through adenylate cyclase. Such relaxation may involve phosphorylation of both the myocyte sarcolemma (188,324) and cytoplasmic proteins, particularly myosin light-chain kinase. Cyclic AMP-dependent phosphorylation of myosin light-chain kinase appears to inhibit its ability to phosphorylate and thereby increase the Ca^{2+} sensitivity of myosin (28,29,213,339,340). It is uncertain whether or not relaxation also involves the phosphorylation state of the membranes of intracellular Ca^{2+} storage sites (249,369).

As the idea that adenosine is the sole chemical mediator of coronary resistance has lost some of its momentum, a number of laboratories have initiated studies aimed at defining under what conditions and to what extent adenosine participates in coronary regulation. Although some of this evidence is available only in the form of preliminary communications, it is already clear that there are conflicts that future research will have to reconcile. For example, in the dog, β-adrenergic stimulation of $M\dot{V}O_2$ by norepinephrine elicits release of adenosine into coronary venous blood, whereas electrical pacing to similar levels of $M\dot{V}O_2$ and coronary blood flow does not (231). This experiment suggests that whether or not adenosine mediates a coronary flow response might depend on the kind of stimulus to the response. However, experiments using theophylline to block coronary adenosine receptors have led to a different conclusion than studies of adenosine release. Theophylline reduces the hyperemic response to pacing tachycardia (189,218) but has no effect on either the rise in tissue adenosine levels or the rise in coronary flow rate produced by norepinephrine administration (301). Studies in isolated buffer-perfused rodent hearts have shown that adenosine and certain of its analogs modulate the stimulatory effects on cardiac performance, metabolism, and coronary flow of agonists such as norepinephrine, dopamine, and histamine (326,386). Detailed biochemical studies have suggested that adenosine exerts these effects through adenylate cyclase inhibitory A1 receptors and that the coronary flow response is secondary to this effect on cardiocyte metabolism (326,386). However, in blood-perfused *in situ* dog hearts, intracoronary infusion of adenosine deaminase to destroy adenosine in the cardiac interstitial space reduces the coronary hyperemic response to isoproterenol infusion, but this effect is accounted for by a corresponding reduction in $M\dot{V}O_2$ (275). Although ischemia stimulates adenosine release (268), intracoronary adenosine deaminase infusions do not change coronary resistance distal to a critical stenosis (138). Intracoronary adenosine deaminase fails to modify either dynamic or static autoregulatory responses to changes in coronary perfusion pressure (91,162).

INTRAMURAL CORONARY BLOOD VOLUME

That the coronary circulation has capacitative as well as resistive properties has been recognized for many years (154,387). Only in the past decade, however, has it been possible to do the kinds of experiments that lead to a full appreciation of just how importantly capacitative effects influence the dynamics of coronary flow.

Blood in the coronary vessels constitutes a sizable fraction of the volume of the heart wall. One can estimate this volume, V, from indicator dilution estimates of mean coronary transit time, $\bar{t}$, and an independent estimate of coronary flow rate, Q, because these variables are related to each other through the fundamental equation $V = Q\bar{t}$. Such estimates made in open-chest dogs show that the volume of blood contained in the perfusion field of the left coronary artery is, at a perfusion pressure of 70 mm Hg, 11.0 ml/100 g (247). Owing to the fact that the left coronary artery of the dog supplies the left atrium and also part of the right ventricle in addition to the entire left ventricle (154,254), this figure somewhat overestimates the blood volume of the left ventricle. Coronary blood volume varies concordantly with perfusion pressure; in the study cited earlier, raising perfusion pressure to 170 mm Hg increased intramural blood volume to 17.8 ml/100 g. Because coronary sinus pressure fell, those authors believed that the increase in coronary blood volume occurred mainly on the arterial side of the circulation. As one would expect, pharmacological vasodilation at a constant perfusion pressure likewise increases coronary blood volume, but in this instance the increase in blood volume appears to involve both the arterial and venous sides of the circulation (173). The availability of flow meters and techniques for chronic catheterization of coronary arteries and veins (111) make possible studies of the regulation of coronary blood volume in conscious animals, yielding information that will be of great interest.

Dynamic changes in coronary blood volume within each cardiac cycle influence coronary flow in ways that are not evident from the steady-state measurements described earlier, which average out systolic and diastolic fluctuations. As shown in Fig. 5, coronary arterial inflow is primarily diastolic, whereas coronary venous outflow is almost exclusively systolic. This means that coronary blood volume increases during each diastole and decreases during each systole. Such volume changes are only moderate. For example, in a dog whose heart rate is 60/min and whose coronary flow is 60 ml/100 g, the change in coronary blood volume between systole and diastole will be approximately 1 ml/100 g, or 8 to 9% of the total. Just how this increment in blood volume is distributed among the anatomical elements of the coronary vascular bed is unknown.

That the coronary circulation has both resistive and capacitative properties means that these two properties interact. Indeed, the most powerful models of the physical attributes of the coronary circulation are those that, recognizing this interaction, represent it by electrical analogs, i.e., by R-C circuits (88,100,113,219,349,385). The behavior of the coronary circulation as a vascular waterfall and the throttling effect of systole are two prominent manifestations of the interaction of coronary resistance and capacitance.

Coronary Vascular Waterfalls

The term *vascular waterfall* describes circulations in which tissue pressure, P_T, rather than venous pressure, P_V, is the back-pressure that opposes arterial pressure, P_A. In such a system, resistance is calculated as $(P_A - P_T)/Q$ rather than by the usual equation $(P_A - P_V)/Q$. The vascular waterfall concept was developed to explain

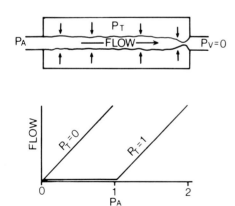

FIG. 10. Hydraulic model of a vascular waterfall **(top)** and a hypothetical pressure-flow curve describing its behavior **(bottom).** Model consists of a collapsible tube containing fluid at a pressure P_A that is surrounded by an extraluminal collapsing force P_T. The outflow pressure, P_V, in this example is zero. The pressure-flow curve shows that if P_T is zero, flow varies directly with P_A. However, if $P_T > 0$, flow through the tube will not commence until P_A just exceeds P_T. (From ref. 100, with permission.)

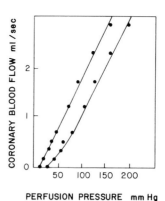

FIG. 11. Coronary pressure-flow curves from an open-chest anesthetized dog, illustrating the kind of evidence used to support the vascular waterfall hypothesis. The curve at *left* is from an arrested heart, that on the *right* from a beating heart. In both, pharmacological vasodilation abolished autoregulatory tone. Note that in the absence of systolic extravascular compression, flow is linearly pressure-dependent and ceases at a pressure distinctly higher than zero. In the beating heart, flow is linearly dependent on perfusion pressure if this pressure is higher than ventricular systolic pressure, but alinear if pressure is lower than systolic ventricular pressure. The alinear portion of the curve is interpreted as evidence that flow ceases in vessels whose distending pressure is less than local intramyocardial tissue pressure. (From ref. 100, with permission.)

pulmonary blood flow, wherein alveolar pressure rather than pulmonary venous pressure determines resistance (289,290). A mechanical model of a vascular waterfall is shown in Fig. 10; its essential features are a collapsible vessel surrounded by a tissue pressure that exceeds the venous pressure.

Downey and Kirk (100) were the first to recognize that the relationship between coronary flow and perfusion pressure contains evidence for vascular waterfalls. In open-chest dogs whose coronary autoregulatory tone was abolished by vasodilation with adenosine, they found that during vagal asystole, the mean coronary flow rate varied directly with perfusion pressure and that such pressure-flow curves had a positive intercept on the pressure axis (Fig. 11). If the hearts were beating, the entire pressure-flow curve was displaced toward a higher pressure. If perfusion pressure exceeded left ventricular cavitary pressure, the pressure-flow curve paralleled that of the asystolic heart, but below this pressure the relationship was concave upward. They interpreted the curvilinear portion of the curve as evidence for a gradient of tissue pressure, the inflection point representing the highest pressure attained during systole, and the intercept on the pressure axis being the lowest pressure attained during diastole. Both pressures exceeded that in the right atrium, hitherto considered to be the back-pressure in the coronary circuit. Accordingly, they concluded that the coronary circulation behaves as though it were composed of a series of vascular waterfalls.

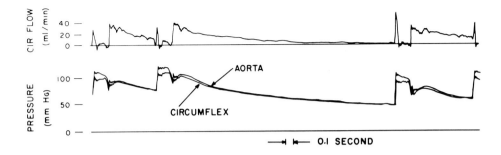

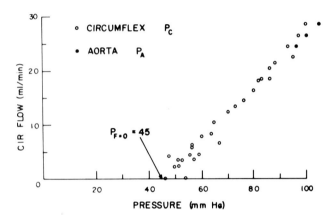

FIG. 12. Epicardial coronary artery pressure-flow relationships in a conscious dog, showing that when autoregulation and α-adrenergic vasoconstrictor tone are present, flow may cease in an epicardial artery at relatively high perfusion pressures. **Top:** Left circumflex (CIR) coronary flow rate, aortic and circumflex coronary artery pressures. **Bottom:** Pressure-flow relationship during the long diastole shown in the flow curve demonstrating a stop-flow pressure of 45 mm Hg. (From ref. 33, with permission.)

Bellamy (33) extended the inquiry into the existence of coronary vascular waterfalls by analyzing phasic flow curves obtained from conscious animals. Figure 12 illustrates the salient result of this study: When diastole is prolonged, flow in an epicardial branch may stop when perfusion pressure is surprisingly high, 45 mm Hg in this example. Analysis of the diastolic pressure-flow relationships during vasodilation caused by an interval of ischemia or by intracoronary adenosine infusion showed, by linear extrapolation of such curves to the pressure axis, that the "stop-flow" pressure[1] was considerably lower, approximately 20 mm Hg. He concluded that these experiments supported the existence of a coronary vascular waterfall and that the waterfall pressure was the correct back-pressure to use when calculating coronary vascular resistance.

Bellamy's report stimulated a great deal of research that has modified his conclusions to some degree. As yet these investigations have not given a complete and unambiguous picture of the dynamic interaction of coronary resistance and capacitance. Consequently, one cannot decide whether a vascular waterfall model or, alternatively, a model based on the concept of a "critical

closing pressure" (63) best accounts for coronary pressure-flow relationships. Estimating the zero-flow pressure by linear extrapolation may lead to an overestimate if the pressure-flow relationship is curvilinear, as found by some (112,206), but not all, investigators (89,90, 100,113,349). Bellamy's recognition that coronary autoregulatory tone contributes importantly to the stop-flow pressure has been confirmed in detail (89,200,206). Passive collapse of intramural arteries as a consequence of a falling diastolic perfusion pressure tends to propel blood in these vessels forward, while at the same time the decrease in vessel caliber tends to raise resistance and retard the emptying of the epicardial vessels. Thus, flow through capillaries probably continues even after it has stopped in more proximal vessels (88,89,113,206). Experiments in which autoregulatory tone was abolished by pharmacological coronary vasodilation and capacitance effects were minimized by constant-pressure perfusion have indicated that the minimum diastolic stop-flow pressure is on the order of 5 to 15 mm Hg (88,89,113,206). Such a figure agrees reasonably well with the rather imperfect estimates of diastolic tissue pressure that are currently available (see pages 1005–1008) and also with the diastolic pressures measured distal to a completely occluded coronary artery (111,154) or measured by solid-state sensors implanted in the myocardium (352,353). Augmenting intramyocardial tissue pressure by elevating left ventricular diastolic pressure significantly raises coronary stop-flow pressure

---

[1] We prefer the terms *stop-flow pressure* or *zero-flow pressure*, because unlike the term *critical closing pressure*, they do not imply actual physical closure of vessels. Vital microscopy does not support the notion of vessel collapse (364); indeed, there is histological evidence that collagen struts between myocytes and coronary microvessels may oppose the compressive effect of intramyocardial pressure (67).

(6,7,13,112), an observation that has obvious implications concerning coronary perfusion in heart failure.

Attempts to represent the coronary circulation by electrical analogs based on experiments in the laboratories of the proponents of each model have yet to arrive at a consensus. Two recent reviews discuss the evidence favoring the two major types of models, the intramyo-cardial pump (capacitative) model (347) or, alternatively, the vascular waterfall (resistive) model (205). There has been some success in integrating resistive and capacitative effects in the same model (219). There is vigorous debate (101,350) over the operating characteristics of these models, particularly the value of the time constant for capacitative discharge (resistance multiplied by capaci-tance, a product whose unit is time). The outcome of this debate has important implications; a long time constant tends to diminish the validity of late diastolic coronary resistance as an index of beat-to-beat changes in coronary tone (84). To date, the interpretations of stop-flow pressure measurements have apparently not taken into account the longitudinal gradient of arterial pressure identified by direct pressure measurements in coronary microvessels (264,365). Such pressure gradients could have important consequences on pressure-flow relationships and might account for the fact that the rather small change in diastolic ventricular pressure caused by atrial systole produces such a large flow reduction during the atrial cove (34).

Clearly, sorting out the interaction of resistance and capacitance will continue to tax the ingenuity of inves-tigators whose goal is to understand myocardial perfusion at the microcirculatory level, but whose experiments constrain them to interpret observations made at the rather remote vantage point of the epicardial vessels.

"Concealed" Systolic Backflow

The decrease in left coronary inflow during systole has been interpreted as primarily resistive (the result of extramural coronary vascular compression) (154) or capacitative (the result of retrograde expulsion of blood from intramural vessels) (387). Given the evidence that the coronary circulation has both resistive and capaci-tative properties, both views would seem to have an element of truth. Spaan et al. (349) have drawn attention to this possibility in a study of the effect of coronary stenosis on systolic coronary flow rate. The experiment consisted of perfusing the left coronary artery of a dog through a circuit containing an adjustable stenosis. Pressure proximal to the stenosis could be varied such that the mean coronary perfusion pressure was constant. As shown in Fig. 13, application of stenosis raised systolic perfusion pressure and lowered diastolic perfusion pressure. Diastolic coronary flow tended to fall, whereas the systolic flow rate increased nearly to diastolic levels.

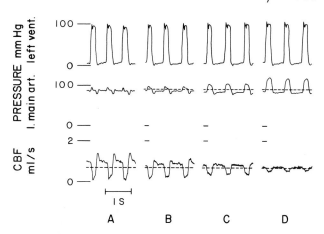

FIG. 13. Evidence that the typically low rate of antegrade systolic coronary flow in an epicardial coronary artery is due to concealed backflow from intramural coronary arteries. See text for discussion. (From ref. 349, with permission.)

These authors interpreted this result as evidence that the stenosis, by raising systolic perfusion pressure, acted as a resistance opposing backflow. This analysis predicts that lowering systolic coronary perfusion pressure should promote systolic backflow; this is indeed the case (348).

TRANSMURAL CORONARY FLOW DISTRIBUTION

Estimates of coronary flow rates at various depths in the left ventricular myocardium by means of either particulate or diffusible indicators have established a consensus: Normally, myocardial perfusion is very nearly uniform across the heart wall. There is evidence, albeit imperfect, for a substantial gradient of systolic extravas-cular compression that diminishes from endocardium to epicardium. More recent work has suggested that there are also gradients of intramyocardial pressure in diastole. Relatively uniform perfusion, despite such gra-dients of resistance, implies that there must be one or more compensatory mechanisms that preserve flow to the deeper layers of the heart wall. Thus, intramyocardial pressure is a fundamental determinant of coronary flow distribution, and for this reason it is worth devoting some attention to the experimental evidence that char-acterizes it. Subsequently we shall consider the possible compensatory mechanisms that interact with tissue pres-sure to determine flow distribution.

Intramyocardial Pressure

Van der Meer et al. (366) have classified the methods for measuring intramyocardial pressure (IMP) as "closed," "open," and "perfusion." As originally de-scribed by Johnson and Di Palma, the closed method consists of implanting in the heart wall a fluid-filled segment of blood vessel that is closed at one end and attached to manometer at the other. The vessel is then inflated to a pressure between 60 mm Hg and several hundred millimeters of mercury. The difference between systolic and diastolic pressures at any degree of inflation is taken to be the IMP (185). The open method consists of measuring pressure sensed by a fluid-filled needle or catheter inserted directly into the heart wall. Pressure is then measured in a droplet of fluid injected into the muscle (155). In the open method, the pressure sensor communicates directly with the cardiac interstitium, whereas in the closed method the sensor is separated from the interstitium by a membrane, i.e., the wall of the implanted vessel segment. The perfusion method consists of implanting a collapsible tube, usually a blood vessel segment, in the myocardium and measuring pressures in and flow rate through the tube as fluid is pumped through the system (26). Flow commences when perfusion pressure exceeds the minimum IMP and becomes continuous throughout the cardiac cycle when perfusion pressure exceeds the highest IMP. During the past decade several investigators have measured IMP by means of solid-state pressure sensors implanted in the myocardium (11). Because the sensor is in direct contact with the interstitial space, this technique is a variant of the open method.

Almost immediately after publication of Johnson and Di Palma's measurements it was recognized that the closed method is subject to serious artifacts (155). The material properties of the vessel segment alter the pressure transmitted to the manometer such that, depending on caliber, wall thickness, and pressure inflating the vessel, IMP may be several times higher than that in the aorta during systole and, in some circumstances, throughout the cardiac cycle. The first observation is incompatible with the fact that coronary flow is antegrade during systole (156), and an IMP exceeding that in the aorta throughout the cardiac cycle is incompatible with coronary flow altogether. Pressures recorded by the open method depend on the size of the fluid droplet (155). Brandi and McGregor (51) sought to circumvent the droplet size artifact by measuring steady-state infusion pressures as fluid was infused through a plastic tube inserted directly into the myocardium. Extrapolation of perfusion pressure to zero flow rate, i.e., zero "droplet" size, estimated the IMP. Restricting droplet size to volumes as small as 0.5 mm³ and waiting for this volume to be dissipated before making pressure measurements is a variant of this stratagem (210). The absolute values of IMP estimated by the perfusion method appear to depend on whether the implanted vessel segment is an artery or a vein and whether flow is measured proximal or distal to the vascular segment (368). The IMP sensed by solid-state devices is said by some (209), but not others (353), to depend on the

orientation of the device relative to local myofiber orientation.

An unavoidable artifact introduced by the instrumentality of measurement is common to all methods for measuring IMP. Any sensor occupies space and, as a consequence, alters local conditions such that the volume element of tissue under observation may not represent the myocardium generally. Insertion of a measuring device must injure some muscle fibers and stretch others, thus altering their contractile properties. Disruption of the blood supply to fibers immediately adjacent to a sensor seems inescapable. Without exception, reports that have asserted that tissue damage was minimal or absent (if this is mentioned at all) have not included histological documentation. Finally, myofiber orientation varies continuously across the myocardial wall (357). The contraction and relaxation of the heart must certainly impart a torque to implanted devices that will vary according to the depth of implantation. Such a torque could cause the sensor to move discordantly with respect to surrounding structures, generating an artifactual pressure in its own right and possibly further damaging the tissue under study. One can only conclude that measurements of *absolute* IMP are closer to the realm of faith than fact.

Despite these shortcomings, independent evidence from other kinds of experiments shows that measurements of IMP have a substantial capacity to predict the behavior of the coronary circulation. Accordingly, it is possible that the various sources of artifact listed earlier collectively constitute a systematic error that is not so large as to vitiate such measurements altogether. Figure 14, taken from a recent report by Stein et al. (352), illustrates how one can use independent evidence to judge the validity of IMP measurements. The tissue pressure measurements shown in this figure were obtained by means of miniature solid-state sensors mounted near the tips of steel needles. The sensors were inserted into the left ventricular free wall to depths of 4 and 10 mm in order to monitor subepicardial and subendocardial pressures, respectively. The phasic relationships of the pressures measured at these sites, and also in the aorta and ventricular cavity, generate testable predictions about coronary flow and its transmural distribution. For the sake of clarity we shall discuss systole and diastole separately. Because there is no way to know if the results of this study are more nearly correct than the observations of others, we shall try to point out conflicts with the literature (Table 2).

According to Fig. 14, peak subepicardial IMP during systole is lower than aortic pressure but subendocardial IMP exceeds that in the aorta. Such a subendocardial-to-subepicardial gradient agrees with all previous studies (11,25,27,87,135,185,198,209–211,368). A subepicardial pressure lower than aortic pressure predicts the fact that systolic coronary flow is normally antegrade and also

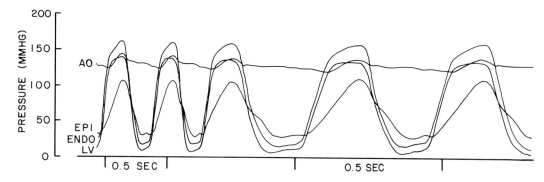

FIG. 14. Recordings of aortic (AO), left ventricular (LV), and intramyocardial pressures obtained in the superficial (EPI) and deeper (ENDO) layers of the left ventricular wall by miniature solid-state sensors. See text for discussion. (From ref. 352, with permission.)

predicts the results of experiments showing that ^{86}Rb or radiomicrosphere distribution is predominantly to the subepicardium when coronary perfusion is restricted to systole (102,171). It is uncertain whether systolic IMP in the subendocardium exceeds that in the aorta and whether or not, as a consequence, the subendocardium is ischemic during systole. Although some IMP measurements show that subendocardial IMP exceeds aortic pressure (11,25,135,185,198,210,211,295), others do not (27,51,87,103,195,320). The aforementioned studies (99,168) of regional flow distribution during exclusively systolic coronary perfusion show that although flow to

the deeper layers is diminished, it is clearly not zero. However, evidence that intramural flow may continue after it has ceased in the epicardial coronary arteries (see pages 1002–1005) admits the possibility that indicator particles entering the coronary arteries during systole may not have come to rest in the tissue until diastole, when the relationship of deep and superficial IMPs may have been different.

Figure 14 further shows that during diastole, IMP in the subepicardium is lower than in the subendocardium, which in turn is higher than that in the ventricular cavity. Thus, the gradient of IMP found in systole is

TABLE 2. *Estimates of left ventricular intramyocardial pressure*

	Systolic			Diastolic		
Peak Endo > AO	Endo/Epi	Epi > AO	>LV cavitary	Endo/Epi	Refs.
Closed method						
Yes	>1	Sometimes	NR	NR	186
No	NR	NR	NR	NR	107
Usually no	NR	NR	Yes, 12–40 mm Hg	NR	319
No	>1	Yes	NR	<1	90
Yes	NR	NR	NR	NR	294
Open method						
Yes	>1	Yes	Yes, 10–20 mm Hg	NR	210,211
Yes	>1	Yes	NR	NR	199
No	NR	NR	NR	NR	52
Perfusion method						
Yes	>1	NR	Yes, 6–20 mm Hg	NR	366
No	>1	Yes	Yes, 10–30 mm Hg	NR	27
Yes	>1	Yes	NR	NR	25
NR	NR	NR	13 ± 3 mm Hg	NR	291
Yes	>1	Yes	NR	NR	138
NR	NR	NR	Yes, 5.6 mm Hg	<1	23,24
Solid-state sensors						
Yes	>1	Yes	NR	NR	11
No, ≤	NR	NR	NR	NR	196
Equal	>1	Yes	NR	NR	209
Yes	>1	Yes	Yes	<1	350,351

NR = not reported.

reversed in diastole, an observation in accord with those of other investigations (23,24,87).

Studies of radiomicrosphere deposition in hearts under maximum pharmacological coronary vasodilation, a maneuver that minimizes the contribution of transmural gradients of autoregulatory vascular tone, have shown that flow slightly favors the subepicardium (6,7,14, 17,20,97,217,238,250,307,308). Such a result supports the notion of a diastolic IMP gradient diminishing from subepicardium to subendocardium whose effects outweigh the preferential flow in the subepicardium during systole, but only to the extent that radiomicrosphere deposition truly reflects local blood flow.

A second line of evidence from studies of radiomicrosphere distribution during coronary perfusion restricted to diastole tests the prediction that this intervention, by reducing systolic flow to the subepicardium, will raise the subendocardial/subepicardial flow ratio. Such is not the case; the ratio is unchanged (239). Because systolic coronary flow is but a minor fraction of stroke coronary flow, it is perhaps possible that the effect of subtracting its contribution is below the limit of sensitivity of the radiomicrosphere method.

That diastolic IMP exceeds left ventricular intracavitary pressure enjoys strong independent support. As shown in Fig. 15, recordings of flow into coronary arteries perfused directly from the cavity of the left ventricle, i.e., only in systole, show backflow in diastole (99), evidence that IMP exceeds ventricular cavitary pressure during this phase of the cardiac cycle. Pressure-flow curves recorded in epicardial coronary arteries further support the notion that IMP exceeds left ventricular pressure. In the presence of maximum coronary vasodilation by drugs to reduce intrinsic vascular resistance to a minimum, IMP becomes a major component of coronary resistance. Pressure-flow curves, such as the example shown in Fig. 11, indicate that flow ceases at a

pressure greater than that in the cavity of the left ventricle. While studies such as this estimate a minimum IMP, they do not define its location within the heart wall.

Vascularity

The cross-sectional area of the terminal vascular bed is a static or structural determinant of minimum coronary vascular resistance, which obtains when all the capillaries are perfused. Comparisons of coronary microvascular and aortic pressures in beating hearts have shown that there is already a substantial pressure drop at the level of the smaller arterioles (264,365), which means that vessels proximal to precapillary sphincters also contribute to resistance. Transmural gradients of small arterial as well as capillary density thus could be one of the mechanisms compensating for the transmural gradient of extravascular compression. Evidence bearing on the existence of gradients of vascularity depends, to an important degree, on experimental design and methodology.

Table 3 summarizes the literature on capillary density and "terminal vascular volume." The 1971 review of Rakušan (300) summarized reports up to that time, which showed that depending on the species studied and methodology employed, myocardial capillary densities ranged between 2,000 and 5,000/mm². So wide a range doubtless owes to experimental artifacts, such as failure to fill capillaries by postmortem injection, shrinkage of tissue during preparation for microscopic examination, failure to section the tissue exactly perpendicular to the long axis of the capillaries, inability to identify a capillary because it lacks a red cell in the particular section, difficulty in discriminating between capillaries and other microvessels, and, finally, selection bias arising from regional variations in the fraction of relatively avascular interfascial tissue contained in the sample under study.

The 1974 study of Bassingthwaighte et al. (31), which circumvented or made allowance for the sorts of errors listed earlier, reported a capillary density of 2,830 ± 610/ mm² in dog hearts, but did not explicitly address the question of how density might vary transmurally. Studies employing fluorescein-labeled IgG to mark the capillaries of rat hearts have shown that the capillary density in subendocardium is slightly (9%), though not significantly, lower than in the subendocardium under normoxic conditions and is identical during hypoxia (371). Histological studies have confirmed both the magnitude and polarity of such a capillary density gradient (133,134,355).

Wüsten et al. (395) studied transmural variations in small artery blood volume in dog hearts injected postmortem with a suspension of 15-μm radiomicrospheres and $BaSO_4$ in gelatin. This experimental approach ex-

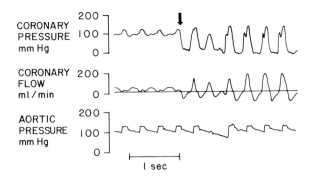

FIG. 15. Demonstration that diastolic intramyocardial pressure exceeds that in the cavity of the left ventricle. In this open-chest dog, a coronary branch was perfused from the aorta or, at the arrow, directly from the cavity of the left ventricle. Note that during perfusion from the ventricle, there is coronary backflow during diastole, evidence that intramyocardial pressure exceeds that in the left ventricle. (From ref. 99, with permission.)

TABLE 3. *Myocardial capillary density and small vessel blood volume*

Anatomical (capillary density)

Species	Technique	Capillary density/mm^2	Refs.
Various, including man	Various	2,000–5,000	299
Dog	Silastic cast, correct for shrinkage	2,830 ± 610	32
Rat	Histology	Endo 2,816 ± 72 Epi 3,885 ± 71	136
Dog	Histology	Endo 3,147 ± 140 Epi 3,637 ± 143	137
Man	Histology	Endo 2,014 ± 38 Epi 2,436 ± 59	353
Rat	Histology	Endo 3,220 ± 120 Epi 3,520 ± 150	369

Indicator dilution (small vessel blood volume)

Species	Tracer(s) & methods	Results			Refs.
Rat	^{51}Cr-RBC mixed 15 min, ^{131}I-albumin mixed 3 min		*Male*	*Female*	118
		Arterial Hct	41.5 ± 0.22	40.9 ± 0.3	
		Cardiac muscle Hct	27.1	32.6	
		Cardiac blood volume (ml/100 g)	0.262	0.238	
Dog	^{51}Cr-RBC + ^{131}I-albumin; sample 2 min	Deep/superficial ratio: RBC 1.42, plasma 1.34			200
Dog	^{131}I-PVP, ^{3}H$_2$O	Vascular volume 5.7 ± 0.2 ml/100 g			45
Dog	^{131}I-albumin; sample 1.5 min	Vascular volume 5.22 ml/100 g			78
Dog	Exsanguinate 30 min after ^{51}Cr-RBV, 10 min after ^{131}I-albumin	RBC vol. 1.98 ± 0.02 ml/100 g; plasma vol. 4.87 ± 0.37 ml/100 g; tissue Hct 29; blood Hct 42			341
Dog	^{59}Fe-siderophilin sample 5–6 min (volumes are ml/100 g)		*epi*	*endo*	181
		Base	5.98	6.93	
		Control	6.57	7.63	
		Apex	6.80	7.94	
		Asphyxia raised volume to 12.4 ml/100 g and abolished gradients			
Rat	Alkaline phosphatase activity per 100 g tissue	Epi 6.38 ± 0.48 U Endo 7.40 ± 0.38 U			99
Dog	^{59}Fe-siderophilin & ^{51}Cr-RBC; sample after 5 min (volumes ml/100 g)		*Normoxic*	*Hypoxic*	79
		Epi	6.1 ± 1.4	10.2 ± 2.6	
		Endo	7.1 ± 2.0	12.6 ± 2.9	
Dog	Radiomicrosphere-BaSO$_4$ = gelatin perfusion; count areas free of major vessels (arterial volume ml/100 ml)	Epi 2.21 ± 0.16 Endo 4.80 ± 0.56			393

ploits the fact that the viscosity of $BaSO_4$-gelatin is such that these suspensions fill only arteries and cannot penetrate into capillaries. Pieces of left ventricle that were shown by X-ray to be devoid of major epicardial or intramural vessels were then counted by gamma-photon spectroscopy, and the vascular volume was calculated by reference to the specific activity of the injectate. Small vessel blood volume increased across the heart wall, from 2.21 ± 0.16 ml/100 g in the subepicardium to 4.80 ± 0.56 ml/100 g in the subendocardium. Parallel studies evaluated transmural variations in capillary density by means of radiomicrosphere deposition, an approach that assumes that the probability of deposition is a function of local capillary density. Electrical fibrillation and maximum pharmacological coronary vasodilation minimized extravascular compression and intrinsic vascular tone, respectively, both of which could have altered the percentage of open capillaries. Radiomicrosphere deposition was a linear function of myocardial depth, the subendocardial/subepicardial ratio averaging 1.62 ± 0.28. If one assumes a constant ratio of capillary-to-small-artery cross-sectional area, such an endocardial/epicardial ratio is consistent with the results of Schlessinger mass studies. Calculating cross-sectional area as vascular volume to the 2/3 power, the subendocardial/subepicardial ratio of small artery cross section is $(4.80/2.21)^{2/3}$, or 1.67, nearly identical with the ratio estimated by use of radiomicrospheres.

A number of investigators have applied indicator dilution methods to estimate the volume of the terminal vascular bed. Such estimates do not, of course, measure only capillary volume but the volumes of the arteries and veins as well. Such estimates are quite sensitive to the choice of indicator and to assumptions about how a particular indicator distributes in tissue.

The first study of regional variations in terminal vascular volume, that of Myers and Honig (258), provides a frame of reference for critical analysis of subsequent studies of this sort. These investigators recognized the possibility that the ratio of red cell volume to plasma volume in the heart ("tissue hematocrit") might differ from that in the major vessels and so made separate measurements of the volumes of distribution of ^{51}Cr-labeled red cells and ^{131}I-albumin, a plasma marker. They also recognized that albumin might escape from the vascular space during equilibration, and thus this tracer might overestimate the true plasma volume. Preliminary experiments showed that such was indeed the case; apparent tissue hematocrit decreased with time, being 80% of the arterial value 2 min after albumin injection and only 50% 30 min after albumin injection. Such a result is entirely consistent with studies showing that ^{131}I-albumin readily penetrates into the cardiac interstitium and can be recovered in cardiac lymph (8,9). As a compromise between a time sufficient for complete mixing of the albumin in the blood and its loss from the vascular space, these investigators sampled heart muscle 2 min after albumin injection. Direct comparisons showed that red cell volume was 41% and plasma volume was 23% larger in the subendocardium than in the subepicardium. The disparity between the two estimates could well be due to escape of ^{131}I-albumin from the vascular space.

Subsequent indicator dilution estimates of terminal vascular volume sometimes employed a single indicator, usually ^{131}I-albumin or ^{59}Fe-transferrin, and equilibration times equal to or several times longer than the 2 min used by Myers and Honig. Some of these studies measured an overall terminal vascular volume (44,75,114,342), and others searched for regional variations in this volume (76,179,199). The estimates of vascular volume ranged between 5.2 and 7.9 ml/100 g LV wet weight; such volumes are similar to those estimated morphometrically in dog heart (123). The experiments designed to detect a transmural gradient of terminal vascular volume did indeed find one; it decreased from subendocardium to subepicardium. Asphyxia or hypoxia significantly increased small vessel blood volume and abolished the transmural gradient (76,179,371).

Is it possible to reconcile anatomical studies showing that capillary density diminishes from epicardium to endocardium with indicator dilution studies pointing to a transmural gradient of vascularity of opposite polarity? One must base judgments on the experiments themselves, what they actually measure, their artifacts, and the assumptions made in their interpretation.

The anatomical study of Vetterlein et al. (371) counted capillaries directly and seems relatively free of artifacts and assumptions. An intravascular marker, fluorescein-labeled IgG, was used to stain capillaries, not to measure a volume of distribution, and appropriate controls showed that this marker did indeed fill all capillaries. Tissue shrinkage during fixation was taken into account, and the sampling protocol seems free of selection bias. The major inference to be drawn from this study, namely, that the anatomical component of coronary resistance is transmurally uniform, entails only the assumption that neither the average number of capillaries served by a resistance vessel nor the caliber of these capillaries varies according to depth in the myocardial wall. Information on this point apparently does not exist. The histological studies that corroborated Vetterlein's observations did not correct for tissue shrinkage. This artifact will affect the absolute value of capillary density, but this is a systematic error that should not greatly influence the transmural gradient.

Studies employing barium-gelatin mass injections to estimate small arterial volume, like capillary counts, estimate the cross-sectional area of the terminal vascular bed indirectly. The experiments of Wusten et al. (395) did not specifically include anatomical studies to assess the extent to which the barium-gelatin mixture filled all of the smaller arterioles. The radiomicrosphere experiments that appeared to independently corroborate the BaSO₄-gelatin injection studies may not be so independent after all; the investigators actually measured deposition of radiomicrospheres added to the injection mass. Given the tendency of radiomicrospheres to follow paths of least branching and least resistance (126), it is possible that the results better reflect the hydrodynamic properties of the radiomicrospheres than the cross-sectional area of the vascular bed under study.

Indicator dilution methods that measure a small vessel blood volume are more convenient than capillary counting, but provide the least reliable estimate of the anatomical component of vascular resistance. This volume is the sum of the volumes of arterioles, true resistance vessels, capillaries, and venules. There is no evidence that defines a relationship between this volume and the cross-sectional area of the resistance vessels. Most such estimates employ plasma indicators with the tacit assumption that the indicator remains confined to the vascular space. Experiment shows that in the case of albumin this is not so (8). Transferrin, another popular "plasma" marker, is probably no better than albumin. The molecular mass and diffusion coefficient of transferrin, 76,000 daltons and 5.9×10^{-7} cm²·sec, are not greatly different from those of albumin, 69,000 daltons and 6.1×10^{-7} cm²·sec (343), and so the two proteins probably escape from the vascular space at approximately the same rate. There is evidence that the permeability of capillaries to macromolecules is greater in subendocardial than in subepicardial capillaries (5); this could also contribute to transmural differences in apparent plasma volume. Perhaps the use of larger proteins, such as IgM, which has a molecular mass greater than 700,000 daltons, would circumvent the problem of escape of indicator from the vascular compartment.

Plasma Skimming

Single-pass indicator dilution curves show that the mean coronary transit time of ¹³¹I-albumin is longer than that of ⁵¹Cr-labeled red cells (400). Because loss of albumin from the vascular space is negligible under these experimental conditions, this means that these blood components partition in the coronary microcirculation, the cellular elements tending to follow paths of higher flow velocity. Vital microscopy shows that partitioning occurs within the individual microvessels, wherein a cuff of slower-moving plasma surrounds a column of cells moving more rapidly through the center of the vessel. This phenomenon is called axial streaming.

Owing to axial streaming, plasma at the vascular wall tends to enter side branches in preference to cells, a process known as plasma skimming. Plasma skimming is unimportant in vessels larger than about 0.25 mm in diameter, but increases as an inverse function of vessel caliber below this size. Geometrical factors such as the angulation of a branch and the disparity between its caliber and that of the parent vessel increase plasma skimming. Vasomotor state also influences plasma skimming, vasodilation tending to reduce it.

The major consequence of plasma skimming is a reduction in microvascular hematocrit. Indeed, detecting skimming experimentally depends on demonstrating, in the absence of arteriovenous shunting, a difference between microvessel and large vessel hematocrits. A study of microvascular hematocrit and red cell flow in hamster cremaster muscle (203) has illustrated some of these points. When the muscle was at rest, capillary hematocrit averaged 10%, whereas large vessel hematocrit was 50%. Red cells moved through these capillaries at a velocity of approximately 200 μm/sec. Vasodilation produced by the combination of electrical stimulation of the muscle and superfusion with 0.1-mM adenosine raised both capillary hematocrit, to 40%, and red cell velocity, to approximately 460 μm/sec.

Owing to the technical difficulties arising from tissue motion, vital microscopy has not been used to obtain evidence for plasma skimming in the heart. However, several studies of small vessel hematocrit have addressed this question. Because an estimate of tissue hematocrit requires separate estimates of red cell volume and plasma volume, the measurements are sensitive to the shortcomings and technical errors inherent in these indicator dilution methods. Escape of plasma marker from the circulation during the equilibration introduces a large element of ambiguity into such measurements. Published reports (76,114,258,299,342) show that the ratio of tissue hematocrit to large vessel hematocrit falls significantly as a function of the time elapsed between injection of the plasma tracer, either ¹³¹I-albumin or ⁵⁹Fe-transferrin, and the time of tissue sampling (Fig. 16). The experiments of Myers and Honig (258), which were least affected by this artifact, suggested that cardiac muscle hematocrit differs from large vessel hematocrit by no more than 10% and is uniform transmurally. However, these authors conceded that cumulative experimental errors limited the precision of their measurements such that a true difference of 10% might have escaped detection. A difference this large would constitute physiologically significant plasma skimming.

An accurate estimate of cardiac small vessel hematocrit is important for reasons quite apart from its implications for plasma skimming. Calculations of regional myocardial oxygen consumption are based on microspectrophotometric measurements of arteriolar and venular oxyhemoglobin percentage *saturation* (see pages 1013–1015), not oxyhemoglobin *concentration*, and so it is necessary to assume some value of blood hemoglobin

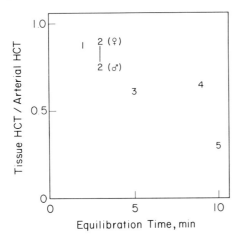

FIG. 16. Dependence of "tissue" hematocrit (HCT) on the time allowed for equilibration of plasma tracer. Numbers 1–5 refer to estimates reported, respectively, in refs. 258, 114, 76, 299, and 340. Note that the ratio of tissue HCT to large vessel HCT decreases systematically with time. See text for further discussion.

content. Such an assumption is, in effect, an assumption about small vessel hematocrit, and it will introduce an error proportional to the difference between assumed and actual small vessel hematocrits.

Autoregulation

Autoregulation, the intrinsic capacity of a blood vessel to adjust its caliber to maintain constant tissue perfusion in the face of changes in perfusion pressure, is a potentially important determinant of the transmural distribution of coronary flow. Three studies have now provided convincing evidence for a transmural gradient of autoregulatory capacity that is strongest in the superficial layers of the heart wall.

All studies assessing regional autoregulatory capacity have employed the same experimental technique, namely, radiomicrosphere measurements of regional blood flow at various levels of coronary perfusion pressure. Figure 17, a composite of observations from the first study of this sort (161), compares the relationships of blood flow to the innermost and outermost layers of the left ventricular free wall as coronary perfusion pressure was lowered by means of mechanical constriction of a major coronary branch. In this example, lowering perfusion pressure to about 70 mm Hg expended the autoregulatory reserve in the subendocardium; below this pressure, subendocardial flow was pressure dependent. By contrast, autoregulation maintained flow to the subepicardium down to perfusion pressures of about 40 mm Hg; flow fell precipitously if pressure was lowered further. Obviously, an autoregulatory curve based on measurements of flow in a major epicardial artery, such as that shown in Fig. 6B, is a composite of the regionally variable autoregulatory capacities.

Autoregulation may fail at perfusion pressures above, as well as below, those that constitute the "autoregulatory range." Boatwright et al. (45) compared transmural differences in the ability to autoregulate at high coronary perfusion pressures. Raising perfusion pressure to 150 mm Hg from a control level of 102 mm Hg produced little change in flow to either the inner or outer third of the left ventricular free wall, the control and high-pressure endocardial/epicardial ratios being 0.90 and 0.94, respectively. Larger increases in pressure, to 197 and 211 mm Hg, increased flow to the subendocardium disproportionately, so that the endocardial/epicardial flow ratio increased significantly to 1.36 and 1.46, respectively. Thus, it seems that the autoregulatory range of subendocardial vessels is narrower, at both the high and low ends, than that of the subepicardial vasculature.

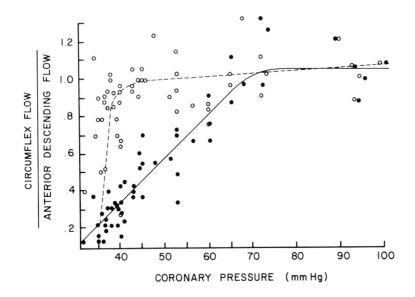

FIG. 17. Variation in autoregulatory capacity as a function of depth in the left ventricular wall. Ratio of epicardial (*open circles*) and endocardial (*filled circles*) flow in the circumflex bed, in which perfusion pressure was varied, to flow in the anterior descending bed, which served as a control. See text for discussion. (This figure is a composite of Figs. 6 and 7 of ref. 161.)

Rouleau et al. (311) studied pressure–regional flow relationships over a range of pressures that exceeded the autoregulatory range at either end (30–260 mm Hg). Because these authors reported indices of perfusion pressure rather than pressure measurements directly, these observations are not directly comparable to those of the other two studies. However, their observations qualitatively confirm that as coronary perfusion pressure is lowered, autoregulatory reserve is expended first in the subendocardium. The demonstration that at perfusion pressures below the autoregulatory range, vasodilation with adenosine raised subepicardial but not subendocardial flows confirms this observation.

Ignorance of the mechanisms that generate and modulate autoregulatory tone precludes a full interpretation of these experiments and leaves many questions unanswered. Is it possible that the aorta–small coronary artery pressure gradients observed in epicardial coronary arteries (264,365) are much smaller than those between aorta and subendocardial arteries, i.e., that the stimulus to myogenic contraction in the subendocardial vessels is smaller? Do subendocardial and subepicardial vessels differ according to sensitivity to stretch or excitation–contraction coupling? Are there transmural gradients of vasodilatory metabolites that influence the ability of a vessel to autoregulate? One attribute of vasodilators, at least those applied experimentally, is that they abolish autoregulation. Are there, as one study would suggest (306), regional differences in the sensitivity of coronary microvessels to endogenous vasoregulatory metabolites, i.e., differences in receptor number or affinity or differences of receptor–effector coupling?

Vasodilatory Metabolites

The metabolic hypothesis of coronary flow regulation posits that a cardiac myocyte elaborates vasodilatory metabolites in proportion to its rate of energy expenditure. Through the action of such metabolites on coronary resistance vessels, the myocyte in effect regulates its own blood supply. Systolic shortening and tension development are greater in subendocardium than subepicardium (358), and consequently the rate of energy expenditure must be greater in the subendocardium. The metabolic hypothesis predicts a parallel gradient of the rate at which myocytes release vasodilators. Of the several candidate metabolites that might effect vasoregulation, there is at present experimental evidence concerning transmural concentration gradients for only three: oxygen, carbon dioxide, and adenosine.

The experimental approaches used to investigate intramyocardial PO_2 include polarographic electrodes inserted into the heart wall, microspectrophotometric assays of capillary or venular oxyhemoglobin saturation in sections of quick-frozen heart muscle, and mass spectro-

graphic analysis of the gas composition in plastic tubes embedded in the heart wall (Table 4). Each method has important technical shortcomings. Insertion of a microelectrode or an even larger gas sampling tube into the myocardium must certainly damage local structures and, in particular, disrupt local blood flow. Unless the electrode current is kept small, oxygen reduction will exceed diffusion such that the electrode will sense the PO_2 in a field of oxygen depletion surrounding the electrode tip that is lower than that of the interstitial space generally. The location of the electrode tip is uncertain, perhaps lying within the interstitial space, within blood vessels, or, in the case of electrodes having tip diameters of only a few microns, possibly even within cells.

Microspectrophotometric methods require rapid freezing of the muscle samples to arrest oxygen usage. This can be accomplished by clamping the tissue between cooled metal blocks (176) or by immersing the sample in liquefied propane (381) or liquid N_2 (53). Clamp freezing is rapid, but it distorts the tissue such that measurements of oxyhemoglobin saturation are possible only in capillaries. Cooling of tissue immersed in liquefied

TABLE 4. *Estimates of intramyocardial oxygen tension and oxyhemoglobin saturation*

	Epicardium	Endocardium	Refs.
Pt electrode (PO_2 in mm Hg)			
	40.8 ± 6.2	22.6 ± 4.5	200
	18 ± 2.3	10.1 ± 1.8	247
	23–27; did not attempt to correlate with depth		192
	No PO_2 gradient; wide variation at any depth		330
	One-third of values 0–5, some up to 80		331
	25.7 ± 2.5 (8–33)	16.5 ± 1.9 (1–22)	381
	25.6 ± 2.5	21.3 ± 2.2	374
	5–65, median 31; did not attempt to correlate with depth		340
Reflectance spectroscopy (% Hb saturation)			
	51.7 ± 3.5	33.8 ± 3.0	134
	19.5 ± 2.3	18.4 ± 2.4	245
Transmission spectroscopy (% Hb saturation)			
	Modal value 20–30 (25%), 30–40 (20%), 40–50 (18%)		163
	53 ± 16	41 ± 19	178
	36.8 ± 2.4	22.1 ± 1.1	380
	34–38	29–31	54
	31.0	20.3	370
Mass spectroscopy (PO_2 in mm Hg)			
	PO_2 18 ± 5 and PCO_2 40 ± 14 1–2 mm below heart surface		53
	34.3 ± 3.7	25.3 ± 3.8	396

gas is relatively slow; core temperatures may not reach 0°C for 10 to 30 sec after immersion (392). Even though the heart may cease to beat during cooling, oxygen consumption could be near the basal rate of 2 to 3 ml/ min per 100 g (204,207,226) during at least the initial part of cooling and accordingly might lower the oxyhemoglobin saturation. Finally, spectrophotometry estimates oxyhemoglobin saturation, not PO_2 directly.

Despite these shortcomings, these three experimental approaches independently arrive at a consensus: There is an intramyocardial gradient of PO_2 that decreases from epicardium to endocardium (Table 4). The errors inherent in each method are systematic, and even though the values of PO_2 or oxyhemoglobin saturation may not be absolutely correct, they lead to a conclusion that is at least probably directionally correct.

Both the polarographic and microspectrophotometric methods show that local PO_2 and oxygen extraction vary over rather wide ranges at a given depth in the heart wall. Thus, intramyocardial PO_2 is better represented by a frequency histogram than by a "mean" PO_2. Such frequency histograms exhibit a modal value that is in reasonable agreement with coronary sinus PO_2 or oxyhemoglobin saturation.

Because coronary flow rate and myocardial oxygen extraction often vary reciprocally, the evidence for local PO_2 and extraction heterogeneity could be a reflection of the time-dependent spatial heterogeneity of myocardial perfusion inferred from indicator dilution studies, the so-called twinkling phenomenon (31,397). Studies of time-dependent flow and PO_2 changes support such a relationship. Analysis of the time course of washout of ^{133}Xe or ^{131}I-iodoantipyrine from beating hearts shows that the time-concentration curves are not monoexponential. Rather, the slope of such a curve is initially high, but decreases with time by sixfold to 10-fold (30). Because the slope is a clearance rate and the clearance of these tracers is proportional to flow, such a result means that there are regions within the heart whose perfusion rates differ by sixfold to 10-fold (30). Radiomicrosphere studies of regional flow are statistical in nature. Typical experiments (115,338,397) consist of injecting a mixture of several types of radiomicrospheres and calculating the mean and variance of all regional flow estimates. In a separate group of dogs, each radiomicrosphere is injected sequentially, and the mean and variance of these flow estimates are calculated. The null hypothesis, i.e., that regional flows do not vary with time, predicts that the means and variances will be similar. Such is not the case; the variance of the flow estimates based on radiomicrospheres injected sequentially is always significantly higher than that for a single injection of a mixture of microspheres. The results of one such study suggest that flow to individual regions varies by as much as 10-fold and is cyclical, the periodicity ranging between 30 and 90 sec (338).

Because microspectrophotometry examines local cardiac oxygen extraction at a single point in time, this technique cannot, of course, give information about time-dependent processes. However, PO_2 electrodes that are left in place after insertion into the heart wall should be able to monitor changes in tissue PO_2 over time. Losse et al. (223) did just that, monitoring PO_2 in the left ventricular free wall by means of platinum electrodes having tip diameters between 35 and 275 μm, average polarizing currents less than 1 nA, and 95% response times of about 7 sec. Observations employing several such electrodes and extending over several minutes showed that local PO_2 indeed oscillates, the usual amplitude of PO_2 change being 5 to 10 torr. Occasional animals exhibited cyclical oscillations having periods between 20 and 150 sec. About 25% of such recordings showed PO_2 oscillations that were of larger amplitude and were more protracted: 20 to 40 torr and 120 to 360 sec.

It is remarkable that these experiments show dynamic changes in regional perfusion and oxygen metabolism, because the volumes of tissue under study, upward of 1 g (115), must contain a very large number of perfusion domains served by individual precapillary sphincters. Even though capillary sphincters are thought to be bistable, operating in either an open or shut mode (152), one would expect this behavior to average out when a large population of sphincters is considered. That such is not the case has important implications for future research. Are such large-scale inhomogeneities concerted and thus evidence for a higher-order control mechanism, say neural activity? Are there concordant changes in myofiber function, and, if so, do the flow changes determine local cardiac function or vice versa? Why does flow heterogeneity persist during pharmacological vasodilation (338), a situation in which one would expect most of the precapillary sphincters to be open?

Weiss combined radiomicrosphere estimates of local blood flow rate with microspectrophotometric measurements of local oxygen extraction to calculate rates of oxygen usage at various depths in the myocardial wall (377–382). These calculations, which apparently assumed the absence of plasma skimming, showed that the oxygen consumption rate was about 40% higher in subendocardium than in subepicardium, 11.7 versus 8.3 ml/min per 100 g. Although that study did not report regional flow data explicitly, one can obtain these data by backcalculation from data on oxygen consumption and arteriovenous oxygen extraction. Comparison of the endocardial/epicardial flow and extraction ratios, 1.13 and 1.25, respectively, suggests that enhanced oxygen extraction in the subendocardium is a more important mechanism for meeting oxygen needs than is flow. Uncertainty as to the mechanism by which PO_2 might affect coronary resistance limits interpretation of the physiological meaning of the transmural gradient of

PO$_2$. It is not known if the transmural gradient of flow that seems to favor the subendocardium reflects subepicardial vasoconstriction due to a higher average PO$_2$ or that due to hypoxic vasodilation in the deeper layers, or a combination of both factors. Additionally, whether hypoxic vasodilation is a direct effect of oxygen on the resistance vessels or an indirect effect mediated by vasodilatory metabolites released from hypoxic myocytes is likewise unknown.

We can find only one report of measurements of PCO$_2$ at different levels in the heart wall, that of Yokoyama et al. (398), who employed mass spectroscopic analysis of the gas composition in probes implanted 2 and 10 mm from the epicardial surface. Under control conditions, PCO$_2$ sensed by the deeper probe was insignificantly higher than that sensed by the subepicardial probe, 34.5 ± 2.6 (SEM) versus 31.5 ± 2.6 mm Hg. From this single experiment it is difficult to see how local PCO$_2$ could contribute to the distribution of coronary flow across the heart wall.

Foley et al. (120) compared adenosine contents in the endocardial and epicardial halves of transmural left ventricular tissue samples and found that the levels were identical when coronary perfusion was normal. The subsequent findings that the interstitial adenosine compartment may constitute no more than 10% of the cardiac pool (276) and that the bulk of myocardial adenosine is intracellular and thus does not participate in vasoregulation complicate interpretation of this experiment. Until a reliable method for measuring interstitial adenosine becomes available, the possibility that a gradient of interstitial adenosine concentration participates in transmural flow regulation remains an open question.

Neural Factors

In addition to the important contribution the cardiac sympathetics make to overall coronary flow regulation (117,281), transmurally nonuniform α-adrenergic coronary vasoconstriction appears to influence the distribution of blood flow within the heart wall. In dogs under unselective β-receptor blockade with propranolol and maximum coronary vasodilation with adenosine to abolish autoregulatory tone, stellate ganglion stimulation reduced the subepicardial perfusion rate but did not change subendocardial perfusion (183). However, stimulation of adrenergic receptors with phenylephrine, norepinephrine, or tyramine decreased regional flows uniformly. Such a result suggests that neither the density nor the properties of coronary α-receptors varied transmurally. As these authors and others (142) have found, the coronary vasoconstriction produced by a combination of β-adrenergic blockade and stellate stimulation affects flow to the deep and superficial layers of the ventricular

wall equally. As Johanssen and his colleagues have suggested, it is possible that the effect of adenosine on coronary flow distribution during stellate stimulation may reflect presynaptic inhibition of neurotransmitter release (196).

MYOCARDIAL REACTIVE HYPEREMIA

Myocardial reactive hyperemia, the exuberant vasodilation caused by an interval of coronary occlusion, is at once one of the most familiar and yet enigmatic responses of the coronary circulation. First described in the dog heart (193), myocardial reactive hyperemia has been demonstrated in every species in which it has been looked for, including man (58,116,237). The intensity of myocardial reactive hyperemia is perhaps the most prominent attribute of this response. The coronary flow rate at the peak of the response may reach levels five or, rarely, even 10 times control. Reactive hyperemia in other vascular beds is much less intense than in the heart; in the kidney, an example of the opposite extreme, reactive hyperemia may be barely perceptible.

Phasic recordings of coronary flow and perfusion pressure during a typical reactive hyperemic response (Fig. 18) show that coronary flow does not attain a maximum rate until several beats after release of the coronary occluder. The reason for the retardation of maximum flow is uncertain. Explanations that have been offered include viscoelastic creep in the walls of the resistance vessels (267) and gradual filling of intramural blood vessels depleted of their blood volume during the ischemic interval (36). Records of phasic reactive hyperemia flow also show that vasodilation increases both systolic and diastolic stroke flow, though not synchronously. Rather, the systolic flow rate reaches its zenith earlier and returns to control levels sooner than the diastolic flow rate. Interpreted in light of evidence that systolic coronary flow is distributed primarily to the epicardium (99,168), such a result suggests that the hyperemic response abates rather quickly in the superficial layers of the heart and that the latter portion of the response primarily reflects flow in the subendocardial half of the ventricular wall. Such an interpretation is consistent with evidence that autoregulatory capacity is greater in the subepicardium than in the subendocardium (see pages 1012–1013).

Figure 18 also contains preliminary observations on coronary venous outflow during reactive hyperemia. Although one cannot make too much of these observations, it is of interest that venous outflow increases during reactive hyperemia and that the maximum venous outflow rate appears to occur one to two beats later than the maximum rate of diastolic coronary inflow.

The historical evolution of thinking about reactive hyperemia has strongly influenced the direction of re-

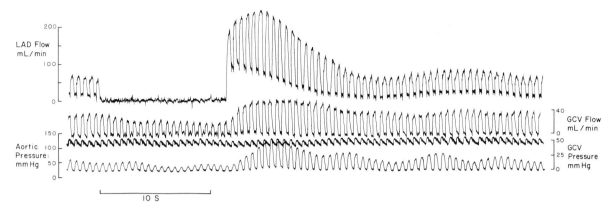

FIG. 18. Phasic recordings of the left anterior descending (LAD) coronary artery and great cardiac vein (GCV) flows and also aortic and GCV pressures during the reactive hyperemic response to an 11.5-sec LAD occlusion. Note that during reactive hyperemia, systolic arterial flow peaks earlier than diastolic flow. That venous outflow is not zero during arterial occlusion owes to the fact that in this open-chest dog, the GCV drained myocardium outside the perfusion field of the coronary artery. (From an unpublished experiment in the authors' laboratory performed by Dr. Noboyuki Yamada.)

search in this field. Well before its demonstration in the coronary circulation, reactive hyperemia was the subject of considerable attention from physiologists interested in blood flow to skeletal muscle. Perhaps influenced by the concept of the oxygen debt incurred during exercise, these investigators analyzed skeletal muscle reactive hyperemia in terms of a "flow debt," the volume of flow that would have occurred had there not been an interval of arterial occlusion, and a "repayment" of this debt through flow in excess of the control rate during the ensuing hyperemia. Because these skeletal muscle experiments showed that repayment matched flow debt, the conclusion followed naturally that reactive hyperemia is in essence a response to a metabolic perturbation. Coffman, whose physiological training was in the peripheral circulation, carried out the first quantitative studies of myocardial reactive hyperemia (73,74). Quite understandably, he analyzed the response in terms of a flow debt and its repayment. The strong emphasis on metabolism in Coffman's two seminal studies has had an abiding influence on thinking about myocardial reactive hyperemia. However, experiments in the past decade, many of them not dealing with reactive hyperemia at all, have revealed inconsistencies and ambiguities in the experimental support for the hypothesis that myocardial reactive hyperemia is purely metabolic in origin.

A single mechanism to explain reactive hyperemia would be esthetically satisfying, but we are instead faced with three plausible mechanisms: metabolic, myogenic, and capacitative. At present there is no way to discriminate between metabolic and myogenic vasodilation during the reactive hyperemic responses to coronary occlusions lasting a number of heartbeats. Ischemia during the interval of coronary occlusion certainly elicits release of vasodilatory metabolites such as adenosine. However, arterial occlusion also causes a rapid fall in

coronary intraluminal pressure, precisely the stimulus for myogenic relaxation. As we shall see, other mechanisms may also make subtle contributions during the course of a myocardial reactive hyperemia response, but separating metabolic from myogenic coronary relaxation remains the central problem for all but the very shortest occlusions. A new ambiguity arises when the duration of coronary occlusion is exceedingly short, one heartbeat or less. Here the problem is one of discriminating between vasodilation due to a change in metabolism, that due to a change in myogenic tone, and that due to a change in intramural coronary blood volume.

A unifying hypothesis, namely, that myocardial reactive hyperemia is the resultant of interaction of vasodilatory metabolites, myogenic relaxation, and changes in coronary capacitance, seems to best account for the experimental observations. The sections that follow describe the evidence to support this hypothesis.

Metabolic Vasodilation

The term *metabolic coronary vasodilation* implies the release of vasodilatory metabolites by cardiac cells (40). In the case of reactive hyperemia, ischemia seems to be the stimulus for production and release of these metabolites. However, ischemia could act directly on the metabolism of the coronary resistance vessels to induce relaxation. Finally, endothelial cells exposed to hypoxia may elaborate vasodilators (65) that could mediate reactive hyperemia. Further experiments will be necessary to evaluate the two alternative hypotheses.

Four lines of evidence support a role for vasodilatory metabolites in reactive hyperemia. First, there is a metabolic debt, and this is repaid. Second, the duration and volume of reactive hyperemia flow are proportional to the duration of coronary occlusion. Third, interventions that alter the rate of myocardial energy expenditure change the intensity of reactive hyperemia concordantly. Finally, the coronary sinus concentration of adenosine, an endogenous vasodilator, increases during reactive hyperemia.

The idea that reactive hyperemia serves to repay a metabolic debt is certainly in keeping with the facts that cardiac function is strongly oxygen-dependent and that functional recovery after a temporary coronary occlusion is complete. Experimental proof of repayment of a metabolic debt, which would support a metabolic cause for reactive hyperemia, has proved exceedingly difficult to obtain. Such investigations have focused on repayment of an oxygen debt, but in so doing have ignored, of course, the fact that ischemia at least temporarily increases anaerobic glycolysis, as evidenced by the release of lactate during reactive hyperemia (74,273,396). Thus, an oxygen debt does not truly represent the total energy deficit incurred during ischemia. Although replenishing glycogen stores requires ATP, the rate of restitution is too slow to materially affect the arteriovenous oxygen difference and so is not included in experimental estimates of the debt/repayment ratio.

Early studies showing that oxygen debt is overpaid employed integrated coronary sinus blood samples to estimate oxygen extraction for calculation of $M\dot{V}O_2$ (74,273). This approach contains a conceptual error, namely, the application of a technique that is valid for steady-state measurements to a situation in which flow and oxygen extraction vary rapidly and not necessarily concordantly. In pointing out this error, Ruiter et al. (315) critically analyzed other errors inherent in estimating oxygen consumption during reactive hyperemia. Such calculations require measurements of instantaneous capillary blood flow and transcapillary oxygen extraction. Because the coronary circulation lacks arteriovenous shunts, and because the mean coronary flow rate changes relatively slowly during reactive hyperemia, measurements of epicardial coronary flow represent the capillary flow rate reasonably well. However, estimating capillary oxygen extraction, which perforce must be inferred from measurements of oxyhemoglobin saturation in one of the larger epicardial veins, requires somewhat arbitrary assumptions about the transit time and dispersion of red cells as they traverse the coronary venous system. Monitoring oxyhemoglobin saturation by means of an optical oxyhemoglobin saturation sensor mounted on the tip of a catheter inserted into the coronary sinus reduced, but did not abolish, the dispersive artifact. Venous oxygen saturation curves (Fig. 19) show an initial dip from levels similar to those that obtain before occlusion, followed by a rise to levels approaching that of arterial blood, and then a gradual return to control. Because myocardial PO_2 is probably zero after the first few seconds of ischemia, the initial decrease in venous oxygen saturation doubtless represents the flushing out

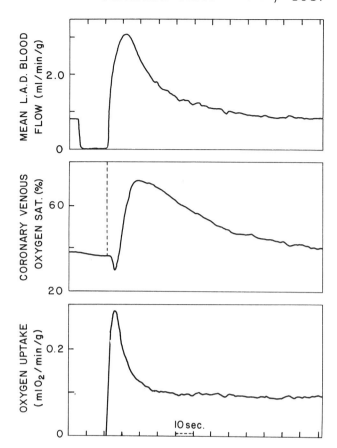

FIG. 19. Oxygen metabolism during myocardial reactive hyperemia following a 15-sec occlusion of the left anterior descending (LAD) coronary artery. See text for discussion. (From ref. 315.)

of blood that spent the ischemic interval in vessels distal to the coronary exchange vessels. The consequence of this artifact is an underestimate of $M\dot{V}O_2$. Ruiter did not try to correct for this artifact, probably because to do so would require arbitrary assumptions about the true shape of the time-saturation curve. Nevertheless, his estimate of the oxygen repayment/debt ratio, 0.87 ± 0.83 (SD), is not statistically significantly different from exact repayment.

Although reactive hyperemia overpays the "flow debt" severalfold, it is clear that the extra flow is not absolutely required to restore the heart to its preischemic state. As mentioned earlier, transcoronary oxygen extraction is reduced during most of the period of reactive hyperemia, prima facie evidence that oxygen supply exceeds demand. Indeed, the calculated $M\dot{V}O_2$ curve of Fig. 18 shows that $M\dot{V}O_2$ returns to the control level well before the end of the hyperemic response. Consonant with this observation, two laboratories (18,110) have shown that if reactive hyperemia is allowed to proceed until the flow debt is repaid and then flow is restricted to the control rate for a period equal to the anticipated period of reactive hyperemia, the ultimate release of constriction evokes only a minor hyperemic response.

In a subsequent study, Giles and Wilcken showed that when reactive hyperemia flow is restricted, it is possible to abolish the terminal hyperemic response altogether if the coronary constriction is maintained until the aorticocoronary pressure gradient disappears (140). They interpreted this result as evidence that reactive hyperemia is a myogenic response rather than a metabolic response. These authors also found that allowing an initial period of uninhibited reactive hyperemia is not absolutely necessary for recovery from ischemia. Restricting postischemic flow to levels only a few percent higher than control throughout the entire postischemic interval greatly prolonged the period of postischemic vasodilation, as judged by a persistent aorticocoronary pressure gradient, but coronary vascular resistance ultimately returned to the control value, and release of the occluder elicited no hyperemic response.

Unfortunately, none of the foregoing studies included measurements of cardiac oxygen extraction, which are essential for unambiguous interpretations. For example, even though $M\dot{V}O_2$ is greatly increased early in a reactive hyperemic response, one should not infer that one repays the oxygen debt by permitting unrestricted flow until repayment of the flow debt and then restricting flow. Figure 19 shows that this is not so. Less than half of the oxygen debt is repaid by the time flow debt is fully repaid. It is plausible that enhanced oxygen extraction during the interval of restricted flow accounts for much of the repayment of oxygen debt. Likewise, without evidence that oxygen extraction has already returned to control, one cannot be sure that the persistence of an aorticocoronary pressure gradient during restricted flow really represents myogenic relaxation.

Both the duration and the volume of reactive hyperemia flow increase concordantly with the length of coronary occlusion, even when the period of occlusion is as long as several minutes. The simplest explanation for this observation is that ischemia promotes release of vasodilatory metabolites and that the return of coronary flow to preischemic levels represents dissipation of these metabolites. Although myogenic relaxation is not instantaneous, it probably reaches completion relatively quickly and thus cannot explain why reactive hyperemia continues to increase as the period of coronary occlusion is extended to tens or, ultimately, hundreds of seconds.

The hypothesis that reactive hyperemia is metabolic in origin predicts that interventions that alter the rate of cardiac energy expenditure will cause concordant changes in the intensity of reactive hyperemia. Pauly et al. (283) showed that in open-chest dogs, imposing pacing tachycardia or paired ventricular pacing during 30- or 60-sec coronary occlusions increased reactive hyperemia flow in proportion to the number of heartbeats during the ischemic interval. Prior β-adrenergic blockade with propranolol significantly blunted the effect of pacing

(284). Almost simultaneous studies in conscious dogs by Bache et al. (16) confirmed and extended this observation. In those experiments, ventricular pacing at 120 beats/min constituted the control state, and paired ventricular pacing at 240 beats/min was the intervention. Paired pacing that was begun before coronary occlusion and was continued throughout the reactive hyperemic responses to 1- to 7-sec coronary occlusions significantly augmented reactive hyperemia flow. Measurements of $M\dot{V}O_2$ showed that the increase in reactive hyperemia flow due to paired pacing was proportional to the effect of this intervention on $M\dot{V}O_2$. In a subset of experiments, confining paired pacing to the ischemic interval increased reactive hyperemia significantly more than when pacing was continued throughout reactive hyperemia. Such a result is surprising, because one would expect that elevating $M\dot{V}O_2$ during recovery from an oxygen debt would, if anything, retard recovery. It is likely that this result owes to the fact that because of paired pacing, coronary flow returned to a steady-state level higher than that when pacing stopped at the end of coronary occlusion. Owing to the method used to calculate reactive hyperemia flow, such an elevation of control flow rate will reduce the volume of hyperemic flow (272).

Solid evidence implicates the participation of adenosine in the genesis of reactive hyperemia. Ischemia stimulates the time-dependent accumulation of this nucleoside in heart muscle (268) and its release into the coronary venous effluent during reactive hyperemia (314). Intracoronary infusion of adenosine deaminase catalytic subunits reduces reactive hyperemia volume by about a third following coronary occlusions lasting between 5 and 30 sec (319). The enzyme reduces peak reactive hyperemia flow only after very short (5-sec) coronary occlusions; the reduction in flow volume following longer occlusions owes primarily to shortening of the duration of the hyperemic response.

Theophylline, a specific antagonist at adenosine receptors (322), competitively antagonizes the coronary vasoactivity of adenosine (1,2,59). This purine reduces reactive hyperemia flow to the same extent as adenosine deaminase, and the combination of the enzyme plus theophylline has no more effect than either agent alone (319). Thus, it appears that adenosine supports only part of postischemic vasodilation.

For several years there was disagreement whether or not theophylline actually curtails reactive hyperemia. A number of investigations showed that theophylline at doses that reduced the vasoactivity of exogenous adenosine had no effect on reactive hyperemia, whereas similar experiments in the hands of others showed that reactive hyperemia was blunted (Table 5). The failure to inhibit reactive hyperemia now appears to be a matter of inadequate dosage. Those experiments in which theophylline reduced reactive hyperemia employed direct

TABLE 5. *Effect of theophylline on myocardial reactive hyperemia*

Preparation	Theophylline dose	Adenosine response	Coronary occlusion	Reduction of reactive hyperemia	Refs.
Conscious dog, EMF	8 mg/kg i.v.	NR	15 sec 90 sec	13% 11%	191
Open-chest dog, EMF	100 mg i.v.	−58%	30–120 sec	No reduction	44
Open-chest cat, TC	7 mg/kg i.v.	−101%	NR	Reduction, but not quantified	372
Open-chest dog, EMF	5 or 10 mg i.c.	−41%	10–20 sec	39%[a]	80
Conscious dog, EMF	10 mg/kg i.v.	−65%	4–8 sec	No reduction	112
Open-chest dog, EMF	0.2 mg/min i.c.	−87%	60 sec	No reduction	113
Open-chest dog, EMF	10 mg i.v. plus 0.2 mg/min i.c.	−82%	8 sec	19%[a]	144
Open-chest dog, EMF	0.025 mg/ml coronary blood	−80%	4 beats 10 beats 25 beats	1% 20%[a] 21%[a]	333
Open-chest dog, EMF	0.05–0.1 mM in coronary plasma	−83%	5 sec 10 sec 20 sec 30 sec	26%[a] 36%[a] 27%[a] 32%[a]	318

EMF = electromagnetic flow meter; TC = thermal conductivity meter; i.v. = intravenous; i.c. = intracoronary; NR = not reported.
[a] Statistically significant reduction.

intracoronary infusion of the drug at rates that produced blood concentrations between 0.05 and 0.1 mM. By contrast, most of the experiments that failed to show an effect employed intravenous administration of the drug; the coronary artery concentration is unknown. The ability of theophylline to antagonize the vasoactivity of adenosine during normoxic coronary perfusion may not predict the extent to which the drug inhibits vasodilation during recovery from ischemia, wherein acidosis may potentiate the effect of adenosine and inhibit that of theophylline (240,241). The experiments of Schutz et al. (334) deserve special comment. These investigators found that theophylline had no effect on reactive hyperemia after coronary occlusions for four heartbeats, but it significantly inhibited the responses to 10- and 25-beat occlusions. Such a result supports the idea that adenosine plays a significant role only in reactive hyperemic responses to relatively long occlusions and that other mechanisms or other vasodilatory metabolites mediate the responses to short occlusions.

Several years ago we reported that left ventricular adenosine content falls during reactive hyperemia in parallel with the return of coronary flow to preocclusion levels (277). A dose-response curve constructed from measurements of coronary flow at the time of tissue sampling and the adenosine content of the samples had

a slope significantly different from the dose-response curve of exogenous adenosine. We interpreted this discrepancy as evidence that adenosine was not exclusively responsible for reactive hyperemia. Subsequent demonstration that most of the cardiac adenosine pool is intracellular and thus does not participate in coronary vasomotion (276) and also evidence that adenosine uptake by endothelial cells might importantly modify the apparent vasoactivity of exogenous adenosine (262,263) vitiate this interpretation. Whether or not this experiment at all supports a role for adenosine awaits information about how the interstitial and intracellular adenosine compartments change during ischemia and reperfusion.

Information about the compartmentalization of adenosine is also needed to interpret the experiment by Downey et al. (98) showing that coronary flow rate during 3 min of perfusion with deoxygenated blood (hypoxia) produces a coronary flow response significantly larger than that attained at the peak of reactive hyperemia following a coronary occlusion (ischemia) of comparable length. Myocardial adenosine content rose during ischemia to levels nearly 20 times control, but decreased by half during hypoxia. The authors' conclusion that hypoxic vasodilation reflects a direct effect of oxygen lack on coronary resistance vessels may be correct, but this experiment does not exclude the possibility that during hypoxia the extracellular adenosine compartment is large enough to account for the observed flow rate.

Myogenic Relaxation

Coronary occlusion may cause ischemia, but it also causes a fall in transmural coronary pressure differential, the stimulus to myogenic relaxation. Subsequent release of the occlusion imposes a step increase in perfusion pressure on a bed that is relaxed. It is thus little wonder that the time course of a reactive hyperemic response resembles that of the dynamic response to a step increase in perfusion pressure (compare Figs. 6A and 18). However, such a superficial similarity between the two kinds of flow responses scarcely serves to identify the mechanism of vascular relaxation. Accordingly, one must seek other kinds of evidence for a myogenic contribution to reactive hyperemia.

Two types of experiments can be used to test the hypothesis that reactive hyperemia is myogenic. The first type compares the flow response to a period of hypoxic perfusion at the prevailing coronary artery pressure with the reactive hyperemia flow elicited by a comparable period of coronary occlusion. As the reasoning goes, hypoxic perfusion does not change the coronary transmural pressure differential, and so any difference from reactive hyperemia must owe to myogenic relaxation. The second type of experiment employs coronary occlusions thought to be too short to cause significant ischemia, i.e., those lasting two heartbeats or less.

Kelley and Gould (194) compared the reactive hyperemic responses to 10- or 15-sec coronary occlusions with the flow responses to comparable periods of coronary perfusion with highly deoxygenated blood delivered at a pressure identical with aortic pressure. Coronary flow rose substantially during hypoxic perfusion, then promptly returned to control levels when perfusion with oxygenated blood resumed. Flow in excess of the control rate had a volume less than a third that of reactive hyperemia flow following the same period of coronary occlusion. The experiments of Sugishita et al. (359) employed perfusion with Krebs-Henseleit buffer for 180 sec. Flow in excess of the control rate during recovery had a volume 31% that of reactive hyperemia after 180 sec of coronary occlusion.

Although these experiments suggest that removing the stimulus to myogenic relaxation reduces the flow response to hypoxia, these authors acknowledged that the washout of vasodilatory metabolites during hypoxic perfusion could also account for their observations. As pointed out previously, in blood-perfused *in situ* dog hearts, hypoxic perfusion lowered cardiac muscle adenosine content, whereas a comparable period of occlusion

markedly elevated adenosine levels (98). Hypoxic perfusion of isolated guinea pig hearts likewise stimulated release of adenosine (328).

Giles and Wilcken showed that very brief coronary occlusions, for one or two heartbeats or 0.7 to 1.4 sec at the prevailing heart rates, elicited reactive hyperemic responses that they interpreted as myogenic in origin (110). However, Schwartz et al. (335) showed that even shorter coronary occlusions, 0.2 to 0.4 sec or only a fraction of a single diastole, also elicited perceptible reactive hyperemia, but in that instance the authors favored a metabolic mechanism. Which of the divergent views is correct depends crucially on how rapidly coronary occlusion induces the hypoxic stimulus to production of vasodilatory metabolites. Because neither of these experiments included metabolic observations, both groups resorted to the literature to support their interpretations. Unfortunately, the literature does not give a clear answer whether or not the normoxic transition begins within 2 sec after coronary occlusion.

Calculations of cardiac oxygen stores (267) suggest that myoglobin, if completely saturated, could support cardiac activity for about 6 sec in the conscious dog with a relatively low heart rate. Indeed, in this preparation, coronary occlusions lasting this long are required to elicit lactate release (273). However, in open-chest dogs, cardiac muscle adenosine levels are already substantially elevated after 5 sec of coronary occlusion (268), but at what point in time the adenosine levels begin to rise is unknown.

Measurements of myocardial PO_2 by means of polarographic electrodes inserted to a depth of 3 mm into the left ventricular wall of open-chest dogs show that PO_2 begins to fall almost immediately after coronary occlusion and is 15% lower than control after 1 sec (323). Whether or not this degree of hypoxia is sufficient to evoke metabolite release is unknown. Spectroscopic studies of the effect of coronary occlusion on oxymyoglobin saturation and NAD reduction have good time resolution, 8 msec in a study of isolated nonworking rat hearts perfused at 30°C with buffer (192). Following coronary occlusion, the oxymyoglobin concentration did not begin to fall for 5 sec, and NADH fluorescence did not rise for about 10 sec. Because these hearts were cooler than normal and were not working, the development of hypoxia was doubtless retarded. That the deoxygenation of myoglobin and the appearance of NADH fluorescence were not synchronous owes to experimental design. Oxymyoglobin saturation was monitored by absorption spectroscopy, i.e., by transillumination, which senses the average change in absorbance across the entire heart wall. Fluorimetry monitored NADH concentration changes in only the most superficial layers of the epicardium, which, by virtue of its lower work load, is thought to be less sensitive to oxygen lack. Harden et al. (164) investigated the time course of the normoxic-to-hypoxic transition in isolated, buffer-perfused rabbit hearts by taking motion pictures of these hearts as they were illuminated with ultraviolet light to excite NADH fluorescence. The frame speed of the camera, either 1/heartbeat or 4/heartbeat, and also the ability of the investigator to detect a change in film density set the limits of time resolution in this experiment. When the hearts were doing no external work, coronary occlusion initiated NAD reduction in 2 to 4 sec, but if the hearts were working, this time decreased to 1 to 2 sec. Because NADH fluorescence reports the status of the epicardium, one may speculate that anoxia might have occurred earlier in the deeper layers. However, because physiological buffers are oxygen-poor relative to blood, the sensitivity of these hearts to anoxia could be greater than that of blood-perfused hearts.

In summary, the evidence provided by these metabolic studies admits the possibility that the reactive hyperemia that follows a coronary occlusion of 1 to 2 sec may have a metabolic component, but absolute proof is lacking. Even if metabolic vasodilation is present, there is no certainty that it accounts for the entire reactive hyperemic response. Thus, support for the idea that myogenic vasodilation participates in reactive hyperemia rests mainly on negative evidence, namely, the inability of metabolic vasodilation to fully account for this response.

To extrapolate back in time from such ambiguous evidence to assign a metabolic cause to reactive hyperemia following occlusions for only part of a diastole seems risky. At this time there is simply no experimental evidence that this period of ischemia initiates the normoxic-to-hypoxic transition. This does not necessarily mean that myogenic relaxation accounts for the reactive hyperemia following very brief occlusions. Rather, in the section that follows we offer an alternative explanation for the special case of reactive hyperemia following ischemia for a fraction of a heartbeat.

Intramural Coronary Capacitance

Figure 20 summarizes the salient results of Schwartz's elegant experiments on reactive hyperemia following occlusion for a fraction of one diastole, typifying his observations in both open-chest anesthetized dogs and conscious dogs (335). Coronary occlusion for part of a diastole was followed by a transient (about 50 msec) flow spike that these authors attributed to refilling of capacitance vessels. For the rest of that diastole, D_0, the flow rate was identical with that in beats without a coronary occlusion and did not increase above the control rate until systole of the succeeding beat, S_0. In succeeding beats, both systolic and diastolic flows were elevated. Because heart rate, i.e., diastolic duration, was

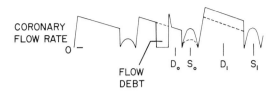

FIG. 20. Diagrammatic representation of myocardial reactive hyperemia following a coronary occlusion lasting for a fraction of a single diastole. Flow debt is calculated on the basis of the flow rate that would have occurred had there not been coronary occlusion (dash line). D_0 and S_0 represent the diastolic and systolic intervals immediately following the interval of inflow occlusion, and D_1 and S_1 the corresponding intervals in the succeeding beat. Note that at the end of coronary occlusion there is a transient flow spike, but the flow rate then returns to the control level for the remainder of D_0 and does not rise above the control rate until S_0. The dash lines in S_0 and D_1 represent the flow rate expected in the absence of a coronary occlusion. See text for further discussion. (Adapted from ref. 335, with permission.)

controlled by surgical heart block and electrical pacing, and the timing and duration of coronary occlusion also varied, the interval between the end of coronary occlusion and the onset of reactive hyperemia varied from as short as 50 msec to as long as 500 msec. Although the stimulus to myogenic relaxation was certainly present, the peripheral coronary pressure falling by 36 mm Hg after only 0.1 sec of occlusion, these authors argued quite reasonably that the highly variable latent period excludes a myogenic response.

We believe that the delayed onset of reactive hyperemia is likewise unmistakable evidence that these hyperemic responses are not metabolic. If coronary occlusion generated the stimulus to metabolic vasodilation, one would expect vasodilation immediately on restoration of flow, i.e., during diastole of the beat in which the occlusion occurred. Just as variable latency argues against a myogenic mechanism, so latency of any duration argues against a metabolic mechanism.

We suggest that a decrease in intramyocardial blood volume brought about by the transient interruption of coronary inflow best accounts for reactive hyperemia after such extremely short coronary occlusions. It is now clear that cardiac intramural blood volume oscillates phasically, a process that has been likened to the charging and discharging of a capacitor (see pages 1002–1005). Coronary inflow during diastole, when venous outflow is zero (186), increases intramural blood volume, which then diminishes as systole ejects blood into the coronary veins and, to a lesser extent, into arterioles. It is the concealed backflow of blood into the arterial side of the coronary circulation, rather than systolic compression of the arterioles, that is responsible for the decrease in the antegrade coronary flow rate in systole (348).

Coronary occlusion during part of a diastole will

reduce the filling of the intramural capacitor and, as a consequence, diminish the amount of blood ejected into the arterial and venous sides of the circulation during the succeeding systole. Such a decrease in concealed backflow manifests itself as increased systolic antegrade flow, and restoration of intramural blood volume as an increase in diastolic antegrade flow. Such a course of events is precisely what is seen following coronary occlusion for only part of a diastole.

We wish to emphasize that our alternative explanation concerns the *intramyocardial* capacitance, not that of the epicardial coronary arteries (95). We agree with Schwartz and associates that epicardial compliance, as evidenced by the momentary flow increase that occurs immediately on release of the coronary occluder, plays a negligible role in these reactive hyperemic responses.

Additional experiments will be necessary to define the role of intramural capacitative changes in reactive hyperemia following coronary occlusions for several heart-beats. To what extent does the increase in systolic coronary flow early in reactive hyperemia reflect a reduction in concealed backflow due to depletion of intramural blood volume, as opposed to metabolic vasodilation of resistance vessels? Does the delayed peak of diastolic reactive hyperemia flow represent the restoration of intramural blood volume? Measurements of phasic venous outflow are technically feasible and might provide the means to a mass balance analysis of coronary capacitative changes. There are, at present, no methods for measuring phasic changes in intramural blood volume directly.

Neural Influences on Reactive Hyperemia

Several studies in conscious instrumented dogs have tested the hypothesis that autonomic nervous influences can modify myocardial reactive hyperemic responses. These studies arrived at strongly divergent conclusions.

An early study (272) showed that atropine, guanethidine, and reserpine did modify reactive hyperemia. However, the effects of these drugs on heart rate and control coronary blood flow rate accounted for the observed changes, suggesting that the drugs acted indirectly through their effects on cardiac metabolism.

Total cardiac denervation, "chemical sympathectomy" by treatment with 6-hydroxydopamine, α-adrenergic blockade with phentolamine, or β blockade with propranolol does not significantly alter the intensity of reactive hyperemia (15).

Two nearly identical studies of the effects of acute decentralization of the stellate ganglia arrived at contradictory conclusions. In both experiments, snares placed central to the stellate ganglia, when pulled, severed the central connections. Depending on the order of decen-

tralization, this permitted comparisons of the effects of right, left, and bilateral stellectomy. In the first such study, Schwartz and Stone (336) found that left stellectomy increased the repayment of flow debt by about a third, whereas right stellectomy did not alter the hyperemic response. α-Adrenergic blockade with phentolamine mimicked the effect of left stellectomy, whereas β-adrenergic blockade with propranolol diminished reactive hyperemia. These authors interpreted these results as evidence for a tonic α-adrenergic constrictor influence on the coronary circulation that limits the flow response to ischemia.

The experiments of Peterson and Bishop (291) differed mainly in the duration of occlusion, 60 sec versus 10 sec in the experiments of Schwartz and Stone. Right, but not left, stellectomy significantly reduced the repayment of flow debt, by about a third. Additional studies with practolol, a selective β_1 antagonist, and propranolol, an unselective β antagonist, discriminated between the effects on cardiac metabolism and direct stimulation of coronary β_2 receptors. Both antagonists reduced the repayment of flow debt significantly, but the effect of propranolol was greater. After left stellectomy, the effects of these drugs were similar to those in intact dogs. These authors concluded that β_2-adrenergic vasodilation makes a major contribution to reactive hyperemia and that the metabolic consequences of β_1 stimulation are less important.

There is no obvious reason why the two experiments that employed selective stellectomy should give results that differ so dramatically from those of earlier studies that examined total cardiac denervation and the effects of some of the same drugs. While it is true that total denervation removes cholinergic as well as adrenergic innervation, the cholinergic influence on coronary vasomotion is considered minor (117,281) and probably does not account for this discrepancy. Likewise, it is difficult to see how lengthening the duration of coronary occlusion from 10 sec to 60 sec would change the nature of the response from α vasoconstriction to direct β_2 vasodilation.

It is not easy to think of an experiment that would reconcile these divergent observations. Perhaps measurements of oxygen consumption rates to more precisely define the metabolic state during each of the interventions would help.

REGULATION OF RIGHT CORONARY FLOW

By contrast with the wealth of information about the control of left ventricular perfusion, relatively little is known about the relationship among performance, metabolism, and perfusion in the right ventricle. The reasons for this dearth of knowledge are mainly anatomical and technical. The right coronary artery of the dog is considerably smaller than the left, and its origin lies in a pad of rather friable periaortic fat, which complicates the implantation of flow meters for long-term studies. In further contrast with the left ventricle, which is supplied solely by the left coronary artery (154), the right ventricle receives a dual blood supply. In the normal dog, the right coronary artery perfuses the central portion of the right ventricular free wall; blood flow to the paraseptal zone, about a third of total right ventricular perfusion, is from branches of the left coronary artery (154,254). Perhaps the greatest obstacle to studying the control of right ventricular perfusion is that the venous drainage of this chamber is as complicated as the arterial supply. Up to five "major" anterior cardiac veins and a number of minor veins drain the free wall of this chamber directly into the right atrium. One or more tributaries may drain the infundibular region by way of the great cardiac vein. Even the major anterior cardiac veins are small, usually 1 mm or less in diameter, and they are thin-walled; so sampling of their contents during acute experiments requires considerable dexterity. As yet, no one has devised a method for collecting anterior cardiac vein blood in a chronic animal preparation.

Simultaneous measurements of the rates of right and left ventricular perfusion by means of radiomicrospheres (251,254) or by electromagnetic flow meters on coronary branches (215,224) have shown that blood flow per unit tissue mass is lower in the right than in the left ventricle. Right ventricular perfusion is transmurally very nearly uniform (169,251,254). Flow to the infundibular portion of the right ventricle is slightly higher than to the remainder of the chamber (254); such a result is consistent with theoretical and experimental evidence that the work load of the infundibulum is higher than that of the rest of the right ventricle (10). Temporary occlusion of the right coronary artery elicits a reactive hyperemic response (224). Direct comparisons in a given animal show that longer right coronary artery occlusions are necessary to elicit a peak reactive hyperemia flow response, 60 sec versus 30 sec in a left coronary branch (215). Presumably, this difference owes to a lower rate of energy expenditure in the right ventricle. The minimum coronary resistance attained at the peak of a maximum hyperemic response is higher in the right than in the left coronary circulation, 0.45 versus 0.25 PRU, respectively (215).

As pointed out earlier, phasic flow in the right coronary artery differs from that in a left coronary branch, the systolic flow rate being nearly as high as that during diastole (Fig. 2A). Indeed, the right coronary flow curve often bears a striking resemblance to the aortic pressure curve. The relatively high systolic flow rate probably means that right ventricular systolic intramural pressure

is too low to effectively oppose coronary inflow pressure. When right coronary flow is artificially confined to systole, the transmural flow gradient is normal (169), additional evidence that intramyocardial pressure is a much less important determinant of right than of left ventricular perfusion. Measurements of right ventricular intramyocardial pressure to directly test this inference are desirable.

$\dot{M}VO_2$ in the right ventricle is lower than in the left, a difference consistent with the respective work loads of the two chambers. The lower rate of right ventricular perfusion clearly accounts for at least part of the difference in $\dot{M}VO_2$, but whether or not the two ventricles differ additionally according to the extent of transcoronary oxygen extraction is an unsettled question. Microspectrophotometric measurements of oxyhemoglobin saturation in the intramural venules suggest that oxygen extraction is equally high in the two ventricles and is regionally and transmurally uniform in the right ventricle (381). Such an observation means that the circulations of the two ventricles respond to a change in oxygen demand in much the same way, i.e., mainly through a change in coronary flow rather than oxygen extraction. By contrast, measurements of the oxygen content of anterior cardiac veins are consistently higher than those of blood drawn simultaneously from the coronary sinus, and anterior cardiac vein saturation falls when the right ventricular work load is augmented by constriction of the pulmonary artery (46,215). Such observations lead to the fundamentally different conclusions that the right ventricle has a larger "extraction reserve" than the left and that physiologically significant changes in oxygen extraction as well as changes in coronary flow adjust right ventricular $\dot{M}VO_2$ to work load. At present there seems no way to reconcile these divergent results.

In the few instances in which sampling blood from more than one anterior cardiac vein was technically feasible, the oxygen content sometimes varied substantially from one vein to another. Raising right ventricular work load by pulmonary artery constriction tended to abolish the between-vein difference in chemical composition (215). Such a result contrasts with observations that the chemical composition of coronary sinus tributaries is regionally uniform and changes concordantly during interventions that alter flow or $\dot{M}VO_2$ of the entire left ventricle (273). The variability of anterior cardiac venous blood composition is consistent with the observation that regional right ventricular perfusion is more heterogeneous than in the left ventricle (254), perhaps reflecting regional differences in right ventricular work rate (10). A direct correlation of the oxygen content in several anterior cardiac veins with flow to the drainage field of each would furnish valuable information about the regulation of right ventricular perfusion.

Little else is known about the mechanisms that control right ventricular perfusion or the extent to which the right coronary circulation exhibits autoregulation. Analysis of right coronary pressure-flow relationships supports a waterfall mechanism in the right ventricle (35). Vasodilatory metabolites that might regulate right coronary flow remain to be identified and their importance assessed. The neural contributions to right coronary flow are essentially unexplored. It is only a slight exaggeration to say that almost any experiment already done on the left coronary circulation would yield, if done on the right, important new information about the fundamental mechanisms of coronary regulation. Experimental designs that directly compare the right and left coronary circulations in a given animal are particularly appropriate.

Acute Right Ventricular Pressure Overload

Several studies exploring the pathogenesis of the cardiac dysfunction caused by pulmonary embolism have provided a fairly detailed picture of right ventricular perfusion during acute pressure overload (92,93,118,119, 143,144,232–234,351). Collectively, these studies illustrate interplay of the physical determinants of coronary perfusion and are particularly instructive when contrasted with the coronary flow adjustments evoked by left ventricular pressure overload.

Experiments in conscious dogs by Gold and Bache (143) are typical of most acute right ventricular overload studies. Cuff occlusion of the pulmonary artery that

raised right ventricular systolic pressure to levels somewhat lower than aortic systolic pressure raised right ventricular diastolic pressure moderately but did not affect left ventricular hemodynamics. A further increase in the degree of pulmonary artery obstruction raised right ventricular diastolic pressure still more without further increasing systolic pressure. Because this degree of obstruction compromised cardiac output (54), aortic pressure fell. These authors designated the two states as moderate and severe pulmonary artery constriction, MPAC and SPAC, respectively.

Table 6 is an abstract of salient measurements of pressures and radiomicrosphere estimates of right ventricular perfusion in these experiments. Moderate pulmonary artery constriction raised right ventricular perfusion rate twofold, the resultant of a significant increase in heart rate as well as of afterload, but transmural flow distribution was normal. Severe obstruction reduced right ventricular perfusion rate, particularly in the subendocardium. Restoring coronary perfusion pressure by cuff constriction of the descending aorta returned right ventricular perfusion rate to a level comparable to that during moderate pulmonary artery constriction, relieved the subendocardial ischemia, and somewhat lowered right ventricular diastolic pressure.

To test the hypothesis that the right ventricular dysfunction caused by severe pulmonary artery constriction owes to limited right coronary vasodilator reserve, these investigators next examined the effect of coronary vasodilation by adenosine. In dogs without pulmonary artery obstruction whose hearts were paced at rates comparable to those caused by severe pulmonary artery

TABLE 6. *Right ventricular perfusion during acute pulmonary artery constriction*

Criteria	Control	MPAC	SPAC	Aortic pressure + SPAC	Adenosine	Adenosine + SPAC	Aortic pressure + adenosine + SPAC
Heart rate (beats/min)	98	140	172	170	197	197	173
RV pressure (mm Hg)	36/4	92/9	64/13	88/6	42/2	77/8	87/8
Aortic pressure (mm Hg)	113/63	110/71	77/43	112/71	105/52	75/42	106/65
Mean aortic pressure (mm Hg)	83	87	55	87	68	52	77
RV perfusion (ml/min/g)	0.77	1.69	0.81	1.72	3.92	2.25	2.08
RV Endo/Epi perfusion	1.23	1.36	0.77	1.36	1.24	0.61	1.35

MPAC = moderate pulmonary artery constriction; SPAC = severe pulmonary artery constriction; RV = right ventricular; Endo/Epi = endocardial/epicardial.
From ref. 143.

obstruction, intravenous infusion of adenosine raised right coronary perfusion substantially, to nearly 4 ml/min per gram, clear evidence that there is a large flow reserve in the unstressed right ventricle. However, during severe pulmonary artery obstruction, with its attendant fall in coronary perfusion pressure, adenosine only doubled right ventricular perfusion and failed to correct subendocardial ischemia. When adenosine administration was combined with restoration of coronary perfusion pressure, the right ventricular perfusion rate was only slightly higher than the rate achieved simply by raising perfusion pressure.

While all of these experiments clearly emphasize the importance of arterial and intracavitary pressures as determinants of myocardial perfusion, none explains the paradox of subendocardial ischemia in the face of a largely unexpended coronary vasodilator reserve. The astonishingly modest coronary vasoactivity of adenosine during severe pulmonary artery obstruction is likewise unexplained. The persistent right ventricular subendocardial ischemia caused by pressure overload contrasts sharply with the perfusion response to acute left ventricular pressure overload, wherein subendocardial ischemia is only transitory. Radiomicrosphere estimates of left coronary perfusion showed subendocardial ischemia 5 sec after abrupt elevation of aortic pressure, but not after 30 sec of hypertension, by which time transmural myocardial perfusion rate had risen by 63% from a control value of 1.18 ml/min per gram and transmural flow distribution was normal (375). An explanation for why the two ventricles respond so differently to pressure overload awaits studies of the extent to which a change in right ventricular cavitary pressure affects intramural pressure as well as studies of the capacity of the right coronary circulation to autoregulate.

A subsequent study by Gold et al. (144) searched for the cause of the reduced vasoactivity of adenosine during severe pulmonary artery constriction. Owing to between-animal variation, a subset of dogs had much higher right ventricular systolic pressures at the time aortic pressure began to decline. Perhaps in proportion to this stress, these dogs had significantly higher concentrations of systemic plasma epinephrine and norepinephrine. Both the right and left coronary circulations showed reduced responsiveness to adenosine. α-Adrenergic blockade with phentolamine restored the sensitivity of the left coronary circulation to adenosine, but had no influence on the effect of this nucleoside on right ventricular perfusion. Thus, the well-established ability of α-adrenergically mediated coronary vasoconstriction to overcome adenosine vasodilation (55) seems able to explain the left, but not right, coronary flow response to acute right ventricular overload. Catecholamine release is doubtless reflex in origin, but neither the reflexigenic zone nor the afferent pathway(s) are known. Likewise,

the reason for the refractoriness of the right coronary circulation remains obscure.

Chronic Right Ventricular Pressure Overload

An experiment of nature, congenital pulmonic valvular stenosis, and experimental pulmonary artery obstruction by means of inflatable periarterial cuffs (251,254,255) have provided important insights into the coronary flow response to chronic right ventricular pressure overload. The right coronary artery phasic flow curve for dogs with congenital pulmonic stenosis (Figs. 2B and 2C) exhibits a decrease in systolic flow rate that appears to parallel the degree of right ventricular hypertension and/or hypertrophy (224). Precisely what factors contribute to "left ventricularization" of the right coronary flow pattern are unknown.

A series of investigations by Murray and associates characterized right ventricular perfusion during the development of hypertrophy consequent to chronic pulmonary artery obstruction (251,254–256). These observations are particularly valuable because they were longitudinal, made in dogs in the conscious state, and can be compared with similar studies of pressure overload hypertrophy in the left ventricle. That these studies raise more questions than they answer further enhances their value.

As shown in Table 7, the right ventricular perfusion rate per unit tissue mass increases during the evolution of hypertrophy, ultimately exceeding that of the left ventricle. Experiments suggesting that right ventricular oxygen extraction increases in response to acute pressure overload (215) have suggested that right ventricular $M\dot{V}O_2$ may increase even more than these estimates of perfusion rate would indicate. By contrast, the perfusion rate per unit mass of a left ventricle in stable hypertrophy is normal. The reason for these qualitatively different flow responses of the two ventricles to overload is uncertain. Marcus (235) has pointed out that an increase in wall thickness normalizes wall stress in the hypertrophied left ventricle and has suggested that perhaps the degree of right ventricular hypertrophy is insufficient to compensate for increased wall stress. It is possible that an even longer period of right ventricular overload could produce stable hypertrophy and a normal rate of myocardial perfusion.

In a subsequent study, Murray and Vatner (254) addressed the question whether or not right ventricular hypertrophy reduces coronary vasodilator reserve, which hypertrophy appears to do in the left ventricle (20,236,266). Radiomicrosphere estimates of transmural myocardial perfusion during intravenous infusion of adenosine at a rate that abolished reactive hyperemia yielded an estimate of "minimum" coronary resistance.

TABLE 7. *Right ventricular perfusion during development of right ventricular hypertrophy*

	Normal	4–6 wk	4–5 mo
LV weight/body weight (g/kg)	4.95 ± 0.18	4.81 ± 0.21	4.66 ± 0.36
RV weight/body weight (g/kg)	1.43 ± 0.06	2.07 ± 0.09[a]	3.01 ± 0.23[a]
LV transmural perfusion (ml/min/g)	1.00 ± 0.06	1.01 ± 0.09	1.00 ± 0.19
LV Endo/Epi perfusion ratio	1.17 ± 0.03	1.23 ± 0.07	1.31 ± 0.14
RV transmural perfusion (ml/min/g)	0.67 ± 0.04	0.91 ± 0.07[a]	1.40 ± 0.23[a]
RV Endo/Epi perfusion ratio	1.17 ± 0.04	1.10 ± 0.05	1.14 ± 0.03

[a] Significantly greater than control.
From ref. 251.

In normal dogs, vasodilation reduced right coronary resistance by 89% from a control level of 128 ± 14 to 14.2 ± 1.1 PRU. As a consequence of lower control resistance, vasodilation reduced resistance in the hypertrophied right ventricles by only 55% from a control value of 51 ± 3 to 22.8 ± 4.4 PRU. Thus, hypertrophy appears to reduce coronary vasodilator reserve by a combination of a higher control flow rate and, more important, a higher maximum resistance. One wonders if the same mechanism explains the reduced coronary sensitivity to adenosine in acute and chronic right ventricular overload. In view of the uncertainty over the importance of right ventricular oxygen extraction as a compensatory mechanism, it is premature to conclude that the limited vasodilator reserve of the hypertrophied right ventricle necessarily entails a corresponding reduction in the capacity to deliver oxygen.

The authors of the foregoing study also compared reactive hyperemia responses in normal and hypertrophied right ventricles as a means of further assessing coronary vasodilator reserve. Although this investigation was only tangential to the main thrust of the study, it illustrates how ambiguities in interpretation limit the usefulness of reactive hyperemia responses in assessing the extent of vascular adaptation to hypertrophy (174). The premises underlying such an experimental approach are that minimum resistance is directly related to the anatomical cross-sectional area of the bed under study (i.e., its capillary density) and also that a coronary occlusion of sufficient length is able to elicit maximum coronary vasodilation—in other words, minimum coronary resistance—at the peak of the ensuing hyperemic response. Experiment showed that peak reactive hyperemia flow following a 15-sec coronary occlusion was significantly higher in the hypertrophied ventricles and, because coronary inflow pressures were similar in the two groups of dogs, minimum coronary resistance was lower. Owing to a significant elevation in control flow rate, the volume of reactive hyperemia flow was only slightly larger in the hypertrophied ventricles, and the repayment of flow debt was substantially less. Although a lower minimum resistance might argue that a hypertrophied ventricle has a normal coronary reserve, one must take into account the larger mass of myocardium supplied by the right coronary artery. The ratio of peak hyperemia to the control flow rate, another index of vascular reserve, is not applicable here, because hypertrophy of itself raises the control flow rate per unit mass of tissue. Similarly, the elevated control flow rate confounds interpretation of the reduced volume of hyperemia flow. Finally, it is not certain that a 15-sec coronary occlusion produced comparable stimuli to vasodilation in the normal and hypertrophied ventricles. The evidence that 60 sec of right coronary occlusion is required to evoke a maximum flow response (215) suggests that a 15-sec occlusion probably did not elicit a maximum response in the normal dogs. A threefold larger flow debt in the dogs with hypertrophied ventricles suggests that the stimulus to vasodilation was larger, though one cannot be sure that it was maximum.

ENDOTHELIUM-DEPENDENT VASOMOTION

Furchgott's discovery that endothelial cells mediate the vasodilatory action of acetylcholine (130) is a profoundly important insight into the mechanisms of local blood flow control. Hypotheses that envision local control in terms of vasodilatory metabolites elaborated by parenchymal cells must be modified to recognize that under certain circumstances, endothelial cells may play the primary role in vasoregulation. A recent review (128,305) tentatively defined the horizons of this rapidly progressing field and the instances in which endothelium-mediated vascular responses are or are not physiologically significant.

It is now clear that the effect of acetylcholine on endothelial cells is to evoke release of an extremely labile vasodilator: endothelium-dependent relaxing factor (EDRF). Owing to its lability—estimates of the biological half-life of EDRF range between 6 sec (159) and 20 sec

(121)—EDRF has not been isolated nor characterized chemically. Indirect evidence from experiments employing inhibitors suggests that EDRF may be a lipid, a product of the lipoxygenase pathway and perhaps even a free radical. Thus, agents that antagonize vascular relaxation by acetylcholine include phospholipase A_2 inhibitors such as quinacrine or p-α-dibromoacetophenone, lipoxygenase inhibitors such as 5,8,11,14-eicosatetraynoic acid or nordihydroguiaretic acid, and free radical scavengers such as hydroquinone or methylene blue. Inhibitors of cyclooxygenase or prostaglandin synthase do not antagonize acetylcholine vasodilation. Interpretation of the evidence that EDRF is a lipoxygenase product is complicated by the fact that many C_{10}–C_{22} fatty acids, either saturated or unsaturated, cause vascular relaxation, perhaps through nonspecific effects such as changes in membrane fluidity (68,127). It is interesting that EDRF is a vasodilator, because some other products of the lipoxygenase pathway, leukotrienes C_4 and D_4, are coronary vasoconstrictors (393).

At vascular smooth muscle cells, EDRF stimulates the production of cyclic GMP and causes a change in the pattern of protein phosphorylation that possibly includes a decrease in the phosphorylation of myosin light chains (303,304). Because nitroprusside and 8-bromo cyclic GMP produce similar alterations in protein phosphorylation, it is possible that EDRF and the organic nitrite vasodilators cause relaxation by a common final pathway (302,305). Thus, phosphorylation of myosin light chains and, according to present information, the contractile state of vascular smooth, muscle appear to be under dual control of two phosphorylation cascades, one initiated by activation of adenylate cyclase (see pages 1001–1002), the other by activation of guanylate cyclase.

Acetylcholine is not the only endothelium-dependent vasodilator, nor does EDRF appear to be the only mediator of endothelium-dependent relaxation. Histamine and serotonin, as well as peptides such as bradykinin, substance P, and thrombin, and purines such as ATP and ADP (but not AMP or adenosine) (80) all exert endothelium-dependent vascular relaxation. The extent of relaxation depends on the species, or whether the vessel is an artery or a vein and, in the case of arteries, the anatomical location of the artery. Such variability is consistent with other evidence for endothelial cell heterogeneity (12,83). Prostacyclin appears to mediate relaxation in some instances (64,82,288); whether or not there are still other relaxation factors is unknown.

The endothelium-dependent relaxation exerted by ATP and ADP has two important implications. First, it is evidence that vascular tissue contains, in its endothelial elements, type P2 purinergic receptors in addition to the A2 or R_a subtype of P1 receptors found in smooth

muscle cells. (For a discussion of classification of purinergic receptors, see ref. 61 and 62). Second, and even more important, ATP released from blood platelets during their interaction with damaged endothelial cells may influence the course of thrombosis and its hemodynamic consequences. Because the concentration of ATP in platelet granules is about 1 M, platelet degranulation during aggregation could produce physiologically significant local concentrations of this nucleotide. The dynamics of the chemical events during interaction of platelets with blood vessels whose endothelium is injured or denuded are exceedingly complex. For example, ATP, which is an inhibitor of platelet aggregation, is readily hydrolyzed by ectophosphatases of endothelial cells to form ADP, a promoter of aggregation. Further hydrolysis of ADP gives rise to adenosine, which, like ATP, is a powerful antagonist of platelet aggregation as well as a direct smooth muscle relaxant (285). This account of the role of purines in platelet-endothelial interactions is but a small part of an immensely more complicated picture involving other vasoactive and platelet-activating agents released from platelets such as serotonin and thromboxane A_2, as well as enzymes released from neutrophils such as elastase, which elicits ATP release from endothelial cells (22). A great deal of work will be required to arrive at a full understanding of the role of endothelial cells in the hemodynamic responses to platelet-endothelial cell interactions.

There is now preliminary evidence that endothelial cells may produce vasoconstrictor(s) in addition to EDRFs. Agricola et al. (3) reported that cultured bovine aortic endothelial cells release into the culture medium a powerful constrictor of cow, dog, and pig epicardial coronary arteries. This action is endothelium-independent and is unaffected by cyclooxygenase or lipoxygenase inhibitors. The constrictor substance appears to be a peptide whose molecular mass is approximately 8,500 daltons. Aside from the obvious implications for the pathogenesis of coronary vasospasm, this evidence raises the possibility that this or other endothelially derived peptides may contribute to basal coronary resistance.

There are several reasons why the available evidence has neither established nor excluded a role for EDRF(s) in the moment-to-moment control of myocardial perfusion. First, most of what is known about EDRFs comes from noncoronary vessels. Second, the formidable technical obstacles to studies of vessels as small as the true resistance vessels currently limit this information to vessels 200 μm in diameter or larger (81). The probability that the attributes of endothelial cells differ according to their locations in the vascular tree (12) precludes unqualified extrapolation to resistance vessels of the results of experiments on conductance vessels. However, the short biological half-lives of EDRFs suggest that they exert their effects at the site of formation rather than at some point distal in the circulation. Because the known endothelium-dependent agonists are all potent coronary vasodilators, it is thus possible that the endothelium of the coronary resistance vessels may well have the capacity to produce EDRFs.

Endothelial cells might initiate coronary vascular smooth muscle relaxation in response to physical as well as chemical stimuli. Bassenge and Holtz (175) have described experiments suggesting that the flow rate or, more precisely, the shear rate at the endothelial cell surface may be a stimulus to release of vasodilatory metabolites. Whether or not such shear-dependent vasodilation could account for postischemic epicardial coronary vasodilation (225) is unknown.

ACKNOWLEDGMENTS

The preparation of this chapter was supported by funds from the Ed C. Wright Chair of Cardiovascular Research established by the Suncoast Chapter, Florida AHA Affiliate. We are particularly indebted to Ms. Jo Ella Young for compiling the references, to Mrs. Dianne Peebles for artwork, and to Mrs. Eunice Oliver and Mr. Robert Vomacka for preparation of the manuscript.

REFERENCES

1. Afonso, S. (1970): Inhibition of coronary vasodilating action of dipyridamole and adenosine by aminophylline in the dog. *Circ. Res.*, 26:743–752.
2. Afonso, S., Ansfield, T. J., Berndt, T. B., and Rowe, G. G. (1972): Coronary vasodilator responses to hypoxia before and after aminophylline. *J. Physiol. (Lond.)*, 221:589–599.
3. Agricola, K. M., Rubanyi, G., Paul, R. J., and Highsmith, R. F. (1984): Characterization of a potent coronary artery vasoconstrictor produced by endothelial cells in culture. *Fed. Proc.*, 43:899 (abstract).
4. Anand-Srivastrava, M. B., Franks, D. J., Cantin, M., and Genest, J. (1982): Presence of "R$_a$" and "P"-site receptors for adenosine coupled to adenylate cyclase in cultured vascular smooth muscle cells. *Biochem. Biophys. Res. Commun.*, 108:218–219.
5. Anversa, P., Giacomelli, F., and Wiener, J. (1973): Regional variation in capillary permeability of ventricular myocardium. *Microvasc. Res.*, 6:273–285.
6. Archie, J. P. (1975): Intramyocardial pressure: Effect of preload on transmural distribution of systolic coronary blood flow. *Am. J. Cardiol.*, 35:904–911.
7. Archie, J. P. (1978): Transmural distribution of intrinsic and transmitted left ventricular diastolic intramyocardial pressure in dogs. *Cardiovasc. Res.*, 12:255–262.
8. Areskog, N. H., Arturson, G., and Grotte, G. (1964): Studies on heart lymph. I. Kinetics of ^{131}I-albumin in dog heart-lung preparations. *Acta Physiol. Scand.*, 62:209–217.
9. Areskog, N. H., Arturson, G., Grotte, K. G., and Wallenius, G. (1964): Studies on heart lymph. II. Capillary permeability of the dog's heart, using dextran as a test substance. *Acta Physiol. Scand.*, 62:218–223.
10. Armour, J. A., Pace, J. B., and Randall, W. C. (1970): Interrelationship of architecture and function of the right ventricle. *Am. J. Physiol.*, 218:174–179.
11. Armour, J. A., and Randall, W. C. (1971): Canine left ventricular intramyocardial pressures. *Am. J. Physiol.*, 220:1833–1839.

12. Auerbach, R., Alby, L., Grieves, J., Lindgren, J. C., Morrisey, L. W., Sidley, Y. A., Tu, M., and Watt, S. L. (1982): Monoclonal antibody against angiotensin-converting enzyme: Its use as a marker for murine, bovine, and human endothelial cells. *Proc. Natl. Acad. Sci. U.S.A.*, 79:7891–7895.
13. Aversano, T., Klocke, F. M., Mates, R. E., and Canty, J. M., Jr. (1984): Preload-induced alterations in capacitance-free diastolic pressure-flow relationships. *Am. J. Physiol.*, 246:H410–H417.
14. Bache, R. J., Ball, R. M., Cobb, F. R., Rembert, J. C., and Greenfield, J. C. (1975): Effects of nitroglycerin on transmural myocardial blood flow in the unanesthetized dog. *J. Clin. Invest.*, 55:1219–1228.
15. Bache, R. J., Cobb, F. R., Ebert, P. A., and Greenfield, J. C., Jr. (1975): Neurogenic influences on the coronary vascular response to ischemia in the awake dog. *J. Thorac. Cardiovasc. Surg.*, 69:421–428.
16. Bache, R. J., Cobb, F. R., and Greenfield, J. C. (1973): Effects of increased myocardial oxygen consumption on coronary reactive hyperemia in the awake dog. *Circ. Res.*, 33:588–596.
17. Bache, R. J., Cobb, F. R., and Greenfield, J. C. (1974): Myocardial blood flow distribution during ischemia-induced coronary vasodilation in the unanesthetized dog. *J. Clin. Invest.*, 54:1462–1472.
18. Bache, R. J., Cobb, F. R., and Greenfield, J. C. (1974): Limitation of the coronary vascular response to ischemia in the awake dog. *Circ. Res.*, 35:527–535.
19. Bache, R. J., and Dymek, D. J. (1981): Local and regional regulation of coronary vascular tone. *Prog. Cardiovasc. Dis.*, 24:191–212.
20. Bache, R. J., Vrobel, T. R., Arentzen, C. E., and Ring, W. S. (1981): Effect of maximal coronary vasodilation on transmural myocardial perfusion during tachycardia in dogs with left ventricular hypertrophy. *Circ. Res.*, 49:742–750.
21. Baer, H. P., and Drummond, G. E., editors (1979): *Physiological and Regulatory Functions of Adenosine and Adenine Nucleotides*. Raven Press, New York.
22. Baer, H. P., Drummond, G. I., and Duncan, E. L. (1966): Formation and deamination of adenosine by cardiac muscle enzymes. *Mol. Pharmacol.*, 2:67–76.
23. Baird, R. J., and Adiseshia, M. (1976): The response of diastolic myocardial tissue pressure and regional coronary blood flow to increased preload from blood, colloid, and crystalloid. *Surgery*, 79:644–651.
24. Baird, R. J., Adiseshia, M., and Okumori, M. (1976): The gradient in regional myocardial tissue pressure in the left ventricle during diastole: Its relationship to regional flow distribution. *J. Surg. Res.*, 20:11–16.
25. Baird, R. J., Goldbach, M. M., and de la Rocha, A. (1972): Intramyocardial pressure. The persistence of its transmural gradient in the empty heart and its relationship to myocardial oxygen consumption. *J. Thorac. Cardiovasc. Surg.*, 64:635–646.
26. Baird, R. J., and Manktelow, R. T. (1969): The systolic pressure in the tunnelled portion of a myocardial vascular implant. *J. Thorac. Cardiovasc. Surg.*, 57:714–720.
27. Baird, R. J., Manktelow, R. T., Shah, P. A., and Ameli, F. M. (1970): Intramyocardial pressure. A study of its regional variations and its relationship to intraventricular pressure. *J. Thorac. Cardiovasc. Surg.*, 59:810–823.
28. Barany, M., and Barany, K. (1981): Protein phosphorylation in cardiac and vascular smooth muscle. *Am. J. Physiol.*, 241:H117–H128.
29. Barron, J. T., Barany, M., Barany, K., and Storti, R. V. (1980): Reversible phosphorylation and dephosphorylation of the 20,000-dalton light chain of myosin during the contraction-relaxation-contraction cycle of arterial smooth muscle. *J. Biol. Chem.*, 255:6238–6244.
30. Bassingthwaighte, J. B., Strandell, T. B., and Donald, D. E. (1968): Estimation of coronary blood flow by washout of diffusible indicators. *Circ. Res.*, 23:259–278.
31. Bassingthwaighte, J. B., Yipntsoi, T., and Harvey, R. B. (1974): Microvasculature of the dog left ventricular myocardium. *Microvasc. Res.*, 7:229–249.
32. Belardinelli, L., Rubio, R., and Berne, R. M. (1979): Blockade

of Ca²⁺-dependent rat atrial slow action potentials by adenosine and lanthanum. *Pfluegers Arch.*, 380:19–27.

33. Bellamy, R. F. (1978): Diastolic coronary artery pressure-flow relations in the dog. *Circ. Res.*, 43:92–101.

34. Bellamy, R. F. (1981): Effect of atrial systole on canine and porcine coronary blood flow. *Circ. Res.*, 49:701–710.

35. Bellamy, R. F., and Lowensohn, H. S. (1980): Effect of systole on coronary pressure-flow relations in the right ventricle of the dog. *Am. J. Physiol.*, 238:H481–H486.

36. Bellamy, R. F., Lowensohn, H. S., and Olsson, R. A. (1979): Factors determining delayed peak flow in canine myocardial reactive hyperemia. *Cardiovasc. Res.*, 13:147–151.

37. Belloni, F. L. (1979): The local control of coronary blood flow. *Cardiovasc. Res.*, 13:63–85.

38. Berman, H. J., and Gamble, W. J. (1975): Myocardial oxygen usage: Its measurement, regulation and meaning. *Microvasc. Res.*, 9:127–135.

39. Berne, R. M. (1963): Cardiac nucleotides in hypoxia: Possible role in regulation of coronary blood flow. *Am. J. Physiol.*, 204:317–322.

40. Berne, R. M. (1980): The role of adenosine in the regulation of coronary blood flow. *Circ. Res.*, 47:807–813.

41. Berne, R. M., Rall, T. W., and Rubio, R., editors (1983): *Regulatory Function of Adenosine.* Martinus Nijhoff, Boston.

42. Berne, R. M., and Rubio, R. (1979): Coronary circulation. In: *Handbook of Physiology. The Coronary System,* edited by R. M. Berne and N. Sperelakis, pp. 873–952. American Physiological Society, Washington, D.C.

43. Bittar, N., and Pauly, T. J. (1971): Myocardial reactive hyperemia responses in the dog after aminophylline and lidoflazine. *Am. J. Physiol.*, 220:812–815.

44. Bloor, C. M., and Roberts, L. E. (1965): Effect of intravascular isotope content on the isotopic determination of coronary collateral blood flow. *Circ. Res.*, 16:537–544.

45. Boatwright, R. B., Downey, H. F., Bashour, F. A., and Crystal, G. J. (1980): Transmural variation in autoregulation of coronary blood flow in hyperperfused canine myocardium. *Circ. Res.*, 47:599–609.

46. Boatwright, R. B., Sheji, T., Williams, D. O., and Griggs, D. M., Jr. (1982): Comparison of oxygen, lactate and catecholamine metabolism in the right and left ventricles of the anesthetized, open-chest dog. *Fed. Proc.*, 41:1528 (abstract).

47. Bontemps, F., Van den Berghe, G., and Hers, H. G. (1983): Evidence for a substrate cycle between AMP and adenosine in isolated hepatocytes. *Proc. Natl. Acad. Sci. U.S.A.*, 80:2829–2833.

48. Borgers, M., Schaper, J., and Schaper, W. (1971): Localization of specific phosphatase activities in canine coronary blood vessels and heart muscle. *J. Histochem. Cytochem.*, 19:526–539.

49. Borgers, M., Schaper, J., and Schaper, W. (1971): Adenosine-producing sites in the mammalian heart: A cytochemical study. *J. Mol. Cell. Cardiol.*, 3:287–296.

50. Borgström, P., Grande, P. O., and Mellander, S. (1982): A mathematical description of the myogenic response in the micro-circulation. *Acta Physiol. Scand.*, 116:363–376.

51. Brandi, G., and McGregor, M. (1969): Intramural pressure in the left ventricle of the dog. *Cardiovasc. Res.*, 3:472–475.

52. Brantigan, J. W., Gott, V. L., and Martz, M. N. (1972): A Teflon membrane for measurement of blood and intramyocardial gas tensions by mass spectroscopy. *J. Appl. Physiol.*, 32:276–282.

53. Briden, K. L., and Weiss, H. R. (1981): Effect of moderate arterio-venous shunt on regional extraction, blood flow and oxygen consumption in the dog heart. *Cardiovasc. Res.*, 15:206–213.

54. Brooks, H., Kirk, E. S., Vokonas, P. S., Urschel, C. W., and Sonnenblick, E. H. (1971): Performance of the right ventricle under stress: Relation to right coronary flow. *J. Clin. Invest.*, 50:2176–2183.

55. Buffington, C. W., and Feigl, E. O. (1981): Adrenergic coronary vasoconstriction in the presence of coronary stenosis in the dog. *Circ. Res.*, 48:416–423.

56. Bukoski, R. D., Sparks, H. V., and Mela, L. M. (1983): Rat heart mitochondria release adenosine. *Biochem. Biophys. Res. Commun.*, 113:990–995.

57. Bukoski, R. D., Sparks, H. V., Jr., and Mela-Riker, L. (1984): Adenosine release by rat heart mitochondria: Site of adenosine production. *Fed. Proc.*, 43:307 (abstract).

58. Bünger, R., Haddy, F. J., and Gerlach, E. (1975): Coronary responses to dilating substances and competitive inhibition by theophylline in the isolated perfused guinea pig heart. *Pfluegers Arch.*, 358:218–224.

59. Bünger, R., Haddy, F. J., Querengässer, A., and Gerlach, E. (1976): Studies of potassium induced coronary dilation in the isolated guinea pig heart. *Pfluegers Arch.*, 363:27–31.

60. Bünger, R., Soboll, S., and Permanetter, B. (1983): Effects of norepinephrine on coronary flow, myocardial substrate utilization, and subcellular adenylates. In: *Ca²⁺ Entry Blockers, Adenosine and Neurotumors,* edited by G. F. Merrill and H. R. Weiss, pp. 267–279. Urban and Schwarzenberg, Munich.

61. Burnstock, G. (1972): Purinergic nerves. *Pharmacol. Rev.*, 24:509–581.

62. Burnstock, G., editor (1981): *Receptors and Recognition Series B, Vol. 12, Purinergic Receptors.* Chapman and Hall, London.

63. Burton, A. C. (1951): On the physiological equilibrium of small blood vessels. *Am. J. Physiol.*, 164:319–329.

64. Busse, R., Förstermann, U., Matsuda, H., and Pohl, U. (1984): The role of prostaglandins in the endothelium-mediated vasodilatory response to hypoxia. *Pfluegers Arch.*, 401:77–83.

65. Busse, R., Pohl, U., Kellner, C., and Klemm, U. (1983): Endothelial cells are involved in the vasodilatory response to hypoxia. *Pfluegers Arch.*, 397:78–80.

66. Carew, T. E., and Covell, J. W. (1976): Effect of intramyocardial pressure on the phasic flow in the intraventricular septal artery. *Cardiovasc. Res.*, 10:56–64.

67. Caulfield, J. B., and Borg, T. K. (1979): The collagen network of the heart. *Lab. Invest.*, 40:364–372.

68. Cherry, P. D., Furchgott, R. F., and Zawadzki, J. V. (1983): The endothelium-dependent relaxation of vascular smooth muscle by unsaturated fatty acids. *Fed. Proc.*, 42:619 (abstract).

69. Chilian, W. M., Boatwright, R. B., Shoji, T., and Griggs, D. M. (1981): Evidence against significant resting sympathetic coronary vasoconstrictor tone in the conscious dog. *Circ. Res.*, 49:866–876.

70. Chilian, W. M., and Marcus, M. L. (1982): Phasic coronary blood flow velocity in intramural and epicardial coronary arteries. *Circ. Res.*, 50:775–781.

71. Clanachan, A. S., and Marshall, R. J. (1980): Diazepam potentiates the coronary vasodilator actions of adenosine in anesthetized dogs. *Br. J. Pharmacol.*, 70:66–67.

72. Coburn, R. F. (1977): Oxygen tension sensors in vascular smooth muscle. *Adv. Exp. Med. Biol.*, 78:101–123.

73. Coffman, J. D., and Gregg, D. E. (1960): Reactive hyperemia characteristics of the myocardium. *Am. J. Physiol.*, 199:1143–1149.

74. Coffman, J. D., and Gregg, D. E. (1961): Oxygen metabolism and oxygen debt repayment after myocardial ischemia. *Am. J. Physiol.*, 201:881–887.

75. Corsini, G., Puri, P. S., Duran, P. V. M., and Bing, R. J. (1968): Effect of nicotine on capillary flow and terminal vascular capacity of the heart in normal dogs and circulation. *J. Pharmacol. Exp. Ther.*, 163:353–361.

76. Crystal, G. J., Downey, H. F., and Bashour, F. A. (1981): Small vessel and total coronary blood volume during intracoronary adenosine. *Am. J. Physiol.*, 241:H194–H201.

77. Curnish, R. R., Berne, R. M., and Rubio, R. (1972): Effect of aminophylline on myocardial reactive hyperemia. *Proc. Soc. Exp. Biol. Med.*, 141:593–598.

78. Daly, J. W., Kuroda, Y., Phillis, J. W., Shimizu, H., and Ui, M., editors (1983): *Physiology and Pharmacology of Adenosine Derivatives.* Raven Press, New York.

79. De la Haba, G., and Cantoni, G. L. (1959): The enzymatic synthesis of S-adenosyl-L-homocysteine from adenosine and homocysteine. *J. Biol. Chem.*, 234:603–608.

80. De Mey, J. G., Claeys, M., and Vanhoutte, P. M. (1982): Endothelial-dependent inhibitory effects of acetylcholine, adenosine

triphosphate, thrombin and arachidonic acid in the canine femoral artery. *J. Pharmacol. Exp. Ther.*, 222:166–173.

81. De Mey, J. G., Gray, S. D., and Mulvany, J. J. (1984): Effects of endothelial damage on reactivity of isolated 200 μm arteries. *Fed. Proc.*, 43:737 (abstract).

82. De Mey, J. G., and Vanhoutte, P. M. (1981): Role of the intima in cholinergic and purinergic relaxation of isolated canine femoral arteries. *J. Physiol. (Lond.)*, 316:347–355.

83. De Mey, J. G., and Vanhoutte, P. M. (1982): Heterogeneous behavior of the canine arterial and venous wall. *Circ. Res.*, 51:439–447.

84. Dennison, A. B., Jr., and Green, H. D. (1958): Effects of autonomic nerves and their mediators on coronary circulation and myocardial contraction. *Circ. Res.*, 6:633–643.

85. DePierre, J. W., and Karnovsky, M. L. (1974): Ecto-enzymes of the guinea pig polymorphonuclear leukocyte. I. Evidence for an ecto-adenosine monophosphatase, -adenosine triphosphatase and -*p*-nitrophenyl phosphatase. *J. Biol. Chem.*, 249:7111–7120.

86. DePierre, J. W., and Karnovsky, M. L. (1974): Ecto-enzymes of the guinea pig polymorphonuclear leukocyte. II. Properties and suitability as markers for the plasma membrane. *J. Biol. Chem.*, 249:7121–7129.

87. Dieudonne, J. M. (1967): Tissue-cavitary difference pressure of dog left ventricle. *Am. J. Physiol.*, 213:101–106.

88. Dole, W. P., Alexander, G. M., Campbell, A. B., Hixson, E. L., and Bishop, V. S. (1984): Interpretation and physical significance of diastolic coronary artery pressure-flow relationships in the canine coronary bed. *Circ. Res.*, 55:215–226.

89. Dole, W. P., and Bishop, V. S. (1982): Influence of autoregulation and capacitance on diastolic coronary artery pressure-flow relationships in the dog. *Circ. Res.*, 51:261–270.

90. Dole, W. P., Montville, W. J., and Bishop, V. S. (1981): Dependency of myocardial reactive hyperemia on coronary artery pressure in the dog. *Am. J. Physiol.*, 240:H709–H715.

91. Dole, W. P., Yamada, N., Bishop, V. S., and Olsson, R. A. (1985): Role of adenosine in coronary blood flow regulation after reduction in perfusion pressure. *Circ. Res.*, 56:517–524.

92. Domenech, R. J., and Ayuy, A. H. (1974): Total and regional coronary blood flow during acute right ventricular pressure overload. *Cardiovasc. Res.*, 8:611–620.

93. Domenech, R. J., and De la Prida, J. M. (1975): Mechanical effects of heart contraction on coronary flow. *Cardiovasc. Res.*, 9:509–514.

94. Donald, D. E., and Essex, H. E. (1954): The canine septal coronary artery. An anatomic and electrocardiographic study. *Am. J. Physiol.*, 176:143–154.

95. Douglas, J. E., and Greenfield, J. C., Jr. (1970): Epicardial coronary artery compliance in the dog. *Circ. Res.*, 27:921–929.

96. Dowell, R. T. (1977): Hemodynamic factors and vascular density as potential determinants of blood flow in hypertrophied rat heart. *Proc. Soc. Exp. Biol. Med.*, 154:423–426.

97. Downey, H. F., Bashour, F. A., Boatwright, R. B., Parker, P. E., and Kechejian, S. J. (1975): Uniformity of transmural perfusion in anesthetized dogs with maximally dilated coronary circulation. *Circ. Res.*, 37:111–117.

98. Downey, H. F., Crystal, G. J., Bockman, E. L., and Bashour, F. A. (1982): Nonischemic myocardial hypoxia: Coronary dilation without increased tissue adenosine. *Am. J. Physiol.*, 243:H512–H516.

99. Downey, J. M., and Kirk, E. S. (1974): Distribution of the coronary blood flow across the canine heart wall during systole. *Circ. Res.*, 34:251–257.

100. Downey, J. M., and Kirk, E. S. (1975): Inhibition of coronary blood flow by a vascular waterfall mechanism. *Circ. Res.*, 36:753–760.

101. Downey, J. M., Lee, J., and Chambers, D. (1982): Capacitative time constant of the coronary artery. (abstr) *Circulation* [*Suppl. II*], 66:42.

102. Drury, A. N., and Szent-Györgyi, A. (1929): The physiological activity of adenine compounds with especial reference to their action upon the mammalian heart. *J. Physiol. (Lond.)*, 68:213–237.

103. D'Silva, J. L., Mendel, D., and Winterton, M. C. (1964): Deter-

minants of intramyocardial pressure in the cat. *Am. J. Physiol.*, 207:1117–1122.

104. Eckstein, R. W., Moir, T. W., and Driscol, T. E. (1963): Phasic and mean blood flow in the canine septal artery and an estimate of systolic resistance in deep myocardial vessels. *Circ. Res.*, 12:203–211.

105. Edlund, A., Fredholm, B. B., Patrignani, P., Patrono, C., Wennmalm, A., and Wennmalm, M. (1983): Release of two vasodilators, adenosine and prostacyclin, from isolated rabbit hearts during controlled hypoxia. *J. Physiol. (Lond.)*, 340:487–501.

106. Edwards, M. J., and Maguire, M. H. (1970): Purification and properties of rat heart 5'-nucleotidase. *Mol. Pharmacol.*, 6:641–648.

107. Edwards, N. L., Recker, D., Manfredi, J., Rembecki, R., and Fox, I. H. (1982): Regulation of purine metabolism by plasma membrane and cytoplasmic 5'-nucleotidases. *Am. J. Physiol.*, 243:C270–C277.

108. Eikens, E., and Wilcken, D. E. L. (1973): Myocardial reactive hyperemia in conscious dogs: Effect of dipyridamole and aminophylline on responses to four- and eight-second coronary artery occlusions. *Aust. J. Exp. Biol. Med. Sci.*, 51:617–630.

109. Eikens, E., and Wilcken, D. E. L. (1973): The effect of dipyridamole and of aminophylline on responses to sixty-second coronary artery occlusions in dogs. *Aust. J. Exp. Biol. Med. Sci.*, 51:631–642.

110. Eikens, E., and Wilcken, D. E. L. (1974): Reactive hyperemia in the dog heart. Effect of temporarily restricting arterial inflow and of coronary occlusions lasting one and two cardiac cycles. *Circ. Res.*, 35:702–712.

111. Elliott, E. C., Jones, E. L., Bloor, C. M., Leon, A. S., and Gregg, D. E. (1968): Day-to-day changes in coronary hemodynamics secondary to constriction of circumflex branch of left coronary artery in conscious dogs. *Circ. Res.*, 22:237–250.

112. Ellis, A. K., and Klocke, F. J. (1980): Effects of preload on the transmural distribution of perfusion and pressure-flow relationships in the canine coronary vascular bed. *Circ. Res.*, 46:68–77.

113. Eng, C., Jentzer, J. H., and Kirk, E. S. (1982): The effects of the coronary capacitance on the interpretation of diastolic pressure-flow relationships. *Circ. Res.*, 50:334–341.

114. Everett, N. B., Simmons, B., and Lasher, E. P. (1956): Distribution of blood (Fe^{59}) and plasma (I^{131}) volumes of rats determined by liquid nitrogen freezing. *Circ. Res.*, 4:419–424.

115. Falsetti, H. L., Carroll, R. J., and Marcus, M. L. (1975): Temporal heterogeneity of myocardial blood flow in anesthetized dogs. *Circulation*, 52:848–853.

116. Fedor, J. M., McIntosh, D. M., Rembert, J. C., and Greenfield, J. C. (1978): Coronary and transmural myocardial blood flow responses in awake domestic pigs. *Am. J. Physiol.*, 235:H435–H444.

117. Feigl, E. O. (1983): Coronary physiology. *Physiol. Rev.*, 63:1–205.

118. Fixler, D. E., Archie, J. P., Jr., Ullyot, D. J., Buckberg, G. D., and Hoffman, J. I. E. (1973): Effects of acute right ventricular systolic hypertension on regional myocardial blood flow in anesthetized dogs. *Am. Heart J.*, 85:491–500.

119. Fixler, D. E., Archie, J. P., Jr., Ullyot, D. J., and Hoffman, J. I. E. (1973): Regional coronary flow with increased right ventricular output in anesthetized dogs. *Am. Heart J.*, 86:788–797.

120. Foley, D. H., Miller, W. L., Rubio, R., and Berne, R. M. (1979): Transmural distribution of myocardial adenosine content during coronary constriction. *Am. J. Physiol.*, 236:H833–H838.

121. Förstermann, U., Trogisch, G., and Busse, R. (1985): Species-dependent differences in the nature of endothelium derived vascular relaxing factor. *Eur. J. Pharmacol.*, 106:639–643.

122. Fox, I. H., and Kelley, W. N. (1978): The role of adenosine and 2'-deoxyadenosine in mammalian cells. *Annu. Rev. Biochem.*, 47:655–686.

123. Frank, J. S., and Langer, G. A. (1974): The myocardial interstitium: Its structure and its role in ionic exchange. *J. Cell Biol.*, 60:586–601.

124. Frick, G. P., and Lowenstein, J. M. (1976): Studies of 5'-

nucleotidase in the perfused rat heart. *J. Biol. Chem.*, 251:6372–6378.

125. Frick, G. P., and Lowenstein, J. M. (1978): Vectorial production of adenosine by 5'-nucleotidase in the perfuse rat heart. *J. Biol. Chem.*, 253:1240–1244.
126. Fung, Y. C. (1973): Stochastic flow in capillary blood vessels. *Microvasc. Res.*, 5:34–48.
127. Furchgott, R. F. (1983): Role of endothelium in responses of vascular smooth muscle. *Circ. Res.*, 53:557–573.
128. Furchgott, R. F. (1984): The role of endothelium in the responses of vascular smooth muscle to drugs. *Annu. Rev. Pharmacol. Toxicol.*, 24:175–197.
129. Furchgott, R. F., and Jothianandan, D. (1983): Relation of cyclic GMP levels to endothelium-dependent relaxation by acetylcholine in rabbit aorta. *Fed. Proc.*, 42:619 (abstract).
130. Furchgott, R. F., and Zawadzki, J. V. (1980): The obligatory role of endothelial cells in the relaxation of arterial smooth muscle by acetylcholine. *Nature*, 288:373–376.
131. Gamble, W. J., LaFarge, C. G., Fyler, D. C., Weisul, J., and Monroe, R. G. (1974): Regional coronary venous oxygen saturation and myocardial oxygen tension following abrupt changes in ventricular pressure in the isolated dog heart. *Circ. Res.*, 34:672–681.
132. Gellai, M., Norton, J. M., and Detar, R. (1973): Evidence for direct control of coronary vascular tone by oxygen. *Circ. Res.*, 32:279–289.
133. Gerdes, A. M., Callas, G., and Kasten, F. H. (1979): Differences in regional capillary distribution and myocyte sizes in normal and hypertrophic rat hearts. *Am. J. Anat.*, 156:523–531.
134. Gerdes, A. M., and Kasten, F. H. (1980): Morphometric study of endomyocardium and epimyocardium of the left ventricle in adult dogs. *Am. J. Anat.*, 159:389–394.
135. Gerke, E., Juchelka, W., Mittmann, U., and Schmier, J. (1975): Der intramyokardiale Druck des Hundes in veschiedenen Tiefen, bei Druckbelastung und bei Ischämie des Herzmuskels. *Basic Res. Cardiol.*, 70:537–546.
136. Gerlach, E., Deuticke, B., and Dreisbach, R. H. (1963): Der Nucleotid-abbau im Herzmuskel bei Sauerstoffmangel und seine mögliche Bedeutung für die Coronärdurchblutung. *Naturwissenschaften*, 50:228–229.
137. Gerritsen, M. E., and Printz, M. P. (1981): Sites of prostaglandin synthesis in the bovine heart and isolated bovine coronary microvessels. *Circ. Res.*, 49:1152–1163.
138. Gewirtz, H., Brautigan, D. L., Olsson, R. A., Brown, P., and Most, A. S. (1983): Role of adenosine in the maintenance of coronary vasodilation distal to a severe coronary artery stenosis: Observations in conscious domestic swine. *Circ. Res.*, 53:42–51.
139. Ghai, G., Lowery, T., and Olsson, R. A. (1984): Adenosine receptor coupled adenylate cyclase of cultured coronary endothelial and smooth muscle cells. IUPHAR Satellite Symposium, *Purines: Pharmacology and Physiological Roles*, London, U.K., 6–7 August 1984.
140. Giles, R. W., and Wilcken, D. E. L. (1977): Reactive hyperemia in the dog heart: Evidence for a myogenic contribution. *Cardiovasc. Res.*, 11:64–73.
141. Giles, R. W., and Wilcken, D. E. L. (1977): Reactive hyperemia in the dog heart: Inter-relations between adenosine, ATP and aminophylline and the effect of indomethacin. *Cardiovasc. Res.*, 11:113–121.
142. Giudicelli, J., Berdeaux, A., Tato, F., and Garnier, M. (1980): Left stellate stimulation: Regional myocardial flows and ischemic injury in dogs. *Am. J. Physiol.*, 239:H359–H364.
143. Gold, F. L., and Bache, R. J. (1982): Transmural right ventricular blood flow during acute pulmonary artery hypertension in the sedated dog. *Circ. Res.*, 51:196–204.
144. Gold, F. L., Horwitz, L. D., and Bache, R. J. (1984): Adrenergic coronary vasoconstriction in acute right ventricular hypertension. *Cardiovasc. Res.*, 18:447–454.
145. Goldman, S. J., Dickinson, E. S., and Slakey, L. L. (1983): Effect of adenosine on synthesis and release of cyclic AMP by cultured vascular cells from swine. *J. Cyclic Nucleotid. Prot. Phosphor. Res.*, 9:69–78.
146. Gordon, G. B., Price, H. M., and Blumberg, J. M. (1967): Electron microscopic localization of phosphatase activities within striated muscle fibers. *Lab. Invest.*, 16:422–435.
147. Granata, L., Huvos, A., Pasquè, A., and Gregg, D. E. (1969): Left coronary hemodynamics during hemorrhagic hypotension and shock. *Am. J. Physiol.*, 261:1583–1589.
148. Granata, L., Olsson, R. A., Huvos, A., and Gregg, D. E. (1965): Coronary inflow and oxygen usage following cardiac sympathetic nerve stimulation in unanesthetized dogs. *Circ. Res.*, 16:114–120.
149. Grände, P., Borgström, P., and Mellander, S. (1979): On the nature of basal vascular tone in cat skeletal muscle and its dependence on transmural pressure stimuli. *Acta Physiol. Scand.*, 107:365–376.
150. Grände, P., Lundvall, J., and Mellander, S. (1977): Evidence for a rate-sensitive regulatory mechanism in myogenic microvascular control. *Acta Physiol. Scand.*, 99:432–447.
151. Grände, P., and Mellander, S. (1978): Characteristics of static and dynamic regulatory mechanisms in myogenic microvascular control. *Acta Physiol. Scand.*, 102:231–245.
152. Granger, H. J., Goodman, A. H., and Cook, B. H. (1975): Metabolic models of microcirculatory regulation. *Fed. Proc.*, 34:2025–2030.
153. Gregg, D. E. (1937): Phasic blood flow and its determinants in the right coronary artery. *Am. J. Physiol.*, 119:580–588.
154. Gregg, D. E. (1950): *Coronary Circulation in Health and Disease.* Lea & Febiger, Philadelphia.
155. Gregg, D. E., and Eckstein, R. W. (1941): Measurements of intramyocardial pressure. *Am. J. Physiol.*, 132:781–790.
156. Gregg, D. E., and Fisher, L. C. (1963): Blood supply to the heart. In: *Handbook of Physiology. Circulation*, Sect. 2, Vol. 2, edited by W. F. Hamilton, pp. 1517–1584. American Physiological Society, Washington, D.C.
157. Gregg, D. E., Khouri, E. M., Donald, D. E., Lowensohn, H. S., and Pasyk, S. (1972): Coronary circulation in the conscious dog with cardiac neural ablation. *Circ. Res.*, 31:129–144.
158. Gregg, D. E., Khouri, E. M., and Rayford, C. R. (1965): Systemic and coronary energetics in the resting unanesthetized dog. *Circ. Res.*, 16:102–113.
159. Griffith, T. M., Edwards, D. H., Lewis, M. J., Newby, A. C., and Henderson, A. H. (1984): The nature of endothelium-derived vascular relaxant factor. *Nature*, 308:645–647.
160. Grunewald, W. A., and Lübbers, D. W. (1975): Die Bestimmung der intracapillären HbO2-Sättigung mit einer kryo-mikrofotometrischen Methode angewandt am Myokard des Kaninchens. *Pfluegers Arch.*, 353:255–273.
161. Guyton, R. A., McClenathan, J. H., Newman, G. E., and Michaelis, J. E. (1977): Significance of subendocardial S-T segment elevation caused by coronary stenosis in the dog. *Am. J. Cardiol.*, 40:373–380.
162. Hanley, F. L., Grattan, M. T., Stevens, M. B., and Hoffman, J. I. E. (1984): The role of adenosine in coronary autoregulation. *Fed. Proc.*, 43:308 (abstract).
163. Hanley, F., Messina, L. M., Baer, R. W., Uhlig, P. N., and Hoffman, J. I. E. (1983): Direct measurement of left ventricular interstitial adenosine. *Am. J. Physiol.*, 245:H327–H335.
164. Harden, W. R., Barlow, C. H., Simson, M. B., and Harken, A. H. (1979): Temporal relation between onset of cell anoxia and ischemic contractile failure. *Am. J. Cardiol.*, 44:741–746.
165. Harder, D. R. (1984): Pressure-dependent membrane depolarization in cat middle cerebral artery. *Circ. Res.*, 55:197–202.
166. Harder, D. R., Belardinelli, L., Sperelakis, N., Rubio, R., and Berne, R. M. (1979): Differential effects of adenosine and nitroglycerin on the action potentials of large and small coronary arteries. *Circ. Res.*, 44:176–182.
167. Hershfield, M. S., and Kredich, N. M. (1978): S-adenosylhomocysteine hydrolase is an adenosine-binding protein: A target for adenosine toxicty. *Science*, 202:757–760.
168. Hess, D. S., and Bache, R. J. (1976): Transmural distribution of myocardial blood flow during systole in the awake dog. *Circ. Res.*, 38:5–15.
169. Hess, D. S., and Bache, R. J. (1979): Transmural right ventricular myocardial blood flow during systole in the awake dog. *Circ. Res.*, 45:88–94.

170. Heymann, M. A., Payne, B. D., Hoffman, J. I. E., and Rudolph, A. M. (1977): Blood flow measurements with radionuclide-labeled particles. *Prog. Cardiovasc. Dis.*, 20:55–79.

171. Hilton, S. M. (1959): A peripheral arterial conducting mechanism underlying dilation of the femoral artery and concerned in functional vasodilation in skeletal muscle. *J. Physiol. (Lond.)*, 149:93–111.

172. Hintze, T. H., and Kaley, G. (1977): Prostaglandins and the control of blood flow in the canine myocardium. *Circ. Res.*, 40: 313–320.

173. Hirche, H. J., and Lochner, W. (1962): Messung der Durchblutung und der Blutfullung des coronaren Gefassbettes mit der teststoffinjektions Methode am narkotisierten Hund bei geschlossenem Thorax. *Pfluegers Arch.*, 274:624–632.

174. Hoffman, J. I. E. (1984): Maximal coronary flow and the concept of coronary vascular reserve. *Circulation*, 70:153–159.

175. Holtz, J. Förstermann, U., Pohl, U., Geisler, M., Bassenger, E. (1984): Flow-dependent, endothelium mediated dilation of epicardial coronary arteries in conscious dogs: Effects of cyclooxygenase inhibition. *J. Cardiovasc. Pharmacol.*, 6:1161–1169.

176. Holtz, J., Grunewald, W. A., Manz, R., Restorff, W., and Bassenge, E. (1977): Intracapillary hemoglobin oxygen saturation and oxygen consumption in different layers of the left ventricular myocardiaum. *Pfluegers Arch.*, 370:253–258.

177. Holtz, J., Mayer, E., and Bassenge, E. (1977): Demonstration of alpha-adrenergic coronary control in different layers of canine myocardium by regional myocardial sympathectomy. *Pfluegers Arch.*, 372:187–194.

178. Howard, R. O., Richardson, D. W., Smith, M. H., and Patterson, J. L. (1965): Oxygen consumption of arterioles and venules as studied in the Cartesian diver. *Circ. Res.*, 16:187–196.

179. Howe, B. B., and Winbury, M. M. (1973): Effect of pentrintol, nitroglycerin and propranolol on small vessel blood content of the canine myocardium. *J. Pharmacol. Exp. Ther.*, 187:465–474.

180. Huhmann, W., and Niesel, W. (1967): Untersuchungen über die Bedingungen für die Sauerstoffversorgung des Myokards an perfundierten Rattenherzen. *Pfluegers Arch.*, 294:250–255.

181. Itoh, R. (1982): Studies on some molecular properties of cytosol 5′-nucleotidase from rat liver. *Biochim. Biophys. Acta*, 716:110–113.

182. Jochem, G., and Nawrath, H. (1983): Adenosine activates a potassium conductance in guinea-pig atrial heart muscle. *Experientia*, 39:1347–1349.

183. Johannsen, U. J., Mark, A. L., and Marcus, M. L. (1982): Responsiveness to cardiac sympathetic nerve stimulation during maximal coronary dilation produced by adenosine. *Circ. Res.*, 50:510–517.

184. Johansson, B., and Mellander, S. (1975): Static and dynamic components in the vascular myogenic response to passive changes in length as revealed by electrical and mechanical recordings from the rat portal vein. *Circ. Res.*, 36:76–83.

185. Johnson, J. R., and Di Palma, J. R. (1939): Intramyocardial pressure and its relation to aortic blood pressure. *Am. J. Physiol.*, 125:234–243.

186. Johnson, J. R., and Wiggers, C. E. (1937): The alleged validity of coronary sinus outflow as a criterion of coronary reactions. *Am. J. Physiol.*, 118:38–50.

187. Johnson, P. C. (1977): The myogenic response and the microcirculation. *Microvasc. Res.*, 13:1–18.

188. Jones, A. W., Bylund, D. B., and Forte, L. R. (1984): cAMP-dependent reduction in membrane fluxes during relaxation of arterial smooth muscle. *Am. J. Physiol.*, 246:H306–311.

189. Jones, C. E., Hurst, T. W., and Randall, J. R. (1982): Effect of aminophylline on coronary functional hyperemia and myocardial adenosine. *Am. J. Physiol.*, 243:H480–H487.

190. Juhran, W., Voss, E. M., Dietman, K., and Schaumann, W. (1971): Pharmacological effects of coronary reactive hyperemia in conscious dogs. *Naunyn Schmiedebergs Arch. Pharmacol.*, 269:32–47.

191. Kadatz, R. (1969): Sauerstoffdruck und Durchblutung im gesunden und koronarinsuffizienten Myokard des Hundes und ihre Beeinflussung durch koronarerweiternd Pharmaka. *Arch. Kreislaufforsch.*, 58:263–293.

192. Kanaide, H., Yoshimura, R., Makino, N., and Nakamura, M. (1982): Regional myocardial function and metabolism during acute coronary artery occlusion. *Am. J. Physiol.*, 242:980H–989H.

193. Katz, L. N., and Lindner, E. (1939): Quantitative relationship between reactive hyperemia and the myocardial ischemia which it follows. *Am. J. Physiol.*, 126:283–288.

194. Kelley, K. O., and Gould, K. L. (1981): Coronary reactive hyperemia after brief occlusion and after deoxygenated perfusion. *Cardiovasc. Res.*, 15:615–622.

195. Kelly, D. T., and Pitt, B. (1973): Regional changes in intramyocardial pressure following myocardial ischemia. *Adv. Exp. Med. Biol.*, 39:115–119.

196. Kennedy, C., and Burnstock, G. (1984): Evidence for an inhibitory prejunctional P_1-purinoceptor in the rat portal vein with characteristics of the A_2 rather than of the A_1 subtype. *Eur. J. Pharmacol.*, 100:363–368.

197. Khouri, E. M., Gregg, D. E., and Rayford, C. R. (1965): Effect of exercise on cardiac output, left coronary flow and myocardial metabolism in the unanesthetized dog. *Circ. Res.*, 17:427–437.

198. Kirk, E. S., and Honig, C. (1964): An experimental and theoretical analysis of myocardial tissue pressure. *Am. J. Physiol.*, 207:361–367.

199. Kirk, E. S., and Honig, C. R. (1964): Nonuniform distribution of blood flow and gradients of oxygen tension within the heart. *Am. J. Physiol.*, 207:661–668.

200. Kirkeeide, R., Puschmann, S., and Schaper, W. (1981): Diastolic coronary pressure-flow relationships investigated by induced long-wave pressure oscillations. *Basic Res. Cardiol.*, 76:564–569.

201. Kleber, A. (1984): Extracellular potassium accumulation in acute myocardial ischemia. *J. Mol. Cell. Cardiol.*, 16:389–394.

202. Kline, R. P., and Morad, M. (1978): Potassium efflux in heart muscle during activity: Extracellular accumulation and its implications. *J. Physiol. (Lond.)*, 280:537–558.

203. Klitzman, B., and Duling, B. R. (1979): Microvascular hematocrit and red cell flow in resting and contracting striated muscle. *Am. J. Physiol.*, 237:H481–H490.

204. Klocke, F. J., Kaiser, G. A., Ross, J., Jr., and Braunwald, E. (1965): Mechanism of increase of myocardial oxygen uptake produced by catecholamines. *Am. J. Physiol.*, 209:913–918.

205. Klocke, F. J., Mates, R. E., Canty, J. M., and Ellis, A. K. (1985): Coronary pressure-flow relationships: controversial issues and probable implications. *Circ. Res.*, 56:310–323.

206. Klocke, F. J., Weinstein, I. R., Klocke, J. F., Ellis, A. K., Kraus, D. R., Mates, R. E., Canty, J. M., Anbar, R. D., Romanowski, R. R., Wallmeyer, K. W., and Echt, M. P. (1981): Zero-flow pressures and pressure-flow relationships during single long diastoles in the canine coronary bed before and during maximum vasodilation. *J. Clin. Invest.*, 68:970–980.

207. Kohn, R. M. (1963): Myocardial oxygen uptake during ventricular fibrillation and electromechanical dissociation. *Am. J. Cardiol.*, 11:483–486.

208. Kolassa, N., Pfleger, K., and Rummel, W. (1970): Specificity of adenosine uptake into the heart and inhibition by dipyridamole. *Eur. J. Pharmacol.*, 9:265–268.

209. Koyama, T., Sasajima, T., Yagi, T., Kakiuchi, Y., and Arai, T. (1978): Local pulsatile intramyocardial pressure (IMP) as a vector force: Simultaneous measurements of IMP and tissue oxygen availability. *Recent Adv. Stud. Cardiac Struct. Metab.*, 12:237–243.

210. Kreuzer, H., and Schoeppe, W. (1963): Das Verhalten des Druckes in der Herzwand. *Pfluegers Arch.*, 278:181–198.

211. Kreuzer, H., and Schoeppe, W. (1963): Zur Entstehung der Differenz zwischen systolischem Myokard- und Ventrikeldruck. *Pfluegers Arch.*, 278:199–208.

212. Kukovetz, W. R., Pöch, G., Holzmann, S., Wurm, A., and Rinner, I. (1978): Role of cyclic nucleotides in adenosine-mediated regulation of coronary flow. *Adv. Cyclic Nucleotide Res.*, 9:397–409.

213. Kuriyama, H., Ito, Y., Suzuki, H., Kitamura, K., and Itoh, T. (1982): Factors modifying contraction-relaxation cycle in vascular smooth muscles. *Am. J. Physiol.*, 243:H641–H662.

214. Kusachi, S., Bugni, W. J., and Olsson, R. A. (1984): Forskolin

potentiates the coronary vasoactivity of adenosine in the open chest dog. *Circ. Res.*, 55:116–119.

215. Kusachi, S., Nishiyama, O., Yasuhara, K., Saito, D., Haraoka, S., and Nagashima, H. (1983): Right and left ventricular oxygen metabolism in open-chest dogs. *Am. J. Physiol.*, 243:H761–H766.

216. Kusachi, S., Thompson, R., Bugni, W., and Olsson, R. A. (1983): Ligand selectivity of dog coronary adenosine receptor resembles that of adenylate cyclase stimulatory (R_a) receptors. *J. Pharmacol. Exp. Ther.*, 227:316–321.

217. L'Abbate, A., Marzilli, M., Ballestra, A. M., Camici, P., Trivella, M. G., Pelosi, G., and Klassen, G. A. (1980): Opposite transmural gradients of coronary resistance and extravascular pressure in the working dog's heart. *Circ. Res.*, 14:21–29.

218. Lammerant, J., and Becsei, I. (1975): Inhibition of pacing-induced coronary dilation by aminophylline. *Cardiovasc. Res.*, 9:532–537.

219. Lee, J., Chambers, D. E., Akisuki, S., and Downey, J. M. (1984): The role of vascular capacitance in the coronary arteries. *Circ. Res.*, 55:751–762.

220. Le Roy, E. C., Ager, A., and Gordon, J. L. (1984): Effects of neutrophis elastase and other proteases on porcine aortic endothelial prostaglandin I_2 production, adenine nucleotide release and responses to vasoactive agents. *J. Clin. Invest.*, 74:1003–1010.

221. Liang, C. S., and Lowenstein, J. M. (1978): Metabolic control of the circulation: Effects of acetate and pyruvate. *J. Clin. Invest.*, 62:1029–1038.

222. Lindner, F., and Rigler, R. (1931): Über die Beeinflussung der Weite der Herzkranzgefasse durch Produkte des Zellkernstoffwechsels. *Pfluegers Arch.*, 226:697–708.

223. Lösse, B., Schuchhardt, S., and Niederle, N. (1975): The oxygen pressure histogram in the left ventricular myocardium of the dog. *Pfluegers Arch.*, 356:121–132.

224. Lowensohn, H. S., Khouri, E. M., Gregg, D. E., Pyle, R. L., and Patterson, R. E. (1976): Phasic right coronary artery blood flow in conscious dogs with normal and elevated right ventricular pressures. *Circ. Res.*, 39:760–766.

225. Macho, P., Hintze, T. H., and Vatner, S. F. (1981): Regulation of large coronary arteries by increases in myocardial metabolic demands in conscious dogs. *Circ. Res.*, 49:594–599.

226. McKeever, W. P., Gregg, D. E., and Canney, P. C. (1958): Oxygen uptake of nonworking left ventricle. *Circ. Res.*, 6:612–623.

227. McKenzie, J. E., McCoy, F. P., and Bockman, E. L. (1980): Myocardial adenosine and coronary resistance during increased cardiac performance. *Am. J. Physiol.*, 239:H509–H515.

228. McKenzie, J. E., Steffen, R. P., and Haddy, F. J. (1982): Relationships between adenosine and coronary resistance in conscious exercising dogs. *Am. J. Physiol.*, 242:H24–H29.

229. McKenzie, J. E., Swindall, B. T., Johnston, J., and Haddy, F. J. (1982): Adenosine concentrations in cardiac lymph during administration of isoproterenol. *Physiologist.*, 25:229 (abstract).

230. Madrid-Marina, V., and Fox, I. H. (1984): The kinetic regulation of human placental cytoplasmic 5'-nucleotidase. *Fed. Proc.*, 43:1473 (abstract).

231. Manfredi, J. P., and Sparks, H. V. (1982): Adenosine's role in coronary vasodilation induced by atrial pacing and norepinephrine. *Am. J. Physiol.*, 243:H536–H545.

232. Manohar, M., Bisgard, B. E., Bullard, V., Will, J. A., Anderson, D., and Rankin, J. H. G. (1978): Myocardial perfusion and function during acute right ventricular systolic hypertension. *Am. J. Physiol.*, 235:H628–H636.

233. Manohar, M., Bisgard, B. E., Bullard, V., Will, J. A., Anderson, D., and Rankin, J. H. G. (1979): Regional myocardial blood flow and myocardial function during acute right ventricular pressure overload in calves. *Circ. Res.*, 44:531–539.

234. Manohar, M., Thurmon, J. C., Tranquilli, W. J., Devous, M. D., Sr., Theodorakis, M. C., Shawley, R. V., Feller, D. L., and Benson, J. G. (1981): Regional myocardial blood flow and coronary vascular reserve in unanesthetized young calves with severe concentric right ventricular hypertrophy. *Circ. Res.*, 48:785–796.

235. Marcus, M. L. (1983): *The Coronary Circulation in Health and Disease.* McGraw-Hill, New York.

236. Marcus, M. L., Mueller, T. M., and Eastham, C. L. (1983): Effects of short and long-term left ventricular hypertrophy on coronary circulation. *Am. J. Physiol.*, 241:H358–H362.

237. Marcus, M. L., Wright, C., Doty, D., Eastham, C., Laughlin, D., Krumm, P., Fastenow, C., and Brody, M. (1981): Measurements of coronary velocity and reactive hyperemia in the coronary circulation of humans. *Circ. Res.*, 49:877–891.

238. Mathes, P., and Rival, J. (1971): Effect of nitroglycerin on total and regional coronary blood flow in the normal and ischemic canine myocardium. *Cardiovasc. Res.*, 5:54–61.

239. Mays, A. E., McHale, P. A., and Greenfield, J. C. (1981): Transmural myocardial blood flow in a canine model of coronary artery bridging. *Circ. Res.*, 49:726–732.

240. Merrill, G. F., Haddy, F. J., and Dabney, J. M. (1978): Adenosine, theophylline and perfusate pH in the isolated, perfused guinea pig heart. *Circ. Res.*, 42:225–229.

241. Merrill, G. F., and Young, M. A. (1981): The influence of concurrently administered theophylline, ouabain and hypocapnia on coronary flow pertubations in the perfused guinea pig heart. *Blood Vessels*, 18:1–9.

242. Miller, W. L., Bellardinelli, L., Bacchus, A., Foley, D. H., Rubio, R., and Berne, R. M. (1979): Canine myocardial adenosine and lactate production, oxygen consumption and coronary blood flow during stellate ganglia stimulation. *Circ. Res.*, 45:708–718.

243. Mistry, G., and Drummond, G. I. (1983): Heart microvessels: Presence of adenylate cyclase stimulated by catecholamines, prostaglandins and adenosine. *Microvasc. Res.*, 26:157–169.

244. Moir, T. W., Driscol, T. E., and Eckstein, R. W. (1964): Thebesian drainage in the left heart of the dog. *Circ. Res.*, 14:245–249.

245. Molnar, J. I., Scott, J. B., Frolich, E. D., and Haddy, F. J. (1962): Local effects of various anions and H^+ on dog limb and coronary vascular sesistances. *Am. J. Physiol.*, 203:125–132.

246. Monroe, R. G., Gamble, W. J., LaFarge, C. G., Benoualid, H., and Weisul, J. (1975): Transmural coronary venous O_2 saturations in normal and isolated hearts. *Am. J. Physiol.*, 228:318–324.

247. Morgenstern, C., Holjes, U., Arnold, G., and Lochner, W. (1973): The influence of coronary pressure and coronary flow on intracoronary blood volume and geometry of the left ventricle. *Pfluegers Arch.*, 340:101–111.

248. Moss, A. J. (1968): Intramyocardial oxygen tension. *Cardiovasc. Res.*, 3:314–318.

249. Mueller, E., and Van Breemen, C. (1979): Role of intracellular Ca^{2+} sequestration in β-adrenergic relaxation of a smooth muscle. *Nature*, 281:682–683.

250. Mueller, T. A., Marcus, M. L., Kerber, R. D., Young, J. A., Barnes, R. W., and Abboud, F. M. (1978): Effect of renal hypertension and left ventricular hypertrophy on the coronary circulation in dogs. *Circ. Res.*, 42:543–549.

251. Murray, P. A., Baig, H., Fishbein, M. C., and Vatner, S. F. (1979): Effects of experimental right ventricular hypertrophy on myocardial blood flow in conscious dogs. *J. Clin. Invest.*, 64:421–427.

252. Murray, P. A., Belloni, F. L., and Sparks, H. V. (1979): The role of potassium in the metabolism control of coronary vascular resistance of the dog. *Circ. Res.*, 44:767–780.

253. Murray, P. A., and Sparks, H. V. (1978): The mechanism of K^+-induced vasodilation of the coronary vascular bed of the dog. *Circ. Res.*, 42:35–42.

254. Murray, P. A., and Vatner, S. F. (1980): Fractional contributions of the right and left coronary arteries to perfusion of normal and hypertrophied right ventricles of conscious dogs. *Circ. Res.*, 47:190–200.

255. Murray, P. A., and Vatner, S. F. (1981): Carotid sinus baroreceptor control of right coronary circulation in normal, hypertrophied and failing right ventricles of conscious dogs. *Circ. Res.*, 49:1339–1349.

256. Murray, P. A., and Vatner, S. F. (1981): Reduction of maximal coronary vasodilator capacity in conscious dogs with severe right ventricular hypertrophy. *Circ. Res.*, 48:27–33.

257. Mustafa, S. J., Rubio, R., and Berne, R. M. (1975): Uptake of

adenosine by dispersed chick embryonic cardiac cells. *Am. J. Physiol.*. 228:62–67.

258. Myers, W. W., and Honig, C. R. (1964): Number and distribution of capillaries as determinants of myocardial oxygen tension. *Am. J. Physiol.*, 207:653–660.

259. Namm, D. H. (1973): Myocardial nucleotide synthesis from purine bases and nucleosides. Comparison of the rates of formation of purine nucleotides from various precursors and identification of the enzymatic routes for nucleotide formation in the isolated rat heart. *Circ. Res.*, 33:686–695.

260. Needleman, P., Key, S. L., Isakson, P. C., and Kulkarni, P. S. (1975): Relationship between oxygen tension, coronary vasodilation and prostaglandin biosynthesis in the isolated rabbit heart. *Prostaglandins*, 9:123–134.

261. Nees, S., Gerbes, A. L., Gerlach, E., and Staubesand, J. (1981): Isolation, identification and continuous culture of coronary endothelial cells from guinea pig hearts. *Eur. J. Cell. Biol.*, 24:287–297.

262. Nees, S., Gerbes, A. L., Willershausen-Zönnchen, B., and Gerlach, E. (1980): Purine metabolism in cultured coronary endothelial cells. *Adv. Exp. Med. Biol.*, 122B:25–30.

263. Nees, S., and Gerlach, E. (1983): Adenine nucleotide and adenosine metabolism in cultured coronary endothelial cells: Formation and release of adenine compounds and possible functional implications. In: *Regulatory Function of Adenosine*, edited by R. M. Berne, T. W. Rall, and R. Rubio, pp. 347–360. Martinus Nijhoff, Boston.

264. Nellis, S. H., Liedtke, A. J., and Whitesell, L. (1981): Small coronary vessel pressure and diameter in an intact beating rabbit heart using fixed-position and free-motion techniques. *Circ. Res.*, 49:342–353.

265. Nuutinen, E. M., Nelson, D., Wilson, D. F., and Erecinska, M. (1983): Regulation of coronary blood flow: Effects of 2,4-dinitrophenol and theophylline. *Am. J. Physiol.*, 244:H396–H405.

266. O'Keefe, D. D., Hoffman, J. I., Cheitlin, R., O'Neill, M. J., Allard, J. R., and Shapkin, E. (1978): Coronary blood flow in experimental canine left ventricular hypertrophy. *Circ. Res.*, 43:43–51.

267. Olsson, R. A. (1964): Kinetics of myocardial reactive hyperemia blood flow in the unanesthetized dog. *Circ. Res. [Suppl. 1]*, 14:81–86.

268. Olsson, R. A. (1970): Changes in content of purine nucleoside in canine myocardium during coronary occlusion. *Circ. Res.*, 26:301–306.

269. Olsson, R. A. (1981): Local factors regulating cardiac and skeletal muscle blood flow. *Annu. Rev. Physiol.*, 43:385–395.

270. Olsson, R. A., Davis, C. J., Khouri, E. M., and Patterson, R. E. (1976): Evidence for an adenosine receptor on the surface of dog coronary myocytes. *Circ. Res.*, 39:93–98.

271. Olsson, R. A., Gentry, M. K., and Snow, J. A. (1973): Steric requirements for binding of adenosine to a membrane carrier in canine heart. *Biochim. Biophys. Acta*, 311:242–250.

272. Olsson, R. A., and Gregg, D. E. (1965): Myocardial reactive hyperemia in the unanesthetized dog. *Am. J. Physiol.*, 208:224–230.

273. Olsson, R. A., and Gregg, D. E. (1965): Metabolic responses during myocardial reactive hyperemia in the unanesthetized dog. *Am. J. Physiol.*, 208:231–236.

274. Olsson, R. A., Khouri, E. M., Bedynek, J. L., and McLean, J. (1979): Coronary vasoactivity of adenosine in the conscious dog. *Circ. Res.*, 45:468–478.

275. Olsson, R. A., and Kusachi, S. (1982): Intracoronary adenosine deaminase antagonizes β-adrenergic stimulation of cardiac oxygen usage. *Circulation [Suppl. II]*, 66:154 (abstract).

276. Olsson, R. A., Saito, D., and Steinhart, C. R. (1982): Compartmentalization of the adenosine pool of dog and rat hearts. *Circ. Res.*, 50:617–626.

277. Olsson, R. A., Snow, J. A., and Gentry, M. K. (1978): Adenosine metabolism in canine myocardial reactive hyperemia. *Circ. Res.*, 42:358–362.

278. Olsson, R. A., Snow, J. A., Gentry, M. K., and Frick, G. P. (1972): Adenosine uptake by canine heart. *Circ. Res.*, 31:767–778.

279. Olsson, R. A., and Steinhart, C. R. (1982): Metabolic regulation of coronary blood flow. *Physiologist*, 25:51–55.

280. Overton, W. R. (1982): Creationism in schools: The decision in McLean versus the Arkansas Board of Education. *Science*, 215:934–943.

281. Pace, J. B. (1977): Autonomic control of the coronary circulation. In: *Neural Regulation of the Heart*, edited by W. C. Randall, pp. 315–344. Oxford University Press, New York.

282. Patterson, A. R. P., Jakobs, E. A., Harley, E. R., Fu, N. W., Robins, M. J., and Cass, C. E. (1983): Inhibition of nucleoside transport. In: *Regulatory Function of Adenosine*, edited by R. M. Berne, T. W. Rall, and R. Rubio, pp. 203–230. Martinus Nijhoff, Boston.

283. Pauly, T. J., and Bittar, N. (1971): Myocardial reactive hyperemia responses in the dog after beta receptor block with propranolol. *Cardiovasc. Res.*, 5:440–443.

284. Pauly, T. J., Zarnstorff, W. C., and Bittar, N. (1973): Myocardial metabolic activity as a determinant of reactive hyperemia responses in the dog heart. *Cardiovasc. Res.*, 7:90–94.

285. Pearson, J. D., Carleton, J. S., and Gordon, J. L. (1980): Metabolism of adenine nucleotides by ectoenzymes of vascular endothelial and smooth-muscle cells in culture. *Biochem. J.*, 190:421–429.

286. Pearson, J. D., and Gordon, J. L. (1979): Vascular endothelial and smooth muscle cells in culture selectively release adenine nucleotides. *Nature*, 281:384–386.

287. Pearson, J. D., Slakey, L. L., and Gordon, J. L. (1983): Stimulation of prostaglandin production through purinoceptors on cultured porcine endothelial cells. *Biochem. J.*, 214:273–276.

288. Pearson, J. D., Carleton, J. S., Hutchings, A., and Gordon, J. L. (1978): Uptake and metabolism of adenosine by pig aortic endothelial and smooth-muscle cells in culture. *Biochem. J.*, 170:265–271.

289. Permutt, S., Bromberger-Barnea, B., and Bare, H. N. (1962): Alveolar pressure, pulmonary venous pressure and the vascular waterfall. *Med. Thorac.*, 19:239–260.

290. Permutt, S., and Riley, R. L. (1963): Hemodynamics of collapsible vessels with tone: The vascular waterfall. *J. Appl. Physiol.*, 18:924–932.

291. Peterson, D. F., and Bishop, V. S. (1980): Influences of selective sympathetic denervation on coronary reactive hyperemia in conscious dogs. *J. Auton. Nerv. Syst.*, 2:47–59.

292. Peyster, R. G., and Stuckey, J. H. (1974): Diastolic intramyocardial tissue pressure before, during and after temporary occlusion of the left anterior descending coronary artery. *J. Thorac. Cardiovasc. Surg.*, 67:343–348.

293. Pfleger, K., Volkmer, I., and Kolassa, N. (1969): Hemmung der Aufnahme von Adenosin und Verstärkung seiner Wirkung am isolierten Warmblüterherzen durch coronarwirksame Substanzen. *Arzneim. Forsch.*, 19:1972–1974.

294. Piemme, T. E., and Dexter, L. (1963): Pressure transients occurring in diastole in the central aorta. *Circ. Res.*, 13:585–594.

295. Pifarré, R. (1968): Intramyocardial pressure during systole and diastole. *Ann. Surg.*, 168:871–875.

296. Pina, J. A. E., Correia, M., and Goyri O'Neill, J. (1975): Morphological study on the thebesian veins of the right cavities of the heart in the dog. *Acta Anat.*, 92:310–320.

297. Pitt, B., and Gregg, D. E. (1968): Coronary hemodynamic effects of increasing ventricular rate in the unanesthetized dog. *Circ. Res.*, 22:753–761.

298. Pyle, R. L., Lowensohn, H. S., Khouri, E. M., Gregg, D. E., and Patterson, D. F. (1973): Left circumflex coronary hemodynamics in conscious dogs with congenital subaortic stenosis. *Circ. Res.*, 33:34–38.

299. Rakušan, K. (1971): Vascular capacity and hematocrit in experimental cardiomegaly due to aortic constriction in rats. *Can. J. Physiol. Pharmacol.*, 49:819–823.

300. Rakušan, K. (1971): Quantitative morphology of capillaries of the heart. *Methods Achiev. Exp. Pathol.*, 5:272–286.

301. Randall, J. R., Overn, S. P., and Jones, C. E. (1984): The adenosine antagonist aminophylline attenuates pacing-induced coronary functional hyperemia. *Fed. Proc.*, 43:309 (abstract).

302. Rapoport, R. M., Draznin, M. B., and Murad, F. (1982): Sodium

nitroprusside-induced protein phosphorylation in intact rat aorta is mimicked by 8-bromo cyclic GMP. *Proc. Natl. Acad. Sci. U.S.A.,* 79:6470–6474.

303. Rapoport, R. M., Draznin, M. B., and Murad, F. (1983): Endothelium-dependent vascular relaxation may be mediated through cyclic GMP-dependent protein phosphorylation. *Clin. Res.,* 31: 526a (abstract).

304. Rapoport, R. M., and Murad, F. (1983): Agonist-induced endothelium-dependent relaxation in rat thoracic aorta may be mediated through cGMP. *Circ. Res.,* 52:352–357.

305. Rapoport, R. M., and Murad, F. (1983): Endothelium-dependent and nitrovasodilator-induced relaxation of vascular smooth muscle. *J. Cyclic Nucleotid. Prot. Phosphor. Res.,* 9:281–296.

306. Rembert, J. C., Boyd, L. M., Watkinson, W. P., and Greenfield, J. C. (1980): Effect of adenosine on transmural myocardial blood flow distribution in the awake dog. *Am. J. Physiol.,* 239:H7–H13.

307. Rembert, J. C., Kleinman, L. H., Fedor, J. M., Wechsler, A. S., and Greenfield, J. C. (1978): Myocardial blood flow distribution in concentric left ventricular hypertrophy. *J. Clin. Invest.,* 62: 379–386.

308. Restorff, W. von, Holtz, J., and Bassenge, E. (1977): Exercise induced augmentation of myocardial oxygen extraction in spite of normal coronary dilatory capacity in dogs. *Pfluegers Arch.,* 372:181–185.

309. Rivas, F., Rembert, J. C., Bache, R. J., Cobb, F. R., and Greenfield, J. C., Jr. (1980): Effect of hyperoxia on regional blood flow after coronary occlusion in awake dogs. *Am. J. Physiol.,* 238:H244–H248.

310. Rostgaard, J., and Behnke, O. (1965): Fine structural localization of adenine nucleoside phosphatase activity in the sarcoplasmic reticulum and the T system of rat myocardium. *J. Ultrastruct. Res.,* 12:579–591.

311. Rouleau, J., Boerboom, L. E., Surjadhana, A., and Hoffman, J. I. E. (1979): The role of autoregulation and tissue diastolic pressures in the transmural distribution of left ventricular blood flow in anesthetized dogs. *Circ. Res.,* 45:804–815.

312. Rubio, R., and Berne, R. M. (1969): Release of adenosine by the normal myocardium in dogs and its relationship to the regulation of coronary resistance. *Circ. Res.,* 25:407–415.

313. Rubio, R., Berne, R. M., and Dobson, J. G. (1973): Sites of adenosine production in cardiac and skeletal muscle. *Am. J. Physiol.,* 225:938–953.

314. Rubio, R., Berne, R. M., and Katori, M. (1969): Release of adenosine in reactive hyperemia of the dog heart. *Am. J. Physiol.,* 216:56–62.

315. Ruiter, J. H., Spaan, J. A. E., and Laird, J. D. (1978): Transient oxygen uptake during myocardial reactive hyperemia in the dog. *Am. J. Physiol.,* 235:H87–H94.

316. Sabiston, D. C., Jr., and Gregg, D. E. (1957): Effect of cardiac contraction on coronary blood flow. *Circulation,* 15:14–20.

317. Saebø, J., and Ueland, P. M. (1979): A study on the sequestration of adenosine and its conversion to adenine by the cyclic AMP-adenosine binding protein/S-adenosylhomocysteinase from mouse liver. *Biochim. Biophys. Acta,* 587:333–343.

318. Saito, D., Nixon, D. G., Vomacka, R. B., and Olsson, R. A. (1980): Relationship of cardiac oxygen usage, adenosine content and coronary resistance in dogs. *Circ. Res.,* 47:875–882.

319. Saito, D., Steinhart, C. R., Nixon, D. G., and Olsson, R. A. (1981): Intracoronary adenosine deaminase reduces canine myocardial reactive hyperemia. *Circ. Res.,* 49:1262–1267.

320. Salisbury, P. F., Cross, C. E., and Rieben, P. A. (1962): Intramyocardial pressure and strength of left ventricular contraction. *Circ. Res.,* 10:608–623.

321. Sasaki, T., Abe, A., and Sakagami, T. (1983): Ecto-5′-nucleotidase does not catalyze vectorial production of adenosine in the perfused rat liver. *J. Biol. Chem.,* 258:6947–6951.

322. Sattin, A., and Rall, T. W. (1970): The effect of adenosine and adenine nucleotides on the cyclic adenosine 3′,5′-phosphate content of guinea pig cerebral cortex slices. *Mol. Pharmacol.,* 6:13–23.

323. Sayen, J. J., Sheldon, W. F., Horwitz, O., Kuo, P. T., Pierce, G., Zinsser, H. F., and Mead, J. (1951): Studies of coronary disease in the experimental animal. II. Polarographic determinations of

local oxygen availability in the dog's left ventricle during coronary occlusion and pure oxygen breathing. *J. Clin. Invest.,* 30:932–940.

324. Scheid, C. R., Honeyman, T. W., and Fay, F. S. (1979): Mechanism of β-adrenergic relaxation of smooth muscle. *Nature,* 277:32–36.

325. Scholtholt, J., Nitz, R. E., and Schraven, E. (1972): On the mechanism of the antagonistic action of xanthine derivatives against adenosine and coronary vasodilators. *Arzneim. Forsch.,* 22:1255–1259.

326. Schrader, J., Baumann, G., and Gerlach, E. (1977): Adenosine as inhibitor of myocardial effects of catecholamines. *Pfluegers Arch.,* 372:29–35.

327. Schrader, J., and Gerlach, E. (1976): Compartmentation of cardiac adenine nucleotides and formation of adenosine. *Pfluegers Arch.,* 367:129–135.

328. Schrader, J., Haddy, F. J., and Gerlach, E. (1977): Release of adenosine, inosine and hypoxanthine from the isolated guinea pig heart during hypoxia, flow-autoregulation and reactive hyperemia. *Pfluegers Arch.,* 369:1–6.

329. Schrader, J., Nees, S., and Gerlach, E. (1977): Evidence for a cell surface adenosine receptor on coronary myocytes and atrial muscle cells. *Pfluegers Arch.,* 369:251–257.

330. Schrader, J., Schütz, W., and Bardenheuer, H. (1981): Role of S-adenosylhomocysteine hydrolase in adenosine metabolism in mammalian heart. *Biochem. J.,* 196:65–70.

331. Schuchhardt, S. (1971/72): The intramyocardial oxygen pressure at normoxia and hypoxia. *Cardiology,* 56:125–128.

332. Schuchhardt, S., and Lösse, B. (1973): Static and dynamic behavior of local oxygen pressure in the myocardium. *Bibl. Anat.,* 11:164–168.

333. Schütz, W., Schrader, J., and Gerlach, E. (1981): Different sites of adenosine formation in the heart. *Am. J. Physiol.,* 240:H963–H970.

334. Schütz, W., Zimpfer, M., and Raberger, G. (1977): Effect of aminophylline on coronary reactive hyperemia following brief and long occlusion periods. *Cardiovasc. Res.,* 11:507–511.

335. Schwartz, G. G., McHale, P. A., and Greenfield, J. C. (1982): Hyperemic response of the coronary circulation to brief diastolic occlusion in the conscious dog. *Circ. Res.,* 50:28–37.

336. Schwartz, P. J., and Stone, H. L. (1977): Tonic influence of the sympathetic nervous system on myocardial reactive hyperemia and on coronary blood flow distribution in dogs. *Circ. Res.,* 41: 51–58.

337. Scott, J. B., Frolich, E. D., Hardin, R. A., and Haddy, F. J. (1961): Na$^+$, K$^+$, Ca^{++} and Mg^{++} action on coronary vascular resistance in the dog heart. *Am. J. Physiol.,* 201:1095–1100.

338. Sestier, F. J., Mildenberger, R. R., and Klassen, G. A. (1978): Role of autoregulation in spatial and temporal perfusion heterogeneity of canine myocardium. *Am. J. Physiol.,* 235:H64–H71.

339. Silver, P. J., and DiSalvo, J. (1979): Adenosine 3′:5′-monophosphate mediated inhibition of myosin light chain phosphorylation in bovine aortic actomyosin. *J. Biol. Chem.,* 254:9951–9954.

340. Silver, P. J., Schmidt-Silver, C., and DiSalvo, J. (1982): β-adrenergic relaxation and cAMP kinase activation in coronary arterial smooth muscle. *Am. J. Physiol.,* 242:H177–H184.

341. Skolasinska, K., Harbig, K., Lübbers, D. W., and Wodick, R. (1978): PO$_2$ and microflow histograms of the beating heart in response to changes in arterial PO$_2$. *Basic Res. Cardiol.,* 73:307–319.

342. Smith, E. L., Deavers, S., and Huggins, R. A. (1972): Absolute relative residual organ blood volumes and organ hematocrits in growing beagles. *Proc. Soc. Exp. Biol. Med.,* 140:285–290.

343. Smith, M. H. (1976): Molecular parameters of purified human plasma proteins. In: *Handbook of Biochemistry and Molecular Biology,* Vol. II, edited by G. D. Fasman, pp. 242–258. CRC Press, Cleveland.

344. Snyder, R., Downey, J. M., and Kirk, E. S. (1975): The active and passive components of extravascular coronary resistance. *Cardiovasc. Res.,* 9:161–166.

345. Sobol, B. J., Wanlass, S. A., Joseph, E. B., and Azarshahy, I. (1962): Alteration of coronary blood flow in the dog by inhalation of 100 percent oxygen. *Circ. Res.,* 11:797–802.

346. Soboll, S., and Bünger, R. (1981): Compartmentation of adenine

nucleotides in the isolated working guinea pig heart stimulated by noradrenaline. *Hoppe Seylers Z. Physiol. Chem.*, 362:125–132.

347. Spaan, J. A. E. (1985): Coronary diastolic pressure-flow relation and xero flow pressure explained on the basis of intramyocardial compliance. *Circ. Res.*, 56:293–309.

348. Spaan, J. A. E., Breuls, N. P. W., and Laird, J. D. (1981): Forward coronary flow normally seen in systole is the result of both forward and concealed back flow. *Basic Res. Cardiol.*, 76:582–586.

349. Spaan, J. A. E., Breuls, N. P. W., and Laird, J. D. (1981): Diastolic-systolic coronary flow differences are caused by intramyocardial pump action in the anesthetized dog. *Circ. Res.*, 49:584–593.

350. Spaan, J. A. E., and Laird, J. D. (1981): Coronary vasoconstriction in long diastoles. *Circulation [Suppl. IV]*, 64:39 (abstract).

351. Stein, P. D., Alshabkhoun, S., Hawkins, H. F., and Hyland, J. W. (1969): Right coronary blood flow in acute pulmonary embolism. *Am. Heart J.*, 77:356–362.

352. Stein, P. D., Marzilli, M., Sabbah, H. N., and Lee, T. (1980): Systolic and diastolic pressure gradients within the left ventricular wall. *Am. J. Physiol.*, 238:H625–H630.

353. Stein, P. D., Sabbah, H. N., Marzilli, M., and Blick, E. F. (1980): Comparison of the distribution of intramyocardial pressure across the canine left ventricular wall in the beating heart during diastole and in the arrested heart. *Circ. Res.*, 47:258–267.

354. Steinhausen, M., Tillmanns, H., and Thederan, H. (1978): Microcirculation of the epimyocardial layer of the heart. I. A method for in vivo observation of the microcirculation of superficial ventricular myocardium of the heart and capillary flow pattern under normal and hypoxic conditions. *Pfluegers Arch.*, 378:9–14.

355. Stoker, M. E., Gerdes, A. M., and May, J. F. (1982): Regional differences in capillary density and myocyte size in the normal human heart. *Anat. Rec.*, 202:187–191.

356. Stone, H. L. (1983): Control of the coronary circulation during exercise. *Annu. Rev. Physiol.*, 45:213–227.

357. Streeter, D. D., Spotnitz, H. M., Patel, D. P., Ross, J., and Sonnenblick, E. H. (1969): Fiber orientation in the canine left ventricle during diastole and systole. *Circ. Res.*, 24:339–347.

358. Streeter, D. D., Vaishnav, N., Patel, D. J., Spotnitz, H. M., Ross, J., and Sonnenblick, E. H. (1970): Stress distribution in the canine left ventricle during diastole and systole. *Biophys. J.*, 10:345–363.

359. Sugishita, Y., Kakihana, M., and Murao, S. (1978): Decreased reactive hyperemia after coronary perfusion with nonoxygenated solution. *Am. J. Physiol.*, 234:H625–H628.

360. Sullivan, J. M., and Alpers, J. B. (1971): In vitro regulation of rat heart 5′-nucleotidase by adenine nucleotides and magnesium. *J. Biol. Chem.*, 246:3057–3063.

361. Sybers, H. D., Helmer, P. R., and Murphy, Q. R. (1971): Effects of hypoxia on myocardial potassium balance. *Am. J. Physiol.*, 220:2047–2050.

362. Sybers, R. G., Sybers, H. D., Hellmer, P. R., and Murphy, Q. R. (1965): Myocardial potassium balance during cardioaccelerator nerve and atrial stimulation. *Am. J. Physiol.*, 209:699–701.

363. Thompson, C. I., Rubio, R., and Berne, R. M. (1980): Changes in adenosine and glycogen phosphorylase activity during the cardiac cycle. *Am. J. Physiol.*, 238:H389–H398.

364. Tillmanns, H., Ikeda, S., Hansen, H., Sarma, J. S. M., Fauvel, J., and Bing, R. J. (1974): Microcirculation in the ventricle of the dog and turtle. *Circ. Res.*, 34:561–569.

365. Tillmanns, H., Steinhausen, M., Leinberger, H., Thederan, H., and Kubler, W. (1981): Pressure measurements in the terminal vascular bed of the epimyocardium of rats and cats. *Circ. Res.*, 49:1202–1211.

366. Tomoike, H., Ootsubo, H., Sakai, K., Kikuchi, Y., and Nakamura, M. (1981): Continuous measurement of coronary artery diameter in situ. *Am. J. Physiol.*, 250:H73–H79.

367. Ueland, P. M. (1982): Pharmacological and biochemical aspects of S-adenosylhomocysteine hydrolase. *Pharmacol. Rev.*, 34:223–253.

368. van der Meer, J. J., Reneman, R. S., Schneider, H., and Wieberdink, J. (1970): A technique for estimation of intramyocardial pressure in acute and chronic experiments. *Cardiovasc. Res.*, 4:132–140.

369. Van Breemen, C., and Siegel, B. (1980): The mechanism of α-adrenergic activation of the dog coronary artery. *Circ. Res.*, 46:426–429.

370. Vatner, S. F., Pagani, M., Manders, W. T., and Pasipoularides, A. D. (1980): Alpha adrenergic vasoconstriction and nitroglycerin vasodilation of large coronary arteries in the conscious dog. *J. Clin. Invest.*, 65:5–9.

371. Vetterlein F., Dal Ri, H., and Schmidt, G. (1982): Capillary density in rat myocardium during timed plasma staining. *Am. J. Physiol.*, 242:H133–H141.

372. Vinten-Johansen, J., and Weiss, H. R. (1980): Oxygen consumption in subepicardial and subendocardial regions of the canine left ventricle. The effect of experimental acute valvular aortic stenosis. *Circ. Res.*, 46:139–145.

373. Vlahakes, G. J., Baer, R. W., Uhlig, P. N., Verrier, E. D., Bristow, J. D., and Hoffmann, J. I. E. (1982): Adrenergic influence on the coronary circulation of conscious dogs during maximal vasodilation with adenosine. *Circ. Res.*, 51:371–384.

374. Wadsworth, R. M. (1972): The effects of aminophylline on the increased myocardial blood flow produced by systemic hypoxia or by coronary artery occlusion. *Eur. J. Pharmacol.*, 20:130–132.

375. Walston, A., II, Rembert, J. C., Fedor, J. M., and Greenfield, J. C. (1978): Regional myocardial blood flow after sudden aortic constriction in awake dogs. *Circ. Res.*, 42:419–425.

376. Weiss, H. R. (1974): Control of myocardial oxygenation—effect of atrial pacing. *Microvasc. Res.*, 8:362–376.

377. Weiss, H. R. (1979): Regional oxygen consumption and supply in the dog heart: Effect of atrial pacing. *Am. J. Physiol.*, 236:H231–H237.

378. Weiss, H. R. (1979): Regional oxygen consumption and supply in the rabbit heart—effect of nitroglycerin and propranolol. *J. Pharmacol. Exp. Ther.*, 211:68–73.

379. Weiss, H. R. (1980): Effect of coronary artery occlusion on regional arterial and venous O_2 saturation, O_2 extraction, blood flow and O_2 consumption in the dog heart. *Circ. Res.*, 47:400–407.

380. Weiss, H. R., and Cohen, J. A. (1978): Changes in small vessel blood content of the rat heart induced by hypercapnic, hyperoxic or asphyxic conditions. *Cardiology*, 63:199–207.

381. Weiss, H. R., Neubauer, J. A., Lipp, J. A., and Sinha, A. K. (1978): Quantitative determination of regional oxygen consumption in the dog heart. *Circ. Res.*, 42:394–401.

382. Weiss, H. R., and Sinha, A. K. (1978): Regional oxygen saturation of small arteries and veins in the canine myocardium. *Circ. Res.*, 42:119–126.

383. Weiss, H. R., and Winbury, M. M. (1972): Intracoronary nitroglycerin, pentaerythritol trinitrate and dipyridamole on intramyocardial oxygen tension. *Microvasc. Res.*, 4:273–284.

384. Weiss, H. R., and Winbury, M. M. (1974): Nitroglycerin and chromonar on small-vessel blood content of the ventricular walls. *Am. J. Physiol.*, 226:838–843.

385. Westerhof, N., Sipkema, P., and Van Huis, G. A. (1981): Coronary pressure-flow relations and the vascular waterfall. *Cardiovasc. Res.*, 17:162–169.

386. Wiedmeier, V. T., and Spell, L. H. (1977): Effects of catecholamines, histamine, and nitroglycerin on flow, oxygen utilization, and adenosine production in the perfused guinea pig heart. *Circ. Res.*, 41:503–508.

387. Wiggers, C. J. (1954): The interplay of coronary vascular resistance and myocardial compression in regulating coronary flow. *Circ. Res.*, 2:271–279.

388. Wikman-Coffelt, J., and Coffelt, R. J. (1982): A stimulator-regulated rapid freeze clamp for terminating metabolic processes of the heart during normal physiological working conditions. *IEEE Trans. Biomed. Eng.*, 29:448–452.

389. Wikman-Coffelt, J., Sievers, R., Coffelt, R. J., and Parmley, W. W. (1983): The cardiac cycle: Regulation and energy oscillations. *Am. J. Physiol.*, 245:H354–H362.

390. Wilcken, D. E. L. (1983): Local factors controlling coronary circulation. *Am. J. Cardiol.,* 52:8A–14A.

391. Wolfe, K. B. (1959): Anatomy of the septal artery in dogs' hearts. *Am. J. Surg.,* 97:279–282.

392. Wollenberger, A., Ristau, O., and Schoffa, G. (1960): Eine einfache Technik der extrem schnellen Abkühlung grosserer Gewebestücke. *Pfluegers Arch.,* 270:399–412.

393. Woodman, O. L., and Dusting, G. (1983): Coronary vasoconstriction induced by leukotrienes in the anesthetized dog. *Eur. J. Pharmacol.,* 86:125–128.

394. Worku, Y., and Newby, A. C. (1983): The mechanism of adenosine production in rat polymorphonuclear leucocytes. *Biochem. J.,* 214:325–330.

395. Wüsten, B., Buss, D. D., Deist, H., and Schaper, W. (1977): Dilatory capacity of the coronary circulation and its correlation to the arterial vasculature in the canine left ventricle. *Basic Res. Cardiol.,* 72:636–650.

396. Yazaki, Y., Kuramoto, K., Kimata, S., Ikeda, M., and Nakao, K. (1970): Myocardial metabolism in reactive hyperemia. *Jpn. Circ. J.,* 34:413–418.

397. Yipintsoi, T., Dobbs, W. A., Jr., Scanlon, P. D., Knopp, T. J., and Bassingthwaighte, J. B. (1973): Regional distribution of diffusible tracers and carbonized microspheres in the left ventricle of isolated dog hearts. *Circ. Res.,* 33:573–587.

398. Yokoyama, M., Maekawa, K., Katada, Y., Ishikawa, Y., Azumi, T., Mizutani, T., Fukuzaki, H., and Tomomatsue, T. (1978): Effects of graded coronary constriction on regional oxygen and carbon dioxide tensions in outer and inner layers of the canine myocardium. *Jpn. Circ. J.,* 42:701–709.

399. Zeirler, K. L. (1962): Circulation times and the theory of indicator-dilution methods for determining blood flow and volume. In: *Handbook of Physiology, Circulation,* Sect. 2, Vol. 1, edited by W. F. Hamilton, pp. 585–615. American Physiological Society, Washington, D.C.

400. Ziegler, W. H., and Goresky, C. A. (1971): Transcapillary exchange in the working left ventricle of the dog. *Circ. Res.,* 29:181–207.

—

The Heart and Cardiovascular System,
edited by H. A. Fozzard et al.
Raven Press, New York © 1986.

CHAPTER **49**

Studies of Membrane-Bound and Soluble Adenylate Cyclase

Eva J. Neer

The object of this chapter is not to give recipes for assays of the activity of adenylate cyclase and its components, which can be found in many places in the literature, but to discuss experimental approaches. For instance, suppose an investigator has discovered a new agent that affects cardiac contractility and wants to know if this acts by way of adenylate cyclase, or suppose a physiological manipulation leads to an altered response to hormone and the investigator wants to know if this is because of a changed response of adenylate cyclase to stimulation. This kind of experiment starts with a physiological observation and goes on to enzyme studies. Therefore, the investigator needs a hormone-responsive system in which to measure adenylate cyclase activity. Having established that adenylate cyclase activity is indeed affected, the investigator may want to define which component of the hormone-responsive system is causing the change. In order to do so, the investigator must be able to assay the function of each component individually. One example of successful application of

such an approach is the demonstration that the defect in a genetic disease, pseudohypoparathyroidism, in which there is diminished responsiveness to parathyroid hormone, is a deficiency in the activity of the guanine-nucleotide-binding protein that couples hormone receptors to stimulation of adenylate cyclase (46,102).

If one then wants to relate a functional change to a structural change, one must be able to isolate each component. In that way, one can determine if the change is due to some structural modification of an adenylate cyclase component, a change in the rate of synthesis of components, or a change in membrane insertion. Methods to study the last two problems are just being developed and will be greatly aided by cloning the genes for all the components, as well as by the development of *in vitro* translation systems. In the interval between the writing of this chapter and publication of this book, it is very likely that at least some of these things will have been accomplished and will change research in this field.

CURRENT CONCEPTS OF THE STRUCTURE AND INTERACTIONS OF ADENYLATE CYCLASE COMPONENTS[1]

Hormones of many chemical classes stimulate or inhibit adenylate cyclase through separate receptors. Hormone receptors that stimulate adenylate cyclase are coupled to the enzyme through a guanine-nucleotide-binding protein, called G_s, that is a heterotrimer made up of α, β, and γ subunits (33,62,130,164).[2] The α subunit of G_s, called α_s, contains the guanine-nucleotide-binding site (127). On binding a guanine nucleoside triphosphate, the heterotrimer dissociates to give guanine-nucleotide-liganded α_s and free $\beta \cdot \gamma$ (164). The guanine-nucleotide-liganded α_s associates with the catalytic unit (C) to form the activated complex (129) according to the model shown in Fig. 1. This model is supported by the observations that α_s separated from $\beta \cdot \gamma$ can activate C (129) and that the molecular weight of C increases on activation by G_s (8).

When α_s is activated by nonhydrolyzable analogues of GTP such as Gpp(NH)p or GTPγS, stimulation of C is essentially irreversible unless G_s can interact with an agonist-liganded hormone receptor. In contrast, activation by GTP is quickly terminated by hydrolysis of GTP to GDP on α_s. The α_s component has GTPase activity that is stimulated by agonist-liganded hormone receptors (22,45). Hormone binding to receptors promotes the interaction of receptor with G_s, leading to release of GDP. Release of GDP allows binding of GTP to G_s. The net effect is that agonist-liganded receptors allow more substrate GTP to bind at the active site and so promote more hydrolysis. Hormone-sensitive GTPase activity can be measured either in membranes (24) or in purified G_s after reconstitution with receptors in phospholipid vesicles (17,18).

The α_s protein can be identified in membranes by cholera-toxin-catalyzed ADP-ribosylation. Cholera toxin

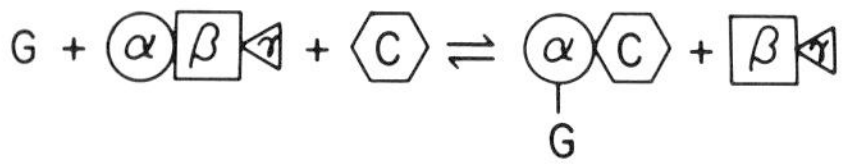

---

[1] A comprehensive review of the biochemistry of adenylate cyclase is that of Ross and Gilman (143). Other useful recent reviews are by Rodbell (139), Smigel et al. (161), Codina et al. (34), Jakobs et al. (79), and Klee et al. (94).

[2] Abbreviations: C: The catalytic unit of adenylate cyclase. G_s: The guanine nucleotide regulatory unit that mediates hormonal stimulation of adenylate cyclase. It is composed of α_s and $\beta \cdot \gamma$ components. α_s: The polypeptide component of G_s that binds guanine nucleotides; it can be ADP-ribosylated by cholera toxin, and it activates the catalytic unit. β: A polypeptide component of both G_i and G_s with a molecular weight of 35,000 to 36,000. γ: A small protein (5–10 kd) of unknown function associated with β. G_i: The guanine nucleotide regulatory unit that mediates hormonal inhibition of adenylate cyclase. It is composed of α, β, and γ units. α_{39}: A 39-kd guanine-nucleotide-binding protein from brain that can be ADP-ribosylated by pertussis toxin. The protein is called G_0 by Sternweis and Robishaw (165). α_{41}: A 41-kd guanine-nucleotide-binding protein that is the predominant substrate for ADP-ribosylation by pertussis toxin. Gpp(NH)p: Guanosine 5'-(β,γ-imino)triphosphate. GTPγS: Guanosine 5'-(3-O-thio)triphosphate. SDS-PAGE: Polyacrylamide-gel electrophoresis in sodium dodecyl sulfate. kd: Kilodalton.

FIG. 1. Activation.

transfers ADP-ribose from NAD to two membrane proteins (51). One protein, with a molecular weight of 42 to 45 kd, is found in all cells. In addition, another cholera toxin substrate, with a molecular weight of 46 to 51 kd, is found in some cell types (87,125). Tryptic peptide mapping shows that these two proteins are extremely similar, and, indeed, the smaller may be derived from the larger (69). Treatment of membranes with cholera toxin leads to persistent activation of adenylate cyclase by GTP to a level similar to that produced by the nonhydrolyzable analogues. This observation suggested the idea that cholera toxin inhibits the GTPase activity of α_s (103). This prediction was confirmed by Cassel and Pfeuffer (23).

Whereas there seems to be general agreement about the mechanism of activation of adenylate cyclase, there is less unanimity on the mechanism of hormonal inhibition. Like the receptors that stimulate adenylate cyclase, the receptors that inhibit adenylate cyclase are coupled to the enzyme by a heterotrimeric guanine-nucleotide-binding protein termed G_i. The α_i component of G_i is a 41-kd protein that was first identified because it was ADP-ribosylated by a toxin from *Bordetella pertussis* (90,91). ADP-ribosylation by pertussis toxin blocks the ability of inhibitory hormones to lower adenylate cyclase activity. A consequence of this is that intracellular cAMP levels may rise after treatment of intact cells with pertussis toxin (58,169). Cholera toxin produces the same end result, but for a different reason. Pertussis toxin treatment also prevents guanine-nucleotide-mediated shifts in inhibitory receptor affinity for agonists (68) and inhibits the GTPase stimulated by those hormones that decrease adenylate cyclase activity (20).

The 41-kd protein, which is the predominant pertussis toxin substrate in most cells, was first purified from rabbit liver (15). Like α_s, the α_i component carries the guanine-nucleotide-binding site and interacts with the same $\beta \cdot \gamma$ that is associated with α_s (111). Like α_s, α_i is a GTPase when reconstituted with a hormone receptor (5). Although they are similar, the α_s and α_i components are different proteins. Binding of guanine nucleotides causes dissociation of α_i from the $\beta \cdot \gamma$ components (31,71,89).

There are at least two possible mechanisms by which hormonal inhibition of adenylate cyclase could occur (Fig. 2). The first model is exactly analogous to hormonal stimulation. The hormone receptor would promote guanine nucleotide binding to α_i, with subsequent dissociation of α_i from $\beta \cdot \gamma$. The guanine-nucleotide-liganded α_i would then interact with the catalytic unit, with the

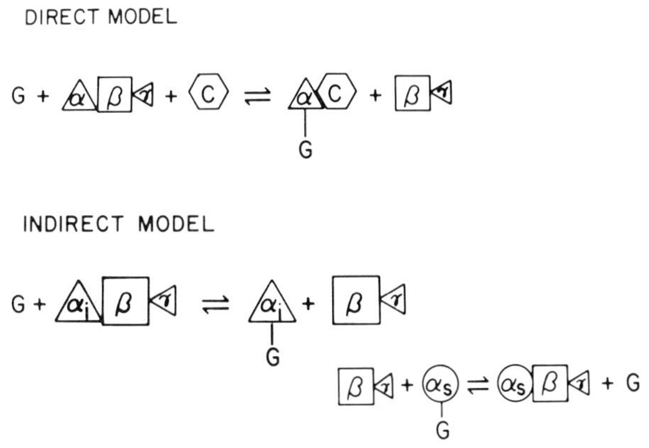

DIRECT MODEL

INDIRECT MODEL

FIG. 2. Inhibition.

consequence that the activity of the catalytic unit would be inhibited.

Another possible mechanism is an indirect one. Because excess $\beta \cdot \gamma$ subunits deactivate the N_s component, any protein in the membrane that liberates free $\beta \cdot \gamma$ will reverse activation of adenylate cyclase. For this mechanism to work, the α_i unit would need to exist in excess of α_s so that it could act as a reservoir for $\beta \cdot \gamma$. The present evidence suggests that at least in liver, brain, and erythrocytes, α_i is in excess over α_s. There is a great deal of evidence in support of the indirect hypothesis of hormonal inhibition, and a number of its predictions have been experimentally verified. For instance, the indirect hypothesis predicts that the pure 41-kd α_i protein should activate adenylate cyclase by binding up the inhibitory $\beta \cdot \gamma$ protein. This, in fact, does occur (89). Several laboratories, including the author's, have tried to show direct inhibition of the resolved adenylate cyclase catalytic unit by G_i. Although some inhibition occurs, it is not enough to explain the results in intact membranes. The difficulty of demonstrating direct inhibition of C by α_i stands in contrast to the ease with which stimulation of catalytic activity can be demonstrated with α_s.

There are also data that cannot be easily explained by the indirect hypothesis. In particular, mutant S49 lymphoma cells that lack the α_s component can nevertheless be inhibited by somatostatin (60,78). In principle, there should be no inhibition of adenylate cyclase in the absence of α_s, according to the indirect model. Furthermore, because the indirect model requires a common subunit, $\beta \cdot \gamma$, inhibition and stimulation should follow competitive kinetics. Hildebrandt and Birnbaumer (60) have shown that this condition seems not to be met. Although it is not yet definitively known which mechanism applies in the membrane, or if perhaps both may be operating simultaneously, the two models provide clear hypotheses to be tested.

In addition to the 41-kd protein, there is a second pertussis toxin substrate of 39 kd that has been purified from brain (124,165). This α_{39} protein is present in many tissues, including heart (70). The α_{39} protein binds guanine nucleotides with the same affinity as α_{41}, associates reversibly with the same $\beta \cdot \gamma$ component, and has intrinsic GTPase activity (70,124). It is less readily ADP-ribosylated than α_{41} (124). Because it can release $\beta \cdot \gamma$ units, it can potentially act as an α_i component. However, it may also be involved in coupling hormone receptors to effectors other than adenylate cyclase. A rapidly growing body of evidence suggests that guanine-nucleotide-binding pertussis toxin substrates may regulate Ca^{2+} fluxes or phosphatidylinositol turnover (14,16,131). One of the major challenges at present is to characterize the proteins involved and to define the mechanisms of their coupling to other enzymes or ion channels.

MEASUREMENT OF HORMONE-STIMULATED ADENYLATE CYCLASE ACTIVITY

Preparation of Tissues

Hormone-responsive adenylate cyclase activity can be measured either in purified membranes or in crude homogenates. Partial purification of membranes is a relatively straightforward procedure and ordinarily enhances the specific activity of adenylate cyclase. However, the stability of hormone responsiveness varies from system to system for reasons that are not entirely clear. In some cases, hormonal responsiveness is lost in the process of preparing membranes, even though the adenylate cyclase activity itself is quite stable. Especially where the amount of tissue available is extremely small, as in embryonic tissue, cultured cells, or biopsy specimens, the most reproducible results may be obtained by simply homogenizing the tissue and assaying the activity in the entirely crude system. A standard buffer for homogenizing is 0.05- to 0.1-M Tris-Cl, pH 7.6 to 8. HEPES buffer may also be used; imidazole buffers often inhibit adenylate cyclase activity. Phosphate buffers are not compatible with the Mg^{2+} required both for assay and to stabilize adenylate cyclase, because insoluble $Mg_3(PO_4)_2$ is formed. Mg^{2+} (5–10 mM) and 1-mM dithiothreitol stabilize the enzyme. EDTA (1 mM) is sometimes included to chelate heavy metals. Sucrose (75–100 mM) makes the membranes more stable to freezing. Addition of protease inhibitors helps to protect the preparation, especially when hormonal inhibition is to be measured, because the α_i proteins seem to be more sensitive to proteolysis than α_s. One such cocktail is 1 μg/ml each of soybean and lima bean trypsin inhibitors and 3 mM benzamidine. However, effective protease inhibitor mixes are difficult to prescribe, because the proteases present depend on the cell type and the preparation procedure. In any case, it is impossible to inhibit them all.

Another complication in assays of membranes or crude homogenates of cardiac tissue may be the presence of adenosine. Adenosine interacts with adenylate cyclase in two ways: The nucleoside may stimulate or inhibit the enzyme through specific membrane receptors, analogous to hormone receptors (R sites), or it may inhibit the enzyme through another site, termed the P site (107), which seems to be on the catalytic unit or on protein closely associated with C (7). The presence of variable amounts of adenosine may give erratic or misleading results. Addition of adenosine deaminase eliminated adenosine's actions at the P site, and methylxanthines blocked actions through the R site. If addition of a methylxanthine depresses adenylate cyclase activity, then the investigator might suspect that endogenous adenosine is stimulating the activity in this preparation. Methylxanthines are also phosphodiesterase inhibitors. If addition of a methylxanthine increases activity, the effect could be due to blockade of adenosine inhibition or prevention of cAMP breakdown. Inhibition through the P site is prevented by adenosine deaminase, which converts adenosine to inosine.

Although very reproducible results can be obtained with crude systems, it is important to take precautions to be sure that the substrate levels are maintained and that the product is not broken down because of the actions of contaminating enzymes. It is essential that the investigator establish very early in a study that the rate of cAMP production is linear with protein concentration and with time. If the substrate concentration is not constant or cAMP is being broken down, misleading results may be obtained.

Assays of Adenylate Cyclase Activity

There are two similar assay systems in widespread use for measuring adenylate cyclase activity. The first assay was described by Krishna, Weiss, and Brodie (96). In this assay, [^{3}H]ATP is separated from [^{3}H]cAMP by chromatography over Dowex 50X2 (AG450WX2, Biorad), columns followed by precipitation of any contaminating AMP with barium sulfate. The other assay is that of Salomon et al. (147), in which [^{32}P]cAMP is separated from [^{32}P]ATP by sequential chromatography over Dowex, followed by Alumina. This procedure is described in detail by Salomon (146). The author's laboratory routinely uses the modified Krishna, Weiss, and Brodie method, which is described in the Appendix. It has several advantages and drawbacks. The [^{3}H]ATP must be purified before use, because otherwise the assay blank is too large (see Appendix). Purification takes 2 to 3 hr for a 5-mCi batch of ATP, which is sufficient for about 2,000 assays. Tritium does not require shielding, and there is no significant radiation exposure. The specific activity of [^{3}H]ATP does not change once a

batch is made. For this reason, using [^{3}H]ATP is an advantage if a laboratory does not do adenylate cyclase assays regularly. Informal comparisons with other groups using the two-column assay suggest that the time required for each is about the same. The relative expense depends on how many assays are done, because [^{32}P]ATP decays rapidly.

Although both assays are routinely used and give excellent results, it is very important when first setting them up to validate the assay explicitly by determining that the radioactive product is indeed cAMP. This can be done by running the assay in the routine manner, collecting the column fraction, which should contain cAMP, lyophilizing the collected fraction, and analyzing it by descending chromatography on Ecteola paper (117). Alternatively, the authenticity of the radioactive product can be verified by HPLC (158,170).

Because crude homogenates and membranes contain ATPases, an ATP-regenerating system made up of creatine kinase and creatine phosphate or pyruvate kinase and phosphoenol pyruvate is usually included in the assay cocktail. However, these enzymes cannot regenerate ATP if it is cleaved between the α and β phosphates by nucleotide pyrophosphatase. Furthermore, the 5'-AMP formed may be further degraded to adenosine by 5'-nucleotidase. As discussed earlier, adenosine can either activate or inhibit adenylate cyclase, depending on the membrane being studied, and can confound results if its presence is not suspected. Finally, pyrophosphatase can hydrolyze Gpp(NH)p or GTP and lower their concentrations. Dithiothreitol inhibits the pyrophosphatase. Its enhancement of adenylate cyclase in liver membranes may be by this mechanism. Including myokinase to catalyze rephosphorylation of 5'-AMP may be necessary to maintain substrate levels. Because the commercially available enzymes used in regenerating systems are not entirely pure, they may introduce contaminants into the assay. An excellent discussion of these problems and their solutions is given by Johnson (83).

Guanine Nucleotide Requirements

It is a fortunate accident that cell membranes are contaminated with relatively large amounts of GTP, because without this, early investigators would not have been able to show hormonal stimulation of adenylate cyclase activity. The ease with which investigators could show appropriate hormone responses in membranes from cells helped to establish the importance of cAMP as a mediator of hormone action and, for some time, obscured the guanylnucleotide requirement (140). However, investigators should not rely on the contaminating levels of GTP to provide sufficient guanine nucleotides to support hormonal activation of adenylate cyclase. Hormonal responses are ordinarily measured in the presence of either GTP or Gpp(NH)p. Which to choose depends on the particular experiment and the properties of the system under study. GTP usually has little effect on basal activity, whereas Gpp(NH)p substantially increases it (108). However, because the increment in hormone-stimulated activity is often larger in the presence of Gpp(NH)p than in the presence of GTP, the signal-to-noise ratio may be more favorable with a nonhydrolyzable analogue. Gpp(NH)p has the advantage that it cannot be hydrolyzed by GTPases, and therefore results will not be affected by changes in bulk cellular GTPase activity. This eliminates at least one variable from consideration when evaluating new systems where hormonal responsiveness of adenylate cyclase has changed. As mentioned earlier, it can be hydrolyzed by pyrophosphatases (76), but usually not to an appreciable extent.

Metal-Ion Requirement

The substrate for the adenylate cyclase reaction is not free ATP but Mg-ATP. Therefore, enough Mg^{2+} must be present to complex all the ATP. However, in addition to this requirement, free Mg^{2+} is an important modulating ligand. The rate of activation of G_s is increased by increasing concentrations of Mg^{2+} (75,164). Furthermore, addition of hormone during activation results in lowering the Mg^{2+} needed for activation of G_s from millimolar to micromolar amounts (27,75,164).

It is important when setting up a new adenylate cyclase assay system to determine the Mg^{2+} concentration needed for maximal hormonal stimulation. In some cases, the Mg^{2+} concentration dependence has a steeply biphasic curve, and stimulation by hormone will be missed if the wrong Mg^{2+} concentration is used (2). Because the free Mg^{2+} concentration is the important variable, the total Mg^{2+} required for optimal hormonal response will vary with the ATP concentration used in the assay.

Mn-ATP is also an excellent substrate for adenylate cyclase, and Mn^{2+} activates the enzyme. However, in some, but not all, tissues, hormonal stimulation is blocked by concentrations of Mn^{2+} greater than 15 mM (81,105).

Relation of Basal Activity to Hormone-Stimulated Activity

The usual way of expressing hormonal stimulation is as a multiple of the basal activity (the basal activity is that measured using Mg-ATP as a substrate and no other activators). It is not evident that this is the best way to think about hormonal activation of adenylate cyclase. Expressing the hormonally stimulated activity

as a multiple of the basal implies that the same population of catalytic units that gives the basal activity is stimulated by hormone to a new level of activity. However, it is also possible that there are two populations of adenylate cyclase molecules, one of which is independent of hormonal stimulation, whereas the other goes from a completely inactive state to an active state. Therefore, it is important to bear in mind that the absolute increment in adenylate cyclase activity may be the important thing, not the activity relative to the basal. Despite many years of work, it is still not at all clear what the basal activity represents. It is unlikely to be simply the activity of the catalytic unit unaffected by any of the regulatory proteins in the membrane. After solubilization of brain adenylate cyclase, a portion of the catalytic activity that represents the basal form can be physically separated from the guanine-nucleotide-sensitive enzyme, suggesting that two populations do exist (122).

Forskolin

Hormonal activation of adenylate cyclase can be enhanced by low concentrations of the plant diterpene forskolin (Calbiochem) (38,153,154,156). This substance, which was used for centuries as a cardiotonic agent in traditional Indian medicine, was found to activate adenylate cyclase from all cells tested, except for sperm. The activation is rapid in onset and fully reversible by washing the cells or membranes. Half-maximal activation usually requires 3 to 20 μM forskolin. In membranes, the activation is usually at least additive and often synergistic with that elicited by Gpp(NH)p. Forskolin can amplify the response to stimulatory hormones severalfold. In some cases, forskolin lowers the apparent K_{act} for hormonal stimulation of adenylate cyclase; in others it affects V_{max} only (10,38,39,106,154).

Cardiac Adenylate Cyclase

Table 1 gives the specific activities determined by several laboratories for cardiac adenylate cyclase from a number of species. The list is not comprehensive and includes only those studies in which the substrate concentration was at the K_m or above. The list illustrates the range of activity to be expected. Hormonal stimulation of cardiac adenylate cyclase is not as great as in some other tissues, for reasons that are not understood. The reader can refer to these sources for specific descriptions of cardiac membrane preparations, as well as to Drummond and Severson (43).

In heart, the pore-forming antibiotic alamethicin has been used to enhance hormonal responsiveness (9,85). The mechanism of this effect is not clear, although

TABLE 1. *Activity of cardiac adenylate cyclase*

Species (reference)	Preparation	°C	Basal	NaF	GTP	Glucagon	Glucagon and GTP	Gpp(NH)p	Isoproterenol	Isoproterenol and Gpp(NH)p
							Adenylate cyclase activity (pmol cAMP/min/mg)			
Cat (92)	Washed, particulate	32.5	20						100	
Guinea pig (4)	Washed, particulate	37	100					1,200		
Rat (49)	Washed, particulate	37	51		67	79	255			
Rabbit (41)	Washed, particulate	24	50					150		220
Guinea pig (115)	Sarcolemma	30	245	700				396		889
Chick (3)	Homogenate	37	49					126	128	363

Jones et al. (85) proposed that alamethicin permeabilizes sealed vesicles from cardiac membrane.

MEASUREMENT OF HORMONE-INHIBITED ADENYLATE CYCLASE ACTIVITY

Hormonal inhibition of adenylate cyclase is technically harder to measure than stimulation and has some different characteristics. The basal activity is often very low to begin with, and it is poorly inhibited by hormones. Inhibition is therefore easier to demonstrate if the enzyme is first activated either by a stimulatory hormone or by forskolin (*vide infra*) or both. Hormonal inhibition of adenylate cyclase is never complete but is usually 40 to 60% of either basal activity or guanine-nucleotide-stimulated activity. The guanine nucleotide requirement for inhibition is different from that for activation. The concentration of GTP is 5 to 10 times greater for half-maximal inhibition of adenylate cyclase than for stimulation. However, low concentrations of nonhydrolyzable analogues must be used, because high concentrations cause irreversible activation of the catalytic unit through α_s. In addition, hormonal inhibition requires or is facilitated by the presence of 20 to 100 mM of sodium ions (1,12,79). The apparent requirement for sodium appears to be the consequence of the fact that high concentrations of GTP are needed to support hormonal inhibition. These concentrations are inhibitory in themselves in many membrane systems and obscure the hormonal effects. Sodium counteracts the inhibitory effect of GTP and so reveals and amplifies the effect of hormones. Inhibition is optimal at low concentrations of magnesium (1–2 mM) and is blocked by higher concentrations. Hormonal inhibition is very sensitive to Mn^{2+} and is usually blocked by 1 mM Mn^{2+} (79).

As discussed earlier, stimulation of adenylate cyclase by Gpp(NH)p and forskolin is usually additive or synergistic. However, forskolin potentiates both hormonal stimulation and inhibition. Therefore, the observation that the response to forskolin and Gpp(NH)p is less than additive suggests the presence of a dually regulated adenylate cyclase (156). When forskolin is used to enhance hormonal inhibition, less than maximal concentrations of forskolin should be used, or else the very large activation of the enzyme by the diterpene will obscure hormonal effects (72,106,160).

EVALUATION IN MEMBRANES OF ACTIVITIES OF INDIVIDUAL COMPONENTS OF ADENYLATE CYCLASE

In order to define the basis of a change in hormone responsiveness, it is necessary to assess the activities of individual adenylate cyclase components. To evaluate a system, it is clearly important to look at the interaction of G_s or G_i with hormone receptors, as well as with the adenylate cyclase enzyme. The functional state of guanine-nucleotide-binding proteins can be determined by quantitating the effects of guanine nucleotides on agonist binding. Measuring guanine nucleotide effects on agonist binding is fundamental to characterizing receptor function. However, I will not deal with measuring the amount or affinity of hormone receptors, because such methods have been described in other chapters in this volume.

Catalytic Unit

There is no certain way to measure the intrinsic activity of the catalytic unit in membranes. Two activities have been taken as measures of the activity of the catalytic unit itself: the activity measured in the presence of manganese, and the activity measured in the presence of forskolin. Manganese activates the isolated catalytic unit in the absence of either G_s or G_i (144,166). In some systems, manganese has been shown to uncouple hormone receptors from activation of adenylate cyclase (105), although this is not a universal finding.

However, the activity measured with Mn^{2+} is influenced by the interaction of C with G_s (7,8). In normal membranes, the ratio of catalytic activity measured with Mn-ATP to activity measured with Mg-ATP is never so high as in S49 cyc membranes or in the resolved catalytic unit. This observation suggests that there is always some coupling of C and G_s in membranes.

Forskolin seems to act directly on the catalytic unit. No effect of forskolin on the function of G_s was found when the effect of forskolin on resolved G_s was studied. However, activation by forskolin is extremely sensitive to interaction of the catalytic unit with G_s, and the activated catalytic unit is much more responsive to forskolin than is the catalytic unit alone (7). Therefore, the activity measured with forskolin is not a simple index of the amount of free catalytic unit available.

In the earlier literature, fluoride activation was taken as a measure of the catalytic unit activity. This is now known to be wrong. Fluoride activates the catalytic unit not directly but through G_s. Therefore, the activity measured with fluoride reflects measuring a function very similar to that which is measured using guanine nucleotides (143).

Stimulatory Guanine Nucleotide Regulatory Unit

If receptor number is unchanged, altered hormone responsiveness of membrane-bound adenylate cyclase could be due to a change in the amount of G_s, in the ability of G_s to interact with receptors, in the ability of G_s to activate the catalytic unit, or in the capacity of the catalytic unit to respond to it. The ability of G_s to interact with hormone receptors can be evaluated by measuring the guanine-nucleotide-induced change in receptor affinity for agonists (see *Chapter* 51). A decreased sensitivity to guanine nucleotides might suggest either a decreased amount or activity of G_s or a defect in the ability of the receptor to interact with it. The receptor can be bypassed in some of the procedures to be described later. However, in membranes it is not always possible to localize unambiguously the site at which the system is perturbed. However, a combination of assays that measure different aspects of G_s function will yield many of the pieces to the puzzle.

Guanine-Nucleotide-Stimulated Adenylate Cyclase

The most straightforward way to measure the activity of G_s is to measure guanine-nucleotide-stimulated ade-

nylate cyclase activity. It is very important to keep two things in mind when setting up the assay: Activation of adenylate cyclase by Gpp(NH)p or GTPγS may be slow. Therefore, to compare preparations, the investigator must either compare the rates of activation or, if a single time point is used, be sure equilibrium has been reached. One obvious way to do this is to measure the accumulation of cAMP as a function of time. If activation continues to increase over the time of the assay, the curve will be concave upward. However, if activation is very slow, the deviation from linearity may be difficult to spot. An alternative and more sensitive design is to incubate the sample with Gpp(NH)p or GTPγS for various times. After preincubation, the adenylate cyclase assay reagents are added, and the rate of cAMP formation is measured over a short time. An example of this procedure is given by Neer et al. (123).

The difficulty with these experiments is not doing them but interpreting them. Suppose an intervention decreases the maximal response to Gpp(NH)p by 50%. Is this due to decreased activity of G_s or increased activity of G_i? Because the proteins share subunits, their interaction must always be considered. Hsia et al. (67) have shown that maximal activation of adenylate cyclase in cultured NG108-15 cells occurs after treatment with both cholera and pertussis toxins, suggesting a tonic inhibitory influence of G_i at least in those cells. One way to try to get around the problem is to take advantage of the sensitivity of the inhibitory system to Mn^{2+}. Mn^{2+} at 1 mM uncouples hormonal inhibition of adenylate cyclase (63) but does not affect G_s coupling to C (7). If an observed difference in responsiveness to Gpp(NH)p or GTP persists with 1 mM Mn^{2+}, then it is likelier to be due to a difference in G_s activities.

It might seem that treating membranes with pertussis toxin would be another way to inactivate the inhibitory system. However, as will be discussed in greater detail later, pertussis toxin treatment does not always block inhibition by Gpp(NH)p even when it blocks hormonal inhibition (37).

GTPase

Cassel and Selinger (24) showed that turkey erythrocytes contain an isoproterenol-stimulated GTPase activity. As would be expected, this GTPase was a very small fraction of the total GTPase activity, even though Cassel and Selinger set up the assay in such a way as to inhibit nonspecific nucleotide hydrolysis. Despite such precautions, it has proved difficult to demonstrate hormonal stimulation of GTP hydrolysis in other cells. However, Lester et al. (98) were able to lower background GTPase activity by treating platelet membranes with N-ethylmaleimide. This lowered the background activity to a sixth of the original level and allowed the investigators to measure a 46% increase in GTP hydrolysis by PGE_1.

The authors verified that *N*-ethylmaleimide did not grossly affect hormonal stimulation of GTPase activity by comparing the GTPases of turkey erythrocytes before and after *N*-ethylmaleimide treatment. However, it is now known that G_i is very sensitive to *N*-ethylmaleimide. Because the G_s and G_i proteins share common subunits, anything that affects one may affect the other. If hormonally activated GTPase can be measured only after alkylation of membranes, then the results should be interpreted with caution.

To be sure that any hormone-dependent increase in GTPase activity is actually due to increased activity of the G_s GTPase, it is important to demonstrate that the hormone dose–response relation is similar to that for adenylate cyclase activation, that the GTPase has a low K_m for GTP (0.1–0.2×10^{-6} M), and that the increase in GTPase activity can be blocked by cholera toxin. Pike and Lefkowitz (138) showed that agonist-induced desensitization of frog and turkey erythrocytes to adrenergic stimulation affected both adenylate cyclase and hormone-sensitive GTPase activities. This confirmed the conclusion that measuring hormonally stimulated GTPase activity is a useful way to assay G_s function.

Because of the problems produced by high background GTPase activity in many tissues, Cassel et al. (21) proposed another assay to measure GTP hydrolysis by measuring the rate at which adenylate cyclase activity is turned off. The enzyme is first activated by hormone and GTP. The activation is stopped either by adding GDPβS [guanosine 5'-*O*-(2-thiodiphosphate)], a nonhydrolyzable GDP analogue (49), or by a hormone antagonist. The rate of decay of adenylate cyclase then reflects the rate of hydrolysis of GTP at the active site of G_s. The rate constant for GTP hydrolysis is 6.2 to 10 min^{-1} for turkey erythrocytes, rat parotid, and rat liver enzymes.

Hormone-Receptor-Stimulated Guanyl Nucleotide Exchange

Because hormone receptors increase the turnover of the G_s-associated GTPase, they should also stimulate release of nucleotides. The procedure to measure release of guanine nucleotides bound to G_s was described by Cassel and Selinger (26). Membranes can be incubated with [^{3}H]GTP or [^{32}P]GTP in the presence of hormone to fill available sites on G_s, then washed free of unbound nucleotide, and incubated with unlabeled GTP in the absence of hormone to displace GTP from nonspecific sites and to decrease the background of the assay. The appropriate hormone agonist is then added to release the bound nucleotides. The hormone-induced release of [^{3}H]GDP is defined as the difference between the amounts of nucleotide displaced by Gpp(NH)p with and without hormone. Release of [^{3}H]GDP should follow the same time course and have the same hormone concentration dependence and specificity as activation of adenylate cyclase.

Pike and Lefkowitz (138) used the assay described by Cassel and Selinger to compare β-adrenergic responses in frog and turkey erythrocytes. They found that in the former, release of [^{3}H]GDP was strictly dependent on hormone stimulation, whereas in frog red cell membranes some [^{3}H]GDP release occurred spontaneously. These authors further found that PGE$_1$ was able to release the nucleotide loaded in the presence of a β-adrenergic agonist. These data suggest that PGE$_1$ and β-adrenergic receptors interact with a common pool of G_s proteins in the membranes. This observation could be generalized to study interactions among stimulatory receptors in any cell.

It should be noted that experiments of this type are very different from simply measuring guanine nucleotide binding to membranes. There are too many guanine-nucleotide-binding proteins that are not related to adenylate cyclase regulation to allow any certainty that the adenylate-cyclase-linked proteins can be identified. In studies of nucleotide exchange, it matters less how much nucleotide is bound, because only that which is released by hormone is considered.

Suidan et al. (167) refined the measurement of guanyl-nucleotide exchange by showing that hormone receptors change the ability of GDPβS to inhibit Gpp(NH)p-stimulated adenylate cyclase activity. Thus, in pineal membranes, β-adrenergic agonists increase the rate of activation of adenylate cyclase by Gpp(NH)p by about 40-fold and decrease the inhibitory potency of GDPβS by 1,000-fold. This reflects the same phenomenon as measured by hormone-stimulated GDP release: the decrease in affinity of G_s for GDP produced by agonist-liganded hormone receptors. In some cells, such as turkey erythrocytes, release of GDP and activation by Gpp(NH)p are strictly dependent on hormone receptor activation, so results can be quite clean. In most others, some activation by Gpp(NH)p occurs without hormone receptors, although at a slower rate, and there is some slow release of GDP. Thus, the signal-to-noise ratio may not be favorable. By measuring the change in inhibitory potency of GDPβS, the capacity of receptors to facilitate a functional exchange between GDPβS and Gpp(NH)p can be evaluated and compared even in those cells in which coupling of G_s to receptors is not very tight.

ADP-Ribosylation by Cholera Toxin

One of the earliest ways developed to measure the amount of N_s was to use the enzymatic activity of cholera toxin. Cholera toxin catalyzes the transfer of ADP-ribose from NAD to membrane proteins with molecular weights of 42 to 52 kd (44,50,52). Most membranes have only the lower-molecular-weight form of cholera toxin substrate (42–46 kd), whereas others have both this lower-molecular-weight form and another substrate with a molecular weight of 47 to 52 kd (80,125). The component of G_s can be readily ribosylated in membranes, but can be modified after solubilization only if a protein factor is added (157). In many tissues, ADP-ribosylation requires a poorly defined cytosolic factor in addition to the components of the reaction mixture to be described later. Therefore, initial experiments are often performed on unfractionated homogenates that contain both the membrane-bound substrates and the cytosolic factor. Complete [^{32}P]ADP-ribosylation of G_s typically requires [^{32}P]NAD (5 M), cholera toxin that has been "activated" with dithiothreitol and SDS to liberate the enzymatic A_1 peptide (about 10–20 μg/ml), and GTP or one of its nonhydrolyzable analogues. Thymidine (10 mM) is often added to restrict interference from nuclear poly(ADP-ribose)polymerase. The thymidine blocks the appearance of free poly(ADP-ribose), which would otherwise appear on autoradiograms as a "ladder" of bands from decamers to unmeasurably large. It does allow a small amount of labeling of the poly(ADP-ribose)polymerase itself (M_r = 115,000). ADP-ribosylation is sometimes increased and the background on gels is usually decreased by the addition of ADP-ribose. Finally, a high NADase activity in the cell homogenate will inhibit ADP-ribosylation by destroying the substrate. Isonicotinic acid hydrazide (INH) is an effective inhibitor of NAD glycohydrolases, and inclusion of 1 mM INH can enhance ADP-ribosylation (126).

Although cholera-toxin-catalyzed incorporation of [^{32}P]ADP-ribose into the $α_s$ component can be quantitated, the conditions of the experiment must be very carefully controlled. We have recently shown that the distribution of ADP-ribose between the smaller and larger forms of $α_s$ is variable and can be experimentally manipulated. The smaller-molecular-weight $α_s$ component tends to dominate when total labeling is low for any one of a variety of reasons and may in some cases be the only detectable product. Conversely, the larger $α_s$ band is usually more intensely labeled under conditions that give more complete labeling, and this can be easily achieved by raising the NAD concentration (126).

Nonhydrolyzable analogues of GTP such as GTPγS or Gpp(NH)p enhance ADP-ribosylation by cholera toxin. These guanine nucleotides also dissociate $α_s$ from the $β·γ$ component. However, the enhancement in labeling does not seem to be a result of dissociation of the components, because fluoride, which also dissociates $α_s$ from $β·γ$, does not enhance ADP-ribosylation (51).

Inhibitory Guanine Nucleotide Regulatory Unit and Related Proteins

Guanine Nucleotide Inhibition of Adenylate Cyclase and Related Assays

There are so many similarities in the functions of stimulatory and inhibitory guanine nucleotide regulatory proteins that parallel methods can be used to study both. For example, Michel and Lefkowitz (112) used

[^{3}H]Gpp(NH)p release from membranes to measure the interaction of inhibitory $α_2$-adrenergic receptors with G_i. Nevertheless, there are some methodological differences. Inhibition of adenylate cyclase by hormones and guanine nucleotides is more sensitive to proteolysis, alkylating agents, and organic mercurials than is stimulation (170). Other assays of G_i function are also likely to be sensitive to these agents. For instance, sodium blocks GTP inhibition of adenylate cyclase and also decreases the hormone-sensitive GTPase associated with an inhibitory receptor (95).

ADP-Ribosylation by Pertussis Toxin

Just as cholera toxin was used to quantitate the amount of $α_s$ in membranes, another bacterial toxin, pertussis toxin, can be used to label the $α$ component of G_i. Pertussis toxin transfers ADP-ribose to a 41-kd protein present in most membranes tested (169). In addition, in some membranes, including those from heart, a second labeled band is seen at 39 kd (54,110,124). It is not clear if both proteins are involved in mediating hormonal inhibition of adenylate cyclase or if both the pertussis toxin substrates can also interact with other membrane effectors.

The general conditions for labeling with pertussis toxin are very similar to those developed for cholera toxin. There are a few differences, however. Labeling by pertussis toxin seems to have no requirement for a cytosolic factor and goes equally well in membranes as in solubilized systems. Whereas ADP-ribosylation with cholera toxin can be enhanced by very low concentrations of detergents sufficient to permeabilize membrane vesicles, cholera toxin usually will not ADP-ribosylate solubilized enzyme components. In contrast, pertussis toxin works very well on solubilized substrates. ADP-ribosylation by pertussis toxin requires the presence of ATP and GTP and is strongly inhibited by nonhydrolyzable analogues of GTP such as GTPγS (124). That is because the true substrate for pertussis toxin ADP-ribosylation is not the $α$ component but the $α·β·γ$ complex (104). Because this is the case, pertussis toxin measures not only the quantity of the $α$ component but also that of the $β·γ$ component. If something changes the amount of $β·γ$ so that there is not sufficient $β·γ$ to complex with all the $α$ present in the membrane, the consequence will be decreased ADP-ribosylation of the $α$ protein. This will happen even though the amount of $α$ protein itself has not changed. It is important to bear this possibility in mind when interpreting the effects of perturbations in cell function on the amount of ADP-ribose incorporated into the 41-kd or 39-kd proteins.

STUDIES OF SOLUBILIZED ADENYLATE CYCLASE

To understand in detail how adenylate cyclase works, one must understand its structure. To define the structure and the interaction of components, one needs to dissect the system, isolate and assay the individual components, and eventually reassemble the whole in a functional form. The first step of this process requires the use of detergents to solubilize adenylate cyclase, because the enzyme is firmly membrane-bound in all eukaryotic cells except those from the mature testis (19,119). Depending on the detergent used, the enzyme is solubilized in association with the regulatory components or dissociated from them. In general, nonionic detergents solubilize a complex of catalytic unit and guanine nucleotide regulatory units, whereas ionic detergents such as cholate seem to be more effective detergents when separation of the components is desired.

Although guanine-nucleotide-sensitive adenylate cyclase has been solubilized with several nonionic detergents, Lubrol 12A9 (available from Sigma) has been consistently the most useful. Even this detergent, however, inhibits adenylate cyclase at concentrations required to solubilize it. Therefore, in each system, an empirical balance must be struck between yield of solubilized enzyme and the deleterious effect of the detergent on activity.

Solubilization of the myocardial enzyme was first reported by Levey (100). Approximately 90% of the enzyme activity was solubilized with 1.2% Lubrol PX (which is the same as Lubrol 12A9) in 0.25 M sucrose, 0.2 M Tris-Cl (pH 7.4), and 1 mM EDTA-MgCl$_2$. Drummond and Dunham (41), modified the procedure by adding 1 mM dithiothreitol to the buffer. These authors found a marked inhibition by Lubrol PX unless assays were conducted below 26°C. Homcy et al. (64) used 1% Brij 35, a similar nonionic detergent, in 10 mM Tris-Cl (pH 7.4), 5 mM MgCl$_2$, and 1 mM dithiothreitol to solubilize the enzyme from canine myocardium. The yield of enzyme was not given.

One of the reasons for wide variations from laboratory to laboratory in yield of solubilized enzyme may be the relative crudity of commercially available preparations of detergents. They are synthesized for industrial purposes, not biochemical purposes. An informal survey of the colors of Lubrol PX or Lubrol 12A9 obtained by different laboratories showed that the range is from dark orange to water-clear. We routinely stir new stock 20% solutions (w/v) of Lubrol 12A9 with a mixed-bed resin (Biorad) overnight before using the detergent. The detergent is stored at 4°C. Another problem is that epoxides may form in aqueous solutions of detergents over time and may affect results (99).

Detergent-solubilized adenylate cyclase from most tissues can be stimulated by fluoride and stimulated or inhibited by guanine nucleotides. However, it usually does not respond to hormone. A number of reports over the years have described solubilization of adenylate cyclase that is still responsive to hormone (101). However, none of the methods reported has proved to be generally and reproducibly useful.

One of the purposes of solubilizing an enzyme is to be able to study its structure. A start toward this goal is to determine its size, its shape, and its hydrophobicity. Because nonionic detergents bind to specific hydrophobic regions on proteins, the amount of detergent bound may reveal how much of the protein's surface is hydrophobic and available for interaction with membrane lipids or hydrophobic membrane proteins. Helenius and Simons (59) and Clarke (30) showed that a number of proteins that were known on independent grounds to span the lipid bilayer of the membrane bind large amounts of nonionic detergent (0.2–1.1 mg detergent/mg protein). Soluble proteins bind virtually no detergent, because their hydrophobic amino acids are located in the interior of the molecule. Membrane proteins that associate with a large amount of detergent can do so in two ways: They can insert into detergent micelles, as does glycophorin, or they can combine with individual detergent molecules like the band-3 protein of the erythrocyte membrane (30).

Because adenylate cyclase has not yet been purified to homogeneity, one cannot measure detergent binding directly using radioactively labeled detergent. However, one can exploit the partial specific volume, $\bar{v}$, of detergent to estimate the amount of detergent bound. The partial specific volume for most proteins is 0.73 to 0.74 ml/g, and the partial specific volume of Lubrol 12A9 or Triton X-100 is 0.94 to 0.98 ml/g (53,162). A complex of protein and detergent has a partial specific volume intermediate between these and proportional to the fraction of detergent and protein in the complex. If one measures the partial specific volume of adenylate cyclase, in the presence and absence of detergent, one can calculate the amount of detergent bound, assuming the protein itself has a value for $\bar{v}$ similar to that for a typical protein. The partial specific volume of an impure enzyme can be determined by measuring its rate of sedimentation (relative to marker proteins of known $\bar{v}$) in sucrose density gradients made up in H$_2$O and D$_2$O. The methods for performing such analysis and calculating the results have been described previously (117,118). Adenylate cyclase solubilized from different sources seems to fall into two categories: enzyme that seems to bind very little detergent and to be rather hydrophilic in solution, and enzyme that binds 25 to 30% of its mass in detergent (120). The hydrophobicity of the cardiac enzyme has not yet been determined. The physical basis for the difference in detergent binding is not yet known.

The sucrose density-gradient experiments give not only the partial specific volume but also the sedimentation coefficient of the solubilized adenylate cyclase. By eluting the enzyme from gel filtration columns together with calibrating enzymes of known Stokes radius, the Stokes radius of the enzyme in detergent can be determined. From these three experimentally determined values ($\bar{v}$, sedimentation coefficient, and Stokes radius), the molecular weight of the detergent-protein complex can be calculated, as well as the molecular weight of its protein component (117,118).

In performing these experiments, certain precautions must be observed. First, the density-gradient centrifugation and the gel filtration of the enzyme must be carried out under identical conditions, insofar as is possible, i.e., the same salt concentration, pH, reducing agents, temperature. Second, the detergent used must have a partial specific volume very different from that of a typical protein. Otherwise, the change in $\bar{v}$ due to the contribution of the detergent is very hard to detect. In a detergent whose $\bar{v}$ is similar to those of proteins (cholate, for example), one can determine only the molecular weight of the detergent-protein complex, not the fraction of that complex that is protein. Third, it is important to include the marker proteins in the sample being analyzed by sucrose density-gradient centrifugation or gel filtration. This is much more accurate than running parallel columns or gradients, especially when small differences in sedimentation rates or Stokes radii need to be determined.

Lubrol 12A9, Triton X-100, Brij 56, and Nonidet NP40 are all detergents with high $\bar{v}$ values and low critical micelle concentrations; so they are useful for determination of detergent binding. However, they have certain disadvantages: They have large micelle sizes that elute close to adenylate cyclase from gel filtration columns. Thus, it is difficult to free the enzyme of detergent by gel filtration or by dialysis. These detergents also precipitate in high concentrations of salt, so that one cannot free the enzyme of detergent by precipitating the protein with ammonium sulfate.

Of the ionic detergents, the bile salts and their derivatives have proved the most useful in studies of adenylate cyclase. Both cholate, an ionic detergent, and CHAPS, a zwitterionic detergent, have been used to solubilize adenylate cyclase in a form such that the catalytic unit can be readily separated from the guanine-nucleotide-binding proteins. Very similar methods were independently developed by Strittmatter and Neer (166) and by Ross and Gilman (144) to resolve the catalytic component from bovine cerebral cortex and rabbit liver, respectively.

Strittmatter and Neer (166) solubilized approximately 50% of the enzyme activity in crude bovine cerebral cortical brains with 14 mM cholate and 1.2 M $(NH_4)_2SO_4$. The need for high-ionic-strength buffer emphasizes the fact that solubilization may depend on factors other than the hydrophobic interactions of the detergent with the protein. The high ionic strength may affect the structure of adenylate cyclase, or it may modify the conformation of other proteins in the membrane and so allow access of the detergent to otherwise inaccessible sites. The properties of adenylate cyclase solubilized with cholate and ammonium sulfate are very different from those of the enzyme solubilized with nonionic detergents. After gel filtration over Sepharose 6B equilibrated with cholate, ammonium sulfate, and phospholipids, activity was virtually unmeasurable with Mg^{2+} and ATP, but was activated 8- to 15-fold by addition of Mn^{2+}. It was unresponsive to stimulation by guanine nucleotides. Adenylate cyclase in the membrane or after solubilization with Lubrol is activated only 2- to 3-fold by Mn^{2+} (121).

The requirement for Mn^{2+} to express catalytic activity, together with an absence of response to Gpp(NH)p, suggested that gel filtration in cholate and ammonium sulfate had separated the catalytic unit from the guanine nucleotide regulatory unit. The combination of a Mn^{2+} requirement and a lack of response to guanine nucleotides occurs in other instances: the soluble testicular enzyme, adenylate cyclase from mutant S49 lymphoma cells that lack a functional G_s (19,119,144). The guanine nucleotide regulatory unit can be located in the column effluent by its ability to reconstitute guanine nucleotide responsiveness to the separated catalytic unit. The same factor restores fluoride responsiveness to the catalytic unit. For the reconstitution to take place, cholate must first be removed from the components either by precipitating them with ammonium sulfate (163) or by diluting the column fractions 5- to 10-fold into Tris buffer without detergent or ammonium sulfate (7).

The conditions for separating C from G_s developed by Ross and Gilman (144) differ somewhat from those described earlier. Ross and Gilman precipitated the solubilized preparation with 2 M $(NH_4)_2SO_4$ before gel filtration over Ultrogel AcA34 equilibrated and eluted with 0.1 M Tris-Cl (pH 8), 1 mM EDTA, 0.5 mM dithiothreitol, and 0.5 M $(NH_4)_2SO_4$/12 mM Na cholate. Their column buffer did not include Mg^{2+} or phospholipids. We found the enzyme to be more stable when phospholipids were included. However, their inclusion makes it impossible to study the effects of specific lipids on activity or reconstitution as Ross (142) went on to do.

This laboratory has used the same method to separate the catalytic unit of canine myocardial adenylate cyclase from G_s as was used for bovine cerebral cortex (*unpublished data*). The gel filtration was carried out in phospholipids, and the catalytic unit thus prepared was stable at $-70°C$ for many months. Ten to twenty grams of tissue are sufficient to produce enough catalytic unit for a very large number of reconstitution experiments. If the catalytic unit is to be used only as a means of assaying G_s activity, there is no particular advantage to using cardiac catalytic unit that has about one-tenth the activity of catalytic unit from bovine cerebral cortex or caudate nucleus. Catalytic unit from bovine cerebral cortex or caudate nucleus has been used to reconstitute G_s activity from rat testes, canine heart, and rat kidney. Therefore, the abilities of the catalytic unit and guanine nucleotide regulatory unit to interact seem to have been extremely well preserved over evolution.

Other methods for preparing catalytic unit have been described, although they have been used less than the cholate/ammonium sulfate method. Bitonti et al. (11) reported separation of catalytic unit from G_s after solubilization with CHAPS detergent. Drummond and Dunham (40) reported partial separation of catalytic and G_s units after DEAE chromatography of Lubrol-solubilized skeletal muscle adenylate cyclase. Pfeuffer and Helmreich (134) separated pigeon erythrocyte C from G_s by GTP affinity chromatography. For reasons that are not clear, the method has been useful only with avian erythrocytes.

PURIFICATION OF ADENYLATE CYCLASE COMPONENTS

Catalytic Unit

The catalytic unit of adenylate cyclase is notoriously unstable and has therefore been difficult to purify. Homcy et al. (64) reported substantial purification of myocardial adenylate cyclase using affinity chromatography. An important step in the purification was hydrophobic chromatography over a dodecyl-Sepharose column that removed many hydrophobic proteins. Following hydrophobic chromatography, the adenylate cyclase remained soluble without detergents, making subsequent purification steps more effective.

A promising ligand for purification of adenylate cyclase has been described by Pfeuffer and Metzger (135). They purified myocardial adenylate cyclase using an immobilized forskolin derivative as an affinity ligand.

Adenylate cyclase probably makes up no more than 0.01% of plasma membrane proteins, so that complete purification is a formidable task. It is not known what the specific activity of a purified preparation ought to be. We have been able to measure specific activities of 0.1 μmol cAMP/mg/min by activating the catalytic unit with G_s, Mn^{2+}, and forskolin. By protein staining of an SDS polyacrylamide gel, the sample is barely distinguishable from the total solubilized protein. Therefore, the specific activity of entirely pure, activated adenylate cyclase should be at least 1 μmol cAMP/mg/min. Assuming a polypeptide molecular weight of 150,000, the turnover number would be 150 moles product per mole of enzyme per minute at that specific activity. Thus, pure adenylate cyclase should have a turnover number similar to those of other enzymes. Some reported purifications of adenylate cyclase yield enzymes with turnover numbers of less than 1 mol product per mole of enzyme per minute. In those cases, the author must establish firmly that the protein isolated is, indeed, adenylate cyclase, because a low level of activity could come from an amount of enzyme too small to be detected on as SDS polyacrylamide gel.

Measurement of G_s Activity in Solution

Once the G_s unit has been solubilized from the membrane, its activity can be measured by reconstitution with the catalytic unit either in cyc-S49 lymphoma cell mutant membranes (145) or with resolved catalytic unit prepared as described earlier. The G_s protein has been solubilized from many sources (liver, brain, turkey erythrocytes, human erythrocytes, heart) with several kinds of detergents. For purification of G_s, which will be described later, the most commonly used detergent is cholate.

Reconstitution of the catalytic unit with the G_s unit does not require that the proteins be put into lipid vessels. The interaction between α_s and the catalytic unit seems to be a simple protein-protein interaction. In order to activate the catalytic unit, the G_s unit must be liganded either with guanine nucleotides or with fluoride. Activation of solubilized G_s by guanine nucleotides does not occur instantaneously. Just as there is a lag in activation of the catalytic unit by guanine nucleotides in membranes, so there is a time dependence to the activation of G_s in solution. An important early experiment in setting up reconstitution assays is to determine the time required for maximum activation of G_s. This can vary from a few minutes at 30°C to 1 hr in the case of G_s solubilized from brain (125). The rate of activation of G_s depends on several factors. Activation is speeded by increasing the magnesium concentration (57). The rate can also be increased by adding ammonium sulfate (125). Although the maximal level of activity depends on the concentration of guanine nucleotides, the rate of activation is independent of the guanine nucleotide concentration (127).

One interfering factor in an assay of G_s activity in crude supernatants is the fact that the detergent that solubilizes G_s also solubilizes adenylate cyclase activity. In some cases, this activity is much less than that contributed by the catalytic unit and can be blanked out simply by doing assays with and without added catalytic unit. For instance, cholate at low ionic strength solubilizes very little adenylate cyclase activity from brain, so that cholate extracts can easily be assayed directly. In contrast, Lubrol 12A9 solubilizes both G_s and a large amount of catalytic adenylate cyclase activity. This must be separated from G_s before the extract can be conveniently assayed. Because the sizes of adenylate cyclase and G_s are quite different, the separation is easily achieved by gel filtration over Sepharose 6B (125).

It is very important to remember that the G_s unit does not have an intrinsic activity, but is acting to stimulate a second protein. What is actually being measured is the activity of the catalytic unit. The reaction is a bimolecular one and depends both on the concentration of G_s and on the concentration of the catalytic unit. Activation of the catalytic unit can be used as a way of quantitating the amount of G_s activity that is present in an extract, provided the conditions are very carefully standardized. If a single preparation of the catalytic unit is used, then relative amounts of G_s can be determined and will be proportional to the activation of the catalytic unit. However, different preparations of catalytic unit respond with slightly different concentration dependences and reach slightly different maximal levels of activation. Therefore, it is difficult to compare increments in adenylate cyclase activity from preparation to preparation.

A better way to calculate the activation of the catalytic unit by G_s is to measure the rates of activation of different amounts of the catalytic unit by different concentrations of G_s. This method is decribed in detail by Sternweis et al. (164). For such data to be meaningful, it is essential to know that the guanine nucleotide regulatory unit has been completely activated by either fluoride or nonhydrolyzable guanine nucleotides before the start of the assay. These conditions should be determined by the kinetic experiments described earlier.

Measurement of G_i in Solution

The detergents that solubilize G_s also solubilize the inhibitory guanine-nucleotide-binding protein (G_i). Assaying the activity of G_i in solution is more difficult than assaying the activity of G_s. Direct recombination of α_i with catalytic unit does not lead to inhibition (J. W. Winslow and E. J. Neer, *unpublished data*). The α_i activity can be measured by reconstituting into platelet membranes that have previously been treated with pertussis toxin to inactivate the endogenous α_i activity. This assay is well described by Katada et al. (88). In principle, any membrane in which all endogenous α_i can be ADP-ribosylated by pertussis toxin could act as an acceptor for solubilized α_i.

Because ADP-ribosylation by pertussis toxin proceeds very well in the presence of detergent (in contrast to ADP-ribosylation catalyzed by cholera toxin), the amount of α_i could be quantitated by this means. However, the true substrate for ADP-ribosylation is not α_i but the $\alpha_i \cdot \beta \cdot \gamma$ complex. Therefore, the amount of ADP-ribose incorporated depends not only on the amount of α_i but also on the amount of $\beta \cdot \gamma$ present. The relative amounts of α_i and $\beta \cdot \gamma$ have not been measured in many tissues, but where they have been estimated it seems that there are enough or more than enough $\beta \cdot \gamma$ subunits to interact with all the α_i present (70).

In brain, but not in other tissues, the 39-kd pertussis toxin substrate makes up approximately 0.5% of total membrane protein. In this tissue, therefore, binding of GTPγS can be used as a way to measure the amount of the 39-kd protein. Compared with this very large amount of the 39-kd protein, the other guanine-nucleotide-binding proteins are present in small quantities and do not contribute greatly to the binding assay. Nonneural tissues seem to contain much less of the pertussis toxin substrates than does brain, and therefore direct guanine nucleotide binding as a measure of these proteins becomes difficult to interpret.

Measurement of $\beta \cdot \gamma$ Activity in Solution

The activity of $\beta \cdot \gamma$ in solution can be measured in one of two ways. $\beta \cdot \gamma$ inhibits activation of G_s by guanine nucleotides. This observation can form the basis for a quantitative assay (128). The rate of activation of a standard preparation of G_s is determined with and without increasing dilutions of a solution containing $\beta \cdot \gamma$. In crude solution, $\beta \cdot \gamma$ activity can be measured only after incubation in 10 mM MgCl$_2$, 10 mM NaF, and 20 μM AlCl$_3$ at 30°C for 30 min. This treatment presumably dissociates $\beta \cdot \gamma$ from the components. By comparing the effect on activation of G_s of the unknown solution with the effect of pure $\beta \cdot \gamma$ at known concentration, the amount of $\beta \cdot \gamma$ in the test solution can be determined.

Another assay for $\beta \cdot \gamma$ activity depends on the observation that $\beta \cdot \gamma$ enhances ADP-ribosylation of α_i. In this situation, pure α_i is used as the substrate, and ADP-ribosylation is measured as a function of increasing amounts of an unknown solution. In such an assay, the endogenous α_i in the crude $\beta \cdot \gamma$ extract would be ribosylated as well as the pure substrate. If the endogenous ADP-ribosylation is high compared with the amount of ADP-ribose that can be incorporated into the purified protein, then the signal-to-noise ratio will become unacceptably large.

Purification of G_s and G_i

The procedures to purify both of these proteins will be discussed together, because the same general methods are used to purify both. The methods published for the purification of these proteins have all been variants of the procedure originally described by Northup et al. (130) and Sternweis et al. (164) for purification of G_s from rabbit liver. G_s was solubilized with cholate and fractionated by DEAE Sephacel chromatography and gel filtration. An extremely important step in the purification is hydrophobic chromatography over heptylamine Sepharose. This resin is not available commercially and must be synthesized by the method of Shalteil (158). The synthesis involves cyanogen bromide activation of Sepharose CL4B, followed by coupling with heptylamine. Once made, the resin can be used many times after regeneration with urea (164). The hydrophobic chromatography step is followed by two or three further ion-exchange or gel-filtration separations. Procedures for purifying G_s and G_i, either with or without activating ligands, have already been described in great detail (33,35,56,57,124,125). In our experience in purifying the proteins from bovine brain, it was very helpful to add a DEAE-Sephacel column before the heptylamine Sepharose step (125).

It is very important that the cholate be purified prior to use for purification, because as supplied by the manufacturer it contains a number of impurities. We routinely make 10 liters of a 3 to 4% solution of Tris cholate. This is passed over a 5 × 30-cm DEAE-Sephacel column that has been equilibrated with 0.05 M Tris-HCl, pH 8. Because cholate is an ionic detergent, it binds to the DEAE-Sephacel, and much more than a column volume must go through before cholate begins to be eluted. The effluent is periodically tested by adding HCl to a small sample. Cholate precipitates in acid, and it is readily apparent when it is beginning to elute from the column. All the rest of the cholate is then collected in a single batch. A tarry brown material accumulates at the top of the column. The cholate is precipitated by adding HCl to bring the pH of the solution down to 4. It is collected by filtration and washed several times with ether, which is then to evaporate.

The guanine-nucleotide-binding proteins have been purified after activation by fluoride or in the unliganded form. There are advantages to both procedures. Activation by fluoride tends to dissociate the α_s and $\beta \cdot \gamma$ subunits. Nevertheless, for reasons that are not well understood, the final product always has both α_s and $\beta \cdot \gamma$ components in it. Activation also dissociates the G_i proteins, but unlike the situation with α_s it is relatively easy to purify these individually. Because the affinity of α_{39} for $\beta \cdot \gamma$ is less than the affinity of α_{41} for $\beta \cdot \gamma$, the former is easier to obtain in large quantities uncontaminated by $\beta \cdot \gamma$ than is the latter (71). Although a ligand may stabilize α_s and α_i, it must be removed for further studies, and this means that an additional step must be added. One way to deactivate G_s is to pass it over hydroxyl apatite, as described by Northup et al. (130). Although this is very effective at producing deactivation, in brain it also leads to unacceptably large losses of activity. Fluoride can be removed from α_{41}, α_{39}, and $\beta \cdot \gamma$ simply by passage over a Sephadex G25 (Pharmacia) column.

The specific activity of G_s depends on the amount of C in the assay. Sternweis et al. (164) measured the amount of fully activated G_s needed to activate the C in different amounts of cyc membrane. Adenylate cyclase activity was plotted against G_s concentration. The curves were consistent with a simple bimolecular reaction in which

$$G_s + C \rightleftharpoons G_s \cdot C$$

Sternweis et al. (164) then derived the relationship between the initial slopes of the curves and the amount of functional catalytic unit present. A plot of the inverse of the initial slope against the inverse of the maximal activity (V_{max}) for each amount of C gave a straight line. Extrapolating the curve to infinite C concentration ($1/V_{max} = 0$) gives a specific activity of G_s (μmol min^{-1} mg^{-1}) that is independent of the amount of C in a particular assay.

One factor in determining the specific activity of pure G_s is an accurate measure of activity. An accurate determination of the protein is equally important and sometimes harder to get. If the total yield after a large preparation is a few hundred micrograms (as is typical for G_s), the investigator is loathe to sacrifice a large amount to a Lowry protein determination (109). The most sensitive way to obtain an accurate measure is to submit a sample to total acid hydrolysis and automated amino acid analysis. The mass of the amino acids measured is summed to give the total protein. About 2 to 3 μg of protein is sufficient for the determination. It is important to submit a buffer blank for analysis when using this method.

GTPase Activity of Purified Components

As described earlier, membranes that contain hormone-sensitive adenylate cyclase also contain a hormone-sensitive GTPase. The GTPase is a property of the guanine nucleotide regulatory units and can be inhibited by treatment with cholera toxin or pertussis toxin. It would be expected, therefore, that the purified solubilized components would have GTPase activity. In fact, all of the components do have this activity. Measuring the GTPase activity of purified components is a much simpler matter than measuring the GTPase activity of crude preparations, because all the contaminating GTPases have been separated away. Therefore, the assay mix can be much simpler and consists of 0.2 to 0.5 μM GTP and 2 to 10 mM magnesium, and a buffer to keep the pH between 7.6 and 8. The α_s component has no measurable GTPase as purified, because the Lubrol 12A9 used in the last step is a strong inhibitor of enzymatic activity (18). However, enzymatic activity can be measured after reconstitution of α_s into lipid vesicles, and the GTPase activity can be increased if, in addition, a hormone receptor is included in the vesicles. The GTPase activity of the α_{39} protein can be measured in Lubrol and in cholate without any reconstitution. The activity of α_{41} from brain is much lower than the activity of α_{39}. The α_{41} protein from liver has been reconstituted into the vesicles, and the GTPase activity is both measurable and enhanced by hormone receptors. Although easily measurable, the GTPase activities of all the components under all circumstances are very low compared with those of other enzymes. The turnover number ranges from 0.2 to 2 mol of substrate cleaved per mole of enzyme per minute. The reason for this slowness of the reaction is not known, but it may be related to the fact that the basic function of the GTPase is regulatory, and it is not intended rapidly to break down GTP and to use the energy of hydrolysis for other metabolic ends.

Reconstitution of Purified Components

Activation of C by G_s does not require insertion of the protein into lipid vesicles. However, reconstitution of hormonal responsiveness seems to require that the proteins be assembled in the proper orientation in lipid vesicles. The first reconstitution of a hormone receptor with G_s was described for the β-adrenergic receptor (29) with the components still in membranes. Pederson and Ross (132) showed that purified hepatic G_s could be coupled to partially purified β-adrenergic receptors in lipid vesicles. Brandt et al. (17) went on to show that pure turkey erythrocyte β-adrenergic receptors could increase the GTPase activity of pure G_s from rabbit liver when the two were inserted into lipid vesicles.

The general protocol for reconstitution is that the pure proteins in detergent are mixed with lipids in detergent and the detergent is then slowly removed to allow the proteins and lipids to reassemble. Brandt et al. (17) made vesicles from dimyristoylphosphatidylcholine and polar lipids extracted from turkey red blood cell membranes. The original mixture also contained Lubrol 12A9, deoxycholate, and cholate. The detergent was removed by gel filtration over Sephadex G50.

A different method for removing detergent was used by Cerione et al. (28) to reconstitute hormone-sensitive adenylate cyclase activity. Pure β-adrenergic receptors from guinea pig lung, pure G_s from human erythrocyte membranes, and partially purified catalytic unit solubilized from bovine caudate nucleus (resolved from receptors and G_s by gel filtration) were mixed with soybean phosphatidylcholine and octylglucoside. The mixture also contained digitonin and cholate, which were carried over with the proteins. The detergents were removed on an Extracti-gel (Pierce Chemical Co.) column. The eluates were incubated with 12% polyethyleneglycol (6,000–8,000), diluted 10-fold with 100 mM NaCl, 10 mM Tris-Cl, and 1 mM dithiothreitol and centrifuged at $250,000 \times g$ for 1.5 hr to pellet the protein-containing vesicles. Isoproterenol increased adenylate cyclase activity twofold over that measured with GTP alone. The effect was stereospecific and was blocked by alprenolol.

These successful reconstitutions show the feasibility of reassembling the hormone response system from purified components. The approach allows the investigator to control the stoichiometry of the components and to define the minimum number of polypeptides needed for hormonal regulation of the enzyme.

ACKNOWLEDGMENTS

Supported by grants GM34571 from NIH and BC380A from the American Cancer Society.

REFERENCES

1. Aktories, K., Schultz, G., and Jakobs, K. H. (1979): Inhibition of hamster fat cell adenylate cyclase by prostaglandin E_1 and epinephrine: Requirement for GTP and sodium ions. *FEBS Lett.*, 107:100–104.
2. Abramowitz, J., and Birnbaumer, L. (1982): Properties of the hormonally responsive rabbit lutal adenylize cyclase: Effects of guanine nucleotides and magnesium ion on stimulation by gonadotropin and catecholamines. *Endocrinology*, 110:773–781.
3. Alexander, R. W., Galper, J. B., Neer, E. J., and Smith, T. W. (1982): $\gamma\beta$-adrenergic receptor in developing chick heart. *Biochem. J.*, 204:825–830.
4. Alvarez, R., and Bruno, J. J. (1977): Activation of cardiac adenylate cyclase: Hormonal modification of the magnesium ion requirement. *Proc. Natl. Acad. Sci. USA*, 74:92–95.
5. Asano, T., Katada, T., Gilman, A. G., and Ross, E. M. (1984): Activation of the inhibitory GTP-binding protein of adenylate cyclase, G_i, by β-adrenergic receptors in reconstituted phospholipid vesicles. *J. Biol. Chem.*, 259:9351–9354.
6. Baker, S. P., and Potter, L. T. (1981): A minor component of the binding of [^{3}H]guanine-5'-yl imidodiphosphate to cardiac membranes associated with the activation of adenylate cyclase. *J. Biol. Chem.*, 256:7925–7931.
7. Bender, J. L., and Neer, E. J. (1983): Properties of the adenylate cyclase catalytic unit from caudate nucleus. *J. Biol. Chem.*, 258: 2432–2439.
8. Bender, J., Wolf, L. G., and Neer, E. J. (1984): Interaction of forskolin with resolved adenylate cyclase components. *Adv. Cyclic Nucleotide Prot. Phosph. Res.*, 17:101–109.
9. Besch, H. R., Jr., Jones, L. R., Fleming, J. W., and Watanabe, A. M. (1977): Parallel unmasking of latent adenylate cyclase and (Na$^+$,K$^+$)-ATPase activities in cardiac sarcolemmal vesicles. *J. Biol. Chem.*, 252:7905–7908.
10. Birnbaumer, L., Stengel, D., Desmier, M., and Hanoune, J. (1983): Forskolin regulation of liver membrane adenylyl cyclase. *Eur. J. Biochem.*, 136:107–112.
11. Bitonti, A., Moss, J., Hjelmeland, L., and Vaughan, M. (1982): Resolution and activity of adenylate cyclase components in a zwitterionic cholate derivative [3[(3-cholamidopropyl)dimethylammonio]-1-propane sulfonate]. *Biochemistry*, 21:3650–3653.
12. Blume, A. J., Lichtentein, D., and Boone, G. (1979): Coupling of opiate receptors to adenylate cyclase: Requirement for Na$^+$ and GTP. *Proc. Natl. Acad. Sci. USA*, 76:5626–5630.
13. Bockaert, J., Cantau, B., and Sebben-Perez, M. (1984): Hormonal inhibition of adenylate cyclase, a crucial role for Mg^{2+}. *Mol. Pharmacol.*, 26:180–186.
14. Bokoch, G. M., and Gilman, A. G. (1984): Inhibition of receptor-mediated release of arachidonic acid by pertussis toxin. *Cell*, 39: 301–308.
15. Bokoch, G. M., Katada, T., Northup, J. K., Ui, M., and Gilman, A. G. (1984): Purification and properties of the inhibitory guanine nucleotide-binding regulatory component of adenylate cyclase. *J. Biol. Chem.*, 259:3560–3567.
16. Bradford, P. G., and Rubin, R. P. (1985): Pertussis toxin inhibits chemotactic factor-induced phospholipase C stimulation and lysosomal enzyme secretion in rabbit neutrophils. *FEBS Lett.*, 183:317–320.
17. Brandt, D. R., Asano, T., Pedersen, S. E., and Ross, E. M. (1983): Reconstitution of catecholamine-stimulated guanosinetriphosphatase activity. *Biochemistry*, 22:4357–4362.
18. Brandt, D. R., and Ross, E. M. (1985): GTPase activity of the stimulatory GTP-binding regulatory protein of adenylate cyclase, G_s. *J. Biol. Chem.*, 260:266–272.
19. Braun, T., and Dods, R. (1975): Development of a Mn^{2+}-sensitive, "soluble" adenylate cyclase in rat testis. *Proc. Natl. Acad. Sci. USA*, 72:1097–1101.
20. Burns, D. L., Hewlett, E. L., Moss, J., and Vaughan, M. (1983): Pertussis toxin inhibits enkephalin stimulation of GTPase of NG108-15 cells. *J. Biol. Chem.*, 258:1435–1438.
21. Cassel, D., Eckstein, F., Lowe, M., and Selinger, Z. (1979): Determination of the turn-off reaction for the hormone-activated adenylate cyclase. *J. Biol. Chem.*, 254:9835–9838.
22. Cassel, D., Levkovitz, H., and Selinger, Z. (1977): The regulatory GTPase cycle of turkey erythrocyte adenylate cyclase. *J. Cyclic Nucleotide Res.*, 3:393–406.
23. Cassel, D., and Pfeuffer, T. (1978): Mechanism of cholera toxin action: Covalent modification of the guanyl nucleotide-binding protein of the adenylate cyclase system. *Proc. Natl. Acad. Sci. USA*, 75:2669–2673.
24. Cassel, D., and Selinger, Z. (1976): Cathecholamine-stimulated GTPase activity in turkey erythrocyte membranes. *Biochim. Biophys. Acta*, 452:538–551.
25. Cassel, D., and Selinger, Z. (1977): Mechanism of adenylate cyclase activation by cholera toxin: Inhibition of GTP hydrolysis at the regulatory site. *Proc. Natl. Acad. Sci. USA*, 74:3307–3311.
26. Cassel, D., and Selinger, Z. (1978): Mechanism of adenylate cyclase activation through the β-adrenergic receptor: Catecholamine-induced displacement of bound GDP by GTP. *Proc. Natl. Acad. Sci. USA*, 75:4155–4159.
27. Cech, S. Y., Broaddus, W., and Maguire, M. E. (1980): Adenylate

cyclase: The role of magnesium and other divalent cations. *Mol. Cell. Biochem.,* 33:67–92.

28. Cerione, R. A., Sibley, D. R., Codina, J., Benovic, J. L., Winslow, J., Neer, E. J., Birnbaumer, L., Caron, M. G., and Lefkowitz, R. J. (1984): Reconstitution of a hormone-sensitive adenylate cyclase system. *J. Biol. Chem.,* 259:9979–9982.

29. Citri, Y., and Schramm, M. (1982): Probing of the coupling site of the β-adrenergic receptor. Competition between different forms of the guanyl nucleotide binding protein for interaction with the receptor. *J. Biol. Chem.,* 257:13257–13262.

30. Clarke, S. (1975): The size and detergent binding of membrane proteins. *J. Biol. Chem.,* 250:5459–5469.

31. Codina, J., Hildebrandt, J. D., Birnbaumer, L., and Sekura, R. D. (1984): Effects of guanine nucleotides and Mg²⁺ on human erythrocyte Nᵢ and Nₛ, the regulatory components of adenylyl cyclase. *J. Biol. Chem.,* 259:11408–11418.

32. Codina, J., Hildebrandt, J., Iyengar, R., Birnbaumer, L., Sekura, R. D., and Manclark, C. R. (1983): Pertussis toxin substrate, the putative Nᵢ component of adenylyl cyclases, is an αβ heterodimer regulated by guanine nucleotide and magnesium. *Proc. Natl. Acad. Sci. USA,* 80:4276–4280.

33. Codina, J., Hildebrandt, J. D., Sekura, R. D., Birnbaumer, M., Bryan, J., Manclark, C. R., Iyengar, R., and Birnbaumer, L. (1984): Nₛ and Nᵢ, the stimulatory and inhibitory regulatory components of adenylyl cyclases. Purification of the human erythrocyte, proteins without the use of activating regulatory ligands. *J. Biol. Chem.,* 259:5871–5886.

34. Codina, J., Hildebrandt, J., Sunyer, T., Sekura, R. D., Manclark, C. R., Iyengar, R., and Birnbaumer, L. (1984): Mechanisms in vectorial receptor-adenylate cyclase signal transduction. *Adv. Cyclic Nucleotide Prot. Phosph. Res.,* 17:111–126.

35. Codina, J., Rosenthal, W., Hildebrandt, J. D., Sekura, R. D., and Birnbaumer, L. (1984): Updated protocols and comments on the purification without use of activating ligands of the coupling proteins Nₛ and Nᵢ of the hormone sensitive adenylyl cyclase. *J. Recept. Res.,* 4:411–442.

36. Cooper, D. M. F., Londos, C., and Rodbell, M. (1980): Adenosine receptor-mediated inhibition of rat cerebral cortical adenylate cyclase by a GTP-dependent process. *Mol. Pharmacol.,* 18:598–601.

37. Cote, T. E., Frey, E. A., and Sekura, R. D. (1984): Altered activity of the inhibitory guanyl nucleotide-binding component (Nᵢ) induced by pertussis toxin. *J. Biol. Chem.,* 259:8693–8698.

38. Daly, J. W., Padgett, W., and Seamon, K. B. (1982): Activation of cyclic AMP-generating systems in brain membranes and slices by the diterpene forskolin: Augmentation of receptor-mediated responses. *J. Neurochem.,* 38:532–544.

39. Darfler, F. J., Mahan, L. C., Koachman, A. M., and Insel, P. A. (1982): Stimulation by forskolin of intact S49 lymphoma cells involves the nucleotide regulatory protein of adenylate cyclase. *J. Biol. Chem.,* 257:11901–11907.

40. Drummond, G. I., and Dunham, J. (1978): Properties of detergent-dispersed myocardial adenylate cyclase. *Arch. Biochem. Biophys.,* 189:63–75.

41. Drummond, G. I., and Dunham, J. (1978): Adenylate cyclase in cardiac microsomal fractions. *J. Mol. Cell. Cardiol.,* 10:317–331.

42. Drummond, G. I., Sano, M., and Nambi, P. (1980): Skeletal muscle adenylate cyclase: Reconstitution of a fluoride and guanylnucleotide sensitivity. *Arch. Biochem. Biophys.,* 201:286–295.

43. Drummond, G. I., and Severson, D. L. (1974): Preparation and characterization of adenylate cyclase from heart and skeletal muscle. *Methods Enzymol.,* 38:143–149.

44. Enomoto, K., and Gill, D. M. (1980): Cholera toxin activation of adenylate cyclase. *J. Biol. Chem.,* 255:1252–1258.

45. Eckstein, F., Cassel, D., Levkovitz, H., Lowe, M., and Selinger, Z. (1979): Guanosine 5'-O-(2-thiodiphosphate): An inhibitor of adenylate cyclase stimulation by guanine nucleotides and fluoride ions. *J. Biol. Chem.,* 254:9829–9834.

46. Farjel, Z., Brickman, A. S., Kaslow, H. R., Brothers, V. M., and Bourne, H. R. (1980): Defect of receptor-cyclase coupling protein in pseudohypoparathyroidism. *N. Engl. J. Med.,* 303:237–242.

47. Florio, V. A., and Sternweis, P. C. (1985): Reconstitution of resolved muscarinic cholinergic receptors with purified GTP-binding proteins. *J. Biol. Chem.,* 260:3477–3483.

48. Franklin, P. H., and Hoss, W. (1984): Opiates stimulate low-Kₘ GTPase in brain. *J. Neurochem.,* 43:1132–1135.

49. Fricke, R. F., Queener, S. F., and Clark, C. M., Jr. (1980): Cardiac adenylate cyclase: Kinetics of synergistic activation by guanosine-5'-triphosphate (GTP) and glucagon. *J. Mol. Cell. Cardiol.,* 12:595–608.

50. Gill, D. M. (1982): In: *ADP-Ribosylation Reactions,* edited by O. Hayaishi and K. Ueda, pp. 593–621. Academic Press, New York.

51. Gill, D. M., and Meren, R. (1983): A second guanyl nucleotide-binding site associated with adenylate cyclase. *J. Biol. Chem.,* 258:11908–11914.

52. Gill, D. M., and Meren, R. (1978): ADP-ribosylation of membrane proteins catalyzed by cholera toxin: Basis of the activation of adenylate cyclase. *Proc. Natl. Acad. Sci. USA,* 75:3050–3054.

53. Greenwald, H. L., and Brown, G. L. (1954): The unusual viscosity of water solutions of alkylaryl polyoxyethylene ethanols. *J. Phys. Chem.,* 58:825–828.

54. Halvorsen, S. W., and Nathanson, N. M. (1984): Ontogenesis of physiological responsiveness and guanine nucleotide sensitivity of cardiac muscarinic receptors during chick embryonic development. *Biochemistry,* 23:5813–5821.

55. Hanski, E., and Garty, N. B. (1983): Activation of adenylate cyclase by sperm membranes: The role of guanine nucleotide binding proteins. *FEBS Lett.,* 162:447–452.

56. Hanski, E., and Gilman, A. G. (1982): The guanine nucleotide-binding regulatory component of adenylate cyclase in human erythrocytes. *J. Cyclic Nucleotide Res.,* 8:323–336.

57. Hanski, E., Sternweis, P. C., Northup, J. K., Dromerick, A. W., and Gilman, A. G. (1981): The regulatory component of adenylate cyclase. Purification and properties of the turkey erythrocyte protein. *J. Biol. Chem.,* 256:12911–12919.

58. Hazeki, O., and Ui, M. (1981): Modification by islet-activating protein of receptor-mediated regulation of cyclic AMP accumulation in isolated rat heart cells. *J. Biol. Chem.,* 256:2856–2862.

59. Helenius, A., and Simons, K. (1972): The binding of detergents to lipophilic and hydrophobic proteins. *J. Biol. Chem.,* 247:3656–3661.

60. Hildebrandt, J. D., and Birnbaumer, L. (1983): Inhibitory regulation of adenylyl cyclase in the absence of stimulatory regulation. Requirements and kinetics of guanine nucleotide-induced inhibition of the Cyc⁻ S49 adenylyl cyclase. *J. Biol. Chem.,* 258:13141–13147.

61. Hildebrandt, J. D., Codina, J., and Birnbaumer, L. (1984): Interaction of the stimulatory and inhibitory regulatory proteins of the adenylyl cyclase system with the catalytic component of Cyc⁻ S49 cell membranes. *J. Biol. Chem.,* 259:13178–13185.

62. Hildebrandt, J. D., Codina, J., Risinger, R., and Birnbaumer, L. (1984): Identification of a γ subunit associated with the adenylyl cyclase regulatory proteins Nₛ and Nᵢ. *J. Biol. Chem.,* 259:2039–2042.

63. Hoffman, B. B., Yim, S., Tsai, B. S., and Lefkowitz, R. J. (1981): Preferential uncoupling by manganese of alpha adrenergic receptor mediated inhibition of adenylate cyclase in human platelets. *Biochem. Biophys. Res. Commun.,* 100:724–731.

64. Homcy, C., Wrenn, S., and Haber, E. (1978): Affinity purification of cardiac adenylate cyclase: Dependence on prior hydrophobic resolution. *Proc. Natl. Acad. Sci. USA,* 75:59–63.

65. Howlett, A. C., and Gilman, A. G. (1980): Hydrodynamic properties of the regulatory component of adenylate cyclase. *J. Biol. Chem.,* 255:2861–2866.

66. Howlett, A. C., Sternweis, P. C., Macik, B. A., Van Arsdale, P. M., and Gilman, A. G. (1979): Reconstitution of catecholamine-sensitive adenylate cyclase. *J. Biol. Chem.,* 254:2287–2295.

67. Hsia, J., Moss, J., Hewlett, E., and Vaughan, M. (1984): Requirement for both choleragen and pertussis toxin to obtain maximal activation of adenylate cyclase in cultured cells. *Biochem. Biophys. Res. Commun.,* 119:1068–1074.

68. Hsia, J., Moss, J., Hewlett, E. L., and Vaughan, M. (1984): ADP-ribosylation of adenylate cyclase by pertussis toxin. *J. Biol. Chem.,* 259:1086–1090.

69. Hudson, T., and Johnson, G. (1980): Peptide mapping of adenylate cyclase regulatory proteins that are cholera toxin substrates. *J. Biol. Chem.,* 255:7480–7486.

70. Huff, R. M., Axton, J. M., and Neer, E. J. (1985): Physical and immunological characterization of a guanine nucleotide binding protein from bovine cerebral cortex. *J. Biol. Chem.,* 260:10864–10871.

71. Huff, R. M., and Neer, E. J. (1986): Subunit interactions of native and ADP-ribosylated α_{39} and α_{41}, two guanine nucleotide binding proteins from bovine cerebral cortex. *J. Biol. Chem.*, 261:(in press).

72. Insel, P. A., Stengel, D., Ferry, N., and Hanoune, J. (1982): Regulation of adenylate cyclase of human platelet membranes by forskolin. *J. Biol. Chem.*, 257:7485–7490.

73. Iyengar, R. (1981): Hysteretic activation of adenylyl cyclases. II. Mg ion regulation of the activation of the regulatory component as analyzed by reconstitution. *J. Biol. Chem.*, 256:11042–11050.

74. Iyengar, R., and Birnbaumer, L. (1981): Hysteretic activation of adenylyl cyclases. I. Effect of Mg ion on the rate of activation by guanine nucleotides and fluoride. *J. Biol. Chem.*, 256:11036–11041.

75. Iyengar, R., and Birnbaumer, L. (1982): Hormone receptor modulates the regulatory component of adenylyl cyclase by reducing its requirement for Mg^{2+} and enhancing its extent of activation by guanine nucleotides. *Proc. Natl. Acad. Sci. USA*, 79:5179–5183.

76. Jacobs, S., Bennett, V., and Cuatrecasas, P. (1976): Kinetics of irreversible activation of adenylate cyclase of fat cell membranes by phosphonium and phosphoramidate analogs of GTP. *J. Cyclic Nucleotide Res.*, 2:205–223.

77. Jakobs, K., and Aktories, K. (1981): The hamster adipocyte adenylate cyclase system regulation of enzyme stimulation and inhibition by manganese and magnesium. *Biochimica*, 676:51–58.

78. Jakobs, K. H., Aktories, K., and Schultz, G. (1983): A nucleotide regulatory site for somatostatin inhibition of adenylate cyclase in S_{49} lymphoma cells. *Nature (Lond.)*, 303:177–179.

79. Jakobs, K. H., Aktories, K., and Schultz, G. (1984): Mechanisms and components involved in adenylate cyclase inhibition. *Adv. Cyclic Nucleotide Prot. Phosph. Res.*, 17:135–144.

80. Johnson, G., Kaslow, H., and Bourne, H. (1978): Genetic evidence that cholera toxin substrates are regulatory components of adenylate cyclase. *J. Biol. Chem.*, 253:7120–7123.

81. Johnson, R. A. (1982): Mn^{2+} does not uncouple adenosine "R_a" receptors from the liver adenylate cyclase. *Biochem. Biophys. Res. Commun.*, 105:347–353.

82. Johnson, R. A. (1980): Stimulatory and inhibitory effects of ATP-regenerating systems on liver adenylate cyclase. *J. Biol. Chem.*, 255:8252–8258.

83. Johnson, R. A. (1980): Stimulatory and inhibitory effects of ATP-regenerating systems on liver adenylate cyclase. *J. Biol. Chem.*, 255:8252–8258.

84. Johnson, R. A., Jakobs, K. H., and Shultz, G. (1985): Extraction of the adenylate cyclase-activating factor of bovine sperm and its identification as a trypsin-like protease. *J. Biol. Chem.*, 260:114–121.

85. Jones, L. R., Maddok, S. W., and Besch, H. R., Jr. (1980): Unmasking effect of alamethicin on the (Na^+,K^+)-ATPase, β-adrenergic receptor-coupled adenylate cyclase, and cAMP-dependent protein kinase activities of cardiac sarcolemmal vesicles. *J. Biol. Chem.*, 255:9971–9980.

86. Kahn, R. A., and Gilman, A. G. (1984): ADP-ribosylation of G_s promotes the dissociation of its α and β subunits. *J. Biol. Chem.*, 259:6235–6240.

87. Kaslow, H. R., Johnson, G. L., Brothers, V. M., and Bourne, H. R. (1980): A regulatory component of adenylate cyclase from human erythrocyte membranes. *J. Biol. Chem.*, 255:3736–3741.

88. Katada, T., Bokoch, G. M., Smigel, M. D., Ui, M., and Gilman, A. G. (1984): The inhibitory guanine nucleotide-binding regulatory component of adenylate cyclase. *J. Biol. Chem.*, 259:3586–3595.

89. Katada, T., Northup, J. K., Bokoch, G. M., Ui, M., and Gilman, A. G. (1984): The inhibitory guanine nucleotide-binding regulatory component of adenylate cyclase. Subunit dissociation and guanine nucleotide-dependent hormonal inhibition. *J. Biol. Chem.*, 259:3578–3585.

90. Katada, T., and Ui, M. (1982): ADP-ribosylation of the specific membrane protein of C6 cells by islet-activating protein associated with modification of adenylate cyclase activity. *J. Biol. Chem.*, 257:7210–7216.

91. Katada, T., and Ui, M. (1982): Direct modification of the membrane adenylate cyclase system by islet-activating protein due to ADP-ribosylation of a membrane protein. *Proc. Natl. Acad. Sci. USA*, 79:3129–3133.

92. Kaumann, A. J., and Birnbaumer, L. (1974): Studies on receptor-mediated activation of adenylyl cyclases. *J. Biol. Chem.*, 249:7874–7885.

93. Keenan, A. K., Gal, A., and Levitzki, A. (1982): Reconstitution of the turkey erythrocyte adenylate cyclase sensitivity to L-epinephrine upon re-insertion of the Lubrol solubilized components into phospholipid vesicles. *Biochem. Biophys. Res. Commun.*, 105:615–623.

94. Klee, W., Koski, G., Tocque, B., and Simonds, W. F. (1984): On the mechanism of receptor-mediated inhibition of adenylate cyclase. *Adv. Cyclic Nucleotide Prot. Phosph. Res.*, 17:153–160.

95. Koski, G., Streaty, R. A., and Klee, W. A. (1982): Modulation of sodium sensitive GTPase by partial opiate agonists. *J. Biol. Chem.*, 257:14035–14040.

96. Krishna, G., Weiss, B., and Brodie, B. B. (1968): A simple sensitive method for the assay of adenylate cyclase. *J. Pharmacol. Exp. Ther.*, 163:379–385.

97. Larner, A. C., and Fleming, J. W. (1984): Hormone-sensitive adenylate cyclase, assay of the individual components. In: *Methods in Diabetes Research, Vol. I, Laboratory Methods, part A*, edited by J. Larner and S. Pohl. Wiley, New York.

98. Lester, H. A., Steer, M. L., and Levitzki, A. (1982): Prostaglandin-stimulated GTP hydrolysis associated with activation of adenylate cyclase in human platelet membranes. *Proc. Natl. Acad. Sci. USA*, 79:719–723.

99. Lever, M. (1977): Peroxides in detergents as interfering factors in biochemical analysis. *Anal. Biochem.*, 83:274–284.

100. Levey, G. S. (1970): Solubilization of myocardial adenyl cyclase. *Biochem. Biophys. Res. Commun.*, 38:86–92.

101. Levey, G. S., and Klein, I. (1972): Solubilized myocardial adenylate cyclase. *J. Clin. Invest.*, 51:1578–1582.

102. Levine, M. A., Downs, R. W., Singer, M., Marx, S. J., Aurbach, G. D., and Spiegel, A. M. (1980): Deficient activity of guanine nucleotide regulatory protein in erythrocytes from patients with pseudohypoparathyroidism. *Biochem. Biophys. Res. Commun.*, 94:1319–1324.

103. Levinson, S., and Blume, A. (1977): Altered guanine nucleotide hydrolysis as basis for increased adenylate cyclase activity after cholera toxin treatment. *J. Biol. Chem.*, 252:3766–3774.

104. Lim, L. K., Sekura, R. D., and Kaslow, H. R. (1985): Adenosine nucleotides directly stimulate pertussis toxin. *J. Biol. Chem.*, 260:2585–2588.

105. Limbird, L. E., Hickey, A. R., and Lefkowitz, R. J. (1979): Unique uncoupling of the frog erythrocyte adenylate cyclase system by manganese. *J. Biol. Chem.*, 254:2677–2683.

106. Litosch, I., Hudson, T. H., Mills, I., Li, S.-Y., and Fain, N. (1982): Forskolin as an activator of cyclic AMP accumulation and lipolysis in rat adipocytes. *Mol. Pharmacol.*, 22:109–115.

107. Londos, C., and Wolff, J. (1977): Two distinct adenosine-sensitive sites on adenylate cyclase. *Proc. Natl. Acad. Sci. USA*, 74:5482–5486.

108. Londos, C., Salomon, Y., Lin, M. C., Harwood, J. P., Schramm, M., Wolff, J., and Rodbell, M. (1974): 5'-guanylylimidodiphosphate, a potent activator of adenylate cyclase systems in eukaryotic cells. *Proc. Natl. Acad. Sci. USA*, 71:3087–3090.

109. Lowry, O. H., Rosebrough, N. J., Farr, A. L., and Randall, R. J. (1951): Protein measurement with the folin phenol reagent. *J. Biol. Chem.*, 193:265–275.

110. Malbon, C. C., Mangano, T. J., and Watkins, D. C. (1985): Heart contains two substrates ($M_r = 40,000$ and 41,000) for pertussis toxin-catalyzed ADP-ribosylation that co-purify with N_s. *Biochem. Biophys. Res. Commun.*, 128:809–815.

111. Manning, D. R., and Gilman, A. G. (1983): The regulatory components of adenylate cyclase and transducin. A family of structurally homologous guanine nucleotide-binding proteins. *J. Biol. Chem.*, 258:7059–7063.

112. Michel, T., and Lefkowitz, R. J. (1982): Hormonal inhibition of adenylate cyclase: Alpha$_2$ adrenergic receptors promote release of [^{3}H]guanylylimidodiphosphate from platelet membranes. *J. Biol. Chem.*, 257:13557–13563.

113. Moss, J., Burns, D., Chang, P., Cutilletta, A., and Vaughan, M. (1982): Characterization of the GTP-binding component of adenylate cyclase system in isolated myocardial muscle cells. *J. Mol. Cell. Cardiol. [Suppl. 3]*, 14:71–75.

114. Moss, J., and Vaughan, M. (1977): Choleragen activation of solubilized adenylate cyclase: Requirement for GTP and protein

activator for demonstration of enzymatic activity. *Proc. Natl. Acad. Sci. USA,* 74:4396–4400.

115. Narayanan, N., and Sulakhe, P. (1977): 5'guanylylimidodiphosphate-activated adenylate cyclase of cardiac sarcolemma displays higher affinity for magnesium ions. *Mol. Pharmacol.,* 13:1033–1047.

116. Narayanan, N., and Sulakhe, P. V. (1978): Stimulatory and inhibitory effects of guanyl-5'-yl imidodiphosphate on adenylate cyclase activity of cardiac sarcolemma. *Arch. Biochem. Biophys.,* 185:72–81.

117. Neer, E. J. (1974): The size of adenylate cyclase. *J. Biol. Chem.,* 249:6527–6531.

118. Neer, E. J. (1978): Size and detergent binding of adenylate cyclase from bovine cerebral cortex. *J. Biol. Chem.,* 253:1498–1502.

119. Neer, E. J. (1978): Physical properties of water-soluble and detergent-solubilized adenylate cyclase from mature rat testis. *J. Biol. Chem.,* 253:5808–5812.

120. Neer, E. J. (1978): Multiple forms of adenylate cyclase. *Adv. Cyclic Nucleotide Res.,* 9:69–83.

121. Neer, E. J. (1979): Interaction of soluble brain adenylate cyclase with manganese. *J. Biol. Chem.,* 254:2089–2096.

122. Neer, E. J. (1982): Studies of solubilized adenylate cyclase. In: *Cell Regulation by Intracellular Signals,* edited by S. Swillens and J. Dumont, pp. 31–45. Plenum Press, New York.

123. Neer, E. J., Echeverria, D., and Knox, S. (1980): Increase in the size of soluble brain adenylate cyclase with activation by guanosine 5'-(β,γ-imino)triphosphate. *J. Biol. Chem.,* 255:9782–9789.

124. Neer, E. J., Lok, J. M., and Wolf, L. G. (1984): Purification and properties of the inhibitory guanine nucleotide regulatory unit of brain adenylate cyclase. *J. Biol. Chem.,* 259:14222–142229.

125. Neer, E. J., and Salter, R. S. (1981): Reconstituted adenylate cyclase from bovine brain. Functions of subunits. *J. Biol. Chem.,* 256:12102–12107.

126. Neer, E. J., Wolf, L. G., and Gill, D. M. (1986): The stimulatory guanine nucleotide regulatory unit of adenylate cyclase from bovine cerebral cortex: ADP-ribosylation and purification. *(Submitted.)*

127. Northup, J. K., Smigel, M. D., and Gilman, A. G. (1982): The guanine nucleotide activating site of the regulatory component of adenylate cyclase. Identification by ligand binding. *J. Biol. Chem.,* 257:11416–11423.

128. Northup, J. K., Sternweis, P. C., and Gilman, A. G. (1983): The subunits of the stimulatory regulatory component of adenylate cyclase. Resolution, activity and properties of the 35,000 dalton protein. *J. Biol. Chem.,* 258:11361–11368.

129. Northup, J. K., Smigel, M. D., Sternweis, P. C., and Gilman, A. G. (1983): The subunits of the stimulatory regulatory component of adenylate cyclase. Resolution of the activated 45,000-dalton (α) subunit. *J. Biol. Chem.,* 258:11369–11376.

130. Northup, J. K., Sternweis, P. C., Smigel, M. D., Schleifer, L. S., Ross, E. M., and Gilman, A. G. (1980): Purification of the regulatory component of adenylate cyclase. *Proc. Natl. Acad. Sci. USA,* 77:6516–6520.

131. Okajima, F., and Ui, M. (1984): Conversion of adrenergic mechanism from an α- to a β-type during primary culture of rat hepatocytes. Accompanying decreases in the function of the inhibitory guanine nucleotide regulatory component of adenylate cyclase identified as the substrate of islet-activating protein. *J. Biol. Chem.,* 259:15464–15469.

132. Pederson, S. E., and Ross, E. M. (1982): Functional reconstitution of β-adrenergic receptors and the stimulatory GTP-binding protein of adenylate cyclase. *Proc. Natl. Acad. Sci. USA,* 79:7228–7232.

133. Pfeuffer, T. (1977): GTP-binding proteins in membranes and the control of adenylate cyclase activity. *J. Biol. Chem.,* 252:7224–7234.

134. Pfeuffer, T., and Helmreich, E. J. M. (1975): Activation of pigeon erythrocyte membrane adenylate cyclase by guanylnucleotide analogues and separation of a nucleotide binding protein. *J. Biol. Chem.,* 250:867–876.

135. Pfeuffer, T., and Metzger, H. (1982): 7-O-Hemisuccinyl-deacetyl forskolin-Sepharose: A novel affinity support for purification of adenylate cyclase. *FEBS Lett.,* 146:369–375.

136. Reference deleted in proof.

137. Pike, L. J., and Lefkowitz, R. J. (1980): Activation and desensitization of β-adrenergic receptor-coupled GTPase and adenylate cyclase of frog and turkey erythrocyte membranes. *J. Biol. Chem.,* 255:6860–6867.

138. Pike, L. J., and Lefkowitz, R. J. (1981): Correlation of β-adrenergic receptor-stimulated [³H]GDP release and adenylate cyclase activation. *J. Biol. Chem.,* 256:2207–2212.

139. Rodbell, M. (1980): The role of hormone receptors and GTP-regulatory proteins in membrane transduction. *Nature,* 284:17–22.

140. Rodbell, M., Birnbaumer, L., Pohl, S. L., and Krans, M. J. (1970): The glucagon-sensitive adenyl cyclase system in plasma membranes of rat liver. *J. Biol. Chem.,* 245:1877–1882.

141. Ross, E. M. (1981): Physical separation of the catalytic and regulatory proteins of hepatic adenylate cyclase. *J. Biol. Chem.,* 256:1949–1953.

142. Ross, E. M. (1982): Phosphatidylcholine-promoted interaction of the catalytic and regulatory proteins of adenylate cyclase. *J. Biol. Chem.,* 257:10751–10758.

143. Ross, E. M., and Gilman, A. G. (1980): Biochemical properties of hormone-sensitive adenylate cyclase. *Annu. Rev. Biochem.,* 44:533–564.

144. Ross, E. M., and Gilman, A. G. (1977): Resolution of some components of adenylate cyclase necessary for catalytic activity. *J. Biol. Chem.,* 252:6966–6969.

145. Ross, E. M., Howlett, A. C., Ferguson, K. M., and Gilman, A. G. (1978): Reconstitution of hormone-sensitive adenylate cyclase activity with resolved components of the enzyme. *J. Biol. Chem.,* 253:6401–6412.

146. Salomon, Y. (1979): Adenylate cyclase assay. *Adv. Cyclic Nucleotide Res.,* 10:35.

147. Salomon, Y., Londos, E., and Rodbell, M. (1974): A highly sensitive adenylate cyclase assay. *Anal. Biochem.,* 58:541–548.

148. Reference deleted in proof.

149. Shaltiel, S. (1974): Hydrophobic chromatography. *Methods Enzymol.,* 34:126–140.

150. Sanders, R. B., Thompson, W. J., and Robison, G. A. (1977): Epinephrine- and glucagon-stimulated cardiac adenylyl cyclase activity. *Biochim. Biophys. Acta,* 498:10–20.

151. Seamon, K., and Daly, J. W. (1981): Activation of adenylate cyclase by the diterpene forskolin does not require the guanine nucleotide regulatory protein. *J. Biol. Chem.,* 256:9799–9801.

152. Seamon, K. B., and Daly, J. W. (1981): Forskolin: A unique diterpene activator of cyclic AMP-generating systems. *J. Cyclic Nucleotide Res.,* 7:201–224.

153. Seamon, K. B., and Daly, J. W. (1982): Guanosine 5'-(β,γ-imido)triphosphate inhibition of forskolin-activated adenylate cyclase is mediated by the putative inhibitory guanine nucleotide regulatory protein. *J. Biol. Chem.,* 257:11591–11596.

154. Seamon, K. B., Vaillancourt, R., Edwards, M., and Daly, J. W. (1984): Binding of [³H]forskolin to rat brain membranes. *Proc. Natl. Acad. Sci. USA,* 81:5081–5085.

155. Seamon, K. B., and Wetzel, B. (1984): Interaction of forskolin with dually regulated adenylate cyclase. *Adv. Cyclic Nucleotid Prot. Phosph. Res.,* 17:91–100.

156. Schleifer, L. S., Kahn, R. A., Hanski, E., Northup, J. K., Sternweis, P. C., and Gilman, A. G. (1982): Requirements for cholera toxin-dependent ADP-ribosylation of the purified regulatory component of adenylate cyclase. *J. Biol. Chem.,* 257:20–23.

157. Schulz, D. W., and Mailman, R. B. (1984): An improved, automated adenylate cyclase assay utilizing preparative HPLC: Effects of phosphodiesterase inhibitors. *J. Neurochem.,* 42:764–774.

158. Shalteil, S. (1974): Hydrophobic chromatography. *Methods Enzymol.,* 34:126–140.

159. Shreeve, S. M., Roeske, W. R., and Venter, J. C. (1984): Partial functional reconstitution of cardiac muscarinic cholinergic receptor. *J. Biol. Chem.,* 259:12398–12402.

160. Siegl, A. M., Daly, J. W., and Smith, J. B. (1982): Inhibition of aggregation and stimulation of cyclic AMP generation in intact human platelets by the diterpene forskolin. *Mol. Pharmacol.,* 21:680–687.

161. Smigel, M., Katada, T., Northup, J. K., Bokoch, G. M., Ui, M., and Gilman, A. G. (1984): Mechanisms of guanine nucleotide-mediated regulation of adenylate cyclase activity. *Adv. Cyclic Nucleotide Prot. Phosph. Res.,* 17:1–18.

162. Steele, J. C. H., Tanford, C., and Reynolds, J. A. (1978): Determination of partial specific volumes for lipid-associated proteins. *Methods Enzymol.*, 48:11–23.

163. Stengel, D., and Hanoune, J. (1981): The catalytic unit of Rani sperm adenylate cyclase can be activated through the guanosine nucleotide regulatory component and prostaglandin receptors of human erythrocytes. *J. Biol. Chem.*, 255:2861–2866.

164. Sternweis, P. C., Northup, J. K., Smigel, M. D., and Gilman, A. G. (1981): The regulatory component of adenylate cyclase. *J. Biol. Chem.*, 256:11517–11526.

165. Sternweis, P. C., and Robishaw, J. D. (1984): Isolation of two proteins with high affinity for guanine nucleotides from membranes of bovine brain. *J. Biol. Chem.*, 259:13806–13813.

166. Strittmatter, S., and Neer, E. J. (1980): Properties of the separated catalytic and regulatory units of brain adenylate cyclase. *Proc. Natl. Acad. Sci. USA*, 77:6344–6348.

167. Suidan, H., Tamir, A., and Tolkovsky, A. (1983): A simple test for enhanced guanyl nucleotide exchange in brain adenylate cyclase systems activated by neurotransmitters. *J. Biol. Chem.*, 258:10524–10529.

168. Sunyer, T., Codina, J., and Birnbaumer, L. (1984): GTP hydrolysis by pure N_i, the inhibitory regulatory component of adenylyl cyclases. *J. Biol. Chem.*, 259:15447–15451.

169. Ui, M., Katada, T., Murayama, T., Kurose, H., Yajima, M., Tamura, M., Nakamura, T., and Nogimori, K. (1984): Islet-activating protein, pertussis toxin: A specific uncoupler of receptor-mediated inhibition of adenylate cyclase. *Adv. Cyclic Nucleotide Res.*, 17:145–152.

170. Yamamura, H., Lad, P. M., and Rodbell, M. (1977): GTP stimulates and inhibits adenylate cyclase in fat cell membranes through distinct regulatory processes. *J. Biol. Chem.*, 252:7964–7966.

APPENDIX

Adenylate Cyclase Assay Protocol[3]

Section I: Reagents

Dowex resin (AG 50W-X2, Biorad).

Prepare 2.5 lb resin as follows: Add 2 liters 2-M NaOH, stir, then filter in Buchner funnel, and wash with distilled water until the pH of the eluent is neutral. Add the resin to 1 liter 6-N HCl. Wash as before until pH of eluent is about 6. The final form of the resin is H^+.

Pour a 4-cm-high column, in 5.75-inch Pasteur pipettes, carefully measuring height from top of a glass-wool plug. The columns should be calibrated before using a new batch of resin by determining the elution volume of [^{14}C]cAMP on three 4-cm-high Dowex columns, using 200-μl samples of diluting solution (*vide infra*). Store columns at room temperature in a closed jar containing a little distilled water.

Solutions.

All solutions are prepared beforehand, but not combined until time of assay. All are stored at $-20°$C.

Amount to add to final volume of 100 ml	Concentration in stock solution	Concentration in adenylate cyclase assay
1.2 g Tris-Cl 0.4 g Tris-OH	0.1 M	About 50–100 mM; 30 mM Tris comes from the stock solution; note that more is contributed by the sample, etc.
0.6 g BSA	0.6%	0.08%
4 ml of 1-M MgCl$_2$	40 mM	5.3 mM

Adjust pH to 7.6 if necessary. Aliquot into 10-ml quantities and store at $-20°$C. Add 40 mg cAMP/10 ml (7.2 mM) before use. A bottle may be thawed and frozen many times. The cAMP is 1 mM in final assay.

ATP-regenerating system.

Creatine kinase and creatine phosphate are from Boehringer-Mannheim. Make up 10 ml at a time, divide into 0.2-ml aliquots, and store at $-20°$C.

	Amount to add to 10 ml 0.05-M Tris-Cl (pH 7.6)	Final concentration in assay
Creatine kinase	67 mg (25 U/mg)	1 U/ml
Creatine phosphate	491 mg	10 mM

Combine and bring volume up to 10 ml with 0.05-M Tris-Cl (pH 7.6). Adjust pH with 1-M Tris-OH.

[^{3}H]ATP.

Purification of [^{3}H]ATP is essential to obtain low blanks. Pour a 25-ml (1-cm-diameter) Dowex AG 50W-X2 column in H$_2$O. Before applying sample, wash the resin with 25 ml distilled water to remove excess yellow dye. To avoid contaminating a fraction collector, the fractions are collected manually. Apply 5 mCi [^{3}H]ATP (Amersham or NEN). Rinse vial with 0.5 ml H$_2$O and apply to column. Portions of 0.5 ml H$_2$O are applied to the top of the column, and the 0.5 ml effluent is collected. The column will not run dry; so it is not necessary to apply the portions of H$_2$O rapidly. Collect 25 tubes, place 1 μl from each fraction into 0.1 ml H$_2$O, add 1 ml scintillation fluid, and count for 1 min. Pool peak fractions, leaving out the trailing back region.

The [^{3}H]ATP solution then needs to be brought up to an ATP concentration that will give a specific activity of 80 to 100 cpm/pmole. Make a 200- to 300-mM solution of unlabeled ATP. Check the concentration by diluting a sample into 0.05-M Tris (pH 7) and measuring the optical density (O.D.) at 259 nanometers. Add unlabeled ATP to [3H]solution slowly, and check specific activity by diluting, reading O.D., and counting a sample until the desired specific activity is reached.

Diluting solution, [14C]cAMP stop solution.

Diluting solution contains [14C]cAMP and a relatively high concentration of unlabeled ATP. [14C]cAMP is used to account for recovery of [3H]cAMP from columns. Diluting solution should contain 1,500 to 2,000 cpm/0.1 ml. An excess of unlabeled ATP effectively stops the reaction, because the specific activity of cAMP formed after its addition will be too low to detect. Make 200-ml aliquot into 15-ml quantities and store at $-20°C$.

223-mM ATP: 1.2 g in 100 ml 0.05-M Tris-Cl (pH 7.6)

3.4-mM cAMP:
            0.11 g in 100 ml 0.05-M Tris-Cl (pH 7.6)

Adjust each to pH 7.6 with 1-M Tris-OH and then combine. Add [14C]cAMP to make a final solution with 1,500 to 2,000 cpm/0.1 ml.

Precipitating solutions.

The Dowex column does not separate cAMP perfectly from AMP or ADP, which can be precipitated with $BaSO_4$. Make up solutions in quantity and store them at room temperature.

Saturated Ba(OH)₂ solution.

Add 70 g $Ba(OH)_2$ to 500 ml boiling distilled water; let cool.

Zinc solution.

Dissolve 25 g $ZnSO_4$ in 500 ml 0.1-M Tris-Cl (pH 7.6). The pH will be about 5.6. Do not adjust to 7 or a precipitate will form. The buffering capacity of other assay components is sufficient that the supernatant after adding $Ba(OH)_2$ should be neutral.

Scintillation fluid.

We use Ultrafluor (National Diagnostics), which gives a low cross-talk of 14C into the 3H channel. Other brands may be used provided the cross-talk is not greater than 20%.

Section II: Procedures

1. Sample volume: 50 μl containing 5 to 70 μg protein. To this add 20 μl of assay solution that contains

            10 μl stock solution

            5 μl regenerating system

            5 μl [3H]ATP solution

(or an amount needed to give the desired final concentration of ATP; make up volume with 0.05-M Tris, pH 7.6, if it is less than 5 μl). Mix enough assay solution for all tubes. Always make up enough mix for one or two tubes more than needed in order to cover any losses on the outsides of micropipettes.

2. Incubate 10 min at 30°C with shaking. Place on ice and add 0.1 ml diluting solution (containing carrier [14C]cAMP and ATP to stop the reaction and to determine recoveries). Boil 1 min. Chill on ice.

3. Add 0.3 ml distilled water to each sample, and apply each sample to an individual Dowex column for separation of ATP from cAMP. Before application, make sure the elution position of cAMP is known for that specific batch of Dowex resin (test as described in the preceding Dowex section). Note that ATP does not stick to column and comes off first.

4. Typically we wash the sample onto the column with 0.8 ml distilled water. Exact wash volumes must be determined for each batch of resin. Then we run 2 ml distilled water and collect into a waste pan. Finally we apply 1 ml distilled water and collect into clear plastic centrifuge tubes placed under each column. This last 1 ml contains the cAMP.

5. To the 1 ml collected, add 0.1 ml $ZnSO_4$ solution, then 0.1 ml of $Ba(OH)_2$ solution, and swirl the tube. Spin 2 min at 2,000 rpm to pellet the precipitate. Repeat $ZnSO_4$ and $Ba(OH)_2$ additions without disturbing pellet. Spin 5 min at 2,000 rpm. The resulting supernatant should be transferred at once into scintillation fluid.

6. Take up 1 ml of supernatant and count it in 10 ml scintillation fluid for 10 min. Make sure to have [3H]ATP and diluting solution standards counting at the same time. One can now determine the amount of [3H]ATP converted to cAMP per sample. To find the specific activity of adenylate cyclase, one needs to know the amount of protein assayed.

7. Dowex columns can be regenerated for reuse. Fill each column to the top (greater than bed volume) with 1-M NaOH. Wash two times as before with distilled water. Then add 1-N HCl three times. Finally, wash again four times with distilled water, and columns are ready to reuse.

The Heart and Cardiovascular System,
edited by H. A. Fozzard et al.
Raven Press, New York © 1986.

CHAPTER 50

Identification and Characterization of Alpha-Adrenergic Receptors

Robert M. Graham and Stephen M. Lanier

It is precisely in the manifold character of the possibilities of combination that I see a special advantage and peculiar possibilities of development. When once we are acquainted with the majority of . . . receptors . . . , which will be a long piece of work, occupying many hands and heads, we shall have the most far-reaching possibilities of simultaneous attack by various agencies.

P. Ehrlich (88)

HISTORICAL PERSPECTIVE

Receptor Concept

Based on studies of the agonist and antagonist interplay of pilocarpine and atropine as they affect salivary gland flow in the cat, Langley (212) formulated what was probably the first expression of the "receptor concept." Thus, he stated, "there is some substance or substances in the nerve endings or gland cell with which both atropin and pilocarpin are capable of forming compounds . . . according to some law of which their relative mass and chemical affinity for the substance are factors." Langley was undoubtedly influenced by similar studies on the sweat gland of the foot of the cat by Luchsinger (232) that led the latter to conclude that "there exists

between pilocarpin and atropin a true mutual antagonism, their actions summing themselves algebraically like wave crests and hollows, like plus and minus. The final result depends simply and solely upon the relative number of molecules of the poisons present." Nevertheless, it was with considerable insight that Langley additionally implicated an interaction between "poison" and some substance on the nerve endings or gland cells.

In subsequent studies on the actions of nicotine and curare on striated muscle, Langley (213) extended this concept. In those investigations he clearly demonstrated that as "both nicotine and curari abolish the effect of nerve stimulation, but do not prevent contraction from being obtained by direct stimulation of the muscle, or by a further adequate injection of nicotine, it may be inferred that neither the poisons nor the nervous impulse act directly on the contractile substance of the muscle, but on some accessory substance. Since this accessory substance is the recipient of stimuli, which it transfers to the contractile material, we may speak of it as the 'receptive substance' of the muscle."

Langley further perceived the general applicability of his theory: "Thus there is evidence that the majority of substances which are ordinarily supposed to act upon nerve-endings (as nicotine, curari, atropine, pilocarpine, strychnine) act upon the receptive substances of cells. And as adrenalin, an internal secretion, acts upon a receptive substance, it is probable that secretin, thyroid-ine, and the internal secretion formed by the generative organs, also act on receptive substances, although in these cases the cells may be unconnected with nerve fibres." In light of this latter statement by Langley, it is of interest that in the same year Starling (344) coined the term "hormone" (from ὁρμάω, "I excite" or "arouse") during a Croonian lecture on "The Chemical Correlation of the Functions of the Body" to describe "the chemical messengers which, speeding from cell to cell along the blood stream, may coordinate the activities and growth of different parts of the body."

The receptor concept (Table 1) was further advanced at about the same time by Ehrlich (86), who, struck by the high degree of specificity of antibodies, postulated the existence of specific "side-chains" in the cell proto-plasm. These side chains, he suggested, had a unique chemical and steric architecture with which only anti-bodies of the appropriate shape and chemical composi-tion could combine. Moreover, he assumed that all cells had these side chains, which were essential for their life processes ("Corpora non agunt nisi fixata"), and that their compositions and shapes differed for different cell types. Thus, he suggested, chemotherapeutic drugs could be fashioned to combine specificity with side chains of a parasite and yet, at the same time, fit poorly the side chains of host tissues. Indeed, in his 1905 paper, Langley (213) referred to this theory: "The relation between the receptive and the contractile substance is clearly very close, and, on the general lines of Ehrlich's immunity theory, it might be supposed that a receptive substance is a side-chain molecule of the molecule of contractile

TABLE 1. *Major developments in the receptor concept*

Pharmacological concepts (ref.)	Contributions from physical chemistry (ref.)
Side-chain theory: Ehrlich, 1909 (87) Receptive substance: Luchsinger, 1877; Langley 1878, 1905 (212, 213, 232)	Law of mass action: Guldberg and Waage, 1864 (146) Lock-and-key fit of enzyme and substrate: Fisher, 1894 (101) Enzyme kinetics: Henri, 1902; Michaelis and Menten, 1913; Briggs and Haldane, 1925; Lineweaver and Burk, 1934 (38, 154, 230, 249)
Hormone: Starling, 1905 (344) Occupancy theory: Hill, 1909; Shackell, 1924; Clark, 1933; Gaddum, 1926 (60, 110, 158, 321)	
Adrenergic-receptor classification: Ahlquist, 1948 (5)	Adsorption isotherm: Langmuir, 1918 (214) Bimolecular interactions: Scatchard, 1949 (309)
Intrinsic activity: Ariens, 1954 (13) Efficacy: Stephenson, 1956 (346) Spare receptors: Nickerson, 1956 (270)	
Receptor reserve: Ariens et al. 1960; Van Rossum and Ariens, 1962; Furchgott, 1964 (14, 107, 376) Rate theory: Paton, 1961; Paton and Rang, 1966 (273, 274)	Induced-fit theory: Koshland, 1958 (194)
	Allosteric transition model: Monod et al., 1965; Rubin and Changeux, 1966 (255, 301) Ligand-induced cooperative models: Koshland et al., 1966 (195) Allosteric linkage: Wyman, 1967 (396)
Radioligand binding: Lin and Goodfriend, 1970; Lefkowitz et al., 1970 (222, 229) Two-state model: Colquhoun, 1973 (64) Adrenergic receptor binding: Levitzki et al., 1974; Aurbach et al., 1974; Lefkowitz et al., 1974; Greenberg et al., 1976; Williams and Lefkowitz, 1976 (18, 14, 221, 224, 390)	Enzyme-inhibitor relationship: Cheng and Prusoff, 1973 (54)
	Partitioning theory: Jencks, 1975 (180) Floating-receptor hypothesis: Cuatrecasas and Hollenberg, 1976 (73)

Adapted from ref. 78.

substance." Finally, to the "certain specific component parts of the cell side-chains" to which "destructive toxins" are absorbed, Ehrlich (87) gave the name "receptors."

Hill (158), Shackell (321), Gaddum (110), and Clark (58–60) established receptor theory on a firm quantitative basis, resulting in the formulation of a general theory of drug action: the "occupancy" theory. Thus, according to Clark (60), the drug-receptor interaction closely follows Langmuir's adsorption isotherm (214), derived from considerations of the law of mass action (146), and holds that the intensity of pharmacological effects is directly proportional to the number of receptors occupied by the drug. Clearly, this and subsequent considerations of drug-receptor interactions were heavily influenced by crucial conceptual advances in other fields such as immunology, enzymology, and physical chemistry (Table 1). Considerations of the theory of drug action can therefore be similarly applied to those encompassing enzyme kinetics and inhibition formulated by Henri (154), Michaelis and Menten (249), Briggs and Haldane (38), and Lineweaver and Burk (230).

Although the occupancy theory had broad applicability, it became clear that some drugs never elicit a maximal response even at infinite concentrations ("partial agonists"), whereas others apparently elicit a maximal biological response while occupying only a fraction of the total receptors available. Such considerations led to the concepts of "intrinsic activity" (13) or "efficacy" (346) and of "spare receptors" (270) or reserve receptors (14,107,376), and subsequently to formulation of the "rate" theory of drug-receptor interaction (273).

Paton (273) conceived of receptor activation as a quantal event associated with the moment of interaction between drug and receptor. Occupation of the receptor after this resulted in blockade, whereas dissociation of the agonist from the receptor rendered it again available for activation. A rapid dissociation rate, therefore, implied high efficacy, whereas a slow dissociation rate resulted in prolonged occupancy and antagonism. Partial agonists, according to the rate theory, have intermediate dissociation rate constants.

Differences between the occupancy theory and rate theory can be reconciled in terms of a piano-playing analogy. With the occupancy theory, a note is sounded every time a key is depressed, and the intensity of the sound generated is directly proportional to the number of keys depressed. With the rate theory, a note is sounded the instant a key is touched, and the intensity of the sound is proportional to the rapidity with which a key can be depressed.

As compared with the concept of the receptor as a rigid structure that binds drug as a "key in a lock" (101), a more dynamic picture of the receptor molecule, wherein conformational changes are involved in the link between drug binding and effect, gradually emerged in

the sixties, leading to two-state (64,255) and cooperative models (195) of receptor-drug or enzyme-substrate interaction. These models postulate that the receptor can exist in two interconvertible states, a ground state (which is the more abundant) and an excited state, that are in equilibrium with each other. A biological response is initiated by the agonist binding to the excited state, thus displacing the equilibrium in favor of receptor activation. By contrast, an antagonist binds only to the ground state, thus preventing formation of the excited state.

More recently, refinements of these models have led to the "floating-receptor" hypothesis (73), wherein an agonist modulates the dominant aggregative state of a multisubunit receptor or enzyme protein, and to the "partitioning" theory (104,180). This theory predicts that the efficacy of an agonist can be interpreted in terms of the free energy of binding that is partitioned between the productive binding energy used to induce a biologically effective conformational change in the receptor, and the nonproductive binding, typical of antagonists, that is expressed as tightness of binding. The latter theory is supported by thermodynamic analyses of agonist and antagonist binding to receptors (383). Such evaluations demonstrate a large decrease in enthalpy with agonist binding, as would be anticipated with a change in receptor conformation, whereas interaction with antagonists appears to be largely entropy-driven (281,327,383,384).

Adrenergic Receptors

Dale (75) extended Langley's concept of a receptive mechanism to the mechanism of action of the sympathetic nervous system. In his classic paper on the sympatholytic and adrenolytic actions of ergot alkaloids he recognized that what he called the "sympathetic myoneuronal junction" was synonymous with Langley's "receptive substance for adrenaline," and he used this mechanism to explain the fact that the ergot alkaloids prevented only the motor (excitatory) actions of adrenaline, but had no effects on the inhibitory actions of adrenaline or on the exitatory actions of barium or pituitrin.

However, it was a serendipitous finding that led to Sir Henry's discovery of ergot's alpha-adrenergic blocking properties. Dale, while working at the Wellcome Laboratories (Herne Hill, U.K.), was involved in evaluating the pharmacology of ergots. One of his routine tasks at that time was to bioassay adrenal extracts (Wellcome adrenaline preparations). This was done by determining pressor effects in the cat. Because this work was of a routine nature, it was usually performed at the end of the day after the regular experiments. After administering the adrenaline-containing solutions into cats that had received ergot during the normal day's experiments, Dale found that instead of the rise in blood pressure that adrenal extracts normally produced, he observed a fall in blood pressure. Being an astute investigator, Sir Henry reasoned that the ergot, in some way, might be modifying the effects of adrenaline, and after additional experiments he concluded that pretreatment with ergot affected the pressor response of adrenaline by blockade of its vasoconstrictor effects.

This, then, was the first demonstration of the ability of any drug to produce blockade of some of adrenaline's effects. And in retrospect was the first demonstration of drug antagonism due to alpha-adrenergic receptor blockade, although Sollman and Brown, in their publication of 1905 (337), which followed Dale's initial presentation but which preceded Dale's 1906 publication (75), presumably independently observed that adrenaline could cause vasodilatation after ergot pretreatment.

Throughout the 1920s and 1930s, Cannon, Rosenblueth, and associates (47) performed a number of studies that more clearly delineated the mechanisms involved in autonomic neurotransmission. In their classic experiments of 1921, Cannon and Uridil (48) established that a chemical mediator is liberated at neuroeffector junctions in response to sympathetic nerve stimulation, and in subsequent studies they obtained evidence that the responses to this mediator (sympathin) differed qualitatively from those observed with adrenine (adrenaline). However, they challenged Langley's hypothesis that the differing effects observed with a single substance such as adrenaline, stimulatory in some tissues and inhibitory in others, were due to differing "receptive substances" in the responsive cells (47). They suggested, rather, that there was one receptor, which in different effector cells released one or the other of two different effector substances, and they called these effectors sympathin E (exitatory) and sympathin I (inhibitory).

This concept remained unchallenged and was accepted as physiological "law" until Ahlquist's elegant studies (5) were published in 1948. Using six different sympathomimetic amines (*l*-epinephrine, *dl*-epinephrine, *dl*-norepinephrine, *dl*-methylnorepinephrine, *dl*-methylepinephrine, *dl*-isoproterenol), he examined their effects on seven different tissues (heart, blood vessels, intestine, uterus, ureter, dilator pupillae, and nictitating membrane) of three to four different species (dog, cat, rat, and rabbit). He concluded from these studies that there is "one order of potency—*dl*-isoproterenol > *l*-epinephrine > *dl*-methylepinephrine > *dl*-epinephrine > *dl*-norepinephrine—on the following functions: vasodilation, inhibition of the uterus and myocardial stimulation." "The variations in activity," he suggested, "could be due to any or all of three factors: a) quantitative differences in potency, b) qualitatively different effects, or c) differences due entirely to the experimental methods used. If the last two factors are controlled as much as possible by the selection of the amines and by using suitable experimental techniques, then the variations in

activity are presumably due to actual differences in the receptors involved."

On the basis of these studies, Ahlquist termed one type of receptor "alpha," which was associated with most of the excitatory functions and with at least one inhibitory function (intestinal smooth-muscle relaxation), and the other type "beta," which was associated with most of the inhibitory functions and with one important excitatory function (cardiac stimulation). Because of the opposing effects associated with each type of receptor, he correctly suggested that the customary signs, E (excitatory) and I (inhibitory), could not be applied universally and, therefore, that the concept of sympathin E and I was incorrect.

Ahlquist's classification was initially received with skepticism and was not definitively accepted until it was confirmed with the development of the beta-adrenergic antagonists dichloroisoproterenol (329) and propranolol (28). However, it is now widely recognized that Ahlquist's classification has had enormous impact on the pharmacological and clinical applications of the receptor concept, and alpha- and beta-adrenergic receptors have now been identified and characterized in a wide variety of both sympathetically innervated and noninnervated organs and tissues (129).

Radioligand Binding Studies

Like other hormone receptors, adrenergic receptors have two functions in mediating the actions of the sympathetic nervous system. First, they function as discriminators by their selective recognition and binding of catecholamines. Second, once activated, they are responsible for initiating a sequence of events that results in the physiological response to catecholamines. Conventional pharmacological studies can probe the latter of these functions but can provide only limited information on the mechanisms whereby receptors can discriminate between biological molecules and how receptors transmit information into the interior of the cell.

In the late sixties and early seventies, a new approach to the study of hormone receptors was developed in which radioactive adrenergic ligands (radioligands) were used as probes to directly identify and study the receptor binding sites (222,229). This technique allows the receptors to be quantitated, their specificity to be defined, the kinetics of their interactions with ligands to be examined, and specific information about their roles as transducers of information from the catecholamine signal to the cellular machinery to be deduced. Additionally, alterations in the numbers or characteristics of receptors in various physiological and pathological states can be directly examined.

Early attempts to label alpha-adrenergic receptors with radiolabeled antagonists, such as [^{3}H]norepinephrine, were unsuccessful (102,257,361,400), probably because of the low specific activity (25–50 mCi/mmol) of the available radioligands and the use of intact strips of tissue rather than membrane preparations as the source of receptors (membrane preparations allowing the attainment of higher receptor concentrations and possibly the elimination of some drug and hormone uptake processes present in intact tissue).

Successful labeling of alpha-adrenergic receptors using radiolabeled adrenergic ligands was not reported until 1976. Lefkowitz and associates (390–392) took advantage of the fact that hydrogenation of naturally occurring ergot alkaloids results in compounds that are highly potent alpha-adrenergic antagonists. The product of catalytic reduction of alpha-ergocryptine with tritium gas, [³H]dihydroergocryptine, allowed specific labeling of alpha-adrenergic receptors sites. Independently, Snyder and associates (140,373) reported successful identification of alpha-adrenergic receptors using the radiolabeled antagonist [³H]WB-4101 {2-([2′,6′-dimethoxy]phenoxy-ethanolamino)methylbenzodioxan} and the radiolabeled agonists [³H]clonidine, [³H]epinephrine, and [³H]nor-epinephrine. Another radioligand, [³H]dihydroazapetine, was also used in an attempt to label alpha-adrenergic binding sites, but the sites labeled did not have affinity for alpha-adrenergic agonists (303).

CLASSIFICATION OF ALPHA-ADRENERGIC RECEPTORS

Background

The earliest method of classifying receptors related to Ehrlich's notion of "chemoreceptors" and was based on receptor desensitization (88). Ehrlich found that if a batch of trypanosomes was exposed to increasing doses of an arsenical, it eventually became refractory to all arsenicals. He attributed this refractoriness to loss of chemoreceptors for arsenicals. By applying similar desensitization procedures to other trypanocidal drugs, he subdivided them into three classes, each acting on a separate chemoreceptor.

On the basis of such studies he suggested a procedure for discovering new receptors. Thus, he argued, if trypanosomes had been desensitized to the three known types of trypanocidal drugs and were then found to be sensitive to a new drug, then the new drug must be acting on a fourth receptor.

This method, though ingenious, has not been widely used, perhaps because later studies showed receptor desensitization to be rather less specific than Ehrlich believed. In more recent times, classification of receptors has relied on the comparative efficacies of agonists and antagonists.

Classification by agonists has been widely used in relation to adrenergic receptors and led to the initial subdivision of these receptors into alpha and beta sub-

types (5). Subclassification of beta receptors into beta₁ and beta₂ subtypes by Lands et al. (204) and Furchgott (108) was also based on studies with agonists. In both cases, classification has involved the assumption that agonists acting on similar receptors will show similar activity ratios in different tissues. This assumption may not necessarily be correct if it is considered that the effects of agonists are dependent on both their affinity and their efficacy (intrinsic activity) (13,14,346). A more precise procedure would be determination of agonist affinities instead of activities. Although this is readily possible with radioligand binding studies, such calculations from conventional pharmacological procedures require complex measurements (311,376). For this reason, the most widely accepted basis for receptor classification has become comparison of the affinity constants for competitive antagonists, which can be readily determined from both pharmacological data (16,209) and radioligand binding data (167). However, even with the use of "antagonist" data, various pitfalls and complexities of receptor subtype analyses need to be recognized, as detailed, for example, by McGrath (237) and Kenakin (192).

More recently, Wikberg (388) and Fain and Garcia-Sainz (97) have suggested what might be considered as a biochemical approach, based on the observation that the biochemical mechanism of signal transduction for the alpha₁ receptor involves primarily an increase in intracellular calcium and increased turnover of phosphatidylinositol, whereas alpha₂-receptor effects are mediated by inhibition of adenylate cyclase. Although a subclassification based on biochemical mechanisms may eventually prove to be useful, at present our knowledge of signal transduction pathways is still limited, and numerous exceptions to and complexities (169) in the foregoing receptor-coupled responses are still being elucidated (a detailed discussion of signal transduction mechanisms will be presented later).

Pharmacological Studies

At the time of Ahlquist's experiments (5), the known adrenolytic drugs, such as the irreversibly acting haloalkylamines, dibenamine, and phenoxybenamine, various ergot derivatives, and the imidazoline antagonists phentolamine and tolazoline, all appeared to specifically block alpha-receptor responses, and a subclassification of alpha receptors into alpha₁ and alpha₂ types was not proposed until some 25 years later (206). This subclassification was initially suggested on an anatomical basis to differentiate classic postjunctional alpha receptors (alpha₁) from prejunctional release-modulating receptors (alpha₂).

The concept of release-modulating receptors stemmed from initial observations in isolated, perfused cat spleen that the alpha blocker phenoxybenzamine increased the overflow of norepinephrine into the perfusate (40). Earlier studies by Trendelenberg (366) and Dixon (82) can now be interpreted on the basis of a prejunctional modulating mechanism, and studies by Monnier and Bacq (254) with piperoxane and yohimbine were a prelude to both the detection of prejunctional alpha receptors and the alpha$_1$- and alpha$_2$-receptor subclassification. However, the observation by Brown and Gillespie (40) was initially interpreted as indicating that the alpha receptor of the effector organ was an important site of loss for the released transmitter, although it is of interest that in 1960 Paton (272) proposed the adrenergic nerve endings as a site of action of phenoxybenzamine, which Brown (39) considered "a most attractive heresay . . . because the idea that a blocking agent of any sort should act on the nerve endings" he regarded "as having gone out rather earlier this century."

Accordingly, Brown and Gillespie (40) reasoned that when the alpha receptors of the effector cell were occupied by the blocking agent, the released transmitter would not be able to combine with the receptors, and thus the overflow would increase without changes in transmitter release. Because phenoxybenzamine is a potent inhibitor of neuronal uptake of norepinephrine (uptake 1), as well as extraneuronal uptake (uptake 2), it was subsequently suggested that the increase in transmitter overflow was due to uptake blockade and therefore reduced metabolism of norepinephrine. This view was challenged when it was shown that uptake blockers, which do not interact with alpha receptors, did not increase transmitter overflow. Furthermore, quantitative analysis of the transmitter overflow obtained in the presence of phenoxybenzamine revealed that in addition to inhibiting norepinephrine uptake, phenoxybenzamine increased the output of the neurotransmitter (205). A similar conclusion was reached by Starke and associates (338), who demonstrated that phenoxybenzamine and phentolamine increased transmitter overflow in concentrations that did not inhibit either neuronal or extraneuronal uptake. Moreover, DePotter et al. (79) reported that phenoxybenzamine increased the release of dopamine beta-hydroxylase during nerve stimulation. Because this enzyme, which is co-released with norepinephrine from the postganglionic sympathetic neuronal storage granule, is not subject to uptake and does not interact with alpha receptors, it followed that neurotransmitter release, per se, must be increased by alpha-adrenergic antagonists.

Initially, these observations led to the suggestion that the amount of transmitter output might be controlled transsynaptically by the response of the effector cells (339). According to this hypothesis, alpha-adrenergic antagonists increased transmitter output by reducing the tissue response. However, this view was abandoned when it was shown that alpha-adrenergic antagonists increased transmitter overflow even in tissues in which

the response was mediated by adrenergic receptors of the beta type (236,338).

On the basis of these and other studies (206, 288,339,386) it became apparent from experiments with isolated perfused organs and brain slices, and more recently with conscious animals (135,137), that norepinephrine and other catecholamines, as well as imidazoline agonists, acted at an adrenergic receptor to inhibit the stimulated release of norepinephrine stored in central and peripheral noradrenergic nerve terminals, and alpha antagonists prevented this inhibitory effect. It should be noted, however, that a physiological role for prejunctional alpha receptors in modulation of neurotransmitter release is not universally accepted (11,12,184) and has been the topic of considerable debate (208,211,349). Moreover, in some vascular beds, investigators have been unable to demonstrate prejunctional control of norepinephrine release by alpha-adrenergic receptors (296).

Although the release-modulating receptor or autoreceptor has the general pharmacological characteristics of an alpha-adrenergic receptor, differences emerged between this receptor and the postjunctional alpha receptor. Thus, imidazoline agonists, such as clonidine, tramzoline, and oxymetazoline, the catecholamine agonist alpha-methylnorepinephrine, and the antagonist piperoxan, tolazoline, yohimbine, and its diastereoisomer rauwolscine are more potent at the release-modulating or alpha$_2$ receptor, whereas the agonists phenylephrine, methoxamine, and cirazoline and the antagonists prazosin and phenoxybenzamine, the benzodioxane derivative WB-4101, and the phenylethylamine BE-2254 {2-(β-[4-hydroxyphenyl]ethylaminomethyl)tetralon} are selectively potent at the classic postjunctional or alpha$_1$ receptor.

In addition to these differences in potencies of alpha-adrenergic agents at prejunctional and postjunctional receptors, it became apparent that in some tissues, alpha receptors, which are anatomically postjunctional, behaved functionally as prejunctional receptors, insofar as the potency series for various agonists and antagonists at these receptors was similar to that for prejunctional receptors. Moreover, alpha receptors in tissues that are not sympathetically innervated may behave functionally as either prejunctional or postjunctional alpha receptors (129). Because an anatomical classification clearly was not relevant in these tissues, a functional classification of alpha receptors into alpha$_1$ and alpha$_2$ subtypes was proposed (24) and is now widely accepted (237,388).

The terminal noradrenergic axon has been proposed as the location of prejunctional alpha receptors. In agreement with this view, alpha-adrenergic modulation of norepinephrine release has been observed irrespective of the anatomical environment of the axons (e.g., exocrine glands, smooth muscle and cardiac muscle, adipose tissue, brain), after atrophy of innervated effector cells (100), and in experiments with synaptosomes (i.e., fragments of terminal axons torn from their normal environment) (263). However, most radioligand binding studies have failed to locate alpha receptors on noradrenergic axons (355,371). Similarly, experiments demonstrating alpha₂-receptor modulation of norepinephrine release in brain slices (358) cannot be said to prove conclusively that alpha₂ receptors with this function reside on norepinephrine terminal membranes. And it is possible that this alpha₂ effect results from glial-neuronal interactions or short neuronal circuits in the vicinity of the norepinephrine synapse, involving alpha₂ receptors not located on norepinephrine terminals (340). Finally, there is now direct evidence for prejunctional heteroreceptors (i.e., receptors on prejunctional sympathetic nerve endings that are not sensitive to norepinephrine, the transmitter released from these nerves, but to transmitters released from nerves that synapse on the prejunctional sympathetic nerve terminals, e.g., acetylcholine acting on prejunctional muscarinic receptors) (201). However, prejunctional autoreceptors (i.e., receptors on prejunctional sympathetic nerves sensitive to the released neurotransmitter) have not been demonstrated (9,202). Indeed, more and more evidence has been accumulating over the last few years to suggest that autoreceptors may not be located prejunctionally (210,237).

More recently it has been proposed that both alpha₁- and alpha₂-adrenergic receptors may exist postjunctionally in vascular smooth muscle and mediate the same response: vasoconstriction. Evidence for this concept has come from studies in at least four species: rat (83,362), cat (21), rabbit (239), and dog (211). However, not all vascular beds appear to have postjunctional alpha₂- as well as alpha₁-adrenergic receptors (85,342).

Because alpha₁-selective antagonists more potently inhibit vasoconstrictor responses resulting from sympathetic nerve stimulation than those resulting from exogenously administered norepinephrine, it has been suggested that alpha₁ receptors might predominate intrasynaptically, whereas alpha₂ receptors may have a predominant extrasynaptic location (207,208). This difference in the locations of postjunctional alpha₁ and alpha₂ receptors may explain the long-standing observation that some alpha₂-adrenergic antagonists, previously termed adrenolytic agents, more effectively block responses to exogenous epinephrine and norepinephrine (254), whereas other antagonists (sympatholytic agents) are more effective at blocking responses resulting from neurogenically released neurotransmitter. However, Drew and Whiting (85) have observed that in contrast to the responses to nerve stimulation in some tissues that are blocked by low doses of the alpha₁-selective antagonist prazosin, responses to stimulation of cat splanchnic nerve are not. This finding suggests that at least some prazosin-insensitive receptors (presumably alpha₂ receptors) are innervated and thus are likely intrasynaptic.

The exact locations and functions of postjunctional alpha₁- and alpha₂-adrenergic receptors, therefore, remain unclear. It is possible that there are considerable species and tissue differences in their distributions and relative concentrations. Other factors, such as the size of the neuroeffector junction, which varies from as little as 40 to 60 nm in some capillaries to 2 μm in rabbit pulmonary artery (25), and the location of the adrenergic nerve terminal plexus within the adventitio-medial layers of the blood vessel, may also influence the responses to neurogenically released and exogenously administered alpha-adrenergic agonists (208). Finally, the possibility that there are subtypes, in addition to alpha₁ and alpha₂ receptors, cannot be excluded. Indeed, recent evidence from both pharmacological studies (77,157,280) and radioligand binding studies (56; S. M. Lanier, H.-J. Hess, R. M. Graham, and C. J. Homcy, *unpublished observations*) suggests that subtypes of alpha₂-adrenergic receptors may exist.

At present, receptors are classified as being different when, for a given drug, the drug-receptor dissociation constants (or, in other words, the affinities) differ. These constants can be determined directly from the ability of an unlabeled drug in question to inhibit receptor binding by a labeled congener (*vide infra*). Affinities can also be determined in functional experiments in which the biological response of the tissue is used as an indication of the drug-receptor interaction. For antagonists, the dissociation constant can be readily determined by Schild (310) analysis and is equal to the antagonist concentration that shifts the log concentration–response curve to the right by a factor of 2. Determination of agonist affinities is less straightforward. In general, responses elicited by an agonist are not directly related to the number of receptors occupied, but rather are unknown functions of receptor occupancy. What is determined in most functional studies is not the affinity of an agonist, but its potency, which is proportional to the EC_{50} value, i.e., the concentration that produces 50% of the maximal effect obtainable with the agonist.

On the basis of these considerations, alpha₁-adrenergic receptors can be defined, from both functional and binding studies in a variety of tissues, as those for which the affinities of antagonists decline in the order shown in Table 2, and alpha₂-adrenergic receptors are defined as those for which the affinities of antagonists decline in the opposite order. Of course, this definition can be based on a different series of antagonists (although, at present, the foregoing series is probably the most discriminant) and does not exclude the possibility that a further receptor subtype may exist that has yet a different potency series, and at which a theoretical antagonist(s), yet to be developed, would have higher affinity than at alpha₁ or alpha₂ receptors.

Definition of alpha-receptor subtypes from the standpoint of agonists is even more problematic. From studies

TABLE 2. *Relative potencies of antagonists at alpha$_1$- and alpha$_2$-adrenergic receptors*

Alpha$_1$	Prazosin
	Corynanthine
	WB-4101
	Phenoxybenzamine
	Phentolamine
	Mianserin
	Tolazoline
	Piperoxan
	Yohimbine
	Rauwolscine
Alpha$_2$	Idazoxan

Adapted from ref. 129.

reported thus far, it appears that at alpha$_1$ receptors, (−)norepinephrine has a greater affinity and potency than (−)alpha-methylnorepinephrine, whereas at alpha$_2$ receptors it has lesser affinity and potency than (−)alpha-methylnorepinephrine. Additionally, at alpha$_2$ receptors, clonidine has much higher affinity and potency than (−)phenylephrine, whereas at alpha$_1$ receptors it has higher affinity than phenylephrine, but a lower (or, at best, similar) potency. The situation with clonidine is complicated, because under particular experimental conditions it behaves as an antagonist rather than an agonist. This phenomenon is characteristic of partial-agonist compounds such as clonidine (243,244). Such agents stimulate receptors to produce a response when added alone, but antagonize the effects of full agonists when added before the agonist. Nevertheless, with the recent availability of subtype-selective agonists, classification of alpha receptors based on functional responses to these agents should be less problematic. Presently the most discriminant potency series for agonists is that shown in Table 3.

Ultimately, ability to discriminate between receptor subtypes will depend on demonstration of structural and chemical differences in their binding sites, following isolation and purification of the receptor macromolecules (169). The availability of these purified receptor proteins may also permit development of binding-site- and non-binding-site-directed antibodies, which may provide, in addition to the existing functional tests for discriminating between receptors, an immunological basis for identifying receptor subtypes (132,169).

Gamma Receptors

A third type of adrenergic receptor, the gamma receptor, was proposed by Furchgott (106) on the basis of the finding that neither the alpha-adrenergic antagonists phentolamine and dibenamine nor the beta-adrenergic antagonist dichloroisoproterenol effectively blocked the inhibitory effects of norepinephrine and epinephrine on

isolated rabbit duodenum. However, Ahlquist and Levy (6) subsequently showed in intact dogs that a combination of an alpha and a beta antagonist was effective and postulated that activation of either receptor subtype can elicit an inhibitory response. Because this observation was subsequently confirmed by Furchgott (107) in isolated rabbit duodenum, the proposal of a gamma-adrenergic receptor was withdrawn.

More recently, a third or gamma subtype of alpha-adrenergic receptors has again been proposed, predicated on the findings of electrophysiological studies in arteriolar preparations (159,199). In these studies, excitatory junctional potentials (EJPs) have been recorded in response to low-frequency stimulation of sympathetic nerves to blood vessels that are resistant to blockade by a variety of alpha-adrenergic antagonists (10). In the absence of antagonists to block the EJPs, it is premature to ascribe these phenomena to a new type of receptor. Nevertheless, the responses observed clearly represent measurements based on the transmitter–end-organ interaction and thus should not be dismissed.

Radioligand Binding Studies

The results of binding experiments with radiolabeled alpha-adrenergic agents support the concept of alpha$_1$ and alpha$_2$ subtypes (45,163,313,393). The radiolabeled ergot alkaloid [^{3}H]dihydroergocryptine was the first ra-

TABLE 3. *Relative potencies of agonists at alpha$_1$- and alpha$_2$-adrenergic receptors*

Alpha$_1$	Methoxamine
	Amidephrine
	Cirazoline
	Phenylephrine
	Norepinephrine
	Epinephrine
	Alpha-methylnorepinephrine
	Dopamine
	6-*F*-norepinephrine
	Clonidine
	p-Aminoclonidine
	M7[a]
	UK-14,304[b]
	TL-99[c]
	BHT-920[d]
Alpha$_2$	BHT-933[e]

[a] 2-*N*,*N*-dimethylamino-5,6-dihydroxy-1,2,3,4-tetrahydronaphthalene.
[b] 5-Bromo-6-(2-imidazolin-2-ylamino)quinoxaline.
[c] 2-*N*,*N*-dimethylamino-6,7-dihydroxy-1,2,3,4-tetrahydronaphthalene.
[d] 2-Amino-6-allyl-5,6,7,8-tetrahydro-4*H*-thiazolo(4,5-*d*)azepine.
[e] 2-Amino-6-allyl-4,5,7,8-tetrahydro-6*H*-oxazolo(5,4-*d*)azepine.
Adapted from ref. 209.

dioligand used to study alpha-adrenergic receptors. Initially, the high- and low-affinity sites detected by this radioligand and by the radiolabeled agonist [³H]clonidine were interpreted as agonist- and antagonist-specific sites (138,140,277). Subsequent studies clearly demonstrated that [³H]dihydroergocryptine labels alpha₁- and alpha₂-adrenergic receptors with equal affinity (45,160,248,313), whereas [³H]clonidine selectively labels alpha₂-adrenergic receptors (45,356).

Following these early studies, the characterization of alpha-adrenergic receptors has been extensively investigated in a wide variety of tissues, including brain, kidney, heart, ileum, lung, platelets, liver, uterus, fat cells, salivary glands, and blood vessels, as well as in various cultured cell lines (15,22,32,33,113,160–162, 171,178,247,306,307,313,316,318,323,326,348,355, 371,393), as reviewed by Bylund and U'Prichard (45).

Subtype analysis of alpha-adrenergic receptors with the nonselective radioligand [³H]dihydroergocryptine required construction of competition curves determined with subtype-selective agents such as prazosin, which possesses a 6,000- to 10,000-fold selectivity for the alpha₁-adrenergic receptor (46,131,163,360), and yohimbine or its diastereoisomer rauwolscine, which possess approximately 500-fold selectivity for alpha₂ receptors (163,342). Nevertheless, by computer modeling of such competition curves, not only could the subtypes of alpha-adrenergic receptors be defined, but also the proportion of each subtype could be evaluated and the subtype selectivity of the competing agents confirmed. For example, in the human platelet, the competition curves for [³H]dihydroergocryptine with prazosin, yohimbine, and the nonselective antagonist phentolamine were found to be steep and monophasic, indicating the presence of one homogeneous class of receptors. Because yohimbine competed more potently than prazosin, whereas phentolamine was of intermediate potency, the alpha receptor of the platelet could be identified as an alpha₂ receptor. By contrast, in rabbit uterus, the prazosin and yohimbine competition curves were biphasic, indicating the presence of both alpha₁ and alpha₂ receptors. The alpha₁ receptor composed approximately 40% of the total receptor population and had higher affinity for prazosin and lower affinity for yohimbine, whereas the alpha₂ receptor composed approximately 60% of the total receptors and had higher affinity for yohimbine than for prazosin. The competition curve for phentolamine, on the other hand, was steep and monophasic, indicating that phentolamine, like [³H]dihydroergocryptine, does not discriminate between alpha₁ and alpha₂ receptors, having approximately equal affinities for both subtypes (163). Similar experiments with mammalian kidney indicated the presence of both alpha₁ and alpha₂ receptors at a ratio of approximately 1:3 (313). These findings were confirmed with the availability

of subtype-selective radioligands such as [³H]prazosin for the alpha₁ receptor (141) and [³H]yohimbine for the alpha₂ receptor (74), which additionally allowed direct and precise quantitation of each receptor subtype (313).

ALPHA-ADRENERGIC RADIOLIGANDS

Agonists

A number of radiolabeled agonists have been developed as radioligands for analysis of alpha-receptor subtypes (Table 4). These include [³H]epinephrine, [³H]norepinephrine, [³H]clonidine (336), [³H]para-aminoclonidine (299), [³H]guanfacine (363), [³H]lofexidine (365), and [³H]UK-14,304 (231). However, subtype analysis with these radioligands may be complex, because it is likely that they label only a fraction of the alpha₂-receptor population and that this fraction may vary with the ligand and tissue under consideration. This may be related to the fact that the affinity of agonists for alpha₂ receptors appears to be modulated by guanine nucleotides (129,163,169) (vide infra). In the absence of guanine nucleotides, alpha₂ receptors exhibit two states of different affinities for agonists. ³H-labeled agonists such as [³H]epinephrine and [³H]norepinephrine, which are full agonists, bind only to that fraction of alpha₂ receptors in the high-affinity state. With partial agonists, such as [³H]clonidine, the situation is even more complex, because it can label both high- and low-affinity states of the alpha₂ receptor (163), although under certain experimental conditions only binding to the high-affinity state occurs (163,370). Additionally, although there is general agreement on the rank order of potencies of competing adrenergic agents in different tissues, many discrepancies exist in their absolute affinity values (341).

These various complexities of binding studies performed with radiolabeled agonists make interpretations regarding receptor subtypes difficult with these agents and have led to considerable debate about subtype analysis of alpha receptors in some tissues (91,163). Additionally, such studies with radiolabeled agonists initially led to the notion of discrete "agonist" and "antagonist" states of the receptor (91,140,371). It is of interest that on the basis of considerations of receptor binding theory, Furchgott (109) predicted that this interpretation of discrete agonist and antagonist binding sites was incorrect, and it is now clear that differences between agonist and antagonist binding can best be explained on the basis of the readily demonstrable high-affinity nucleotide-sensitive agonist state of membrane alpha₂ receptors. Parenthetically, a high-affinity temperature-dependent and nucleotide-dependent state has been demonstrated more recently for the alpha₁-adrenergic receptor (72,233,315,318). The implications of this site will be discussed later.

TABLE 4. *Alpha-adrenergic receptor agonist radioligands*

Radioligand	Receptor subtype labeled	Specific activity (Ci/mmol)	Comment
[^{3}H]epinephrine	α_1, α_2	10–120	Binding may be complex; mainly labels high-affinity state with K_d of 1–10 nM
[^{3}H]norepinephrine	α_1, α_2	20–40	Lower affinity than epinephrine at α_2 receptors
[^{3}H]clonidine	α_2	27	Partial agonist; binds with K_d of 1–3 nM at α_2 receptors
[^{3}H]p-aminoclonidine	α_2	40–60	Affinity may be higher (K_d = 0.3–2 nM) than that of clonidine; partial agonist
[^{3}H]guanfacine	α_2	24	Usefulness may be limited by high nonspecific binding
[^{3}H]UK-14,304	α_2	84	Not yet widely evaluated; specific binding may be low in the absence of Mn^{2+}; K_d = 1.4 nM

Antagonists

In addition to [^{3}H]prazosin and [^{3}H]yohimbine, a number of other radiolabeled antagonists have been developed and proposed as subtype-selective ligands for alpha$_1$ and alpha$_2$ receptors (Table 5). These include [^{3}H]WB-4101 (45,185), [^{125}I]BE-2254 (93,94,123), [^{3}H]E-643 (151), [^{125}I]CP63,789 {2-[4-(4-amino-3-[^{125}I]iodoben-zoyl)piperazin-1-yl]-4-amino-6,7-dimethoxyquinazoline} (136,320), and [^{125}I]A55453 {4-amino-6,7-dimethoxy-2-[4-[5-(4-amino-3-[^{125}I]iodophenyl)pentanoyl]-1-piperazinyl]quinazoline} (220) for the alpha$_1$-adrenergic receptor, and [^{3}H]rauwolscine (269,278), [^{3}H]lisuride (45), [^{3}H]idazoxan, and [^{125}I]CP68,489 {17α-hydroxy-20α-yohimban-16β-(N-4-[^{125}I]iodoaminophenethyl)carboxamide} (215,216) for the alpha$_2$-adrenergic receptor.

TABLE 5. *Alpha-adrenergic receptor antagonist radioligands*

Radioligand	Receptor subtype labeled	K_d (nM)	Specific activity (Ci/mmol)	Comment
[^{3}H]prazosin	α_1	0.05–1.75	12–80	Most widely used for characterization of α_1 receptors
[^{3}H]WB-4101	α_1	0.17–3	25	May not label α_1 receptors selectively in peripheral tissues
[^{3}H]E-643	α_1	0.59	50	Not yet widely evaluated
[^{125}I]BE-2254	α_1	0.1	2,175	May bind to nonreceptor sites
[^{125}I]CP63,789	α_1	0.1–0.6	2,175	Not yet widely evaluated
[^{125}I]A55453	α_1	0.08	2,175	Not yet widely evaluated
[^{3}H]phenoxybenzamine	α_1, α_2	1	3.3–45	May bind to nonspecific and non-α-receptor sites
[^{3}H]phentolamine	α_1, α_2	12	23	Usefulness limited by low affinity and nonselectivity
[^{3}H]dihydroergocryptine	α_1, α_2	1–10	23	Usefulness limited by nonselectivity
[^{3}H]yohimbine	α_2	1–11	81.6	Widely evaluated; selectivity for α_2 receptors less than that of rauwolscine
[^{3}H]rauwolscine	α_2	1–4	81.6	Widely evaluated
[^{3}H]idazoxan	α_2	1	30–50	Subtype characterization may be limited by partial α_1- and α_2-agonist properties
[^{125}I]CP68,489	α_2	2	2,175	First radioiodinated ligand for α_2 receptors

[³H]WB-4101 has been suggested to label exclusively alpha$_1$-adrenergic receptors, with a dissociation constant (K_d) between 0.1 and 0.9 μM (45). However, although selective labeling of alpha$_1$ receptors can be demonstrated in central nervous system tissue, its selectivity in peripheral tissues has been questioned. For example, in rat uterus, [³H]WB-4101 binds with similar affinities to alpha$_1$ and alpha$_2$ receptors (163), and in human platelets, which lack detectable alpha$_1$ receptors, [³H]WB-4101 binds potently to alpha$_2$ receptors, although its K_d value in this tissue is still about 10-fold greater than in tissues in which it labels alpha$_1$ receptors (74). Similarly, in bovine retina, [³H]WB-4101 appears to label alpha$_2$ receptors (27).

[¹²⁵I]BE-2254 is an aminotetralone derivative that has been shown to selectively label alpha$_1$-adrenergic receptors in membranes from cerebral cortex and various peripheral tissues, with K_d values in the 0.1-nM range (93,94,123). However, in guinea pig brain membranes, this radioligand appears to bind with high affinity to a nonalpha-adrenergic receptor site (2).

[¹²⁵I]CP63,789 and [¹²⁵I]A55453 are arylamine analogs of the selective alpha$_1$-adrenergic antagonist prazosin that bind reversibly and with high affinity to alpha$_1$-adrenergic receptors and identify similar binding-site concentrations to the parent radioligand, [³H]prazosin (220,319,320). Because of their high specific radioactivity (2,175 Ci/mmol), these compounds are especially useful where the yield of receptor-containing tissue is necessarily limited. Additionally, by diazotization and reaction with sodium azide, these compounds can be readily converted to photoaffinity probes. These radiolabeled arylazide analogs can then be covalently coupled to the receptor binding site by activation with ultraviolet light and used to investigate the molecular characteristics of the receptor (vide infra).

Rauwolscine is a diastereoisomer of yohimbine that binds with somewhat higher affinity and more selectively to alpha$_2$-adrenergic receptors and can be radiolabeled to fairly high specific radioactivity (80 Ci/mmol). The radioligand [³H]rauwolscine is thus particularly useful for characterization of alpha$_2$ receptors in a variety of tissues (260,278).

[³H]Lisuride is an ergoline derivative that binds with high affinity to brain alpha$_2$-adrenergic receptors (45). However, its usefulness is probably limited, because, in common with other ergots, it also interacts with high affinity at other brain monoaminergic receptors.

[³H]Idazoxan (RX781094) is a recently available radioligand that binds with high affinity and selectivity to alpha$_2$ receptors. However, despite the clearly demonstrated alpha$_2$-adrenergic receptor antagonist properties of idazoxan (51,84), it has recently been shown also to possess partial-agonist properties at some alpha$_2$ (271) and alpha$_1$ (225) receptors, which may complicate receptor-subtype analyses with this agent.

[¹²⁵I]CP68,489 is a p-aminophenethylamine derivative of rauwolscine that binds with high affinity to alpha$_2$-adrenergic receptors (215). It is the first high-affinity high-specific-radioactivity (2,175 Ci/mmol) probe available for direct study of alpha$_2$-adrenergic receptors and thus should be particularly useful in situations in which the yield of receptor-containing material is low. Additionally, by diazotization and reaction with sodium azide, it can be converted to the arylazide, which should be a useful photoaffinity probe for molecular characterization of alpha$_2$-adrenergic receptors.

Other radioligands that have been used to characterize alpha-adrenergic receptors include [³H]dihydroergocryptine and [³H]dihydroazapetine (vide supra), as well as [³H]phentolamine (235,345) and [³H]phenoxybenzamine (143,198,290). These compounds bind nonselectively to both alpha$_1$- and alpha$_2$-adrenergic receptors. Their usefulness is therefore generally limited to investigations of alpha receptors in tissues that contain predominantly only one alpha-receptor subtype, such as platelets. Phentolamine, tritiated to a specific activity of 23 Ci/mmol, has been applied to investigations of platelet alpha$_2$-adrenergic receptors, and appropriate binding characteristics have been demonstrated. However, at these sites it binds with relatively low affinity (K_d 12 nM). Phentolamine has also been labeled with ¹²⁵I, although the radioiodinated product did not bind appropriately to cerebral cortex membranes (2).

Phenoxybenzamine, by virtue of its alkylating properties, can be used as an affinity probe that covalently binds to alpha-adrenergic receptors. This property of phenoxybenzamine, which results in irreversible inactivation of the receptor binding site, has been used to advantage to investigate questions of receptor turnover and metabolism (147,238,242).

The usefulness of phenoxybenzamine as a radioligand following tritiation was initially limited by its low specific radioactivity (3·3 Ci/mmol), although some success at characterizing rat hepatic membrane alpha$_1$-adrenergic receptors was reported with this compound (44). More recently, a higher-specific-activity (45 Ci/mmol) compound has been developed and used to characterize both alpha$_1$ (198) and alpha$_2$ (290) receptors. Nevertheless, although in general the pharmacological specificity of [³H]phenoxybenzamine binding correlates with the binding of subtype-selective ligands (198), [³H]phenoxybenzamine should be used with caution, because it also interacts covalently with a number of other monoaminergic receptors, such as muscarinic cholinergic (31), opiate (297), and dopaminergic (223) receptors, as well as with nonspecific plasma membrane sites (198). It has been suggested that its specificity can be enhanced by using it in very low concentrations (197). However, even with the compound of higher specific radioactivity, identification of the extremely low concentrations of receptor sites present in most tissues is likely to be problematic and may necessitate initial purification of the receptor proteins (290).

BIOCHEMICAL MECHANISMS OF SIGNAL TRANSDUCTION

Alpha$_1$-Adrenergic Receptors

General Features of Alpha$_1$-Receptor Signaling

Although the mechanism(s) of signal transduction associated with alpha$_1$-adrenergic receptor remained elusive activation for many years, recent studies have provided significant insights (Fig. 1). In contrast to beta-adrenergic and alpha$_2$-adrenergic receptors, which are coupled to the membrane-bound enzyme adenylate cyclase (Fig. 1), activation of alpha$_1$-adrenergic receptors does not alter intracellular levels of cAMP. Rather, the mobilization of calcium from intracellular vesicles and/or the influx of extracellular calcium appear to be linked closely to activation of the alpha$_1$-receptor, as well as other calcium-mobilizing receptors, such as acetylcholine (muscarinic), vasopressin, angiotensin II, dopamine (D$_2$), histamine (H$_1$), thromboxane, thrombin, platelet-activating factor, and various chemoattractant and growth-factor receptors. As detailed next, this change in intracellular calcium likely results from a receptor-mediated degradation of membrane phospholipids.

Role of Calcium

Activation of alpha$_1$-adrenergic receptors leads to a rapid rise in cytosolic free calcium that precedes the physiological response (Table 6) (52,53). The increased available free calcium exerts its effects intracellularly mainly by binding to the ubiquitous calcium-dependent regulatory protein calmodulin. The calcium-calmodulin complex thus formed alters the activities of a variety of enzymes and other cellular proteins, which leads to the various physiological responses observed in different tissues.

In smooth muscle from many tissues, such as blood vessels, uterus, vas deferens, iris, piloerector muscles, bladder trigone and sphincter, ureter, esophagus, and gastrointestinal sphincters, activation of alpha$_1$-adrenergic receptors leads to contraction (41). In these tissues, myosin light-chain kinase is activated by the calcium-calmodulin complex (4), leading to phosphorylation of myosin light chains. Phosphorylation of myosin light chains permits actin activation of myosin ATPase and the cross-bridge formation between actin and myosin that leads to contraction (4,302).

The rise in cytosolic calcium induced by alpha$_1$-adrenergic receptor activation of vascular and most smooth muscle is derived initially from release of calcium from intracellular stores such as sarcoplasmic reticulum

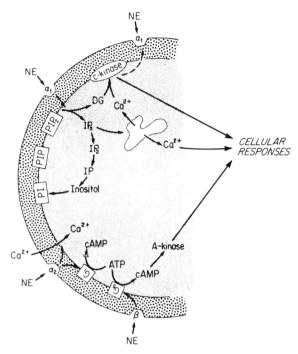

FIG. 1. Alpha$_1$-, alpha$_2$-, and beta-adrenergic-receptor-coupled signal transduction mechanisms leading to cellular responses. Binding of an agonist to the alpha$_1$ receptor is postulated to activate an enzyme that hydrolyzes phosphatidylinositol-4,5-bisphosphate (PIP$_2$) to form myoinositol-1,4,5-trisphosphate (IP$_3$) and diacylglycerol (DG). Availability of IP$_3$ leads to intracellular Ca^{2+} release, which can then activate cellular responses such as actin-myosin coupling or, together with DG, may promote protein kinase C (C-kinase) activation. C-kinase activation may limit (*broken line*) further signal transduction via the alpha$_1$-adrenergic receptor. Resynthesis of PIP$_2$ involves conversion of IP$_3$ to inositol by sequential removal of three phosphate groups to form inositol bisphosphate (IP$_2$), then inositol phosphate (IP), and finally inositol. A cytosine nucleotide derivative, cytosine diphosphatediacylglycerol (not shown), combines with inositol to produce phosphatidylinositol (PI), which is phosphorylated to yield PIP and then PIP$_2$. Activation of alpha$_2$- or beta-adrenergic receptors inhibits or stimulates, respectively, the membrane-bound enzyme adenylate cyclase (not shown); responses are mediated by independent inhibitory (G$_i$) and stimulatory (G$_s$) guanine-nucleotide-binding regulatory proteins. Increased adenylate cyclase activity promotes hydrolysis of adenosine triphosphate (ATP) to cyclic adenosine monophosphate (cAMP), which is then available to activate cAMP-dependent protein kinase (A-kinase). (From ref. 169, with permission.)

and plasma membranes. This initial phasic component of alpha$_1$-adrenergic-receptor-mediated vasoconstriction is thus independent of calcium influx and is resistant to calcium-channel blockade (237). The trigger for release of calcium from sarcoplasmic reticulum may be an initial receptor-coupled release of calcium from the internal surface of the plasma membrane adjacent to the receptor (41). A more slowly developing calcium-influx-dependent tonic component of the vasoconstrictor response resulting from increased membrane calcium permeability (36,81), follows the initial phasic compo-

TABLE 6. *Target tissues and responses of alpha-adrenergic receptors*

Receptor subtype	Tissue	Response
Alpha$_1$-adrenergic	Smooth muscle: vascular, uterus, trigone, pilomotor, ureter, sphincters (gastrointestinal and bladder), eye (iris), radial, vas deferens	Contraction
	Smooth muscle (gastrointestinal)	Relaxation
	Liver[a]	Glycogenolysis, gluconeogenesis, ureogenesis
	Myocardium	Increased force of contraction
	Central nervous system	Increased locomotor activity, neurotransmission
	Salivary glands	Secretion (K$^+$, H$_2$O)
	Kidney (proximal tubule)	Gluconeogenesis
	Adipose tissue	Glycogenolysis
Alpha$_2$-adrenergic	Sympathetic nerve terminal	Inhibition of norepinephrine release
	Vascular smooth muscle	Contraction
	Platelets	Aggregation, granule release
	Central nervous system	Sedation, inhibition of sympathetic outflow, neurotransmission
	Adipose tissue	Inhibition of lipolysis
	Eye	Decreased intraocular pressure
	Endothelium	Release of vasodilator substance
	Jejunum	Inhibition of secretion
	Kidney	Inhibition of renin release
	Pancreatic islet cells	Inhibition of insulin release
	Cholinergic neurones and cell bodies of noradrenergic neurons	Inhibition of firing
	Melanocytes	Inhibition of MSH-induced granule dispersion

[a] Applies mainly to the rat; in humans, beta$_2$-adrenergic responses predominate.
Data from refs. 129 and 131.

nent. This increase in calcium permeability may result from the opening of receptor-operated calcium channels (36), because the tonic vasoconstrictor response can be inhibited by calcium-channel blockers (237,364). It has been suggested that the existence of receptor reserve or the number of receptors activated determines the relative contributions of the calcium-influx-dependent and independent components of the vasoconstrictor response (305). However, this contention has recently been disputed (364).

By contrast, alpha$_1$-adrenergic receptor activation in most gastrointestinal smooth muscle, apart from that mentioned earlier, leads to relaxation. The exact mechanism leading to this inhibitory response is unknown; however, increased binding of calcium to the inner surface of the plasma membrane, leading to the opening of a potassium channel and increased potassium and chloride conductances, may be involved (41). This membrane binding of calcium may be secondary to release of this ion from internal stores. In salivary and lacrimal glands, a similar mechanism involving an initial

release of calcium from intracellular stores, followed by calcium influx and the opening of potassium channels, leading to increased plasma membrane permeability to potassium, is likely responsible for the efflux of potassium and H$_2$O associated with alpha$_1$-adrenergic receptor activation in these tissues (286).

In liver, alpha$_1$-adrenergic stimulation leads to a variety of metabolic responses, including glycogenolysis, gluconeogenesis, ureogenesis, increased amino acid transport, alterations in potassium fluxes and respiration, and inhibition of glycogen synthesis and lipogenesis (95,96). Alpha$_1$-adrenergic-receptor-mediated glycogenolysis, which is seen in many species, but is of minor importance in humans, in whom beta-adrenergic control predominates, is the most widely studied of these responses. Breakdown of liver glycogen results from the receptor-mediated rise in cytosolic calcium, which allosterically activates phosphorylase *b* kinase (57) via its calmodulin-containing gamma subunit. This enzyme, in turn, converts phosphorylase *b* to the more active form, phosphorylase *a*. With the activation of phosphorylase, glycogen is converted to glucose-1-phosphate and subsequently to glucose.

The increase in cytosolic free calcium that accompanies alpha$_1$-adrenergic receptor activation in liver is discernible within 1 sec (52) and is clearly derived from intracellular stores, particularly endoplasmic reticulum and mitochondria (19,30,264,291,292). Associated with the increase in cytosolic calcium there is an initial efflux of calcium from the liver, which then apparently alters the kinetics of calcium transfer, such that an elevated cytosolic calcium is maintained without net influx or efflux of the ion. Whereas the initial release of calcium into the cytosol from intracellular organelles is likely associated with receptor-coupled phosphoinositide breakdown (*vide infra*), two mechanisms have been postulated to account for alpha$_1$-adrenergic-receptor-mediated alterations in transmembrane fluxes; calcium channels in the membrane may be opened (291,292), or Ca^{2+}-Mg^{2+}-ATPase/Ca^{2+}-pump activity of the membrane that extrudes calcium from the cell may be inhibited (285).

In addition to glycogenolysis, hepatic alpha$_1$-adrenergic receptor activation leads to gluconeogenesis and inhibition of glycogen synthesis. Stimulation of gluconeogenesis results from effects at several sites, including stimulation of mitochondrial pyruvate carboxylation (8,114), phosphorylation, and inactivation of pyruvate kinase (50,115), and increased transfer of reducing equivalents across mitochondrial membranes by the glycerol-3-phosphate dehydrogenase system (385,398). Inhibition of glycogen synthesis, on the other hand, results from inactivation of glycogen synthase (351).

Activation of alpha$_1$-adrenergic receptors in renal cortical tissue also leads to gluconeogenesis by a calcium-dependent mechanism (193), although the details of this process remain undefined. By contrast, stimulation of alpha$_1$ receptors in adipose tissue activates phosphorylase and inactivates glycogen synthase by calcium-dependent pathways that are likely similar to those in liver (217,218). In adipose tissue, alpha$_1$-adrenergic receptors are generally less important in most species than beta$_1$- and alpha$_2$-adrenergic receptors, which in this tissue are the predominant receptors mediating lipolysis (98).

Alpha$_1$-adrenergic receptors are also found in myocardial tissue, where their activation leads to an increased inotropic response, prolongation of the action potential, reduced automaticity in Purkinje fibers and sinus node (70), and increased phosphofructokinase-mediated glucose uptake and flux (61,275). These responses are likely mediated by receptor-coupled increases in cytosolic calcium (70). Alpha$_1$-adrenergic receptor activation has also been shown to stimulate hypertrophy of cultured neonatal rat heart cells, a response that was found to be blocked by addition of the protein synthesis inhibitor cycloheximide (325). Whether or not this effect is due to Ca^{2+} release has not been determined, however, and preliminary evidence in cultured adult heart cells suggests

that norepinephrine-induced receptor activation does not cause hypertrophy (127).

Role of Membrane Phospholipids

Initially, a phospholipid mechanism for signal transduction of calcium-mobilizing receptors was believed to involve phosphodiesteratic cleavage of the membrane-bound phospholipid phosphatidylinositol (PI), to yield diacylglycerol and a mixture of inositol-1:2-cyclic phosphate and inositol-1-phosphate (IP) (252). These products of the cleavage reaction were then thought to increase intracellular calcium by an ionophore-like action. More recently, Berridge (23) and, subsequently, Streb et al. (350) and Joseph et al. (183) have provided plausible evidence that activation of calcium-mobilizing receptors results in breakdown of the polyphosphoinositide phosphatidylinositol-4,5-bisphosphate (PIP$_2$) to release diacylglycerol and myoinositol-1,4,5-trisphosphate (IP$_3$). Furthermore, IP$_3$ can selectively release Ca^{2+} from non-mitochondrial vesicular stores, possibly endoplasmic reticulum (181). On the basis of these observations, the finding of appropriate temporal changes in IP$_3$, and considerations of the IP$_3$-induced calcium changes with respect to its kinetics, concentration–response curve, and specificity, several reports have postulated that IP$_3$ is the second messenger for the alpha$_1$-adrenergic (183) and other calcium-mobilizing (350) receptors.

Similar findings have now been reported from studies with various types of cells, including insulin- and prolactin-secreting tumor cells, neutrophils, and vascular smooth-muscle cells [for a review, see Joseph (181)], and with hepatocytes, pancreatic islet cells, and blowfly salivary gland used in studies mentioned earlier (23,183,350). In rat hepatocytes, Kunos (197) has questioned the role of IP$_3$ as a mediator of intracellular calcium release, because the breakdown of PIP$_2$ to IP$_3$ depends on extracellular calcium and requires a much higher concentration of agonist than is required for increases in phosphorylase activity or calcium release (293).

The enzymes involved in the PI-IP$_3$ cascade have not yet been clearly identified. Of particular interest is the enzyme catalyzing the hydrolysis of PIP$_2$ to IP$_3$, presumably a PIP$_2$-specific membrane-bound phosphodiesterase. Phospholipase C, a cytosolic enzyme, was initially thought to be an unlikely candidate for this reaction, because it is not membrane-bound and requires calcium for activation. However, Hoffman and Majerus (164) recently reported isolation of two distinct PI-specific phospholipase-C enzymes, one of which specifically hydrolyzed only phosphatydlinositol-4-phosphate (PIP) and PIP$_2$ after calcium depletion with the chelator EGTA. This finding suggests that cleavage of PIP and PIP$_2$ occurs prior to increases in Ca^{2+} (240). Further, once intracellular calcium rises, PI breakdown by calcium-dependent phospholipase C may predominate, because PI is quantitatively the major potential substrate for this enzyme. A predominantly membrane-bound and magnesium-dependent phosphatase, specific for IP$_3$, has more recently been isolated from rat liver (181). This enzyme presumably catalyzes the degradation of IP$_3$ and inositol-4,5-bisphosphate (IP$_2$) and may explain the observation that following the rapid phase of IP$_3$-induced calcium release there is a gradual reuptake of the divalent cation (181). Thus, as would be expected for a second messenger, the cell appears to possess enzymes capable of promoting both the production of IP$_3$ and its degradation to IP$_2$ and phosphate (62,182).

Another recent suggestion by several groups is that the mechanism of signal transduction for alpha$_1$-adrenergic receptors may involve more than one pathway (37,112,181,258). In certain situations, responses to alpha$_1$-adrenergic agonists can be clearly dissociated from those of other calcium-mobilizing hormones, such as vasopressin and angiotensin II (72,112). For example, in isolated hepatocytes, the phorbol ester 12-O-tetradecanoylphorbol-13-acetate (TPA) can attenuate the metabolic effects of alpha$_1$-adrenergic agonists without altering the response to vasopressin or angiotensin II (71,72).

The phorbol ester TPA, a diterpene tumor-promoting agent, activates the calcium- and phospholipid-dependent enzyme "C kinase" in vitro. This activation is believed to reflect the structural similarity between TPA and diacylglycerol (269), which bind specifically and with high affinity to the enzyme. Diacylglycerol, as discussed earlier, is produced by hydrolysis of PIP$_2$ and is believed to be the endogenous activator of C kinase. This enzyme phosphorylates protein substrates at seryl and threonyl residues. Because covalent modification of proteins by phosphorylation is a common mechanism for their inactivation, it is likely that the selective attenuation of alpha$_1$-adrenergic responses by TPA (72) is due to C-kinase-induced phosphorylation of a protein very proximal in the signal transduction pathway. Because TPA stimulates phosphorylation of insulin and somatomedin-C receptors (172), it has been suggested that the alpha$_1$-receptor protein may itself be phosphorylated by TPA (72). Indeed, evidence in support of this postulate is the recent demonstration that TPA rapidly promotes phosphorylation of alpha$_1$-adrenergic receptors in DDT$_1$ cells (a cell line derived from hamster vas deferens smooth muscle) (219). Further, this effect is temporally related to the ability of TPA to attenuate norepinephrine-stimulated inositol phospholipid turnover.

Thus, in hepatocytes, activation of protein kinase C could be part of a feedback system for alpha$_1$-adrenergic receptors, a control mechanism that may also be applicable to other related receptors (e.g., the M$_1$ muscarinic receptor) (111). Blockade of alpha$_1$-adrenergic responses by phorbol esters has also been observed in other models, such as rat aorta (76) and rat hippocampal

slices (200). However, preliminary evidence from studies with rabbit thoracic aorta strips suggests that in this system, phorbol esters mimic alpha$_1$-adrenergic responses, and that the resulting activation of protein kinase C leads to intermediary activation of a lipoxygenase pathway (253,399).

At least two major mechanisms for signal transduction may therefore be operative. Initially, IP$_3$ is formed rapidly and leads to calcium mobilization. This response is probably common to all calcium-mobilizing receptors. Subsequently, with the availability of increased calcium, as well as diacylglycerol, protein kinase C may be activated and either selectively limit or mimic alpha$_1$-adrenergic-receptor-mediated responses.

Role of cGMP

Increased production of cGMP has also been proposed as a mediator of alpha$_1$-receptor responses. However, the role of cGMP and the mechanism that leads to increased levels of this cyclic nucleotide still are not clearly understood. Calcium directly stimulates guanylate cyclase, although arachidonic acid peroxide and prostaglandin endoperoxide are more likely to be the in vivo activators of this enzyme (128).

Haslam et al. (150) have suggested that cGMP may act as a negative messenger, because sodium nitroprusside, a potent vasodilator and platelet inhibitor, induces cGMP formation. Similarly, Schultz et al. (314) have demonstrated that both sodium nitroprusside and the cGMP analog 8-bromo-cGMP cause smooth-muscle relaxation. Nevertheless, alpha-adrenergic- and muscarinic-agonist-induced contractions are associated with enhanced levels of cGMP, as well as inositol phospholipid breakdown. Nishizuka (269) has interpreted these findings to indicate that in those cells in which cGMP generation inhibits the transmission of "positive signals," cAMP and cGMP do not act antagonistically, but similarly inhibit receptor-induced degradation of inositol phospholipids. These nucleotides may thereby act as a control mechanism to limit the "positive" or vasoconstrictor stimulus.

Involvement of a Guanine-Nucleotide-Binding Protein

Whether or not the alpha$_1$-adrenergic receptor is coupled to its signal transduction mechanism by a guanine-nucleotide-binding protein is presently unclear. Nevertheless, it is of interest that a guanine-nucleotide-binding protein has been implicated in the gating of Ca^{2+} by receptors (125). Preliminary studies by Haslam and Davidson (149) also suggest a role for guanine-nucleotide-binding proteins in the activation of platelets by thrombin. Thus, guanine-nucleotide-binding proteins, including G$_i$ or perhaps G$_o$, the newest member of the family described very recently by Sternweiss and Robishaw (347) and Neer et al. (267), may well be involved in the signal transduction pathways for the alpha$_1$-adrenergic and other calcium-mobilizing receptors. Alternatively, several lines of evidence (182) suggest that a novel guanine-nucleotide-binding protein, tentatively designated G$_p$, which is also subject to ADP-ribosylation by pertussis toxin (62), may be involved in the coupling of receptors to inositol phospholipid breakdown. More direct evidence for involvement of a guanine-nucleotide-binding protein in alpha$_1$-adrenergic receptor signaling is the recent finding by Blackmore et al. (29) that in rat hepatocytes, AlF$_4^-$, which is known to modulate the activities of other G proteins (G$_1$, G$_s$, and T$_c$), mimics the effects of calcium-mobilizing hormones.

Alpha$_2$-Adrenergic Receptors

Activation of alpha$_2$-adrenergic receptors leads to a variety of responses (Table 6) and, as in the case of muscarinic receptors in the heart (174,380) and opiate receptors in neuroblastoma-glioma (NG 108-15) cultured cells (322), inhibits stimulation of adenylate cyclase (Fig. 1). This, in turn, limits the availability of intracellular cAMP in a variety of tissues, including platelets, adipose tissue, liver, pancreatic islets, and NG 108-15 cells (7,42,69,177,190) (Fig. 1). Binding of ligands to alpha$_2$-adrenergic receptors and, in some tissues, responses to alpha$_2$ agonists correlate with this inhibitory activity (177). Thus, like beta-adrenergic (Fig. 1) and other cAMP-dependent receptors, such as those for dopamine (D$_1$ or D$_2$), histamine (H$_1$), ACTH, and prostaglandin E$_2$, signal transfer for alpha$_2$-adrenergic receptors may involve agonist-induced coupling to adenylate cyclase by a guanine-nucleotide-binding protein. Additionally, GTP is required for alpha$_2$-agonist-induced inhibition of adenylate cyclase, GTP decreases the affinity of alpha$_2$-adrenergic receptors for agonists, and regulation of receptor affinity by guanine nucleotides correlates with agonist efficacy in modulating catalytic activity (174).

Despite these similarities with the adenylate-cyclase-activating receptor, it is now clear that the coupling protein for the alpha$_2$-adrenergic receptor, G$_i$, is distinct from that for adenylate-cyclase-stimulating receptors, G$_s$ (35,69,187–189,283,312,331,399). G$_s$ and G$_i$ are both multisubunit proteins (heterotrimers) with two common subunits: beta (MW = 35,000) and gamma (MW = 8,000). However, the molecular weights of the alpha subunits differ: 45,000 for G$_s$ and 41,000 for G$_i$. Furthermore, the alpha subunit of G$_s$ (G$_s$-alpha) is a substrate for ADP-ribosylation by cholera enterotoxin, whereas G$_i$-alpha is a substrate for ADP-ribosylation by islet-activating protein, a toxin secreted by *Bordetella pertussis*. ADP-ribosylation by this latter toxin eliminates, or at least reduces, the attenuating effects of alpha$_2$-adrenergic agonists on adenylate cyclase activity.

Details of this alpha$_2$-agonist-induced attenuation of adenylate cyclase remain unclear. However, Gilman (118) has presented plausible evidence to implicate the following scheme: Activation of G$_s$-coupled receptors leads to dissociation of the alpha- and beta-subunit complex of G$_s$. In the absence of G$_i$-coupled receptor activation, G$_s$-alpha is available to stimulate adenylate cyclase. However, when G$_i$-coupled receptors are activated, the alpha- and beta-subunit complex of G$_i$ dissociates. Because the concentration of G$_i$ is greatly in excess of G$_s$, the homologous 35,000-dalton beta subunit of G$_i$ released by this process prevents G$_s$-alpha-induced stimulation of adenylate cyclase by binding and thus inactivating G$_s$-alpha. According to this scheme, G$_i$-alpha is a "passive bystander," acting as an antiinhibitor of adenylate cyclase. It is also possible that G$_i$-alpha plays an active role in the regulation of other alpha-adrenergic functions, just as guanine-nucleotide-binding proteins have roles independent of interaction with adenylate cyclase. For example, it has been suggested that insulin affects a plasma membrane kinase and cAMP phosphodiesterase through a specific guanine nucleotide regulatory protein (155,156).

A particularly interesting system that also involves a guanine-nucleotide-binding regulatory protein, termed transducin (T$_c$), is visual transduction. On absorption of light by the visual pigment of the retina, rhodopsin, which is embedded in specialized membrane regions of the photoreceptor, leads to the exchange by T$_c$ (like G$_s$ and G$_i$) of GTP for GDP. The T$_c$-GTP complex thus formed activates a cGMP phosphodiesterase that in turn mediates hydrolysis of cGMP (20,26,105). Marked similarities have also been noted between the gene products of the ras gene (contained in a significant proportion of human tumor cell lines and chemically induced rodent tumors) and the guanine-nucleotide-binding proteins responsible for inhibition and stimulation of adenylate cyclase (268). It is likely, in this setting, that the ras-gene product couples the activation of growth-factor receptors to intracellular events leading to cell proliferation and tumorigenesis.

Such considerations call into question the possibility that not all alpha$_2$-adrenergic responses are mediated by inhibition of adenylate cyclase activity. Connolly and Limbird (67), for example, have postulated that the effects of epinephrine on platelet function may result from modulation of a sodium-sensitive process independent of the alpha$_2$-adrenergic receptor/adenylate cyclase system. Indeed, preliminary evidence by Sweatt and Limbird (354) suggests that alpha$_2$-adrenergic receptor activation in the platelet is coupled to the receptor-mediated secretory response by a membrane Na$^+$/H$^+$ antiport exchange system. Similarly, Ullrich and Wolheim (369) have provided evidence that epinephrine inhibits insulin release from intact isolated rat pancreatic islet cells, at a step distal to generation of cAMP. Finally, with respect to the classic alpha₂-adrenergic receptor of prejunctional sympathetic terminals, there is as yet no evidence to show that inhibition of adenylate cyclase decreases norepinephrine release. Electrophysiological studies indicate that stimulation of prejunctional alpha₂ receptors leads to hyperpolarization (353,357), a response that may be mediated by activation of the sodium pump, i.e., Na^+-K^+ ATPase. As a result, calcium efflux is enhanced (63), thereby limiting calcium availability for excitation-secretion coupling. Nevertheless, in adipocytes from humans, hamsters, and some other species, alpha₂-adrenergic-receptor-mediated inhibition of lipolysis (98,203) can clearly be attributed to decreases in cAMP, because cAMP-dependent protein kinase phosphorylates and activates hormone-sensitive triglyceride lipase in this tissue.

FACTORS MODULATING LIGAND BINDING

As our understanding of the molecular mechanisms involved in adrenergic receptor-effector coupling has increased, it has become evident, particularly with the adenylate cyclase system, that several regulatory factors influence receptor-coupled signal transduction across the lipid bilayer. Evidence from radioligand binding studies using membrane-bound and solubilized alpha-adrenergic receptors indicates that guanine nucleotides, as well as certain monovalent and divalent cations, produces agonist-specific alterations in receptor affinity at both alpha₁- and alpha₂-adrenergic receptors. These effects have been studied in greater detail at alpha₂-adrenergic receptors, which are coupled in a negative manner to adenylate cyclase. Although alpha₁-adrenergic receptors were not considered to be coupled to adenylate cyclase, recent studies indicate that a guanine-nucleotide-binding protein may also be involved in signal transduction for this alpha-receptor subtype (vide supra) and that guanine nucleotides and certain cations also influence agonist binding to receptor. Radioligand binding techniques have also been used to investigate the potential role of changes in alpha-receptor number or affinity in the phenomena of denervation supersensitivity and agonist-induced desensitization, as well as in the altered effector cell responsiveness to adrenergic agonists that is observed in certain pathological states, such as thyrotoxicosis or hypoadrenalism. In these latter conditions, perturbations in adrenergic-receptor mechanisms result as secondary responses to primary alterations in other hormonal systems.

The majority of studies addressing alpha-adrenergic receptor regulation have been primarily phenomenological, and in only a few instances have the mechanisms involved been clearly elucidated. The findings of these studies are summarized in this section, and, where possible, the molecular mechanisms involved are discussed.

Alpha₁-Adrenergic Receptors

Guanine Nucleotides

In contrast to studies of alpha₂-adrenergic receptors (vide infra), studies aimed at demonstrating a role for guanine nucleotides in the regulation of agonist affinity states at alpha₁-adrenergic receptors have produced conflicting results. A guanine-nucleotide-induced decrease in agonist affinity was observed in early studies with hepatic membranes using the nonselective radioligand [³H]dihydroergocryptine. However, this finding was interpreted as indicating a nucleotide effect not at alpha₁-adrenergic receptors but at the small population of hepatic alpha₂ receptors (117,166). In contrast, a nucleotide-mediated effect on agonist binding to alpha₁-adrenergic receptors was suggested from binding studies with liver membranes in which the radiolabeled agonists [³H]epinephrine and [³H]norepinephrine (91,116,117) and, more recently, the alpha₁-selective antagonist [³H]prazosin (126) were used as radioligands.

Recent findings by Lynch et al. (233) provide a plausible explanation for these apparently discrepant findings. These investigators demonstrated that the ability to identify a guanine-nucleotide-induced shift in agonist affinity at hepatic membrane alpha₁-adrenergic receptors relates to the method of membrane preparation. Thus, a shift in agonist affinity is apparent if chelators of endogenous cations (particularly calcium) are used stringently, and if the membranes are washed vigorously to prevent retention of endogenous nucleotides, an observation subsequently confirmed by others (72,317). On the basis of these and other findings, it was postulated that a calcium-sensitive protease promotes uncoupling of the alpha₁-adrenergic receptor from its guanine-nucleotide-binding protein and thus obscures demonstration of high-affinity agonist binding (234).

Monovalent and Divalent Cations

The influences of monovalent and divalent cations on agonist and antagonist affinity states have not been as clearly defined at alpha₁- as at alpha₂-adrenergic receptors. Nevertheless, the results of the available studies are generally consistent and indicate that sodium decreases and magnesium increases the affinity of agonists (Tables 7 and 8). However, neither cation significantly influences antagonist affinity or receptor number. Although the divalent cation calcium does not influence antagonist affinity or the number of binding sites identified, in rat liver it appears to convert high-affinity agonist binding sites to sites with low affinity (233,234). As discussed earlier, this effect of calcium may be due to activation of a calcium-sensitive protease that prevents identification of high-affinity agonist interaction by uncoupling the receptor from its guanine-nucleotide-binding protein.

TABLE 7. *Modulation of radioligand binding to alpha-adrenergic receptors by sodium*

Tissue	Receptor subtype	Radioligand	B_{max}^a (%Δ)	Affinity		$[Na^+]$ (mM)	Refs.
				$K_d(\Delta)^b$	$IC_{50}(\Delta)^c$		
Rat renal cortex	α_1	[³H]prazosin	0	0	+2(E)	100	332
Rat heart[d]	α_1	[³H]prazosin	0	0	+3(NE)	150	122
					+2(NE)		
Rat cerebral cortex[d]	α_1	[³H]prazosin	0	0	+3.0(E)	150	121
Solubilized rat cerebral cortex	α_1	[³H]prazosin	n.d.	n.d.	+(E)[j]	150	145
					+13(NE)		
Rabbit platelet membranes	α_2	[³H]DHEC	0	0	+16(E)	100	367
Human platelet membranes	α_2	[³H]yohimbine	+22	−1.5	+10(E)	120	228
Human platelet membranes	α_2	[³H]yohimbine	n.d.	n.d.	+4(E)	100	262
Intact human platelet[e]	α_2	[³H]yohimbine	n.d.	n.d.	+6(E)	100	262
Intact human platelet[f]	α_2	[³H]yohimbine	0	+1.4	+2(E)	—	261
Intact human platelet[g]	α_2	[³H]DHEC	0	+3	0(E)	150	90
Rat renal cortex	α_2	[³H]yohimbine	+40	0	+3(E)(NE)	100	332
Rat cerebral cortex[h]	α_2	[³H]rauwolscine	+50	0	n.d.	—	81
Solubilized human platelet	α_2	[³H]yohimbine	+22	−1.8	n.d.	120	228
Rat cerebral cortex[i]	α_2	[³H]yohimbine	+50	0	+10(NE)	200	55
Rat cerebral cortex[i]	α_2	[³H]yohimbine	+40	0	+10(E)	200	395
Rat renal cortex	α_2	[³H]yohimbine	0	0	+10(E)	200	395
					+50(E)		
Human platelet membranes	α_2	[³H]p-aminoclonidine	−60	+10	+220(NE)	130	256
Guinea pig renal cortex	α_2	[³H]clonidine	0	+6	n.d.	100	352
Rat cerebral cortex	α_2	[³H]guanfacine	−65	0	n.d.	150	179

[a] Percentage change in receptor density as determined by Scatchard analysis of equilibrium binding studies performed in the absence and presence of the indicated concentration of sodium; +/−/0 indicate increase, decrease, and no change in receptor density, respectively.

[b] Fold change in radioligand affinity determined by Scatchard analysis, as in footnote a; + indicates an increase in the dissociation constant (K_d), but a decrease in affinity; −/0 indicate an increase or no change in affinity, respectively.

[c] Fold change in the affinity of competing agonist (norepinephrine or epinephrine), as determined from the concentration of the agonist producing 50% inhibition of radioligand binding. Values are derived from competitive inhibition studies performed in the presence or absence of the indicated concentration of sodium; +/0 indicate a decrease or no change in receptor affinity for the competing agent, respectively.

[d] Effect of sodium required presence of magnesium.

[e] In this study, extracellular sodium was replaced with sucrose.

[f] In this study, intracellular $[Na^+]$ was increased by use of the sodium ionophore monensin. In contrast, decreasing intracellular $[Na^+]$ by replacement of extracellular sodium with n-methyl-D-glucamine resulted in a twofold increase in the affinity for epinephrine.

[g] In this study, extracellular sodium was replaced with NH_4^+.

[h] In this study, [³H]rauwolscine binding could be resolved into two sites of high and low affinity. Sodium increased the number of high-affinity binding sites.

[i] The increase in receptor density can be attributed to retention of endogenous catecholamines, as discussed in the text.

[j] Degree of affinity change not quantitated.

Abbreviations: n.d., not determined; NE, norepinephrine, E, epinephrine; DHEC, dihydroergocryptine.

Alpha₂-Adrenergic Receptors

Guanine Nucleotides

As discussed earlier, in a number of tissues, alpha₂-adrenergic receptors are coupled in an inhibitory fashion to adenylate cyclase. Analogous to the situation for receptors coupled positively to adenylate cyclase (397), inhibition of the enzyme by alpha₂-receptor activation requires guanine nucleotides. However, 10-fold-higher concentrations of guanine nucleotides are required in this situation, as compared with receptors that stimulate adenylate cyclase activity (175). At alpha₂-adrenergic receptors, guanine nucleotides also produce concentra-

tion-dependent reductions in receptor affinity for agonists, but not antagonists. In the absence of guanine nucleotides, agonist inhibition curves are shallow (Hill coefficients <1; see *Chapter* 10 for a discussion of Hill plots) and best fit a two-site model of high- and low-affinity states. Addition of guanine nucleotides results in a steepening of the agonist competition curve (Hill coefficient = 1) due to loss of high-affinity sites (165). The degree of this shift is directly related to the intrinsic activity of the agonist (368). Thus, marked shifts are observed with full agonists, but shifts are not as prominent with partial agonists.

In equilibrium binding studies with radiolabeled agonists, Scatchard plots may be curvilinear. This is due

TABLE 8. *Modulation of radioligand binding to alpha-adrenergic receptors by magnesium*[a]

Tissue	Receptor subtype	Radioligand	B_{max} (%Δ)	Affinity		[Mg^{2+}] (mM)	Refs.
				K_d(Δ)	IC$_{50}$(Δ)		
Rat cerebral cortex	α_1	[^{3}H]prazosin	0	0	−4(E)	10	122
Rat heart	α_1	[^{3}H]prazosin	0	0	−3(NE)	10.5	122
Rat liver	α_1	[^{3}H]prazosin	0	n.d.	−2(E)	10	126
Rabbit platelet membranes	α_2	[^{3}H]DHEC	0	0	−4(E)	1.25	367
Human platelet membranes	α_2	[^{3}H]DHEC	n.d.	n.d.	−5(E)	8.5	368
Human platelet membranes	α_2	[^{3}H]yohimbine	n.d.	n.d.	−2.5(E)	8	262
Human platelet membranes	α_2	[^{3}H]yohimbine	n.d.	+2	−2(E)	5	372
Human platelet membranes	α_2	[^{3}H]yohimbine	0	+1.7	n.d.	5	74
Rat cerebral cortex	α_2	[^{3}H]yohimbine	−40	0	n.d.	10	298
Intact human platelet	α_2	[^{3}H]DHEC	−22	0	0(E)	1	90
Intact human platelet	α_2	[^{3}H]yohimbine	0	+3	n.d.	1	90
Guinea pig renal cortex[b]	α_2	[^{3}H]clonidine	0	−2	n.d.	0.1	352
Rat cerebral cortex[b]	α_2	[^{3}H]guanfacine	−65	0	n.d.	5	179

[a] See Table 7 for explanation of symbols and abbreviations.
[b] Result obtained with manganese.

to identification of both high- and low-affinity states of the receptor by the agonist radioligand (300). In general, the lower-affinity component cannot be adequately characterized, because extremely high concentrations of radioligand are required to appropriately saturate these sites. In these studies with agonist radioligands, the numbers of high-affinity binding sites are consistently less than the total numbers of sites identified with radiolabeled antagonists. This is likely due to the fact that antagonists bind with similar affinities to the entire population of receptors, although some investigators have recently contested this notion. Rather, it has been suggested that multiple affinity states of the alpha$_2$-adrenergic receptor may exist, termed super high, high, and low (372), and that different antagonists and agonists recognize all of these sites with variable affinities (308).

Radiolabeled agonists, such as [^{3}H]epinephrine and [^{3}H]clonidine, have also been used to investigate the role of guanine nucleotides in regulating alpha$_2$-receptor affinity for agonists. The findings of these studies indicate that guanine nucleotides reduce specific binding of the radioligand by increasing the rate of dissociation and by decreasing the number of detectable high-affinity sites (91,179,235,374). However, the number of binding sites identified may be influenced by the intrinsic activity of the agonist radioligand, and this must be considered when comparing [^{3}H]clonidine, a partial agonist, with [^{3}H]epinephrine or [^{3}H]norepinephrine, which are both full agonists.

The degree of guanine-nucleotide-induced shift in agonist competition curves may vary in different tissues. Although in all instances guanine nucleotides do produce a steepening of the agonist competition curve, the resultant curve may still have a Hill coefficient significantly less than 1. This suggests that other regulators of agonist affinity may be involved. Alternatively, the differences

between various tissues may relate to the heterogeneity of membrane structure and/or to differences in membrane preparation. As will be discussed later, certain cations can markedly affect agonist affinity, either directly or by interacting antagonistically or synergistically with guanine nucleotides.

In some instances, guanine nucleotides can also influence antagonist binding. In general, increased numbers of binding sites are observed with little change in affinity (37,395). This increase may be due to release of endogenous agonist that is presumably "locked" to the receptor binding site when endogenous guanine nucleotides are washed away during membrane preparation. With the release of this tightly bound agonist, the number of sites that can be identified with the antagonist radioligand is then increased (37,55).

Monovalent and Divalent Cations

Depending on the tissue and experimental conditions, sodium can either enhance or inhibit the ability of alpha$_2$-adrenergic receptor activation to decrease adenylate cyclase activity (176). Like guanine nucleotides, sodium consistently reduces alpha$_2$-adrenergic receptor affinity for agonists, but not antagonists (Table 7). The effect of sodium is specific, because it is observed with a number of different sodium salts, whereas other monovalent cations (potassium and lithium) are much less effective (228,367).

The sensitivity of alpha$_2$ receptors to this sodium effect appears to be directly related to the intrinsic affinity of the agonist used (367). Further evidence of a role for sodium in regulating receptor affinity for agonists is the finding that sodium decreases the specific binding of agonist radioligands (Table 7). Whether this is due to a decrease in the affinity of the total receptor population or to a decrease in the number of high-affinity binding sites is presently unclear.

The effect of sodium on agonist affinity at alpha$_2$-adrenergic receptors appear to be qualitatively somewhat different from that observed with guanine nucleotides. In studies with platelets, computer-assisted analyses of agonist competition curves indicate that, in contrast to the characteristic guanine-nucleotide-induced loss of the high-affinity component of agonist binding, sodium reduces the numbers of both high- and low-affinity sites without altering the biphasic nature of the agonist competition curve (250). This does not appear to be the case in all tissues. In rat renal cortex, for example, sodium apparently decreases the number of sites with high affinity for epinephrine, in addition to decreasing agonist affinity at the low-affinity binding sites (332). Furthermore, the agonist-specific loss in affinity produced by guanine nucleotides, but not sodium, is greater in the presence of magnesium (250). Although both guanine nucleotides and sodium are capable of producing an agonist-specific decrease in receptor affinity, the observations that guanine nucleotides and sodium act differently and that their effects are not additive suggest that guanine nucleotides and sodium regulate agonist affinity by distinct mechanisms. Indeed, studies by Limbird (226) indicate that these mechanisms can be dissociated. Specifically, in platelet membranes, the effect of guanine nucleotides, but not sodium, is lost after exposure to the sulfhydryl blocking agent *n*-ethylmaleimide (1 mM), exposure to heat (45°C for 20 min), or digitonin solubilization. This suggests that sodium acts at a site distinct from the guanine-nucleotide-binding protein, possibly at the receptor molecule itself. However, these studies do not exclude the possibility that sodium may act on a subunit of the guanine-nucleotide-binding protein G$_i$ (e.g., β subunit) that is not directly involved in the binding of guanine nucleotides and thus is insensitive to the foregoing perturbations.

The effect of sodium on receptor binding is most often studied in broken cell preparations in which it is impossible to ascertain if the cation acts at an extracellular or intracellular site. Nevertheless, it is apparent from such studies with membrane preparations that the concentration of sodium producing 50% of the maximal decrease in agonist affinity is in the range of 5 to 15 mM (228). Extracellular sodium is maintained at a constant level of approximately 140 mM. Therefore, if the sodium regulatory site were external, it is likely that all receptors would be in a sodium-locked state of low affinity for agonists. In contrast, because the concentration of sodium inside the cell is in the range of 10 to 30 mM, alterations in the intracellular concentration of this ion are more likely to influence receptor affinity for agonists. Studies by Motulsky and Insel (261) suggested that the sodium binding site is indeed intracellular. In intact human platelets it was found that elevation of

intracellular sodium by use of the sodium ionophore monensin or the Na$^+$-K$^+$-ATPase inhibitor ouabain decreased receptor affinity for agonists. In contrast, preparation of platelets in a sodium-free buffer (which reduces intracellular sodium by twofold) increased receptor affinity for agonists.

In rat kidney (332), human platelets (228), and rat cerebral cortex (55,81,395), sodium may also influence the binding of antagonists at alpha$_2$-adrenergic receptors. Again, this may relate to release of endogenously retained ligand and to variations in membrane preparations, as discussed earlier for guanine nucleotides. This is illustrated by studies in the cerebral cortex indicating that the numbers of binding sites identified with radiolabeled antagonist are doubled in the presence of guanine nucleotides and sodium (55,395). In both of these studies, preparation of cerebral cortex membranes with a hypertonic sucrose buffer resulted in a receptor density of 50 fmoles/mg protein. Following addition of sodium, GTP, or GTP plus sodium, receptor density increased 100, 80, and 130%, respectively. Alternatively, after membrane preparation with hypotonic buffer, the receptor density was 2.5 times higher and was not altered by sodium and/or guanine nucleotides (55). Quantitation of endogenous catecholamines indicated retention of these amines with hypertonic sucrose membrane preparation, presumably because the nerve terminals were not effectively lysed. It is likely, therefore, that the increases in receptor density observed with sodium and/or guanine nucleotides resulted from enhanced dissociation of tightly bound endogenous catecholamines. With hypotonic buffer preparation, the synaptosomes were apparently lysed, and no endogenous agonist was retained. Nevertheless, this phenomenon was not observed with rat renal cortical membranes, which may relate to the comparatively fewer neuronal structures in this tissue (55,395). This does not rule out a direct effect of sodium on alpha$_2$-adrenergic receptor affinity for antagonists (228,332), however, and emphasizes the importance of careful membrane preparation, as well as the heterogeneity of membrane structures in different tissues.

As discussed in *Chapter* 51, in addition to guanine nucleotides, certain divalent cations are required for stimulation or inhibition of adenylate cyclase following receptor activation. Magnesium, for example, appears to be required to form a high-affinity state of the receptor for agonists, which is then able to interact with the catalytic unit of adenylate cyclase (153). However, magnesium can often exert biphasic effects not only on agonist affinity but also on adenylate cyclase activity; higher concentrations of the divalent cation antagonize the ability of guanine nucleotides to stimulate adenylate cyclase and also reduce receptor affinity for agonists.

In most tissues studied, divalent cations (magnesium and manganese) increase the affinity for agonists and have no effect on or produce a slight decrease in antagonist affinity (Table 8). The effect of magnesium is temperature-dependent, as is the decrease in agonist affinity observed with guanine nucleotides (120). Computer-assisted analyses of agonist competition curves resulting from studies with human platelet membranes indicate that magnesium steepens the normally biphasic curve by increasing the number of alpha$_2$-adrenergic receptors in the high-affinity state (250). Thus, magnesium appears to exert effects opposite to those of guanine nucleotides; indeed, in some tissues, the presence of magnesium is required for identification of a guanine nucleotide shift. In general, manganese exerts the same effects as magnesium and in some tissues is considerably more potent (298,299).

In studies with agonist radioligands, magnesium and/or manganese have produced marked increases in specific binding of the radioligands (Table 8). These increases in binding appear to be due to increases in both affinity and receptor density. When examined, it has been found that magnesium apparently increases affinity by decreasing the rate of dissociation and also by increasing the rate of association (120,124). Again, the effect of this divalent cation is biphasic, with low concentrations (1–10 mM) increasing agonist binding, and higher concentrations (100 mM) decreasing agonist binding. The effects of higher magnesium concentrations are also observed with other divalent cations and may be due to nonspecific oxidative reactions at the receptor.

The effects of divalent cations on antagonist binding are not well understood. In both human platelets and rat cerebral cortex, magnesium (10 mM) has been shown to decrease the binding of [^{3}H]yohimbine, which may be due to either loss of affinity or loss of receptor density. In the rat cerebral cortex, similar effects were observed with manganese and calcium (299). In rat and pig lung and submandibular gland, magnesium also produced dose-dependent reductions in [^{3}H]-yohimbine binding that were due to decreases in receptor affinity (99).

Results of studies with agonist radioligands and the effects of magnesium on central nervous system membrane receptors (124,298,372,375) are complex and not well-defined. For example, antagonist competition curves resulting from studies with agonist radioligands exhibit Hill coefficients significantly less than 1 and are steepened by addition of magnesium, resulting in an increase in antagonist K_i (308). Whether this effect of magnesium is due to an alteration in receptor affinity for the radioligand or the competing unlabeled antagonist is not clear. Nevertheless, it has been suggested from the findings of such studies that multiple forms of the alpha$_2$-adrenergic receptor may exist that display different affinities (super high, high, and low) for various agonists and antagonists (308,372). These conclusions are based on consideration of similar findings observed in studies of cardiac muscarinic and pituitary dopamine (D$_2$)

receptors, both of which are coupled in an inhibitory fashion to adenylate cyclase (89,382).

ALPHA-ADRENERGIC RECEPTOR REGULATION

Background

The responses of various effector tissues mediated by adrenergic receptors can be influenced, over a period of time, by local concentrations of catecholamines, a phenomenon termed "homologous receptor regulation." With elevated levels of catecholamines, effector cell responsiveness can be attenuated ("down-regulation"). On the other hand, decreases in catecholamines can lead to potentiation of adrenergic-receptor-mediated responses, an effect termed "up-regulation" or supersensitivity. Alterations in effector cell responsiveness to catecholamines can also result from changes in unrelated hormones, such as thyroid hormones or corticosteroids, a phenomenon termed "heterologous regulation." As indicated, heterologous or homologous regulation usually occurs gradually over a period of hours to several days.

These alterations in effector tissue responsiveness can have important therapeutic implications, because prolonged drug administration can result in undesirable increases or decreases in adrenergic-receptor-mediated effects. However, the physiological relevance of homologous or heterologous regulation and the role of such alterations in tissue responsiveness in various disease states have not been clearly defined. Moreover, in many instances it is not clear if changes in catecholamine-elicited responses involve specific alterations in receptor affinity, density, or coupling mechanism or merely represent generalized nonspecific modulation of effector cell responsiveness, involving a variety of receptor systems.

Nevertheless, the molecular basis for these effects at the level of the receptor and its coupled transduction mechanism has been the subject of intense investigation, particularly for beta-adrenergic-receptor-mediated responses (148). The mechanisms involved in similar alterations at alpha-adrenergic receptors have not been as well studied, and conflicting results have often been reported. Much of the data available is largely phenomenological, because careful, comprehensive, and detailed investigations of both receptor alterations (density, antagonist and agonist affinities) and associated changes in coupled functional responses are infrequently undertaken. As shown in Tables 9 and 10, few studies have attempted to address the following questions that likely are the minimal criteria required to elucidate the mechanisms involved in homologous and heterologous receptor regulation: (a) What is the time course of receptor alteration, and are observed changes reversible? (b) Are the observed effects quantitatively related to the magnitude of the particular perturbation (dose-related), and has the perturbation (e.g., catecholamine infusion) indeed produced the desired effect (i.e., elevated plasma catecholamines)? (c) Do the observed effects represent a specific alteration in the adrenergic receptor system, or can they be attributed to nonspecific modification of effector cell membrane structure? For example, are other plasma membrane proteins (5'-nucleotidase, Na^+-K^+ ATPase) or other receptor systems (e.g., muscarinic cholinergic) also altered? (d) Are the observed effects agonist-specific, and can they be prevented by receptor-specific antagonists? (e) If the receptor alterations involve changes in agonist affinity, can various modulators of agonist affinity (guanine nucleotides, sodium, magnesium) be implicated?

Investigations of homologous or heterologous regulation of alpha-adrenergic receptors are also limited by our poor understanding of the effector coupling mechanisms. The precise details of many of the complex molecular mechanisms involved in the receptor-mediated effector response, even under physiological conditions, and the techniques to evaluate these mechanisms are unavailable. For example, only very recently has evidence been provided for mediation of alpha$_1$-receptor responses by a coupled guanine-nucleotide-binding protein. Virtually nothing is known about the molecular properties of this putative nucleotide-binding protein, let alone the stoichiometry of its coupling to the receptor or its interaction with the intracellular components of the response mechanism (*vide supra*). Until such components of the receptor-mediated response, as well as the receptor protein per se, are clearly defined, isolated, and characterized and are available for functional reconstitution, our ability to define the molecular basis for alterations in effector responsiveness will remain limited.

A more pragmatic issue in evaluating alterations in effector organ responsiveness and the involvement of changes in receptor density or affinity concerns extrapolation of findings derived from studies with tissues that are readily obtainable, such as platelets, to alterations in vascular smooth-muscle cells, for example, which are not readily available for study. Such extrapolations require careful validation, because rarely are they well substantiated and, indeed, in many instances may be entirely invalid.

Homologous Regulation of Alpha₁ Receptors

Pharmacological and physiological studies of alpha-receptor-mediated vascular smooth-muscle contraction indicate that removal of endogenous agonist by chemical or surgical denervation leads to increases in effector cell responsiveness to catecholamines and other alpha agonists. The increased responsiveness observed after such perturbations can be attributed in many instances to

decreased metabolism of norepinephrine, because neuronal uptake is either eliminated or substantially reduced. However, nonspecific alterations in receptor effector mechanisms may also be involved in certain tissues (103) (Table 9). Abel et al. (1) and Nasseri et al. (266) have fairly convincingly demonstrated that in the rat vas deferens, changes in alpha₁-receptor density or agonist and antagonist affinities are not involved in the enhanced responsiveness observed after surgical denervation or reserpine treatment. Unaltered antagonist and agonist affinities have also been demonstrated when responses of denervated preparations have been evaluated pharmacologically (304,359).

Studies of denervation supersensitivity have also been performed in other tissues, including kidney, uterus, and brain. However, evidence for or against a role for receptor alterations in these tissues remains inconclusive. Such studies in the central nervous system are complicated by the marked neuronal heterogeneity of brain tissue. Nevertheless, a study by Menkes et al. (246) suggested that increased alpha₁-receptor density without changes in agonist or antagonist affinity may mediate the increased responsiveness of lateral geniculate neurons following catecholamine depletion with 6-hydroxydopamine. These investigators showed that enhanced responsiveness to norepinephrine occurred gradually over a period of days and that the effect was specific, because responses to carbachol (muscarinic agonist) or serotonin were not altered. Neuronal uptake apparently was not involved, because responses to methoxamine and phenylephrine, alpha₁ agonists that are poor substrates for the norepinephrine uptake system, remained unchanged.

Decreased alpha₁-receptor density was demonstrated in several studies in which agonist levels were increased either by *in vivo* infusion or *in vitro* incubation of cells with catecholamines (Table 9). However, the significance of this finding is unclear, because the specificity and reversibility of the response was not defined, and/or because associated alterations in receptor-coupled effector responses were not evaluated.

Heterologous Regulation of Alpha₁ Receptors

Heterologous receptor regulation of alpha₁-adrenergic-receptor-mediated responses has been evaluated in liver from adult rats, in which increased glycogenolysis can be mediated by either alpha₁- or beta-adrenergic receptors (Table 9). Under physiological conditions, the increase in glycogenolysis produced by epinephrine or norepinephrine is mediated by alpha₁-adrenergic receptors. However, after thyroidectomy (284) or adrenalectomy (126), the epinephrine-induced increase in glycogenolysis switches to a beta-adrenergic-receptor-mediated response. In thyroidectomized animals this phenomenon is associated with decreased alpha₁-receptor density without changes in receptor affinity for agonists or antagonists.

TABLE 9. Regulation of alpha$_1$-adrenergic receptors

Tissue	Perturbation[a]	B_{max}[b] (%Δ)	Affinity[c] $K_d(\Delta)$	Affinity[c] $IC_{50}(\Delta)$	Functional correlate[d]	Temporal change[e]	Reversibility	Specificity[f]	Refs.
Homologous									
Rat kidney	NE/E infusion[i]	−50	0	n.d.	n.d.	+	n.d.	+	335
Rat kidney	T.P.[i]	−66	0	n.d.	n.d.	n.d.	n.d.	+	334
Rat liver	T.P.[i]	0	0	n.d.	n.d.	n.d.	n.d.	+	334
Rat lung	R.P.[i]	−75	0	n.d.	n.d.	n.d.	n.d.	+	334
MDCK cells	E incubation	−80	0	n.d.	+	+	+	+	245
Rabbit aortic smooth-muscle cells	NE incubation	−41	0	0	+	n.d.	n.d.	n.d.	33
		−70	0	n.d.	n.d.	+	n.d.	+	387
		−80[g]	0	n.d.	+	+	n.d.	n.d.	65
Rat mesenteric artery	E infusion	−50	0	0	n.d.	n.d.	n.d.	n.d.	66
	Denervation	0	−2	−8	n.d.	+	n.d.	n.d.	66
Rat vas deferens[h]	Denervation[i]	0	0	0	+	+	n.d.	n.d.	1,266
Rat caudal artery[h]	Denervation	0	0	n.d.	+	+	n.d.	n.d.	266
Rat submaxillary gland	Denervation	0	0	n.d.	+	n.d.	n.d.	n.d.	92
Rat submaxillary gland	Denervation	+60	0	0	+	n.d.	n.d.	+	44
Rat thalamus	Denervation	+45	0	0	+	+	n.d.	+	246
Rat kidney	Denervation[i]	+19	n.d.	0	n.d.	n.d.	n.d.	+	394
Heterologous									
Rat liver	Adrenalectomy	−24	0	+[i]	+	n.d.	+	+	126
		0	n.d.	0	+	n.d.	n.d.	+	49
	Thyroidectomy	−40	0	0	+	n.d.	+	n.d.	284

[a] Denervation was produced either surgically or by treatment with reserpine or 6-OH dopamine.

[b] Percentage change in receptor density produced by the perturbation indicated. Receptor density was determined as described in Table 7.

[c] Fold change in K_d or IC_{50} produced by the perturbation (see Table 7).

[d] + indicates that an appropriate functional response (e.g., vasoconstriction in vascular tissue or phosphorylase activation in rat liver) associated with alpha$_1$-adrenergic receptor activation was evaluated and identified.

[e] + indicates that the effects of the perturbation on changes in receptor density or affinity were evaluated and found to be temporally related.

[f] + indicates that changes in other adrenergic receptors (e.g., alpha$_2$, beta) were investigated and were not observed, or that the effects of the perturbation on receptor binding could be specifically blocked (e.g., with phentolamine).

[g] In this study, the effects of NE were found to be dose-related. This is the only study in which this parameter was investigated.

[h] Changes in the investigated functional response were not specific for alpha$_1$-adrenergic receptors.

[i] In these studies, the effects of the perturbation were verified by appropriate quantitation of catecholamine levels.

[j] Indicates loss of high-affinity agonist binding sites.

Abbreviations: NE, norepinephrine; E, epinephrine; T.P., transplanted pheochromocytoma.

Both the functional and receptor alterations can be partially reversed by administration of *l*-triiodothyronine. In adrenalectomized animals, a decrease in alpha$_1$-receptor-mediated glycogenolysis is also observed, but in this situation it is apparently associated with loss of high-affinity agonist binding sites. This is manifested by a loss in the ability of guanine nucleotides to induce a leftward shift in agonist competition curves. Again, these changes can be partially reversed by subsequent administration of cortisol.

Homologous Regulation of Alpha$_2$ Receptors

Alpha$_2$-adrenergic receptors were originally characterized by their prejunctional effects at adrenergic nerve terminals. However, attempts to specifically identify prejunctional alpha$_2$-adrenergic receptors by radioligand binding techniques have met with little success (*vide supra*). If alpha$_2$-adrenergic receptors were located solely at presynaptic sites, destruction of adrenergic neurons would be expected to eliminate alpha$_2$-receptor binding sites. However, chemical sympathectomy with 6-hydroxydopamine has variously been reported to result in a slight decrease, no change, or an increase in the number of central nervous system membrane binding sites identified with alpha$_2$-selective radioligands (142,152,259). One interpretation of these findings is that alpha$_2$-adrenergic receptors located postsynaptically may up-regulate in the face of the associated decreased agonist levels and therefore obscure any changes in presynaptic receptors. Because alpha$_2$-receptor-mediated inhibition of neurotransmitter release cannot be evaluated after reserpine or 6-hydroxydopamine treatment, the significance of these findings, in the absence of such a functional correlate, remains unclear.

In rat submandibular gland, depletion of neurotransmitter stores by reserpine or guanidine, or alpha$_2$-receptor blockade with yohimbine, increased the number of binding sites detected with the alpha$_2$-agonist radioligand [^{3}H]clonidine (44). However, in these studies, no specific binding was observed with the alpha$_2$ agonist [^{3}H]para-aminoclonidine or antagonist [^{3}H]yohimbine. Furthermore, the effect of reserpine to increase [^{3}H]clonidine binding was evident after only 3 hr of reserpine administration, which contrasts with the relatively longer time required for reserpine to deplete neurotransmitter stores. Also, an alteration in the effect of alpha$_2$-adrenergic receptor activation on cAMP or potassium release could not be demonstrated in that study. Increased [^{3}H]-clonidine binding after superior cervical ganglionectomy has been observed in rat submaxillary gland (92,282) and in rat vas deferens following reserpine treatment (381). Again, no functional response mediated by these putative alpha$_2$ receptors could be demonstrated, and in the vas deferens, specific binding of [^{3}H]rauwolscine was not observed (1).

Down-regulation of alpha$_2$-adrenergic receptors in response to elevated levels of agonist has been studied primarily in blood platelets (Table 10). In an early investigation, Cooper et al. (68) showed that *in vitro* exposure of intact human platelets to epinephrine (100 μM) decreased the number of [^{3}H]dihydroergocryptine binding sites, which was accompanied by decreased ability of epinephrine to promote platelet aggregation.

However, Karliner et al. (186) subsequently demonstrated that this apparent down-regulation of platelet alpha$_2$-adrenergic receptors was likely an artifact due to masking of the binding sites by retained epinephrine. In a more recent study, Hollister et al. (168) reported that increases in plasma catecholamine concentrations associated with standing exercise or infusion of norepinephrine or epinephrine resulted in a decrease in the affinity of platelets for agonists, with no change in receptor number or antagonist affinity. Incubation of human platelets with epinephrine also produced an agonist-specific decrease in receptor affinity and a diminished ability of epinephrine to induce platelet aggregation. However, considerably higher concentrations of the catecholamines were required to produce an effect in these *in vitro* studies.

Results obtained in isolated human adipocytes also suggest that epinephrine exposure may cause a loss of high-affinity binding sites for agonists. Incubation of adipocytes with 10-μM epinephrine (3 hr) decreased the binding of [^{3}H]para-aminoclonidine (which labels high-affinity agonist sites) without altering the number of [^{3}H]yohimbine binding sites (43). However, the ability of epinephrine to inhibit cAMP generation was not altered in these studies, despite the 40% loss of [^{3}H]para-aminoclonidine binding sites. Similar results have been reported in human subcutaneous fat cells and hamster adipocytes, in which *in vitro* incubation with clonidine reduced the number of [^{3}H]clonidine binding sites by 30 to 40%, but [^{3}H]yohimbine binding and alpha$_2$-

TABLE 10. *Regulation of alpha$_2$-adrenergic receptors* [a]

Tissue	Perturbation	B_{max} (%Δ)	Affinity $K_d(\Delta)$	Affinity $IC_{50}(\Delta)$	Functional correlate	Temporal change	Reversibility	Specificity	Refs.
Homologous									
Rat kidney	NE/E infusion[c]	0	0	n.d.	n.d.	n.d.	n.d.	+	335
Rat kidney	T.P.[c]	0	0	n.d.	n.d.	n.d.	n.d.	+	334
Human platelets	Posture/exercise[c]	0	0	+3.4	n.d.	+	n.d.	n.d.	168[b]
	NE/E infusion[c]	0	0	+3	n.d.	+	n.d.	n.d.	168
	NE/E incubation	0	0	+2	+	n.d.	n.d.	+	168[b]
	E incubation	−40	0	n.d.	+	+	n.d.	n.d.	68[b]
		0	+2	0	n.d.	+	+	n.d.	186[b]
Human adipocytes	E incubation	0	0	n.d.	+	n.d.	n.d.	+	43
	Clonidine incubation	0	0	n.d.	+	n.d.	n.d.	n.d.	379
Hamster adipocytes	Clonidine incubation	0	0	n.d.	+	n.d.	n.d.	n.d.	379
	Clonidine infusion	0	0	n.d.	+	n.d.	n.d.	n.d.	379
	E infusion	0	0	n.d.	+	n.d.	n.d.	+	276
Heterologous									
Rabbit uterus	Estrogen	+250	0	0	+	+	+	+	294[b,d]
		+550	0	0	+	n.d.	n.d.	+	162
Rabbit platelets	Estrogen	−40	0	n.d.	n.d.	+	n.d.	n.d.	295

[a] See Tables 7 and 9 for explanation of symbols and abbreviations.
[b] The effects of the perturbations on receptor density or affinity were found to be dose-related in these studies.
[c] Perturbations in these studies were verified by appropriate quantitation of catecholamine levels.
[d] An increase in receptor density was identified with estrogen treatment and was associated with increased contractile responsiveness of the tissue. However, this functional response is likely mediated by alpha$_1$-adrenergic receptors, whereas the change in receptor density was subsequently shown to be due to an increase in alpha$_2$- but not alpha$_1$-adrenergic receptors (162).

receptor-mediated inhibition of cAMP generation were unaltered (379).

Heterologous Regulation of Alpha₂ Receptors

Few, if any, studies have provided convincing evidence for heterologous regulation of alpha$_2$-adrenergic receptors (Table 10). For example, increases or no change in numbers of platelet alpha$_2$-adrenergic receptors have been reported in women taking oral contraceptives (279). However, no changes were observed in platelet alpha$_2$ receptors during the menstrual cycle or with pregnancy (279). In studies of white fat cells, administration of triiodothyronine decreased the number of sites identified with the nonselective antagonist [^{3}H]dihydroergocryptine (119). Although not evaluated, the binding of this ligand was presumably to alpha$_2$-adrenergic receptors, because the alterations in binding were associated with diminished ability of epinephrine to inhibit adenylate cyclase.

MOLECULAR CHARACTERIZATION OF ALPHA-ADRENERGIC RECEPTORS

Alpha₁-Adrenergic Receptors

Solubilization, Purification, and Biophysical Characterization

To date, most studies directed at solubilization and molecular characterization of the alpha$_1$-adrenergic receptor have employed rat hepatic plasma membranes. This tissue is particularly suitable for such studies, because membranes can be obtained in highly purified form, and the specific activity of hepatic alpha$_1$-adrenergic receptors is about 10-fold higher than that in most other tissues. Also, alpha$_1$-adrenergic receptors are the predominant subtype in this tissue, being about four times more abundant than alpha$_2$-adrenergic receptors.

Initial attempts to characterize the binding of solubilized rat hepatic alpha$_1$-adrenergic receptors with the nonselective antagonist [^{3}H]dihydroergocryptine were unsuccessful, probably because of the lipophilicity of this radioligand (143). Prelabeling with [^{3}H]dihydroergocryptine before solubilization, or use of the nonionic detergent digitonin, instead of the ionic detergent Lubrol-PX, did not enhance the identification of a solubilized receptor protein (143). For this reason, Guellaen et al. (143) covalently labeled the receptor with the irreversible antagonist [^{3}H]phenoxybenzamine before solubilization with Lubrol-PX and investigation of its biophysical properties.

For reasons detailed earlier, the specificity of [^{3}H]phenoxybenzamine binding to alpha$_1$-adrenergic receptors may be problematic, although it has been suggested that this can be enhanced by using very low concentrations of the radioligand (197). Nevertheless, identification of the extremely low concentrations of receptor sites present in most tissues may then be difficult, given the relatively low specific activity (3·3–45 Ci/mmol) of this radioligand. An additional problem with the use of [^{3}H]phenoxybenzamine is that prelabeling of membrane receptors before solubilization precludes investigation of the binding characteristics of the solubilized protein, because its binding site has been irreversibly occupied by the radioprobe. Other investigators, therefore, have attempted to solubilize the membrane-bound receptor in active form.

Several ionic and nonionic detergents have been investigated using a variety of solubilization protocols and various detergent-to-protein ratios (133,134). Only the nonionic detergent digitonin reproducibly released the membrane-bound receptors in a form that could be identified by direct radioligand binding assay. The binding characteristics of the digitonin-solubilized preparation were identical with those of hepatic membranes, and the binding of the alpha$_1$-selective radioligand [^{3}H]-prazosin was of high affinity and saturable. When the specificity of [^{3}H]prazosin binding to the solubilized preparation was examined in competition studies with a variety of adrenergic ligands, affinities comparable to those determined with particulate preparations were observed, and the stereoisomer potency ratio of agonists was conserved. These findings thus indicate that the alpha$_1$-adrenergic receptor binding site of hepatic membranes can be solubilized, with retention of its binding characteristics.

Digitonin has subsequently been used to solubilize membrane-bound alpha$_1$-adrenergic receptors from a variety of tissues and species; e.g., rat kidney and rabbit liver (K. R. Schwarz, C. J. Homcy, and R. M. Graham, *unpublished observations*). In addition, Wikberg et al. (389) have since reported successful solubilization of rat hepatic alpha$_1$-adrenergic receptors using a combination of digitonin, glycerol, and sonication. Interestingly, the protein solubilized by this technique demonstrated increased affinity for the agonists norepinephrine and epinephrine.

With the ability to solubilize the alpha$_1$-adrenergic receptor in active form, its purification (approximately 70,000-fold) to apparent homogeneity has been achieved with sequential affinity and gel-filtration chromatography (134). The affinity-chromatography step of this procedure required the synthesis of a novel analog of the highly selective alpha$_1$-adrenergic antagonist prazosin that could be immobilized on a solid-phase support. More recently, Leeb-Lundberg et al. (219) have reported partial purification of smooth-muscle-cell alpha$_1$-adrenergic receptors using a related, but distinct, prazosin-analog affinity resin.

Biophysical characterization of the purified receptor protein has been confined to evaluation of the receptor-protein/detergent complex, because the hydrodynamic properties of digitonin preclude determination of protein/ detergent stoichiometry. Nevertheless, the Stokes radius, sedimentation coefficient, and frictional ratio of the purified receptor protein have been determined (134). The values obtained from these studies differ from those for the solubilized [³H]phenoxybenzamine-binding protein reported by Guellaen et al. (143). This difference may relate to the limitations of receptor identification by [³H]phenoxybenzamine labeling, discussed earlier, as well as to the divergent physicochemical properties of the different detergents used in these studies, namely, Lubrol-PX (143) and digitonin (134).

The subunit characteristics of the alpha₁-adrenergic receptor have been investigated after [³H]phenoxybenzamine labeling of the membrane receptor (144, 198,324), after purification (134), and, more recently, after covalent labeling of membranes with high-specific-activity selective photoaffinity probes for the alpha₁-adrenergic receptor (220,319,320). Subunit molecular masses were determined from gel electrophoresis studies. Guellaen et al. (144) reported a subunit of 45,000 daltons for the [³H]phenoxybenzamine-binding protein of rat hepatic membranes. Using [³H]phenoxybenzamine of higher specific activity, Kunos et al. (198) more recently reported identification of a major 80,000-dalton band as well as a minor 58,000-dalton subunit, whereas Shreeve et al. (324) reported a subunit of 85,000 daltons and an isoelectric point of 4.6. Because these studies were performed with membranes prepared in the presence of multiple protease inhibitors, it is likely that the 45,000-dalton peptide identified by Guellaen et al. (144), in the absence of such inhibitors, is a proteolytic fragment. Similar considerations may also apply to the 59,000-dalton peptide identified after purification of the alpha₁-adrenergic receptor protein (134). Nevertheless, this subunit retains hormone-binding activity, because specific [³H]prazosin binding was identified following elution and renaturation of the purified receptor protein from polyacrylamide gels.

Using high-specific-activity radioiodinated photoaffinity probes, Seidman et al. (319,320) and Leeb-Lundberg et al. (220) identified a major subunit of approximately 80,000 daltons, as well as a subunit of 58,000 to 59,000 daltons and smaller species, in membranes from several tissues and species.

Using the photoaffinity probe developed by Seidman et al. (319,320), Lynch et al. (233,234) have more recently provided convincing evidence that the major subunit of the alpha₁-adrenergic receptor is approximately 80,000 daltons and that the smaller species (particularly the 58,000–59,000-dalton peptide) are proteolytic fragments. Thus, if appropriate protease inhibitors were used to block the effects of calcium-sensitive proteases, a predominant 78,000-dalton peptide could be identified. Less stringent protease inhibition caused the loss of the 78,000-dalton peptide and the appearance of smaller proteins (233,234).

The structure of the rat hepatic membrane alpha₁-adrenergic receptor has also been investigated using target size analysis performed by radiation inactivation (377). The results of these studies indicated an average molecular mass for the holoreceptor of 160,000 daltons. Based on this finding, or a molecular mass of 147,000 daltons deduced from the biophysical properties of the purified receptor (134), it is probable that the alpha₁-adrenergic receptor protein contains more than one subunit.

Structural Properties

Studies with the purified rat hepatic alpha₁-adrenergic receptor protein indicate a resilient tertiary structure that is likely stabilized by a disulfide bond. Thus, complete binding activity can be recovered after lyophilization of the receptor protein and renaturation out of guanidine (133,134,170). Binding activity is also resistant to high concentrations of the reducing agent, dithiothreitol (DTT). However, if the receptor protein is first denatured and then treated with DTT, or is reduced and then alkylated with iodoacetamide, binding activity cannot be recovered after renaturation (170). These findings indicate that the receptor binding site contains a disulfide bond that is inaccessible to solvent but is nonetheless critical for ligand binding. Strong hydrophobic interactions, stabilizing the binding site of the alpha₁-adrenergic receptor, are also likely, because full binding activity can be observed with urea solubilization (170).

In addition to a disulfide bond, studies with rat brain (287) and rat kidney (333) membranes suggest that the alpha₁-adrenergic receptor also contains a sulfhydryl group within or close to its recognition site.

Alpha₂-Adrenergic Receptors

Molecular characterization of alpha₂-adrenergic receptors has not progressed as rapidly as similar studies of alpha₁- and beta-adrenergic receptors (vide supra) (169). However, recently, several groups have made progress with solubilization, purification, and biochemical characterization of this alpha-adrenergic receptor subtype from human platelets and from the adrenocarcinoma cell line 494 (173,289,290,330,331). In addition, the alpha₂-adrenergic receptor of rat brain has been solubilized and its binding properties characterized (241,328). Several pharmacological and physiological studies suggest that alpha₂-adrenergic receptors exhibit heterogeneity in different tissues and species, both in terms of agonist/ antagonist recognition properties and in terms of receptor-effector coupling responses (55,191,365). Substantiation of such receptor heterogeneity by isolation, purification, and molecular characterization of the receptor proteins may thus have important therapeutic implications for the management and understanding of cardiovascular disease states and may potentially provide a basis for development of more selective ligands.

Solubilization, Purification, and Biophysical Characterization

Alpha$_2$-adrenergic receptors have been solubilized, with retention of binding activity, from human platelets (330), the adrenocortical carcinoma 494 cell line (173,265), rat brain (196,241,328), and rat kidney cortex (S. M. Lanier et al., *unpublished observations*) with the zwitterionic detergent 3-[(3-cholamidopropyl)dimethyl-ammonio-1-propane sulfonate] (CHAPS) and with the plant glycoside digitonin. Digitonin (0.5–1%) has proved to be most effective for kidney and platelet receptors, allowing approximately 40 to 60% of membrane-bound receptors to be solubilized. However, as noted for a number of other receptors, different batches of digitonin are quite variable with regard to effectiveness in solubilization. Other detergents such as deoxycholate, Lubrol-PX, Triton-X100, and chenodeoxycholate are considerably less effective in solubilizing the receptor protein in a form that permits its identification by radioligand binding techniques.

In general, the solubilized alpha$_2$-adrenergic receptor protein displays binding characteristics similar to those of the membrane-bound form. One important difference between digitonin and CHAPS is that solubilization of alpha$_2$-adrenergic receptors with the former, but not the latter, detergent results in a receptor preparation that exhibits low affinity for agonists. Studies by Smith and Limbird (330) indicate that the low agonist affinity of the digitonin-solubilized alpha$_2$-adrenergic receptor from human platelets is due to loss of a membrane component (G$_i$) that confers guanine nucleotide sensitivity on agonist binding (330). With agonist pretreatment of platelet or brain membranes, guanine nucleotide sensitivity is retained with digitonin solubilization, and agonist affinity is higher (196,330). The digitonin-solubilized agonist-occupied receptor also exhibits a higher sedimentation coefficient than the unoccupied or antagonist-occupied receptor (251,330) and can be distinguished from the receptor solubilized in the absence of agonist pretreatment by ion-exchange chromatography (227). Thus, it appears that solubilization with digitonin disrupts the interaction between the receptor and G$_i$, or a component of G$_i$ responsible for the high agonist affinity and guanine nucleotide sensitivity. In contrast, solubilization of brain membranes with CHAPS does not alter the affinity of the solubilized receptor for agonists, and sensitivity to guanine nucleotides is retained (241,328).

Alpha$_2$-adrenergic receptors from both platelets and the adrenocortical carcinoma 494 cell line have been partially purified using affinity chromatography as the principal technique (173,290). Regan et al. (290) used a 3-benzazepine alpha$_2$-receptor antagonist coupled to Sepharose CL-4B and achieved a 600-fold purification of the human platelet alpha$_2$-adrenergic receptor. A similar degree of purification (1,000-fold) of solubilized alpha$_2$-adrenergic receptor from the adrenocortical carcinoma 494 cell line has been reported with affinity chromatography with a para-aminoclonidine-Sepharose resin, followed by HPLC gel-exclusion chromatography. However, the pharmacological characteristics of this partially purified protein have not been fully defined.

A Stokes radius of 6.6 nm and an isoelectric point (pI) of 5.6 to 5.8 (241) have been determined from gel-filtration and isoelectric-focusing studies of the solubilized rat brain alpha$_2$-adrenergic receptor. This contrasts with a pI of 4.6 reported for the solubilized human platelet alpha$_2$-adrenergic receptor (324).

High-affinity agonist binding of both rat membrane and CHAPS-solubilized alpha$_2$-adrenergic receptor preparations is abolished by the sulfhydryl blocking agent *n*-ethylmaleimide (241,287). This suggests that a reactive sulfhydryl group is involved in the interaction between G$_i$ and receptor. Both antagonist binding and agonist binding of the membrane and CHAPS-solubilized receptor also appear to be sensitive to inactivation by organic mercurial agents, suggesting a reactive sulfhydryl group in or near the ligand recognition site of the receptor (241,287).

Affinity Labeling Studies

Developments in high-affinity radioiodinated probes, which can be used to covalently label receptor binding sites, have proved useful in identification and characterization of a number of hormone and neurotransmitter receptors. Atlas and Steer (17) have reported development of an affinity probe for the alpha$_2$-adrenergic receptor, but it is not available in radiolabeled form. At present, only tritiated ligands are available for molecular characterization studies of the alpha$_2$-adrenergic receptor. [^{3}H]phenoxybenzamine has been used for affinity labeling of partially purified, solubilized platelet alpha$_2$-adrenergic receptors, although specific labeling of membrane preparations with this compound apparently was not possible (290). Gel electrophoresis studies of this [^{3}H]phenoxybenzamine-labeled protein indicate an apparent molecular mass of 61,000 daltons, although in some experiments a specifically labeled 80,000-dalton peptide was also identified. Shreeve et al. (324) have reported a predominant 85,000-dalton peptide from studies in which platelet membranes were initially labeled with [^{3}H]-phenoxybenzamine. These investigators suggested that the inconsistently labeled 60,000-dalton band represents a proteolytic product. [^{3}H]para-azidoclonidine has been used as a photoaffinity probe to label the partially purified alpha$_2$-adrenergic receptor from adrenocarcinoma cell line 494. The results of those studies indicated specific labeling of a peptide with a molecular mass of 67,000 daltons (173). Finally, radiation inactivation studies indicate a molecular mass of 160,000 daltons for the holoreceptor of human platelets (378). Given the subunit sizes reported for the alpha$_2$ receptor, it is likely that the native protein is composed of more than one subunit.

ACKNOWLEDGMENTS

We thank Debra Rollins for typing the manuscript, Charles Homcy, Hans-Jürgen Hess, Kurt Schwarz, Christine Seidman, and Laureen Sena, who participated in the research, and Edgar Haber for continued support and encouragement.

Studies reported here were supported in part by NIH grant NS-19583, American Heart Association (AHA) grant 83-1242, with funds from the Massachusetts Affiliate, and a grant from the R. J. Reynolds Company. R.M.G. is an Established Investigator of the AHA (grant 82-240), and S.M.L. is the recipient of an AHA research fellowship (Massachusetts Affiliate no. 13-404-845) and a National Research Service Award, no. F32 HL07127-01.

REFERENCES

1. Abel, P. W., Johnson, R. D., Martin, T. I., and Minneman, K. P. (1985): Sympathetic denervation does not alter the density or properties of alpha$_1$-adrenergic receptors in rat vas deferens. *J. Pharmacol. Exp. Ther.*, 233:570–577.
2. Adams, A., and Jarrott, B. (1982): Development of a radioiodinated ligand for characterising alpha$_1$-adrenoceptors. *Life Sci.*, 30:945–952.
3. Adams, A., and Jarrott, B. (1984): A non-alpha-adrenoceptor binding site for [^{125}I]BE2254 in guinea pig brain membranes. *Biochem. Pharmacol.*, 33:2154–2158.
4. Adelstein, R. S., and Eisenberg, E. (1980): Regulation and kinetics of the actin-myosin-ATP interaction. *Annu. Rev. Biochem.*, 49:921–956.
5. Ahlquist, R. P. (1948): A study of the adrenotropic receptors. *Am. J. Physiol.*, 153:586–600.
6. Ahlquist, R. P., and Levy, B. (1959): Adrenergic receptor mechanism of canine ileum. *J. Pharmacol. Exp. Ther.*, 127:146–149.
7. Aktories, K., Schultz, G., and Jakobs, K. H. (1979): Inhibition of hamster fat cell adenylate cyclase by prostaglandin E$_1$ and epinephrine: Requirement for GTP and sodium ions. *FEBS Lett.*, 107:100–104.
8. Allan, E. H., Chisholm, A. B., and Titheradge, M. A. (1983): Hormonal stimulation of mitochondrial pyruvate carboxylatino in filipin-treated hepatocytes. *Biochem. J.*, 212:417–426.
9. Alonso, F. G., Cena, V., Garcia, A. G., Kirpekar, S. M., and Sanchez-Garcia, P. (1982): Presence and axonal transport of cholinoceptor, but not adrenoceptor sites on a cat noradrenergic neurone. *J. Physiol. (Lond.)*, 333:595–618.
10. Angus, J. A. (1982): Sympathetic vasoconstriction—no role for alpha-adrenoceptors. *Trends Pharmacol. Sci.*, 12:464–465.
11. Angus, J. A., Bobik, A., Jackson, G. P., Kopin, I. J., and Korner, P. I. (1984): Role of auto-inhibitory feed-back in cardiac sympathetic transmission assessed by simultaneous measurements of changes in ^{3}H-efflux and atrial rate in guinea-pig atrium. *Br. J. Pharmacol.*, 81:201–214.
12. Angus, J. A., and Korner, P. I. (1980): Evidence against presynaptic

13. Ariens, E. J. (1954): Affinity and intrinsic activity in the theory of competitive inhibition. *Arch. Int. Pharmacodyn. Ther.*, 99:32–41.
14. Ariens, E. J., Van Rossum, J. M., and Koopman, P. C. (1960): Receptor-reserve and threshold phenomena. I. Theory and experiments with autonomic drugs tested on isolated organs. *Arch. Int. Pharmacodyn. Ther.*, 127:459–463.
15. Arnett, C. D., and Davis, J. N. (1979): Denervation-induced changes in alpha- and beta-adrenergic receptors of the rat submandibular gland. *J. Pharmacol. Exp. Ther.*, 211:394–400.
16. Arunlakshann, O., and Schild, H. O. (1959): Some quantitative uses of drug antagonists. *Br. J. Pharmacol. Chemother.*, 14:48–58.
17. Atlas, D., and Steer, M. L. (1982): Clonidine *p*-isothiocyanate, an affinity label for alpha$_2$-adrenergic receptors on human platelets. *Proc. Natl. Acad. Sci. USA*, 79:1378–1382.
18. Aurbach, G. D., Fedak, S. A., Woodard, C. J., Palmer, J. S., Hauser, D., and Troxler, T. (1974): The beta-adrenergic receptor: Stereospecific interaction of iodinated beta-blocking agents with a high affinity site. *Science*, 186:1223–1224.
19. Babcock, D. F., Chen, L. J., Yip, B. P., and Lardy, H. A. (1979): Evidence for mitochondrial localization of the hormone-responsive pool of Ca^{2+} in isolated hepatocytes. *J. Biol. Chem.*, 254:8117–8120.
20. Baehr, W., Morita, E. A., Swanson, R. J., and Applebury, M. L. (1982): Characterization of bovine rod outer segment G-protein. *J. Biol. Chem.*, 257:6452–6460.
21. Bentley, S. M., Drew, G. M., and Whiting, S. B. (1977): Evidence for two distinct types of postsynaptic alpha-adrenoceptor. *Br. J. Pharmacol.*, 61:116P–117P.
22. Berlan, M., and Lafontan, M. (1980): Identification of alpha$_2$-adrenergic receptors in human fat cell membranes by [^{3}H]clonidine binding. *Eur. J. Pharmacol.*, 67:481–484.
23. Berridge, M. J. (1983): Rapid accumulation of inositol trisphosphate reveals that agonists hydrolyse polyphosphoinositides instead of phosphatidylinositol. *Biochem. J.*, 212:849–858.
24. Berthelsen, S., and Pettinger, W. A. (1977): A functional basis for classification of alpha-adrenergic receptors. *Life Sci.*, 21:595–606.
25. Bevan, J. A. (1979): Evidence for restriction of presynaptic alpha-receptors to the intrasynaptic neuronal membrane. In: *Presynaptic Receptors*, edited by S. Z. Langer, K. Starke, and M. L. Dubocovich, pp. 49–52. Pergamon Press, Oxford.
26. Bitensky, M. W., Wheeler, G. L., Aloni, B., Vetury, S., and Matuo, Y. (1978): Light- and GTP-activated photoreceptor phosphodiesterase: Regulation of a light activated GTPase and identification of rhodopsin as the phosphodiesterase binding site. *Adv. Cyclic Nucleotide Res.*, 9:553–572.
27. Bittiger, H., Heid, J., and Wigger, N. (1980): Are only alpha$_2$-adrenergic receptors present in bovine retina? *Nature*, 287:645–647.
28. Black, J. W., Crowther, A. F., Smith, L. H., Shanks, R. G., and Dornhorst, A. C. (1964): A new adrenergic beta-receptor antagonist. *Lancet*, 1:1080–1084.
29. Blackmore, P. F., Bocchino, S. B., Waynick, L. E., and Exton, J. H. (1985): Role of a guanine nucleotide-binding regulatory protein in the hydrolysis of heptocyte phosphatidylinositol 4,5-bisphosphate by calcium-mobilizing hormones and the control of cell calcium. Studies utilizing aluminum fluoride. *J. Biol. Chem.*, 260:14477–14483.
30. Blackmore, P. F., Dehaye, J.-P., and Exton, J. H. (1979): Studies on alpha-adrenergic activation of hepatic glucose output: The role of mitochondrial calcium release in alpha-adrenergic activation of phosphorylase in perfused rat liver. *J. Biol. Chem.*, 254:6945–6950.
31. Blazso, G., and Minker, E. (1980): Alkylation of ganglionic cholinergic receptors with haloalkyl amines. *Acta Pharm. Hung.*, 50:137–144.
32. Bobik, A. (1982): Identification of alpha-adrenoceptor subtypes in dog arteries by [^{3}H]yohimbine and [^{3}H]prazosin. *Life Sci.*, 30:219–228.
33. Bobik, A., Campbell, J. H., and Little, P. (1985): Desensitization

of the alpha$_1$-adrenoceptor system in vascular smooth muscle. *Biochem. Pharmacol.,* 33:1143–1145.

34. Bodnar, L., Hoopes, M. T., Gec, M., Ito, H., Roth, G. S., and Baum, B. J. (1983): Multiple transduction mechanisms are likely involved in calcium-mediated exocrine secretory events in rat parotid cells. *J. Biol. Chem.,* 258:2774–2777.

35. Bokoch, G. M., Katada, T., Northup, J. K., Ui, M., and Gilman, A. G. (1984): Purification and properties of the inhibitory guanine nucleotide-binding regulatory component of adenylate cyclase. *J. Biol. Chem.,* 259:3560–3567.

36. Bolton, T. B. (1979): Mechanisms of action of transmitters and other substances on smooth muscle. *Physiol. Rev.,* 59:606–718.

37. Boyer, J. L., Garcia, A., Posadas, C., and Garcia-Sainz, J. A. (1984): Differential effect of pertussis toxin on the affinity state for agonists or renal alpha$_1$- and alpha$_2$-adrenoceptors. *J. Biol. Chem.,* 259:8076–8079.

38. Briggs, G. E., and Haldane, J. B. S. (1925): A note on the kinetics of enzyme action. *Biochem. J.,* 19:663–672.

39. Brown, G. L. (1960): Release of sympathetic transmitter by nerve stimulation. In: *Adrenergic Mechanisms,* edited by J. R. Vane, G. E. W. Wolstenholme, and M. O'Connor, p. 127. Churchill, London.

40. Brown, G. L., and Gillespie, J. S. (1957): The output of sympathetic transmitter from the spleen of the cat. *J. Physiol. (Lond.).,* 138: 81–102.

41. Bulbring, E. H., Ohashi, H., and Tomita, T. (1981): Adrenergic mechanisms. In: *Smooth Muscle: An Assessment of Current Knowledge,* edited by E. Bulbring, A. F. Brading, A. W. Jones, and T. Tomita, pp. 219–248. University of Texas Press, Austin.

42. Burns, T. W., and Langley, P. E. (1975): The effect of alpha- and beta-adrenergic receptor stimulation and adenylate cyclase activity of human adipocytes. *J. Cyclic Nucleotide Res.,* 1:321–328.

43. Burns, T. W., Langley, P. E., Terry, B. E., and Bylund, D. B. (1982): Studies on desensitization of adrenergic receptors of human adipocytes. *Metabolism,* 31:288–293.

44. Bylund, D. B., Martinez, J. R., and Pierce, D. L. (1982): Regulation of autonomic receptors in rat submandibulor gland. *Mol. Pharmacol.,* 21:27–35.

45. Bylund, D. B., and U'Prichard, D. C. (1983): Characterization of alpha$_1$- and alpha$_2$-adrenergic receptors. *Int. Rev. Neurobiol.,* 24:343–431.

46. Cambridge, D., Davey, M. J., and Massingham, R. (1977): Prazosin, a selective antagonist of post-synaptic alpha-adrenoceptors. *Br. J. Pharmacol.,* 59:514P–515P.

47. Cannon, W. B., and Rosenblueth, A. (1937): *Autonomic Neuroeffector Systems.* Macmillan, New York.

48. Cannon, W. B., and Uridil, J. E. (1921): Studies on the conditions of activity in endocrine glands. VIII. Some effects on the denervated heart of stimulating the nerves of the liver. *Am. J. Physiol.,* 58: 353–364.

49. Chan, T. M., Blackmore, P. F., Steiner, K. E., and Exton, J. H. (1979): Effects of adrenalectomy on hormone action in hepatic glucose metabolism. *J. Biol. Chem.,* 254:2428–2433.

50. Chan, T. M., and Exton, J. H. (1978): Studies on alpha-adrenergic activation of hepatic glucose output: Studies on alpha-adrenergic inhibition of hepatic pyruvate kinase and activation of gluconeogenesis. *J. Biol. Chem.,* 253:6393–6400.

51. Chapleo, C. B., Doxey, J. C., Myers, P. L., and Roach, A. G. (1981): RX781094, a new potent, selective antagonist of alpha$_2$-adrenoceptors. *Br. J. Pharmacol.,* 74:842P.

52. Charest, R., Blackmore, P. F., Berthon, B., and Exton, J. H. (1983): Changes in free cytosolic Ca^{2+} in hepatocytes following alpha$_1$-adrenergic stimulation. *J. Biol. Chem.,* 258:8769–8773.

53. Charest, R., Prpic, V., Exton, J. H., and Blackmore, P. F. (1985): Stimulation of inositol trisphosphate formation in hepatocytes by vasopressin, epinephrine and angiotensin II and its relationship to changes in cytosolic-free Ca^{2+}. *Biochem. J.,* 227:79–90.

54. Cheng, Y., and Prusoff, W. H. (1973): Relationship between the inhibition constant (K_I) and the concentration of inhibitor which causes 50% inhibition (I_{50}) of an enzymatic reaction. *Biochem. Pharmacol.,* 22:3099–3108.

55. Cheung, Y.-D., Barnett, D. B., and Nahorski, S. F. (1984): Interactions of endogenous and exogenous norepinephrine with

alpha$_2$-adrenoceptor binding sites in rat cerebral cortex. *Biochem. Pharmacol.,* 33:1293–1298.

56. Cheung, Y.-D., Nahorski, S. R., Rhodes, K. F., and Waterfall, J. F. (1983): Studies of the alpha$_2$-adrenoceptor affinity and the alpha$_2$- to alpha$_1$-adrenoceptor selectivity of some substituted benzoquinolizine using receptor-binding techniques. *Biochem. Pharmacol.,* 33:1566–1568.

57. Chrisman, T. D., Jordan, J. E., and Exton, J. H. (1982): Purification of rat liver phosphorylase kinase. *J. Biol. Chem.,* 257: 10798–10804.

58. Clark, A. J. (1926): The reaction between acetylcholine and muscle cells. *J. Physiol. (Lond.).,* 61:530–546.

59. Clark, A. J. (1926): The antagonism of acetyl choline by atropine. *J. Physiol. (Lond.).,* 61:547–556.

60. Clark, A. J. (1933): *The Mode of Action of Drugs on Cells.* E. Arnold, London.

61. Clark, M. G., and Patten, G. S. (1984): Adrenergic regulation of glucose metabolism in rat heart. A calcium-dependent mechanism mediated by both alpha- and beta-adrenergic receptors. *J. Biol. Chem.,* 259:15204–15211.

62. Cockcroft, S., and Gomperts, B. D. (1985): Role of guanine nucleotide binding protein in the activation of polyphosphoinositide phosphodiesterase. *Nature,* 314:534–536.

63. Cohen, J., Eckstein, L., and Gutman, Y. (1980): The mechanism of alpha-adrenergic inhibition of catecholamine release. *Br. J. Pharmacol.,* 71:135–142.

64. Colquhoun, D. (1973): The relation between classical and cooperative models for drug action. In: *Drug Receptors,* edited by H. P. Rang, pp. 149–182. Macmillan, New York.

65. Colucci, W. S., Brock, T. A., Atkinson, W. J., Alexander, R. W., and Gimbrone, M. A. (1985): Cultured vascular smooth muscle cells: An *in vitro* system for study of alpha-adrenergic receptor coupling and regulation. *J. Cardiovasc. Pharmacol.,* 7:S79–S87.

66. Colucci, W. S., Gimbrone, M. A., and Alexander, R. W. (1981): Regulation of the postsynaptic alpha-adrenergic receptor in rat mesenteric artery: Effects of chemical sympathectomy and epinephrine treatment. *Circ. Res.,* 48:104–111.

67. Connolly, T. M., and Limbird, L. E. (1983): The influence of Na$^+$ on the alpha$_2$-adrenergic receptor system of human platelets. A method for removal of extraplatelet Na$^+$: Effect of Na$^+$ removal on aggregation, secretion, and cAMP accumulation. *J. Biol. Chem.,* 258:3907–3912.

68. Cooper, B., Handin, R. I., Young, L. H., and Alexander, R. W. (1978): Agonist regulation of the human platelet alpha-adrenergic receptor. *Nature,* 274:703–706.

69. Cooper, D. M. F., Schlegel, W., Lin, M. C., and Rodbell, M. (1979): The fat cell adenylate cyclase system. Characterization and manipulation of its bimodal regulation of GTP. *J. Biol. Chem.,* 254:8927–8931.

70. Corr, P. B., and Sharma, A. D. (1984): Alpha-adrenergic-mediated effects on myocardial calcium. In: *Calcium Antagonists and Cardiovascular Disease,* edited by L. H. Opie, pp. 193–204. Raven, New York.

71. Corvera, S., and Garcia-Sainz, J. A. (1984): Phorbol esters inhibit alpha$_1$-adrenergic stimulation of glycogenolysis in isolated rat hepatocytes. *Biochem. Biophys. Res. Commun.,* 119:1128–1133.

72. Corvera, S., Schwarz, K. R., Graham, R. M., and Garcia-Sainz, J. A. (1986): Phorbol esters inhibit alpha$_1$-adrenergic effects and decrease the affinity of liver cell alpha$_1$-adrenergic receptors for (-)-epinephrine. *J. Biol. Chem.,* 261:520–526.

73. Cuatrecasas, P., and Hollenberg, M. D. (1976): Membrane receptors and hormone secretion. *Adv. Protein Chem.,* 30:251–451.

74. Daiguji, M., Meltzer, H. Y., and U'Prichard, D. C. (1981): Human platelet alpha$_2$-adrenergic receptors: Labeling with [^{3}H]yohimbine, a selective antagonist ligand. *Life Sci.,* 28:2705–2717.

75. Dale, H. H. (1906): On some physiological actions of ergot. *J. Physiol. (Lond.).,* 34:163–206.

76. Danthuluri, N. R., and Deth, R. C. (1984): Phorbol ester-induced contraction of arterial smooth muscle and inhibition of alpha-adrenergic response. *Biochem. Biophys. Res. Commun.,* 125: 1103–1109.

77. DeJonge, A., Santing, P. N., Timmermans, P. B. M. W. M., and Van Zweiten, P. A. (1981): A comparison of peripheral pre- and

postsynaptic alpha$_2$-adrenoceptors using meta-substituted imidazolidines. *J. Auton. Pharmacol.*, 1:377–383.

78. DeMeyts, P., and Rousseau, G. G. (1980): Receptor concepts. A century of evolution. *Circ. Res.*, 46:I-3-I-9.

79. DePotter, W. P., Chubb, I. W., Put, A., and DeSchaepdryver, A. F. (1971): Facilitation of the release of noradrenaline and dopamine-beta-hydroxylase at low stimulation frequencies by alpha-blocking agents. *Arch. Int. Pharmacodyn.*, 193:191–197.

80. Deth, R., and Van Breeman, C. (1974): Relative contributions of Ca^{2+} influx and cellular Ca^{2+} release during drug induced activation of the rabbit aorta. *Pfluegers Arch.*, 348:13–22.

81. Diop, L., Dausse, J. P., and Meyer, P. (1983): Specific binding of [^{3}H]rauwolscine to alpha$_2$-adrenoceptors in rat cerebral cortex: Comparison between crude and synaptosmal plasma membranes. *J. Neurochem.*, 41:710–715.

82. Dixon, W. E. (1924): Nicotin, Conur, Piperidin, Lupetidin, Cytisin, Lobeln, Sparetein, Gelsemin. Mittel, welche auf bestimmte Nervenzellen wirken. In: *Handbuch der experimentellen Pharmakologie, Vol. 2,* edited by A. Heffter, pp. 656–736. Springer-Verlag, Berlin.

83. Docherty, J. R., and McGrath, J. C. (1980): A comparison of pre- and post-junctional properties of several alpha-adrenergic receptor agonists in the cardiovascular system and anococcygeus muscle of the rat. *Naunyn Schmiedebergs Arch. Pharmacol.*, 312:107–116.

84. Doxey, J. C., Roach, A. G., and Smith, C. F. C. (1983): Studies on RX781094, a selective potent specific antagonist of alpha$_2$-adrenoceptors. *Br. J. Pharmacol.*, 78:489–505.

85. Drew, G. M., and Whiting, S. B. (1979): Evidence for two distinct types of postsynaptic alpha-adrenoceptor in vascular smooth muscle *in vivo. Br. J. Pharmacol.*, 67:207–215.

86. Ehrlich, P. (1907): Chemotherapeutiche Trypanosomen—Studien. *Berlin Klin. Wochenschr.*, 3:183–192.

87. Ehrlich, P. (1909): Ueber den jetzugen Stand der Chemotherapie. *Ber. Dtsch. Chem. Ges.*, 42:17–47.

88. Ehrlich, P. (1913): Chemotherapeutics: Scientific principles, methods and results. *Lancet*, 2:445–451.

89. Elhart, F. J., Roeske, W. R., and Yamamura, H. I. (1980): Regulation of muscarinic receptor binding by guanine nucleotides and *N*-ethylmaleimide. *J. Supramol. Struct.*, 14:149–162.

90. Elliot, J. M., and Grahme-Smith, D. G. (1982): The effects of monovalent and divalent cations on the alpha-adrenoceptor of intact human platelets. *Br. J. Pharmacol.*, 77:277–283.

91. El-Refai, M. R., Blackmore, P. H., and Exton, J. H. (1979): Evidence for two alpha-adrenergic binding sites in liver plasma membranes. *J. Biol. Chem.*, 254:4375–4386.

92. Elverdin, J. C., Luchelli-Fortis, M. A., Stefano, F. J. E., and Perec, C. J. (1984): Alpha$_1$-adrenoceptors mediate secretory responses to norepinephrine in innervated and denervated rat submaxillary glands. *J. Pharmacol. Exp. Ther.*, 229:261–266.

93. Engel, G., and Hoyer, D. (1981): [^{125}I]BE2254, a new high affinity radioligand for alpha$_1$-adrenoceptors. *Eur. J. Pharmacol.*, 73:221–224.

94. Engel, G., and Hoyer, D. (1982): [^{125}Iodo]BE2254, a new radioligand for alpha$_1$-adrenoceptors. *J. Cardiovasc. Pharmacol.*, 4:S25–S29.

95. Exton, J. H. (1981): Molecular mechanisms involved in alpha-adrenergic responses. *Mol. Cell. Endocrinol.*, 23:233–264.

96. Exton, J. H. (1985): Mechanisms involved in alpha-adrenergic phenomena. *Am. J. Physiol.*, 248:E633–E647.

97. Fain, J. N., and Garcia-Sainz, J. A. (1980): Role of phosphatidylinositol turnover in alpha$_1$ and adenylate cyclase inhibition in alpha$_2$-effects of catecholamines. *Life Sci.*, 26:1183–1194.

98. Fain, J. N., and Garcia-Sainz, J. A. (1983): Adrenergic regulation of adipocyte metabolism. *J. Lipid Res.*, 24:945–966.

99. Feller, D. J., and Bylund, D. B. (1984): Comparison of alpha$_2$-adrenergic receptors and their regulation in rodent and porcine species. *J. Pharmacol. Exp. Ther.*, 228:275–282.

100. Filinger, E. J., Langer, S. Z., Perec, C. J., and Stefano, F. J. E. (1978): Evidence for the presynaptic location of the alpha-adrenoceptors which regulate noradrenaline release in the rat submaxillary gland. *Naunyn Schmiedebergs Arch. Pharmacol.*, 304:21–26.

101. Fisher, E. (1894): Einfluss der Configuration auf die Wirkung der Enzyme. *Ber. Dtsch. Chem. Ges.*, 27:2985–3005.

102. Fiszer de Plazas, S., and DeRobertis, E. (1972): Isolation of a proteolipid from spleen capsule binding (±)[^{3}H]norepinephrine. *Biochim. Biophys. Acta,* 266:246–254.

103. Fleming, W. W. (1976): Variable sensitivity of excitable cells: Possible mechanisms and biological significance. *Rev. Neurosci.*, 2:43–90.

104. Franklin, T. J. (1980): Binding energy and the activation of hormone receptors. *Biochem. Pharmacol.*, 29:853–856.

105. Fung, B. K. K., Hurley, J. B., and Stryer, L. (1981): Flow of information in the light-triggered cyclic nucleotide cascade of vision. *Proc. Natl. Acad. Sci. USA,* 78:152–156.

106. Furchgott, R. F. (1959): The receptors for epinephrine and norepinephrine (adrenergic receptors). *Pharmacol. Rev.*, 11:429–441.

107. Furchgott, R. F. (1964): Receptor mechanisms. *Annu. Rev. Pharmacol.*, 4:21–50.

108. Furchgott, R. F. (1967): The pharmacological differentiation of adrenergic receptors. *Ann. N.Y. Acad. Sci.*, 139:553–570.

109. Furchgott, R. F. (1978): Pharmacological characterization of receptors: Its relation to radioligand-binding studies. *Fed. Proc.*, 37:115–120.

110. Gaddum, J. H. (1926): The action of adrenalin and ergotamine on the uterus of the rabbit. *J. Physiol. (Lond.).*, 61:141–150.

111. Garcia-Sainz, J. A. (1985): Alpha$_1$-adrenergic and M$_1$-muscarinic actions and signal propazation. *Trends Pharmacol. Sci.*, 6:349–350.

112. Garcia-Sainz, J. A., and Corvera, S. (1983): Alpha$_1$-adrenergic action: Only calcium? *Trends Pharmacol. Sci.*, 12:489.

113. Garcia-Sainz, J. A., Hollingsworth, P. J., and Smith, C. B. (1981): Alpha$_2$-adrenoceptors on human platelets: Selective labeling by [^{3}H]clonidine and [^{3}H]yohimbine and competitive inhibition by antidepressant drugs. *Eur. J. Pharmacol.*, 74:329–341.

114. Garrison, J. C., and Borland, M. K. (1979): Regulation of mitochondrial pyruvate carboxylation and gluconeogenesis in rat hepatocytes via an alpha-adrenergic, adenosine 3',5'-monophosphate-independent mechanism. *J. Biol. Chem.*, 254:1129–1133.

115. Garrison, J. C., Borland, M. K., Florio, V. A., and Twible, D. A. (1979): The role of calcium ion as a mediator of the effects of angiotensin II, catecholamines, and vasopressin on the phosphorylation and activity of enzymes in isolated hepatocytes. *J. Biol. Chem.*, 254:7147–7156.

116. Geynet, P., Borsodi, A., Ferry, N., and Hanoune, J. (1980): Proteolysis of rat liver plasma membranes cancel the guanine nucleotide sensitivity of agonist binding to the alpha-adrenoceptor. *Biochem. Biophys. Res. Commun.*, 97:947–954.

117. Geynet, P., Ferry, N., Borsodi, A., and Hanoune, J. (1981): Two distinct alpha$_1$-adrenergic receptor sites in rat liver: Differential binding of (-)[^{3}H]norepinephrine, [^{3}H]prazosin and [^{3}H]dihydroergocryptine. Effects of guanine nucleotides and proteolysis: Implications for a two-site model of alpha-receptor regulation. *Biochem. Pharmacol.*, 30:1665–1675.

118. Gilman, A. G. (1984): Guanine nucleotide-binding regulatory proteins and dual control of adenylate cyclase. *J. Clin. Invest.*, 73:1–4.

119. Giudicelli, Y., Lacasa, D., and Agli, B. (1980): White fat cell alpha-adrenergic receptors and responsiveness in altered thyroid status. *Biochem. Biophys. Res. Commun.*, 94:1113–1122.

120. Glossmann, H., and Hornung, R. (1980): Alpha$_2$-adrenoceptors in rat brain. The divalent cation site. *Naunyn Schmiedebergs Arch. Pharmacol.*, 314:101–109.

121. Glossmann, H., and Hornung, R. (1980): Alpha-adrenoceptors in rat brain: Sodium changes in the affinity of agonists for prazosin sites. *Eur. J. Pharmacol.*, 61:407–408.

122. Glossmann, H., Hornung, R., and Presek, P. (1980): The use of ligand binding for the characterization of alpha-adrenoceptors. *J. Cardiovasc. Pharmacol. [Suppl. 3]*, 2:303–324.

123. Glossmann, H., Lubbecke, F., and Bellemann, P. (1981): [^{125}I]HEAT, a selective, high-affinity, high-specific activity ligand for alpha$_1$-adrenoceptors. *Naunyn Schmiedebergs Arch. Pharmacol.*, 318:1–9.

124. Glossmann, H., and Presek, P. (1979): Alpha-noradrenergic receptors in brain membranes: Sodium, magnesium and guanyl nucleotides modulate agonist binding. *Naunyn Schmiedebergs Arch. Pharmacol.*, 306:67–73.

125. Gomperts, B. D. (1983): Involvement of guanine nucleotide-

binding protein in the gating of Ca^{2+} by receptors. *Nature*, 306: 64–66.

126. Goodhardt, M., Ferry, N., Geynet, P., and Hanoune, J. (1982): Hepatic alpha₁-receptors show agonist-specific regulation by guanine nucleotides. *J. Biol. Chem.*, 257:11577–11583.

127. Gordon, P. R., Mercer, W. E., Lauva, I. K., Marino, T. A., and Cooper, G. (1985): Adrenergic stimulation of isolated cardiac muscle cells. *Circulation*, 72:325.

128. Graff, G., Stephenson, J. H., Glass, D. B., Haddox, M. K., and Goldberg, N. D. (1978): Activation of soluble splenic cell guanylate cyclase by prostaglandin endoperoxides and fatty acid hydroperoxides. *J. Biol. Chem.*, 253:7662–7676.

129. Graham, R. M. (1981): The physiology and pharmacology of alpha- and beta-blockade. *Cardiovasc. Med.* [*Special Suppl. April*], pp. 7–22.

130. Graham, R. M. (1984): Alpha-adrenergic receptor involvement in antihypertensive therapy and circulatory homeostasis. In: *Selective Alpha-blockade in the Treatment of Cardiovascular Disease, Vol. 29*, edited by J. Shaw, pp. 51–62. Excerpta Medica, Amsterdam.

131. Graham, R. M. (1984): Selective alpha₁-adrenergic antagonists: Therapeutically relevant antihypertensive agents. *Am. J. Cardiol.*, 53:16A–20A.

132. Graham, R. M., Hess, H.-J., Haber, E., and Homcy, C. J. (1982): Antibodies to the alpha₁- and alpha₂-selective antagonists prazosin and yohimbine as probes of the alpha-adrenergic binding sites. *Hypertension*, 4:183–187.

133. Graham, R. M., Hess, H.-J., and Homcy, C. J. (1982): Solubilization and purification of the alpha₁-adrenergic receptor using a novel affinity resin. *Proc. Natl. Acad. Sci. USA*, 79:2186–2190.

134. Graham, R. M., Hess, H.-J., and Homcy, C. J. (1982): Biophysical characterization of the purified alpha₁-adrenergic receptor and indentification of the hormone binding subunit. *J. Biol. Chem.*, 257:15174–15178.

135. Graham, R. M., and Pettinger, W. A. (1979): Effect of prazosin and phentolamine on arterial pressure, heart rate and renin activity: Evidence in the conscious rat for the functional significance of the presynaptic alpha-receptor. *J. Cardiovasc. Pharmacol.*, 1:497–502.

136. Graham, R. M., Seidman, C. E., Sena, L., Hess, H.-J., and Homcy, C. J. (1984): [¹²⁵I]amino- and [¹²⁵I]azido-benzoyl analogs of prazosin: High specific activity radioligands and affinity probes for the alpha₁-adrenergic receptor. *New England Nuclear Product News*, 4:8.

137. Graham, R. M., Stephenson, W. H., and Pettinger, W. A. (1980): Pharmacological evidence for a functional role of the prejunctional alpha-adrenoceptor in noradrenergic neurotransmission in the conscious rat. *Naunyn Schmiedebergs Arch. Pharmacol.*, 311: 129–138.

138. Greenberg, D. A., and Snyder, S. H. (1978): Pharmacological properties of [³H]dihydroergokryptine binding sites associated with alpha-noradrenergic receptors in rat brain membranes. *Mol. Pharmacol.*, 14:38–49.

139. Greenberg, D. A., U'Prichard, D. C., Sheehan, P., and Snyder, S. H. (1978): Alpha-noradrenergic receptors in brain: Differential effects of sodium on binding of [³H]agonists and [³H]antagonists. *Brain Res.*, 140:378–384.

140. Greenberg, D. A., U'Prichard, D. C., and Snyder, S. H. (1976): Alpha-noradrenergic receptor binding in mammalian brain: Differential labelling of agonist and antagonist states. *Life Sci.*, 19: 69–76.

141. Greengrass, P., and Brenner, R. (1979): Binding characteristics of [³H]prazosin to rat brain alpha-adrenergic receptors. *Eur. J. Pharmacol.*, 55:323–326.

142. Grob, G., Gothert, M., Glapu, U., Engel, G., and Schumann, H. J. (1985): Lesioning of serotoninergic and noradrenergic nerve fibres of the rat brain does not decrease binding of [³H]clonidine and [³H]rauwolscine to cortical membranes. *Naunyn Schmiedebergs Arch. Pharmacol.*, 328:229–235.

143. Guellaen, G., Aggerbeck, M., and Hanoune, J. (1979): Characterization and solubilization of the alpha-adrenoceptor of rat liver plasma membranes labeled with [³H]phenoxybenzamine. *J. Biol. Chem.*, 254:10761–10768.

144. Guellaen, G., Goodhardt, M., Barouki, R., and Hanoune, J.

(1982): Subunit structure of rat liver alpha₁-adrenergic receptor. *Biochem. Pharmacol.*, 31:2817–2820.

145. Guicheney, P., Rappuport, A., and Marcel, D. (1983): Solubilization of active brain alpha₁-adrenoceptors by a zwitterionic detergent. *J. Neurochem.*, 41:56–61.

146. Guldberg, C. M., and Waage, P. (1864): Studies over affiniteten. In: *The Law of Mass Action*, edited by O. Bastiansen, pp. 7–17. Univesitetsforlaget, Oslo.

147. Hamilton, C., Dalrymple, H., and Reid, J. (1982): Recovery *in vivo* and *in vitro* of alpha-adrenoceptor responses and radioligand binding after phenoxybenzamine. *J. Cardiovasc. Pharmacol.*, 4: S125–S128.

148. Harden, T. K. (1983): Agonist-induced desensitization of the beta-adrenergic receptor-linked adenylate cyclase. *Pharmacol. Rev.*, 35:5–32.

149. Haslam, R. J., and Davidson, M. M. L. (1984): Roles of Ca^{2+}, GTP, diglyceride and protein phosphorylation in the secretion of 5-HT from permeabilized platelets. *Fed. Proc.*, 43:736 (abstract).

150. Haslam, R. J., Salama, S. E., Fox, J. E. B., Lynham, J. A., and Davidson, M. M. L. (1980): Roles of cyclic nucleotides and of protein phosphorylation in the regulation of platelet function. In: *Platelets: Cellular Response Mechanisms and Their Biological Significance*, edited by A. Rotman, F. A. Meyer, C. Gitler, and A. Sildeberg, pp. 213–231. Wiley, New York.

151. Hata, F., Kondo, E., Kondo, S., Kagawa, K., and Ishide, H. (1982): Characteristics of [³H]E-643 binding to alpha-adrenoceptors. *Jpn. J. Pharmacol.*, 32:181–187.

152. Hedler, L., Stamm, G., Weitzell, R., and Starke, K. (1981): Functional characterization of central alpha-adrenoceptors by yohimbine diastereoisomers. *Eur. J. Pharmacol.*, 70:43–52.

153. Heidenreich, K. A., Weiland, G. A., and Molinoff, P. B. (1982): Effects of magnesium and N-ethylmaleimide on the binding of [³H]hydroxybenzylisoproterenol to beta-adrenergic receptors. *J. Biol. Chem.*, 257:804–810.

154. Henri, V. (1902): Theorie generale de l'action de quelques diastases. *C. R. Acad. Sci. (Paris)*, 135:916–919.

155. Heyworth, C. M., Rawal, S., and Houslay, M. D. (1983): Guanine nucleotides can activate the insulin-stimulated phosphodiesterase in liver plasma membranes. *FEBS Lett.*, 154:87–91.

156. Heyworth, C. M., Wallace, A. V., and Houslay, M. D. (1983): Insulin and glucagon regulate the activation of two distinct membrane-bound cyclic AMP phosphodiesterases in hepatocytes. *Biochem. J.*, 214:99–110.

157. Hicks, P. E. (1981): Antagonism of pre- and postsynaptic alpha-adrenoceptors by BE2254 (HEAT) and prazosin. *J. Auton. Pharmacol.*, 1:391–397.

158. Hill, A. V. (1909): The mode of action of nicotine and curari, determined by the form of the contraction curve and the method of temperature coefficients. *J. Physiol. (Lond.).*, 39:361–372.

159. Hirst, G. D. S., and Neild, T. O. (1981): Localization of specialized noradrenline receptors at neuromuscular junctions on arterioles of the guinea pig. *J. Physiol. (Lond.).*, 313:343–350.

160. Hoffman, B. B., DeLean, A., Wood, C. L., Schocken, D. D., and Lefkowitz, R. J. (1979): Alpha-adrenergic receptor subtypes: Quantitative assessment of ligand binding. *Life Sci.*, 24:1739–1746.

161. Hoffman, B. B., Dukes, D. F., and Lefkowitz, R. J. (1981): Alpha-adrenergic receptors in liver membranes: Delineation with subtype selective radioligands. *Life Sci.*, 28:265–272.

162. Hoffman, B. B., Lavin, T. N., Lefkowitz, R. J., and Ruffolo, R. R. (1981): Alpha-adrenergic receptor subtypes in rabbit uterus: Mediation of myometrial contraction and regulation by estrogens. *J. Pharmacol. Exp. Ther.*, 219:290–295.

163. Hoffman, B. B., and Lefkowitz, R. J. (1980): Radioligand binding studies of adrenergic receptors: New insights into molecular and physiological regulation. *Annu. Rev. Pharmacol. Toxicol.*, 20: 581–608.

164. Hoffman, B. B., and Majerus, P. W. (1982): Identification and properties of two distinct phosphatidylinositol-specific phospholipase C enzymes from sheep seminal vesicular glands. *J. Biol. Chem.*, 257:6461–6469.

165. Hoffman, B. B., Michel, T., Brenneman, T. B., and Lefkowitz, R. J. (1982): Interactions of agonists with platelet alpha₂-adrenergic receptors. *Endocrinology*, 110:926–932.

166. Hoffman, B. B., Mullikin-Kilpatrick, D., and Lefkowitz, R. J.

(1980): Heterogeneity of radioligand binding to alpha-adrenergic receptor: Analysis of guanine nucleotide regulation of agonist binding in relation to receptor subtypes. *J. Biol. Chem.*, 255: 4645–4652.

167. Hollenberg, M. D., and Cuatrecasas, P. (1979): Distinction of receptor from nonreceptor interactions in binding studies. In: *The Receptors. A Comprehensive Treatise,* edited by R. D. O'Brien, pp. 193–214. Plenum, New York.

168. Hollister, A. S., Fitzgerald, G. A., Nadeau, J. H. J., and Robertson, D. (1983): Acute reduction in human platelet alpha$_2$-adrenoceptor affinity for agonist by endogenous and exogenous catecholamines. *J. Clin. Invest.*, 72:1498–1505.

169. Homcy, C. J., and Graham, R. M. (1985): Molecular characterization of adrenergic receptors. *Circ. Res.*, 56:635–650.

170. Homcy, C. J., Graham, R. M., Haber, E., and Hess, H.-J. (1982): Characterization of the purified mammalian alpha- and beta-adrenergic receptors reveals homologous molecular properties. *Clin. Res.*, 30:482A.

171. Hornung, R., Presek, P., and Glossman, H. (1979): Alpha-adrenoceptors in rat brain: Direct identification with prazosin. *Naunyn Schmiedebergs Arch. Pharmacol.*, 308:223–230.

172. Jacobs, S., Sahyoun, N. E., Saltiel, A. R., and Cuatrecasas, P. (1983): Phorbol esters stimulate the phosphorylation of receptors for insulin and somatomedin C. *Proc. Natl. Acad. Sci. USA*, 80: 6211–6213.

173. Jaiswal, R. K., and Sharma, R. K. (1985): Purification and biochemical characterization of alpha$_2$-adrenergic receptor from the rat adrenocortical carcinoma. *Biochem. Biophys. Res. Commun.*, 130:58–64.

174. Jakobs, K. H. (1979): Inhibition of adenylate cyclase by hormones and neurotransmitters. *Mol. Cell. Endocrinol.*, 16:147–156.

175. Jakobs, K. H., Aktories, K., Minuth, M., and Schultz, G. (1985): Inhibition of adenylate cyclase. In: *Advances in Cyclic Nucleotide and Protein Phosphorylation Research,* edited by D. M. F. Cooper and K. B. Seamon, pp. 137–149. Raven Press, New York.

176. Jakobs, K. H., Minuth, M., and Aktories, K. (1984): Sodium regulation of hormone-sensitive adenylate cyclase. *J. Receptor Res.*, 4:443–458.

177. Jakobs, K. H., Saur, W., and Schultz, G. (1976): Reduction of adenylate cyclase activity in lysates of human platelets by the alpha-adrenergic component of epinephrine. *J. Cyclic Nucleotide Res.*, 2:381–392.

178. Jarrott, B., Louis, W. J., and Summers, R. J. (1979): The characteristics of [3H]clonidine binding to an alpha-adrenoceptor in membranes from guinea-pig kidney. *Br. J. Pharmacol.*, 65: 663–670.

179. Jarrott, B., Louis, W. J., and Summers, R. J. (1982): [3H]guanfacine: A radioligand that selectively labels high affinity alpha$_2$-adrenoceptor sites in homogenates of rat brain. *Br. J. Pharmacol.*, 75:401–408.

180. Jencks, W. P. (1975): Binding energy, specificity and enzymic catalysis: The circle effect. *Adv. Enzymol.*, 43:219–410.

181. Joseph, S. K. (1984): Inositol trisphosphate: An intracellular messenger produced by Ca^{2+} mobilizing hormones. *Trends Biochem. Sci.*, 9:420–421.

182. Joseph, S. K. (1985): Receptor-stimulated phosphoinositide metabolism: A role for GTP-binding proteins? *Trends Biochem. Sci.*, 10:297–298.

183. Joseph, S. K., Thomas, A. P., Williams, R. J., Irvine, R. F., and Williamson, J. R. (1984): Myo-inositol-1,4,5-trisphosphate. A second messenger for the hormonal mobilization of intracellular Ca^{2+} in liver. *J. Biol. Chem.*, 259:3077–3081.

184. Kalsner, S., and Chan, C. C. (1979): Adrenergic antagonists and the presynaptic receptor hypothesis in vascular tissue. *J. Pharmacol. Exp. Ther.*, 211:257–264.

185. Kapur, H., Ruout, B., and Snyder, S. H. (1979): Binding to alpha-adrenergic receptors: Differential pharmacological potencies and binding affinities of benzodioxanes. *Eur. J. Pharmacol.*, 57: 317–328.

186. Karliner, J. S., Motulsky, H. J., and Insel, P. A. (1982): Apparent "down-regulation" of human platelet alpha$_2$-adrenergic receptors is due to retained agonist. *Mol. Pharmacol.*, 21:36–43.

187. Katada, T., Bokoch, G. M., Northup, J. K., Ui, M., and Gilman, A. G. (1984): The inhibitory guanine nucleotide-binding regulatory component of adenylate cyclase. Properties and function of the purified protein. *J. Biol. Chem.*, 259:3568–3577.

188. Katada, T., Bokoch, G. M., Smigel, M. D., Ui, M., and Gilman, A. G. (1984): The inhibitory guanine nucleotide-binding regulatory component of adenylate cyclase. Subunit dissociation and the inhibition of adenylate cyclase in S49 lymphoma cyc⁻ and wild type membranes. *J. Biol. Chem.*, 259:3586–3595.

189. Katada, T., Northup, J. K., Bokoch, G. M., Ui, M., and Gilman, A. G. (1984): The inhibitory guanine nucleotide-binding regulatory component of adenylate cyclase. Subunit dissociation and guanine nucleotide-dependent hormonal inhibition. *J. Biol. Chem.*, 259: 3578–3595.

190. Katada, T., and Ui, M. (1981): Islet-activating protein. A modifier of receptor-mediated regulation of rat islet adenylate cyclase. *J. Biol. Chem.*, 256:8310–8317.

191. Kawahara, R. S., and Bylund, D. B. (1985): Solubilization and characterization of putative alpha$_2$-adrenergic receptors from the human platelet and the rat cerebral cortex. *J. Pharmacol. Exp. Ther.*, 233:603–610.

192. Kenakin, T. P. (1983): Receptor classification by selective agonists: Coping with circularity and circumstantial evidence. *Trends Pharmacol. Sci.*, 7:291–295.

193. Kessar, P., and Saggerson, E. D. (1982): Effect of alpha-adrenergic agonists on gluconeogenesis and ⁴⁵Ca efflux in rat kidney tubules. *Biochem. Pharmacol.*, 31:2331–2337.

194. Koshland, D. E., Jr. (1958): Application of a theory of enzyme specificity to protein synthesis. *Proc. Natl. Acad. Sci. USA*, 44: 98.

195. Koshland, D. E., Jr., Nemethy, G., and Filmer, D. (1966): Comparison of experimental binding data and theoretical models in proteins containing subunits. *Biochemistry*, 5:365–385.

196. Kremenetzky, R., and Atlas, D. (1984): Solubilization and reconstitution of alpha$_2$-adrenergic receptors from rat and calf brain. *Eur. J. Biochem.*, 138:573–577.

197. Kunos, G. (1984): The hepatic alpha$_1$-adrenoceptor. *Trends Pharmacol. Sci.*, 5:380–383.

198. Kunos, G., Kan, W. H., Greguski, R., and Venter, J. C. (1983): Selective affinity labeling and molecular characterization of hepatic alpha-adrenergic receptors with [3H]phenoxybenzamine. *J. Biol. Chem.*, 258:326–332.

199. Kuriyama, H., and Makita, Y. (1983): Modulation of noradrenergic transmission in the guinea-pig mesenteric artery. An electrophysiological study. *J. Physiol. (Lond.).*, 335:609–627.

200. Labarca, R., Janowsky, A., Patel, J., and Paul, S. M. (1984): Phorbol esters inhibit agonist-induced [3H]inositol-1-phosphate accumulation in rat hippocampal slices. *Biochem. Biophys. Res. Commun.*, 123:703–709.

201. Laduron, P. M. (1980): Axoplasmic transport of muscarinic receptor. *Nature*, 26:287–288.

202. Laduron, P. M. (1985): Presynaptic heteroreceptors in regulation of neuronal transmission. *Biochem. Pharmacol.*, 34:467–470.

203. Lafontan, M., and Berlan, M. (1981): Alpha-adrenergic receptors and the regulation of lipolysis in adipose tissue. *Trends Pharmacol. Sci.*, 2:126–129.

204. Lands, A. M., Arnold, A., McAuliff, J. P., Luduena, F. P., and Brown, T. G. (1967): Differentiation of receptor systems activated by sympathomimetic amines. *Nature*, 214:597–598.

205. Langer, S. Z. (1970): The metabolism of [3H]noradrenaline release by electrical stimulation from the isolated nictitating membrane of the cat and from the vas deferens of the rat. *J. Physiol. (Lond.).*, 208:515–546.

206. Langer, S. Z. (1974): Presynaptic regulation of catecholamine release. *Br. J. Pharmacol.*, 23:1793–1800.

207. Langer, S. Z. (1981): Presence and physiological role of presynaptic inhibitory alpha$_2$-adrenoreceptors in guinea pig atria. *Nature*, 294:671–672.

208. Langer, S. Z., and Armstrong, J. M. (1984): Prejunctional receptors and the cardiovascular system: Pharmacological and therapeutic relevance. In: *Cardiovascular Pharmacology,* edited by M. Antonaccio, pp. 197–213. Raven Press, New York.

209. Langer, S. Z., and Hicks, P. E. (1984): Alpha-adrenoceptor subtypes in blood vessels: Physiology and pharmacology. *J. Cardiovasc. Pharmacol. [Suppl. 4]*, 6:547–558.

210. Langer, S. Z., and Schepperson, N. B. (1982): Recent developments

in vascular smooth muscle pharmacology: The post-synaptic alpha$_2$-adrenoceptor. *Trends Pharmacol. Sci.*, 3:440–444.

211. Langer, S. Z., Shepperson, N. B., and Massingham, R. (1981): Preferential noradrenergic innervation of alpha$_1$-adrenergic receptors in vascular smooth muscle. *Hypertension*, 3:I-112–I-118.

212. Langley, J. N. (1878): On the physiology of the salivary secretion. *J. Physiol. (Lond.)*, 1:339–369.

213. Langley, J. N. (1905): On the reaction of cells and of nerve-endings to certain poisons, chiefly as regards the reaction of striated muscle to nicotine and to curari. *J. Physiol. (Lond.)*, 33:374–413.

214. Langmuir, I. (1918): The adsorption of gases on plane surfaces of glass, mica and platinum. *J. Am. Chem. Soc.*, 40:1361–1403.

215. Lanier, S. M., Graham, R. M., Hess, H.-J., and Homcy, C. J. (1985): Synthesis and characterization of a novel radioiodinated probe for the alpha$_2$-adrenergic receptor. *Fed. Proc.*, 44:494.

216. Lanier, S. M., Hess, H.-J., Grodski, A., Graham, R. M., and Homcy, C. J. (1986): Synthesis and characterization of a high-affinity radioiodinated probe for the alpha$_2$-adrenergic receptor. *Mol. Pharmacol., (in press)*.

217. Lawrence, J. C., Jr., and Larner, J. (1977): Evidence for alpha-adrenergic activation of phosphorylase and inactivation of glycogen synthase in rat adipocytes. *Mol. Pharmacol.*, 13:1060–1075.

218. Lawrence, J. C., Jr., and Larner, J. (1978): Effects of insulin, methoxamine, and calcium on glycogen synthase in rat adipocytes. *Mol. Pharmacol.*, 14:1079–1091.

219. Leeb-Lundberg, L. M. F., Cotecchia, S., Komasney, J. W., DeBarnadis, J. F., Lefkowitz, R. J., and Caren, M. G. (1985): Phorbol esters promote alpha$_1$-adrenergic receptor phosphorylation and receptor uncoupling from inositol phospholipid metabolism. *Proc. Natl. Acad. Sci. USA*, 82:5651–5655.

220. Leeb-Lundberg, L. M. F., Dickinson, K. E. J., Heald, S. L., Wikberg, J. E. S., Hagen, P. G., DeBernardis, J. F., Winn, M., Arendsen, D. L., Lefkowitz, R. J., and Caron, M. G. (1984): Photoaffinity labeling of mammalian alpha$_1$-adrenergic receptors. Identification of the ligand binding subunit with a high affinity radioiodinated probe. *J. Biol. Chem.*, 259:2579–2587.

221. Lefkowitz, R. J., Mukherjee, C., Coverstone, M., and Caron, M. G. (1974): Stereospecific [^{3}H](-)-alprenolol binding sites, beta-adrenergic receptors and adenyl cyclase. *Biochem. Biophys. Res. Commun.*, 69:703–710.

222. Lefkowitz, R. J., Roth, J., Pricer, W., and Pastan, I. (1970): ACTH receptors in the adrenal: Specific binding of ACTH-[^{125}I] and its relation to adenyl cyclase. *Proc. Natl. Acad. Sci. USA*, 65:745–752.

223. Lehmann, J., and Lanager, S. Z. (1981): Phenoxybenzamine blocks dopamine autoreceptors irreversibly: Implications for multiple dopamine receptor hypothesis. *Eur. J. Pharmacol.*, 75:247–254.

224. Levitzki, A., Atlas, D., and Steer, M. L. (1974): The binding characteristics and number of beta-adrenergic receptors on the turkey-erythrocyte. *Proc. Natl. Acad. Sci. USA*, 71:4246–4248.

225. Limberger, N., and Starke, K. (1983): Partial agonist effect of 2-[2-(1,4-benzodiaxanyl)]-2-imidazoline (RX781094) at presynaptic alpha$_2$-adrenoceptors in rabbit ear artery. *Naunyn Schmiedebergs Arch. Pharmacol.*, 324:75–78.

226. Limbird, L. (1984): GTP and Na$^+$ modulate receptor-adenyl cyclase coupling and receptor-mediated function. *Am. J. Physiol.*, 247:E59–E68.

227. Limbird, L. E., MacMillan, S. T., and Kalinoski, D. L. (1985): The resolution of agonist alpha$_2$-adrenergic receptor complexes from unoccupied receptors or antagonist alpha$_2$-receptor complexes using DEAE chromatography. *J. Cyclic Nucl. Prot. Phosphorylation Res.*, 10:75–82.

228. Limbird, L. E., Speck, J. L., and Smith, S. K. (1982): Sodium ion modulates agonist and antagonist interactions with the human platelet alpha$_2$-adrenergic receptor in membrane and solubilized preparations. *Mol. Pharmacol.*, 21:609–617.

229. Lin, S. Y., and Goodfriend, T. L. (1970): Angiotensin receptors. *Am. J. Physiol.*, 218:1319–1328.

230. Lineweaver, H., and Burk, D. (1934): The determination of enzyme dissociation constants. *J. Am. Chem. Soc.*, 56:658–666.

231. Loftus, D. J., Stolk, J. M., and U'Prichard, D. C. (1984): Binding

of the imidazoline UK-14,304, a putative full alpha$_2$-adrenoceptor agonist, to rat cerebral cortex membranes. *Life Sci.*, 35:61–69.

232. Luchsinger, B. (1877): Die Wirkungen von Pilocarpin und Atropin auf die Schweissdrussen der Katze. Ein Beitrag zur Lehre vom doppelseitigen Antagonismus zweier Gifte. *Pfluegers Arch.*, 15:482–492.

233. Lynch, C. J., Charest, R., Blackmore, P. F., and Exton, J. H. (1985): Studies on the hepatic alpha$_1$-adrenergic receptor. Modulation of guanine nucleotide effects by calcium temperature and age. *J. Biol. Chem.*, 260:1593–1600.

234. Lynch, C. J., Sobo, G. E., and Exton, J. H. (1985): An endogenous Ca^{2+}-sensitive protease converts the hepatic alpha$_1$-adrenergic receptor to guanine nucleotide insensitive forms. *Biochem. Biophys. Acta, (in press)*.

235. Lynch, C. J., and Steer, M. L. (1981): Evidence for high and low affinity alpha$_2$-receptor. *J. Biol. Chem.*, 256:3298–3303.

236. McCulloch, M. W., Rand, M. J., and Story, D. F. (1972): Inhibition of ^{3}H-noradrenaline release from sympathetic nerves of guinea-pig atria by a presynaptic adrenoceptor mechanism. *Br. J. Pharmacol.*, 46:523P–524P.

237. McGrath, J. C. (1982): Evidence for more than one type of postjunctional alpha-adrenoceptor. *Biochem. Pharmacol.*, 31:467–484.

238. McKernan, R. M., and Campbell, I. C. (1982): Measurement of alpha-adrenoceptor "turnover" using phenoxybenzamine. *Eur. J. Pharmacol.*, 80:279–280.

239. Madjar, H., Docherty, J. R., and Starke, K. (1980): An examination of pre- and post-synaptic alpha-adrenergic receptors in the auto-perfused rabbit hindlimb. *J. Cardiovasc. Pharmacol.*, 2:619–627.

240. Majerus, P. W., Neufeld, E. J., and Wilson, D. B. (1984): Production of phosphoinositide-derived messengers. *Cell*, 37:701–703.

241. Matsui, H., Asakura, M., Tsukamoto, T., Imafuku, J., Ino, M., Saitoh, N., Miyamura, S., and Hasegawa, K. (1985): Solubilization and characterization of rat brain alpha$_2$-adrenergic receptor. *J. Neurochem.*, 44:1625–1632.

242. Mauger, J.-P., Sladeczek, F., and Bockaert, J. (1982): Characteristics and metabolism of alpha$_1$-adrenergic receptors in a nonfusing muscle cell line. *J. Biol. Chem.*, 257:875–879.

243. Medgett, I. C., McCulloch, M. W., and Rand, M. J. (1978): Partial agonist action of clonidine on prejunctional and postjunctional alpha-adrenoceptors. *Naunyn Schmiedebergs Arch. Pharmacol.*, 304:215–221.

244. Medgett, I. C., and Rand, M. J. (1981): Dual effects of clonidine on rat prejunctional alpha-adrenoceptors. *Clin. Exp. Pharmacol. Physiol.*, 8:503–507.

245. Meier, K. E., Sperling, D. M., and Insel, P. A. (1985): Agonist-mediated regulation of alpha$_1$- and beta$_2$-adrenergic receptors in cloned MDCK cells. *Am. J. Physiol.*, 249:C69–C77.

246. Menkes, D. B., Gallager, D. W., Reinhard, J. F., and Aghajanian, G. K. (1983): Alpha$_1$-adrenoceptor denervation supersensitivity in brain: Physiological and receptor binding studies. *Brain. Res.*, 272:1–12.

247. Miach, P. J., Dausse, J.-P., Cardot, A., and Meyer, P. (1980): [^{3}H]prazosin binds specifically to alpha$_1$-adrenoceptors in rat brain. *Naunyn Schmiedebergs Arch. Pharmacol.*, 312:23–26.

248. Miach, P. J., Dausse, J.-P., and Meyer, P. (1978): Direct biochemical demonstration of two types of alpha-adrenoreceptor in rat brain. *Nature*, 274:492–494.

249. Michaelis, L., and Menten, M. L. (1913): Die Kinetic der Invertinwirkung. *Biochem. Z.*, 49:333–369.

250. Michel, T., Hoffman, B. B., and Lefkowitz, R. J. (1980): Differential regulation of the alpha$_2$-adrenergic receptor by Na$^+$ and guanine nucleotides. *Nature*, 288:709–711.

251. Michel, T., Hoffman, B. B., Lefkowitz, R. J., and Caron, M. G. (1981): Different sedimentation properties of agonist- and antagonist-labelled platelet alpha$_2$-adrenergic receptors. *Biochem. Biophys. Res. Commun.*, 100:1131–1136.

252. Michell, R. H. (1975): Inositol phospholipids and cell surface receptor function. *Biochem. Biophys. Acta*, 415:81–147.

253. Miyake, R., Yokoyama, M., Kaibuchi, K., Takai, Y., and Nishizuka, Y. (1985): Phosphoinositide metabolism and its regulation by cyclic nucleotides in vascular smooth muscle. *Circulation*, 72:323.

254. Monnier, A. M., and Bacq, Z. M. (1935): Recherches sur la physiologie et la pharmacologie du systeme nerveux autonome XVI—Dualite du mechanisme de la transmission neuro-musculaire de l'excitation chez le muscle lisse. *Arch. Intern. Physiol.,* 40:485–510.

255. Monod, J., Wyman, J., and Changeux, J. P. (1965): On the nature of allosteric transitions: A possible model. *J. Mol. Biol.,* 12:88–118.

256. Mooney, J. J., Horne, W. L., Handin, R. J., Schildkraut, J. J., and Alexander, R. W. (1982): Sodium inhibits both adenylate cyclase and high-affinity [³H]labeled *p*-aminoclonidine binding to alpha₂-adrenergic receptors in purified human platelet membranes. *Mol. Pharmacol.,* 21:600–608.

257. Moran, J. F., May, A., Kimelberg, H., and Triggle, D. J. (1967): Studies on the noradrenergic alpha-receptor. I. Techniques of receptor isolation. The distribution and specific of action of *N*-(2-bromoethyl)-*N*-ethyl-1-naphthylmethylamine, a competitive antagonist of noradrenaline. *Mol. Pharmacol.,* 3:15–27.

258. Morgan, N. G., Blackmore, P. F., and Exton, J. H. (1983): Age-related changes in the control of hepatic cyclic AMP levels by alpha₁- and beta₂-adrenergic receptors in male rats. *J. Biol. Chem.,* 258:5103–5109.

259. Morris, M. J., Elghazi, J. L., Pausse, J. P., and Meyer, P. (1981): Alpha₁- and alpha₂-adrenoceptors in rat cerebral cortex: Effect of frontal lobotomy. *Naunyn Schmiedebergs Arch. Pharmacol.,* 316: 42–44.

260. Motulsky, H. J., and Insel, P. A. (1982): [³H]dihydroergocryptine binding to alpha-adrenergic receptors of human platelets. A reassessment using the selective radioligands [³H]prazosin, [³H]yohimbine and [³H]rauwolscine. *Biochem. Pharmacol.,* 31: 2591–2597.

261. Motulsky, H. J., and Insel, P. A. (1983): Influence of sodium on the alpha₂-adrenergic receptor system of human platelets. Role of intraplatelet Na⁺ in receptor binding and function. *J. Biol. Chem.,* 258:3913–3919.

262. Motulsky, H. J., Shattil, S. J., and Insel, P. A. (1980): Characterization of alpha₂-adrenergic receptors in human platelets using [³H]yohimbine. *Biochem. Biophys. Res. Commun.,* 97:1562–1570.

263. Mulder, A. H., de Langen, C. D. J., de Regt, V., and Hogenboom, F. (1978): Alpha-receptor-mediated modulation of the ³H-noradrenaline release from rat brain cortex synaptosomes. *Naunyn Schmiedebergs Arch. Pharmacol.,* 303:193–196.

264. Murphy, E., Coll, K., Rich, L., and Williamson, J. R. (1980): Hormonal effects on calcium homeostasis in isolated hepatocytes. *J. Biol. Chem.,* 255:6600–6608.

265. Nambi, P., Aiyar, N. V., and Sharma, R. K. (1982): Solubilization of epinephrine-specific alpha₂-adrenergic receptors from adrenocortical carcinoma. *FEBS Lett.,* 140:98–102.

266. Nasseri, A., Barakeh, J. F., Abel, P. W., and Minneman, K. P. (1985): Reserpine-induced postjunctional supersensitivity in rat vas deferens and caudal artery without changes in alpha-adrenergic receptors. *J. Pharmacol. Exp. Ther.,* 234:350–357.

267. Neer, E. J., Lok, J. M., and Wolf, L. G. (1984): Purification and properties of the inhibitory guanine nucleotide regulatory unit of brain adenylate cyclase. *J. Biol. Chem.,* 259:14222–14229.

268. Newbold, R. (1984): Mutant ras proteins and cell transformation. *Nature,* 310:628–629.

269. Nishizuka, Y. (1984): The role of protein kinase C in cell surface signal transduction and tumour promotion. *Nature,* 308:693–698.

270. Nickerson, M. (1956). Receptor occupancy and tissue response. *Nature,* 178:697–698.

271. Paciorek, P. M., and Shepperson, N. B. (1983): Alpha₁-adrenoceptor agonist activity of alpha₂-adrenoceptor antagonists in the pithed rat preparation. *Br. J. Pharmacol.,* 79:12–14.

272. Paton, W. D. M. (1960): Release of sympathetic neurotransmitter by nerve stimulation (commentary). In: *Adrenergic Mechanisms,* edited by J. R. Vane, G. E. W. Wolstenholme, and M. O'Connor, pp. 124–127. Churchill, London.

273. Paton, W. D. M. (1961): A theory of drug action based on the rate of drug-receptor combination. *Proc. R. Soc. Lond.* [*Biol.*], 154:21–32.

274. Paton, W. D. M., and Rang, H. P. (1966): A kinetic approach to the mechanism of drug action. *Adv. Drug Res.,* 3:57.

275. Patten, G. S., Filsell, O. H., and Clark, M. G. (1982): Epinephrine regulation of phosphofructokinase in perfused rat heart: A calcium ion-dependent mechanism mediated via alpha-receptors. *J. Biol. Chem.,* 257:9480–9486.

276. Pecquery, R., Leneveu, M. C., and Giudicelli, Y. (1984): *In vivo* desensitization of the *β*, but not the alpha₂-adrenoceptor-coupled adenylate cyclase system in hamster white adipocytes after administration of epinephrine. *Endocrinology,* 114:1576–1583.

277. Peroutka, S. J., Greenberg, D. A., U'Prichard, D. C., and Snyder, S. H. (1978): Regional variation in *α*-adrenergic receptor interactions of [³H]dihydroergocryptine in calf brain: implications for a two-site model of receptor function. *Mol. Pharmacol.,* 14:403–412.

278. Perry, B. D., and U'Prichard, D. C. (1981): [³H]rauwolscine (alpha-yohimbine): A specific antagonist radioligand for brain alpha₂-adrenergic receptors. *Eur. J. Pharmacol.,* 76:461–464.

279. Peters, J. R., Elliot, J. M., and Grahame-Smith, D. G. (1979): Effect of oral contraceptives on platelet noradrenaline and 5-hydroxytryptamine receptors and aggregation. *Lancet,* 2:933–936.

280. Pichler, L., Hortnagl, H., and Kobinger, W. (1982): B-HT958, a new alpha-adrenoceptor agonist with a high pre/postsynaptic activity ratio. *Naunyn Schmiedebergs Arch. Pharmacol.,* 320: 110–114.

281. Pike, L. J., and Lefkowitz, R. F. (1978): Agonist-specific alterations in receptor binding affinity associated with solubilization of turkey erythrocyte membrane beta-adrenergic receptors. *Mol. Pharmacol.,* 14:370–375.

282. Pimoule, C., Briley, M. S., and Langer, S. Z. (1980): Short-term surgical denervation increases [³H]clonidine binding in rat salivary gland. *Eur. J. Pharmacol.,* 63:85–87.

283. Pinkett, M. O., Jaworski, C. J., Evain, D., and Anderson, W. B. (1980): Limited proteolysis eliminates guanine nucleotide inhibition of choleragen-activated adenylate cyclase. Possible basis for proteolytic stimulation of cyclic AMP production. *J. Biol. Chem.,* 255:7716–7721.

284. Preiksaitis, H. G., Kan, W. H., and Kunos, G. (1982): Decreased alpha₁-adrenoceptor responsiveness and density in liver cells of thyroidectomized rats. *J. Biol. Chem.,* 257:4321–4327.

285. Prpic, V., Green, K. C., Blackmore, P. F., and Exton, J. H. (1984): Vasopressin-, angiotensin II-, and alpha-adrenergic-induced inhibition of Ca²⁺ by transport by rat liver plasma membrane vesicles. *J. Biol. Chem.,* 259:1382–1385.

286. Putney, J. W., Jr. (1979): Stimulus-permeability coupling: Role of calcium in receptor regulation of membrane permeability. *Pharmacol. Rev.,* 30:209–245.

287. Quenneday, M.-C., Bockaert, J., and Rouot, B. (1984): Direct and indirect effects of sulfhydryl blocking agents on agonist and antagonist binding to central alpha₁- and alpha₂-adrenoceptors. *Biochem. Pharmacol.,* 33:3923–3928.

288. Rand, M. J., Story, D. F., Allen, G. S., Glover, A. B., and McCulloch, W. (1973): Pulse-to-pulse modulation of noradrenaline release through a prejunctional alpha-receptor auto-inhibitory mechanism. In: *Frontiers in Catecholamine Research,* edited by E. Usdein and S. H. Snyder, pp. 579–581. Pergamon Press, New York.

289. Regan, J. W., Barden, N., Lefkowitz, R. J., Caron, M. G., DeMarinis, R. M., Krog, A. J., Holden, K. G., Matthews, W. D., and Hieble, J. P. (1982): Affinity chromatography of human platelet alpha₂-adrenergic receptors. *Proc. Natl. Acad. Sci. USA,* 79:7223–7227.

290. Regan, J. W., DeMarinis, R. M., Caron, M. G., and Lefkowitz, R. J. (1984): Identification of the subunit binding site of alpha₂-adrenergic receptors using [³H]phenoxybenzamine. *J. Biol. Chem.,* 259:7864–7869.

291. Reinhart, P. H., Taylor, W. M., and Bygrave, F. L. (1984): The contribution of both extracellular and intracellular calcium to the action of alpha-adrenergic agonists in perfused rat liver. *Biochem. J.,* 220:35–42.

292. Reinhart, P. H., Taylor, W. M., and Bygrave, F. L. (1984): The role of calcium ions in the mechanism of action of alpha-adrenergic agonists in rat liver. *Biochem. J.,* 223:1–13.

293. Rhodes, D., Prpic, V., Exton, J. H., and Blackmore, P. F. (1983): Stimulation of phosphatidylinositol 4,5-bisphosphate hydrolysis in hepatocytes by vasopressin. *J. Biol. Chem.,* 258:2770–2773.

294. Roberts, J. M., Goldfein, R. D., Tsuchiya, A. M., Goldfein, A., and Insel, P. A. (1979): Estrogen treatment decreases alpha-adrenergic binding sites on rabbit platelets. *Endocrinology,* 104: 722–728.

295. Roberts, J. M., Insel, P. A., and Goldfein, A. (1981): Regulation of myometrical adrenoceptors and adrenergic response by sex steroids. *Mol. Pharmacol.,* 20:52–58.

296. Robie, N. W. (1980): Evaluation of presynaptic alpha-receptor function in the canine renal vascular bed. *Am. J. Physiol.,* 239: H422–H426.

297. Robson, L. E., and Kosterlitz, H. W. (1979): Specific protection of the binding sites of D-Ala^2-D-Leu^4-enkephalin (delta receptors) and dihydromorphine (mu receptors). *Proc. R. Soc. Lond. [Biol.],* 205:425–432.

298. Rouot, B., Quenneday, M. C., and Schwartz, J. (1982): Characteristics of the [^{3}H]yohimbine binding on rat brain alpha$_2$-adrenoceptors. *Naunyn Schmiedebergs Arch. Pharmacol.,* 321: 253–259.

299. Rouot, B. M., and Snyder, S. H. (1979): [^{3}H]para-amino-clonidine: A novel ligand which binds with high affinity to alpha-adrenergic receptors. *Life Sci.,* 25:769–774.

300. Rouot, B. M., U'Prichard, D. C., and Snyder, S. H. (1980): Multiple alpha$_2$-adrenergic receptor sites in rat brain: Selective regulation of high-affinity [^{3}H]clonidine binding by guanine nucleotides and divalent cations. *J. Neurochem.,* 34:374–384.

301. Rubin, M., and Changeux, J. P. (1966): On the nature of allosteric transitions: Implications of non-exclusive ligand binding. *J. Mol. Biol.,* 21:265–274.

302. Ruegg, J. C. (1982): Vascular smooth muscle: Intracellular aspects of adrenergic receptor contraction coupling. *Experientia,* 38: 1400–1404.

303. Ruffolo, R. R., Fowble, J. W., Miller, D. D., and Patil, P. N. (1976): Binding of [^{3}H]dihydroazapetine to alpha-adrenoceptor-related proteins from rat vas deferens. *Proc. Natl. Acad. Sci. USA,* 73:2730–2734.

304. Ruffolo, R. R., Morgan, E. L., and Messick, K. (1984): Possible relationship between receptor reserve and the differential antagonism of alpha$_1$- and alpha$_2$-adrenoceptor-mediated pressor-responses by calcium-channel antagonists in the pithed rat. *J. Pharmacol. Exp. Ther.,* 230:587–594.

305. Ruffolo, R. R., and Patil, P. W. (1979): Kinetics of alpha-adrenoceptor blockade by phentolamine in the normal and denervated rabbit aorta and rat vas deferens. *Blood Vessels,* 16: 135–143.

306. Sabol, S. L., and Nirenberg, M. (1979): Regulation of adenylate cyclase of neuroblastoma × glioma hybrid cells by alpha-adrenergic receptors. I. Inhibition of adenylate cyclase mediated by alpha-receptors. *J. Biol. Chem.,* 254:1913–1920.

307. Sabol, S. L., and Nirenberg, M. (1979): Regulation of adenylate cyclase of neuroblastoma × glioma hybrid cells by alpha-adrenergic receptors. II. Longlived increase of adenylate cyclase activity mediated by alpha-receptors. *J. Biol. Chem.,* 254:1921–1926.

308. Salama, A. I., Lin, L. L., Repp, L. D., and U'Prichard, D. C. (1982): Magnesium reduces affinities of antagonists at rat cortex alpha$_2$-adrenergic receptors labeled with [^{3}H]clonidine: Evidence for heterogeneity of alpha$_2$-receptor conformations with respect to antagonists. *Life Sci.,* 30:1305–1311.

309. Scatchard, G. (1949): The attraction of proteins for small molecules and ions. *Ann. N.Y. Acad. Sci.,* 51:660–672.

310. Schild, H. O. (1947): pA$_2$, a new scale for the measurement of drug antagonism. *Br. J. Pharmacol.,* 2:189–206.

311. Schild, H. O. (1972): Receptor classification with special reference to beta-adrenergic receptors. In: *Drug Receptors,* edited by H. P. Rang, pp. 29–36. University Park Press, Baltimore.

312. Schlegel, W., Cooper, D. M. F., and Rodbell, M. (1980): Inhibition and activation of fat cell adenylate cyclase by GTP is mediated by stuctures of different size. *Arch. Biochem. Biophys.,* 201:678–682.

313. Schmitz, J. M., Graham, R. M., Sagalowsky, A., and Pettinger, W. A. (1981): Renal alpha$_1$- and alpha$_2$-adrenergic receptors: Biochemical and pharmacological correlations. *J. Pharmacol. Exp. Ther.,* 219:400–406.

314. Schultz, K. D., Schultz, K., and Schultz, G. (1977): Sodium nitroprusside and other smooth muscle-relaxants increase cyclic GMP levels in rat ductus deferens. *Nature,* 265:750–751.

315. Schwarz, K. R., Carter, E. A., Graham, R. M., and Homcy, C. J. (1985): High-affinity agonist binding sites at alpha$_1$-adrenergic receptors: The physiologically relevant state for catecholamine action. *Clin. Res.,* 33:226A.

316. Schwarz, K. R., Carter, E. A., Homcy, C. J., and Graham, R. M. (1985): Regulation of adrenergic agonist affinity states. *Fed. Proc.,* 44:1628.

317. Schwarz, K. R., Lanier, S. M., Carter, E. A., Homcy, C. J., and Graham, R. M. (1985): Rapid reciprocal changes in adrenergic receptors in intact isolated hepatocytes during primary cell culture. *Mol. Pharmacol.,* 27:200–209.

318. Schwarz, K. R., Lanier, S. M., Carter, E. A., Homcy, C. J., and Graham, R. M. (1985): Transient high-affinity binding of agonists to alpha$_1$-adrenergic receptors of intact liver cells. *FEBS Lett.,* 187:205–210.

319. Seidman, C. E., Hess, H.-J., Homcy, C. J., and Graham, R. M. (1984): Synthesis and characterization of a radioiodinated photoaffinity probe for the alpha$_1$-adrenergic receptor. *Hypertension [Suppl. I],* 6:7–11.

320. Seidman, C. E., Hess, H.-J., Homcy, C. J., and Graham, R. M. (1984): Photoaffinity labeling of the alpha$_1$-adrenergic receptor using an ^{125}I-labeled aryl azide analogue of prazosin. *Biochemistry,* 23:3765–3770.

321. Shackell, E. (1924): The relation of dosage to effect. *J. Pharmacol. Exp. Ther.,* 24:53–65.

322. Sharma, S. K., Klee, W. A., and Nirenberg, M. (1977): Opiate-dependent modulation of adenylate cyclase. *Proc. Natl. Acad. Sci. USA,* 74:3365–3369.

323. Shattil, S. J., McDonough, M., Turnbull, J., and Insel, P. A. (1981): Characterization of alpha-adrenergic receptors in human platelets using [^{3}H]clonidine. *Mol. Pharmacol.,* 19:179–183.

324. Shreeve, S. M., Fraser, C. M., and Venter, J. C. (1985): Molecular comparison of alpha$_1$- and alpha$_2$-adrenergic receptors suggests that these proteins are structurally related "isoreceptors." *Proc. Natl. Acad. Sci. USA,* 82:4842–4846.

325. Simpson, P. (1985): Stimulation of hypertrophy of cultured neonatal rat heart cells through an alpha$_1$-adrenergic receptor and induction of beating through an alpha$_1$- and beta$_1$-adrenergic receptor interaction. Evidence for independent regulation of growth and beating. *Circ. Res.,* 56:884–894.

326. Skomedal, T., Aass, H., and Osnes, J.-B. (1985): Specific binding of [^{3}H]prazosin to myocardial cells isolated from adult rats. *Biochem. Pharmacol.,* 33:1897–1906.

327. Sladeczek, F., Bockaert, J., and Mauger, J.-P. (1983): Differences between agonist and antagonist binding to alpha$_1$-adrenergic receptors in intact and broken-cell preparations. *Mol. Pharmacol.,* 24:392–397.

328. Sladeczek, F., Bockaert, J., and Rouot, B. (1984): Solubilization of brain alpha$_2$-adrenoceptor with a zwitterionic detergent: Preservation of agonist affinity and its sensitivity to GTP. *Biochem. Biophys. Res. Commun.,* 119:1116–1121.

329. Slater, I. H., and Powell, C. E. (1957): Blockade of adrenergic inhibitory receptor sites by 1-(3',4'-dichlorophenyl)-2-isopropyl-aminoethanol hydrochloride. *Fed. Proc.,* 16:336.

330. Smith, S. K., and Limbird, L. E. (1981): Solubilization of human platelet alpha-adrenergic receptors: Evidence that agonist occupancy of the receptors stabilizes receptor-effector interactions. *Proc. Natl. Acad. Sci. USA,* 78:4026–4030.

331. Smith, S. K., and Limbird, L. E. (1982): Evidence that human platelet alpha-adrenergic receptors coupled to inhibition of adenylate cyclase are not associated with the subunit of adenylate cyclase ADP-ribosylated by cholera toxin. *J. Biol. Chem.,* 257: 10471–10478.

332. Snavely, M. D., and Insel, P. A. (1982): Characterization of alpha-adrenergic receptor subtypes in rat renal cortex: Differential regulation of alpha$_1$- and alpha$_2$-receptors by guanyl nucleotides and Na$^+$. *Mol. Pharmacol.,* 22:532–546.

333. Snavely, M. D., and Insel, P. A. (1983): Different roles for thiol groups in renal alpha$_1$- and alpha$_2$-adrenergic receptors. *Fed. Proc.,* 42:1876.

334. Snavely, M. D., Mahan, L. C., O'Connor, D. T., and Insel, P. A. (1983): Selective "down-regulation" of adrenergic receptor subtypes in tissues from rats with pheochromocytoma. *Endocrinology,* 113:354–361.

335. Snavely, M. D., Ziegler, M. G., and Insel, P. A. (1985): Subtype

selective "down-regulation" of rat renal cortical alpha- and beta-adrenergic receptors by catecholamines. *Endocrinology,* 117:2182–2189.

336. Snyder, S. H., U'Prichard, D. C., and Creese, I. (1979): Catecholamine receptor binding in brain. In: *Catecholamines: Basic and Clinical Frontiers,* edited by E. Usdin, J. J. Kopin, and J. D. Barchas, pp. 534–541. Pergamon Press, Oxford.

337. Sollman, T., and Brown, E. D. (1905): Intravenous injection of ergot. Effects on the mammalian circulation. *J.A.M.A.,* 45:229–240.

338. Starke, K. (1971): Influence of alpha-receptor stimulants on noradrenaline release. *Naturwissenschaften,* 58:420.

339. Starke, K. (1977): Regulation of noradrenaline release by presynaptic receptor systems. *Rev. Physiol. Biochem.,* 77:1–124.

340. Starke, K. (1979): Presynaptic modulation of catecholamine release in the central nervous system: Some open questions. In: *Presynaptic Receptors,* edited by S. Z. Langer, K. Starke, and M. L. Dubocovich, pp. 129–136. Pergamon Press, Oxford.

341. Starke, K. (1981): Alpha-adrenoceptor subclassification. *Rev. Physiol. Biochem. Pharmacol.,* 88:199–236.

342. Starke, K., and Docherty, J. R. (1980): Recent developments in alpha-receptor research. *J. Cardiovasc. Pharmacol.,* 2:S269–S286.

343. Starke, K., Montel, H., and Schumann, H. J. (1971): Influence of cocaine and phenoxybenzamine on noradrenaline uptake and release. *Naunyn Schmiedebergs Arch. Pharmacol.,* 270:210–214.

344. Starling, E. H. (1905): The chemical correlation of the functions of the body. *Lancet,* 2:339–341.

345. Steer, M. L., Khorana, J., and Galgoci, B. (1979): Quantitation and characterization of human platelet alpha-adrenergic receptors using [³H]phentolamine. *Mol. Pharmacol.,* 16:719–728.

346. Stephenson, R. P. (1956): A modification of receptor theory. *Br. J. Pharmacol.,* 11:379–383.

347. Sternweiss, P. C., and Robishaw, J. D. (1984): Isolation of two proteins with high affinity for guanine nucleotides from membrane of bovine brain. *J. Biol. Chem.,* 259:13806–13813.

348. Story, D. F., Briley, M. S., and Langer, S. Z. (1979): The effects of chemical sympathectomy with 6-hydroxydopamine on alpha-adrenoceptor and muscarinic cholinoceptor binding in rat heart ventricle. *Eur. J. Pharmacol.,* 57:423–426.

349. Story, D. F., McCulloch, M. W., Rand, M. J., and Stanford-Starr, C. A. (1981): Conditions required for the inhibitory feedback loop in noradrenergic transmission. *Nature,* 293:62–65.

350. Streb, H., Irvine, R. F., Berridge, M. J., and Schulz, I. (1983): Release of Ca²⁻ from a nonmitochondrial intracellular store in pancreatic acinar cells by inositol-1,4,5-trisphosphate. *Nature,* 306:67–69.

351. Strickland, W. G., Blackmore, P. F., and Exton, J. H. (1980): The role of calcium in alpha-adrenergic inactivation of glycogen synthase in rat hepatocytes and its inhibition by insulin. *Diabetes,* 29:617–622.

352. Summers, R. J. (1980): [³H]clonidine binding to alpha-adrenoceptors in membranes prepared from regions of guinea pig kidney. Alteration by monovalent and divalent cations. *Br. J. Pharmacol.,* 71:57–63.

353. Svensson, T. H., Bunney, B. S., and Aghajanian, G. K. (1975): Inhibition of both noradrenergic and serotonergic neurons in brain by the alpha-adrenergic agonist clonidine. *Brain Res.,* 92:291–306.

354. Sweatt, J. D., and Limbird, L. E. (1985): Inhibitors of Na⁺/H⁺ exchange block epinephrine- and ADP-induced stimulation of human platelet phospholipase C by blockade of arachidonic acid release at a prior step. *Circulation,* 72:322.

355. Tanaka, T., and Starke, K. (1979): Binding of ³H-clonidine to an alpha-adrenoceptor in membranes of guinea-pig ileum. *Naunyn Schmiedebergs Arch. Pharmacol.,* 309:207–215.

356. Tanaka, T., and Starke, K. (1980): Antagonist/agonist-preferring alpha-adrenoceptors or alpha₁/alpha₂-adrenoceptors? *Eur. J. Pharmacol.,* 63:191–194.

357. Taokimasa, T., Morita, K., and North, A. (1981): Opiates and clonidine prolong calcium-dependent after-hyperpolarizations. *Nature,* 294:162–163.

358. Taube, H. D., Starke, K., and Borowski, E. (1977): Presynaptic receptor systems on the noradrenergic neurones of rat brain. *Naunyn Schmiedebergs Arch. Pharmacol.,* 299:123–141.

359. Taylor, J., and Green, R. D. (1971): Analysis of reserpine-induced supersensitivity in aortic strips of rabbits. *J. Pharamcol. Exp. Ther.,* 177:127–135.

360. Terai, M., Takenaka, T., and Maeno, H. (1983): Measurements of pharmacological and [³H]ligand binding in adrenergic receptors. In: *Methods in Biogenic Amine Research,* edited by S. Parvez, T. Nagatsu, I. Nagatsu, and H. Parvez, pp. 1–28. Elsevier, New York.

361. Tesner, V. K., Cook, D. A., and Marks, G. S. (1971): Studies of the chemical nature of the alpha-adrenergic receptor. V. Validity of the receptor protection approach. *Biochem. Pharmacol.,* 20:597–603.

362. Timmermans, P. B. M. W. M., Kwa, H. Y., and Van Zweiten, P. A. (1979): Possible subdivision of postsynaptic alpha-adrenergic receptors mediating pressor responses in the pitted rat. *Naunyn Schmiedebergs Arch. Pharmacol.,* 310:189–193.

363. Timmermans, P. B. M. W. M., Schoop, A. M. C., and Van Zweiten, P. A. (1982): Binding characteristics of [³H]guanfacine to rat brain alpha-adrenoceptors. Comparison with [³H]clonidine. *Biochem. Pharmacol.,* 31:899–905.

364. Timmermans, P. B. M. W. M., Thoolen, J. J. M. C., Mathy, M. J., Wilffert, B., de Jonge, A., and Van Zweiten, P. A. (1985): Effects of the irreversible alpha-adrenoceptor antagonists phenoxybenzamine and benextramine on the effectiveness of nifedipine in inhibiting alpha₁- and alpha₂-adrenoceptor mediated vasoconstriction in pithed rats. *Naunyn Schmiedebergs Arch. Pharmacol.,* 329:404–413.

365. Timmermans, P. B. M. W. M., and Van Zweiten, P. A. (1982): Alpha₂-adrenoceptors: Classification, localization, mechanisms and targets for drugs. *J. Med. Chem.,* 25:1389–1401.

366. Trendelenberg, P. (1917): Physiologische und pharmakologische Versuche über die Dunndarmperistaltik. *Naunyn Schmiedebergs Arch. Pharmacol.,* 81:55–129.

367. Tsai, B. S., and Lefkowitz, R. J. (1978): Agonist-specific effects of monovalent and divalent cations on adenylate cyclase-coupled alpha-adrenergic receptors in rabbit platelets. *Mol. Pharmacol.,* 14:540–548.

368. Tsai, B. S., and Lefkowitz, R. J. (1979): Agonist-specific effects of guanine nucleotides on alpha-adrenergic receptors in human platelets. *Mol. Pharmacol.,* 16:61–68.

369. Ullrich, S., and Wolheim, C. B. (1984): Islet cyclic AMP levels are not lowered during alpha₂-adrenergic inhibition of insulin release. Studies with epinephrine and forskolin. *J. Biol. Chem.,* 259:4111–4115.

370. U'Prichard, D. C., Bechtel, W. D., Rouot, B. M., and Snyder, S. H. (1979): Multiple apparent alpha-noradrenergic receptor binding sites in rat brain: Effect of 6-hydroxydopamine. *Mol. Pharmacol.,* 16:47–60.

371. U'Prichard, D. C., Greenberg, D. A., and Snyder, S. H. (1977): Binding characteristics of a radiolabeled agonist and antagonist at central nervous system alpha-noradrenergic receptors. *Mol. Pharmacol.,* 13:454–473.

372. U'Prichard, D. C., Mitrius, J. C., Kahn, D. J., and Perry, B. D. (1983): The alpha₂-adrenergic receptor: Multiple affinity states and regulation of a receptor inversly coupled to adenylate cyclase. In: *Molecular Pharmacology of Neurotransmitter Receptors,* edited by T. Segawat, pp. 53–72. Raven Press, New York.

373. U'Prichard, D. C., and Snyder, S. H. (1977): [³H]epinephrine and [³H]norepinephrine binding to alpha-noradrenergic receptors in calf brain membranes. *Life Sci.,* 20:527–534.

374. U'Prichard, D. C., and Snyder, S. H. (1978): Guanyl nucleotide influences on [³H]ligand binding to alpha-noradrenergic receptors in calf brain membranes. *J. Biol. Chem.,* 253:3444–3452.

375. U'Prichard, D. C., and Snyder, S. H. (1980): Interactions of divalent cations and guanine nucleotides at alpha₂-noradrenergic receptor binding sites in bovine brain mechanisms. *J. Neurochem.,* 34:385–394.

376. Van Rossum, J. M., and Ariens, E. J. (1962): Receptor-reserve and threshold phenomena. II. Theories on drug action and a quantitative approach to spare receptors and threshold values. *Arch. Int. Pharmacodyn. Ther.,* 136:385–394.

377. Venter, J. C., Horne, P., Eddy, B., Greguski, R., and Fraser, C. M. (1984): Alpha₁-adrenergic receptor structure. *Mol. Pharmacol.,* 26:196–205.

378. Venter, J. C., Schaber, J. S., U'Prichard, D. C., and Fraser, C. M. (1983): Molecular size of the human platelet alpha₂-

adrenergic receptor as determined by radiation inactivation. *Biochem. Biophys. Res. Commun.,* 116:1070–1075.

379. Villeneuve, A., Carpene, C., Berlan, M., and Lafontan, M. (1985): Lack of desensitization of alpha$_2$-mediated inhibition of lipolysis in fat cells after acute and chronic treatment with clonidine. *J. Pharmacol. Exp. Ther.,* 233:433–440.

380. Watanabe, A. M., McConnaughey, M. M., Strawbridge, R. A., Fleming, J. W., Jones, L. R., and Besch, H. R. (1978): Muscarinic cholinergic receptor modulation of beta-adrenergic receptor affinity for catecholamine. *J. Biol. Chem.,* 253:4833–4836.

381. Watanabe, Y., Lai, R. T., Maeda, H., and Yoshida, H. (1982): Reserpine and sympathetic denervation cause an increase of postsynaptic alpha$_2$-adrenoceptors. *Eur. J. Pharmacol.,* 80:105–108.

382. Wei, J. W., and Sulakhe, P. V. (1981): Requirement for sulfhydryl groups in the differential effects of magnesium ion and GTP on agonist binding of muscarinic cholinergic receptor sites in rat atrial membrane fraction. *Naunyn Schmiedebergs Arch. Pharmacol.,* 314:51–59.

383. Weiland, G. A., Minneman, K. P., and Molinoff, P. B. (1979): Fundamental difference between the molecular interactions of agonists and antagonists with the beta-adrenergic receptor. *Nature,* 281:114–117.

384. Weiland, G. A., Minneman, K. P., and Molinoff, P. B. (1980): Thermodynamics of agonist and antagonist interactions with mammalian beta-adrenergic receptors. *Mol. Pharmacol.,* 18:341–350.

385. Wernette, M. E., Ochs, R. S., and Lardy, H. A. (1981): Ca^{2+} stimulation of rat liver mitochondrial glycerophosphate dehydrogenase. *J. Biol. Chem.,* 256:12767–12771.

386. Westfall, T. C. (1977): Local regulation of adrenergic neurotransmission. *Physiol. Rev.,* 57:659–728.

387. Wikberg, J. E. S., Akers, M., Caron, M. G., and Hagen, P. O. (1983): Norepinephrine-induced "down-regulation" of alpha$_1$-adrenergic receptors in cultured rabbit aortic smooth muscle cells. *Life Sci.,* 33:1409–1417.

388. Wikberg, J. E. S. (1979): The pharmacological classification of adrenergic alpha$_1$- and alpha$_2$-receptors and their mechanisms of action. *Acta Physiol. Scand.,* 468:1–99.

389. Wikberg, J. E. S., Lefkowitz, R. J., and Caron, M. G. (1983): Solubilization of rat liver alpha$_1$-adrenergic receptors. Agonist

390. Williams, L. T., and Lefkowitz, R. J. (1976): Alpha-adrenergic receptor identification by [^{3}H]dihydroergocryptine binding. *Science,* 192:791–793.

391. Williams, L. T., and Lefkowitz, R. J. (1977): Molecular pharmacology of alpha-adrenergic receptors: Utilization of [^{3}H]dihydroergocryptine in the study of pharmacological receptor alterations. *Mol. Pharmacol.,* 13:304–313.

392. Williams, L. T., Mullikin, D., and Lefkowitz, R. J. (1977): Identification of alpha-adrenergic receptors in uterine smooth muscle by [^{3}H]dihydroergocryptine binding. *J. Biol. Chem.,* 251:6915–6923.

393. Wood, C. L., Arnett, C. D., Clarke, W. R., Tsai, B. S., and Lefkowitz, R. J. (1979): Subclassification of α-adrenergic receptors by direct binding studies. *Biochem. Pharmacol.,* 28:1277–1282.

394. Woodcock, E. A., Morris, M. J., McLeod, J. K., and Johnston, C. I. (1985): Specific increase in renal alpha$_1$-adrenergic receptors following unilateral renal denervation. *J. Receptor Research,* 5:133–146.

395. Woodcock, E. A., and Murley, B. (1982): Increased central alpha$_2$-adrenergic receptors measured with [^{3}H]yohimbine in the presence of sodium ion and guanylnucleotides. *Biochem. Biophys. Res. Commun.,* 105:252–258.

396. Wyman, J. (1967): Allosteric linkage. *J. Am. Chem. Soc.,* 89:2202–2218.

397. Yamamura, H., Lad, P. M., and Rodbell, M. (1977): GTP stimulates and inhibits adenylate cyclase in fat cell membranes through distinct regulatory processes. *J. Biol. Chem.,* 252:7964–7966.

398. Yip, B. P., and Lardy, H. A. (1981): The role of calcium in the stimulation of gluconeogenesis by catecholamines. *Arch. Biochem. Biophys.,* 212:370–377.

399. Yokoyama, M., Miyake, R., Awano, K., Kashiki, M., Kawashima, S., and Fukuzaki, H. (1985): Vascular contractions induced by TPA (12-O-tetradecanoylphorbol-13-acetate): Possible involvement of a lipooxygenase pathway and protein kinase C. *Circulation,* 72:322.

400. Yong, M. S., and Nickerson, M. (1973): Dissociation of alpha-adrenergic receptor protection from inhibition of [^{3}H]phenoxybenzamine binding in vascular tissue. *J. Pharmcol. Exp. Ther.,* 186:100–108.

specific alteration in receptor binding affinity. *Biochem. Pharmacol.,* 32:3171–3178.

The Heart and Cardiovascular System,
edited by H. A. Fozzard et al.
Raven Press, New York © 1986.

CHAPTER 51

The Beta-Adrenergic Receptor/Adenylate Cyclase System

J. Peter Longabaugh, Dorothy E. Vatner, and Charles J. Homcy

HISTORICAL BACKGROUND

Adrenergic receptors compose a class of cell surface proteins that bind catecholamines and mediate the initial steps of signal transduction across the plasma membrane. In this chapter we are specifically concerned with the beta-adrenergic receptor. It is linked to intracellular enzyme systems via two other membrane elements, the stimulatory guanyl nucleotide binding protein (G_s) and adenylate cyclase. What follows is a historical perspective of how these elements were discovered and what their individual chemical and physical properties are. Further, we shall describe beta receptor, G_s, and cyclase interactions, how these interactions may be regulated, and how alterations in this system are important in pathophysiologic states. It is interesting to note that our current understanding results from invaluable contributions from various disciplines, such as physiology, pharmacology, cell biology, protein chemistry, and molecular biology.

The influence of extracellular substances on intracellular events has long been recognized. Langley (65) first

developed the concept of receptors and circulating effectors in the late nineteenth and early twentieth centuries. Simultaneously, Starling (115) was making his landmark contributions in the field of homeostatic mechanisms and coined the word "hormone" in 1905. Although Cannon had firmly established the existence of "sympathen," later proved to be norepinephrine, as the chemical mediator at sympathetic nerve terminals, it remained for Ahlquist (4) to demonstrate that catecholamines exert their effects by exciting two distinct receptor systems, termed alpha and beta. His initial observations suggested that alpha activation, for example, generally leads to smooth-muscle contraction, as evidenced by vasoconstriction or uterine contraction, whereas beta stimulation produces the opposite effect of relaxing smooth muscle as well as increasing inotropy and chronotropy. He also pointed out that catecholamines stimulate their "receptors" in a differential way such that a rank order of potency can be assigned. For example, isoproterenol is more potent than epinephrine, which is generally more potent than norepinephrine in evoking a beta effect, whereas isoproterenol is essentially ineffective in producing alpha-adrenergic activation, with nor-epinephrine and epinephrine being generally equipotent.

The initial observation of how adrenergic stimulation can affect intracellular metabolism was made in the 1940s. It was noted that liver cells, when exposed to epinephrine, activated an enzyme, glycogen phosphory-lase, that initiated glycogenolysis. Subsequently it was found that a small molecule was produced when isolated liver membranes were exposed to epinephrine in the presence of adenosine triphosphate (ATP). This molecule can cause glycogen phosphorylase activation and was identified as 3′5′-cyclic adenosine monophosphate (cAMP) in 1959 by Sutherland (128). Those experiments not only established the identity of a ubiquitous intracel-lular regulatory molecule but also clearly localized to the plasma membrane the molecular machinery by which an extracellular signal could be sensed and a corresponding intracellular signal could be generated. Identification and characterization of this machinery progressed slowly until 1970. By that time, the development of relatively simple membrane systems from avian red cells and the avail-ability of a vast array of highly specific and potent agonists and antagonists allowed the ligand binding assay to be-come a critically important tool. Suffice it to say that in the past two decades our knowledge of the beta receptor and its coupling to intracellular events has fairly exploded.

CYCLASE AND RECEPTOR ARE TWO DISTINCT ENTITIES

Because the receptor and adenylate cyclase activities are localized to the plasma membrane, as determined by the experiments described earlier, the next step was to show that they are independent protein moieties. This was accomplished more or less simultaneously by several groups using various methods. These have been nicely reviewed by Ross and Gilman (100). Initial experiments by Schramm (104) demonstrated that in-activation of adenylate cyclase in erythrocytes did not alter ligand binding characteristics of the beta receptor. Other treatments destroyed ligand binding activity but did not alter adenylate cyclase (103). The best evidence came from three lines of experimentation. Orley and Schramm (90) extended their work to cell fusion studies (Fig. 1). A heterokaryon was constructed with Sendai virus between turkey red blood cells whose adenylate cyclase had been inactivated, but which contained func-tional beta receptor, and Friend erythroleukemia cells that lacked beta receptor but possessed adenylate cyclase. Within a very short period of time after fusion, the adenylate cyclase of the leukemia cells that had not been coupled to a beta receptor in the native state could be activated by a beta-adrenergic agonist acting through the receptor "donated" by the turkey cells. As noted by Ross and Gilman (100), this experiment was also an

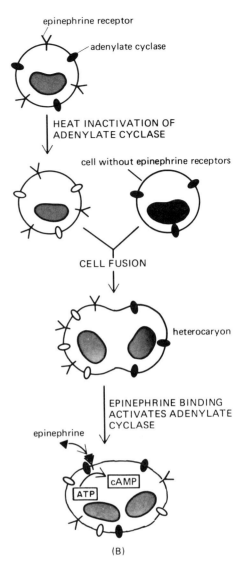

FIG. 1. Cell fusion experiment in which one of the participants lacks adenylate cyclase and the other lacks adrenergic receptor. Within minutes of fusion the adenylate cyclase of one cell is functionally coupled to the receptor of the other and can be stimulated by agonist. This suggests that ade-nylate cyclase and the receptor are separate molecular entities. (Reprinted from Alberts, B., Bray, D., Lewis, J., Raff, M., Roberts, K., and Watson, J. D. (1983): *Molecular Biology of the Cell.* Garland Publishing, New York & London, p. 738.)

important validation of the fluid-mosaic model of the plasma membrane, which predicts that receptors as well as other membrane proteins are mobile within the lipid bilayer.

Complementary data supporting the distinct molecular identities of beta receptor and adenylate cyclase were published by Limbird and Lefkowitz (72). They were able to solubilize these membrane components using digitonin and physically separate the ligand binding activity from the enzyme activity by size-exclusion chro-matography. Cerione and others recently refined this work (23). They were able to purify the solubilized beta receptor to virtual homogeneity and then insert it into *Xenopus laevis* (African clawed toad) erythroyctes that lack beta receptor in the native state. These "transplanted" receptors, when occupied by an agonist, were able to stimulate the erythrocyte adenylate cyclase, much as in the fusion experiments of Orley and Schramm, except in a more defined system (Fig. 2). Ideally, one would like to see purified receptor and purified adenylate cyclase interact in a completely artificial membrane. However, as will be described in depth later, other components are necessary.

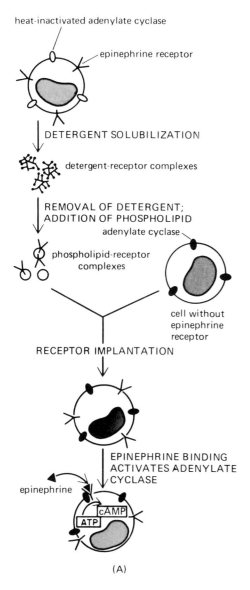

(A)

FIG. 2. Reconstitution study. Adrenergic receptors are solubilized, purified, and then reconstituted into cells that lack receptor but possess active adenylate cyclase, resulting in coupling between the two. This confirms the independent nature of the receptor and the enzyme. (Reprinted from Alberts, B., Bray, D., Lewis, J., Raff, M., Roberts, K., and Watson, J. D. (1983): *Molecular Biology of the Cell.* Garland Publishing, New York & London, p. 738.)

TECHNIQUES

The molecular characteristics of what were then thought to be two distinct proteins have been intensely investigated. Before reviewing these data, we shall briefly review several techniques whose development has been indispensable.

Ligand Binding Assay

The ability to assay for receptors directly, rather than indirectly through measurement of receptor-mediated events, was the major advance in allowing the beta-receptor protein to be purified and characterized (54). The ligand binding assay depends on the ability of the receptor protein to bind labeled ligand. The bound ligand and free ligand are then separated and quantitated. The critical aspect of such an assay is to verify that the bound ligand is the true measurement of the amount of receptor protein. Thus, certain criteria must be satisfied. The binding must be saturable, rapid, and reversible and must demonstrate an order of potency for a variety of beta-adrenergic agonists and antagonists that follows their functional efficacies.

Many labeled ligands are now available for study of the beta-adrenergic receptor (Table 1). These include both tritiated and iodinated probes. Certain of their chemical properties make them more or less desirable as receptor ligands. Because the concentrations of beta-adrenergic receptors are low in most membrane preparations (50–400 fmoles/mg membrane protein), the labeled ligand must bind with high affinity, with a dissociation constant in the nanomolar range or less. For the same reason, the probe must also be labeled to a high specific activity. One can calculate that for a receptor concentration in the femtomolar range, it is necessary to have a ligand labeled to a specific activity of at least 20 Ci/mmole. [^{125}I]derivatized ligands can be separated from the parent compound, and thus a specific activity equal to that of atomic iodine itself (approximately 2,200 Ci/mmol) can be achieved.

If nonspecific binding of the ligand to the membrane preparation or to the other materials used in the assay is sufficiently high (generally greater than 50% of total binding), the validity of the data must be questioned. The degree of nonspecific binding usually correlates with the ligand's hydrophobicity. The two most commonly employed ligands for beta-adrenergic receptor binding studies are [^{3}H]dihydroalprenolol ([^{3}H]DHA) and [^{125}I]cyanopindolol ([^{125}I]CYP). Unlike ^{125}I-labeled ligands, those labeled with ^{3}H have a much longer shelf life and thus for certain kinds of studies may be a reasonable compromise in terms of their utility and overall cost. The iodinated probes, because of their 50- to 100-fold-greater specific activity, as compared with ^{3}H-labeled ligands, offer a definite advantage for assays in which the receptor concentration is low.

TABLE 1. *Beta-adrenergic receptor ligands*

Radioligand	Maximum specific radioactivity (Ci/mmole)	Approximate ks (pM)	Specificity
Antagonists			
1-^{3}H dihydroalprenolol (1-^{3}H DHA)	120	500–2,000	Beta$_1$ = Beta$_2$
d1-^{3}H propranolol (d1-^{3}H PRO)	30	1,000–10,000	
1-^{3}H propranolol (1-^{3}H PRO)	30	1,000–10,000	
d1-^{3}H carazolol (d1-^{3}H CAR)	40	30–200	
1-^{3}H carazolol (1-^{3}H CAR)	24	10	
1-^{3}H bupranolol (1-^{3}H BUP)	18	650	
d1-^{125}I iodohydroxybenzylpindolol (d1-^{125}I HYP)	2,200	10–10,000	
d1-^{125}I iodocyanopindolol (d1-^{125}I CYP)	2,200	40–100	
d1-^{125}I iodopindolol (dl-^{125}I PIN)	2,200	130	
1-^{125}I iodopindolol (1-^{125}I PIN)	2,200	90	
Agonists			
d1-^{3}H hydroxybenzylisoproterenol (d1-^{3}H HBI)	20	1,000–10,000	B$_2$ > B$_1$
1-^{3}H epinephrine (1-^{3}H EPI)	145	80,000	
1-^{3}H norepinephrine (1-^{3}H NEP)	60		
d1-^{3}H isoproterenol (d1-^{3}H ISO)	15	150,000	

Reprinted from Stiles, G. L., Caron, M. G., and Lefkowitz, R. J. (1984): Beta-adrenergic receptors: biochemical mechanisms of physiological regulation. *Physio. Rev.*, 64:661–734.

Following incubation of the probe with the membrane preparation, separation of bound ligand from free ligand is most commonly achieved by vacuum filtration on glass-fiber filters. This method is rapid and does not allow time for bound ligand to dissociate. Furthermore, the degree of nonspecific binding to this kind of filter (as opposed to nonspecific binding to membranes) is low (generally less than 1–2% of the total bound).

A newer ligand, [^{3}H]CG, is more hydrophilic than previously available antagonists. This property has proved useful in whole-cell binding assays. Whereas hydrophilic ligands can freely cross the plasma membrane and label internalized receptors, this ligand, because of its more polar properties, is excluded by the plasma membrane and therefore behaves as a selective marker of the externalized receptor species. It has proved useful in gaining insight into the process of homologous desensitization (*vide infra*). It appears that during this process, receptors internalize and can no longer be labeled by [^{3}H]CG, but are still available for [^{125}I]CYP binding that has gained access to the cell interior.

As will be discussed, the beta receptor has also been solubilized in active form with the nonionic detergent digitonin. The solubilized receptor can be most simply assayed by one of two techniques that allow large numbers of samples to be processed. In the first method, free ligand is separated from receptor-bound ligand by size-exclusion chromatography on either Sephadex G25 or G50 columns (19). The receptor, with bound ligand, is collected in the void volume, while unbound ligand is retained. In the second procedure, the receptor, with

bound ligand, is coprecipitated with a carrier protein such as bovine gamma globulin after addition of polyethylene glycol (PEG) (8,000 MW) to a final concentration of 10%. The mixture is then poured over GF/C filters using the same filtration procedure as for membrane preparations. The only difference is that the washing buffer includes 8% PEG. Details of these techniques can be found in several of the references cited. Further information on the ligand binding assay itself, including data handling and interpretation, can be found in *Chapter* 10.

Solubilization

In order for one to use the classic techniques in biochemistry for analysis, e.g., electrophoresis, analytical and preparative centrifugation, and column chromatography, the protein in question must be in solution rather than embedded in a membrane. Solubilization, per se, is not difficult. However, one must also ensure that the activity characteristics of these proteins, i.e., enzyme activity or ligand binding, are retained for these studies to be meaningful. As mentioned earlier, digitonin has been the most useful agent in solubilizing the active beta receptor (68), although other agents have been used with varying degrees of success. Cholate and deoxycholate, both bile acid salts, are the standards for use with the other components of this system, G$_s$ and adenylate cyclase. A nonionic detergent, NP-40, and derivatives of cholic acid have recently also shown promise (68).

S49 Mouse Lymphoma Cells

Another invaluable tool has been the S49 mouse lymphoma cell line and its genetic variants (11). The parent cell line is remarkable in that it possesses a complete beta-receptor/adenylate cyclase system and also is killed by high intracellular levels of cAMP, which can be generated by incubation with beta agonists. Because of this, variants may be found in much the same fashion as in the classic technique of selecting genetic mutants of bacteria. A cell that survives beta-agonist treatment must be defective in some aspect of the mechanism that links agonist binding to the receptor with synthesis of cAMP or in distal effector mechanisms, e.g., protein kinase. One particular variant, cyc-, is deficient in G_s.

Reconstitution

Reconstitution requires the availability of solubilized, active membrane components. These can be "transplanted" into "recipient" membranes. Initially, crude solubilized membrane preparations were used to donate various components to native membranes, as in Fig. 2. As work has progressed, this technique has been refined so that purified components can be inserted into native membranes or even into "artificial" membranes consisting of phospholipid vesicles (22). A stringent set of criteria has been developed to evaluate the efficacy and validity of such reconstitution techniques and should be applied to each new system as it is developed. First, the donated components must be physically integrated into the membrane, as demonstrated by cosedimentation with the membrane. The components of a reconstituted membrane must also retain the same activity that they individually possess in the native membrane. For example, the receptor must demonstrate its usual ligand binding characteristics, and the adenylate cyclase should respond to its independent activators such as Mn^{2+}. Last, the reconstituted system must display the properties that result from interactions of its components, i.e., the binding of agonists to the receptor must stimulate the adenylate cyclase in the same manner as in the native membrane. The power of this technique will be more evident as its use is described in succeeding sections.

BETA RECEPTOR

Distribution and Subtypes

The beta receptor is widely distributed and can be identified in almost all tissues and cell types. Table 2 lists the relative concentrations of the two beta-receptor subtypes found in various tissues. On the basis of

TABLE 2. Beta₁- and beta₂-adrenergic receptor subtypes in various tissues

Tissue and species	Ratio of β_1- to β_2-adrenergic receptors	Refs.
Heart		
Frog	20:80(LV)[a]	47
Rat	100:0(LV)	47
Guinea pig	77:23(RA)	36
	100:0(LV)	36
	100:0(LV)	49
Rabbit	72:28(RA)	14
	92:8(RV)	14
	93:7(LV)	14
	82:18(LA)	14
Cat	78:22(RA)	49
	98:2(LV)	49
Dog	85:15(LV)	76
Human	74:26(RA)	123
	86:14(LV)	123
Lung		
Rat	20:80	32,33
	25:75	101
	15:85	79
Hamster	4:96	8
Guinea pig	20:80	36
Rabbit	80:20	32
	60:40	101
Dog	5:95	76

[a] LA, left atrial tissue; LV, left ventricular tissue; RA, right atrial tissue; RV, right ventricular tissue.

pharmacologic studies it initially appeared that only one beta-receptor subtype existed in a particular tissue or cell type. However, more sensitive ligand binding techniques have demonstrated that this concept is not valid. These studies, which employ subtype-selective drugs in competition binding studies with a labeled ligand, can detect a second receptor subtype when it accounts for as little as 10% of the total. However, such an approach is limited in assigning specific or different actions to the receptor subtypes. Furthermore, it cannot determine if one cell type in a specific tissue has both beta-1 and beta-2 receptors on its surface, or if the heterogeneity can be explained by the presence of different cell types in any particular organ. An example here will be illustrative. It is now clear from several studies of heart muscle in different species that both atrium and ventricle contain both beta-1 and beta-2 receptors in various proportions, with the former typically constituting anywhere from 50 to 80% of the total. These results are based on ligand binding studies. Controversy has developed as to whether or not the beta-1 or beta-2 receptor subtypes selectively mediate inotropy or chronotropy. Various studies have suggested that there are relatively high concentrations of the beta-2 subtype in the SA and AV nodes, consistent with certain physiologic data that have argued for a predominant beta-2 subtype in regulating the sympathetic component of heart rate (17,18). In contrast, Ablad et al. (3) have developed evidence in explanted human cardiac tissue that both beta-1 and beta-2 receptors can mediate increased inotropy, as evidenced by studies with isolated atrial appendage. The beta-1:beta-2 receptor ratio in this tissue has been reported to be approximately 4:1 based on ligand binding studies (122). However, at least two types of data make this interpretation less than certain. Muntz et al. (86) showed by autoradiography that the beta-2 receptor in myocardium may reside exclusively in arteriolar smooth muscle, because the beta-1-selective ligand metoprolol was less effective in competing for these sites than for [³H]dihydroalprenolol binding to cardiocytes. A second piece of data stems from *in vitro* studies performed with isolated myocytes. Using culture techniques that can enrich the population in myocytes as compared with fibroblast and endothelial cells, Buxton and Brunton (15) have shown that myocytes may selectively contain the beta-1 subtype, and the beta-2-receptor population may be contributed to by other cell types. These data emphasize the difficulty in relating the results of ligand binding studies, which employ impure membrane preparations, to functional data.

Molecular Characterization

Solubilization and Purification

Like other intrinsic membrane proteins, the beta-adrenergic receptor requires a detergent to release it from the membrane bilayer. Of the entire class of nondenaturing nonionic detergents, only digitonin, similar in structure to the bile acids, has permitted detection of the solubilized species by direct ligand binding techniques (19,54). It is still not clear which factors are responsible for the masking of ligand binding when membranes are solubilized with other detergents, such as NP-40 or Lubrol. These detergents routinely release other membrane proteins in active form. Digitonin, however, is not an optimal detergent in which to characterize the biophysical properties of the solubilized receptor (28,116). In particular, its partial specific volume is similar to that of hydrophilic proteins, thus preventing determination of the amount of bound detergent. Digitonin additionally forms large-molecular-weight micelles, making hydrodynamic characterization of solubilized membrane proteins difficult. Moreover, the critical micellar concentration is quite low, and therefore it is difficult to remove the detergent by dialysis. Its chemical properties in solution have not been well defined and likely differ from batch to batch. The detergent is also poorly soluble in aqueous buffer and often spontaneously precipitates even when present in low concentrations.

Despite these difficulties, both the beta-1 and beta-2 receptors have been purified to homogeneity. This, however, remains an onerous task because of the extremely low concentration of the receptor present in most tissues. Typically, membrane preparations contain 50 to 400 fmoles/mg, whereas in highly purified plasma membranes, concentrations as high as 1 to 2 pmoles/mg may be obtained. The strategy for receptor purification relies on the technique of affinity chromatography. This approach takes advantage of the unique specificity of the receptor protein in binding beta-adrenergic ligands. Thus, high-affinity ligands susceptible to covalent modification can be attached to a solid support such as agarose (20,54). The solubilized receptor preparation then can be selectively adsorbed to the resin, while contaminating proteins are washed away. The receptor is then specifically eluted by incubating the resin with a competing ligand such as alprenolol. Additional steps are required in that only a 200- to 500-fold purification can be achieved with affinity chromatography. Purification to homogeneity requires an additional 500- to 1,000-fold increase in specific activity, which has been achieved most efficiently by employing high-performance gel-filtration chromatography in addition to affinity chromatography.

Several laboratories have now completely purified the beta-adrenergic receptor, both the beta-1 and beta-2, from mammalian (7,30,54) and nonmammalian (107, 108,140) sources. The results are fairly consistent. For all mammalian species, it appears that the receptor consists of a single 62- to 67-kd peptide with one ligand binding site per molecule. This finding has been confirmed by photoaffinity labeling of the membrane-bound receptor, which identifies a peptide of molecular mass identical with that of the purified receptor. However, it is still not clear how the receptor exists within the membrane bilayer. For example, the intact receptor may be a monomer or dimer. Following solubilization in digitonin, the receptor behaves on size-exclusion gel-filtration columns as a protein of approximately 150 kd (54). Because the holoreceptor is a hydrophobic membrane protein and likely does not behave as a globular structure in solution, its absolute mass cannot be directly calculated by comparing its hydrodynamic properties (Stokes's radius and partial specific volume) to those of standard hydrophilic proteins that do not bind detergent and are generally more compact. Hydrodynamic data do, however, suggest that the intact receptor contains not more than two of the hormone-binding subunits.

Glycosylation

As with other membrane proteins (89,118), the receptor is known to be glycosylated. This has been shown in several different ways. First, the solubilized receptor will bind to lectin affinity resins, particularly wheat germ hemagglutinin (89,118). Second, tunicamycin, an antibiotic that inhibits glycosylation of proteins in the Golgi, results in the appearance of a receptor protein with increased mobility on SDS gel, i.e., as a protein of smaller molecular weight (34). This is consistent with the known effects of carbohydrate moieties on the migration of proteins in SDS polyacrylamide gels. Third, treatment with endoglycosidase F or H, enzymes that cleave extended carbohydrate chains at a locus near their point of attachment to the protein backbone, reduces the apparent molecular mass of the hormone-binding subunit from approximately 65 to 67 kd to approximately 40 to 45 kd (118).

The role and significance of glycosylation in receptor function, metabolism, or processing are not yet clear. However, as with other hormone receptors, there is evidence that this type of posttranslational modification is a maturation step that is important in routing the receptor to its plasma membrane residence. Doss et al. (34) have provided preliminary evidence for this proposal by finding that the appearance of newly synthesized beta receptors is blocked in tunicamycin-treated astrocytoma cells.

The availability of purified receptor preparations and affinity-labeled receptors has allowed preliminary comparisons of receptor subtype structures to be made. The laboratories of Caron and Lefkowitz (7,122) and Malbon (44) have compared peptides obtained by limited proteolytic digestion of either purified or photolabeled mammalian beta-1 and beta-2 receptors. Peptides of different molecular masses were detected, suggesting that differences in their primary amino acid structures exist, as one might expect. Moreover, they also differ in carbohydrate composition (7,118); the significance of this latter finding remains unclear. There is evidence, however, to support the fact that differences in glycosylation do not play a role in the specificity of ligand binding (89).

It is clear that further insight into the structure-function relationship of the beta-receptor molecule will be gained only when complete sequence data for this protein become available. In this way, domains such as membrane spanning regions can be assigned and comparisons between subtypes and species made with more certainty.

SH and S-S Groups

The availability of relatively selective chemical reagents that can either alkylate sulfhydryl groups or reduce disulfide bonds has allowed determination of their roles in receptor activation. For the beta-2 receptor, at least, and likely for the beta-1 receptor as well, there appears to be a disulfide bond that plays a role in maintaining

the integrity of the ligand binding site (139; C. J. Homcy, *unpublished observations*). Exposure to increasing concentrations of the reducing agent dithiothreitol progressively inactivates receptor units without altering the affinity of the remaining molecules. Loss of receptor activity affects both agonist and antagonist binding. The location and importance of such a disulfide bond in maintaining a correct tertiary structure have not been further elucidated.

ADENYLATE CYCLASE

Structure

From data already discussed, it is clear that the binding of agonist to the beta receptor influences intracellular events via the action of adenylate cyclase. Characterization of the physical properties of the receptor has progressed more rapidly than that for the protein associated with adenylate cyclase catalytic activity. The primary problem lies in its exquisite lability when solubilized. Some data are available for adenylate cyclase, obtained from many types of tissue, and these have been nicely summarized by Ross and Gilman (100). Most studies show that the native protein has a molecular mass of approximately 190 kd. Strittmatter and Neer (126), as well as Ross (98), have succeeded in solubilizing and separating adenylate cyclase from related membrane components. Finally, Schlegel et al. (102) performed target-size analysis in which an electron beam was used to inactivate adenylate cyclase. By comparing the time course over which enzymatic activity was lost with that for an enzyme of known size, and using other assumptions that have proved valid in other cases, they were able to confirm the data yielded by more classic techniques. Again, the data are limited, because the enzyme has only recently been purified by Pfeuffer (93). He was able to achieve a 10,000-fold purification of the enzyme by passing a solubilized crude preparation over a forskolin affinity column. The data from that study yielded a molecular mass of 150 kd. It is likely that the larger masses noted in earlier studies resulted from an unrecognized complex between adenylate cyclase and the alpha component of G_s.

Enzymatic Activity

Study of the enzymatic activity of adenylate cyclase, however, has been exceedingly fruitful. This activity may be functionally linked to several receptor types in the same membrane, and therefore the enzyme can be stimulated by a variety of agonists, e.g., isoproterenol, prostaglandin E, and glucagon. The enzyme can also be stimulated to synthesize cAMP directly with manganese ion (Mn^{2+}), using adenosine triphosphate (ATP) as the substrate. This requires only the presence of the enzyme itself. Finally, there are several compounds that will stimulate adenylate cyclase in the absence of receptor, but only if adenylate cyclase can interact with a third entity, G_s, the regulatory protein. Most of the compounds are analogues of guanosine triphosphate (GTP), and there is GTP itself, which Rodbell et al. (96) demonstrated in 1971 to be critical to agonist-stimulated adenylate cyclase activity. Fluoride ion (F^-) in millimolar concentrations (the GTP analogues must be present in only micromolar concentrations) can also stimulate the enzyme (100). Elucidation of how these compounds act in a stimulatory fashion forms a cornerstone for our understanding of the workings of the beta-receptor/adenylate cyclase system. The reader is referred to *Chapter* 49 for a more complete discussion of adenylate cyclase.

STIMULATORY GUANYL NUCLEOTIDE BINDING PROTEIN

Discovery

It is clear that there are at least two components to the beta-adrenergic system, namely, the receptor and adenylate cyclase. However, a third component, G_s, has been identified more recently, and we shall trace that history here. As noted, Rodbell demonstrated the essential nature of guanyl nucleotides in regulating interactions between the receptor and adenylate cyclase (96). Using these data, as well as observations of the kinetics of receptor-stimulated adenylate cyclase, Levitzki and colleagues proposed that a third component, a "guanyl nucleotide effector," might be involved (68). In 1975, Bourne et al. (11), on the basis of studies of genetic mutants of the S49 lymphoma cell, suggested that a third component was necessary. Their arguments were theoretical and were based on indirect evidence only, but nevertheless represent remarkable contributions.

More direct evidence of the existence of a separate regulatory component came from several lines of investigation. Pfeuffer (92) was the first to demonstrate that the GTP binding activity and adenylate cyclase enzyme activity could be physically separated. Using a GTP-Sepharose affinity column, he was able to retain GTP-binding proteins while eluting the adenylate cyclase activity. The eluted activity was not responsive to GTP analogues by itself, but this property could be restored on recombination with materials specifically bound to the affinity resin. Furthermore, of many species of GTP-binding protein, he identified a 42-kd polypeptide that could associate with adenylate cyclase. Simultaneously, Ross and Gilman (99) were able to solubilize membrane components of cells that lacked beta receptor but had adenylate cyclase that could be activated by GTP analogues as well as nonadrenergic receptor agonists, e.g., prostaglandin E (PGE). The solubilized components

were inserted into a unique variant of the S49 lymphoma cell, the cyc- strain mentioned earlier that had beta-receptor as well as adenylate cyclase activity (as demonstrated by Mn^{2+} stimulation) but lacked the ability to be stimulated by beta agonists or GTP analogues. On reconstitution of the donor and acceptor, fairly complete restoration of beta-agonist and guanyl nucleotide stimulation of adenylate cyclase was achieved. Both types of experiments strongly suggest a third component distinct from receptor and adenylate cyclase that is integral to the coupling of receptor to adenylate cyclase and that possesses GTP binding characteristics. Ross and Gilman's studies (99), in conjunction with Braun and Levitzki's kinetic data (12), also suggest that G_s, as well as the adenylate cyclase, can interact with adrenergic as well as nonadrenergic receptors in the same membrane.

Subsequently, Cassel and Pfeuffer (21), as well as Gill and Meren (41), showed that G_s could be covalently modified using the A peptide of cholera toxin as the enzyme and nicotine adenine dinucleotide (NAD) as the substrate. The modification involves the transfer of an adenosine diphosphate (ADP) ribosyl group to an arginine residue on the G protein. Using [alpha-^{32}P]NAD, both groups demonstrated the presence of a 42-kd polypeptide on SDS polyacrylamide gels. The degree of covalent modification of this polypeptide correlated directly with G_s-mediated adenylate cyclase stimulation. It had long been known that increased intracellular levels of cAMP in intestinal mucosal cells were responsible for the secretory diarrhea seen with cholera toxin. This work, in addition to confirming the existence of G_s, established the molecular pathophysiology of the disease associated with *Vibrio cholerae* infection. Thus, in historical perspective, we have identified the major components of the beta-receptor membrane system, namely, the receptor, G_s, and adenylate cyclase. The reader is cautioned about the multiplicity of terms in the primary literature. G_s protein is referred to variously as the G protein, the G/F protein, the nucleotide regulatory protein, N-protein, N_s protein, and the regulatory subunit of adenylate cyclase. Adenylate cyclase itself has been called the catalytic subunit and the C protein.

Structural Analysis of G_s

Structural analysis of the G protein has been made possible by its purification. Many investigators have published methods for doing this. They can generally be divided into those that require guanyl nucleotides or fluoride for stabilization of G_s and those that do not. Northup et al. (88) have published a seven-step procedure that results in a 2,000-fold purification from membrane protein with a recovery of 3%. Codina et al. (29) described a method that is more arduous and yields significantly less protein but does not require guanyl nucleotides or fluoride. At this writing, G_s appears to be a heterotrimer of three subunits, alpha (45 kd), beta (35 kd), and gamma (8 kd), that have been described only in the past two years (42). The holoprotein then should have a mass of approximately 88 kd. This has been predicted by hydrodynamic data (100). G_s is relatively heat-stable compared with adenylate cyclase and likewise is relatively resistant to N-ethylmaleimide. The observation that G_s can under certain conditions be inactivated by an agent that alkylates sulfhydryl groups is important when one considers the functional nature of this protein (*vide infra*). Clearly, G_s does have a sulfhydryl group that is important in maintaining its functional integrity. It is also known from other studies that the catalytic unit of adenylate cyclase has a sensitive S-H group, as evidenced by its inactivation with N-ethylmaleimide (117).

Function

The alpha subunit of G_s appears to carry the "activity" ascribed to the protein. It possesses the guanyl nucleotide binding site and in fact can hydrolyze bound GTP to GDP (42). Furthermore, it acts to alter receptor binding characteristics (*vide infra*) and therefore presumably has a receptor binding site. It is the site of cholera toxin action and therefore can be ADP-ribosylated. Finally, when suitably activated, it can stimulate adenylate cyclase, and it possesses a recognition site for this protein (42). The significance of these various activities and the relationships between the alpha subunit and other subunits will be discussed next. What follows is a distillate of contributions by many investigators, and the authors regret any inadvertent failure to cite key reports.

INTERACTIONS AMONG RECEPTOR, G_s, AND CYCLASE

Receptor-G_s

The receptor and G_s interact in a reciprocal fashion. Clearly, binding of agonist to the receptor causes activation of G_s so that it can stimulate adenylate cyclase. Conversely, the G_s can alter the receptor's affinity for agonists, depending on whether G_s has GTP or GDP (hydrolyzed *in situ* from GTP) or no nucleotide bound to it (105). Specifically, when the beta receptor binds agonist in the absence of GTP, a relatively high average affinity is observed. If these data are modeled to two sites, one obtains high- and low-affinity constants. However, if the binding study is performed in the presence of GTP, only one affinity is measured, which is the same as the lower affinity observed in the absence of GTP. This phenomenon, the "GTP binding shift" is demonstrated in Fig. 3. The molecular mechanisms responsible for it are not well worked out, but one theory will be discussed in a later section. The interactions

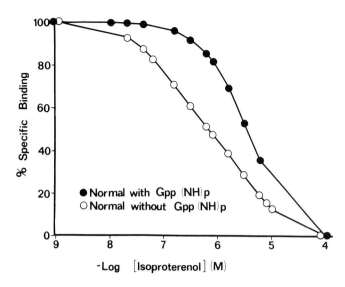

FIG. 3. Guanyl nucleotide–beta-adrenergic receptor agonist binding shift. Competition analysis in the absence of a guanyl nucleotide yields a curve with a relatively shallow slope and can be modeled to two sites of low and high affinity. When a guanyl nucleotide is included in the binding assay, the curve becomes steeper and is shifted to the right. In this case, only one low affinity site can be modeled.

inducing the GTP binding shift were reproduced by Cerione et al. (22) in a totally defined system constructed by reconstitution of purified receptor and purified G_s in an artificial membrane consisting of phospholipid vesicles. That study indicated that the components described here are necessary and sufficient to account for the behavior observed in the native membrane.

G_s-Cyclase

The interaction between adenylate cyclase and G_s is not so well understood, largely owing to difficulties in manipulating the former. It is clear that G_s is necessary for maximal adenylate cyclase activity and that this occurs only if G_s is associated with GTP or nonhydrolyzable analogues such as Gpp(NH)p, or with F^-. Magnesium ion is required for this interaction and binds at or near the adenylate cyclase catalytic site (42).

Collision Coupling Model

With these observations in hand, one can construct what is the currently accepted model of the receptor-cyclase system; here we shall review the key data that support it. It is referred to as the collision coupling model and has been presented in many forms, but the key features are as described in Fig. 4. The reader should be aware that the alpha subunit of G_s alone, rather than the holoprotein, may be the participant here. Later we shall discuss the relevance of the beta and gamma

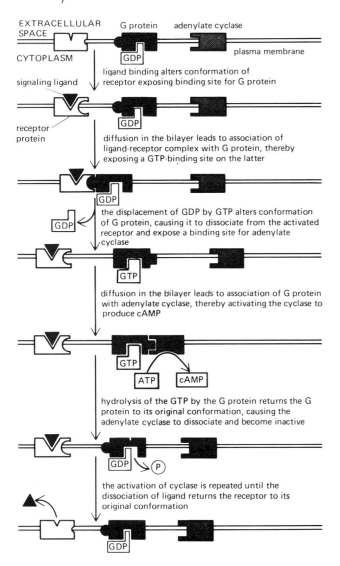

FIG. 4. Collision coupling model of the interaction of the various components of the beta-adrenergic receptor–adenylate cyclase system. The three components are shown as independent moieties although another version of the model suggests that the G protein is permanently associated with adenylate cyclase. (Reprinted from Alberts, B., Bray, D., Lewis, J., Raff, M., Roberts, K., and Watson, J. D. (1983): *Molecular Biology of the Cell.* Garland Publishing, New York & London, p. 740.)

subunits. Beginning arbitrarily at a point where no ligand is bound, the three proteins are independently floating in the lipid bilayer. The G protein has GDP bound to it, and adenylate cyclase is "inactive." On binding of hormone (H) to receptor (R), this HR complex can then interact with G_s. In doing so, G_s can then exchange a GTP for the existing GDP, which then allows it to dissociate from the HR complex. This G_s-GTP complex is the *activated* form of G protein and can stimulate adenylate cyclase. Stimulation of adenylate cyclase can occur continuously, resulting in the production of more than one molecule of cAMP, until G_s

"shuts itself off" by hydrolyzing the bound GTP to GDP. The HR complex can itself cause activation of many molecules of G_s. In Fig. 5, then, one sees that this model offers a two-stage amplification process.

Functional data already discussed provide the best support for this model. Interaction between receptor and G_s is best evidenced by the GTP binding shift. Reconstitution of pure G_s and receptor, first accomplished by Pederson and Ross (91) and further refined by Cerione (22), has clearly established that G_s is necessary and sufficient (when associated with GTP) to account for this phenomenon. Further, Limbird et al. (71) were able to identify a receptor/G-protein complex that was formed only in the presence of beta agonists and could be dissociated in the presence of GTP or a nonhydrolyzable analogue. This validates the propositions (a) that the receptor and G protein can interact in the presence of agonists and (b) that the binding of GTP to G_s is crucial in allowing it to dissociate from the receptor and then "find" an adenylate cyclase to stimulate. An early observation that G_s (alpha subunit) interacts with adenylate cyclase was made by Pfeuffer (92). He demonstrated that these proteins were bound together in detergent solutions but could be physically separated on a GTP-Sepharose affinity column. Clearly, maximal adenylate cyclase activity is achieved only when G_s is present. In most systems, manganese stimulation of cyclase is less than 20% of that achieved with Gpp(NH)p or fluoride, which act only via G_s. Other support for the model involves a kinetic theory that is beyond the scope of this chapter; it was proposed in embryonic form first by Braun and Levitzki (12) and revised to its current status by many others. Gilman (42) and Schramm and Selinger (105) have recently published excellent reviews.

Current Controversies

Stoichiometry

When one considers the potential amplification characteristics of this system, the stoichiometry of these interactions becomes important. How many G_s proteins can be activated by a hormone-receptor complex, and how many are available? In turn, what is the numeric relationship between G_s and adenylate cyclase? It has long been known that maximal stimulation of adenylate cyclase by isoproterenol in some systems occurs at much lower concentrations than are necessary to fully occupy all of the beta receptors (141). That gave rise to the idea that beta receptors are present in excess of what is needed to interact optimally with existing G_s; thus a "spare-receptor" theory for the beta receptor. Amplification of the signal within the beta-receptor system is perhaps better considered as only one mechanism by

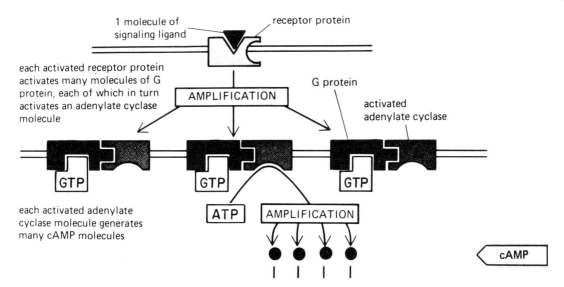

FIG. 5. Possible amplification characteristics of the beta-adrenergic receptor–adenylate cyclase system. Each receptor-ligand complex can activate many G proteins that can then activate adenylate cyclase and result in the production of many molecules of cAMP. (Reprinted in part from Alberts, B., Bray, D., Lewis, J., Raff, M., Roberts, K., and Watson, J. D. (1983): *Molecular Biology of the Cell.* Garland Publishing, New York & London, p. 750.)

which sensitivity to very low concentrations of extracellular agonist can be maximized. Another way is to have "excess" receptors. If one considers hormone binding to receptor in light of the laws of mass action, it is apparent that an increase in the number of receptors will shift the equilibrium to a state that favors formation of hormone-receptor complexes. This phenomenon has been demonstrated by Vatner and associates, who showed that the neonatal canine heart had a 50% increase in beta-receptor number. This resulted in a *reduction* in the concentration of agonist necessary to stimulate adenylate cyclase to half of its maximum activity (EC_{50}) (135), as seen in Fig. 6. Thus, having excess beta

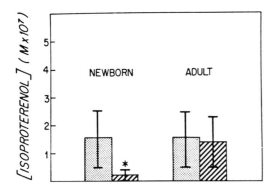

FIG. 6. Binding constants and activation constants for cardiac membranes in newborn and adult dogs. While the binding constants are the same, the activation constant is significantly lower in the newborn. This is accounted for by a 50% increase in the number of beta-adrenergic receptors in the newborn. The net result is that a lower concentration of ligand, in this case isoproterenol, is needed to achieve the same level of activation of adenylate cyclase.

receptors can, in fact, improve the sensitivity of the system.

Resolution of the question of stoichiometry will also require rejection of the notion that the system can be perceived as existing by itself in the membrane as an exclusive entity. In fact, a great deal of evidence is accumulating that the activation of one receptor system can influence the activity of another. This has profound implications in regard to regulatory phenomena and is exemplified by interactions between the alpha-2 and beta systems (*vide infra*). More complete elucidation of these mechanisms must await the development of new techniques to study the behavior of these systems. Two types of approaches have already proved invaluable. One involves reconstitution of purified components into artificial lipid vesicles. This has already been accomplished with the beta receptor and G_s (22). With the recent purification of adenylate cyclase (93), presumably a reconstituted system including all three of the components can be constructed. One should recall that even in the "purest" native membrane systems, these proteins account for less than 0.1% of the total. The completely defined, artificial membrane offers the opportunity to validate the proposed models for the beta-receptor-cyclase system. Furthermore, one can vary the concentration of each of the components independently and thereby better address the question of stoichiometry.

The other approach involves working with membranes that are part of a living system. An example is provided by ligand binding data on whole cells, which have already offered new insights into receptor function. Inactivation analysis, described briefly in a previous section, can be performed on whole cells and may also provide data that are more relevant to the living system.

G_s Structure–Function Relationships

Other questions exist with regard to the significance of the alpha-beta-gamma heterotrimer of G protein. This becomes important when one considers that all of the activity discussed to this point may reside in the alpha subunit. It appears, as delineated by Gilman (42), that the heterotrimer is an inactive form of the G protein. It is only when the alpha subunit is dissociated that it becomes active, leaving a beta-gamma complex behind (Fig. 7). The regulation of this dissociation then might logically be considered next. It is likely to be complex. First, it is known that GTP can cause this dissociation. This creates a problem in the collision coupling model. If the alpha subunit is in fact the entity that binds to the HR complex, it should, by the model presented (Fig. 3), have GDP bound to it first, and only as a consequence of binding to receptor should it exchange a GTP for the existing GDP. However, if the alpha subunit is already dissociated from the holoprotein by GTP (before interacting with receptor), then GTP should be bound to it (Fig. 4). This question has not yet been settled.

G_s-Cyclase Regulatory Phenomena

Further, it is known that in some cases alpha-2 receptors are linked to adenylate cyclase via an inhibitory G protein (G_i) that is analogous to the stimulatory G protein (G_s) we have described earlier. G_i is a heterotrimer, with the beta and gamma subunits being identical with those of G_s. The alpha subunit of G_i is distinct from that of G_s and has the unusual property of being ADP-ribosylated by pertussis toxin in a fashion analogous to the modification of the G_s alpha by cholera toxin. The analogy between G_s and G_i breaks down when one

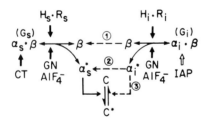

FIG. 7. Model for regulation of adenylate cyclase by stimulatory and inhibitory hormones. H, hormone; R, receptor; CT, cholera toxin; GN, guanyl nucleotide analogue; AlF_4^-, the presumed active complex of fluoride; s, stimulatory; i, inhibitory. Dissociation of G_s results in stimulation of C (adenylate cyclase) by the alpha subunit. Dissociation of G_i results in inhibition of enzyme activity by release of the beta gamma subunit (gamma subunit not shown) which can then bind to the alpha subunit of G_s and thereby inactivate it. (Reprinted from Gilman, A. G. (1984): Guanine nucleotide-binding regulatory proteins and dual control of adenylate cyclase. *J. Clin. Invest.*, 73:1–4.)

considers the proposed mechanism by which G_i inhibits adenylate cyclase (42). One might suppose that the G_i alpha subunit binds to adenylate cyclase and turns it off. However, it may be that occupation of alpha-2 receptors with agonists allows the G_i heterotrimer to dissociate, thus freeing beta-gamma complexes that can then tie up free G_s alpha subunits and prohibit them from activating adenylate cyclase (Fig. 7).

It is also known that cholera toxin causes dissociation of the G_s-protein heterotrimer by ADP ribosylation (42). Clearly this is a pathophysiologic process, but work reported by Moss and colleagues suggests that endogenous enzymes exist in at least some systems that catalyze the same covalent modification (81), and there are others that reverse the process (80). It is possible that ADP ribosylation by native enzymes is a relevant control mechanism and that it causes release of the alpha subunit from the inactive heterotrimer (Fig. 5). Regulation of the entire system also occurs at the level of the beta receptor; this will be discussed later.

Molecular Events in Receptor-G_s Interactions

Another area of interest can be generally described as the study of intramolecular events, such as changes in conformation, that are responsible for the behavior that these proteins exhibit. Mention was made earlier that binding of G_s to receptor can alter the hormone binding affinities of the receptor under certain conditions, the so-called GTP binding shift (Fig. 3). If the receptor binds G protein without available GTP, a relatively high average affinity of receptor for agonists is measured. However, if GTP is present, the average affinity of receptor for a given agonist is decreased. Presumably this is caused by binding of GTP to G_s. Schramm used this observation as a cornerstone for his "locking hypothesis" (Fig. 8), which states that the receptor and G_s with bound GDP (possibly only the G_s alpha subunit) undergo mutual conformational changes when they interact in the presence of agonists (105). The receptor is thought to undergo a conformational change from a low-affinity state to a high one (this initial step is speculative). Additionally, the receptor and/or G_s change their conformations such that their affinity for each other is increased (HR-G_s complex is "locked"), and the guanyl nucleotide binding site is exposed so that GTP can move in to replace GDP. Once this last step occurs, a second conformational change occurs such that the receptor and G_s become unlocked, as do the receptor and hormone. Thus, an explanation for the GTP binding shift is forwarded. Schramm supported this model by noting that the locked state of the HR G_s complex can be "trapped" by modifying the G protein with an agent that alkylates a sulfhydryl group important to the integrity of the guanyl nucleotide binding site (Fig. 7). This refers to the fact that the receptor now maintains a confor-

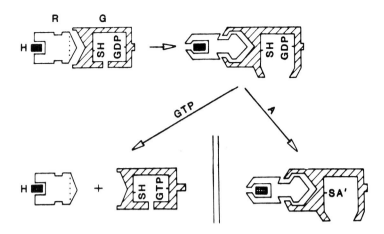

FIG. 8. Locking hypothesis. The low affinity HR complex (**upper left**) can with G protein form an HRG complex where the receptor has a high affinity for the hormone and is also tightly bound to G (**upper right**). This interaction exposes the GDP/GTP binding site as well as a sulfhydryl group. Normally, the complex is dissociated when GDP is released and GTP replaces it (**lower left**) but the high affinity complex can be "trapped" by modifying the sulfhydryl group with an alkylating agent, A (**lower right**). (Reprinted from Schramm, M., and Selinger, Z. (1984): Message transmission; receptor controlled adenylate cyclase system. *Science*, 225:1350–1356.)

mation in which agonist dissociation is relatively slow, as if the receptor is held in a high-affinity or coupled state, i.e., hormone, receptor, and G_s are trapped as an activated complex. Based on kinetic measurements, Heidenrich et al. (50) have put forth a similar hypothesis. Additional experiments have also pinpointed the action of *N*-ethylmaleimide to a sulfhydryl group on G_s itself, because after alkylation, functional receptor can be detected in subsequent reconstitution studies, although G_s is then found to be inactive (92,105). Furthermore, a locked HR complex can be obtained in the absence of G protein by modifying the lipid environment in which the receptor exists by adding detergent.

RECEPTOR REGULATION

It is the dynamic behavior of the beta-adrenergic receptor that is its most intriguing feature. Following exposure to an agonist, the receptor eventually becomes refractory to additional activation, and a state of desensitization is achieved. It is important to emphasize that although a host of literature demonstrates various effects of other hormones or processes on beta-receptor density or on signal transduction itself, the relevance and quantitative significance of these mechanisms *in vivo* have been poorly defined. For the sake of clarity, it is easiest to discuss factors that affect receptor density, receptor-cyclase coupling, or both. However, at this time, the discussion on receptor regulation is best illustrated by the concept of desensitization, because an understanding of its mechanism likely holds the key to unraveling the processes that control catecholamine-mediated signal transduction.

Homologous Desensitization

Homologous desensitization refers to the process whereby the cell becomes selectively refractory to a hormone that initially stimulated adenylate cyclase activity (48). It is usually rapid (occurring within minutes),

in contrast to the slower time course of the heterologous form (*vide infra*). Several lines of evidence indicate that it is not cAMP-mediated; specifically, it cannot be reproduced by agents that increase intracellular cAMP, such as dibutyl cAMP or phosphodiesterase inhibitors.

The phenomenon of desensitization was first recognized in studies in intact animals. Mickey and associates showed that cardiac beta-receptor numbers were considerably reduced following infusion of isoproterenol into laboratory animals. The loss of beta receptors paralleled a fall in chronotropic response to a given dose of isoproterenol (78). Most of our information concerning the mechanism of desensitization, however, has come from cell culture models. The initial event is an uncoupling of the receptor from adenylate cyclase, i.e., stimulatory activity is lost, and later there is loss of cell surface receptors for the hormone (55,56,73,130,143). A general model that accounts for these observations is as follows: The beta-receptor proteins themselves are situated within the lipid bilayer as distinct species that interact with hormone and G_s, which couples the receptor protein to the catalytic unit of adenylate cyclase (105). On binding, presumably after interaction with at least one G_s molecule, there is a rapid conversion from the native form of the receptor to one incapable of forming a ternary complex with G_s, as determined by loss of high-affinity agonist binding sites (48,55,56,143). It is postulated, but has not been proved, that this event is likely due to covalent modification of the receptor protein. Recently, Lefkowitz and associates have suggested that receptor phosphorylation may represent an early step in the homologous form of desensitization (110). Beta agonists promote receptor phosphorylation both in frog erythrocytes and in S49 lymphoma cells, each of which undergoes the homologous form of desensitization. Even in the cyc- and kin- variants of the S49 cell line, which lack G_s and cAMP-dependent protein kinase, respectively, receptor phosphorylation can be detected (66). This is consistent with previous observations that the homologous form of desensitization is not mediated by a cAMP-dependent reaction. It is likely, then, that a non-cAMP-dependent protein kinase exists that phosphorylates the beta receptor following agonist activation. The exact steps in this process have yet to be defined.

Following phosphorylation, the receptor protein is probably internalized and either degraded or reprocessed, as indicated by evidence from several laboratories (48,56,124,130,143). Chuang and Costa (25) were the first to suggest this possibility, using the frog erythrocyte as a model system to demonstrate that [³H]DHA binding sites appeared in the cytosol after exposure of the cells to isoproterenol. This provided evidence that a biochemical pathway similar to that mediating internalization of protein hormone receptors might be involved; however, the details of these events still remain sketchy. This process was subsequently confirmed by others, who also demonstrated that the internalized beta receptor can be detected in low-density vesicles within the cytosol (130,143). The initial processes of uncoupling and internalization are rapid, beginning within 1 to 2 min after binding of agonists. In addition to being responsible for loss of adenylate cyclase activation, internalization and/or sequestration may also explain the apparent low-affinity agonist binding that is seen in whole-cell binding assays. Because hydrophilic catecholamines cannot freely cross the plasma membrane to compete with the binding of lipophilic ligands such as [³H]DHA, the internalized receptors are partitioned from agonist, and a falsely low affinity is measured (130). Subsequent loss of receptors, as detected by ligand binding studies in intact cells, may result from lysosomal degradation of the internalized species, a processing pathway that regulates the activity of a variety of membrane proteins (48).

Heterologous Desensitization

Heterologous desensitization refers to that process whereby a generalized refractoriness develops such that the catalytic unit of adenylate cyclase can no longer be fully stimulated following its initial activation, whether by Gpp(NH)p or by any of several hormone types that may normally activate it (48). This can be contrasted with the more selective process of homologous desensitization of the receptor whereby the decrease in adenylate cyclase responsiveness appears only on rechallenge with a beta agonist and is associated with a decrease in functional receptor number. In heterologous desensitization, changes in receptor numbers are not relevant (32,48,112).

An increase in the level of intracellular cAMP itself is responsible for the heterologous form of desensitization (32,40). A useful model system has been the turkey erythrocyte. In this cell, dibutyryl cAMP will eventually make the cell refractory to beta-receptor-mediated cyclase stimulation, as well as to other agents that activate adenylate cyclase, including NaF and guanylyl nucleo-

tides (112). With the availability of receptor purification and affinity-labeling techniques, significant inroads into understanding this process have been made. Stadel et al. (114) first made the observation that following exposure of turkey erythrocytes to dibutyryl cAMP, an alteration in the mobility of the photolabeled receptor was apparent on SDS gels. In subsequent experiments, this group demonstrated that the partially purified receptor became phosphorylated during the desensitization process, and that accounted for its altered electrophoretic mobility. Subsequent work has shown that the purified receptor can be directly phosphorylated by cAMP-dependent protein kinase (114). Furthermore, the phosphorylated receptor shows an intrinsic reduction in its ability to couple with G_s and activate adenylate cyclase activity, as demonstrated by reconstitution experiments wherein the phosphorylated receptor is introduced into the membranes of Xenopus laevis erythrocytes that lack beta receptor but possess G_s and cyclase catalytic activity (6). Reconstitution with purified G_s has yielded similar results (127). It appears that phosphorylation of serine and/or threonine groups in the receptor molecule is not limited to the action of a cAMP-dependent protein kinase. Several groups have now reported that desensitization in the avian erythrocyte can also be effected by the action of the newly discovered enzyme protein kinase C (60,109). This enzyme normally is stimulated by activation of the polyphosphatidylinositol pathway, whereby hydrolysis of this class of membrane lipids leads to release of inositol trisphosphate (IP₃) and diacylglycerol (9). IP₃ leads to the release of intracellular calcium stores (57,125). The increased intracellular calcium levels and diacylglycerol act in concert to stimulate protein kinase C, which is a membrane-associated enzyme (53) (see Chapter 51). It is also known that the class of tumor-promoting diterpenes known as phorbol esters can substitute for diacylglycerol and directly stimulate protein kinase C (87). When avian erythrocytes are treated with this agent, phosphorylation of the beta receptor and a concomitant decrease in isoproterenol-mediated cyclase responsiveness occur (60,109). There is no evidence yet whether or not this pathway has physiologic relevance. Because polyphosphatidylinositol breakdown is stimulated by several different hormones, it is tempting to speculate that this mechanism could regulate beta-receptor activity in certain tissues.

The concomitant reductions in all cyclase-activity parameters [hormone, NaF, and Gpp(NH)p] that occur during heterologous desensitization also suggest another mechanism for this effect: that the function of G_s itself may be modified. Data exist to support this hypothesis. For example, Kassis and Fishman (59) have reported that G_s solubilized from PGE-sensitized fibroblasts is less effective than native G_s in reconstitution of hormone responsiveness into S49 cyc- membranes. As emphasized by Harden (48), these techniques are not entirely quantitative, however, and the results cannot be considered conclusive. Furthermore, it is likely that the same mechanism of heterologous desensitization does not occur in all cell types. The reader is referred to recent reviews for a more detailed perspective on these issues.

IN VIVO ALTERATIONS OF RECEPTOR/ ADENYLATE CYCLASE SYSTEM

An area that has been relatively slow to develop has been that relating biochemical changes in the beta-receptor/adenylate cyclase system to physiologic and pathophysiologic states. In this last section we shall review data that suggest linkages between the two.

Developmental Changes

The sympathetic innervation of the newborn heart has been shown to be incomplete (38). Beta-adrenergic receptor density is increased in the newborn, possibly in response to a state of incomplete innervation, and then decreases with maturation (95,97). Increased adenylate cyclase responsiveness to isoproterenol is also observed, as compared with that in adult dogs, which suggests normal coupling of the receptor to cyclase. But when physiologic responsiveness in neonatal dogs is studied, a blunted response of left ventricular (LV) dP/dt to catecholamines is observed. In 6-week-old puppies, an intermediate inotropic response is seen (95). Changes in adenylate cyclase and organ responsiveness to catecholamine stimulation suggest that the pronounced increase in neonatal receptor density is a specific, adaptive change to a blunted effector mechanism in adrenergic modulation. The exact nature of the cellular impairment of the heart's response to catecholamines in immature animals remains speculative, but it is clearly distal to adenylate cyclase in the cellular activation sequence. This increase in receptor density in the neonatal heart is one mechanism whereby compensation for an inherent depression in adrenergic responsiveness can occur.

With aging, cardiac function is diminished because of decreased responsiveness to catecholamines (46). Using Wistar rats, Guarnieri and associates proposed that the reduced inotropic response to catecholamines in senescent tissue may involve impaired mobilization of calcium. In rat heart (64), a 50% increase in beta-receptor density was reported, but there were decreases in basal and isoproterenol-stimulated adenylate cyclase activity. That study also demonstrated an age-related defect in the cardiac beta-receptor/cyclase system. In senescent rats, a decrease in the rate of regeneration of beta receptors was shown (94). This was based on studies of senescent Sprague-Dawley rats using bromoacetyl alprenolol methane. This drug binds to and irreversibly blocks beta receptors. Paired with Scatchard analysis of

[³H]DHA binding in heart, lung, and brain, this group showed a marked reduction in receptor density that was not reversed until 1 month after treatment in aged rats, as compared with 10 days in younger rats. The recovery of binding was presumed to be due to synthesis of new beta receptors. Thus, at both ends of the spectrum of development, the neonatal and the senescent animal, one finds reduced responses to catecholamines and an increased beta-adrenergic receptor density. These studies indicate the importance of examining not only the beta-receptor/cyclase system but also biochemical machinery distal to it, as well as the physiologic responsiveness of the heart to catecholamines, in order to interpret the meaning of changes in beta-receptor density.

Altered Hormone States

Thyroid

Hyperthyroidism resembles a hyperadrenergic state, but catecholamine levels are not increased. Thus, the speculation has been made that thyroid hormone in some way regulates adrenergic receptors. The effects of an excess or lack of thyroid hormone availability on cardiac beta receptors have been well documented (26,27,63,77,119,120,131,132,144).

In hyperthyroid states produced by injections of l-thyroxine (T_4) or l-triiodothyronine (T_3), most studies have shown increases in cardiac beta-receptor density (26,27,61,77,119,132). This is associated with significant increases in maximal isoproterenol-responsive adenylate cyclase activity (27,61,132) and cellular cAMP accumulation (131). Interestingly, a parallel increase in the rate of development of contractile force in ventricular strips in response to isoproterenol has been reported (61). In these studies, receptor affinity was unchanged. However, Stiles and Lefkowitz (119) reported a significant increase in receptor density and a decrease in K_d for isoproterenol in hyperthyroid rats. This increase was probably due to a shift in the normal distribution of high- and low-affinity beta receptors for agonists to a pattern with predominantly high-affinity receptors.

In hypothyroid states, produced either by surgical ablation or by administration of propylthiouracil, beta-receptor numbers were consistently decreased by 30 to 40% (26,77,144), but there was no change in receptor affinity or in the number of high-affinity agonist binding sites. However, reduction in the maximal isoproterenol response in hypothyroid rats has been reported (27). Similarly, rat atria in hypothyroid hearts display reduced chronotropic and inotropic responses to isoproterenol (63), but contractility is restored on administration of thyroid hormone. Thus, studies in animals have supported the notion that thyroid hormone regulates adrenergic receptor function in the heart by altering receptor density as well as by changing the coupling efficiency of receptor to adenylate cyclase.

Pheochromocytoma.

Humans with pheochromocytoma are chronically exposed to elevated catecholamine levels and exhibit decreases in beta-receptor densities in leukocytes, as measured by ligand binding with [³H]DHA (45,67). Rats with transplanted pheochromocytomas have decreases in beta-receptor numbers in the heart, as measured by ligand binding with [¹²⁵I]CYP (106,111,142). Snavely et al. (111) also showed that the decline in beta-receptor number was specific for the beta-1 receptor, and there was no change in beta-receptor content in the lung (predominantly beta-2) in these animals. Furthermore, there was no change in beta-receptor affinity in animals with pheochromocytoma. These results indicate that rats with pheochromocytoma have beta-receptor subtype- and tissue-specific down-regulation. Pheochromocytoma is an example of down-regulation secondary to excess endogenous catecholamines. The down-regulation in this case can be thought of as a protective mechanism to dampen the cardiac response to excessive catecholamines.

Exogenous agonist administration.

The concept of down-regulation or desensitization by excess hormone is also supported by studies of leukocyte receptors in human subjects treated with terbutaline, an antiasthmatic agent that is somewhat specific for the beta-2 receptor. Galant et al. (39) and Tashkin et al. (129) showed that tissues in such subjects had markedly reduced numbers of beta receptors as compared with those of controls. Decreases in beta-receptor numbers have also been noted in cardiac tissue of laboratory animals that have been given chronic infusions of isoproterenol (78). Thus, exogenous as well as endogenous beta agonists can down-regulate the beta receptor.

Up-regulation of beta receptors may play a role in abnormalities of sympathetic cardiac regulation.

Apparent beta-adrenergic hypersensitivity is seen with chronic exposure to beta-receptor antagonists. Propranolol administration yields significant increases in beta-receptor densities in rat cerebral cortex and heart and human leukocytes (1,44). Acute withdrawal of chronic propranolol therapy from patients has precipitated a syndrome suggesting hypersensitivity. Aarons et al. (1) showed that beta-receptor density remained increased for several days after discontinuation of the drug, permitting a transient beta-receptor supersensitivity. Whether this syndrome is due to an actual increase in number of receptors or an altered responsiveness with the same number of receptors is unknown. An alternative explanation for the withdrawal syndrome is persistence of increased synaptic release of catecholamines. During propranolol therapy, one could postulate heightened afferent sympathetic nervous activity due to blocked end-organ receptors. Abrupt withdrawal might then produce a period of continued increased catecholamine release for a given stimulus, causing the hypersensitive state seen clinically.

Myocardial Ischemia

One hour of experimental myocardial ischemia in dogs has been shown to produce an increase in receptor density in ischemic tissue that is associated with marked decreases in tissue catecholamine levels (83). One interpretation is that up-regulation of the beta receptor is due to reduced innervation and lower myocardial catecholamine levels. The reduced innervation may result from ischemic insult to local sympathetic nerves. These investigators also examined a canine model with 1 hr of coronary artery occlusion followed by 15 min of reperfusion during which isoproterenol was infused. The receptor density, cAMP content, and conversion of phosphorylase b to a were increased in the previously ischemic portion of the heart as compared with nonischemic myocardium. This suggests that receptor up-regulation in response to ischemia translated into increased physiologic responsiveness to catecholamines (83,85). In a recent study, Maisel et al. (75) also observed increased receptor density in guinea pigs with left anterior descending coronary artery occlusion for 15 to 90 min. They demonstrated that after 30 min of occlusion, sarcolemma beta-receptor density increased by 45%. They also studied the intracellular pool of beta receptors that appears to be contained in small membrane-bound lipid vesicles within the myocardial cytosol. They were able to show that the increase in the number of sarcolemma receptors was concomitant with a decrease in the intracellular pool of beta receptors, suggesting that those in the intracellular pool were transferred to the sarcolemma. The study of beta-receptor changes in ischemia is incomplete. However, it is interesting to speculate that the increased beta-receptor density in the presence of acute myocardial ischemia contributes to arrhythmogenesis and sudden death.

Hypertension and Myocardial Hypertrophy

Most studies of alterations in beta receptors in hypertension have been conducted in rodents with renovascular hypertension (5,10,40,145) or in spontaneously hypertensive rat models (69,84). In these studies, beta-receptor numbers were either normal (40,69) or depressed

(5,10,145), with normal antagonist affinity. In rats with aortic banding, Limas (70) showed increased beta-receptor numbers, whereas Cervoni et al. (24) demonstrated no change. In addition, Kumano et al. (62) found increased beta-receptor density and no change in affinity in renal-hypertensive rats, but decreased receptor density in spontaneously hypertensive rats, again with no change in affinity.

In dogs with left ventricular hypertrophy secondary to aortic banding, physiologic responsiveness to catecholamines is essentially normal (33). In the left ventricle, beta-receptor density is increased, but antagonist affinity declines. The decrease in beta-receptor affinity in the presence of chronic pressure overload and resulting left ventricular hypertrophy may be responsible for offsetting the increases in receptor number, resulting in the "normal" inotropic responsiveness of the hypertrophied ventricle to catecholamines. It is important to note that increased beta-receptor density and reduced affinity were only observed in the left ventricle. The right ventricle, which served as an internal control, showed no derangements in receptor density or affinity. Similarly, there were no changes in the hemodynamic parameters of that chamber. Basal adenylate cyclase activity, Gpp(NH)p-stimulated activity, and EC_{50} for isoproterenol-stimulated adenylate cyclase were not altered. Plasma norepinephrine levels were similar to those in control animals, but myocardial norepinephrine levels were depressed in aortic-banding-induced LV hypertrophy (LVH).

In order to determine if these alterations in beta-receptor density and affinity were unique to the model of aortic-banding-induced LVH, dogs with LVH induced by chronic hypertension were studied (134). This model was different not only in the stimulus used to produce hypertrophy but also in that all manipulations and observations were made in adult hypertensive animals. Despite these differences, both models of LVH are characterized by nearly identical increases in beta-receptor density and reductions in affinity. These data suggest that pressure-overload hypertrophy in dogs, whether induced by mechanical obstruction or by systemic hypertension, results in similar increases in beta-receptor density and decreases in receptor affinity.

Congestive Heart Failure

Several disorders of autonomic cardiovascular control have been described in experimental animals and patients with heart failure (2,35,52). Prior studies examining beta-adrenergic receptor regulation in heart failure have reported divergent results. Karliner et al. (58) found increased beta-receptor numbers in a guinea pig heart-failure model, whereas Bristow et al. (13) found the reverse in end-stage heart failure in humans. A recent investigation in a chronic pressure-overload model of

heart failure in the dog indicates that several alterations in the beta-receptor/cyclase system occur (136).

In this last study, animals that had developed hypertrophy in response to aortic banding eventually developed left ventricular decompensation. Beta-receptor numbers increased, and decreased affinity for [^{3}H]DHA (antagonist) was observed in the decompensated state, similar to the hypertrophic state described earlier. Although the increases in receptor numbers could be a secondary response to depletion of local catecholamine stores, it is difficult to reconcile the persistent alterations in antagonist affinity. This phenomenon is not an artifact of the binding procedure employed, as evidenced by recent studies using identical biochemical techniques in canine hearts following chronic surgical denervation (135). In that model it was demonstrated that increases in receptor numbers of similar magnitudes occur without any alteration in affinity for [^{3}H]DHA. Taken together, these observations suggest that the receptor protein present in the left ventricle in animals with LV hypertrophy and LV failure may differ from that in normal animals. This may be similar to the expression of new gene products for a variety of myocardial proteins, including myosin (74), creatine phosphokinase (137), and lactate dehydrogenase (37,146), that occurs with the development of hypertrophy. Such a protein may have small differences in its primary amino acid structure, possibly occurring within an epitope of the ligand binding site itself. Alternatively, a posttranslation modification such as phosphorylation might be responsible for differences in antagonist affinity.

The canine model for heart failure also has changes in agonist binding that are distinct from those of antagonist binding. Previous work has demonstrated that the beta receptor can exist in two affinity states for agonist. It is the high-affinity form of the receptor that is functionally coupled to G_s, as noted in previous sections, and thus has been considered to be the physiologically relevant form of the receptor. To determine which form of the receptor exists in dogs with LV failure, agonist competition curves were generated in the presence and absence of Gpp(NH)p. In the absence of guanylyl nucleotides, the curve is more shallow and can be modeled to two sites, one of low and one of high affinity for isoproterenol. With the addition of Gpp(NH)p, all the receptors are converted into a low-affinity state, as seen in Fig. 3 (136). The curve shifts to the right, becomes steeper, and follows a typical mass-action relationship for a single site of low affinity. Computer modeling of these curves demonstrated major differences between normal and heart-failure animals. Experimental data indicate that in the absence of GTP, only 11% of the total receptor population is in a high-affinity or coupled state in heart-failure animals, as compared with 51% for normal animals, as seen in Fig. 9. Additional changes in the receptor/cyclase system have been noted. When

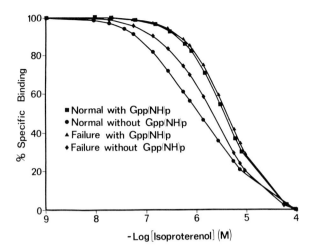

FIG. 9. Guanyl nucleotides binding shifts in cardiac membranes of dogs with heart failure and normal controls. Although the curves in the presence of guanyl nucleotides are superimposable, the curves without guanyl nucleotides are markedly different. See text for details.

adenylate cyclase is simulated with isoproterenol, a 50% reduction in maximum cyclase activity is observed. This reduction is also seen when cyclase is stimulated with fluoride or with Gpp(NH)p, which act via G_s and do not involve the beta receptor. Although changes in receptor number or affinity could explain the isoproterenol data, they cannot explain why receptor-independent cyclase stimulation is reduced.

A possible mechanism underlying the observed reduction in the fraction of high-affinity receptors in heart failure, as well as the reduction in receptor-independent stimulation of adenylate cyclase, is a deficiency or abnormality of G_s. These findings imply that G_s could be functionally deficient in the hearts of failure animals. There is precedent in other systems to suggest that alterations in G_s might play a significant role in the molecular pathophysiology of disease. Such an abnormality occurs in one form of pseudohypoparathyroidism in which decreased concentrations of high-affinity beta-receptor agonist binding sites in erythrocytes have been documented (51). This occurs in association with an apparent quantitative deficiency in the concentration of G_s. In certain other pathophysiologic states, such as hypothyroidism, or in adrenalectomized animals, similar findings of decreased fractions of high-affinity agonist binding sites (31,120) have been noted. Although data on agonist binding shifts and Gpp(NH)p- or fluoride-stimulated adenylate cyclase provide indirect evidence for abnormalities in G_s as playing a role in myocardial failure, more direct evidence will be necessary to strengthen this hypothesis.

In summary, simple demonstration of alterations in cellular receptor content should not necessarily lead one to the conclusion that these represent the primary event responsible for the observed physiologic phenomena.

The value of ligand binding assays in delineating the role of alterations in receptor concentrations on physiologic functions depends on several critical factors. Certain criteria should be met before a causal relationship can be considered to exist. First, demonstration in the same animal model that the observed physiologic effect is associated with an alteration in receptor activity, as determined by binding assays in tissue obtained from these animals, will provide a stronger argument for causal relationships. Second, the experimental design must ensure that a change in receptor concentration is not an artifact of the tissue preparation, particularly when impure plasma membranes are employed as a source of receptors. Determination that the concentrations of other unrelated membrane-bound proteins do not vary in a manner directionally similar to the receptor concentration will be a reasonable control. Third, distal effector mechanisms, e.g., adenylate cyclase activity, would be expected to vary in their responsiveness to hormone concentration in association with changes in receptor number or affinity if the latter processes are biochemically relevant. For example, during ontogeny, the immature heart can be shown to be poorly responsive to inotropic effects of catecholamines. However, receptor concentrations in these animals are actually severalfold greater than in the adult, and, as expected, adenylate cyclase responsiveness is enhanced. The defect in the neonates apparently lies distal to cAMP generation, possibly in a phosphorylation step mediated by a cAMP-dependent kinase. The criteria listed herein are offered to assist the reader in critically evaluating any experimental protocol that suggests that an alteration in receptor number or affinity is the primary event leading to a pathophysiologic state.

REFERENCES

1. Aarons, R., Nies, A., Gal, J., and Hagstrand, L. (1980): Elevation of beta adrenergic receptor density in human lymphocytes after propranolol administration. *J. Clin. Invest.*, 65:949–957.
2. Abboud, F. M., Fozzard, H. A., Gilmore, J. P., and Reis, D. J. (editors) (1981): *Disturbances in Neurogenic Control of the Circulation.* Williams & Wilkins, Baltimore.
3. Ablad, B., Carlsson, B., Carlsson, E., Dahlof, C., Ek, L., and Hultberg, E. (1974): Cardiac effects of beta-adrenergic receptor antagonists. *Adv. Cardiol.*, 12:290–302.
4. Ahlquist, R. P. (1948): Study of adrenotropic receptors. *Am. J. Physiol.*, 153:586–600.
5. Ayobe, M. H., and Tarazi, R. C. (1983): Beta-receptors and contractile reserve in left ventricular hypertrophy. *Hypertension*, 5:192–197.
6. Benovic, J. L., Pike, L. J., Cerione, R. A., et al. (1985): Phosphorylation of the mammalian beta-adrenergic receptor by cyclic AMP-dependent protein kinase: Regulation of the rate of receptor phosphorylation and dephosphorylation by agonist occupancy and effects on coupling of the receptor to the stimulatory guanine nucleotide regulatory protein. *J. Biol. Chem.*, 260:7094–7101.
7. Benovic, J. L., Shorr, R. G. L., Lefkowitz, R. J., and Caron, M. G. (1984): Mammalian beta-2 adrenergic receptor: Purification and characterization. *Biochemistry*, 23:4510–4518.
8. Benovic, J. L., Stiles, G. L., and Lefkowitz, R. J. (1983): Photoaffinity labelling of mammalian beta-adrenergic receptors:

Metal-dependent proteolysis explains apparent heterogeneity. *Biochem. Biophys. Res. Commun.,* 110:504–511.

9. Berridge, M. J. (1983): Rapid accumulation of inositol trisphosphate reveals that agonists hydrolyse polyphosphoinositides instead of phosphatidylinositol. *Biochem. J.,* 212:849–858.

10. Bobik, A., and Korner, P. (1981): Cardiac beta adrenoceptors and adenylate cyclase in normotensive and renal hypertensive rabbits during changes in autonomic activity. *Clin. Exp. Hypertens.,* 3:257–280.

11. Bourne, H. R., Coffino, P., and Tomkins, G. M. (1975): Selection of a variant lymphoma cell deficient in adenylate cyclase. *Science,* 187:750–752.

12. Braun, S., and Levitzki, A. (1979): The attenuation of epinephrine dependent adenylate cyclase. *Mol. Pharmacol.,* 16:737–748.

13. Bristow, M. R., Ginsburg, R., Minobe, W., Cubicciotti, R. S., Sageman, W. S., Lurie, K., Billingham, M. E., Harrison, D. C., and Stinson, E. B. (1982): Decreased catecholamine sensitivity and beta-adrenergic-receptor density in failing human hearts. *N. Engl. J. Med.,* 307:205–211.

14. Brodde, O. E., Leifet, F. J., and Krehl, H. J. (1982): Coexistence of beta-1 and beta-2 adrenoceptors in the rabbit heart: Quantitative analysis of the regional distribution by (−)[³H]dihydroalprenolol binding. *J. Cardiovasc. Pharmacol.,* 4:34–43.

15. Buxton, I. O., and Brunton, L. L. (1985): Direct analysis of beta-adrenergic receptor subtypes on intact adult ventricular myocytes of the rat. *Circ. Res.,* 56:126–132.

16. Cannon, W. B., and Rosenthal, A. (1973): *Autonomic Neuroeffector Systems.* Macmillan, New York.

17. Carlsson, E., Ablad, B., Brandstrom, A., and Carlsson, B. (1972): Differentiated blockade of the chronotropic effects of various adrenergic stimuli in the cat heart. *Life Sci.,* 11:953–958.

18. Carlsson, E., Dahlof, C., Hedberg, A., Person, H., and Tangstrand, B. (1977): Differentiation of cardiac chronotropic and inotropic effects of beta-adrenoceptor agonist. *Naunyn Schmiedebergs Arch. Pharmacol.,* 300:101–105.

19. Caron, M. G., and Lefkowitz, R. J. (1976): Solubilization and characterization of the beta-adrenergic receptor binding site of frog erythrocytes. *J. Biol. Chem.,* 251:2374–2384.

20. Caron, M. G., Srinivasan, Y., Pitha, J., Kociolek, K., and Lefkowitz, R. J. (1979): Affinity chromatography of the beta-adrenergic receptor. *J. Biol. Chem.,* 254:2923–2927.

21. Cassel, D., and Pfeuffer, T. (1978): Mechanism of cholera toxin action: Covalent modification of the guanyl nucleotide binding protein of the adenylate cyclase system. *Proc. Natl. Acad. Sci. (USA),* 75:2669–2673.

22. Cerione, R. A., Codina, J., Benovic, J. L., Lefkowitz, R. J., Birnbaumer, L., and Caron, M. G. (1984): The mammalian beta-2 receptor: Reconstitution of functional interactions between pure receptor and pure stimulatory nucleotide binding protein of the adenylate cyclase system. *Biochemistry,* 23:4519–4525.

23. Cerione, R. A., Strulovici, B., Benovic, J. L., Lefkowitz, R. J., and Caron, M. G. (1983): Pure beta-adrenergic receptor: The single polypeptide confers catecholamine responsiveness to adenylate cyclase. *Nature,* 306:562–566.

24. Cervoni, P., Herzlinger, H., Lai, F. M., and Tanikella, T. (1981): A comparison of cardiac reactivity and beta-adrenoceptor number and affinity between aorta-coarcted hypertensive and normotensive rats. *Br. J. Pharmacol.,* 74:517–523.

25. Chuang, D. M., and Costa, E. (1979): Evidence for internalization of the recognition site of beta-adrenergic receptors during receptor subsensitivity induced by (−)isoproterenol. *Proc. Natl. Acad. Sci. (USA),* 76:3024–3028.

26. Ciaraldi, T., and Marinett, G. V. (1977): Thyroxine and propylthiouracil effects in vivo on alpha and beta adrenergic receptors in rat heart. *Biochem. Biophys. Res. Commun.,* 74:984–991.

27. Ciaraldi, T. P., and Marinett, G. V. (1978): Hormone action at the membrane level. VIII. Adrenergic receptors in rat heart and adipocytes and their modulation by thyroxine. *Biochim. Biophys. Acta,* 54:334–346.

28. Clarke, S. (1975): The size and detergent binding of membrane proteins. *J. Biol. Chem.,* 250:5459–5469.

29. Codina, J., Rosenthal, W., Hildebrandt, J. D., Birnbaumer, L., and Sekura, R. D. (1985): Purification of Ns and Ni, the coupling proteins of hormone-sensitive adenylyl cyclases without interven-

tion of activation regulatory ligands. *Methods Enzymol.,* 109:446–465.

30. Cubero, A., and Malbon, C. C. (1984): The fat cell beta-adrenergic receptor: Purification and characterization of a mammalian beta-1 adrenergic receptor. *J. Biol. Chem.,* 259:1344–1351.

31. Davies, A. O., DeLean, A., and Lefkowitz, R. J. (1981): Myocardial beta-adrenergic receptors from adrenalectomized rats: Impaired formation of high affinity agonist-receptor complexes. *Endocrinology,* 108:720–722.

32. Dickinson, K. E. J., and Nahorski, S. R. (1981): Identification of solubilized beta-1 and beta-2 adrenoceptors in mammalian lung. *Life Sci.,* 29:2527–2533.

33. Dickinson, K., Richardson, A., and Nahorski, S. R. (1981): Homogeneity of beta-2 adrenoceptors on rat erythrocytes and reticulocytes: A comparison with heterogeneous rat lung beta-adrenoceptors. *Mol. Pharmacol.,* 19:194–204.

34. Doss, R. C., Harden, T. K., and Perkins, J. P. (1982): Role of protein glycosylation in the synthetic processing of beta-adrenergic receptors. *Fed. Proc.,* 41:1534.

35. Eckberg, D. L., Drabinsky, M., and Braunwald, E. (1971): Defective cardiac parasympathetic control in patients with heart disease. *N. Engl. J. Med.,* 285:877–883.

36. Engle, G., Hoyer, D., Berthold, R., and Wagner, H. (1981): (+)[¹²⁵I]cyanopindolol, a new ligand for beta-adrenoceptors: Identification and quantitation of subclasses of beta-adrenoceptors in guinea pig. *Naunyn Schmiedebergs Arch. Pharmacol.,* 317:277–285.

37. Fox, A. C., and Reed, G. E. (1969): Changes in lactate dehydrogenase composition of hearts with right ventricular hypertrophy. *Am. J. Physiol.,* 216:1026–1033.

38. Friedman, W. F., Pool, P. E., Jacobowitz, D., Segren, S. F., and Braunwald, E. (1968): Sympathetic innervation of the developing rabbit heart; biochemical and histochemical comparisons of fetal, neonatal, and adult myocardium. *Circ. Res.,* 23:25–32.

39. Galant, S. P., Duriseti, L., Underwood, S., and Insel, P. A. (1978): Decreased beta-adrenergic receptors on polymorphonuclear leukocytes after adrenergic therapy. *N. Engl. J. Med.,* 299:933–936.

40. Giachetti, A., Clark, T. L., and Berti, F. (1982): Subsensitivity of cardiac beta-adrenoceptors in renal hypertensive rats. *J. Cardiovasc. Pharmacol.,* 1:467–471.

41. Gill, D. M., and Meren, R. (1978): ADP-ribosylation of membrane proteins catalyzed by cholera toxin: Basis of the activation of adenylate cyclase. *Proc. Natl. Acad. Sci. (USA),* 75:3050–3054.

42. Gilman, A. G. (1984): Guanine nucleotide-binding regulatory proteins and dual control of adenylate cyclase. *J. Clin. Invest.,* 73:1–4.

43. Glaubiger, S., and Lefkowitz, R. (1977): Elevated beta-adrenergic receptor number after chronic propranolol treatment. *Biochem. Biophys. Res. Commun.,* 78:720–725.

44. Graziano, M. P., Moxham, C. P., and Malbon, C. C. (1985): Purified rat hepatic beta adrenergic receptor. *J. Biol. Chem.,* 260:7665–7674.

45. Greenacre, J. K., and Connolly, M. E. (1978): Desensitization of the beta-adrenoceptor of lymphocytes from normal subjects and patients with pheochromocytoma. *Br. J. Clin. Pharmacol.,* 5:191.

46. Guarnieri, T., Filburn, C. R., Zitnik, G., Roth, G. S., and Lakatta, E. G. (1980): Contractile and biochemical correlates of beta-adrenergic stimulation of the aged heart. *Am. J. Physiol.,* 239:H501–H508.

47. Hancock, A. A., DeLean, A. L., and Lefkowitz, R. J. (1980): Quantitative resolution of beta-adrenergic subtypes by selective ligand binding: Application of a computerized model fitting technique. *Mol. Pharmacol.,* 16:1–9.

48. Harden, T. K. (1983): Agonist-induced desensitization of the beta-adrenergic receptor-linked adenylate cyclase. *Pharmacol. Rev.,* 35:5–32.

49. Hedberg, A., Minneman, K. P., and Molinoff, P. B. (1980): Differential distribution of beta-1 and beta-2 adrenergic receptors in cat and guinea pig heart. *J. Pharmacol. Exp. Ther.,* 212:503–508.

50. Heidenreich, K. H., Weiland, G. A., and Molinoff, P. B. (1982): Effects of magnesium and N-ethyl maleimide on the binding of

[³H]hydroxybenzyl isoproterenol to beta adrenergic receptor. *J. Biol. Chem.*, 257:804.

51. Heinsimer, J. A., Davies, A. O., Downs, R. W., Levine, M. A., Spiegel, A. M., Drezner, M. K., DeLean, A., Wreggett, K. A., Caron, M. G., and Lefkowitz, R. J. (1984): Impaired formation of beta-adrenergic receptor–nucleotide regulatory protein complexes in pseudohypoparathyroidism. *J. Clin. Invest.*, 73:1335–1343.

52. Higgins, C. B., Vatner, S. F., Eckberg, D. L., and Braunwald, E. (1972): Alterations in the baroreceptor reflex in conscious dogs with heart failure. *J. Clin. Invest.*, 51:715–724.

53. Homcy, C. J., and Graham, R. M. (1985): Molecular characterization of adrenergic receptors. *Circ. Res.*, 56:636–650.

54. Homcy, C. J., Rockson, S. G., Countaway, J., and Egan, D. (1983): Purification and characterization of the mammalian beta-2 adrenergic receptor. *Biochemistry*, 22:660–668.

55. Hoyer, D., Reynolds, E. E., and Molinoff, P. B. (1984): Agonist-induced changes in the properties of beta-adrenergic receptors on intact S49 lymphoma cells: Time dependent changes in the affinity of the receptor for agonist. *Mol. Pharmacol.*, 25:209–218.

56. Insel, P. A., Mahan, L. C., Motulsky, H. J., Stoolman, L. M., and Koachman, A. M. (1983): Time-dependent decreases in binding affinity of agonists for beta-adrenergic receptors of intact S49 lymphoma cells: A mechanism of desensitization. *J. Biol. Chem.*, 258:13597–13605.

57. Joseph, S. K., Thomas, A. P., Williams, R. J., Irvine, R. F., and Williamson, J. R. (1984): Myoinositol-1,4,5-trisphosphate: A second messenger for the hormonal mobilization of intracellular Ca(2+) in liver. *J. Biol. Chem.*, 259:3077–3081.

58. Karliner, J. S., Barnes, P., Brown, M., and Dollery, C. (1980): Chronic heart failure in the guinea pig increases cardiac alpha- and beta-adrenoceptors. *Eur. J. Pharmacol.*, 67:115–118.

59. Kassis, S., and Fishman, P. H. (1982): Different mechanisms of desensitization of adenylate cyclase by isoproterenol and prostaglandin E₄ in human fibroblasts: Role of regulatory components in desensitization. *J. Biol. Chem.*, 257:5312–5318.

60. Kelleher, D. J., Pessin, J. E., Ruoho, A. E., and Johnson, G. L. (1984): Phorbol ester induces desensitization of the beta-adrenergic receptor in turkey erythrocytes. *Proc. Natl. Acad. Sci. (USA)*, 81:4316–4320.

61. Krawietz, W., Werdan, K., and Erdmann, E. (1982): Effect of thyroid status on beta-adrenergic receptor, adenylate cyclase activity and guanine nucleotide regulatory unit in rat cardiac and erythrocyte membranes. *Biochem. Pharmacol.*, 31:2463.

62. Kumano, K., Upsher, M. E., and Khairallah, P. A. (1983): Beta adrenergic receptor response coupling in hypertrophied hearts. *Hypertension*, 5:175–183.

63. Kunos, G., Mucci, L., and O'Regan, S. (1980): The influence of hormonal and neuronal factors on rat heart adrenoceptors. *Br. J. Pharmacol.*, 71:371.

64. Kusiak, J. W., and Pitha, J. (1983): Decreased response with age of the cardiac cathecolamine sensitive adenylate cyclase system. *Life Sci.*, 33:1679–1686.

65. Langley, J. N. (1878): On the physiology of the salivary secretion. II. On the mutual antagonism of atropin and pilocarpin having a special reference to their relations in the sub-maxillary gland of the cat. *J. Physiol. (Lond.)*, 1:339–369.

66. Lefkowitz, R. J., and Caron, M. G. (1985): Adrenergic receptors: Molecular mechanisms of clinically relevant regulation. *Clin. Res.*, 33:395–406.

67. Lefkowitz, R. J., Wessels, M. R., and Stadel, J. M. (1980): Hormone receptors and cyclic AMP: Their role in target cell refractoriness. *Curr. Top. Cell. Regul.*, 17:205.

68. Levitzki, A. (1985): Reconstitution of membrane receptor systems. *Biochim. Biophys. Acta*, 892:127–153.

69. Limas, C. J. (1979): Increased number of beta-adrenergic receptors in the myocardium of spontaneously hypertensive rats. *Biochem. Biophys. Res. Commun.*, 83:710–714.

70. Limas, C., and Limas, C. J. (1978): Reduced number of beta-adrenergic receptors in the myocardium of spontaneously hypertensive rats. *Biochem. Biophys. Res. Commun.*, 83:710–714.

71. Limbird, L. E., Gill, D. M., and Lefkowitz, R. J. (1980): Agonist-promoted coupling of the beta-adrenergic receptor with the guanine nucleotide regulatory protein of adenylate cyclase system. *Proc. Natl. Acad. Sci. (USA)*, 77:775–779.

72. Limbird, L. E., and Lefkowitz, R. J. (1977): Resolution of beta-adrenergic receptor binding and adenylate cyclase activity by gel exclusion chromatography. *J. Biol. Chem.*, 252:799–802.

73. Linden, J., Patel, A., Spanier, A. M., and Weglicki, W. B. (1984): Rapid agonist-induced decrease of ¹²⁵I-pindolol binding to beta-adrenergic receptors relationship to desensitization of cyclic AMP accumulation in intact heart cells. *J. Biol. Chem.*, 259:15115–15122.

74. Lompre, A., Schwartz, D., D'Albis, A., Lacombe, G., Van Thien, N., and Swynghedauw, B. (1979): Myosin isoenzyme redistribution in chronic heart overload. *Nature*, 282:105–107.

75. Maisel, A. S., Motulsky, H. J., and Insel, P. A. (1985): Externalization of beta-adrenergic receptors promoted by myocardial ischemia. *Science*, 230:183–186.

76. Manalan, A. S., Besch, H. R., and Watanabe, A. M. (1981): Characterization of [³H](±)carazolol binding to beta-adrenergic receptors, application to study of beta-adrenergic receptor subtypes in canine ventricular myocardium and lung. *Circ. Res.*, 49:326–336.

77. McConnaughey, M. M., Jones, L. R., Watanabe, A. M., Besch, H. R., Jr., Williams, L. T., and Lefkowitz, R. J. (1979): Thyroxine and propylthiouracil effects on alpha- and beta-adrenergic receptor number, ATPase activities, and sialic acid content of rat cardiac membrane vesicles. *J. Cardiovasc. Pharmacol.*, 1:609–623.

78. Mickey, J., Tate, R., and Lefkowitz, R. J. (1975): Subsensitivity of adenylate cyclase and decreased beta-adrenergic receptor binding after chronic exposure to (−)-isoproterenol in vitro. *J. Biol. Chem.*, 250:5727–5729.

79. Minneman, K. P., Hegstrand, L. R., and Molinoff, P. B. (1979): Simultaneous determination of beta-1 and beta-2 adrenergic receptors in tissues containing both receptor subtypes. *Mol. Pharmacol.*, 16:34–46.

80. Moss, J., Jacobson, M. K., and Stanley, S. J. (1985): Reversibility of arginine specific mono(ADP-ribosyl)ation: Identification in erythrocytes of an ADP-ribose-L-arginine cleavage enzyme. *Proc. Natl. Acad. Sci. (USA)*, 82:5603–5607.

81. Moss, J., Stanley, S. J., and Oppenheimer, N. J. (1979): Substrate specificity and partial purification of stereospecific NAD- and guanidine-dependent ADP ribosyltransferase from avian erythrocytes. *J. Biol. Chem.*, 254:8891–8894.

82. Motulsky, H. J., and Insel, P. A. (1982): Adrenergic receptors in man. Direct identification, physiological regulation, and clinical alterations. *N. Engl. J. Med.*, 307:18.

83. Mukherjee, A., Bush, L. R., McCoy, K. E., Duke, R. J., Hagler, H., Buja, L. M., and Willerson, J. T. (1982): Relationship between beta-adrenergic receptor numbers and physiological responses during experimental canine myocardial ischemia. *Circ. Res.*, 50:735–741.

84. Mukherjee, A., Graham, R. M., Sagalowsky, A. I., Pettinger, W., and McCoy, K. E. (1980): Myocardial beta-adrenergic receptors in the stroke-prone spontaneously hypertensive rat. *J. Mol. Cell. Cardiol.*, 12:1263–1272.

85. Mukherjee, A., Wong, T. M., Buja, L. M., Lefkowitz, R. J., and Willerson, J. T. (1979): Beta adrenergic and muscarinic cholinergic receptors in canine myocardium. *J. Clin. Invest.*, 64:1423–1428.

86. Muntz, K. H., Olson, E. G., Larriviere, G. R., D'Souza, S., Mukherjee, A., Willerson, J. T., and Buja, L. M. (1984): Autoradiographic characterization of beta-adrenergic receptors in coronary blood vessels and myocytes in normal and ischemic myocardium of the canine heart. *J. Clin. Invest.*, 73:349–357.

87. Nishizuka, Y. (1984): The role of protein kinase C in cell surface signal transduction and tumour promotion. *Nature*, 308:693–698.

88. Northup, J. K., Sternweis, P. C., Smigel, M. D., Schleifer, L. S., Ross, E. M., and Gilman, A. G. (1980): Purification of the regulatory component of adenylate cyclase. *Proc. Natl. Acad. Sci. (USA)*, 77:6516–6520.

89. Olivier, P. C., Diroei-Trautmann, O., Delavier-Klutchko, C., and Strosberg, A. D. (1985): The oligosaccharide moiety of the beta-1 adrenergic receptor from turkey erythrocytes has a biantennary, N-acetyllactosamine-containing structure. *Biochemistry*, 24:3765–3770.

90. Orley, J., and Schramm, M. (1976): Coupling of catecholamine receptor from one cell with adenylate cyclase from another cell by cell fusion. *Proc. Natl. Acad. Sci. (USA)*, 73:4410–4417.

91. Pederson, S. E., and Ross, E. M. (1982): Functional reconstitution of beta-adrenergic receptors and the stimulatory GTP-binding protein of adenylate cyclase. *Proc. Natl. Acad. Sci. (USA)*, 79:7228–7232.

92. Pfeuffer, T. (1977): GTP binding proteins in membranes and the control of adenylate cyclase activity. *J. Biol. Chem.*, 252:7224–7234.

93. Pfeuffer, E., Dreher, R. M., Metzger, H., and Pfeuffer, T. (1985): Catalytic unit of adenylate cyclase: Purification and identification by affinity crosslinking. *Proc. Natl. Acad. Sci. (USA)*, 82:3086–3090.

94. Pitha, J., Hughes, B. A., Kusiak, J. W., Dax, E. M., and Baker, S. P. (1982): Regeneration of beta-adrenergic receptors in senescent rats: A study using an irreversible binding antagonist. *Proc. Natl. Acad. Sci. (USA)*, 79:4424–4427.

95. Rockson, S. G., Homcy, C. J., Quinn, P., Manders, W. T., Haber, E., and Vatner, S. F. (1981): Cellular mechanisms of impaired adrenergic responsiveness in neonatal dogs. *J. Clin. Invest.*, 67:319–327.

96. Rodbell, M., Krnas, H. M., Pohl, S. L., and Birnbaumer, L. (1971): The glucagon sensitive adenyl cyclase system in plasma membranes of rat liver. *J. Biol. Chem.*, 246:1872–1876.

97. Roeske, W. R., and Wildenthal, K. (1981): Responsiveness to drug and hormones in the murine model of cardiac ontogenesis. *Pharmacol. Ther.*, 14:55–66.

98. Ross, E. M. (1981): Physical separation of the catalytic and regulatory proteins of hepatic adenylate cyclase. *J. Biol. Chem.*, 256:1949–1953.

99. Ross, E. M., and Gilman, A. G. (1977): Reconstitution of catecholamine-sensitive adenylate cyclase activity: Interactions of solubilized components with receptor-replete membranes. *Proc. Natl. Acad. Sci. (USA)*, 74:3715–3719.

100. Ross, E. M., and Gilman, A. G. (1980): Biochemical properties of hormone sensitive adenylate cyclase. *Annu. Rev. Biochem.*, 49:533–564.

101. Rugg, E. L., Barnett, D. B., and Nahorski, S. R. (1978): Coexistence of beta-1 and beta-2 adrenoceptors in mammalian lung: Evidence from direct binding studies. *Mol. Pharmacol.*, 14:996–1005.

102. Schlegel, W., Kempner, E., and Rodbell, M. (1979): Activation of adenylate cyclase in hepatic membranes involves interactions of the catalytic unit with multimeric complexes of regulatory proteins. *J. Biol. Chem.*, 254:5168–5176.

103. Schramm, M. (1976): Blocking of catecholamine activation of adenylate cyclase by N,N'-dicyclohexyl carbodiimide in turkey erythrocytes. *J. Cyclic Nucleotide Res.*, 2:347–358.

104. Schramm, M., and Naim, E. (1970): Adenyl cyclase of rat parotid gland. *J. Biol. Chem.*, 245:3225–3231.

105. Schramm, M., and Selinger, Z. (1984): Message transmission: Receptor controlled adenylate cyclase system. *Science*, 225:1350–1356.

106. Shenkman, L., Saito, M., Feh, F., and Goldstein, M. (1979): Reduced number of cardiac beta-adrenergic receptors in rat pheochromocytoma. *Clin. Res.*, 27:595A (abstract).

107. Shorr, R. G. L., Lefkowitz, R. J., and Caron, M. G. (1981): Purification of the beta-adrenergic receptor: Identification of the hormone binding subunit. *J. Biol. Chem.*, 256:5820–5826.

108. Shorr, R. G. L., Strohsacker, M. W., Lavin, T. N., Lefkowitz, R. J., and Caron, M. G. (1982): The beta₁-adrenergic receptor of the turkey erythrocyte: Molecular heterogeneity revealed by purification and photoaffinity labelling. *J. Biol. Chem.*, 257:12341–12350.

109. Sibley, D. R., Nambi, P., Peters, J. R., and Lefkowitz, R. J. (1984): Phorbol esters promote beta-adrenergic receptor phosphorylation and adenylate cyclase desensitization in duck erythrocytes. *Biochem. Biophys. Res. Commun.*, 121:973–979.

110. Sibley, D. R., Strasser, R. H., Caron, M. G., and Lefkowitz, R. J. (1985): Homologous desensitization of adenylate cyclase is associated with phosphorylation of the beta-adrenergic receptor. *J. Biol. Chem.*, 260:3883–3886.

111. Snavely, M. D., Mahan, L. C., O'Connor, D. T., and Insel, P. A. (1983): Selective down-regulation of adrenergic receptor subtypes in tissues from rats with pheochromocytoma. *Endocrinology*, 113:354–361.

112. Stadel, J. M., DeLean, A., Mullikin-Kilpatrick, D. D., Sawyer, D. O., and Lefkowitz, R. J. (1981): Catecholamine-induced desensitization in turkey erythrocytes: cAMP-mediated impairment of high affinity agonist binding alteration in receptor number. *J. Cyclic Nucleotide Res.*, 7:37–47.

113. Stadel, J. M., Shorr, R. G. L., Limbird, L. E., and Lefkowitz, R. J. (1981): Evidence that a beta-adrenergic receptor-associated guanine nucleotide regulatory protein conveys guanosine 5'-O-(3-thiotriphosphate)-dependent adenylate cyclase activity. *J. Biol. Chem.*, 256:8718–8723.

114. Stadel, J. M., Nambi, P., Shorr, R. G. L., Sawyer, D. F., Caron, M. G., and Lefkowitz, R. J. (1983): Catecholamine-induced desensitization of turkey erythrocyte adenylate cyclase is associated with phosphorylation of the beta-adrenergic receptor. *Proc. Natl. Acad. Sci. (USA)*, 80:3173–3177.

115. Starling, E. H. (1905): The chemical correlation of the functions of the body. *Lancet*, 2:339–341.

116. Steele, J. C. H., Tanford, C., and Reynolds, A. J. (1978): Determination of partial specific volumes for lipid associated problems. *Methods Enzymol.*, 48:11–29.

117. Sternweis, P. C., and Gilman, A. G. (1979): Reconstitution of catecholamine-sensitive adenylate cyclase: Reconstitution of the uncoupled variant of the S40 lymphoma cell. *J. Biol. Chem.*, 254:3333–3340.

118. Stiles, G. L., Benovic, J. L., Caron, M. G., and Lefkowitz, R. J. (1984): Mammalian beta-adrenergic receptors: Distinct glycoprotein populations containing high mannose or complex type carbohydrate chains. *J. Biol. Chem.*, 259:8655–8663.

119. Stiles, G. L., and Lefkowitz, R. J. (1981): Thyroid hormone modulation of agonist–beta-adrenergic receptor interactions in the rat heart. *Life Sci.*, 28:2529–2536.

120. Stiles, G. L., Stadel, J. M., DeLean, A., and Lefkowitz, R. J. (1981): Hypothyroidism modulates beta adrenergic receptor-adenylate cyclase interactions in rat reticulocytes. *J. Clin. Invest.*, 68:1450–1455.

121. Stiles, G. L., Strasser, R. H., Caron, M. G., and Lefkowitz, R. J. (1983): Mammalian beta-adrenergic receptors: Structural differences in beta-1 and beta-2 subtypes revealed by peptide map. *J. Biol. Chem.*, 258:10689–10694.

122. Stiles, G. L., Strasser, R. H., Lavin, T. N., Jones, L. R., Caron, M. G., and Lefkowitz, R. J. (1983): The cardiac beta-adrenergic receptor: Structural similarities of beta-1 and beta-2 receptor subtypes demonstrated by photoaffinity labelling. *J. Biol. Chem.*, 258:8443–8449.

123. Stiles, G. L., Taylor, S., and Lefkowitz, R. J. (1983): Human cardiac beta-adrenergic receptors: Subtype heterogeneity delineated by direct radioligand binding. *Life Sci.*, 33:467–473.

124. Strader, C. D., Sibley, D. R., and Lefkowitz, R. J. (1984): Association of sequestered beta-adrenergic receptors with the plasma membrane: A novel mechanism for receptor down regulation. *Life Sci.*, 35:1601–1610.

125. Streb, H., Irvine, R. F., Berridge, M. J., and Schulz, I. (1983): Release of Ca(2-) from a nonmitochondrial intracellular store in pancreatic acinar cells by inositol-1,4,5-trisphosphate. *Nature*, 306:67–69.

126. Strittmatter, S., and Neer, E. J. (1980): Properties of the separated catalytic and regulatory units of brain adenylate cyclase. *Proc. Natl. Acad. Sci. (USA)*, 77:6344–6348.

127. Strulovici, B., Cerione, R. A., Kilpatrick, B. F., et al. (1984): Direct demonstration of impaired functionality of a purified desensitized beta-adrenergic receptor in a reconstituted system. *Science*, 225:837–840.

128. Sutherland, E. W. (1972): Studies on the mechanism of hormone action. *Science*, 177:401–408.

129. Tashkin, D. P., Conolly, M. E., Deutsch, R. I., et al. (1982): Subsensitization of beta-adrenoceptors in airways and lymphocytes of healthy and asthmatic subjects. *Am. Rev. Respir. Dis.*, 125:185–193.

130. Toews, M. L., Waldo, G. L., Harden, T. K., and Perkins, J. P. (1984): Relationship between an altered membrane form and a low affinity form of the beta-adrenergic receptor occurring during

catecholamine-induced desensitization. *J. Biol. Chem.*, 259:11844–11850.

131. Tsai, J. S., and Chen, A. (1978): Effect of L-triiodothyroxine on (−)[³H]dihydroalprenolol binding and cyclic-AMP response to (−)adrenaline in cultured heart cells. *Nature*, 275:138.

132. Tse, J., Wrenn, R. W., and Kuo, J. F. (1980): Thyroxine induced changes in characteristics and activities of beta-adrenergic receptors and adenosine 3′5′-monophosphate and guanosine 3′5′-monophosphate systems in the heart may be related to reported catecholamine supersensitivity in hyperthyroidism. *Endocrinology*, 107:6.

133. Vatner, D. E., Homcy, C. J., Sit, S. P., and Vatner, S. F. (1984): Effects of pressure overload, left ventricular hypertrophy on beta-adrenergic receptors and responsiveness to catecholamines. *J. Clin. Invest.*, 73:1473–1482.

134. Vatner, D. E., Kirby, D. A., Homcy, C. J., and Vatner, S. F. (1985): Beta adrenergic and cholinergic receptors in hypertension induced hypertrophy. *Hypertension*, 7:155–160.

135. Vatner, D. E., Lavallee, M., Amon, J., Finizola, A., Homcy, C. J., and Vatner, S. F. (1985): Mechanisms of supersensitivity to sympathomimetic amines in the chronically denervated heart of the conscious dog. *Circ. Res.*, 57:55–64.

136. Vatner, D. E., Vatner, S. F., Fujii, A. M., and Homcy, C. J. (1985): Loss of high affinity cardiac beta-adrenergic receptors in dogs with heart failure. *J. Clin. Invest.*, 76:2259–2264.

137. Vatner, D. E., Vatner, S. F., Sit, S. P., and Ingwall, J. S. (1982): Alteration of creatine kinase and its isozymes in response to pressure overload. *Physiologist*, 25:191.

138. Vauquelin, S., Bottari, C., Andre, B., Jacobson, D., and Strosberg, D. A. (1980): Interaction between beta-adrenergic receptors and

quanine nucleotide sites in turkey erythrocyte membranes. *Proc. Natl. Acad. Sci. (USA)*, 77:3801.

139. Vauquelin, G., Bottari, S., Kanarek, L., and Strosberg, A. D. (1979): Evidence for essential disulfide bonds in beta-1-adrenergic receptors of turkey erythrocyte membranes. *J. Biol. Chem.*, 254:4462–4467.

140. Vauquelin, G., Geynet, P., Hanoune, J., and Strosberg, A. D. (1977): Isolation of adenylate cyclase free beta-adrenergic receptors from turkey erythrocyte membranes by affinity chromatography. *Proc. Natl. Acad. Sci. (USA)*, 74:3710–3714.

141. Venter, J. C. (1979): High efficiency coupling between beta-adrenergic receptors and cardiac contractility: Direct evidence for "spare" beta-adrenergic receptors. *Mol. Pharmacol.*, 16:429–440.

142. Vlachakis, N. D., Kogusov, E., Ransom, F., Woodcock, E., and Alexander, N. (1982): Catecholamines and cardiac beta-adrenoceptors in rats with transplanted pheochromocytoma. *Clin. Res.*, 30:259A (abstract).

143. Waldo, G. L., Northup, J. K., Perkins, J. P., and Harden, T. K. (1983): Characterization of an altered membrane form of the beta-adrenergic receptor produced during agonist-induced desensitization. *J. Biol. Chem.*, 258:13900–13908.

144. Williams, L. T., Lefkowitz, R. J., Watanabe, A. M., Hathaway, D. R., and Besch, H. R., Jr. (1977): Thyroid hormone regulation of beta-adrenergic receptor number. *J. Biol. Chem.*, 252:2787–2789.

145. Woodcock, E. A., and Johnston, C. I. (1980): Changes in tissue alpha- and beta-adrenergic receptors in renal hypertension in the rat. *Hypertension*, 2:156–161.

146. York, J. W., Penney, D. G., Weeks, T. A., and Stagno, P. A. (1976): Lactate dehydrogenase changes following several cardiac hypertrophic stresses. *J. Appl. Physiol.*, 40:923–926.

The Heart and Cardiovascular System,
edited by H. A. Fozzard et al.
Raven Press, New York © 1986.

CHAPTER 52

Sympathetic Mechanisms Regulating Myocardial Contractility in Conscious Animals

Alan M. Fujii and Stephen F. Vatner

The sympathetic nervous system is the primary mediator of the left ventricular inotropic response to stress. Sympathetic activation increases the release of endogenous catecholamines, which results in an elevation in arterial pressure by increasing peripheral resistance, heart rate, and myocardial contractility mediated by stimulation of α- and β-adrenergic receptors. Parasympathetic activation decreases arterial pressure by decreasing heart rate, cardiac output, and peripheral resistance. Discussion of the parasympathetic nervous system will be limited to its role in modulating the sympathetic nervous system, because the primary goal of this chapter is to describe left ventricular inotropic responses to sympathetic activation by physiologic stresses and the responses to β-adrenergic stimulation by sympathomimetic amines. In particular, we shall discuss left ventricular inotropic responses to sympathetic activation, produced by administration of specific agonists, including the neurotransmitter norepinephrine, and physiologic activation, as occurs during exercise, reflex activation, and in response to hypotensive hemorrhage. Modulation of the left ventricular inotropic response to sympathetic neural activation and to exogenously administered sympathomimetic amines by the parasympathetic nervous system

and by the absence of intrinsic innervation will also be reviewed.

EXERCISE

Maximal exercise is one of the most severe physiologic stresses that the cardiovascular system encounters (97,106). In dogs, during severe dynamic exercise (Fig. 1), the heart rate rapidly increases by threefold or fourfold to over 300 beats/min, and left ventricular dP/dt rises by a similar amount to 12,000 to 15,000 mm Hg/sec (101). In normal humans, heart rate may increase to 200 beats/min (64,81). Approximately half of the chronotropic response is due to β-adrenergic stimulation, because prior β-adrenergic receptor blockade limits the increase in heart rate by approximately one-half, the other half being due to withdrawal of parasympathetic tone (101). Prior cholinergic receptor blockade does not alter the left ventricular inotropic response, indicating negligible parasympathetic tone during maximal exercise (111). In contrast, prior β-adrenergic receptor blockade nearly eliminates the inotropic response (Fig. 2), indicating that nearly all of the inotropic response is due to

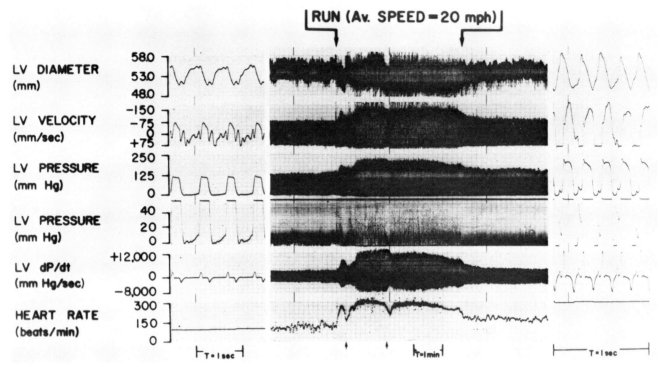

FIG. 1. Representative effects of severe exercise on phasic left ventricular (LV) diameter (epicardial), velocity, pressure, diastolic pressure, dP/dt, and heart rate. Phasic waveforms at rapid paper speed in the control period (**left**) can be contrasted with those during severe exercise (**right**). Arrows denote times when the dog paused to urinate. Note that end-diastolic diameter fell and then rapidly increased when severe exertion was resumed. (From ref. 101, with permission.)

β-adrenergic receptor stimulation (101). The marked increase in heart rate tends to limit increases in left ventricular diastolic dimensions during exercise and masks the functioning of the Frank-Starling mechanism. Utilization of the Starling mechanism to enhance the left ventricular inotropic response during exercise is best demonstrated in intact animals when heart rate is maintained constant (101). Autonomic mechanisms appear important in mediating the rapid onset of the initial response to dynamic exercise, because these changes are delayed in animals after cardiac denervation (24,25). Thus, exercise elicits multiple responses, including sym-

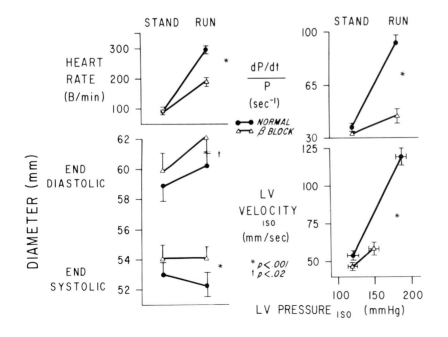

FIG. 2. Average values (±SE) for 7 conscious dogs standing at rest and during severe steady-state exercise studied during spontaneous rhythm before and after β-adrenergic receptor blockade with propranolol (1.0 mg/kg). The values attained during severe exercise that were significantly different are noted. Note that pretreatment with propranolol nearly eliminated the increase in $dP/dt/P$ and shortening velocity induced by severe exercise. (From ref. 101, with permission.)

pathetic activation and withdrawal of parasympathetic tone, to ensure optimal cardiac efficiency. The large positive left ventricular inotropic response to exercise appears to override the usual opposing cardiovascular reflexes (94).

Cardiovascular reflexes with sympathetic efferent pathways also play a role in regulating the left ventricular inotropic state, although the magnitude of this response is much less than that generated by exercise. Reflex control of myocardial function will be discussed next.

REFLEX CONTROL OF MYOCARDIAL CONTRACTILITY

Reflex responses arise from a variety of chemoreceptors and mechanoreceptors that transmit information centrally (57). The efferent information is conveyed peripherally via sympathetic and parasympathetic nerves, and by catecholamines and other secreted hormones, to induce changes in the cardiovascular system (78,89,115).

Cardiovascular Reflex Control in Anesthetized and Conscious Animals

When interpreting human and animal studies dealing with sympathetic regulation of left ventricular contractility, it is important to recognize that base-line contractility and responsiveness to sympathetic activation and sympathomimetic amines can be profoundly altered by general anesthesia and recent surgery. Barbiturates, the most common anesthetic agents used in animal experimentation, depress most aspects of autonomic reflex control (100), reduce myocardial contractility, and increase the base-line heart rate (62). In acute animal preparations, increased sympathetic tone in response to the stress of surgery can be superimposed on the effects of barbiturates (62,99,112). In conscious dogs, β-adrenergic receptor blockade with propranolol induces only small decreases in heart rate and left ventricular dP/dt (98), indicating low sympathetic tone. On the other hand, cholinergic blockade with atropine methylbromide causes a marked increase in heart rate, but little change in left ventricular dP/dt (110), indicating a high resting parasympathetic tone, with little effect on contractility. Accordingly, in this review, descriptions of sympathetic mechanisms regulating the left ventricular inotropic state will emphasize data from studies of conscious, chronically instrumented animals.

Arterial Baroreflex

Arterial baroreflex modulation of left ventricular inotropy is not nearly as pronounced as its influence on heart rate and arterial pressure. In conscious, chronically instrumented dogs, electrical stimulation of the carotid sinus nerve, the afferent limb of the arterial baroreflex, produces no significant decrease in left ventricular $dP/dt/P$ (102). Because under physiologic conditions in normal conscious dogs and humans sympathetic tone is very low, it is difficult to demonstrate withdrawal of sympathetic tone to the heart. On the other hand, it is clear that unloading of the arterial baroreceptors in anesthetized dogs increases the inotropic state of the left ventricle because of an increase in sympathetic tone (32,84). In conscious, chronically instrumented dogs, unloading of the carotid and aortic arterial baroreceptors with intravenous nitroglycerin results in a 25 to 30% increase in left ventricular dP/dt, when heart rate is allowed to increase (39,107). The reflex rise in left ventricular dP/dt is slightly less when heart rate is maintained constant. Bilateral carotid occlusion (Fig. 3), with antagonistic input from the aortic baroreceptors, increased left ventricular dP/dt by only 12% when heart rate was held constant (102). Thus, in a conscious dog with a high resting parasympathetic tone and low resting sympathetic tone, unloading the arterial baroreceptors induces a modest positive inotropic response, whereas loading the baroreceptors has little negative effect on the left ventricular inotropic state.

Chemoreflex

Arterial chemoreceptors are located in the carotid and aortic bodies and are stimulated by a fall in arterial P_{O_2}, a rise in P_{CO_2}, or a fall in pH (12). Arterial chemoreceptors are also stimulated by hemorrhage and increased sympathetic activity (4,43,93). Arterial che-

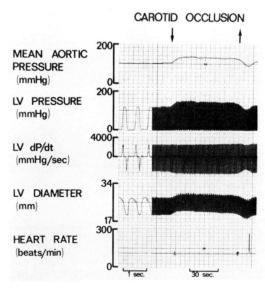

FIG. 3. Effects of bilateral carotid occlusion on mean aortic pressure, LV pressure, dP/dt, and diameter in a conscious dog with heart rate held constant by pacing. Carotid occlusion increased pressure, but increased dP/dt only slightly. (From ref. 108, with permission.)

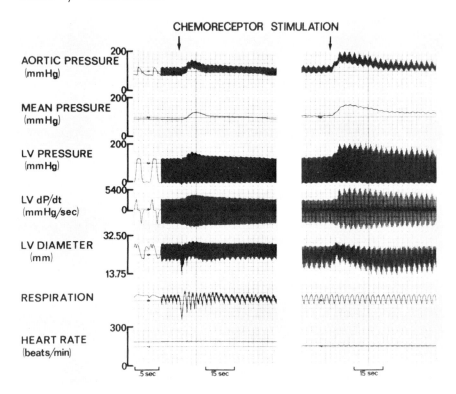

CHEMORECEPTOR STIMULATION

AORTIC PRESSURE (mmHg)

MEAN PRESSURE (mmHg)

LV PRESSURE (mmHg)

LV dP/dt (mmHg/sec)

LV DIAMETER (mm)

RESPIRATION

HEART RATE (beats/min)

FIG. 4. Effects of carotid chemoreceptor stimulation on phasic and mean aortic pressure, LV pressure, dP/dt, diameter, respiration (as monitored by a pneumograph), and heart rate are compared in the same conscious dog with spontaneous respiration (**left**) and with respiration controlled (**right**). Respiration was controlled with a mechanical ventilator after skeletal muscle paralysis with succinylcholine. Heart rate was held constant by pacing. Carotid chemoreceptor stimulation markedly increased respiration, as well as aortic and LV pressures and LV dP/dt. In the right-hand panel, with ventilation controlled, the same carotid chemoreceptor stimulus induced larger increases in pressure and LV dP/dt. (From ref. 108, with permission.)

moreceptor stimulation induces secondary reflex hyperventilation (16–19,88). Hyperventilation secondarily elicits the pulmonary inflation reflex, which exerts an opposing negative inotropic effect (3,16). The pulmonary inflation reflex may even completely mask the positive inotropic effect of chemoreflex activation. In conscious

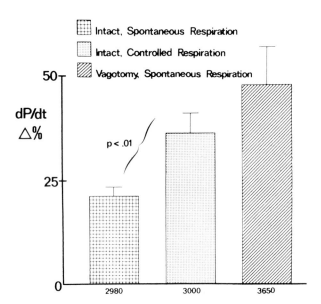

FIG. 5. Effects of carotid chemoreceptor reflex stimulation on LV dP/dt are compared in intact dogs with spontaneous respiration, intact dogs with controlled respiration, and dogs with spontaneous respiration after bilateral vagotomy. Control values are noted at the bases of the bars. Carotid chemoreceptor reflex stimulation induced greater increases in dP/dt either when respiration was controlled in intact dogs or after vagotomy with spontaneous respiration. (From ref. 108, with permission.)

dogs, carotid chemoreceptor stimulation with nicotine induces a 21% increase in left ventricular dP/dt that is eliminated by β-adrenergic receptor blockade. In conscious, mechanically ventilated dogs pretreated with succinylcholine to suppress the pulmonary inflation reflex, carotid chemoreceptor stimulation results in a 36% increase in left ventricular dP/dt (Fig. 4). Carotid chemoreceptor stimulation after elimination of the pulmonary inflation reflex by bilateral cervical vagotomy (Fig. 5) results in a 48% increase in left ventricular dP/dt (80,108,109). Thus, in conscious dogs, stimulation of the arterial chemoreceptors results in a sympathetically mediated positive inotropic response that is inhibited by the pulmonary inflation reflex. However, the magnitude of the positive inotropic response to these extensively investigated reflexes is small when compared with the inotropic response to maximal dynamic exercise, which can increase left ventricular dP/dt by threefold to fourfold.

It should be kept in mind that there are several other mechanoreceptor and chemoreceptor reflexes that are important in regulating the cardiovascular system (26,27). However, the extent to which these other reflexes regulate the left ventricular inotropic state, particularly in the conscious animal, has not been established. Hemorrhage, which will be discussed next, represents one physiologic condition in which several of these cardiovascular reflexes are activated.

HEMORRHAGE

Hemorrhage severe enough to reduce arterial pressure would be expected to elicit autonomic reflexes that

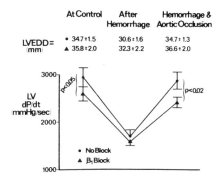

FIG. 6. Effects of hemorrhage (30 ml/kg) on LV *dP/dt* are compared in the same 6 conscious dogs, with heart rate held constant by pacing, studied in the presence (*triangles*) and absence (*circles*) of selective β_1-adrenergic receptor blockade. LV end-diastolic diameter (**top**) was returned to the prehemorrhage control level by inflation of an aortic occluder. With hemorrhage (30 ml/kg), LV end-diastolic diameter and LV *dP/dt* fell under both conditions (**middle**). When LV end-diastolic diameter was returned to the control level (**right**), LV *dP/dt* returned almost precisely to the control level in those dogs without β_1-adrenergic receptor blockade. (From ref. 38, with permission.)

would activate the sympathetic nervous system to increase arterial pressure and maintain peripheral perfusion. In anesthetized animals, hemorrhage increases sympathetic neural activity (10) and circulating catecholamines (36) and unloads the arterial baroreceptors, to produce important inotropic effects (21,32,84). In conscious animals, however, although hemorrhage increases heart rate and peripheral vascular resistance (10,47,96), there is surprisingly little increase in the left ventricular inotropic state (38). With hemorrhage, left ventricular *dP/dt* increases by only 10% during the initial normotensive phase of hemorrhage and subsequently declines. After 30 ml/kg blood loss, left ventricular *dP/dt* decreases by 1,246 ± 120 from 3,338 ± 126 mm Hg/sec. Even when left ventricular preload and

afterload are returned to control levels by aortic constriction (Fig. 6) there is no demonstrable increase in left ventricular *dP/dt*. This lack of a positive inotropic response was found to occur in the presence of plasma norepinephrine concentrations that increased by 1,108 ± 206 from 437 ± 106 pg/ml and plasma epinephrine concentrations that increased by 1,475 ± 266 from 342 ± 79 pg/ml. Thus, hypotensive hemorrhage (30 ml/kg, blood loss) decreased all indices of left ventricular contractility while plasma concentrations of norepinephrine and epinephrine increased by twofold to fourfold (38). The increases in plasma norepinephrine and epinephrine during hemorrhage were two to five times greater than the respective changes during exercise, whereas the changes in left ventricular *dP/dt* were directionally opposite. It is important to keep in mind that levels of circulating catecholamines do not indicate the concentration of norepinephrine at the synaptic cleft.

The difference in left ventricular inotropic responses to catecholamines released during hemorrhage and during exercise may be explained, in part, by differential activation of sympathetic nerves to the heart and peripheral vascular beds. Woodman and colleagues (117) found that during hypotensive hemorrhage (30 ml/kg, blood loss) there was a net removal of circulating catecholamines by the heart such that the fractional extraction of norepinephrine [100 × (arterial − coronary sinus concentration)/(arterial concentration)] changed from −52 ± 22% (a net secretion of norepinephrine) to 66 ± 9%. The fractional extraction of epinephrine increased from 16 ± 6% to 73 ± 8% (Figs. 7 and 8). In contrast, moderate treadmill exercise induced increases in net secretions of both norepinephrine and epinephrine by the heart (63,67,117,118). During hemorrhage, net extraction, rather than secretion, of catecholamines by the heart supports the concept that there is little increase in cardiac sympathetic tone with this stimulus. In addition, left ventricular inotropic responses to hemorrhage

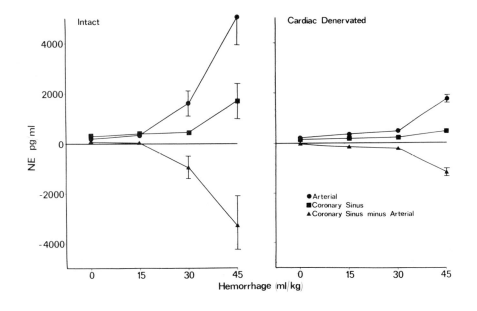

FIG. 7. Effects of hemorrhage on arterial and coronary sinus norepinephrine concentrations are compared in intact (**left**) and cardiac-denervated (**right**) dogs. The difference between coronary sinus and arterial levels is also plotted. With hemorrhage, increases in arterial norepinephrine were greater than increases in coronary sinus norepinephrine (i.e., there was net uptake of norepinephrine).

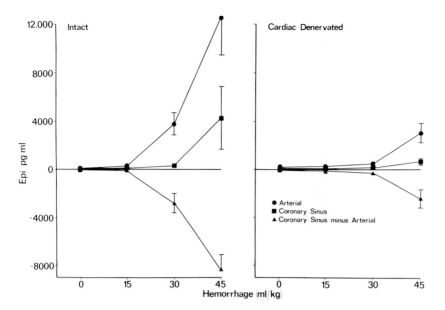

FIG. 8. Effects of hemorrhage on arterial and coronary sinus epinephrine concentrations are compared in intact (**left**) and cardiac-denervated (**right**) dogs. The difference between coronary sinus and arterial levels is also plotted. With hemorrhage, increases in arterial epinephrine were greater than increases in coronary sinus epinephrine (i.e., there was net uptake of epinephrine).

in dogs after cardiac denervation were similar to responses in intact animals, as were fractional extractions of catecholamines (117). Similar left ventricular inotropic and catecholamine extraction data in intact dogs and in dogs after cardiac denervation further support the contention that sympathetic mechanisms play little role in regulating cardiac performance during hemorrhage (38). Thus, unlike dynamic exercise, hemorrhage does not appear to induce a major increase in sympathetic tone to the heart in conscious dogs. It is interesting to consider that there is little teleologic utility of increasing sympathetic tone to a heart with a low preload and afterload, a circumstance in which increasing the force of contraction has limited potential for increasing stroke volume.

Hypotensive hemorrhage does increase sympathetic activity to the peripheral vascular system, inducing a potent vasoconstriction in the mesenteric and iliac beds, while the renal vascular bed remains largely unaffected (96). In fact, hypotensive hemorrhage induces a decrease in renal sympathetic nerve activity (69). Thus, hemorrhage induces nonuniform activation of the sympathetic nervous system, with more intense drive to the gastrointestinal and muscular beds and less to the heart and kidney.

These data would suggest that circulating catecholamines may not have an important role in regulating the left ventricular inotropic state. Accordingly, experiments were conducted to determine the importance of circulating catecholamines in regulation of myocardial contractility.

CIRCULATING AND NEURALLY RELEASED CATECHOLAMINES

The importance of circulating catecholamines in regulation of the left ventricular inotropic state is controver-

sial. Plasma catecholamine concentration has been widely used as an indicator of sympathetic neural activity (11,14,15) and has been shown to correlate with increases in arterial pressure and heart rate (14,20,61). The left ventricular inotropic responses to sympathetic stimulation, however, are not adequately explained by levels of circulating plasma catecholamines.

To investigate this apparent incongruity, infusions of norepinephrine and epinephrine were administered to conscious, chronically instrumented dogs, and simultaneous arterial plasma catecholamine levels were measured (119). No significant increase in left ventricular *dP/dt* was observed until the plasma norepinephrine or epinephrine concentration exceeded 1,000 pg/ml, a level well above those that occur with modest sympathetic neural activation. Higher plasma catecholamine levels induced a linearly related increase in left ventricular *dP/dt* (Fig. 9). Note that whereas infusion of either norepi-

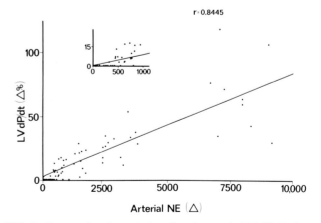

FIG. 9. Regression line relating the change in LV *dP/dt* from control to the change in plasma norepinephrine (NE) content during intravenous infusion of NE (0.01–0.50 µg/kg/min). Inset depicts the same regression at a slightly expanded scale. Values for regression: $r = 0.8445$, slope = 0.25, $p < 0.01$. (From ref. 119, with permission.)

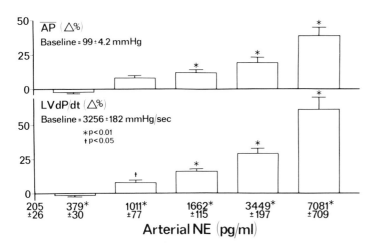

FIG. 10. Effects of stepwise norepinephrine (NE) infusion (0.01–0.5 µg/kg/min) on mean arterial pressure (AP) and LV dP/dt. Plasma NE content is shown at the bottom of the graph for each infusion rate. Significant changes from base-line value are indicated: *$p < 0.01$; †$p < 0.05$. (From ref. 119, with permission.)

FIG. 11. Effects of stepwise epinephrine (Epi) infusion (0.01–0.5 µg/kg/min) on mean arterial pressure (AP) and LV dP/dt. Plasma Epi content is shown at the bottom of the graph for each infusion rate. Significant changes from base-line value are indicated: *$p < 0.01$; †$p < 0.05$. (From ref. 119, with permission.)

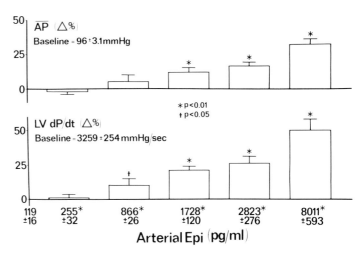

nephrine or epinephrine at a dosage of 0.5 µg/kg/min increased left ventricular dP/dt by only 50%, the plasma norepinephrine concentration increased to 7,081 ± 709 pg/ml (Fig. 10), and the epinephrine (Fig. 11) concentration increased to 8,011 ± 593 pg/ml during their respective infusions. In contrast, left ventricular dP/dt nearly doubled during moderate treadmill exercise, whereas plasma norepinephrine concentration increased by only 563 ± 128 from 183 ± 21 pg/ml, and epinephrine concentration by 292 ± 50 from 125 ± 31 pg/ml. Neither norepinephrine nor epinephrine infusions, at rates that raised plasma catecholamine concentrations to levels observed during moderate treadmill exercise, exceeded the threshold level for an increase in left ventricular contractility. Thus, dynamic exercise is associated with relatively minor increases in plasma catecholamines and large increases in myocardial contractility.

These studies indicate that the concentration of neurotransmitter at the effector site is critical and that circulating levels of catecholamines do not necessarily reflect the amount of neurotransmitter at the cleft. It is also important to remember that release of norepinephrine at the terminal may be modulated by the parasympathetic nervous system.

SYMPATHETIC-PARASYMPATHETIC INTERACTION

The close anatomic relationship of the postganglionic vagal and sympathetic nerve endings (13,44) facilitates the peripheral interactions that occur (37,54,55,87,113) in the modulation of the left ventricular inotropic response to sympathetic stimulation. The principal type of peripheral interaction is called "accentuated antagonism" (55), in which the inhibitory effects of vagal activity on the left ventricular inotropic state are accentuated as the level of sympathetic activity is raised (56,58). Presynaptic and postsynaptic mechanisms may be involved in this sympathetic-parasympathetic interaction.

Several receptor subtypes are located on postganglionic presynaptic sympathetic nerve endings in the heart. The presynaptic muscarinic cholinergic receptor inhibits release of norepinephrine during sympathetic neural activity (71,95). In anesthetized dogs, the rate of norepinephrine overflow into the coronary sinus blood, induced by cardiac sympathetic nerve stimulation, is substantially diminished by simultaneous efferent vagal stimulation (50,51,56). Vagal suppression of norepinephrine release explains, in part, attenuation of the inotropic response to sympathetic stimulation and the occurrence of only a weak negative inotropic effect of vagal stimulation when there is low background sympathetic activity (55).

Sympathetic-parasympathetic interaction may be mediated postsynaptically at the level of the cardiac effector cell. Blockade of muscarinic receptors with atropine in conscious, chronically instrumented dogs markedly augments the positive inotropic responses (Fig. 12) to infusions of sympathomimetic amines (110). Augmentation of the positive inotropic response can be abolished by prior vagotomy. This demonstrates a vagally mediated antagonism of the inotropic effects of circulating catecholamines. Attenuation of the positive inotropic effects of catecholamines and other β-adrenergic receptor agonists by acetylcholine and choline esters has also been demonstrated in anesthetized animals (9,42,49,66,114). Postsynaptic muscarinic antagonism of the β-adrenergically mediated inotropic response is due to combined inhibition of catecholamine-induced increases in adenylate cyclase activity and attenuation of cyclic AMP effects. Thus, muscarinic agonists may decrease the amount of cyclic AMP production induced by β-adrenergic stimulation and decrease the efficacy of the cyclic AMP that is produced.

Although sympathetic-parasympathetic interactions are readily demonstrable using direct electrical stimulation of nerves in anesthetized animals, the physiologic importance of such an interaction has yet to be demonstrated. In physiologic situations it is unusual for high sympathetic and parasympathetic activities to coexist. In conscious animals, for example, there is no further augmentation of the inotropic response to maximal dynamic exercise with addition of cholinergic blockade (111), because there is a concomitant withdrawal of parasympathetic tone. Even under conditions in which high sympathetic tone and high parasympathetic tone

do coexist, such as with chemoreceptor activation (80,109), the inotropic response is not augmented by prior cholinergic blockade. Thus, an important physiologic sympathetic-parasympathetic interaction in intact conscious animals remains to be demonstrated.

Left ventricular inotropic responses to sympathetic neural activation or to exogenously administered sympathomimetic amines in the innervated heart can be very different from the inotropic responses of the left ventricle in pathologic conditions. In particular, there may be an alteration in sympathetic neural responsiveness and/or an alteration in myocardial tissue responsiveness to β-adrenergic receptor stimulation.

MODULATION OF β-ADRENERGIC MECHANISMS BY CARDIAC DENERVATION

The recent development of ligand binding techniques, used to study the β-adrenergic receptor complex, has stimulated intense interest in delineating the biochemical mechanisms involved in altering the myocardial inotropic and chronotropic responses to β-adrenergic receptor stimulation (52,53). There are many potential mechanisms by which the inotropic or chronotropic responsiveness of the left ventricle to β-adrenergic receptor stimulation may be altered. For example, the density or affinity of the β receptors may be altered, access of hormone to the β-adrenergic receptor complex may be changed, or the intracellular efficacy of the β-adrenergic receptor complex may be altered.

Although several biochemical studies have described desensitization of the β-adrenergic receptor mechanism after chronic catecholamine exposure, there are few physiologic data, particularly in conscious animals, to correlate with the cellular mechanisms. On the other hand, many more data are available regarding the opposite phenomenon, i.e., denervation-induced supersensitivity to catecholamines.

Recent clinical success with cardiac transplantation (29,45) has revived interest in studying myocardial function after cardiac denervation and in understanding the mechanisms involved in denervation supersensitivity (6). It is well-known that the denervated heart responds remarkably well to the stress of severe dynamic exercise (24,25) by invoking the Starling mechanism (24,65,77) and by exhibiting greater dependence on circulating catecholamines to augment myocardial contractility (23). The inotropic response may be due, in part, to greater amounts of norepinephrine at the receptor site, because there is little neuronal uptake after cardiac denervation (22). In addition, there is an increase in β-adrenergic receptor density (31,74,105).

Several investigators found that inotropic responses to norepinephrine were increased in animals after cardiac denervation (22,72). Vatner and colleagues (105) found a nearly threefold increase in the inotropic response to

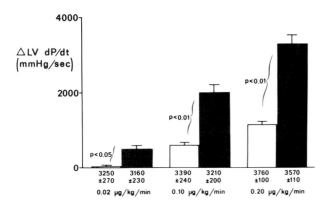

FIG. 12. Steady-state effects of 10-min intravenous infusions of graded doses of norepinephrine on LV *dP/dt* in conscious intact dogs before (*open bars*) and after muscarinic blockade (*closed bars*). Control values (±SE) are shown at the bases of the bars. Muscarinic blockade augmented the increase in LV *dP/dt* induced by each dose of norepinephrine. (From ref. 110, with permission.)

norepinephrine (0.2 μg/kg) in dogs with cardiac denervation that persisted even after elimination of autonomic reflex buffering with prior ganglionic, α_1-adrenergic, and cholinergic receptor blockades (Fig. 13). The inotropic responses to isoproterenol after cardiac denervation, however, were similar to those in innervated hearts (22,72). The apparent paradox in the augmented inotropic response to norepinephrine, but not to isoproterenol, can be explained if one remembers that in intact animals the chronotropic or inotropic response to isoproterenol is the sum of the direct effect of the drug and the added reflex action. After elimination of autonomic reflexes with ganglionic blockade in conscious dogs, Vatner and colleagues (105) found 40% and 32% greater increases in left ventricular (LV) dP/dt and 51% and 36% greater increases in heart rate in response to isoproterenol (0.1 and 0.2 μg/kg) in the dogs with cardiac denervation than in intact dogs. Similar results were observed with prenalterol, a selective β_1-adrenergic receptor agonist. Prenalterol (4 μg/kg) induced a 42% greater increase in LV dP/dt and a 24% greater increase in heart rate in the denervated dogs, as compared with the responses in intact dogs. The augmented inotropic and chronotropic responses to prenalterol were nearly identical to those obtained with isoproterenol (Fig. 14). The augmentation of inotropic responses to isoproterenol and prenalteral correspond with the 40 to 50% increase in β-adrenergic receptor density and unchanged receptor affinity in the myocardium of dogs after cardiac denervation (Fig. 15).

Vatner et al. (105) found an enhanced coupling of the β-adrenergic receptors in the denervated animals to adenylate cyclase. There was also a reduction in the EC_{50} (50% maximal cyclase stimulation by isoproterenol) in the dogs after cardiac denervation (cardiac denervated, 0.22 ± 0.05 μM vs normals 0.54 ± 0.25). This decrease in EC_{50} would have been predicted in the setting of a 50% increase in receptor concentration (92). The biochemical data for the β-adrenergic receptor-adenylate cyclase activity in the dogs with cardiac denervation still

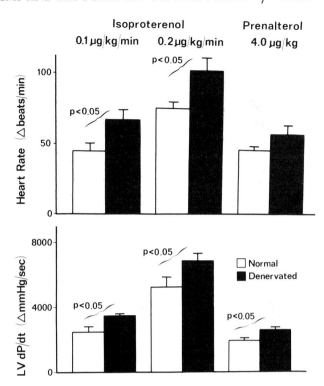

FIG. 14. Effects of isoproterenol and prenalterol on heart rate and LV dP/dt, in the presence of ganglionic and cholinergic receptor blockades, are compared in conscious normal dogs and in conscious dogs after cardiac denervation. The increases in LV dP/dt were significantly greater in dogs with cardiac denervation for isoproterenol at 0.1 μg/kg/min (40%) and 0.2 μg/kg/min (32%), and prenalterol at 4 μg/kg/min (41%). (From ref. 105, with permission.)

did not explain the large, two- to threefold increase in the inotropic responsiveness to norepinephrine. Although norepinephrine is actively taken up by presynaptic nerve terminals (40), neither prenalterol nor isoproterenol is inactivated by nerve terminal uptake mechanisms in the

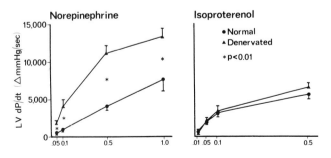

FIG. 13. Increases in LV dP/dt with bolus injections of norepinephrine and isoproterenol are compared for 7 normal conscious dogs with all reflexes intact and 5 conscious dogs with cardiac denervation. Increases in LV dP/dt were markedly greater in dogs with cardiac denervation in response to norepinephrine, but not to isoproterenol. (From ref. 105, with permission.)

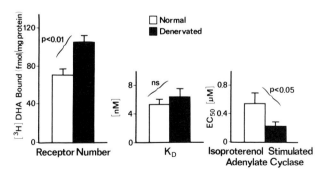

FIG. 15. β-Adrenergic receptor number (**left**), as determined by ^{3}H-DHA binding (1.0–30 nM), receptor affinity (K_D) (**middle**), and EC_{50} from adenylate cyclase (**right**) are compared in membrane preparations from intact and denervated hearts. β-Adrenergic receptor density in denervated hearts increased significantly (50%), while receptor affinity was not different. The EC_{50} for adenylate cyclase was also different in the membrane preparations from denervated hearts. (From ref. 105, with permission.)

intact animal (41,105). After pretreatment with desmethylimipramine to block norepinephrine uptake, Vatner and colleagues (105) found only a 10 to 21% greater augmentation of the inotropic and chronotropic response to norepinephrine in the dogs after cardiac denervation when they were compared with intact animals. Thus, the greater augmentation of the inotropic response to norepinephrine may be explained primarily by elimination of catecholamine uptake mechanisms by cardiac denervation.

Thus, the combination of physiologic and biochemical data suggests that there are five possible mechanisms for the denervation supersensitivity phenomenon: (a) increased amounts of catecholamines at the receptor cell because of reduced sympathetic uptake of norepinephrine, which is by far the most important mechanism, (b) increased β-adrenergic receptor density, (c) reduced efferent vagally mediated inhibition of the myocardial contractile response to catecholamines (110), (d) decreased muscarinic cholinergic receptor density to inhibit the cellular response to β-adrenergic stimulation, and (e) absence of arterial baroreflex buffering, because the efferent nerves are absent from the denervated heart.

Clearly, modulation of left ventricular inotropic responsiveness to β-adrenergic receptor stimulation is complex, because several interrelated mechanisms are involved. To understand the nature of these interrelated mechanisms, it is important that future multidisciplinary collaborative studies correlate the biochemical findings with the physiologic responses.

β-ADRENERGIC RESPONSES IN PRESSURE-OVERLOAD LEFT VENTRICULAR HYPERTROPHY

The inotropic responsiveness of the hypertrophied left ventricle to β-adrenergic receptor stimulation is controversial (1,2,73,76,82,83). Although it is generally agreed that myocardial hypertrophy is the major mechanism by which the left ventricle compensates for a chronic pressure-overload lesion, allowing the ventricle to function in a normal inotropic state (33–35,85,86,91), the natural history of pressure-overload hypertrophy is progressive deterioration of myocardial function and eventual development of heart failure (7,68,75,79,90). It has been postulated that a reduction in inotropic responsiveness to sympathetic stimulation may contribute to the gradual decline in left ventricular function and the eventual development of heart failure. However, in conscious dogs with severe pressure-overload left ventricular hypertrophy, inotropic responses to β-adrenergic receptor stimulation are normal (28,103). In conscious, chronically instrumented dogs with severe left ventricular hypertrophy [(LV free-wall weight)/(body weight) = 7.0 ± 0.4 versus 4.0 ± 0.4 g/kg in control dogs], norepinephrine (0.4 μg/kg/min) increased left ventricular

pressure from 224 ± 16 to 305 ± 22 mm Hg, mean arterial pressure from 90 ± 2 to 132 ± 4 mm Hg, mean systolic wall stress from 224 ± 11 to 307 ± 24 g/cm^2, and dP/dt from $3,246 \pm 156$ to $5,619 \pm 345$ mm Hg/sec. In the control dogs, norepinephrine (0.4 μg/kg/min) increased left ventricular pressure from 121 ± 2 to 177 ± 9 mm Hg, mean arterial pressure from 97 ± 2 to 143 ± 9 mm Hg, mean systolic wall stress from 194 ± 14 to 299 ± 22 g/cm^2, dP/dt from $3,363 \pm 123$ to $5,174 \pm 343$ mm Hg/sec. The inotropic responses to infusions of norepinephrine were normal in the dogs with left ventricular hypertrophy, whether the isovolumic index of contractility (dP/dt) or ejection-phase indices of contractility were used to assess responses, because wall stresses increased similarly in the two groups (Fig. 16). The inotropic responses in the dogs with left ventricular hypertrophy were normal even when prenalterol, a specific β_1-adrenergic receptor agonist with little effect on afterload, was used (Fig. 17).

Biochemical studies of β-adrenergic receptors in hypertrophied left ventricle have produced conflicting results (1,5,8,30,46,48,59,60,70,116). Biochemical studies from this laboratory have shown increases in β-adrenergic number and decreases in β-adrenergic receptor affinity (Fig. 18) in dogs with severe compensated pressure-overload left ventricular hypertrophy (104,105). The increases in β-adrenergic receptor density were associated

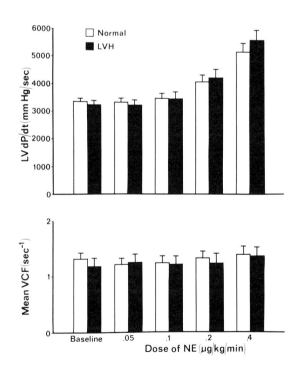

FIG. 16. Absolute values for LV dP/dt during graded infusions of norepinephrine (NE) **(top)** and values for mean velocity of circumferential fiber shortening (VCF) during infusions of NE **(bottom)**. LV dP/dt increased similarly in control dogs and in dogs with LV hypertrophy. VCF remained relatively constant in both groups because of the concomitant increases in afterload induced by the peripheral vascular effects of NE.

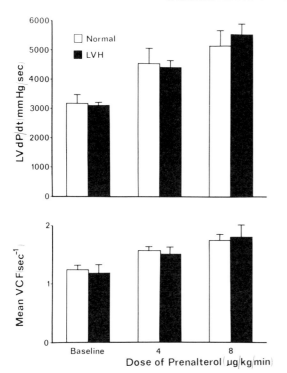

FIG. 17. Values for LV dP/dt during graded infusions of prenalterol (**top**) and values for mean velocity of circumferential fiber shortening (VCF) (**bottom**). LV dP/dt and VCF increased similarly in control dogs and in dogs with LV hypertrophy. Afterload remained relatively constant, because prenalterol is a specific β_1-adrenergic receptor agonist with little direct effect on the peripheral vasculature.

with normal plasma concentrations of circulating catecholamines, but reduced tissue catecholamine levels in the left ventricle, and reduced maximal adenylate cyclase activity (105). These offsetting biochemical changes associated with pressure-overload left ventricular hypertrophy may explain the maintenance of a normal inotropic response to sympathomimetic amines in the conscious dogs studied. Thus, the left ventricular inotropic response to β-adrenergic receptor stimulation may be difficult to

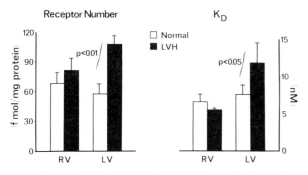

FIG. 18. β-Adrenergic receptor concentrations and affinity constants (K_D) are compared in the right and left ventricles of normal dogs ($N = 11$) and dogs with LV hypertrophy ($N = 8$). Note that the marked increases in both receptor number and K_D are observed only in the LV of dogs with LV hypertrophy. (From ref. 103, with permission.)

predict from biochemical assessment of β-adrenergic receptor density alone. Clearly, future biochemical studies need to be combined with physiologic studies to interpret the relevance of the findings from each discipline.

SUMMARY

In this review, some of the issues and controversies involved in the question of modulation of the myocardial inotropic state by neurally released catecholamines and exogenously administered sympathomimetic amines have been discussed. Whereas it is generally recognized that sympathetic mechanisms are of major importance in controlling the myocardial inotropic state, it is also important to recognize that the sympathetic nervous system is only one of several redundant mechanisms regulating cardiac performance. Studies in humans with transplanted hearts (65,77) and in animals with cardiac denervation (24,25) have clearly shown that relatively normal responses to stress, including exercise, can be achieved even in the absence of the sympathetic nervous system. This is accomplished in part by increased responsiveness to circulating catecholamines during exercise. However, in the absence of both neural and humoral adrenergic mechanisms, the cardiac response to exercise is depressed (23).

It is also surprising that either direct or reflex activation of the sympathetic nerves induces relatively small increases (20–40%) in the left ventricular inotropic state, as compared with the threefold to fourfold increase associated with maximal dynamic exercise. Studies of left ventricular inotropic responses to hemorrhage and exercise show surprisingly poor correlation with concentrations of circulating plasma catecholamines. These data suggest that plasma catecholamine concentrations are not always indicative of the catecholamine concentration at the β-adrenergic receptor complex and that other factors, such as sympathetic-parasympathetic interaction, may modulate inotropic responses to catecholamines. The development of biochemical ligand-binding techniques to evaluate the β-adrenergic receptor complex should provide a means of examining the mechanisms to explain physiologic observations. As is apparent from the sections describing studies in dogs after cardiac denervation or pressure-overload hypertrophy, both biochemical and physiologic studies must be performed before the mechanisms involved in modulation of the inotropic response to catecholamines can be understood. The biochemical and physiologic changes may be antagonistic, additive, or even synergistic. It is clear that future studies dealing with sympathetic control of the left ventricular inotropic state in pathologic states will require collaboration between physiologists, biochemists, and molecular biologists. It is this type of knowledge, involving an understanding of physiologic processes at multiple levels, that will be critical to a full understanding of sympathetic regulation of left ventricular function in physiologic and pathologic conditions.

ACKNOWLEDGMENTS

Supported in part by USPHS grants HL-33065, HL-33107, HL-33743, and RR-00168. Dr. Fujii was supported by Clinical Investigator Award HL-01542.

REFERENCES

1. Ayobe, M. H., and Tarazi, R. E. (1983): Beta-receptors and contractile reserve in left ventricular hypertrophy. *Hypertension (Suppl. I)*, 5:192.
2. Ayobe, M. H., and Tarazi, R. E. (1984): Reversal of changes in myocardial β-receptors and inotropic responsiveness with regression of cardiac hypertrophy in renal hypertensive rats (RHR). *Circ. Res.*, 54:125.
3. Bernthal, T., Greene, W., Jr., and Revzin, A. M. (1951): Role of carotid chemoreceptors in hypoxic cardiac acceleration. *Proc. Soc. Exp. Biol. Med.*, 76:121–124.
4. Biscoe, T. J. (1971): Carotid body: Structure and function. *Physiol. Rev.* 51:437–495.
5. Bobik, A., and Korner, P. (1981): Cardiac beta adrenoreceptors and adenylate cyclase in normotensive and renal hypertensive rabbits during changes in autonomic activity. *Clin. Exp. Hyperten.*, 3:257–280.
6. Cannon, W. B. (1939): A law of denervation. *Am. J. Med. Sci.*, 198:737–750.
7. Carabello, B. A., Green, L. H., Grossman, W., Cohn, L. H., Koster, J. K., and Collin, J. J. (1980): Hemodynamic determinants of prognosis of aortic valve replacement in critical aortic stenosis and advanced congestive heart failure. *Circulation*, 62:42.
8. Cervoni, P., Herzlinger, H., Lai, F. M., and Tanikella, T. (1981): A comparison of cardiac reactivity and β-adrenoceptor number and affinity between aorta—coarcted hypertensive and normotensive rats. *Br. J. Pharmacol.*, 74:517–523.
9. Chamales, M. H., Gourley, R. D., and Williams, B. J. (1975): Effect of acetylcholine on changes in contractility, heart rate and phosphorylase activity produced by isoprenaline, salbutamol, and aminophylline in the perfused guinea pig heart. *Br. J. Pharmacol.*, 53:531–538.
10. Chien, S. (1967): Role of the sympathetic nervous system in hemorrhage. *Physiol. Rev.*, 47:214–288.
11. Christensen, N. J., and Brandsborg, O. (1973): The relationship between plasma catecholamine concentration and pulse rate during exercise and standing. *Eur. J. Clin. Invest.*, 3:299–306.
12. Coleridge, J. C. G., and Coleridge, H. M. (1979): Chemoreflex regulation of the heart. In: *Handbook of Physiology, Sec. 2, The Cardiovascular System, Vol. 2, The Heart*, edited by R. M. Berne, N. Speralakis, and S. R. Geiger, pp. 653–676. American Physiological Society, Bethesda.
13. Cooper, T. (1965): Terminal innervation of the heart. In: *Nervous Control of the Heart*, edited by W. C. Randall, pp. 130–153. Williams & Wilkins, Baltimore.
14. Cousineau, D., Ferguson, R. J., De Champlain, J., Gauthier, P., Cote, P., and Bourassa, M. (1977): Catecholamines in coronary sinus during exercise in man before and after training. *J. Appl. Physiol.*, 43:801–806.
15. Cryer, P. E. (1980): Physiology and pathophysiology of the human sympathoadrenal neuroendocrine system. *N. Engl. J. Med.*, 303:436–444.
16. Daly, M. de B., and Hazzledine, J. L. (1963): The effects of artificially induced hyperventilation on the primary cardiac reflex response to stimulation of the carotid bodies in the dog. *J. Physiol. (Lond.)*, 168:872–889.
17. Daly, M. de B., and Scott, M. J. (1958): The effects of stimulation of the carotid body chemoreceptors on heart rate in the dog. *J. Physiol. (Lond.)*, 144:148–166.
18. Daly, M. de B., and Scott, M. J. (1962): An analysis of the primary cardiovascular reflex effects of stimulation of the carotid body chemoreceptors in the dog. *J. Physiol. (Lond.)*, 162:555–573.
19. Daly, M. de B., and Scott, M. J. (1963): The cardiovascular responses to stimulation of the carotid body chemoreceptors in the dog. *J. Physiol. (Lond.)*, 165:179–197.
20. De Champlain, J., Farley, L., Cousineau, D., and Van Ameringen, M. (1976): Circulating catecholamine levels in human and experimental hypertension. *Circ. Res.*, 38:109–114.
21. DeGeest, H., Levy, M. N., and Zieski, H. (1964): Carotid sinus baroreceptor reflex effects upon myocardial contractility. *Circ. Res.*, 15:327–342.
22. Dempsey, P. J., and Cooper, T. (1968): Supersensitivity of the chronically denervated feline heart. *Am. J. Physiol.*, 215:1245–1249.
23. Donald, D. E., Ferguson, D. A., and Milburn, S. E. (1968): Effect of beta-adrenergic receptor blockade on racing performance of greyhounds with normal and with denervated hearts. *Circ. Res.*, 22:127–134.
24. Donald, D. E., and Shepherd, J. T. (1963): Response to exercise in dogs with chronic cardiac denervation. *Am. J. Physiol.*, 205:393–400.
25. Donald, D. E., and Shepherd, J. T. (1964): Initial cardiovascular adjustment to exercise in dogs with chronic cardiac denervation. *Am. J. Physiol.*, 207:1325–1329.
26. Donald, D. E., and Shepherd, J. T. (1976): Cardiopulmonary receptors with vagal afferents: Location, fibre type and physiologic role. In: *Cardiac Receptors*, edited by R. Hainsworth, C. Kidd, and R. J. Linden, pp. 421–435. Cambridge University Press, Cambridge.
27. Donald, D. E., and Shepherd, J. T. (1978): Reflexes from the heart and lungs. Physiological curiosities or important regulatory mechanisms? *Cardiovasc. Res.*, 12:449–469.
28. Fujii, A. M., Mirsky, I., Serur, J., Als. A., and Vatner, S. F. (1986): Normal inotropic response of the hypertrophied left ventricle to specific β₁ adrenergic stimulation in conscious dogs. *J. Am. Coll. Cardiol.*, 7:122A (abstract).
29. Gaudiani, V. A., Stinson, E. B., Alderman, E., Hunt, S. A., Schroeder, J. S., Perlroth, M. G., Bieber, C. P., Oyer, P. E., Reitz, B. A., Jamieson, S. W., Christopherson, L., and Shumway, N. E. (1981): Long-term survival and function after cardiac transplantation. *Ann. Surg.*, 194:381–385.
30. Giachetti, A., Clark, T. L., and Berti, F. (1979): Subsensitivity of cardiac β-adrenoceptors in renal hypertensive rats. *J. Cardiovasc. Pharmacol.*, 1:467–471.
31. Glaubiger, G., Tsai, B. S., Lefkowitz, R. J., Weiss, B., and Johnson, E. M., Jr. (1978): Chronic guanethidine treatment increases cardiac beta adrenergic receptors. *Nature*, 273:240–242.
32. Glick, G. (1971): Importance of the carotid sinus baroreceptors in the regulation of myocardial performance. *J. Clin. Invest.*, 50:1116–1123.
33. Graham, T. P., Jarmakani, J. M., Canent, R. V., and Anderson, P. A. W. (1971): Evaluation of left ventricular contractile state in childhood: Normal values and observations with pressure overload. *Circulation*, 44:1043.
34. Grossman, W., Jones, D., and McLaurin, L. P. (1975): Wall stress and patterns of hypertrophy in man. *J. Clin. Invest.*, 56:64.
35. Gunther, S., and Grossman, W. (1979): Determinants of ventricular function in pressure-overload hypertrophy in man. *Circulation*, 59:679.
36. Hall, R. C., and Hodge, R. L. (1971): Changes in catecholamine and angiotensin levels in cat and dog during hemorrhage. *Am. J. Physiol.*, 221:1305–1309.
37. Higgins, C. B., Vatner, S. F., and Braunwald, E. (1973): Parasympathetic control of the heart. *Pharmacol. Rev.*, 25:119–155.
38. Hintze, T. H., and Vatner, S. F. (1982): Cardiac dynamics during hemorrhage: Relative unimportance of adrenergic inotropic responses. *Circ. Res.*, 50:705–713.
39. Hintze, T. H., and Vatner, S. F. (1983): Comparison of effects of nifedipine and nitroglycerin on large and small coronary arteries and cardiac function in conscious dogs. *Circ. Res. [Suppl. I]*, 52:139–146.

40. Hertting, G. (1964): The fate of norepinephrine (NE) at the sympathetic nerve endings. *Acta Neuroveg. (Wien)*, 26:267–270.

41. Hertting, G. (1984): The fate of ^{3}H-isoproterenol in the rat. *Biochem. Pharmacol.*, 13:1119–1128.

42. Hollenberg, M., Carriere, S., and Barger, A. C. (1965): Biphasic action of acetylcholine on ventricular myocardium. *Circ. Res.*, 16:527–536.

43. Howe, A., and Neil, E. (1972): Arterial chemoreceptors. In: *Handbook of Sensory Physiology, Enteroceptors, Vol. 3, Pt. 1*, edited by E. Neil, pp. 47–80. Springer-Verlag, Berlin.

44. Jacobowitz, D., Cooper, T., and Barner, H. B. (1967): Histochemical and chemical studies of the localization of adrenergic and cholinergic nerves in normal and denervated cat hearts. *Circ. Res.*, 20:289–298.

45. Jamieson, S. W., Stinson, E. B., and Shumway, N. E. (1979): Cardiac transplantation in 150 patients at Stanford University. *Br. Med. J.*, 1:93–95.

46. Karliner, J. S., Barnes, P., Brown, M., and Dollery, C. (1980): Chronic heart failure in the guinea pig increase cardiac α_1- and β-adrenoceptors. *Eur. J. Pharmacol.*, 67:115–118.

47. Kirchheim, H. R. (1976): Systemic arterial baroreceptor reflexes. *Physiol. Rev.*, 56:100–176.

48. Kumano, K., Upsher, M. E., and Khairallah, P. A. (1983): Beta adrenergic receptor response coupling in hypertrophied hearts. *Hypertension [Suppl.]*, 5:176–183.

49. La Raia, P. J., and Sonnenblick, E. H. (1971): Autonomic control of cardiac AMP. *Circ. Res.*, 28:377–384.

50. Lavallee, M., De Champlain, J., Nadeau, R. A., and Yamaguchi, N. (1978): Muscarinic inhibition of endogenous myocardial catecholamine liberation in the dog. *Can. J. Physiol. Pharmacol.*, 56:642–649.

51. Lavallee, M., De Champlain, J., and Nadeau, R. A. (1980): Reflexly induced inhibition of catecholamine release through a peripheral muscarinic mechanism. *Can. J. Physiol. Pharmacol.*, 58:1334–1341.

52. Lefkowitz, R. J., Mukherjee, C., Coverstone, M., and Caron, M. G. (1974): Stereospecific [^{3}H](-)-alprenolol binding sites, β-adrenergic receptors and adenylate cyclase. *Biochem. Biophys. Res. Commun.*, 60:703–709.

53. Lefkowitz, R. J., Stadel, J. M., and Caron, M. G. (1983): Adenylate cyclase-coupled beta-adrenergic receptors: Structure and mechanisms of desensitization. *Annu. Rev. Biochem.*, 52:159–186.

54. Levy, M. N. (1977): Parasympathetic control of the heart. In: *Neural Regulation of the Heart*, edited by W. C. Randall, pp. 95–129. Oxford University Press, New York.

55. Levy, M. N. (1978): Neural control of the heart: Sympathetic-vagal interactions. In: *Cardiovascular System Dynamics*, edited by J. Baan, A. Noordergraaf, and J. Raines, pp. 365–370. MIT Press, Cambridge.

56. Levy, M. N., and Blattberg, B. (1976): Effect of vagal stimulation on the overflow of norepinephrine into the coronary sinus during cardiac sympathetic nerve stimulation in the dog. *Circ. Res.*, 38:81–85.

57. Levy, M. N., and Martin, P. J. (1979): Neural control of the heart. In: *Handbook of Physiology, Section 2: The Cardiovascular System, Vol. 1*, edited by R. M. Berne, N. Sperelakis, and S. R. Geiger, pp. 581–620. American Physiological Society, Bethesda.

58. Levy, M. N., Ng, M., Martin, P., and Zieske, H. (1966): Sympathetic and parasympathetic interactions on the left ventricle of the dog. *Circ. Res.*, 19:5–10.

59. Limas, C. J. (1979): Increased number of β-adrenergic receptors in the hypertrophied myocardium. *Biochim. Biophys. Acta*, 588:174–178.

60. Limas, C., and Limas, C. J. (1978): Reduced number of β-adrenergic receptors in the myocardium of spontaneously hypertensive rats. *Biochem. Biophys. Res. Commun.*, 83:710–714.

61. Louis, W. J., Doyle, A. E., and Anavekar, S. (1973): Plasma norepinephrine levels in essential hypertension. *N. Engl. J. Med.*, 288:590–601.

62. Manders, W. T., and Vatner, S. F. (1976): Effects of sodium pentobarbital anesthesia on left ventricular function and distribution of cardiac output in dogs, with particular reference to the mechanism for tachycardia. *Circ. Res.*, 39:512–517.

63. Manhem, P., Lecerof, H., and Hokfelt, B. (1978): Plasma catecholamine levels in the coronary sinus, the left renal vein and peripheral vessels in healthy males at rest and during exercise. *Acta Physiol. Scand.*, 104:364–369.

64. McArdle, W. D., Foglia, G. F., and Patti, A. V. (1967): Telemetered cardiac response to selected running events. *J. Appl. Physiol.*, 23:566.

65. McLaughlin, P. R., Kleiman, J. H., Martin, R. P., Doherty, P. W., Reitz, B., Stinson, E. B., Daughters, G. T., Ingels, N. B., and Alderman, E. L. (1978): The effect of exercise and atrial pacing on left ventricular volume and contractility in patients with innervated and denervated hearts. *Circulation*, 58:476–483.

66. Meester, W. D., and Harman, H. F. (1967): Blockade of the positive inotropic actions of epinephrine and theophylline by acetylcholine. *J. Pharmacol. Exp. Ther.*, 158:241–247.

67. Miura, Y., Haneda, T., Sata, T., Miyazawa, K., Sakuma, H., Kobayashi, K., Minai, K., Shirato, K., Honna, T., Takishima, T., and Yoshinaga, K. (1976): Plasma catecholamine levels in the coronary sinus, aorta and femoral vein of subjects undergoing cardiac catheterization at rest and during exercise. *Jpn. Circ. J.*, 40:929–934.

68. Mirsky, I., Pfeffer, J. M., Pfeffer, M. A., and Braunwald, E. (1983): The contractile state as the major determinant in the evolution of left ventricular dysfunction in the spontaneously hypertensive rat. *Circ. Res.*, 53:767.

69. Morita, H., and Vatner, S. F. (1985): Effects of hemorrhage on renal nerve activity in conscious dogs. *Circ. Res.*, 57:788–793.

70. Mukherjee, A., Graham, R. M., Sagalowsky, A. I., Pettinger, W., and McCoy, K. E. (1980): Myocardial beta-adrenergic receptors in the stroke-prone spontaneously hypertensive rat. *J. Mol. Cell. Cardiol.*, 12:1263–1272.

71. Muscholl, E. (1980): Peripheral muscarinic control of norepinephrine release in the cardiovascular system. *Am. J. Physiol.*, 239:H713–H720.

72. Nadeau, R. A., De Champlain, J., and Tremblay, G. M. (1971): Supersensitivity of the isolated rat heart after chemical sympathectomy with 6-hydroxydopamine. *Can. J. Physiol. Pharmacol.*, 49:36–44.

73. Newman, W. H., and Webb, J. G. (1980): Adaptation of left ventricle to chronic pressure overload: Response to inotropic drugs. *Am. J. Physiol.*, 239:H134.

74. Nomura, Y., Kajiyama, H., and Segawa, T. (1980): Hypersensitivity of cardiac beta-adrenergic receptors after neonatal treatment of rats with 6-hydroxydopa. *Eur. J. Pharmacol.*, 66:225–232.

75. O'Kane, H. O., Geha, A. S., Kleiger, R. E., Abe, T., Salaymeh, M. T., and Malik, A. B. (1973): Stable left ventricular hypertrophy in the dog. *J. Thorac. Cardiovasc. Surg.*, 65:264.

76. Pfeffer, M. A., Pfeffer, J. M., and Frohlick, E. D. (1974): Hemodynamics of the spontaneously hypertensive rat: Effects of isotroterenol (37946). *Proc. Soc. Exp. Biol. Med.*, 145:1025.

77. Pope, S. E., Stinson, E. B., Daughters, G. T., Schroeder, J. S., Ingels, N. B., and Alderman, E. L. (1980): Exercise response of the denervated heart in long-term cardiac transplant recipients. *Am. J. Cardiol.*, 46:213–218.

78. Randall, W. C., Wechsler, J. S., Pace, J. B., and Szentivanyi, M. (1968): Alterations in myocardial contractility during stimulation of the cardiac nerves. *Am. J. Physiol.*, 214:1205–1212.

79. Ross, J., and Braunwald, E. (1968): Aortic stenosis. *Circulation [Suppl. V]*, 38:61.

80. Rutherford, J. D., and Vatner, S. F. (1978): Integrated carotid chemoreceptor and pulmonary inflation reflex control of peripheral vasoactivity in conscious dogs. *Circ. Res.*, 43:200–208.

81. Saltin, B., and Astrand, P. (1967): Maximal oxygen uptake in athletes. *J. Appl. Physiol.*, 23:353.

82. Saragoca, M., and Tarazi, R. C. (1981): Impaired cardiac contractile response to isoproterenol in the spontaneously hypertensive rat. *Hypertension*, 3:380.

83. Saragoca, M. A., and Tarazi, R. C. (1981): Left ventricular hypertrophy in rats with renovascular hypertension: Alterations in cardiac function and adrenergic responses. *Hypertension [Suppl. II]*, 3:171.

84. Sarnoff, S. J., Gilmore, J. P., Brockman, S. R., Mitchell, J. H., and Linden, R. J. (1960): Regulation of ventricular contraction

by the carotid sinus: Its effect on atrial and ventricular dynamics. *Circ. Res.*, 8:1123–1136.

85. Sasayama, S., Franklin, D., and Ross, J. (1977): Hyperfunction with normal inotropic state of the hypertrophied left ventricle. *Am. J. Physiol.*, 232:H418.

86. Sasayama, S., Ross, J., Franklin, D., Bloor, C. M., Bishop, S., and Dilley, R. B. (1976): Adaptations of the left ventricle to chronic pressure overload. *Circ. Res.*, 38:172.

87. Schwegler, M. (1974): Sympathetic-parasympathetic interactions on the ventricular myocardium; possible role of cyclic nucleotides. *Basic Res. Cardiol.*, 69:215–221.

88. Scott, M. J. (1966): The effects of hyperventilation on the reflex cardiac response from the carotid bodies in the cat. *J. Physiol. (Lond.)*, 186:307–320.

89. Shipley, R. E., and Gregg, D. E. (1945): The cardiac response to stimulation of the stellate ganglia and cardiac nerves. *Am. J. Physiol.*, 143:396–401.

90. Smith, N., McAnulty, J. H., and Rahimtoola, S. H. (1978): Severe aortic stenosis with impaired left ventricular function and clinical heart failure: Results of valve replacement. *Circulation*, 58:255.

91. Spann, J. F., Bove, A. A., Natarajan, G., and Kreulen, T. (1980): Ventricular performance, pump function and compensatory mechanisms in patients with aortic stenosis. *Circulation*, 62:576.

92. Stiles, G. L., Caron, M. G., and Lefkowitz, R. J. (1984): β-Adrenergic receptors; biochemical mechanisms of physiological regulation. *Physiol. Rev.*, 64:661–743.

93. Torrance, R. W. (1974): Arterial chemoreceptors. In: *MTP International Review of Science, Respiratory Physiology, Ser. 21, Vol. 2*, edited by J. G. Widdicombe, pp. 247–271. University Park Press, Baltimore.

94. Vanhoutte, P., Lacroix, E., and Leusen, I. (1966): The cardiovascular adaptation of the dog to the muscular exercise. Role of the arterial pressoreceptors. *Arch. Int. Physiol. Biochem.*, 74:201.

95. Vanhoutte, P. M., and Levy, M. N. (1980): Prejunctional cholinergic modulation of adrenergic neurotransmission in the cardiovascular system. *Am. J. Physiol.*, 238:H275–H281.

96. Vatner, S. F. (1974): Effects of hemorrhage on regional blood flow distribution in dogs and primates. *J. Clin. Invest.*, 54:225–235.

97. Vatner, S. F. (1984): Neural control of the heart and the coronary circulation during exercise. In: *Nervous Control of Cardiovascular Function*, edited by W. C. Randall, pp. 414–424. Oxford University Press, London.

98. Vatner, S. F., Baig, H., Manders, W. T., Ochs, H., and Pagani, M. (1977): Effects of propranolol on regional myocardial function, electrograms and blood flow in conscious dogs with myocardial ischemia. *J. Clin. Invest.*, 60:353–360.

99. Vatner, S. F., and Braunwald, E. (1975): Cardiovascular control mechanisms in the conscious state. *N. Engl. J. Med.*, 293:970–976.

100. Vatner, S. F., Franklin, D., and Braunwald, E. (1971): Effects of anesthesia and sleep on circulatory response to carotid sinus nerve stimulation. *Am. J. Physiol.*, 220:1249–1255.

101. Vatner, S. F., Franklin, D., Higgins, C. B., Patrick, T., and Braunwald, E. (1972): Left ventricular response to severe exertion in untethered dogs. *J. Clin. Invest.*, 51:3052–3060.

102. Vatner, S. F., Higgins, C. B., Franklin, D., and Braunwald, E. (1972): Extent of carotid sinus regulation of the myocardial contractile state in conscious dogs. *J. Clin. Invest.*, 51:995–1008.

103. Vatner, D. E., Homcy, C. J., Sit, S. P., Manders, W. T., and Vatner, S. F. (1984): Effects of pressure overload left ventricular hypertrophy on beta-adrenergic receptors and responsiveness to catecholamines. *J. Clin. Invest.*, 73:1473–1482.

104. Vatner, D. E., Kirby, D. A., Homcy, C. J., and Vatner, S. F. (1985): Beta adrenergic and cholinergic receptors in hypertension-induced hypertrophy. *Hypertension*, 7:55–60.

105. Vatner, D. E., Lavallee, M., Amano, J., Finizola, A., Homcy, C. J., and Vatner, S. F. (1985): Mechanisms of supersensitivity to sympathomimetic amines in the chronically denervated heart of the conscious dog. *Circ. Res.*, 57:55–57.

106. Vatner, S. F., and Pagani, M. (1976): Cardiovascular adjustments to exercise: Hemodynamics and mechanisms. *Prog. Cardiovasc. Dis.*, 19:91–108.

107. Vatner, S. F., Pagani, M., Rutherford, J. D., Millard, R. W., and Manders, W. T. (1978): Effects of nitroglycerin on cardiac function and regional blood flow distribution in conscious dogs. *Am. J. Physiol.*, 234:H244–H252.

108. Vatner, S. F., and Rutherford, J. D. (1978): Control of the myocardial contractile state by carotid chemo- and baroreceptor and pulmonary inflation reflexes in conscious dogs. *J. Clin. Invest.*, 61:1593–1601.

109. Vatner, S. F., and Rutherford, J. D. (1981): Interaction of carotid chemoreceptor and pulmonary inflation reflexes in circulatory regulation in conscious dogs. *Fed. Proc.*, 40:2188–2193.

110. Vatner, S. F., Rutherford, J. D., and Ochs, H. R. (1979): Baroreflex and vagal mechanisms modulating left ventricular contractile responses to sympathomimetic amines in conscious dogs. *Circ. Res.*, 44:195–207.

111. Vatner, S. F., Rutherford, J. D., Priano, L. L., Manders, W. T., and Ochs, H. R. (1978): Parasympatholytic augmentation of inotropic response to infused but not neurally released norepinephrine. *Fed. Proc.*, 37:833 (abstract).

112. Vatner, S. F., and Smith, N. T. (1974): Effects of halothane on left ventricular function and distribution of regional blood flow in dogs and primates. *Circ. Res.*, 34:155–167.

113. Watanabe, A. M. (1984): Cellular mechanisms of muscarinic regulation of cardiac function. In: *Nervous Control of Cardiovascular Function*, edited by W. C. Randall, pp. 130–164. Oxford University Press, London.

114. Watanabe, A. M., and Besch, H. R., Jr. (1975): Interaction between cyclic adenosine monophosphate and cyclic guanosine monophosphate in guinea pig ventricular myocardium. *Circ. Res.*, 37:309–317.

115. Wiggers, C. J., and Katz, L. N. (1920): The specific influence of the accelerator nerves on the duration of ventricular systole. *Am. J. Physiol.*, 53:49–64.

116. Woodcock, E. A., and Johnston, C. I. (1980): Changes in tissue alpha- and beta-adrenergic receptors in renal hypertension in the rat. *Hypertension*, 2:156–161.

117. Woodman, O. L., Amano, J., Hintze, T. H., and Vatner, S. F. (1986): Augmented catecholamine uptake by the heart during hemorrhage in the conscious dog. *Am. J. Physiol.*, 250: H76–H81.

118. Yamaguchi, N., De Champlain, J., and Nadeau, R. (1975): Correlation between the response of the heart to sympathetic stimulation and the release of endogenous catecholamines into the coronary sinus of the dog. *Circ. Res.*, 36:662–668.

119. Young, M. A., Hintze, T. H., and Vatner, S. F. (1985): Correlation between cardiac performance and plasma catecholamine levels in conscious dogs. *Am. J. Physiol.*, 248:H82–H88.

The Heart and Cardiovascular System,
edited by H. A. Fozzard et al.
Raven Press, New York © 1986.

CHAPTER 53

Myocardial Ischemia, Hypoxia, and Infarction

Keith A. Reimer and Robert B. Jennings

DEFINITIONS AND CLINICAL IMPORTANCE

Ischemia

Myocardial ischemia has become, in the last several decades, a widespread cause of morbidity and the number-one cause of mortality in the economically developed countries of the Western world. Although the relative importance of coronary deaths has declined gradually during the past decade, approximately 25% of all deaths in the United States were attributed to "heart attacks" in 1982 (6). About half of such deaths occurred suddenly, apparently due to arrhythmias, usually in the setting of underlying coronary atherosclerotic disease. Although the immediate causes of such arrhythmias often are uncertain, a significant proportion occur in the setting of acute myocardial ischemia or infarction. Moreover, the non-sudden "heart attack" deaths, which usually occur following hospitalization, occur as a consequence of myocardial infarction.

The myocardium depends on oxygen delivered by the arterial blood to support high-energy phosphate (HEP) production by oxidative phosphorylation in mitochondria. The latter is the only metabolic process that can provide sufficient chemical energy to support the continuous contractile function of the heart. When the amount of oxygen delivered to the myocardium is insufficient to meet the requirements for mitochondrial respiration, the myocardium begins to produce some, albeit markedly reduced, amounts of HEP by anaerobic glycolysis. Lactate, the end product of anaerobic glycolysis, accumulates. Thus, myocardial ischemia has been defined as an imbalance between the supply of oxygenated blood and the oxygen requirements of the myocardium; major hallmarks of ischemia include reduction in contractile function and the presence of anaerobic glycolysis, as evidenced by accumulation of its metabolic products.

The degree of imbalance between oxygen supply and demand is variable and necessitates qualification of the degree of ischemia as mild, moderate, or severe. Complete abolition of blood flow to a region of myocardium is termed "total ischemia". When ischemia is of sufficient severity and persists long enough, myocytes become "irreversibly injured" and undergo cellular necrosis. Myocyte necrosis caused by myocardial ischemia defines "myocardial infarction." Ischemia is termed "relative" when an imbalance between oxygen supply and demand results from increased myocardial metabolic requirements even though coronary blood flow is maintained. Angina pectoris of the exertional type may be due to relative ischemia. On the other hand, many cases of nonexertional angina and most cases of myocardial infarction are consequences of an absolute reduction in myocardial blood flow. This chapter will be limited, for the most part, to a discussion of severe, absolute ischemia and its eventual result, myocardial infarction.

When myocardial ischemia is confined to a region of the heart but does not affect the entire heart, the term "regional ischemia" is used. In contrast, if the entire heart becomes ischemic, as would occur in cases of severe systemic hypotension or by virtue of aortic cross-clamping necessitated by various cardiac surgical procedures, the term "global ischemia" is employed. Global ischemia, like regional ischemia, can be qualified as to severity based on the degree of blood flow deficit.

Hypoxia/Anoxia

Hypoxia is defined as a supply of oxygen insufficient to meet the oxygen requirements of the tissue. Hypoxia, like ischemia, may range from mild to severe. Complete lack of oxygen is termed "anoxia." Hypoxia is an important component of ischemia. Myocardial hypoxia in its pure form, i.e., without reduced coronary blood flow, occurs at high altitudes, in severe anemia, or in certain types of poisoning; however, it is an infrequent clinical problem. Moreover, when hypoxia is severe, as may be the case with asphyxia or carbon monoxide poisoning, the cerebral consequences often overshadow the cardiac consequences. However, persistent albeit more mild degrees of hypoxia, which can be caused by a variety of conditions, including cyanotic congenital heart disease or severe anemia, can cause progressive cardiac damage and cardiac failure.

Comparison and Contrast of Ischemia and Hypoxia

Many different experimental models have been used to gain knowledge about the myocardial consequences of ischemia and hypoxia. High-flow hypoxia in perfused hearts has been used by many investigators to study various aspects of ischemia. It is important, when interpreting the results of such studies, to recognize that ischemia and hypoxia are not synonymous and that the consequences of hypoxia are not necessarily the same as the consequences of ischemia. Hypoxia is an important, perhaps the most important, component of ischemia. However, reduction of myocardial perfusion results not only in hypoxia but also in a reduced supply of metabolic substrates and reduced removal of catabolites. The distinction between ischemia and hypoxia is most dramatically illustrated by contrasting the potential for energy production via anaerobic glycolysis in ischemia versus anoxia (422,426). In severe or total ischemia, lactate accumulates and tissue acidosis increases. These changes are accompanied by a marked slowing of the rate of anaerobic glycolysis (268,511). The reduced rate of glycolysis is not due to substrate depletion, because glycolysis slows while abundant supplies of glycogen and

glycolytic intermediates are present in the tissue (268,426). The mechanism is thought to be inhibition of glyceraldehyde-3-phosphate dehydrogenase by lactate and NADH, and perhaps also inhibition of phospho-fructokinase by lactate and H^+, and declining availaby of pyruvate (423,510). In contrast, in hypoxia, when lactate accumulation and cellular acidosis are prevented by continued perfusion, anaerobic glycolysis continues at an accelerated rate, so long as substrate (endogenous glycogen or exogenous glucose) remains available (426,511). The consequence of this difference is that in anoxia, HEPs are depleted slowly or not at all, and contractile function is better maintained than in severe ischemia (511,609).

MODELS FOR STUDY

A large number of different experimental models have been developed to study the consequences of myocardial ischemia or hypoxia. The proper choice of an experimental model depends first and foremost on the purpose of one's proposed studies. To understand the importance of some of the differences among various experimental models used to study myocardial ischemia or hypoxia, it is useful to consider, in broad general terms, certain features that may be involved in the biology of ischemia and infarction (Fig. 1) (487). In ischemia, the insufficiency of energy production or the accumulation of catabolites or both quickly inhibit cellular functions, including contractile function and a variety of transport and synthetic functions. Initially, the inhibition of cellular functions is reversible, but eventually damage occurs to some critical subcellular organelle(s) that is irreversible; the myocyte undergoes coagulation necrosis, followed by an inflammatory response, macrophage removal of the dead myocyte, and replacement by scar. Ischemic damage of the microvasculature also occurs; the latter further stimulates the inflammatory response. Whether or not microvascular injury exacerbates the severity of ischemia by impeding perfusion via collateral arterial anastomoses is unknown. In addition, the inflammatory response, per se, might further damage myocytes and/ or capillaries, for example, via production of free radicals (500). However, this hypothesis also is unproven.

If reperfusion occurs, either spontaneously or through experimental or clinical intervention, the consequences depend on the state of the myocardium at the time reperfusion occurs. For example, if reperfusion is established when myocytes and microvasculature are still in the "reversible" phase of injury, cell death is prevented, and cellular ultrastructure and metabolic and contractile functions eventually recover. Conversely, if myocytes have been "irreversibly" injured, restoration of blood flow results not in cellular recovery but rather in explosive swelling of the myocytes, massive calcium overload, and disruption of the myofibrillar apparatus (267,484). These

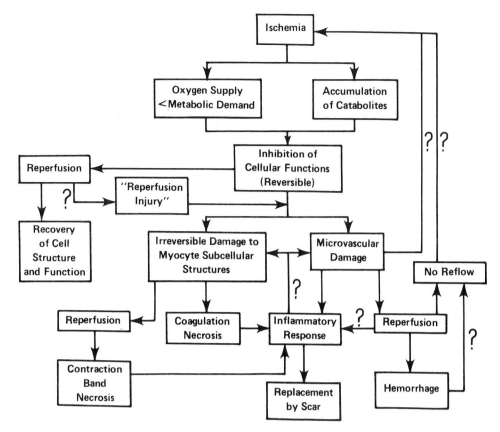

FIG. 1. Components of myocardial ischemia, infarction, and repair. Myocardial infarction is a dynamic process in which cardiac myocytes undergo necrosis and eventual replacement by scar. Myocyte necrosis occurs as a direct consequence of ischemic injury. In addition, microvascular damage occurs; it is uncertain whether or not and in what circumstances microvascular damage exacerbates ischemia. The inflammatory response is essential for the eventual repair of an infarct. It is possible, but unproven, that the inflammatory response may exacerbate myocyte cell injury and contribute to overall infarct size. (From ref. 478, with permission.)

changes are evident at the light-microscopic level as "contraction-band necrosis." Reperfusion should be uniform if the microvasculature is still intact at the onset of reperfusion. On the other hand, if severe microvascular injury has occurred, reperfusion of an occluded artery may result in heterogeneous reperfusion of the myocardium. Thus, microvascular damage could result in persistent or even progressive myocardial ischemia despite reopening of the occluded artery.

Although contraction-band necrosis and microvascular damage may occur during reperfusion, it is not known if they are important contributing factors to ultimate myocardial infarct size (267,481). A currently popular, albeit yet unproven, concept is that some myocytes, only reversibly injured by ischemia up to the moment of reperfusion, are killed by the restoration of arterial blood flow to the tissue ("reperfusion injury") (147,280,502). If this hypothesis is correct, some ischemic myocytes that die despite reperfusion might be salvageable if the reperfusion conditions are appropriately modified.

To the extent that the complex interactions among myocytes and between myocytes and other tissue ele-

ments such as leukocytes or endothelial cells are important components of myocardial ischemic injury, results from experimental studies of ischemia in vivo would be more applicable than results from studies of isolated cells. For example, possible myocyte damage from free radicals produced by endothelial cells or leukocytes would be eliminated from an isolated myocyte preparation. Thus, by reproducing only certain components of myocardial ischemic injury, important steps in the pathogenesis of cell death might be removed from the experimental setting.

For another example, disruption of the plasmalemma has been observed at the onset of irreversible ischemic cell injury in vivo (261,266,276). In contrast, such membrane disruption often has not been detected in in vitro models of myocardial hypoxic injury (276). One possible reason for this difference between ischemia in vivo and hypoxia in vitro may be a greater degree of cell swelling during ischemia than in hypoxia. During ischemia in vivo, large osmotic forces may be caused by intracellular retention of metabolic end-products because the extracellular space is small and prevents removal of such catabolites. In contrast, with isolated cells, incubated slices, or isolated perfused hearts, an essentially infinite extracellular space permits diffusion of intracellular metabolites and electrolytes into the medium or effluent (272,580).

On the other hand, events within a single box shown in Fig. 1 often can be studied in a setting where interpretation of results is not clouded by the possible interaction of many other factors that may contribute to injury *in vivo*. For example, injurious agents, either exogenous metabolic inhibitors or endogenous catabolites, can be delivered to isolated cells in precise dosage without the need for an intact vasculature to deliver the agent; the extracellular environment can be precisely controlled and can be altered quickly during the course of an experiment; interventions can be studied in isolated cells that could not be studied *in vivo* because of systemic toxicity. Some additional advantages and limitations of various models will be considered in the following paragraphs.

Ischemia

Global (and Total) Ischemia In Situ

Successful completion of many cardiac surgical procedures requires temporary creation of a bloodless surgical field with an arrested heart. This is achieved during cardiopulmonary bypass by cross-clamping the aorta and thereby eliminating all coronary flow. Global (and total) ischemia, produced by identical procedures in experimental animals, particularly dogs, has been widely used to study the metabolic and functional consequences of temporary total ischemia. Such models have also been widely used to optimize cardioplegic solutions and surgical techniques with the aim of preserving myocardial integrity and postischemic functional recovery.

Regional Ischemia In Vivo

Temporary or permanent occlusion of one or more coronary arteries to create regional ischemia is commonly employed to reproduce the major features of myocardial ischemia or infarction, as observed clinically in patients with coronary disease. Several species of animals have been used for such studies, and the relative merits of each have been widely debated. For example, some humans have few collateral anastomoses between major coronary arteries; an acute coronary occlusion would be expected to cause severe, transmural ischemia. It has been argued that pigs (135,364) or nonhuman primates (96,634), which also have few collateral anastomoses, would most closely represent patients of this type. On the other hand, some patients, particularly those with long-standing coronary atherosclerotic disease, do develop extensive collateral connections. The functional

importance of such connections is readily apparent from postmortem observations; total atherosclerotic coronary occlusions with little scarring of the region of myocardium supplied by the occluded artery are common findings. This may be analogous to the situation in the dog heart, which normally has preformed collateral anastomoses, where coronary occlusion causes severe subendocardial ischemia, but often causes only moderate or mild ischemia in the subepicardial zone of the ischemic region (29,37,475).

Smaller animals such as rats have also been used extensively for studies of regional myocardial ischemia and infarction. The rat model has been advocated for screening for possible therapeutic efficacy of interventions designed to limit myocardial infarct size (128,142,338,450). A major advantage of the rat model is its low cost and simplicity as compared with models using larger animal species. However, because of the small size of rat hearts, base-line variables that influence infarct size, such as the total amount and local distribution of collateral blood flow, cannot be readily measured or controlled. Additionally, the small size of rat coronary arteries make temporary occlusion and reperfusion technically difficult. Because of this, most studies utilizing rats do not allow reperfusion, but rather have permanent occlusions. The inherent variability of the model and the inability to correct for base-line variables limit the precision of results that can be obtained from this model; the applicability to patients of results obtained from smaller species has not been established.

It also must be recognized that the experimental procedures for inducing regional ischemia in any species will not reproduce precisely all of the features of coronary occlusion and myocardial infarction seen clinically. For example, in dogs, the most commonly used species for cardiovascular studies, myocardial infarction often is induced by sudden occlusion of a major coronary artery. This most closely mimics sudden occlusion of a previously normal or mildly diseased coronary artery by thromboembolism (a relatively uncommon cause of myocardial infarction). The prior existence of severe narrowing of the occluded vessel and the coexistence of severe disease in other coronary vessels are not reproduced in the usual experimental setting. Moreover, sudden occlusion by an arterial snare does not reproduce the potentially gradual or intermittent development of an intracoronary thrombus. Reproduction of such clinical features of disease may be an advantage for certain experimental questions. Conversely, for many experimental questions, reproduction of such clinical details would be inappropriate. For example, the results of studies to establish therapeutic interventions that could limit infarct size are most precise when the onset, severity, and duration of ischemic injury are clearly defined, even though such well-defined conditions do not always occur in the clinical setting.

Complex animal models have been developed to reproduce other features of acute myocardial ischemia and infarction. For example, awake-animal models have been utilized in order to study the consequences of myocardial ischemia in the setting of intact cardiovascular physiology, including sympathetic and parasympathetic reflexes (284,338,482,492). Such studies are essential to learn to what degree the pathophysiologic responses to ischemia or cardiac sensitivity to drugs are altered by anesthetic agents or an open thoracotomy. A disadvantage of such models is the high cost in time and effort required. For example, awake-animal models often entail initial surgery for placement of coronary snares and/or monitoring devices, with follow-up care and training, before the actual experimental study can be done.

In some models, coronary occlusions have been done via catheterization followed by balloon occlusion (87) or coronary embolization (71) or by electrical induction of thrombi (499). These occlusion techniques have the advantage of avoiding the damage to the coronary vessels and adjacent nerves that might be caused by direct dissection. However, embolic methods have the disadvantage that the initial site of occlusion is difficult to control, and an embolus may migrate distally during the ischemic period. Also, coronary catheterization requires the availability of fluoroscopic equipment. Induction of an intracoronary thrombus mimics the most common cause of acute myocardial ischemia and infarction in humans; to the extent that gradual versus sudden occlusion or activated platelets (399) influence the ischemic process, use of a thrombosis model could contribute to our understanding of myocardial ischemia in humans. Conversely, as noted previously, the duration and severity of ischemia are difficult to monitor in such models.

Intact-animal preparations (either anesthetized or awake) are essential for a variety of types of studies. For example, studies of the determinants of myocardial infarct size, the effects of therapy on infarct size, the long-term functional or metabolic consequences of brief episodes of ischemia, factors that influence arrhythmogenesis, etc., can be done only in an intact-animal preparation. However, the creation of regional ischemia *in vivo* is accompanied by inherent variables that must be considered. For example, coronary occlusion in dogs does not cause total ischemia to the entire vascular region of the occluded artery, because collateral flow occurs by way of interarterial anastomoses. The severity of ischemia varies among individual animals and from area to area within the ischemic region of a given animal. Studies of the metabolic, structural, or functional consequences of ischemia can be interpreted only if the severity of ischemia is controlled, or at least known.

In summary, each animal model has advantages and limitations that must be considered in relation to specific experimental questions that are posed. Relative to the pathophysiology of myocardial ischemia and infarction, it seems likely that some patients' hearts are more like those of pigs or baboons, and others resemble those of dogs. For many experimental questions, open-chest animal models suffice and have the advantage of relative simplicity; some experimental questions can be answered only using an awake-animal model.

Total or Low-Flow Ischemia In Vitro

The acute consequences of myocardial ischemia often are studied more easily by selecting an isolated heart model. In such models, uniform, total ischemia (no collateral perfusion) can be readily created. The simplest *in vitro* models of ischemia consist of excised nonperfused hearts (218,358) or portions of myocardium, retained at controlled temperature in a humid environment (268,483). The progression of metabolic or ultrastructural changes within the ischemic myocardium can be readily followed in such a preparation. Ischemia thus can be studied as an isolated entity, without the superimposed influences of hemodynamic and neurophysiologic variables (an advantage or disadvantage, depending on the nature of the experimental question).

The isolated, blood-perfused myocardial septum (27,555) has been used to combine the advantages of uniform, controlled severity of ischemia with the capability of following short-term postischemic recovery and to assess the effects of altered blood electrolytes or of pharmacologic interventions. Metabolic and electrolyte changes can be monitored by comparing concentrations in arterial and venous blood effluents. Blood perfusion permits adequate myocardial oxygenation during preischemic and postischemic periods, but the presence of the cellular elements of blood also may cause unwanted difficulties, e.g., microvascular obstruction by thrombi. In addition, a donor source of blood is required.

Isolated perfused hearts from small mammals, in particular rabbits and rats, have been widely used for studies of myocardial metabolism and functional, metabolic, or structural responses to myocardial injury. These isolated heart preparations are classified generally as either nonworking or working heart models. The suitability of either model for studies of myocardial ischemia or hypoxia has been reviewed (107,373,608, Chapter 7). Briefly, various versions of the "Langendorf" preparations are nonworking models in that the left ventricle does not eject perfusate into the aortic root; coronary flow is provided by retrograde aortic perfusion at constant pressure that keeps the aortic valve closed. In contrast, in working heart preparations, as first developed by Neely et al. (421), perfusate is supplied via a cannula in the left atrium; left ventricular contraction provides pulsatile antegrade aortic and coronary flow. Aortic and coronary flow and aortic pressure can be measured; left atrial pressure or flow or aortic pressure can be controlled, thereby permitting control of cardiac external work and/or permitting calculation of pressure–volume function curves.

With either type of model, the isolated hearts are by definition denervated, but nevertheless contract spontaneously. Faster heart rates can be obtained by pacing. Most investigators have used a buffered solution (commonly Krebs-Henseleit bicarbonate buffer) with added substrate, usually glucose. Other substrates such as pyruvate and free fatty acids also can be employed. Perfusate temperature, pH, electrolyte content, and substrate availability can all be readily controlled. Metabolic pathways can be studied by measuring the output of metabolites into the effluent. Similarly, the degree of myocardial damage can be assessed by light or electron microscopy or by monitoring the release of large intracellular proteins, such as myoglobin or creatine kinase. The use of a non-blood solution circumvents perfusion problems that would arise due to platelet microaggregation or fibrin deposits in the microcirculation. By gassing the perfusate with 95% oxygen, high oxygen tension can be achieved. Nevertheless, such oxygenated buffers have only limited oxygen-carrying capacity. In addition, unless colloid content is replaced, interstitial myocardial edema occurs. Total or low-flow global ischemia can be induced in isolated perfused models by simply clamping the aortic or left atrial inflow cannulas.

Whereas these models have several advantages, including simplicity of design and easy control of hemodynamic variables and perfusate composition, isolated perfused models differ from intact hearts in a variety of respects, including denervation and removal of cellular blood elements, which may contribute to ischemic injury *in vivo*. In addition, alterations in myocardial composition during an initial equilibration period could alter the subsequent cellular response to ischemia in important ways. For example, if perfusion during an initial equilibration period results in the development of interstitial edema, the effect of ischemia on myocyte osmolarity or electrolyte content could be substantially modified (272). Moreover, interstitial edema may contribute to nonuniform perfusion in studies of postischemic recovery. Studies of postischemic recovery may be limited by nonuniform reperfusion, caused by microvascular compression, not only from interstitial edema but also because of the onset of contracture rigor (243,244). The latter can be prevented and perfusion better maintained if diastolic ventricular volume is maintained by placing a fluid-filled balloon into the left ventricular cavity prior to the initiation of ischemic or hypoxic conditions (161).

It also is important to recognize that with all models using isolated hearts, studies of postischemic recovery are limited to acute functional or biochemical recovery. Long-term studies such as those involving measurement of infarct size or the time course of biochemical and functional recovery require an intact animal. With any *in vitro* model, "irreversible" injury can be defined only in a relative sense, dictated by the short-term stability of the experimental preparation. Reversible and irreversible injury, which we define in terms of cellular viability, cannot be evaluated in absolute biologic terms *in vitro*. For example, although myocytes that have been lethally injured cannot recover contractile function, failure to fully recover contractile function immediately following ischemic or hypoxic myocardial injury does not necessarily imply that some cells have been killed. Viable myocytes may fail to contract or may contract weakly for a variety of reasons.

Hypoxia

Hypoxia is obviously an important component of ischemia, and much has been gained from studies of the effects of hypoxia on cardiac muscle. The most commonly employed experimental models have utilized isolated perfused hearts as described in the previous section.

Alternatively, vascular changes that could influence perfusability can be avoided by using thin slices of myocardium (162,194,276), fetal mouse hearts in culture (251,317), or isolated fetal or adult cardiac myocytes (*vide infra*) that do not depend on an intact vasculature for oxygenation. However, the accuracy of metabolite or electrolyte data obtained from myocardial slices is reduced by unavoidable damage of surface myocytes during slice preparation. Slice thickness is critical; diffusion of oxygen to the slice center will be inadequate if the slice is too thick (56), whereas the proportion of damaged myocytes will be excessive if the slice is too thin.

Isolated cardiac myocytes have become increasingly popular for experimental studies to elucidate mechanisms of cell injury (5,58,378,411,456,457,487,547). Isolated cardiac myocytes, by definition, have been physically separated from all other types of cells with which they ordinarily interact in an intact, functioning heart. Thus, isolated myocytes, similar to all isolated *in vitro* preparations, have lost their normal neurohumoral modulation; sympathetic neural innervation is abolished, and even catecholamine-containing nerve endings are removed. Also, intravascular cellular elements such as leukocytes and platelets are eliminated. In addition, isolated myocytes differ from those in intact working hearts in that they are under no stimulus to perform external work; moreover, they are not subject to the possible traumatic effects of work done on them by other working myocytes. In other words, the possible consequences of repetitive stretch and compression of an ischemic region of myocardium imposed by nonischemic functional tissue in an *in vivo* model of regional ischemia cannot be a factor in isolated myocytes. With isolated myocytes, interactions between the microvasculature and the myocyte also are eliminated. Thus, metabolic pathways requiring the interaction of myocytes and microvasculature are eliminated. For example, the degradation of adenine nucleotides in ischemic myocardium results in accumulation of hypoxanthine and xanthine. The final steps of this degradation are promoted by the enzymes nucleoside phosphorylase and xanthine oxidase, respectively. Nucleoside phosphorylase (174,514) and perhaps xanthine oxidase are localized in endothelial cells or pericytes, but are absent from cardiac myocytes. Another important difference between isolated myocytes and intact myocardium is that intact myocardium has a limited extracellular volume into which metabolic end-products and intracellular potassium can diffuse (in the absence of vascular perfusion), whereas isolated myocytes are bathed in a medium that, for practical purposes, is infinite. This difference may affect intracellular concentrations of electrolytes and metabolites during energy-deficient conditions.

In addition to the loss of interactions between cardiac myocytes and other tissue components, isolated myocytes may have altered properties because of the process of isolation per se (118,119,155,221). For example, myocyte isolation requires treatment of the tissue with a variety of digestive enzymes, such as collagenase or hyaluronidase, in order to remove the collagen struts and other constituents of the extracellular matrix that compose the skeletal framework of the heart. In addition, myocytes must be separated from their attachments to each other at the intercalated discs (656). This usually is accomplished by brief exposure to a calcium-free solution. Exposure to digestive enzymes alters and usually removes the glycocalyx (basal lamina) of the sarcolemma. In addition, it is unclear whether or not mixtures of proteolytic enzymes may alter protein constituents of the plasmalemma and thereby alter the functions of ion channels, cell surface receptors, etc. Thus, the isolated myocyte may prove to be an inappropriate model for studies of some sarcolemmal functions.

The removal of calcium to separate intercalated discs must be precisely controlled in order to minimize the development of calcium intolerance, i.e., the cellular equivalent of the calcium-paradox phenomenon (164,193,660). A proportion of calcium-intolerant myocytes may be an inevitable consequence of subjecting adult cardiac myocytes to even a brief calcium-free period. In addition, whereas removal of calcium causes separation of macula and fascia adherens junctions of intercalated discs, the nexuses (gap junctions), which are the sites of electrochemical coupling between cardiac myocytes, do not separate, but rupture, especially during calcium repletion; the complete nexus is retained by one cell, whereas a hole is created in the cell membrane of the other (287,390).

Either neonatal or adult cardiac myocytes are used for experimental studies. Either can be studied immediately after isolation or can be maintained in culture and studied later (344,455,504). Myocytes maintained in culture for several days have the opportunity to repair sublethal injury induced by the isolation procedures. However, cultured cardiac myocytes may become contaminated with an overgrowth of proliferating fibroblasts; precautions are required to prevent or to control this problem (38,76,241). Neonatal myocytes are more easily maintained in culture, but they have a variety of structural and functional differences from adult myocytes (229). For example, they contain relatively few myofibrils and depend chiefly on glycolytic energy production (117,504). The latter may alter the metabolic response of these cells to injury.

BIOLOGY OF MYOCARDIAL ISCHEMIA AND INFARCTION

Etiology in Humans

Underlying Coronary Disease

In virtually all people who develop myocardial ischemia, coronary vascular disease exists as an underlying anatomic substrate; moreover, in most people with long-standing coronary artery narrowing, the cause is atherosclerotic. Less frequent causes of chronic coronary stenosis include inflammatory disease, such as polyarteritis nodosa, rheumatic or rheumatoid arteritis, or thromboangiitis obliterans (Buerger's disease). Coronary deposits of amyloid or epicardial tumors rarely may cause progressive obstruction of myocardial arteries. Narrowing of the coronary ostia may be caused by atherosclerosis of the aortic root or, less commonly, by syphilitic aortitis.

Causes of Sudden Onset of Ischemia

The majority of myocardial infarcts involve myocardium supplied by a single coronary artery. When studied post-mortem in the acute phase, a majority (but not all) of such infarcts can be related to recent occlusion of a coronary artery, usually by thrombosis superimposed on preexisting atherosclerotic disease (100,337,495,562). In many cases of coronary thrombosis, the thrombi contain fragments of atherosclerotic plaque. Disruption of the endothelial surface, with consequent hemorrhage into the plaque and rupture of plaque contents into the residual coronary lumen, can be found in association with nearly all coronary thrombi if serial histologic sections are examined (Fig. 2). Based on such observations, several investigators have postulated that the immediate cause of coronary thrombosis is almost always

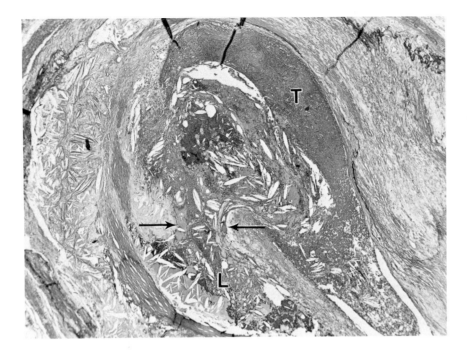

FIG. 2. Cross section of an occluded coronary artery from a patient who died of myocardial infarction. There is disruption of the fibrous cap (*arrows*) of a partially occlusive atherosclerotic plaque that has permitted expulsion of necrotic debris from the underlying lipid pool (L) into the residual lumen of the artery. This plaque rupture is associated with thrombotic (T) occlusion of the remaining lumen.

the prior disruption of the atherosclerotic plaque (72,99,131,154,490).

Myocardial infarction also may be caused by thromboemboli in the presence or absence of underlying atherosclerotic narrowing. The source of coronary emboli may be mural thrombi of the left atrium or ventricle, valvular vegetations in the setting of infectious endocarditis, or nonbacterial thrombotic (marantic) endocarditis. Atrial fibrillation is a common predisposing cause of atrial thrombi; ventricular mural thrombi can be associated with any cause of endocardial injury or turbulent flow, including congestive cardiomyopathies or previous myocardial infarction.

In a significant minority of fatal cases of myocardial infarction there is no postmortem anatomic explanation for the initiation of the infarct. In such cases the coronary artery normally supplying the region of infarct either may be open or may be occluded by atherosclerotic plaque antedating the myocardial infarct (337). In the latter situation it must be presumed that myocardial infarction was precipitated by interference with blood flow through collateral arterial anastomoses. In either case, the absence of an acute coronary event requires the postulate that the infarct was caused by a dynamic event, i.e., a transient obstruction of coronary blood flow that initiated the infarct but was no longer demonstrable at the time of autopsy (182). A likely cause of dynamic coronary occlusion is thrombosis or embolism, with subsequent spontaneous thrombolysis (438). Alternatively, in recent years, coronary artery spasm alone, or in conjunction with platelet aggregation, has become a recognized cause of acute myocardial ischemia (148,380,433).

The frequency of spontaneous coronary thrombolysis is unknown. However, in recent years, with the advent of emergency coronary bypass surgery, or more commonly emergency coronary angiography for the purpose of identifying lesions amenable to thrombolytic therapy, coronary thrombi have been observed in association with 80 to 90% or more of acute myocardial infarcts. For example, DeWood et al. (111) reported coronary thrombi in 87% of patients studied angiographically within 4 hr of the onset of symptoms. This incidence of occlusive thrombi observed in living patients studied acutely is higher than the incidence observed in most postmortem studies (range 21–91%) (496). Moreover, in the studies of DeWood et al. (111), the incidence of thrombi decreased with increasing duration of symptoms. These clinical studies suggest that thrombosis is a more frequent cause of myocardial infarction than had previously been suspected. In addition, the decreasing incidence of thrombi with increasing duration of symptoms is circumstantial evidence favoring spontaneous thrombolysis.

Coronary spasm, if prolonged, might cause myocardial infarction. In addition, the possible interactions among endothelial injury, platelet microaggregation, release of prostaglandins and other vasoactive substances, and coronary spasm have sparked considerable interest (379). However, the relative frequency of coronary vasospasm as a cause of acute myocardial infarction remains unknown.

Hemodynamic disturbances that cause increased myocardial metabolic demands or reduced coronary perfusion pressure or both also may cause myocardial infarction. Subendocardial myocardial infarcts often are unassociated with coronary thrombi and may be the consequence of hemodynamic disturbances superimposed on severe coronary atherosclerotic disease. Circumferential subendocardial infarcts may be caused by transient hypotension in the presence or absence of generalized atherosclerotic coronary disease. Anatomic causes of reduced coronary perfusion pressure include aortic stenosis or insufficiency and hypertrophic cardiomyopathy with aortic outflow obstruction.

Location and Time Course of Myocyte Necrosis

It is now generally accepted that following coronary occlusion, ischemic myocytes do not die instantaneously, mildly ischemic myocytes may survive indefinitely, and within the region that does undergo infarction, not all myocytes die simultaneously (475,485). These concepts are crucially important; they form the basis for experimental and clinical efforts to design therapy that can limit myocardial infarct size (227). However, the time course of ischemic cell death during myocardial infarction cannot be easily established in humans. Thus, the duration of time during which therapy could conceivably limit myocardial infarct size can be estimated only crudely from indirect assessments of infarct size or cardiac function in large clinical trials, or from more direct studies of the time course of myocardial infarction in the experimental animal. Thus, the following paragraphs will review the location and time course of ischemic cell death in experimental animals and the physiologic basis for this time course.

Experimental Coronary Occlusion in Dogs

In dogs, as well as in humans, the subendocardial zone of the myocardial wall is more susceptible to myocardial infarction (337,475,485). This increased susceptibility may be related to a more severe degree of ischemia in this zone following coronary occlusion or to greater metabolic requirements of the subendocardial zone, or both. In order to understand the basis for such transmural differences, it is necessary to understand the major determinants of myocardial metabolic requirements and of myocardial blood flow.

Determinants of myocardial metabolic rate and coronary blood flow.

The energy requirements of the myocardium include requirements for basal metabolism, for electrical activation, i.e., membrane depolarization and repolarization, and for the performance of internal and external mechanical work. The energy required for mechanical work includes the energy required to develop and maintain systolic tension, as well as the energy required to deactivate the contractile system (53,54). Basal oxygen requirements, e.g., the requirements of an electrically

arrested, normothermic heart on cardiopulmonary bypass, have been estimated to be about 0.7 to 2.0 ml O_2/min/100 g (45,366), or 20% of total myocardial oxygen consumption (MVO_2) in a beating heart (8–15 ml/min/100 g). In addition to this basal oxygen demand, the energy requirement of electrical activation is about 0.5 ml/min/100 g, i.e., about 5% of total oxygen requirements. This estimate was obtained by pacing, at different rates, hearts that were perfused with blood devoid of ionized calcium (312). Contractile work thus accounts for the majority of myocardial oxygen consumption. However, contractile work and consequently total myocardial energy requirements vary greatly. In general terms, the three major determinants of myocardial oxygen demand are heart rate, myocardial wall tension, and the intrinsic contractile state of the myocardium (Fig. 3) (427,524,574,575). Wall tension is related (by the law of Laplace) to more readily measurable parameters, i.e., ventricular volume and ventricular pressure; contractility is often estimated by measuring maximum dP/dt, the maximal rate of increase in systolic pressure.

Under any set of hemodynamic conditions, and at all phases of the cardiac cycle, there is a transmural gradient of wall tension, with tension greatest in the subendocardial region and least in the subepicardial region (15,303,518). For this reason, the energy requirements for contraction of subendocardial myocardium exceed those of subepicardial myocardium (121). In addition, there is evidence that basal oxygen requirements of subendocardial myocardium may exceed those of subepicardial myocardium. For example, recent studies of

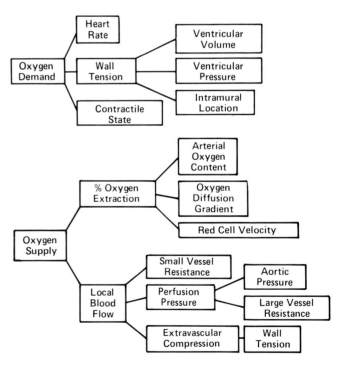

FIG. 3. Major determinants of local metabolic rate (oxygen demand) and myocardial oxygen delivery.

excised transmural slabs of dog heart have shown more rapid ATP depletion from the subendocardial region, even though the experimental preparation eliminated transmural differences in myocardial wall tension and collateral blood flow (357).

Major factors that determine the oxygen supply to any region of myocardium also are illustrated in Fig. 3. In general terms, oxygen supply is determined by the local rate of capillary perfusion and by the amount of oxygen that can be extracted from the blood. Oxygen extraction may vary according to the oxygen content of arterial blood and be affected by the oxygen diffusion gradient and by red cell velocity through the capillaries. However, under normal circumstances oxygen extraction is high, averaging about 75%. Although oxygen extraction can be as high as 90% in extreme conditions, such as hemorrhagic shock, there is insufficient reserve oxygen in capillary blood to cover the major variations in MVO_2 that occur with varying myocardial work loads. Normally, oxygen extraction is fairly constant, and major changes in metabolic demand are met by corresponding changes in the local rate of blood flow, i.e., coronary blood flow is tightly matched to myocardial oxygen needs. This metabolic regulation of coronary blood flow is achieved through control of the vascular resistance of precapillary arterioles. A closely related phenomenon, autoregulation, is the capability of the heart to maintain constant coronary flow (at constant oxygen requirements) despite variation in coronary perfusion pressure (402). The metabolic bases for both metabolic vasoregulation and autoregulation are incompletely understood. Considerable evidence has been amassed favoring a role for either adenosine (33) or K^+ (31) in metabolic vasoregulation. Moreover, it seems unlikely that a single metabolic vasodilator can account for both metabolic vasoregulation and autoregulation (331). Additional putative mediators of either autoregulation and/or vasoregulation include prostaglandins and oxygen tension in the tissue or precapillary arterioles. For autoregulation, a myogenic mechanism also has been proposed. H^+ and PCO_2 have been studied but seem less likely to be involved in either regulatory mechanism (31,542).

If myocardial oxygen requirements are increased markedly, and/or if coronary perfusion pressure is reduced sufficiently, the precapillary resistance vessels become dilated maximally; the limits of vasoregulatory control are exceeded. Under such circumstances of maximum precapillary vasodilation, local microvascular perfusion becomes dependent on the arteriolar perfusion pressure, counterbalanced by extravascular compressive force (8). Arteriolar perfusion pressure is in turn determined by aortic pressure and by the resistance across the larger coronary arteries or, in the case of severe narrowing or occlusion of the native artery, resistance across collateral arterial anastomoses.

Because of systolic microvascular compression, coronary blood flow occurs in a phasic pattern such that diastolic coronary blood flow exceeds systolic flow (519). As noted previously, systolic intramyocardial pressure is greatest in the subendocardial region. Thus, in systole, subendocardial coronary flow is impeded to a greater extent than is subepicardial flow (116,219,523). Nevertheless, because of reduced coronary resistance in the subendocardium, diastolic flow is preferentially shunted to this zone (326); overall blood flow to the subendocardial region normally equals or exceeds subepicardial flow. However, if maximum arteriolar vasodilation occurs, because of coronary stenosis or hypotension, a gradient of coronary blood flow develops in inverse relation to the intramyocardial pressure gradient (14). It has been consistently observed in experimental models of coronary occlusion that if there is collateral blood flow available, it is distributed disproportionately to the subepicardial zone of the ischemic region (Fig. 4) (30,121,475,492,652).

Transmural progression of ischemic cell death.

The time course of ischemic cell death has been most clearly demonstrated by studies in which various periods of temporary coronary occlusion have been followed by reperfusion. In anesthetized, open-chest dogs, even the most severely ischemic myocytes remain viable for at least 15 min (273,275). If reperfusion is established during this time interval, infarction can be prevented, and cellular metabolism, ultrastructure, and contractile function all eventually recover. Beyond 15 min of coronary occlusion in this experimental model, increasing numbers of ischemic myocytes become irreversibly injured, as defined by the fact that reperfusion does not prevent subsequent infarction. By 40 min, much of the subendocardial zone, if severely ischemic, has been irreversibly injured (275,475). Nevertheless, much of the midepicardial and subepicardial region is still viable; reperfusion prevents infarction of these zones. With increasing duration of coronary occlusion, a transmural "wavefront" of cell death progresses from the subendocardium to the subepicardium (Fig. 5) (475,485); if ischemia is uninterrupted, infarcts eventually involve an average of 80% of the ischemic region. Reperfusion at 3 hr can limit the transmural extent of the infarct by about 10%, but by 6 hr, infarcts have reached their full size; infarct size is not influenced by reperfusion at this time (475). A similar temporal evolution of myocardial infarcts, beginning in the subendocardial region, and only later involving the subepicardial region, has been observed in awake as well as anesthetized dogs and in other species, including rabbits, pigs, and baboons (26,85,156,171,310,313,535,625). In all such experimental models of abrupt coronary occlusion, the spatial evolution of infarction is complete in 6 hr or less.

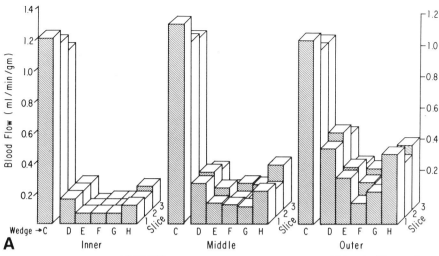

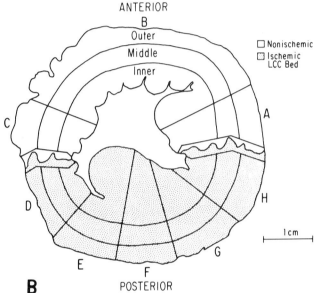

FIG. 4. Three-dimensional distribution of coronary collateral blood flow within the vascular region anatomically supplied by the occluded circumflex coronary artery in anesthetized dogs. The data represent means of collateral blood flow mapped in 7 animals (**A**). In each heart, the anatomic area at risk was identified by postmortem simultaneous perfusion of the occluded circumflex and nonoccluded left main arteries with different-colored dyes. After formalin fixation, the ventricles were cut into four transverse slices (basal slice = slice 1; apical slice = slice 4). Blood flow was mapped in slices 1–3; slice 4 was excluded. Each slice was divided into wedges of nonischemic and ischemic regions as diagrammed in the lower panel. One to three millimeters of tissue was trimmed from the ischemic/nonischemic interfaces to eliminate visible admixture of the two regions. Each wedge was further subdivided into inner, middle, and outer thirds. In the upper panel, nonischemic blood flows in wedges A and B have been eliminated for simplicity; they did not differ substantially from the values illustrated from wedge C. Note that collateral blood flow within any one transmural layer (i.e. inner, middle, or outer) was similar throughout the three central wedges (E, F, and G) of all three slices. However, there was a marked transmural gradient of collateral flow, increasing from the subendocardial layer to subepicardial layer. Mean collateral flow also was slightly higher in lateral and septal than in the three central wedges of each layer; however, analysis of individual samples indicated that these higher means were most likely due to contamination of some samples with nonischemic tissue, despite the careful sampling procedure (**B**). Thus, there is a prominent transmural gradient of collateral flow, but the severity of ischemia is relatively uniform throughout a given layer. [From studies of Long et al. (356).]

It is logical to reason that the transmural wavefront of myocardial cell death after coronary occlusion in dogs is caused by the transmural gradient of collateral blood flow, i.e., that the subendocardial region dies quickly because it is severely ischemic (flow <0.15 ml/min/g) and that the subepicardial region dies more slowly because it often is only moderately ischemic (flow 0.15–0.30 ml/min/g) or mildly ischemic (flow >0.30 ml/min/g) (259). On the other hand, there is evidence that transmural differences in collateral blood flow are not the sole explanation for the transmural wavefront of cell death. In both pigs (156,310,625) and primates (171,336) there is virtually no native collateral blood

flow to the ischemic region; the subepicardial zone is as severely ischemic as the subendocardial region. Nevertheless, analyses of both ultrastructure and infarct location (following reperfusion) in these species indicate the existence of a transmural wavefront of irreversible cellular injury despite the absence of a blood flow gradient. Also, in studies in which myocardium has been made totally ischemic *in vivo* or *in vitro*, ultrastructural and metabolic features of cell injury have occurred more quickly in the subendocardial region than in the subepicardial region, despite the transmural absence of blood flow (123,357). Thus, transmural differences in myocardial work load or basal metabolic needs may

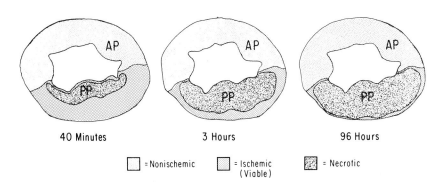

FIG. 5. Progression of cell death versus time after circumflex coronary occlusion in dogs. Necrosis occurs first in the subendocardial myocardium. With longer occlusions, a wavefront of cell death moves from the subendocardial zone across the wall to involve progressively more of the transmural thickness of the ischemic zone. In contrast, the lateral margins in the subendocardial region of the infarct are established as early as 40 min after occlusion and are sharply defined by the anatomic boundaries of the ischemic bed. AP = anterior papillary muscle; PP = posterior papillary muscle. (From ref. 475, with permission.)

contribute to the transmural progression of injury. Recent studies in anesthetized dogs indicate considerable differences between the subendocardial and subepicardial metabolic responses to coronary occlusion (Fig. 6) and suggest that both collateral blood flow and transmural location are independent determinants of these differences (Fig. 7) (412). In the final analysis, the volume of collateral flow determines whether or not myocytes die (*vide infra*). Metabolic factors affect the rate at which cell death occurs.

Lateral boundaries of infarct—relation to vascular area at risk.

There has been much controversy over the existence and width of ischemic gradients at the lateral bound-

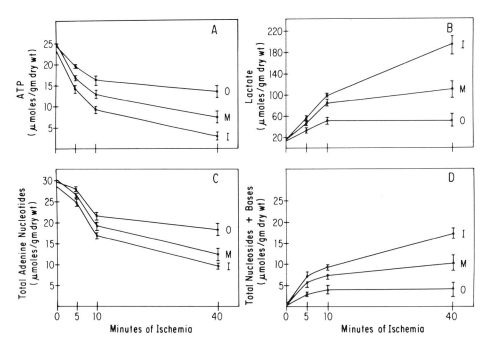

FIG. 6. Time course of metabolic changes during myocardial ischemia plotted by transmural layer (I = inner, subendocardial; M = middle; O = outer subepicardial). Ischemia was induced by circumflex occlusion in anesthetized dogs. Data for different times are based on different groups of dogs; N = 4 to 6; brackets indicate plus or minus one standard error of the mean. **A:** More rapid depletion of ATP in the inner layer, highly significant after 5 min of ischemia ($p < 0.01$). **B:** Tissue lactate accumulation, with the most rapid accumulation in the subendocardium. For all layers there was a progressive increase in lactate content during the first 10 min of ischemia. Between 10 and 40 min there was continued lactate accumulation in the inner and middle layers, but not in the outer layer. **C:** Total adenine nucleotide content (ATP + ADP + AMP). Adenine nucleotide degradation was most rapid in the subendocardium. Note the time lag between ATP depletion (graph A) and adenine nucleotide breakdown. **D:** Total nucleosides and bases, which are the products of adenine nucleotide degradation. Accumulation was fastest in the subendocardium. As with lactate (graph B), nucleoside and base content in the outer layer was maximal by 10 min and was not further increased at 40 min, even though adenine nucleotide breakdown in this layer continued (graph C). [From studies of Murry et al. (412).]

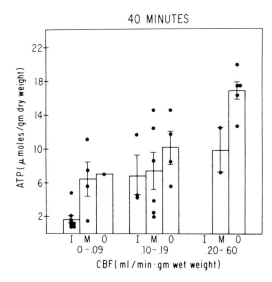

FIG. 7. ATP content after 40 min of ischemia in individual samples of myocardium grouped according to both collateral blood flow and transmural location from which the sample was obtained. (I = inner, subendocardial; M = middle; O = outer, subepicardial). Significant transmural gradients of ATP were detected within the severe (0–0.09 ml/min/g) ($p <$ 0.01) and mild (0.20–0.60 ml/min/g) ($p < 0.05$) ischemia categories. Additionally, analysis of variance showed that for the inner ($p < 0.01$) and outer ($p < 0.05$) layers, samples with high collateral flow had significantly higher ATP levels than those with low collateral flow. Thus, after 40 min of ischemia, ATP content was related both to the amount of collateral flow to the sample and to the transmural location of the sample, independent of flow. [From studies of Murry et al. (412).]

aries of an ischemic region (213). Many studies have shown intermediate values of coronary blood flow (29,212,371,492,533,618), electrophysiologic changes (212, 226,255,256,305), metabolic derangements (34,212, 255,564), functional deficits (593), and ultrastructural or histochemical indices of ischemic cell damage (93, 141,183,442) in samples from the lateral edges of the ischemic region. However, based on more detailed analyses of such observations, the currently favored concept is that there is a sharp transition, an "interface" rather than a "border zone," between ischemic and nonischemic myocardium (Fig. 8) (129,206,231,375,409,475,563,654). The observations of intermediate levels of blood flow deprivation, metabolite alterations, functional depression, etc., most likely have been due to the failure of investigators to precisely identify the interface between ischemic and nonischemic myocardium, or to otherwise correct for the admixture of ischemic and nonischemic tissue in samples. In the latter-mentioned studies, when the ischemic/nonischemic interface has been carefully identified, lateral gradients have been narrow.

It now seems most likely that this sharp transition can be explained on the basis that the important collateral anastomoses between major coronary arteries are on the epicardial surface of the heart (531). The myocardium

is perfused through smaller penetrating branches of these larger surface arteries (Fig. 9). Although both subepicardial and intramural collateral anastomoses have been described in various species (39,254), the functional importance of the latter has been debated (120,129). Recent anatomic studies suggest that the penetrating intramural arteries are essentially end arteries, with few or no interconnections between adjacent capillary beds (Fig. 6) (129). If so, there is no anatomic explanation based on intramural vascular connections for the existence of broad lateral border zones of intermediate severity of ischemia.

However, a narrow border zone of intermediate ischemic injury (34,183) might occur by virtue of interdigitation of ischemic and nonischemic capillary networks, combined with intramyocardial diffusion of oxygen and metabolites over short distances (563). In dogs with coronary occlusion followed by reperfusion as early as 40 min after the onset, the resulting subendocardial infarcts extend to within 1 or 2 mm of the edge of the occluded vascular beds (475). A similar narrow rim of viable myocytes persists even if coronary ligations are permanent (probably because of tissue diffusion of oxygen and metabolites) (475). These results provide direct evidence against the existence of any lateral progression of infarction in the subendocardial zone.

Transmural extent—relation to collateral blood flow.

In dogs, even permanent ligation of a major coronary artery often does not result in complete infarction of

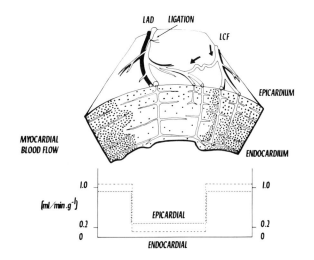

FIG. 8. Myocardial blood flow distribution within adjacent vascular regions following acute coronary occlusion in the dog. The density of dots represents the density of microspheres injected to measure local blood flow during ligation of the LAD artery. Corresponding flow values are illustrated in the lower graph. Some blood flow to the LAD vascular region occurs via epicardial collateral connections (*arrows*) from other arteries such as the circumflex. The lateral interface between vascular regions is irregular but sharply defined. (From ref. 304, with permission.)

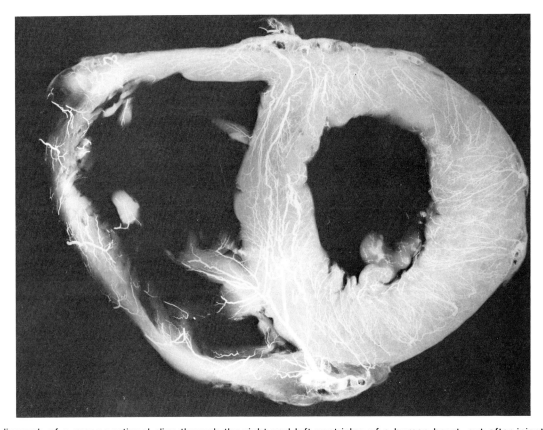

FIG. 9. Radiograph of a cross-sectional slice through the right and left ventricles of a human heart, cut after injection of the coronary arteries with a barium sulfate suspension. Myocardial perfusion occurs through small penetrating branches of the larger epicardial coronary arteries. Major collateral anastomoses between epicardial coronary arteries may occur. In contrast, recent evidence indicates that the smaller penetrating arteries have few, if any, interconnections and are essentially end arteries. By comparing radiographs of the whole heart with those of serial cross-sectional slices, the regions of myocardium supplied by each coronary artery can be defined; myocardial mass can be calculated from planimetric measurements. (From ref. 337, with permission.)

the occluded vascular region (183,475,485,535,625). For example, after circumflex occlusion, there is persistent viable myocardium in the subepicardial zone, averaging about 20% of the ischemic vascular bed (475). In this experimental model, collateral blood flow to the subepicardial zone is quite variable (Fig. 10); the amount of subepicardial sparing is inversely related to the amount of collateral blood flow provided to this zone during the early phase of ischemia (Fig. 11) (475,482). Moreover, some studies have shown a correlation between collateral blood flow and the amount of myocardial necrosis in individual samples of ischemic myocardium (492). In dogs with permanent occlusions, both the size of the ischemic vascular bed and the amount of subepicardial collateral blood flow are major determinants of infarct size (185,186,284,359,475,482,492,521,533). In contrast to dogs, baboons and pigs have few native coronary collateral anastomoses; permanent coronary occlusion is followed by severe transmural ischemia and by solid transmural infarcts (171,310,336,625). Thus, in these species, infarct size is determined primarily by the size of the occluded vascular bed.

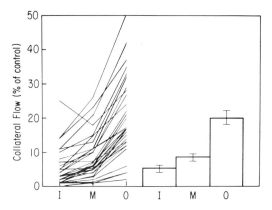

FIG. 10. Transmural distribution of collateral blood flow found 20 min after occlusion of the circumflex coronary artery in 31 dogs. Results from individual dogs are shown on the left, whereas the group means ± SEM are shown on the right. I, M, and O refer to inner (subendocardial), middle, and outer (subepicardial) thirds of the transmural wall of the left ventricle. Subendocardial blood flow was almost always severely depressed (<15%) and averaged 4.5% of control. Subepicardial flow was more variable but always greater (averaged 20% of control) than subepicardial flow. (Adapted from ref. 475.)

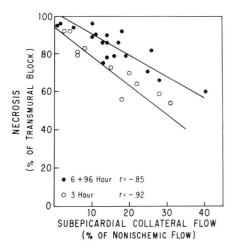

FIG. 11. Relation between transmural extent of necrosis and subepicardial collateral blood flow in dogs with circumflex coronary artery occlusions. Flow was measured 20 min after coronary occlusion, and infarct size was measured histologically after a 4-day survival period. The regression line indicated by the solid dots includes dogs with infarcts caused by permanent coronary ligation and dogs with infarcts reperfused at 6 hr, because reperfusion at the latter time did not influence infarct size. The *open circles* represent infarcts that were reperfused at 3 hr. Each regression line indicates a strong inverse relationship between the transmural extent of the infarct and the amount of collateral blood flow to the subepicardial region. The downward shift of the regression for 3-hr infarcts indicates limitation of infarct size by reperfusion at this time. (From ref. 475, with permission.)

Myocardial Infarction in Humans

Time course.

In humans, as in experimental models, subendocardial myocardium is more susceptible to ischemic injury than is subepicardial myocardium. This concept is supported by the fact that infarcts usually are not completely transmural (337). Most human infarcts observed at autopsy, whether or not Q waves were present in electrocardiograms obtained during life, are most extensive in the subendocardial region, with variable degrees of projection into the subepicardial region (527,627,645). Because the subendocardial region is most susceptible to ischemic injury, it is reasonable to assume that myocardial infarction begins there and later progresses toward the epicardium, as has been demonstrated experimentally. However, a transmural progression of injury has not been proved in humans. Moreover, if a transmural wavefront of injury does occur in patients, the time course of such progression is unknown. As noted earlier, the 3- to 6-hr time limit of salvageability observed in open-chest dogs has been confirmed in closed-chest awake dogs and in nonhuman primates. Thus, it seems likely that a similar time course might apply to the subset of patients with severe myocardial ischemia, caused by sudden proximal occlusion of a major coronary artery, when no previous stimulus for collateral growth had been present. Such a worst-case scenario might result from a coronary embolus, for example. It is plausible, but not proved, that the time course of ischemic cell death could be slower if the degree of ischemia is less severe or if it has a more gradual onset (471). For example, ischemia could be less severe if the involved coronary artery is only partially obstructed, or if prior coronary disease has induced the growth of functionally important collateral interconnections. Moreover, infarction could be expected to develop relatively slowly in patients whose hemodynamic determinants of myocardial oxygen needs are low.

Recent experimental studies in dogs have shown that "preconditioning" myocardium with repetitive brief episodes of ischemia delays adenosine triphosphate (ATP) depletion and the onset of myocardial necrosis in a subsequent longer period of ischemia (413). If such results are applicable to humans, infarcts either caused by or preceded by intermittent coronary spasm or intermittent thrombosis alleviated by spontaneous thrombolysis might develop over a slower time course compared with the time course established in experimental animals with sudden coronary occlusions.

Postmortem studies of the microcirculation in human hearts have shown "end-capillary loops," i.e., capillaries loop back without making connections between vascular regions at the capillary level (130). Likewise, postmortem studies of human myocardial infarcts have shown a close relationship between the lateral boundaries of the infarct and the boundaries of the involved vascular bed, using radiographs of ventricular slices after coronary injection with radiopaque material to identify the vascular bed (337). In these studies, infarct boundaries consistently matched vascular bed boundaries. While such studies of completed infarcts do not rule out a lateral progression of infarct evolution, such results do suggest that the lateral boundaries of an infarct are predetermined by vascular anatomy and that lateral salvage of ischemic myocardium, unlike subepicardial salvage, does not occur spontaneously.

Infarct boundaries—relation to collateral blood flow and vascular area at risk.

The importance of collateral anastomoses in patients with ischemic heart disease has been the subject of much controversy in the past. It is generally accepted that coronary collaterals are present but poorly developed in normal human hearts (22,158). On the other hand, patients with severe coronary artery disease often do have collateral anastomoses that are sufficiently well developed to be visualized by coronary angiography. The functional value of such visible collaterals has been widely debated (80,428). The severity of angina and myocardial dysfunction often has been no better, and the incidence of myocardial infarction no lower, in patients with versus those without demonstrable collaterals (42,82,180,216,458,646). On the other hand, the incidence of Q waves and pump failure has been lower in several studies of patients with myocardial infarcts if collaterals have been visible angiographically (151,203,431,646). From experimental studies it is known that even complete coronary occlusion, if induced gradually, may result in no myocardial infarction at all (190,302). Moreover, it has long been recognized from postmortem studies of human hearts that complete coronary occlusion may be associated with little or no myocardial infarction (20,40,41,567). Such observations are direct and striking evidence for the importance of coronary collateral perfusion for the prevention of infarction or limitation of infarct size. Thus, it is likely that the transmural extent of a human myocardial infarct is determined at least in part by the amount of collateral blood flow to this region (337).

Although postmortem studies of human myocardial infarcts have shown a close correspondence between infarct boundaries and the boundaries of the area at risk (337), preexisting, widespread coronary vascular disease makes the pathophysiology more complex; the area at risk of infarction is not always easily defined. For example, occlusion of a coronary artery may occur gradually, and because collateral anastomoses enlarge, infarction may be prevented. As a result, two anatomic vascular regions may be dependent on flow through a single coronary artery. Occlusion of this artery not only would place its myocardial region at risk but also would jeopardize the collateral dependent vascular region (337) and thereby cause "infarction at a distance" (159). Hemodynamic disturbances also may cause ischemia in two or more vascular regions if severe coronary stenoses exist. Severe hemodynamic disturbances may place the entire ventricle in jeopardy and cause circumferential subendocardial infarction.

Cellular Consequences of Severe Myocardial Ischemia

Myocyte Injury

Much of our understanding of the early cellular consequences of ischemic injury has developed from experimental studies of severely ischemic myocardium. Moderately or mildly ischemic myocardium has been more difficult to characterize, because myocardium with uniformly intermediate degrees of ischemia is not readily attained. Although myocytes are not all equally ischemic, and the severity of ischemia influences the duration of cell survival, it is often assumed that the cellular consequences of myocardial ischemia are the same irrespective of the severity of ischemia, except that the time frame of cellular injury may be decelerated or accelerated. However, just as there are critical qualitative differences between hypoxia and ischemia, there may be critical qualitative differences in the way myocytes respond to moderate versus severe ischemia. In the following paragraphs, some of the early consequences of severe myocardial ischemia will be reviewed. It should not be automatically assumed that all aspects of severe ischemia are of similar importance in moderate ischemia.

Metabolic.

Energy metabolism. Human life is dependent on the continuous, nonstop contractile function of the heart; the average adult heart contracts 100,000 times per day and in so doing pumps 4,300 gallons of blood at systolic pressures of 120 mm Hg. To sustain this activity, myocardium is absolutely dependent on aerobic metabolism for the production of energy in the form of ATP. Myocytes contain very limited reserve stores of HEPs and are dependent on a continuous source of oxygen and metabolic substrate. Myocardium can utilize a variety of substrates, including glucose, ketone bodies, amino acids, and fatty acids; however, fatty acids are the preferred substrate. When presented with both fatty acids and glucose, myocardium preferentially oxidizes fatty acids; glucose is converted to glycogen (424,556,657). During severe exercise, lactate may replace free fatty acids as the principal myocardial substrate (561). In either case, nearly all HEP production occurs through mitochondrial oxidation. The great dependence of the myocardium on mitochondrial metabolism is illustrated by the composition of cardiac myocytes; 30 to 38% of the volume of left ventricular myocytes is occupied by mitochondria (441).

With the cessation of coronary blood flow, the relatively small quantities of oxygen remaining in capillary erythrocytes or attached to myoglobin are rapidly consumed. The decreasing tissue oxygen content (528,529) is reflected by the appearance of cyanosis within the first 5 to 15 sec of moderate to severe ischemia *in vivo*. Without oxygen as the final electron acceptor, all components of the terminal electron transport chain of the mitochondria become reduced. Indeed, cessation of mitochondrial electron transport has been observed by nuclear magnetic resonance spectroscopy 2 sec after the onset of global ischemia in isolated rat hearts (640). The reduction of nicotinamide adenine dinucleotide (NAD) to $NADH_2$ also has been demonstrated to begin within 2 sec after the onset of ischemia (18,19).

Concomitant with the developing inhibition of oxidative mitochondrial metabolism, glycogenolysis and anaerobic glycolysis are accelerated. During the first few seconds, glycogen phosphorylase activity is the rate-limiting step for anaerobic energy production (325,649). However, there is a rapid increase in phosphorylase activity during the first 10 sec of ischemia that is due to a variety of changes, including (a) activation of phosphorylase b by increased adenosine monophosphate (AMP) and inorganic phosphate, (b) decreased inhibition of phosphorylase a because of decreased ATP and glucose-6-phosphate (G-6-P) (436,649), and (c) conversion of phosphorylase b to phosphorylase a (114,325, 389,520,650). The latter conversion is achieved through a sequence of reactions that include β-adrenergic stimulation of adenylate cyclase (242), with consequent increased production of cyclic AMP (416). Cyclic AMP activates a cyclic-AMP-dependent protein kinase, which activates phosphorylase b kinase through phosphorylation. Phosphorylase b kinase, in turn, converts phosphorylase b to phosphorylase a, again through phosphorylation (621). In cardiac and skeletal muscle, phosphorylase b kinase can be activated directly by calcium. This "flash activation" by Ca^{2+} is thought to be an effect of calmodulin, which is a subunit of phosphorylase b kinase in skeletal muscle (81) and probably in cardiac muscle as well (622). During this initial phase of ischemia, the rate of anaerobic glycolysis also is accelerated markedly through activation of phosphofructokinase by the increasing availability of AMP and inorganic phosphate and by declining concentrations of ATP and citrate (647). However, in severe ischemia, the rate of anaerobic glycolysis soon slows markedly because of inhibition of glyceraldehyde-3-phosphate dehydrogenase activity by a combination of increasing concentrations of NADH, H^+, and lactate (397,423). Phosphofructokinase also is inhibited by increasing tissue acidosis and increased citrate levels (247,325,436).

As noted earlier, the rate of energy production from anaerobic glycolysis is greatly dependent on the level of myocardial perfusion (319,426). The rate of anaerobic glycolysis is much greater under conditions of moderate ischemia or high-flow anoxia, because inhibitory concentrations of lactate and H^+ can be washed out of the tissue, and exogenous glucose is supplied to the myocytes. Under any circumstances, anaerobic glycolysis is an inefficient means of creating HEP; two molecules of adenosine diphosphate (ADP) can be phosphorylated to ATP per molecule of glucose converted to lactate (three per glucosyl unit of glycogen), compared with 38 molecules of ATP created by complete oxidation of glucose to carbon dioxide and water. The glycolytic rate can be accelerated to a marked degree in hypoxia; anaerobic glycolysis can produce enough ATP to prevent severe ATP depletion and maintain some contractile function in isolated hypoxic hearts, provided that sufficient glucose is made available (635). Nevertheless, even under conditions of maximum stimulation, anaerobic glycolysis can produce no more than about 7% of the HEP needs of normal working myocardium (319).

Myocardial reserve stores of HEPs are extremely limited. Normal left ventricular myocardium in dogs and humans contains about 8 μmoles of creatine phosphate (CP), 5.8 μmoles of ATP, and 0.8 μmole of ADP per gram of wet weight. Because the HEP bond of ADP can be utilized through the adenylate kinase (myokinase)

reaction ($2ADP \leftrightharpoons 1ATP + 1AMP$), a total of about 20 μmoles of HEP bonds are available per gram wet weight (268). However, this amount of HEP, if completely utilized, is sufficient for much less than a minute of normal myocardial contractile activity.

On the other hand, the rate of utilization of HEP is rapidly reduced in ischemia because contractile function is suppressed. Nevertheless, electrical activity and minimal mechanical activity continue to utilize HEP; other metabolic reactions that consume ATP despite the reduced rate of ATP production may include reactions involved in calcium sequestration by the sarcoplasmic reticulum, the sarcolemmal Na^+-K^+ ATPase, and perhaps a variety of other enzymes such as adenyl cyclase and ATPases involved in lipid catabolism. The various pathways contributing to ATP production and utilization in ischemia are summarized in Fig. 12.

Depletion of HEPs and purine nucleotides. To summarize the preceding section, a major feature of ischemia is that HEP requirements invariably exceed the rate of production. Consequently, the HEP content of ischemic myocardium rapidly declines. Creatine phosphate is almost completely depleted within the first 3 min (49,281); ATP content declines more slowly, but nevertheless is depleted quickly. For example, in severe regional ischemia in anesthetized dogs, ATP decreases to about 35% of control by 15 min and to less than 10% by 40 min (261,474). Similar results have been observed in other experimental models (49,268,281,425).

The utilization of ATP results in a 50% or greater early increase in ADP in severe ischemia *in vivo* (Fig. 13) and a smaller increase in low-flow ischemia in the perfused heart (281,425). However, this increase is transient because of the adenylate kinase reaction. After 10 min of severe ischemia, declining ATP content is paralleled by declining ADP. Moreover, the AMP produced by adenylate kinase is catabolized further (Fig. 14), primarily to adenosine via the enzyme 5'-nucleotidase. This enzyme is located both within the cytosol (546) and in the sarcolemma (515). It is not known whether or not and how much sarcoplasmic adenosine is further catabolized within the myocyte. Adenosine does escape from the myocyte and is further catabolized to inosine, hypoxanthine, and even some xanthine by the enzymes adenosine deaminase, nucleoside phosphorylase, and xanthine oxidase, respectively (268,273,434). Histochemical studies have localized these enzymes primarily to endothelial cells or pericytes (516). In severe or total myocardial ischemia, the decreasing tissue content of adenine nucleotides is stoichiometrically matched by increasing content of nucleosides and bases (Fig. 13) (268,273). When the degree of ischemia is less severe, inosine and hypoxanthine appear in the venous effluent (106).

Thus, because of the aforementioned reactions, ischemia causes not only depletion of HEP bonds but also

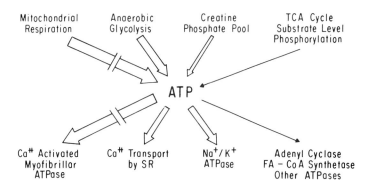

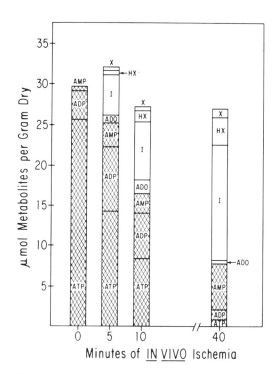

FIG. 12. Principal reactions producing and utilizing HEP in ischemic tissue are illustrated. The width of the arrows indicates the estimated quantitative importance of the various reactions. In severe ischemia, aerobic respiration is abolished. The preexisting stores of HEP, in the form of creatine phosphate (CP) or ATP, are relatively small. Thus, anaerobic glycolysis becomes the principal source of energy, producing 80 to 90% of the HEP bonds that can be utilized by severely ischemic tissue. Substrate-level phosphorylation of α-ketoglutarate in the mitochondria (448) does not require O_2, but the tissue content of substrates that can be shuttled to α-ketoglutarate is small. Energy utilization also is markedly reduced during ischemia. Cardiac contraction, which is mediated by Ca^{2+}-activated myofibrillar ATPase, consumes much of the ATP produced in aerobic myocardium. However, contraction is abolished or severely depressed in areas of severe ischemia. Nevertheless, ATP continues to be required to remove Na^+ from the cell, to keep Ca^{2+} sequestered in the sarcoplasmic reticulum, and for a variety of other cellular processes that may continue to compete for the remaining ATP. (From ref. 266, with permission.)

FIG. 13. Effect of severe ischemia on myocardial adenine nucleotides, nucleosides, and bases during circumflex artery occlusion in dogs. Measurements were made in nonischemic myocardium (0 min) and in the posterior papillary muscle (representative of the severely ischemic subendocardial zone of the occluded circumflex vascular region). ADO = adenosine; I = inosine; H = hypoxanthine; X = xanthine. Note the transient increase in ADP at 5 and 10 min, the progressive decrease in total adenine nucleotides (*shaded parts of bars*), and the stoichiometric recovery of the degraded nucleotides as nucleosides and bases. In more moderately ischemic myocardium, nucleotide catabolites are lost to the circulation (see Fig. 6). (From ref. 264, with permission.)

rapid degradation of the total adenine nucleotide pool (268,281,474,484). For example, during severe ischemia *in vivo,* half of the total adenine nucleotide pool is lost by 10 to 15 min (Fig. 13) (261,474). Total nicotinamide adenine dinucleotide content (NAD + NADH) is relatively stable in the early phase of ischemia but is lost from ischemic myocardium, especially after the myocytes have been lethally injured (268,309).

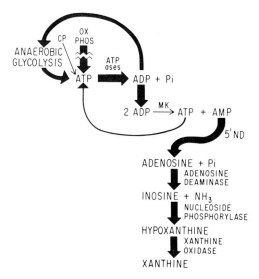

FIG. 14. Major pathways of adenine nucleotide catabolism during myocardial ischemia. The most important routes of ATP and adenine nucleotide degradation are indicated by the heavier arrows. CP = creatine phosphate; ADP = adenosine diphosphate; AMP = adenosine monophosphate; ATP = adenosine triphosphate; MK = adenylate kinase (myokinase); 5'ND = 5'-nucleotidase. (From ref. 269, with permission.)

Accumulation of metabolic end-products. The products of a variety of catabolic pathways progressively accumulate in myocardial ischemia. We have already noted the rapid accumulation of lactate, the end-product of anaerobic glycolysis, and of purine bases as a result of the breakdown of adenine nucleotides. Tissue acidosis increases rapidly (78,79,249,334,367) because of several catabolic processes, including glycolysis, lipolysis, and ATP hydrolysis (176). Ammonia is produced by the deamination of adenosine, amino acids, etc., and has been shown to increase in totally ischemic myocardium (110). Although potentially toxic, some of the ammonia can be detoxified by conversion of pyruvate to alanine through the action of alanine aminotransferase; alanine also accumulates in totally ischemic myocardium (587). The combined effects of the aforementioned catabolite accumulations create a substantial osmotic load within the ischemic myocyte (272,579).

Myocardial cellular acidosis may be a significant factor in the decline of contractile function (78,79,579). While detrimental for the whole organism, the loss of contractility in the ischemic region might be advantageous to the affected myocytes by preserving their HEP content. On the other hand, myocardial acidosis has a variety of potentially deleterious consequences, including inhibition of various metabolic pathways (648), such as enzymes of the glycolytic pathway. As noted earlier, inhibition of anaerobic glycolysis limits the amount of ATP that can be synthesized from glycogen in the early phase of ischemia. Acidosis also has been associated with ultrastructural changes in myocardium, including aggregation of nuclear chromatin and formation of mitochondrial amorphous matrix densities (11).

Lactate also has direct effects on cardiac myocytes that could contribute to the evolution of ischemic injury. For example, it has been observed that a high concentration of lactate alters the action potential and decreases the tension developed by isolated frog atrium (653). A high lactate concentration has been linked to mitochondrial swelling *in vivo* and to decreased phosphorylating capabilities of mitochondria in (lactate-rich) myocardium (10,285). Recently, Neely and Grotoyohann (420) showed that recovery of ventricular function following 30 min of total ischemia in rat hearts was inversely related to the accumulated levels of lactate. If lactate accumulation in ischemia was prevented by a previous period of high-flow hypoxia (to deplete myocardial glycogen), functional recovery following ischemia was improved.

Lipid and protein metabolism. Myocardium contains reserve energy supplies in the form of triglyceride (610). Moreover, myocardial lipolysis has been reported to be increased early in ischemia, apparently through a catecholamine-dependent mechanism (278,292). Under conditions of severe or total ischemia, increased but small quantities of fatty acids, acyl coenzyme A (CoA), and acyl carnitine can accumulate in the myocardium

(462,611). However, oxidation of fatty acids to CO_2 and water is a mitochondrial process and does not occur in the absence of oxygen.

When some oxygen is available because significant quantities of collateral flow are present in *in vivo* ischemia, fatty acid metabolism is more complicated. In zones of moderate or high-flow ischemia, fatty acids may be taken up by the ischemic myocytes from the circulating blood; such uptake may be facilitated because the circulating level of fatty acids often is elevated during myocardial ischemia (614) due to systemic lipolysis induced by increased systemic sympathetic activity and/or reflex-mediated adrenal catecholamine release (365,577,578). In this setting, variable rates of fatty acid oxidation may occur. However, fatty acid uptake exceeds the rate of oxidation because of the limited supply of oxygen; fatty acyl CoA and acyl carnitine accumulate in mildly ischemic myocardium (398). Moreover, because glycerol, the backbone of triglyceride, is readily available from increased quantities of α-glycerol phosphate (an intermediate product of anaerobic glycolysis) (325, 350,436,510), triglycerides also accumulate in mildly ischemic myocardium (55,95,278,538). This accumulation of triglyceride is detectable by light microscopy, where it has been called fatty change or fatty metamorphosis. The accumulated lipids also can be identified by histochemical means (34,626).

Fatty acid metabolism also has been studied in isolated perfused hearts, where delivery of large amounts of various fatty acids bound to albumin is possible in experimental conditions of high-flow anoxia or ischemia. In such circumstances, marked myocardial accumulation of nonesterified free fatty acids, acyl CoA, acyl carnitine, or triglycerides may occur (419,641).

The increased concentrations of fatty acid esters have a number of detrimental consequences for ischemic myocardium (295,349). Fatty acid accumulation may contribute to the cytosolic deficit of HEPs per se, because acyl CoA inhibits adenine nucleotide translocase. This enzyme is located on the inner mitochondrial membrane and is responsible for export of ATP from its site of production at the matrix side of the inner mitochondrial membrane to the outside (232,560). Fatty acids also may have a variety of other cellular consequences (295,349), including inhibition of a variety of enzymes (445); mitochondrial respiration is impaired and oxidative phosphorylation is uncoupled (46). Fatty acids also impair contractile function (352). Moreover, it has been postulated that fatty acids and fatty acid esters, such as lysophospholipids, may act as detergents and thereby disrupt cellular membranes (75,88,296,419).

Arachidonic acid is one of the fatty acids that accumulates in ischemic myocardium early in the phase of injury (74,462). Because it is a major component of phospholipids, arachidonate accumulation is direct evidence for degradation of phospholipids, a major structural component of cellular membranes, in ischemic injury. However, the significance of this early phospholipid degradation is uncertain at the present time; total myocardial phospholipid loss is small in the first 3 hr of ischemia (75,581).

Both protein synthesis and protein degradation are energy-requiring processes; both have been shown to be inhibited during the early phases of ischemia (43, 291,463). However, recent evidence indicates that cellular proteases also become activated during ischemia and may contribute to the degradation of critical structural or enzymatic proteins of the cell. For example, a calcium-activated neutral protease has been isolated from heart muscle (599) that has been postulated to degrade troponin subunits within the first 4 hr after coronary occlusion (600). Similar proteases have been shown to remove Z lines from skeletal muscle myofibrils (62,102,467). Proteolytic degradation of cytoskeletal proteins attached to the plasmalemma hypothetically could result in weakening of the structural supports of the sarcolemma and contribute to plasmalemmal disruption in ischemia (272,580).

Free radicals. Free radicals have been implicated in a large variety of physiologic (e.g., neutrophil-mediated killing of foreign organisms) and pathologic processes (109,152,361). In recent years, considerable attention has been focused on the idea that production of free radicals may be increased in myocardial ischemia (220,465,557). Even more important may be the production of free radicals such as superoxide during post-ischemic reperfusion (*vide infra*). Possible mechanisms for increased free-radical production in ischemia have not been thoroughly elucidated, but a variety of reactions are known to produce free radicals. For example, super-oxide is produced by autoxidation of a variety of small molecules such as thiols, flavins, and catecholamines (152). Free radicals also are produced as by-products of a variety of enzymatic reactions; a notable example is xanthine-oxidase-mediated conversion of hypoxanthine to xanthine (153). Both superoxide and hydroxyl radicals are generated by mitochondrial electron transport (48,113,606); superoxide production is greatest when respiratory chain carriers are highly reduced (607). Superoxide and hydroxyl radicals also can be generated as by-products of microsomal oxidase reactions, some involving the cytochrome P_{450} system (152). Free radicals also can be produced by enzymes of the plasmalemma. A notable example is the production of a free radical by cyclooxygenase-mediated oxidation of arachidonate (381).

Free radicals are highly reactive and can cause detrimental alterations in proteins, nucleic acids, and lipids (152). For example, enzyme conformation may be altered by free-radical-mediated formation of disulfide bonds or methionine sulfoxide (152); free radicals also cause hydroxylation of proline and lysine (602). Lipid perox-idation, with potentially deleterious changes in membranes of the sarcolemma or internal organelles, is known to occur when free radicals react with phospholipids of membranes (61,150); the possible role of lipid peroxidation in myocardial ischemic injury has received particular attention in recent years (391,392,465).

Direct demonstration of increased free-radical production in myocardial ischemia has not been easily achieved; however, Rao et al. (464) have shown increased free-radical production by electron-spin resonance as early as 15 min after coronary occlusion in dogs. Lipid peroxidation, a major consequence of free-radical production, can be assessed by measuring malondialdehyde, a product of lipid peroxidation (322,351,464). Malondialdehyde was increased by 45 min after coronary occlusion in the studies of Rao et al. (464); such data are indirect evidence for increased production of free radicals during ischemia.

Functional.

Contractile failure. It has been known for many years that contractile dysfunction is one of the earliest consequences of ischemia (529,589,592). Indeed, contractile force is measurably suppressed within 6 to 10 sec after the onset of ischemia (205,503). The cause of such rapid functional inhibition remains elusive. Inasmuch as contraction is an energy-dependent process, it would seem logical to attribute contractile failure to a reduced HEP supply. However, this simple explanation most likely is incorrect, because the onset of contractile failure precedes any substantial decline in total tissue ATP content (92,288). If contractile failure is due to insufficient ATP, the insufficiency must be in a particular small pool of ATP, perhaps coupled with a defect in intracellular energy transport (210,324). It has been postulated that ATP depletion at the level of the contractile proteins should produce rigor rather than contractile failure; however, there is evidence for a modulatory role of ATP in the control of passive ion fluxes across cell membranes; a slight decrease in ATP might reduce the influx of Ca^{2+} across the sarcolemma and from the sarcoplasmic reticulum and thereby promote early contractile failure (324). An alternative explanation for contractile failure is the rapidly developing cellular acidosis (579). For example, accumulating hydrogen ions might compete with calcium for the calcium-binding sites on troponin (293). Although acidosis may partially account for early contractile failure in ischemia (253), several studies have shown that the initial contractile failure also precedes a measurable decrease in intracellular pH (253,330,632). Moreover, contractile failure also occurs rapidly during high-flow anoxia *in vitro,* when acidosis develops slowly because of the buffering capacity of the perfusate.

Electrolyte and electrophysiologic changes. Another very early event in ischemia is a net loss of a small fraction of total cellular potassium (69,207). This K^+

loss begins within seconds after the onset of ischemia; extracellular K^+ gradually increases from about 5 mM to 10 to 15 mM during the first few minutes (225,307). The mechanism of this early potassium loss, like the loss of contractile function, is not completely understood. It is well known that maintenance of electrolyte gradients across the cell membrane requires energy-dependent transport processes. However, the early loss of potassium occurs concurrently with the onset of anaerobic glycolysis and contractile failure, prior to any substantial diminution of total myocardial ATP content. Studies of unidirectional potassium flux indicate that the early potassium depletion is due to an increased rate of efflux from the cell; K^+ influx via the Na^+-K^+-ATPase pump is not altered, and intracellular Na^+ is not increased in the earliest phase of ischemia (179,306,466). Shine (554) has shown this K^+ loss to be depolarization-dependent. Inhibition of depolarization results in retention of K^+ during hypoxia. Inasmuch as electroneutrality must be maintained, if net potassium efflux is not accompanied by net sodium influx, it must be accompanied by efflux of anions. The most likely counterbalancing anions include lactate and inorganic phosphate (149,306,307). There is some evidence that cellular efflux of phosphate and lactate does begin in the same time frame as the efflux of K^+ (369,382). This early efflux of K^+ and associated anions may be of benefit to the ischemic myocytes to the extent that it attenuates the intracellular osmotic load imposed by the rapid catabolism of creatine phosphate to creatine and phosphate and of glycogen to intermediates of anaerobic glycolysis (580).

Several electrophysiologic changes can be recorded through microelectrodes on the heart early in ischemia. These changes include both T-Q depression (due to partial diastolic depolarization caused by the reduced K^+ gradient) (149) and ST-segment elevation; these changes summate to produce ST-segment elevation that characteristically develops on surface electrocardiograms within 15 to 30 sec after the onset of ischemia. In addition, ischemia causes shortening of the action-potential duration, slowed intramyocardial conduction, and dispersion of refractoriness (89). The subcellular basis for these changes is not entirely understood; these electrophysiologic changes are thought to be the consequence of one or more of several metabolic or electrolytic changes (230,320,400,437), including extracellular hyperkalemia (548,591,633), intracellular acidosis, local catecholamine release (with production of cyclic AMP) (289), fatty acid (403,582) or lysophospholipid accumulation (90,372,568), and cellular calcium overload (77,417). One or more of these metabolic and/or electrophysiologic consequences of myocardial ischemia presumably provide the subcellular basis for the potentially life-threatening dysrhythmias observed in some people or experimental animals in the early phase of ischemic injury.

Because maintenance of electrolyte gradients is energy-dependent, it seems surprising that more severe changes in electrolyte gradients and cell volume regulation do not occur earlier in ischemia. One explanation for the maintenance of Na^+-K^+-ATPase activity and of relatively normal intracellular sodium content early in ischemia is that membrane ion transport may preferentially utilize glycolytically derived ATP, whereas mitochondrial ATP is required for contractile activity (208,363,395). Similarly, cell volume regulation has been found to be relatively insensitive to metabolic inhibition. For example, slices of anoxic myocardium have been shown to resist cell swelling, perhaps because of continued ion transport or perhaps because of extracellular collagenous restraints (453,454). Moreover, in severe ischemia *in vivo*, cell swelling may also be limited by the limited amount of extracellular fluid present in the tissue (261,273). Nevertheless, ultrastructural studies show that mild cell swelling is an early feature of myocardial ischemia (112,273).

A number of investigators have postulated that ischemia may result in increased cytosolic calcium (297,418,459), either because of increased influx from the extracellular space (555) or sarcoplasmic reticulum or because of insufficient energy for calcium sequestration or extrusion. Such a calcium overload could have serious consequences for the myocyte; calcium activates a variety of proteases, lipases, and phospholipases (134), augments ATP utilization by activating many ATPases (297,418), and inhibits mitochondrial oxidative phosphorylation (605). However, although rapid influx of calcium and massive mitochondrial calcification are well-known consequences of reperfusing severely damaged ischemic myocytes that have sarcolemmal disruption (*vide infra*) (261,316,551), the existence of increased cytosolic calcium entry or cytosolic concentration earlier in the reversible phase of ischemia or hypoxia has not been definitively demonstrated (3,4,271,273).

Neurophysiologic changes. Within the first hour after onset of myocardial ischemia there is progressive release of endogenous norepinephrine from adrenergic nerve terminals within the myocardium (2,239,383,408, 439,541). Simultaneously, the numbers of exposed beta-receptors on membrane fractions of homogenized cardiac myocytes are increased (404,405). The mechanism for this progressive redistribution of norepinephrine out of nerve terminals is unknown; it is known, however, that neuronal reuptake of norepinephrine is an ATP-dependent process (408).

Local release of norepinephrine has a variety of possible consequences. The role of adrenergic stimulation in the activation of anaerobic glycolysis has been mentioned earlier. Also it has been postulated that the redistribution of endogenous catecholamines in acutely ischemic myocardium, perhaps coupled with increased adrenergic sensitivity because of larger numbers of ex-

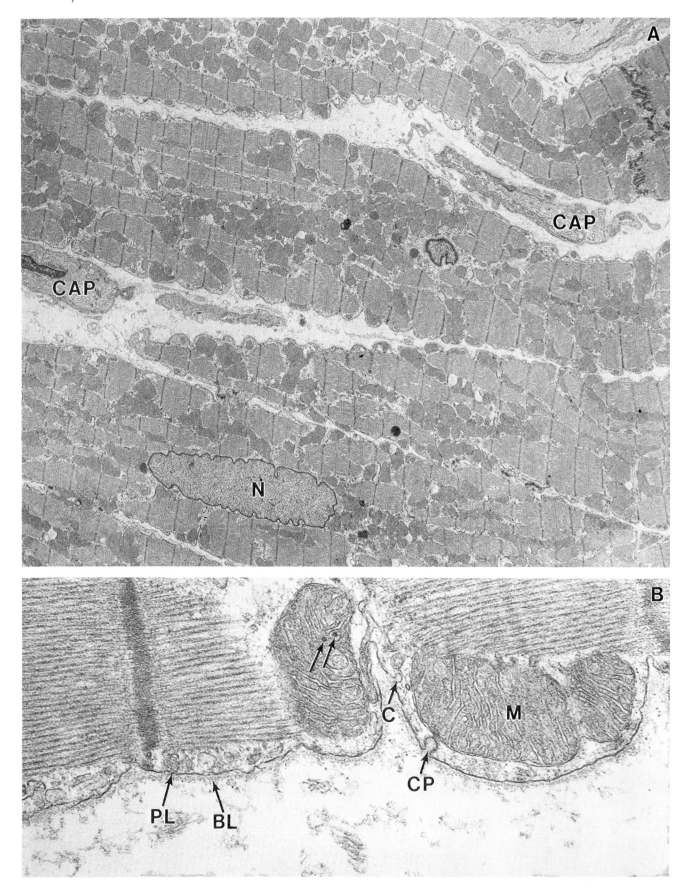

posed receptors, could increase calcium influx to the myocyte. The latter could contribute to both the progression of ischemic cell injury and the increased propensity for cardiac arrhythmias (91).

Structural.

General ultrastructural features of normal canine left ventricular myocardium are illustrated in Fig. 15. During the first 15 min of severe myocardial ischemia in anesthetized dogs, when myocytes still are reversibly injured, the principal ultrastructural changes consist of mild edema of the sarcoplasm and intracellular organelles, including mitochondria, diminution of glycogen deposits, relaxation or stretching of myofibrils, and mild margination of nuclear chromatin (Fig. 16) (258,260,261,273). In addition, mitochondria show loss of the normal matrix granules and may show mild swelling, with disorganization of cristae.

Following longer periods of injury, these changes become much more marked (Figs. 17–20). Nuclear chromatin is aggregated along the nuclear membrane, glycogen becomes severely depleted, mitochondrial swelling and loss of cristae become pronounced, and cell swelling is accentuated. Two additional ultrastructural features distinguish irreversibly injured myocytes from reversibly injured myocytes: Amorphous densities develop within the matrix space of mitochondria, and breaks in the plasmalemma of the sarcolemma become detectable (Figs. 18 and 19) (258,266,276,484).

The speed at which ultrastructural signs of ischemic injury develop is variable, depending on the severity of ischemia and animal species. Nevertheless, the general sequence of changes outlined earlier for canine myocardium has also been observed in other animal models of myocardial ischemia *in vivo* (12,181,314,346,530,590) and in total ischemia *in vitro* (218) (Fig. 21). Quantitative analysis by morphometry has revealed a decrease in the intracellular content of sarcoplasmic reticular membrane, dissolution of gap junctions, and migration of multivesicular bodies to the intercalated discs after 30 to 60 min of ischemia in the isolated working rat heart model (360). Broadening of Z bands is a late change that has been observed after 3 hr or more of coronary occlusion

in dogs and is thought to be associated with loss of myofibrillar proteins, including α-actinin (525).

The exact composition and the cause of formation of the mitochondrial amorphous matrix densities (also referred to as flocculent densities) are unknown. Analytical electron microscopy has failed to demonstrate calcium in these densities (57,202) (in contrast to the granular densities of calcium phosphate to be described later in this chapter that are often found in irreversibly injured myocardium after reperfusion). Mitochondria containing amorphous densities have been isolated and the densities partially purified; it has been reported that they are composed predominantly of lipid (258) or protein (83,252). In isolated perfused heart, the relative number and size of amorphous densities have been observed to correlate with the mitochondrial concentration of acyl carnitine. Based on this observation, it has been hypothesized that amorphous matrix densities may consist of structurally altered membrane-bound proteins, formed by the detergent action of acyl carnitine (137).

Transition from reversible to irreversible injury.

Precise definition of life versus death, when applied to the whole individual, has been the cause of ongoing medicolegal disputes; definition of life versus death of individual cells has been no less difficult. When a cell has been dead for some period of time, classic histologic features of necrosis develop and are paralleled by loss of metabolic activity and dramatic biochemical changes that are universally accepted indices of cell death. However, in myocardial ischemia there is no striking sudden change that marks the point of transition from life to death. Thus, for purposes of study, it has been necessary to consider cellular injury in the less absolute terms of reversible or irreversible injury. As used throughout the preceding paragraphs, reversible injury is injury from which the cells will recover if the cause of injury (ischemia) is removed (reperfusion); irreversible injury is injury that proceeds to necrosis despite removal of the cause of injury (257,275). This concept of reversible versus irreversible injury was developed in the mid-1950s as a framework on which to base studies of the molecular events that cause the myocytes to enter the

FIG. 15. Ultrastructure of control (nonischemic) left ventricular myocardium of the dog. **A:** Several myocytes are shown. Note that the chromatin of the nuclei (N) is evenly distributed. Several capillaries (CAP) are present in the interstitial space. Abundant mitochondria with tightly packed cristae are present between the myofibrils. ×17,000. **B:** High-power view (×51,500) of the sarcolemma. The basal lamina (BL) or glycocalyx and the plasmalemma (PL) are both intact. An early phase of invagination of a pinocytotic vesicle is shown at C. A coated pit is at CP. Note the tightly packed cristae of the mitochondria. Occasional matrix granules (*arrows*) are present. These granules disappear very early in ischemia. Junctional sarcoplasmic reticulum is present adjacent to the mitochondrion with the labeled matrix granules. This and all subsequent electron micrographs in this chapter are of tissue that was fixed in glutaraldehyde with postosmication, except when indicated otherwise in the legends. Thin sections were stained with uranyl acetate and lead citrate. No *en bloc* staining was employed. (From ref. 270, with permission.)

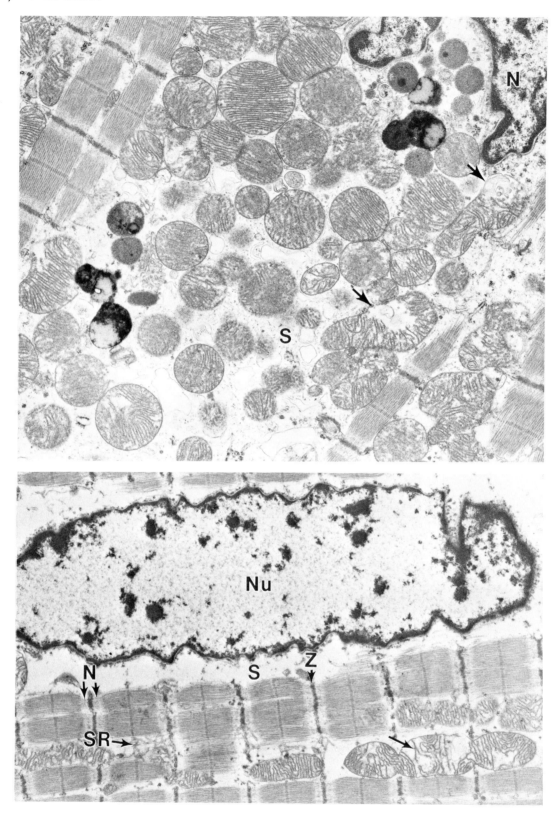

FIG. 16. Top: Fifteen minutes of ischemia with no reperfusion. The typical structural changes induced by 15 min of severe ischemia in the subendocardial myocardium are shown in the top panel and should be contrasted with representative control tissue in Fig. 15 and Fig. 30, panel B. Note that the chromatin of the nucleus (N) is peripherally aggregated. Also, the sarcoplasm (S) of the damaged myocyte is clearer than control because of cellular edema and partial loss of glycogen. There is increased matrix space in some mitochondria, as well as focal swelling (*thick arrows*). The normal matrix granules have disappeared. Although not illustrated here, the sarcolemma was indistinguishable from control at this time. ×15,750. **Bottom:** Micrograph illustrates the most marked ultrastructural changes observed after 15 min of severe low-flow ischemia. The chromatin of the nucleus (Nu) is markedly aggregated peripherally. The sarcoplasm (S) is clear and contains very little glycogen. The myofibrils are relaxed and contain N bands (N) in the prominent I-band region on either side of the Z line (Z). The sarcoplasmic reticulum (SR) is intact. The matrix space of virtually all mitochondria is increased, and the cristae are occasionally disorganized (*arrow*). ×12,500. (From ref. 273, with permission.)

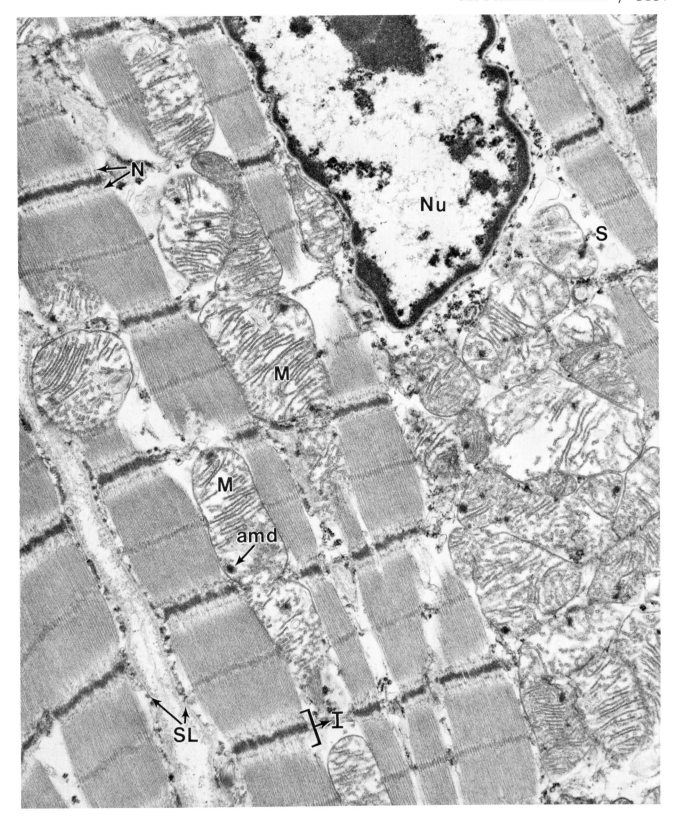

FIG. 17. Irreversibly injured myocyte. This myocyte is representative of myocytes injured by 40 min of low-flow ischemia in the open-chest anesthetized dog. The chromatin of the nucleus (Nu) is aggregated peripherally. Note the clarity of the sarcoplasmic space (S) and the generalized mitochondrial (M) swelling. Prominent amorphous matrix densities (amd) are present in virtually every mitochondrial profile. The myofibrils are relaxed; the I bands (I) are prominent, and an N line is observable in most I bands (N). SL = sarcolemma. ×17,500. (From ref. 24, with permission.)

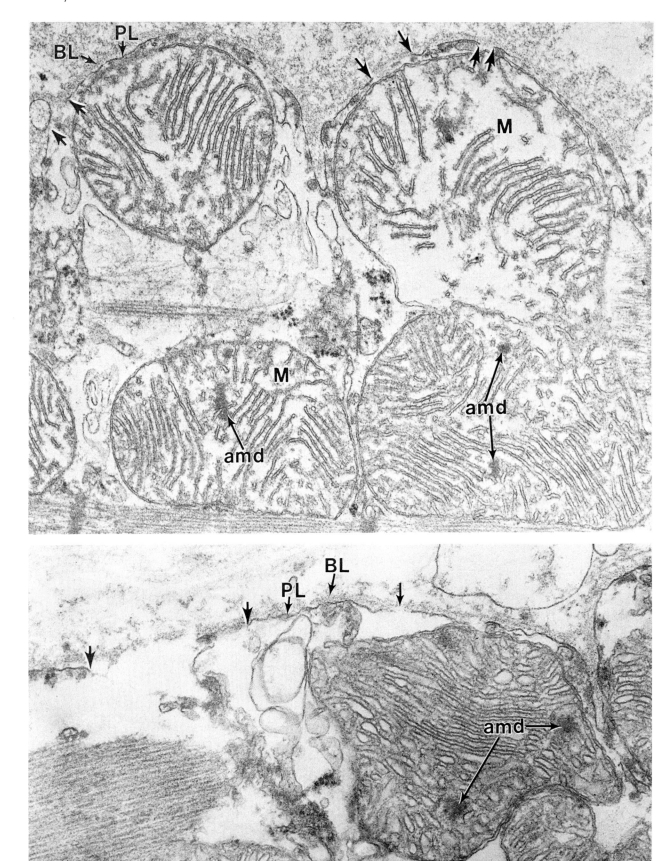

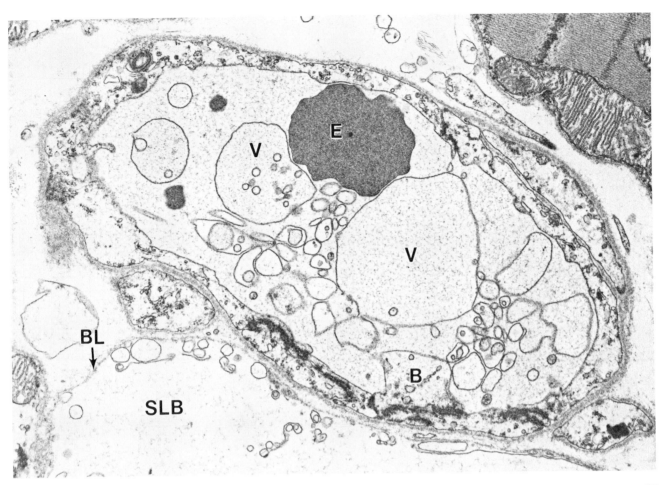

FIG. 19. Changes in a capillary after 3 hr of severe ischemia. Extensive swelling of the endothelium is obvious. Blebs (B) extend from the endothelial cells into the lumen, which is partially obstructed by numerous membrane-bound vesicles (V). The latter are either isolated fragments of endothelial cells or cross sections of endothelial blebs. A crenated erythrocyte (E) is present in the lumen. Pinocytotic vesicles, which are abundant in normal endothelium, disappear in the late phase of irreversible injury. A prominent subsarcolemmal bleb of edema fluid (SLB) is present in an adjacent myocyte. Over much of the bleb, the plasmalemma is broken up into circular profiles; however, the basal lamina (BL) is generally intact. Osmium tetroxide fixation. ×15,000.

irreversible phase (277), i.e., to pass the "point of no return." These early studies showed that the transition to irreversibility occurs after 20 to 60 min of severe ischemia in the dog heart, i.e., long before cell death can be recognized with routine techniques of study such as light microscopy (275). The concept of reversibility versus irreversibility may need to be refined if the act of or manner of restoring myocardial perfusion causes additional cellular injury per se (*vide infra*). Nevertheless,

there is not at present a more precise way to define the transition from life to death.

The initial consequences of myocardial ischemia include inhibition of oxidative metabolism and reduced contractile function. The loss of contractile function is of obvious importance to the well-being of the experimental animal or patient; moreover, restoration of arterial flow is not followed by prompt restoration of contractile function to control levels. Nevertheless, loss

FIG. 18. Characteristic changes in the sarcolemma of severely ischemic left ventricular myocytes that were irreversibly injured by 40 min of *in vivo* ischemia. **Top:** Sarcolemma is distended by two swollen mitochondria (M), each of which contains amorphous matrix densities (amd). In regions where the sarcolemma is intact, a trilaminar plasmalemma (PL) is visible along with the overlying basal lamina (BL). Between the *thick arrows* are prominent breaks in the plasmalemma. In other areas, no identifiable plasmalemma is present. ×150,000. **Bottom:** Relatively small gap in the plasmalemma (*thin arrow*) and another much larger gap (*between the two thick arrows*). Note that the attachment between the plasmalemma and the underlying myofibril at the level of the Z line (Z) is broken. Perfusion fixation with glutaraldehyde and paraformaldehyde followed by postosmication. ×62,500. (From ref. 260, with permission.)

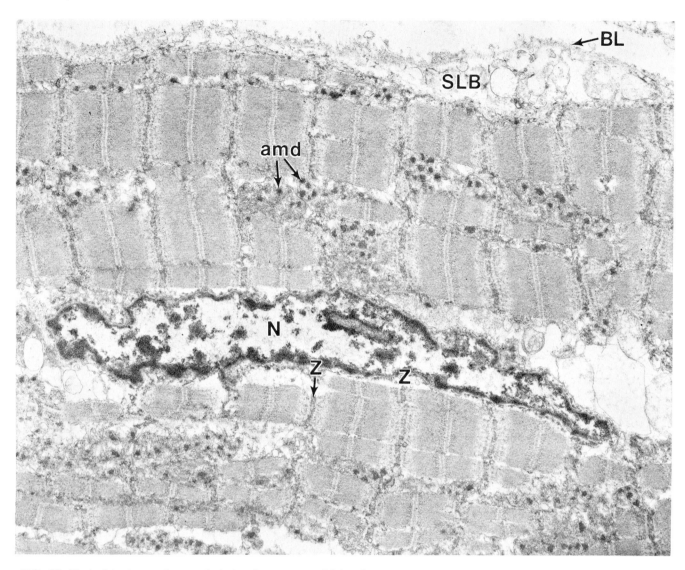

FIG. 20. Typical features of severely ischemic myocytes 24 hr after coronary occlusion. The changes are more severe but qualitatively similar to the changes seen early in the irreversible phase (Figs. 17 and 18). The general architecture of the myofibrils is retained. The Z lines (Z) are generally in register. The mitochondria show large amorphous matrix densities (amd). The plasmalemma no longer is identifiable, but a subsarcolemmal bleb (SLB) and basal lamina (BL) of the sarcolemma are present. The chromatin of the nucleus (N) is maximally aggregated peripherally. ×12,500.

of contractile function does not necessarily imply that the ischemic myocytes have died. Although dead myocytes are, by definition, noncontractile, living myocytes also may lose contractility; therefore, contractile failure cannot be used as an absolute indication of myocyte cell death. One or more other cellular functions, such as maintenance of ionic homeostasis, is crucial for cell survival. The absence of such functions must at some point result not simply in the inactivity of cellular machinery but in the very destruction of that machinery, after which recovery is not possible.

Characteristic features of reversibly and irreversibly injured myocytes. In order to study the pathogenesis of myocardial ischemic cell death, it has been useful to compare and contrast changes present in ischemic cells during the reversible phase of injury with changes present

following the onset of irreversibility. This can be done in the open-chest dog model, for example, by studying the consequences of 10 to 15 min of ischemia (when all myocytes are reversibly injured) (275) versus 40 min of coronary occlusion, which results in uniform irreversible injury of the subendocardial region provided that this region has been *severely* ischemic (275,475). Qualitative differences between reversibly and irreversibly injured myocytes are few. In other words, the metabolic and functional consequences of ischemia reviewed in the preceding paragraphs begin early in the reversible phase of injury. Similarly, many of the ultrastructural changes seen in ischemia, such as cell swelling, glycogen depletion, margination of nuclear chromatin, elongation of myofibrils, etc., can be seen within the first few minutes of ischemia, although these changes become progressively

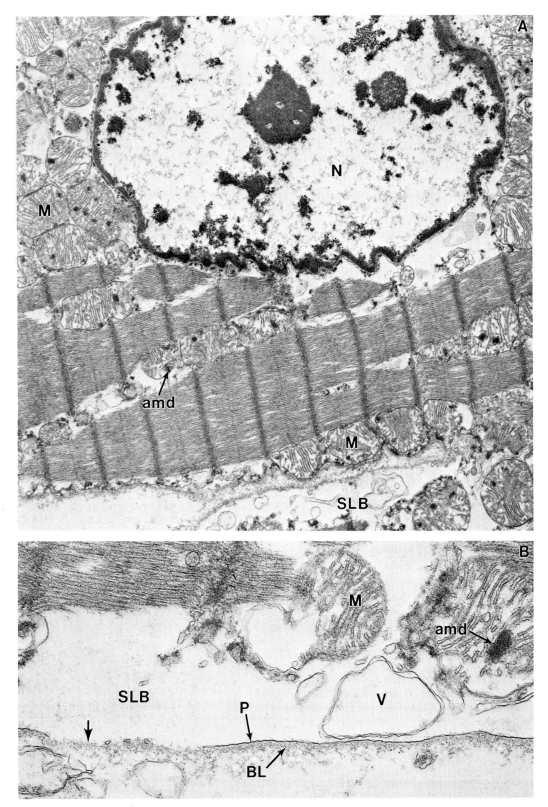

FIG. 21. Typical changes of far-advanced ischemic injury in myocytes after 200 min of total ischemia at 37°C. The changes are indistinguishable from those noted *in vivo* (compare Figs. 17 and 18). **A:** Nuclear chromatin (N) is peripherally aggregated, and all mitochondria (M) contain amorphous matrix densities (amd) and a clear matrix. The sarcolemma is scalloped because of attachments at the Z-band region. In some areas, subsarcolemmal blebs (SLB) have formed by separation of the sarcolemma from the myofibrils by edema fluid. ×41,280. **B:** Typical subsarcolemmal bleb. Note that a portion of the sarcolemma with its basal lamina (BL) and plasmalemma (P) is intact. However, other parts of the bleb are contained by segments of basal lamina without plasmalemma (*thick arrow*). A mitochondrion with a large bleb and a vacuole (V) of uncertain origin (probably mitochondrial swelling) also are present within the swollen myocyte. ×116,800.

more severe in the irreversible phase of injury. However, as noted previously, two ultrastructural changes are distinctive of the irreversible phase of injury—amorphous matrix densities in mitochondria and tiny breaks in the plasmalemma of the sarcolemma (266,484).

Whereas qualitative metabolic differences between reversibly and irreversibly injured myocytes have not been identified, quantitative differences obviously occur and may be of great significance in the pathogenesis of ischemic cell injury. For example, myocardial ATP content, which is reduced to 35% by 15 min, is virtually exhausted by 40 min of severe ischemia in anesthetized dogs (261). Homeostatic processes that might continue with a generalized 65% reduction of ATP content could be abolished with more severe ATP loss from a critical subcellular pool. For example, myofibrillar rigor complexes are prevented as long as ATP content exceeds 10% of control, but myocardial rigor contracture occurs at lower ATP levels (358). In addition, ATP production from anaerobic glycolysis requires ATP to prime the reaction; ATP is consumed in the phosphorylation of fructose-6-phosphate to fructose-1,6-diphosphate. Thus, severe ATP depletion might abolish further ATP production via anaerobic glycolysis. That this occurs is supported by observations that lactate accumulation ceases in ischemic myocardium when ATP supplies are depleted to less than 0.4 μmole per gram wet myocardium, even though glycogen is still present and G-6-P levels are elevated (Fig. 22) (268). If, for example, glycolytic production of ATP is preferentially available for maintenance of ionic gradients (208,363,395), the loss of this seemingly small source of ATP production could conceivably have lethal consequences.

Causes of irreversible injury. The cause of the transition to lethal injury in *in vivo* ischemia has not been estab-

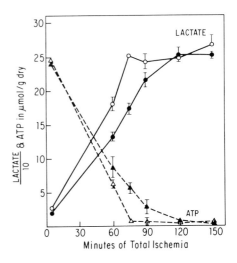

FIG. 22. Lactate accumulation and ATP depletion in totally ischemic dog myocardium. Six hearts have been subgrouped according to rate of ATP depletion; open symbols indicate three hearts with the most rapid ATP depletion; solid symbols indicate three hearts with the slowest rate of ATP depletion. In the hearts with rapid ATP depletion, lactate accumulation also was more rapid, and vice versa. In all hearts, lactate accumulation ceased concomitant with the virtually complete depletion of ATP. (From ref. 268, with permission.)

lished. In very general terms, cell death must be an eventual consequence either of loss of HEPs (261,266) or of progressive accumulation of catabolites, one or more of which may be toxic to the cell. Some representative consequences of these two general features of ischemia are listed in Table 1.

Because HEP is required to provide energy to support many of the complex functions of the myocyte, the hypothesis that depletion of HEP is directly or indirectly related to development of the irreversible state is attrac-

TABLE 1. *Potential causes of irreversibility*[a]

(A) HEP depletion/cessation of anaerobic glycolysis
    Catabolism without resynthesis of macromolecules
    Reduced transsarcolemmal gradients of Na^+ and K^+
        Cell swelling
    Calcium overload
        Activation of phospholipases/proteases
        Impaired mitochondrial function
        Activation of ATPases

(B) Catabolite accumulation [lactate, H^+ (acidosis), fatty acyl derivatives, free radicals, ammonia, inorganic phosphate, etc.]
    Enzyme denaturation
    Membrane damage
    Increased intracellular osmolarity
        Cell swelling

[a] Two major features of ischemia are HEP depletion and catabolite accumulation. Some consequences of each are listed. Cell death may be related to the consequences of one or both general features of ischemic injury. Some effects of ischemia may be related to both HEP depletion and catabolite accumulation. For example, cell swelling may be due both to loss of ATP-dependent ion transport and to intracellular production of low-molecular-weight catabolites.

tive. It is supported by a number of observations, including the fact that reversibly injured myocytes tolerate ATP levels as low as 10 μmoles ATP per gram dry weight (273), whereas irreversibly injured cells invariably have 2 to 5 μmoles ATP per gram dry weight or less (261,266). Furthermore, interventions that delay ATP depletion delay cell death, and vice versa (283,477). However, ATP depletion may need to be present for a period of time before irreversibility supervenes. Thus, the evidence that supports the hypothesis that HEP depletion is related causally to irreversibility is indirect. Proof of the hypothesis will require identification of the reaction or reactions that are inhibited by diminished ATP availability (and therefore cease at or before the transition to irreversible injury) and that are essential for viability (266).

Alternatively, some of the potentially lethal consequences of catabolite accumulation [e.g., H^+, lactate (420), fatty acyl derivatives, and free radicals], and the deleterious effects of increased cytosolic calcium have been reviewed earlier.

Several hypotheses of the pathogenesis of ischemic cell death center on sarcolemmal damage (Fig. 23) (266). At the time that the biochemical counterparts of irreversibility are fully developed, i.e., when ATP levels are less than 10% of control and when anaerobic glycolysis is slowing or has stopped, striking structural and functional evidence of sarcolemmal disruption is found. Breaks in the plasmalemma of the sarcolemma of the myocyte can be observed by electron microscopy (Figs. 18 and 19). These breaks in the plasmalemma are prominent in regions in which the cytoskeletal attachments between the sarcolemma and the underlying myofibrils have been broken. In such areas, the sarcolemma may be separated from the myofibrils by a subsarcolemmal bleb of edema fluid. In these blebs, the plasmalemma often is disrupted totally and is detectable only as small vesicles. The presence of membrane breaks can be detected not only by electron microscopy but also by increases in the inulin diffusible space of thin tissue slices prepared from this tissue and incubated *in vitro* in Krebs-Ringer phosphate (Fig. 24).

Unrestricted entry of extracellular constituents into the myocyte and loss of critical cofactors and low-molecular-weight enzymes from the myocyte to the extracellular space are the early consequences of membrane disruption. Both these phenomena are believed to be incompatible with continued survival of the cell. Increased levels of cytosolic Ca^{2+} caused by release of Ca^{2+} from intracellular stores and/or caused by entry of extracellular Ca^{2+} into the sarcoplasmic space may activate degradative enzymes and impair energy-producing mechanisms of the myocyte (266,271,418); however, loss of enzymes and critical ions such as Mg^{2+} and K^+ produces extensive disruption of the metabolic machinery of the myocyte regardless of the level of sarcoplasmic Ca^{2+}.

The results of the several aforementioned experiments are consistent with the hypothesis that membrane disruption is an event, perhaps *the* event, that signifies that ischemic injury has entered the lethal phase. However, if sarcolemmal disruption is the proximate cause of

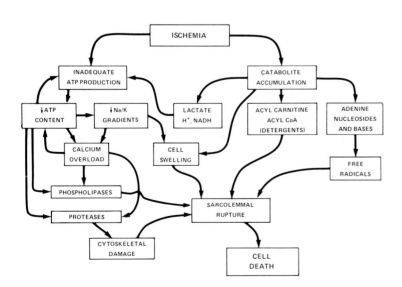

FIG. 23. Some potential pathways leading to sarcolemmal damage, which form the basis for various hypotheses of events leading to irreversible ischemic cell injury. In general terms, two major facets of ischemia are the inadequate production of ATP and the accumulation of potentially noxious catabolites. Declining ATP content could have many adverse consequences including loss of sodium and potassium gradients, calcium overload, and activation of endogenous phospholipases or proteases. The latter could damage the sarcolemma and/or its cytoskeletal supports. Accumulation of catabolites such as lactate, H^+, and NADH inhibit anaerobic glycolysis and thereby inhibit ATP production in ischemia. Products of lipid degradation may act as detergents and damage cell membranes. Adenine nucleosides and bases accumulate and might be a major source of free radicals via the xanthine oxidase reaction. In addition, accumulating catabolites are an intracellular osmotic load which may accentuate cell swelling and facilitate the rupture of already weakened membranes. At the present time the relative importance of these various pathways in the pathogenesis of ischemic cell death has not been established. Moreover, many reactions occur in ischemic myocardium which have been less well studied and are not included on this diagram; it is not even certain that the most important assays are illustrated.

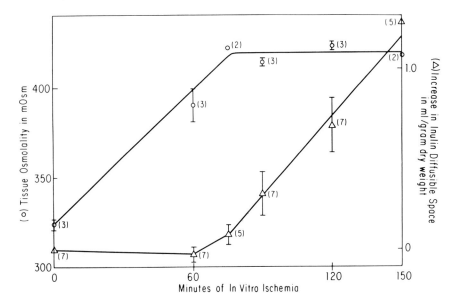

FIG. 24. Relationship between tissue osmolality and plasma membrane damage during total ischemia *in vitro*. Tissue osmolality was measured in myocardial slices prepared from totally ischemic myocardium using vapor-pressure osmometry. Plasma membrane damage was inferred from an increased inulin diffusible space (IDS) after incubation of slices in an oxygenated buffered salt solution containing ^{14}C-inulin; an increased IDS was interpreted to reflect the development of membrane permeability to the large (5,000 M.W.) inulin molecule. The latter normally is confined to the extracellular space. Note that tissue osmolality is increased substantially well before the IDS begins to increase. (From ref. 580, with permission.)

irreversible ischemic injury, the antecedent cause of such disruption has not been elucidated. Several possible mechanisms of membrane damage are diagrammed in Fig. 23.

For example, either ATP depletion or calcium overload could cause membrane damage through activation of plasmalemmal phospholipases. In this regard, it has been reported (74) that arachidonate and other unesterified fatty acids, the by-products of phospholipid degradation, increase significantly in ischemic myocardium between 20 and 60 min. Thus, it would appear that some phospholipid degradation occurs during the transition to irreversibility. However, because the total quantity of phospholipid is minimally changed during this same time period (581), we believe that plasma membrane disruption due to ischemia can occur without significant phospholipid breakdown. Release and activation of lysosomal phospholipases or proteases (68, 104,105,184,235,628,642,643) is currently thought to be a relatively late change that is unlikely to be the primary cause of cell death. The detergent effects of fatty acyl derivatives (295,296,419), which accumulate in moderate-flow ischemia (295,641), also appear to be unlikely mechanisms for disruption of the sarcolemma, at least in zones of total or low-flow ischemia where the accumulation of acyl compounds is rather small.

The possible role of free radicals in inducing irreversible damage to the sarcolemma or other organelles of the myocyte, or to the microvasculature, has been a subject of intense interest in recent years (220,465,557). It seems unlikely that free-radical production of significant degree can occur in zones of low-flow or total ischemia because of the absence of oxygen and because of the presence of abundant quantities of reduced cytochrome oxidase in the mitochondria. The latter protein serves as an avid scavenger of any O_2 present. The roles free radicals play in zones of moderate-flow and high-flow ischemia remain to be established. A detailed

review of evidence for and against the hypothesis that free radicals may cause lethal ischemic myocardial cell injury is beyond the scope of this chapter; suffice it to say that despite much data and debate, the hypothesis that free-radical production is the cause of lethal myocardial ischemic injury has not been proved.

Another potential cause of sarcolemmal disruption and consequent cell death is cell swelling because of osmotic overload (Fig. 24) (272,323,601), coupled with weakening of the sarcolemma, e.g., by proteolytic disruption of its cytoskeletal supports (272,580). With this hypothesis, membrane disruption may be a two-stage process. First, degradation of membrane or cytoskeletal proteins by proteases activated in a low-energy environment must occur, and, second, the cell must swell or contract sufficiently to cause the weakened membrane or its supports to rupture (580).

Both structural damage and functional damage to mitochondria are characteristic of the irreversible phase of ischemic injury. Structural changes have been described earlier and include swelling, cristal disruption, and amorphous matrix densities. Reoxygenation of ischemic myocardium must be followed by resumption of integrated mitochondrial function if the myocytes are to remain viable and recover contractile function. For this reason, many studies have been done to assess the nature and severity of mitochondrial damage induced by ischemia. However, although a variety of mitochondrial functional defects have been observed in ischemic injury (63,262,263,286,354,410,468,507–509,558,576, 598,603), the importance of such mitochondrial damage in the pathogenesis of ischemic cell death has been questioned (266). Reperfusion of ischemic myocardium (*vide infra*) results either in cellular recovery (and at least gradual mitochondrial recovery) (273) or in rapid cell death due to "explosive cell swelling" that is characterized by sarcolemmal disruption, severe cellular swelling accompanied by massive cytosolic calcium overload, and contraction-band necrosis (261,316,639). In the setting of this massive cellular disorganization, excess cytosolic calcium is accumulated by mitochondria and inhibits mitochondrial respiration and oxidative phosphorylation (605). However, it is unknown whether or not mitochondrial damage would preclude myocyte recovery if membrane disruption and calcium overload could be prevented (266).

Microvascular Injury

Whereas we have heretofore emphasized the direct consequences of myocardial ischemia on the affected myocytes, myocardial infarction *in vivo* may involve a complex interplay between myocytes and other elements of the tissue (Fig. 1). For example, the microvasculature also is injured by ischemia (Fig. 19) (9,145,169,260, 315,318,394,638). The nature of microvascular injury has not been as well characterized as has myocyte injury; its pathogenesis is poorly understood. The interrelationship between HEP production and utilization, which may play a major role in myocyte injury, may or may not also be important in the pathogenesis of microvascular injury. Several recent studies have highlighted the potential role of free radicals in microvascular injury (108,279,332). Endothelial injury also may be mediated by fibrin-derived peptides (512).

Obstruction to blood flow through the microvasculature could contribute to myocyte injury by increasing the severity of ischemia. However, the consequences of microvascular injury seem likely to be more important as potential limiting factors for reperfusion of ischemic myocardium; the nature of microvascular obstruction and its consequences will be considered in more detail later, in the reperfusion section of this chapter.

Inflammatory Response and Reparative Phase

Myocardial infarction is a complex, dynamic process in which ischemic cell death is an early event. Dead cardiac myocytes do not regenerate; they must be removed and eventually replaced by scar. Whereas progression of myocardial cell death may go to completion in a matter of minutes or hours, the process of repair requires 4 to 6 weeks under optimum conditions.

Inflammatory Response

Although lysosomal proteases and lipases are released and activated within dead myocytes (and may even contribute to lethality), endogenous degradative enzymes are insufficient to bring about complete dissolution of dead myocytes. Removal of necrotic myocytes depends on the influx of inflammatory cells, including polymorphonuclear neutrophils and macrophages. In the center of large infarcts, both myocytes and the microvasculature undergo necrosis; inflammatory cells initially have no access to the infarct center. In such areas, dead myocytes

persist, retaining their basic structure for days or weeks, until inflammatory cells, initially present on the outer edge of the infarct, can invade the infarct center by direct migration or by ingrowth of new capillaries (Figs. 25 and 26).

The general characteristics of the acute inflammatory response have been studied extensively, especially in regard to infectious disease and traumatic injury (644). The neutrophilic response has been characterized as a process involving margination (concentration toward the endothelial cell), emigration across the capillary wall, and chemotactic attraction to sites of injury. In general terms, chemotactic factors for polymorphonuclear neutrophils are known to include components of the complement pathway, histamine, various kinins, fibrinopeptides, and certain products of bacteria (539,569). Macrophages are attracted by other complement components, bacterial factors, factors from degenerating neutrophils, kallikreins, lymphokines, etc. (624).

The inflammatory response, as it relates specifically to myocardial infarction, has not been as widely studied. In large myocardial infarcts, when much microvascular damage has occurred, an intense neutrophilic response often is observed. In contrast, in smaller infarcts, when most of the microvasculature has been spared, the neutrophilic response may be minimal, and macrophages will be the most notable elements of the early inflammatory response. The specific factors that attract inflammatory cells to myocardial infarcts and that determine the intensity of the inflammatory response are not completely elucidated. However, it is known that subcellular fractions of cardiac muscle can activate the complement system (177,451). More specifically, lysosomal proteases can activate complement; components of this pathway may, in turn, attract neutrophils to the dead myocytes (224). In addition, metabolites of arachidonic acid, such as hydroxyeicosatetraenoic acids (HETEs), are produced by the action of neutrophil lipoxygenases; these substances also are chemotactic for neutrophils (444,569) and may serve to amplify the initial neutrophilic response.

The inflammatory response is essential for resolution and repair of an infarcted area. On the other hand, recent evidence suggests that the inflammatory response also might cause additional injury of still viable myocytes, and thereby increase infarct size. Components of the complement system as well as polymorphonuclear neutrophils accumulate in ischemic myocardium (452,505). Polymorphonuclear neutrophils release a variety of proteases and lipases (636), as well as free radicals, such as the superoxide anion, to the myocardial interstitium (133). Moreover, the inflammatory response begins at and is most intense at the peripheral zone of an infarct where the microvasculature permits access. However, whether or not and to what extent and under what circumstances the inflammatory response does in fact cause additional myocyte necrosis remains open to question (406,500,505).

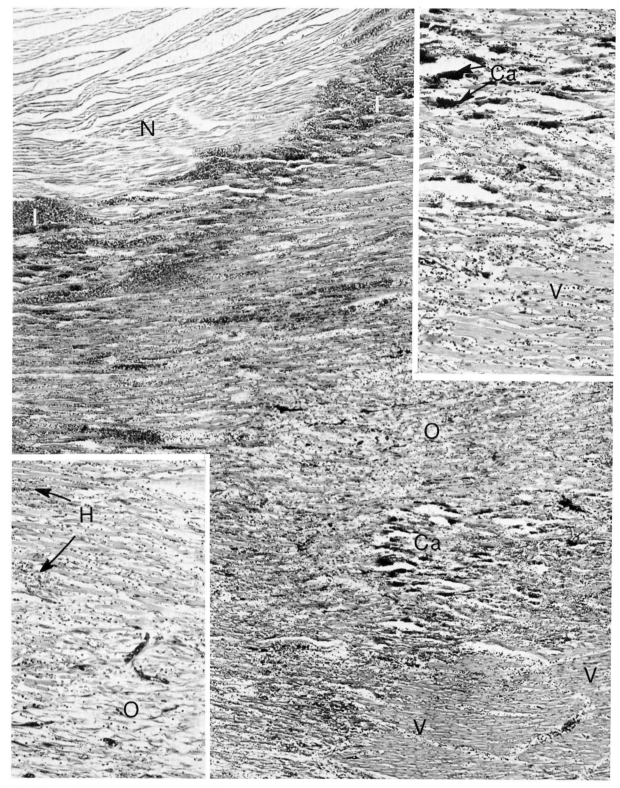

FIG. 25. Characteristic histologic zones of inflammation and repair in a 4-day-old myocardial infarct in a dog. This view is from the center of the circumflex bed and incorporates much of the transmural wall from the subendocardial region (**top**) to subepicardial region (**bottom**). There is a subendocardial central core of coagulation necrosis (N), with separation of fibers due to interstitial and cellular edema, but with relatively little cellular infiltration. This zone is surrounded by a zone with hemorrhage (H) and an intense acute inflammatory response (I). In the peripheral zone, organization (O) has begun and is characterized by macrophages, which have removed some of the necrotic cells, and ingrowth of fibroblasts and capillaries. This is better seen in the lower inset. Some heavily calcified cells (Ca) also are present in the peripheral zone. Some viable muscle (V) survived in the subepicardial region seen at the lower right. This region between the organizing zone of the infarct and viable myocardium is shown at higher power in the upper inset. Stained with hematoxylin and eosin; ×50; insets ×100. (From ref. 476, with permission.)

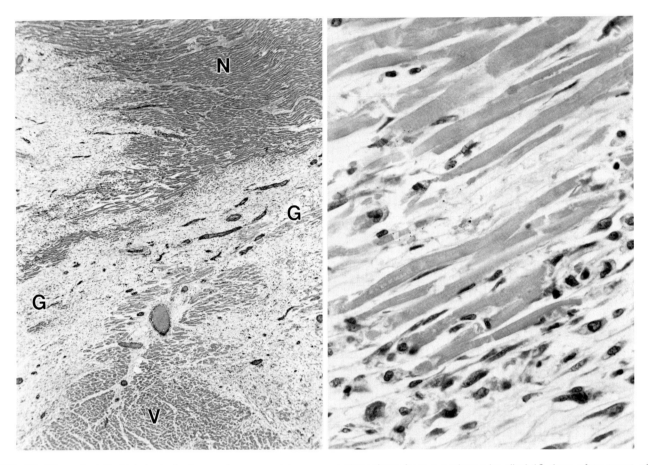

FIG. 26. Characteristic histologic features of an organizing myocardial infarct from a patient who died 13 days after onset of coronary occlusion. **Left:** Infarct consists of a persistent central core of necrotic myocytes (N) surrounded by a peripheral rim of granulation tissue (G). Viable myocardium (V) is present on the subepicardial side of the infarct, around a penetrating artery. ×25. **Right:** Necrotic myocytes flanked by the developing scar. The inflammatory response at this time consists primarily of macrophages digesting the peripheral most necrotic myocytes. Myofibrillar cross-striations are still faintly visible in the remaining necrotic myocytes even at this late stage. Stained with hematoxylin and eosin; ×400.

Reparative Phase

The general process of repair by scar formation also is known, but again, detailed mechanisms of the reparative phase are poorly understood, and the determinants of the quantity and tensile strength of myocardial scars are unknown. The most widely held view is that necrotic myocardium, including its reticular framework (526), is removed and replaced by granulation tissue (new capillaries and fibroblasts), with gradual deposition of both collagen and components of ground substance such as proteoglycans and glycoproteins (35,340,553) (Fig. 26). However, in smaller infarcts, and particularly when the microvasculature has been spared, scar formation may occur by collagen deposition on the original reticular framework in the infarcted region.

Most investigators believe that the major determinant of scar size is infarct size. It also is recognized that myocardial scars may be considerably smaller than the volume of necrotic myocardium that they have replaced (7,476) (and appear even smaller because of compensatory hypertrophy of remaining viable myocardium) (7,513). However, neither the precise relationship be-

tween initial infarct size and ultimate scar size nor variables that affect this relationship are well known. Such knowledge would be of considerable value; whereas infarct size affects cardiac function through loss of contractile mass, the nature of the scar may have additional, independent effects on function. For example, an overly exuberant scar may restrict the contraction of remaining viable myocytes in an ischemic region. Conversely, a weak scar may result in further loss of function because of aneurysmal dilatation of the infarct region; a weak scar may be fatal if cardiac rupture supervenes. It has been reported that exercise has an adverse effect on infarct repair in rats (204).

Gross and Microscopic Patterns of Infarction

The speed of healing of a myocardial infarct depends first and foremost on the size of the infarct and on the extent of microvascular damage. In addition, the rate of healing depends on other less readily characterized factors, such as neutrophil competence. Nevertheless, the sequence of inflammation and repair is sufficiently predictable to permit the age of an infarct to be estimated. The precision with which infarct age can be established is inversely related to age; on the first day or so, infarct age can be established to the nearest 6 to 12 hr; the age of 2-week-old infarcts can be established plus or minus 3 or 4 days; beyond 6 months, scars of different ages often cannot be differentiated. The general sequence of events from which infarct age can be estimated has long been known from the work of Mallory et al. (370) and others (143,355) and is as follows.

Although dramatic metabolic and ultrastructural changes occur early in ischemic injury, myocardial infarction may not be detectable by routine gross or histologic techniques until 6 to 12 hr have elapsed. The earliest gross evidence of infarction often is palor, most likely related to the development of cardiac rigor and the accompanying compression of the microvasculature and expulsion of erythrocytes. In contrast, focal areas of hemorrhage may develop because of microvascular injury. The gross changes become more prominent with time during the first 48 hr. The classic histologic features of coagulation necrosis, consisting of increased cytoplasmic eosinophilia and nuclear karyolysis (dissolution) or pyknosis (shrinkage), may be detectable in some cases within the first 2 to 4 hr, but in some cases may not be detectable as late as 8 to 12 hr. In our experience, because staining intensity may vary, increased eosinophilia best can be recognized when the interface between dead and viable myocytes can be located. For example, because a narrow rim of myocytes below the endocardium often survives an ischemic insult (presumably by diffusion of oxygen and substrates from the left ventricular cavity), increased eosinophilia can be detected with greatest sensitivity by comparing deeper subendocardial myocardium with this superficial layer. Increased eosinophilia is matched by increased acidophilia when connective-tissue stains such as Masson's trichrome stain are used. An additional early feature of myocardial infarction is the development of "wavy fiber change" (47) (due to stretching of ischemic myocytes during life, with undulations developing after death when rigor contracture develops in surrounding areas). Contraction-band necrosis, a second type of necrosis more characteristic of ischemia followed by reperfusion (*vide infra*) (485), may be detected as early as the first hour after the onset of ischemia, if reperfusion has been established. In the absence of reperfusion, contraction-band necrosis can sometimes be seen on the edge of an infarct (573). Although loss of sarcoplasmic cross-striations and karyolysis are often considered to be hallmarks of early necrosis according to standard textbook descriptions, these changes are not absolute; in the center of myocardial infarcts, nuclear outlines and cross-striations may be visible for days or even weeks, so long as unresorbed myocytes persist (Fig. 26, right panel).

Polymorphonuclear neutrophils marginating within the microvasculature sometimes can be observed within the first hour or two of infarction. However, in many cases, the influx of neutrophils cannot be easily detected until 12 to 18 hr after the onset. The number of inflammatory cells increases with time, becoming most prominent by the third day post infarction. Neutrophils that migrate to the site of infarction do not return to the circulation, but undergo lysis at the site of injury. Fragments of disintegrated neutrophils are often detectable by the second day and are most prominent by the third through fifth days. By the fourth or fifth day, the influx of neutrophils has begun to subside, macrophages have become more prominent, and the removal of necrotic myocytes has begun (Fig. 25). The progressive removal of necrotic myocytes is soon followed by ingrowth of new capillary buds and fibroblasts; by the 10th day, the periphery of the infarct is bordered by a distinct rim of granulation tissue (Fig. 26). By gross observation, necrotic myocardium becomes yellow, as compared with the red-brown color of normal myocardium. The peripheral rim of granulation tissue is grossly evident as a hyperemic rim around the infarct (related to the marked vascularity of granulation tissue) (Fig. 27). Between the second and fourth week, much of the necrotic muscle is removed, although the duration of time required for complete removal depends on the initial size of the infarct. As necrotic myocytes are removed, the rim of granulation tissue expands. This removal of necrotic muscle and ingrowth of granulation tissue is referred to as "organization" of the infarct. By about the 12th day, thin collagen fibers begin to be deposited within the young scar. With increasing time, collagen content increases, and the cellularity of the scar gradually decreases. Grossly, the reddish-gray gelatinous character of granulation tissue is replaced by the opaque gray-white color characteristic of a dense collagen scar (Fig. 28). Although some macrophages and mononuclear inflammatory cells may persist for as long as a year or two after infarction, the process of infarct repair is essentially complete by 3 to 6 months. Given this typical sequence of the reparative process, it is possible to estimate, from the gross character and more precisely from microscopic features, the approximate age of an acute or organizing myocardial infarct.

Early Diagnosis of Myocardial Infarction

Because the histologic features of coagulation necrosis develop slowly, much effort has been devoted to establishing methods to enable earlier anatomic recognition of the presence and extent of myocardial infarction. The ultrastructural characteristics of irreversible injury reviewed in previous paragraphs permit early recognition of infarction in experimental studies, but electron microscopy is impractical for assessing the extent of injury

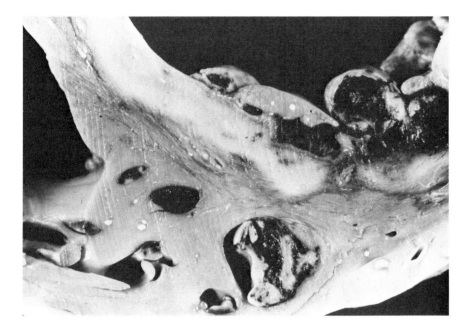

FIG. 27. Cross section of the anterior wall of the right and left ventricles and anterior interventricular septum of a human heart containing an organizing infarct. The section is viewed from the base with the anterior wall toward the bottom. An anteroseptal infarct is present in the subendocardial zone of the anteroseptal region of the left ventricle; this infarct occurred about 10 days prior to the patient's death and is characterized by a central core of necrotic muscle that was yellow-gray, surrounded by a rim of granulation tissue that was dark red. The darker color of this peripheral rim is due to erythrocytes within the proliferating capillaries.

(only a few myocytes can be evaluated in any given sample of tissue; processing multiple samples is extremely time-consuming). Moreover, electron-microscopic evaluation usually is of little value as an aid to early diagnosis of human myocardial infarcts, because changes induced by regional ischemia *in vivo* soon become indistinguishable from identical changes induced by postmortem autolysis, i.e., global, total ischemia. For this reason, a variety of special histologic or histochemical staining techniques have been studied (215), including the periodic-acid-Schiff (PAS) stain for glycogen loss (16,138,300,311,559,655) or entry of PAS-positive diastase-fast plasma proteins into the myocytes (299,655), chemical analysis of tissue potassium/sodium ratios (274,501,543,661), hematoxylin/basic-fuchsin/picric-acid

staining (347,612), tetracycline binding (585), and a host of stains for specific intracellular enzyme activities such as phosphorylase or succinic dehydrogenase (16,215, 300,559,619). For the most part, these staining techniques have not been widely accepted. Under controlled circumstances, each technique may be useful. However, most of these methods are limited either by lack of specificity (failure to differentiate ischemia from postmortem autolysis) or insufficiently early sensitivity.

In contrast, macroscopic methods of staining for dehydrogenase activity have become widely used. The most widely used dehydrogenase stains are para-nitroblue tetrazolium (pNBT) and triphenyl tetrazolium chloride (TTC) (132,144,348,414,534). Each of these two dyes is colorless when oxidized, but turns blue (pNBT) or brick

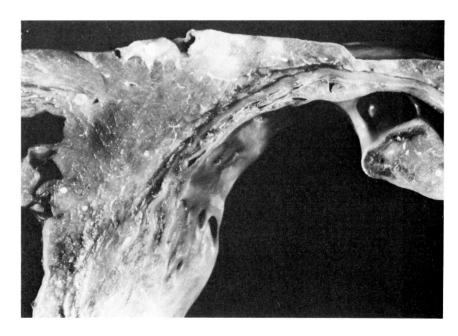

FIG. 28. Cross section of the posteroseptal region of the same human heart. The posterior wall of the left ventricle is markedly thinned, and the myocardium has been replaced by a fibrous scar. This scar is the result of an inferior infarct caused by an occlusion of the right coronary artery months or years prior to the patient's death.

red (TTC) when reduced through the transfer of hydrogen to the dyes from NADH or reduced flavoproteins, catalyzed by endogenous myocardial dehydrogenases. Viable myocardium is capable of reducing either of these dyes, but myocardium that has lost dehydrogenase activity or sufficient concentrations of the cofactors, e.g., NADH (308), remains unstained after addition of the oxidized dyes. Such absence of staining is considered to indicate cell death. Of the two dyes, TTC is the more commonly employed; it is less expensive than pNBT and can be perfused throughout the ischemic region via the coronary arteries, whereas pNBT does not readily traverse the capillary and therefore must be applied to the surfaces of myocardial slices. When used with completed infarcts, or in the setting of reperfused infarcts, these histochemical stains are capable of identifying dead myocardium and demarcating the boundaries of infarcts that might otherwise be poorly differentiated from viable tissue (Fig. 29). Some investigators hold that these histochemical staining techniques permit early diagnosis and even demarcation of the boundaries of infarcts within the first 3 hr after the onset and before histologic diagnosis is possible (144). However, this view remains controversial. Whereas loss of dehydrogenase enzyme activity probably indicates cell death, lethal cell injury precedes loss of such activity, and the presence and extent of early infarction may be underestimated.

Reperfusion of Ischemic Myocardium

The advent of the therapeutic capability for restoring myocardial blood flow to ischemic myocardium, partic-

ularly through application of thrombolytic agents, has sparked widespread clinical and experimental interest regarding myocardial consequences of ischemia and reperfusion (84,168,175,298,328,329,385,488,489,571). In a previous section of this chapter we reviewed the time frame within which reperfusion can limit infarct size in experimental models of infarction. In the present section we shall consider the local consequences of myocardial reperfusion on ischemic myocytes. These consequences depend on the condition of the affected myocytes and adjacent microvasculature at the time reperfusion is established (267,481).

Reversibly Injured Myocytes

As noted earlier, 15 min of severe ischemia induced by occlusion of a coronary artery in a dog results in cellular injury that is reversible, in the sense that no necrosis ensues if reperfusion is established (275). Moreover, moderately ischemic myocytes in the subepicardial zone of an ischemic region may remain reversibly injured for as long as 3 to 6 hr (475,485). However, full metabolic (103,313,474,584) and functional recovery (313,630,651) may require several days, following as little as 5 min of ischemia.

Ultrastructural recovery occurs rapidly. At the end of 15 min of ischemia, characteristic features of reversibly injured myocytes include partial loss of glycogen particles, relaxation of myofibrils, mild margination of nuclear chromatin, mild cell swelling, and mitochondrial changes, including swelling and loss of the normal matrix granules (Fig. 16) (273,484). Observations at 3 min after reper-

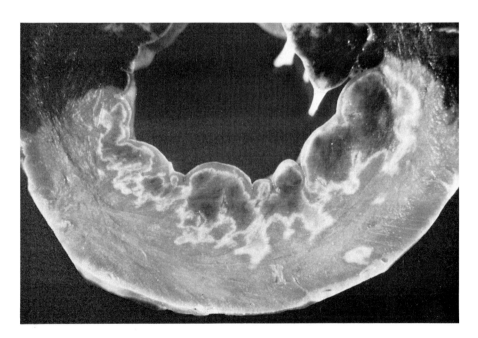

FIG. 29. Subendocardial myocardial infarct in a dog heart, delineated by dehydrogenase staining using triphenyl tetrazolium chloride (TTC). The illustration includes part of a cross-sectional slice of a dog left ventricle, viewed from the apex. Prior to sectioning, the ischemic and nonischemic vascular regions were identified by postmortem coronary perfusion with blue dye (nonischemic) and TTC (ischemic region). In viable subepicardial areas, TTC was reduced by tissue dehydrogenases from its colorless oxidized state to a brick-red color. The lighter subendocardial areas demarcate the infarct, caused by 40 min of circumflex coronary occlusion followed by 4 days of reperfusion. The dark areas within the confines of the infarct are due to hemorrhage. Note that whereas the subepicardial half of the ischemic region was spared by reperfusion, lateral boundaries of viable myocardium within the previously ischemic vascular bed were narrow. (From ref. 481, with permission.)

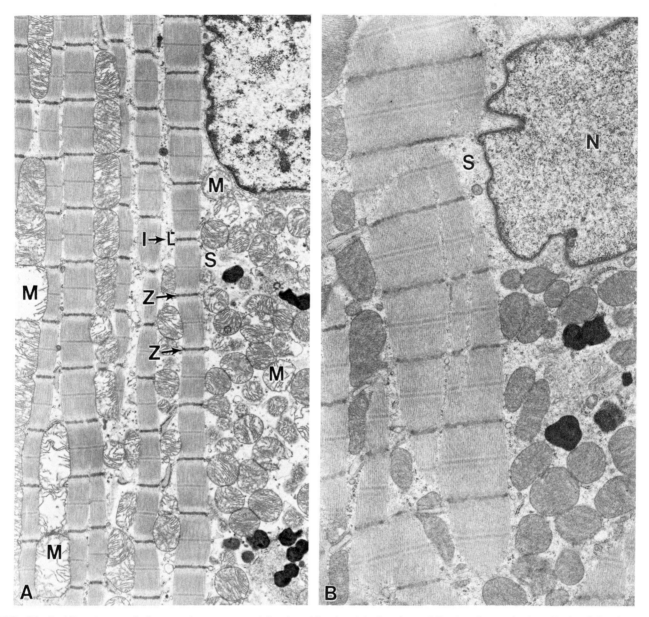

FIG. 30. A: Ultrastructural changes in myocytes following 15 min of ischemia and 3 min of reperfusion. Each of five hearts studied at this time showed features similar to those illustrated. Marked swelling was noted in some mitochondria (M). The remaining mitochondria were less markedly involved. The chromatin of the nucleus is still aggregated peripherally. Compared to control myocardium (panel B), the sarcoplasm (S) is less dense and contains less granular glycogen. The myofibrils are relaxed; they demonstrate large I bands (I), in contrast to the contracted myocytes of control tissue. Z = Z lines. ×7,750. **B:** Nonischemic myocardium from the same dog. The appearance is similar to that shown in Fig. 15. S = sarcoplasm; N = nucleus. ×10,075. (From ref. 273, with permission.)

fusion showed that these changes were still present and that mitochondrial swelling was accentuated (Fig. 30). However, by 20 min after reperfusion, all of these ultrastructural features of injury had disappeared, with the exception of an occasional swollen mitochondrion remaining as a monument to the preceding injury (Figs. 31 and 32). Swollen mitochondria, often engulfed by lysosomes, were seen in occasional myocytes even 4 days after reperfusion. However, most mitochondria quickly recovered; swelling disappeared and normal matrix granules reappeared.

In the same studies, both tissue water and tissue potassium content were increased above control values at 3 min after reperfusion (Fig. 33) (273). The potassium overshoot persisted through 60 min of reperfusion, but was no longer detectable at 24 hr. The tissue edema persisted for 24 hr. Although not marked, and not apparent by qualitative ultrastructural analysis, the increased contents of both potassium and water were suggestive of persistent intracellular edema.

Mitochondrial oxidative phosphorylation recovers rapidly after reperfusion, as evidenced by restoration of

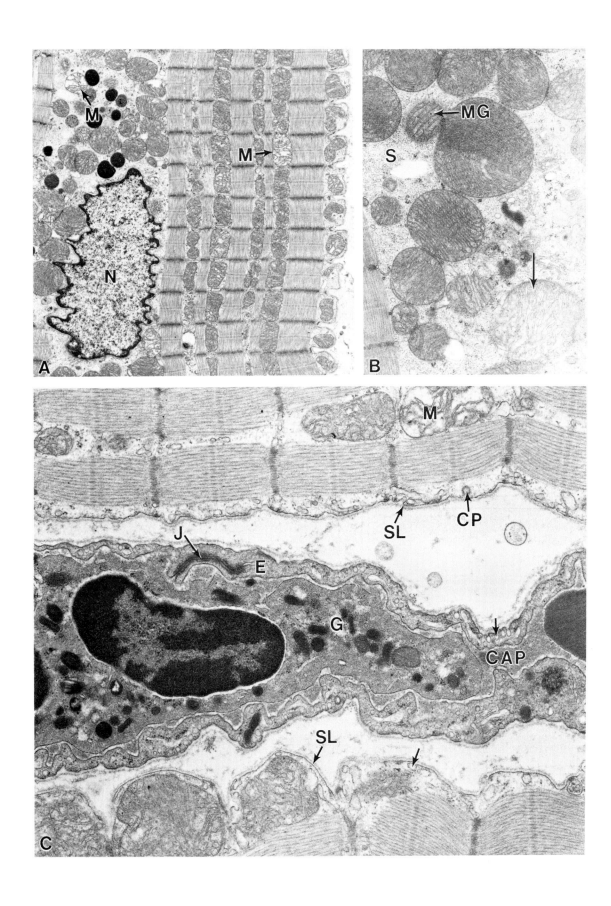

the adenylate charge (474) [(ATP + $\frac{1}{2}$ADP)/(ATP + ADP + AMP)] and creatine phosphate (248,469,584). However, several studies have shown that tissue ATP content does not recover fully for 4 days or longer (Fig. 34) (313,341,474,584,615). The explanation for this prolonged depletion of ATP is that repletion of the adenine nucleotide pool, either by *de novo* or salvage pathways of synthesis, is slow in myocardium (658,659). Adenine nucleotide repletion can be accelerated by infusion of precursors of the synthetic pathways, especially adenosine and ribose (388,623).

Contractile function also recovers slowly, with functional depression present as long as several days following brief periods of occlusion (51,222,313,624,630). The cause of this prolonged functional depression is unknown. One hypothesis is that the functional depression is due to the slow repletion of the ATP of the damaged myocytes to control levels. In some studies, accelerated repletion of ATP, e.g., by infusion of adenosine, has been accompanied by faster functional recovery (198). However, in other studies, functional depression has persisted despite restoration of ATP (234). Additional possible mechanisms for prolonged functional depression include defects in (a) the creatine phosphate shuttle, such that ATP made in the mitochondria is poorly transported to sites of utilization at the myofibril, and (b) the myofibrillar apparatus, including the myosin ATPase per se.

It is noteworthy that in anesthetized dogs with reperfusion after various periods of coronary occlusion, the incidence of ventricular fibrillation (VF) within the first few seconds of reperfusion (reflow VF) is greatest after 15 min, less at 40 min, and rare at 3 hr (Fig. 35). Thus, reflow VF is most likely to occur when the entire ischemic region still is reversibly injured, and it is progressively less likely to occur as the amount of potentially salvageable myocardium decreases (481). Whether or not a similar inverse relationship between the amount of salvageable myocardium and the likelihood of serious arrhythmias exists in patients is unknown; one can speculate that the occurrence of arrhythmias during thrombolytic therapy, while potentially life-threatening, may be a positive indication that reperfusion was achieved and that viable ischemic myocytes still were present at the time.

Irreversibly Injured Myocytes—Intact Vasculature

When an episode of ischemia is sufficiently prolonged to cause irreversible injury of myocytes, the consequences of reperfusion are strikingly different. Reperfusion in this case accelerates the structural disintegration of the myocyte. As seen on electron microscopy, there is explosive cell swelling (261,267,316,481), with formation of large blebs of cytosolic edema beneath the sarcolemma. Such blebs are associated with more marked disruption of the sarcolemma, which may persist only as scattered vesicles along the glycocalyx of the sarcolemma (276). Concomitantly, myofibrils are disrupted, with marked supercontraction of some sarcomeres, interspersed with other sarcomeres that are ripped apart (Fig. 36) (316,485). Corresponding chemical analysis reveals marked increases in myocardial water and sodium content, coupled with marked loss of intracellular ions, including potassium and magnesium (639). Moreover, there is a massive increase in tissue calcium content, coupled with deposition of crystalline granules, composed of calcium and phosphate, in mitochondria (Fig. 36, inset) (316,551,552). Soluble cytosolic constituents, such as the enzyme creatine kinase and other enzymes and cofactors, are rapidly lost and washed to the systemic circulation. All of these changes occur with striking rapidity, being easily observed 2 min after reperfusion.

Explosive cell swelling is thought by some to be due to increased tissue osmolality and preexisting functional or structural defects that permit rapid equilibration of the cytosolic and plasma constituents when the available plasma volume suddenly becomes infinite because of reperfusion (266,276). The massive influx of calcium in this setting is probably related more to the structural damage of the membrane than to more subtle defects in calcium-transport mechanisms, even though such may coexist. The cause of myofibrillar contraction-band formation has not been demonstrated, but probably it is a consequence of the massive calcium overload.

The myofibrillar disruption and contraction-band for-

FIG. 31. Ultrastructural changes in myocytes following 15 min of ischemia and 20 min of reperfusion. **A:** Lower-power view shows that the architecture of the myocytes is well preserved. Myocytes are virtually indistinguishable from typical control myocytes shown in Figs. 15 and 30 (panel B). The chromatin of the nucleus (N) is evenly distributed. An occasional swollen mitochondrion (M) is detected. The myofibrils are contracted. ×6,300. **B:** Higher-power view of typical mitochondria; except for one swollen mitochondrion (*arrow*), they are indistinguishable from control mitochondria. Note that there is abundant glycogen in the sarcoplasm (S). Matrix granules (MG) are present but tiny. ×13,000. **C:** Micrograph shows a granulocyte (G) in the lumen of a capillary (CAP) located between two myocytes. Granulocytes were seen in occasional capillaries of reversibly injured damaged tissue after reperfusion, but were very rare in control tissue. However, no granulocytes were seen in the interstitial space, nor was attachment of granulocytes to endothelial cells observed. The endothelium (E) of the capillary is intact; *arrow* shows the typical pinocytic vesicles of healthy myocardial capillaries; a tight junction (J) also is present in the field. The sarcolemma (SL) of the myocytes is intact and also shows pinocytotic activity at the *arrow* in the lower myocyte. A swollen mitochondrion (M) also is present. However, most mitochondria were similar to control. CP = coated pit. ×22,500. (From ref. 273, with permission.)

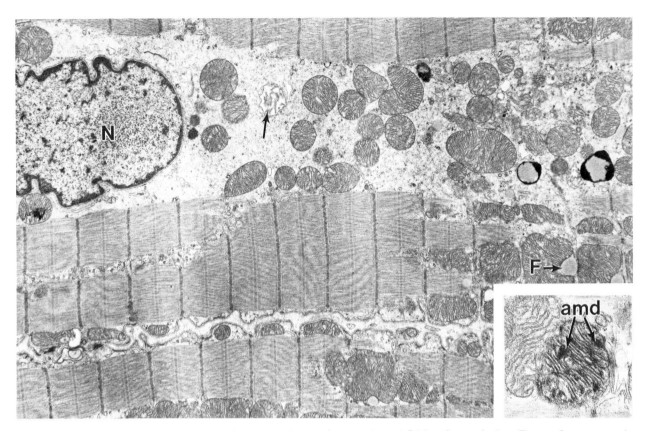

FIG. 32. Ultrastructural features of myocytes following 15 min of ischemia and 24 hr of reperfusion. Except for an occasional swollen (*arrow*) or disrupted mitochondrion (*inset*), these myocytes are indistinguishable from control. The chromatin of the nucleus (N) is evenly distributed. The mitochondrion in the inset was the only damaged mitochondrion in another myocyte. It contains prominent amorphous matrix densities (amd). Glycogen is prominent. Occasional droplets of triglyceride (F) are detectable. However, it is unlikely that this "fatty change" is a true reflection of previous ischemic damage, because control myocardium from the same dog also contained such fat droplets. ×10,750; inset ×22,000. (From ref. 273, with permission.)

mation evident by electron microscopy also are readily visible by routine histology (Fig. 37), especially if sections are evaluated with a connective-tissue stain such as Masson's trichrome stain or Mallory's stain (485). Unlike coagulation necrosis, which may not be recognizable for several hours following the onset of ischemia, contraction-band necrosis can be observed within the first 2 min after reperfusion, provided that ischemia has been of sufficient duration to cause irreversible cell injury (316). Contraction-band necrosis is seen in human hearts following ischemia and reperfusion, the most common settings being cardiac surgery (217) and, more recently, thrombolytic therapy for acute myocardial infarction. It should be noted, however, that contraction-band necrosis is not unique for ischemic injury followed by reperfusion; it is the form of necrosis seen in many experimental or clinical conditions whenever myocytes die in the presence of either continuous or restored perfusion (470). Contraction-band necrosis sometimes may be seen at the edges of non-reperfused myocardial infarcts (573). It also may be induced by catecholamine cardiotoxicity, cardiac electrical shock, in association with cerebral vascular accidents (189), toxic, traumatic, or drug-in-

duced cardiac injury, myocarditis, hypokalemia or hypomagnesemia, hypoxia with reoxygenation (160), and in the calcium-paradox phenomenon (perfusion without calcium, followed by restoration of calcium) (164,660). Contraction-band necrosis has also been referred to by other terms, including "myofibrillar degeneration" (470) and, in the reparative phase, coagulative "myocytolysis" (21). The latter has been particularly confusing, because the term "myocytolysis" more commonly has been used to refer to vacuolar degeneration of sick but still viable cardiac myocytes (59,172).

Irreversibly Injured Myocytes—Damaged Microvasculature

Another aspect of myocardial ischemia is the development of microvascular damage (9,145,169,188,197, 260,313,316,394,638). Restoration of arterial perfusion pressure to damaged arterioles and capillaries may result in accentuated myocardial edema because of increased capillary permeability (362,596,597), or intramyocardial hemorrhage where the vessels are more severely damaged

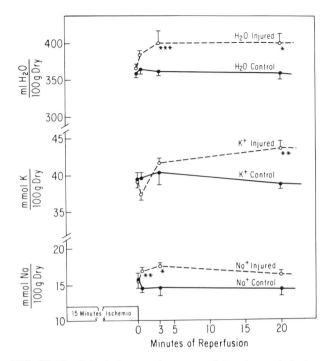

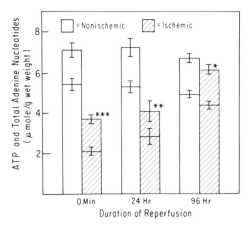

FIG. 34. Myocardial content of ATP and adenine nucleotides after 15 min of severe ischemia in dogs without reperfusion, or with 24 or 96 hr of reperfusion. Fifteen minutes of severe ischemia resulted in loss of 60% of the ATP and 50% of the adenine nucleotide pool. Repletion of the adenine nucleotide pool as slow, being incomplete even 4 days after the acute injury. $*p < 0.05$; $**p < 0.01$; $***p < 0.001$. (From ref. 474, with permission.)

FIG. 33. Persistent changes in myocardial water and electrolytes following 15 min of severe ischemia and reperfusion. The data illustrated are from the subendocardial zones of dog hearts after 15 min of ischemia induced by circumflex coronary occlusion and various periods of reperfusion. Control data are from the nonischemic region of the same hearts. During ischemia per se, tissue water and electrolytes did not change, presumably because of the very low collateral blood flow to the subendocardial zone. Following reperfusion, tissue water and sodium increased promptly and remained elevated. Tissue potassium decreased initially, but then increased above control. Although not illustrated, these changes persist for at least 60 min but are not detectable at 24 hr in this experimental model. (From ref. 273, with permission.)

(Figs. 25, 29, and 38) (52,145,223,475,481,485). On the other hand, where the vasculature has become obstructed, e.g., by extravascular compression due to myocyte edema or contracture (170,209,243,244,353) or to interstitial edema or hemorrhage (157) or to intravascular obstruction by swollen endothelial cells (Fig. 19) (9,316), sticky white cells (126), or platelet-fibrin microthrombi (136), reperfusion may simply not be possible despite reopening of the occluded artery (65,315). This has been termed the "no-reflow" phenomenon.

The possibility that late reperfusion might cause hemorrhage into an infarct that could cause further enlargement of infarct size, deterioration of myocardial function, or anatomic catastrophes such as cardiac rupture has been of considerable clinical concern. However, in experimental studies, when the effects of reperfusion on infarct size were measured directly, the sizes of infarcts that developed following reperfusion were either smaller or the same as the sizes of infarcts that developed in comparable control animals in the absence of reperfusion;

reperfusion has never been shown to increase infarct size, irrespective of the duration of coronary occlusion preceding reperfusion (26,44,66,85,171,178,186,236,313, 387,430,475,485,566). Also, although hemorrhagic in-

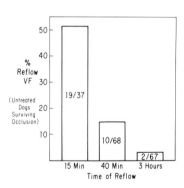

FIG. 35. Incidence of ventricular fibrillation (VF) associated with reperfusion after various periods of proximal occlusion of the circumflex coronary artery in anesthetized open-chest dogs. The dogs listed here are dogs that served as control dogs for a number of different studies over a 5-year period, all using the same experimental protocol as far as surgical procedures, but differing according to duration of occlusion. The number in each column indicates the number of dogs developing reflow VF divided by the total number reperfused after the indicated duration of occlusion. On the average, 10 to 15% of dogs in each group developed VF and died during the occlusion. Of the 172 dogs that survived occlusion, 50% developed VF when reflow was established at 15 min, 15% at 40 min, and 3% at 3 hr. Thus, in this experimental model, the likelihood of reflow VF is inversely related to the amount of potentially salvageable ischemic myocardium. Dogs reperfused early enough to completely prevent infarction nevertheless have the highest mortality. (From ref. 481, with permission.)

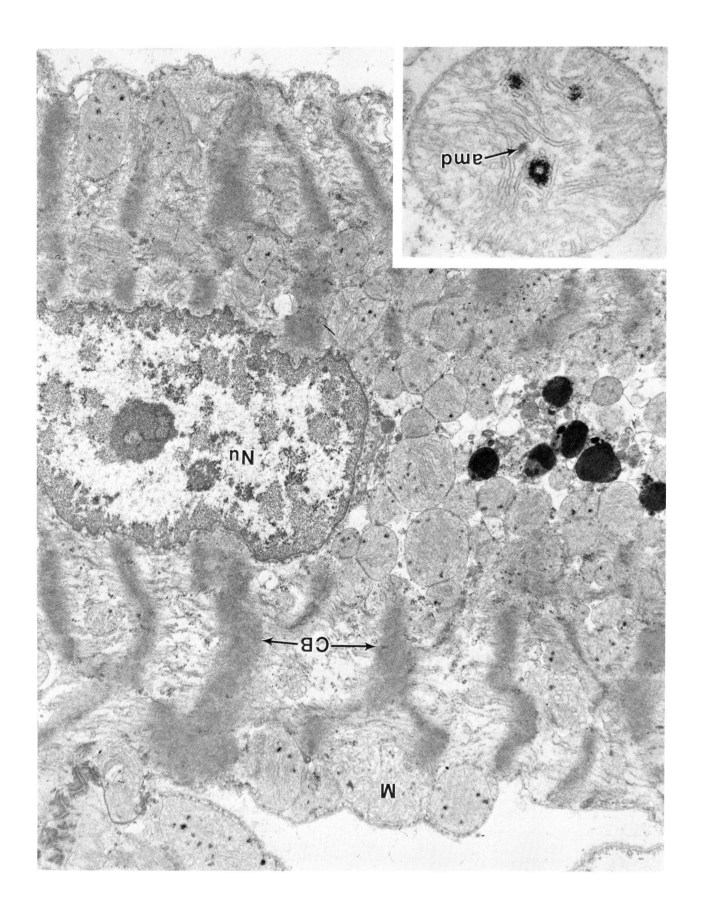

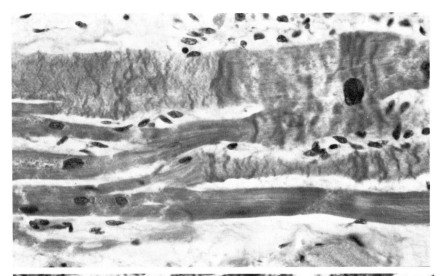

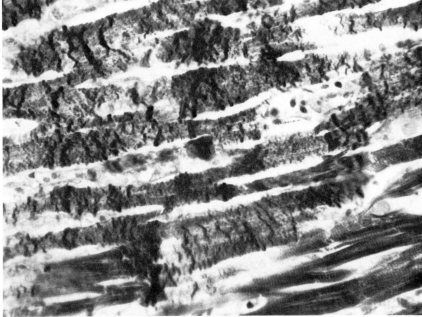

FIG. 37. Typical histologic features of contraction-band necrosis. The myofibrillar disruption and formation of contraction bands observed by electron microscopy (Fig. 36) are readily apparent by light microscopy. **Top:** Stained with hematoxylin and eosin, the necrotic myocytes with contraction bands (**upper right**) are easily distinguished from viable myocytes (**lower left**). **Bottom:** Stained with Heidenhain's variant of Mallory's connective-tissue stain, contraction bands are even more prominent. A few viable myocytes are present in the lower right corner for comparison. In contrast to coagulation necrosis, which may not become detectable for several hours after the onset of myocardial infarction, contraction-band necrosis develops almost immediately on reperfusion of irreversibly injured myocytes. This illustration is from a patient who died 2 hr after coronary bypass surgery. ×350.

farcts have been observed at autopsy following thrombolytic therapy in humans (Fig. 38) (290,386), the clinical experience with thrombolytic therapy to date has generally been favorable. Although reperfusion can increase the amount of hemorrhage within an infarct, several experimental studies have shown that such hemorrhage is primarily confined to the infarct center, where myocytes already are beyond hope of salvage (144,

313,475,485). The finding of myocyte necrosis peripheral (subepicardial) to areas of hemorrhage or no-reflow (Figs. 25 and 29) suggests that microvascular injury occurs more slowly than myocyte damage. Moreover, because the source of myocardial perfusion is from the epicardial surface of the heart, but hemorrhage occurs closer toward the endocardial zone (475,485), it seems unlikely that hemorrhage could limit collateral flow to

FIG. 36. Ultrastructural features of contraction-band necrosis induced by 40 min of *in vivo* ischemia and 20 min of reperfusion. Numerous dense contraction bands (CB) are obvious. Peripheral condensation of nuclear chromatin (Nu) is also apparent, and mitochondria (M) appear swollen and contain both amorphous and granular matrix densities. The inset on the lower left shows a higher-power view of characteristic granular densities of calcium phosphate in mitochondria of these cells. Both amorphous (amd) and granular densities are present. Osmium fixation. ×14,000; inset ×45,000.

still viable subepicardial myocardium. On the other hand, hemorrhage might increase myocardial stiffness early after reperfusion and might be either beneficial (by reducing a systolic bulge) or detrimental (by impeding contractile function of residual viable myocytes).

When the no-reflow phenomenon occurs, the inflammatory response and process of repair occur from the periphery toward the infarct center, as occurs in non-reperfused infarcts. However, the effects of successful reperfusion and/or intramyocardial hemorrhage on the inflammatory response and the process of repair, including the size and strength of the ultimate scar, have not been thoroughly studied.

Reperfusion Injury

The dramatic and immediate aforementioned cellular consequences of reperfusion of irreversibly injured myocytes (explosive cell swelling, enzyme washout, massive calcium overload, and contraction-band necrosis) have been considered by some to be evidence of "reperfusion injury," i.e., myocyte death caused by the reperfusion per se (147,280,502). This concept involves the hypothesis that ischemic cells, although injured, are still potentially viable at the instant of reperfusion but are killed by the added detrimental consequences of reperfusion itself. The alternative hypothesis (266,267) is that myo-

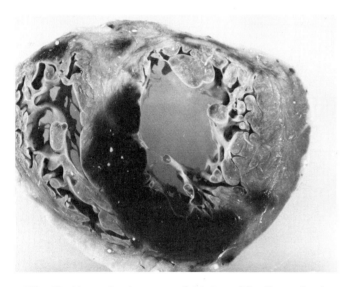

FIG. 38. Hemorrhagic myocardial infarct. The illustration is of a cross section through the ventricles of a heart from a patient who died following myocardial infarction and intracoronary administration of streptokinase. The section is viewed from the basal side (anterior wall at bottom of photo). There is extensive hemorrhage within a nearly transmural anteroseptal infarct (*dark area*). A scar from a prior posteroseptal (inferior) myocardial infarct also is present. (Adapted from ref. 290.)

cytes have suffered severe injury prior to reperfusion and that the dramatic consequences of reperfusion are simply postmortem manifestations of lethal injury that are made possible by the sudden availability of large volumes of plasma water and/or calcium.

On the one hand, it is clear that early reperfusion limits infarct size by salvaging some ischemic myocytes that ultimately die if reperfusion is not initiated. Thus, it is undisputed that for the total population of ischemic myocytes, early reperfusion is better than no reperfusion. However, it has not been proved that some myocytes that do undergo explosive cell swelling might have been able to recover had it not been for some additional insult from reperfusion. Possible mechanisms for reperfusion injury include (a) calcium overload because of altered membrane permeability to calcium, increased Na^+/Ca^{2+} exchange due to increased cytosolic Na^+ (192) and/or insufficient ATP content to handle even a normal calcium influx, (b) a burst of free-radical production, as might occur by xanthine-oxidase-mediated production of superoxide anions during the conversion of large quantities of hypoxathine to xanthine (280), and (c) massive myocyte swelling due to a combination of the osmolar load of ischemia and deficient energy-dependent volume-regulating mechanisms with rupture of the sarcolemma. The principal evidence against the concept of reperfusion injury is that severe mitochondrial damage and damage of the sarcolemma of irreversibly injured myocardial cells can be detected by electron microscopy as early as 30 to 40 min after coronary occlusion and prior to reperfusion in dogs (261,276). Evidence favoring the existence of reperfusion injury includes observations of less myocardial cell injury when reperfusion of ischemic myocardium has been accompanied by free-radical scavengers (280), when reperfusion has been initiated with hypocalcemic blood, followed by gradual restoration of normal blood calcium (147), or when reperfusion has been established with hypertonic blood (146,460).

The oxygen-paradox phenomenon is of interest with respect to reperfusion injury. This phenomenon is observed in isolated buffer-perfused hearts. When such preparations are perfused with hypoxic buffer and then switched back to oxygenated buffer, reoxygenation is followed by explosive cell swelling, contraction-band necrosis, and massive enzyme washout (166,211). Similarly, sudden cellular disruption is observed when anoxic cultured myocytes are reoxygenated (237,498). In this phenomenon, the dramatic sudden cellular dissolution does not require reperfusion, because perfusion is never reduced, but depends solely on the removal and subsequent restoration of oxygen. Although the mechanism of the oxygen paradox is not completely understood, it is known that it is the resumption of oxidative metabolism rather than oxygen per se that initiates the phenomenon; inhibition of cellular respiration with cyanide

(166) or uncoupling oxidative phosphorylation with dinitrophenol (165) prevents the paradox. It has been postulated that the oxygen paradox may occur because of contracture-induced membrane disruption that occurs when mitochondrial ATP production resumes (163). Whether or not the restoration of oxygen via blood reperfusion *in vivo* has parallel consequences vis-à-vis the oxygen paradox *in vitro* is unknown.

Intermittent Ischemia and Reperfusion

The fact that a single brief episode of ischemia may induce prolonged depletion of the adenine nucleotide pool, accompanied by prolonged functional depression, suggests that repetitive brief periods of ischemia, as might occur in patients with angina pectoris, could cause cumulative loss of adenine nucleotides, prolonged functional depression, and perhaps even myocardial infarction. Recent studies, however, have shown that (on the contrary) despite the slow repletion of adenine nucleotides following a single brief episode of myocardial ischemia, cumulative ATP depletion, worsening contractile dysfunction, and lethal cellular injury develop only very slowly, if at all, in the setting of repetitive brief episodes of myocardial ischemia (Fig. 39) (24,173,333,335,486,583). The explanation for this resistance to cumulative effects of repeated episodes of ischemia is not understood at present. The prevention of cumulative loss of ATP and adenine nucleotides could be related to increased availability of HEPs from sources other than the intracellular pool of ATP (e.g., creatine phosphate or anaerobic glycolysis), to depressed HEP demands during subsequent episodes of ischemia, to compartmentation of ATP, or to reduced activity of one or more of the enzymes responsible for degradation of ATP or the adenine nucleotide pool (486). Recently it has been found that repeated brief episodes of ischemia may precondition the myocardium such that infarcts produced by 40 min of coronary occlusion are actually smaller if preceded by four 5-min episodes of transient ischemia (i.e., 60 min of cumulative ischemia) (413). The explanation for this surprising observation also is unknown.

Early and Late Cardiac Complications
of Myocardial Infarction

The morbidity and mortality associated with myocardial infarction in humans can be related in most cases either to inadequate pumping capabilities of the heart (pump failure) or to cardiac arrhythmias. Severe pump failure may occur in the acute phase of myocardial infarction and result in the clinical syndrome known as

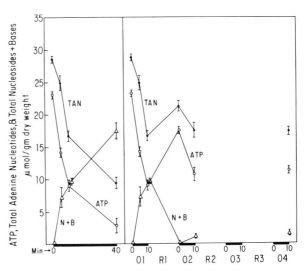

FIG. 39. Myocardial ATP, total adenine nucleotide pool (TAN), and total pool of nucleosides and bases (N + B) during 40 min of continuous ischemia (**left panel**) and during 40 min of cumulative ischemia with intermittent reperfusion (**right panel**). Ischemia was induced by circumflex occlusion in anesthetized dogs. All measurements were made in samples of the severely ischemic subendocardial zone. Data for different times are based on different groups of dogs, N = 4 to 6; brackets indicate plus or minus one standard error of the mean. By 10 min (shown on both panels), ATP was reduced by 61%, and the total adenine nucleotide pool by 41%. By 40 min of sustained ischemia, 87% of the ATP was gone, and only 33% of the adenine nucleotide pool remained. A 20-min period of reperfusion after 10-min ischemia resulted in only partial recovery of ATP. This partial recovery was related to restoration of the adenylate charge, and perhaps to modest early repletion of the adenine nucleotide pool. A second episode of ischemia induced a much slower rate of ATP depletion. Moreover, even after a third and fourth 10-min period of ischemia, ATP and adenine nucleotides were no lower than they were after a single occlusion. The preservation of adenine nucleotides during repetitive occlusions was paralleled by markedly reduced production of nucleosides (adenosine and inosine) and bases (hypoxanthine and xanthine) during repetitive ischemic episodes. (From ref. 486, with permission.)

"cardiogenic shock." Less severe dysfunction may persist long after an acute infarct as congestive heart failure. Usually these forms of heart failure are caused by loss of a substantial quantity of functional myocardium. Cardiac dilatation or papillary muscle dysfunction may cause mitral insufficiency, which also contributes to reduced cardiac performance. In a minority of cases, cardiac dysfunction may be due to specific anatomic complications such as acute infarct expansion or later formation of a ventricular aneurysm. Rupture of some part of the myocardium, e.g., the external wall, interventricular septum, or, rarely, a papillary muscle, may cause sudden and often catastrophic pump failure.

A variety of supraventricular and ventricular cardiac dysrhythmias may complicate myocardial infarction in the acute phase; a propensity for ventricular dysrhythmias may persist chronically and become manifest as recurrent ventricular tachycardia or as sudden death; the latter is thought usually to be caused by ventricular fibrillation. A specific anatomic basis for most types of acute or chronic dysrhythmias has not been identified; however, disturbances of cardiac conduction such as complete heart block or bundle branch block (282) may be caused by necrosis of myocardium within or near a segment of the conduction pathways (28,201). See *Chapters* 55 and 57 for a discussion of the arrhythmias of ischemia.

In general, the aforementioned complications of myocardial infarction, which are so important in the clinical setting, have unfortunately been difficult to reproduce in experimental animals. The notable exception is early ventricular fibrillation, an often undesired event that has prematurely terminated many studies of other aspects of myocardial ischemia. Nevertheless, we shall briefly consider some of the aforementioned complications in the following paragraphs. Two additional cardiac complications of myocardial infarction, namely, pericarditis (301,345) and left ventricular mural thrombosis (13,64), and several systemic complications of myocardial infarction and/or cardiac failure, such as pulmonary systemic emboli, pulmonary edema, and acute "central hemorrhagic necrosis" or chronic "cardiac cirrhosis" of the liver, will not be considered further in this chapter.

Cardiogenic Shock

The majority of deaths from myocardial infarction are due to arrhythmias, many of which occur outside the hospital setting; the most common cause of death among hospitalized patients with myocardial infarction is "pump failure." This gives rise to the clinical syndrome of cardiogenic shock (97) and is a complication that occurs in about 10 to 20% of hospitalized patients with myocardial infarction (536). Postmortem studies of hearts of patients who died from myocardial infarction have shown that, in most cases, there are no distinctive anatomic features that permit differentiation of pump failure versus arrhythmic death (536). However, cardiogenic shock is almost always associated with large areas of myocardial infarction involving at least 30% and often in excess of 40% of the left ventricle (70,440). Unusually prolonged increases of plasma creatine kinase (MB fraction) have been observed in such patients; this observation is consistent with the view that cardiogenic shock per se may cause further myocardial ischemic injury and thereby result in a vicious cycle of progressive cardiac necrosis and dysfunction (196,440). Up to the present time, no reproducible experimental model of cardiogenic shock has been described. For example, in dogs with acute coronary occlusions, creation of an area of ischemia sufficiently large to cause sustained hypoten-

sion is almost invariably accompanied by intractable ventricular fibrillation.

"Ischemic Cardiomyopathy"

In some patients with long-standing ischemic heart disease, often with but sometimes without a clinical history of one or more myocardial infarcts, impaired ventricular contractile function gives rise to the clinical features of a dilated cardiomyopathy. This entity has been termed "ischemic cardiomyopathy" (60,447). Although the term "cardiomyopathy" simply means heart muscle disease, most authorities on the cardiomyopathies restrict the definition of cardiomyopathy to heart muscle disease *excluding* that due to ischemic heart disease (1,98). Thus, "ischemic cardiomyopathy" is a contradiction in terms; the syndrome might better be referred to as "end-stage ischemic heart disease," although the latter term is admittedly more cumbersome than "ischemic cardiomyopathy." Semantics aside, the pathologic counterparts to progressive, often refractory congestive heart failure most often are diffuse, severe coronary atherosclerosis and widespread myocardial scarring due to one or more previous myocardial infarcts (545,616). Chronic heart failure, like cardiogenic shock, has not been widely studied in experimental animals. An experimental model of chronic heart failure has been described, induced in dogs by administering massive intracoronary doses of microspheres (327).

Mitral Regurgitation

A frequent contributing cause of pump failure in myocardial infarction is mitral regurgitation, which has been reported to occur in up to 40% of posterior (inferior) and 13% of anterior myocardial infarcts (522). Necrosis of one of the papillary muscles as well as the adjacent free wall of the heart is the usual anatomic counterpart to this clinical problem (396,449,549,604). However, necrosis of a papillary muscle occurs much more frequently than does clinically apparent mitral insufficiency; thus, papillary muscle necrosis alone probably is not sufficient to cause mitral insufficiency (522). Mitral insufficiency of a mild degree has been reported in 25% of dogs surviving infarction of the posterior papillary muscle and posterior ventricular wall induced by occlusion of the circumflex artery (140).

Infarct Expansion and Ventricular Aneurysm

Marked thinning and lateral expansion of the infarcted region contribute to overall left ventricular dilatation, and perhaps to global left ventricular dysfunction, in one-third or more of patients who die of myocardial infarction during the first 30 days (246). Infarct expansion has been detected clinically, using serial two-dimensional echocardiography, as early as 3 days after the onset of infarction, with progression over a period of days to weeks (124). Infarct expansion also has been observed experimentally in rats (233).

The incidence of ventricular aneurysms following myocardial infarction depends to a large extent on one's definition of an aneurysm; a saccular bulge with a definable neck (angiographically) or a defined external protrusion of a localized area of the left ventricular wall (by postmortem evaluation) occurs in 3 to 4% of cases of myocardial infarction (122). On the other hand, systolic bulging (dyskinesis) of a thinned-out region of the myocardial wall (Fig. 28) undoubtedly occurs much more commonly. Although infarct expansion occurs early, ventricular aneurysms, by the more restricted definition, are often late sequelae of myocardial infarction. For example, in a series of 40 patients described by Davis and Ebert (101), the mean time between initial infarction and detection of a ventricular aneurysm was 2.8 years. Why a small fraction of myocardial scars gradually expand to form aneurysms is unknown. Although large akinetic areas of solid transmural infarction have been produced experimentally (443), chronic ventricular aneurysms have not been reproduced and studied in animal models. In patients, 65 to 80% of ventricular aneurysms involve the anteroapical region of the left ventricle (122,432). Congestive heart failure is present in 30 to 85% of patients with aneurysms and is the most common cause of death (101,122,195). Mural thrombi have been observed in more than half of cases studied post-mortem, but the clinical incidence of systemic thromboemboli is less frequent (5–40% of cases) (101,122,195).

Cardiac Rupture

Cardiac rupture is a catastrophic cause of pump failure that has a variably reported incidence of 5 to 25% of fatal cases of myocardial infarction (25,342,415). External cardiac rupture accounts for the majority of these cases (617), and ventricular septal, papillary muscle, or combined ruptures account for the remainder. Cardiac ruptures occur with greatest frequency during the first week of infarction, corresponding to the time when necrosis and inflammation predominate; rupture is rare beyond the third week, by which time collagen deposition in the developing scar is well under way. The average duration from onset of infarction to rupture has been reported to be about 4 days in several studies of external, septal, or papillary muscle rupture (125,245,613, 617,629); however, as many as one-third of external ruptures have occurred within the first 24 hr in some studies (342). Relatively little is known about the patho-

genesis of cardiac rupture, although several predisposing factors are recognized (25,191,321,342,415,637); rupture usually requires a transmural (although not necessarily large) myocardial infarct and often occurs through first-time infarcts in hearts without a long-standing stimulus for collateral coronary growth. Systemic hypertension and cardiac hypertrophy are frequently mentioned risk factors; whether or not other clinical factors such as physical activity or therapy with digitalis or anticoagulants are risk factors is controversial. Cardiac rupture has been associated with preceding infarct expansion in a recent study (544). Despite the importance of cardiac rupture in the clinical consideration of myocardial infarction, cardiac rupture is apparently not a feature of animal models of myocardial infarction; among the hundreds of myocardial infarcts we have studied in dogs, we have never observed any type of cardiac rupture.

PROTECTION OF ISCHEMIC MYOCARDIUM

Importance and Rationale

Much basic and clinical research effort has been expended in the search for means to delay or prevent myocardial ischemic injury. The potential applications of such therapy include (a) preservation of myocardium during cardiac surgery, when transient periods of myocardial ischemia are necessary parts of the procedure, and (b) prevention or limitation of myocardial infarct size. The idea that human myocardial infarct size could potentially be limited (50,376) received early support from the frequent observation, at autopsy, of infarcts that were smaller than the myocardial region supplied by the occluded coronary artery (627,645). The concept has been confirmed by experimental studies that have documented the fact that ischemic myocytes do not die instantaneously or simultaneously and that infarct size can indeed be limited for a period of time after the onset of ischemia. Given the temporal and spatial biology of infarction reviewed earlier in this chapter, the realistic goal of therapy most likely is conversion of a potentially transmural infarct to one that is subendocardial or at least nontransmural (265,337,475). The most critical aspect of any interventional therapy, if it is to have any chance of success in limiting infarct size, is to minimize the delay between the onset of ischemia and the onset of treatment (265,471). An additional goal of therapy should be to prevent recurrent infarction (infarct extension).

The potential benefits of limiting infarct size in humans have been inferred from many clinical and experimental studies that have demonstrated a direct relationship between infarct size and the incidence and severity of arrhythmic and hemodynamic complications of myocardial infarction. For example, larger infarcts in dogs or rats have been associated with a greater loss of contractility and greater susceptibility to induction of ventricular fibrillation (17,435,450). Large infarcts in patients, as estimated from serial measurements of serum creatine kinase, have been associated with worse cardiac function (240,384), a higher frequency of ventricular ectopic beats (94), and higher short-term mortality (570,594). In autopsy studies of patients who have died in cardiogenic shock, infarct size has often exceeded 40% of the left ventricle (70,440). On the other hand, the transmural extent of infarction, to the degree this can be estimated by the presence or absence of Q waves on the EKG, has not had prognostic importance in most studies (67,368,491,537,586).

General Concepts—Points of Intervention

It is clear that long-term limitation of infarct size and the hoped-for functional benefits of limiting infarct size are absolutely dependent on restoration of adequate coronary blood flow to the ischemic region. Such restoration of coronary blood flow might be achieved by active intervention (i.e., by thrombolytic therapy, angioplasty, or surgical revascularization) or by ischemia-induced natural growth and enlargement of collateral anastomoses. Thus, much clinical and experimental effort has been devoted to developing practical means of achieving early restoration of myocardial blood flow. In addition, however, much effort has been expended to develop ways to directly protect ischemic myocardium in the interval of time before adequate coronary perfusion is restored.

As a basis for limiting infarct size, one could intervene at any one of the general steps illustrated in Fig. 1. Intervening to improve oxygen supply or to reduce metabolic demand is straightforward from the conceptual point of view. Intervening to directly prevent the specific mechanism of cell death is a very desirable aim as well; however, it will be difficult to design effective interventions until we know the mechanism of ischemic cell death. Thus, developing therapies to intervene at a mechanistic level can be done only by trial and error. Such interventions must be selected based on a best guess of what may be a critical step in the transition to irreversibility. Conversely, testing certain interventions to determine whether or not they limit ischemic injury may lead to a better understanding of the pathogenesis of ischemic cell death. Many different categories of drugs have been studied in one or another experimental model of ischemic injury or in clinical trials involving patients with myocardial infarction. To date, although much information has been accumulated, there is no single therapy that has proved effective for limiting infarct size in patients. For more detailed reviews of the extensive experimental evidence for and against the many potential therapies, the reader is referred to several recent books on the subject (214,401,620). Table 2 presents a general

mechanistic classification of a large number of possible modes of intervention that have been studied. This classification may be useful by providing a rational means for selecting new and as yet untested modes of therapy. However, a drawback to such a mechanistic classification is that individual drugs often do not fit into a single categorical niche.

In the general framework of Table 2, the energy utilization of the ischemic cell might be decreased either by reducing the hemodynamic determinants of myocardial energy utilization or by directly inhibiting those reactions within the ischemic cell that continue to consume HEPs. On the other side of the energy production/utilization equation, a large number of suggested therapies have actions that might increase the potential for energy production. The potential for energy production could be increased either by increasing blood flow to the ischemic region or by increasing the oxygen or substrate delivery to the region despite persistent ischemia. Perfusion could be restored directly by emergency revascularization or by lysis of thrombi. Collateral perfusion also might be improved by interventions that would increase diastolic blood pressure, dilate collateral anastomoses, or decrease external compression of the microvasculature. The capacity of ischemic cells to produce energy could be increased, despite persistent ischemia, if blood oxygen or substrate content were increased or if interstitial diffusion of oxygen or substrates could be increased. The accumulation of metabolites could be reduced either by improving perfusion, and thereby facilitating washout, or by inhibiting non-energy-producing catabolic pathways.

Irrespective of the balance between energy production and utilization, some potential therapies are pertinent because they might slow or reverse one or more of the effects of ischemia on cell structure or on the cytosolic milieu of the cell. Agents that could inhibit cell swelling, prevent calcium influx, stabilize cell membranes, or prevent formation of free radicals are general examples of this category of therapy.

If microvascular injury contributes to the progression of myocyte necrosis, interventions that could prevent either endothelial injury or capillary obstruction could be beneficial. Also, if the inflammatory response causes necrosis of myocytes that might otherwise have survived ischemic injury, interventions that interfere with the inflammatory response might prove beneficial.

Testing Potential Therapies

Although limitation of infarct size is a rather simple concept, testing the hypothesis that various interventions are protective has been extraordinarily costly and fraught with difficulties. The major problems have been twofold (478): (a) It is difficult to estimate, and virtually impossible to measure, infarct size in living patients precisely.

TABLE 2. *Potential ways to limit acute necrosis (minimize infarct
size) or prevent subsequent necrosis (prevent infarct extension)*[a]

(A) Decrease energy utilization
   (1) Reduce hemodynamic work
      (a) Reduce heart rate: β-blockade, carotid sinus stimulation
      (b) Reduce contractility: β-blockade, Ca^{2+}-flux inhibition (calcium antagonists), prostaglandins
      (c) Reduce afterload: intraaortic balloon counterpulsation
      (d) Reduce preload: nitrates, digitalis (in the failing heart)
   (2) Reduce cell metabolism directly
      (a) Reduce Ca^{2+} influx: β-blockade, calcium antagonists
      (b) Induce hypothermia

(B) Increase the potential for energy production
   (1) Restore or preserve existing perfusion of ischemic myocardium
      (a) Do emergency revascularization
      (b) Alter coagulation
         (i) Lyse existing thrombi: streptokinase, urokinase, tissue-type plasminogen activator
         (ii) Prevent microthrombi: aspirin, prostaglandins
      (c) Improve or preserve collateral blood flow
         (i) Increase diastolic blood pressure
            (a) Balloon counterpulsation
            (b) α-Adrenergic stimulation: methoxamine, norepinephrine
         (ii) Use vasodilators: calcium antagonists, nitrates, α-adrenergic blockage, prostaglandins, dipyridamole
         (iii) Decrease diastolic wall tension (reduce preload): nitrates
         (iv) Prevent myocardial edema: osmotic agents (mannitol), hyaluronidase
      (d) Do coronary venous retroperfusion or intermittent coronary sinus occlusion
   (2) Increase blood oxygen or substrate content despite persistent ischemia
      (a) Increase oxygen: correct hypoxemia and anemia, hyperbaric oxygen, fluorocarbon blood substitutes
      (b) Increase substrates: glucose-insulin-potassium (GIK), hypertonic glucose, ATP, pyruvate, amino acids, fructose diphosphate, ribose, adenosine
      (c) Enhance tissue diffusion: hyaluronidase

(C) Reduce catabolism
   (1) Inhibit adenine nucleotide catabolism: allopurinol
   (2) Inhibit lipolysis: β-pyridyl carbinol, prostaglandins
   (3) Increase acidosis
   (4) Induce hypothermia

(D) Stabilize cell structure or cytosolic composition
   (1) Reduce electrolyte shifts/prevent cell swelling: β-blockade, Ca^{2+}-flux inhibition (calcium antagonists), osmotic agents (mannitol)
   (2) Stabilize cell membranes (plasmalemma, lysosomes): steroids, prostaglandins
   (3) Prevent free-radical production (allopurinol) or introduce free-radical scavengers (superoxide dismutase)

(E) Prevent microvascular damage or obstruction
   (1) Prevent endothelial swelling: osmotic agents (mannitol)
   (2) Prevent platelet aggregation: prostaglandins
   (3) Prevent free-radical injury: allopurinol, free-radical scavangers (superoxide dismutase)

(F) Reduce inflammatory response
   (1) Antiinflammatory agents: steroids, nonsteroidal antiinflammatory drugs (ibuprofen)

[a] This table presents a classification of mechanisms that could protect ischemic myocardium. For more detailed reviews of an extensive literature regarding the experimental basis for limitation of myocardial infarct size, we refer the reader to several recent books on the subject (214,401,620). The drugs or classes of drugs listed here are included for illustrative purposes. Thus, this table is not meant to be a compendium of all drugs that may have beneficial effects on ischemic myocardium. In addition, inclusion of a therapy on this list does not necessarily imply that direct tests of efficacy have been done or that positive results have been obtained. In fact, no therapy has yet been accepted for general clinical use. Note that many drugs, e.g., β-blockers or calcium antagonists, have more than one potentially beneficial effect.

It is even more difficult to predict how large an infarct would have been had one not intervened with therapy. (b) In order to select potential therapies for study in humans, reliable experimental models to assess efficacy of an intervention are crucial.

Evaluating Efficacy of Interventions in Humans

One of the great impediments to the testing of potential therapies for beneficial effects on ischemic myocardium has been the fact that myocardial infarct size, which can be precisely quantitated by thorough postmortem anatomic studies in experimental animals or in the relatively small subset of patients who die and can be studied at autopsy, cannot be measured precisely in the majority of patients because most survive the acute phase of myocardial infarction, and many of those who die are buried with no autopsy performed. Thus, in clinical studies of interventions designed to limit infarct size, it is generally necessary to rely on very indirect indices of efficacy, such as patient survival or death, or indices of overall cardiac function, frequency of arrhythmias, etc. Moreover, because infarct size varies markedly among patients in the absence of any therapy to limit infarct size, it is necessary to study very large groups of patients in order to detect a therapeutic effect. Thus, clinical trials to test for agents that might limit infarct size are simultaneously extraordinarily costly and disappointingly imprecise in the answers they provide.

For this reason, there has been much effort to develop indirect methods that could provide accurate estimates of myocardial infarct size among smaller groups of living patients. Methods that have been developed to estimate infarct size in humans have utilized measurements of electrocardiographic, enzymatic, and functional changes, or one of several imaging techniques. Changes in the EKG have been quantitatively assessed, using ST-segment elevation measured in multiple precordial leads (238,377,407) or QRS changes (127,139,228,506). The total amount of an intracellular enzyme, such as creatine kinase, released into the circulation can be estimated from multiple determinations of plasma enzyme activity and calculated time–activity curves (187,493,494,497, 550,572,595). The most frequently used enzyme for this purpose is creatine kinase (total activity or MB subfraction). Global or regional cardiac dysfunction can be quantitated using contrast or radionuclide ventriculography (540) or ultrasound (23,393,446,631). Infarcted myocardium also can be differentiated from nonischemic myocardium by various nuclear-medicine methods (32) involving planar imaging techniques (374,517) or transmission (115,565) or emission computerized tomography (86,339,343,429,588). Planar imaging and emission computerized tomographic techniques rely on either exclusion (e.g., thallium 201 or [^{11}C]palmitate) or enhanced uptake [e.g., antimyosin monoclonal antibodies (199) or ^{99m}Tc-labeled pyrophosphate] of radioactive isotopes by the necrotic myocytes. A further review of the history, experimental basis, and accuracy of various methods of estimating myocardial infarct size is available (620).

All of the aforementioned methods provide estimates of infarct size that correlate, to some degree, either with infarct size measured directly or with other indirect estimates of infarct size. Some of these methods, such as estimation of infarct size by time–activity curves of plasma creatine kinase, when applied to large groups of patients, may improve the precision of clinical trials

designed to test the efficacy of a therapy on infarct size (200). On the other hand, it must be kept in mind that all such techniques have substantial variance that precludes accurate measurement of infarct in an individual patient. Thus, there is a continuing need for research to develop and test clinical methods for estimating myocardial infarct size. Much of such developmental work can be done only in experimental animals; however, final validation of the accuracy of estimating infarct size in humans can be done only through detailed comparisons of clinical estimates with actual infarct size measured by postmortem anatomic quantitation (200). The latter type of study is difficult to undertake because of limited availability of postmortem material from patients who have undergone detailed clinical study; moreover, direct comparison of clinical and postmortem measurements may be confounded by myocardial changes during the sometimes long intervals between clinical evaluation and death of the patient.

Achieving an accurate measurement of infarct size in living patients will be only the beginning of the solution to precise evaluation of therapy in humans. Myocardial infarct size varies markedly even in the absence of any therapy. As discussed elsewhere in this chapter, infarct size is determined by several base-line variables; in dogs, the size of the ischemic vascular bed (area at risk) and the amount and local distribution of collateral blood flow within this area at risk are major determinants of infarct size. The area at risk is variable in dogs, even though the same artery is occluded at the same site in most experimental studies; the area at risk must be a much greater variable among patients, because infarction may be caused by an occlusion of any artery at any site. Collateral flow also may be highly variable in patients with coronary vascular disease of variable duration and severity. Thus, there is a great need for methods that can measure the size of the ischemic region and quantitatively map the distribution of blood flow and differentiate between necrotic and still viable myocardium within the ischemic region.

Although there is great need for indirect methods for estimating myocardial infarct size in patients, it is worth pointing out that all of these indirect indices are inappropriate for use as the sole endpoint in experimental animal studies done to test the efficacy of an intervention on infarct size. An imprecise estimate has value when the only alternative is no estimate at all; an imprecise estimate has no value when a direct measurement can be easily done. The once widespread but now declining use of indirect indices of infarct size in experimental studies has surely contributed to the uncertainty that now exists regarding which interventions might or might not be efficacious in limiting infarct size.

Animal Models for Testing Interventions

Simple models of myocardial ischemic injury may be used to evaluate the role of specific metabolic pathways or organelle function in the pathogenesis of ischemic injury or to screen a variety of interventions to identify those with sufficient promise to merit testing in a more complex model. More complex models are necessary to more closely reproduce myocardial infarction as it occurs clinically and to provide a more reliable analysis of the likelihood of clinical efficacy. Appropriate endpoints also must be selected depending on the question posed (478). For example, one might ask whether or not a calcium antagonist would reduce the metabolic demand of ischemic myocardium. An appropriate endpoint would be myocardial HEP content after a given period of ischemia, and the model could be either simple (e.g., an isolated rat heart) or complex. As another example, one might question whether or not a particular cardioplegic solution would improve postischemic contractile function. In this case, a model of global ischemia might be more appropriate than a model of regional ischemia produced by coronary occlusion. The appropriate endpoint would be a measure of contractile function, for example, contractile force at constant preload. Such studies could be done either with isolated hearts or in intact animals. However, if one were to pose the additional question, "Is the postischemic survival of the animal improved?" the answer could be obtained only in an intact and much more complex whole-animal model. If one wanted to know if a calcium antagonist prevented mitochondrial calcification following ischemia and reperfusion, an analysis of tissue calcium content and electron-microscopic evaluation of the injured mitochondria would be appropriate endpoints. However, if the question is "Does this therapy limit infarct size?" the only appropriate endpoint is infarct size itself. Measurement of indices such as myocardial contractile function or HEP content cannot directly answer this question.

Although a variety of indirect methods have been developed to provide means of estimating myocardial infarct size clinically, in experimental studies the most precise way to evaluate infarct size is to measure infarct size post-mortem by direct anatomic methods. Among published anatomic studies, gross staining techniques using triphenyl tetrazolium chloride (TTC) or nitroblue tetrazolium chloride (132,144,348,414,534) have been used more commonly than histologic techniques. Gross staining techniques have the advantage of being less time-consuming and less expensive. However, we prefer histologic methods because positive staining of myocardium with TTC may not necessarily be synonymous with myocyte viability, and because resolution of the complex interdigitations between necrotic and viable areas can be done most reliably by histologic evaluation. However, histologic sizing requires 3- to 4-day survival of the experimental animal and is more tedious than gross methods (475,482).

There is considerable variation in infarct size among untreated control dogs. This variation exists even though details of the experimental procedures, such as site of coronary occlusion, may be precisely controlled. Given this basic characteristic of any biological system, it is essential to identify and measure those variables within the experimental model that are most responsible for the variation in infarct size (478,482). Several studies have shown that variation in infarct size in dogs is related to variation in (a) the size of the ischemic region (area at risk) (284,359,475,533), (b) collateral blood flow to the ischemic region (186,284,475,492,533), and (c) myocardial metabolic demand, which is determined in part by hemodynamic parameters, including heart rate, wall tension, and myocardial contractility (533). Measuring such variables and including them in the analysis of efficacy can markedly improve the precision of experimental studies done to identify ways to limit infarct size (475,478,479,480).

Although in a large randomized study, base-line variables would tend to be balanced among different groups, it is important to control for them statistically in a small study. This is especially true if a significant fraction of the animals are excluded, for example, because of early mortality. For example, in the multicenter "Animal Models for Protecting Ischemic Myocardium" (AMPIM) study (482), variation in the size of the area at risk accounted for over half the variation in infarct size (as percentage of LV), and when collateral flow and rate-pressure product were included in the model, 90% of the variation among controls in an unconscious model and 80% of the variation among control infarcts in a conscious model could be explained.

The area at risk of undergoing infarction has been defined as the anatomic region supplied by the occluded coronary artery (284,337,475), or, alternatively, a "physiologic" risk region (103), defined as the area with moderate or severe ischemia, based on the paucity of myocardial staining by dyes injected in vivo. We prefer an anatomic definition of area at risk (478) because (a) it is a base-line constant, determined by coronary anatomy, that cannot be altered by spontaneous or therapeutically induced fluctuation in collateral blood flow during an experiment, and (b) identification of an anatomic vascular region requires the identification of boundaries between two vascular regions but does not require the arbitrary distinction between severely versus less severely ischemic myocardium based on a graded concentration of injected dyes or particles.

Two methods of identifying the anatomic area are often used: (a) When extensive collateral growth has not been induced, the area at risk can be identified by the boundary between the two different-colored dyes injected post-mortem (Fig. 29) (475). Precise sampling of ischemic and nonischemic areas for blood flow analysis is possible because vascular boundaries are seen directly on the ventricular slices. (b) In the setting of permanent coronary occlusions, new collaterals develop such that dyes in fluid suspension may readily cross the ischemic/non-ischemic interface. For such studies, coronary arteries can be injected post-mortem with barium sulfate suspended in liquid gelatin; after the gelatin solidifies, vascular-bed boundaries can be identified on radiographs of serial slices of the ventricle (Fig. 9) (284,337,409). The radiographic technique allows direct anatomic delineation of vascular-bed boundaries, which are not influenced by collateral growth. The principal limitations of the radiographic techniques are the overlap of vasculature on two-dimensional representation of three-dimensional myocardial slices and the relative imprecision of using X-rays to guide the sampling of myocardium for blood flow analysis.

ACKNOWLEDGMENTS

Many of the ideas presented in this chapter were developed in research studies supported by Grants HL23138 and HL27416 from the National Institutes of Health.

REFERENCES

1. Abelman, W. H. (1984): Classification and natural history of primary myocardial disease. *Prog. Cardiovasc. Dis.,* 26:73–94.
2. Abrahamsson, T., Almgren, O., and Carlsson, L. (1984): Washout of noradrenaline and its metabolites by calcium-free reperfusion after ischaemia: Support for the concept of ischaemia-induced noradrenaline release. *Br. J. Pharmacol.,* 81:22–24.
3. Allen, D. G., and Orchard, C. H. (1983): The effect of hypoxia and metabolic inhibition on intracellular calcium in mammalian heart muscle. *J. Physiol. (Lond.),* 339:102–122.
4. Allen, D. G., and Orchard, C. H. (1984): Measurements of intracellular calcium concentration in heart muscle: The effects of inotropic interventions and hypoxia. *J. Mol. Cell. Cardiol.,* 16:117–128.
5. Altschuld, R. A., Hostetler, J. R., and Brierley, G. P. (1981): Response of isolated rat heart cells to hypoxia, re-oxygenation, and acidosis. *Circ. Res.,* 49:307–316.
6. American Heart Association (1985): *Heart Facts.* AHA, Office of Communications, Dallas.
7. Anversa, P., Beghi, C., Kikkawa, Y., and Olivetti, G. (1985): Myocardial response to infarction in the rat. Morphometric measurement of infarct size and myocyte cellular hypertrophy. *Am. J. Pathol.,* 118:484–502.
8. Archie, J. P., Jr. (1978): Transmural distribution of intrinsic and transmitted left ventricular diastolic intramyocardial pressure in dogs. *Cardiovasc. Res.,* 12:255–262.
9. Armiger, L. C., and Gavin, J. B. (1975): Changes in the microvasculature of ischemic and infarcted myocardium. *Lab. Invest.,* 33:51–56.
10. Armiger, L. C., Seelye, R. N., Phil, D., Elswijk, J. G., Carnell, V. M., Benson, D. C., Gavin, J. B., and Herdson, P. B. (1975): Mitochondrial changes in dog myocardium induced by lactate *in vivo. Lab. Invest.,* 33:502–508.
11. Armiger, L. C., Seelye, R. N., Phil, D., Elswijk, J. G., Carnell, V. M., Gavin, J. B., and Herdson, P. B. (1977): Fine structural changes in dog myocardium exposed to lowered pH *in vivo. Lab. Invest.,* 37:237–242.
12. Ashraf, M., and Sybers, H. D. (1975): Scanning electron microscopy of the heart after coronary occlusion. *Lab. Invest.,* 32:157–162.
13. Asinger, R. W., Mikell, F. L., Elsperger, J., and Hodges, M. (1981): Incidence of left ventricular thrombosis after acute transmural myocardial infarction. *N. Engl. J. Med.,* 305:297–302.
14. Bache, R. J., and Schwartz, J. S. (1982): Effect of perfusion pressure distal to a coronary stenosis on transmural myocardial blood flow. *Circulation,* 65:928–935.
15. Baird, R. J., and Ameli, F. M. (1971): The changes in intramyocardial pressure produced by acute ischemia. *J. Thorac. Cardiovasc. Surg.,* 62:87–94.
16. Bajusz, E., and Jasmin, G. (1964): Histochemical studies on the myocardium following experimental interference with coronary circulation in the rat. I. Occlusion of coronary artery. *Acta Histochem.,* 18:222–237.
17. Bakshandeh, K., Kaiser, G. A., and Bolooki, H. (1974): Hemodynamic correlates of the size of myocardial infarct. *Surg. Forum,* 23:152–153.
18. Barlow, C. H., and Chance, B. (1976): Ischemic areas in perfused rat hearts: Measurement by NADH fluorescence photography. *Science,* 193:909–910.
19. Barlow, C. H., Harken, A. H., and Chance, B. (1977): Evaluation of cardiac ischemia by NADH fluorescence photography. *Ann. Surg.,* 186:737–740.
20. Baroldi, G. (1971): Functional morphology of the anastomotic circulation in human cardiac pathology. In: *Functional Morphology of the Heart,* edited by E. Bajusz and G. Jasmin, pp. 438–473. Karger, Basel.
21. Baroldi, G. (1975): Different types of myocardial necrosis in coronary heart disease: A pathophysiologic review of their functional significance. *Am. Heart J.,* 89:742–752.
22. Baroldi, G., Mantero, O., and Scomazzoni, G. (1956): The collaterals of the coronary arteries in normal and pathologic hearts. *Circ. Res.,* 9:223–229.
23. Barzilai, B., Madaras, E. I., Sobel, B. E., Miller, J. G., and Perez, J. E. (1984): Effects of myocardial contraction on ultrasonic backscatter before and after ischemia. *Am. J. Physiol.,* 247:H478–H483.
24. Basuk, W. L., Reimer, K. A., and Jennings, R. B. (1986): Effect of repetitive brief episodes of ischemia on cell volume, electrolytes and ultrastructure. *J. Am. Col. Cardiol., (in press).*
25. Bates, R. J., Beutler, S., Resnekov, L., and Anagnostopoulos, C. E. (1977): Cardiac rupture—challenge in diagnosis and management. *Am. J. Cardiol.,* 40:429–437.
26. Baughman, K. L., Maroko, P. R., and Vatner, S. F. (1981): Effects of coronary artery reperfusion on myocardial infarct size and survival in conscious dogs. *Circulation,* 63:317–323.
27. Bayliss, C. E., Crawford, F. B., and Nsafoah, B. (1977): The interventricular septum: An isolated perfused model for assessing myocardial function. *Can. J. Physiol. Pharmacol.,* 55:1358–1368.
28. Becker, A. E., Lie, K. I., and Anderson, R. H. (1978): Bundle-branch block in the setting of acute anteroseptal myocardial infarction. *Br. Heart J.,* 40:773–782.
29. Becker, L. C., Ferreira, R., and Thomas, M. (1973): Mapping of left ventricular blood flow with radioactive microspheres in experimental coronary artery occlusion. *Cardiovasc. Res.,* 7:391–400.
30. Becker, L. C., Fortuin, N. J., and Pitt, B. (1971): Effect of ischemia and antianginal drugs on the distribution of radioactive microspheres in the canine left ventricle. *Circ. Res.,* 28:263–269.
31. Belloni, F. L. (1979): The local control of coronary blood flow. *Cardiovasc. Res.,* 13:63–85.
32. Berger, H. J., and Zaret, B. L. (1981): Nuclear cardiology. *N. Engl. J. Med.,* 305:799–807, 855–865.
33. Berne, R. M. (1980): The role of adenosine on the regulation of coronary blood flow. *Circ. Res.,* 47:807–813.
34. Biheimer, D. W., Buja, L. M., Parkey, R. W., Bonte, F. J., and Willerson, J. T. (1978): Fatty acid accumulation and abnormal lipid deposition in peripheral and border zones of experimental myocardial infarcts. *J. Nucl. Med.,* 19:276–283.
35. Bing, R. J. (1971/72): Reparative processes in heart muscle following myocardial infarction. *Cardiology,* 56:314–324.
36. Bishop, S. P., and Drummond, J. L. (1979): Surface morphology and cell size measurement of isolated rat cardiac myocytes. *J. Mol. Cell. Cardiol.,* 11:423–433.
37. Bishop, S. P., White, F. C., and Bloor, C. M. (1976): Regional myocardial blood flow during acute myocardial infarction in the conscious dog. *Circ. Res.,* 38:429–438.
38. Blondel, B., Roijen, I., and Cheneval, J. P. (1971): Heart cells in culture: A simple method for increasing the proportion of myoblasts. *Experientia,* 27:356–358.
39. Bloor, C. M. (1974): Functional significance of the coronary collateral circulation. *Am. J. Pathol.,* 76:561–588.
40. Blumgart, H., Schlesinger, M., and Davis, D. (1940): Studies on the relationship of the clinical manifestations of angina pectoris, coronary thrombosis, and myocardial infarction to the pathologic findings. *Am. Heart J.,* 19:1–91.

41. Blumgart, H. L., Schlesinger, M. J., and Zoll, P. M. (1941): Angina pectoris, coronary failure and acute myocardial infarction: The role of coronary occlusions and collateral circulation. *J.A.M.A.*, 116:91–97.

42. Bodenheimer, M. M., Banka, V. S., Hermann, G. A., Trout, R. G., Pasdar, H., and Helfant, R. H. (1977): The effect of severity of coronary artery obstructive disease and the coronary collateral circulation on local histopathologic and electrographic observations in man. *Am. J. Med.*, 63:193–199.

43. Bolli, R., Davenport, N. J., Goldstein, R. E., and Epstein, S. E. (1983): Myocardial proteolysis during acute myocardial ischaemia. *Cardiovasc. Res.*, 17:274–281.

44. Bolooki, H., Kotler, M. D., Lottenberg, L., Dresnick, S., Andrews, R. C., Kipnis, S., and Ellis, R. M. (1975): Myocardial revascularization after acute infarction. *Am. J. Cardiol.*, 36:395–406.

45. Bonhoeffer, K. (1967): Der Sauerstoffverbrauch des normo- und hypothermen Hundeherzens vor und während verschiedener Formen des induzierten Herzstillstandes. *Bibl. Cardiol.*, 18:1–73.

46. Borst, P., Loos, J. A., Christ, E. J., et al. (1962): Uncoupling activity of long-chain fatty acids. *Biochim. Biophys. Acta*, 62:509–518.

47. Bouchardy, B., and Majno, G. (1974): Histopathology of early myocardial infarcts: A new approach. *Am. J. Pathol.*, 74:301–331.

48. Boveris, A. (1977): Mitochondrial generation of superoxide and hydrogen peroxide. *Adv. Exp. Biol. Med.*, 78:67–82.

49. Braasch, W., Gudbjarnason, S., Puri, P. S., Ravens, K. G., and Bing, R. J. (1968): Early changes in energy metabolism in the myocardium following acute coronary artery occlusion in anesthetized dogs. *Circ. Res.*, 23:429–438.

50. Braunwald E. (1967): The pathogenesis and treatment of shock in myocardial infarction. Topic in clinical medicine. *Johns Hopkins Med. J.*, 121:421–429.

51. Braunwald, E., and Kloner, R. A. (1982): The stunned myocardium: Prolonged, postischemic ventricular dysfunction. *Circulation*, 66:1146–1149.

52. Bresnahan, G. F., Roberts, R., Shell, W. E., Ross, J., Jr., and Sobel, B. E. (1974): Deleterious effects due to hemorrhage after myocardial reperfusion. *Am. J. Cardiol.*, 33:82–86.

53. Bretschneider, H. J., Cott, L. A., Hellige, G., Hensel, I., Kettler, D., and Martel, J. (1971): A new hemodynamic parameter consisting of 5 additive determinants for estimation of the O₂-consumption of the left ventricle. In: *Proceedings of International Congress of Physiological Sciences*. Munich, p. 633 (abstract).

54. Bretschneider, H. J., Cott, L. A., Hensel, I., Kettler, D., and Martel, J. (1970): Ein neuer Komplexer haemodynamischer Parameter aus 5 additiven Gliedern zur Bestimmung des O₂-Bedarfs des linken Ventrikels. *Pfluegers Arch.*, 319:R14–R15.

55. Bruce, T. A., and Myers, J. T. (1973): Myocardial lipid metabolism in ischemia and infarction. *Recent Adv. Stud. Cardiac Struct. Metab.*, 3:773–780.

56. Buerk, D. G., and Longmuir, I. S. (1977): Evidence for nonclassical respiratory activity from oxygen gradient measurements in tissue slices. *Microvasc. Res.*, 13:345–353.

57. Buja, L. M., Dees, J. H., Harling, D. F., and Willerson, J. T. (1976): Analytical electron microscopic study of mitochondrial inclusions in canine myocardial infarcts. *J. Histochem. Cytochem.*, 24:508–516.

58. Buja, L. M., Hagler, H. K., Parsons, D., Chien, K., Reynolds, R. C., and Willerson, J. T. (1985): Alterations of ultrastructure and elemental composition in cultured neonatal rat cardiac myocytes following metabolic inhibition with iodoacetic acid. *Lab. Invest.*, 53:397–412.

59. Buja, L. M., Poliner, L. R., Parkey, R. W., Pulido, J. I., Hutcheson, D., Platt, M. R., Mills, L. J., Bonte, F. J., and Willerson, J. T. (1977): Clinicopathologic study of persistently positive technetium-99m stannous pyrophosphate myocardial scintigrams and myocytolytic degeneration after myocardial infarction. *Circulation*, 56:1016–1023.

60. Burch, G. E., Tsui, C. Y., and Harb, J. M. (1972): Ischemic cardiomyopathy. *Am. Heart J.*, 83:340–350.

61. Bus, J. S., and Gibson, J. E. (1979): Lipid peroxidation and its role in toxicology. In: *Reviews in Biochemical Toxicology*, edited by E. Hodgson, J. R. Bend, and R. M. Philpot, pp. 125–149. Elsevier/North Holland, Amsterdam.

62. Busch, W. A., Stromer, M. H., Goll, D. E., and Suzuki, A. (1972): Ca²⁺-specific removal of Z lines from rabbit skeletal muscle. *J. Cell Biol.*, 52:367–381.

63. Bush, L. R., Shlafer, M., Haack, D. W., and Lucchesi, B. R. (1980): Time-dependent changes in canine cardiac mitochondrial function and ultrastructure resulting from coronary occlusion and reperfusion. *Basic Res. Cardiol.*, 75:555–571.

64. Cabin, H. S., and Roberts, W. C. (1980): Left ventricular aneurysm, intraaneurysmal thrombus and systemic embolus in coronary heart disease. *Chest*, 77:586–590.

65. Camilleri, J. P., Nlom, M. O., Joseph, D., Michel, J. B., Barres, D., and Mignot, J. (1983): Capillary perfusion patterns in reperfused ischemic subendocardial myocardium: Experimental study using fluorescent dextran. *Exp. Mol. Pathol.*, 39:89–99.

66. Campbell, C. D., Takanashi, Y., Laas, J., Meus, P., Pick, R., and Replogle, R. L. (1981): Effect of coronary artery reperfusion on infarct size in swine. *J. Thorac. Cardiovasc. Surg.*, 81:288–296.

67. Cannom, D. S., Levy, W., and Cohen, L. S. (1976): The short- and long-term prognosis of patients with transmural and nontransmural myocardial infarction. *Am. J. Med.*, 61:452–458.

68. Carr, F. K., and Goldfarb, R. D. (1980): Ischemia-induced canine myocardial lysosome labilization: The role of endogenous prostaglandins and cyclic nucleotides. *Exp. Mol. Pathol.*, 33:36–42.

69. Case, R. B. (1971/72): Ion alterations during myocardial ischemia. *Cardiology*, 56:245–262.

70. Caulfield, J. B., Leinbach, R., and Gold, H. (1976): The relationship of myocardial infarct size and prognosis. *Circulation*, 53:141–144.

71. Chagrasulis, R. W., and Downey, J. M. (1977): Selective coronary embolization in closed-chest dogs. *Am. J. Physiol.*, 232:H335–H337.

72. Chapman, I. (1965): Morphogenesis of occluding coronary artery thrombosis. *Arch. Pathol.*, 80:256–261.

73. Chien, K. R., Buja, L. M., Mukherjee, A., and Willerson, J. T. (1981): Fatty acyl metabolites and membrane injury in ischemic canine myocardium; dissociation from a sarcolemmal Ca⁺⁺ permeability defect and correlation with mitochondrial dysfunction. *Circulation [Suppl. II]*, 64:153 (abstract).

74. Chien, K. R., Han, A., Sen, A., Buja, L. M., and Willerson, J. T. (1984): Accumulation of unesterified arachidonic acid in ischemic canine myocardium. *Circ. Res.*, 54:313–322.

75. Chien, K. R., Reeves, J. P., Buja, L. M., Bonte, F., Parkey, R. W., and Willerson, J. T. (1981): Phospholipid alterations in canine ischemic myocardium. Temporal and topographical correlations with Tc-99m-PPi accumulation and an *in vitro* sarcolemmal calcium permeability defect. *Circ. Res.*, 48:711–719.

76. Clark, W. A. (1976): Selective control of fibroblast proliferation and its effect on cardiac muscle differentiation in vitro. *Dev. Biol.*, 52:263–282.

77. Clusin, W. T., Buchbinder, M., and Harrison, D. C. (1983): Calcium overload, "injury" current, and early ischaemic cardiac arrhythmias—a direct connection. *Lancet*, 1:272–274.

78. Cobbe, S. M., and Poole-Wilson, P. A. (1980): Tissue acidosis in myocardial hypoxia. *J. Mol. Cell. Cardiol.*, 12:761–770.

79. Cobbe, S. M., and Poole-Wilson, P. A. (1980): The time of onset and severity of acidosis in myocardial ischaemia. *J. Mol. Cell. Cardiol.*, 12:745–760.

80. Cohen, M. V. (1978): The functional value of coronary collaterals in myocardial ischemia and therapeutic approach to enhance collateral flow. *Am. Heart J.*, 95:396–404.

81. Cohen, P., Burchell, A., Foulkes, J. G., Cohen, F. T., Vonoman, T. C., and Nairn, A. C. (1978): Identification of the Ca²⁺-dependent modulator protein as the fourth subunit of rabbit skeletal muscle phosphorylase kinase. *FEBS Lett.*, 92:287–293.

82. Cohn, P. F., Maddox, D. E., Holman, B. L., and See, J. R. (1980): Effect of coronary collateral vessels on regional myocardial blood flow in patients with coronary artery disease: Relation of collateral circulation to vasodilatory reserve and left ventricular function. *Am. J. Cardiol.*, 46:359–364.

83. Collan, Y., McDowell, E., and Trump, B. F. (1981): Studies on the pathogenesis of ischemic cell injury: VI. Mitochondrial flocculent densities in autolysis. *Virchows Arch. [Zellpathol.]*, 35:189–199.

84. Collen, D., and Verstraete, M. (1983): Systemic thrombolytic therapy of acute myocardial infarction. *Circulation*, 68:462–465.

85. Connelly, C., Vogel, W. M., Hernandez, Y. M., and Apstein, C. S. (1982): Movement of necrotic wavefront after coronary artery occlusion in rabbit. *Am. J. Physiol.*, 243:H682–690.

86. Corbett, J. R., Lewis, S. E., Wolfe, C. L., Jansen, D. E., Lewis, M., Rellas, J. S., Parkey, R. W., Rude, R. E., Buja, L. M., and Willerson, J. T. (1984): Measurement of myocardial infarct size by technetium pyrophosphate single-photon tomography. *Am. J. Cardiol.*, 54:1231–1236.

87. Corday, E., Lang, T.-W., Meerbaum, S., Gold, H., Hirose, S., Rubins, S., and Dalmastro, M. (1974): Closed chest model of intracoronary occlusion for study of regional cardiac function. *Am. J. Cardiol.*, 33:49–59.

88. Corr, P. B., Gross, R. W., and Sobel, B. E. (1984): Amphipathic metabolites and membrane dysfunction in ischemic myocardium. *Circ. Res.*, 55:135–154.

89. Corr, P. B., and Sobel, B. E. (1979): The importance of metabolites in the genesis of ventricular dysrhythmia induced by ischemia. I. Electrophysiological considerations. *Mod. Concepts Cardiovasc. Dis.*, 28:43–48.

90. Corr, P. B., and Sobel, B. E. (1979): The importance of metabolites in the genesis of ventricular dysrhythmia induced by ischemia. II. Biochemical factors. *Mod. Concepts Cardiovasc. Dis.*, 28:49–52.

91. Corr, P. B., Witkowski, F. X., and Sobel, B. E. (1978): Mechanisms contributing to malignant dysrythmias induced by ischemia in the cat. *J. Clin. Invest.*, 61:109–119.

92. Covell, J. W., Pool, P. E., and Braunwald, E. (1967): Effects of acutely induced ischemic heart failure on myocardial high energy phosphate stores. *Proc. Soc. Exp. Biol. Med.*, 124:126–131.

93. Cox, J. L., McLaughlin, V. W., Flowers, N. C., and Horan, L. G. (1968): The ischemic zone surrounding acute myocardial infarction. Its morphology as detected by dehydrogenase staining. *Am. Heart J.*, 76:650–659.

94. Cox, J. R., Roberts, R., Ambos, H. D., Oliver, G. C., and Sobel, B. E. (1976): Relations between enzymatically estimated myocardial infarct size and early ventricular dysrhythmia. *Circulation*, 53:150–155.

95. Crass, M. F., III, and Sterrett, P. R. (1975): Distribution of glycogen and lipids in the ischemic canine left ventricle: Biochemical and light and electron microscopic correlates. *Recent Adv. Stud. Cardiac Struct. Metab.*, 10:251–263.

96. Crozatier, B., Ross, J., Jr., Franklin, D., Bloor, C. M., White, F. C., Tomoike, H., and McKown, D. P. (1978): Myocardial infarction in the baboon: Regional function and the collateral circulation. *Am. J. Physiol.*, 235:H413–H421.

97. da Luz, P. L., Weil, M. H., and Shubin, H. (1976): Current concepts on mechanisms and treatment of cardiogenic shock. *Am. Heart J.*, 92:103–113.

98. Davies, M. J. (1984): The cardiomyopathies: A review of terminology, pathology and pathogenesis. *Histopathology*, 8:363–393.

99. Davies, M. J., and Thomas, A. C. (1985): Plaque fissuring—the cause of acute myocardial infarction, sudden ischaemic death, and crescendo angina. *Br. Heart J.*, 53:363–373.

100. Davies, M. J., Woolf, N., and Robertson, W. B. (1976): Pathology of acute myocardial infarction with particular reference to occlusive coronary thrombi. *Br. Heart J.*, 38:659–664.

101. Davis, R. W., and Ebert, P. A. (1972): Ventricular aneurysm: A clinical-pathologic correlation. *Am. J. Cardiol.*, 29:1–6.

102. Dayton, W. R., Goll, D. E., Stromer, M. H., Reville, W. J., Zeece, M. G., and Robson, R. M. (1975): Some properties of a Ca⁺⁺-activated protease that may be involved in myofibrillar turnover In: *Proteases and Biological Control, Cold Spring Harbor Conferences on Biological Control, Vol. 2,* edited by E. Reich, D. B. Rifem, and E. Shaw, pp. 551–577. Cold Spring Harbor Laboratory, Cold Spring Harbor, N.Y.

103. DeBoer, L. W. V., Ingwall, J. S., Kloner, R. A., and Braunwald, E. (1980): Prolonged derangements of canine myocardial purine metabolism after a brief coronary artery occlusion not associated with anatomic evidence of necrosis. *Proc. Natl. Acad. Sci. USA*, 77:5471–5475.

104. Decker, R. S., Poole, A. R., Griffin, E. E., Dingle, J. R., and Wildenthal, K. (1977): Altered distribution of lysosomal cathepsin D in ischemic myocardium. *J. Clin. Invest.*, 59:911–921.

105. Decker, R. S., and Wildenthal, K. (1978): Sequential lysosomal alterations during cardiac ischemia II. Ultrastructural and cytochemical changes. *Lab. Invest.*, 38:662–673.

106. de Jong, J. W., and Goldstein, S. (1974): Changes in coronary venous inosine concentration and myocardial wall thickening during regional ischemia in the pig. *Circ. Res.*, 35:111–116.

107. de Leiris, J., Harding, D. P., and Pestre, S. (1984): The isolated perfused rat heart: A model for studying myocardial hypoxia or ischaemia. *Basic Res. Cardiol.*, 79:313–321.

108. Del Maestro, R. F., Bjork, J., and Arfors, K.-E. (1981): Increase in microvascular permeability induced by enzymatically generated free radicals. II. Role of superoxide anion radical, hydrogen peroxide, and hydroxyl radical. *Microvasc. Res.*, 22:255–270.

109. Del Maestro, R. F., Thaw, H. H., Bjork, J., Planker, M., and Arfors, K. E. (1980): Free radicals as mediators of tissue injury. *Acta Physiol. Scand.*, 492:43–57.

110. Deuticke, B., Gerlach, E., and Dierkesmann, R. (1966): Abbau freier Nukleotide in Herz, Skelettmuskel, Gehirn und Leber der Ratte bei Sauerstoffmangel. *Pfluegers Arch.*, 292:239–254.

111. DeWood, M. A., Spores, J., Notske, R., Mouser, L. T., Burroughs, R., Golden, M. S., and Lang, H. T. (1980): Prevalence of total coronary occlusion during the early hours of transmural myocardial infarction. *N. Engl. J. Med.*, 303:897–902.

112. DiBona, D. R., and Powell, W. J. (1980): Quantitative correlation between cell swelling and necrosis in myocardial ischemia in dogs. *Circ. Res.*, 47:653–665.

113. Dionisi, O., Galeotti, T., Terranova, T., and Azzi, A. (1975): Superoxide radicals and hydrogen peroxide formation in normal and neoplastic tissues. *Biochim. Biophys. Acta*, 403:292–300.

114. Dobson, J. G., and Mayer, S. E. (1973): Mechanism of activation of cardiac glycogen phosphorylase in ischemia and anoxia. *Circ. Res.*, 33:412–420.

115. Doherty, P. W., Lipton, M. J., Berninger, W. H., Skioldebrand, C. G., Carlsson, E., and Redington, R. W. (1981): Detection and quantitation of myocardial infarction in vivo using transmission computed tomography. *Circulation*, 63:597–606.

116. Domenech, R. J., and De La Prida, J. M. (1975): Mechanical effects of heart contraction on coronary flow. *Cardiovasc. Res.*, 9:509–514.

117. Doorey, A. J., and Barry, W. H. (1983): The effects of inhibition of oxidative phosphorylation and glycolysis on contractility and high-energy phosphate content in cultured chick heart cells. *Circ. Res.*, 53:192–201.

118. Dow, J. W., Harding, N. G. L., and Powell, T. (1981): Review: Isolated cardiac myocytes: I. Preparation of adult myocytes and their homology with the intact tissue. *Cardiovasc. Res.*, 15:483–514.

119. Dow, J. W., Harding, N. G. L., and Powell, T. (1981): Review: Isolated cardiac myocytes: II. Functional aspects of mature cells. *Cardiovasc. Res.*, 15:549–579.

120. Downey, H. F., Crystal, G. J., and Bashour, F. A. (1981): Functional significance of microvascular collateral anastomoses after chronic coronary artery occlusion. *Microvasc. Res.*, 21:212–222.

121. Downey, J. M. (1984): Why the endocardium? In: *Therapeutic Approaches to Myocardial Infarct Size Limitation,* edited by D. J. Hearse and D. M. Yellon, pp. 125–138. Raven Press, New York.

122. Dubnow, M. H., Burchell, H. B., and Titus, J. L. (1965): Postinfarction ventricular aneurysm: A clinicomorphologic and electrocardiographic study of 80 cases. *Am. Heart J.*, 70:753–760.

123. Dunn, R. B., and Griggs, D. M., Jr. (1975): Transmural gradients in ventricular tissue metabolites produced by stopping coronary blood flow in the dog. *Circ. Res.*, 37:438–445.

124. Eaton, L. W., Weiss, J. L., Bulkley, B. H., Garrison, J. B., and Weisfeldt, M. L. (1979): Regional cardiac dilatation after acute myocardial infarction. *N. Engl. J. Med.*, 300:57–62.

125. Edwards, B. S., Edwards, W. D., and Edwards, J. E. (1984): Ventricular septal rupture complicating acute myocardial infarction: Identification of simple and complex types in 53 autopsied hearts. *Am. J. Cardiol.*, 54:1201–1205.

126. Engler, R. L., Schmid-Schonbein, G. W., and Pavelec, R. S. (1983): Leukocyte capillary plugging in myocardial ischemia and reperfusion in the dog. *Am. J. Pathol.*, 111:98–111.

127. Essen, R. V., Merx, W., Doerr, R., Effert, S., Silny, J., and Rau, G. (1980): QRS mapping in the evaluation of acute anterior myocardial infarction. *Circulation*, 62:266–276.

128. Evans, R. G., Val-Mejias, J. E., Kulevich, J., Fischer, V. W., and Mueller, H. S. (1985): Evaluation of a rat model for assessing interventions to salvage ischaemic myocardium: Effects of ibuprofen and verapamil. *Cardiovasc. Res.*, 3:132–138.

129. Factor, S. M., Okun, E. M., and Kirk, E. S. (1981): The histological lateral border of acute canine myocardial infarction: A function of microcirculation. *Circ. Res.*, 48:640–649.

130. Factor, S. M., Okun, E. M., Minase, T., and Kirk, E. S. (1982): The microcirculation of the human heart: End-capillary loops with discrete perfusion fields. *Circulation*, 66:1241–1248.

131. Falk, E. (1983): Plaque rupture with severe pre-existing stenosis precipitating coronary thrombosis. Characteristics of coronary atherosclerotic plaques underlying fatal occlusive thrombi. *Br. Heart J.*, 50:127–134.

132. Fallon, J. T. (1979): Simplified method for histochemical demonstration of experimental myocardial infarct. *Circulation*, 60:11–42.

133. Fantone, J. C., and Ward, P. A. (1982): Role of oxygen-derived free radicals and metabolites in leukocyte-dependent inflammatory reactions. *Am. J. Pathol.*, 107:397–418.

134. Farber, J. L., Chien, K. R., and Mittnacht, S. (1981): The pathogenesis of irreversible cell injury in ischemia. *Am. J. Pathol.*, 102:271–281.

135. Fedor, J. M., McIntosh, D. M., Rembert, J. C., and Greenfield, J. C., Jr. (1978): Coronary and transmural myocardial blood flow responses in awake pigs. *Am. J. Physiol. Heart Circ. Physiol.*, 235:H435–444.

136. Feinberg, H., Rosenbaum, D. S., Levitsky, S., Silverman, N. A., Kohler, J., and LeBreton, G. (1982): Platelet deposition after surgically induced myocardial ischemia. An etiologic factor for reperfusion injury. *J. Thorac. Cardiovasc. Surg.*, 84:815–822.

137. Feuvray, D., and Plouet, J. (1981): Relationship between structure and fatty acid metabolism in mitochondria isolated from ischemic rat hearts. *Circ. Res.*, 48:740–747.

138. Fine, G., Morales, A., and Scerpella, J. R. (1966): Experimental myocardial infarction: A histochemical study. *Arch. Pathol.*, 82:4–8.

139. Fioretti, P., Brower, R. W., Lazzeroni, E., Simoons, M. L., Wijns, W., Reiber, J. H. C., Bos, R. J., and Hugenholtz, P. G. (1985): Limitations of a QRS scoring system to assess left ventricular function and prognosis at hospital discharge after myocardial infarction. *Br. Heart J.*, 53:248–252.

140. Fischer, G. C., Wessel, H. U., and Sommers, H. M. (1972): Mitral insufficiency following experimental papillary muscle infarction. *Am. Heart J.*, 83:382–388.

141. Fishbein, M. C., Hare, C. A., Gissen, S. A., Spadaro, J., Maclean, D., and Maroko, P. R. (1980): Identification and quantification of histochemical border zones during the evolution of myocardial infarction in the rat. *Cardiovasc. Res.*, 14:41–49.

142. Fishbein, M. C., Maclean, D. M., and Maroko, P. R. (1978): Experimental myocardial infarction in the rat. Qualitative and quantitative changes during pathologic evolution. *Am. J. Pathol.*, 90:57–70.

143. Fishbein, M. C., Maclean, D., and Maroko, P. R. (1978): The histopathologic evolution of myocardial infarction. *Chest*, 73:843–849.

144. Fishbein, M. C., Meerbaum, S., Rit, J., Lando, U., Kanmatsuse, K., Mercier, J. C., Corday, E., and Ganz, W. (1981): Early phase acute myocardial infarct size quantification: Validation of the triphenyl tetrazolium chloride tissue enzyme staining technique. *Am. Heart J.*, 101:593–600.

145. Fishbein, M. C., Y-Rit, J., Lando, U., Kanmatsuse, K., Mercier, J. C., and Ganz, W. (1980): The relationship of vascular injury and myocardial hemorrhage to necrosis after reperfusion. *Circulation*, 62:1274–1279.

146. Fixler, D. E., Buja, L. M., Wheeler, J. M., and Willerson, J. T. (1977): Influence of mannitol on maintaining coronary flows and salvaging myocardium during ventriculotomy and during prolonged coronary artery ligation. *Circulation*, 56:340–346.

147. Follette, D. M., Fey, K., Buckberg, G. D., Helly, J. J., Jr., Steed, D. L., Foglia, R. P., and Maloney, J. V., Jr. (1981): Reducing postischemic damage by temporary modification of reperfusate calcium, potassium, pH, and osmolarity. *J. Thorac. Cardiovasc. Surg.*, 82:221–238.

148. Folts, J. D., Gallagher, K., and Rowe, G. G. (1982): Blood flow reductions in stenosed canine coronary arteries: Vasospasm or platelet aggregation? *Circulation*, 65:248–255.

149. Fozzard, H. A., and Makielski, J. C. (1985): The electrophysiology of acute myocardial ischemia. *Annu. Rev. Med.*, 36:275–284.

150. Frankel, E. N. (1980): Lipid oxidation. *Prog. Lipid Res.*, 19:1–22.

151. Freedman, S. B., Dunn, R. F., Bernstein, L., Morris, J., and Kelly, D. T. (1985): Influence of coronary collateral blood flow on the development of exertional ischemia and Q wave infarction in patients with severe single-vessel disease. *Circulation*, 71:681–686.

152. Freeman, B. A., and Crapo, J. D. (1982): Biology of disease: Free radicals and tissue injury. *Lab. Invest.*, 47:412–426.

153. Fridovich, I. (1970): Quantitative aspects of production of superoxide anion radical by milk xanthine oxidase. *J. Biol. Chem.*, 245:4053–4057.

154. Friedman, M. (1971): The coronary thrombus: Its origin and fate. *Hum. Pathol.*, 2:81–128.

155. Fry, D. M., Scales, D., and Inesi, G. (1979): The ultrastructure of membrane alterations of enzymatically dissociated cardiac myocytes. *J. Mol. Cell. Cardiol.*, 11:1151–1163.

156. Fujiwara, H., Ashraf, M., Sato, S., and Millard, R. W. (1982): Transmural cellular damage and blood flow distribution in early ischemia in pig hearts. *Circ. Res.*, 51:683–693.

157. Fukuyama, T., Sobel, B. E., and Roberts, R. (1984): Microvascular deterioration: Implications for reperfusion. *Cardiovasc. Res.*, 18:310–320.

158. Fulton, W. F. M. (1963): Arterial anastomoses in the coronary circulation. I. Anatomical features in normal and diseased hearts demonstrated by stereoarteriography. *Scot. Med. J.*, 8:420–434.

159. Fulton, W. F. M. (1964): Anastomotic enlargement and ischaemic myocardial damage. *Br. Heart J.*, 26:1–15.

160. Ganote, C. E. (1983): Contraction band necrosis and irreversible myocardial injury. *J. Mol. Cell. Cardiol.*, 15:67–73.

161. Ganote, C. E., and Humphrey, S. M. (1985): Effects of anoxic or oxygenated reperfusion in globally ischemic, isovolumic, perfused rat hearts. *Am. J. Pathol.*, 120:129–145.

162. Ganote, C. E., Jennings, R. B., Hill, M. L., and Grochowski, E. C. (1976): Experimental myocardial ischemic injury. II. Effect of in vivo ischemia on dog heart slice function in vitro. *J. Mol. Cell. Cardiol.*, 8:189–204.

163. Ganote, C. E., and Kaltenbach, J. P. (1979): Oxygen-induced enzyme release: early events and a proposed mechanism. *J. Mol. Cell. Cardiol.*, 11:389–406.

164. Ganote, C. E., Liu, S. Y., Safavi, S., and Kaltenbach, J. P. (1981): Anoxia, calcium and contracture as mediators of myocardial enzyme release. *J. Mol. Cell. Cardiol.*, 13:93–106.

165. Ganote, C. E., McGarr, J., Liu, S. Y., and Kaltenbach, J. P. (1980): Oxygen-induced enzyme release. Assessment of mitochondrial function in anoxic myocardial injury and effects of the mitochondrial uncoupling agent 2,4-dinitrophenol (DNP). *J. Mol. Cell. Cardiol.*, 12:387–408.

166. Ganote, C. E., Worstell, J., and Kaltenbach, J. P. (1976). Oxygen-induced enzyme release after irreversible myocardial injury. *Am. J. Pathol.*, 84:327–350.

167. Ganz, W., Buchbinder, M., Marcus, H., et al. (1981): Intracoronary thrombolysis in evolving myocardial infarction. *Am. Heart J.*, 101:4–13.

168. Ganz, W., Geft, I., Maddahi, J., Berman, D., Charuzi, Y., Shah, P. K., and Swan, H. J. C. (1983): Nonsurgical reperfusion in evolving myocardial infarction. *J. Am. Coll. Cardiol.*, 1:1247–1253.

169. Gavin, J. B., Seelye, R. N., Nevalainen, T. J., and Armiger, L. C. (1978): The effect of ischaemia on the function and fine structure of the microvasculature of myocardium. *Pathology*, 10:103–111.

170. Gavin, J. B., Thomson, R. W., Humphrey, S. M., and Herdson, P. B. (1983): Changes in vascular morphology associated with the no-reflow phenomenon in ischaemic myocardium. *Virchows Arch.* [*Pathol. Anat.*], 399:325–332.

171. Geary, G. G., Smith, G. T., and McNamara, J. J. (1982): Quantitative effect of early coronary artery reperfusion in baboons:

Extent of salvage of the perfusion bed of an occluded artery. *Circulation,* 66:391–396.

172. Geer, J. C., Crago, C. A., Little, W. C., Gardner, L. L., and Bishop, S. P. (1980): Subendocardial ischemic myocardial lesions associated with severe coronary atherosclerosis. *Am. J. Pathol.,* 98:663–680.

173. Geft, I. L., Fishbein, M. C., Ninomiya, K., Hashida, J., Chaux, E., Yano, J., Y-Rit, J., Genov, T., Shell, W., and Ganz, W. (1982): Intermittent brief periods of ischemia have a cumulative effect and may cause myocardial necrosis. *Circulation,* 66:1150–1153.

174. Geisbuhler, T., Altschuld, R. A., Trewyn, R. W., Ansel, A. Z., Lamka, K., and Brierley, G. P. (1984): Adenine nucleotide metabolism and compartmentation in isolated rat heart cells. *Circ. Res.,* 54:536–546.

175. Gersh, B. J. (1985): Role of thrombolytic therapy in evolving myocardial infarction. *Mod. Concepts Cardiovasc. Dis.,* 54:13–17.

176. Gevers, W. (1977): Generation of protons by metabolic processes in heart cells. *J. Mol. Cell. Cardiol.,* 9:867–873.

177. Giclas, P. C., Pinckard, R. N., and Olson, M. S. (1979): In vitro activation of complement by isolated human heart subcellular membranes. *J. Immunol.,* 122:146–151.

178. Ginks, W. R., Sybers, H. D., Maroko, P. R., Covell, J. W., Sobel, B. E., and Ross, J. (1972): Coronary artery reperfusion. II. Reduction of myocardial infarct size at 1 week after the coronary occlusion. *J. Clin. Invest.,* 51:2717–2723.

179. Goerke, J., and Page, E. (1965): Cat heart muscle in vitro. VI. Potassium exchange in papillary muscles. *J. Gen. Physiol.,* 48:933–948.

180. Goldberg, H. L., Goldstein, J., Borer, J. S., Moses, J. W., and Collins, M. B. (1984): Functional importance of coronary collateral vessels. *Am. J. Cardiol.,* 53:694–699.

181. Goldstein, M. A., and Murphy, D. L. (1983): A morphometric analysis of ischemic canine myocardium with and without reperfusion. *J. Mol. Cell. Cardiol.,* 15:325–334.

182. Gorlin, R. (1983): Dynamic vascular factors in the genesis of myocardial ischemia. *J. Am. Coll. Cardiol.,* 3:897–906.

183. Gottlieb, G. J., Kubo, S. H., and Alonso, D. R. (1981): Ultrastructural characterization of the border zone surrounding early experimental myocardial infarcts in dogs. *Am. J. Pathol.,* 103:292–303.

184. Gottwik, M. G., Kirk, E. S., Hoffstein, S., and Weglicki, W. B. (1975): Effect of collateral flow on epicardial and endocardial lysosomal hydrolases in acute myocardial ischemia. *J. Clin. Invest.,* 56:914–923.

185. Gottwik, M. G., Puschmann, S., Wusten, B., Nienaber, C., Muller, K.-D., Hofmann, M., and Schaper, W. (1984): Myocardial protection by collateral vessels during experimental coronary ligation: A prospective study in a canine two-infarction model. *Basic Res. Cardiol.,* 79:337–343.

186. Gottwik, M., Zimmer, P., Wusten, B., Hofmann, M., Winkler, B., and Schaper, W. (1981): Experimental myocardial infarction in a closed-chest canine model: Observations of temporal and spatial evolution over 24 hours. *Basic Res. Cardiol.,* 76:670–680.

187. Grande, P., Hansen, B. F., Christiansen, C., and Naestoft, J. (1981): Acute myocardial infarct size estimated by serum CK-MB determinations: Clinical accuracy and prognostic relevance utilizing a practical modification of the isoenzyme approach. *Am. Heart J.,* 101:582–586.

188. Grayson, J., Davidson, J. W., Fitzgerald-Finch, A., and Scott, C. (1974): The functional morphology of the coronary microcirculation in the dog. *Microvasc. Res.,* 8:20–43.

189. Greenhoot, J. H., and Reichenbach, D. D. (1969): Cardiac injury and subarachnoid hemorrhage: A clinical, pathological, and physiological correlation. *J. Neurosurg.,* 30:521–531.

190. Gregg, D. E. (1974): The natural history of coronary collateral development. *Circ. Res.,* 35:335–344.

191. Griffith, G. C., Hegde, B., and Oblath, R. W. (1961): Factors in myocardial rupture. *Am. J. Cardiol.,* 8:792–798.

192. Grinwald, P. M. (1982): Calcium uptake during post-ischemic reperfusion in the isolated rat heart: Influence of extracellular sodium. *J. Mol. Cell. Cardiol.,* 14:359–365.

193. Grinwald, P. M., and Nayler, W. G. (1981): Calcium entry in the calcium paradox. *J. Mol. Cell. Cardiol.,* 13:867–880.

194. Grochowski, E. C., Ganote, C. E., Hill, M. L., and Jennings, R. B. (1976): Experimental myocardial ischemic injury. I. A comparison of Stadie-Riggs and free-hand slicing techniques on tissue ultrastructure, water and electrolytes during in vitro incubation. *J. Mol. Cell. Cardiol.,* 8:173–187.

195. Grondin, P., Kretz, J. G., Bical, O., Donzeau-Gouge, P., Petitclerc, R., and Campeau, L. (1979): Natural history of saccular aneurysms of the left ventricle. *J. Thorac. Cardiovasc. Surg.,* 77:57–64.

196. Gutovitz, A. L., Sobel, B. E., and Roberts, R. (1978): Progressive nature of myocardial injury in selected patients with cardiogenic shock. *Am. J. Cardiol.,* 41:469–475.

197. Haack, D. W., Bush, L. R., Shlafer, M., and Lucchesi, B. R. (1981): Lanthanum staining of coronary microvascular endothelium: Effects of ischemia reperfusion, propranolol, and atenolol. *Microvasc. Res.,* 21:362–376.

198. Haas, G. S., DeBoer, L. W. V., O'Keefe, D. D., Bodenhamer, R. M., Geffin, G. A., Drop, L. J., Teplick, R. S., and Daggett, W. M. (1984): Reduction of postischemic myocardial dysfunction by substrate repletion during reperfusion. *Circulation,* 70:65–74.

199. Haber, E., Katus, H. A., Hurrell, J. G., Matsueda, G. R., Ehrlich, P., Zurawski, V. R., Jr., and Khaw, B. (1982): Detection and quantification of myocardial cell death: Application of monoclonal antibodies specific for cardiac myosin. *J. Mol. Cell. Cardiol.* [*Suppl. 3*], 14:139–146.

200. Hackel, D. B., Reimer, K. A., Ideker, R. E., Mikat, E. M., Hartwell, T. D., Parker, C. B., Braunwald, E. B., Buja, M., Gold, H. K., Jaffe, A. S., Muller, J. E., Raabe, D. S., Rude, R. E., Sobel, B. E., Stone, P. H., Roberts, R., and the MILIS Study Group (1984): Comparison of enzymatic and anatomic estimates of myocardial infarct size in man. *Circulation,* 70:824–835.

201. Hackel, D. B., Wagner, G., Ratliff, N. B., Cies, A., and Estes, E. H. (1972): Anatomic studies of the cardiac conducting system in acute myocardial infarction. *Am. Heart J.,* 83:77–81.

202. Hagler, H. K., Sherwin, L., and Buja, L. M. (1979): Effect of different methods of tissue preparation on mitochondrial inclusions of ischemic and infarcted canine myocardium. *Lab. Invest.,* 40:529–544.

203. Hamby, R. I., Aintablian, A., and Schwartz, A. (1976): Reappraisal of the functional significance of the coronary collateral circulation. *Am. J. Cardiol.,* 38:305–309.

204. Hammerman, H., Schoen, F. J., and Kloner, R. A. (1983): Short-term exercise has a prolonged effect on scar formation after experimental acute myocardial infarction. *J. Am. Coll. Cardiol.,* 2:979–982.

205. Harden, W. R., III, Barlow, C. H., Simson, M. B., and Harken, A. H. (1979): Temporal relation between onset of cell anoxia and ischemic contractile failure. *Am. J. Cardiol.,* 44:741–746.

206. Harken, A. H., Simson, M. B., Haselgrove, J., Wetstein, L., Harden, W. R., and Barlow, C. H. (1981): Early ischemia after complete coronary ligation in the rabbit, dog, pig, and monkey. *Am. J. Physiol.,* 241:H202–H210.

207. Harris, A. S. (1966): Potassium and experimental coronary occlusion. *Am. Heart J.,* 71:797–802.

208. Hasin, Y., and Barry, W. H. (1984): Myocardial metabolic inhibition and membrane potassium uptake. *Am. J. Physiol.,* 247:H322–H329.

209. Hauschild, U., Baghirzade, M. F., and Kirsch, U. (1970): Compression of capillaries as a result of ischemia. *Virchows Arch.* [*Pathol. Anat.*], 351:205–224.

210. Hearse, D. J. (1979): Oxygen deprivation and early myocardial contractile failure: A reassessment of the possible role of adenosine triphosphate. *Am. J. Cardiol.,* 44:1115–1121.

211. Hearse, D. J., Humphrey, S. M., Nayler, W. G., Slade, A., and Border, D. (1975): Ultrastructural damage associated with reoxygenation of the anoxic myocardium. *J. Mol. Cell. Cardiol.,* 7:315–324.

212. Hearse, D. J., Opie, L. H., Katzeff, I. E., Lubbe, W. F., Van Der Werff, T. J., Peisach, M., and Boulle, G. (1977): Characterization of the "border zone" in acute regional ischemia in the dog. *Am. J. Cardiol.,* 40:716–726.

213. Hearse, D. J., and Yellon, D. M. (1981): The "border zone" in evolving myocardial infarction: Controversy or confusion? *Am. J. Cardiol.,* 47:1321–1334.

214. Hearse, D. J., and Yellon, D. M. (editors) (1984): *Therapeutic*

Approaches to Myocardial Infarct Size Limitation, Raven Press, New York.

215. Hecht, A. (1971): Enzyme histochemistry of heart muscle in normal and pathologic conditions. *Methods Achiev. Exp. Pathol.,* 5:384–435.

216. Helfant, R. H., Vokonas, P. S., and Gorlin, R. (1971): Functional importance of the human coronary collateral circulation. *N. Engl. J. Med.,* 284:1277–1281.

217. Henson, D. E., Najafi, H., Callaghan, R., Coogan, P., Julian, O. C., and Eisenstein, R. (1969): Myocardial lesions following open heart surgery. *Arch. Pathol.,* 88:423–430.

218. Herdson, P. B., Kaltenbach, J. P., and Jennings, R. B. (1969): Fine structural and biochemical changes in dog myocardium during autolysis. *Am. J. Pathol.,* 57:539–557.

219. Hess, D. S., and Bache, R. J. (1976): Transmural distribution of myocardial blood flow during systole in the awake dog. *Circ. Res.,* 38:5–15.

220. Hess, M. L., Manson, N. H., and Okabe, E. (1982): Involvement of free radicals in the pathophysiology of ischemic heart disease. *Can. J. Physiol. Pharmacol.,* 60:1382–1389.

221. Hewett, K., Legato, M. J., Danilo, P., Jr., and Robinson, R. B. (1983): Isolated myocytes from adult canine left ventricle: Ca^{2+} tolerance, electrophysiology, and ultrastructure. *Am. J. Physiol.,* 245:H830–H839.

222. Heyndrickx, G. R., Baig, H., Nellens, P., Leusen, I., Fishbein, M. C., and Vatner, S. F. (1978): Depression of regional blood flow and wall thickening after brief coronary occlusions. *Am. J. Physiol.,* 234:H653–H659.

223. Higginson, L. A. J., Beanlands, D. S., Nair, R. C., Temple, V., and Sheldrick, K. (1983): The time course and characterization of myocardial hemorrhage after coronary reperfusion in the anesthetized dog. *Circulation,* 67:1024–1031.

224. Hill, J. H., and Ward, P. A. (1971): The phlogistic role of C3 leukotactic fragments in myocardial infarcts of rats. *J. Exp. Med.,* 133:885–900.

225. Hill, J. L., and Gettes, L. S. (1980): Effect of acute coronary artery occlusion on local myocardial extracellular K^+ activity in swine. *Circulation,* 61:768–777.

226. Hillis, L. D., Askenazi, J., Braunwald, E., Radvany, P., Muller, J. E., Fishbein, M. C., and Maroko, P. R. (1976): Use of changes in the epicardial QRS complex to assess interventions which modify the extent of myocardial necrosis following coronary artery occlusion. *Circulation,* 54:591–598.

227. Hillis, L. D., and Braunwald, E. (1977): Myocardial ischemia. *N. Engl. J. Med.,* 296:971–978, 1034–1041, 1093–1096.

228. Hinohara, T., Hindman, N. B., White, R. D., Ideker, R. E., and Wagner, G. S. (1984): Quantitative QRS criteria for diagnosing and sizing myocardial infarcts. *Am. J. Cardiol.,* 53:875–878.

229. Hirakow, R., and Gotoh, T. (1975): A quantitative ultrastructural study of developing rat heart. In: *Developmental and Physiological Correlates of Cardiac Muscle,* edited by M. Lieberman and T. Sano, pp. 37–49. Raven Press, New York.

230. Hirche, H., Franz, C., Bos, L., Bissig, R., Lang, R., and Schramm, M. (1980): Myocardial extracellular K^+ and H^+ increase and noradrenaline release as possible cause of early arrhythmias following acute coronary artery occlusion in pigs. *J. Mol. Cell. Cardiol.,* 12:579–593.

231. Hirzel, H. O., Sonnenblick, E. H., and Kirk, E. S. (1977): Absence of a lateral border zone of intermediate creatine phosphokinase depletion surrounding a central infarct 24 hours after acute coronary occlusion in the dog. *Circ. Res.,* 41:673–683.

232. Ho, C. H., and Pande, S. V. (1974): On the specificity of the inhibition of adenine nucleotide translocase by long chain acyl-coenzyme A esters. *Biochim. Biophys. Acta,* 369:86–94.

233. Hochman, J. S., and Bulkley, B. H. (1982): Expansion of acute myocardial infarction: an experimental study. *Circulation,* 65:1446–1450.

234. Hoffmeister, H. M., Mauser, M., and Schaper, W. (1984): Failure of postischemic ATP repletion by adenosine to improve regional myocardial function. In: *Coronary Sinus,* edited by W. Mohl, E. Wolner, and D. Glogar, pp. 148–152. Steinkopff, Darmsdadt.

235. Hoffstein, S., Gennaro, D. E., Weissmann, G., Hirsch, J., Streuli, F., and Fox, A. C. (1975): Cytochemical localization of lysosomal enzyme activity in normal and ischemic dog myocardium. *Am. J. Pathol.,* 79:193–200.

236. Hofmann, M., Hofmann, M., Genth, K., and Schaper, W. (1980): The influence of reperfusion on infarct size after experimental coronary artery occlusion. *Basic Res. Cardiol.,* 75:572–582.

237. Hohl, C., Ansel, A., Altschuld, R., and Brierley, G. P. (1982): Contracture of isolated rat heart cells on anaerobic to aerobic transition. *Am. J. Physiol.,* 242:H1022–H1030.

238. Holland, R. P., and Brooks, H. (1977): TQ-ST segment mapping: Critical review and analysis of current concepts. *Am. J. Cardiol.,* 40:110–129.

239. Holmgren, S., Abrahamsson, T., Almgren, O., and Eriksson, B.-M. (1981): Effect of ischaemia on the adrenergic neurons of the rat heart: A fluorescence histochemical and biochemical study. *Cardiovasc. Res.,* 15:680–689.

240. Hori, M., Inoue, M., Fukui, S., Shimazu, T., Mishima, M., Ohgitani, N., Minamino, T., and Abe, H. (1979): Correlation of ejection fraction and infarct size estimated from the total CK released in patients with acute myocardial infarction. *Br. Heart J.,* 41:433–440.

241. Horres, C. R., Lieberman, M., and Purdy, J. E. (1977): Growth orientation of heart cells on nylon monofilament: Determination of the volume to surface area ratio and intracellular potassium concentration. *J. Membr. Biol.,* 34:313–329.

242. Hough, F. S., and Gevers, W. (1975): Catecholamine release as mediator of intracellular activation in ischemic perfused rat hearts. *S. Afr. Med. J.,* 49:538–543.

243. Humphrey, S. M., Gavin, J. B., and Herdson, P. B. (1980): The relationship of ischemic contracture to vascular reperfusion in the isolated rat heart. *J. Mol. Cell. Cardiol.,* 12:1397–1406.

244. Humphrey, S. M., Thomson, R. W., and Gavin, J. B. (1981): The effect of an isovolumic left ventricle on the coronary vascular competence during reflow after global ischemia in the rat heart. *Circ. Res.,* 49:784–791.

245. Hutchins, G. M. (1979): Rupture of the interventricular septum complicating myocardial infarction: Pathological analysis of 10 patients with clinically diagnosed perforations. *Am. Heart J.,* 97:165–173.

246. Hutchins, G. M., and Bulkley, B. H. (1978): Infarct expansion versus extension: Two different complications of acute myocardial infarction. *Am. J. Cardiol.,* 41:1127–1132.

247. Ichihara, K., and Abiko, Y. (1982): Crossover plot study of glycolytic intermediates in the ischemic canine heart. *Jpn. Heart J.,* 23:817–828.

248. Ichihara, K., and Abiko, Y. (1984): Rebound recovery of myocardial creatine phosphate with reperfusion after ischemia. *Am. Heart J.,* 108:1594–1597.

249. Ichihara, K., Haga, N., and Abiko, Y. (1984): Is ischemia-induced pH decrease of dog myocardium respiratory or metabolic acidosis? *Am. J. Physiol.,* 246:H652–H657.

250. Idell-Wenger, J. A., Grotyohann, L. W., and Neely, J. R. (1978): Coenzyme A and carnitine distribution in normal and ischemic hearts. *J. Biol. Chem.,* 253:4310–4318.

251. Ingwall, J. S., DeLuca, M., Sybers, H. D., and Wildenthal, K. (1975): Fetal mouse hearts: A model for studying ischemia. *Proc. Natl. Acad. Sci. USA,* 72:2809–2813.

252. Itkonen, P., and Collan, Y. (1983): Mitochondrial flocculent densities in ischemia, digestion experiments. *Acta Pathol. Microbiol. Immunol. Scand.,* 91:463–468.

253. Jacobus, W. E., Pores, I. H., Lucas, S. K., Weisfeldt, M. L., and Flaherty, J. T. (1982): Intracellular acidosis and contractility in the normal and ischemic heart as examined by PNMR. *J. Mol. Cell. Cardiol.,* 14:13–20.

254. James, T. N. (1970): The delivery and distribution of coronary collateral circulation. *Chest,* 58:183–203.

255. Janse, M. J., Cinca, J., Morena, H., Fiolet, J., Klever, A., DeVries, G. P., Becker, A., and Durrer, D. (1979): The "border zone" in myocardial ischemia. An electrophysiological, metabolic and histochemical correlation in the pig heart. *Circ. Res.,* 44:576–588.

256. Janse, M. J., and Wilms-Schopman, F. (1982): Effect of changes in perfusion pressure on the position of the electrophysiologic border zone in acute regional ischemia in isolated perfused dog and pig hearts. *Am. J. Cardiol.,* 50:74–82.

257. Jennings, R. B. (1970): Editorial: Myocardial ischemia—observations, definitions and speculations. *J. Mol. Cell. Cardiol.,* 1:345–349.

258. Jennings, R. B., and Ganote, C. E. (1974): Structural changes in myocardium during acute ischemia. *Circ. Res.*, 34–35:156–172.

259. Jennings, R. B., Ganote, C. E., and Reimer, K. A. (1975): Ischemic tissue injury. *Am. J. Pathol.*, 81:179–198.

260. Jennings, R. B., and Hawkins, H. K. (1980): Ultrastructural changes of acute myocardial ischemia. In: *Degradative Processes in Heart and Skeletal Muscle*, edited by K. Wildenthal, pp. 295–346. Elsevier/North Holland, Amsterdam.

261. Jennings, R. B., Hawkins, H. K., Lowe, J. E., Hill, M. L., Klotman, S., and Reimer, K. A. (1978): Relation between high energy phosphate and lethal injury in myocardial ischemia in the dog. *Am. J. Pathol.*, 92:187–214.

262. Jennings, R. B., Herdson, P. B., and Sommers, H. M. (1969): Structural and functional abnormalities in mitochondria isolated from ischemic dog myocardium. *Lab. Invest.*, 20:548–557.

263. Jennings, R. B., Kaltenbach, J. P., and Sommers, H. M. (1967): Mitochondrial metabolism in ischemic injury. *Arch. Pathol.*, 84:15–19.

264. Jennings, R. B., Murry, C. E., Steenbergen, C., and Reimer, K. A. (1986): The acute phase of regional ischemia. In: *Acute Myocardial Infarction: Emerging Concepts of Pathogenesis and Treatment*, edited by R. H. Cox, Praeger, New York.

265. Jennings, R. B., and Reimer, K. A. (1974): Salvage of ischemic myocardium. *Mod. Concepts Cardiovasc. Dis.*, 43:125–130.

266. Jennings, R. B., and Reimer, K. A. (1981): Lethal myocardial ischemic injury. *Am. J. Pathol.*, 102:241–255.

267. Jennings, R. B., and Reimer, K. A. (1983): Factors involved in salvaging ischemic myocardium: Effect of reperfusion of arterial blood. *Circulation*, 68:25–36.

268. Jennings, R. B., Reimer, K. A., Hill, M. L., and Mayer, S. E. (1981): Total ischemia in dog hearts, in vitro. I. Comparison of high energy phosphate production, utilization, and depletion, and of adenine nucleotide catabolism in total ischemia in vitro vs. severe ischemia in vivo. *Circ. Res.*, 49:892–900.

269. Jennings, R. B., Reimer, K. A., Jones, R. N., and Peyton, R. B. (1983): High energy phosphates, anaerobic glycolysis and irreversibility in ischemia. In: *Myocardial Injury*, edited by J. J. Spitzer, pp. 403–419. Plenum, New York.

270. Jennings, R. B., Reimer, K. A., Kinney, R. B., Steenbergen, C., Jr., Sharov, V. G., Jones, R. N., and Peyton, R. B. (1986): Sarcolemmal damage in ischemia. In: *Sixth Joint US-USSR Symposium on Myocardial Metabolism*, edited by A. Katz and V. Smirnov. Gordon & Breach, New York.

271. Jennings, R. B., Reimer, K. A., and Steenbergen, C. (1985): Myocardial ischemia and reperfusion: role of calcium. In: *Control and Manipulation of Calcium Movement*, edited by J. R. Parratt, pp. 273–302. Raven Press, New York.

272. Jennings, R. B., Reimer, K. A., and Steenbergen, C., Jr. (1986): Editorial: Myocardial ischemia revisited. The osmolar load, membrane damage, and reperfusion. *J. Mol. Cell. Cardiol.*, (in press).

273. Jennings, R. B., Schaper, J., Hill, M. L., Steenbergen, C., and Reimer, K. A. (1985): Effect of reperfusion late in the phase of reversible ischemic injury. Changes in cell volume, electrolytes, metabolites, and ultrastructure. *Circ. Res.*, 56:262–278.

274. Jennings, R. B., Sommers, H. M., Kaltenbach, J. P., and West, J. J. (1964): Electrolyte alterations in acute myocardial ischemic injury. *Circ. Res.*, 14:260–269.

275. Jennings, R. B., Sommers, H. M., Smyth, G. A., Flack, H. A., and Linn, H. (1960): Myocardial necrosis induced by temporary occlusion of a coronary artery in the dog. *Arch. Pathol.*, 70:68–78.

276. Jennings, R. B., Steenbergen, C., Jr., Kinney, R. B., Hill, M. L., and Reimer, K. A. (1983): Comparison of the effect of ischaemia and anoxia on the sarcolemma of the dog heart. *Eur. Heart J.*, 4:123–137.

277. Jennings, R. B., and Wartman, W. B. (1957): Reactions of the myocardium to obstruction of the coronary arteries. *Med. Clinics N. Amer.*, 1–15.

278. Jesmok, G. J., Wartlier, D. C., Gross, G. J., and Hardman, H. F. (1978): Transmural triglycerides in acute myocardial ischaemia. *Cardiovasc. Res.*, 12:659–665.

279. Johnson, A. R., Revtyak, G., and Campbell, W. B. (1985): Arachidonic acid metabolites and endothelial injury: Studies with cultures of human endothelial cells. *Fed. Proc.*, 44:19–24.

280. Jolly, S. R., Kane, W. J., Bailie, M. B., Abrams, G. D., and Lucchesi, B. R. (1984): Canine myocardial reperfusion injury. Its reduction by the combined administration of superoxide dismutase and catalase. *Circ. Res.*, 54:277–285.

281. Jones, C. E., Thomas, J. X., Parker, J. C., and Parker, R. E. (1976): Acute changes in high energy phosphates, nucleotide derivatives, and contractile force in ischaemic and nonischaemic canine myocardium following coronary occlusion. *Cardiovasc. Res.*, 10:275–282.

282. Jones, M. E., Terry, G., and Kenmure, A. C. F. (1977): Frequency and significance of conduction defects in acute myocardial infarction. *Am. Heart J.*, 94:163–167.

283. Jones, R. N., Reimer, K. A., Hill, M. L., and Jennings, R. B. (1982): Effect of hypothermia on changes in high-energy phosphate production and utilization in total ischemia. *J. Mol. Cell. Cardiol.* [*Suppl. 3*], 14:123–130.

284. Jugdutt, B. I., Hutchins, G. M., Bulkley, B. H., and Becker, L. C. (1979): Myocardial infarction in the conscious dog: Three-dimensional mapping of infarct, collateral flow and region at risk. *Circulation*, 60:1141–1150.

285. Kahles, H., Gebhard, M. M., Mezger, V. A., Nordbeck, H., Preuse, C. J., and Spieckermann, P. G. (1979): The role of ATP and lactic acid for mitochondrial function during myocardial ischemia. *Basic Res. Cardiol.*, 74:611–620.

286. Kahles, H., Göring, G. G., Nordbeck, H., Preusse, C. J., and Spieckermann, P. G. (1977): Functional behaviour of isolated heart muscle mitochondria after in situ ischemia. Polarographic analysis of mitochondrial oxidative phosphorylation. *Basic Res. Cardiol.*, 72:563–574.

287. Kameyama, M. (1983): Electrical coupling between ventricular paired cells isolated from guinea-pig heart. *J. Physiol. (Lond.)*, 336:345–357.

288. Kanaide, H., Yoshimura, R., Makino, N., and Nakamura, M. (1982): Regional myocardial function and metabolism during acute coronary artery occlusion. *Am. J. Physiol.*, H980–H989.

289. Kanayama, H., Ban, M., Ogawa, K., and Satake, T. (1982): Myocardial concentration of norepinephrine and cyclic AMP in ventricular fibrillation during acute myocardial ischemia. *J. Cardiovasc. Pharmacol.*, 4:1018–1023.

290. Kao, K. J., Hackel, D. B., and Kong, Y. (1984): Hemorrhagic myocardial infarction after streptokinase treatment for acute coronary thrombosis. *Arch. Pathol. Lab. Med.*, 108:121–124.

291. Kao, R., Rannels, E., and Morgan, H. E. (1976): Effects of anoxia and ischemia on protein synthesis in perfused rat hearts. *Circ. Res.*, 38:124–130.

292. Karwatowski-Krynska, E., and Bereswicz, A. (1983): Effect of locally released catecholamines on lipolysis and injury of the hypoxic isolated rabbit heart. *J. Mol. Cell. Cardiol.*, 15:523–536.

293. Katz, A. M. (1973): Effects of ischemia on the contractile processes of heart muscle. *Am. J. Cardiol.*, 32:456–460.

294. Katz, A. M. (1982): Membrane-derived lipids and the pathogenesis of ischemic myocardial damage. *J. Mol. Cell. Cardiol.*, 14:627–632.

295. Katz, A. M., and Messineo, F. C. (1981): Lipid-membrane interactions and the pathogenesis of ischemic damage in the myocardium. *Circ. Res.*, 48:1–16.

296. Katz, A. M., and Messineo, F. C. (1982): Fatty acid effects on membranes: Possible role in the pathogenesis of ischemic myocardial damage. *J. Mol. Cell. Cardiol.*, 14:119–122.

297. Katz, A. M., and Reuter, H. (1979): Cellular calcium and cardiac cell death. *Am. J. Cardiol.*, 44:188–190.

298. Kennedy, J. W., Ritchie, J. L., Davis, K. B., and Fritz, J. K. (1983): Western Washington randomized trial of intracoronary streptokinase in acute myocardial infarction. *N. Engl. J. Med.*, 309:1477–1482.

299. Kent, S. P. (1967): Diffusion of plasma proteins into cells: A manifestation of cell injury in human myocardial ischemia. *Am. J. Pathol.*, 50:623–638.

300. Kent, S. P., and Diseker, M. (1955): Early myocardial ischemia. Study of histochemical changes in dogs. *Lab. Invest.*, 4:398–405.

301. Khan, A. H. (1975): Pericarditis of myocardial infarction: Review of the literature with case presentation. *Am. Heart J.*, 90:788–794.

302. Khouri, E. M., Gregg, D. E., and McGranahan, G. M. (1971): Regression and reappearance of coronary collaterals. *Am. J. Physiol.*, 220:655–661.

303. Kirk, E. S., and Honig, C. R. (1964): An experimental and theoretical analysis of tissue pressure. *Am. J. Physiol.*, 207:361–367.

304. Kirk, E. S., and Jennings, R. B. (1982): Pathophysiology of myocardial ischemia. In: *The Heart*, ed. 5, edited by J. W. Hurst, pp. 976–1008. McGraw-Hill, New York.

305. Kjekshus, J. K., Maroko, P. R., and Sobel, B. E. (1972): Distribution of myocardial injury and its relation to epicardial ST-segment changes after coronary artery occlusion in the dog. *Cardiovasc. Res.*, 6:490–499.

306. Kleber, A. G. (1983): Resting membrane potential, extracellular potassium activity, and intracellular sodium activity during acute global ischemia in isolated perfused guinea pig hearts. *Circ. Res.*, 52:442–450.

307. Kleber, A. G. (1984): Extracellular potassium in acute ischemia. *J. Mol. Cell. Cardiol.*, 16:389–394.

308. Klein, H. H., Puschmann, S., Schaper, J., and Schaper, W. (1981): The mechanism of the tetrazolium reaction in identifying experimental myocardial infarction. *Virchows Arch. [Pathol. Anat.]*, 393:287–297.

309. Klein, H. H., Schaper, J., Puschmann, S., Nienaber, C., Kreuzer, H., and Schaper, W. (1981): Loss of canine myocardial nicotinamide adenine dinucleotides determines the transition from reversible to irreversible ischemic damage of myocardial cells. *Basic Res. Cardiol.*, 76:612–621.

310. Klein, H. H., Schubothe, M., Nebendahl, K., and Kreuzer, H. (1984): Temporal and spatial development of infarcts in porcine hearts. *Basic Res. Cardiol.*, 79:440–447.

311. Klionsky, B. (1960): Myocardial ischemia and early infarction. A histochemical study. *Am. J. Pathol.*, 36:575–591.

312. Klocke, F. J., Braunwald, E., and Ross, J., Jr. (1966): Oxygen cost of electrical activation of the heart. *Circ. Res.*, 18:357–365.

313. Kloner, R. A., Ellis, S. G., Lange, R., and Braunwald, E. (1983): Studies of experimental coronary artery reperfusion: Effects on infarct size, myocardial function, biochemistry, ultrastructure and microvascular damage. *Circulation*, 68:8–15.

314. Kloner, R. A., Fishbein, M. C., Hare, C. M., and Maroko, P. R. (1979) Early ischemic ultrastructural and histochemical alterations in the myocardium of the rat following coronary artery occlusion. *Exp. Mol. Pathol.*, 30:129–143.

315. Kloner, R. A., Ganote, C. E., and Jennings, R. B. (1974): The "no-reflow" phenomenon after temporary coronary occlusion in the dog. *J. Clin. Invest.*, 54:1496–1508.

316. Kloner, R. A., Ganote, C. E., Whalen, D., and Jennings, R. B. (1974): Effect of a transient period of ischemia on myocardial cells: II. Fine structure during the first few minutes of reflow. *Am. J. Pathol.*, 74:399–422.

317. Kloner, R. A., and Ingwall, J. S. (1980): The cultured fetal mouse heart as a model for studying myocardial ischemic necrosis. *Exp. Mol. Pathol.*, 32:317–335.

318. Kloner, R. A., Rude, R. E., Carlson, N., Maroko, P. R., DeBoer, L. W. V., and Braunwald, E. (1980): Ultrastructural evidence of microvascular damage and myocardial cell injury after coronary artery occlusion: Which comes first? *Circulation*, 62:945–952.

319. Kobayashi, K., and Neely, J. R. (1979): Control of maximum rates of glycolysis in rat cardiac muscle. *Circ. Res.*, 44:166–175.

320. Kodama, I., Wilde, A., Janse, M. J., Durrer, D., and Yamada, K. (1984): Combined effects of hypoxia, hyperkalemia and acidosis on membrane action potential and excitability of guinea-pig ventricular muscle. *J. Mol. Cell. Cardiol.*, 16:247–259.

321. Kohn, R. M. (1959): Mechanical factors in cardiac rupture. *Am. J. Cardiol.*, 4:279–281.

322. Kramer, J. H., Mak, I. T., and Weglicki, W. B. (1984): Differential sensitivity of canine cardiac sarcolemmal and microsomal enzymes to inhibition by free radical-induced lipid peroxidation. *Circ. Res.*, 55:120–124.

323. Krieger, W. J. G., ter Welle, H. F., Fiolet, J. W. T., and Janse, M. J. (1984): Tissue osmolality, metabolic response, and reperfusion in myocardial ischemia. *Basic Res. Cardiol.*, 79:562–571.

324. Kubler, W., and Katz, A. M. (1977): Mechanism of early "pump" failure of the ischemic heart: Possible role of adenosine triphosphate depletion and inorganic phosphate accumulation. *Am. J. Cardiol.*, 40:467–471.

325. Kübler, W., and Spieckermann, P. G. (1970): Regulation of glycolysis in the ischemic and the anoxic myocardium. *J. Mol. Cell. Cardiol.*, 1:351–377.

326. L'Abbate, A., Marzilli, M., Ballestra, A. M., Camici, P., Trivella, M. G., Pelosi, G., and Klassen, G. A. (1980): Opposite transmural gradients of coronary resistance and extravascular pressure in the working dog's heart. *Cardiovasc. Res.*, 14:21–29.

327. LaFarge, C. G., Carr, J. E., Coleman, S., and Bernhard, W. F. (1972): The maintenance of circulatory competence during chronic microsphere-induced myocardial failure. *J. Thorac. Cardiovasc. Surg.*, 64:652–658.

328. Laffel, G. L., and Braunwald, E. (1984): Thrombolytic therapy. A new strategy for the treatment of acute myocardial infarction. *N. Engl. J. Med.*, 311:710–717.

329. Laffel, G. L., and Braunwald, E. (1984): Thrombolytic therapy. A new strategy for the treatment of acute myocardial infarction. *N. Engl. J. Med.*, 311:770–776.

330. Lai, F., and Scheuer, J. (1975): Early changes in myocardial hypoxia: Relations between mechanical function, pH and intracellular compartmental metabolites. *J. Mol. Cell. Cardiol.*, 7:289–303.

331. Laird, J. D., Breuls, P. N., van der Meer, P., and Spaan, J. A. E. (1981): Can a single vasodilator be responsible for both coronary autoregulation and metabolic vasodilation? *Basic Res. Cardiol.*, 76:354–358.

332. Lamb, F. S., and Webb, R. C. (1984): Vascular effects of free radicals generated by electrical stimulation. *Am. J. Physiol.*, 247:H709–H714.

333. Lange, R., Ingwall, J. S., Hale, S. L., Alker, K. J., and Kloner, R. A. (1984): Effects of recurrent ischemia on myocardial high energy phosphate content in canine hearts. *Basic Res. Cardiol.*, 79:469–478.

334. Lange, R., Kloner, R. A., Zierler, M., Carlson, N., Seiler, M., and Khuri, S. F. (1983): Time course of ischemic alterations during normothermic and hypothermic arrest and its reflection by on-line monitoring of tissue pH. *J. Thorac. Cardiovasc. Surg.*, 86:418–434.

335. Lange, R., Ware, J., and Kloner, R. A. (1984): Absence of a cumulative deterioration of regional function during three repeated 5 or 15 minute coronary occlusions. *Circulation*, 69:400–408.

336. Lavalee, M., and Vatner, S. F. (1984): Regional myocardial blood flow and necrosis in primates following coronary occlusion. *Am. J. Physiol.*, 246:H635–H639.

337. Lee, J. T., Ideker, R. E., and Reimer, K. A. (1981): Myocardial infarct size and location in relation to the coronary vascular bed at risk in man. *Circulation*, 64:526–534.

338. Lepran, I., Koltai, M., Siegmund, W., and Szekeres, L. (1983): Coronary artery ligation, early arrhythmias, and determination of the ischemic area in conscious rats. *J. Pharmacol. Meth.*, 9:219–230.

339. Lerch, R. A., Ambos, H. D., Bergmann, S. R., Welch, M. J., Ter-Pogossian, M. M., and Sobel, B. E. (1981): Localization of viable, ischemic myocardium by positron-emission tomography with ¹¹C-palmitate. *Circulation*, 64:689–699.

340. Lerman, R. H., Apstein, C. W., Kagan, H. M., Osmers, E. L., Chichester, C. O., Vogel, W. M., Connelly, C. M., and Steffee, W. P. (1983): Myocardial healing and repair after experimental infarction in the rabbit. *Circ. Res.*, 53:378–388.

341. Levitsky, S., and Feinberg, H. (1975): Biochemical changes of ischemia. *Ann. Thorac. Surg.*, 20:21–29.

342. Lewis, A. J., Burchell, H. B., and Titus, J. L. (1969): Clinical and pathologic features of postinfarction cardiac rupture. *Am. J. Cardiol.*, 23:43–53.

343. Lewis, S. E., Devous, M. D., Sr., Corbett, J. R., Izquierdo, C., Nicod, P., Wolfe, C. L., Parkey, R. W., Buja, L. M., and Willerson, J. T. (1984): Measurement of infarct size in acute canine myocardial infarction by single-photon emission computer tomography with technetium-99m pyrophosphate. *Am. J. Cardiol.*, 54:193–199.

344. Libby, P. (1984): Long-term culture of contractile mammalian heart cells in a defined serum-free medium that limits non-muscle cell proliferation. *J. Mol. Cell. Cardiol.*, 16:803–811.

345. Lichstein, E., Arsura, E., Hollander, G., Greengart, A., and Sanders, M. (1982): Current incidence of postmyocardial infarction (Dressler's) syndrome. *Am. J. Cardiol.*, 50:1269–1271.

346. Lichtig, C., and Brooks, H. (1975): Myocardial ultrastructure and

function during progressive early ischemia in the intact heart. *J. Thorac. Cardiovasc. Surg.,* 70:309–315.

347. Lie, J. T., Holley, K. E., Kampa, W. R., and Titus, J. L. (1971): New histologic method for morphologic diagnosis of early stages of myocardial ischemia. *Mayo Clin. Proc.,* 46:319–327.

348. Lie, J. T., Pairolero, P. C., Holley, K. E., and Titus, J. L. (1975): Macroscopic enzyme-mapping: Verification of large, homogeneous, experimental myocardial infarcts of predictable size and location in dogs. *J. Thorac. Cardiovasc. Surg.,* 69:599–604.

349. Liedtke, A. J. (1981): Alterations of carbohydrate and lipid metabolism in the acutely ischemic heart. *Prog. Cardiovasc. Dis.,* 23:321–336.

350. Liedtke, A. J., Hughes, H. C., and Neely, J. R. (1976): Effects of excess glucose and insulin on glycolytic metabolism during experimental myocardial ischemia. *Am. J. Cardiol.,* 38:17–27.

351. Liedtke, A. J., Mahar, C. Q., Ytrehus, M. K., and Mjos, O. D. (1984): Estimates of free-radical production in rat and swine hearts: Method and application of measuring malondialdehyde levels in fresh and frozen myocardium. *Basic Res. Cardiol.,* 79: 513–518.

352. Liedtke, A. J., Nellis, S. H., and Mjos, O. D. (1984): Effects of reducing fatty acid metabolism on mechanical function in regionally ischemic hearts. *Am. J. Physiol.,* 247:H387–H394.

353. Lipasti, J. A., Alanen, K. A., and Nevalainen, T. J. (1982): Effect of hypertonic mannitol on microvascular function in hypoxic and reoxygenated rat myocardium. *Cardiovasc. Res.,* 16:283–287.

354. Lochner, A., Opie, L. H., Owen, P., Kotze, J. C. N., Bruyneel, K., and Gevers, W. (1975): Oxidative phosphorylation in infarcting baboon and dog myocardium: Effects of mitochondrial isolation and incubation media. *J. Mol. Cell. Cardiol.,* 7:203–217.

355. Lodge-Patch, I. (1951): The ageing of cardiac infarcts, and its influence on cardiac rupture. *Br. Heart J.,* 13:37–42.

356. Long, J. B., Reimer, K. A., and Jennings, R. B. (1985): Distribution of collateral blood flow after circumflex coronary occlusion in dogs. *Fed. Proc.,* 44:821 (abstract).

357. Lowe, J. E., Cummings, R. G., Adams, D. H., and Hull-Ryde, E. A. (1983): Evidence that ischemic cell death begins in the subendocardium independent of variations in collateral flow or wall tension. *Circulation,* 68:190–202.

358. Lowe, J. E., Jennings, R. B., and Reimer, K. A. (1979): Cardiac rigor mortis in dogs. *J. Mol. Cell. Cardiol.,* 11:1017–1031.

359. Lowe, J. E., Reimer, K. A., and Jennings, R. B. (1978): Experimental infarct size as a function of the amount of myocardium at risk. *Am. J. Pathol.,* 90:363–379.

360. McCallister, L. P., Trapukdi, S., and Neely, J. R. (1979): Morphometric observations on the effects of ischemia in the isolated perfused rat heart. *J. Mol. Cell. Cardiol.,* 11:619–630.

361. McCord, J. M., and Fridovich, I. (1978): The biology and pathology of oxygen radicals. *Ann. Intern. Med.,* 89:122–127.

362. McDonagh, P. F., Goldman, N., and Laks, H. (1982): The effects of global myocardial ischemia followed by reperfusion on transcoronary exchange during cardiopulmonary bypass. *Microcirculation,* 2:243–270.

363. McDonald, T. F., and MacLeod, D. P. (1973): Metabolism and the electrical activity of anoxic ventricular muscle. *J. Physiol. (Lond.),* 229:559–582.

364. McDonough, K. H., Dunn, R. B., and Griggs, D. M., Jr. (1984): Transmural changes in porcine and canine hearts after circumflex artery occlusion. *Am. J. Physiol.,* 246:H601–H607.

365. McGrath, B. P., Lim, S. P., Leversha, L., and Shanahan, A. (1981): Myocardial and peripheral catecholamine responses to acute coronary artery constriction before and after propranolol treatment in the anaesthetized dog. *Cardiovasc. Res.,* 15:28–34.

366. McKeever, W. P., Gregg, D. E., and Canney, P. C. (1958): Oxygen uptake of the nonworking left ventricle. *Circ. Res.,* 6: 612–623.

367. McNamara, J. J., Soeter, J. R., Suehiro, G. T., Anema, R. J., and Smith, G. T. (1974): Surface pH changes during and after myocardial ischemia in primates. *J. Thorac. Cardiovasc. Surg.,* 67:191–194.

368. Madias, J. E., Chahine, R. A., Gorlin, R., and Blacklow, D. J. (1974): A comparison of transmural and nontransmural acute myocardial infarction. *Circulation,* 49:498–507.

369. Mainwood, G. W., and Worsley-Brown, P. (1975): The effects of extracellular pH and buffer concentration on the efflux of lactate from frog sartorius muscle. *J. Physiol. (Lond.),* 250:1–22.

370. Mallory, G. K., White, P. D., and Salcedo-Salgar, J. (1939): The speed of healing of myocardial infarction. A study of the pathologic anatomy in seventy-two cases. *Am. Heart J.,* 18:647–671.

371. Malsky, P. M., Vokonas, P. S., Paul, S. J., Robbins, S. L., and Hood, W. B. (1977): Autoradiographic measurement of regional blood flow in normal and ischemic myocardium. *Am. J. Physiol.,* 232:576–583.

372. Man, R. U. K., Slater, T. L., Pelletier, M. P., and Choy, P. C. (1983) Alterations of phospholipids in ischemic canine myocardium during acute arrhythmia. *Lipids,* 18:677–681.

373. Manning, A. S., Hearse, D. J., Dennis, S. C., Bullock, G. R., and Coltart, D. J. (1980): Myocardial ischaemia: An isolated, globally perfused rat heart model for metabolic and pharmacological studies. *Eur. J. Cardiol.,* 11:1–21.

374. Marcus, M. L., and Kerber, R. E. (1977): Present status of the ^{99m}technetium pyrophosphate infarct scintigram. *Circulation,* 56: 335–339.

375. Marcus, M. L., Kerber, R. E., Ehrhardt, J., and Abboud, F. M. (1975): Three dimensional geometry of acutely ischemic myocardium. *Circulation,* 52:254–263.

376. Maroko, P. R., Kjekshus, J. K., Sobel, B. E., Watanabe, T., Covell, J. W., Ross, J., Jr., and Braunwald, E. (1971): Factors influencing infarct size following experimental coronary artery occlusion. *Circulation,* 43:67–82.

377. Maroko, P. R., Libby, P., Covell, J. W., Sobel, B. E., Ross, J., Jr., and Braunwald, E. (1972); Precordial S-T segment elevation mapping: An atraumatic method for assessing alterations in the extent of myocardial ischemic injury: The effects of pharmacologic and hemodynamic interventions. *Am. J. Cardiol.,* 29:223–230.

378. Marsh, J. D. (1983): The cultured heart cell: A useful model for physiological and biochemical investigation. *Int. J. Cardiol.,* 3: 465–468.

379. Maseri, A., and Chierchia, S. (1982): Coronary artery spasm: Demonstration, definition, diagnosis, and consequences. *Prog. Cardiovasc. Dis.,* 25:169–192.

380. Maseri, A., L'Abbate, A., Baroldi, G., Chierchia, S., Marzilli, M., Ballestra, A. M., Severi, S., Parodi, O., Biagini, A., Distante, A., and Pesola, A. (1978): Coronary vasospasm as a possible cause of myocardial infarction. *N. Engl. J. Med.,* 299:1271–1277.

381. Mason, R. P., Kalyanaraman, B., Tainer, B. E., and Eling, T. E. (1980): A carbon-centered free radical intermediate in the prostaglandin synthetase oxidation of arachidonic acid: Spin trapping and oxygen uptake studies. *J. Biol. Chem.,* 255:5012–5022.

382. Mather, P. P., and Case, R. B. (1973): Phosphate loss during reversible myocardial ischemia. *J. Mol. Cell. Cardiol.,* 5:375–393.

383. Mathes, P., and Gudbjarnason, S. (1971): Changes in norepinephrine stores in the canine heart following experimental myocardial infarction. *Am. Heart J.,* 18:211–219.

384. Mathey, D., Bleifeld, W., Hanrath, P., and Effert, S. (1974): Attempt to quantitate relation between cardiac function and infarct size in acute myocardial infarction. *Br. Heart J.,* 36:271–279.

385. Mathey, D. G., Kuck, K. H., Titsner, V., Krebber, H. J., and Bleifeld, W. (1981): Nonsurgical coronary artery recanalization in acute transmural myocardial infarction. *Circulation,* 63:489–497.

386. Mathey, D. G., Schofer, J., Kuck, K.-H., Beil, U., and Kloppel, G. (1982): Transmural, haemorrhagic myocardial infarction after intracoronary streptokinase. Clinical, angiographic, and necropsy findings. *Br. Heart J.,* 48:546–551.

387. Mathur, V. S., Guinn, G. A., and Burris, W. H., III (1975): Maximal revascularisation (reperfusion) in intact conscious dogs after 2 to 5 hours of coronary occlusion. *Am. J. Cardiol.,* 36: 252–261.

388. Mauser, M., Hoffmeister, H. M., Nienaber, C., and Schaper, W. (1985): Influence of ribose, adenosine, and "AICAR" on the rate of myocardial adenosine triphosphate synthesis during reperfusion after coronary artery occlusion in the dog. *Circ. Res.,* 56:220–230.

389. Mayer, S. E., Williams, B. J., and Smith, J. M. (1967): Adrenergic mechanisms in cardiac glycogen metabolism. *Ann. N.Y. Acad. Sci.,* 139:686–702.

390. Mazet, F., Wittenberg, B. A., and Spray, D. C. (1985): Fate of intercellular junctions in isolated adult rat cardiac cells. *Circ. Res.,* 56:195–204.

391. Mead, J. F. (1976): Free radical mechanisms of lipid damage and consequences for cellular membranes. *Free Radicals Biol.,* 1:51–68.

392. Meerson, F. Z., Kagan, V. E., Kozlov, Y. P., Belkina, L. M., and Arkhipenko, Y. V. (1982): The role of lipid peroxidation in pathogenesis of ischemic damage and the antioxidant protection of the heart. *Basic Res. Cardiol.,* 77:465–485.

393. Meltzer, R. S., Woythaler, J. N., Buda, A. J., Griffin, J. C., Kernoff, R., Harrison, D. C., Popp, R. L., and Martin, R. P. (1980): Non-invasive quantification of experimental canine myocardial infarct size using two-dimensional echocardiography. *Eur. J. Cardiol.,* 11:215–225.

394. Meneely, G. R. (1974): The capillary factor in myocardial infarction. *Am. J. Cardiol.,* 34:581–587.

395. Mercer, R. W., and Dunham, P. B. (1981): Membrane-bound ATP fuels the Na/K pump. Studies on membrane-bound glycolytic enzymes on inside-out vesicles from human red cell membranes. *J. Gen. Physiol.,* 78:547–568.

396. Mittal, A. K., Langston, M., Cohn, K. E., Selzer, A., and Kerth, W. J. (1971): Combined papillary muscle and left ventricular wall dysfunction as a cause of mitral regurgitation. *Circulation,* 44:174–180.

397. Mochizuki, S., and Neely, J. R. (1979): Control of glyceraldehyde-3-phosphate dehydrogenase in cardiac muscle. *J. Mol. Cell. Cardiol.,* 11:221–236.

398. Moore, K. H., Radloff, J. F., Hull, F. E., and Sweeley, C. C. (1980): Incomplete fatty acid oxidation by ischemic heart: β-hydroxy fatty acid production. *Am. J. Physiol.,* 239:H257–H265.

399. Moore, S. (1976): Platelet aggregation secondary to coronary obstruction. *Circulation,* 53:66–69.

400. Morena, H., Janse, M. J., Fiolet, J. W. T., Krieger, W. J. G., Crijns, H., and Durrer, D. (1980): Comparison of the effects of regional ischemia, hypoxia, hyperkalemia, and acidosis on the intracellular and extracellular potentials and metabolism in the isolated porcine heart. *Circ. Res.,* 46:634–646.

401. Morganroth, J., and Moore, E. N. (editors) (1984): *Interventions in the Acute Phase of Myocardial Infarction,* Martinus Nijhoff, Boston.

402. Mosher, P., Ross, J., McFate, P. A., and Shaw, R. F. (1964): Control of coronary blood flow by an autoregulatory mechanism. *Circ. Res.,* 14:250–259.

403. Most, A. S., Capone, R. J., and Mastrofrancesco, P. A. (1977): Free fatty acids and arrhythmias following acute coronary artery occlusion in pigs. *Cardiovasc. Res.,* 11:198–205.

404. Mukherjee, A., McCoy, K. E., Duke, R. J., Hogan, M., Hagler, H., Buja, L. M., and Willerson, J. T. (1982): Relationship between beta adrenergic receptor numbers and physiological responses during experimental canine myocardial ischemia. *Circ. Res.,* 50:735–741.

405. Mukherjee, A., Wong, T. M., Buja, L. M., Lefkowitz, R. J., and Willerson, J. T. (1979): Beta adrenergic and muscarinic cholinergic receptors in canine myocardium: Effects of ischemia. *J. Clin. Invest.,* 64:1423–1428.

406. Mullane, K. M., Read, N., Salmon, J. A., and Moncada, S. (1984): Role of leukocytes in acute myocardial infarction in anesthetized dogs: Relationship to myocardial salvage by anti-inflammatory drugs. *J. Pharmacol. Exp. Ther.,* 228:510–522.

407. Muller, J. E., Maroko, P. R., and Braunwald, E. (1975): Evaluation of precordial electrocardiographic mapping as a means of assessing changes in myocardial ischemic injury. *Circulation,* 52:16–27.

408. Muntz, K. H., Hagler, H. K., Boulas, H. J., Willerson, J. T., and Buja, L. M. (1984): Redistribution of catecholamines in the ischemic zone of the dog heart. *Am. J. Pathol.,* 114:64–78.

409. Murdock, R. H., Jr., Harlan, D. M., Morris, J. J., III, Pryor, W. W., Jr., and Cobb, F. R. (1983): Transitional blood flow zones between ischemic and non-ischemic myocardium in the awake dog. Analysis based on distribution of the intramural vasculature. *Circ. Res.,* 52:451–459.

410. Murfitt, R. R., Stiles, J. W., Powell, W. J., Jr., and Sanadi, D. R. (1978): Experimental myocardial ischemia characteristics of isolated mitochondrial subpopulations. *J. Mol. Cell. Cardiol.,* 10:109–123.

411. Murphy, E., Aiton, J. F., Horres, C. R., and Lieberman, M. (1983): Calcium elevation in cultured heart cells: Its role in cell injury. *Am. J. Physiol.,* 245:C316–C321.

412. Murry, C. E., Reimer, K. A., Hill, M. L., Yamasawa, I., and Jennings, R. B. (1985): Collateral blood flow and transmural location: Independent determinants of ATP in ischemic canine myocardium. *Fed. Proc.,* 44:823 (abstract).

413. Murry, C. E., Reimer, K. A., Long, J. B., and Jennings, R. B. (1985): Preconditioning with ischemia protects ischemic myocardium. *Circulation [Suppl. 3],* 72:119 (abstract).

414. Nachlas, M. M., and Shnitka, T. K. (1963): Macroscopic identification of early myocardial infarcts by alterations in dehydrogenase activity. *Am. J. Pathol.,* 42:379–405.

415. Naeim, F., Maza, L. M., and Robbins, S. L. (1972): Cardiac rupture during myocardial infarction. *Circulation,* 45:1231–1239.

416. Namm, D. H., and Mayer, S. E. (1968): Effects of epinephrine on cardiac cyclic 3',5'-AMP, phosphorylase kinase and phosphorylase. *Mol. Pharmacol.,* 4:61–69.

417. Nayler, W. G. (1981): The heart cell: Some metabolic aspects of cardiac arrhythmias. *Acta Med. Scand. [Suppl.],* 647:17–31.

418. Nayler, W. G. (1981): The role of calcium in the ischemic myocardium. *Am. J. Pathol.,* 102:262–270.

419. Neely, J. R., and Feuvray, D. (1981): Metabolic products and myocardial ischemia. *Am. J. Pathol.,* 102:282–291.

420. Neely, J. R., and Grotoyohann, L. W. (1984): Role of glycolytic products in damage to ischemic myocardium. Dissociation of adenosine triphosphate levels and recovery of function of reperfused ischemic hearts. *Circ. Res.,* 55:816–824.

421. Neely, J. R., Liebermeister, H., Battersby, E. J., and Morgan, H. E. (1967): Effect of pressure development on oxygen consumption by isolated rat hearts. *Am. J. Physiol.,* 212:804–814.

422. Neely, J. R., Liedtke, A. J., Whitmer, J. T., and Rovetto, M. J. (1975): Relationship between coronary flow and adenosine triphosphate production from glycolysis and oxidative metabolism. In: *Recent Advances in Studies on Cardiac Structure and Metabolism, Vol. 8, The Cardiac Sarcoplasm,* edited by P. E. Roy and P. Harris, pp. 301–321. University Park Press, Baltimore.

423. Neely, J. R., and Morgan, H. E. (1974): Relationship between carbohydrate and lipid metabolism and the energy balance of heart muscle. *Annu. Rev. Physiol.,* 36:413–459.

424. Neely, J. R., Rovetto, M. J., and Oram, J. F. (1972): Myocardial utilization of carbohydrate and lipids. *Prog. Cardiovasc. Dis.,* 15:289–329.

425. Neely, J. R., Rovetto, M. J., Whitmer, J. T., and Morgan, H. E. (1973): Effects of ischemia on function and metabolism of the isolated working rat heart. *Am. J. Physiol.,* 225:651–658.

426. Neely, J. R., Whitmer, J. T., and Rovetto, M. J. (1975): Effect of coronary blood flow on glycolytic flux and intracellular pH in isolated rat hearts. *Circ. Res.,* 37:733–741.

427. Neill, W. A., Levine, H. J., Wagman, R. J., and Gorlin, R. (1963): Left ventricular oxygen utilization in intact dogs: Effect of systemic hemodynamic factors. *Circ. Res.,* 12:163–169.

428. Newman, P. E. (1981): The coronary collateral circulation: Determinants and functional significance in ischemic heart disease. *Am. Heart J.,* 102:431–445.

429. Nichols, A. B., Moore, R. H., Cochavi, S., Pohost, G. M., and Strauss, W. H. (1980): Quantification of myocardial infarction by computer-assisted positron emission tomography. *Cardiovasc. Res.,* 14:428–434.

430. Nienaber, C., Gottwik, M., Winkler, B., and Schaper, W. (1983): The relationship between the perfusion deficit, infarct size and time after experimental coronary artery occlusion. *Basic Res. Cardiol.,* 78:210–226.

431. Nohara, R., Kambara, H., Murakami, T., Kadota, K., Tamaki, S., and Kawai, C. (1983): Collateral function in early acute myocardial infarction. *Am. J. Cardiol.,* 52:955–959.

432. Olearchyk, A. S., Lemole, G. M., and Spagna, P. M. (1984): Left ventricular aneurysm. *J. Thorac. Cardiovasc. Surg.,* 88:544–553.

433. Oliva, P. B., and Breckinridge, J. C. (1977): Arteriographic evidence of coronary arterial spasm in acute myocardial infarction. *Circulation,* 56:366–374.

434. Olsson, R. A. (1970): Changes in content of purine nucleoside in canine myocardium during coronary occlusion. *Circ. Res.,* 26:301–306.

435. Opherk, D., Finke, R., Mittmann, U., Muller, J. H., Wirth,

R. H., and Schmier, J. (1977): The influence of the size of acute ischaemic myocardial lesions on coronary reserve and left ventricular function in the dog. *Basic Res. Cardiol.*, 72:402–410.

436. Opie, L. H. (1976): Effects of regional ischemia on metabolism of glucose and fatty acids. Relative rates of aerobic and anaerobic energy production during myocardial infarction and comparison with effects of anoxia. *Circ. Res.*, 38:52–74.

437. Opie, L. H., Nathan, D., and Lubbe, W. F. (1979): Biochemical aspects of arrhythmogenesis and ventricular fibrillation. *Am. J. Cardiol.*, 43:131–148.

438. O'Reilly, R. J., and Spellberg, R. D. (1974): Rapid resolution of coronary arterial emboli: Myocardial infarction and subsequent normal coronary arteriograms. *Ann. Intern. Med.*, 81:348–359.

439. Paessens, R., and Borchard, F. (1980): Morphology of cardiac nerves in experimental infarction of rat hearts. I. Fluorescence microscopical findings. *Virchows Arch.* [*Pathol. Anat.*], 386:265–278.

440. Page, D. L., Caulfield, J. B., Kastor, J. A., DeSanctis, R. W., and Sanders, C. A. (1971): Myocardial changes associated with cardiogenic shock. *N. Engl. J. Med.*, 285:133–137.

441. Page, E., and McCallister, L. P. (1973): Quantitative electron microscopic description of heart muscle cells. Application to normal, hypertrophied and thyroxin-stimulated hearts. *Am. J. Cardiol.*, 31:172–181.

442. Page, E., and Polimeni, P. I. (1977): Ultrastructural changes in the ischemic zone bordering experimental infarcts in rat left ventricles. *Am. J. Pathol.*, 86:81–104.

443. Pairolero, P. C., McCallister, B. D., Hallerman, F. J., Titus, J. L., and Ellis, F. H. (1970): Experimental left ventricular akinesis. Results of excision. *J. Thorac. Cardiovasc. Surg.*, 60:683–693.

444. Palmer, R. M. J., Stepney, R. J., Higgs, G. A., and Eakins, K. E. (1980): Chemokinetic activity of arachidonic acid lipoxygenase products on leukocytes of different species. *Prostaglandins*, 20:411–418.

445. Pande, S. V., and Mead, J. F. (1968): Inhibition of enzyme activities by free fatty acids. *J. Biol. Chem.*, 243:6180–6185.

446. Pandian, N. G., Koyanagi, S., Skorton, D. J., Collins, S. M., Eastham, C. L., Kieso, R. A., Marcus, M. L., and Kerber, R. E. (1983): Relations between 2-dimensional echocardiographic wall thickening abnormalities, myocardial infarct size and coronary risk area in normal and hypertrophied myocardium in dogs. *Am. J. Cardiol.*, 52:1318–1325.

447. Pantely, G. A., and Bristow, J. D. (1984): Ischemic cardiomyopathy. *Prog. Cardiovasc. Dis.*, 27:95–114.

448. Penney, D. G., and Cascarano, J. (1970): Anaerobic rat heart: Effects of glucose and tricarboxylic acid-cycle metabolites on metabolism and physiological performance. *Biochem. J.*, 118:221–227.

449. Perloff, J. K., and Roberts, W. C. (1972): The mitral apparatus. Functional anatomy of mitral regurgitation. *Circulation*, 46:227–239.

450. Pfeffer, M. A., Pfeffer, J. M., Fishbein, M. C., Fletcher, P. J., Spadaro, J., Kloner, R. A., and Braunwald, E. (1979): Myocardial infarct size and ventricular function in rats. *Circ. Res.*, 44:503–512.

451. Pinckard, R. N., Olson, M. S., Giclas, P. C., Terry, R., Boyer, J. T., and O'Rourke, R. A. (1975): Consumption of classical complement components by heart subcellular membranes in vitro and in patients after acute myocardial infarction. *J. Clin. Invest.*, 56:740–750.

452. Pinckard, R. N., O'Rourke, R. A., Crawford, M. H., Grover, F. S., McManus, L. M., Ghidoni, J. J., Storrs, S. B., and Olson, M. S. (1980): Complement localization and mediation of ischemic injury in baboon myocardium. *J. Clin. Invest.*, 66:1050–1056.

453. Pine, M. B., Bing, O. H. L., Brooks, W. W., and Abelmann, W. H. (1978): Changes in in vitro myocardial hydration and performance in response to transient metabolic blockage in hypertonic, isotonic, and hypotonic media. *Cardiovasc. Res.*, 12:569–577.

454. Pine, M. B., Caulfield, J. B., Bing, O. H. L., Brooks, W. H., and Abelmann, W. (1979): Resistance of contracting myocardium to swelling with hypoxia and glycolytic blockade. *Cardiovasc. Res.*, 13:215–224.

455. Piper, H. M., Probst, I., Schwartz, P., Hutter, F. J., and Spieck-

ermann, P. G. (1982): Culturing of calcium stable adult cardiac myocytes. *J. Mol. Cell. Cardiol.*, 14:397–412.

456. Piper, H. M., Schwartz, P., Hutter, J. F., and Spieckermann, P. G. (1984): Energy metabolism and enzyme release of cultured adult rat heart muscle cells during anoxia. *J. Mol. Cell. Cardiol.*, 16:995–1007.

457. Piper, H. M., Schwartz, P., Spahr, R., Hutter, J. F., and Spieckermann, P. G. (1985): Anoxic injury of adult cardiac myocytes. *Basic Res. Cardiol.*, 80:37–42.

458. Plotnick, G. D., Fisher, M. L., Lerner, B., Carliner, N. H., Peters, R. W., and Becker, L. C. (1983): Collateral circulation in patients with unstable angina. *Chest*, 82:719–725.

459. Poole-Wilson, P. A., Harding, D. P., Bourdillon, P. D. V., and Tones, M. A. (1984): Calcium out of control. *J. Mol. Cell. Cardiol.*, 16:175–187.

460. Powell, W. J., Jr., DiBona, D. R., Flores, J., Frega, N., and Leaf, A. (1976): Effects of hyperosmotic mannitol in reducing ischemic cell swelling and minimizing myocardial necrosis. *Circulation*, 53:45–49.

461. Powers, E. R., DiBona, D. R., and Powell, W. J., Jr. (1984): Myocardial cell volume and coronary resistance during diminished coronary perfusion. *Am. J. Physiol.*, 247:H467–H477.

462. Prinzen, F. W., Van der Vusse, G. J., Arts, T., Roemen, T. H. M., Coumans, W. A., and Reneman, R. S. (1984): Accumulation of nonesterified fatty acids in ischemic canine myocardium. *Am. J. Physiol.*, 247:H264–H272.

463. Rannels, D. E., Kao, R., and Morgan, H. E. (1976): Effect of cardiac ischemia on protein degradation. *Circulation*, 53:30–31.

464. Rao, P. S., Cohen, M. V., and Mueller, H. S. (1983): Production of free radicals and lipid peroxides in early experimental myocardial ischemia. *J. Mol. Cell. Cardiol.*, 15:713–716.

465. Rao, P. S., and Mueller, H. S. (1983): Lipid peroxidation and acute myocardial ischemia. In: *Myocardial Injury*, edited by J. J. Spitzer, pp. 341–367. Plenum, New York.

466. Rau, E. E., Shine, K. I., and Langer, G. A. (1977): Potassium exchange and mechanical performance in anoxic mammalian myocardium. *Am. J. Physiol.*, 232:H85–H94.

467. Reddy, M. K., Etlinger, J. D., Rabinowitz, M., Fischman, D. A., and Zak, R. (1975): Removal of Z-lines and α-actinin from isolated myofibrils by a calcium-activated neutral protease. *J. Biol. Chem.*, 250:4278–4284.

468. Regitz, V., Paulson, D. J., Hodach, R. J., Little, S. E., Schaper, W., and Shug, A. L. (1984): Mitochondrial damage during myocardial ischemia. *Basic Res. Cardiol.*, 79:207–217.

469. Reibel, D. K., and Rovetto, M. J. (1978): Myocardial ATP synthesis and mechanical function following oxygen deficiency. *Am. J. Physiol.*, 234:H620–H624.

470. Reichenbach, D. D., and Benditt, E. P. (1970): Catecholamines and cardiomyopathy: The pathogenesis and potential importance of myofibrillar degeneration. *Hum. Pathol.*, 1:125–150.

471. Reimer, K. A. (1980): Myocardial infarct size. Measurements and predictions. *Arch. Pathol. Lab. Med.*, 104:225–230.

472. Reimer, K. A. (1982): Overview of potential mechanisms. In: *Myocardial Infarction: Measurement and Intervention*, edited by G. S. Wagner, pp. 387–395. Martinus Nijhoff, Boston.

473. Reimer, K. A. (1985): The relationship between coronary blood flow and reversible and irreversible ischemic injury. In: *Acute Coronary Care: Principles and Practice*, edited by R. M. Califf and G. S. Wagner, pp. 9–20. Martinus Nijhoff, Boston.

474. Reimer, K. A., Hill, M. L., and Jennings, R. B. (1981): Prolonged depletion of ATP and of the adenine nucleotide pool due to delayed resynthesis of adenine nucleotides following reversible myocardial ischemic injury in dogs. *J. Mol. Cell. Cardiol.*, 13:229–239.

475. Reimer, K. A., and Jennings, R. B. (1979): The "wavefront phenomenon" of myocardial ischemic cell death. II. Transmural progression of necrosis within the framework of ischemic bed size (myocardium at risk) and collateral flow. *Lab. Invest.*, 40:633–644.

476. Reimer, K. A., and Jennings, R. B. (1979): The changing anatomic reference base of evolving myocardial infarction. Underestimation of myocardial collateral blood flow and overestimation of experimental anatomic infarct size due to tissue edema, hemorrhage and acute inflammation. *Circulation*, 60:866–876.

477. Reimer, K. A., and Jennings, R. B. (1984): Verapamil in two

reperfusion models of myocardial infarction: Temporary protection of severely ischemic myocardium without limitation of ultimate infarct size. *Lab. Invest.*, 51:655–666.

478. Reimer, K. A., and Jennings, R. B. (1984): Can we really quantitate myocardial cell injury? In: *Therapeutic Approaches to Myocardial Infarct Size Limitation*, edited by D. J. Hearse and D. M. Yellon, pp. 163–184. Raven Press, New York.

479. Reimer, K. A., and Jennings, R. B. (1985): Failure of the xanthine oxidase inhibitor allopurinol to limit infarct size after ischemia and reperfusion in dogs. *Circulation*, 71:1069–1075.

480. Reimer, K. A., and Jennings, R. B. (1985): Effects of calcium-channel blockers on myocardial preservation during experimental acute myocardial infarction. *Am. J. Cardiol.*, 55:107B–115B.

481. Reimer, K. A., and Jennings, R. B. (1985): Effects of reperfusion on infarct size: experimental studies. *Eur. Heart J.* [Suppl. E], 6: 97–108.

482. Reimer, K. A., Jennings, R. B., Cobb, F. R., Murdock, R. H., Greenfield, J. C., Jr., Becker, L. C., Bulkley, B. H., Hutchins, G. M., Schwartz, R. P., Jr., Bailey, K. R., and Passamani, E. R. (1985): Animal models for protecting ischemic myocardium: Results of the NHLBI Cooperative Study. Comparison of unconscious and conscious dog models. *Circ. Res.*, 56:651–665.

483. Reimer, K. A., Jennings, R. B., and Hill, M. L. (1981): Total ischemia in dog hearts in vitro. II. High energy phosphate depletion and associated defects in energy metabolism, cell volume regulation, and sarcolemmal integrity. *Circ. Res.*, 49:901–911.

484. Reimer, K. A., Jennings, R. B., and Tatum, A. H. (1983): Pathobiology of acute myocardial ischemia: Metabolic, functional and ultrastructural studies. *Am. J. Cardiol.*, 52:72A–82A.

485. Reimer, K. A., Lowe, J. E., Rasmussen, M. M., and Jennings, R. B. (1977): The wavefront phenomenon of ischemic cell death. 1. Myocardial infarct size vs. duration of coronary occlusion in dogs. *Circulation*, 56:786–794.

486. Reimer, K. A., Murry, C. E., Yamasawa, I., Hill, M. L., and Jennings, R. B. (1986): Repetitive brief periods of myocardial ischemia cause no cumulative loss of adenine nucleotides or myocardial infarction. *Am. J. Physiol.* (in press).

487. Reimer, K. A., Steenbergen, C., and Jennings, R. B. (1985): Isolated cardiac myocytes: Is their response to injury relevant to our understanding of ischemic injury, in vivo? *Lab. Invest.*, 53: 369–372.

488. Rentrop, K. P. (1985): Thrombolytic therapy in patients with acute myocardial infarction. *Circulation*, 71:627–631.

489. Rentrop, K. P., Cohen, M., and Hosat, S. T. (1984): Thrombolytic therapy in acute myocardial infarction: Review of clinical trials. *Am. J. Cardiol.*, 54:29E–31E.

490. Ridolfi, R. L., and Hutchins, G. M. (1977): The relationship between coronary artery lesions and myocardial infarcts: Ulceration of atherosclerotic plaques precipitating coronary thrombosis. *Am. Heart J.*, 93:468–486.

491. Rigo, P., Murray, M., Taylor, D. R., Weisfeldt, M. L., Strauss, H. W., and Pitt, B. (1975): Hemodynamic and prognostic findings in patients with transmural and nontransmural infarction. *Circulation*, 51:1064–1070.

492. Rivas, F., Cobb, F. R., Bache, R. J., and Greenfield, J. C., Jr. (1976): Relationship between blood flow to ischemic regions and extent of myocardial infarction. Serial measurement of blood flow to ischemic regions in dogs. *Circ. Res.*, 38:439–447.

493. Roberts, R., Ambos, H. D., and Sobel, B. E. (1983): Estimation of infarct size with MB rather than total CK. *Int. J. Cardiol.*, 2: 479–489.

494. Roberts, R., and Ishikawa, Y. (1983): Enzymatic estimation of infarct size during reperfusion. *Circulation*, 68:83–89.

495. Roberts, W. C. (1972): Relationship between coronary thrombosis and myocardial infarction. *Mod. Concepts Cardiovasc. Dis.*, 41: 7–10.

496. Roberts, W. C., and Buja, L. M. (1972): The frequency and significance of coronary arterial thrombi and other observations in fatal acute myocardial infarction. A study of 107 necropsy patients. *Am. J. Med.*, 52:425–443.

497. Roe, C. R. (1977): Validity of estimating myocardial infarct size from serial measurements of enzyme activity in the serum. *Clin. Chem.*, 23:1807–1812.

498. Roeske, W. R., Deluca, M., and Ingwall, J. S. (1978): Factors influencing enzyme release from cultured fetal mouse hearts deprived of oxygen and glucose. *J. Mol. Cell. Cardiol.*, 10:907–919.

499. Romson, J. L., Haack, D. W., and Lucchesi, B. R. (1980): Electrical induction of coronary artery thrombosis in the ambulatory canine: A model for in vivo evaluation of anti-thrombotic agents. *Thromb. Res.*, 17:841–853.

500. Romson, J. L., Hook, B. G., Kunkel, S. L., Abrams, G. D., Schork, A., and Lucchesi, B. R. (1983): Reduction of the extent of ischemic myocardial injury by neutrophil depletion in the dog. *Circulation*, 67:1016–1023.

501. Rose, A. G., Opie, L. H., and Bricknell, O. L. (1976): Early experimental myocardial infarction: Evaluation of histologic criteria and comparison with biochemical and electrocardiographic measurements. *Arch. Pathol. Lab. Med.*, 100:516–521.

502. Rosenkranz, E. R., and Buckberg, G. D. (1983): Myocardial protection during surgical coronary reperfusion. *J. Am. Coll. Cardiol.*, 1:1235–1246.

503. Ross, J., Jr., and Franklin, D. (1976): Analysis of regional myocardial function, dimensions, and wall thickness in the characterization of myocardial ischemia and infarction. *Circulation*, 53:88–92.

504. Ross, P. D., and McCarl, R. L. (1984): Oxidation of carbohydrates and palmitate by intact cultured neonatal rat heart cells. *Am. J. Physiol. Heart Circ. Physiol.*, 246:H389–H397.

505. Rossen, R. D., Swain, J. L., Michael, L. H., Weakley, S., Giannini, E., and Entman, M. L. (1985): Selective accumulation of the first component of complement and leukocytes in ischemic canine heart muscle. A possible initiator of an extra myocardial mechanism of ischemic injury. *Circ. Res.*, 57:117–130.

506. Roubin, G. S., Shen, W. F., Kelly, D. T., and Harris, P. J. (1983): The QRS scoring system for estimating myocardial infarct size; clinical, angiographic and prognostic correlations. *J. Am. Col. Cardiol.*, 2:38–44.

507. Rouslin, W. (1983): Mitochondrial complexes I, II, III, IV, and V in myocardial ischemia and autolysis. *Am. J. Physiol.*, 244: H743–H748.

508. Rouslin, W., and Millard, R. W. (1981): Mitochondrial inner membrane enzyme defects in porcine myocardial ischemia. *Am. J. Physiol.*, 240:H308–H313.

509. Rouslin, W., and Ranganathan, S. (1983): Impaired function of mitochondrial electron transfer complex I in canine myocardial ischemia: Loss of flavin mononucleotide. *J. Mol. Cell. Cardiol.*, 15:537–542.

510. Rovetto, M. J., Lamberton, W. F., and Neely, J. R. (1975): Mechanisms of glycolytic inhibition in ischemic rat hearts. *Circ. Res.*, 37:742–751.

511. Rovetto, M. J., Whitmer, J. T., and Neely, J. R. (1973): Comparison of the effects of anoxia and whole heart ischemia on carbohydrate utilization in isolated working rat hearts. *Circ. Res.*, 32:699–711.

512. Rowland, F. N., Donovan, M. J., Picciano, P. T., Wilner, G. D., and Kreutzer, D. L. (1984): Fibrin-mediated vascular injury. Identification of fibrin peptides that mediate endothelial cell retraction. *Am. J. Pathol.*, 117:418–428.

513. Rubin, S. A., Fishbein, M. C., and Swan, H. J. C. (1983): Compensatory hypertrophy in the heart after myocardial infarction in the rat. *J. Am. Coll. Cardiol.*, 1:1435–1441.

514. Rubio, R., and Berne, R. M. (1980): Localization of purine and pyrimidine nucleoside phosphorylases in heart, kidney and liver. *Am. J. Physiol.*, 239:H721–H730.

515. Rubio, R., Berne, R. M., and Dobson, J. G. (1973): Sites of adenosine production in cardiac and skeletal muscle. *Am. J. Physiol.*, 225:938–953.

516. Rubio, V. R., Wiedmeier, T., and Berne, R. M. (1972): Nucleoside phosphorylase: Localization and role in the myocardial distribution of purines. *Am. J. Physiol.*, 222:550–555.

517. Rude, R. E., Parkey, R. W., Bonte, F. J., Lewis, S. E., Twieg, D., Buja, L. M., and Willerson, J. T. (1980): Clinical implications of the technetium-99m stannous pyrophosphate myocardial scintigraphic "doughnut" pattern in patients with acute myocardial infarcts. *Circulation*, 59:721–730.

518. Sabbah, H. N., and Stein, P. D. (1982): Effect of acute regional ischemia on pressure in the subepicardium and subendocardium. *Am. J. Physiol.*, 242:H240–H244.

519. Sabiston, D. C., and Gregg, D. E. (1957): Effect of cardiac contraction on coronary blood flow. *Circulation*, 15:14–20.
520. Sakai, K., and Abiko, Y. (1981): Acute changes of myocardial norepinephrine and glycogen phosphorylase in ischemic areas after coronary ligation in dogs. *Jpn. Circ. J.*, 45:1250–1255.
521. Sakai, K., Tomoike, H., Ootsubo, H., Kikuchi, Y., and Nakamura, M. (1982): Preocclusive perfusion area as a determinant of infarct size in a canine model. *Cardiovasc. Res.*, 16:408–416.
522. Sanders, C. A., Armstrong, P. W., Willerson, J. T., and Dinsmore, R. E. (1971): Etiology and differential diagnosis of acute mitral regurgitation. *Prog. Cardiovasc. Dis.*, 14:129–152.
523. Sanders, M., White, F. C., Peterson, T. M., and Bloor, C. M. (1978): Characteristics of coronary blood flow and transmural distribution in miniature pigs. *Am. J. Physiol.*, 235:H601–H609.
524. Sarnoff, S. J., Braunwald, E., Welch, G. H., Jr., Case, R. B., Stainsby, W. N., and Marcruz, R. (1958): Hemodynamic determinants of the oxygen consumption of the heart with special reference to the tension time index. *Am. J. Physiol.*, 192:148–156.
525. Sashida, H., Uchida, K., and Abiko, Y. (1984): Changes in cardiac ultrastructure and myofibrillar proteins during ischemia in dogs, with special reference to changes in Z lines. *J. Mol. Cell. Cardiol.*, 16:1161–1172.
526. Sato, S., Ashraf, M., Millard, R. W., Fujiwara, H., and Schwartz, A. (1983): Connective tissue changes in early ischemia of porcine myocardium: An ultrastructural study. *J. Mol. Cell. Cardiol.*, 15: 261–275.
527. Savage, R. M., Wagner, G. S., Ideker, R. E., Podolsky, S. A., and Hackel, D. B. (1977): Correlation of postmortem anatomic findings with electrocardiographic changes in patients with myocardial infarction. Retrospective study of patients with typical anterior and posterior infarcts. *Circulation*, 55:279–285.
528. Sayen, J. J., Peirce, G., Katcher, A. H., and Sheldon, W. F. (1961): Correlation of intramyocardial electrocardiograms with polarographic oxygen and contractility in the nonischemic and regionally ischemic left ventricle. *Circ. Res.*, 9:1268–1279.
529. Sayen, J. J., Sheldon, W. F., Peirce, G., and Kuo, P. T. (1958): Polerographic oxygen, the epicardial electrocardiogram and muscle contraction in experimental acute regional ischemia of the left ventricle. *Circ. Res.*, 6:779–798.
530. Schaper, J., Mulch, J., Winkler, B., and Schaper, W. (1979): Ultrastructural, functional, and biochemical criteria for estimation of reversibility of ischemic injury: A study on the effects of global ischemia on the isolated dog heart. *J. Mol. Cell. Cardiol.*, 11: 521–541.
531. Schaper, W. (1971): Pathophysiology of coronary circulation. *Prog. Cardiovasc. Dis.*, 14:275–296.
532. Schaper, W. (1971): *The Collateral Circulation of the Heart*, pp. 29–50. North Holland, Amsterdam.
533. Schaper, W. (1979): Residual perfusion of acutely ischemic heart muscle. In: *The Pathophysiology of Myocardial Perfusion*, edited by W. Schaper, pp. 345–378. Elsevier/North Holland, New York.
534. Schaper, W., Frenzel, H., and Hort, W. (1979): Experimental coronary artery occlusion. I. Measurement of infarct size. *Basic Res. Cardiol.*, 74:46–53.
535. Schaper, W., Frenzel, H., Hort, W., and Winkler, B. (1979): Experimental coronary artery occlusion. II. Spatial and temporal evolution of infarcts in the dog heart. *Basic Res. Cardiol.*, 74: 233–239.
536. Scheidt, S., Ascheim, R., and Killip, T., III (1970): Shock after acute myocardial infarction. A clinical and hemodynamic profile. *Am. J. Cardiol.*, 26:556–564.
537. Scheinman, M. M., and Abbott, J. A. (1973): Clinical significance of transmural versus nontransmural electrocardiographic changes in patients with acute myocardial infarction. *Am. J. Med.*, 55: 602–607.
538. Scheuer, J., and Brachfeld, N. (1966): Myocardial uptake and fractional distribution of palmitate-I-C^{14} by the ischemic dog heart. *Metabolism*, 15:945–954.
539. Schifferman, E. (1982): Leukocyte chemotaxis. *Annu. Rev. Physiol.*, 44:553–568.
540. Schneider, R. M., Roberts, K. B., Morris, K. G., Stanfield, J. A., and Cobb, F. R. (1984): Relation between radionuclide angiographic regional ejection fraction and left ventricular regional ischemia in awake dogs. *Am. J. Cardiol.*, 53:294–301.
541. Schomig, A., Dart, A. M., Dietz, R., Mayer, E., and Kubler, W. (1984): Release of endogenous catecholamines in the ischemic myocardium of the rat. Part A: Locally mediated release. *Circ. Res.*, 55:689–701.
542. Schubert, R. W., Whalen, W. J., and Nair, P. (1978): Myocardial Po$_2$ distribution: Relationship to coronary autoregulation. *Am. J. Physiol.*, 234:H361–H370.
543. Schultz, T. C., and Skinner, J. M. (1981): The post-mortem myocardial potassium sodium ratio in detection of infarction. *Pathology*, 13:313–316.
544. Schuster, E. H., and Bulkley, B. H. (1979): Expansion of transmural myocardial infarction: A pathophysiologic factor in cardiac rupture. *Circulation*, 60:1532–1538.
545. Schuster, E. H., and Bulkley, B. H. (1980): Ischemic cardiomyopathy; a clinicopathologic study of fourteen patients. *Am. Heart J.*, 100:506–512.
546. Schutz, W., Schrader, J., and Gerlach, E. (1981): Different sites of adenosine formation in the heart. *Am. J. Physiol.*, 240:H963–H970.
547. Schwartz, P., Piper, H. M., Spahr, R., and Spieckermann, P. G. (1984): Ultrastructure of cultured adult myocardial cells during anoxia and reoxygenation. *Am. J. Pathol.*, 115:349–361.
548. Senges, J., Seller, H., Brachmann, J., Braun, W., Mayer, E., Rizos, I., and Kubler, W. (1984): Role of some components of ischemia in the genesis of spontaneous ventricular arrhythmias. *Basic Res. Cardiol.*, 79:68–74.
549. Shelburne, J. C., Rubenstein, D., and Gorlin, R. (1969): A reappraisal of papillary muscle dysfunction. *Am. J. Med.*, 46: 862–871.
550. Shell, W. E., Kjekshus, J. K., and Sobel, B. E. (1971): Quantitative assessment of the extent of myocardial infarction in the conscious dog by means of analysis of serial changes in serum creatine phosphokinase activity. *J. Clin. Invest.*, 50:2614–2625.
551. Shen, A. C., and Jennings, R. B. (1972): Myocardial calcium and magnesium in acute ischemic injury. *Am. J. Pathol.*, 67:417–440.
552. Shen, A. C., and Jennings, R. B. (1972): Kinetics of calcium accumulation in acute myocardial ischemic injury. *Am. J. Pathol.*, 67:441–452.
553. Shetlar, M. R., Shetlar, C. L., and Kischer, C. W. (1979): Healing of myocardial infarction in animal models. *Tex. Rep. Biol. Med.*, 39:339–355.
554. Shine, K. J. (1981): Ionic events in ischemia and anoxia. *Am. J. Pathol.*, 102:256–261.
555. Shine, K. I., Douglas, A. M., and Ricchiuti, N. V. (1978): Calcium, strontium, and barium movements during ischemia and reperfusion in rabbit ventricle. Implications for myocardial preservation. *Circ. Res.*, 43:712–720.
556. Shipp, J. C., Opie, L. H., and Challoner, D. (1961): Fatty acid and glucose metabolism in the perfused heart. *Nature*, 189:1018–1019.
557. Shlafer, M., Kane, P. F., Wiggins, V. Y., and Kirsh, M. M. (1982): Possible role for cytotoxic oxygen metabolites in the pathogenesis of cardiac ischemic injury. *Circulation*, 66:85–92.
558. Shlafer, M., Kirsh, M., Lucchesi, B. R., Slater, A. D., and Warren, S. (1981): Mitochondrial function after global cardiac ischemia and reperfusion: Influences of organelle isolation protocols. *Basic Res. Cardiol.*, 76:250–266.
559. Shnitka, T. K., and Nachlas, M. M. (1963): Histochemical alterations in ischemic heart muscle and early myocardial infarction. *Am. J. Pathol.*, 42:507–527.
560. Shug, A. L., and Shrago, E. (1973): A proposed mechanism for fatty acid effects on energy metabolism of the heart. *J. Lab. Clin. Med.*, 81:214–218.
561. Siess, M. (1980): Some aspects on the regulation of carbohydrate and lipid metabolism on cardiac tissue. *Basic Res. Cardiol.*, 75: 47–56.
562. Silver, M. D., Baroldi, G., and Mariani, F. (1980): The relationship between acute occlusive coronary thrombi and myocardial infarction studied in 100 consecutive patients. *Circulation*, 61:219–227.
563. Simson, M. B., Harden, W., Barlow, C., and Harken, A. H. (1979): Visualization of the distance between perfusion and anoxia along an ischemic border. *Circulation*, 60:1151–1155.
564. Sladek, T., Fikuka, J., Dolezel, S., Vasku, J., Hartmannova, B.,

and Travnickova, J. (1984): The border zone of the early myocardial infarction in dogs; its characteristics and viability. *Basic Res. Cardiol.,* 79:344–349.

565. Slutsky, R. A., Peck, W. W., Mancini, J., Mattrey, R. F., and Higgins, C. B. (1984): Myocardial infarct size determined by computed transmission tomography in canine infarcts of various ages and in the presence of coronary reperfusion. *J. Am. Coll. Cardiol.,* 3:138–142.

566. Smith, G. T., Soeter, J. R., Haston, H. H., and McNamara, J. J. (1974): Coronary reperfusion in primates. Serial electrocardiographic and histologic assessment. *J. Clin. Invest.,* 54:1420–1427.

567. Snow, P., Jones, A., and Daber, R. (1955): Coronary disease: A pathological study. *Br. Heart J.,* 17:503–510.

568. Snyder, D. W., Crafford, W. A., Glashow, J. L., Rankin, D., Sobel, B. E., and Corr, P. B. (1981): Lysophosphoglycerides in ischemic myocardium effluents and potentiation of their arrhythmogenic effects. *Am. J. Physiol.,* 241:H700–H707.

569. Snyderman, R., and Goetzl, E. (1981): Molecular and cellular mechanisms of leukocyte chemotaxis. *Science,* 213:830–837.

570. Sobel, B. E. (1976): Infarct size, prognosis, and causal contiguity. *Circulation,* 53:146–149.

571. Sobel, B. E., Geltman, E. M., Tiefenbrunn, A. J., Jaffe, A. S., Spadaro, J. J., Ter-Pogossian, M. M., Collen, D., and Ludbrook, P. A. (1984): Improvement of regional myocardial metabolism after coronary thrombolysis induced with tissue-type plasminogen activator or streptokinase. *Circulation,* 69:983–990.

572. Sobel, B. E., and Shell, W. E. (1972): Serum enzyme determinations in the diagnosis and assessment of myocardial infarction. *Circulation,* 45:471–482.

573. Sommers, H. M., and Jennings, R. B. (1964): Experimental acute myocardial infarction. Histologic and histochemical studies of early myocardial infarcts induced by temporary or permanent occlusion of a coronary artery. *Lab. Invest.,* 13:1491–1503.

574. Sonnenblick, E. H., Ross, J., and Braunwald, E. (1968): Oxygen consumption of the heart—newer concepts of its multifactorial determination. *Am. J. Cardiol.,* 22:328–336.

575. Sonnenblick, E. H., Ross, J., Covell, J. W., Kaiser, G., and Braunwald, E. (1965): Velocity of contraction as a determinant of myocardial oxygen consumption. *Am. J. Physiol.,* 209:919–927.

576. Sordahl, L. A., and Stewart, M. L. (1980): Mechanism(s) of altered mitochondrial calcium transport in acutely ischemic canine hearts. *Circ. Res.,* 47:814–820.

577. Staszewska-Barczak, J. (1971): The reflex stimulation of catecholamine secretion during the acute stages of myocardial infarction in the dog. *Clin. Sci.,* 41:419–439.

578. Staszewska-Barczak, J., and Ceremuzynski, L. (1968): The continuous estimation of catecholamine release in the early stages of myocardial infarction in the dog. *Clin. Sci.,* 34:531–539.

579. Steenbergen, C., Delleuw, G., Rich, T., and Williamson, J. R. (1977): Effects of acidosis and ischemia on contractility and intracellular pH of rat heart. *Circ. Res.,* 41:849–858.

580. Steenbergen, C., Hill, M. L., and Jennings, R. B. (1985): Volume regulation and plasma membrane injury in aerobic, anaerobic, and ischemic myocardium in vitro. Effect of osmotic cell swelling on plasma membrane integrity. *Circ. Res.,* 57:864–875.

581. Steenbergen, C., and Jennings, R. B. (1984): Relationship between lysophospholipid accumulation and plasma membrane injury during *in vitro* ischemia in dog heart. *J. Mol. Cell. Cardiol.,* 16:605–621.

582. Sugiyama, S., Miyazaki, Y., Kotaka, K., Kato, T., Suzuki, S., and Ozawa, T. (1982): Mechanism of free fatty acid-induced arrhythmias. *J. Electrocardiol.,* 15:227–232.

583. Swain, J. L., Sabina, R. L., Hines, J. J., Greenfield, J. C., and Holmes, E. W. (1984): Repetitive episodes of brief ischaemia (12 min) do not produce a cumulative depletion of high energy phosphate compounds. *Cardiovasc. Res.,* 18:264–269.

584. Swain, J. L., Sabina, R. L., McHale, P. A., Greenfield, J. C., Jr., and Holmes, E. W. (1982): Prolonged myocardial nucleotide depletion after brief ischemia in the open-chest dog. *Am. J. Physiol.,* 242:H818–H826.

585. Sybers, H. D., Ashraf, M., Braithwaite, J. R., and Lok, M. P. (1972): Early myocardial infarction. A fluorescent method of detection. *Arch. Pathol.,* 93:49–54.

586. Szklo, M., Goldberg, R., Kennedy, H. L., and Tonascia, J. A. (1978): Survival of patients with nontransmural myocardial infarction: A population-based study. *Am. J. Cardiol.,* 42:648–652.

587. Taegtmeyer, H., Ferguson, A. G., and Lesch, M. (1977): Protein degradation and amino acid metabolism in autolyzing rabbit myocardium. *Exp. Mol. Pathol.,* 26:52–62.

588. Tamaki, S., Kambara, H., Kadota, K., Suzuki, Y., Nohara, R., Kawai, C., Tamaki, N., and Torizuka, K. (1984): Improved detection of myocardial infarction by emission computed tomography with thallium-201. Relation to infarct size. *Br. Heart J.,* 52:621–627.

589. Tatooles, C. J., and Randall, W. C. (1961): Local ventricular bulging after acute coronary occlusion. *Am. J. Physiol.,* 201:451–456.

590. Taylor, I. M., Shaikh, N. A., and Downar, E. (1984): Ultrastructural changes of ischemic injury due to coronary artery occlusion in the porcine heart. *J. Mol. Cell. Cardiol.,* 16:79–94.

591. Taylor, R. R. (1971): Myocardial potassium and ventricular arrhythmias following reperfusion of ischaemic myocardium. *Aust. N.Z. J. Med.,* 2:114–120.

592. Tennant, R., and Wiggers, C. J. (1935): The effect of coronary occlusion on myocardial contraction. *Am. J. Physiol.,* 112:351–361.

593. Theroux, P., Franklin, D., Ross, J., Jr., and Kemper, W. S. (1974): Regional myocardial function during acute coronary artery occlusion and its modifications by pharmacologic agents in the dog. *Circ. Res.,* 35:896–908.

594. Thompson, P. L., Fletcher, E. E., and Katavatis, V. (1979): Enzymatic indices of myocardial necrosis: Influence on short- and long-term prognosis after myocardial infarction. *Circulation,* 59:113–119.

595. Thygesen, K., Horder, M., Petersen, P. H., and Nielsen, B. L. (1983): Limitation of enzymatic models for predicting myocardial infarct size. *Br. Heart J.,* 50:70–74.

596. Tillisch, J. H., and Gaynor-Berk, R. (1983): The effects of ischemia on myocardial vascular flow and permeability. *J. Mol. Cell. Cardiol.,* 15:105–112.

597. Tilton, R. G., Williamson, E. K., Cole, P. A., Larson, K. B., Kilo, C., and Williamson, J. R. (1985): Coronary vascular hemodynamic and permeability changes during reperfusion after no-flow ischemia in isolated, diltiazem-treated rabbit hearts. *J. Cardiovasc. Pharmacol.,* 7:424–436.

598. Toleikis, A., Dzeja, P., Praskevicius, A., and Jasaitis, A. (1979): Mitochondrial functions in ischemic myocardium. I. Proton electrochemical gradient, inner membrane permeability, calcium transport and oxidative phosphorylation in isolated mitochondria. *J. Mol. Cell. Cardiol.,* 11:57–76.

599. Toyo-Oka, T., and Masaki, T. (1979): Calcium-activated neutral protease from bovine ventricular muscle. *J. Mol. Cell. Cardiol.,* 11:769–786.

600. Toyo-Oka, T., and Ross, J., Jr. (1981): Ca^{2+} sensitivity change and troponin loss in cardiac natural actomyosin after coronary occlusion. *Am. J. Physiol.,* 240:H704–H708.

601. Tranum-Jensen, J., Janse, M. J., Fiolet, J. W. T., Krieger, W. J. G., D'Alnoncourt, C. N., and Durrer, D. (1981): Tissue osmolality, cell swelling and reperfusion in acute regional myocardial ischemia in the isolated porcine heart. *Circ. Res.,* 49:364–381.

602. Trelstad, R. L., Lawley, K. R., and Holmes, L. B. (1981): Nonenzymatic hydroxylations of proline and lysine by reduced oxygen derivatives. *Nature,* 289:310–312.

603. Trump, B. F., Mergner, W. J., Kahng, M. W., and Saladino, A. J. (1976): Studies on the subcellular pathophysiology of ischemia. *Circulation,* 53:17–26.

604. Tsakiris, A. G., Rastelli, G. C., Amorin, D. S., Titus, J. L., and Wood, E. (1970): Effect of experimental papillary muscular damage in mitral valve closure in intact anaesthetized dogs. *Mayo Clin. Proc.,* 45:275–285.

605. Tsokos, J., and Bloom, S. (1977): Effects of calcium on respiration and ATP content of isolated, leaky, heart muscle cells. *J. Mol. Cell. Cardiol.,* 9:823–836.

606. Turrens, J. F., and Boveris, A. (1980): Generation of superoxide anion by NADH dehydrogenase of bovine heart mitochondria. *Biochem. J.,* 191:421–427.

607. Turrens, J. F., Freeman, B. A., Levitt, J. G., and Crapo, J. D. (1982): The effect of hyperoxia on superoxide production by lung

submitochondrial particles. *Arch. Biochem. Biophys.,* 217:401–410.

608. Tyers, G. F. O., and Morgan, H. E. (1975): Isolated heart perfusion techniques for rapid screening of myocardial preservation methods. *Ann. Thorac. Surg.,* 20:56–65.

609. Van Der Laarse, A., Altona, J. C., Zoet, A. C. M., Oemrawsingh, P., and Dijkman, P. R. M. (1984): A comparative study on ischaemia- or anoxia-induced impairment of myocytic structure and cardiac function in the isolated, isovolumicly-contracting, perfused rat heart. *Cardiovasc. Res.,* 12:768–778.

610. Van der Vusse, G. J., and Reneman, R. S. (1983): Glycogen and lipids (endogenous substrates). In: *Cardiac Metabolism,* edited by A. J. Drake-Holland, and M. I. M. Noble, pp. 215–237. Wiley, London.

611. Van der Vusse, G. J., Roemen, T. H. M., Prinzen, F. W., Coumans, W. A., and Reneman, R. S. (1982): Uptake and tissue content of fatty acids in dog myocardium under normoxic and ischemic conditions. *Circ. Res.,* 50:538–546.

612. Van Reempts, J., Borgers, M., and Reneman, R. S. (1976): Early myocardial ischaemia: Evaluation of the histochemical haematoxylin-basic fuchsin-picric acid (BFP) staining technique. *Cardiovasc. Res.,* 10:262–267.

613. Van Tassel, R. A., and Edwards, J. E. (1972): Rupture of heart complicating myocardial infarction: Analysis of 40 cases including nine examples of left ventricular false aneurysm. *Chest,* 61:104–116.

614. Vetter, N. J., Adams, W., Strange, R. C., and Oliver, M. F. (1974): Initial metabolic and hormonal response to acute myocardial infarction. *Lancet,* 1:284–288.

615. Vial, C., Font, B., Goldschmidt, D., Pearlman, A. S., and Delaye, J. (1978): Regional myocardial energetics during brief periods of coronary occlusion and reperfusion: comparison with ST-segment changes. *Cardiovasc. Res.,* 12:470–476.

616. Virmani, R., and Roberts, W. C. (1980): Quantification of coronary arterial narrowing and of left ventricular myocardial scarring in healed myocardial infarction with chronic, eventually fatal, congestive cardiac failure. *Am. J. Med.,* 68:831–838.

617. Vlodaver, Z., and Edwards, J. E. (1977): Rupture of ventricular septum or papillary muscle complicating myocardial infarction. *Circulation,* 55:815–822.

618. Vokonas, P. S., Malsky, P. M., Paul, S. J., Robbins, S. L., and Hood, W. B. (1978): Radioautographic studies in experimental myocardial infarction: Profiles of ischemic blood flow and quantification of infarct size in relation to magnitude of ischemic zone. *Am. J. Cardiol.,* 42:67–75.

619. Wachstein, M., and Meisel, E. (1955): Succinic dehydrogenase activity in myocardial infarction and in induced myocardial necrosis. *Am. J. Pathol.,* 31:353–365.

620. Wagner, G. S. (editor) (1982): *Myocardial Infarction: Measurement and Intervention.* Martinus Nijhoff, Boston.

621. Walsh, D. A., Perkins, J. P., Bronstrom, C. O., Ho, E. S., and Krebs, E. G. (1971): Catalysis of the phosphorylase kinase activation reaction. *J. Biol. Chem.,* 246:1968–1976.

622. Walsh, M. P., LePeuch, C. J., Vallet, B., Cavadore, J. C., Demaille, J. G. (1980): Cardiac calmodulin and its role in the regulation of metabolism and contraction. *J. Mol. Cell. Cardiol.,* 12:1091–1101.

623. Ward, H. B., St. Cyr, J. A., Cogordan, J. A., Alyono, D., Bianco, R. W., Kriett, J. M., and Foker, J. E. (1984): Recovery of adenine nucleotide levels after global myocardial ischemia in dogs. *Surgery,* 96:248–255.

624. Ward, P. A., Hugli, J. E., and Chenoweth, D. (1979): Complement and chemotaxis. In: *Chemical Messengers of the Inflammatory Process,* edited by J. C. Houck, pp. 153–178. Elsevier/North Holland, Amsterdam.

625. Warltier, D. C., Zyvoloski, M. G., Gross, G. J., and Brooks, H. L. (1982): Subendocardial versus transmural myocardial infarction: Relationship to the collateral circulation in canine and porcine hearts. *Can. J. Physiol. Pharmacol.,* 60:1700–1706.

626. Wartman, W. B., Jennings, R. B., Yokoyama, H. O., and Clabaugh, G. F. (1956): Fatty change of the myocardium in early experimental infarction. *Arch. Pathol.,* 62:318–323.

627. Wartman, W. B., and Souders, J. C. (1950): Localization of myocardial infarcts with respect to the muscle bundles of the heart. *Arch. Pathol.,* 50:329–346.

628. Wattiaux, R., and Wattiaux-De Coninck, S. (1984): Effects of ischemia on lysosomes. *Int. Rev. Exp. Pathol.,* 26:85–106.

629. Wei, J. Y., Hutchins, G. M., and Bulkley, B. H. (1979): Papillary muscle rupture in fatal acute myocardial infarction. A potentially treatable form of cardiogenic shock. *Ann. Intern. Med.,* 90:149–153.

630. Weiner, J. M., Apstein, C. S., Arthur, J. H., Pirzada, F. A., and Hood, W. B., Jr. (1976): Persistence of myocardial injury following brief periods of coronary occlusion. *Cardiovasc. Res.,* 10:678–686.

631. Weiss, J. L., Bulkley, B. H., Hutchins, G. M., and Mason, S. J. (1981): Two-dimensional echocardiographic recognition of myocardial injury in man: Comparison with postmortem studies. *Circulation,* 63:401–408.

632. Weiss, J., Couper, G. S., Hiltbrand, B., and Shine, K. I. (1984): Role of acidosis in early contractile dysfunction during ischemia: Evidence from pH_o measurements. *Am. J. Physiol.,* 247:H760–H767.

633. Weiss, J., and Shine, K. I. (1982): $[K^+]_o$ accumulation and electrophysiological alterations during early myocardial ischemia. *Am. J. Physiol.,* 243:H318–H327.

634. Weisse, A. B., Kearney, K., Narang, R. M., and Regan, T. J. (1976): Comparison of the coronary collateral circulation in dogs and baboons after coronary occlusion. *Am. Heart J.,* 92:193–200.

635. Weissler, A. M., Kruger, F. A., Baba, N., Scarpelli, D. G., Leighton, R. F., and Gallimore, J. K. (1968): Role of anaerobic metabolism in the preservation of functional capacity and structure of anoxic myocardium. *J. Clin. Invest.,* 47:403–416.

636. Weissman, G., Smolen, J., and Korchak, H. (1980): Release of inflammatory mediators from stimulated neutrophils. *N. Engl. J. Med.,* 303:27–34.

637. Wessler, S., Zoll, P. M., and Schlesinger, M. J. (1952): The pathogenesis of spontaneous cardiac rupture. *Circulation,* 6:334–351.

638. West, P. N., Connors, J. P., Clark, R. E., Weldon, C. S., Ramsey, D. L., Roberts, R., Sobel, B. E., and Williamson, J. R. (1978): Compromised microvascular integrity in ischemic myocardium. *Lab. Invest.,* 38:677–684.

639. Whalen, D. A., Hamilton, D. G., Ganote, C. E., and Jennings, R. B. (1974): Effect of a transient period of ischemia on myocardial cells. I. Effects on cell volume regulation. *Am. J. Pathol.,* 74:381–397.

640. Whitman, G., Kieval, R., Wetstein, L., Seeholzer, S., McDonald, G., and Harken, A. (1983): The relationship between global myocardial redox state, and high energy phosphate profile. A phosphorous-31 nuclear magnetic resonance study. *J. Surg. Res.,* 35:332–339.

641. Whitmer, J. T., Idell-Wenger, J. A., Rovetto, M. J., and Neely, J. R. (1978): Control of fatty acid metabolism in ischemic and hypoxic hearts. *J. Biol. Chem.,* 253:4305–4309.

642. Wildenthal, K. (1978): Editorial: Lysosomal alterations in ischemic myocardium; Result or cause of myocellular damage? *J. Mol. Cell. Cardiol.,* 10:595–603.

643. Wildenthal, K., Decker, R. S., Poole, A. R., Griffin, E. E., and Dingle, J. T. (1978): Sequential lysosomal alterations during cardiac ischemia. I. Biochemical and immunohistochemical changes. *Lab. Invest.,* 38:656–661.

644. Wilkinson, P. C. (1974): *Chemotaxis and Inflammation.* vi, p. 214. Churchill Livingstone, London.

645. Wilkinson, R. S., Schaefer, J. A., and Abildskov, J. A. (1963): Electrocardiographic and pathologic features of myocardial infarction in man. *Am. J. Cardiol.,* 11:24–35.

646. Williams, D. O., Amsterdam, E. A., Miller, R. R., and Mason, D. T. (1976): Functional significance of coronary collateral vessels in patients with acute myocardial infarction: Relation to pump performance, cardiogenic shock and survival. *Am. J. Cardiol.,* 37:345–351.

647. Williamson, J. R. (1966): Glycolytic control mechanisms. II. Kinetics of intermediate changes during the aerobic-anoxic transition in perfused rat heart. *J. Biol. Chem.,* 241:5026–5036.

648. Williamson, J. R., Schaffer, S. W., Ford, C., and Safer, B. (1976): Contribution of tissue acidosis to ischemic injury in the perfused rat heart. *Circulation,* 53:3–14.

649. Wollenberger, A., and Krause, E. (1968): Metabolic control

characteristics of the acutely ischemic myocardium. *Am. J. Cardiol.*, 22:349–359.

650. Wollenberger, A., Krause, E. G., and Heier, G. (1969): Stimulation of 3′,5′-cyclic AMP formation in dog myocardium following arrest of blood flow. *Biochem. Biophys. Res. Commun.*, 36:664–670.

651. Wood, J. M., Hanley, H. G., Entman, M. L., Hartley, C. J., Swain, J. A., Busch, U., Chang, C., Lewis, R. M., Morgan, W. J., and Schwartz, A. (1979): Biochemical and morphological correlates of acute experimental myocardial ischemia in the dog. IV. Energy mechanisms during very early ischemia. *Circ. Res.*, 44:52–61.

652. Wusten, B., Flameng, W., Schaper, W., and Carl, M. (1974): The distribution of myocardial flow. I. Effects of experimental coronary occlusion. *Basic Res. Cardiol.*, 69:422–434.

653. Yatani, A., Fujino, T., Kinoshita, K., and Goto, M. (1981): Excess lactate modulates ionic currents and tension components in frog atrial muscle. *J. Mol. Cell. Cardiol.*, 13:147–161.

654. Yellon, D. M., Hearse, D. J., Crome, R., Grannell, J., and Wyse, R. K. H. (1981): Characterization of the lateral interface between normal and ischemic tissue in the canine heart during evolving myocardial infarction. *Am. J. Cardiol.*, 47:1233–1239.

655. Yokoyama, H. O., Jennings, R. B., Clabaugh, G. F., and Wartman, W. B. (1955): Histochemical studies of early experimental myocardial infarction. *Arch. Pathol.*, 59:347–354.

656. Yokoyama, H. O., Jennings, R. B., and Wartman, W. B. (1961): Intercalated disks of dog myocardium. *Exp. Cell Res.*, 23:29–44.

657. Zierler, K. L. (1976): Fatty acids as substrates for heart and skeletal muscle. *Circ. Res.*, 38:459–463.

658. Zimmer, H. G., and Gerlach, E. (1978): Stimulation of myocardial adenine nucleotide biosynthesis by pentoses and pentitols. *Pfluegers Arch.*, 376:223–227.

659. Zimmer, H. G., Trendelenbrug, C., Kammermeier, H., and Gerlach, E. (1973): De novo synthesis of myocardial adenine nucleotides in the rat. Acceleration during recovery from oxygen deficiency. *Circ. Res.*, 32:635–642.

660. Zimmerman, A. N. E., Daems, W., Hulsmann, W. C., Snijder, J., Wisse, E., and Durrer, D. (1967): Morphological changes of heart muscle caused by successive perfusion with calcium-free and calcium-containing solutions (calcium paradox). *Cardiovasc. Res.*, 1:201–209.

661. Zugibe, F. T., Bell, P., Jr., Conley, T., and Standish, M. L. (1966): Determination of myocardial alterations at autopsy in the absence of gross and microscopic changes. *Arch. Pathol.*, 81:409–411.

The Heart and Cardiovascular System,
edited by H. A. Fozzard et al.
Raven Press, New York © 1986.

CHAPTER 54

Reentry Rhythms

Michiel J. Janse

In the normally activated heart, the impulse generated in the sinus node stops after sequential activation of atria and ventricles, because it is surrounded by refractory tissue that it has just excited and because it meets the inexcitable fibrous annulus. A new impulse must arise in the sinus node before the chambers of the heart are subsequently activated, and there is a fairly long interval of quiescence between the end of the refractory period following one activation and the beginning of the next one. Under special conditions, the impulse may not die out after complete activation of the heart but may persist to reexcite atria or ventricles after the end of the refractory period. This is called reentrant excitation. Reentrant excitation as a cause of cardiac arrhythmias has been studied since the second decade of this century. The early literature has been admirably reviewed by Garrey (73) and by Rytand (175). Excellent reviews and books covering later studies are available (33,82,84,85,117,148,166,188,225,229). The characteristics of reentrant excitation and the conditions necessary for initiation and maintenance of reentrant excitation were well defined by 1914. For many decades, however, reentry as a cause for arrhythmias was considered by many a theoretical possibility, and only some 50 years later did it become generally accepted that reentry could be responsible for a wide variety of clinically observed arrhythmias. The reason for this is that, as Wit and

Cranefield wrote: "difficult as it is to doubt that circus movement causes arrhythmias, it is just as difficult to prove that it does" (225).

HISTORICAL NOTES

Throughout the years, two causes for tachycardia have been considered: enhanced impulse formation and reentrant excitation. In 1887, McWilliam suggested for the first time that disturbances in impulse conduction could be a mechanism for tachyarrhythmias:

Apart from the possibility of rapid spontaneous discharges of energy by the muscular fibers, there seems to be another probable cause for continued and rapid movement. The peristaltic contractions traveling along such a structure as that of the ventricular wall must reach adjacent bundles at different points of time, and since these bundles are connected with one another by anastomosing branches the contraction would naturally be propagated from one contracting fiber to another over which the contraction wave had already passed. . . . Hence the movement would tend to go on until the excitability of the muscular tissue had been lowered, so that it failed to respond with a rapid series of contractions (134).

It is clear that McWilliam envisaged the possibility that myocardial fibers could be reexcited as soon as their refractory period had ended by an irregularly propagating impulse and that the resulting tachyarrhythmia could be terminated when reexcitation failed because of reduced excitability. However, some 30 years elapsed before the concept of reentry as a mechanism for cardiac arrhythmias became more firmly established by the experiments of two independent investigators who published at about the same time: Mines and Garrey (72,145,146). Both Mines and Garrey were inspired by experiments on a rather surprising preparation, the subumbrella tissue of a jellyfish, by Mayer (131–133).

> If we cut off the marginal sense organs of the scyphomedusa Cassiopea (Xamachana), the disk becomes paralysed and does not pulsate in sea-water. The disk will pulsate in sea-water, however, if we make either a single ring or a series of concentric broken ring-like cuts through the muscular tissue of the subumbrella. Then upon momentarily stimulating the disk in any manner, it suddenly springs into rapid, rhythmical pulsation so regular and sustained as to recall the movement of clock work (131).

In one preparation, the impulse kept on circling for 11 days (133).

> This single wave going constantly in one direction around the circuit may maintain itself for days traveling at a uniform rate. The circuit must, however be long enough to allow each point to rest for an appreciable interval of time before the return of the wave. . . . The point which was stimulated and from which the contraction-wave first arises is of no importance in maintaining the rhythmical movement than is any other point in the ring . . . the wave is not reinforced and sent forth anew every time it returns to its place of origin, but is maintained by each and every part of the ring in succession as it passes (132).

Mayer proved his statement by isolating the site where the wave originated from the rest of the ring by cuts, without terminating the circus movement. Although Mayer also performed experiments in strips cut from the ventricle of turtle heart, he did not consider circus movement as a cause for cardiac arrhythmias, because he thought that the complete organ was constructed in such a way as to make reentrant excitation impossible. Mines worked with ringlike preparations from atria and ventricles from dog hearts, from atria of large rays, and with atrioventricular preparations from the turtle heart in which both chambers were connected by two connections. He not only confirmed Mayer's observations but also recognized one of the essential requirements for the initiation of a reentrant rhythm, namely the presence of an area of unidirectional block, caused by differences in refractory periods in adjacent regions.

> In such a preparation a single stimulus applied to any point in the ring starts a wave in each direction. The waves meet on the opposite side of the ring and die out. But by the application of several stimuli in succession it is sometimes possible to start a wave in one direction only while the tissue on the other side of the point stimulated is still refractory. Such a wave moves round the ring sufficiently slowly for the refractory phase to have passed off in each part of the ring when the wave approaches it (145).

Mines also made the important observation that extra stimuli could terminate the circus movement:

> while the cycle was being regularly repeated (i.e. during continuous circulation of the impulse), the application of an external stimulus to either of the chambers, if out of phase with the cycle, stopped the contractions, showing that they were not originated by an automatic rhythm in any part of the preparation, but were due to a wave of excitation passing slowly round and round the ring of tissues (145).

Mines was the first to consider reentrant excitation as a cause for arrhythmias occurring in man. In 1913 he wrote: "I venture to suggest that a circulating mechanism of this type may be responsible for some cases of paroxysmal tachycardia as observed clinically" (145). One year later, having read a paper published in 1913 by Kent (110) in which a human heart was described with an extra connection between atria and ventricles on the right side of the heart, Mines repeated his view:

> I now repeat this suggestion in the light of the new histological demonstration by Stanley Kent that the muscular connection between auricles and ventricles in the human heart is multiple. Suppose that for some reason an impulse from the auricle reached the main A-V bundle but failed to reach this "right lateral" connection. It is possible then that the ventricle would excite the ventricular end of this lateral connection, not finding it refractory as normally it would at such a time. The wave spreading then to the auricle might be expected to circulate around the path indicated (146).

This was written 16 years before Wolff, Parkinson, and White published their paper "Bundle Branch Block with Short PR Interval in Healthy Young People Prone to Paroxysmal Tachycardia" (233) and 18 years before Holzmann and Scherf postulated for the first time that the abnormal electrocardiogram described by Wolff, Parkinson, and White was caused by ventricular activation via both the normal conducting system and an accessory atrioventricular connection (86). It was not until the 1960s that clinical studies utilizing multiple intracardiac recording and stimulation and the recording of extracellular electrograms directly from the surface of the heart during cardiac surgery confirmed that Mines's predictions were true in every detail (48,49).

In 1914, Garrey made observations similar to those of Mines on ringlike preparations and became convinced that reentrant excitation was the basis for fibrillation. Garrey wrote that the nature of fibrillation lies in the existence of "blocks of transitory character and shifting location" in a series of ringlike circuits of "multiple complexity" (72). He was able to induce fibrillation with a single stimulus, just as he could start circus movement in a ring. When he cut fibrillating myocardium into large pieces of equal sizes, each of them continued to fibrillate. This was convincing proof that fibrillation could not be due to a single, rapidly firing focus. An important contribution of Garrey was that he proved that a minimal mass of tissue is required to maintain fibrillation. Small pieces of tissue ceased to fibrillate when Garrey isolated them from fibrillating atria or ventricles: "The larger the mass, the greater the probability that each impulse will circulate until it reaches tissue which has once contracted but has passed out of the refractory state" (72). This explained the earlier observations of McWilliam (134) that ventricular fibrillation occurred much more easily in large hearts than in small ones and that fibrillation in hearts of small mammals may stop spontaneously, whereas it usually does not terminate by itself in larger hearts, such as the dog heart. Garrey realized that the circus movement in fibrillation was much more complex than in a single ring: "the impulse is diverted into different paths weaving and intercoursing through the tissue mass, crossing and recrossing old paths again to course over them or to stop short as it impinges on some barrier of refractory tissue" (73). He was the first to consider that reentry could occur without the involvement of an anatomical obstacle around which the circulating wave front could circulate, and he thought that differences in refractory periods would create temporal barriers for conduction, necessary to maintain circus movement: "natural rings are not essential for maintenance of circus contractions" (73).

The criteria for demonstrating that an arrhythmia is based on reentry were formulated by Mines in his 1913 and 1914 articles and can be summarized as follows:

1. An area of unidirectional block must be demonstrated.
2. The movement of the excitatory wave should be observed to progress through the pathway, to return to its point of origin, and then again to follow the same pathway. Even when it can be shown that the excitation wave propagates in the sequence expected of a circus movement, one cannot rule out spontaneous impulse formation in one point of the ring. Mines was fully aware of this pitfall:

Ordinary graphic records either mechanical or electrical are of no value in attesting occurrence of a true circulating excitation since the records show a rhythmic series of waves and do not discriminate between a spontaneous series of beats and a wave of excitation which continues to circulate because it always finds excitable tissue ahead of it. The chief error to be guarded against is that of mistaking a series of automatic beats originating in one point of the ring and traveling in one direction only owing to complete block close to the point of origin of the rhythm on one side of this point (146).

As will become apparent, most of the studies in which the sequence of activation during arrhythmias was determined provided at best incomplete maps, and only in very few studies was Mines's last, and probably most important, criterion met.

3. "The best test for circulating excitation is to cut through the ring at one point. If the impulse continues to arise in the cut ring, circus movement as a cause can be ruled out" (146).

Most of the experimental work on reentrant arrhythmias has been concentrated on the first two of Mines's

criteria. In particular, it was attempted to document the spread of activation during an arrhythmia, because, as Lewis (124) wrote in 1920, "What is not described by those who postulate the view of circus movement in the intact heart, is the path by which the re-entrant tract is affected." Initially, Lewis was quite skeptical about the validity of the circus movement concept, and "leaned to the view that irritable foci in the muscle underlay tachycardia and fibrillation" (126), a view also expressed in the first edition of his famous book *The Mechanism and Graphic Registration of the Heart Beat* (124). However, in this book, an addendum dated May 1920 was added, stating: "In observations, recently completed and as yet unpublished, we have observed much direct evidence to show that atrial flutter consists essentially of a single circus movement . . . the hypothesis which Mines and Garrey have advocated now definitely holds the field." These bold statements were based on a study of 2 dogs in which atrial flutter was induced by faradic stimulation, or by driving the atria at increasingly faster rates (127). The pathway of excitation during atrial flutter (lasting only 35 min) was reconstructed based on measuring the intervals between intrinsic deflections in several extracellular electrograms recorded directly from the atrial surface around the orifices of the caval veins. During one tachycardia cycle, activity propagated from the inferior vena cava along the crista terminalis, turned around the orifice of the superior vena cava, and appeared again behind the orifice of the inferior vena cava, and then the same pathway was resumed. The complete reentrant circuit was not traced, because no measurements were made from the tissue on the left side of the caval veins. However, assuming that the duration of the tachycardia cycle was equal to the time needed to complete the reentry circuit, calculated and measured arrival times at the various recording sites were in good agreement. Furthermore, by comparing the activation sequence during flutter and during stimulation at the inferior vena cava, it was found that in the latter case the left atrium was excited much earlier than during flutter. Although these experiments fell short of meeting the criteria of Mines (unidirectional block during initiation of the flutter was not demonstrated, the complete pathway of excitation was not mapped, and it was not attempted to terminate the arrhythmia by cutting through the supposed pathway), they were the first attempts to document reentry in the intact heart and were of great influence on later studies.

Lewis wrote at length about the theoretical aspects of circus movement and clearly formulated that the reentrant circuit is "governed by three factors, which in themselves are often closely interdependent: 1) the length of the muscle path, 2) the rate at which the wave travels, 3) the duration of the refractory state at any given point" (125). Although he considered an anatomical obstacle necessary for reentrant excitation to occur, he came close, as we shall see later, to defining the conditions necessary for reentrant circuits that are wholly determined by the functional properties of the tissue involved. The work of Lewis and co-workers marked the beginning of extensive efforts to determine the activation sequence in the chambers of the heart during arrhythmias. It is a sobering thought that despite considerable technical advances made since, there are still many uncertainties concerning the exact pathways during reentrant arrhythmias. This is largely because of the fact that for many decades after Lewis's classic studies, mapping experiments were performed using extracellular recordings made sequentially at multiple sites in the heart. To reconstruct the pathways of excitation from subsequent recordings, one had to assume that these remained constant from beat to beat. Whereas this is true for certain types of reentrant arrhythmias, it certainly is not the case during atrial or ventricular fibrillation. Only recently has it become possible to record simultaneously from a substantial number of sites in the heart, so that the activation sequence during complex reentrant arrhythmias can be analyzed.

UNIDIRECTIONAL BLOCK

The occurrence of unidirectional block, one of the essential requirements for initiation of a reentrant rhythm, may be due to regional differences in recovery of excitability and to differences in cellular connections.

Unidirectional Block Due to Nonuniform Recovery of Excitability

When an impulse propagates through tissue in which differences in the durations of refractory periods exist, propagation may fail in regions with the longest refractory periods. These regions will be available for reexcitation, provided that the appropriate conditions exist for the impulse, propagating through areas where excitability has more fully recovered, to return to the site of block. Because in normal working myocardium and conducting fibers there is, even at fast heart rates, a substantial diastolic interval during which excitability is normal, such a situation is most likely to occur during propagation of a premature impulse. Such a premature impulse may occur spontaneously (and could in principle be caused by reentry elsewhere in the heart) or be induced by premature electrical stimulation. Mines, the first to consider unidirectional block based on differences in refractory periods, initiated a circulating reentrant rhythm by rapid stimulation. Both in experimental studies and in clinical studies, reentrant rhythms are most often initiated by premature stimulation. The nature of a spontaneous premature impulse that initiates reentrant rhythms "spontaneously" is most often neglected; yet it is as necessary a requirement for reentrant rhythms as the electrophysiological properties allowing a premature

impulse to set a self-sustaining reentrant rhythm in motion. Reentry, induced by premature stimulation, is facilitated because refractory periods shorten at short cycle lengths (99,136), and therefore the pathways over which the impulse must propagate to return to the site of unidirectional block are shortened as well. Moreover, because of electrotonic current flow from unexcited cells, repolarization in the last cells to be activated is enhanced, and action potentials and refractory periods of cells proximal to the site of unidirectional block are shortened (139,176). The degree of nonuniformity in refractory periods necessary for the occurrence of unidirectional block following premature stimulation may be quite small. In isolated rabbit left atria, refractory periods were measured at multiple sites (4). The differences between shortest and longest refractory periods were on the order of 30 msec. When premature stimuli were delivered at the border of two areas with different refractory periods, the minimal difference necessary for unidirectional block of a properly timed premature stimulus was between 11 and 16 msec (4). It was therefore concluded that the physiological dispersion in refractory periods in the atrium was sufficient to create areas of unidirectional block during propagation of a premature impulse. Reentrant tachycardias could indeed be induced in these experiments by properly placed and timed premature stimuli. Reentry was facilitated in these experiments by adding carbachol to the perfusion fluid, so that refractory periods were shortened to about 50 msec. In normal ventricular myocardium, refractory periods are much longer, even at fast heart rates. In the normal canine left ventricle, the differences between longest and shortest refractory period are on the order of 40 msec (78,92). Despite this dispersion in refractory periods, no areas of block were found during application of five successive premature stimuli, each delivered at the shortest possible coupling interval, and no reentrant rhythms could be induced (92). However, by changing local temperature in the ventricles, large variations in dispersion of refractory periods can be induced, and in this situation, reentrant rhythms can be initiated by premature stimulation (118,202). It appears that there is a critical dispersion in refractory periods, ranging from 95 to 145 msec in different experiments, at which a single premature stimulus, delivered at the site of the shortest refractory period, is able to induce repetitive activity in the canine left ventricle (118). As argued by Allessie et al. (4), differences between shortest and longest refractory periods are not the decisive indicators for the risk of developing reentry. Apart from conduction velocity, and the duration of the refractory period, the dimension of the area of unidirectional block is important. When, even in the presence of large disparities in refractory periods, the sites of prolonged refractoriness are small, reentry will not occur. Temporal differences in recovery of excitability may occur as a consequence of the activation sequence of a previous impulse, even when no differences in duration of refractory periods exist. In a computer model, consisting of a homogeneous sheet of elements with identical refractory periods, unidirectional block occurred when a properly timed premature stimulus was applied in the wake of a uniformly propagating wave front. The premature stimulus elicited a wave front that was blocked in the antegrade direction (the direction in which the previous wave front was propagating), but was conducted retrogradely, where the elements were in a more advanced stage of recovery, and started a circus movement (197).

Reentrant arrhythmias occurring on the basis of temporal differences in recovery of excitability, where the unidirectional block is transient, are dependent on the critical timing of a premature depolarization. Permanent unidirectional block not dependent on differences in refractory periods may be caused by differences in cellular connections or by asymmetrical damage and depression of electrophysiological properties of myocardial tissue.

Geometrical Factors Causing Unidirectional Block

When a thin bundle of cells inserts into a large muscle mass, the junction of the two structures may provide a site for unidirectional block. An impulse may be conducted through the small strand, but the efficacy of the wave front may be insufficient to bring a large volume of cells to threshold at the insertion point with the large muscle mass. Conduction in the reverse direction would be possible, because the "strength" of the wave front arriving over the large muscle mass toward the small bundle would be more than sufficient to excite it. Such a situation has been thought to exist at the junction of the terminal Purkinje fibers with the myocardium, where the junction is thought to be a "funnel," where the narrow portion is the Purkinje fiber and the conical part the progressively increasing muscle fibers (140). Under normal conditions, propagation in both antegrade and retrograde directions is possible, albeit with different delays, conduction in the Purkinje-muscle direction having a longer delay than conduction in the opposite direction (130). However, in the presence of elevated extracellular potassium concentrations, with partial inactivation of the rapid sodium channels, block occurs in the Purkinje-muscle direction while conduction in the muscle-Purkinje direction is still possible (140). Recent studies have shown that the interface between Purkinje and muscle fibers is better represented by a three-dimensional model of overlying two-dimensional sheets, rather than by a strand of "terminal" Purkinje fibers inserting into a three-dimensional ventricular muscle mass (199). Activation of the ventricular muscle layer from the Purkinje layer occurs only at specific junctional sites, where a considerable resistive barrier exists between the two cell layers. In in vitro preparations under normal conditions, it was shown that propagation from ventricular muscle to Purkinje cells was possible at certain sites where propagation from Purkinje to muscle did not occur (160). The reason for unidirectional block between Purkinje and muscle layers may be due to differences in excitability of the two layers, to differences in thicknesses of the layers (where the muscle layer would present a larger "load" on the Purkinje layer than vice versa), and to increased coupling resistance at sites showing unidirectional block (108). When atrial tissue is dissected in such a way that a narrow bridge inserts into a larger mass of atrial tissue, unidirectional block occurs at the junction of the narrow bridge with the larger area (38). This experimental model has its counterpart in the preexcitation syndrome, where a thin accessory atrioventricular bundle inserts into a large ventricular muscle mass, and where permanent unidirectional block in the atrioventricular direction may occur, while conduction in the opposite direction is still possible (159,214). In such patients, who during sinus rhythm have no electrocardiographic evidence for existence of an accessory atrioventricular pathway, a ventricular premature beat, finding the atrioventricular node refractory, may initiate a reentrant tachycardia by being conducted toward the atria via the "concealed" accessory pathway.

Thus, sites where the cross-sectional area of interconnected cells suddenly increases may be sites for unidirectional block. An example from an analog model, simulating a branching site of a bundle of myocardial cells, is shown in Fig. 1. Two strands merge into a final common exit pathway. None of the strands can by itself excite the other strand or the exit path. Only when both strands are stimulated can the exit pathway be activated, even when the excitation waves do not arrive simultaneously at the junction. In the example shown, with a time lag of 60 msec between the arrivals of the two wave fronts, the action potentials in the two input pathways show double components. The prepotential in the middle tracing is an electrotonic reflection of the earlier action potential in the upper tracing. The secondary hump in the repolarization phase of the first action potential is an electrotonic reflection of the upstroke of the second action potential. When the delay increases to 90 msec, the exit path can no longer be excited.

The importance of geometrical factors causing unidirectional block and reentry in tissue with uniform membrane properties has been experimentally investigated by Spach et al. (186,187). From these studies it emerged that, indeed, branching sites, or junctions of separate muscle bundles, formed areas of a low safety factor for propagation where unidirectional block could easily occur [the safety factor for propagation may be defined as the ratio of the current that can be provided

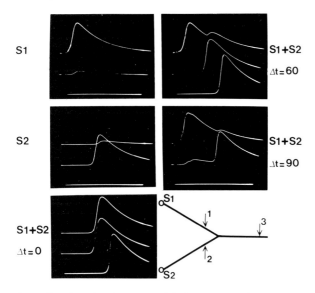

FIG. 1. Simulated action potentials in a converging geometry to demonstrate the occurrence of block at a branching site. Only when S₁ and S₂ were both stimulated did propagation to the exit path occur. (From ref. 198, with permission.)

by the proximal cells to the current required to bring distal cells to threshold (108)]. An example is shown in Fig. 2, from an experiment on an isolated canine atrial preparation. Extracellular recording electrodes were placed on the crista terminalis (C) and on an extension of the limbus that crossed the crista (L). Stimuli were delivered at the crista, and premature stimuli were applied at progressively shorter coupling intervals. In the graph (B), the times of local excitation are indicated for each of the recording electrodes. The electrogram recorded from electrode 3 showed two components, one associated with activation of the crista, the other with excitation of the limbus. As the coupling interval decreased from 1,000 to 310 msec, there was a gradual and small increase in arrival time at each site (see B). However, when the coupling interval was shortened from 275 to 270 msec, an abrupt increase in the time of arrival of excitation in the limbus occurred. This was caused by block across the junction of crista and limbus and a longer route of the propagating wave front to reach the limbus. At a coupling interval of 220 msec, conduction block occurred at the crista, but activity did spread from the crista to the pectinate muscles, reached the limbus with delay, and reexcited the crista. Failure of conduction in the crista was apparently not due to differences in refractory periods of the tissues involved, the refractory periods of crista and limbus being 200 and 202 msec, respectively (186). Although in this example, block did occur at the junction of two bundles, the unidirectional block that finally permitted reentry of the crista occurred in the crista itself. This may be related to differences in coupling between cells in the direction parallel to their long fiber axis and in the transverse direction.

The influence of the way myocardial cells are connected to each other on the propagation of the impulse is apparent when conduction velocity in the general fiber direction is compared with conduction velocity in the transverse direction (27,45,170,187). The transverse velocity is only about one-third of the conduction velocity in the longitudinal direction, and this difference is adequately explained by the differences in intracellular and extracellular resistances in both directions (24). One would intuitively expect conduction block to occur more easily in the transverse than in the longitudinal direction. This would provide an explanation for functional longitudinal dissociation, where a wave front traveling along a bundle with uniformly reduced excitability (e.g., an early premature impulse) would be blocked in the transverse direction, but would still propagate in the longitudinal direction. In a computer simulation, where excitable elements with uniform electrophysiological properties were connected to each other, and coupling resistance in the transverse direction was higher than in the longitudinal direction, conduction of a premature impulse did indeed fail in the transverse direction, and succeeded in the longitudinal direction (196). It is therefore quite surprising that Spach et al. (187) postulated just the opposite. In their studies, transverse conduction had a larger margin of safety than longitudinal conduction. A premature impulse elicited in the crista terminalis was blocked in the longitudinal direction, but conduction continued in a transverse direction. Eventually, a more distal site in the crista terminalis was excited, and activity propagated retrogradely in the longitudinal direction to induce a reentrant return extrasystole (187). The reasons for the discrepancy between the experimental results and the computer simulation are not clear. On the one hand, electrophysiological characteristics of the computer model may be too far removed from reality; on the other hand, in the experimental situation regional differences in excitability may have been present and may have complicated the results.

Unidirectional Block Based on Asymmetrical Depression of Conduction and Excitability

Asymmetry in a region of depressed excitability can result in unidirectional block. This was first postulated in 1895 by Engelmann (58), who locally applied cold and poison to frog sartorious muscle to produce unidirectional block. Various experimental techniques have been used to cause localized depression of excitability, such as local hyperkalemia (32,181), focal cooling (44), local crushing (44,181), and application of depolarizing current (219). A schematic representation of longitudinal dissociation based on asymmetrical depression of electrophysiological properties is shown in Fig. 3, reproduced from the classic article of Schmitt and Erlanger (181). In a strip of ventricular muscle from the turtle heart,

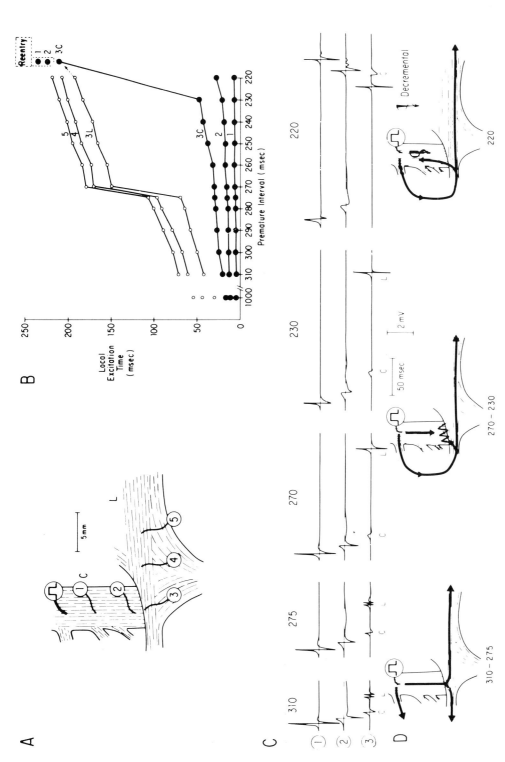

FIG. 2. Reentry caused by the complex structure of canine atrial myocardium. **A:** Locations of the stimulating electrode (square wave) and the recording electrodes on the crista terminalis (C) and the limbus of the fossa ovalis (L) where the local excitation times were measured for induced premature impulses, shown graphically in **B.** *Filled circles* are activation times for the crista, *open circles* for the limbus. Extracellular electrograms recorded from sites 1, 2, and 3 are shown in **C.** The numbers above the recorded signals represent the interval (in msec) between the last regular stimulus and the premature stimulus. The patterns of excitation are indicated by solid lines with arrows in **D.** Note abrupt delay of activation of the limbus at a coupling interval of 270 msec, caused by block at the junction of crista and limbus, and excitation of the limbus via an alternate path. At a coupling interval of 220 msec, block occurs in the crista, in the direction parallel to the long fiber axis, and reentry occurs. (From ref. 186, with permission.)

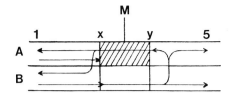

FIG. 3. Schematic representation of reentry in a linear bundle with a region of asymmetrical depressed tissue, as proposed by Schmitt and Erlanger (181). The *shaded area* is a zone of unidirectional block. The impulse propagating from left to right blocks at *x*, in region A, but conducts slowly in B beyond this area. There the impulse crosses over to A via lateral connections and propagates slowly back through the depressed zone *y-x*, to reexcite the left part of the bundle.

part of the segment at M was subjected to injury by pressure, and KCl was applied locally. As a result, conduction between *x* and *y* was "greatly slowed" in layer A, whereas layer B was less affected. An impulse arriving from A was blocked, but was very slowly conducted in layer B. The time needed to traverse the distance *xy* was 2.5 sec! Because of this delay in transmission, the region *xy* in layer A recovered from refractoriness, and the impulse returned to reexcite the region proximal to the site of unidirectional block.

Another way in which asymmetrical depression of excitability may lead to unidirectional block is schematically depicted in Fig. 4. This scheme is based on experiments in isolated sheep Purkinje fibers in which unidirectional block was produced by asymmetric cooling or crushing (44). The region of greatest injury shows an abrupt rise in threshold for excitation; the region of lesser injury shows a more gradual rise. Between *x* and *y*, cells are inexcitable. An impulse traveling in a "retrograde" direction encounters the zone of inexcitable cells abruptly (at *y*), and the amplitude of the action potential decays with distance. Depending on the length of the inexcitable gap and the threshold for excitation of the cells at the opposite end of the lesion, the electrotonically transmitted response may just be sufficient to initiate a regenerative response at point *x* and to ensure retrograde transmission. By contrast, an impulse traveling in the opposite ("antegrade") direction encounters a gradually rising threshold, resulting in decremental conduction of the active wave front and a progressive decrease in action potential amplitude. At point *x*, where cells become inexcitable, the action potential amplitude is therefore much smaller than the response of the retrograde impulse at point *y*. The electrotonically transmitted impulse is not large enough when reaching point *y* to excite the cells at that point, and thus antegrade conduction fails. In other words, conduction fails when a wave front meets the least depressed side of an injured segment first, and successful conduction occurs in the direction in which the propagating wave encounters the most depressed side first (44,198). It is of interest to

note that in 1896 Engelmann (59) concluded that an impulse conducts more easily from rapidly conducting tissues to slowly conducting tissues than in the reverse direction.

ROLE OF SLOW CONDUCTION

The early investigators realized that one of the conditions making reentry possible was that the impulse had to be delayed sufficiently in an alternate pathway to allow the elements proximal to a site of unidirectional pathway to allow the elements proximal to a site of unidirectional block to recover from refractoriness. Reentry would therefore be facilitated when conduction was slower than normal. (Reentry in tissue where conduction is already slow under normal conditions, the sinoatrial and atrioventricular nodes, will be discussed separately.) Several factors determine the speed at which an action potential is propagated in atrial, ventricular, and Purkinje fibers. Among these are the magnitude of the inward current flowing through the fast Na$^+$ channels

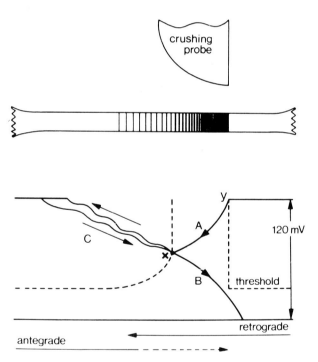

FIG. 4. Schematic representation of unidirectional block in a Purkinje fiber with asymmetric injury produced by crush (*upper part*). The lower part illustrates the influence of the injury on excitability threshold and contrasts the amplitudes of the antegrade (C-*x*-B) and retrograde (A-*x*-C) wave fronts at corresponding points. At *y*, the transition between normal cells and inexcitable, injured cells is abrupt. C represents decremental or augmental conduction, depending on direction, through a transitional zone of partial injury; *x* represents the point of transition between partially excitable cells and inexcitable cells (*x-y*). A and B represent electrotonic transmission through inexcitable cells. The retrograde wave front succeeds in conducting across, while the antegrade wave front fails. (From ref. 44, with permission.)

during the action potential upstroke and the rapidity with which this current reaches its maximum. The magnitude of the Na^+ inward current depends on the fraction of Na^+ channels that open when the cell is excited and on the concentration differences of Na^+ across the cell membrane (168,205). The fraction of Na^+ channels available for opening is determined by the level of membrane potential at which an action potential is initiated (205) and also by the time elapsed after an action potential upstroke (75). Directly following the upstroke, cardiac cells are inexcitable because of inactivation of Na^+ channels. During repolarization, removal of inactivation allows increasingly larger Na^+ currents to flow through partially reactivated channels. Amplitude and upstroke velocity of premature action potentials initiated during repolarization are reduced, and conduction velocity is low. As already described, reentry may occur during propagation of a premature impulse in a region with different action potential durations, because of block and slow conduction. Reentry may also occur in cardiac fibers with persistent low levels of membrane potential. At levels between -60 and -70 mV, about 50% of Na^+ channels are inactivated (67). Also, at these resting potential levels, recovery from inactivation following an action potential is markedly prolonged and extends beyond complete repolarization (75). In partially depolarized fibers, reentry may occur even with normally propagated responses when local differences in membrane potential give rise to slow conduction in some regions and to conduction block in more depressed areas. The chance for reentry during premature activation is even greater in such tissue. Although it is generally true that reductions in action potential amplitude and upstroke velocity may reduce conduction velocity, this is not the case in all circumstances. When cardiac fibers (other than those in sinoatrial and atrioventricular nodes) are gradually depolarized by stepwise increases in extracellular K^+ concentration, there is a small range of membrane potentials at which action potentials with smaller amplitudes and reduced upstroke velocities actually propagate faster than in control conditions. This is due to the fact that current requirements to bring unexcited cells to threshold are reduced because of the smaller difference between reduced membrane potential and unchanged threshold potential (42,165).

When the Na^+ channels are inactivated at membrane potentials below -50 mV, the slow inward current can still be activated and, especially in the presence of catecholamines, can give rise to regenerative depolarizations (22,194). The propagated responses that are primarily due to inward current via partially inactivated fast Na^+ channels are sometimes referred to as "depressed fast responses," and those that are dependent solely on the slow inward current are known as "slow responses." True slow responses propagate very slowly, and they have been implied to underlie the occurrence of reentrant

arrhythmias (29). Because conduction depends on local current circuits, by which one cell excites the other by bringing its membrane potential to threshold, the coupling resistance between cells is another factor determining conduction velocity, in addition to the magnitude and rapidity of local inward current and the potential difference between membrane potential and threshold potential. When coupling resistance increases, conduction velocity decreases. Coupling resistance increases as intracellular calcium increases and also when intracellular pH decreases (39,208). This may occur in various conditions, such as exposure to ouabain (207) and hypoxia (231). Only a marked increase in coupling resistance will produce a sizable reduction in conduction velocity, because conduction velocity is proportional to the square root of longitudinal internal resistance (207). The importance of tissue anisotropy caused by differences in coupling resistance in the directions perpendicular and parallel to the fiber axis as a factor causing unidirectional block and reentry has already been discussed.

DIFFERENT FORMS OF REENTRY

Reentry Involving an Anatomical Obstacle

The simplest model of reentry in cardiac tissue was introduced by Mines (145) in 1913 and is illustrated in Fig. 5. In both parts A and B, excitation is propagated only in one direction. In A, "if the rate of propagation is rapid as compared with the duration of the wave, the whole circuit will be in the excited state at the same time, and the excitation wave will die out." When, however, "the wave is slower and shorter . . . the excited state will have passed off at the region where the excitation started before the wave of excitation reaches this point of the circle at the completion of revolution." "Under these circumstances, the wave of excitation may spread a second time over the same tract of tissue" (145). Thus, in an anatomically defined circuit, Mines recognized that both the duration of the refractory period and the conduction velocity determined whether or not reentrant excitation would occur. An important feature of this model of circus movement is the existence of an excitable gap (the white part of the circle in Fig. 5B) between the crest of the excitation wave and its tail of relative refractoriness (dotted area). This implies that impulses originating outside the reentrant circuit may enter it and influence the reentrant rhythm. Because the normal pacemakers of the heart are likely to be "overdrive-suppressed" during a circus movement tachycardia, such impulses are usually initiated artificially, either by electrical stimulation or mechanically ("chest thump"). The effects of such premature impulses on a reentrant circuit with an excitable gap are illustrated in Fig. 6. In both instances (a_1 and b_1) a premature impulse reaches the reentrant circuit when it is relatively refractory. In

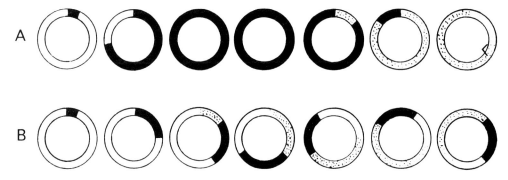

FIG. 5. Mines's diagram to explain that reentry will occur if conduction is slowed and the refractory period duration is decreased. A stimulated impulse leaves in its wake absolutely refractory tissue (*black area*) and relatively refractory tissue (*stippled area*). In both **A** and **B**, the impulse conducts in one direction only. In A, because of fast conduction and a long refractory period, the tissue is still absolutely refractory when the impulse has returned to its site of origin. In B, because of slow conduction and a short refractory period, the tissue has recovered excitability by the time the impulse has reached the site of origin, and the impulse continues to circulate. (From ref. 145, with permission.)

a_1, the circuit is entered at the end of its relative refractory period, and the impulse penetrates in both directions. In the "retrograde" pathway, it meets the oncoming circulating wave front, and both waves extinguish themselves. However, because the premature impulse also invades the "antegrade" pathway, the arrhythmia is not terminated but only "reset" (Fig. 6a$_2$). In b$_1$, the premature wave front reaches the circuit when it is

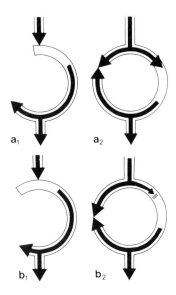

FIG. 6. Schematic representation of the effect of a premature impulse on a reentrant circuit with an excitable gap. The *dotted area* is the relatively refractory part of the circuit, the *black area* the absolutely refractory part. In a$_1$, a premature impulse reaches the circuit in its relatively refractory "tail." In a$_2$, a moment later, the premature impulse has invaded the circuit in two directions, blocking the retrograde wave front coming up through the circuit and advancing in the antegrade pathway, thus changing the phase of the tachycardia ("resetting"). In b$_1$, the premature impulse reaches the circuit when it is less excitable. It blocks the retrograde wave front and cannot excite the antegrade path (b$_2$). Thus, tachycardia is terminated. (From ref. 97, with permission.)

less excitable, so that it fails to be conducted in the antegrade pathway. It is able to propagate into the retrograde pathway, where it meets cells that are progressively more excitable. By blocking the circulating wavefront, the circus movement tachycardia is terminated (Fig. 6b$_2$). When the heart is paced at a regular rate that is faster than the intrinsic rate of the circus movement, the situation depicted in Fig. 6a$_1$ and 6a$_2$ may be perpetuated: The first paced impulse (when properly timed) blocks the circulating wave front but also enters the antegrade pathway and continues in the circuit. The next paced beat blocks the retrograde wave front but again enters the antegrade path. The heart therefore follows the pacing rate, but on stopping the pacing, the original tachycardia continues. This is called "transient entrainment" (129). Overdrive pacing may, of course, also result in termination of the tachycardia, according to the principle depicted in Fig. 6b$_1$ and b$_2$.

Several variations of the reentry model involving an anatomical obstacle exist. In 1920, Lewis and co-workers (127) induced atrial flutter in dogs by faradic stimulation of the atria or by pacing the atria at rapid rates. By direct recording of extracellular electrograms from the tissue around the caval veins (but not, however, from the tissue on the left side of the caval orifices), they obtained evidence for a circus movement around the caval orifices, with a supposed area of bidirectional block in the tissue between the two orifices. This type of reentrant circuit is schematically illustrated in Fig. 7B. The important difference from the model described by Mines is that as soon as the excitable gap becomes longer than the perimeter of the smallest obstacle, the circulating impulse may short-circuit the circuit. This can have two effects: Either the tachycardia is terminated or, when the impulse continues to circulate around the larger of the two obstacles, the rate suddenly increases. Lewis realized the importance of the excitable gap: "a wave may be supposed to circulate around both cavae

MINES   LEWIS   MOE

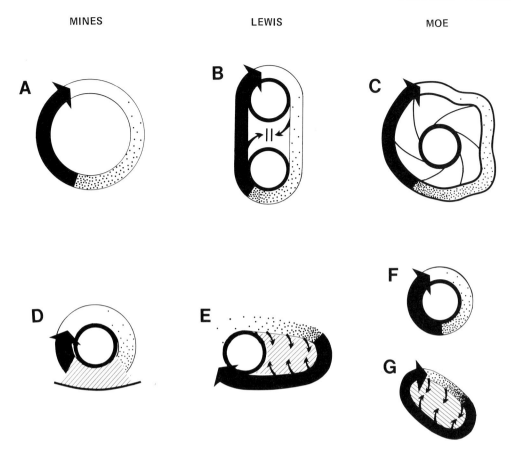

FIG. 7. Schematic representation of various types of circus movement reentry. The *arrows* represent the crest of the circulating wave front, and in its wake are the areas of absolute refractoriness (*black areas*) and relative refractoriness (*dotted areas*). **A:** Circus movement around a gross anatomical obstacle, as introduced by Mines. **B:** Circus movement around the orifices of two veins, separated by a zone of bidirectional block, as suggested by Lewis to be responsible for atrial flutter. **C:** Model of circus movement introduced by Moe and co-workers, in which the impulse is thought to circulate in a loop composed of bundles having a greater conduction velocity than the tissue around it. **D** and **E:** Types of circus movement based on a combination of an anatomical obstacle and an adjacent area of diseased tissue exhibiting depressed conduction (*hatched areas*). **F:** Circus movement around a relatively small obstacle has become possible because of shortening of the refractory period and a decrease in conduction velocity, resulting in a shortening of the wavelength of the impulse. **G:** Circus movement without involvement of an anatomical obstacle. (From ref. 6, with permission.)

while the gap between its crest and wake is considerable; the crest of the wave will fail to take the path between the two cavae if, as it passes the intercaval muscle, its wake in the other side has not retreated from this region" (125). He also wrote that "when shorter or larger paths become available, the length of the refractory period is in sole control of the rate of beating" (125), emphasizing that even in the presence of an anatomical obstacle, functional properties determined the length of the reentrant circuit. Later studies, in which the tissue between the caval veins was crushed to create an artificial anatomical obstacle and in which more detailed mapping was performed, confirmed the findings of Lewis et al. (80,111,120,173). The question still remained whether or not naturally occurring obstacles in the atria were large enough for sustained reentry to occur. When anisotropy of conduction in the atria is taken into account, the need for a large anatomical obstacle diminishes (164). For example, when conduction velocity in

a loop of muscle bundles is twice as large as in the surrounding tissues, the effective perimeter of a natural orifice within the loop is doubled (6). This situation is depicted in Fig. 7C. In the original publication from Moe's laboratory (164) it was supposed that specialized intranodal atrial pathways would provide such loops having a high conduction velocity. As discussed earlier, anisotropy provided by differences in cellular coupling could also lead to differences in conduction velocity, where conduction in the longitudinal direction of an atrial muscle bundle may be two to three times faster than in the transverse direction (24,187).

Allessie and co-workers (6) postulated some more variations of circus movement involving an anatomical obstacle (Fig. 7D and 7E), where the length of the circuit could be reduced when an area of depressed conduction was present. Circus movement can be permanent provided the perimeter of the obstacle exceeds the wavelength of the impulse. The wavelength is defined as the distance traveled during a period of time equal to the refractory period. Wavelength (in cm) can be expressed as conduction velocity (cm/sec) times refractory period (sec) (221). The wavelength can be shortened by a shortening of the refractory period or by a decrease in conduction velocity, or by both. When wavelength is shortened, the anatomical obstacle necessary to sustain circus movement obviously becomes smaller as well (Fig. 7F).

Reentry Without an Anatomical Obstacle: The Leading-Circle Model

Allessie et al. (3–5) were able to induce circus movement tachycardia in small pieces of isolated left atria

from rabbit hearts by a properly timed premature stimulus. In this preparation, no anatomical obstacles are present, and the reentrant circuit is completely defined by the electrophysiological properties of the tissue involved. Figure 8 shows activation maps obtained during regular pacing of the isolated preparation (basic beat), during the induced premature beat that initiated the tachycardia, and during the first cycle of the tachycardia. Also shown is a map indicating the durations of the refractory periods at several sites during a regularly driven basic rhythm. During regular pacing, spread of activity occurred in a more or less radial way from the central stimulating electrode. However, the distance between isochrones was not uniform, conduction being

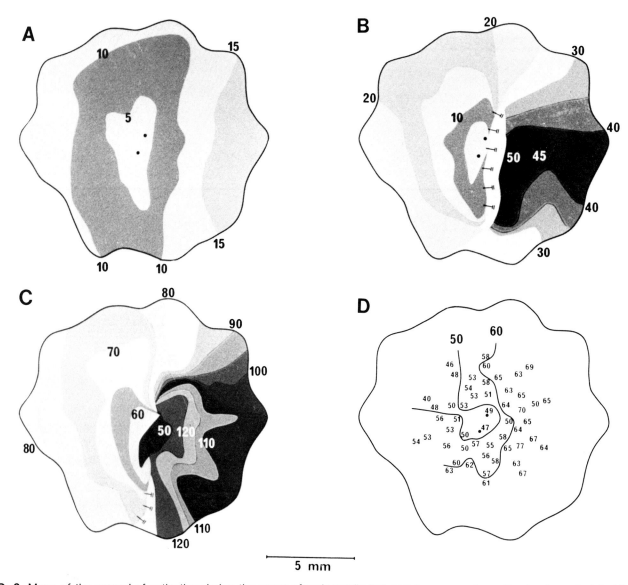

FIG. 8. Maps of the spread of activation during the onset of tachycardia induced by a premature stimulus in an isolated left atrial preparation from rabbit heart. The sites at which premature stimuli elicited tachycardia are indicated by *dots*. The activation times (in msec) given at the outer borders of the maps refer to the moment of the basic stimulus [**A:** basic beat (interval 500 msec)] and the moment of the premature stimulus [**B:** premature beat (delay 56 msec) and **C:** first cycle of the tachycardia]. *Double bars* indicate conduction block. **D:** refractory period durations determined at multiple sites (in msec). (From ref. 4, with permission.)

faster in the vertical direction than in the horizontal direction, suggesting that the long axis of the atrial fibers was predominantly oriented in a vertical direction. The premature impulse propagated in the direction of sites with shorter refractory periods and was blocked in the direction in which refractory periods were longer (if anisotropy due to fiber orientation had been a factor in causing block, it would seem that in this case block occurred in a direction transverse to the long fiber axis). Activity spread in two directions around the arc of conduction block, until the two wave fronts merged 50 msec after the premature stimulus. This wave front succeeded in reexciting the tissue proximal to the zone of block, the stimulation site being activated after 60 msec (the duration of the refractory period was in these experiments shortened by the addition of carbachol to the superfusion fluid). Although during the initiation of tachycardia, usually two wave fronts propagated around the zone of unidirectional block, during sustained tachycardia, a single circus movement was most often present. Figure 9 shows the activation map during stable tachycardia in another experiment, together with microelectrode recordings made from the center of the reentrant circuit. Under the influence of carbachol, action potential duration had greatly shortened, but the refractory period

was less affected and outlasted the duration of the action potential ("post-repolarization refractoriness"). Fibers A and D were located on the perimeter of the circulating wave front. The difference in activation times of A and D was about half the revolution time of the circulating wave. The fibers in the center (fibers 1–5) were activated in a centripetal manner. From A, fibers 1, 2, 3, and 4 were activated in that order. Amplitude, upstroke velocity, and duration of the responses gradually decreased, until somewhere between 4 and 5 the centripetal wavelet became extinguished. From the opposite side of the circuit, fibers 5, 4, and 3 were subsequently excited, and again conduction was decremental and the wavelet died out between 3 and 2. From these studies, the leading-circle concept was formulated. The leading circle was defined as "the smallest possible pathway in which the impulse continues to circulate, and in which the stimulating efficacy of the wavefront is just enough to excite the tissue ahead which is still in its relative refractory phase" (5). The length of the circuit is equal to the wavelength of the impulse and can in principle be defined as the product of conduction velocity and refractory period. However, because the crest of the wave front impinges on the relative refractory tail of the previous wave, the circulating wave travels through

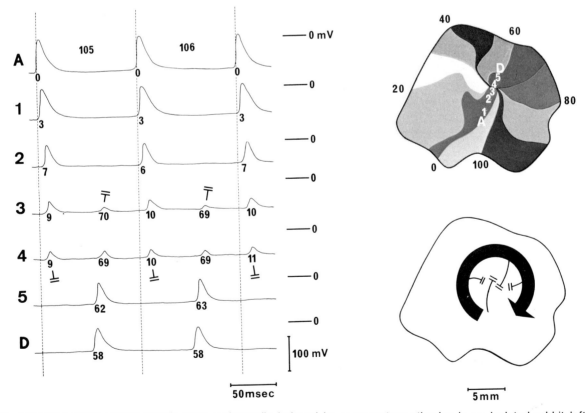

FIG. 9. Activation maps during steady-state tachycardia induced by a premature stimulus in an isolated rabbit left atrium (**upper right**). On the **left** are transmembrane potentials recorded from seven fibers located on a straight line through the center of the circus movement. Note that the central area is activated by centripetal wavelets and that the fibers in the central area show double responses of low amplitude. Both responses are unable to propagate beyond the center, thus preventing the impulse from short-cutting the circuit. **Lower right:** the activation pattern is schematically indicated, showing the leading circuit and the converging centripetal wavelets. Block is indicated by *double bars.* (From ref. 5, with permission.)

partially refractory tissue. Therefore, conduction velocity is reduced. Moreover, it is difficult to give a single value for the refractory period. In fact, during circus movement in the leading-circle model, refractory period and conduction velocity are interdependent. Allessie and co-workers used a curve derived from the classic strength-interval curve to indicate the relationship between stimulating efficacy of the impulse and revolution time of the leading circle (Fig. 10). When the stimulating efficacy of the wave front (which was considered to be primarily determined by the amplitude and upstroke velocity of the action potential) is diminished, revolution time increases. This was verified experimentally by application of tetrodotoxin (TTX) during tachycardia, resulting in a decrease in the rate of the tachycardia (5). A decrease in the duration of the refractory period, effected by addition of carbachol, should, and did, result in a shortening of revolution time and therefore in an increase in the rate. Cooling of the preparation, which resulted in a lengthening of the refractory period and a decrease in stimulating efficacy, lengthened the revolution time (Fig. 10C). When the stimulating efficacy was reduced by an increase in heart rate, which also gradually

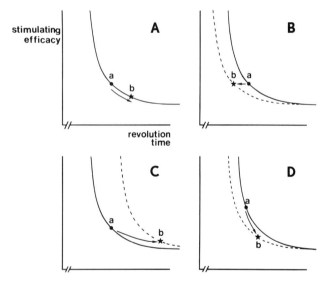

FIG. 10. Modified strength-interval curves to explain changes in rate in the leading-circle model of circus movement tachycardia. *Ordinate*, stimulus strength is replaced by stimulating efficacy of the circulating wave front. *Abscissa*, the interval is replaced by revolution time of the circulating wave. **A:** A decrease in stimulating efficacy causes a lengthening of the revolution time of the leading circle from *a* to *b*. **B:** A shortening of the refractory period results in a shortening of the revolution time. **C:** Tachycardia is slowed by a combination of a decrease in stimulating efficacy and lengthening of refractory period. **D:** At a sudden increase in rate (i.e., at the onset of tachycardia), the stimulating efficacy of the impulse is gradually decreasing, while the refractory period shortens. The net effect on the cycle length of the tachycardia depends on the relative degrees of these changes. In this case, revolution time lengthened from *a* to *b*. (From ref. 5, with permission.)

shortened the refractory periods, the effect depended on the degree at which each factor was altered. When circus movement tachycardia was initiated in the left atrium of the rabbit, the cycle length of the tachycardia initially increased and reached a stable value after about 100 beats. This was presumably due to progressive decreases in action potential amplitude and upstroke velocity, which had a greater effect on revolution time than the concomitant shortening of the refractory period (Fig. 10D). It is, of course, conceivable that cycle length decreases during the initial beats of a reentrant rhythm of the leading-circle type, when the shortening of the refractory period dominates over the reduction in stimulating efficacy. The main differences between the simple reentry model of Mines and the leading-circle-type model are summarized in Fig. 11.

The leading-circle model of reentry such as occurs in normal atrial myocardium, where electrophysiological properties are fairly uniform, obviously does not have a gap of fully excitable tissue. As put forward by Frame and Hoffman (63), when within a functionally determined reentrant circuit large differences in refractoriness occur, there may exist an excitable gap in the region of the loop where the refractory period is shortest. The practical consequence of this is that some types of reentrant tachycardias based on the leading-circle model may not be influenced by premature impulses initiated outside the reentrant circuit, whereas in the presence of an excitable gap, termination of tachycardia or resetting and entrainment may occur.

A distinction has been made between orderly reentry and random reentry (85). Orderly reentry occurs over relatively fixed reentrant pathways and results in a regular rhythm. During random reentry, propagation occurs over reentrant pathways that continuously change their size and location with time, and the resulting rhythm is irregular. Even though reentry of the leading-circle type is the basis for random reentry, the reentrant impulse seldom follows the same pathway more than once. During random reentry, several independent wave fronts are present, and as a rule, a particular area is reexcited by another wave front than the one by which it was activated before. The experimental evidence for random reentry will be discussed more fully in the sections on atrial and ventricular fibrillation.

Reflection

Reflection is a form of reentry occurring in a one-dimensional structure, where the impulse is conducted to-and-fro over the same pathway. The earliest experiments on "reflected contractions" were performed on the same preparation used to establish the concept of circus movement reentry: the jellyfish. In 1903, Bethe (12) used a strip of the umbrella of the Medusa with a "rim body" (Randkoerper) at one end. Stimulation of

1. FIXED LENGTH OF
   CIRCUIT.

2. USUALLY EXCITABLE
   GAP BETWEEN HEAD
   AND TAIL OF IMPULSE.

2. INVERSE RELATION
   REVOLUTION TIME AND
   CONDUCTION VELOCITY.

1. CIRCUIT LENGTH
   DEPENDENT ON
   COND.VEL.REFR.PER.

2. NO GAP OF FULL
   EXCITABILITY.

3. REVOLUTION TIME
   PROPORTIONAL TO
   LENGTH REFRACTORY
   PERIOD.

4. SHORTCUT OF CIRCUIT
   POSSIBLE.

FIG. 11. Differences in characteristics of circus movement reentry in an anatomically defined circuit and a functionally defined circuit. (Adapted from ref. 5.)

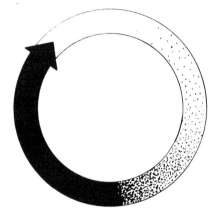

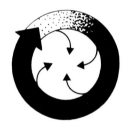

the other end resulted in propagation of the impulse toward the rim body, where it initiated not one but two impulses, the second of which was reflected back over the strip. When the rim body was removed, the retrograde wave failed to appear. Bethe wrote that such a mechanism of "reflected contraction" could be observed in the heart from which the sinus node was removed. The early literature on this phenomenon, which has been called "pseudoreflection," was thoroughly reviewed by Scherf and Cohen (178). They considered the Schmitt and Erlanger explanation for reflection (Fig. 3) unlikely and suggested that "an impulse traveling into an area with damaged fibers leads to the formation of after potentials and oscillatory potentials which may reach threshold value and thus initiate the formation of a new impulse which is conducted back to the point of origin." The key feature of pseudoreflection is that a propagated response induces two responses at one end of a strand of tissue, the second of which is retrogradely conducted over the same strand. It depends on "triggered activity," where a propagated action potential is followed by either an early or a delayed afterdepolarization, from which one or a series of repetitive focal responses may arise (29,30).

In "true" reflection, only one response occurs at the distal end of the preparation, and the experiments conducted to study this form of reexcitation usually

involve a linear bundle of tissue in which two excitable ends are separated by an area of depressed conduction. One form of reflection is the type of reentry described by Schmitt and Erlanger, illustrated in Fig. 3. A fundamentally different mechanism has been proposed, where antegrade and retrograde transmissions occur through the same fibers (29,32). The basis for this proposition was the experimental finding that a fast action potential upstroke interrupting a slow, low-voltage response in the depressed segment occurred after the fast action potential upstroke observed in the tissue beyond the depressed segment (32). Later experiments on reflection (9,10,91,174) used essentially a three-compartment tissue bath where a zone of conduction block was created in the central segment. This was accomplished either by making the central zone inexcitable by superfusion with a solution containing a high K^+ concentration or by electrical insulation of the extracellular spaces of the two outer compartments by perfusing the central compartment with isotonic sucrose. In the latter case, an external shunt resistor connecting the outer compartments replaces the extracellular space of the central compartment, and by varying this resistance, a high-resistance block between the two outer segments can be created. The essential feature of both experimental conditions is that the central compartment can transmit electrotonic potentials only. The proposed mechanism for reflection in these latter studies was that the electrotonic potential, transmitted through the inexcitable or high-resistance gap, excited the distal elements with a delay. The active response in the distal tissue caused an electrotonic potential, which was transmitted in the reverse direction over the same blocked segment and reexcited the proximal elements. (A variation of reflection could occur when the block in the central segment is unidirectional; electrotonic transmission then occurs only in an antegrade direction, and the retrograde impulse actively propagates back through the same tissue.) Interpretation of the experimental results is complicated by two factors. In the case of Purkinje fibers, displaying automaticity, subthreshold depolarizations caused by electrotonic transmission through an inexcitable or high-resistance gap will influence the automatic mechanism. When they occur early in the spontaneous cycle of an automatic pacemaker, the spontaneous discharge will be delayed; when they fall late in the cycle, the next spontaneous depolarization will be accelerated (89,90,152,193,204). A properly timed action potential, arriving at an inexcitable or high-resistance gap, may therefore initiate an action potential in the distal tissue with a delay that is a combination of electrotonic transmission time and acceleration of phase four depolarization. This delay may be long enough to allow repolarization of the proximal cells and produce reflection (10). A second difficulty arises with the question whether inhomogeneities exist within the gap or at the boundaries of the depressed segment with the normally excitable tissues. When asymmetric depression is present in the gap, micro-reentry of the Schmitt-Erlanger type (Fig. 3) may occur. When inhomogeneities exist at the boundaries, transmission between proximal and distal excitable segments may not be purely electrotonic, but instead may be a mixture of electrotonic spread and slow conduction in a transitory region where excitability gradually returns to normal (10). The essential requirement for reflection is that the delay across the gap be long enough to allow the proximal cells to repolarize, so that the retrogradely transmitted electrotonic potential can reexcite these cells at the end of their refractory period. Figure 12 shows the results of a computer simulation in which two excitable elements were connected via a high-resistance gap [essentially the same phenomena occur when an inexcitable element is interposed between two or more excitable elements (95)]. Element number one was stimulated and produced an action potential. In the left panel, the second element showed only a subthreshold depolarization, but in the right panel, where coupling resistance was slightly decreased, the second element produced an action potential, preceded by a slow prepotential. The delay between the two active responses was the longest that could be achieved. During this delay, the membrane capacity of the second element was discharged by depolarizing

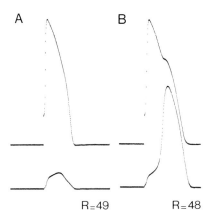

FIG. 12. Computer simulation of interaction of two excitable elements across a high-resistance gap. **A:** the coupling resistance R (in arbitrary units) is just too high to permit propagation from the stimulated element (*upper trace*) to the second element (*lower trace*). **B:** at a slightly lower value of the coupling resistance, the second element is activated. Its activation corresponds with a hump in the repolarization phase of the first element. The latency between the activation of both elements represents the longest obtainable delay. (From ref. 196, with permission.)

current supplied by the first cell, until threshold was reached. The latency could not outlast the duration of the action potential of the first cell. The reason for this is simply that during the period of latency, depolarizing current flows from the first to the second cell, and therefore the membrane potential of the first cell must during this time be more positive. The second element can fire, if it fires at all, only well before the first element has repolarized. The only effect on the first element is a hump during the plateau phase that lengthens the duration of the proximal action potential. Exactly the same action potential configurations were obtained in experiments in which feline and canine ventricular trabeculae were placed in a three-compartment bath in which the central compartment was superfused with solutions containing very high levels of K^+ (25–35 mM) (174). In computer simulation studies (95) it was necessary to produce an extra delay in the distal elements to produce reflection that resulted in a premature action potential in the proximal elements. This was achieved by adding pacemaking properties to the distal elements. *In vitro* studies on tissue without pacemaking properties (right ventricular trabeculae or epicardial muscle strips) showed that delay produced by a nonhomogeneously depressed zone could result in reflection, causing closely coupled premature action potentials in proximal cells (174). Figure 13 shows transmembrane potentials recorded from an epicardial strip of muscle, where the proximal (P) and distal (D) ends were superfused with normal Tyrode solution, while the central segment (a gap 1 mm in width) was superfused with a solution containing 35 mM K^+. The action potential of the proximal cells brought the distal cells to threshold after

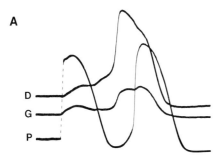

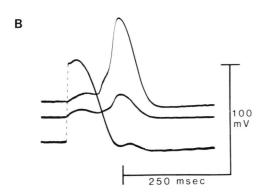

FIG. 13. Transmembrane potentials recorded from a strip of feline epicardial ventricular muscle placed in a three-compartment tissue bath. Proximal (P) and distal (D) segments were superfused with normal Tyrode solution. The middle segment 1 mm in width was superfused with a solution containing 35 mM K^+ ("inexcitable gap," G). The preparation was stimulated at the proximal end with a basic cycle length of 1 sec. In **A**, the distal element is activated with sufficient delay to allow reflection across the inexcitable gap, and reexcitation of the proximal segment occurs. (From ref. 174, with permission.)

a delay of 120 msec, at which time the proximal cells had repolarized. The action potentials of the distal cells produced a second electrotonic potential in the gap, which succeeded in eliciting a premature action potential in the proximal segment (panel A) or, at other times, produced only a subthreshold depolarization at the end of repolarization (panel B). Similar recordings were made when the central segment was superfused with high-K^+ solutions containing tetrodotoxin and verapamil to prevent any regenerative responses to occur in the central gap. It can clearly be seen that the electrotonic depolarization reflecting the time course of the proximal action potential did not bring the distal cells to threshold, but a second, slow depolarization did so. The reason for this extra delay was most likely due to the existence of a transitory zone of reduced excitability between the inexcitable gap and the fully excitable distal and proximal cells. At the boundary of the gap, because of diffusion of K^+, fibers close to the boundary will be exposed to relatively high levels of K^+, and fibers farther away to lower, but still elevated, concentrations. Therefore, both depressed fast responses and slow responses may occur

at the boundary, either of which could be responsible for the second slow depolarization that precedes the distal action potential. The important result of these studies is that propagation across a small (1–2 mm) segment of inexcitable tissue is discontinuous and can result in delays on the order of 100 to 200 msec (10,174), which is long enough to allow proximal cells to recover their excitability and be available for reexcitation. Such a situation may exist in hearts with regional ischemia, where local inhomogeneities (due, for example, to local variations in extracellular K^+ concentrations) (81) may give rise to conditions similar to those present in the *in vitro* studies. It would obviously be very difficult to prove the reality of reflection models in the intact heart. The potential sites for reflection are many, and because of their small dimensions, they could easily escape detection.

REENTRY IN THE SINUS NODE

Slow conduction has been recognized for a long time as a factor promoting reentry. The sinus node would therefore seem to be a natural site for reentry, because conduction velocity within the sinus node may be as low as 5 cm/sec (162). Already in 1943 it was suggested that the sinus node could participate in a reentrant circuit (11). Several studies, using microelectrode recordings from isolated preparations, have provided evidence that reentry can indeed occur in the sinus node (2,16,77,116,192). In most of these, the atrium was paced, and after a properly timed premature stimulus, a nonstimulated "echo beat" followed the activation initiated by the premature stimulus. In one study, the preparation was beating spontaneously, and after each 15th spontaneous beat, a single premature stimulus delivered to the atrium produced an echo beat (2). In none of the experimental studies has a sustained circus movement been demonstrated in the sinus node, the only manifestation of sinus node reentry being as single echo beat. Han and co-workers (77) made subsequent microelectrode recordings at 18 different sites during the time period in which the echo beat could reproducibly be initiated. The activation sequence of the impaled cells in the sinus node was different during conduction of the premature beat, as compared with the sequence during regular atrial pacing. Conduction block occurred in some cells; others were activated much later than expected. Although circus movement could not be proved because of the limited number of recording sites, the findings were in agreement with the concept of functional longitudinal dissociation occurring during propagation of an atrial premature impulse, possibly based on differences in refractoriness within the sinus node. The most complete study was the one by Allessie and Bonke (2) in which moments of activation during a sinus echo were determined of 130 sinus node fibers (from subsequent microelectrode recordings) and 32 adjacent atrial sites (from simultaneously recorded atrial extracellular electrograms). A circus movement could be demonstrated, located in the center of the sinus node (i.e., the area where during spontaneous sinus rhythm the im-

pulses were generated). The dimension was very small, the diameter being on the order of 1 to 2 mm. Figure 14 shows in diagrammatic fashion the pathway of the induced atrial premature impulse and the resulting sinus echo. In the lower part of the sinus node, entrance block

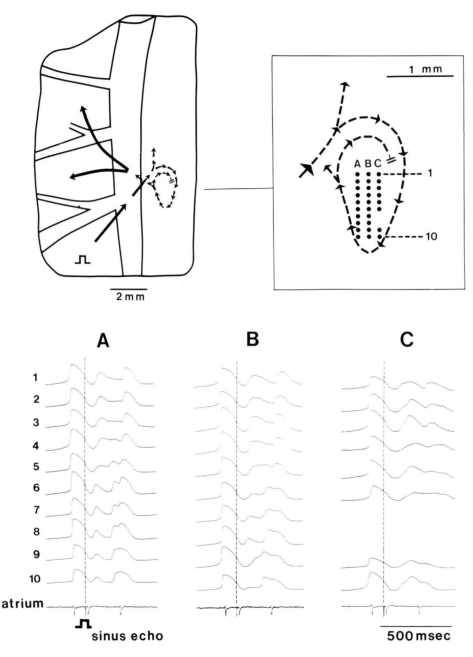

FIG. 14. Electrical activity in the center of a reentrant circuit in the sinus node. A premature stimulus applied to the atrium close to the sinus node results in a sinus echo that reexcites the atrium. **Upper panels:** localization and dimensions of the reentrant circuit. Three rows of recording sites (A, B, and C) in the center of the circuit are indicated. Each *dot* represents a successful impalement of a sinus node fiber. The distance between rows was 150 μm; the distance between recording points in a row was 100 μm. **Lower panels:** transmembrane potentials at the corresponding points. These were not simultaneously recorded, but successively with a single microelectrode during repeated induction of identical sinus echoes. Each tracing starts with the last action potential of a series of 15 normal sinus beats. The *broken vertical line* indicates the moment of the stimulus applied to the atrium. During sinus rhythm, action potentials were completely normal. During the circuitous pathway of the impulse around the area recorded from, strong electrotonic interactions become apparent. The circulating wave front exerts an electrotonic depolarizing effect on the fibers in the center, leading either to a prolonged depolarization (fibers 1–5) or to fusion responses (fibers 6–10). (From ref. 2, with permission.)

occurred (arrows pointing from left to right, ending in a double bar). However, the premature wavefront was conducted in the upper part of the node, then traveled downward around the zone of block to emerge 225 msec after the premature stimulus at the border between sinus node and atrium to reexcite the atrium. Also shown are microelectrode recordings from the center of the reentrant circuit. During the circus movement, the circulating wave front exerted a depolarizing influence on fibers in the vortex, leading either to markedly prolonged action potentials or to fusion responses. During spontaneous sinus rhythm, the fibers in the center of the circuit showed completely normal action potentials. No evidence was found for anatomically separated pathways serving as a preexisting reentrant circuit. On the contrary, the electrotonic interactions between fibers in the center and fibers that conducted the impulse around the center strongly suggested that there was electrical continuity across the center of the circuit. As already mentioned, in none of the experimental studies, which were all performed on normal tissue, was a sustained circus movement in the sinus node observed. Clinical evidence exists that certain types of supraventricular tachycardia may be based on sinus reentry (34,158,163). It is possible that in the presence of abnormal, diseased sinus node tissue, the chances for persisting circus movement are enhanced.

REENTRY IN THE ATRIUM

Atrial Flutter

Atrial flutter is a supraventricular tachycardia that in man is defined on the basis of electrocardiographic characteristics. The atrial rate is higher than 240/min (209), but the upper and lower limits of atrial rate are not well defined in various studies (218). In the electrocardiogram, so-called flutter waves are seen that are equally spaced and have equal contours and amplitudes. The flutter waves cause a characteristic continuous activity of the base line. When direct electrograms are recorded from the atrial surface during surgery, cycle length, polarity, morphology, and amplitude of the electrograms are uniform (218). Similar arrhythmias can be induced in dogs by rapid atrial stimulation, and atrial flutter was the first arrhythmia in which mapping experiments supported the concept of circus movement (127). Rosenblueth and Garcia Ramos (173) extended the observations of Lewis and co-workers. By crushing the tissue between the orifices of the two caval veins, thus increasing the dimension of the anatomical obstacle, they easily induced flutter by rapid atrial stimulation. They were able to fulfill Mines's third criterion: By extending the lower limit of the obstacle to the atrioventricular groove, so that the obstacle was no longer surrounded on all sides by excitable tissue, the flutter

was terminated and could no longer be induced. More elaborate mapping studies by Kimura et al. (111) and Hayden et al. (80) provided additional evidence that a large circus movement around an anatomical obstacle could produce flutter. The main characteristics of experimental flutter were (a) that the arrhythmia could be induced and terminated by electrical stimulation, (b) that the pathway of excitation (although not mapped in great detail) was in agreement with that expected for circus movement, and (c) that cutting through the pathway abolished the arrhythmia.

The study of Hayden et al. (80) included 2 dogs with spontaneous flutter, but it is unknown if any anatomical abnormalities were present in these animals. Boineau et al. (15) performed extensive mapping in a dog with spontaneous atrial flutter. In addition to showing circus movement, he found an area of slow conduction in a hypoplastic region in the right atrium lateral to the superior vena cava that was considered to be the site of unidirectional block, necessary for initiation of circus movement reentry. In most cases the anatomical obstacle included the orifices of the caval veins. However, as Lewis had already indicated (127), the circulating wave could in some instances not circulate around the cavae, but "in some other ring of muscle such as that surrounding the mitral orifice." Recent experiments (64) partially confirmed Lewis's suggestion. When an incision was made extending from superior to inferior vena cava, with an additional branching incision from inferior vena cava, extending parallel to the atrioventricular groove toward the right atrial appendage, flutter could be initiated and terminated by electrical stimulation, which was based on circus movement in the tricuspid ring.

If, indeed, atrial flutter is caused by a large circus movement around an anatomical obstacle, one would expect an excitable gap to be present, permitting resetting and termination of the arrhythmia by premature stimuli. Clinical experience in this respect varies. Wellens (209,212) was unable to terminate atrial flutter by premature stimulation and concluded that the arrhythmia was caused either by a focal mechanism or by a small reentrant circuit located low in the atrium. The same conclusion was reached after intraoperative atrial mapping in a patient with atrial flutter (215). Other investigators reported similar results (106,201). In some clinical studies, however, it was found that single premature stimuli could "reset" the flutter, and in rare cases even terminate it (41,88). The width of the excitable gap was estimated at 14 to 25% of the cycle length of the flutter (88). Thus, clinical studies provide evidence variously arguing against and in favor of the existence of large reentrant circuits with a sizable excitable gap. Atrial flutter in humans, and also in dogs, can occur in different types (15,218). In man, type I and type II have been distinguished (218). The main difference was that type I was influenced by stimulation from the high right atrium, and type II was not. Also, the rate of type I flutter was slower. Both the size of the excitable gap and the distance from site or stimulation to reentrant circuit determine whether or not a reentrant rhythm is influenced by extra stimuli. Failure to influence an arrhythmia by extra stimuli does not rule out reentry. It is therefore quite possible that reentry of types F and G, schematically depicted in Fig. 7, can both occur and can be the cause of atrial flutter in man.

Evidence for a leading-circle type of reentry underlying flutter was provided by Allessie et al. (6). Endocardial mapping of the atria was performed in isolated dog hearts, perfused with blood according to the Langendorff technique. Recordings were made from 960 electrodes (simultaneous recordings could be made from 192 different sites). Flutter was induced by rapid atrial pacing, after addition of acetylcholine to the blood. In all cases, an intraatrial circus movement of the leading-circle type was demonstrated. Cycle lengths of the flutter varied in the different hearts from 65 to 145 msec, and lengths of the reentrant circuits from 5 to 10 cm. No site of special preference was found; the circuits could be anywhere in either left or right atrium. Although in these experiments the wavelength was reduced by shortening of the refractory period by acetylcholine, the conclusion seems warranted that in the atrium a wide spectrum of reentrant circuits may occur. The presence of anatomical obstacles, or areas of depressed conduction and excitability, will facilitate the occurrence of reentry. Given the proper conditions, resulting in a reduction in wavelength, intraatrial reentry can occur without involvement of an anatomical obstacle.

Atrial Fibrillation

Atrial fibrillation in dogs can be induced in various ways. Garrey (72) used strong faradic shocks applied to the atrium and demonstrated that the resulting fibrillation, although often short-lived, was not sustained from the site where it had been initiated. After induction of fibrillation by faradizing an atrial appendage, he removed the appendage and observed that the appendage became quiescent, but the atria continued to fibrillate. Another way to induce atrial fibrillation is local application of aconitine (177). Although the resulting rhythm is the same, as far as rate and irregularity are concerned, as fibrillation induced by other means, this type of fibrillation is dependent for its continuation on the site where aconitine was applied. After clamping off the appendage, after application of aconitine, from the rest of the atria, sinus rhythm was promptly restored in the atrium, while the clamped-off appendage showed a fast, regular tachycardia (149). This experiment demonstrated that the arrhythmia was due to a focus that fired so rapidly that uniform excitation of the atria was no longer possible.

When areas of conduction block develop at multiple sites, with different dimensions, and when sites and dimensions change from beat to beat, the excitation pattern of the atria becomes irregular, and cycle lengths in different parts of the atria will vary. This kind of fibrillation may best be described as "fibrillatory conduction" (7). Moe and Abildskov (149) also studied the kind of fibrillation produced by Garrey. They found that atrial fibrillation induced by rapid stimulation of the atrial appendage quickly stopped spontaneously, but when combined with vagal stimulation, fibrillation persisted for as long as vagal stimulation was maintained. When during this type of fibrillation the appendage was clamped off, fibrillation ceased in the appendage and continued in the rest of the atrium. This arrhythmia could be called true fibrillation. To explain the characteristics of this type of fibrillation, the multiple-wavelet hypothesis was formulated (147,149). The key element of this hypothesis is that the

> wave front becomes fractionated as it divides about islets or strands of refractory tissue, and each of the daughter wavelets may now be considered as independent offspring. Such a wavelet may accelerate or decelerate as it encounters tissue in a more or less advanced state of recovery. It may become extinguished as it encounters refractory tissue; it may divide again or combine with a neighbor; it may be expected to fluctuate in size and change in direction. Its course, though determined by the excitability or refractoriness of surrounding tissue, would appear to be as random as Brownian motion. Fully developed fibrillation would then be a state in which many such randomly wandering wavelets coexist (149).

Moe (147) emphasized that although the multiple-wavelet hypothesis was perhaps only a variation of the circus movement theory, "it seems unlikely that repeated passage of an impulse through a constant or slightly wavering route could be a stable process, consistent with continuation for months or years." In maintained atrial fibrillation, "the circuits must be multiple, changing in position, shape, size and number with each successive excitation" (147). Moe also stated that "direct test of the hypothesis is difficult, if not impossible in living tissue." At that time, simultaneous recording from a sufficient number of atrial sites to document the complex excitation pattern was impossible. Moe and associates developed a computer model to simulate atrial fibrillation (155). The key feature of the model was a nonhomogeneous distribution of refractory periods in otherwise identical elements. Premature stimulation at sites with short refractory periods initiated a self-sustaining rhythm that was rapid and irregular. The rhythm was sustained by "irregular drifting eddies which varied in position, number and size" (155). The average number of individually wandering wavelets varied between 23 and 40. The arrhythmia could be terminated by prolonging the refractory period.

Direct test of the multiple-wavelet hypothesis was performed by Allessie and co-workers (7). They inserted two egg-shaped multipolar electrodes into the atrial cavities of isolated, Langendorff-perfused dog hearts. Each electrode contained 480 recording terminals, equally spaced at distances of 3 mm. Simultaneous recordings could be made from 192 terminals. Atrial fibrillation was induced by a single premature stimulus, while acetylcholine was continuously administered to the perfusion fluid. Fibrillation was maintained as long as acetylcholine was infused, but terminated spontaneously as soon as the infusion was stopped. During maintained fibrillation, excitations of right and left atria were mapped consecutively. The presence of multiple independent wavelets was demonstrated. Conduction velocity of the wavelets varied between 20 and 90 cm/sec. The widths of the wavelets could be as small as a few millimeters, but broad wave fronts propagating uniformly over large segments of the atria were observed as well. Each individual wavelet existed for a short time, not longer than several hundred milliseconds. Extinction of a wavelet could be caused by fusion or collision with another wavelet, by reaching the border of the atria, or by meeting refractory tissue. New wavelets could be formed by division of a wave at a local area of conduction block, or by an offspring of a wave, traveling toward the other atrium. The major difference between the excitation pattern during this type of atrial fibrillation and the rhythm in the computer model of Moe and associates was that the number of wavelets was much smaller. It was estimated that the critical number of wavelets in both atria necessary to maintain fibrillation was between three and six. Although no evidence for rapidly discharging foci was found, this possibility could not be excluded: "the basic mechanism would be the presence of multiple wandering wavelets, but the statistical chance of termination of fibrillation by simultaneous cancellation of wavelets could be reduced to zero by the additional support of one or more sites of impulse formation" (7).

It may be questioned whether atrial fibrillation induced by rapid or premature stimulation, with or without concomitant vagal stimulation or administration of acetylcholine, is the same arrhythmia as spontaneously occurring atrial fibrillation. Autocorrelograms and histograms of the ventricular rhythms of patients with atrial fibrillation, and of dogs with spontaneous atrial fibrillation, show the same random pattern of successive R-R intervals (17,141,191). In contrast, in dogs with artificially induced atrial fibrillation, the autocorrelogram of the ventricular rhythm may show a nonrandom distribution of ventricular cycles (191), in which the occurrence of "long cycles tends to favour the occurrence of subsequent long cycles" (150). It has been argued that a nonrandom distribution of ventricular cycles cannot be attributed to true atrial fibrillation, which is a random process, but requires additional sources of (focal?) activity (191).

REENTRY IN THE ATRIOVENTRICULAR JUNCTION

Reentry Utilizing Accessory Atrioventricular Pathways

In 1914, Mines (146) predicted that circus movement should occur in hearts with multiple atrioventricular (AV) connections following a properly timed premature impulse, but it took many years before his views were commonly accepted. Some of the milestones that mark the way from hypothesis to clinical application are the following. In 1915, Wilson (223) described a patient, suffering from recurrent attacks of tachycardia, with the electrocardiographic characteristics of what is now called the Wolff-Parkinson-White (WPW) syndrome, namely a short P-R interval and a broad QRS complex with an abnormal initial deflection. In 1930, Wolff, Parkinson, and White reported on 11 such patients, all young and healthy apart from their attacks of tachycardia (233). In 1932, Holzmann and Scherf (86) were the first to propose that muscular bundles linking atrium and ventricle could account for the electrocardiographic characteristics. In 1933, Wolferth and Wood (232) suggested that the tachycardias might be due to reentry. In 1943, Wood and co-workers (235) reported on the presence of abnormal AV connections in a boy with the WPW syndrome who had died of paroxysmal tachycardia. In 1967, Durrer and Roos (48) recorded directly from the surface of the heart during surgery in a patient with the WPW syndrome and demonstrated a site of early ventricular excitation on the lateral base of the right ventricle. In the same year, Burchell et al. (20) confirmed these findings and were able to temporarily ablate the accessory pathway. Also in 1967, Durrer et al. (49) used programmed electrical stimulation to initiate and terminate circus movement tachycardia in patients with the WPW syndrome, and this marked the beginning of many clinical studies employing electrical stimulation to elucidate arrhythmia mechanisms and to guide antiarrhythmic therapy in many different types of tachycardias (212). The first successful surgical interruption of the anomalous AV connection, resulting in permanent cessation of tachycardias and normalization of the electrocardiograms, was performed in 1968 (25).

The usual way in which tachycardia is initiated is by a properly timed atrial or ventricular premature beat that is blocked in one of the two AV connections. The reentrant pathway consists of atrium, AV node, ventricular conduction system, ventricular myocardium, and accessory pathways. Usually, conduction from atrium to ventricle during circus movement tachycardia is via the AV node, conduction from ventricle to atrium via the accessory pathway. However, variations are possible. The many possible AV connections can be classified according to the European study group for preexcitation (8) into (a) accessory AV pathways, which directly connect atrial and ventricular myocardium, (b) nodo-ventricular accessory pathways, connecting the AV node with ventricular myocardium, (c) fasciculo ventricular accessory pathways, which form a link between the penetrating part or the branching part of the AV bundle (the bundle of His), and (d) AV nodal bypass tracts, which are pathways connecting the atrium either with the penetrating AV bundle (atriofascicular bypass tracts) or with ventricular myocardium. In one heart, multiple accessory pathways may exist. It is therefore not surprising that many variations of Mines's type of reentrant circuit are possible, and it is no surprise that 15 different ways of initiating circus movement tachycardia in patients with accessory pathways have been described (211). For more details concerning reentrant arrhythmias in such patients, the reader is referred to the articles by Gallagher and co-workers (68) and by Wellens (210,212). In man, there are no other arrythmias in which the criteria of Mines have been more completely fulfilled.

Reentry in the AV Node

Reentry in the AV node was considered in a clinical case report in 1915 by White (220), in which during AV dissociation, idioventricular beats were sometimes propagated back to the atrium, to be followed by a QRS complex. When such "reciprocation" occurred and an inverted P wave was sandwiched between two QRS complexes, there was an inverse relation between retrograde conduction time (long R-P interval) and antegrade conduction time (short P-R interval). The explanation given was that during retrograde conduction only part of the AV node was capable of conducting the impulse to the atrium, another part being still refractory. Conduction to the atrium was slow enough so that the part with the longer refractory period could recover and be available for antegrade conduction. The sum of retrograde and antegrade conduction times would be sufficient to allow recovery of excitability in the lower node and His bundle so that reexcitation of the ventricles would occur. The first experimental study on this form of reciprocal rhythm was performed by Scherf and Shookhoff in 1926 (179), and their findings and interpretation were similar. They induced a series of ventricular extrasystoles in a dog heart in which AV conduction was impaired by administration of quinine hydrochloride. The last extrasystole was conducted with delay to the atria and returned to the ventricles, causing a ventricular premature beat. This beat was called "return extrasystole" ("umkehr Extrasystole" or "reciprocal beat"). The concept of "functional longitudinal dissociation" within the AV node was introduced in that report. Because the

P-R interval of the return extrasystole was inversely related to the preceding R-P interval, it was concluded that at least part of the conduction path was used by the impulse in both directions. These experiments were later extended by Moe and co-workers (154) and by Rosenblueth (172), who introduced the term "echoes."

The early studies were devoted to ventricular echoes; reciprocation in the other direction, in which an impulse originating in the sinus node or in the atrium turns back in the AV node to reexcite the atrium, received attention at a later stage (113). This could have been due to difficulties in differentiating an atrial echo from an atrial or junctional premature beat with blocked propagation to the ventricles (183).

When techniques for intracardiac recording and stimulation during cardiac catheterization were developed, allowing recording and stimulation from various sites in the atria and His bundle in man (49,76), many reports on both atrial and ventricular echoes appeared (13,167,183,184). Echo beats could be induced by premature stimulation in hearts with no apparent AV conduction disturbances, so that the phenomenon of functional longitudinal dissociation can be considered to be a normal physiological mechanism (184). Analysis of time intervals between signals recorded from ventricles, His bundle, and atrium sometimes led to the conclusion that at least three functionally different pathways existed in the AV node (112,183). Animal experiments in which the echo phenomenon was studied in a similar way, by analyzing input-output relations of the AV node, also supported the idea that echoes can be induced in normal hearts by appropriately timed premature stimuli (137,144,154). The chances for AV nodal reentry are obviously increased when conduction through the node is impaired, be it by disease or drugs.

In patients with spontaneous reciprocal tachycardia it has been possible to induce repetitive AV nodal reentry by premature stimulation of the atria (13,28,167), but in humans with normal AV nodal function, repetitive reentry cannot be induced. In animal experiments it has in a few instances been possible to induce repetitive AV nodal reciprocation (97,138,151,227), and some of the publications are case reports (97,151).

The studies providing the most direct evidence that reentry can occur within the AV node are those in which echo beats or reciprocating tachycardia occurred during microelectrode recording in the AV node of isolated rabbit preparations (97,138,161,203,227). The experiments of Mendez and Moe (138) gave the first direct evidence that the upper part of the AV node is functionally and spatially dissociated into two pathways, called alpha and beta pathways. Somewhere in the lower node these paths are joined together to form a final common pathway that connects to the bundle of His. An atrial premature beat can be blocked in the alpha pathway while being conducted via the beta path. On

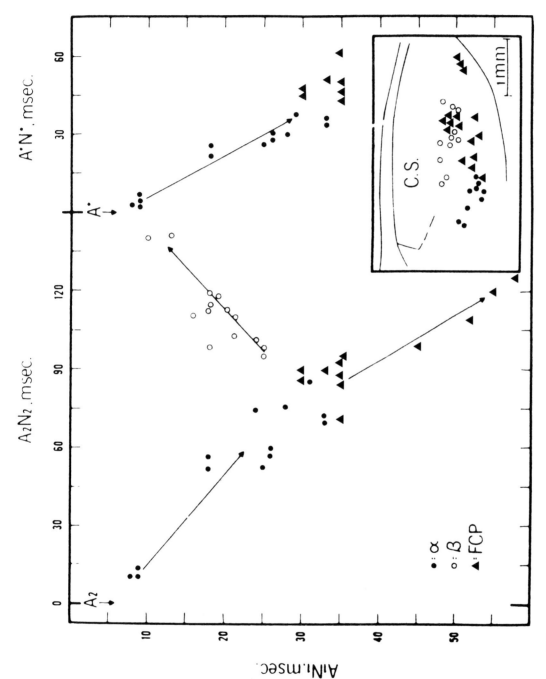

FIG. 15. Anatomical and temporal relationship of 35 fibers in rabbit AV node during an echo beat. On the *vertical axis*, the activation time of each cell is indicated during propagation of a basic beat driven from the atrium $(A_1 N_1)$. Although expressed in time, it can be regarded as an arbitrary distance scale, going from atrium to His bundle. On the *horizontal axis*, the activation times of the same cells are indicated during a premature atrial impulse $(A_2 N_2)$, the resulting echo $(A^* N^*)$ and the abortive re-echo. The **inset** shows anatomical positions of the recording points (CS = coronary sinus). *Filled circles* indicate cells belonging to the alpha pathway (antegrade pathway), *open circles* are cells in the beta pathway (retrograde pathway), and *triangles* are cells in the final common pathway (FCP) leading to the His bundle. (From ref. 138, with permission.)

reaching the junction, the alpha pathway is retrogradely invaded, and the impulse can reexcite the atrium as an echo. The echo can again penetrate the beta pathway, and the sequence can repeat itself, leading to circus movement tachycardia. Variations are possible, for example, an "abortive" echo, in which retrograde activity in the alpha path fails to reach the atrium, or failure of the atrial echo to conduct antegradely in the beta path. Figure 15 shows the anatomical and temporal relationship of 35 different AV nodal fibers, successively impaled with a single microelectrode during repeated induction of an atrial echo in an isolated rabbit heart preparation. On the vertical axis, the position of each cell is indicated during propagation of a regularly driven beat from the atrium (A_1N_1). Although expressed in time, the vertical axis can be regarded as an arbitrary distance scale, going from atrium to His bundle. On the horizontal axis, the activation times of the same cells during conduction of a premature atrial impulse (A_2N_2) and of the resulting atrial echo are indicated. In this experiment, the atrial echo did reach the final common path again, but failed to conduct to the His bundle, and also failed to retro-

gradely invade the alpha path. However, in a "surprising number of preparations, two or more complete circuits were recorded," and "in some episodes, eight or ten complete circuits were sustained" (138). Wit and co-workers (227) were able to induce repetitive reentry in 6 of 40 isolated rabbit heart preparations, lasting from 20 to 500 cycles. Whenever this occurred, the tachycardia could be repeatedly terminated and initiated by premature stimulation. Janse et al. (97) recorded by means of a "brush" electrode consisting of 10 microelectrodes from 54 AV nodal cells both during regular driving of the atrium and during sustained tachycardia. The tachycardia did not terminate spontaneously, but could be repeatedly and reproducibly initiated and terminated by premature stimuli. Figure 16 shows simultaneous recordings from a cell in the alpha pathway (N_1, or "retrograde pathway") and from a cell in the beta pathway (N_2, or "antegrade pathway"). During tachycardia, a stimulator gave off stimuli to the right atrium at a regular rate, most of which fell in the refractory period of the atrium, but which sometimes excited the atrium prematurely. In the diagram, the hatched line

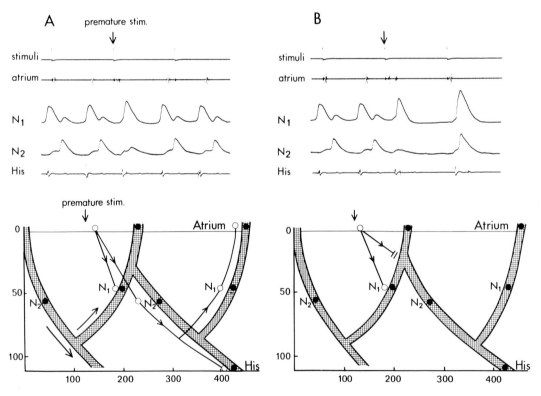

FIG. 16. Effect of premature beats applied during tachycardia caused by reentry in the rabbit AV node. **A:** "Resetting" of tachycardia by a stimulus applied 145 msec after the atrial complex. **B:** Termination of tachycardia by a premature stimulus applied 135 msec after the atrial complex. **Upper panels** show stimuli, atrial and His bundle electrograms, and transmembrane potentials from a cell belonging to the retrograde pathway (N_1) and a cell of the antegrade pathway (N_2). During tachycardia, stimuli were applied at a fixed rate to the atrium, most of them falling in the atrial refractory period, and some of them exciting the atrium prematurely. In the diagram, the *vertical axis* is a time scale indicating the moments of activation of N_1 and N_2 during a basic beat driven from the atrium. The *horizontal axis* indicates the activation times of N_1 and N_2 during steady-state tachycardia (*hatched bars, filled circles*) and during the interpolated atrial premature beats (*open circles*). (See text for discussion.) (From ref. 97, with permission.)

schematically depicts the activation sequence during tachycardia, and the solid circles depict the activation times of N_1 and N_2. Superimposed on this sequence are the moments of activation of N_1 and N_2 following the atrial premature stimuli. In panel A, the atrial premature impulse excited cell N_2 prematurely (open circles) and reached cell N_1 almost simultaneously with the retrograde front coming up from the node. Tachycardia was thus "reset." The premature impulse reached the circuit when it was relatively refractory, so that its propagation into the antegrade pathway was slower than during steady-state tachycardia. Therefore, although the next complexes are earlier than would have been expected if the premature impulse had no effect at all, the interval following the premature beat is longer than the steady-state tachycardia cycle. In fact, confusion with a compensatory pause (indicating a focal mechanism) is possible. In panel B, a slightly earlier premature impulse fails to excite the antegrade path (N_2) but can propagate into the retrograde path and excite N_1 before the arrival of the retrograde front. The two fronts collide, and the circuit is extinguished. In the last beat of panel B, the atrium follows the stimulator, and during normal AV nodal propagation, N_1 and N_2 are now nearly simultaneously excited. Although these studies strongly support the concept of intranodal reentry being responsible for echoes and tachycardia, it must be emphasized that in the studies employing microelectrodes, recordings have been made from very few cells. The reentrant pathway has by no means been mapped completely; in the study of Janse et al. (97), action potentials were recorded from only two cells in the antegrade pathway. Nor has it been possible to interrupt the circuit and terminate echoes or tachycardia. Therefore, the possibility of triggered activity cannot be excluded (197,225).

Functional dissociation in the AV node is presumed to be the result of differences in refractory periods of alpha and beta pathways, but this has never been directly demonstrated. No anatomical delineation of alpha and beta pathways has been found, although the AV node has two atrial "inputs," one via the crista terminalis, the other via the interatrial septum, and these could serve as alpha and beta pathways (96). The question whether or not part of the atrium is a necessary part of the circuit has not been completely settled, and arguments pro (137,185,227) and con (104,144) can be found. It is quite possible that the complex architecture of the upper AV node, with different coupling resistances in different directions, and with many branching sites, could lead to functional dissociation based on tissue anisotropy rather than on differences in refractory periods. The findings illustrated in Fig. 15, where action potentials of antegrade and retrograde pathways are in electrotonic contact, support the notion that the two pathways are not anatomically separated and are not electrically insulated from each other.

REENTRY IN THE HIS-PURKINJE SYSTEM
Macro-reentry

Functional dissociation within the AV node need not be the only cause for the occurrence of atrial echoes. When differences in refractory periods exist between right and left bundle branches, a premature impulse (originating in atrium, AV node, or His bundle) may be blocked in one of the branches and conducted in the other. The branch where block occurs may be retrogradely invaded by activity traveling from one side of the interventricular septum to the other, and reexcitation of the tissue proximal to the block may occur. Moe et al. (153) obtained evidence that a premature impulse, induced in the canine His bundle, could be blocked in the right bundle branch and that retrograde activation of the right bundle occurred via conduction from the left side of the septum, sometimes resulting in an atrial echo. Especially at slow heart rates, even an atrial premature beat could induce an atrial echo in this way, because it could traverse the AV node before the refractory period in one of the bundle branches had ended (83,153). Several clinical cases of ventricular tachycardia, where, for example, it was found that an atrial premature beat could terminate the tachycardia (216), or in which surgical interruption of the anterior division of the left bundle abolished the arrhythmia (190), were interpreted as being due to macro-reentry involving the bundle branches. Direct recording from the suggested reentrant pathway was, of course, impossible in these patients, and the success of surgery may also have been due to other surgical interventions that were simultaneously carried out, such as aneurysmectomy.

Premature stimulation of the ventricles may induce another type of macro-reentry involving the bundle branches. Because the refractory period of the bundle branches is longer than that of ventricular myocardium (92,156), a premature stimulus delivered to the right side of the septum may fail to retrogradely excite the right bundle. The impulse will be conducted through the septal myocardium, activate the left bundle after some delay, travel toward the His bundle, cross over to the right bundle, and excite the distal part of the right bundle 100 to 170 msec after the premature stimulus (92). Reexcitation of the right ventricular myocardium was not observed in the study of Janse (92), but was demonstrated by Lyons and Burgess (128), who recorded from six different sites of the canine specialized conducting system. These authors proved that the occurrence of a nonstimulated ventricular response following an induced ventricular premature beat was due to reentry via the long pathway described, not due to local reentry or triggered activity, by sectioning the right bundle (or by blocking conduction in it by long anodal pulses), which prevented the phenomenon. They observed on occasion two loops of reentrant activation, but could not produce longer runs of successive reentrant impulses. Similar reentry has been found in humans during right ventricular stimulation (1). Most often, a single reentrant ventricular impulse occurs, but sometimes reentry is observed for three successive beats. Longer runs have not been observed (57,61,62). This form of reentry in the His-Purkinje system (most commonly called "bundle branch reentry" or "V_3 phenomenon") occurs in about 50% of so-called normal patients, i.e., patients who have no history or evidence of arrhythmias, electrolyte imbalance, or ischemia (40,62). It may therefore be considered to be a physiological response to premature stimulation of the ventricles. Its characteristics include the following: (a) the His bundle deflection in the extracellular His bundle electrogram precedes the reentrant complex V_3; (b) the time from prematurely induced ventricular response (V_2) to retrogradely activated His bundle response (H_2) is prolonged; (c) the interval between H_2 and V_3 is normal or prolonged; (d) the QRS configuration of V_3 is similar to that of the paced beats.

Micro-reentry

Short refractory periods (on the order of 30 msec) have been found to occur in Purkinje fibers just proximal to a site of unidirectional block between Purkinje fiber and ventricular myocardium, caused by premature stimulation of a free-running Purkinje fiber (176). Very slow conduction, on the order of 5 cm/sec, has been observed in isolated Purkinje fibers exposed to medium containing high K^+ concentrations (226,228). The combination of very slow conduction and very short refractory periods can lead to a micro-reentrant circuit with a circumference of only 1 or 2 cm. Wit et al. (228) demonstrated sustained circus movement in closed loops of fibers of the specialized ventricular conducting system of canine and bovine hearts. The isolated preparations consisted of both Purkinje fibers and ventricular myocardium, and conduction in part of the preparation (or sometimes in the entire preparation) was depressed by exposure to 15 mM K^+ and 5×10^{-6} M epinephrine. A premature stimulus caused unidirectional block in one part of the loop, and conduction in the other part was slow enough to outlast the refractory period and cause sustained reentry in a circuit 2 to 3 cm in length. In this experimental model, resting membrane potential was reduced to a level low enough to inactivate the fast sodium channels, and in the presence of epinephrine, slow responses, dependent only on inward current via the slow channels, were elicited. Because in acute myocardial ischemia, where myocardial fibers are exposed to elevated extracellular K^+ concentrations and to norepinephrine, a similar situation might exist, it has been speculated that such micro-reentrant circuits may occur in intact hearts with acute regional myocardial ischemia.

REENTRY IN ACUTELY ISCHEMIC VENTRICULAR MYOCARDIUM

Within a few minutes following occlusion of a coronary artery, conduction velocity in the ischemic myocardium decreases, and activation, especially of the ischemic subepicardium, becomes delayed (14,26,47,180,200,222). The increase in activation delay coincides with the spontaneous occurrence of ventricular tachycardia and fibrillation (180,222). This, and the finding of fragmented deflections in bipolar or multipolar extracellular recordings that bridged the diastolic interval between normally conducted beats and ectopic beats, or between successive beats of a tachycardia (14,47,52,55,180,200), has been interpreted as an indication that reentry is the mechanism underlying the arrhythmias caused by ischemia and infarction. Many studies in which recovery of excitability was studied with the extra-stimulus technique (where the shortest interval preceding a successful premature stimulus is determined) reported that refractory periods of ischemic myocardium shortened (18,50,78,119,123, 157,169,195). Furthermore, several studies found an increased dispersion of refractory periods during acute ischemia (78,123,157). Thus, conditions for reentry (slow conduction, short refractory periods, and inhomogeneities in recovery of excitability in adjacent areas) apparently are present in acutely ischemic myocardium.

Measurements of conduction velocity in ischemic myocardium are scarce, because it is difficult to obtain accurate information on the spread of activity in a three-dimensional structure such as the left ventricular wall in acute ischemia, where conditions change rapidly. Preliminary data, obtained by simultaneous recording from 100 extracellular electrodes positioned at 1-mm distances on the epicardial surface of the left ventricle of isolated, Langendorff-perfused porcine hearts, indicated that the lowest conduction velocities in ischemic myocardium were on the order of 20 cm/sec (in the direction parallel to the long axis of the fibers) and 10 cm/sec (in the transverse direction), compared with control values on the order of 50 and 20 cm/sec, respectively (114). These values were considerably higher than the conduction velocity of the slow response (induced during coronary perfusion of the same hearts with a solution containing 18 mM K^+ and epinephrine), where values of 10 cm/sec (longitudinal direction) and 5 cm/sec (transverse direction) were found (114).

Determination of refractory period duration in ischemic myocardium by the classic extra-stimulus technique presents several problems. First, the current requirement for stimulation rapidly increases in ischemic myocardium, and the use of strong current intensities for determination of local refractory periods may give rise to erroneous results, because tissue at a considerable distance from the stimulating electrode, with shorter refractory periods, may be excited rather than the tissue close to the site of stimulation (93). Second, action potentials of ischemic cells frequently alternate with respect to amplitude and duration, and refractory period duration then changes from beat to beat (94). Third, recovery of excitability in partially depolarized ischemic cells lags behind completion of repolarization ("post-repolarization refractoriness") (43,56,122,182), and amplitude and upstroke velocity of premature action potentials vary considerably with time elapsed after full repolarization. The smallest responses will not be able to propagate; somewhat larger action potentials will propagate more slowly than regularly paced beats. Generally speaking, because of post-repolarization refractoriness, recovery of excitability is delayed rather than shortened in ischemic myocardium (43,93). Because conduction velocity of premature responses and recovery of excitability are interrelated, it is difficult to predict the length of a reentrant pathway in ischemic myocardium by the product of "the" conduction velocity and "the" refractory period. However, a rough estimate of a

reentrant circuit of the leading-circle type would give a circuit of fairly large dimensions, given the fact that refractory period duration is prolonged and conduction velocity is not extremely reduced; a reasonable estimate would be the product of 20 cm/sec and 400 msec, which results in a pathway length of 8 cm.

Mapping experiments, in which simultaneous recordings were made from 60 epicardial or intramural sites (98) during spontaneous ventricular tachycardias occurring between 2 and 10 min after coronary artery ligation, showed that indeed circus movement reentry occurs in such large circuits (Fig. 17). A conspicuous feature of reentry in ischemic myocardium is that the position of the area of refractory tissue around which the circulating wave propagates often changes from beat to beat. This is to be expected, because ischemic cells, which at short intervals between activations fail to produce an action potential, may show large action potentials after a long pause (43). Therefore, cells that during one beat are inexcitable and belong to the vortex of a reentrant

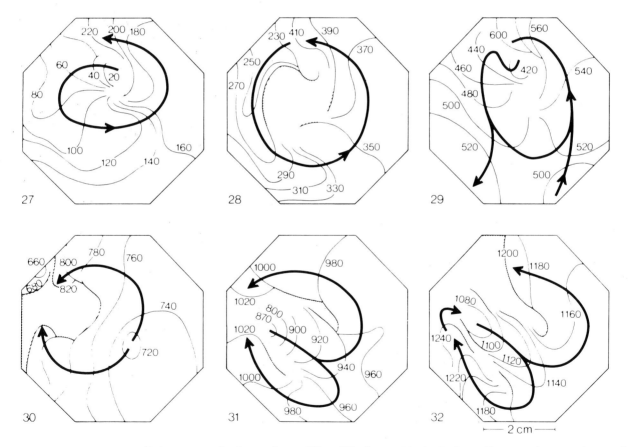

FIG. 17. Activation patterns of six consecutive beats (beats 27 to 32) of a ventricular tachycardia, occurring spontaneously 5 min after occlusion of the left anterior descending coronary artery in an isolated, perfused pig heart. Sixty electrograms were simultaneously recorded from the epicardial surface of the left ventricle within the octagonal surface depicted. Numbers at the isochrones are in msec; time zero was arbitrarily chosen. Shaded areas are zones of block. Arrows indicate general direction of spread of excitation. Note how the reentrant circuit changes its position and dimension from beat to beat. No reentrant activity could be demonstrated between beat 29 and beat 30; the source of earliest activity during beat 30 (720-msec isochrone) is unknown. Note figure-8 type of reentry in beats 30 and 31. In beat 31, two wave fronts circle around two separate areas of block to unite in a final common pathway. In beat 32, one of these wave fronts is blocked, and reentry is due to a single circulating wave. (Adapted from ref. 98.)

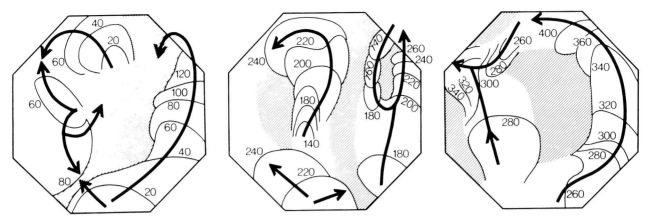

FIG. 18. Activation patterns of three successive "beats" during ischemia-induced ventricular fibrillation in an isolated perfused pig heart. Note presence of multiple independent wave fronts. Both collision and fusion of wave fronts occur, and occasionally a complete circus movement occurs. (From ref. 98, with permission.)

circuit may participate in propagation of the circulating wave in the next beat. Although activation patterns during ventricular tachycardia often showed only one circulating wave front, other forms of reentry were found as well. For example, frequently, two circulating wave fronts were present, circling around two separate areas of block, one in a clockwise direction, the other in a counterclockwise direction, both wave fronts finally uniting in a final common pathway (Fig. 17). Because of the fact that the reentrant circuit or circuits during ventricular tachycardia changed their positions from beat to beat, fulfillment of Mines's third criterion seems an impossible task in the setting of acute ischemia.

A totally different pattern of excitation was found when ventricular tachycardia degenerated into ventricular fibrillation (Fig. 18). During fibrillation, multiple independent wavelets were present, and multiple islets of conduction block that shifted their positions from beat to beat. Wave fronts could be blocked, or would extinguish themselves by collision, but summation of wave fronts could also occur. No detailed maps, such as have been made during atrial fibrillation, are available for ventricular fibrillation, and because of the three-dimensional structure of the left ventricular wall, simultaneous recording from a much larger number of sites is needed to fully describe the activation pattern of ventricular fibrillation. As yet, no estimate can be given concerning the number of independent wave fronts necessary to maintain fibrillation, nor can it be excluded that in ventricular fibrillation a rapidly discharging focus or foci coexists with reentrant excitation or "fibrillatory conduction."

Complete circus movement was mapped during ventricular fibrillation induced by premature stimulation of the canine right ventricle, made locally hypothermic (36). Diameters of the circuits varied from 8 to 30 mm, which is smaller than those of circuits found in acutely ischemic myocardium. It is conceivable that ventricular fibrillation in the very early phase of myocardial ischemia

begins as a reentrant tachycardia, although the spontaneous ventricular depolarizations that initiate the reentrant rhythm may be due to other mechanisms (95,98). Centrifugal wavelets from the reentrant circuits would be rapidly propagated via the specialized conducting system toward normal myocardium. This would be activated at a rapid rate, and because of the shifts of the reentrant circuit in the ischemic myocardium, activation of various portions of the nonischemic myocardium may at certain moments become out of phase. Because of this, and because of the shortening of the refractory period in the normal tissue, reentrant wavelets of smaller diameter than those in the ischemic zone may be set up. It has been shown that during the transitory phase from ventricular tachycardia to fibrillation, induced by sudden reperfusion after coronary artery occlusion in the dog, the nonischemic myocardium is rapidly activated (at frequencies of 500 to 600/min) and that initially this occurs in an orderly fashion (87). It has also been shown that following destruction of the Purkinje system by intracavitary application of phenol, ischemia-induced ventricular tachycardia caused by reentry in the ischemic tissue does not degenerate into ventricular fibrillation. Rather, the ventricles are activated at fairly slow rates, corresponding to the revolution times of the reentrant circuits in the ischemic myocardium, which are on the order of 350 msec (M. J. Janse, *unpublished observations*). Although much more detailed mapping is necessary to prove the hypothesis, it is conceivable that the Purkinje system is a necessary link between ischemic and normal myocardium for fibrillation to occur and that ischemia-induced fibrillation is possible only when multiple-wavelet reentry can develop in the nonischemic ventricular myocardium.

REENTRY IN INFARCTED MYOCARDIUM

The animal species most often studied for arrhythmias caused by myocardial infarction is the dog, in which several experimental models have been developed. Complete occlusion of a coronary artery, performed in two stages, where during the first 20 min the artery is constricted but not completely occluded, has been used since the pioneering studies of Harris (79). During several weeks following this procedure, ventricular tachycardias can be induced by premature stimuli (51, 52,109,234). Another infarct model in which ventricular tachycardias can be induced is based on occlusion and subsequent reperfusion, after 2 hr, of a coronary artery (69,109,142,143). In both types of infarcts, the occurrence of inducible ventricular tachycardia is dependent on the site of stimulation and on the size of the infarction. The highest incidence of induced tachycardia occurs when stimuli are applied to the left ventricle within 2 cm of the infarct border (142). Tachycardia is most easily induced in infarcts that comprise an area larger than 30% of the left ventricle (69,109). The infarcts that result from the different procedures are different. Complete occlusion produces a nearly transmural region of necrosis, with thin rims of surviving cells on endocardial and epicardial surfaces and with a sharp lateral border. In contrast, when the occluded artery is reperfused after 2 hr, the infarct is not homogeneously necrotic. Viable myocardium with normal histologic characteristics is found interposed among the necrotic myocardium throughout the infarct, giving it a mottled aspect (109,142,143). Sustained ventricular tachycardias are induced in a much greater percentage of experiments in the occlusion-reperfusion infarct model than in hearts with infarcts produced by permanent coronary artery occlusion (109,142), and this may be related to the different anatomy.

Experiments in which recordings were made simultaneously from multiple sites provided direct evidence for reentrant excitation. Both in infarcts caused by permanent occlusion (53,54,135,224) and in infarcts caused by occlusion and reperfusion (224), induced tachycardias were caused by reentry in the surviving rim of epicardial muscle overlying the infarct. It appears that tachycardia cannot be induced when the surviving rim is smaller than a few cell layers, or thicker than about 100 cells (70). Induced premature impulses can be blocked in the subepicardium of the infarcted area, and conduction through the surviving muscle layer is slow enough (around 10 cm/sec) to allow recovery of excitability in the tissue proximal to the zone of unidirectional block (224). Often, the reentrant circuit has a figure-8 configuration, where two circulating wave fronts propagate around two separate areas of block. These two wave fronts coalesce into a common wave front that travels between the two zones of block before reexciting the myocardium on the other sides of the blocks (54,135). Mines's third criterion was met in the study of El-Sherif et al. (54), who were able to terminate the tachycardia by cryoablation of the common reentrant

pathway immediately proximal to the site of earliest excitation. Localized cooling of the point of earliest excitation (the "exit" of the circuit) did not interrupt reentry, but shifted the reentrant circuit and prolonged the cycle length of the tachycardia. Other workers also could terminate induced sustained tachycardia by cooling a specific epicardial area (74). In contrast to the reentrant circuits in acutely ischemic myocardium, the reentrant circuits in the surviving subepicardium are relatively fixed. This suggests that the circuits are not solely determined by functional properties of the surviving cells, but also by anatomical factors. Indeed, it appears that the slow conduction within the surviving subepicardium is not due to a depression of upstroke characteristics but rather to the marked tissue anisotropy. In a 5-day-old canine infarct, conduction velocity in the surviving rim of subepicardial fibers was 35 cm/sec in the direction parallel to fiber orientation and 8 cm/sec in the transverse direction. Transmembrane action potentials were abnormally short, but resting membrane potential and maximum upstroke velocity were close to normal (71). At this stage, the surviving subepicardial fibers (also called the subepicardial border zone) were uniformly arranged in a thin layer. An induced premature impulse was blocked in the longitudinal direction, as in the experiments of Spach and co-workers (187) on normal atrial myocardium, and was slowly conducted tangentially and perpendicularly to the long fiber axis around the zone of block, to reexcite the tissue proximal to the block (71). With time, the structure of the epicardial border zone changes. By 2 weeks, fibrosis occurs, and muscle bundles are separated along their longitudinal axes, leaving fewer side-to-side connections between the bundles (71). A similar structure was found in resected subendocardial preparations that were the regions of origin of recurrent ventricular tachycardia in patients with chronic infarcts (60). Extracellular electrograms recorded from endocardial regions of healed infarcts in humans often show multiple deflections of low amplitude separated by isoelectric intervals (115,206). Such so-called fragmented electrograms are, however, not specifically recorded from sites where tachycardias originate (23). They have also been recorded from surviving intramural fibers (35,46) and in the epicardial border zone (71) of canine infarcts. The appearance of fragmented electrograms in the epicardial border zone coincides with the appearance of connective tissue that separates the muscle bundles and distorts their orientation (71). Transmembrane action potentials recorded from sites where fragmented electrograms were recorded in isolated, superfused preparations excised from hearts with chronic infarcts are completely normal. The slow, inhomogeneous conduction observed in these preparations was therefore due to the nonuniform tissue anisotropy and poor coupling between cells, not to depression of action potential upstroke characteristics (71).

The relationship between fragmented extracellular electrograms and reentry remains to be elucidated. It is noteworthy that in the canine infarct it becomes more difficult or even impossible to induce ventricular tachycardias as time progresses, that is to say, when fibrous tissue appears in the epicardial border zone and electrograms become fragmented (109,142,234).

There are insufficient data available to establish whether or not the surviving cells in the subendocardium or the surviving intramural fibers form reentrant pathways. In one study, ventricular fibrillation could reproducibly be induced by two successive premature stimuli only when applied to the subendocardium of the infarcted zone in dogs with chronic infarcts produced several months to 1 year previously. Extracellular recordings from multipolar intramural needles showed localized, fragmented activity, bridging the interval between premature impulse and first ectopic complex (46). Although such findings are suggestive for reentry, they offer no proof.

Reentrant excitation can easily be induced by premature stimuli in subendocardial Purkinje fibers in large infarct preparations isolated from hearts 24 to 72 hr after coronary artery occlusion and superfused *in vitro* (21,66,121). An important reason for this is that Purkinje fibers overlying an infarct have abnormally prolonged action potentials (65) and form the site of unidirectional block, whereas conduction of the premature impulse is maintained in fibers with shorter action potentials. Repetitive activity has been observed in such preparations following premature stimulation, but the pathway of (reentrant?) activity has not been mapped. Because the electrophysiological characteristics of surviving Purkinje fibers normalize with time, it is uncertain which role these fibers play in arrhythmias that occur later after coronary occlusion.

It is difficult to extrapolate findings in the animal models used for studying arrhythmias in the chronic phase of myocardial infarction to the ventricular arrhythmias occurring in man with chronic myocardial infarction. There is evidence that the site of origin of recurrent ventricular tachycardia, occurring spontaneously weeks or months after the acute phase of myocardial infarction, is the subendocardium. These arrhythmias can be abolished by surgical resection of relatively small areas of subendocardial tissue overlying the infarct (100). Mapping studies during surgery showed that the site of earliest excitation during sustained and nonsustained ventricular tachycardia is in the subendocardium (37,100,102,189). Several other observations suggest that the tachycardia originates in a small area. Thus, supraventricular stimuli applied during tachycardia could capture the ventricles and produce normal QRS complexes without any effect on the tachycardia (103). No complete reentrant circuit has, however, been mapped in these patients. Most of the evidence that the tachy-cardias are reentrant in nature is indirect and consists of the fact that the tachycardias can be reproducibly induced and terminated by premature stimuli (213,217) and of the finding of localized, fragmented continuous activity in subendocardial catheter recordings during the initiation of tachycardia, and during the arrhythmia itself (101). The direct evidence for reentry in patients with recurrent ventricular tachycardia in the chronic phase of myocardial infarction is rather meager. The Philadelphia group, with long experience in endocardial mapping, may in this respect be quoted:

> In rare cases, a sequential pattern of activation is present around an aneurysm, with each electrical signal at every point being dependent on activation of the prior site. In the four patients in whom we have observed this phenomenon, digital pressure at multiple sites along the loop of sequential activity resulted in termination of the tachycardia. This is the closest we have come in man to recording, at least in gross terms, reentrant activity (105).

Such large reentrant circuits in patients with ventricular tachycardia appear to be the exception rather than the rule.

SOME CHARACTERISTICS OF REENTRANT TACHYCARDIAS

The only way to prove beyond doubt that an arrhythmia is due to reentry is to fulfill the criteria of Mines, i.e., to demonstrate unidirectional block, to map the complete reentrant pathway, and to terminate the arrhythmia by interrupting the reentrant circuit. Even in arrhythmias in experimental animals or in isolated preparations this is often difficult, if not impossible, and in patients such direct proof has been obtained only in tachycardias in patients with accessory AV pathways. In the absence of direct proof, circumstantial evidence for reentry may be obtained by observing certain characteristics, particularly when an arrhythmia is reproducibly induced and terminated by premature stimuli (212). Because repetitive rhythms caused by delayed afterdepolarizations can be initiated and terminated by single premature stimuli (230), the fact that an arrhythmia can be induced and abolished by programmed stimulation is in itself not enough evidence for reentry. Characteristics of triggered activity have been summarized by Rosen and Reder (171), and criteria to differentiate reentry from triggered activity in clinical arrhythmias have been discussed by Brugada and Wellens (19). Although the latter authors emphasized that it is often difficult, if not impossible, to establish the arrhythmia mechanism, the following characteristics may be helpful in the diagnosis of reentry: (a) When a tachycardia is initiated by a premature stimulus, an inverse relationship between the coupling interval of the premature stimulus and the interval between premature response and first complex of the tachycardia (the echo interval) speaks in favor of reentry (13,19,103,213). The progressive increase in echo interval on a decrease in coupling interval of the premature stimulus initiating the tachycardia is caused by slowing of conduction in part of the reentrant circuit. It is considered one of the most reliable criteria for reentry. On the basis of this criterion, tachycardias were reentrant in nature in 417 of 425 patients in whom tachycardias could reproducibly be induced by premature stimuli (19). Shortening of the echo interval on increasing prematurity of the test stimulus, however, does not rule out reentry (19). Thus, a sudden shortening of the reentrant pathway leads to a shortening of the echo interval, and this was observed in tachycardias in which the antegrade pathway was an accessory AV connection and the retrograde pathway could change from left to right bundle branch (19). It is also possible that the increase in conduction time in the retrograde pathway, caused by increasing prematurity of the test stimulus, is offset by a decrease in conduction time in the antegrade pathway, so that the sum of both conduction times may shorten, rather than lengthen. One cause for this is, for example, the disappearance of concealed conduction of the induced premature impulse in the antegrade pathway, so that antegrade conduction of the reentering impulse is improved (19). (b) When a premature stimulus abolishes tachycardia, this occurs abruptly in a reentrant rhythm, without any additional ectopic complexes following the premature stimulus, as is often the case in triggered arrhythmias (19,171,213). However, "delayed" termination has on occasion been observed in a reentrant tachycardia in a patient with accessory AV connections (19). (c) The site where premature stimuli are delivered is of importance in inducing reentrant rhythms. They should ideally be applied at the boundary of regions with different refractory periods (118). The greatest chance for inducing reentrant tachycardia occurs when the basic stimuli are applied close to the part of the reentrant circuit with the shortest refractory period, and premature stimuli to the part with the longest refractory period (212). When stimuli are given too far from the reentrant circuit, tachycardia may not be induced. Therefore, failure to induce tachycardia by premature stimulation at certain sites, and inducibility at other sites, is one of the characteristics of reentry. (d) Reentrant tachycardias can be induced only at a certain range of basic heart rates (212). As described by Wit and co-workers (228), reentry may be induced at a very slow heart rate, may become less frequent or may disappear at a moderate rate, reappear at faster rates, and vanish at very fast rates. The explanation is that increases in heart rate may either improve or abolish conduction through a depressed area. Improvement of conduction in a depressed area with an increase from a very slow to a moderate rate has been ascribed to postexcitatory hyperpolarization (31). A further increase in rate may increase the conduction delay through the depressed zone, thus permitting reentry, or, at very high rates, the

impulse may not invade the depressed area at all, thereby abolishing reentry. Because triggered activity may also be induced at certain basic heart rates, the rate dependence of induction of arrhythmias is not a useful criterion to differentiate between the two mechanisms.

REFERENCES

1. Akhtar, M., Damato, A. N., Batsford, W. P., Ruskin, J. N., Ogunkelu, J. B., and Vargas, G. (1974): Demonstration of re-entry within the His-Purkinje system in man. *Circulation,* 50: 1150–1162.
2. Allessie, M. A., and Bonke, F. I. M. (1979): Direct demonstration of sinus node re-entry in the rabbit heart. *Circ. Res.,* 44:557–569.
3. Allessie, M. A., Bonke, F. I. M., and Schopman, F. J. G. (1973): Circus movement in rabbit atrial muscle as a mechanism of tachycardia. *Circ. Res.,* 33:54–62.
4. Allessie, M. A., Bonke, F. I. M., and Schopman, F. J. G. (1976): Circus movement in rabbit atrial muscle as a mechanism of tachycardia. II. The role of non-uniform recovery of excitability in the occurrence of unidirectional block as studied with multiple microelectrodes. *Circ. Res.,* 39:168–177.
5. Allessie, M. A., Bonke, F. I. M., and Schopman, F. J. G. (1977): Circus movement in rabbit atrial muscle as a mechanism of tachycardia. III. The "leading circle" concept: A new model of circus movement in cardiac tissue without the involvement of an anatomical obstacle. *Circ. Res.,* 41:9–18.
6. Allessie, M. A., Lammers, W. J. E. P., Bonke, F. I. M., and Hollen, J. (1984): Intra-atrial reentry as a mechanism for atrial flutter induced by acetylcholine and rapid pacing in the dog. *Circulation,* 70:123–135.
7. Allessie, M. A., Lammers, W. J. E. P., Bonke, F. I. M., and Hollen, J. (1985): Experimental evaluation of Moe's multiple wavelet hypothesis of atrial fibrillation. In: *Cardiac Arrhythmias,* edited by D. P. Zipes and J. Jalife, pp. 265–276. Grune & Stratton, New York. (*in press*).
8. Anderson, R. H., Becker, A. E., Brechenmacher, C., Davies, M. J., and Rossi, L. (1975): Ventricular preexcitation. A proposed nomenclature for its substrates. *Eur. J. Cardiol.,* 3:27–36.
9. Antzelevitch, C., Jalife, J., and Moe, G. K. (1980): Characteristics of reflection as a mechanism of reentrant arrhythmias and its relationship to parasystole. *Circulation,* 61:182–191.
10. Antzelevitch, C., and Moe, G. K. (1981): Electrotonically mediated delayed conduction and reentry in relation to "slow responses" in mammalian ventricular conducting tissue. *Circ. Res.,* 49:1129–1139.
11. Barker, P. S., Wilson, F. V., and Johnston, F. D. (1943): Mechanism of auricular paroxysmal tachycardia. *Am. Heart J.,* 26:435–445.
12. Bethe, A. (1903): *Allgemeine Anatomie und Physiologie des Nervensystems,* pp. 427–432. George Thieme, Leipzig.
13. Bigger, J. T., and Goldreyer, B. N. (1970): The mechanism of supraventricular tachycardia. *Circulation,* 42:673–688.
14. Boineau, J. P., and Cox, J. L. (1973): Slow ventricular activation in acute myocardial infarction. A source of reentrant premature ventricular contraction. *Circulation,* 48:703–713.
15. Boineau, J. P., Schuessler, R. B., Mooney, C. R., Miller, C. B., Wylds, A. C., Hudson, R. D., Borremans, J. M., and Brockens, C. W. (1980): Natural and evoked atrial flutter due to circus movement in dogs. *Am. J. Cardiol.,* 45:1167–1181.
16. Bonke, F. I. M., Bouman, L. N., and Schopman, F. J. G. (1971): Effect of an early atrial premature beat on activity of the intraatrial node and atrial rhythm in the rabbit. *Circ. Res.,* 29: 704–715.
17. Bootsma, B. K., Hoelen, A. J., Strackee, J., and Meijler, F. L. (1970): Analysis of R-R intervals in patients with atrial fibrillation at rest and during exercise. *Circulation,* 41:783–794.
18. Brooks, C. M., Gilbert, J. L., Greenspan, M. E., Lange, G., and Mazzella, H. M. (1960): Excitability and electrical response of ischemic heart muscle. *Am. J. Physiol.,* 198:1143–1147.
19. Brugada, P., and Wellens, H. J. J. (1983): The role of triggered

activity in clinical arrhythmias. In: *Frontiers of Electrocardiography,* edited by M. Rosenbaum and M. Elizari, pp. 195–216. Martinus Nijhoff, The Hague.

20. Burchell, H. B., Fry, R. L., Anderson, M. W., and McGoon, D. C. (1967): Atrioventricular and ventriculo-atrial excitation in Wolff-Parkinson-White syndrome (type B). Temporary ablation at surgery. *Circulation,* 36:663–672.
21. Cardinal, R., and Sasyniuk, B. (1978): Electrophysiological effects of bretyllium tosylate on subendocardial Purkinje fibers from infarcted hearts. *J. Pharmacol. Exp. Ther.,* 204:159–174.
22. Carmeliet, E., and Vereecke, J. (1969): Adrenaline and the plateau phase of the cardiac action potential. *Pfluegers Arch.,* 379:300–315.
23. Cassidy, D. M., Vassallo, J. A., Buxton, A. E., Doherty, J. U., Marchlinsky, F. E., and Josephson, M. E. (1984): The value of catheter mapping during sinus rhythm to localize site of origin of ventricular tachycardia. *Circulation,* 69:1103–1110.
24. Clerc, L. (1976): Directional differences of impulse spread in trabecular muscle from mammalian heart. *J. Physiol. (Lond.),* 255:335–346.
25. Cobb, F. R., Blumenschein, S. D., Sealy, W. C., Boineau, J. P., Wagner, G. S., and Wallace, A. G. (1968): Successful surgical interruption of the bundle of Kent in a patient with Wolff-Parkinson-White syndrome. *Circulation,* 38:1018–1029.
26. Conrad, L. L., Cuddy, E., and Bayley, R. H. (1959): Activation of the ischemic ventricle and acute peri-infarction block in experimental coronary occlusion. *Circ. Res.,* 7:555–564.
27. Corbin, L. V., and Scher, A. M. (1977): The canine heart as an electrocardiographic generator. Dependence on cardiac cell orientation. *Circ. Res.,* 41:58–67.
28. Coumel, P., Cabrol, C., Fabiato, A., Gourgon, R., and Slama, R. (1967): Tachycardia permanente par rhythme reciprogue. *Arch. Mal. Coeur,* 60:1830–1864.
29. Cranefield, P. F. (1975): *The Conduction of the Cardiac Impulse. The Slow Response and Cardiac Arrhythmia.* Futura, Mt. Kisco, N.Y.
30. Cranefield, P. F. (1977): Action potentials, after potentials and arrhythmias. *Circ. Res.,* 41:416–423.
31. Cranefield, P. F., and Hoffman, B. F. (1971): Conduction of the cardiac impulse. II. Summation and inhibition. *Circ. Res.,* 28:220–233.
32. Cranefield, P. F., Klein, H. O., and Hoffman, B. F. (1971): Conduction of the cardiac impulse. I. Delay, block and one-way block in depressed Purkinje fibers. *Circ. Res.,* 28:199–219.
33. Cranefield, P. F., Wit, A. L., and Hoffman, B. F. (1973): Genesis of cardiac arrhythmias. *Circulation,* 47:190–204.
34. Curry, P. V. L., and Krikler, D. M. (1977): Paroxysmal reciprocating sinus tachycardia. In: *Reentrant Arrhythmias,* edited by H. E. Kulbertus, pp. 39–62. MTP Press, Lancaster.
35. Daniel, T. M., Boineau, J. P., and Sabiston, D. C. (1971): Comparison of human ventricular activation with a canine model in chronic myocardial infarction. *Circulation,* 44:74–89.
36. De Bakker, J. M. T., Henning, B., and Merx, W. (1979): Circus movement in canine right ventricle. *Circ. Res.,* 45:374–378.
37. De Bakker, J. M. T., Janse, M. J., Van Capelle, F. J. L., and Durrer, D. (1983): Endocardial mapping by simultaneous recording of endocardial electrograms during cardiac surgery for ventricular aneurysm. *J. Am. Coll. Cardiol.,* 2:947–953.
38. De la Fuente, D., Sasyniuk, B. I., and Moe, G. K. (1971): Conduction through a narrow isthmus in isolated canine atrial tissue. A model of the WPW syndrome. *Circulation,* 44:803–809.
39. De Mello, W. C. (1975): Effect of intracellular injection of calcium and strontium in cell communication in heart. *J. Physiol. (Lond.),* 250:231–245.
40. Dhatt, M. S., Akhtar, M., Reddy, P., Gomes, J. A., Lau, S. H., Caracta, A. R., and Damato, A. (1977): Modification and abolition of re-entry within the His-Purkinje system in man by diphenylhydantoin. *Circulation,* 56:720–726.
41. Disertori, M., Inama, G., Vergara, G., Guarnierio, M., Del Favero, A., and Furlanello, F. (1983): Evidence of a reentry circuit in the common type of atrial flutter in man. *Circulation,* 67:435–440.
42. Dominguez, G., and Fozzard, H. A. (1970): Influence of extracellular K$^+$ concentration on cable properties and excitability of sheep cardiac Purkinje fibers. *Circ. Res.,* 26:565–574.

43. Downar, E., Janse, M. J., and Durrer, D. (1977): The effect of acute coronary artery occlusion on subepicardial transmembrane potentials in the intact porcine heart. *Circulation,* 56:217–224.
44. Downar, E., and Waxman, M. B. (1976): Depressed conduction and unidirectional block in Purkinje fibers. In: *The Conduction System of the Heart,* edited by H. J. J. Wellens, K. I. Lie, and M. J. Janse, pp. 393–409. Lea & Febiger, Philadelphia.
45. Draper, M. H., and Mya-Tu, M. (1959): A comparison of the conduction velocity in cardiac tissues of various mammals. *Q. J. Exp. Physiol.,* 44:91–109.
46. Durrer, D., Van Dam, R. T., Freud, G. E., and Janse, M. J. (1971): Re-entry and ventricular arrhythmias in local ischemia and infarction of the intact dog heart. *Proc. Kon. Ned. Akad. Wetenschappen (Amsterdam)* [Series C], 74:321–334.
47. Durrer, D., Formijne, P., Van Dam, R. T., Buller, J., Van Lier, A. A. W., and Meijler, F. L. (1961): The electrocardiogram in normal and abnormal condition. *Am. Heart J.,* 61:303–314.
48. Durrer, D., and Roos, J. P. (1967): Epicardial excitation of the ventricles in a patient with Wolff-Parkinson-White syndrome. *Circulation,* 35:15–21.
49. Durrer, D., Schoo, L., Schuilenburg, R. M., and Wellens, H. J. J. (1967): The role of premature beats in the initiation and termination of supraventricular tachycardia in the Wolff-Parkinson-White syndrome. *Circulation,* 36:644–662.
50. Elharrar, V., Foster, P. R., Jirak, T. L., Gaum, W. E., and Zipes, D. P. (1977): Alterations in canine myocardial excitability during ischemia. *Circ. Res.,* 40:98–105.
51. El-Sherif, N., Hope, R. R., Scherlag, B. J., and Lazzara, R. (1977): Re-entrant ventricular arrhythmias in the late myocardial infarction period. I. Conduction characteristics in the infarction zone. *Circulation,* 55:686–702.
52. El-Sherif, N., Hope, R. R., Scherlag, B. J., and Lazzara, R. (1977): Re-entrant ventricular arrhythmias in the late myocardial infarction period. II. Patterns of initiation and termination of reentry. *Circulation,* 55:702–719.
53. El-Sherif, N., Mehra, R., Gough, W. B., and Zeiler, R. H. (1982): Ventricular activation pattern of spontaneous and induced rhythms in canine one-day-old myocardial infarction. Evidence for focal and reentrant mechanism. *Circ. Res.,* 51:152–166.
54. El-Sherif, N., Mehra, R., Gough, W. B., and Zeiler, R. H. (1983): Reentrant ventricular arrhythmias in the late myocardial infarction period. Interruption of reentrant circuits by cryothermal techniques. *Circulation* 68:644–656.
55. El-Sherif, N., Scherlag, B. J., and Lazzara, R. (1975): Electrode catheter recording during malignant ventricular arrhythmia following acute myocardial ischemia. Evidence for re-entry due to conduction delay and block in ischemic myocardium. *Circulation,* 51:1003–1014.
56. El-Sherif, N., Scherlag, B. J., Lazzara, R., and Samet, P. (1974): Pathophysiology of tachycardia- and bradycardia-dependent block in the canine proximal His-Purkinje system after acute myocardial ischemia. *Am. J. Cardiol.,* 33:529–540.
57. Engel, T. R., Meister, S. G., and Frankl, W. S. (1978): Ventricular extrastimulation in the mitral valve prolapse syndrome, evidence for ventricular reentry. *J. Electrocardiol.,* 11:137–142.
58. Engelmann, T. W. (1895): Ueber reciproke und irreciproke Reizleitung mit besonderer Beziehung auf das Herz. *Pfluegers Arch.,* 61:275–284.
59. Engelmann, T. W. (1896): Versuche ueber irreciproke Reizleitung in Muskelfasern. *Pfluegers Arch.,* 62:400–414.
60. Fenoglio, J. J., Jr., Pham, T. D., Harken, A. H., Horowitz, L. N., Josephson, M. E., and Wit, A. L. (1983): Recurrent sustained ventricular tachycardia: Structure and ultrastructure of subendocardial regions in which tachycardia originates. *Circulation,* 68:518–533.
61. Fisher, J. D., Cohen, H. L., Mehra, R., Altschuler, H., Escher, D. J. W., and Furman, S. (1977): Cardiac pacing and pacemakers. II. Serial electrophysiologic-pharmacologic testing for control of recurrent tachycarrhythmias. *Am. Heart J.,* 93:658–668.
62. Fleischmann, D. W., Dop, T., and De Bakker, J. M. T. (1977): Evidence of re-entry within the His-Purkinje system in man during extrasystolic stimulation of the right ventricle: Macroversus micro-reentry. In: *Reentrant Arrhythmias,* edited by H. E. Kulbertus, pp. 256–270. MTP Press, Lancaster.
63. Frame, L. H., and Hoffman, B. F. (1984): Mechanisms of

tachycardia. In: *Tachycardias,* edited by B. Surawicz, C. P. Reddy, and E. Prystowsky, pp. 7–36. Martinus Nijhoff, The Hague.

64. Frame, L. H., Page, R. L., Boyden, P. A., and Hoffman, B. F. (1983): A right atrial incision that stabilizes reentry around the triuspid ring. *Circulation* [*Suppl. III*], 68:361.

65. Friedman, P. L., Stewart, J. R., Fenoglio, J. J., Jr., and Wit, A. L. (1973): Survival of subendocardial Purkinje fibers after extensive myocardial infarction in dogs: In vitro and in vivo correlation. *Circ. Res.,* 33:597–611.

66. Friedman, P. L., Stewart, J. R., and Wit, A. L. (1973): Spontaneous and induced cardiac arrhythmias in subendocardial Purkinje fibers surviving extensive myocardial infarction in dogs. *Circ. Res.,* 33:612–626.

67. Gadsby, D. C., and Wit, A. L. (1981): Electrophysiologic characteristics of cardiac cells and the genesis of cardiac arrhythmias. In: *Cardiac Pharmacology,* edited by R. G. Wilkersen, pp. 229–241. Academic Press, New York.

68. Gallagher, J. J., Kasell, J., Sealy, W. C., Pritchett, E. L. C., and Wallace, A. G. (1978): Epicardial mapping in the Wolff-Parkinson-White syndrome. *Circulation,* 57:854–866.

69. Gang, E. S., Bigger, J. T., Jr., and Livelli, F. D., Jr. (1982): A model for chronic ischemic arrhythmias: The relation between electrically inducible ventricular tachycardia, ventricular fibrillation threshold and infarct size. *Am. J. Cardiol.,* 50:469–477.

70. Gardner, P. I., Ursell, P. C., Fenoglio, J. J., Jr., Allessie, M. A., Bonke, F. I. M., and Wit, A. L. (1981): Structure of the epicardial border in canine infarct is a cause of reentrant excitation. *Circulation* [*Suppl. IV*], 64:320.

71. Gardner, P. I., Ursell, P. C., Pham, T. D., Fenoglio, J. J., Jr., and Wit, A. L. (1984): Experimental chronic ventricular tachycardia: Anatomic and electrophysiologic substrates. In: *Tachycardias: Mechanisms, Diagnosis and Treatment,* edited by M. E. Josephson and H. J. J. Wellens, pp. 29–60. Lea & Febiger, Philadelphia.

72. Garrey, W. E. (1914): The nature of fibrillary contraction of the heart—its relation to tissue mass and form. *Am. J. Physiol.,* 33:397–414.

73. Garrey, W. E. (1924): Auricular fibrillation. *Physiol. Rev.,* 4:215–250.

74. Gessman, L. J., Agarwal, J. B., Endo, T., and Helfant, R. H. (1983): Localization and mechanisms of ventricular tachycardia by ice mapping 1 week after the onset of myocardial infarction in dogs. *Circulation,* 68:657–666.

75. Gettes, L. S., and Reuter, H. (1974): Slow recovery from inactivation of inward currents in mammalian myocardial fibers. *J. Physiol. (Lond.),* 240:703–724.

76. Giraud, G., Puech, P., Latour, H., and Hertault, J. (1960): Variations de potentiel liees a l'active du systeme de conduction auriculoventriculaire chez l'homme (enregistrement electrocardiographique endocavitaire). *Arch. Mal. Coeur,* 53:757.

77. Han, J., Malozzi, A. M., and Moe, G. K. (1968): Sinoatrial reciprocation in the isolated rabbit heart. *Circ. Res.,* 22:355–362.

78. Han, J., and Moe, G. K. (1964): Nonuniform recovery of excitability of ventricular muscle. *Circ. Res.,* 14:44–60.

79. Harris, A. S. (1950): Delayed development of ventricular ectopic rhythms following experimental coronary occlusion. *Circulation,* 1:1318–1328.

80. Hayden, W. G., Hurley, E. J., and Rytand, D. A. (1967): The mechanism of canine atrial flutter. *Circ. Res.,* 20:496–505.

81. Hill, J. L., and Gettes, L. S. (1980): Effect of acute coronary artery occlusion on local myocardial extracellular K⁺ activity in swine. *Circulation,* 61:768–778.

82. Hoffman, B. F. (1960): Physiological basis of disturbances of cardiac rhythm and conduction. *Prog. Cardiovasc. Dis.,* 2:319–333.

83. Hoffman, B. F., Cranefield, P. F., and Stuckey, J. H. (1961): Concealed conduction. *Circ. Res.,* 9:194–203.

84. Hoffman, B. F., and Cranefield, P. F. (1964): Physiologic basis of cardiac arrhythmias. *Am. J. Med.,* 37:670–684.

85. Hoffman, B. F., and Rosen, M. R. (1981): Cellular mechanisms for cardiac arrhythmias. *Circ. Res.,* 49:1–15.

86. Holzmann, M., and Scherf, D. (1932): Ueber Elektrokardiogramme mit verkuertzte Vorhof-Kammer-Distanz un positiven P-Zachen. *Zeitschr. Kon. Med.,* 121:404–423.

87. Ideker, R. E., Klein, G. J., Harrison, L., Smith, W. M., Kasell, J., Reimer, K. A., Wallace, A. G., and Gallagher, J. J. (1981): The transition to ventricular fibrillation induced by reperfusion after acute ischemia in the dog: A period of organized epicardial activation. *Circulation,* 63:1371–1379.

88. Inoue, H., Matsuo, H., Takayanagi, K., and Murao, S. (1981): Clinical and experimental studies of the effects of atrial extrastimulation and rapid pacing on atrial flutter cycle. *Am. J. Cardiol.,* 48:623–631.

89. Jalife, J., and Moe, G. K. (1976): Effect of electrotonic potentials on pacemaker activity of canine Purkinje fibers in relation to parasystole. *Circ. Res.,* 39:801–808.

90. Jalife, J., and Moe, G. K. (1979): A biological model of parasystole. *Am. J. Cardiol.,* 43:761–772.

91. Jalife, J., and Moe, G. K. (1981): Excitation, conduction and reflection of impulses in isolated bovine and canine Purkinje fibers. *Circ. Res.,* 49:233–247.

92. Janse, M. J. (1971): The effects of changes in heart rate in the refractory period of the heart. PhD thesis, University of Amsterdam.

93. Janse, M. J., Capucci, A., Coronel, R., and Fabius, M. A. W. (1985): Variability of recovery of excitability in the normal canine and the ischemic porcine heart. *Eur. Heart J.,* 6(Suppl. D):41–52.

94. Janse, M. J., and Downar, E. (1977): The effect of acute ischemia on transmembrane potentials in the intact heart. The relation to re-entrant arrhythmias. In: *Reentrant Arrhythmias,* edited by H. E. Kulbertus, pp. 195–209. MTP Press, Lancaster.

95. Janse, M. J., and Van Capelle, F. J. L. (1982): Electrotonic interactions across an inexcitable region as a cause of ectopic activity in acute regional myocardial ischemia. A study in intact porcine and canine hearts and computer models. *Circ. Res.,* 50:527–537.

96. Janse, M. J., Van Capelle, F. J. L., Anderson, R. H., Touboul, P., and Billette, J. (1976): Electrophysiology and structure of the atrioventricular node of the isolated rabbit heart. In: *The Conduction System of the Heart,* edited by H. J. J. Wellens, K. I. Lie, and M. J. Janse, pp. 298–315. Martinus Nijhoff, The Hague.

97. Janse, M. J., Van Capelle, F. J. L., Freud, G. E., and Durrer, D. (1971): Circus movement within the AV node on a basis for supraventricular tachycardia as shown by multiple microelectrode recording in the isolated rabbit heart. *Circ. Res.,* 28:403–414.

98. Janse, M. J., Van Capelle, F. J. L., Morsink, H., Kleber, A. G., Wilms-Schopman, F. J. G., Cardinal, R., Naumann d'Alnoncourt, C., and Durrer, D. (1980): Flow of "injury" current and patterns of excitation during early ventricular arrhythmias in acute regional myocardial ischemia in isolated porcine and canine hearts. Evidence for 2 different arrhythmogenic mechanisms. *Circ. Res.,* 47:151–165.

99. Janse, M. J., Van der Steen, A. B. M., Van Dam, R. T., and Durrer, D. (1969): Refractory period of the dog ventricular myocardium following sudden changes in frequency. *Circ. Res.,* 24:251–262.

100. Josephson, M. E., Harken, A. H., and Horowitz, L. N. (1979): Endocardial excision: A new surgical technique for treatment of recurrent ventricular tachycardia. *Circulation,* 60:1460–1439.

101. Josephson, M. E., Horowitz, L. N., and Farshidi, A. (1978): Continuous local electrical activity: A mechanism of recurrent ventricular tachycardia. *Circulation,* 57:659–665.

102. Josephson, M. E., Horowitz, L. N., Farshidi, A., Spear, J. F., Kastor, J. A., and Moore, E. N. (1978): Recurrent sustained ventricular tachycardia. 2. Endocardial mapping. *Circulation,* 57:440–447.

103. Josephson, M. E., Horowitz, L. N., Farshidi, A., Spielman, S. R., Michelson, E. L., and Greenspan, A. M. (1978): Sustained ventricular tachycardia: Evidence for protected localized reentry. *Am. J. Cardiol.,* 42:416–426.

104. Josephson, M. E., and Kastor, J. A. (1976): Paroxysmal supraventricular tachycardia. Is the atrium a necessary link? *Circulation,* 54:430–435.

105. Josephson, M. E., Marchlinski, F. E., Buxton, A. E., Waxman, H. L., Doherty, J. H., Kienzle, M. G., and Falcone, R. (1984): Electrophysiologic basis for sustained ventricular tachycardia. Role of reentry. In: *Tachycardias: Mechanism, Diagnosis, Treatment,* edited by M. E. Josephson and H. J. J. Wellens, pp. 305–324. Lea & Febiger, Philadelphia.

106. Josephson, M. E., Scharf, D. L., Kastor, J. A., and Kitchen, J. G. (1977): Atrial endocardial activation in man: Electrode catheter technique for endocardial mapping. *Am. J. Cardiol.*, 39:972–981.

107. Joyner, R. W. (1982): Effects of the discrete pattern of electrical coupling on propagation through an electrical synsytimus. *Circ. Res.*, 50:192–200.

108. Joyner, R. W., Overholt, E. D., Ramza, B., and Veenstra, R. D. (1984): Propagation through electrically coupled cells: Two inhomogeneously coupled cardiac tissue layers. *Am. J. Physiol.*, 247:H596–H609.

109. Karagueuzian, H. S., Fenoglio, J. J., Jr., Weiss, M. B., and Wit, A. L. (1979): Protracted ventricular tachycardia induced by premature stimulation of the canine heart after coronary artery occlusion and reperfusion. *Circ. Res.*, 44:833–846.

110. Kent, A. F. S. (1913): Observations on the auriculo-ventricular junction of the mammalian heart. *Q. J. Exp. Physiol.*, 7:193–197.

111. Kimura, E., Kato, K., Murao, S., Ajisaka, H., Koyama, S., and Omiya, Z. (1954): Experimental studies on the mechanism of the auricular flutter. *Tohoku J. Exp. Med.*, 60:197–207.

112. Kistin, A. D. (1963): Multiple pathways of conduction and reciprocal rhythm with interpolated ventricular premature systoles. *Am. Heart J.*, 65:162–179.

113. Kistin, A. D. (1965): Atrial reciprocal rhythm. *Circulation*, 32:687–707.

114. Kleber, A. G., and Janse, M. J. (1982): Conduction velocity in acutely ischemic myocardium. *Circulation [Suppl. II]*, 66:157 (abstract).

115. Klein, H., Kard, R. B., Kouchoukos, N. T., Zorn, G., Jr., James, T. N., and Waldo, A. L. (1982): Intraoperative electrophysiologic mapping of the ventricles during sinus rhythm in patients with a previous myocardial infarction. *Circulation*, 66:847–853.

116. Klein, H. O., Singer, D. H., and Hoffman, B. F. (1973): Effects of atrial premature systoles on sinus rhythm in the rabbit. *Circ. Res.*, 28:480–491.

117. Kulbertus, H. E. (editor) (1977): *Reentrant Arrhythmias, Mechanisms and Treatment.* MTP Press, Lancaster.

118. Kuo, C. S., Munakata, K., Pratap Reddy, C., and Surawicz, B. (1983): Characteristics and possible mechanisms of ventricular arrhythmias dependent on the dispersion of action potential durations. *Circulation*, 67:1356–1367.

119. Kupersmith, J., Antman, E. M., and Hoffman, B. F. (1975): In vivo electrophysiological effects of lidocaine in canine acute myocardial infarction. *Circ. Res.*, 36:84–91.

120. Lanari, A., Lambutini, A., and Ravin, A. (1956): Mechanism of experimental atrial flutter. *Circ. Res.*, 4:282–287.

121. Lazzara, R., El-Sherif, N., and Scherlag, B. J. (1973): Electrophysiological properties of canine Purkinje cells in one-day-old myocardial infarction. *Circ. Res.*, 33:722–734.

122. Lazzara, R., El-Sherif, N., and Scherlag, B. J. (1975): Disorders of cellular electrophysiology produced by ischemia of the canine His bundle. *Circ. Res.*, 36:444–454.

123. Levites, R., Haft, J. L., Calderon, J., and Venkatachalapathy, J. (1976): Effects of procainamide on the dispersion of recovery of excitability during coronary occlusion. *Circulation*, 53:982–984.

124. Lewis, T. (1920): *The Mechanism and Graphic Registration of the Heart Beat.* Shaw & Sons, London.

125. Lewis, T. (1925): *The Mechanism and Registration of the Heart Beat*, ed. 3. Shaw & Sons, London.

126. Lewis, T., Feil, S., and Stroud, W. D. (1918): Observations upon flutter and fibrillation. I. *Heart*, 7:127–130.

127. Lewis, T., Feil, S., and Stroud, W. D. (1920): Observations upon flutter and fibrillation. II. The nature of auricular flutter. *Heart*, 7:191–346.

128. Lyons, C. J., and Burgess, M. J. (1979): Demonstration of reentry within the canine specialized conduction system. *Am. Heart J.*, 98:595–603.

129. MacLean, W. A. H., Plumb, V. J., and Waldo, A. L. (1981): Transient entrainment and interruption of ventricular tachycardia. *Pace*, 4:358–365.

130. Matsuda, K., Kamiyama, A., and Hoshi, T. (1967): Configuration of the transmembrane potential of the Purkinje-ventricular fiber junction and its analysis. In: *Electrophysiology and Ultrastructure of the Heart*, edited by T. Sano, J. Mizuhira, and K. Matsuda, pp. 177–188. Grune & Stratton, New York.

131. Mayer, A. G. (1906): Rhythmical pulsation in scyphomedusae. Publication 47 of the Carnegie Institution, pp. 1–62. Carnegie Institution, Washington.

132. Mayer, A. G. (1908): Rhythmical pulsation in scyphomedusae. II. Papers from the Marine Biological Laboratory at Tortugas, pp. 115–131. Carnegie Institution, Washington.

133. Mayer, A. G. (1916): Nerve conduction and other reactions in Cassiopea. *Am. J. Physiol.*, 39:375–393.

134. McWilliam, J. (1887): Fibrillar contraction of the heart. *J. Physiol. (Lond.)*, 8:296–310.

135. Mehra, R., Zeiler, R. H., Gough, W. B., and El-Sherif, N. (1983): Reentrant ventricular arrhythmias in the late myocardial infarction period. 9. Electrophysiologic anatomic correlation of reentrant circuits. *Circulation*, 67:11–24.

136. Mendez, C. Gruhzit, C. C., and Moe, G. K. (1956): Influence of cycle length upon refractory period of auricular, ventricles and AV node in the dog. *Am. J. Physiol.*, 184:287–295.

137. Mendez, C., Han, J., Garcia de Jalon, P. D., and Moe, G. K. (1965): Some characteristics of ventricular echoes. *Circ. Res.*, 16:562–581.

138. Mendez, C., and Moe, G. K. (1966): Demonstration of a dual A-V nodal conduction system in the isolated rabbit heart. *Circ. Res.*, 19:378–393.

139. Mendez, C., Mueller, W. J., Meredith, J., and Moe, G. K. (1969): Interaction of transmembrane potentials in canine Purkinje fibers and of Purkinje fiber–muscle junction. *Circ. Res.*, 24:361–372.

140. Mendez, C., Mueller, W. J., and Urguiaga, X. (1970): Propagation of impulses across the Purkinje fiber–muscle junctions in the dog heart. *Circ. Res.*, 26:135–150.

141. Meijler, F. L., Strackee, J., Van Capelle, F. J. L., and Du Perron, J. C. (1968): Computer analysis of the RR interval-contractility during random stimulation at the isolated heart. *Circ. Res.*, 22:695–702.

142. Michelson, E. L., Spear, J. F., and Moore, E. N. (1980): Electrophysiologic and anatomic correlation of sustained ventricular tachyarrhythmias in a model of chronic myocardial infarction. *Am. J. Cardiol.*, 45:583–590.

143. Michelson, E. L., Spear, J. F., and Moore, E. N. (1981): Further electrophysiologic and anatomic correlates in a canine model of chronic myocardial infarction susceptible to the initiation of sustained ventricular tachyarrhythmias. *Anat. Rec.*, 201:55–65.

144. Mignone, R. J., and Wallace, A. G. (1966): Ventricular echoes. Evidence for dissociation of conduction and reentry within the A-V node. *Circ. Res.*, 19:638–649.

145. Mines, G. R. (1913): On dynamic equilibrium in the heart. *J. Physiol. (Lond.)*, 46:349–382.

146. Mines, G. R. (1914): On circulating excitations in heart muscles and their possible relation to tachycardia and fibrillation. *Trans. R. Soc. Can. [Section IV]*, pp. 43–52.

147. Moe, G. K. (1962): On the multiple wavelet hypothesis of atrial fibrillation. *Arch. Int. Pharmacodyn. Ther.*, 140:183–188.

148. Moe, G. K. (1975): Evidence for reentry as a mechanism for cardiac arrhythmias. *Rev. Physiol. Biochem. Pharmacol.*, 72:56–66.

149. Moe, G. K., and Abildskov, J. A. (1959): Atrial fibrillation on a self-sustaining arrhythmia independent of focal discharge. *Am. Heart J.*, 58:59–70.

150. Moe, G. K., and Abildskov, J. A. (1964): Observations on the ventricular dysrhythmia associated with atrial fibrillation in the dog heart. *Circ. Res.*, 14:447–460.

151. Moe, G. K., Cohen, W., and Vick, R. L. (1963): Experimentally induced paroxysmal A-V nodal tachycardia in the dog. *Am. Heart J.*, 65:87–92.

152. Moe, G. K., Jalife, J., Mueller, W. J., and Moe, B. (1977): A mathematical model of parasystole and its application to clinical arrhythmias. *Circulation*, 56:968–979.

153. Moe, G. K., Mendez, C., and Han, J. (1965): Aberrant A-V impulse propagation in the dog heart: A study of functional bundle branch block. *Circ. Res.*, 16:261–286.

154. Moe, G. K., Preston, J. B., and Burlington, H. J. (1956): Physiologic evidence for a dual A-V transmission system. *Circ. Res.*, 4:357–375

155. Moe, G. K., Rheinboldt, W. C., and Abildskov, J. A. (1964): A computer model of atrial fibrillation. *Am. Heart J.*, 67:200–220.

156. Myerburg, R. J., Steward, J. W., and Hoffman, B. F. (1970):

Electrophysiological properties of the canine peripheral A-V conducting system. *Circ. Res.,* 26:361–378.

157. Naimi, S., Avitall, B., Mieszala, B. S., and Levine, H. J. (1977): Dispersion of effective refractory period during abrupt reperfusion of ischemic myocardium in dogs. *Am. J. Cardiol.,* 39:407–412.

158. Narula, O. S. (1974): Sinus node reentry. A mechanism for supraventricular tachycardia. *Circulation,* 50:1114–1128.

159. Neuss, H., Schlepper, M., and Thormann, J. (1975): Analysis of re-entry mechanism in three patients with concealed Wolff-Parkinson-White syndrome. *Circulation,* 51:75–81.

160. Overholt, E. D., Joyner, R. W., Veenstra, R. D., Rawling, D., and Wiedmann, R. (1984): Unidirectional block between Purkinje and ventricular layers of papillary muscles. *Am. J. Physiol.,* 247: H584–H595.

161. Paes de Carvalho, A. (1961): Cellular electrophysiology of the atrial specialized tissues. In: *The Specialized Tissues of the Heart,* edited by A. Paes de Carvalho, W. C. de Mello, and B. F. Hoffman, pp. 115–133. Elsevier, Amsterdam.

162. Paes de Carvalho, A., De Mello, W. C., and Hoffman, B. F. (1959): Electrophysiological evidence for specialized fiber types in rabbit atrium. *Am. J. Physiol.,* 196:483–488.

163. Pahlajani, D. B., Miller, R. A., and Serratto, M. (1975): Sinus node reentry and sinus node tachycardia. *Am. Heart J.,* 90:305–311.

164. Pastelin, G., Mendez, R., and Moe, G. K. (1978): Participation of atrial specialized conduction pathways in atrial flutter. *Circ. Res.,* 42:386–393.

165. Peon, J., Ferrier, G. R., and Moe, G. K. (1978): The relationship of excitability to conduction velocity in canine Purkinje tissue. *Circ. Res.,* 43:125–135.

166. Pick, A., and Langendorf, R. (1979): *Interpretation of Complex Arrhythmias.* Lea & Febiger, Philadelphia.

167. Puech, P. (1970): La conduction reciproque par le noeud de Tawara. Bases experimentales et aspects cliniques. *Ann. Cardiol. Angeiol. (Paris),* 19:21–40.

168. Reuter, H. (1979): Properties of two inward membrane currents in heart. *Annu. Rev. Physiol.,* 41:413–424.

169. Reynolds, E. W., Van der Ark, C. R., and Johnston, F. D. (1960): Effects of acute myocardial infarction on electrical recovery and transmural temperature gradient in left ventricular wall of dogs. *Circ. Res.,* 8:730–737.

170. Roberts, D. E., Hersh, L. T., and Scher, A. M. (1979): Influence of cardiac fiber orientation on wavefront voltage, conduction velocity and tissue resistivity in the dog. *Circ. Res.,* 44:701–712.

171. Rosen, M. R., and Reder, R. F. (1981): Does triggered activity have a role in the genesis of cardiac arrhythmias? *Ann. Intern. Med.,* 94:794–801.

172. Rosenblueth, A. (1958): Ventricular "echoes." *Am. J. Physiol.,* 195:53–60.

173. Rosenblueth, A., and Garcia Ramos, J. (1947): Studies on flutter and fibrillation. II. The Influence of artificial obstacles on experimental auricular flutter. *Am. Heart J.,* 33:677–684.

174. Rozanski, G. J., Jalife, J., and Moe, G. K. (1984): Reflected reentry in nonhomogeneous ventricular muscle as a mechanism of cardiac arrhythmias. *Circulation,* 69:163–173.

175. Rytand, D. A. (1966): The circus movement (entrapped circuit wave) hypothesis and atrial flutter. *Ann. Intern. Med.,* 65:125–159.

176. Sasyniuk, B. I., and Mendez, C. (1971): A mechanism for reentry in canine ventricular tissue. *Circ. Res.,* 28:3–15.

177. Scherf, D. (1947): Studies on auricular tachycardia caused by aconitine administration. *Proc. Soc. Exp. Biol. Med.,* 64:233–239.

178. Scherf, D., and Cohen, J. (1964): *The Atrioventricular Node and Selected Cardiac Arrhythmias,* pp. 230, 259. Grune & Stratton, New York.

179. Scherf, D., and Shookhoff, C. (1926): Experimentelle Untersuchungen ueber die "Umkehr-Extrasystole" (reciprocating beat). *Wien Arch. Inn. Med.,* 12:501–529.

180. Scherlag, B. J., El-Sherif, N., Hope, R. R., and Lazzara, R. (1974): Characterization and localisation of ventricular arrhythmias resulting from myocardial ischemia and infarction. *Circ. Res.,* 35:372–383.

181. Schmitt, F. O., and Erlanger, J. (1928): Directional differences in the conduction of the impulse through heart muscle and their

182. Schuetz, E. (1936): Elektrophysiologie des Herzens bei einphasischer Ableitung. *Ergeb. Physiol.,* 38:493–620.

183. Schuilenburg, R. M., and Durrer, D. (1968): Atrial echo beats in the human heart elicited by induced atrial premature beats. *Circulation,* 37:680–693.

184. Schuilenburg, R. M., and Durrer, D. (1969): Ventricular echo beats in the human heart elicited by induced ventricular premature beats. *Circulation,* 40:337–347.

185. Schuilenburg, R. M., and Durrer, D. (1972): Further observations in the ventricular echo phenomenon elicited in the human heart. Is the atrium part of the echo pathway? *Circulation,* 45:629–638.

186. Spach, M. S., Miller, W. T., Jr., Dolber, P. C., Kootsey, J. M., Sommer, J. R., and Mosher, C. E. (1982): The functional role of structural complexities in the propagation of depolarization in the atrium of the dog. Cardiac conduction disturbances due to discontinuities of effective axial resistivity. *Circ. Res.,* 50:175–191.

187. Spach, M. S., Miller, W. T., Jr., Geselowitz, D. B., Barr, R. C., Kootsey, J. M., and Johnson, E. A. (1981): The discontinuous nature of propagation in normal canine cardiac muscle. Evidence for recurrent discontinuities of intracellular resistance that affect the membrane currents. *Circ. Res.,* 48:39–54.

188. Spear, J. F., and Moore, E. N. (1982): Mechanisms of cardiac arrhythmias. *Annu. Rev. Physiol.,* 44:485–497.

189. Spielman, S. R., Michelson, E. L., Horowitz, L. N., Spear, J. F., and Moore, E. N. (1978): The limitation of epicardial mapping as a guide to the surgical therapy of ventricular tachycardia. *Circulation,* 57:666–670.

190. Spurrell, R. A. J., Sowton, E., and Deuchar, D. C. (1973): Ventricular tachycardia in 4 patients evaluated by programmed electrical stimulation of heart and treated in 2 patients by surgical division of anterior radiation of left bundle-branch. *Br. Heart J.,* 35:1014–1025.

191. Strackee, J., Hoelen, A. J., Zimmerman, A. N. E., and Meijler, F. L. (1971): Artificial atrial fibrillation in the dog. An artifact? *Circ. Res.,* 28:441–445.

192. Strauss, H. C., and Geer, M. R. (1977): Sinoatrial node reentry. In: *Reentrant Arrhythmias,* edited by H. E. Kulbertus, pp. 27–38. MTP Press, Lancaster.

193. Trautwein, W., and Kassebaum, D. G. (1961): On the mechanisms of spontaneous impulse generation in the pacemaker of the heart. *J. Gen. Physiol.,* 45:317–330.

194. Tsien, R. W. (1983): Calcium channels in excitable cell membranes. *Annu. Rev., Physiol.,* 45:341–358.

195. Tsuchida, T. (1965): Experimental studies of the excitability of ventricular musculature in infarcted region. *Jpn. Heart J.,* 6:152–164.

196. Van Capelle, F. J. L. (1983): Slow conduction and cardiac arrhythmias. PhD thesis, University of Amsterdam.

197. Van Capelle, F. J. L., and Durrer, D. (1980): Computer simulation of arrhythmias in a network of coupled excitable elements. *Circ. Res.,* 47:454–466.

198. Van Capelle, F. J. L., and Janse, M. J. (1976): Influence of geometry on the shape of the propagated action potential. In: *The Conduction System of the Heart,* edited by H. J. J. Wellens, K. I. Lie, and M. J. Janse, pp. 316–335. Stenfert Kroese, Leiden.

199. Veenstra, R., Joyner, R. W., and Rawling, D. (1984): Purkinje and ventricular activation sequences of canine papillary muscle: Effects of quinidine and calcium on Purkinje-ventricular conduction delay. *Circ. Res.,* 54:500–515.

200. Waldo, A. L., and Kaiser, G. A. (1973): A study of ventricular arrhythmias associated with acute myocardial infarction in the canine heart. *Circulation,* 47:1222–1228.

201. Waldo, A. L., MacLean, W. A. H., Karp, R. B., Kouchoucos, N. T., and James, J. N. (1977): Entrainment and interruption of atrial flutter with atrial pacing. Studies in man following open heart surgery. *Circulation,* 56:737–745.

202. Wallace, A. G., and Mignone, R. J. (1966): Physiologic evidence concerning the reentry hypothesis for ectopic beats. *Am. Heart J.,* 72:60–70.

203. Watanabe, Y., and Dreifus, L. S. (1965): Inhomogeneous conduction in the A-V node. A model for re-entry. *Am. Heart J.,* 70:505–514.

204. Weidmann, S. (1951): Effect of current flow on the membrane potential of cardiac muscle. *J. Physiol. (Lond.),* 115:227–236.

205. Weidmann, S. (1955): The effect of the cardiac membrane potential on the rapid availability of the sodium carrying system. *J. Physiol. (Lond.),* 127:213–224.

206. Weiner, I., Mindich, B., and Pitcon, R. (1982): Determinants of ventricular tachycardia in patients with ventricular aneurysms: Results of intraoperative epicardial and endocardial mapping. *Circulation,* 65:856–861.

207. Weingart, R. (1977): The actions of ouabain on intercellular coupling and conduction velocity in mammalian ventricular muscle. *J. Physiol. (Lond.),* 264:341–365.

208. Weingart, R., and Reber, W. (1979): Influence of internal pH on Ri of Purkinje fibers from mammalian heart. *Experientia,* 35: 929.

209. Wellens, H. J. J. (1971): *Electrical Stimulation of the Heart in the Study and Treatment of Tachycardia.* Stenfert Kroese, Leiden.

210. Wellens, H. J. J. (1976): The electrophysiological properties of the accessory pathway in the Wolff-Parkinson-White syndrome. In: *The Conduction System of the Heart,* edited by H. J. J. Wellens, K. I. Lie, and M. J. Janse, pp. 567–587. Stenfert Kroese, Leiden.

211. Wellens, H. J. J. (1977): Modes of initiation of circus movement tachycardia in 139 patients with the Wolff-Parkinson-White syndrome studied by programmed electrical stimulation. In: *Reentrant Arrhythmias,* edited by H. E. Kulbertus, pp. 153–169. MTP Press, Lancaster.

212. Wellens, H. J. J. (1978): Value and limitations of programmed electrical stimulation of the heart in the study and treatment of tachycardias. *Circulation,* 57:845–853.

213. Wellens, H. J. J., Duren, D. R., and Lie, K. I. (1976): Observation on mechanisms of ventricular tachycardia in man. *Circulation,* 43:237–244.

214. Wellens, H. J. J., and Durrer, D. (1975): The role of an accessory atrioventricular pathway in reciprocal tachycardia. *Circulation,* 52:58–72.

215. Wellens, H. J. J., Janse, M. J., Van Dam, R. T., and Durrer, D. (1971): Epicardial excitation of the atria in a patient with atrial flutter. *Br. Heart J.,* 33:233–237.

216. Wellens, H. J. J., Lie, K. I., and Durrer, D. (1974): Further observation on ventricular tachycardia as studied by electrical stimulation of the heart. *Circulation,* 49:647–653.

217. Wellens, H. J. J., Schuilenburg, R. M., and Durrer, D. (1972): Electrical stimulation of the heart in patients with ventricular tachycardia. *Circulation,* 46:216–226.

218. Wells, J. L., MacLean, W. A. H., James, T. N., and Waldo, A. L. (1979): Characterization of atrial flutter: Studies in man after open heart surgery using fixed atrial electrodes. *Circulation,* 60: 665–673.

219. Wennemark, J. R., Ruesta, V. J., and Brody, D. A. (1968): Microelectrode study of delayed conduction in the canine right bundle branch. *Circ. Res.,* 23:753–769.

220. White, P. D. (1915): A study of atrioventricular rhythm following auricular flutter. *Arch. Intern. Med.,* 16:517–535.

221. Wiener, N., and Rosenblueth, A. (1946): The mathematical formulation of the problem of conduction of impulses in a network of connected excitable elements, specifically in cardiac muscle. *Arch. Inst. Cardiol. Mex.,* 16:205–265.

222. Williams, D. O., Scherlag, B. J., Hope, R. R., and Lazzara, R. (1974): The pathophysiology of malignant ventricular arrhythmias during acute myocardial ischemia. *Circulation,* 50:1163–1172.

223. Wilson, F. N. (1915): A case in which the vagus influenced the form of the ventricular complex of the electrocardiogram. *Arch. Intern. Med.,* 16:1008–1027.

224. Wit, A. L., Allessie, M. A., Bonke, F. I. M., Lammers, W., Smeets, J., and Fenoglio, J. J., Jr. (1982): Electrophysiologic mapping to determine the mechanisms of experimental ventricular tachycardia initiated by premature impulses. *Am. J. Cardiol.,* 49: 166–185.

225. Wit, A. L., and Cranefield, P. F. (1978): Re-entrant excitation as a cause of cardiac arrhythmias. *Am. J. Physiol.,* 235:H1–H17.

226. Wit, A. L., Cranefield, P. F., and Hoffman, B. F. (1972): Slow conduction and reentry in the ventricular conduction system. I. Return extrasystoles in canine cardiac Purkinje fibers. *Circ. Res.,* 30:11–22.

227. Wit, A. L., Goldreyer, B. N., and Damato, A. N. (1971): An in vitro model of paroxysmal supraventricular tachycardia. *Circulation,* 43:862–875.

228. Wit, A. L., Hoffman, B. F., and Cranefield, P. F. (1972): Slow conduction and reentry in the ventricular conducting system. I. Return extrasystole in canine Purkinje fibers. *Circ. Res.,* 30:1–10.

229. Wit, A. L., Rosen, M. R., and Hoffman, B. F. (1974): Electrophysiology and pharmacology of cardiac arrhythmias. I. Relationship of normal and abnormal electrical activity of cardiac fibers to the genesis of arrhythmia. B. Reentry. *Am. Heart J.,* 88:664–806.

230. Wit, A. L., Wiggins, J. R., and Cranefield, P. F. (1976): Some effects of electrical stimulation on impulse initiation in cardiac fibers; Its relevance for the determination of mechanisms of clinical cardiac arrhythmia. In: *The Conduction System of the Heart,* edited by H. J. J. Wellens, K. I. Lie, and M. J. Janse, pp. 163–181. Martinus Nijhoff, The Hague.

231. Wojtczak, J. (1979): Contractures and increase in internal longitudinal resistance of cow ventricular muscle induced by hypoxia. *Circ. Res.,* 44:88–95.

232. Wolferth, C. C., and Wood, F. C. (1933): The mechanism of production of short PR-intervals and prolonged QRS complexes in patients with presumably undamaged hearts: Hypotheses of an accessory pathway of auriculo-ventricular conduction (bundle of Kent). *Am. Heart J.,* 8:297–311.

233. Wolff, L., Parkinson, J., and White, P. D. (1930): Bundle branch block with short PR interval in healthy young people prone to paroxysmal tachycardia. *Am. Heart J.,* 5:685–704.

234. Wolff, G. A., Veith, F., and Lown, B. (1968): A vulnerable period for ventricular tachycardia following myocardial infarction. *Cardiovasc. Res.,* 2:111–121.

235. Wood, F. C., Wolferth, C. C., and Geckeler, G. D. (1943): Histologic demonstration of accessory muscular communication between auricle and ventricle in case of short P-R interval and prolonged QRS complex. *Am. Heart J.,* 25:454–462.

The Heart and Cardiovascular System,
edited by H. A. Fozzard et al.
Raven Press, New York © 1986.

CHAPTER **55**

Abnormal Automaticity and Related Phenomena

Robert F. Gilmour, Jr., and Douglas P. Zipes

Although all cardiac cells are capable of spontaneous impulse generation, a single synchronous rhythm occurs in the normal heart because of an intrinsic hierarchy of pacemaker activity. Impulses generated by the most rapidly depolarizing pacemaker, the sinus node, initiate a myocardial activation sequence that discharges subsidiary pacemakers before they reach threshold and ensures properly timed contraction of atrial and ventricular myocardium. In the event that the sinus node is unable to generate spontaneous activity or sinus nodal impulses fail to propagate to surrounding atrial cells, subsidiary atrial or atrioventricular (AV) nodal pacemakers having slower intrinsic spontaneous discharge rates assume control of the heart rhythm, ensuring that ventricular systole is maintained. If atrial or AV nodal pacemaker activity is suppressed, more slowly depolarizing pacemakers in the His-Purkinje system may discharge and maintain ventricular activation. Subsidiary pacemakers provide a useful backup to the sinus node; yet inappropriate spontaneous activity by latent pacemakers may produce cardiac arrhythmias and attendant hemodynamic dysfunction.

In this chapter we review present concepts concerning the role of abnormal automaticity in the genesis of cardiac arrhythmias. The chapter is divided into discussions of arrhythmias due to (a) alteration of normal automatic mechanisms, (b) abnormal automatic mechanisms, (c) interactions between automatic foci, and (d) interactions between automaticity and conduction. An-

other important aspect of abnormal impulse formation, triggered activity, is discussed by Wit and Rosen in *Chapter 60.* In each section, experimental findings are introduced first, followed by descriptions of potentially related clinical arrhythmias. Because other chapters in this volume review the ionic bases automaticity and the influences of drugs and hypoxia (see *Chapters 1, 30,* and *56*), descriptions of the physiological properties of the different pacemakers will be brief, and the reader is referred to the relevant chapters for more thorough discussion.

ALTERED NORMAL AUTOMATICITY

Experimental Observations

Sinus Node

The normal spontaneous discharge rate of the sinus node [60–100 beats per minute (bpm)] may be accelerated or decelerated by interventions such as drugs, cardiac disease, or changes in autonomic nervous system tone. The mechanism for automatic discharges under these circumstances may remain normal; i.e., the same ionic pacemaker currents that mediate normal spontaneous diastolic depolarization may be responsible for diastolic depolarization following a given intervention, except that the kinetics or magnitude of the currents will be altered. Alternatively, ionic currents normally not involved in the formation of spontaneous impulses may become pacemaker currents and alter the sinus rhythm by abnormal mechanisms. Because the identity of the current(s) responsible for normal diastolic depolarization in the sinus node presently is unsettled (86), it is difficult to determine whether changes in sinus rhythm are due to alteration of normal automatic mechanisms or to the emergence of abnormal mechanisms, although generally it is assumed that most sinus arrhythmias are due to altered normal automaticity.

Spontaneous diastolic depolarization reflects a progressively increasing net gain of positive charge by the sinus nodal cell. This may result from either (a) a time-dependent decrease in an outward current (such as the potassium current I_K, also called I_{x1}) (86) in the presence of a steady background inward current or (b) a time-dependent increase in an inward current (such as the calcium current I_{Ca} or the pacemaker current I_f) in the presence of a steady outward current. Diastolic depolarization has been ascribed to both mechanisms, and it is not clear at the present time which of the two predominates or whether both may be important under certain circumstances. It does seem clear, however, that the upstroke of sinus nodal action potentials is mediated primarily by inward calcium current (87,125). Accordingly, sinus nodal automaticity is suppressed by calcium channel blockers such as verapamil, diltiazem, and nifedipine (64,125) and is enhanced by agents that increase calcium current, such as catecholamines (93,125).

Although the calcium channel blockers verapamil, nifedipine, and diltiazem all reduce the spontaneous discharge rate of the sinus node if given in sufficient concentrations *in vitro*, their effects on sinus rhythm *in vivo* vary (64,81), partly because of the fact that their so-called use-dependent actions on calcium channels in the sinus node differ, as do their potencies as peripheral vasodilators. With regard to the use-dependent effects of these drugs, several reports have indicated that the calcium channel blocking effects of verapamil and diltiazem are more apparent at high rates of stimulation and at less negative membrane potentials, implying that the drugs bind to inactivated calcium channels (66,73,79). In contrast, dihydropyridine derivatives such as nifedipine have less marked use-dependent effects (67,73,99), which may reduce their negative chronotropic actions during normal sinus rhythm. In addition, the dihydropyridine derivatives reduce blood pressure to a greater extent than verapamil and diltiazem and thereby elicit reflex sympathetic tone that may actually increase heart rate (64,81).

Sympathetic stimulation appears to increase the sinus discharge rate at least in part by initiating a cascade of metabolic events that culminates with an increase in calcium current (93,114). As a first step, β-adrenergic agonists bind to a specific sarcolemmal membrane receptor (the β receptor) and produce a conformational change in the receptor that facilitates the dissociation of two subunits of a regulatory protein to which the receptor is coupled. The subsequent interaction between one of the regulatory protein subunits and adenylate cyclase increases the activity of the cyclase and the formation of cyclic AMP. Cyclic AMP then binds to the regulatory subunit of a cyclic AMP-dependent protein kinase and promotes the phosphorylation of a membrane protein by the catalytic subunit of the kinase. Presumably, membrane phosphorylation induces a conformational change in the calcium channel and thereby increases the probability that the channel will open following an appropriate level of membrane depolarization. Thus, the gradual activation of calcium current that purportedly contributes to the latter half of diastolic depolarization in the sinus node (122) may be accelerated by agents such as isoproterenol.

Although acetylcholine may reduce the sinus nodal discharge rate by decreasing calcium current (29,108), it is more likely that the negative chronotropic effects of acetylcholine are due to increased potassium conductance and hyperpolarization of the membrane potential (8,46). *In vivo,* stimulation of parasympathetic nerves suppresses sinus nodal automaticity, and this effect predominates over the positive chronotropic effects of sympathetic nerve stimulation (74,124). In fact, vagal stimulation produces a greater absolute reduction of sinus nodal discharge rate in the presence of elevated sympathetic tone (74,124), a phenomenon known as accentuated antagonism (74). Antagonism of sympathetic effects by stimulation of parasympathetic nerves probably involves inhibition of norepinephrine release from prejunctional nerves by acetylcholine (70,74,83), as well as acetylcholine-induced reductions of adenylate cyclase activity and cyclic AMP generation in postjunctional membranes (see *Chapter* 71). Continuous or phasic vagal stimulation usually slows the sinus nodal discharge rate, but properly timed phasic stimulation of the vagus nerves also may accelerate sinus nodal automaticity (9,75), a phenomenon that will be described in detail in the section on phase-response relationships. In addition, sinus nodal automaticity may be accelerated transiently following a period of vagal stimulation (postvagal tachycardia) (9).

Subsidiary Atrial Pacemakers

Latent pacemaking cells appear to be present within several regions of the atria, including the coronary sinus (118), the inferior right atrium at its junction with the inferior vena cava (6,58,59,97), Bachmann's bundle (58,59), the AV valves (4,120), and atrial "plateau" fibers (43). Boineau et al. (6) have proposed that the sinus node is but one region of pacemaker cells within an atrial pacemaker complex and that at least two other pacemaking regions, located cranially and caudally to the sinus node, are present. Although under normal circumstances the dominant spontaneous rhythm appears to arise from the sinus node, atrial activation actually may be multicentric, and thus the resultant atrial activation wave front may represent the sum of several different wave fronts originating from the various pacemaker centers. During stimulation of parasympathetic nerves, the dominant spontaneous discharge rate often shifts to the caudal pacemaking area, whereas during sympathetic stimulation the dominant spontaneous discharge rate occurs in the cranial pacemaking area (6,35). Other investigators also have observed similar shifts in pacemaker activity during vagal stimulation or following application of acetylcholine to the sinus nodal area *in vitro* (7,106). Whether the shift in pacemaker dominance during autonomic nerve stimulation is due to different intrinsic responsiveness of the various pacemakers to acetylcholine and norepinephrine or to uneven distribution of the nerves is unclear.

Recent reports by Randall and co-workers (58,59,97) have suggested that disease or surgical excision of the sinus nodal region may unmask right atrial pacemakers located inferiorly to the atrial pacemaker complex. Conscious dogs in which the sinus node has been excised frequently develop P waves and spontaneous rhythms that originate from the junction of the inferior right atrium and inferior vena cava (58,59), although infusion of isoproterenol or left stellate ganglion stimulation may shift the dominant pacemaker site to the region of Bachmann's bundle (58). *In vitro* studies of the inferior right atrium indicate that the latent pacemakers are suppressed to a greater extent than the sinus node by periods of rapid pacing and by cholinergic stimulation (97). Beta-receptor stimulation is required for emergence of spontaneous activity, but the maximal spontaneous discharge rate of the latent pacemakers under sympathetic stimulation is less than that of the sinus node. Therefore, in the presence of normal sinus node function, latent pacemaker activity in the inferior right atrium is suppressed by overdrive activation and by the predominance of vagal tone. If sinus nodal function becomes depressed, however, the latent pacemakers may gain control of atrial rhythm and produce various arrhythmias because of their inappropriate responses to changes in autonomic tone.

The ionic mechanisms for latent pacemaker activity in the atrial pacemaker complex and inferior right atrium have not been established. The disparate effects of autonomic nerve stimulation on the spontaneous discharge rates of the various pacemakers suggest that several mechanisms may occur, although, again, the distribution of sympathetic and parasympathetic nerves may account for these effects. In addition, triggered activity has been demonstrated *in vitro* in the region of the mitral and tricuspid valves (4,120), but the contribution of triggered impulses arising from these areas to cardiac rhythm *in vivo* remains to be determined.

AV Node

It has been known for some time that ablation of atrial pacemakers results in a spontaneous rhythm that can be localized to the region of the AV junction. However, the exact location of pacemaking cells within the AV nodal region still has not been demonstrated conclusively, and it is likely that several potential pacemakers exist. For example, automaticity has been recorded from the region of the AV node nearest the His bundle (the NH region of the rabbit AV node) (89,109,119,121) and in the midportion of the AV node (the N region) if the AV node has been separated surgically from atrial muscle (68,119). The intrinsic spontaneous activity of the N region is similar to that of the sinus node and is abolished by acetylcholine and Mn^{2+} (68,119), whereas spontaneous activity generated in the NH region of the AV node is slower and is incompletely suppressed by acetylcholine (119).

The studies of isolated AV nodal tissues raise the possibility that AV junctional tachyarrhythmias such as nonparoxysmal junctional tachycardia may originate from the midportion of the AV node, provided the node has been isolated from the electrotonic effects of atrial muscle or from sites closer to the His bundle. Tachycardias due to automaticity occurring in the midportion of the AV node should be more rapid and more susceptible to vagally induced slowing than those originating from the more distal regions of the node, an expectation that is in agreement with studies in an intact canine model by Urthaler, James, and co-workers (56,111). However, Tse (110) has proposed that a group of fibers located between atrial muscle and the AV node (the paranodal fibers) have the most rapid intrinsic spontaneous discharge rate in the canine AV nodal region under the conditions of adrenergic drive. Thus, automaticity in the paranodal fibers may be responsible for junctional rhythms, provided vagal tone is low, because these fibers also appear to be more sensitive to acetylcholine than those of the AV node (110).

Action potentials within the N portion of the AV node, like those in the sinus node, are suppressed by verapamil and other calcium channel blockers and have relatively low amplitudes and upstroke velocities (64,68,126). These observations and recent preliminary voltage clamp data suggest that ionic currents in the AV node are similar to those in the sinus node (85), although the anatomical diversity of cell types in the AV node (56,102) may confound the interpretation of macroscopic current recordings.

Ventricle

In isolation, cells of the His-Purkinje system exhibit spontaneous diastolic depolarization and automaticity at spontaneous discharge rates (15–60 bpm) that are considerably slower than those of the sinus and AV junctional pacemakers. Ventricular muscle cells normally do not exhibit spontaneous diastolic depolarization or automaticity. However, recent studies (76) suggest that the pacemaker current I_f may be present in myocardial cells. Reduction of potassium conductance by Ba^{2+} (30,76) or amantadine (98) seemingly can unmask I_f and produce ventricular automaticity (Fig. 1). Thus,

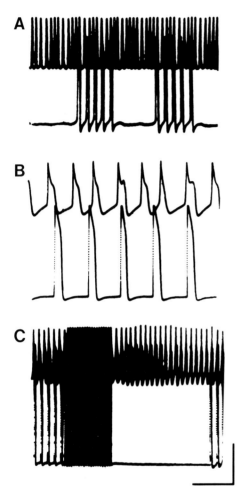

FIG. 1. Automaticity induced in a Purkinje fiber–papillary muscle preparation by superfusion with 0.25 mM BaCl$_2$. Prior to superfusion with BaCl$_2$, the preparation had been superfused with 8.0 mM CaCl$_2$ Tyrode solution to produce irreversible unidirectional block from Purkinje fiber to papillary muscle and subsequently had been superfused with 2.0 mM CaCl$_2$ Tyrode solution. **A:** BaCl$_2$ induced depolarization and sustained automaticity in the Purkinje fiber (*upper recording*) and intermittent spontaneous activity in the papillary muscle (*lower recording*) that was not accompanied by a significant loss of maximum diastolic membrane potential. **B:** Purkinje fiber automaticity did not propagate to papillary muscle, but spontaneous papillary muscle action potentials propagated to the Purkinje fiber when they occurred outside of the Purkinje fiber refractory period (i.e., unidirectional block was present). **C:** Following simultaneous overdrive pacing of Purkinje fiber and papillary muscle, automaticity was suppressed only in papillary muscle. Vertical calibration, 50 mV. Horizontal calibration, 10 sec for panels A and C and 2 sec for panel B. (From ref. 30, with permission.)

under certain circumstances, normally polarized ventricular muscle cells may develop spontaneous action potentials, particularly if they are uncoupled from more rapidly depolarizing Purkinje fibers, but the significance of these observations for ventricular automaticity *in vivo* has not been determined.

Although the spontaneous discharge rate of latent pacemakers in the His-Purkinje system normally is too slow to compete with the sinus node, Purkinje fiber automaticity may be enhanced by some of the metabolic and electrophysiologic consequences of myocardial ischemia and infarction (24,71,72). For example, the spontaneous discharge rate of a normal Purkinje fiber increases as the fiber is depolarized (18,47). Depolarization from −90 to −75 mV can increase the spontaneous discharge rate from 12 bpm to 60 bpm (18), but the mechanism for diastolic depolarization probably remains normal, and the increase in spontaneous discharge rate is due predominantly to a reduction in the time required to depolarize from the lower maximum diastolic potential to threshold. Several studies of subacutely infarcted canine ventricle have shown that some surviving subendocardial Purkinje fibers have moderately reduced maximum diastolic potentials and enhanced spontaneous activity (1,24,38,72). It is not known if the partial depolarization of these Purkinje cells is due to residual membrane damage and altered ionic permeabilities or if the maximum diastolic potential has been reduced because of electrotonic interactions with surrounding muscle cells that are more depolarized. In the latter case, enhanced Purkinje fiber automaticity may result from normal automatic mechanisms and contribute to arrhythmias occurring in these animals 1 to 5 days following acute myocardial infarction (44,45,101). Enhanced automaticity in partially depolarized human ventricular cells also has been observed in preparations of endocardial resections and aneurysms studied *in vitro* (31,103), but the relationship between phenomena occurring in the isolated preparations and arrhythmias occurring *in situ* remains to be established.

The emergence of Purkinje fiber automaticity following myocardial infarction may be facilitated by the creation of entrance block in depolarized or inexcitable myocardium surrounding the Purkinje focus and protection of the focal automaticity from overdrive excitation during sinus rhythm (24,72). Of course, slow conduction and inexcitable zones may cause exit block as well (24,72). Purkinje fiber automaticity also may be enhanced by catecholamines released during ischemia (11), particularly because the positive chronotropic effects of catecholamines appear to be greater in Purkinje fibers surviving myocardial infarction than in normal Purkinje fibers (38), possibly because of denervation supersensitivity (124). However, enhanced Purkinje fiber automaticity can occur when catecholamine release has subsided *in vivo* or in the presence of propranolol *in vitro* (72).

Although enhanced Purkinje fiber automaticity has been reported frequently in subacutely or chronically infarcted myocardium, automaticity in acutely ischemic ventricular myocardium appears to be unchanged (101) or suppressed (34,71). Suppression of automaticity may be due to activation of the background potassium conductance and marked cellular depolarization (86) induced by extracellular accumulation of potassium (40). Cooling and other factors also may contribute to suppression of automaticity, since the spontaneous discharge rate of hamster ventricular transplant cells studied *in situ* decreased prior to a significant loss of maximum diastolic potential (34).

Related Arrhythmias

Sinus Node

Identification of automaticity as a cause of clinically occurring arrhythmias traditionally has been based on a lack of evidence for a reentrant mechanism; i.e., if the arrhythmia could not be initiated or terminated by a single properly timed premature stimulus, it was presumed to be automatic. However, recent studies have shown that single stimuli may initiate and terminate certain forms of automaticity (31,51), as well as triggered activity (see *Chapter* 60). Therefore, at the present time there are no totally acceptable criteria for identifying arrhythmias due to enhanced normal automaticity. As will be discussed below, however, certain arrhythmias are more likely to be due to enhanced automaticity than to reentry.

Sinus tachycardia (sinus rates exceeding 100 bpm) or bradycardia (sinus rates less than 60 bpm) may be precipitated by various physiological stimuli, drugs, and disease states (for review, see ref. 123), but the mechanisms for diastolic depolarization and action potential generation probably are normal under these circumstances; they simply have been enhanced or suppressed. Sinus rhythm also may show cyclic variations in response to respiration or to digitalis intoxication and may become irregular or cease entirely (arrest) as a result of infarction, degenerative cellular changes, drug toxicity, and excessive vagal tone (e.g., hypersensitive carotid sinus syndrome). However, discriminating sinus arrhythmias due to changes in the spontaneous discharge rate from those due to sinoatrial exit block can be difficult.

Subsidiary Atrial Pacemakers

Acceleration of the spontaneous discharge rate of subsidiary atrial pacemakers by a variety of disease states and by drugs such as digitalis and alcohol may produce automatic atrial tachycardias, although it is difficult to eliminate micro-reentry (2) as a cause of these arrhythmias *in vivo*. In patients, suspected automatic atrial tachycardias are associated with P waves and atrial activation sequences that differ from those seen during normal sinus rhythm, and with constant P-wave morphology during the tachycardia. In contrast, most forms of reentrant atrial tachycardia exhibit a different morphology of the initial and subsequent P waves in the tachycardia, because of different atrial activation sequences (36). Automatic atrial tachycardias usually cannot be terminated by vagal stimulation, premature atrial stimulation, or verapamil (123).

Subsidiary atrial pacemakers also may contribute to the wandering pacemaker syndrome, in which the sinus rate gradually decelerates over several beats in association with a change in the P-wave morphology. As the spontaneous discharge rate of the sinus node slows, latent atrial pacemakers may escape and assume control of the rhythm. Discharge of subsidiary pacemakers during more marked transient slowing of the sinus node discharge rate may produce premature atrial complexes.

AV Junction

In the presence of severe sinus bradycardia or block of sinus-initiated impulses proximal to the AV node, automatic foci in the AV junction can escape and produce single complexes or a sustained AV junctional escape rhythm at a rate of 35 to 60 bpm. Following the first AV escape complex, the automatic rate of the AV junction often increases slightly (the so-called rhythm of development or warm-up phenomenon) and then becomes fairly regular. Acceleration of the intrinsic spontaneous discharge rate of the AV junction to rates of 70 to 130 bpm following open-heart surgery, inferior myocardial infarction, myocarditis, or digitalis administration may initiate a nonparoxysmal AV junction tachycardia. The onset and termination of this type of junctional tachycardia usually are gradual (hence nonparoxysmal), and the tachycardia rate is slowed by enhanced vagal tone or is accelerated by vagolytic agents.

Ventricle

Ventricular arrhythmias such as parasystole, accelerated idioventricular rhythms, and some forms of repetitive monomorphic ventricular tachycardia are more likely to be due to enhanced automaticity than to reentry (123). In addition, experimental electrophysiological studies, as discussed previously, have suggested that premature ventricular complexes and ventricular tachycardia following myocardial infarction also may be due to enhanced normal automaticity in subendocardial Purkinje fibers (44,45,101).

Several investigators have suggested that overdrive pacing and premature stimulation can be useful for identifying ventricular arrhythmias due to enhanced normal automaticity, abnormal automaticity, or triggered activity (41,94,113). For example, following a period of overdrive pacing, normal automaticity in Purkinje fibers should be suppressed, whereas slow response-mediated automaticity arising from depolarized Purkinje fibers should be less affected, similar to normal automaticity in other slow response-dependent regions such as the sinus node (see section on Overdrive Suppression of Automaticity and Conduction, below). Depending on the overdrive pacing cycle length, triggered activity will be enhanced, unchanged, or suppressed (14). Attempts to differentiate triggered rhythms from automaticity based on their responses to overdrive pacing have been made in humans (94), but more data are needed to determine if the response of these arrhythmias to overdrive pacing will be a useful diagnostic indicator. Successful differentiation of enhanced normal automaticity from abnormal automaticity may have important therapeutic consequences, because sodium channel blockers would be more likely to suppress enhanced normal automaticity, whereas calcium channel blockers would be more likely to suppress depolarization-induced automaticity.

ABNORMAL AUTOMATICITY

Experimental Observations

Sinus Node

Although the spontaneous discharge rate of the sinus node may become irregular under various circumstances, as discussed earlier, the ionic mechanisms responsible for diastolic depolarization and action potential generation probably remain normal, albeit modified. To our knowledge there are no documented examples of sinus node automaticity that are due to abnormal ionic mechanisms. It should be emphasized, however, that the considerable disagreement concerning the identity of normal sinus nodal pacemaker currents (86) makes determination of a potentially abnormal pacemaker mechanism a quixotic undertaking at the present time.

Subsidiary Atrial Pacemakers and the AV Junction

Identification of abnormal automaticity in the subsidiary atrial pacemakers and the AV junction also is difficult, if not impossible, at the present time, because the mechanisms for normal automaticity in these regions have not been defined. A potential abnormality of impulse formation in atrial and distal AV nodal pacemakers is triggered activity, which differs from abnormal automaticity in that it requires an antecedent depolarizing stimulus or action potential for initiation (see *Chapter 60*). One such triggering stimulus is the delayed afterdepolarization, which occurs following the induction of the transient inward current (I_{ti}) by elevated intracellular

calcium concentration (60). It is possible that under certain pathological conditions or during digitalis intoxication, I_{ti} may contribute to automaticity in the sinus and AV nodes. However, the manifestation of I_{ti} in the sinus and AV nodes simply may be altered diastolic depolarization, rather than an identifiable delayed afterdepolarization.

Ventricle

In isolation, normal cardiac Purkinje fibers usually have relatively slow spontaneous discharge rates, whereas atrial and ventricular muscle fibers are quiescent. However, depolarization of these cells by disease or various experimental maneuvers can accelerate existing spontaneous activity or induce automaticity in previously quiescent cells (18,39,47,48,62,63,90) (Fig. 2). In some respects, depolarization-induced automaticity in Purkinje fibers and ventricular myocardium resembles normal automaticity in the sinus node. For example, the spontaneous discharge rates of the two types of automaticity are similar, and the spontaneous action potentials are suppressed by calcium channel blockers and maneuvers that increase potassium conductance (18,37,47,48,63), but are not significantly affected by sodium channel blockers (18,37,47,62) (Fig. 3A). Conversely, agents that increase calcium current, such as β-adrenergic agonists, accelerate depolarization-induced automaticity (47,48,90). As in the sinus node, the identity of the pacemaker current in depolarized Purkinje fibers and myocardium has not been determined conclusively, and evidence that decay of I_k (39,48,63) and activation of I_{Ca} (90) contribute to spontaneous diastolic depolarization in these cells has been presented.

The spontaneous discharge rates attained by depolarized Purkinje and ventricular muscle cells may be determined not only by the membrane potential of the cell but also by the composition of the external environment and the mass and membrane potential of myocardium surrounding the depolarized area. Small strips (2–3 mm) of normally polarized Purkinje fibers and myocardium subjected to more or less uniform depolarization usually display a continuous curvilinear relationship between membrane potential and spontaneous discharge rate at membrane potentials in the range of −75 to −20 mV (18,47,62) (Fig. 3B). In contrast, focally depolarized regions of Purkinje fibers and ventricular muscle (20,96) or Purkinje fibers subjected to a low extracellular potassium environment (90) discharge spontaneously at membrane potentials greater than −70 mV and less than −50 mV, but become quiescent at voltages within the range of −50 to −70 mV. It is possible that the membrane potential range of −50 to −70 mV is a crossover region for activation of the pacemaker currents I_f and I_k (which may mediate diastolic depolarization at the more negative and less negative membrane potentials, respectively) (86). Because of the relatively small amount

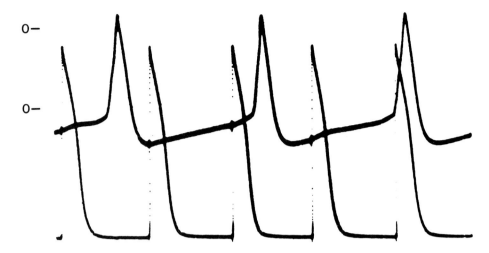

FIG. 2. Automaticity at reduced membrane potentials in diseased human ventricular myocardium. The upper recording was obtained from an area bordering the infarcted zone of an endocardial resection. The lower recording was obtained from more normally appearing myocardium in another area of the resection. Maximum diastolic potentials in the upper and lower recordings were −67 mV and −84 mV, respectively. The abnormal area exhibited spontaneous activity, whereas the normal area was quiescent (not shown). Pacing the normal area at a cycle length of 1,000 msec produced action potentials that did not propagate to the abnormal zone, nor did spontaneous action potentials in the abnormal zone propagate to the normal zone. Vertical calibration, 50 mV. Horizontal calibration, 2 sec.

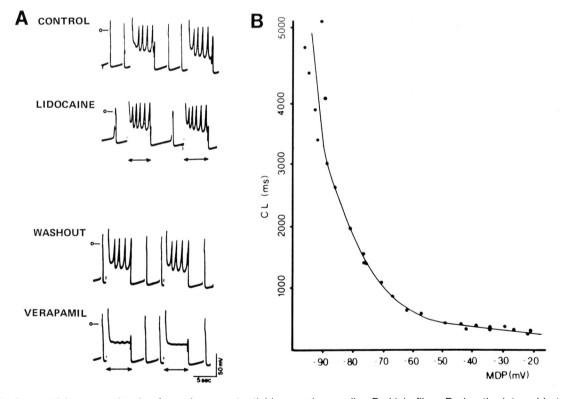

FIG. 3. A: Automaticity at two levels of membrane potential in a canine cardiac Purkinje fiber. During the interval between the arrowheads, the fiber was depolarized from −85 mV to −50 mV using current injection across a sucrose gap. Lidocaine (3 mg/liter) slowed the spontaneous discharge rate and reduced the amplitude of action potentials arising from −85 mV, but did not affect action potentials or automaticity at −50 mV. After washout of lidocaine, exposure to verapamil (3 μM) suppressed automaticity at −50 mV, but not at −85 mV. **B:** Relationship between the maximum diastolic membrane potential (*abscissa*) and the cycle length of spontaneous discharges (*ordinate*) in a canine Purkinje fiber similar to that shown in panel A. Marked shortening of the spontaneous cycle length occurred as the membrane potential was reduced from −90 to −60 mV, with lesser shortening of the cycle length as the membrane potential was reduced further to −20 mV. (From ref. 18, with permission.)

of pacemaker current activated in this range of membrane potentials, spontaneous activity may be aborted by the repolarizing electrotonic effects of more polarized surrounding myocardium or by the reduction of inward current induced by sustained depolarization. Therefore, the occurrence of abnormal automaticity in Purkinje fibers or myocardium depolarized by ischemia or infarction may depend on the membrane potential of the depolarized area and the degree of electrotonic interaction between the depolarized area and surrounding myocardium.

Related Arrhythmias

Supraventricular

Differentiation between clinical arrhythmias due to abnormal automaticity and those due to enhanced normal automaticity, triggered activity, or reentry usually is not possible. Experimental studies in which the sinus rate was determined during maximally effective stimulation of the stellate ganglia suggest that heart rates greater than 200 bpm are not due to enhanced normal automaticity (42,92). However, these tachyarrhythmias still may be due to either abnormal automaticity or reentry. In addition, a heart rate of less than 200 bpm does not exclude abnormal automaticity or reentry as a cause of the rhythm (41,42). Given these diagnostic limitations, abnormal automaticity may be responsible for some examples of atrial flutter and tachycardia or AV junctional tachycardia, although it is more likely that most of these atrial tachyarrhythmias are due to macroscopic or microscopic reentry (123).

Ventricular

Definitive criteria for diagnosis of ventricular arrhythmias due to abnormal automaticity also are lacking. The presence of spontaneous activity in depolarized specimens of diseased human atrium (78,103) and ventricle (15,31,103,105) suggests that abnormal automaticity may occur *in vivo* and cause arrhythmias. However, the spontaneous discharge rates of the isolated preparations usually are too slow to account for clinically occurring atrial or ventricular tachycardias. Perhaps endogenous factors that are absent from the *in vitro* environment, such as sympathetic innervation, histamine, and stretch, may increase the spontaneous discharge rate of these fibers to rates at which a tachycardia can be precipitated, but this remains to be determined.

INTERACTIONS BETWEEN AUTOMATIC FOCI

Experimental Observations

Phase-Response Relationship

Because normal myocardium largely behaves as a functional syncytium, spontaneous discharges generated by the cell with the most rapid rate of diastolic depolarization propagate to and activate neighboring cells before they spontaneously depolarize to threshold. As a result, a synchronous cardiac rhythm occurs. However, the presence of conduction block between two areas of myocardium can allow the areas to generate spontaneous activities at different rates. If the two areas remain coupled to one another via intercellular connections, spontaneous action potentials initiated in each area will generate current that flows passively across the zone of conduction block. Transfer of sufficient electrotonic current from one spontaneously active area to the other may induce subthreshold responses in each of the areas that alter their respective discharge rates.

Electrotonic interactions between ectopic foci can produce complex rhythm disturbances, but these arrhythmias may be predicted on the basis of general properties of biological oscillators (3,82,117). One such property is the phase-response relationship, a common example of which is shown in Fig. 4. In this type-0 phase-response curve (the average slope of the relationship is zero), subthreshold depolarizing impulses that invade a focal area in early diastole delay the next expected spontaneous discharge of the pacemaker, whereas subthreshold impulses that invade the focal area at late diastolic intervals accelerate the next expected discharge. A sharp transition from delay to acceleration occurs at an intermediate diastolic interval. The amount of pacemaker acceleration or delay is proportional to the amplitude of the subthreshold response (53–55), which in turn is determined by the amplitude and duration of action potentials generated by myocardium surrounding the pacemaker focus and by the coupling resistance between the pacemaker site and surrounding myocardium.

The ionic basis for pacemaker acceleration and delay by subthreshold stimuli has not been determined, but it seems likely that depolarizing stimuli delivered during early diastole reactivate outward repolarizing potassium current and thereby retard diastolic depolarization (12,55). This may be particularly important in the sinus node and depolarized Purkinje fibers and ventricular myocardium, where time-dependent decay of I_k is thought to be responsible for the early portion of diastolic depolarization (39,86,87). In addition, subthreshold stimuli may partially reset time- and voltage-dependent activation of inward currents contributing to diastolic depolarization (12), such as I_{Ca} in the sinus node and depolarized ventricular tissues (87,90,122) and I_f for normally polarized Purkinje fibers (17). In contrast, depolarizing stimuli delivered during late diastole probably contribute to the depolarization needed to reach the activation threshold for sodium or calcium channels.

Hyperpolarizing subthreshold stimuli also modulate pacemaker activity, as demonstrated in Fig. 5. In this example, a type-1 phase-response relationship occurs (the average slope of the relationship is one). Stimuli

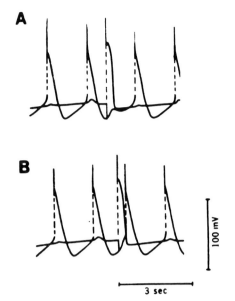

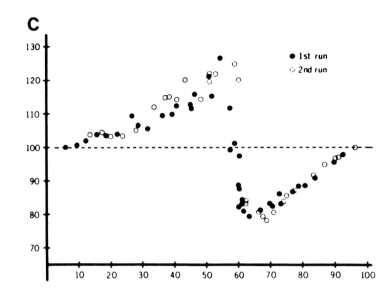

FIG. 4. Phase-dependent acceleration and delay of Purkinje fiber automaticity induced by subthreshold depolarizations. The Purkinje fiber was mounted in a three-chamber bath. The left segment of the fiber was superfused with low-potassium (2 mM) Tyrode solution containing epinephrine (0.1 μg/ml) to induce automaticity. The middle segment was superfused with isotonic sucrose solution to create an area of inexcitable cells, and the right segment was superfused with normal Tyrode solution. Stimulation of the right segment of the fiber produced action potentials that propagated to the border with the middle segment, at which point active propagation ceased because of the inexcitable gap. However, the middle segment acted as a conduit for passive flow of current from right to left segments. Thus, action potentials in the right segment generated an electrotonic potential that produced subthreshold depolarizations in the left segment. **A:** Action potentials were recorded from the right (*upper recording*) and left (*lower recording*) segments of the fiber. The control spontaneous cycle length of the left segment was 1,500 msec. Stimulation of the right segment of the fiber 800 msec after the left segment had discharged spontaneously produced a subthreshold depolarization in the left segment and prolonged the cycle length of the next spontaneous discharge to 1,850 msec (a 23% increase). **B:** Stimulation of the right segment 1,000 msec after the left segment had discharged spontaneously shortened the spontaneous cycle length to 1,230 msec (an 18% decrease). **C:** Complete phase-response curves for the experiment shown in panels A and B. Two different runs are shown. *Ordinate:* percentage increase or decrease in the spontaneous cycle length of the left segment (control cycle length = 100%). *Abscissa:* percentage of the control left segment spontaneous cycle length at which the right segment was stimulated. The spontaneous cycle length was maximally prolonged (by 26%) or shortened (by 20%) by subthreshold depolarizations that entered the left segment after approximately 50% and 60% of diastole had elapsed, respectively. (From ref. 54, with permission.)

delivered during the early phases of diastole accelerate the next expected spontaneous discharge, whereas those delivered later in diastole produce a progressive delay in the next spontaneous discharge. In this experiment, increasing the duration of the stimulus shifted the curve upward (less acceleration and more delay), but increasing the intensity of the hyperpolarizing stimulus may increase the amount of acceleration, particularly for stimuli of short duration (53). The acceleration of spontaneous activity by hyperpolarizing pulses delivered in early diastole is associated with a steeper slope of diastolic depolarization, which may be due to hyperpolarization-induced inactivation of outward potassium current and concomitant unmasking of inward background or pacemaker currents (12,55,88). In addition, hyperpolarization of cells having low maximum diastolic potentials, such as those in the sinus node and depolarized Purkinje fibers, may recruit pacemaker current (17,88). Although hyperpolarization in the later phases of diastole also increases the slope of diastolic depolarization, this effect is counteracted by the increased time required to depolarize from the more negative membrane potential to

threshold. Hyperpolarization-induced acceleration of diastolic depolarization also may be offset by increasing the duration of the hyperpolarizing pulse and forcing the membrane potential to remain below threshold.

The phase-resetting effects of hyperpolarizing current pulses are similar in many respects to the effects of acetylcholine-induced hyperpolarization and may explain acceleration and deceleration of sinus nodal automaticity by vagal stimulation *in vitro* (55) and *in vivo* (9,74,75). In the intact animal or human, each systolic pulse stimulates the aortic and carotid baroreceptors and induces bursts of vagal discharges that may modify the sinus rhythm (74). Changes in the ventricular rate produced, for example, by premature ventricular complexes will alter systolic blood pressure and modulate the effects of the vagus on sinus rhythm. This feedback loop between the ventricular and sinus rhythms can induce complex arrhythmias that appear to be irregular but are in fact the result of a predictable phase-response relationship between the vagus and the sinus node (80).

Strong, continuous vagal stimulation produces sustained hyperpolarization in the sinus node and slows

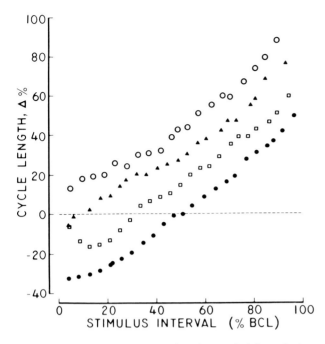

FIG. 5. Phase-dependent acceleration and delay of sinus nodal automaticity by hyperpolarizing current pulses. A thin strip of sinus nodal tissue was mounted in a three-chamber bath. The left segment of the preparation was superfused with normal Tyrode solution, and the middle segment was superfused with isotonic sucrose solution to produce an area of inexcitable cells. The right segment was superfused with Tyrode solution containing 20 mM KCl to depolarize the cells and facilitate current injection. The spontaneous cycle length of the left segment was 480 msec. *Ordinate:* percentage change in spontaneous cycle length. *Abscissa:* percentage of the spontaneous cycle at which the current pulses were delivered. The symbols represent RC current pulses of 24.4 µA in strength and time constants of 150 msec (*filled circles*), 200 msec (*open squares*), 250 msec (*filled triangles*), and 300 msec (*open circles*). Using current pulses having a time constant of 150 msec, the spontaneous cycle length was shortened by pulses delivered early in diastole and prolonged by pulses delivered later in diastole. Increasing the time constant of the current pulses reduced the amount of pacemaker acceleration and increased pacemaker delay. (From ref. 55, with permission.)

the sinus rate, irrespective of the diastolic phase during which it is induced (similar to the upper curve in Fig. 5). On cessation of vagal stimulation, a transient sinus tachycardia may ensue, apparently because the acceleratory effects of acetylcholine on phase four depolarization are no longer offset by continuous hyperpolarization (9,55). Thus, depending on the intensity and timing of vagal discharges, the sinus rate may be accelerated or delayed on a beat-to-beat basis or for relatively long periods of time.

Delivery of a subthreshold depolarizing or hyperpolarizing stimulus of the appropriate duration and intensity at a precise time in diastole [the singular point (117), which usually is near the phase marking the transition from pacemaker delay to pacemaker acceleration] com-

pletely suppresses, or annihilates, spontaneous activity (5,31,51) (Fig. 6). Annihilated foci may remain quiescent until an external stimulus initiates an action potential and restores pacemaker activity. Annihilation of spontaneous activity apparently involves reducing net transmembrane current flow nearly to zero (5,12). In highly polarized cells such as those of the His-Purkinje system, the magnitude and "inertia" of inward and outward currents at membrane potentials other than the resting membrane potential probably are too large to balance precisely, although two levels of stable membrane potentials can be produced under certain circumstances (13,26,116). At less negative maximum diastolic potentials, inward and outward currents are reduced in magnitude and may be closer to equilibrium. Thus, small changes in either are more likely to move the membrane potential to a singular, or null, point.

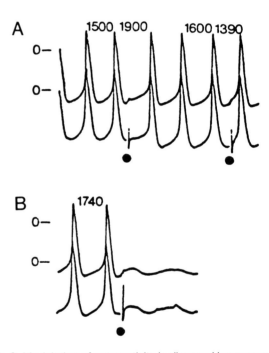

FIG. 6. Modulation of automaticity in diseased human ventricle by subthreshold current pulses. **A:** Action potentials recorded from two sites along the same ventricular trabeculum. Current pulses of 30 msec duration (indicated by the dots) were injected through the lower recording microelectrode. The interval between spontaneous discharges is given above each interval. Injection of a current pulse relatively early in diastole (680 msec after the preceding action potential upstroke; left dot) produced a subthreshold depolarization at the upper recording site and delayed the next spontaneous discharge by 400 msec. Delivery of a current pulse later in diastole (950 msec after the preceding action potential upstroke; right dot) accelerated the next discharge by 210 msec, relative to the preceding spontaneous cycle. **B:** Same preparation as panel A. Delivery of a current pulse at the singular point (930 msec after the preceding action potential upstroke) abolished pacemaker activity. Vertical calibration, 50 mV. Horizontal calibration, 2 sec. (From ref. 31, with permission.)

Entrainment

The experiments described above demonstrate the effects of a single subthreshold stimulus on the cycle length of the next expected pacemaker discharge. Repeated delivery of subthreshold stimuli may force the pacemaker to discharge continuously at a rate that is faster or slower than its intrinsic rate, a process known as entrainment (3,50). Consequently, subthreshold stimuli exchanged between two pacemakers may induce mutual entrainment of the foci. For example, if one pacemaker having a rapid intrinsic spontaneous discharge rate is coupled via an inexcitable segment of tissue to another pacemaker having a slower intrinsic rate, electrotonic currents flowing across the inexcitable segment may modulate diastolic depolarization in both foci and produce a mean spontaneous discharge rate that is some intermediate value between the two intrinsic discharge rates. Increasing the coupling resistance between the two pacemakers reduces the electrotonic influence of each pacemaker on the other and disrupts entrainment. Depending on the coupling resistance, various arrhythmias or complete desynchronization of the two pacemaker activities may occur (50).

Related Arrhythmias

It appears possible, on the basis of experimental results and computer simulations of phase-resetting behavior, that interactions between automatic foci may account for a wide spectrum of cardiac arrhythmias (50,82), including some arrhythmias previously attributed to reentry. Retrospective analyses of clinical electrocardiograms previously purported to represent phenomena such as exit block indicate that modulated parasystole may account for the phenomena equally well (82), and clinical reports of arrhythmias due to complex interactions between automatic foci are beginning to appear. For example, pacemaker acceleration, delay, and annihilation have been observed recently in humans (10,25,84). However, the contribution of phase-resetting phenomena to clinical arrhythmias probably is underappreciated at the present time. As more is learned about the clinical occurrence of arrhythmias involving more than one automatic focus, it may be necessary to revise concepts concerning the major arrhythmia presently attributed to interactions between automatic foci: parasystole.

Classically, parasystole has been considered to be a relatively benign arrhythmia characterized by interactions between two pacemakers having stable, but different, spontaneous discharge rates (61). Intermittent or constant entrance block protects one focus from being reset by impulses initiated in the other, whereas the other focus is subject to resetting if a parasystolic impulse arrives after its refractory period has expired. Exit block from

the parasystolic focus also may occur and may vary the number of ectopic atrial or ventricular complexes. As originally defined, parasystolic discharges occur at intervals that are multiples of a basic interval, and variation in the spontaneous discharge interval constitutes evidence against a parasystolic mechanism being responsible for a given arrhythmia. As discussed above, however, one pacemaker may entrain, accelerate, or delay the spontaneous discharges of another pacemaker. Therefore, variable coupling of spontaneous discharges may be an intrinsic manifestation of parasystole, rather than evidence against its existence.

INTERACTIONS BETWEEN AUTOMATICITY AND CONDUCTION

Experimental Observations

Deceleration-Dependent Conduction Block

One purported example of an interaction between automaticity and conduction is deceleration-dependent conduction block, also called phase four block or bradycardia-dependent block (95). Based on studies of depolarized Purkinje fibers, Singer et al. (104) postulated that during a long diastolic interval secondary to sinus bradycardia or AV block, spontaneous diastolic depolarization in latent pacemakers of the His-Purkinje system would partially inactivate fast sodium channels. As a result, the next impulse to invade the His-Purkinje system might be blocked because of reduced Purkinje fiber action potential amplitude, upstroke velocity, and excitability. Direct measurements of the current necessary to produce excitation in Purkinje cells at the various membrane potentials attained during diastolic depolarization have shown, however, that excitability actually increases as the membrane depolarizes, despite a reduction of action potential amplitude and upstroke velocity (33,91). Evidently, inactivation of fast sodium channels is offset by other factors such as a reduction in the difference between the membrane potential and the threshold potential (91), an increase in membrane resistance and the membrane space constant (115), and progressive activation of the pacemaker and steady-state sodium "window" currents (17,86).

Recently, an alternate explanation for deceleration-dependent conduction block has been proposed (52), based on the observation that action potential amplitude and excitability are reduced at long diastolic intervals in continuously depolarized Purkinje fibers (33,52) and atrial muscle (77) that exhibit little or no phase four depolarization (Fig. 7). The progressive reductions of action potential amplitude and excitability during diastole are associated with an increased propensity for conduction block, suggesting that it is the diastolic interval per se, rather than spontaneous depolarization during dias-

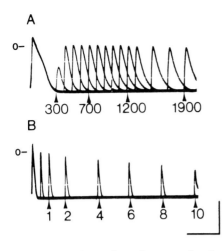

FIG. 7. Biphasic time-dependent changes of action potential amplitude in the middle segment of a Purkinje fiber mounted in a three-chamber bath. The left, middle, and right segments of the fiber were superfused with normal Tyrode solution, Tyrode solution containing 16 mM KCl at a pH of 6.7 and a PO_2 less than 40 mm Hg, and Tyrode solution containing 6 mM KCl, respectively. **A:** Following the last stimulus of a train of 20 stimuli delivered to the left segment of the fiber (basic cycle length = 500 msec), single stimuli were delivered to the right segment at coupling intervals that varied from 300 to 1,900 msec. The middle segment action potential elicited by the last stimulus of the train is shown to the left, and the action potentials elicited by stimulation of the right segment at various coupling intervals are superimposed to the right. Action potential amplitude was low at short coupling intervals (300 msec) and increased to a maximum at intermediate coupling intervals (700 msec). At coupling intervals greater than 1,200 msec, action potential amplitude began to decline. **B:** Same format as panel A, except that the time scale has been expanded to show the decline of action potential amplitude as the coupling interval was prolonged from 1 to 10 sec. Vertical calibration, 50 mV. Horizontal calibration, 400 msec for panel A and 2 sec for panel B.

tole, that determines the success or failure of conduction in depressed His-Purkinje or atrial tissue. However, diastolic depolarization might contribute to deceleration-dependent conduction block if the spontaneously depolarizing region were located proximal to a zone of continuously depolarized tissue. Following a long diastolic interval, low-amplitude, slowly rising action potentials in the spontaneously depolarizing region might not be able to overcome reduced excitability in the continuously depolarized region, and conduction block would occur.

The mechanisms for deceleration-dependent reductions of Purkinje fiber excitability and action potential amplitude are uncertain at present. Recent observations (32) indicate that 4-aminopyridine, an inhibitor of the transient or early outward current (65), prevents the decline of Purkinje fiber action potential amplitude after long diastolic intervals, whereas agents that decrease background potassium conductance ($CsCl_2$) (49) or increase calcium current (isoproterenol) (93) do not. These results suggest that the time-dependent reduction of

action potential amplitude may be due to more complete recovery of the transient outward current, rather than to reduction of inward calcium current.

Overdrive Suppression of Automaticity and Conduction

It has been appreciated for some time that the spontaneous discharge rate of a normal cardiac pacemaking cell is slowed temporarily following a period of rapid pacing, a phenomenon known as overdrive suppression of automaticity (112,113). Overdrive suppression of automaticity appears to result from intracellular accumulation of sodium during prolonged periods of rapid stimulation. Elevated levels of intracellular sodium increase the turnover rate of the sodium pump, and because the pump exchanges three intracellular sodium ions for two extracellular potassium ions, the maximum diastolic membrane potential becomes more negative (16,27). Thus, the time required for the cell to reach threshold is increased, and the spontaneous discharge rate is slowed until the intracellular sodium concentration returns to previous levels. Pacemakers having a relatively large influx of sodium during each action potential, such as those in the His-Purkinje system, are suppressed to a greater extent following overdrive stimulation than are pacemakers whose action potentials are largely dependent on calcium influx, such as the sinus node.

Under the appropriate circumstances, conduction also may be suppressed following a period of rapid pacing (overdrive suppression of conduction) (19,21,33,69,107). This phenomenon appears to be related to biphasic changes of action potential amplitude and excitability in depolarized Purkinje cells (33,107), as shown previously in Fig. 7. If the intensity of stimuli delivered to the depressed segment of Purkinje tissue is low (for example, if action potentials generated in myocardium surrounding the depressed zone have relatively low action potential amplitude), then conduction through the depressed zone will most likely occur only at intermediate coupling intervals or pacing rates, when action potential amplitude and excitability in the depressed zone are maximal. However, if the intensity of the stimuli delivered to the depressed zone is increased, then conduction may be possible at shorter and longer coupling intervals, despite the lower action potential amplitude.

In the example of overdrive suppression of conduction shown in Fig. 8, a Purkinje fiber was mounted in a three-chamber bath, and the experimental conditions were altered to produce anisotropic conduction across a depressed segment of cells located in the middle chamber. Under these conditions, conduction block occurred while pacing the right side of the fiber at cycle lengths less than 450 msec. However, it was possible to achieve 1:1 conduction through the depressed zone at shorter cycle lengths by pacing cells on the left side of the fiber, which

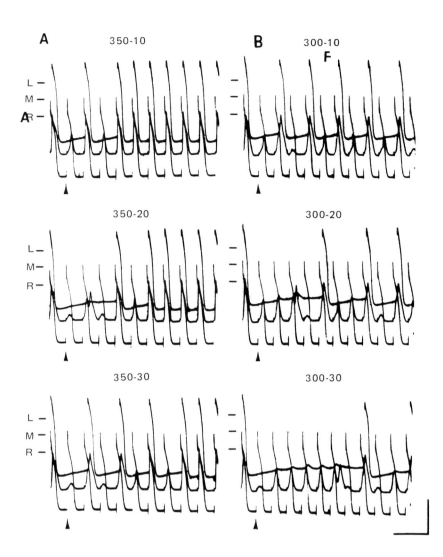

A   350-10
B   300-10

350-20   300-20

350-30   300-30

FIG. 8. Overdrive suppression of conduction in a canine Purkinje fiber mounted in a three-chamber bath. The preparation was similar to that described in Fig. 7. The upper, middle, and lower recordings in each set of recordings were obtained from the left (L), middle (M), and right (R) segments of the fiber, respectively. The horizontal lines to the left of each recording represent zero potential. **A:** Following delivery of a train of 10, 20, or 30 stimuli at a cycle length of 350 msec to the left segment of the fiber (upper, middle, and lower sets of recordings, respectively), the right segment was paced at a cycle length (450 msec) that had produced 1:1 right-to-left conduction prior to overdrive pacing. Action potentials produced by the last stimulus of the train are shown to the left, and the beginning of right segment pacing is indicated by the arrows. As the number of overdrive pacing stimuli was increased from 10 to 30, the time to the first conducted action potential and the time to restoration of 1:1 right-to-left conduction increased. **B:** Same experiment and stimulation protocol as panel A, except that the cycle length of overdrive pacing was reduced to 300 msec. Shortening the cycle length of overdrive pacing further increased the time to the first conducted action potential and the time to restoration of 1:1 conduction (not shown). Vertical calibration, 50 mV. Horizontal calibration, 1 sec. (From ref. 33, with permission.)

had larger action potential amplitudes. Pacing at the shorter cycle lengths produced cumulative reductions of action potential amplitude in the depressed zone, and on return to pacing of the right side of the fiber at the same cycle length that previously had produced 1:1 conduction, action potential amplitude in the depressed segment temporarily remained low, and block occurred. With time, action potential amplitude in the depressed zone normalized, and 1:1 conduction was restored.

Action potential propagation through a region of depressed Purkinje cells may depend not only on the "intensity" of the stimulus provided by cells located proximal to the depressed zone and on action potential amplitude and excitability of cells within the depressed zone but also on the excitability of cells located distal to the depressed zone. Because the excitability of the latter cells increases as the diastolic membrane potential becomes less negative (33,91), changes in the rate of spontaneous diastolic depolarization following periods of rapid or slow pacing can affect conduction through

this region of cells. For example, Fig. 9 demonstrates that following a period of rapid pacing, conduction block was associated with reduced action potential amplitude and excitability in the depressed zone and hyperpolarization and concomitant reduction of excitability in cells located distal to the depressed zone; i.e., overdrive suppression of conduction involved overdrive suppression of automaticity. On the other hand, the occurrence of conduction block at both short and long coupling intervals was reduced following pacing at slow rates, despite low action potential amplitude in the depressed zone, because excitability in the distal region was augmented by less pacing-induced hyperpolarization and a steeper slope of diastolic depolarization.

The examples given above suggest that conduction through a region of depolarized His-Purkinje tissue may involve changes of action potential amplitude and excitability both in the depolarized region and in surrounding myocardium and that these changes may be modulated by the extent of diastolic depolarization.

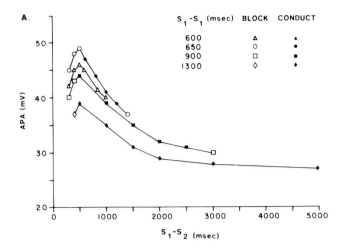

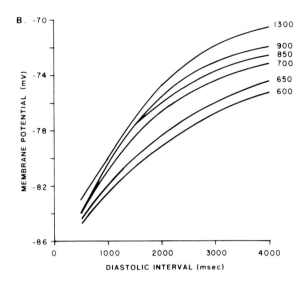

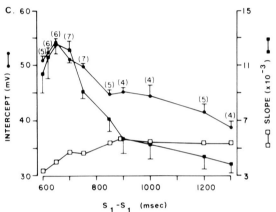

FIG. 9. Interaction between time-dependent changes of action potential amplitude in the middle segment and diastolic membrane potential in the left segment of a Purkinje fiber mounted in a three-chamber bath. The preparation was similar to that described in Fig. 7. **A:** Relationship between action potential amplitude in the middle segment of the fiber (APA; *ordinate*) and the coupling intervals of stimuli delivered to the right segment (S_1-S_2; *abscissa*) after delivery of a train of 20 stimuli to the left segment at cycle lengths of 600, 650, 900, and 1,300 msec (*legend,* **upper right**). Filled symbols indicate action potentials that conducted to the left segment, and unfilled symbols indicate action potentials that blocked. **B:** Recordings of diastolic depolarization in the left segment of the fiber following delivery of 20 stimuli to the left segment at the indicated cycle lengths. **C:** Relationship between the preceding left segment pacing cycle length (S_1-S_1; *abscissa*) and (a) the maximum action potential amplitude in the middle segment produced by stimulation of the right segment at a coupling interval of 500 msec (*intercept, filled circles; left ordinate*), (b) the rate of decline of action potential amplitude in the middle segment as the coupling interval was increased from 500 to 2,000 msec (− *slope, filled squares; right ordinate*) and, (c) the rate of diastolic depolarization in the left segment of the fiber (+ *slope, unfilled squares; right ordinate*). Intercepts and slopes of linear decline of action potential amplitude and membrane potential were calculated from the data in panels A and B, respectively, for S_1-S_2 = 500 to 2,000 msec ($r > 0.97$ for all lines). Data for action potential amplitude are expressed as means + SD. SD values for membrane potential data are omitted because the number of points sampled ($N = 4$) was arbitrary. These data suggest that relatively large amplitude action potentials in the middle segment of the fiber were unable to conduct to the left segment after periods of rapid pacing (e.g., S_1-S_1 = 600 msec) because the membrane potential of the left segment was too far from threshold. After pacing at intermediate cycle lengths (650–900 msec), conduction from the middle to the left segment occurred when action potential amplitude in the middle segment was high and the membrane potential in the left segment was closer to threshold. However, as the coupling interval was prolonged, action potential amplitude declined at a more rapid rate than membrane potential approached threshold, and block occurred at long coupling intervals. The rate of decline in action potential amplitude after pacing at the slower rates (1,300 msec) apparently paralleled the rate of diastolic depolarization, and conduction was maintained over a wider range of coupling intervals. (From ref. 33, with permission.)

Even if the membrane potential of the depolarized region is constant during diastole, phase four depolarization in surrounding myocardium may alter excitability and action potential amplitude and thereby affect conduction. Consequently, diastolic depolarization increases the excitability of cells located proximal and distal to the depressed zone, but decreases action potential amplitude and upstroke velocity. Increased excitability favors conduction, whereas decreased action potential amplitude and upstroke velocity reduce the likelihood of conduction, particularly through the continuously

depolarized zone. It remains to be determined if similar phenomena occur in other regions of the heart that demonstrate diastolic depolarization.

Entrance and Exit Block

Unidirectional block in tissue surrounding a relatively slowly depolarizing pacemaker protects the pacemaker from overdrive suppression and permits spontaneous discharges generated by the pacemaker to depolarize adjacent cells and initiate an arrhythmia. Several mechanisms have been proposed to explain comcomitant entrance block and exit conduction, including differential refractoriness in the automatic focus and surrounding tissue and reduced excitability of the spontaneously depolarizing cells (100). Recently, Ferrier and Rosenthal (20,96) demonstrated that entrance and exit block in focally depolarized regions of isolated Purkinje fibers and ventricular myocardium were related to the membrane potentials of the depolarized area and surrounding cells. Cells depolarized to membrane potentials near −50 mV generated spontaneous activity that propagated to more normally polarized surrounding tissue, although premature action potentials elicited in the normally polarized areas did not activate the automatic focus. More severe depolarization of the focal area reduced the amplitude of spontaneous action potentials and produced exit block. Exit conduction was restored under these circumstances if phase four depolarization in the normally polarized area was enhanced.

Thus, the production of entrance or exit block in focally depolarized preparations appeared to involve an interplay between the action potential amplitude and excitability of two regions of cells having different membrane potentials. Low excitability in the depolarized area during early diastole facilitated entrance block during premature stimulation, whereas higher excitability in surrounding cells permitted exit conduction. Reduction of action potential amplitude in the depolarized area produced exit block, but the block could be overcome by increasing the excitability of surrounding tissue. Similar phenomena have been observed in diseased canine and human ventricular myocardium (31,103) (Fig. 10). In the example shown in Fig. 10, action potentials elicited in normally polarized myocardium surrounding a spontaneously active depolarized area activated the focus only when they arrived late in diastole, as the focus was nearing threshold for a spontaneous discharge. Increasing the stimulation rate of the normally polarized area produced premature activation of the focal area and progressively greater degrees of entrance block.

Figure 10 also demonstrates phase resetting of diastolic depolarization by subthreshold depolarization of the focal area. Impulses that invaded the focal area early in diastole were not able to capture the focus; instead, they reset diastolic depolarization and delayed the approach of membrane potential to threshold. Consequently, 1:1 conduction was possible at a pacing cycle length of 1,200 msec (Fig. 10A), but 3:1 block occurred at a pacing cycle length of 600 msec (Fig. 10E), instead of

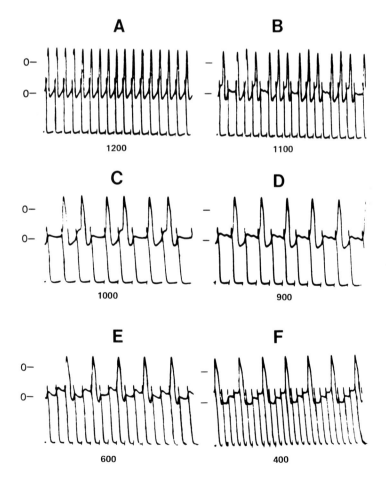

FIG. 10. Frequency-dependent entrance block into a spontaneously depolarizing region of diseased human ventricle. In panels A to F, normal myocardium surrounding an automatic focus was stimulated at progressively shorter cycle lengths, indicated beneath each panel (in msec). As the cycle length of pacing was shortened, the degree of entrance block into the focal area increased. Action potentials in normal myocardium appeared to produce electrotonic depolarizations in the focal region. Subthreshold depolarizations that occurred in the focal area during early or mid-diastole reset diastolic depolarization and failed to capture the focus. Subthreshold depolarizations that occurred later in diastole accelerated phase four depolarization and captured the focus. Vertical calibration, 50 mV. Horizontal calibration, 4 sec in panels A and B and 2 sec in panels C–F. (From ref. 31, with permission.)

the expected 2:1 block. In contrast, subthreshold depolarizations that invaded the focus in late diastole accelerated the approach to threshold (as, for example, in the second of the two captured action potentials in Fig. 10C). These results confirm those of Ferrier and Rosenthal and illustrate the potentially complex rhythm disturbances that may result from interactions between automaticity and conduction.

Injury Currents

Automaticity also may be initiated or modulated by the flow of injury current (57). Injury currents are induced when a region of myocardium is depolarized relative to a neighboring region and a potential gradient between the two groups of cells is established. Several disparities in cellular electrical properties may produce such a gradient, such as different resting membrane potentials, action potential amplitudes, and action potential durations. Current will flow from the region having the more depolarized membrane potential to the region with the more negative membrane potential, be it during diastole, the action potential upstroke, or the terminal portion of the action potential repolarization. For a potential gradient to be maintained, however, the two regions must be separated by an inexcitable zone to prevent equalization of membrane potential and action potential duration.

Circular flow of injury current across the borders of ischemic or infarcted myocardium and more normally polarized cells may induce sustained depolarization in the border zone and elicit automaticity similar to that shown in Fig. 3. Depending on the extent of depolarization, therefore, an automatic tachycardia could be induced via enhanced normal automaticity or abnormal automaticity. Once initiated, spontaneous activity might then be modulated by current flow across the inexcitable zone, as described above for phase resetting. In addition, a single spontaneous action potential could provide the premature impulse needed to initiate a reentrant rhythm. However, the production of spontaneous activity by injury currents *in vivo* remains to be demonstrated conclusively, and the initiation of arrhythmias by this mechanism is hypothetical at present.

Related Arrhythmias

Several rate-related arrhythmias, such as acceleration- and deceleration-dependent bundle branch block (22,95), may involve interactions between automaticity and conduction. As discussed above, pacing at rapid or slow rates reduces action potential amplitude and excitability in depressed Purkinje cells and facilitates the production of conduction block. Under these circumstances, spontaneous diastolic depolarization either may ameliorate conduction block by increasing the excitability of tissue distal to the depressed area or may exacerbate block by reducing action potential amplitude and upstroke velocity in tissue proximal to the depressed area. Interactions between automaticity and conduction also may modulate changes in conduction that follow periods of rapid or slow heart rates. For example, bundle branch block produced during a ventricular tachycardia has been shown to persist temporarily after the ventricular rate has returned to normal (21,22), possibly because of residual reductions of action potential amplitude and excitability in depressed cells and suppression of phase four depolarization in more normally polarized cells. A similar mechanism might explain overdrive suppression of AV conduction (69). In contrast, bundle branch block that occurs during normal sinus rhythm can normalize during sinus bradycardia and temporarily remain normal as the sinus rate accelerates back to the previous rate (28). Under these circumstances, the decrease in heart rate may increase excitability in depressed cells and enhance phase four depolarization and excitability in normal cells, and these effects may persist transiently after restoration of normal sinus rhythm.

Entrance and exit block can be fixed phenomena or can be modulated by the changes in membrane potential and excitability induced by spontaneous activity in an automatic focus. Obviously, block of impulses in cells adjacent to an automatic focus may modulate a wide variety of cardiac rhythms caused by normal and abnormal automaticity. Because the production of exit and entrance block may occur within a feedback loop involving interactions between automaticity and conduction, it may be difficult to determine whether conduction block has modified the spontaneous rhythm or whether the rhythm has modified block. It is possible, therefore, to attribute arrhythmias having fixed or variable coupling, paroxysmal or nonparoxysmal onset and termination, and inducibility or noninducibility by programmed stimulation to modified abnormal automaticity. In short, arrhythmias caused by abnormal automaticity may be indistinguishable from those reentry or triggered activity, given the available clinical diagnostic tools.

REFERENCES

1. Allen, J. D., Brennan, F. J., and Wit, A. L. (1978): Actions of lidocaine on transmembrane potentials of subendocardial Purkinje fibers surviving in infarcted canine hearts. *Circ. Res.*, 43:470–481.
2. Allessie, M. E., Bonke, F. I. M., and Schopman, F. J. G. (1977): Circus movement in rabbit atrial muscle as a mechanism of tachycardia. III. The "leading circle" concept: A new model of circus movement in cardiac tissue without the involvement of an anatomic obstacle. *Circ. Res.*, 41:9–18.
3. Aschoff, J. (1965): *Circadian Clocks.* North Holland, Amsterdam.
4. Bassett, A. L., Fenoglio, J. J., Jr., Wit, A. L., Myerburg, R. J., and Gelband, H. (1976): Electrophysiological and ultrastructural characteristics of the canine tricuspid valve. *Am. J. Physiol.*, 230: 1366–1373.

5. Best, E. N. (1979): Null space in the Hodgkin-Huxley equations. A critical test. *Biophys. J.,* 27:87–104.

6. Boineau, J. P., Schuessler, R. B., Roeske, W. R., Miller, C. B., Wylds, A. C., and Hill, D. A. (1985): Autonomic organization of the atrial pacemaker complex. In: *Cardiac Electrophysiology and Arrhythmias,* edited by D. P. Zipes and J. Jalife, pp. 151–158. Grune & Stratton, New York.

7. Bouman, L. N., Gerlings, E. D., Biersteker, P. A., and Bonke, F. I. M. (1968): Pacemaker shift in the sino-atrial node during vagal stimulation. *Pfluegers Arch.,* 302:255–267.

8. Brooks, C. M., and Lu, H.-H. (1972): *The Sinoatrial Pacemaker of the Heart.* Charles C Thomas, Springfield, Ill.

9. Brown, G., and Eccles, J. (1934): The action of a single vagal volley on the rhythm of the heart beat. *J. Physiol. (Lond.),* 82: 211–241.

10. Castellanos, A., Luceri, R. M., Moleiro, F., Kayden, D. S., Trohman, R. G., Zaman, L., and Myerburg, R. J. (1984): Annihilation, entrainment and modulation of ventricular parasystolic rhythms. *Am. J. Cardiol.,* 54:317–322.

11. Ceremuzynski, L., Stazewska-Barczak, J., and Herbaczynska-Cedro, K. (1969): Cardiac rhythm disturbances and the release of catecholamines after coronary occlusion in dogs. *Cardiovasc. Res.,* 3:190–197.

12. Clay, J. R., Guevara, M. R., and Shrier, A. (1984): Phase resetting of the rhythmic activity of embryonic heart cell aggregates. Experiment and theory. *Biophys. J.* 45:699–714.

13. Cohen, I. S., Falk, R. T., and Kline, R. P. (1982): Voltage-clamp studies on the canine Purkinje strand. *Proc. R. Soc. Lond.,* B217–236.

14. Cranefield, P. F. (1977): Action potentials, afterpotentials and arrhythmias. *Circ. Res.,* 41:415–423.

15. Dangman, K. H., Danilo, P., Jr., Hordof, A. J., Mary-Rabine, L., Reder, R. G., and Rosen, M. R. (1982): Electrophysiologic characteristics of human ventricular and Purkinje fibers. *Circulation,* 65:362–368.

16. Deitmer, J. W., and Ellis, D. (1978): The intracellular sodium activity of cardiac Purkinje fibers during inhibition and reactivation of the Na-K pump. *J. Physiol. (Lond.),* 283:241–259.

17. DiFrancesco, D. (1981): A new interpretation of the pacemaker current in calf Purkinje fibres. *J. Physiol. (Lond.),* 314:359–376.

18. Elharrar, V., and Zipes, D. P. (1980): Voltage modulation of automaticity in cardiac Purkinje fibers. In: *The Slow Inward Current and Cardiac Arrhythmias,* edited by D. P. Zipes, J. C. Bailey, and V. Elharrar, pp. 357–373. Martinus Nijhoff, The Hague.

19. El-Sherif, N., Scherlag, B. J., and Lazzara, R. (1975): Differential effect of atrial and ventricular pacing on the induction of paroxysmal AV block in the ischemic His Purkinje system. *Clin. Res.,* 33:3A.

20. Ferrier, G. R., and Rosenthal, J. E. (1980): Automaticity and entrance block induced by focal depolarization of mammalian ventricular tissues. *Circ. Res.,* 47:238–248.

21. Fisch, C. (1984): Bundle branch block after ventricular tachycardia: A manifestation of "fatigue" or "overdrive suppression." *J. Am. Coll. Cardiol.,* 3:1562–1564.

22. Fisch, C., Zipes, D. P., and McHenry, P. L. (1973): Rate-dependent aberrancy. *Circulation,* 48:714–724.

23. Fozzard, H. A., and Hiraoka, M. (1973): The positive dynamic current and its inactivation properties in cardiac Purkinje fibers. *J. Physiol. (Lond.),* 234:569–586.

24. Friedman, P. L., Stewart, J. R., and Wit, A. L. (1973): Spontaneous and induced cardiac arrhythmias in subendocardial Purkinje fibers after extensive myocardial infarction in dogs. *Circ. Res.,* 33:612–625.

25. Furuse, A., Matsuo, H., and Saigusa, M. (1981): Effects of intervening beats on ectopic cycle length in a patient with ventricular parasystole. *Jpn. Heart J.,* 22:201–209.

26. Gadsby, D. C., and Cranefield, P. F. (1977): Two levels of resting potential in cardiac Purkinje fibers. *J. Gen. Physiol.,* 70:725–746.

27. Gadsby, D. C., and Cranefield, P. F. (1979): Electrogenic sodium extrusion in cardiac Purkinje fibers. *J. Gen. Physiol.,* 73:819–837.

28. Gardberg, M., and Rosen, T. L. (1958): Observations on conduction in a case of intermittent left bundle branch block. *Am. Heart J.,* 55:677–680.

29. Giles, W., and Noble, S. J. (1976): Changes in membrane current in bullfrog atrium produced by acetylcholine. *J. Physiol. (Lond.),* 261:103–123.

30. Gilmour, R. F., Jr., Evans, J. J., and Zipes, D. P. (1984): Preferential interruption of impulse transmission across Purkinje-muscle junctions by interventions that depress conduction. In: *Cardiac Electrophysiology and Arrhythmias,* edited by D. P. Zipes and J. Jalife, pp. 287–300. Grune & Stratton, New York.

31. Gilmour, R. F., Jr., Heger, J. J., Prystowsky, E. N., and Zipes, D. P. (1983): Cellular electrophysiological abnormalities of diseased human ventricular myocardium. *Am. J. Cardiol.,* 51:137–144.

32. Gilmour, R. F., Jr., Salata, J. J., and Davis, J. R. (1986): Effects of 4-aminopyridine on rate-related depression of cardiac action potentials. *Am. J. Physiol. (in press).*

33. Gilmour, R. F., Jr., Salata, J. J., and Zipes, D. P. (1985): Rate-related suppression and facilitation of conduction in isolated canine cardiac Purkinje fibers. *Circ. Res.,* 57:35–45.

34. Gilmour, R. F., Jr., and Zipes, D. P. (1982): Electrophysiological response of vascularized hamster atrial transplants to ischemia. *Circ. Res.,* 50:599–609.

35. Goldberg, J. M. (1975): Intra-SA-nodal pacemaker shifts induced by autonomic nerve stimulation in the dog. *Am. J. Physiol.,* 229: 1116–1123.

36. Goldreyer, B. N., Gallagher, J. J., and Damato, A. N. (1973): The electrophysiologic demonstration of ectopic atrial tachycardia in man. *Am. Heart J.,* 85:205–215.

37. Grant, A. O., and Katzung, B. G. (1976): The effects of quinidine and verapamil on electrically induced automaticity in the ventricular myocardium of guinea pigs. *J. Pharmacol. Exp. Ther.,* 196:407–419.

38. Han, J., and Cameron, J. S. (1985): Effects of epinephrine on automaticity of Purkinje fibers from infarcted ventricles. In: *Cardiac Electrophysiology and Arrhythmias,* edited by D. P. Zipes and J. Jalife, pp. 331–335. Grune & Stratton, New York.

39. Hauswirth, O., Noble, D., and Tsien, R. W. (1969): The mechanism of oscillatory activity at low membrane potentials in cardiac Purkinje fibers. *J. Physiol. (Lond.),* 200:255–265.

40. Hill, J. L., and Gettes, L. S. (1980): Effect of acute coronary artery occlusion on extracellular K$^+$ activity in swine. *Circulation,* 61:678–778.

41. Hoffman, B. F. (1983): Experiments on abnormal automaticity. In: *Frontiers of Cardiac Electrophysiology,* edited by M. B. Rosenbaum and M. V. Elizari, pp. 144–157. Martinus Nijhoff, The Hague.

42. Hoffman, B. F., and Rosen, M. R. (1981): Cellular mechanisms for cardiac arrhythmias. *Circ. Res.,* 49:1–15.

43. Hogan, P. M., and Davis, L. D. (1968): Evidence for specialized fibers in the canine atrium. *Circ. Res.,* 23:387–396.

44. Hope, R. R., Scherlag, B. J., El-Sherif, N., and Lazzara, R. (1976): Hierarchy of ventricular pacemakers. *Circ. Res.,* 39:883–888.

45. Horowitz, L. N., Spear, J. F., and Moore, E. N. (1975): Subendocardial origin of ventricular arrhythmias in 24-hour-old experimental myocardial infarction. *Circulation,* 53:56–63.

46. Hutter, O. F., and Trautwein, W. (1956): Vagal and sympathetic effects on the pacemaker fibers in the sinus venosus of the heart. *J. Gen. Physiol.,* 39:715–733.

47. Imanishi, S. (1971): Calcium-sensitive discharges in canine Purkinje fibers. *Jpn. J. Physiol.,* 21:443–463.

48. Imanishi, S., and Surawicz, B. (1976): Automatic activity in depolarized guinea pig ventricular myocardium: Characteristics and mechanisms. *Circ. Res.,* 39:751–759.

49. Isenberg, G. (1976): Cardiac Purkinje fibers: Cesium as a tool to block inward rectifying potassium currents. *Pfluegers Arch.,* 365: 99–106.

50. Jalife, J. (1984): Mutual entrainment and electrical coupling as mechanisms for synchronous firing of rabbit sino-atrial pacemaker cells. *J. Physiol. (Lond.),* 356:221–243.

51. Jalife, J., and Antzelevitch, C. (1979): Phase resetting and annihilation of pacemaker activity in cardiac tissue. *Science,* 206: 695–697.

52. Jalife, J., Antzelevitch, C., LaManna, V., and Moe, G. K. (1983): Rate-dependent changes in excitability of depressed cardiac Pur-

kinje fibers as a mechanism of intermittent bundle branch block. *Circulation*, 67:912–922.

53. Jalife, J., Hamilton, A. J., LaManna, V. R., and Moe, G. K. (1980): Effects of current flow on pacemaker activity of the isolated kitten sinoatrial node. *Am. J. Physiol.*, 238:H307–H316.

54. Jalife, J., and Moe, G. K. (1976): Effect of electrotonic potentials on pacemaker activity of canine Purkinje fibers in relation to parasystole. *Circ. Res.*, 39:801–808.

55. Jalife, J., and Moe, G. K. (1979): Phasic effects of vagal stimulation on pacemaker activity of the isolated sinus node of the cat. *Circ. Res.*, 45:595–607.

56. James, T. N., Isobe, J. H., and Urthaler, F. (1979): Correlative electrophysiological and anatomical studies concerning the site of origin of escape rhythm during complete atrioventricular block in the dog. *Circ. Res.*, 45:108–119.

57. Janse, M. J., van Capelle, F. J. L., Morsink, H., Kleber, A. G., Wilms-Schopman, F., Cardinal, R., Nauman d'Aloncourt, C., and Durrer, D. (1980): Flow of "injury" current and patterns of excitation during early ventricular arrhythmias in acute regional myocardial ischemia in isolated porcine and canine hearts: Evidence for two different arrhythmogenic mechanisms. *Circ. Res.*, 47:151–165.

58. Jones, S. B., Euler, D. E., Hardie, E. L., Randall, W. C., and Brynjolfsson, G. (1978): Comparison of SA nodal and subsidiary atrial pacemaker function and location in the dog. *Am. J. Physiol.*, 234:H471–H476.

59. Jones, S. B., Euler, D. E., Randall, W. C., Brynjolfsson, G., and Hardie, E. L. (1980): Atrial ectopic foci in the canine heart: Hierarchy of pacemaker automaticity. *Am. J. Physiol.*, 7:H788–H793.

60. Kass, R. S., Lederer, W. J., Tsien, R. W., and Weingart, R. (1978): Role of calcium ions in transient inward currents and after contractions induced by strophanthidin in cardiac Purkinje fibres. *J. Physiol. (Lond.)*, 271:187–208.

61. Katz, L. N., and Pick, A. (1956): *Clinical Electrocardiography. Part I. The Arrhythmias*, pp. 182–184. Lea & Febiger, Philadelphia.

62. Katzung, B. G. (1975): Effects of extracellular calcium and sodium on depolarization-induced automaticity in guinea pig papillary muscle. *Circ. Res.*, 37:118–127.

63. Katzung, B. G., and Morgenstern, J. A. (1977): Effects of extracellular potassium on ventricular automaticity and evidence for a pacemaker current in mammalian ventricular myocardium. *Circ. Res.*, 40:105–111.

64. Kawai, C., Konishi, T., Matsuyama, E., and Okasaki, H. (1981): Comparative effects of three calcium antagonists, diltiazem, verapamil and nifedipine, on the sinoatrial and atrioventricular nodes. *Circulation*, 63:1035–1042.

65. Kenyon, J. L., and Gibbons, W. R. (1979): 4-aminopyridine and the early outward current in sheep cardiac Purkinje fibers. *J. Gen. Physiol.*, 73:139–157.

66. Kohlhardt, M., Bauer, B., Krause, H., and Fleckenstein, A. (1972): Differentiation of the transmembrane Na and Ca channels in mammalian cardiac fibers by the use of specific inhibitors. *Pfluegers Arch.*, 335:309–322.

67. Kohlhardt, M., and Fleckenstein, A. (1977): Inhibition of the slow inward current by nifedipine in mammalian ventricular myocardium. *Naunyn Schmiedebergs Arch. Pharmacol.*, 298:267–272.

68. Kokubun, S., Nishimura, M., Noma, A., and Irisawa, H. (1980): The spontaneous action potential of rabbit atrioventricular node cells. *Jpn. J. Physiol.*, 30:529–540.

69. Langendorf, R., and Pick, A. (1971): Artificial pacing of the human heart. Its contribution to the understanding of arrhythmias. *Am. J. Cardiol.*, 28:516–525.

70. Lavallee, M., de Champlain, J., Nadeau, R. A., and Yamaguchi, N. (1978): Muscarinic inhibition of endogenous myocardial catecholamine liberation in the dog. *Can. J. Physiol. Pharmacol.*, 56:642–649.

71. Lazzara, R., El-Sherif, N., and Scherlag, B. J. (1973): Electrophysiological properties of Purkinje cells in one-day-old myocardial infarction. *Circ. Res.*, 42:740–749.

72. Lazzara, R., El-Sherif, N., and Scherlag, B. J. (1974): Early and late effects of coronary artery occlusion on canine Purkinje fibers. *Circ. Res.*, 35:391–399.

73. Lee, K. S., and Tsien, R. W. (1983): Mechanism of calcium channel blockade by verapamil, D600, diltiazem, and nitrendipine in single dialyzed heart cells. *Nature*, 302:790–794.

74. Levy, M. N., and Martin, P. J. (1979): Neural control of the heart. In: *Handbook of Physiology, Section 2, The Cardiovascular System*, Vol. 1, edited by R. M. Berne, pp. 581–620. American Physiological Society, Bethesda.

75. Levy, M. N., Martin, P. J., Iano, T., and Zieske, H. (1969): Paradoxical effects of vagal nerve stimulation on heart rate in dogs. *Circ. Res.*, 25:303–314.

76. Malecot, C., Coraboeuf, E., and Coulombe, A. (1984): Automaticity of ventricular fibers induced by low concentrations of barium. *Am. J. Physiol.*, 247:H429–H439.

77. Masuda, M. O., and Paes de Carvalho, A. (1982): Rate and rhythm dependency of propagation from normal myocardium to a Ba^{++}, K^+-induced slow response zone in rabbit left atrium. *Circ. Res.*, 50:419–427.

78. Mary-Rabine, L., Hordof, A. J., Danilo, P., Jr., Malm, J. R., and Rosen, M. R. (1980): Mechanisms for impulse initiation in isolated human atrial fibers. *Circ. Res.*, 47:267–277.

79. McDonald, T. F., Pelzer, D., and Trautwein, W. (1980): On the mechanism of slow calcium channel block in the heart. *Pfluegers Arch.*, 385:175–179.

80. Michaels, D. C., Slenter, V. A. J., Salata, J. J., and Jalife, J. (1983): A model of vagus-sinoatrial node interactions. *Am. J. Physiol.*, 245:H1043–H1053.

81. Millard, R. W., Lathrop, D. A., Grupp, G., Ashraf, M., Grupp, I. L., and Schwartz, A. (1982): Differential cardiovascular effects of calcium channel blocking agents: Possible mechanisms. *Am. J. Cardiol.*, 49:499–506.

82. Moe, G. K., Jalife, J., Mueller, W. J., and Moe, B. (1977): A mathematical model of parasystole and its application to clinical arrhythmias. *Circulation*, 56:968–979.

83. Muscholl, E. (1980): Peripheral muscarinic control of norepinephrine release in the cardiovascular system. *Am. J. Physiol.*, 239:H713–H720.

84. Nau, G. T., Aldariz, A. E., Acunzo, R. S., Halpern, M. S., Davidenko, J. M., Elizari, M. V., and Rosenbaum, M. B. (1982): Modulation of parasystolic activity by non-parasystolic beats. *Circulation*, 66:462–469.

85. Nishimura, M., Kokubun, S., Noma, A., Irisawa, H., and Watanabe, Y. (1981): Membrane current systems in the rabbit atrioventricular node. The first voltage clamp study. *Am. J. Cardiol.*, 47:429.

86. Noble, D. (1984): The surprising heart: A review of recent progress in cardiac electrophysiology. *J. Physiol. (Lond.)*, 353:1–50.

87. Noma, A., Yanagihara, K., and Irisawa, H. (1977): Inward current of the rabbit sino-atrial node cell. *Pfluegers Arch.*, 372:43–51.

88. Noma, A., Yanigihara, K., and Irisawa, H. (1977): Inward current activated during hyperpolarization in the rabbit sinoatrial node. *Pfluegers Arch.*, 385:11–19.

89. Paes de Carvalho, A., and de Almeida, D. F. (1960): Spread of activity through the atrioventricular node. *Circ. Res.*, 8:801–809.

90. Pappano, A., and Carmeliet, E. E. (1979): Epinephrine and the pacemaking mechanism at plateau potentials in sheep cardiac Purkinje fibers. *Pfluegers Arch.*, 382:17–26.

91. Peon, J., Ferrier, G. R., and Moe, G. K. (1978): The relationship of excitability to conduction velocity in canine Purkinje tissue. *Circ. Res.*, 43:125–135.

92. Randall, W. C. (1977): Sympathetic control of the heart. In: *Neural Regulation of the Heart*, edited by W. C. Randall, pp. 45–94. Oxford University Press, London.

93. Reuter, H. (1980): Effects of neurotransmitters on the slow inward current. In: *The Slow Inward Current and Cardiac Arrhythmias*, edited by D. P. Zipes, J. C. Bailey, and V. Elharrar, pp. 205–219. Martinus Nijhoff, The Hague.

94. Rosen, M. R., Fisch, C., Hoffman, B. F., Danilo, P., Jr., Lovelace, D. E., and Knoebel, S. B. (1980): Can accelerated atrioventricular junction escape rhythms be explained by delayed afterdepolarizations? *Am. J. Cardiol.*, 45:1272–1284.

95. Rosenbaum, M. B., Elizari, M. V., Lazzari, J. O., Halpern, M. S., Nau, G. I., and Levi, R. J. (1973): The mechanism of intermittent

bundle branch block. Relationship to prolonged recovery, hypopolarization and spontaneous diastolic depolarization. *Chest,* 63: 666–677.

96. Rosenthal, J. E., and Ferrier, G. R. (1983): Contribution of variable entrance and exit block in protected foci to arrhythmogenesis in isolated ventricular tissues. *Circulation,* 67:1–8.

97. Rozanski, G. J., Lipsius, S. L., and Randall, W. C. (1983): Functional characteristics of sinoatrial and subsidiary pacemaker activity in the canine right atrium. *Circulation,* 6:1378–1387.

98. Salata, J. J., Jalife, J., Megna, J. L., and Alperovich, G. (1982): Amantidine-induced diastolic depolarization and automaticity in ventricular muscle. *Circ. Res.,* 51:722–732.

99. Sanquinetti, M. C., and Kass, R. S. (1944): Voltage-dependent block of calcium channel current in the calf cardiac Purkinje fiber by dihydropyridine calcium channel antagonists. *Circ. Res.,* 55:336–348.

100. Scherf, D., and Schott, A. (1956): *Extrasystole and Allied Arrhythmias.* Grune & Stratton, New York.

101. Scherlag, B. J., El-Sherif, N., Hope, R., and Lazzara, R. (1974): Characterization and localization of ventricular arrhythmias resulting from myocardial ischemia and infarction. *Circ. Res.,* 35: 372–383.

102. Sherf, L., James, T. N., and Woods, W. T. (1985): Function of the atrioventricular node considered on the basis of observed histology and fine structure. *J. Am. Coll. Cardiol.,* 5:770–780.

103. Singer, D. H., Baumgarten, C. M., and Ten Eick, R. E. (1981): Cellular electrophysiology of ventricular and other dysrhythmias: Studies on diseased and ischemic heart. *Prog. Cardiovasc. Dis.,* 24:97–156.

104. Singer, D. H., Lazzara, R., and Hoffman, B. F. (1967): Interrelationship between automaticity and conduction in Purkinje fibers. *Circ. Res.,* 21:537–558.

105. Spear, J. F., Horowitz, L. N., Hodess, A. B., MacVaugh, H., III, and Moore, E. N. (1979): Cellular electrophysiology of human myocardial infarction. I. Abnormalities of cellular activation. *Circulation,* 59:247–256.106.

106. Spear, J. F., Kronhaus, K. D., Moore, E. N., and Kline, R. P. (1979): The effect of brief vagal stimulation on the isolated rabbit sinus node. *Circ. Res.,* 32:75–88.

107. Takahashi, N., Gilmour, R. F., Jr., and Zipes, D. P. (1984): Overdrive suppression of conduction in the canine His-Purkinje system after occlusion of the anterior septal artery. *Circulation,* 70:495–505.

108. Ten Eick, R. E., Nawrath, H., McDonald, T. F., and Trautwein, W. (1976): On the mechanism of the negative inotropic effect of acetylcholine. *Pfluegers Arch.,* 361:207–213.

109. Tse, W. W. (1973): Evidence of presence of automatic fibers in the canine atrioventricular node. *Am. J. Physiol.,* 225:716–725.

110. Tse, W. W. (1985): Adrenergic potentiation on spontaneous activity of canine paranodal fibers. *Am. J. Physiol.,* 247:H415–H421.

111. Urthaler, F., Katholi, C. R., Macy, J., Jr., and James, T. N. (1979): Electrophysiological and mathematical characteristics of the escape rhythm during complete AV block. *Cardiovasc. Res.,* 8:173–186.

112. Vassalle, M. (1970): Electrogenic suppression of automaticity in sheep and dog Purkinje fibers. *Circ. Res.,* 27:361–377.

113. Vassalle, M. (1977): The relationship among cardiac pacemakers: Overdrive suppression. *Circ. Res.,* 41:269–277.

114. Watanabe, A. M., Lindemann, J. P., Jones, L. R., Besch, H. R., Jr., and Bailey, J. C. (1981): Biochemical mechanisms mediating neural control of the heart. In: *Disturbances in Neurogenic Control of the Circulation,* edited by F. M. Abboud, H. A. Fozzard, J. P. Gilmore, and D. J. Reis, pp. 189–203. Waverly, Baltimore.

115. Weidmann, S. (1951): Effect of current flow on the membrane potential of cardiac muscle. *J. Physiol. (Lond.),* 115:227–236.

116. Wiggins, J. R., and Cranefield, P. F. (1976): Two levels of resting potential in canine cardiac Purkinje fibers exposed to sodium free solutions. *Circ. Res.,* 39:466–474.

117. Winfree, A. T. (1970): Integrated view of resetting a circadian clock. *J. Theor. Biol.,* 28:327–374.

118. Wit, A. L., and Cranefield, P. F. (1977): Triggered and automatic activity in the canine coronary sinus. *Circ. Res.,* 41:435–445.

119. Wit, A. L., and Cranefield, P. F. (1981): Mechanisms of impulse initiation in the atrioventricular junction and the effects of acetylstrophanthidin. *Am. J. Cardiol.,* 47:405.

120. Wit, A. L., Fenoglio, J. J., Wagner, B. M., and Bassett, A. L. (1973): Electrophysiological properties of cardiac muscle in the anterior mitral valve leaflet and the adjacent atrium in the dog. Possible implications for the genesis of atrial dysrhythmias. *Circ. Res.,* 32:731–745.

121. Woods, W. T., Sherf, L., and James, T. N. (1982): Structure and function of specific regions in the canine atrioventricular node. *Am. J. Physiol.,* 243:H41–H50.

122. Yanagihara, K., Noma, A., and Irisawa, H. (1980): Reconstruction of sinoatrial node pace-maker potential based on voltage clamp experiments. *Jpn. J. Physiol.,* 30:841–857.

123. Zipes, D. P. (1983): Specific arrhythmias: Diagnosis and treatment. In: *Heart Disease: A Textbook of Cardiovascular Medicine,* edited by E. Braunwald, pp. 683–743. W. B. Saunders, Philadelphia.

124. Zipes, D. P., Barber, M. J., Takahashi, N., and Gilmour, R. F., Jr. (1985): Recent observations on autonomic innervation of the heart. In: *Cardiac Electrophysiology and Arrhythmias,* edited by D. P. Zipes and J. Jalife, pp. 181–189. Grune & Stratton, New York.

125. Zipes, D. P., and Fischer, J. C. (1974): Effects of agents which inhibit the slow channel on sinus node automaticity and atrioventricular conduction in the dog. *Circ. Res.,* 34:184–192.

126. Zipes, D. P., and Mendez, M. (1973): Action of manganese ions and tetrodotoxin on atrioventricular nodal transmembrane potentials in isolated rabbit hearts. *Circ. Res.,* 39:76–82.

The Heart and Cardiovascular System,
edited by H. A. Fozzard et al.
Raven Press, New York © 1986.

CHAPTER 56

Mechanisms of Action of Antiarrhythmic Drugs: A Matrical Approach

Morton F. Arnsdorf and J. Andrew Wasserstrom

Cardiac arrhythmias constitute a major public health threat, and their treatment remains a difficult challenge to physicians. The last three decades have witnessed explosive growth in our knowledge of the cellular electrophysiology underlying the normal heart beat, arrhythmogenesis, and the actions of antiarrhythmic and other drugs. The purpose of this chapter is to construct an intellectual framework that will bridge the gap between basic science and clinical science. This intellectual framework will be based on biophysical theory and should allow critical assessment of extrapolations from the basic laboratory to the clinical situation.

MATRIX VERSUS HIERARCHY

One of us (M.F.A.) proposed that the normal active and passive cellular electrophysiologic determinants of excitability form a matrix that can be altered by arrhythmogenic influences, antiarrhythmic drugs, or a combination of factors (6). In this chapter we shall consider more formally the matrical concept. To this end we propose to investigate two hypotheses. The first hypothesis is that there is a normal matrix of electrophysiologic properties that can be altered by arrhythmogenic influences. Second, the normal matrix or the matrix altered by arrhythmogenic influences interacts in one or more ways with an antiarrhythmic drug and results in yet another matrical configuration. From these hypotheses it follows that (a) arrhythmogenic influences and antiarrhythmic drugs affect one or more component of cardiac excitability, (b) net excitability after one or more interventions depends on the balance of the active and passive cellular properties, (c) alterations in the determinants of excitability induced by an intervention change at different rates, (d) virtually identical final states of excitability result from different combinations of altered determinants, and (e) the traditionally considered mechanisms of arrhythmogenesis such as abnormal propagation with reentry and abnormal automaticity are the end result of altered active and passive cellular properties that reside in the perturbed matrix that determines cardiac excitability.

We have pointed out elsewhere that traditional classifications are based on a *hierarchy* of predominant drug actions (6). The power of a *matrical approach* is that it is much more broadly descriptive, and it ultimately can be quantified. The final shape of the matrix, that is, the antiarrhythmic drug effect, depends on the response of the normal matrix and the matrix altered by pathophysiologic influences to one or more influences of a drug or drugs. The matrical approach considers the complex interplay between the nature of the disease itself, the variety of drug actions, and the resulting drug efficacy in terms of the whole disease state that in fact determines the arrhythmia. Further, it extends some of our earlier ideas regarding the importance of altered excitability in the development of clinical arrhythmias to the presumed actions of arrhythmogenic interventions (2,3). Some day, we shall wish to fit each determinant of the active and passive properties of excitability into a matrix capable of describing and predicting electrophysiologic phenomena, but at present we lack the scientific information for such mathematical precision.

COMPONENTS OF THE MATRIX

Essential to this discussion is the concept that the heart beat arises from tightly regulated control of ionic flow through channels in the cardiac membrane, the myoplasm, the gap junctions that link and allow communication between cells, and the extracellular space. This tightly regulated system allows the coordinated spread of excitation and contraction that is required for an efficient cardiac output. Cardiac excitability is determined by active and passive cellular properties. The active properties, or sources, are the active generator properties that include the voltage- and time-dependent cellular mechanisms responsible for normal depolarization and repolarization. The passive properties, or sinks, include the determinants of the resting potential and the linear and nonlinear cable properties caused by the resistance and capacitance of the membranes. Each major determinant fits into the normal or altered matrix. Drug actions on the source and sink are many, and some of the important actions are included in Table 1.

The strategy is to develop a matrical framework based on biophysical theory. Experimental work in electrophysiology, arrhythmogenesis, and pharmacology will be woven into the discussion to illustrate methods, to test our hypotheses, and to suggest future approaches.

BASIC CONCEPTS OF CARDIAC EXCITABILITY

At the risk of redundancy with other chapters in this book, it is necessary to review the electrophysiologic concepts that will be used to create the matrical approach to an understanding of antiarrhythmic drugs developed in later sections.

Normal Heart Beat

We have previously defined cardiac excitability as the process by which cells undergo single and sequential regenerative depolarization and repolarization, communicate with each other, and propagate in a normal or abnormal manner (5,6). Cardiac excitability depends on the interaction between active and passive cellular properties. Weidmann (190,191,193) early on called attention to active and passive cellular properties that underlie excitability in cardiac tissue. Active properties, the source, are characterized by a response out of proportion to the stimulus. Active properties include the liminal length and the voltage- and time-dependent membrane ionic conductances that control the ionic currents responsible for normal and abnormal depolarization, repolarization, and automaticity. Ultrastructurally and biochemically, the ionic-channel proteins span the relatively impermeable lipid bilayer; they connect and are influenced by both the internal and external environments; they can have high and low affinities for drugs and other ligands and can be defined by their physiologic functions, their molecular components, and their physical shapes. It is the active properties that are

TABLE 1. *Arrhythmogenic and drug actions on sources and sinks*

I. Direct effects
   A. Action on source: active cellular properties
      1. Biologic statement of Ohm's law: driving force $\times$ conductance
         a. Driving force:[a] $V_m - E_i$
         b. Conductance: g_i
            (1) Gates and channels
               (a) Activation
               (b) Inactivation
               (c) Repolarization and reactivation
   B. Action on sink: passive cellular properties
      1. Ionic activities, pumps; transmembrane and intercellular gradients
         a. Intracellular influences
         b. Extracellular influences, as, for example, ionic accumulation and depletion
         c. Both, as, for example, in equilibrium potential (E_i)
      2. Resistance–capacitance and cable properties
      3. Intercellular communication
         a. Influenced by central and autonomic nervous systems
   C. Source, sink, excitability, and conduction
      1. Relationship of IA and IB to excitability, including liminal length
      2. Relationship of IA and IB to conduction

II. Indirect effects
   A. Types
      1. Central nervous system
      2. Autonomic nervous system
      3. Interrelationships between 1 and 2 such as reflex mechanisms
      4. Hormonal influences
      5. Hemodynamic
      6. Drug interactions such as synergism, antagonism, altered protein binding, displacement from receptors, etc.
   B. Action on source
      1. As in IA
   C. Action on sink
      1. As in IB
   D. Source, sink, excitability, and conduction
      1. As in IC

[a] V_m, transmembrane voltage; E_i and g_i, equilibrium potential and conductance, respectively, for ion i.
Adapted from Arnsdorf (6).

unique to the excitable cell. Passive properties, the sink, are characterized by a response proportional to the stimulus. Passive properties include the determinants of the resting potential, such as intracellular and extracellular ionic activities, the gradients of which are maintained by energy-requiring pumps, and both linear and nonlinear cable properties. Impulse formation and propagation of the action potential depend on both passive and active properties. Amphipathic compounds, some of which are related to the ischemic process, can insert into the bilayer and affect the active and passive properties—alterations that, in turn, can be influenced by drugs and other interventions. Electrophysiologic events are complex. Noble's analysis (147) in 1962 used two currents to describe the action potential, whereas more recent analyses (80,82,139,181) have required three or more inward and four or more outward currents, as well as complex controls for the passive and active membrane properties that regulate ionic flow.

Electrophysiologic events also trigger and control contractility through release of calcium into the cytoplasm and by influencing intracellular ionic activities. Electrophysiologic events and contraction of the heart, then, are closely interrelated and are mutually interdependent. Intuitively, disease states and drugs should affect the mechanisms that regulate normal cardiac excitability, and this, in turn, should influence contractility. Conversely, contractility should also affect cardiac excitability.

New methodologies have opened exciting approaches to the study of cardiac excitability and its determinants. The preparations used include the very small, such as vesicles, single cells, and patches of membrane that avoid certain aspects of multicellular preparations (such as cable properties and the influence of the extracellular space) that can complicate the interpretation of experimental observations. The preparations also include the multicellular, such as atrial, Purkinje, and ventricular tissues. The heart, after all, is multicellular, and it is important to study interactions between active and passive properties in such.

The further development of a working, experimental definition of cardiac excitability in terms of active and passive properties requires technically demanding electrophysiologic methods. The "standard" techniques that have dominated the drug literature have employed extracellular stimulation and have been limited largely to phenomenologic and descriptive data. Methods are now available for controlling transmembrane voltage (including intracellular constant current application and voltage clamping), for measuring intracellular and extracellular ionic activities utilizing ion-sensitive microelectrodes, for controlling voltage in single myocytes, for voltage-clamping membrane patches, for internal dialysis of single cells, for ligand- and voltage-sensing dyes, and for assessing the interrelationship between the electrophysiologic event and contractility.

Structure and Passive Cellular Properties

The membrane of the cardiac cell is a thin, lipid bilayer that separates the aqueous phase of the inside of the cell from that of the outside (79,164,168,169). Many components of the bilayer have a hydrophobic portion that is oriented toward the interior of the lipid membrane and a charged hydrophilic portion that is oriented toward the internal or external aqueous phase, a situation termed amphipathicity. This amphipathicity of membrane lipids is responsible in large part for the orientation and interactions of membrane lipids within the membrane. The glycocalyx, a material that stains for sugars and is often associated with collagen, covers the plasmalemma. The plasmalemma, in turn, covers the myocardial cell surface, the invaginations of the transverse tubules, and the vesicular caveolae. Transverse tubules introduce surface membrane deep into the cell and produce an extracellular compartment with limited diffusion that is important to the accumulation or depletion of ions and metabolites. Ventricular cells have transverse tubules, whereas other cardiac tissues are generally thought to be devoid of these structures.

Large proteins are found in the membrane, including such structures as (Na^+,K^+)-ATPase and ion-channel proteins that span the plasma membrane and connect the aqueous environments inside and outside the cell. Other proteins may be inserted in one layer or another. There seems to be asymmetry in the distribution of the proteins of the inner and outer surfaces, with a specific type of protein occupying only one and not the other location. Even the proteins that span the membrane do so anisotropically.

The plasma membrane can store charge because some lipids of the bilayer can be polarized; that is, it acts as a capacitor. A lipid bilayer would almost completely prevent the flow of ions and water through the membrane, but the plasma membrane is permeable to ions and water under certain conditions. This permeability is controlled by specialized structures, including aqueous channels of the ion-channel proteins that extend through

the membrane, and protein carriers that either extend or shuttle from the inside to the outside of the membrane. The lipid bilayer, then, is largely responsible for the capacitative component of the membrane; the protein channels and other carriers are largely responsible for the resistive components of the membrane.

In 1954, Sjöstrand and Andersson (167) used electron microscopy to demonstrate that cardiac cells were bound by membranes without direct cytoplasmic connection between cells, thereby demolishing the concept that the heart was an anatomic syncytium. Between the atrioventricular node and the ventricular myocardium exists a specialized conduction system that consists of the His bundle, the fascicles and bundle branches, and terminal ramifications. The cell type of the specialized conduction system is the Purkinje cell. The Purkinje cells form multicellular bundles and often appear as free-running strands. Individual Purkinje cells are 30 to 40 μm in diameter and 100 μm in length; they are connected through low-resistance gap junctions, are packed 2 to 30 cells in cross section, and have a connective-tissue sheath. The Purkinje cell has little in the way of sarcoplasmic reticulum, transverse tubules, or contractile proteins; so some of the confounding geometric factors can be minimized. The packing of the cells results in clefts between the cells that have restricted access to the outside environment, resulting in accumulation and depletion of ions in that space. Use of thin strands and careful selection of species can minimize the influence of the extracellular clefts. The relatively uncomplicated structure of Purkinje fibers has allowed insight into the communication between cells and the effects of passive membrane properties on the electrical signal. Details of the passive properties can be found in a recent review (5) and in Chapter 1. Information relevant to antiarrhythmic drugs will be considered further in a later section on passive cellular properties.

A series of these capacitive and resistive components representing an idealized membrane is shown in Fig. 1B. The current flow (i_m) through any one of these units (e.g., element A-B) consists of a capacitive current (i_c) through capacitor c_m and an ionic current (i_{ion}) through resistor r_m:

$$i_m = i_c + i_{ion} \qquad [1]$$

where the units for i_m are A/cm. Equation 1 approximates the surface of the plasma membrane, but the situation is more complex in the presence of transverse tubules and other invaginations and clefts. The membrane that faces the extracellular clefts contributes series capacitance (c_s) and resistance (r_s) to those of the outer membrane, as expressed in the electrical analogue in panel C of Fig. 1. Three-dimensional geometry adds further complexity (73,112,149).

Given the conditions of an idealized membrane, i_c is determined by the capacitance of a unit length of this

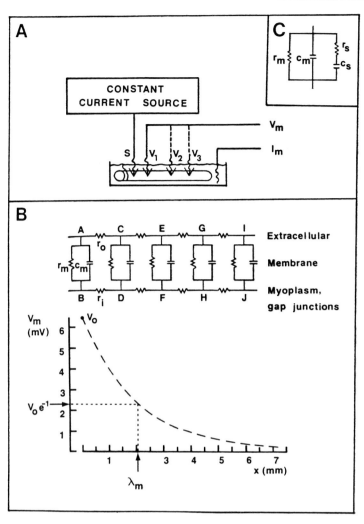

FIG. 1. A: Experimental arrangement for cable analysis. Constant current is injected intracellularly through a microelectrode positioned near the ligated end of a cardiac Purkinje fiber (S), so that all current will pass longitudinally in one direction to the right. The response in V_m is recorded by microelectrodes positioned at several points along the cable-like preparation (V_1, V_2, V_3, etc.). Measurements of current (I) are obtained from the bath ground. B: Electrical analogues of the passive properties of the extracellular space, membrane, and combined myoplasm/gap junctions are shown. Below, V_m is plotted as a function of the distance (x) between the stimulating and recording microelectrodes. Abbreviations are as in the text. C: A more complex electrical analogue that includes series resistance and capacitance (r_s and c_s, respectively). (From ref. 6, with permission.)

membrane, c_m, which is expressed as F/cm and controls the rate at which the transmembrane voltage (V_m) changes:

$$i_c = c_m(dV_m/dt) \qquad [2]$$

Active Cellular Properties and Control of Ionic Currents

As mentioned, the membrane is more permeable to ions and water than would be expected for a lipid bilayer. Ohm's law states that the ionic current will be directly related to the transmembrane voltage, V_m, and inversely related to the membrane resistance for a unit length of membrane, r_m, expressed as $\Omega \cdot$ cm. Therefore,

$$i_{\text{ion}} = V_m/r_m \qquad [3]$$

and, combining Eqs. 1 through 3,

$$i_m = c_m(dV_m/dt) + (V_m/r_m) \qquad [4]$$

Not only is the membrane more permeable to ions and water than would be expected for a lipid bilayer, it is *selectively* permeable. Different ionic species pass through transmembrane channels that are controlled by

gates that open and close in response to voltage and/or time and, in some cases, in response to ligand binding. The control of these currents can be described in terms of driving force and membrane conductance. The *driving force* depends on the maintenance of ionic distribution across the membrane by ionic pumps (*vide infra*). *Membrane conductance* is the reciprocal of resistance (i.e., $g_m = 1/r_m$) and represents the ease with which an ionic species can flow through a membrane channel. For ion y, the driving force is the difference between V_m and the equilibrium potential (E_y), or

$$i_y = \underbrace{g_y}_{\text{conductance}} \underbrace{(V_m - E_y)}_{\text{driving force}} \qquad [5]$$

Equation 5 is a form of Ohm's law with an important addition. Whereas Ohm's law is linear, the relationship between voltage and resistance (or conductance) is usually nonlinear, because the conductance term depends on voltage and/or time, on ionic concentrations, and in some cases on ligand binding. With this qualification, Eq. 5 can be considered the *biological statement of Ohm's law* (5–7).

As will be considered in a later section on ionic concentrations, activities, and pumps, energy-requiring pumps maintain the ionic gradients between the inside and outside of the cell. The pumps may also affect V_m and the equilibrium potential. The equilibrium potential, then, depends on the ionic activities and on the ionic pumps.

The net ionic current (i_{ion}) is determined by movements of the component ionic currents through channels in the membrane. The currents of importance in this discussion are the following: the potassium current (i_K); the sodium current (i_{Na}) that is carried through the "rapid" tetrodotoxin-sensitive channel; and the "slow," "secondary," or "calcium" inward current (i_{si}) that is carried predominantly by Ca^{2+} and to a lesser extent by Na^+ through a channel that is distinct from that of the "rapid" inward sodium current; all the others are included in the term i_x. The net ionic current (i_{ion}), then, is

$$i_{ion} = i_K + i_{Na} + i_{si} + i_x \qquad [6]$$

Positive currents that flow from the outside to the inside of the cell add positive charge to the interior and make V_m less negative; that is, they *depolarize* the cell. Positive currents that flow from the inside to the outside of the cell remove positive charge from the interior of the cell and make V_m more negative; that is, they *hyperpolarize* or, if already depolarized, *repolarize* the cell. The important inward currents in our discussion are i_{Na} and i_{si}, and the important outward currents are potassium currents. Anionic currents, such as chloride, have opposite effects, but are relatively unimportant except during the spike of the action potential.

Combining Eqs. 5 and 6, we have the following description of the total ionic current, the component currents, and the conductances, as well as the driving forces behind the component currents:

$$i_{ion} = g_K(V_m - E_K) + g_{Na}(V_m - E_{Na})$$
$$+ g_{si}(V_m - E_{si}) + g_x(V_m - E_x) \qquad [7]$$

where the abbreviations are as before.

More detailed considerations of the active cellular properties of importance to the actions of antiarrhythmic drugs appear in later sections.

Intracellular Constant-Current Application and Voltage Clamping

At this point it is useful to briefly mention methodology, because much of the discussion in later sections refers to techniques. The use of intracellularly applied current for perturbation of V_m has been fundamental to advances in our knowledge of the active and passive properties relevant to cardiac excitability. Referring to Eq. 5, control of V_m and measurement of i_y in the presence of an unchanged or measurable E_y will allow direct calculation of g_y and identification of influences that contribute to the nonlinearity of current–voltage relationships. Two types of techniques primarily have been used: intracellular constant-current application and voltage clamping.

Intracellular Constant-Current Application

In the resting cell, negative charges are stored along the inside of the cell membrane and are balanced by positive charges outside the membrane. When constant current is applied intracellularly using the experimental approach shown in panel A of Fig. 1, the capacitive charge of the bilayer is filled first, so that V_m is not altered instantaneously. The experimental record in Fig. 2 shows experimental recordings obtained during intra-

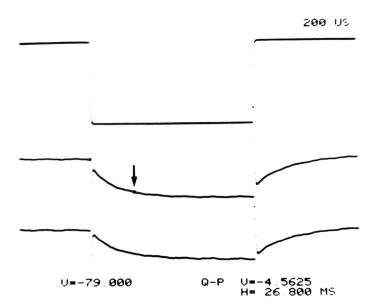

200 US

U=-79.000   Q-P   U=-4.5625
                      H= 26.800 MS

FIG. 2. Experimental recordings obtained during intracellular application of constant current in a long sheep Purkinje fiber. The upper recording is the transmembrane current, which is a constant step function. The middle and lower recordings are V_m at impalements proximal and distal, respectively, to the stimulating microelectrode. A nearly exponential change in V_m occurs in response to the current step because of the resistance and capacitance characteristics of the membrane. The amplitude of deflection in the middle trace is larger than that in the lower trace because the recording microelectrode is closer to the stimulating microelectrode in the former. The time (τ_m) constant was determined by positioning one cursor at V_r immediately before current onset and the second at the point where V_m reached 84% of its final value after the onset of current (*arrow*). The resting potential appears at the lower left (−79 mV). The coordinates of the cursor indicated by the arrow, as compared with the cursor position immediately before current onset, are given at the lower right. τ_m = 26.8 msec. (From ref. 5, with permission.)

cellular application of constant current in a long Purkinje fiber. Note that because of the resistance–capacitance (RC) properties, the response in V_m to the constant current is not linear. The steady-state response in V_m to intracellular application of small hyperpolarizing or depolarizing constant currents is ohmic in the range of V_r and allows estimation of membrane conductance. In the range between the resting potential and threshold, the constant-current–voltage relationship becomes quite nonlinear because of inward rectification of potassium currents (Fig. 3). As will be discussed, inward rectification results from K^+ being able to enter the cell more easily than it exits.

The resistance and capacitance characteristics of the tissue affect the response in the membrane voltage in time, and the time required for V_m to reach a certain percentage of its final value after current onset or offset is termed the time constant (τ_m). The percentage of final value used is 84% in a long cable-like structure and 63% in short fibers (85). Experimental determination of τ_m in a long Purkinje fiber is shown in Fig. 3. The time constant can be expressed as

$$\tau_m = r_m c_m \qquad [8]$$

The power of this technique is that intracellular constant-current application gives information on V_m at various distances (x) from the point of stimulation in time and gives a method of determining τ_m. With this information, characteristics of the flow of current from source to sink can be determined. This is discussed in detail in Chapter 1 and will be briefly reviewed in a later section on passive cellular properties.

Voltage Clamping

Referring to Eq. 5, a method that produces a constant V_m should allow recording of the currents and determination of the conductance. A step response in V_m cannot be obtained by using a constant intracellularly applied current (Fig. 2). A step response in V_m requires variable intracellular current application. One approach uses two microelectrodes in a short Purkinje fiber. The preparation is kept short so as to minimize the influence of current being drained away into neighboring cells. V_m is monitored through one microelectrode and is used to control the output of current from an amplifier. Using a negative-feedback system, variable current is passed intracellularly through the second microelectrode, sufficient and with the proper characteristics to maintain V_m constant. This experimentally controlled current must balance the capacitive and ionic movements that normally change V_m and provide uniform control of the membrane. Another method employs a sucrose gap in which the current is passed through a sucrose-bathed segment of the preparation, but the principle of applying a variable current to maintain a constant V_m is the same. Currents revealed by voltage clamping in multicellular preparations are shown in Fig. 4. An example of drug effect on a specific current is shown in Fig. 21.

The problems of current sources that are not ideal, imperfect spatial control of the preparation because of its complex ultrastructure, and a number of other factors have left us far from the ideal in multicellular preparations (82). However, recent studies in single cells and patches of membrane have been approaching the ideal and will be discussed in later sections.

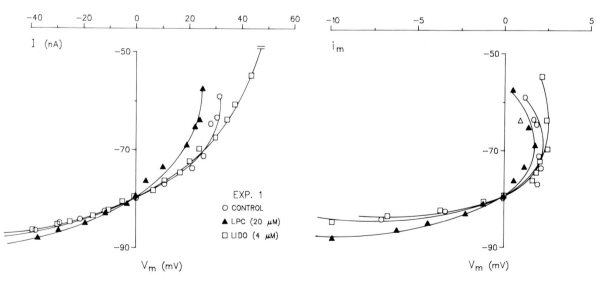

FIG. 3. Current–voltage relationship derived from application of intracellular *constant current* of 100-msec duration. The constant-current–voltage relationship demonstrates the nonlinear relationship between stimulus and response in the subthreshold range of potential before and after lysophosphatidylcholine (LPC), a putative toxic metabolite of ischemia. **A:** *I* vs. V_m. **B:** i_m vs. V_m, where i_m is the mathematically derived current density. Tangents to the curves allow estimation of slope conductance, in this case at $i_m = 0$. (From ref. 14, with permission of the American Heart Association.)

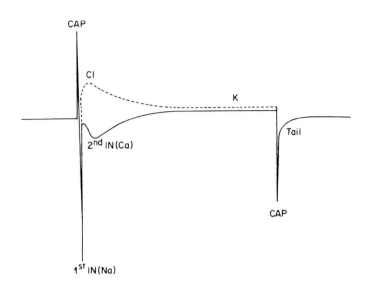

FIG. 4. Diagram of currents seen during a step change in V_m using *voltage clamping* in cardiac tissue. The beginning and end of the voltage step are associated with a capacitive current. By convention, a net inward current is negative and a net outward current is positive. Before the capacitive current is complete, a large inward-current transient occurs representing the sodium current, 1st IN(Na) or i_{Na}, if the voltage step is positive to −55 or −60 mV. This current is inactivated in a few milliseconds. A second inward current, 2nd IN(Ca), follows that is the so-called slow inward current, i_{si}, and is carried primarily by Ca^{2+}. This current inactivates with a slower time course and is followed by an outward current (K) that is carried primarily by K^+. Although somewhat controversial, depolarizations more positive than −20 mV produce an outward transient, Cl, that is thought to be carried by both potassium and chloride ions. At voltage offset, a declining current (Tail) is seen after the capacitive current. The tail results from currents flowing from ionic conductances that had been activated during the voltage step and take time to inactivate. The current may be inward or outward and is usually due to calcium or potassium currents. (From ref. 82, with permission of the American Heart Association.)

IONIC CONCENTRATIONS, ACTIVITIES, AND PUMPS

Equilibrium Potentials

Ordinarily we refer to the free-ion *concentration* in an aqueous solution. However, ions in solution, particularly in physiologic solutions, are not truly "free" of electrostatic interactions. We therefore refer to the *activity* of the ion in solution as a better reflection of its contribution to electrochemical potentials. Solutions of electrolytes show diminished activity with greater concentration or ionic strength. The idea of an "active" ion is all the more important where extensive binding occurs; for example, Ca^{2+} binding inside the cell to various proteins, and Ca^{2+}-buffering compartments (e.g., sarcoplasmic reticulum, sarcolemma, contractile proteins). The intracellular activity of Ca^{2+}, a_{Ca}^i, under these conditions is a much more accurate determinant of its contribution to electrochemical potentials than either Ca^{2+} concentration or content. The activity of an ion is calculated as a function of the activity coefficient at a constant ionic strength multiplied by the concentration.

Ionic gradients across the semipermeable cardiac membrane result in a potential difference between the interior and exterior of the cell. The intracellular potassium concentration ($[K^+]_i$) is about 30 times the extracellular potassium concentration ($[K^+]_o$). K^+, therefore, tends to leak out of the cell down the concentration gradient. The extracellular calcium and sodium concentrations are greater than the intracellular concentrations, and these ions tend to leak into the cell.

Energy-requiring ionic pumps, located in the outer cell membrane and perhaps in the transverse tubules, maintain the normal balance between intracellular and extracellular ionic concentrations. (Na^+,K^+)-ATPase drives the Na^+-K^+ exchange mechanism. ATP, Mg^{2+}, and Na^+ are required at the inner surface and K^+ is required at the outer surface for activation of the pump. The coupling ratio of Na^+ pumped out and K^+ pumped in is usually 3:2. This means that the pump is electrogenic, which results in a few millivolts more negativity than if the pump were neutral. (Na^+,K^+)-ATPase is inhibited by digitalis, Ca^{2+}, low $[K^+]_o$, and compounds with sulfhydryl groups, such as mercurial diuretics and ethacrynic acid. (Na^+,K^+)-ATPase activity can be increased by catecholamines (188) and by increased $[Na^+]_i$. There have been reports of an energy-requiring sarcolemmal Ca^{2+}-ATPase (63,118). There is a Ca^{2+}-Na^+ equilibrium exchange of one intracellular Ca^{2+} for two to four extracellular Na^+ (172) (see *Chapter 26*). The energy for this means of Ca^{2+} extrusion comes from the downhill Na^+ gradient, and therefore it is also dependent on (Na^+,K^+)-ATPase. Protein transport mechanisms also exist for the neutral exchange of ions, such as chloride, and exchange of small organic molecules.

The interrelationships of these ionic influences are of particular interest. A low $[K^+]_o$ reduces the activity of (Na^+,K^+)-ATPase, leading to increases in $[Na^+]_i$ and $[Ca^{2+}]_i$, meaning that the sodium electrochemical gradient is dependent on potassium. Pump activity is increased by an increased $[Na^+]_i$ and by an increase in $[K^+]_o$.

The unequal distribution of charge across the semipermeable membrane results in a potential difference. This potential can be calculated for a given ionic species (y) by using the Nernst equation:

$$E_y = \frac{RT}{zF} \ln \frac{[y]_o}{[y]_i} \qquad [9]$$

where $[y]_o$ and $[y]_i$ are the extracellular and intracellular concentrations (or, more properly, the activities) of y, z is the valence, R is the gas constant (8.314 V C $°K^{-1}$ mol^{-1}), T is the absolute temperature [$T(°$ Kelvin$) =$ $273.16 + T(°$ centigrade$)$], and F is Faraday's constant (9.648×10^{-4} C mol^{-1}). The Nernst equation calculates the potential required to oppose the concentration gradient. The equilibrium potentials at physiologic concentrations for the major ionic species calculated in this manner are approximately as follows: E_{Na}, +60 mV; E_K, +94 mV; E_{Ca}, +130 mV; E_{Cl}, −80 mV. These numbers vary somewhat in different tissues.

As has been mentioned, intracellular ionic activities, rather than bulk ionic concentrations, are more accurately the measurements of electrophysiologic interest. This has been underscored by recent investigations indicating that large fractions of intracellular potassium and sodium are sequestered (131,132). Lee and Fozzard (131), for example, estimated that in rabbit ventricular muscles, about 18% of intracellular potassium and about 79% of intracellular sodium are sequestered. Recent evidence suggests that intracellular ionic activities, which, in part, determine the equilibrium potential, are also voltage-dependent (114,130).

Resting Potential and Effects of Extracellular Potassium

The interior of the quiescent cell is negative as compared with the extracellular potential. V_m in the quiescent cardiac cell is termed the resting potential, V_r. Estimates of the equilibrium potential for potassium, E_K, as calculated from the Nernst equation, closely approximate V_r in normal tissues for $[K^+]_o$ greater than 4.0 mM. That is,

$$V_r \simeq E_K = \frac{RT}{zF} \ln \frac{[K^+]_o}{[K^+]_i} \qquad [10]$$

with the values for the constants as before. Concentrations are used in Eq. 10 and are most commonly employed in the literature. Activities are more accurate and are used in Fig. 5.

V_r is dominated by the intracellular and extracellular potassium activities, because membrane potassium conductance, g_K, is 20 to 100 times higher than any of the other conductances. Because E_K dominates V_r at $[K^+]_o$ over 4.0 mM, the Nernst equation predicts that the cell will depolarize some 59 to 61 mV, depending on conditions, for every unit increase in log $[K^+]_o$. As seen in Fig. 5, the approximation is very close if intracellular potassium activities rather than concentrations are used for sodium-free solutions (163). Increasing $[K^+]_o$ also increases g_K. Depolarization and an increase in g_K have important effects on many electrophysiologic properties of the cell, including inactivation of the sodium system, which in turn will influence excitability, depolarization, repolarization, and impulse propagation.

Below a $[K^+]_o$ of 4.0 mM or an external potassium activity of about 3.2 mM, the prediction of the Nernst equation diverges from the experimental observation of V_r. In hypokalemia, g_K decreases, and the relative contribution of g_{Na} (and perhaps g_{si}) increases. The divergence between V_r and E_K actually increases the driving force (Eq. 5). A simplified version of the Goldman-Hodgkin-Katz constant-field equation approximates this situation:

$$V_r = \frac{RT}{F} \ln \frac{[K^+]_o + (P_{Na}/P_K)[Na^+]_o}{[K^+]_i + (P_{Na}/P_K)[Na^+]_i} \qquad [11]$$

where P is the coefficient of ionic permeability for each ion. P_{Na}/P_K is approximately 0.01 to 0.05 for myocardial cells.

Arrhythmogenic Influences, Antiarrhythmic Drugs, and Ionic Activities

One possible arrhythmogenic consequence of ischemia may be accumulation of lysophosphatidylcholine (LPC)

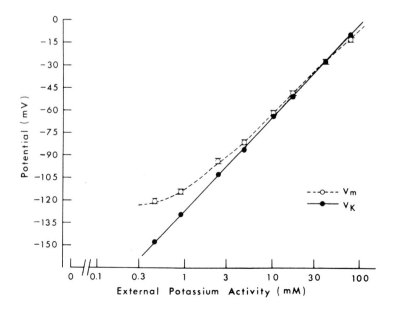

FIG. 5. Resting membrane potential (*open circles, dash line*) in Purkinje fibers as a function of the external potassium activity in sodium-free superfusing solutions. The equilibrium potential for potassium, here termed V_K and represented by the filled circles and the solid line, was calculated from the measured intracellular potassium activity. Note the deviation from prediction at about 4 mM. (From ref. 163, with permission of the American Heart Association.)

(52). This arrhythmogenic influence may also affect intracellular ionic activities. We have investigated the effects of LPC on intracellular sodium (a_{Na}^i) and potassium (a_K^i) activities using microelectrodes filled with liquid ion exchanger. During the initial stages of exposure to LPC, V_r became progressively less negative until it attained a level of about −30 mV. Input resistance increased, but there was little change in a_{Na}^i or a_K^i, suggesting that during that phase the (Na^+,K^+)-ATPase pump was not influenced and membrane integrity was not lost. After prolonged exposure, membrane input resistance began to decrease, a_{Na}^i increased, and a_K^i decreased, suggesting some disruption in membrane integrity.

We have also shown that antiarrhythmic drugs affect contractility, possibly by altering intracellular ionic activities (187). The hypothesis tested was that antiarrhythmic drugs reduce sodium current during phase 0 and the plateau and thereby decrease a_{Na}^i and a_{Ca}^i,

which should correlate with a decrease in twitch tension. To this end, the effects of tetrodotoxin (TTX, a relatively specific fast-channel blocker), encainide, propranolol, and lidocaine on action-potential parameters, a_{Na}^i, and twitch tension were studied in Purkinje fibers. The results showed that all the drugs, including clinically relevant concentrations of the therapeutic agents, decreased $\dot{V}_{max}$, overshoot, action-potential duration, a_{Na}^i, and twitch tension (Fig. 6). The temporal correlations suggest that our hypothesis is correct although effects on action potential morphology may also contribute to this negative inotropy. A representative experiment is shown in Fig. 7.

Very little is known about the effects that drugs have on the determinants of the resting potential. Some information on the effects on a_{Na}^i was mentioned in the previous section. Figure 8 shows an experiment in which V_r was measured as a function of $[K^+]_o$ in sodium-deficient Tyrode solution (8). Sodium-deficient Tyrode

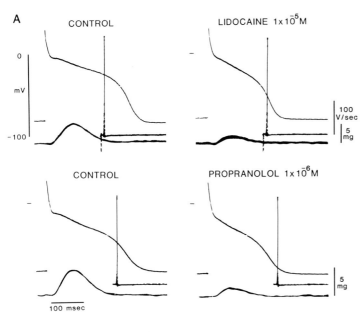

FIG. 6. Effects of lidocaine and propranolol on transmembrane action potentials (**A**) and a_{Na}^i (**B**) in sheep Purkinje fibers stimulated at 1 Hz. **A:** Top trace represents the transmembrane potential; middle trace shows the maximum rate of depolarization ($\dot{V}_{max}$); bottom trace illustrates twitch tension. Lidocaine (1×10^{-5} M) was added to the superfusate, resulting in a shortening of the action-potential duration, a reduction in plateau amplitude, a slight decrease in $\dot{V}_{max}$, and a negative inotropic effect. In another fiber, propranolol (1×10^{-6} M) produced similar electrophysiologic and mechanical effects. **B:** Measurements of a_{Na}^i were obtained in fibers treated similarly to those in part A. Because of the slow response of the Na^+-sensitive microelectrode, the stimulus was terminated until a stable value of a_{Na}^i could be determined. In the top left panel, a_{Na}^i was 7.2 mM under control conditions. Lidocaine (2×10^{-5} M) caused a decrease in a_{Na}^i to 6.5 mM after 15 min of exposure to drug. This effect was reversed and a_{Na}^i recovered after washout of lidocaine for 25 min. In another fiber, propranolol caused a decrease in a_{Na}^i from 8.4 mM to 7.4 mM (**bottom panels**). (From J. A. Wasserstrom, *unpublished observations*.)

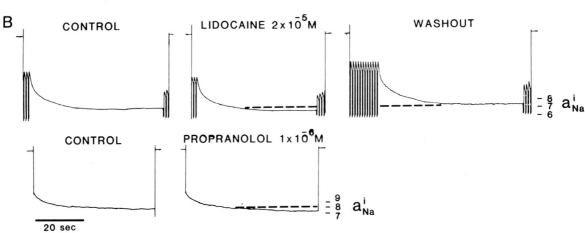

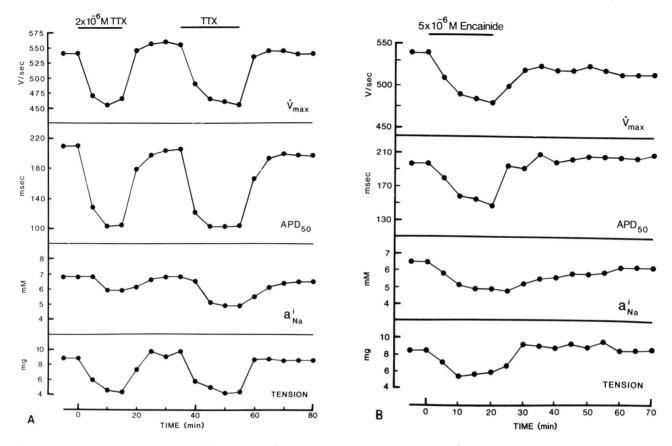

FIG. 7. A: Time course of effects of TTX (2×10^{-6} M) on maximal upstroke velocity ($\dot{V}_{max}$), action-potential duration at 50% of repolarization (APD$_{50}$), a^i_{Na}, and twitch tension in a sheep Purkinje fiber. **B:** Time course of effects of encainide (5×10^{-6} M) on $\dot{V}_{max}$, APD$_{50}$, a^i_{Na}, and twitch tension in a sheep Purkinje fiber. (From ref. 86, with permission.)

was used to further minimize the effects of the background inward sodium current. The presumption was that resting ionic flow could be approximated by $g_K(V_m - E_K)$. Under control conditions (Fig. 8), V_m approximated E_K (the latter determined from the experimental slope, heavy line, which was slightly less steep than that calculated from the Nernst equation, thin line) at $[K^+]_o$ above 4.0 mM. As $[K^+]_o$ was lowered below 4.0 mM, increasing divergence was noted between V_m and E_K because of a decrease in the membrane conductance, presumably primarily to the outward flow of potassium ions. It is clear from Fig. 8 that the driving force for the potassium ion, $(V_m - E_K)$, increased as $[K^+]_o$ was lowered below 4.0. After lidocaine, statistically significant hyperpolarization occurred when $(V_m - E_K)$ was significantly greater than zero, that is, at $[K^+]_o$ less than 2.7. The magnitude of the hyperpolarization was positively correlated with the magnitude of the driving force. These results could be interpreted as indicating an increase in the conductance of the outward potassium current or a decrease in the background inward current, although efforts were made to minimize the effects of the latter. Kabela (119) reported that lidocaine enhanced the efflux of ^{42}K from canine Purkinje fibers at a $[K^+]_o$ of 5.0 mM; he attributed this to increased K^+ conductance.

Whatever the underlying mechanism, lidocaine can hyperpolarize the membrane, and the action is strongest in the depolarized preparation (8,9).

Changes in intracellular ions may play important roles in the arrhythmogenic mechanisms underlying digitalis toxicity. The mechanisms for generation of these arrhythmias have been extensively studied *in vitro*. Elimination of these arrhythmias using therapeutic antiarrhythmic agents has revealed a number of possible sites of action for antiarrhythmic drugs. The following scheme illustrates our present understanding of the consequences of excessive (Na$^+$,K$^+$)-ATPase inhibition from cardiac glycoside toxicity:

$$(Na^+,K^+)\text{-ATPase inhibition}$$
$$\downarrow$$
$$\uparrow a^i_{Na} \rightarrow \uparrow a^i_{Ca} \rightarrow Ca^{2+} \text{ overload of SR}$$
$$\downarrow$$
$$\text{oscillatory } Ca^{2+} \text{ release from SR}$$
$$\downarrow \qquad\qquad \downarrow$$

transient   aftercontraction
depolarization

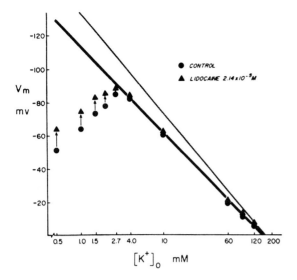

FIG. 8. Resting transmembrane voltage (V_m) in sodium-deficient Tyrode solution during the control period (*circles*) and after lidocaine (*triangles*) is plotted as a function of $[K^+]_o$ on a logarithmic scale. The arrows show the direction of change. The heavy line is a regression line determined from experimental results at $[K^+]_o$ of 10, 60, 90, and 120 mmole/liter that has been extrapolated both to the abscissa and toward the ordinate. The thin line represents E_K as calculated from the Nernst equation. Significant hyperpolarization occurs after application of lidocaine at $[K^+]_o$ of 2.7 mM or less. (From ref. 8, with permission.)

cosides. These agents all decrease twitch tension, either by decreasing a_{Na}^i (86,188) or by reducing Ca^{2+} release from SR (27). The actions of these agents to reduce a_{Ca}^i and/or Ca^{2+} release from the SR, which is responsible for the negative inotropic effects, may then relieve the state of Ca^{2+} overload and oscillatory release of Ca^{2+} from SR. An additional effect to reduce a_{Na}^i by blocking Na^+ channels under conditions of Ca^{2+} overload has also been suggested to occur with lidocaine (74). The effects of these agents on a_{Na}^i have been measured in both normal tissues and tissues in which (Na^+,K^+)-ATPase has been inhibited and a_{Na}^i raised to quite high levels. However, therapeutic concentrations of these agents have been shown to have no effect on a_{Na}^i in the presence of glycoside-inhibited (Na^+,K^+)-ATPase in vitro (188,189). These findings suggest that elimination of the arrhythmias with phenytoin, quinidine, and lidocaine occurs not by reversal of the accumulation of intracellular Na^+ and Ca^{2+} but rather, at least in part, as a drug effect on Ca^{2+} metabolism. The TDs and aftercontractions that occur as a result of calcium overload are abolished in part as a consequence of drug action to interfere with Ca^{2+} release from the SR and/or to reduce a_{Ca}^i. The interactions between antiarrhythmic drugs and arrhythmias due to Ca^{2+} overload are discussed in detail in a later section.

PASSIVE CELLULAR PROPERTIES

Intercellular Communication and Cable Properties

Passive properties account for the behavior of the sink. Passive properties are characterized by a response proportional to the stimulus. In 1952, Weidmann (190) conducted a series of experiments in which he studied the transmission characteristics of Purkinje fibers. He applied subthreshold depolarizing and hyperpolarizing currents intracellularly through one microelectrode and recorded V_m at various points along the length of Purkinje fibers through other recording microelectrodes in the manner depicted in panel A of Fig. 1. Weidmann observed a graded drop in V_m with distance from the point of stimulation. An example of such a drop is shown in Fig. 2. Weidmann found that such a change in V_m as a function of distance could be described quite well by uniform cable theory, a topic that is considered in detail in Chapter 1 and in a recent review (5). Weidmann concluded that because the electrotonic potential could be recorded across several cells within the length of Purkinje fiber between the site of current application and the site of V_m recording, the resistance to ionic flow between cells must be low. Moreover, the magnitude of the change in V_m was quite ohmically, that is, linearly, related to small intracellularly applied depolarizing and hyperpolarizing currents—characteris-

where SR is the sarcoplasmic reticulum. The inability of the SR to sequester adequate high levels of intracellular Ca^{2+} produces oscillations in Ca^{2+} release from the SR that produce membrane depolarizations through Ca^{2+} activation of a nonspecific transient inward current (i_{ti}). In glycoside toxicity, these actions occur also in the presence of membrane depolarization as a consequence of inhibition of (Na^+,K^+)-ATPase. Loss of intracellular K^+ produces a loss in membrane potential, and gain in intracellular Na^+ exchanges from external calcium via the Na^+-Ca^{2+} equilibrium exchange process. Thus, the phenomena associated with calcium overload occur at relatively low maximum diastolic potentials.

The arrhythmogenic and antiarrhythmic effects of intracellular ionic changes underlie glycoside-induced arrhythmias and their suppression with antiarrhythmic drugs. As described earlier, accumulation of a_{Na}^i occurs secondary to (Na^+,K^+)-ATPase inhibition. The Na^+-Ca^{2+} exchange process then loads the cell with Ca^{2+}. Excessive overload causes an oscillatory release of Ca^{2+} from the sarcoplasmic reticulum (SR) that underlies i_{ti}, transient depolarizations (TD), and aftercontractions. The suppression of resulting arrhythmias generated by TD reaching threshold is also dependent on intracellular ionic changes. Wasserstrom and Ferrier (186) demonstrated that phenytoin and quinidine in therapeutic concentrations reduced the amplitude of TDs and aftercontractions in Purkinje fibers exposed to cardiac gly-

tics that favored low-resistance electrical coupling rather than chemical coupling.

Weidmann (192) also used cable theory to calculate the theoretical distribution of ^{42}K within and between ventricular cells and found that observation correlated closely with prediction in that ^{42}K diffused freely between cells. He found the upper limit for resistance between cells to be 3 $\Omega \cdot$ cm, almost 700-fold less than for the outer cell membrane.

The gap junction is the low-resistance structure responsible for electrical communication, and it primarily determines the longitudinal or inside resistance (resistor r_i in Fig. 1). The gap junction permits intercellular communication and mediates transport of small molecules and ions between cells (60,121,138,150,174). The gap junction consists of a geometric array of subunits grouped about a central channel that form a "connexon." The connexon extends from the myoplasm through the inner hydrophilic layer, the hydrophobic lipid bilayer, and the outer hydrophilic layer of the membrane into the gap between the cells, where it meets the connexon extending from the neighboring cell. The central channels of the connexons are continuous and connect the interiors of the two cells.

The communicating cardiac cells resemble telegraph cable in that they have a low-resistance core (the myoplasm and normally low-resistance gap junctions) that is surrounded by insulation of relatively high resistance (the cell membrane). The electrical analogue is as appears in Fig. 2: The insulation leaks, and current is lost through the membrane, and therefore less current flows longitudinally through the myoplasm and gap junctions. Equations modified for nerve (27,98) and heart (190,193)

were found to describe experimental observations rather well. The terms in the modified cable equations can be assessed experimentally, permitting determination of membrane resistance (R_m), the longitudinal resistance term (R_i), membrane capacitance (C_m), the time constant (τ_m) that describes the charging of the capacitor and the effects of membrane resistance, and the length constant (λ_m) that describes the interactions between cells in terms of the distance over which one cell may electronically influence another. Geometric considerations influence electrotonic interaction and other passive properties.

Effects of Arrhythmogenic Interventions and Antiarrhythmic Drugs

Cellular uncoupling at the gap juntion, rather than formation of a new membrane, seems to underlie the "healing-over" capability of cardiac cells (17,19,59–62). Ischemia changes the geometric characteristics of the gap junction (17). Closing of the gap junction with injury isolates the damaged cells, thereby preventing leakage of the contents of normal neighboring cells through the gap junction to the injured cell and then to the outside, and eliminates current flow that may be arrhythmogenic. A decreased pH, or intracellular injection of calcium, as well as some metabolic poisons and digitalis, can increase R_i at the gap junctions and, in some instances, cause cellular uncoupling (56,60, 101,138,150). R_i decreases somewhat on elevating $[K^+]_o$ from 4.0 to 7.0 mM (67).

Arrhythmogenic influences can affect cable properties. As an example, LPC accumulates in the ischemic heart and extracellular fluids and is thought to have clinically

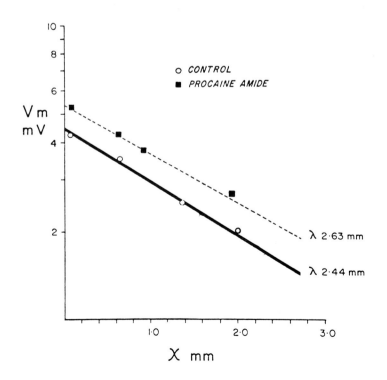

FIG. 9. Effects of procainamide on voltage at the point of the stimulating microelectrode (V_0) and on membrane length constant (λ_m) in a long Purkinje fiber. V_0 is the value of V_m at zero distance, that is, the points on the y axis intercepted by the solid and interrupted lines. The intracellular hyperpolarizing constant current was held at 13.8 nA during both the control and drug periods. Transmembrane responses were recorded at various distances from the stimulating microelectrode along the fiber (x). As compared with the control, procainamide increased V_0 from 4.4 to 5.4 mV and λ_m from 2.44 to 2.63 mm. (From ref. 9, with permission of the American Heart Association.)

relevant electrophysiologic actions (52). We have found that LPC, at low concentrations, increases V_0, V_0/I_0, τ_m, R_i, and R_m, with the balance between R_i and R_m determining λ_m (14). An arrhythmogenic intervention, then, can alter the normal matrix of the passive cellular properties.

Very little information exists regarding the effects of antiarrhythmic drugs on passive properties. It is instructive to consider an example of drug effects on passive properties. A number of years ago, we studied the effects of procainamide on cable properties in cardiac Purkinje fibers (10). The experimental arrangement is shown in panel A of Fig. 1. A plot of V_m versus x for one experiment is shown in Fig. 9. Extrapolation to $x = 0$ gives a value for the voltage at the point of the stimulating microelectrode, V_0, and the length or space constant, λ_m, is defined as the distance (x) over which V_m falls to e^{-1} (about 37%) of its value at V_0. As compared with the control, procainamide increased V_0 from 4.4 to 5.4 mV and λ_m from 2.44 to 2.63 mm. From these measurements and knowledge of τ_m and the transmembrane-applied intracellular current (I_0), the remainder of the cable properties can be determined. Procainamide increased V_0/I_0, τ_m, and R_m. Lidocaine had opposite effects on V_0, λ_m, V_0/I_0, τ_m, and R_m (19).

We studied the effects of lidocaine, procainamide, a β-adrenoreceptor blocker, tolamolol, and encainide on R_i in normal Purkinje fibers and found no change (9–11,15). Lidocaine and tolamolol decreased R_m and λ_m, whereas procainamide and encainide increased R_m and λ_m. Decreases in R_m and τ_m would result in electrotonic currents, producing a smaller change in V_m for a given current than normal and having a lesser effect than normal on tissues at a distance, actions that would be antiarrhythmic. Increases in R_m and λ_m would have the opposite effect, thereby enhancing the influence of electrotonic currents. Such an action could be arrhythmogenic if such currents brought adjacent tissue to threshold and caused regenerative repolarization, or it could be antiarrhythmic if the electrotonic interaction caused discontinuous propagation across an area of unidirectional block.

ACTIVE CELLULAR PROPERTIES IN TISSUES DEPENDENT ON i_{Na} FOR PHASE 0: THE SOURCE IN FAST-RESPONSE TISSUES

Subthreshold Potentials; Threshold; Charge- and Strength-Duration Relationships; Liminal Length

Within a few millivolts of the steady state that characterizes the resting potential, a stimulus produces a response in V_m proportional to the stimulus. With further depolarization by intracellular constant-current application, the nonlinear character of the current–voltage relationship becomes apparent as V_{th} is approached (Fig. 3). The nonlinear behavior is due to the rectifier properties of the membrane. At a certain point, the response in excitable cells is regenerative and out of proportion to the stimulus. This point has often been called the *threshold voltage* or, more simply, the *threshold*. As will be seen, the concept of describing the threshold in terms of a transmembrane voltage is oversimplified, because excitability depends on both active and passive cellular properties.

In 1907, Lapicque (128) observed the current required to produce a response in nerve to be greater for stimuli of short duration than for stimuli of long duration. The rheobasic current was the smallest current, regardless of duration, that could cause a regenerative response. The relationship between the current strength and the duration of the stimulus was described by Lapicque as

$$I_{th} = I_{rh}/[1 - e^{t/\tau}] \qquad [12]$$

where I_{th} is the current required to provoke a regenerative response, I_{rh} is the rheobasic current, t is the duration of I_{th}, and τ approximates the membrane time constant. The data suggested that the charge threshold, $I_{th} \times t$, was relatively constant, and the relationship could be interpreted in terms of a constant threshold and a simple RC circuit. In 1952, Hodgkin and Huxley (97) developed the concept of voltage- and time-dependent activation and inactivation variables for sodium conductances, and Noble and Stein (148) and Cooley and Dodge (48), among others, concluded that the threshold was the situation in which depolarizing inward current equaled repolarizing outward current, with the kinetics of the former being more rapid than those of the latter.

Dominguez and Fozzard (67) studied the relationship between the strength and duration of the intracellularly applied constant currents required to produce regenerative responses in sheep Purkinje fibers. They found that the time constant of the strength–duration curve in heart muscle was shorter than was the membrane time constant and that the voltage that defined the threshold varied with the duration of the stimulus, implying that excitability was a complex function that included passive cellular properties. In 1972, Fozzard and Schoenberg (85) applied the concept of *liminal length,* first proposed by Rushton (158) in 1937 in nerve, to the results in short and long Purkinje preparations. The liminal length is that length of tissue that must be raised above threshold so that the inward depolarizing current from that region will be greater than the repolarizing influences of adjacent tissues. It can be represented as

$$\text{liminal length} = \frac{0.855 Q_{th}}{2(\pi)^{3/2} a C_m \lambda_m V_{th}} \qquad [13]$$

where Q_{th} is the charge threshold, a is the radius, and the other terms are as previously defined. This work indicated that cable properties not only are important in the passive cell but also, to a great extent, define the conditions under which regenerative depolarization can occur. Unfortunately, the error in determining the liminal length experimentally is large and limits its use in studying the effects of arrhythmogenic influences and antiarrhythmic drugs. The concept, however, is useful. These concepts, as well as a discussion of the effects of arrhythmogenic interventions and antiarrhythmic drugs on these properties, will be pursued further in a later section.

Channels and Gating

Membrane channels have evolved to be highly selective and to take part in positive- and negative-feedback systems so as to generate very specific processes. Selec-

tivity means that a certain type of channel selects the type or types of ions that are allowed to pass through. In some tissues, the regenerative action potential depends on the inrush of sodium ions (i_{Na}) through a kinetically rapid channel that is blocked by tetrodotoxin. The rapid kinetics have led to the terminology "fast-response" or i_{Na}-dependent tissues. Such i_{Na}-dependent tissues are found in the atrium, the Purkinje fibers of the specialized infranodal conduction system, and ventricular muscle. The characteristics of these tissues are listed in Table 2.

Two subunits of the sodium channel have been identified (26). The 270,000-dalton unit undergoes phosphorylation by a cAMP-dependent protein kinase (53). Channels have been incorporated into liposomal vesicles (88,178) and into planar bilayers (51,92,126,143).

TABLE 2. *Characteristics of so-called fast- and slow-response cardiac tissues*

	Fast-response tissues	Slow-response tissues
Geographic location	Working and specialized atrial tissues; infranodal specialized conduction system (Purkinje fibers); ventricular muscle; accessory AV bypass tracts (Kent bundles, etc.)	SA and AV nodes; perhaps valves; coronary sinus; injured tissues in which i_{Na}-dependent converted to i_{si}-dependent phase 0
Passive membrane properties		
Normal resting potential (V_r)	Approximately −80 to −95 mV	Approximately −40 to −65 mV
Subthreshold membrane conductance	Primarily components of g_K, particularly g_{K_1}	Probably a component of g_K
Active membrane properties		
"Threshold" voltage	Approximately −60 to −75 mV	Approximately −40 to −60 mV i_{si} (mixed current with both Ca^{2+} and Na^+)
Current responsible for phase-0 depolarization	i_{Na}	
Activation and inactivation kinetics of channel responsible for phase-0 depolarization	Fast	Slow
Maximal rise velocity of phase 0 (dV/dt_{max} or $\dot{V}_{max}$)	300–1,000+ V/sec	1–50 V/sec
Peak overshoot	Approximately +20 to +40 mV	−5 to +20 mV
Overall amplitude of action potential	Approximately +90 to +135 mV	Approximately −30 to +70 mV
Refractoriness and reactivation	Partial reactivation during phase 3; complete reactivation in normal tissue 10 to 50 msec after return to normal V_r	Partial and complete reactivation returns after (>100 msec) attainment of V_r
Relationship of rate to		
(a) Action-potential duration	Marked change	Slight change
(b) Refractory-period duration	Steep curve	"Flat" curve
(c) Threshold	Independent	Varies directly with frequency
(d) Conduction velocity	Independent	Decays with frequency
Supernormal excitability	Often present	Never seen
Conduction velocity	0.5 to 5 m/sec	0.01 to 0.1 m/sec
Safety factor	High	Low
Characteristics conducive to reentry	Only with inactivation of the sodium system	Present even in normally i_{si}-dependent tissues
Automaticity	Yes; normally depends on decreasing i_{K_2} and/or increasing i_f	Yes; normally depends on increasing i_f
Automaticity depressed by physiologic increases in $[K^+]_o$	Yes	No

From Arnsdorf (6), with permission.

The channels open and close to permit or prevent flow of the selected ionic species, a process that is called gating. The probability of a gate being open or closed depends on voltage and time. The sensors for a voltage-sensitive channel are charges that move in response to the electric field of the cardiac membrane, and the movements of these charges have been recorded and measured. Hille (95) has reviewed in some detail the possible mechanisms for channel gating and has concluded that a rotating or sliding gate is the most probable. Figure 10 has utilized a sliding gate.

Hodgkin-Huxley Model

Traditionally, this process has been described in terms of the Hodgkin-Huxley model, which includes time- and voltage-dependent activation and inactivation vari-ables. The Hodgkin-Huxley model rather well describes the behavior of the sodium current in nerve and, with modifications, approximates such behavior in heart (35,95). A modification of Eq. 5 is useful in describing control of the sodium current in terms of conductance and driving force. In nerve, Hodgkin and Huxley (97) proposed the relationship

$$i_{Na} = \bar{g}_{Na}m^3h(V_m - E_{Na}) \qquad [14]$$

where i_{Na} is the sodium current per unit area, $\bar{g}_{Na}$ is the maximal sodium conductance, m and h are dimensionless activation and inactivation variables that, as will be discussed later, can be conceptualized as "on" and "off" gates, respectively, and E_{Na} is the equilibrium potential for sodium.

Equation 14 describes the maximal sodium conductance as determined by two variables that change with

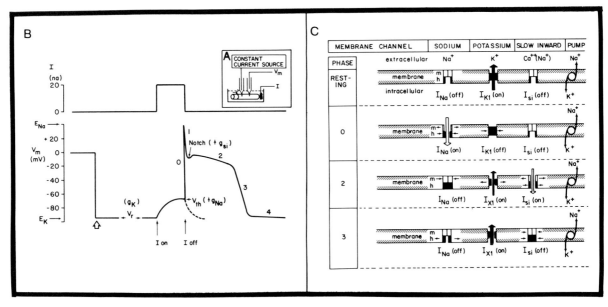

FIG. 10. A (inset): A microelectrode for injecting current into a cell is impaled near the ligated end of the Purkinje preparation and is used for intracellular current application. The second microelectrode records V_m. The bath collects a voltage signal that is proportional to the current, I. B: Oscilloscopic representations of I and V_m are depicted. When the microelectrode is in the extracellular space, V_m is zero. With impalement of the tissue, V_m falls from 0 to −95 mV (open, white arrow), which is the resting potential, V_r. At physiologic extracellular K$^+$ concentrations, V_r approximates the potassium equilibrium potential, E_K, as would be predicted by the Nernst equation. Depolarizing current (I_{on}) causes V_m to become more positive and to approach the threshold voltage, V_{th}, for regenerative phase-0 depolarization. If the liminal-length requirements are not met, V_m decays exponentially because of the passive-membrane resistive–capacitive properties, as shown by the dashed line following I_{off}. Membrane conductance for both the resting membrane and the subthreshold voltage range is determined primarily by the membrane potassium conductance, g_K. If the liminal-length requirements are met, an action potential results, and the overshoot approaches the equilibrium potential for sodium, E_{Na}. The phases of the action potential are shown, as are the conductances of particular importance to each phase (g_K, g_{Na}, g_{si}). C: The gates that control passage of the sodium, potassium, and slow inward currents are depicted diagrammatically for the resting membrane and phases 0, 2, and 3. At rest, the membrane conductance, particularly g_{K_1} (voltage-dependent, time-independent), dominates. During depolarization, the "on" or m gate opens and the "off" or h gate closes. Because the m gate is kinetically faster than the "off" or h gate, brisk depolarization causes the influence of the "on" gate to predominate, sodium rushes into the cell, and rapid phase-0 depolarization results. Voltage-dependent i_{K_1} turns off. During phase 2, the plateau results from inactivation of i_{Na}, activation of depolarizing i_{si}, and rectification of K$^+$ current, favoring depolarization rather than repolarization. During rapid repolarization (phase 3), i_{si} largely turns off, K$^+$ rectification is reversed, and the outward K$^+$ current (in some schemes called i_{x_1}) increases, which together favor rapid repolarization back to the resting potential.

voltage. The rapid-activation variable (m) can be thought of as an "on" gate that opens during depolarization, and the slow-inactivation variable (h) as an "off" gate that closes during depolarization. With depolarization, the kinetics of the opening "on" gate are faster than those of the closing "off" gate. Rapid depolarization, therefore, results in the "on" gate opening before the "off" gate closes, allowing sodium to rush into the cell and produce the rapid upstroke (phase 0) of the action potential. A positive-feedback system is created in which, as the cells depolarize, more m gates open and i_{Na} further increases. The positive-feedback system is responsible for the regenerative process. The maximal rate of rise of phase 0 is often termed $\dot{V}_{max}$ and has normal values of 100 to 200 V/sec in atrial and ventricular muscle and 200 to 1,000 V/sec in Purkinje cells. V_m moves toward E_{Na}, which is about +40 mV.

The "off" or h gate closes very slowly following rapid movement of V_m from V_r to threshold and interferes little with the inrush of sodium ions once the regenerative inrush of i_{Na} begins. After the peak of the action potential and during the plateau, enough time has elapsed so that the h closes completely. The sodium system, therefore, is *inactivated,* regardless of the state of the "on" gate. Such inactivation is the basis of the refractory period and can be absolute or partial.

As has been discussed, V_r is a function of $[K^+]_o$ or, more accurately, the potassium activity. Hyperkalemia, then, depolarizes the cell. This will produce varying degrees of inactivation of the sodium system. There are many channels, and each is either open or shut, but together they reflect the inactivation of the sodium system. Referring to the panel in Fig. 11 in which the channel reflects the composite sodium system rather than an individual channel that is either open or shut, at a $[K^+]_o$ of 4.0 mM and a V_r of −96 mV, the h or "off" gate is open and the m or "on" gate is closed at rest. Brisk depolarization activates and opens the m or "on" gate of the sodium channel; sodium ions rush unimpeded into the cell. If V_r is less negative than normal, say −71 mV at a $[K^+]_o$ of 10 mM in the middle panel, steady-state restriction of the composite voltage-dependent sodium system by "off" or h gates occurs. With activation, the partial closure of the h gate reduces sodium conductance and limits the amount of sodium current that can pass through the channel. At an even higher $[K^+]_o$ of 16 mM, V_r is −59 mV, the "off" or h gate is essentially completely closed, and the sodium system is essentially completely inactivated. Although the "on" or m gate may open during activation, the channel is obstructed by the closed h gate. With hyperkalemia, not only is the g_{Na} term reduced, but so is the driving force, because V_m is now less negative than at a normal $[K^+]_o$. For example, at $[K^+]_o$ of 16 mM, the driving force is approximately 100 mV, as compared with about 130 mV at a $[K^+]_o$ of 4.0 mM. Because both the conductance and the driving force are decreased, so, too, must i_{Na} be decreased. If the sodium system is completely inactivated, phase-0 depolarization may become dependent on i_{si}. If depolarization is slow rather than rapid, the time may be sufficient to partially or completely inactivate the sodium system: a type of voltage-dependent inactivation of the sodium system that has been called *accommodation.*

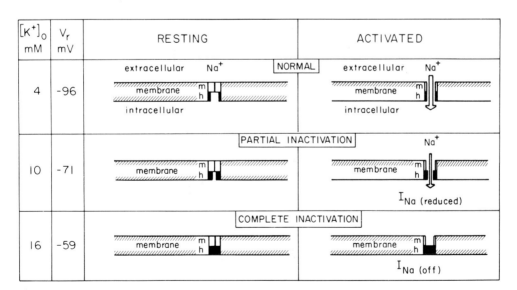

FIG. 11. Effects of external potassium concentration ($[K^+]_o$) on the resting potential (V_r), the voltage-dependent states of the resting and activated "off" (h) and "on" (m) gates, and the resultant ionic sodium current. Three situations are depicted: normal (**top**), partial inactivation (**middle**), and complete inactivation (**lower**). This is a composite channel reflecting the state of the sodium system. In reality, the gate is not partly shut. Rather, there are many gates; some are open and others are not. (From ref. 7, with permission.)

Equation (14) suggests that the sodium channel can be opened by movement of three particles, each with a probability m of being in the right place. The probability of inactivation is $1 - h$. This form was chosen, in part, to simplify calculations, in that the kinetics could be presented as the product of independent variables of the first order. Inactivation and the dependence of the sodium system on V_m also have been used to advantage in physiologic and pharmacologic studies as part of what has been termed "membrane responsiveness". In such studies, the maximum rate of rise of phase 0, $\dot{V}_{max}$, has been used commonly as an indirect measure of i_{Na}. The basis for using $\dot{V}_{max}$ as an approximation of i_{Na} is considered in Chapter 1 and, within limits, is useful. When plotted as a function of V_m at the time of activation by a premature depolarization introduced during phase 3, an S-shaped relationship results that provides an estimate of the magnitude of the h variable at the activation voltage during phase 3. The effects of lidocaine at three concentrations on membrane responsiveness in a canine Purkinje fiber at $[K^+]_o$ of 3.0 mM are shown in Fig. 12 (29). Note in panel A that the higher concentrations of lidocaine (5×10^{-5} and $1 \times$

10^{-4} M) decreased the peak $\dot{V}_{max}$ and shifted the curve rightward and downward, whereas the lower concentration of 1×10^{-5} M actually increased peak $\dot{V}_{max}$, and the curve was steeper. Although not stated, the increased $\dot{V}_{max}$ may have resulted from lidocaine-induced hyperpolarization of the resting membrane, with some removal of inactivation. Panel B shows that the effect of $\dot{V}_{max}$ was reversible.

The sodium-channel cycle, according to the Hodgkin-Huxley scheme, is shown diagrammatically in Fig. 10, the states are depicted in Fig. 13, and a computer simulation of these channel states by Hondeghem and Katzung (104) is presented in Fig. 14. The resting state (R) predominates in normally polarized tissues, where V_r approximates E_K; the activated state (A) occurs transiently on brisk depolarization, with opening of the "on" or m gate before significant closing of the kinetically slower "off" or h gate; the inactivated state (I) is predominant at more positive potentials when the "on" gate inactivates and the "off" or h gate is closed. The R, A, and I states correspond to the phases in panel C of Fig. 11 labeled resting, 0, and 2.

As will be discussed in a later section, evidence is

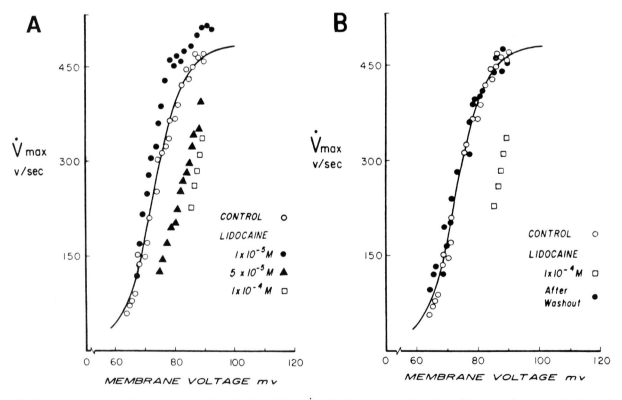

FIG. 12. Membrane responsiveness in a canine Purkinje fiber. $\dot{V}_{max}$ is plotted as a function of the membrane activation voltage during repolarization phase 3. The conditions are as indicated. **A:** Effects of three concentrations of lidocaine on membrane responsiveness. The control shows the typical S-shaped curve; 1×10^{-5} M shifts the curve to the left, makes it steeper, and increases peak $\dot{V}_{max}$; at 5×10^{-5} M, peak $\dot{V}_{max}$ was depressed, and the curve was shifted downward and to the right; at 1×10^{-4} M, there was further depression in peak $\dot{V}_{max}$, and the curve was yet more to the right. Note also the change in the minimal V_m at which a response was elicited. **B:** Reversibility of lidocaine-induced depression of membrane responsiveness. These measurements were made 1 hr after washout had started. (From ref. 29, with permission.)

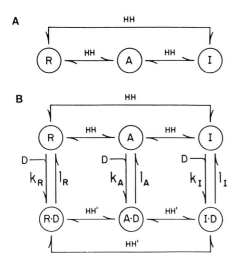

FIG. 13. States of the sodium channel in the absence of drug and in the presence of drug. **A:** Absence of drug. The resting state (R) predominates in normally polarized tissues near E_K. The activated state (A) occurs on brisk depolarization with opening of the "on" or m gate before significant closing of the kinetically slower "off" or h gate. The inactivated state (I) is predominant at more positive potentials when the "off" or h gate is closed. Hodgkin-Huxley parameters are indicated by HH. During the course of the cardiac cycle, the R, A, and I states correspond to the phases in panel C of Fig. 11 labeled resting, 0, and 2. **B:** Presence of drug. Drug molecules can associate (*down arrow*) or dissociate (*up arrow*) with the channels in all three states. The drug-associated channels are R-D, A-D, and I-D. Their Hodgkin-Huxley parameters are shifted to more positive potentials (HH'); so the channels behave as if they are at a less negative transmembrane voltage than in the control. (From ref. 104, with permission.)

accumulating that drugs can associate preferentially with certain states. This has become important in the modulated-receptor hypothesis and other such schemes of drug actions.

Newer Approaches and Concepts

Voltage clamping, as mentioned earlier, permits V_m to be controlled while the current flow across a membrane is measured, permitting calculation of membrane conductance for a given ionic species. V_m must be changed very rapidly to avoid any changes in membrane properties that may be sensitive to voltage. Voltage clamping had been used for many years in multicellular cardiac preparations, but the multicellular structure of cardiac tissues made it impossible to gain sufficiently rapid and uniform control of V_m to permit a measure of i_{Na}. New techniques allow direct measurement of i_{Na}. Small groups of cells, single cells, and even small patches of membrane can be directly studied electrophysiologically. The interested reader is referred to the recent review by Fozzard et al. (84) and to other chapters in this book on these new approaches. A brief summary

of these approaches is in order, because they are becoming increasingly important in the study of antiarrhythmic drugs.

Small Multicellular Preparations

Voltage-clamp techniques have been employed in small multicellular preparations or aggregates of cells by a number of investigators (44,47,68–70). Although the multicellular nature of the preparations still produced some problems, these studies demonstrated that i_{Na} could be activated within a millisecond and that the Hodgkin-Huxley model was imperfect.

Single Cardiac Cells

Single heart cells can be isolated with enzymatic dispersion, which destroys the collagen that holds the cells together. These single cells can be voltage-clamped, and both the intracellular and extracellular ionic milieus can be manipulated, thereby providing a rather complete assessment of the factors included in Eq. 5, including the determinants of the equilibrium potential. Lee et al. (134) and Brown et al. (32,33) have used suction pipettes

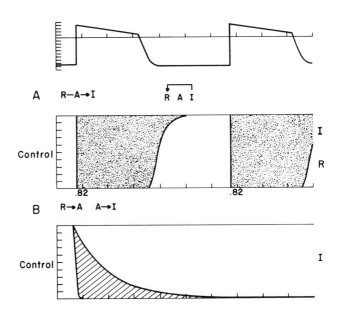

FIG. 14. Computer simulations of channel states during the action potential. **A:** The horizontal axis is 500 msec. The rapid conversion from resting (*white area*) through activated (too brief to be noted at this time scale) to inactivated state (*stippled*) is depicted by the sharp barrier. The maximum normalized sodium conductance is 0.82, less than unity because a few channels are inactivated before the rest of the channels open. **B:** The time scale on the horizontal axis is enlarged, representing 2.4 msec during phase 0 of the first action potential in **A.** The cross-hatched area represents the fraction of channels in the activated state. (From ref. 104, with permission.)

for this purpose. Two suction pipettes have been used on a single ventricular cell, with one used to record V_m and the other used for passing current. The pipette seals to the cell surface, and then the membrane at the tip of the pipette is broken with pressure, permitting equilibration of the interior of the cell with whatever solution is in the pipette. Hume and Giles (106) used a similar method in atrial cells of the bullfrog. Kostyuk (124) used a flow-through polyethylene suction pipette for voltage clamping and internally perfusing single neuronal cells. Similar methods have been used on single rat ventricular myocytes (31), human atrial cells (35), and single canine cardiac Purkinje cells (83,141).

Patch Clamping

Patch clamping is an exciting new technique for measuring the electrophysiologic characteristics of individual ionic channels. In the method of Hamill et al. (91), a small pipette with a tip 1 to 2 μm in diameter is placed against the membrane, suction is applied, and a high-resistance seal (a gigaohm seal or gigaseal) results. The pipette can be used to record from the channels in the small sealed patch while it remains part of the intact cell (cell-attached patch), or the patch can be torn away from the cell (excised patch). Excised patches can be used inside-out or outside-in. The voltage and ionic content of the glass pipette are controlled. Unitary events can be recorded directly, and channel behavior is easily distinguished. This technique has been used for studying cardiac sodium channels (36,89,127,161,180). These studies indicate that the sodium-channel density is low, perhaps 2 to 10/μm². The squid axon, in comparison, has 200 to 500/μm² (135). A single sodium channel with an open time of 1 msec and a conductance of 15 pS will allow the passage of about 1,000 Na⁺.

Grant et al. (89) used patch clamping in rabbit myocytes. These investigators found that the probability of channel opening as well as the channel open time increased with depolarization; single-channel current amplitude ranged from 0.6 to 1.9 pA, and sodium channels could be distinguished from calcium channels by their inactivation-voltage range and response to cadmium. They found only two conductance states: open and closed. First-event latency histograms suggested multiple closed states.

Hodgkin-Huxley and Newer Data

In the Hodgkin-Huxley model, activation and inactivation are processes that instantly change rate as a function of V_m, and inactivation as well as recovery from inactivation are considered single exponentials. Nerve cells have a time lag in activation suggesting intermediate states between the resting and open states, but the voltage clamps in heart cells are not yet fast

enough to test for this. A number of investigators have observed at least two time constants to i_{Na} decay (33,83,152) and a sigmoidal recovery from inactivation (33,84), which suggest more than one inactivated state. As mentioned, Grant et al. (89) have presented first-event latency histograms that suggest multiple closed states. Moreover, a very long phase of recovery from inactivation has been described as a function of duration of depolarization and drugs that affect sodium channels (43,69).

Such findings suggest the type of model shown in Fig. 15. In the resting cell, the channel is in a closed (C) state. With depolarization, the channel may go to the open (O) state or to the inactivated (I) state. A latency of opening after depolarization that is not correlated with gating current suggests that there may be several closed states (C_1 to C_n). The channel either opens or inactivates. Activation (C_n to O) is slow, with a time constant of 1 or 2 msec; inactivation (O to I) is rapid, with a time constant of 0.5 msec, and is not very voltage-dependent. At least two inactive states seem to exist (I_1 and I_2). The maximal i_{Na} also depends on how many channels are directly inactivated (C to I), and the recovery from inactivation is represented by I to one of the C states.

Repolarization

Normal Repolarization and Antiarrhythmic Drugs

Repolarization in fast-response tissues is also a regenerative process. Phase 1 depends on inactivation of g_{Na} and, in Purkinje fibers, perhaps on activation of a current carried by K⁺ and/or Cl⁻. In phase 2, the less negative V_m opens the channel for i_{si}, the mixed Ca²⁺-Na⁺ current (Fig. 10, panel C). Because i_{si} is an inward positive current, it contributes to depolarization and helps to maintain the plateau. It was found that low doses of tetrodotoxin (TTX) shorten the plateau without affecting $\dot{V}_{max}$, suggesting a sodium current during the

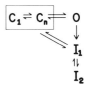

FIG. 15. State model for Na⁺ channels based on data from single-cell and patch-clamp studies. The channel of the resting cell is in a closed (C) state, and the latency of opening after depolarization that is not correlated with gating current suggests that there may be multiple closed states (C_1 to C_n). With depolarization the channel may go to the open (O) or to the inactivated (I) state. There seem to be at least two inactivated states (I_1 and I_2). The recovery from inactivation is represented by the transition of one of the I states to one of the C states. (From ref. 84, with permission of the American Heart Association.)

plateau different from that responsible for phase 0 (49). Subsequently, others confirmed the presence of a TTX-sensitive inward current during the plateau (39,45). This finding has been interpreted in several ways. Possibly the steady-state TTX-sensitive "window" sodium current in cardiac Purkinje fibers arises from voltage-dependent and time-independent sodium channels (18). Alternatively, perhaps there is a voltage- and time-independent channel that provides a background inward current that affects both the resting and plateau potentials. Hyperpolarization of V_r has been observed after TTX (49) and removing $[Na^+]_o$ (163). TTX also reduces intracellular sodium activity (Fig. 7 and 58,114,184,187). Yet another explanation would be a second population of sodium channels that inactivate with time constants of several hundred milliseconds and that would be sensitive to low concentrations of TTX, a suggestion supported by the observations of Gintant et al. (87). Currents of this magnitude could also be generated by transport processes such as electrogenic (Na^+,K^+)-ATPase, the Na^+-Ca^{2+} exchange system, and perhaps other transport systems such as Na^+-H^+.

During phase 2, the driving force for K^+ increases, and potassium conductance decreases in the outward direction while increasing in the inward direction. The result is that K^+ enters the cell more easily than it exits, a mechanism that also maintains the plateau. This phenomenon has been called *anomalous* or *inward rectification*. The anomaly is that conductance decreases with depolarization and sharply increases with hyperpolarization. Part of the rectification is essentially instantaneous (less than 1 msec), but another part develops with a time constant of many milliseconds up to half a second.

During phase 3, the rapid-repolarization phase, there is a rapid return to the resting potential that results from inactivation of i_{si}, reversal of the process of inward rectification, and activation of a repolarizing outward potassium current, a process called delayed or outward rectification. It is almost as if there is a repolarization "threshold" at about -30 mV in Purkinje fibers at which phase 3 occurs. The increasing negativity of V_m produces another positive-feedback system for these repolarizing processes. During phase 3, enough of the sodium system is normally reactivated that another action potential can be electrically induced. Failure of normal repolarization affects excitability and propagation.

It is difficult to design experiments to study the currents involved in maintaining the plateau and in the repolarization process. Traditionally, quinidine, procainamide, and disopyramide are said to increase the action-potential duration and refractory periods, whereas lidocaine, phenytoin, propranolol, mexiletine, and tocainide shorten the action-potential duration and refractory periods in normal tissues (Fig. 6A).

Voltage-clamp techniques suggest that lidocaine increases outward current by inhibiting an inward current. Colatsky (45) found that lidocaine shortened and quinidine lengthened the action-potential duration in rabbit Purkinje fibers. He found the TTX-sensitive inward current during the plateau to be decreased by lidocaine and attributed this to the mechanisms by which the holding current became progressively more outward. Quinidine seemed to have little effect on this current, but it influenced delayed (outward) rectification. Carmeliet and Saikawa (39) performed similar experiments in sheep Purkinje fibers and found that lidocaine, quinidine, and procainamide inhibited the TTX-sensitive plateau current. Quinidine and procainamide were said to shorten the action-potential duration in this tissue. In contrast to the findings in the study by Colatsky, procainamide and quinidine shifted the current–voltage relationship to the outward direction at the level of the plateau. The reasons for the differences between these two tissues remain unclear.

Abnormal Repolarization and Its Normalization by Antiarrhythmic Drugs

Repolarization may fail to occur normally. This may result in abnormal prolongation of the action-potential duration or even in two stable steady states. The latter is shown in Fig. 16, in which we exposed a cardiac Purkinje fiber to lysophosphatidylcholine (LPC), a putative toxic metabolite of ischemia, before and after application of lidocaine (162). The result of the LPC superfusion was a preparation with two stable and quiescent steady states, one at a nearly normal V_r and the other at the plateau. Intracellular current application could shift the preparation from one stable steady state to another (panel B), and lidocaine could "normalize" the action potential (panel C). Arnsdorf and Mehlman (13) showed in fibers with two stable steady states due to injury that lidocaine, phenytoin, and propranolol could facilitate attainment of the repolarization threshold with normalization of the action potential, resulting in one steady-state potential at V_r and essentially normal propagation. Neither disopyramide nor procainamide normalized the action potential. Lidocaine, phenytoin, and propranolol in combination with disopyramide or procainamide could facilitate normal repolarization even when disopyramide and procainamide alone failed to do so (4,13).

Failed repolarization may also lead to triggered sustained rhythmic activity, as shown in panels A and B of Fig. 17 from Arnsdorf (4). After application of lidocaine (panel C), the action potential was normalized, and with washout of lidocaine, the action potential lengthened, and triggered sustained rhythmic activity returned. Tolamolol, a β-adrenoreceptor blocker, was also found capable of normalizing the action potential (11).

Procainamide, however, could not normalize the ac-

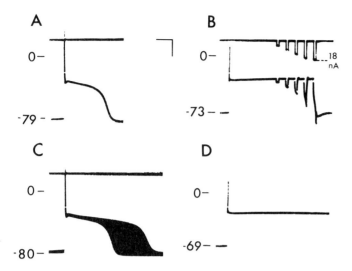

FIG. 16. Failed repolarization. Two stable and quiescent equilibria induced by LPC, with normalization of the action potential by lidocaine. **A:** Control with V_r of −79 mV and action-potential duration of 290 msec. **B:** After application of LPC, one steady state was observed at a V_r of −73 mV, and a second was observed at the plateau potential. Intracellular hyperpolarizing constant currents of increasing strength were applied, with 18 nA finally causing attainment of the repolarization "threshold" and a return to V_r. If current were not applied, V_m would remain at the plateau indefinitely. **C:** Lidocaine progressively shortened the action-potential duration to a normal value of 300 msec and somewhat hyperpolarized the resting cell, with V_r becoming −80 mV. **D:** Washout of lidocaine during continued LPC superfusion caused a return to two stable steady states and a less negative V_r. (From ref. 162, with permission.)

tion potential (4). Figure 18 shows the effect of a combination of procainamide and lidocaine on such a preparation. Triggered sustained rhythmic activity was present in the control situation. In the control, not shown, V_r was −73 mV. After procainamide, V_r was unchanged, the overall amplitude of the nondriven action potentials prior to determination decreased, the threshold for regenerative repolarization was no longer attained, and a quiescent steady state at −40 mV resulted (Fig. 18A). Superfusion with procainamide was continued, and lidocaine was added to the superfusate, after which the plateau steady state was abolished, and essentially normal action potentials resulted (panel B of Fig. 18), with a V_r of −80 mV, an overshoot of +36 mV, $\dot{V}_{max}$ of 580 V/sec, and an action-potential duration of 410 msec while driven at a cycle length of 1,200 msec. Note that this is an example of lidocaine making V_r more negative. Panel C shows superimposed stimulated action potentials at a cycle length of 1,200 msec as lidocaine was washed out but procainamide superfusion was maintained. The progressive beat-to-beat increases in action-potential duration are apparent. After 46 paced beats, the tissue settled at the plateau state of −38 mV, although it could be returned to a V_r of

−72 mV by small hyperpolarizing intracellular current. Shortly thereafter, triggered sustained rhythmic activity was observed, and the situations at 10, 30, and 45 min after the beginning of lidocaine washout are shown in panels D to F. After 45 min, the activity terminated at a steady state of −35 mV.

Action-Potential Duration, Refractoriness, and Cycle Length

Inactivation of the sodium system lessens and reactivation increases during phase 3 of the action potential. In terms of the Hodgkin-Huxley model, the h gate opens as V_m becomes progressively negative. Until h opens, i_{Na} is off, and the muscle is absolutely refractory. At about −40 mV, the h gate begins to open, the channel is still partially inactivated, and the conductance for i_{Na} is low. Normally, the h gate is open within 50 msec of the return to a normal V_r. Reactivation can also be interpreted according to the data from patch-clamping and single-cell studies, or from state diagrams based on studies such as those in Figs. 10 and 13. Without doubt, the interpretation will shift from the classic Hodgkin-Huxley to this newer type of data as soon as sufficient work has been done.

A fundamental property of the action potential is the manner in which its duration changes with the frequency of excitation. In fast-response tissues, increments in the rate of stimulation, within certain limits, abbreviate the action-potential duration and tissue refractoriness. The relative refractory period in fast-response tissues usually ends with the trailing foot of the action potential. The most important determinant of the refractory period is the length of the immediately preceding cycle. This mechanism underlies the long–short cycle aberration of conduction pathways observed during atrial fibrillation (the Ashman phenomenon) or during atrial premature beats. Hyperkalemia will abbreviate and hypokalemia prolong the action-potential duration. A low temperature and a low calcium concentration will increase the action-potential duration.

Strength–interval curves are used to assess the characteristics of refractoriness and excitability *in vitro* using intracellular current application through microelectrodes and both *in vivo* and *in vitro* using extracellular stimulation (Fig. 19). Following a series of regularly stimulated action potentials or depolarization (S_1), the current required to just produce a regenerative response, or, in some cases, the just-subthreshold current, is determined in the quiescent fiber or in late diastole with a single stimulus (S_2). The S_1-S_2 interval is progressively decreased, and the threshold requirements are determined for S_2. As S_2 falls on the descending shoulder of the action potential, threshold requirements rise steeply, and this is termed the relative refractory period. Further shortening of the S_1-S_2 interval places S_2 in the absolute

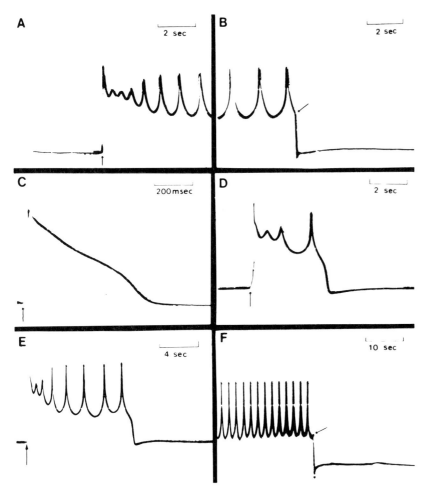

FIG. 17. Effects of lidocaine on triggered sustained rhythmic activity in a cardiac Purkinje fiber. **A** and **B:** In the control situations, the electrically induced action potential triggered oscillatory activity at a low membrane voltage that increased in amplitude and eventuated in nondriven sustained action potentials. The triggered sustained rhythmic activity persisted indefinitely until terminated by a hyperpolarizing intracellular current that permitted attainment of the repolarization threshold and a return to V_r (*arrow* in **B**). The hyperpolarizing current in this instance was applied 45 min after initiation of the sustained rhythmic activity. **C:** Lidocaine caused almost immediate attainment of the repolarization threshold and normalization of the action potential. **D–F:** After washout of lidocaine, triggered sustained rhythmic activity rapidly reappeared. (From ref. 11, with permission.)

refractory period, a zone in which an action potential cannot be provoked regardless of the intensity of the stimulus. Clinically, the intensity of the current is limited to avoid damage to the tissue, and this constraint has led to two other definitions: the functional and the effective refractory periods. These are determined by using some multiple of late-diastolic threshold (usually 1.5 or 2 × threshold) and noting the tissue response to the stimuli. The tissue responses to the stimuli S_1-S_2 are termed R_1-R_2. As the S_1-S_2 is shortened progressively, the R_1-R_2 shortens to a minimum. The functional refractory period is defined as the shortest attainable R_1-R_2 interval. The minimum S_1-S_2 that produces R_1-R_2 is termed the effective refractory period. It should be apparent from Fig. 19 that the membrane-activation voltage (MAV) and the apparent refractory period will vary significantly if defined by a current that is one, two, or three times the late-diastolic current threshold. Premature action potentials that arise during the relative refractory period typically show a diminished upstroke velocity and a slower conduction velocity because of partial inactivation of the sodium system, features fundamental to arrhythmogenesis. In fast-response tissues, the strength–interval curves at various frequencies will show no change in late-diastolic threshold. The ascending

limb will be moved to the left with each increment in the frequency of stimulation.

Observations on Antiarrhythmic Drugs That Prolong Action-Potential Duration

The effects of some drugs on prolonging the action potential are so pronounced that the action-potential duration has been used as the basis for classification in one of the hierarchical classifications (185). The limitations of this approach are obvious when one considers the several drugs that significantly lengthen the action-potential duration. Procainamide, quinidine, and disopyramide are known primarily as blockers of the fast sodium channels, but they also have less well understood effects on prolonging the action potential. As discussed elsewhere, some evidence suggests that quinidine produces this prolongation by decreasing the repolarizing potassium current i_{x_1}. Amiodarone, bretyllium, and sotalol are other drugs that have important effects on repolarization and on the recovery of excitability. Amiodarone is a new agent whose clinical success has been widely accepted, and much of its action was attributed initially to prolongation of the action-potential duration. Its dramatic prolongation of the cardiac action potential

50mV

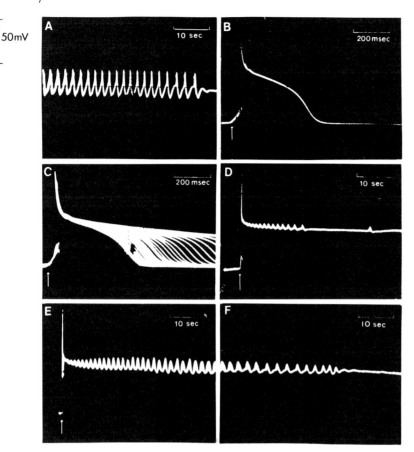

FIG. 18. Effects of a combination of drugs on triggered sustained rhythmic activity. **A:** The situation after procainamide, with termination of triggered activity at a quiescent steady state of −40 mV. **B:** Superfusion with procainamide was continued, and lidocaine was added, with abolition of the plateau steady state and normalization of the action potential. **C:** Superimposed action potentials driven at a cycle length of 1,200 msec. As lidocaine was washed out and procainamide superfusion maintained, the action-potential durations progressively increased, eventually with the establishment of two steady states, one at V_r and the second at the plateau. **D–F:** Situations at 10, 30, and 45 min after lidocaine washout and during continued procainamide superfusion. Between 45 and 60 min, −35 mV became the only stable steady state in this fiber in that hyperpolarizing intracellular currents failed to return the membrane to V_r. (From ref. 4, with permission.)

may be important in its antiarrhythmic action. Amiodarone is known to produce inactivation as well as activation block, so that full recovery of sodium channels will greatly outlast the action-potential duration. Bretyllium tosylate also increases the action-potential duration and has an antiadrenergic effect. Sotalol is a β-adrenoreceptor blocker that prolongs the action-potential duration, with little effect on $\dot{V}_{max}$ in fast-response tissues.

The net effect of prolonging the action potential will be to reduce the likelihood of an active response that is adequate to produce normal or even abnormal conduc-

tion. This prolonged refractoriness and depression of excitability will thus reduce the likelihood of either fast or slow responses. These prolonged voltage-, drug-, and time-dependent kinetics of the fast sodium system will act directly to prolong the time for adequate recovery of the fast system to produce any type of automatic or reentrant activation.

One of the conditions that promotes slow responses and slow activation is a dispersion of refractoriness at low membrane potentials in abnormal tissues. The wide variability in refractoriness thus establishes slow routes

FIG. 19. Diagrammatic representation of an action potential (AP) and the strength–interval curve (SIC). The horizontal interrupted lines indicate the positions of stimuli of one, two, and three times late-diastolic-current threshold. The vertical lines connect the same points in time on both the SIC and AP, thereby defining the apparent refractory period (RP) and the membrane-activation voltage (MAV). As the multiple of late-diastolic-current threshold increases, the position on the SIC is upward and to the left, the apparent RP is shorter, and the MAV is less negative. (From ref. 3, with permission.)

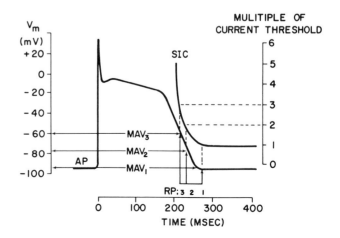

of conduction for extrasystoles, thus promoting establishment of reentrant loops. By causing a uniform and dramatic lengthening of the action potential in the abnormal zones, these agents may abolish preexisting conditions for reentrant activation simply by eliminating the conditions for slow, diffuse reentrant activation.

Antiarrhythmic Drugs and Active Cellular Properties in Fast-Response Tissues

Several examples of drug effects on sodium channels have already been mentioned to illustrate basic electrophysiologic principles. We now turn to a more systematic discussion of the interactions between antiarrhythmic drugs and sodium channels.

Evidence for Voltage- and Time-Dependent Drug Interactions with Fast Sodium Channels

Weidmann demonstrated that local anesthetics such as cocaine and quinidine reduced the maximum rate of depolarization of phase 0 ($\dot{V}_{max}$), which is often a useful indirect index of the sodium current (191). He also found a shift of the steady-state inactivation or h curve to more negative potentials. This action was found to occur with a number of local anesthetic drugs, including other common antiarrhythmic agents such as lidocaine (29,30,40,57,166), phenytoin (176), and procainamide (10,99,116,157). At that time it was thought that the mechanism of sodium-channel block was nonspecific incorporation of drug into the lipid bilayer that altered sodium-channel kinetics. The degree of block was considered to be a result of the physicochemical properties of these drugs, including pK, lipophilicity, size, molecular weight, and the like. Subsequent work confirmed these experimental findings in various cardiac tissues. The reduction in $\dot{V}_{max}$ seemed to be an action common to these clinically effective antiarrhythmic agents, and thus Vaughan Williams and associates defined these agents as possessing class-1 antiarrhythmic actions (185). Others, however, believed that other actions were sufficiently dissimilar to warrant the division of these drugs into at least two groups (2,12,100).

Weidmann also discovered that the reduction in $\dot{V}_{max}$ at all membrane potentials could be reversed at all membrane potentials by previously hyperpolarizing the cell (191). Not only was $\dot{V}_{max}$ restored toward control, but excitability also rapidly recovered. The mechanisms suggested for the amelioration of the drug-induced block by hyperpolarization were two: either a voltage-induced speeding of recovery from inactivation or a voltage-dependent displacement of the drug from its receptor.

Subsequently, Johnson and McKinnon (117) demonstrated that this interaction between antiarrhythmic drug and the sodium channel depended on the frequency of stimulation. They found that $\dot{V}_{max}$ in ventricular myocardium was depressed by quinidine in a time- and use-dependent manner, that is, only when stimulation frequency was relatively rapid. Conversely, the degree of block decreased as stimulation frequency was decreased. Extrasystoles that were induced after complete repolarization of the action potential showed a depressed $\dot{V}_{max}$ in the presence of quinidine, as compared with extrasystoles in control conditions. Chen et al. (40) showed that the sodium channels, as assessed by $\dot{V}_{max}$, did recover from block in the presence of quinidine and lidocaine during electrical diastole, but the process took time and was voltage-dependent. These and other studies implied that therapeutic concentrations of antiarrhythmic drugs produced very little block of sodium channels in normal resting or stimulated fibers in a normal physiologic milieu. Frequency-dependent block would be most prominent under the highest rates of beating, as would occur during a rapid arrhythmia; thus, drug action was more prominent in the abnormal circumstance of rapid rhythm or early extrasystoles and less prominent at physiologic rates. This suggested that the degree of block declined between action potentials, and the longer the time period between action potentials, the greater and more complete the decay of block. In addition, there was a voltage dependence of this effect such that hyperpolarization seemed to relieve the degree of block of the sodium channels. Conversely, depolarization of the resting potential with high potassium or voltage promoted block and decreased the availability of sodium channels in the presence of drug. Thus, for example, therapeutic concentrations of phenytoin and lidocaine that had little effect on $\dot{V}_{max}$ in normal potassium solutions markedly reduced $\dot{V}_{max}$ in the presence of extracellular potassium sufficiently high to decrease the resting potential (115,166). Referring again to Fig. 11, the drugs were effective during the situation marked as partial inactivation. Thus, Hondeghem et al. (102) and Hope et al. (105) proposed that certain drugs exerted important antiarrhythmic effects by selectively inhibiting sodium channels in tissues depolarized by hypoxia or ischemia.

State Dependence and the Modulated- and Guarded-Receptor Hypotheses

On the basis of these and similar studies, Hille (94) and Hondeghem and Katzung (103) in 1977 independently proposed that the voltage- and use-dependent blockade of sodium channels caused by local anesthetic antiarrhythmic agents could be explained by a model based on the channel state, which is in itself voltage-dependent. As already discussed, Figs. 13 and 14 show a Hodgkin-Huxley kinetic scheme for the three states of the channel: rested, activated, and inactivated. As seen in panel B of Fig. 13, drugs can associate with channels in each state, and each state is associated with a different set of association and dissociation rate constants.

The receptor, then, is modulated by the state of the channel. The drug preferentially interacts with one or more modulations of the receptor. This *modulated-receptor hypothesis* allows predictive statements that can be tested. For example, this hypothesis suggests that drugs that have the greatest affinity for the open or activated state of the channel will also show the most sensitivity to frequency of channel opening. In addition, an apparent voltage shift of the inactivation relation is suggested, because inhibited sodium channels behave as if they are at a potential that is less negative than the measured membrane potential.

As will be discussed, channel states have characteristic sets of rate constants for each drug. Starmer et al. (175) have proposed the *guarded-receptor hypothesis,* in which each sodium channel has a constant-affinity binding site for all antiarrhythmic drugs, but accessibility to this site is controlled by the activation and inactivation gates.

Antiarrhythmic Drugs and Their Affinities

Panels A of Figs. 13 and 14 show the normal sequence of sodium-channel opening and closing during the car-

diac cycle in the absence of drug. All channels are in the rested state (R) when the cell is at its resting or maximum diastolic potential. Activation (A) occurs following a suprathreshold depolarization, and channels open. This activated state lasts less than 2 msec, and it is during this period that sodium inward current flows. After the brief period of activation, channels become inactivated (I) for the duration of the plateau, and on repolarization the channels recover rather quickly to the rested state.

Panel A of Fig. 20 shows the effect of an agent that has its highest affinity for the activated or open state of the sodium channel. In the presence of such a drug, the affinity of the sodium channels for the drug is very high during the open state, and drugs bind to and inhibit a large proportion of the channels during this period of activation (A to A-D). This shifts the activated state of the channel to the drug-bound activated state, A-D, which no longer can conduct sodium ions, and an abrupt increase in drug-blocked channels occurs immediately. The $\dot{V}_{max}$ of the first action potential might

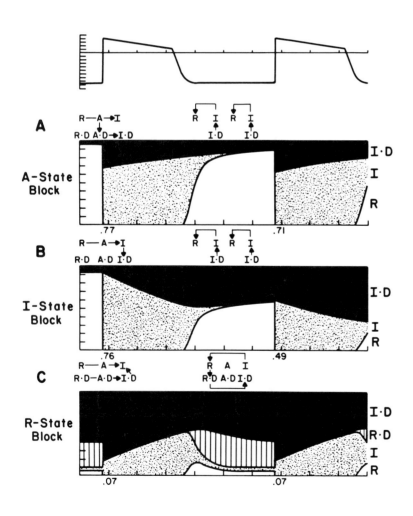

FIG. 20. Computer simulation of channel states in the presence of prototypic drugs: activated-state blocker (**A**); inactivated-state blocker (**B**); rested-state blocker (**C**). Simulated action potentials are at the top. The channels are resting, R (*white area*), inactivated, I (*stippled area*), inactivated and drug-associated block, I-D (*dark area*), resting and drug-associated block, R-D (*vertical stripes*). Activated blocked channels, A-D, exist too briefly to be seen at this time base. **A:** Activated-state blocker. Drug-induced block occurs during the upstroke of the action potential, that is, A to A-D. Note that there is conversion of A-D to I-D. During the plateau and in diastole, the channels unblock and become drug-free inactivated channels (I-D to I). This is indicated by the decreasing dark (I-D) and increasing white (I) areas. On repolarization and a return to diastole, the inactivated channels return to the resting or R state. Whether or not $\dot{V}_{max}$ of the next beat is attenuated depends on the unblocking rate and the diastolic time. **B:** Inactivated-state blocker. Channels are inactivated during the plateau and change from A to I. Inactivated-state blockers bind during the low potentials of the plateau (I to I-D). Graphically, this is depicted as decreasing stippled area (I) and increasing dark area (I-D). The channel also unblocks during diastole and returns to the rested state (I-D to I to R). Because there is more time for block and less time for recovery, $\dot{V}_{max}$ decreases from 0.76 to 0.49. $\dot{V}_{max}$ depends on the length of plateau to determine blocking and the duration of diastole to determine unblocking. **C:** Rested-state blocker. If a drug associates with rested channels (*vertical stripes*), few channels are available to become activated. $\dot{V}_{max}$ is very low at 0.07. Channels unblock only during the plateau, but they are also inactivated at such a low voltage. Inexcitability will result because little or no sodium current can flow. (From ref. 104, with permission.)

reflect some of this inhibition of the sodium current, partly because some channels block during the initial portion of the upstroke of phase 0 before $\dot{V}_{max}$ is attained. During the plateau, channels follow the kinetic scheme to the inactivated (A to I) and inactivated drug-bound pools (A-D to I-D). Because drug affinity for the inactivated channels is low, there is an exponential decrease in the drug-bound inactivated pool in favor of the inactivated pool (I-D to I). Thus, at the end of the action potential, the normal course of drug-free inactivated channels can recover to the rested-state drug-free channels (I to R) as membrane potential returns to resting level. Those channels, however, that are blocked by drug in the inactivated state remain inactivated, because the voltage shift seen by the drug-bound channels makes those channels behave as if they were 25 mV more positive. With subsequent action potentials, channels blocked in the drug-blocked inactivated (I-D) state continue to accumulate until finally at the end of a train of action potentials a steady-state level of blockade of $\dot{V}_{max}$ is reached. Thus, one of the major characteristics of activated-state blockade is that during the plateau phase of the action potential, when inactivation of the sodium channels is maximum, recovery of blocked channels is incomplete but does progress quite close to the preactivated control state; that is, blockade of channels declines during the inactivation phase of the plateau.

In contrast to the actions of an activated-state blocker, a drug that affects the inactivated state of the channel has quite different blocking properties. This is depicted in panel B of Fig. 20. Most of the binding of the drug to the channels will occur during the plateau of the action potential when the channels go from the activated to the inactivated state (A to I to I-D). The process is then reversed during diastole; unblocking occurs (I-D to I), and the inactivated unblocked channels return in part to the rested state (I to R). However, the inactivated blocked channels behave as if the membrane were depolarized even at resting potential, because of the voltage shift, and therefore do not undergo the ordinary essentially full removal of inactivation to the rested drug-bound state. Instead, the relaxation of block occurs slowly, with a time constant characteristic of the drug dissociation from the inactivated channel. The $\dot{V}_{max}$ of the next action potential is therefore markedly reduced compared with the first action potential of the train. Under these circumstances, the recovery from blockade occurs only during diastole, and thus a long train of action potentials will promote a large steady-state block if the frequency is high enough to prevent a great deal of dissociation during diastole. Whereas in the case of the activated-state blocker the recovery from block begins immediately after the activation phase of the action potential, recovery during inactivation block cannot occur until full repolarization has been achieved, and thus steady-state block will be influenced by rate as well as action-potential duration.

A third possibility is for a drug to affect the channel receptor in the rested state. This would be the drug-associated state (R-D) in Fig. 13, and the simulation is shown in panel C of Fig. 20. Under these conditions, a large fraction of the channels would be bound to drug and blocked in the rested state prior to activation. As a consequence of the voltage shift, many of these channels move to the inactivated blocked state, and consequently $\dot{V}_{max}$ of the first action potential is maximally reduced after a long period of rest. It is theoretically possible to reduce the amount of blockade by rapid stimulation in order to minimize the diastolic interval with a drug of this type. These drugs would not be considered therapeutic agents, but would be considered cardiac poisons. They will not be discussed further.

The effects of voltage on the degree of blocked channels in any state are obviously very important to the net number of sodium channels available for the upstroke of the action potential. If the blocked inactivated channels see an apparent shift of 25 mV in the hyperpolarizing direction, this suggests that a hyperpolarization of 25 mV is required in order to cause full recovery of the drug-bound inactivated channels to recover fully to the drug-bound rested state, from which they can quickly unblock to the rested state. Conversely, an even lower resting membrane potential potentiates the accumulation of block by causing more trapping in the drug-bound inactivated state. In this case, the $\dot{V}_{max}$ of the first action potential will be even more inhibited in the depolarized preparation, and progressive block will occur with repetitive activation. In addition, as mentioned earlier, the accumulation of blockade that occurs in a train of action potentials is limited by the degree of recovery that can occur between periods of maximum affinity of drug for receptor that occur as a function of channel state. Therefore, the degree of block at slow heart rates will be less than that achieved at faster rates. Not only will steady-state block be greater at higher rates, but an early extrasystole will show greater block of its $\dot{V}_{max}$ the earlier it occurs after the regular action potential. Therefore, the earlier the extrasystole, the less time for recovery from block, and therefore the greater depression of Na inward current.

Recent studies indicate that quinidine, procainamide, and amiodarone have the highest affinities for the activated state and therefore primarily block the sodium channels in their open state, whereas lidocaine, mexiletine, and tocainide have the highest affinities for the inactive state and therefore primarily block sodium channels during their closed, inactive state (25,37,46,50,54). Referring to panel B of Fig. 13, the drugs with high affinities for the activated state would produce drug-associated channel (A-D), and the drugs with high affinities for the inactivated state would produce drug-associated channel (I-D).

The modulated-receptor hypothesis assumes that local anesthetic receptors bind drugs with an affinity that varies with the channel state, and a number of examples of use dependence and frequency dependence of different local anesthetic antiarrhythmic agents have been mentioned. Voltage-clamp studies by Bean et al. (25) and others have shown that indeed the affinity of the receptor does appear to vary with voltage. Each channel state has a characteristic set of rate constants for each drug. One possible explanation for the differences in the apparent rate constants for the drug has been proposed by Starmer et al. (175) in a *guarded-receptor hypothesis.* This hypothesis suggests that the sodium channel has a constant-affinity binding site for all antiarrhythmic drugs. However, access to this site is controlled by the activation and inactivation gates. The channel receptor is poorly accessible when the *m* gates are closed, but when the *m* gates are open, drug molecules dissolved in the lipid bilayer can access the receptor, whereas charged hydrophilic drug molecules must gain access to the receptor when both the *m* and *h* gates are open. Thus, the gates regulate access of the drug to a receptor that has a fixed affinity for drug. Future work will have to be performed in order to determine which of these two models of drug-channel interaction more closely reflects reality.

It is clear that the lumping together of all sodium-channel blockers, or "membrane-stabilizing drugs," or "local anesthetic agents" is no longer tenable. Whether these drugs should be placed within a single group with a number of subgroups or in separate groups in consideration of other actions, particularly on passive properties, will be a matter for discussion in the next several years.

Implications of a State-Dependent Hypothesis

The modulated-receptor hypothesis helps explain, in part, why certain antiarrhythmic agents work in specific cardiac tissues, whereas others do not. For example, quinidine depresses $\dot{V}_{max}$ in atrial as well as Purkinje fibers and ventricular cells, but lidocaine has very little if any effect on atrial cells. The explanation of this difference lies in the fact that the two drugs have different state-dependent blocking characteristics. Lidocaine acts primarily in the inactivated state, which is very short in the brief action potential of the atrial cell. In addition, for reasons to be described later, the duration of the atrial action potential may in fact be shortened further by lidocaine, which would decrease its effectiveness to create inactivated-state blockade. Quinidine, on the other hand, acts primarily on the activated state and thus will effectively block atrial tissues with their short action-potential durations as easily as it blocks ventricular tissues with their longer action-potential durations. action-potential durations.

The channel-state requirements of block also explain why many of these local anesthetic agents have little effect on nerve and muscle action potentials. In nerve, for example, the depolarization phase is very quick, and there is a very brief repolarization phase during an action potential that lasts no more than 2 to 3 msec in all. Thus, there is very little time for inactivated-state block to occur, and agents such as lidocaine would be very ineffective in producing blockade in nerve.

The effect of decreasing the sodium inward current by these local anesthetics also has the effect of reducing the action-potential duration. This action occurs as a result of inhibition of the residual Na^+ current that flows through the so-called Na^+ window current during the plateau of the action potential, a topic that was discussed earlier. Nearly all of the local anesthetics that shorten the action-potential duration do so by this mechanism. These agents include lidocaine, phenytoin, aprinidine, and many other such agents. A consequence of this action to reduce the action-potential duration is to shorten the period of inactivation and thus reduce the degree of inactivation-dependent block by these same agents. It has also been proposed that agents such as lidocaine shorten the action potential by increasing potassium conductance (i_{x_1}). However, it is clear that either or both mechanisms shorten the action potential and decrease the degree of inactivated-state block. Lidocaine and phenytoin also are known to produce hyperpolarization of depolarized fibers. This, too, would contribute to a shortening of the time in the inactivated state and thus also decrease the degree of inactivated-state block. Thus, for these agents, other processes that control additional electrophysiologic characteristics, aside from the rapid upstroke, may actually influence channel-state-dependent block.

Quinidine has other actions that may alter its effectiveness on activated-state block. Quinidine prolongs the action-potential duration in most tissues, presumably as a consequence of decreasing i_{x_1} or the repolarizing potassium current (46). This topic was discussed in detail earlier. An increase in the action-potential duration may promote the inactivated-state block that occurs with quinidine. Similar actions may be important to the efficacy of other agents that prolong the action potential. In addition, at a given frequency of stimulation, the shorter period of diastole will also decrease the recovery of the fast sodium system.

The combination of effects on activated- versus inactivated-state block and the effects on action-potential durations make it very difficult to predict the excitability of early extrasystoles. Thus, the modulated-receptor hypothesis alone would predict that quinidine, because of its block of activated sodium channels, also has a slow recovery from inactivated-state block, so that block is still evident immediately following repolarization. Lidocaine, however, has very rapid recovery from inactivated-state block following an action potential, so that the recovery of $\dot{V}_{max}$ is very rapid once full repolarization has been achieved in lidocaine. Therefore, quinidine would be the more effective blocking agent for early extrasystoles. Man and Dressel (142) found that lidocaine and tocainide increased conduction times for extrasystoles applied 250 to 400 msec after the preceding QRS complex, whereas procainamide and quinidine increased conduction times throughout electrical diastole.

In spite of these direct predictions from the modulated-receptor hypothesis, there are other considerations that influence the actual ability of these two agents to block extrasystoles *in vivo*. Lidocaine shortens and quinidine usually prolongs the action-potential duration, so that an extrasystole fixed in time after the first stimulus would find a lidocaine action potential fully repolarized after, say, 250 msec, whereas a quinidine action potential would still be repolarizing in phase 3. Thus, although on a voltage basis the fiber exposed to lidocaine might be more responsive than that exposed to quinidine, an extrasystole occurring at the end of an action potential would be better blocked by quinidine than by lidocaine, primarily as a result of the fact that repolarization is not fully achieved at that time.

This question of the relation between refractory period and action-potential duration has been one of much concern and interest over the years. Nearly all agents that affect the fast sodium channel also increase the ratio of change in refractory period to that in action potential duration ($\Delta RP/\Delta APD$), that is to say, even though a drug such as lidocaine shortens the action potential, it also produces a relative prolongation of the refractory period, thus increasing this ratio. Quinidine, on the other hand, increases this ratio by increasing the refractory period more than the action-potential duration, thus exerting additive effects to suppress refractoriness and excitability. In the setting of an arrhythmia, the effectiveness of one agent over another would depend on a variety of circumstances, including action-potential duration, membrane potential, and the general health of the tissue. Thus, in atrium, for example, quinidine prolongs the action potential and would be expected to suppress early extrasystoles of atrial origin, whereas lidocaine would have very little if any effect at all on atrial early activation. In the ventricle or in the His-Purkinje system, lidocaine shortens the action potential and relatively increases the refractory period. Quinidine, on the other hand, usually increases the action-potential duration and increases the refractory period. Thus, the ability of either drug to suppress an early extrasystole would depend on where in the cardiac cycle the extrasystole might occur. If it occurred very early during phase-3 repolarization, both drugs would be expected to suppress the extrasystole. If the spontaneous beat occurred later, when full repolarization was achieved in lidocaine-exposed tissue but prior to full repolarization in quinidine-exposed tissue, then quinidine would be

expected to have a greater suppressant effect than lidocaine. However, the degrees of suppression for the two different drugs would be quite different if an equal voltage were chosen for the initiation of the extrasystole, as, for example, in studies of membrane responsiveness. The suppression of excitability in relation to the changes in action-potential duration was recognized a number of years ago as possibly playing an important role in suppression of reentrant arrhythmias that required an extrasystole to serve as a triggering mechanism. This may yet prove to be an important consequence of the modulated-receptor hypothesis and the interaction of local anesthetic agents with fast sodium channels.

In this context, let us return to the concept of *membrane responsiveness,* which has already been introduced. To recapitulate, one of the ways of evaluating the relation between membrane voltage and $\dot{V}_{max}$ in intact tissues has been to generate h_∞ curves via membrane-responsiveness and steady-state activation techniques. If antiarrhythmic drugs affect the sodium channel differently, they should have different effects on the inactivation curve. Agents such as procainamide and quinidine suppress $\dot{V}_{max}$ at all membrane potentials studied. This is predicted by the modulated-receptor hypothesis because of their ability to produce activation block and slow recovery of this block during repolarization.

At times, lidocaine and phenytoin can increase $\dot{V}_{max}$, a finding that contradicts the modulated-receptor hypothesis. An example is shown in Fig. 12. The explanation for this discrepancy apparently lies in other actions of the drug within the electrophysiologic matrix aside from its action on the inactivated sodium channel. For example, lidocaine and phenytoin can decrease the slope of phase-4 depolarization. The membrane potential at which activation occurs for the normal duty-cycle action potential, therefore, will be more negative, and its degree of inactivation will be less than before exposure to the drug. Lidocaine may also hyperpolarize tissues (8,9,29,30). This is most pronounced in depolarized tissues, but may occur in normal tissues as well so long as there is a driving force for the potassium ion, as in Fig. 8. This results in voltage-dependent removal of inactivation that is independent of the direct effect of the drug. These two effects will summate to increase the takeoff potential at which the duty-cycle action potential is initiated, thus increasing Na^+-channel availability. This example illustrates the multiple effects of a drug and cautions against overly simplistic hierarchical schemes based on single mechanisms.

Small Preparations, Single Cells, and Individual Channels

We have thus far discussed studies that involve $\dot{V}_{max}$ as an indicator of Na^+ current blockade and the involvement of Na^+ channel blockade in the antiarrhythmic actions of local anesthetic agents. As was discussed earlier, sodium currents and single sodium channels can now be studied. Measurement of sodium channels in heart has been hampered by limitations of the voltage-clamp technique. It has been only recently that suitable preparations and physiologic conditions have been developed to measure sodium currents in isolated cardiac fibers. Bean et al. (25) used very short segments of rabbit Purkinje fibers to measure sodium currents and the effects of quinidine and lidocaine on sodium currents obtained at low temperatures and in low extracellular sodium. Colatsky (45) found that high concentrations of lidocaine produced no tonic block of sodium current, but a relatively rapid train of 500-msec pulses reduced sodium current by 63%. In addition, the rate of onset of block increased with increasing drug concentration. These results are close to those obtained in $\dot{V}_{max}$ measurements. Colatsky (46) also showed little resting block with 13.5 μM quinidine, but a large use-dependent block with very short pulses (50 msec). Use-dependent block also decreased if the holding potential was made more negative. Repetitive stimulation produced greater block than a single pulse of equivalent duration, suggesting that the affinity of quinidine was greater for the activated state than for the inactivated state of the sodium channel. In addition, the steady-state inactivation curve was shifted to more negative potentials, although there may have been a technical problem in the protocol, which did not allow enough time for full recovery at the voltages used. Nevertheless, all these findings are consistent with those described earlier for $\dot{V}_{max}$ measurements.

The use of isolated myocytes obtained by enzymatic dissociation from mammalian hearts has enabled investigators to perform measurements of sodium current under other, more carefully controlled, physiologic conditions. There is always the worry, however, that the isolation procedure itself may alter membrane characteristics, specifically ion-channel properties. Lee et al. (134) measured sodium currents in isolated rat myocytes in the presence of lidocaine and quinidine. They observed considerable tonic block of inward sodium current by both quinidine and lidocaine, with little additional frequency-dependent block at higher driving frequency. This is in contrast to the results obtained in multicellular preparations, where block is principally use-dependent, as described earlier. Sanchez-Chapula and Josephson (159) also showed an enhanced affinity of phenytoin for activated sodium channels. The blocking actions of lidocaine and phenytoin were voltage-dependent between -90 and -30 mV. Drug effects on the kinetics of onset and of recovery of block were similar to those observed in multicellular preparations.

Patch-clamp techniques allow examination of the electrical behavior of single membrane channels and will provide new insight into the molecular basis of blockade of sodium channels. In addition, reconstitution experiments of sodium channels into lipid bilayers will also provide additional information about individual channel behavior and binding of local anesthetic agents to specific receptor sites in the channel. The resolution promised by these techniques was unthinkable even 10 years ago, and the next 10 years will probably see the molecular mechanisms revealed for the interaction of local anesthetic antiarrhythmic agents with fast sodium channels in the heart.

Physicochemical Determinants of the Actions of Sodium-Channel Blockers

The chemical properties of local anesthetic agents determine their rates of block and recovery of the sodium channel. Courtney (54) examined the rate of block development for a group of sodium-channel blockers and β-adrenergic blockers in rabbit atria and found that the rate of block development correlated well with molecular weight but poorly with lipid solubility. In addition, the rate of block onset increased with increasing drug concentrations. Campbell (37) also showed that the rate of onset of block was more rapid with low molecular weight compounds than with high-molecular-weight compounds. Thus, together these studies suggest that the rate of block onset is correlated best with molecular weight, but not with lipid solubility, and increases with increasing drug concentrations.

These same investigators have examined the effects of the recovery of $\dot{V}_{max}$ as a function of the physicochemical properties of these sodium-channel blockers. They found a good correlation between molecular weight and the half-time of recovery of $\dot{V}_{max}$ for drugs with very different chemical configurations. Physical size may play an important role in removal of a drug from its receptor. Greater lipid solubility also promoted the recovery from block. The pK_a and pH were corrected for lipid solubility. There was a greater correlation between the effective lipid distribution and shorter recovery times. Ehring et al. (72) demonstrated that for 10 derivatives of lidocaine and procainamide, the recovery-rate constant was an inverse function of molecular weight and the log of the partition coefficient. These are, of course, only general rules of thumb, and Moyer and Hondeghem (144) showed that small changes in molecular structure could produce drastic changes in the kinetics of several aprindine derivatives. Thus, differences in molecular weight, pK_a, and lipid solubility could not account for this small change in molecular structure having large changes in the kinetics of recovery from aprindine blockade. It therefore appears to be a very complicated relation between chemical structure and the ability of these agents to produce and recover from block.

The state of ionization of this family of tertiary

amines to which most of these antiarrhythmic local-anesthetic drugs belong is determined primarily by extracellular pH. Grant et al. (90) found that when extracellular pH was lowered, the time constant of recovery from block was doubled, an effect that was absent when internal pH was lowered. They also demonstrated that recovery of $\dot{V}_{max}$ during exposure to quinidine was also slowed at lower pH. These investigators concluded that the reduction in the rate of recovery of $\dot{V}_{max}$ during acidosis resulted from protonation of the channel-receptor-bound quinidine. Addition of a positive charge to the drug-bound receptor prevented release of the drug from the receptor into the hydrophobic membrane. This problem would be particularly acute for highly lipid-soluble drugs, whose exit depends primarily on the hydrophobic-membrane pathway. This reduction in the rate of recovery of $\dot{V}_{max}$ in the presence of low pH would produce an enhancement of the blocking effects of these antiarrhythmic agents. This explains why recovery from block with permanently charged lidocaine analogues was extremely slow. In addition, acidosis increased the steady-state reduction in $\dot{V}_{max}$ in Purkinje fibers, an effect that also could be explained by the depolarization induced by the acidosis.

Drug Actions and Interactions

One of the most interesting predictions of the modulated-receptor and other state-dependent hypotheses is that despite all the different characteristics of the various sodium-channel blocking agents, the fact that these agents bind to a common site would predict dramatic and possibly clinically useful interactions and competitions for drugs at this site. For example, combined use of two antiarrhythmic agents, each of which has unacceptable secondary actions, should permit a reduction in the dose of each. The combination should permit very potent antiarrhythmic actions. The utility of this type of combination would depend entirely on the kinetics of binding and dissociation to the various channel states. Thus, combination therapy would be most effective in drugs whose actions complement one another rather than necessarily overlap. One successful example of this combination therapy has been the use of lidocaine and mexiletine to prevent arrhythmias that were refractory to either agent alone. In addition, it should also be possible to find agents that serve as competitive inhibitors for one another, and, indeed, bupivacaine, which is a very potent sodium-channel blocker with a high incidence of cardiac toxicity, may be displaced by lidocaine, which has a more avid binding to the receptor. It has been experimentally demonstrated that lidocaine may displace bupivacaine from blockade of the sodium channel (41), and this would predict that clinically induced bupivacaine toxicity might be reversed

at least partially by the use of an agent such as lidocaine. This exciting field of drug interactions and the possible use of low concentrations in adjunct Na^+ channel blocker therapies may prove to be very important in future treatment of clinical arrhythmias.

Matrices and Active Cellular Properties in Fast-Response Tissues

The various state-dependent hypotheses allow further subgrouping into a matrix or matrices. Illustrations have been presented that the state of the sodium channel may depend on voltage and use and that these determinants, in turn, will be influenced by passive membrane properties. Resting potential, depolarization, repolarization, activation, inactivation, and reactivation are intimately involved in the electrophysiologic events of the normal and abnormal heart beat. Arrhythmogenic influences may alter both active and passive properties. The situation that a drug encounters, then, may be quite different during ischemia, depending on the electrophysiologic characteristics of the substrate. The studies of Courtney, Hondeghem, Katzung, and others cited earlier on lipophilicity, molecular weight, and structure, when coupled with physiologic effects, may be of predictive importance in the design of new drugs.

It is therefore of less importance to know the hierarchy of the various drug actions in normal tissues than to view the effectiveness of the drug as a balance between the nature of the arrhythmogenic abnormality and the particular electrophysiologic characteristics of the drug itself. Thus, in a disease state in which the arrhythmia arises as a consequence of altered conduction or excitability of fast response, the efficacy of the drug is determined by a multitude of factors. These include the characteristics of drug binding to its receptor in the channel, which is influenced by the condition of the affected tissue, and the consequences of channel blockade, which is also affected by the pathophysiology of the tissue, as well as how these affect the passive spread of current and so on. Similarly, arrhythmias involving abnormal automaticity are affected by agents that alter the approach and level of threshold. However, these drug actions are also complex functions of the nature of the disease, both electrophysiologically and anatomically, as well as the particular variety of drug effects on the electrotonic spread of excitatory current, drug blockade of ionic channels, and the resulting alterations in intracellular ionic constituents, to mention but a few. We must reconsider our knowledge of drug actions on fast Na channels in light of new understanding of the subtle interactions between the nature of the arrhythmia itself and how the disease state affects the normal electrophysiologic matrix.

ACTIVE CELLULAR PROPERTIES IN TISSUES DEPENDENT ON i_{si} FOR PHASE 0: SLOW-RESPONSE TISSUES

Channels

Phase-0 depolarization may depend on the slow or secondary inward current, i_{si}, rather than on i_{Na}. The normal mechanism of excitation for both the sinoatrial (SA) and atrioventricular (AV) nodes is dependent on i_{si}. The channel of this mixed Ca^{2+}-Na^+ current is kinetically slower than the channel for i_{Na} and is little influenced by potent blockers of the rapid sodium channel such as TTX. The slow inward current has been called a mixed current, because Na^+ can support action potentials that are inhibited by verapamil and Mn^{2+}, but removal of $[Na^+]_o$ in the presence of $[Ca^{2+}]_o$ little affects i_{si}. The channel, therefore, can carry a rather large sodium current, but, in the presence of extracellular calcium, does not. Hess and Tsien (93) studied single guinea pig ventricular cells and found the channel to be occupied almost continuously by one or more calcium ions that bind very strongly to the channel. This results in the strongly bound Ca^{2+} in the channel electrostatically repulsing other ions, thereby limiting the permeability of Na^+ and other ionic species. Further, Ca^{2+} at the outer site repulses Ca^{2+} at the inner site, driving the latter into the cell. Once double Ca^{2+} occupancy occurs, high throughput rates are favored by the repulsion between calcium ions. The calcium current, therefore, would be expected to increase as a function of $[Ca^{2+}]_o$, which it does. This model of a multi-ion, single-file pore seems to fit the observations better than do other models such as one-ion pores or the two-site model of Kostyuk et al. (125). Patch clamps demonstrate that calcium channels may have one of two conductance states: open or closed. Single-channel current has been observed to be between 0.5 and 1.2 pA, using barium as the carrier near a V_m of 0 mV. Extrapolating to 2 mM Ca^{2+} reduces this by perhaps a factor of 70.

Activation and Inactivation

Voltage-clamp studies have been useful in defining the kinetic properties of the slow channel, and the appearance of i_{si} during voltage clamping is shown diagrammatically in Fig. 4 and experimentally in Fig. 21. Slow-response fibers have a less negative resting potential of around −60 mV, a potential at which the sodium system is essentially completely inactivated. The slow channel is voltage-dependent. The probability of an individual cardiac channel being open ranges from 0 to nearly 1 (154); the channels are activated over a range of V_m of about 50 mV, with half activation between −20 and +10 mV, and activation may be sigmoidal (183). Activation of the slow channel requires a greater depolarization and is slower than that of the fast channel. In addition, phosphorylation of a membrane protein, perhaps part of the channel, may influence

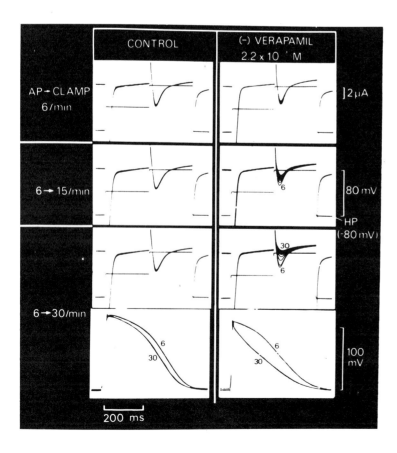

FIG. 21. Effects of stimulation during control (**left column**) and after (−)verapamil (**right column**) on the slow inward current (**top three panels**) and on the action-potential morphology (**bottom panel**) in cat ventricular myocardium. In the voltage-clamp studies, a prestep is used to inactivate the sodium channels. The prestep is followed by the test step to induce the slow inward current, i_{si}, which is the prominent downward deflection in the current trace that follows the test-voltage step. Twelve consecutive clamp cycles are superimposed after the voltage clamp was applied. In the middle and lower panels, cycle frequency was increased after the first voltage-clamp cycle to 15/min and 30/min, respectively. The action potentials in the lower panel were recorded before frequency change and after voltage-clamp conditions were terminated. Note the marked frequency-dependent change in i_{si} after (−)verapamil. (From ref. 71, with permission.)

the availability of calcium channels for voltage activation (173).

With maintained depolarization of the cell, calcium conductance, g_{Ca}, decreases. This inactivation depends on both voltage and time and extends into electrical diastole. This characteristic limits the number of impulses that can traverse the AV node and protects the ventricles in atrial fibrillation and flutter. Inactivation in heart muscle may also be due in part to an increase in intracellular calcium concentration.

Channel kinetics have been considered in Hodgkin-Huxley terms, where the activation variable is d and the inactivation variable is f, analogous to the m and h variables of the sodium channel. Conceptually, this is useful, but it has a number of limitations that have been reviewed by Tsien (183) and Hille (95). The delay in activation is fairly well described by d^2, analogous to the m^3 of sodium channels.

The calcium channel can respond to cyclic nucleotides, epinephrine and norepinephrine, angiotensin II, histamine, acetylcholine, β-adrenoreceptor agonists, and drugs (173,183). Isoproterenol lengthens the mean open time of calcium channels and decreases the intervals between the bursts of channel opening, while little influencing the absolute conductance (155).

The myoplasmic calcium concentration normally is low and is maintained by the Na^+-Ca^{2+} exchange mechanism in the plasmalemma and ATP-dependent pumps in the sarcoplasmic reticulum and mitochondria. $[Ca^{2+}]_i$ is in the range of 10^{-7} M or so. Activation of a calcium channel leads to the development of i_{si}, and a local 20-fold or so increase in $[Ca^{2+}]_i$ may occur that can initiate several types of responses, including contraction, gating (as mentioned earlier in the modulation of potassium and calcium channels), and, in the nerve, secretion of neurotransmitters, which may have effects on myocardial channels.

Tissues that normally were i_{Na}-dependent may have their sodium systems inactivated either by depolarization of the quiescent cell or by a failure of normal repolarization; the tissue may develop action potentials that are dependent on i_{si}. An example of i_{si}-dependent action potentials following the failure of normal repolarization is shown in Figs. 17 and 18 (4). Other characteristics of slow-response tissues are found in Table 2.

Action-Potential Duration, Refractoriness, and Cycle Length

In slow-response tissues, the relative refractory period extends into electrical diastole. This results in a relatively "flat" curve for the relationship of the rate of stimulation to the refractory-period duration. The relationship of rate to the action-potential duration is less marked than for fast-response tissues. In contrast to fast-response tissues, the late diastolic threshold tends to rise with rapid stimulation.

Calcium-Channel Antagonists

Much of the recent effort in the study of agents that block calcium channels has been directed toward characterization of the interactions of these agents with i_{si} and, more recently, individual calcium channels. Important groups of drugs include the following: verapamil and its derivatives, such as D-600, which are chemically related to papaverine; diltiazem, which is a benzothiazipine; nifedipine and its derivatives, such as nisoldipine, nicardipine, and nitrendipine, which are dihydropyridines.

One of the interesting theories proposed to explain the antiarrhythmic effectiveness of these agents was suggested by Fleckenstein (78), who hypothesized that many cardiac arrhythmias may be the result of abnormal calcium influx through the calcium channels. Thus, the effectiveness of these agents in treating the diseased state might be a result of their ability to "normalize" this excessive calcium influx. This is an interesting postulate because of the growing awareness of the role of changes in intracellular ions, particularly calcium ion, in conduction and automatic arrhythmias. Increases in $[Ca^{2+}]_i$ are known to increase intercellular resistance via gap-junctional pathways, thus having dramatic effects on cellular conduction. Likewise, increases in $[Ca^{2+}]_i$ are known to affect sarcoplasmic reticular release of calcium. Changes in $[Ca^{2+}]_i$ are known to affect other ionic conductances across the membrane, thus altering the automatic and other electrophysiologic properties of the cell membrane.

Evidence for Voltage- and Time-Dependent Drug Interactions with Calcium Channels

Verapamil, its derivatives, and diltiazem interact with the calcium channel in a manner similar to that observed with sodium-channel blockers and the sodium channel in that they show voltage- and time-dependent blockade as well as voltage-dependent recovery from blockade (22,23,71,122,123,137,140,145,146,182).

A voltage-clamp study by Ehara and Daufmann (71) on the effects of (−)verapamil on i_{si} in isolated cat ventricular myocardium is shown in Fig. 21. Double-clamp steps were used at rates of 6/min, 15/min, and 30/min, both under control conditions (left column) and after (−)verapamil, 2.2×10^{-6} M (right column). The action potentials in the lower panels were recorded before frequency change and after voltage-clamp conditions were terminated. Note that (−)verapamil little reduced i_{si} at the slow rate of 6/min. At rates of both 15/min and 30/min there was a progressive decrease in i_{si} (middle and lower panels). Increasing the rate from 6 to 15/min reduced the peak i_{si} by about 50%; increasing the rate further from 6 to 30/min reduced the peak i_{si} by 90%. The effect on the action-potential morphology is apparent in the lower panel. D-600 (140) and diltiazem (104) show similar use-dependent blockade.

Nifedipine initially was thought to show little use-dependent blockade (20,21,24). Sanguinetti and Kass (160) used voltage-clamp protocols to demonstrate volt-age-sensitive use-dependence for several dihydropyridine derivatives. They chose to examine the effects of nisoldipine, nitrendipine ($pK_a < 3.5$), and nicardipine ($pK_a = 7$). These agents showed no use-dependent block of Ca^{2+}-channel current at low frequencies (less than 0.5 Hz), but a marked use-dependence at higher frequencies. In addition, the holding potential greatly influenced this use-dependent blockade of Ca^{2+} channels such that depolarization greatly promoted current blockade by these dihydropyridine derivatives. These results suggest that the use-dependent blockade of Ca^{2+}-channel current by these agents is very sensitive to voltage as a result of preferential binding of drug to the inactivated state of the channel. In addition, the degree of ionization of each particular dihydropyridine derivative (and, for that matter, other Ca^{2+}-channel-blocking agents, including verapamil and diltiazem) greatly influences its ability to block Ca^{2+} channels at any given pH. Thus, under both normal and pathologic conditions, the degree of Ca^{2+}-channel block by any of these agents will be influenced by ambient pH. These results suggest an explanation for the disparity between results with these agents under various experimental conditions using different stimulation frequencies, pH, and the pK_a of the particular agent tested.

$\dot{V}_{max}$ in fast-response tissues is not affected by nifedipine and only by very high doses of verapamil or diltiazem. Raschak (153) has provided evidence that it is the (+) enantiomer of racemic verapamil that affects the fast sodium channels. The plateau in fast-response tissues, of course, is determined in part by i_{si}, so the repolarization phase may be affected, as seen in the lower panel of Fig. 21.

State Dependence

Kanaya et al. (120) have shown that diltiazem produces a use-dependent blockade, and the affinity for the inactivated channels is much higher for diltiazem than for the open activated channels. Thus, a similar sort of analysis may be applied to the interaction between calcium channels and calcium-channel antagonists, as has been proposed in the modulated-receptor hypothesis for the interaction of local anesthetics and fast Na^+ channels.

It therefore seems that we may apply our understanding of the modulated-receptor hypothesis to the interaction between these various calcium-channel antagonists

and the calcium channel. Current research efforts have been directed toward a further understanding of the cellular mechanisms of the interaction of the agent with the receptor and the channel. If calcium-blocking agents do interact with the inactivated state of the channel and produce an apparent voltage shift in the hyperpolarizing direction of the drug-bound channel, then the number of excitable channels is greatly reduced in slow-response tissues. This occurs as a result of fewer channels available for excitability and for maintenance of conduction via passive current spread.

A number of inorganic ions block the calcium current. These include Mn^{2+}, Mg^{2+} at high concentrations, Ni^+, and Co^{2+}. There is some evidence to suggest that the inorganic and organic calcium-channel blockers act at different sites. One site relies on the presence of extracellular calcium, and thus in the absence of extracellular calcium the organic agents such as diltiazem or verapamil will have no blocking effect on calcium current carried by a conducting ion such as Ba^{2+}. Beta-adrenoreceptor agonists, histamine, and methylxanthines may increase the number of available calcium channels. Thus, a multiplicity of sites that may be up- and down-regulated may serve to complicate our application of the modulated-receptor hypothesis to the interaction between calcium-channel blockers and their receptor sites in the calcium channel.

PROPAGATION OF THE ACTION POTENTIAL

In Chapter 1 we discussed in some detail the manner in which sources and sinks affect propagation. To avoid redundancy, only a few major points of particular importance to the consideration of antiarrhythmic drugs will be made here.

After the liminal-length requirements are fulfilled in a fast-response fiber, i_{Na} rushes into the cell, displacing the negative charges stored on the inside of the membrane and depolarizing the cell. Depolarization produces positive feedback in voltage-dependent sodium conductance (g_{Na}), which further increases. The local V_m is now more positive than in neighboring portions of the cell, producing a driving force for the longitudinal current in the myoplasm and through gap junctions. K^+ is the major carrier of the longitudinal current, and its flow is regulated primarily by the resistance and capacitance at the gap junctions and, to a lesser extent, by impedances in the myoplasm. The longitudinal current displaces negative charge off the interior of the membrane, depolarizes adjacent elements toward threshold, and thereby increases membrane g_{Na}. The circuit is completed by a capacitive current flow across the membrane and, finally, by current flow in the extracellular space.

Source

If the local electrotonic currents generated by one element or portion of the cell are insufficient to meet the liminal-length requirements of neighboring elements, only local electronic effects result. If the liminal-length requirements are met, g_{Na}-dependent regenerative depolarization occurs after the neighboring element is raised above threshold. Propagation of the action potential results. The fulfillment of liminal-length requirements or the attainment of threshold can be considered the propagated event, with the action potential a local membrane phenomenon (81). If propagation and conduction are viewed in this way, the relationship between the active (the source) and passive (the sink) electrophysiologic properties becomes apparent.

A source, such as a generator or battery, can be added to the electrical analogue in Fig. 1. This source supplies electromotive force. Such a source could provide the active generator property involved in the sodium current, i_{Na}. If this cellular element is made very small, the pure membrane case applies, and the maximal rate of rise of phase 0 of the action potential ($\dot{V}_{max}$) is proportional to the ionic current. As elements are linked together, the relationship of $\dot{V}_{max}$ to i_{Na} is less certain, because it is now influenced by the state of the passive and active properties of neighboring membranes, gap junctions, and cells. In Chapter 1 we presented the mathematical arguments that led to the following approximate equivalence:

$$\dot{V}_{max} = \frac{i_{ion}}{c_m} \qquad [15]$$

If c_m is constant and i_{ion} is equivalent to i_{Na}, $\dot{V}_{max}$ will be expected to correlate with the intensity of the sodium current. It has been difficult to analytically describe the relationship between $\dot{V}_{max}$ and θ, although it would be expected that an increased inward ionic current would be associated with increased θ and $\dot{V}_{max}$. Hunter et al. (107) suggested that conduction velocity did not depend greatly on the maximal sodium conductance and was approximately equivalent to the square root of $\dot{V}_{max}$. Singer et al. (165) reported a correlation between $\dot{V}_{max}$ and conduction velocity θ in Purkinje fibers for depolarizations from different membrane-activating voltages. Given the many assumptions of one-dimensional cable theory and the difficulty in extending linear theory to multidimensional systems, it is interesting that the proportional relationship between $\dot{V}_{max}$ and θ so frequently holds. Because it is difficult to measure i_{Na} directly in multicellular preparations, $\dot{V}_{max}$ has been used as an indirect measure of this current. Perturbations that decrease driving force, inactivate sodium channels, or otherwise decrease i_{Na} generally are associated with a decreased $\dot{V}_{max}$ and a decreased conduction velocity.

The predominant ionic current in this example is i_{Na}, but in slow-response tissues it will be i_{si}. The $\dot{V}_{max}$ of slow-response tissues is very low, as is the conduction velocity. A very low $\dot{V}_{max}$, however, does not identify a slow-response tissue, because depressed or inactivated fast-response tissues can have similar rates of rise and conduction velocities.

Sink

The local action potential is the source that electrotonically influences the neighboring elements (Fig. 1), filling the capacitance of the adjacent resting element. This current source also causes the slow exponentially rising increase in V_m or "foot" that occurs immediately before the rapid depolarization of phase 0 of the propagating action potential (179). The time constant for the foot can be easily derived by plotting the rise in V_m as a function of time. As derived earlier in Chapter 1,

$$\tau_{foot} = \left(\frac{\lambda_m}{\theta}\right)^2 \frac{1}{\tau_m} \qquad [16]$$

and

$$\tau_{foot} = \frac{1}{\theta^2 r_i c_m} = \frac{a}{2\theta^2 R_i C_m} \qquad [17]$$

This inverse correlation between conduction velocity and the foot has been demonstrated in sheep Purkinje fibers (67). The important existing literature relating r_i to θ has been reviewed in Chapter 1. Failure of transmission of impulses has been observed in cardiac tissues when presumably r_i has been manipulated by a variety of techniques. Among the most interesting was a report by DeMello indicating that digitalis glycosides could cause the uncoupling of cells (60).

Discontinuous Propagation

Considerations of structure suggest that discontinuous propagation may be important in cardiac tissues. It has been appreciated for some time that the velocity of propagation may vary with direction (42,161,170,171). Spach et al. (170,171) observed that propagations in atrial and ventricular muscle differed at different angles relative to the orientation of cells. In conditions in which active and passive properties could not have changed, propagation in the direction of the long axis of the cellular structure was relatively rapid as compared with conduction transverse to the long axis. Unexpectedly, longitudinal conduction was associated with a slower $\dot{V}_{max}$ and longer τ_{foot} than was transverse propagation (Fig. 22). Directional dependence of velocity and extracellular potentials was also observed at branch sites and at more complex muscular junctions (Fig. 23). Continuous-cable theory would not predict such dependences on angles, orientation, and direction.

The discontinuous structure of cardiac muscle may be responsible for the observed discontinuities of propagation. To explain such observations, Spach et al. (170,171) have developed the $\bar{R}_a$ hypothesis, where $\bar{R}_a$ is the "effective axial resistivity" representing the resistivity in the direction of propagation rather than the resistivity along the long axis of the fibers. $\bar{R}_a$ includes the influences of cellular geometry, intracellular and

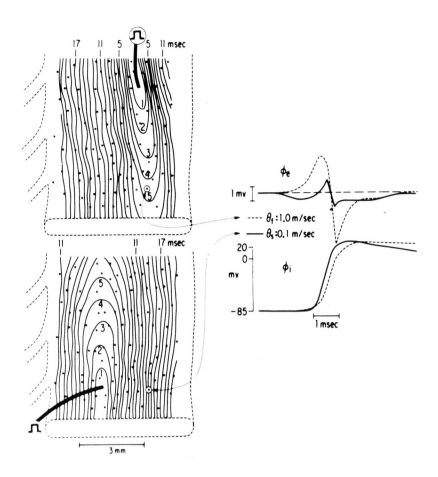

FIG. 22. Directional effects on the action potential in the crista terminalis. The points of stimulation are indicated by the square wave, and the sites of extracellular recording by the dots. The intracellular (ϕ_i) and extracellular (ϕ_e) potentials on the right were recorded at the site indicated when activation proceeded in the longitudinal (**left, top**) and transverse (**left, bottom**) directions. Isochrone activation maps were constructed from the extracellular recordings. Conduction velocity was calculated as the distance traveled normal to the isochrone per unit time. Note that when the velocity of propagation is low (θ_s for transverse propagation), $\dot{V}_{max}$ is higher and τ_{foot} is lower than in the situation for the more rapid longitudinal propagation (θ_f). (From ref. 171, with permission of the American Heart Association.)

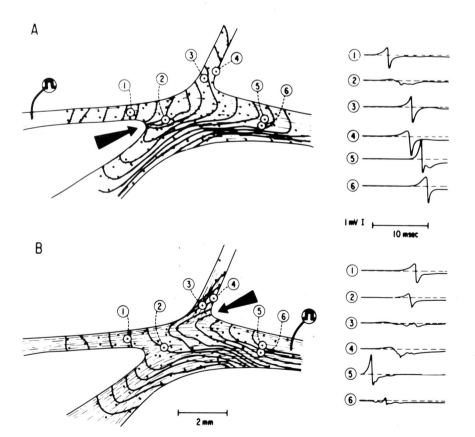

FIG. 23. Directional dependence of velocity and extracellular potentials at branch sites in pectinate muscle bundles. The square waves indicate the site of extracellular stimulation, and the points are the extracellular recording sites from which the activation maps were prepared. The extracellularly recorded waveforms on the right were obtained from the numbered points. (From ref. 170, with permission of the American Heart Association.)

extracellular resistivities, and cellular packing. The term, then, includes the influences imparted by the extent, distribution, and conductances of couplings between cells and other structural units. Substituting $\bar{R}_a$ for r_i in the cable equation and including geometrical terms to convert to membrane current per unit length, we have

$$\frac{\pi a^2 \partial^2 V_m}{\bar{R}_a \partial x^2} = c_m \frac{\partial V_m}{\partial t} + i_{\text{ion}}$$ [18]

Axial currents and propagation velocities were calculated from modifications of this equation, and computed extracellular waveforms at the junction of two uniform cables having different values of $\bar{R}_a$ did reproduce the type of results seen experimentally at tissue junctions.

Safety Factor

The liminal-length concept includes the statement that a certain amount of activating charge (current in time) is required to overcome the repolarizing influences of adjacent tissues to produce a propagated action potential. The term "safety factor" means the excess in the activating charge over that just required to produce a regenerative propagated response or, in other words, the excess of source over sink. The AV node has a low safety factor, and propagation commonly fails. Purkinje fibers of the specialized His-bundle branch system have a high safety factor, and conduction rarely fails.

Source

Hodgkin (96) has calculated a relationship between the density of sodium channels and conduction velocity in unmyelinated nerve. A greater density of sodium channels will increase the maximal i_{Na} and favor propagation, but will also require more gating charges that act as an extra capacitance and slow conduction velocity. The calculations produced an optimal density of channels, a figure that corresponds to the channel density determined experimentally. We anticipate that the same general principles will apply to heart muscle.

Normal fast-response tissues have a higher driving force, greater current flow, and faster reactivation than slow-response tissues, which depend on i_{si}. Steady-state or slow depolarization of a fast-response cell can partially inactivate the sodium system, an action that by reducing the source will tend to decrease the safety factor. These characteristics of the source are consistent with the commonly observed failure of propagation in the AV node and injured tissues, as well as with the relatively unusual failure of propagation in fast-response tissues such as the atrium, His-bundle-branch/Purkinje system, and ventricles.

Sink

The sink is much greater in highly branched tissues such as the AV node, as compared with cable-like

Purkinje fibers, and so the safety factor will be lower in the former and higher in the latter. Spach et al. (170,171) observed in fast-response tissues that propagation velocity was high in the direction of the long axis of cells and low in the transverse direction, and the difference was attributed to electrical coupling. Unexpectedly, they found using increasingly premature extrastimuli that uniform propagation became first decremental and then ceased in the direction with the highest velocity originally, while propagation persisted in the direction that originally had the lower conduction velocity (Fig. 23). The safety factor in "discontinuous" structures was higher when the conduction velocity was lower, and vice versa, which contrasts to the opposite effects in "continuous" structures such as cables when the active and passive membrane properties are changed. The implications of such findings in diseased and ischemic tissues remain to be investigated.

Antzelevitch and Moe (1) demonstrated the potential importance of electrotonic effects. This is shown in Fig. 24. The model consists of a Purkinje fiber in a three-compartment bath. The central segment of tissue was superfused with a solution intended to mimic ischemia that had $[K^+]_o$ of 15 to 20 mM and produced conduction delays as long as 350 msec across the 1.5-mm gap. The gap segment consisted essentially of an inexcitable cable; so conduction must have been electrotonically mediated. Current, however, could flow from the proximal to the distal compartment through the gap junctions in the inexcitable cable in the middle compartment and, if of sufficient intensity, could fulfill the liminal-length characteristics of the distal tissue, resulting in a regenerative action potential. Moreover, electrotonic interaction, rather than depressed i_{Na}- or i_{si}-dependent action potentials, could be responsible for slow conduction. These investigators also demonstrated, using an "ion-free" solution and control of local-circuit current flow through a variable resistance placed within an external shunt pathway, that external resistivity was also of importance in electrotonic currents crossing the gap and influencing the distal segment. Janse and Van Capelle (113) have provided evidence in canine and porcine hearts that ectopic activity in acute regional myocardial ischemia can arise from electrotonic interactions across an inexcitable region.

Antiarrhythmic Drugs, Local-Circuit Currents, Propagation, and Margin of Safety

As seen in Fig. 25, reentrant pathways can be abolished by production of bidirectional block in the depressed segment (panel C) or abolition of the area of unidirectional block (panel D).

The effects of drugs on passive and active cellular properties in tissues that normally depend on i_{Na} for phase-0 depolarization were considered in previous sections. Because little is known regarding the effects of

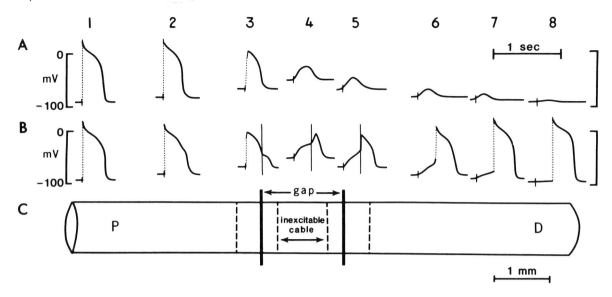

FIG. 24. Representation of the ischemic-gap preparation that demonstrates the importance of electrotonic interaction in bridging an area of inexcitable cable and activating the distal segment. The experimental arrangement is shown in **C.** An impulse is initiated by stimulating the proximal segment (P). The middle compartment is depolarized with a solution high in $[K^+]_o$, so that the sodium system is inactivated and no action potentials occur, including those dependent on i_{si}. Events in the distal segment (D) are assessed by recording V_m with microelectrodes. Because of the inexcitable segment, an impulse arising from stimulation of the proximal segment will propagate to the border of the block and stop there. Electrotonic influences due to local-circuit current will flow axially along the inexcitable cable, generating an electrotonically mediated depolarization that may (**B**) or may not (**A**) bring the distal segment to threshold. (From ref. 1, with permission of the American Heart Association.)

most antiarrhythmic drugs on passive properties, some of what follows is necessarily speculative. Procainamide (9) and encainide (15) would tend to reduce local-circuit currents by inhibiting the source and making the threshold less negative, but would increase the effects at a distance by increasing membrane resistance and the length constant. Although not studied, quinidine presumably would have a similar action on local-circuit currents. Lidocaine would render local-circuit currents less effective by decreasing membrane resistance in the subthreshold range and by shortening the length constant. The source would be effective only if voltage-dependent mechanisms came into play.

Procainamide, quinidine, disopyramide, and encainide decrease conduction velocity in isolated preparations, in experimental animals, and in the clinic. Lidocaine, phenytoin, and tocainide in concentrations achieved clinically do not depress conduction velocity in normal tissue, but will depress conduction in depolarized and ischemic tissues. Lidocaine may further depress conduction by decreasing the length constant and membrane resistance. The opposite would be true for procainamide, which might be expected to enhance discontinuous propagation, but this is purely speculative. Lidocaine, by increasing potassium conductance in the resting membrane, can hyperpolarize the cell, remove inactivation, and improve conduction (30). In a canine model of reentrant arrhythmias in the late myocardial infarction period, El-Sherif et al. (76) used a composite electrode for recording electrical activity and showed that lidocaine prolonged refractoriness and depressed conduc-

tion in the reentrant pathways, thereby interrupting the arrhythmia.

Normalization of action potentials can restore conduction when before there was none, as in Fig. 16, and can abolish slow conduction due to slow-response action potentials, as in Figs. 17 and 18. Lidocaine, phenytoin, propranolol, and tolamolol may have such a normalization action. As shown in Fig. 18, procainamide can favor a steady state at a low V_m that will lead either to slow responses or to inexcitability.

The effects of the calcium antagonists on the source have already been discussed. Verapamil, D-600, and diltiazem act directly on the channel and have a use-dependence. The effects on passive properties are largely unknown. These and other calcium antagonists reduce conduction velocity in i_{si}-dependent tissues, thereby interrupting reentrant circuits by producing bidirectional block in the depressed segment. The margin of safety in normal and abnormal i_{si}-dependent tissues is abnormally low, and drugs that antagonize the slow channel will further reduce the margin of safety. Using the canine model of reentrant ventricular arrhythmias in late myocardial infarction discussed earlier, El-Sherif and Lazzara (75) found verapamil and its derivative, D-600, to improve conduction in the reentrant pathways. No slow-response activity was observed, and these authors concluded that the drugs improved the depressed sodium channel. The mechanism is unclear, but it may be related to local release of catecholamines.

Beta-adrenoreceptor antagonists may have some effect on i_{Na}, with propranolol perhaps having the greatest

A. NORMAL

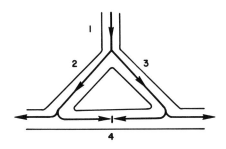

B. UNIDIRECTIONAL BLOCK WITH REENTRY

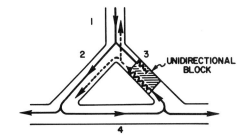

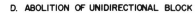

C. PRODUCTION OF BIDIRECTIONAL BLOCK

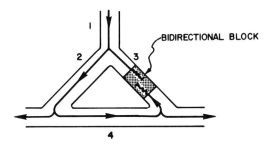

D. ABOLITION OF UNIDIRECTIONAL BLOCK

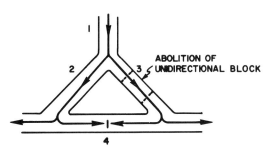

FIG. 25. Postulated effects of antiarrhythmic drugs on reentry using the Schmitt-Erlanger model of reentry at the junction of Purkinje fibers and ventricular muscle. **A:** Normally, an impulse travels from the central Purkinje fiber (1) through two Purkinje branches (2,3) and activates the ventricular tissue (4). This will produce a normal QRS complex on the surface EKG. **B:** As the result of ischemia or other disease, an area of unidirectional block is established in branch 3 while the impulse conducts normally down Purkinje branch 2 to activate the ventricular tissue (4). From the ventricular tissue, the impulse conducts in a retrograde manner slowly through the depressed segment. As indicated by the interrupted lines, if the bifurcation and remainder of the pathway in limb 2 have recovered their excitability, the impulse may reactivate and reenter this pathway, once again reaching the ventricular tissue. This will produce a premature ventricular beat on the surface EKG. Conceivably, not only a reentrant beat but also continuous reentry, with establishment of sustained reentrant ventricular tachycardia, could result. It may also travel retrogradely up the central Purkinje branch (1). **C:** The reentrant loop is abolished by converting unidirectional block to bidirectional block. **D:** The reentrant loop is abolished by abolishing the area of unidirectional block.

effect, pindolol some effect, and timolol, metoprolol, nadolol, and atenolol little or no effect. In general, the β-adrenoreceptor blocking effect has been considered paramount; so it would affect transmission and the margin of safety in the AV node. Virtually nothing is known about the effects on the sink, although tolamolol (11) decreases membrane resistance and shortens the length constant in Purkinje fibers.

Bretylium has little influence on i_{Na} directly (28,38,151,194). Its effects on passive properties are unknown, but it may improve conduction in ischemic tissue, perhaps mediated by local release of catecholamines.

The digitalis glycosides have complicated actions, and a number of these have already been discussed. In therapeutic doses, the primary effect on conduction is through the vagotonic action and perhaps lesser withdrawal of sympathetic tone. This slows AV nodal conduction and increases AV nodal refractoriness. Digitalis excess, however, may influence conduction in i_{Na}-dependent tissue by depressing the sodium system and by producing afterpotentials. This is seen in Fig. 27.

AUTOMATICITY

True spontaneous or automatic activity arises in the absence of direct external causes. Automaticity may be physiologic, as in the SA node and the lower-escape pacemakers, or pathologic, as in states of accelerated, depressed, or abnormal pacemaker function. The pacemaker may be enhanced or depressed by external factors such as catecholamines, acetylcholine, electrolytes, drugs, thyroid hormone, and other factors.

Automaticity may be triggered rather than spontaneous. In triggered automaticity, nondriven action potentials are initiated by one or more driven action potentials. Examples are seen in Figs. 17 and 18.

Membrane Factors in Tissues with i_{si}-Dependent Phase-0 Depolarization

Although the mechanism of automaticity in the SA node has not yet been fully elucidated, pacemaker activity results from a changing balance between positive inward currents that favor depolarization and positive outward currents that favor repolarization (109). The depolarizing current of importance for the action potential is i_{si}, with Na^+ perhaps playing a more important role than it does in the AV node. Brown and DiFrancesco (34) characterized an inward current in the SA node that is activated on hyperpolarization; thus the term i_h. Subsequently a similar inward current was reported to be activated on hyperpolarization in Purkinje fibers; it is called i_f (66). These contribute a time-dependent depolarization during diastole in pacemaker tissues. In addition, a time-dependent decrease in an outward current, probably potassium, has been observed at low V_m in the rabbit SA node. The slow channel in the SA node is inhibited by the usual slow-channel antagonists such as verapamil, D-600, and Mn^{2+}. Beta-adrenoreceptor stimulation increases the pacemaker activity, whereas β-adrenoreceptor blockade, acetylcholine, and many slow-channel blockers slow the pacemaker. Pacemaker cells in the SA node accelerate or decelerate mutually by the electrotonic effects of their action potentials; that is, fast pacemaker cells tend to accelerate slower pacemaker cells, and slow pacemaker cells tend to decelerate rapid pacemaker cells (55). The maximum diastolic potential of the SA nodal pacemaker is quite insensitive to changes in $[K^+]_o$. The AV node has a slow channel through which a mixed Ca^{2+}-Na^+ current flows, and the AV node may show pacemaker activity (110).

Pathologic automaticity can occur at low V_m where the sodium system is partially or completely inactivated. Although the ionic mechanisms have not been fully defined, they again seem to reflect a balance between inward depolarizing and outward repolarizing currents, with i_{si} being the inward current and probably K^+ being the outward ionic species. Such activity has been observed in the simian mitral valve, in tissues near the canine coronary sinus, and in depolarized fast-response fibers. Often some type of triggering is involved.

Membrane Factors in Tissues with i_{Na}-Dependent Phase-0 Depolarization

The heart beat is generally controlled by the SA node, because it is normally the fastest pacemaker. Impulses generated by the SA node sequentially excite the atrium, the AV node, the His bundle, the fascicular and bundle systems, the terminal Purkinje fibers, and the ventricular tissue. Failure or substantial slowing of the sinus node and conduction defects that prevent the normal transmission from the sinus node to the ventricles usually lead to the appearance of a lower-escape pacemaker that will then assume control of the heart. Such escape pacemakers have intrinsic rates slower than the normal SA node and may arise in the atrium, the junction (His bundle and AH region of the AV node), the subjunction (fascicles, bundle branches), and the terminal Purkinje fibers. The so-called "idioventricular" escape rhythm probably originates in the terminal Purkinje fibers rather

than in the ventricle, although pathologic pacemakers may arise in the ventricular tissue.

The pacemaker cell is characterized by ceaseless spontaneous activity due to slow diastolic depolarization (phase 4) beginning at the maximal diastolic V_m and continuing until the attainment of threshold results in an i_{Na}-dependent phase-0 depolarization (Fig. 26A). The rate of spontaneous pacemaker discharge depends on the maximum diastolic V_m, the rate of rise of phase 4, and the liminal length or threshold. If diastolic depolarization is rapid, phase 0 will depend on i_{Na}. If diastolic depolarization is slow, the sodium system may be inactivated by accommodation, and phase 0 may be a depressed response or one that is dependent on i_{si}.

There are several views as to the cause of pacemaker activity in i_{Na}-dependent tissues. It has been supposed that pacemaker activity is due to a time-dependent decrease in a repolarizing potassium current, i_{K_2}, in the presence of a relatively constant inward current, the result being a net depolarizing current (Fig. 26B) and depolarization-induced inactivation of the voltage-dependent potassium conductance, i_{K_1}. DiFrancesco (64,65) suggests that a time-dependent inward current that activates on hyperpolarizations negative to -50 mV may be involved in generation of the pacemaker potential in fast-response fibers. Of interest, DiFrancesco suggests that i_f in Purkinje fibers is a mixed current, carried in part by Na^+ and in part by K^+.

Triggered Sustained Rhythmic Activity

An action potential may trigger membrane activity. Examples of triggered sustained rhythmic activity in the

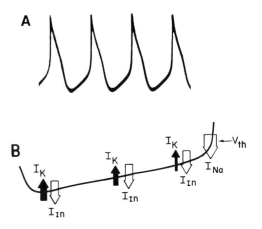

FIG. 26. Spontaneous automaticity in a cardiac Purkinje fiber. **A:** Recording of ceaseless pacemaker activity. Phase 4 shows slow diastolic depolarization between the maximum diastolic transmembrane voltage and threshold. **B:** Phase 4 results from a changing balance between inward depolarizing (i_{in}) and outward repolarizing (i_K) currents. Traditionally, it has been thought that i_K decreases with time, leading to a net increase in the inward depolarizing current. Some evidence suggests that depolarization results from activation of an inward current, i_f, which is not shown. (From ref. 7, with permission.)

situation of failed repolarization have been shown in Figs. 17 and 18.

Afterpotentials and triggered activity may occur at virtually any level of V_m and may depend on i_{Na}, i_{si}, and perhaps other currents such as the so-called transient inward current (i_{ti}) that is normally latent or small but may be large enough to produce sustained rhythmic activity in diseased tissue and in digitalis intoxication. Numerous pathologic, physiologic, and pharmacologic states and interventions can induce afterpotentials, including stretch, hypoxia, electrolyte change, aconitine, veratrine, and digitalis (*vide infra*). The amplitude of transient depolarizations (TDs) is increased by catecholamines. Often, TDs are increased in amplitude by increasing the stimulation frequency and by making extrasystoles increasingly premature. This overdrive enhancement is in contrast to the suppression of true automatic pacemakers by rapid stimulation, a phenomenon called overdrive suppression.

Cardiac Glycosides: Special Case

High concentrations of cardiac glycosides enhance automaticity, induce triggerable membrane activity, and alter excitability. Triggered membrane activity has been observed after digitalis in atrial, Purkinje, and ventricular tissues. On the basis of studies in Purkinje fibers, four

mechanisms for such sustained membrane activity have been suggested: (a) a drug-induced decrease in i_{K_2} without a change in voltage activation (16), (b) inhibition of the electrogenic sodium pump, thereby reducing the time-dependent outward current (111), (c) enhancement of a Ca^{2+} current (76a), (d) enhancement or induction of a depolarizing transient inward current, i_{ti} (129). Most experimental evidence, however, suggests that digitalis little affects i_{si} (77,129), except perhaps indirectly by leading to an accumulation of intracellular calcium. Sustained rhythmic activity after digitalis may be primarily due to an increase in i_{ti}. The ionic mechanism of i_{ti} is unclear (*vide supra*), but it seems to be quite distinct from either i_{si} or i_{K_2}. This current is very small or latent and is enhanced or induced by the cardiac glycosides. Nondriven sustained activity may result from phasic i_{ti} activity.

The difference between i_{K_2} and i_{ti} may explain, in part, the effects of repetitive drive on automatic pacemaker activity unrelated to digitalis and the afterpotentials observed after cardiac glycosides. As mentioned, repetitive drive suppresses normal automaticity and enhances that due to digitalis excess. Increasing the frequency of stimulation may produce extrasystoles (panel A of Fig. 27) or even a sustained rhythm (Fig. 28). As shown in panel B of Fig. 27, repetitive stimulation may potentiate afterpotentials, which in turn produce conduction disturbances.

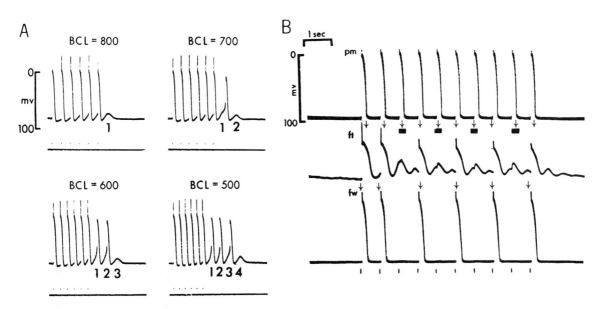

FIG. 27. Triggered activity due to acetylstrophanthidin (AS) in cardiac tissues. **A:** Effects of a sequence of trains of beats at progressively shorter cycle lengths are shown in the presence of a toxic dose of acetylstrophanthidin in a Purkinje fiber. The top trace is the V_m recording; the lower trace is the pattern of stimulation. At a basic cycle length (BCL) of 800 msec, a single subthreshold afterdepolarization results after stimulation is terminated. At basic cycle lengths of 700, 600, and 500 msec, one, two, and three suprathreshold afterdepolarizations occur, respectively, resulting in regenerative action potentials. The last triggered action potential, in turn, is followed by a subthreshold afterdepolarization. **B:** Conduction defects due to acetylstrophanthidin-induced afterdepolarizations. Simultaneous intracellular recordings were made in a preparation consisting of a papillary muscle (pm) to which was attached a false tendon (ft), which in turn connected to a segment of free wall (fw). Extracellular stimulation was delivered to the papillary muscle. The first two action potentials successfully propagate through the false tendon to the free-wall segment. The third papillary response is blocked at the crest of a large afterdepolarization in the Purkinje fiber. This is followed by a stable 2:1 conduction ratio. (From ref. 77, with permission.)

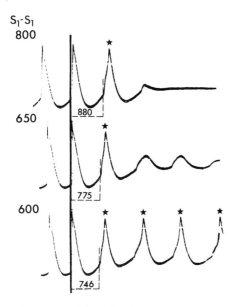

FIG. 28. Triggered activity following exposure to ouabain in a sheep Purkinje fiber. The vertical bar indicates the last driven beat. Beats marked with stars are regenerative action potentials that result from suprathreshold afterdepolarizations. At basic cycle lengths (S_1-S_1) of 800 and 650 msec, a single regenerative beat is observed, but the oscillatory afterpotentials are more pronounced at the higher frequency. After a stimulated rate at the even shorter cycle length of 600 msec, a triggered sustained rhythm results.

The arrhythmogenic role of TDs, also called oscillatory afterpotentials and delayed afterdepolarizations, has received increasing attention as an important mechanism for triggered arrhythmias resulting from cardiac glycoside toxicity. Wasserstrom and Ferrier (186) demonstrated that the TD (and the associated aftercontraction) amplitude is sensitive to transmembrane voltage. Dog Purkinje fibers and ventricular muscle both demonstrated a depolarization-induced increase in TD amplitude. Conversely, hyperpolarization of the transmembrane potential reduced TDs and aftercontraction amplitudes. These results suggest that depolarizing influences of $[K^+]_o$ accumulation and ischemia will promote automaticity resulting from TDs reaching threshold, whereas hyperpolarizing influences (antiarrhythmic drugs, low $[K^+]_o$) will be antiarrhythmic. This possible antiarrhythmic action of hyperpolarization was subsequently examined for several local-anesthetic antiarrhythmic agents. Inhibition of (Na^+,K^+)-ATPase with toxic concentrations of cardiac glycosides causes some depolarization that is often reversed by such agents as lidocaine and phenytoin. This latter agent is widely known to be particularly effective in the treatment of cardiac glycoside arrhythmias. Figure 29 shows the effects on the amplitude of the TDs of changing membrane potential by extracellular current injection. In the top panels, acetylstrophanthidin had been added to the superfusate. A stable TD (panel A) was enhanced by depolarization (panel B). Maximum diastolic potential was reduced, and a very much larger

TD is evident. In panels C and D, phenytoin had been added to the superfusate for 15 min at a concentration of 3 mg/liter, and there was a slight hyperpolarization of the maximum diastolic potential and a diminution in the amplitude of the TD. When depolarizing current was again applied to the same maximum diastolic potential, TD amplitude was greatly diminished in the presence of phenytoin. Panels E and F show more extensive reduction of the TD after 30 min of exposure to phenytoin. Figure 30 shows the complete range of transmembrane potentials that could be obtained with this current-passage technique. With the glycoside alone, TDs (in this case denoted as OAP amplitude) increased with depolarization and decreased with hyperpolarization. The circled value is that obtained at the resting potential. Shortly after administration of phenytoin, TD

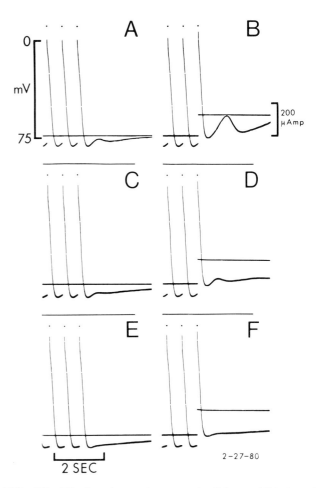

FIG. 29. Effects of membrane potential on AS-induced transient depolarizations before and during exposure of the tissue to phenytoin. In each panel, the top trace is the stimulus marker, the lower horizontal trace is the current record, and the remaining trace is a record of transmembrane potential. A and B: Recorded from a false tendon exposed to AS (1.6×10^{-7} M). C and D: Recorded after exposure of this preparation to phenytoin (1.2×10^{-5} M) for 15 min. E and F: Effects of exposing the tissue to phenytoin for 50 min. Upstrokes were retouched. (From ref. 186, with permission.)

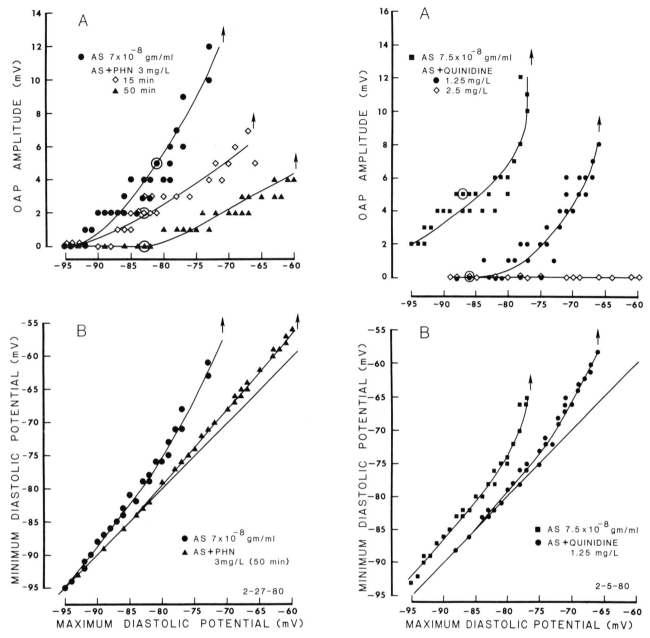

FIG. 30: Effects of phenytoin on the voltage dependence of transient depolarization (oscillatory afterpotentials) induced by AS (1.6×10^{-7} M) in a canine false tendon. **A:** Curves show the relationship between the amplitude of the oscillatory afterpotential and the maximum diastolic potential before exposure of the tissue to phenytoin (1.2×10^{-5} M) (*circles*), after exposure for 15 min (*diamonds*), and after exposure for 50 min (*triangles*). The point on each curve that corresponds to the spontaneous maximum diastolic potential is circled. Arrows indicate the points at which oscillatory afterpotentials reached threshold. **B:** Curves show the relationship between the transmembrane potential at the peak of the oscillatory afterpotential (minimum diastolic potential) and the maximum diastolic potential before exposure of the tissue to phenytoin (*circles*) and after exposure for 50 min (*triangles*). The data are from the same experiment shown in **A,** and the arrows again indicate achievement of threshold. (From ref. 186, with permission.)

FIG. 31. Effects of quinidine on the voltage dependence of transient depolarizations (oscillatory afterpotentials) induced by AS (1.7×10^{-7} M) in a false tendon. **A:** Curves show the relationship between the amplitude of oscillatory afterpotentials and the maximum diastolic potential before exposure of the tissue to quinidine (*squares*), after exposure to 1.6×10^{-6} M (*circles*), and after exposure to 3.2×10^{-6} M (*diamonds*). The circled points correspond to the spontaneous maximum diastolic potentials, and the arrows indicate the points at which oscillatory afterpotentials reached threshold. **B:** Transmembrane potential at the peak of the oscillatory afterpotentials (minimum diastolic potential) is plotted as a function of the maximum diastolic potential (same experiment as in **A**). The relationships are shown for data collected before (*squares*) and after exposure of the tissue to quinidine (1.6×10^{-6} M) (*circles*). Arrows indicate points at which oscillatory afterpotentials reached threshold. (From ref. 186, with permission.)

amplitude was reduced at all membrane potentials tested, and after 30 min there was a further reduction in TD amplitude, although pronounced depolarizations could still elicit measurable TD. The arrows in this figure denote TDs that reached threshold. The bottom graph illustrates the minimum diastolic potential. The minimum diastolic potential at which the arrows occurred is an indicator of threshold potential. Both in the absence and presence of phenytoin, the V_{th} was constant, about -57 mV. These results suggest that phenytoin has a very rapid and primary action to reduce the arrhythmogenic character of TDs by reducing their amplitude without altering V_{th}.

The effects of quinidine sulfate were examined under similar conditions. Figure 31 shows the effects of quinidine on TD amplitude and V_{th}. In the top graph, the glycoside had effects similar to those obtained in the previous illustration; namely, depolarization increased and hyperpolarization decreased TD amplitude. When quinidine was added to the superfusate, there was some decrease in TD amplitude at all membrane potentials. After prolonged exposure, TD amplitude was greatly diminished. Notice that maximum diastolic potential decreased by 1 to 2 mV. When TD amplitude was normalized to indicate V_{th} (lower panel), there was a dramatic positive shift in the minimum diastolic potential at which an automatic beat could be elicited. This indicates that there was a dramatic shift in V_{th} in the positive direction, i.e. a decrease in excitability. Nearly identical results were obtained with procainamide and lidocaine (*unpublished observations*). These results suggest that although these agents may decrease TD amplitude and in that way exert antiarrhythmic actions, these latter three agents also produce a rapid and dramatic shift in excitability. The result is that a TD of similar amplitude will be less likely to reach threshold and produce automaticity in the presence of such agents as lidocaine and quinidine. It is interesting that phenytoin does not seem to share this effect on V_{th}. These results indicate that although one action of these antiarrhythmic agents may be to directly decrease TD amplitude, another important antiarrhythmic action *in vivo* may involve changes in excitability and achievement of V_{th} by arrhythmogenic stimulus of the TD.

One explanation for this direct action on reducing TD amplitude is that decreasing Na$^+$ influx through the Na$^+$ channels might decrease a^i_{Na} under conditions of (Na$^+$,K$^+$)-ATPase inhibition. Reducing a^i_{Na} would eliminate [Ca^{2+}]$_i$ overload, which is ultimately responsible for the oscillatory release of Ca^{2+}, TD, i_{ti}, and aftercontractions. Direct measurements of a^i_{Na} with intracellular Na$^+$-sensitive microelectrodes permits a quantitative evaluation of this putative antiarrhythmic action of these agents. Eisner et al. (74) demonstrated that very high concentrations of lidocaine (0.3 mM) were necessary to reduce a^i_{Na}, Ca^{2+} overload, i_{ti}, and aftercontractions

under voltage-clamp conditions. Wasserstrom (*unpublished observations*) also measured the effects of antiarrhythmic agents on a^i_{Na}, TDs, and aftercontractions under conditions of (Na$^+$,K$^+$)-ATPase inhibition with glycosides. Figure 32 shows the results of one such experiment in which a sheep Purkinje fiber was exposed to toxic concentrations of acetylstrophanthidin (AS). After AS was added to the superfusate, a^i_{Na} and twitch tension increased markedly. At an a^i_{Na} of about 13 mM, TDs and aftercontractions appeared. Twitch tension increased to a maximum and then declined. Once relatively stable aftercontractions, TDs, and a^i_{Na} were obtained, lidocaine was added to the superfusate at several concentrations. TDs and aftercontractions decreased despite the lack of any change in a^i_{Na}. Similar results were obtained with quinidine. These experiments suggest that despite pronounced "antiarrhythmic" actions to reduce TD amplitude, these agents did not alter a^i_{Na} in the presence of maintained inhibition of (Na$^+$,K$^+$)-ATPase. The ability of these agents to reduce the arrhythmogenic stimulus to the TD must lie at another stage of the Ca^{2+}-overload cycle.

One possible mechanism for this antiarrhythmic action to reduce TD amplitude concerns a quite different aspect of the action of these agents. Wasserstrom and Ferrier (186) demonstrated that these agents have profound negative inotropic actions in dog Purkinje fibers. Figure 7 shows an example of the effects of TTX and encainide on a^i_{Na}, $\dot{V}_{max}$, action-potential duration, and twitch tension. These agents immediately reduced all of these characteristics, with similar time courses. However, during washout, there were obvious differences in the recoveries of a^i_{Na} and tension. Similar results have been obtained with quinidine and phenytoin, suggesting a direct action on excitation-contraction coupling independent of their effects on the action potential. Despite the modest decrease in a^i_{Na} of about 1 mM caused by antiarrhythmic agents in sheep Purkinje fibers (86,87), there is a second direct action on contraction that washes out more slowly than the effects on action potential and a^i_{Na}. The notion that these agents have direct negative inotropic effects at the level of Ca^{2+} release from SR was suggested by Bianchi and Bolton (27) for the negative inotropic actions of quinidine and other local-anesthetic agents in skeletal muscle. In addition, all of these agents decrease the action-potential duration, which will further decrease Ca^{2+} influx through the slow inward current. These data suggest that local-anesthetic antiarrhythmic agents may very well reduce TD amplitude by a direct action on Ca^{2+} influx and/or intracellular metabolism. This is also supported by voltage-clamp experiments showing that these agents have direct depressant effects on i_{si} in cardiac tissues.

The results of these studies suggest a multiplicity of actions of local-anesthetic antiarrhythmic agents to prevent cardiac glycoside arrhythmias. They suggest that

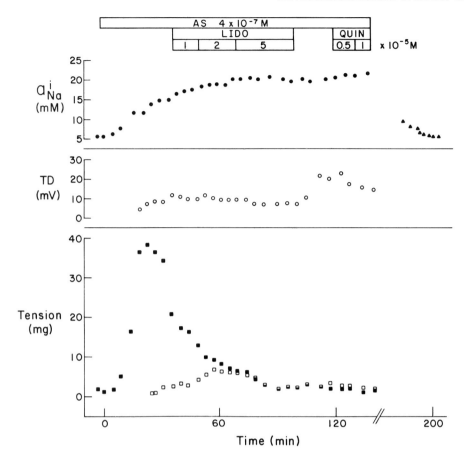

FIG. 32. Effects of lidocaine and quinidine on a^i_{Na}, aftercontractions (ACs), transient depolarization, and twitch tension in a stimulated (1 Hz) sheep Purkinje fiber. After exposure to AS, a^i_{Na} and twitch tension (*solid squares*) increased. When a^i_{Na} increased to about 12 mM, TDs and ACs (*open squares*) appeared. As Ca^{2+} overload increased, as evidenced by AC and TD, twitch tension fell. Lidocaine was added to the superfusate containing glycoside. The highest concentration of lidocaine caused tension, TD, and AC to diminish. These changes occurred without any alteration in a^i_{Na}. After washout of lidocaine, TD and to some extent AC recovered. Quinidine was then added to the superfusate, again causing a fall in TD (and to some extent AC) without any change in a^i_{Na}. (*Unpublished observations.*) For details of methods, see Wasserstrom et al. (188).

an important action may be an effect directly on V_{th}. Subsequent decreases in $[Ca^{2+}]_i$ will then relieve calcium overload and thus cause a reduction in TD amplitude.

MATRICAL APPROACH

Coda

We now wish to draw together the themes of the preceding sections into a matrical approach toward the mechanisms of arrhythmogenesis and the actions of antiarrhythmic drugs. We have proposed two major hypotheses. First, there is a normal matrix of electrophysiologic properties that can be altered by arrhythmogenic influences. Second, the normal matrix or the matrix deformed by arrhythmogenic influences may interact in one or more ways with an antiarrhythmic drug, resulting in yet another matrical configuration. In either instance, arrhythmogenic influences and antiarrhythmic drugs may affect one or more components of excitability; alterations in the determinants of excitability may change at different rates; and net excitability after one or more interventions depends on the balance between active and passive cellular properties. Drawing on information already presented and some additional data, we shall examine each premise conceptually and by means of experimental examples.

Hypothesis 1: There Is a Normal Matrix of Electrophysiologic Properties That Can Be Altered by Arrhythmogenic Influences

Arrhythmogenic Mechanisms

Traditionally, arrhythmogenic mechanisms have been classified in terms of abnormal propagation, particularly reentry, and automaticity. In actuality, *abnormal propagation with reentry and the various types of abnormal automaticity are the end results of altered active and passive cellular properties that reside in perturbed matrices of cardiac excitability.*

The conditions required for reentry depend on anatomy, source, sink, conduction velocity, and refractoriness. Alterations in the source or sink produce a segment that blocks conduction in one direction (unidirectional block) but permits conduction in another. If the impulse persists and conduction is sufficiently slow, it may activate again previously activated tissue that has recovered its excitability. Assuming the type of Schmitt-Erlanger model depicted in Fig. 33, which was discussed in Chapter 1, an estimate of the length of the reentrant loop is

$$L_c = \theta \times RP_r \qquad [19]$$

where L_c is the length of the reentrant circuit, θ is the slowest conduction velocity, and RP_r is the refractory period of the tissue to be reexcited. In the Purkinje fiber, a type of fiber specialized for conduction, θ is about 3 m/sec, and RP_r is about 300 msec; so L_c will be 1 m. If θ is reduced to 0.01 m/sec or less, then L_c is in millimeters, which is realistic anatomically. This circuit may be functional or anatomic, may occur in supraventricular or ventricular tissues, and may occur within a single Purkinje fiber or involve a large circuit such as in bundle branch reentry. The action potentials of the SA and AV nodes depend on i_{si} for phase 0 and normally have slow conduction velocities (Table 2); so these structures may be used as the area of unidirectional block in reentrant beats and sustained rhythms. In fast-response tissues, conduction velocity will be decreased by a reduction in the maximal sodium conductance because of (a) loss of integrity or blockade of the channels, (b) altered kinetics of the activation, inactivation, and reactivation, (c) abnormal refractoriness, (d) inhibition of the ionic pumps, and (e) accommodation. The sink, particularly r_o and r_i, importantly determines conduction velocity. There are several important factors: tissue geometry; the length of the depressed segment; conductances in the membrane, within the myoplasm, across gap junctions, and outside cells; the length constant; the passive determinants of liminal length; and the resultant influence of electrotonic interactions and the margin of safety.

Normally, the refractory state lessens during phase 3 and is over by the return to V_r in fast-response tissues. Drugs and injury may alter the repolarization process and the recovery of refractoriness. Injury, for example, (a) may markedly prolong the action-potential duration, (b) may produce tissue that fails to repolarize normally and has two stable steady states, one at the resting potential and the other at the plateau potential, or (c) in either of these situations may result in slow conduction and/or sustained rhythmic activity during the low voltage of the plateau (Figs. 17 and 18). Myocardial injury or disease may produce a nonuniform recovery of excitability, so that tissues with different levels of refractoriness may be juxtaposed. This dispersion of refractoriness establishes functional pathways conducive to reentry, as well as boundary currents that may depolarize neighboring tissues. In tissues that depend on i_{si}, the refractory period extends beyond the recovery of the diastolic potential, an action important in limiting the transmission of impulses through the AV node in atrial flutter and fibrillation.

Ceaseless pacemaker activity characterizes the automatic cell. This pacemaker activity, in turn, depends on the changing balance between depolarizing and repolarizing currents during phase 4, the maximum diastolic potential, and the liminal-length requirements or threshold required for the production of an action potential. True automatic activity occurs in the absence of a direct external cause, but it may be influenced by catecholamines, drugs, electrolytes, thyroid hormone, and the like. An action potential may trigger membrane activity that has been termed enhanced diastolic depolarization, oscillatory action potentials, low-amplitude potentials, transient depolarizations, afterpotentials, afterhyperpolarizations, and afterdepolarizations. Pathologic, physiologic, and pharmacologic states or interventions may induce afterpotentials, including stretch, hypoxia, ion imbalance, aconitine, veratrine, and digitalis. Triggered activity can be initiated and terminated by a single beat. It therefore has somewhat confused the classic clinical definition of reentry that for many years included the ability of the arrhythmia to be initiated and terminated by a single extrasystole (195).

The simplicity of Eq. 19 is seductive, and it is understandable that we cling to the underlying concept of reentry that has served us so well. The same is true for the descriptive approach to automaticity. So long as the phenomenologic bases of such descriptions are understood, this traditional approach serves a useful purpose, because they occur and can be documented. In the final analysis, it is evident that the situation is much more complex. Alterations in one or more of the matrices that determine the source and sink and interactions between these matrices determine the success or failure of transmission, altered automaticity, and changed excitability.

Perturbation of the Normal Matrix by Arrhythmogenic Influences

In an earlier section, we defined cardiac excitability as the process by which cells undergo single and sequential regenerative depolarization and repolarization, communicate with each other, and propagate in a normal or abnormal manner. Then we reviewed the passive and active cellular properties that determine net excitability. Most simply put, the thesis has been that net excitability is determined by the interaction of source and sink.

One way of determining experimentally the ease of exciting a tissue is by determining constant-current-voltage relationships to investigate the subthreshold range of V_m and by determining strength–duration relationships. We have utilized lysophosphatidylcholine (LPC) as a model for the effect of an ischemic metabolite on cardiac excitability. In Chapter 1 we discussed the fact that some recent studies on excitability do not fit comfortably in the traditional arrhythmogenic categories of abnormal impulse formation or altered impulse propagation. The example used was that LPC altered the relationship between the charge necessary to fulfill the liminal-length requirements for a regenerative action potential and $\dot{V}_{max}$ of the action potential, even though the membrane activation voltage remained unchanged. Such a change would affect conduction.

Figure 3 shows a constant-current–voltage relationship before and after LPC. In that experiment at that point in time, V_r, V_{th}, and the shape of the curves had not yet been affected by LPC. The curve, however, became shifted to the left for depolarizing currents, the two curves crossed over, and a given hyperpolarizing current produced a larger V_m deflection, reflecting an increase in slope resistance.

The phenomenon of altered excitability is shown in Fig. 33, which shows the effects of LPC on V_r, the apparent threshold voltage, V_{th}, and the current required to reach threshold, I_{th}, as determined by intracellular application of constant current (14). The transmembrane-current trace is at the top, and the current duration was 100 msec; the V_m recording is at the bottom. In panels A–C, the V_m recording shows a maximal just-subthreshold response superimposed on a just-suprathreshold response. In panel D, five responses are superimposed. In the control, panel A, I_{th} was 48 nA, V_r was −79 mV, and V_{th} was −68 mV. After LPC, in panel B, excitability increased, as manifested by a 25% decrease in I_{th} without a change in either V_r or V_{th}. With continued exposure of the preparation to LPC, in panel C, excitability decreased, as evidenced by the increase in I_{th} to a value above that in the control. V_r was unchanged, but V_{th} was less negative. In panel D, continued superfusion with LPC is seen to result in inexcitability regardless of the intracellularly applied current.

Excitability can be more broadly assessed by using strength–duration relationships. Figure 34 shows the effects of LPC on the nonnormalized and normalized strength–duration curve after two concentrations of LPC. Note in panel A that as compared with the control, the nonnormalized strength–duration curve was shifted downward after the lower concentration of LPC (triangles), indicating that less current at a given duration was

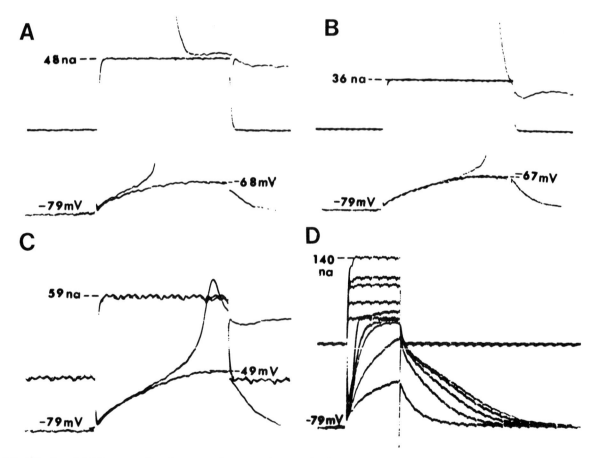

FIG. 33. Effects of LPC on resting transmembrane voltage (V_r), threshold voltage (V_{th}), and the current required to attain threshold (I_{th}). Current was applied intracellularly through one microelectrode, and V_m was recorded through a second microelectrode. The current trace is at the top, the V_m recording at the bottom. **A–C:** V_m recording shows a maximal just-subthreshold response. **D:** Five responses are superimposed. The current duration in all panels was 100 msec. **A:** Control. **B:** Increased excitability after LPC, with a 25% decrease in I_{th} despite no change in V_r or V_{th}. **C:** Decreased excitability as the LPC concentration was increased, as reflected by an increase in I_{th} to above control values. Note that V_r was unchanged but that V_{th} was less negative. **D:** Superfusion with LPC continued. Inexcitability regardless of the current applied intracellularly eventually resulted, despite an unchanged V_r. (From ref. 14, with permission of the American Heart Association.)

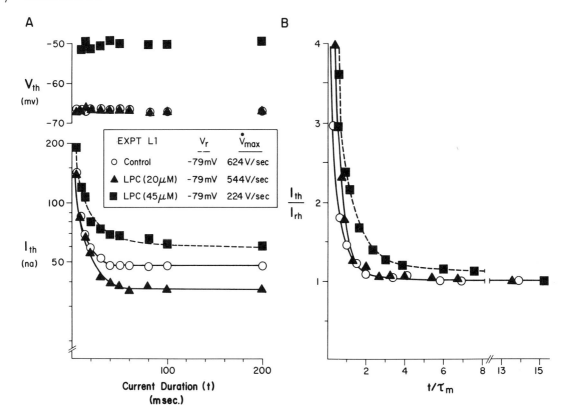

FIG. 34. Nonnormalized (**A**) and normalized (**B**) charge–duration relationships in the control period and after application of LPC at two concentrations. Threshold voltage (V_{th}) is plotted as a function of current duration in the upper portion of **A**. (From ref. 14, with permission of the American Heart Association.)

required to reach threshold; that is, the tissue was "more excitable" in classic terms. The explanation for increased excitability is to be found in the effects of LPC on passive properties. Cable analysis showed LPC to significantly increase input resistance, R_m, τ_m, and λ_m; current–voltage relationships showed LPC to decrease chord and slope conductances over the subthreshold range. Note that excitability increased despite a drop in the maximal rate of rise of phase 0, $\dot{V}_{max}$, a measure that was used as an indirect index of sodium conductance in this multicellular preparation.

At a higher concentration of LPC, the curve was shifted upward, and V_m fell further, indicating "decreased excitability." Note that V_r remained the same in all conditions; V_{th} was the same during the control and low-LPC-concentration periods, but became less negative during exposure to the high concentration of LPC. Normalization of the strength–duration curve (panel B) minimizes the changes in the shape of the curve caused by altered passive membrane properties, but it does not obscure and may even enhance those changes caused by altered active-generator properties [see discussion by Arnsdorf and Sawicki (14)]. The normalized curves suggest that increased excitability after a low concentration of LPC (triangles) was due primarily to altered

passive membrane properties, but that rather prominent changes in the sodium system favoring decreased excitability were already present for short-duration stimuli despite the rather small reduction in the $\dot{V}_{max}$ of the propagated action potential. At a higher concentration of LPC (squares), the curves no longer were superimposable, suggesting that altered active-generator properties were the primary determinants in decreasing excitability.

With this experimental description in mind, we turn to the extremely simplified conception of the normal and perturbed electrophysiologic matrix presented in Fig. 35. Only a few determinants of excitability are included: the resting potential (V_r), threshold voltage (V_{th}), sodium conductance (g_{Na}), membrane resistance (R_m), the length constant (λ_m), and, as a measure of overall excitability, the liminal length (LL). These have been chosen to make a point about the resting potential and its several determinants, active-generator properties and the relevant gates, passive cellular properties that determine transmembrane and longitudinal current flow, and the net excitability. The bonds between the determinants suggest interactions and mutual dependences. The normal state is depicted by the hexagon. The changes in the determinants and in the matrix after LPC are shown during the phases of increased and

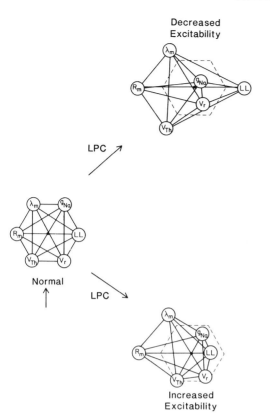

FIG. 35. A simple matrix perturbed by an arrhythmogenic influence. The determinants include resting potential (V_r), threshold voltage (V_{th}), sodium conductance (g_{Na}), membrane resistance (R_m), length constant (λ_m), and, as a measure of overall excitability, liminal length (LL). Each, in turn, has its own determinants, but these contain broad descriptions of the resting potential and its several determinants, active generator properties and the relevant gates, passive cellular properties that determine transmembrane and longitudinal current flow, and the net excitability. The bonds between the determinants suggest interactions and mutual dependences. After a perturbation, the normal state is depicted by the hexagon. A shift toward the center of the hexagon indicates a decrease in the quantity; a shift away from the center of the hexagon indicates an increase in the quantity. LPC either increases (*lower panel*) or decreases (*upper panel*) excitability. Increased excitability is depicted by a decrease in the liminal-length requirement, as indicated by a shift in LL toward the center of the hexagon; increased excitability is depicted by a shift in LL away from the center of the hexagon. Increased excitability is due primarily to increased R_m and λ_m despite small changes in V_r and V_{th} and an actual decrease in g_{Na}. Decreased excitability results primarily from a decreased g_{Na} due to direct effects and a less negative V_r and from a more positive V_{th} despite persistently increased R_m and λ_m.

decreased excitability. These six determinants form a conceptually useful picture, but each term has its own determinants, which in turn are controlled by yet other factors. In the final analysis, such complexity can be expressed only by a mathematical model.

Hypothesis 2: The Normal Matrix or the Matrix Deformed by Arrhythmogenic Influences May Interact with Antiarrhythmic Drugs, Resulting in Yet Another Matrical Configuration

General Principle

Arrhythmogenic influences can alter both active and passive properties. The situation that a drug encounters, then, may be quite different during ischemia, depending on the electrophysiologic characteristics of the substrate. The studies of Courtney, Hondeghem, Katzung, and others cited earlier dealing with lipophilicity, molecular weight, and structure, when coupled with physiologic effect, may be of predictive importance in the design of new drugs. The various state-dependent hypotheses allow further subgrouping within the overall matrix. Illustrations have been presented that the state of the sodium channel may depend on voltage and use and that these determinants in turn will be influenced by passive membrane properties. The resting potential, depolarization, repolarization, activation, inactivation, and reactivation are intimately involved in the electrophysiologic events of the normal and abnormal heart beat.

It is therefore of less importance to know the hierarchy of the various drug actions in normal tissues than to view the effectiveness of the drug as a balance between the nature of the arrhythmogenic abnormality and the particular electrophysiologic characteristics of the drug itself. Thus, in a disease state in which the arrhythmia arises as a consequence of altered conduction or excitability of the fast response, the efficacy of the drug is determined by a multitude of factors. These include the characteristics of drug binding to its receptor in the channel (which are influenced by the condition of the affected tissue), the consequences of channel blockade (which are also affected by the pathophysiology of the tissue), how these affect the passive spread of current, and so on. Similarly, arrhythmias involving abnormal automaticity are affected by agents that alter the approach and level of threshold. However, these drug actions are also complex functions of the nature of the disease, both electrophysiologically and anatomically, as well as the particular variety of drug effects on the electrotonic spread of excitatory current, drug blockade of ionic channels and the resulting alterations in intracellular ionic constituents, to mention but a few. We must reconsider our knowledge of drug actions on fast Na channels in light of new understanding of the subtle interactions between the nature of the arrhythmia itself and how the disease state affects normal cardiac function and drug action in and of itself.

Quite clearly, whether or not the use-, voltage-, and state-dependent actions of an antiarrhythmic drug are of importance in a given arrhythmia depends on whether or not the matrix of the drug well matches the matrix of the arrhythmogenic substrate. For example, the matrix of a normally i_{Na}-dependent tissue must be deformed by depolarization so as to inactivate the sodium channels and allow i_{si}-dependent activity to appear before there is any fit with the calcium antagonists, and the rate must be sufficient to bring into play the exquisite time dependence of calcium antagonists.

Automaticity can also be viewed from the perspective of the matrix. Different tissues as well as different electrophysiologic mechanisms may be involved in the generation of automatic dysrhythmias. Thus, the effects of antiarrhythmic agents will be determined by the tissue involved, its membrane potential, and its channel properties. In addition, the discussion of the various mechanisms by which antiarrhythmic agents may abolish arrhythmias resulting from Ca^{2+} overload addresses another complicated issue. Transient depolarizations appear to be arrhythmogenic by spontaneously depolarizing affected areas to their voltage threshold. Antiarrhythmic agents, therefore, may effectively eliminate the resulting automaticity by the many cellular actions (channel blockade, intracellular ion alterations, interference with Ca^{2+}-release mechanisms, etc.) described earlier. These may occur in concert with alterations in excitability achieved through changes in the cellular passive properties. Thus, the suggestion that these agents exert their antiarrhythmic actions through a singular action appears to disregard the subtle interactions involved in drug actions and the mechanism underlying the arrhythmia. The model of automatic arrhythmias induced by transient depolarizations provides some insight into the complexity of these interactions and interrelations, and it is safe to assume that other mechanisms of arrhythmias and their pharmacologic treatment may be similarly connected.

Drug Effects on the Normal Matrix and on the Matrix Perturbed by Arrhythmogenic Influences

Very little information exists concerning the effects of antiarrhythmic drugs on these determinants of excitability. The importance of the balance of active and passive properties in determining net excitability is shown in strength–duration curves before and after application of procainamide and lidocaine (Fig. 36). In the upper portion of each panel, the threshold voltage (V_{th}) is plotted as a function of current duration (t). In

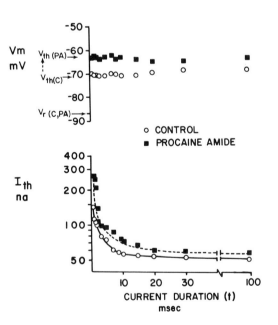

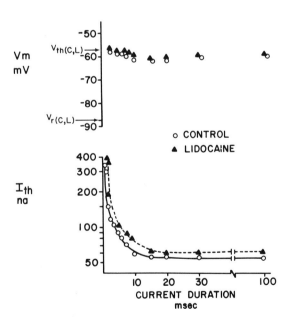

FIG. 36. Effects of procainamide (**A**) and lidocaine (**B**) on strength–duration curves as assessed by the microelectrode technique of intracellular constant-current application and transmembrane voltage recording in cardiac Purkinje fibers. In the upper portion of each panel, the threshold voltage (V_{th}) is plotted as a function of the current duration. In the lower panel, the strength–duration curve is depicted, with the threshold current (I_{th}) plotted as a function of the current duration. As compared with the control, both procainamide and lidocaine shifted the strength–duration curve upward, indicating that the threshold-current requirement increased after the intervention. Neither drug affected V_r, but procainamide made V_{th} less negative, whereas lidocaine little influenced V_{th}. Cable analysis and current–voltage analysis revealed that procainamide increased and lidocaine decreased membrane resistance at rest and in the subthreshold potential range. (From refs. 9 and 10, with permission of the American Heart Association.)

the lower portion of each panel, the strength–duration curve is shown with I_{th} plotted as a function of current duration (t). Both procainamide and lidocaine shifted the strength–duration curve upward, indicating that the threshold-current requirement increased after interventions. In classic terms, such a shift indicates a less excitable membrane. Although I_{th} was increased by both drugs, procainamide decreased excitability by making V_{th} less negative (a term that depends on g_{Na}), despite an actual increase in membrane resistance, whereas lidocaine little affected V_{th} but decreased membrane resistance in the subthreshold range. Cable analysis showed that procainamide increased and lidocaine decreased the length constant, so that the sink would also be altered differently by the two drugs.

More recently, we studied the effects of encainide on active and passive determinants of excitability that were tracked in time with a rapid, on-line, computerized data-analysis system (15). The drug produced multiphasic changes in cardiac excitability, the final state depending on the balance between altered passive and active membrane properties. Encainide enhanced excitability by increasing membrane and slope resistance without altering the nonlinearities of the constant-current–voltage relationship. It could decrease excitability by a number of mechanisms, including (a) depression of the sodium system, (b) decreasing the membrane resistance without altering the nonlinearities of the subthreshold-current–voltage relationship, (c) altering the nonlinearities of the constant-current–voltage relationship, and (d) a combination of these actions. During washout of the drug, excitability could remain altered despite a return to normal in descriptive parameters such as $\dot{V}_{max}$, overshoot, and action-potential duration.

In unpublished studies, we have found that quinidine often decreases the current required to produce a regenerative response in normal tissues. This occurs despite no change in V_r, a somewhat less negative V_{th}, and a decrease in $\dot{V}_{max}$. Increased membrane slope and chord resistance, as determined by cable analysis and constant-current–voltage relationships, seem to be primarily responsible.

In Fig. 37, the deformations of the normal matrix are shown for procainamide, lidocaine, and quinidine, with the first two resulting in decreased and the last in increased excitability.

Sequential changes in the matrix are shown in the very complicated experiment depicted in Fig. 38, in which three periods are shown: control; the phase of increased excitability caused by LPC, as manifested by a 22% decrease in I_{th}; after lidocaine during continued LPC superfusion. At a current duration of 100 msec for the intracellularly applied current ($t = 100$ msec), LPC had little effect on V_r or V_{th}, but it decreased I_{th} from 55 to 43 nA (-22%), reduced $\dot{V}_{max}$ from 816 V/sec to 693 V/sec (-15%), and increased R_m, as determined by cable analysis, from 1,242 $\Omega \cdot cm^2$ to 1,528 $\Omega \cdot cm^2$ ($+23\%$). As compared with the control, the nonnormalized strength–duration curve (I_{th} versus t in panel A) was shifted downward, indicating that less current at a

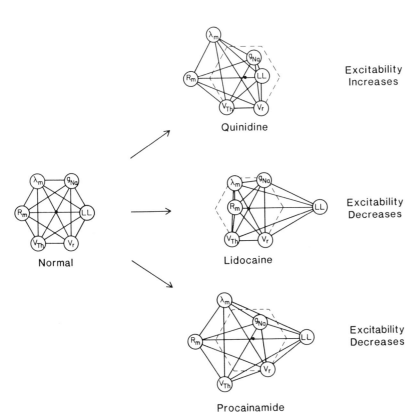

FIG. 37. A simple matrix perturbed by antiarrhythmic drugs. The conventions are the same as in Fig. 36. In normal tissues, procainamide and lidocaine both decrease excitability, as indicated by LL moving away from the normal hexagon, but the mechanisms differ. Procainamide decreases excitability by decreasing g_{Na} due to direct effects and by making V_{th} more positive, despite persistently increased R_m and λ_m, with little change in V_r. Lidocaine decreases excitability by decreasing R_m, with little change in the other determinants. Quinidine often increases excitability in normal tissues, as indicated by LL moving toward the center of the hexagon, primarily by increasing R_m and λ_m, despite little change in V_r and V_{th} and an actual decrease in g_{Na}.

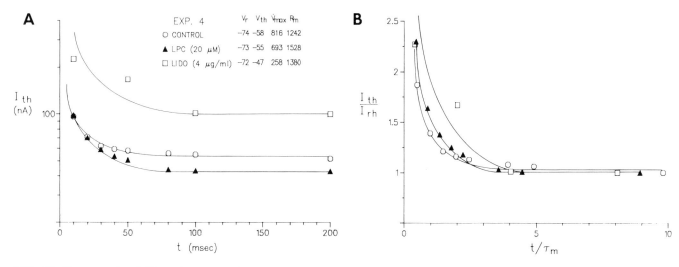

FIG. 38. Nonnormalized (**A**) and normalized (**B**) strength–duration curves during the three test periods: control; the phase of increased excitability after LPC; and after lidocaine. (From ref. 162, with permission.)

given duration was required to reach threshold; that is, the tissue was more excitable in classic terms. As compared with the LPC period, application of lidocaine during continued LPC superfusion little affected V_r, caused V_{th} to become less negative at −47 mV (−15%), further reduced $\dot{V}_{max}$ to 256 V/sec (−63%), and reduced R_m to 1,380 $\Omega \cdot cm^2$ (−9%).

The strength–duration curves in panel A of Fig. 38 were normalized (I_{th}/I_{rh} versus t/τ_m) and appear in panel B. The rationale is that an alteration in R_m tends to produce changes of the same magnitude in I_{th}, I_{rh}, and τ_m (9,10,14,67,85,148); normalization, therefore, will tend to cancel out the effects of the passive property R_m on the curve, and as a result, nonnormalized curves that have been shifted due to alterations in R_m should be essentially superimposable after normalization. The latter has been the case in a number of studies (9,10,14,67). Normalization will not correct for alterations in current–voltage nonlinearities, for changes in the maximum sodium conductance or in the voltage-dependent activation and inactivation variables, or for differing liminal-length requirements resulting from changes in active membrane properties (85,148). Shifted nonnormalized curves, for any of these reasons, then, will not be superimposable after normalization, and experimental studies support such theoretical considerations (10,14). In this particular case, constant-current–voltage relationships were not significantly changed.

Referring to panel B of Fig. 38, the normalized strength–duration curves for the control and LPC periods were essentially superimposable at values of t/τ_m of 1.5 or more. At values less than 1.5, the curves diverged, with the slope for LPC showing a steeper rise for short stimuli than the control. The normalized strength–duration curves, then, suggest that increased excitability after LPC reflected changes primarily in passive membrane properties, but that changes in the sodium system that favored decreased excitability were present for short-

duration stimuli. After application of lidocaine during continued LPC perfusion, the normalized curve superimposed on both the control and LPC curves for t/τ_m greater than 4.0, but diverged from these curves for lesser values. This suggests that lidocaine not only countered the changes induced by LPC on R_m but also further depressed the sodium system, the net result being a preparation that was less excitable than in either the control or LPC period. Cable analysis showed that during the phase of enhanced excitability, LPC increased R_m, whereas lidocaine largely reversed this LPC-induced change. The same was observed for the effect on the length constant.

The phase of increased excitability after LPC is followed by a phase of decreased excitability. During the phase of decreased excitability, lidocaine's action was expressed largely through its depressant effect on the sodium system rather than through its effects on cable properties. Here, the matrix had been deformed, and a minor action during the phase of increased excitability became the predominant action during the phase of decreased excitability.

In Fig. 39, the normal matrix is perturbed by lidocaine alone and by LPC alone, the latter resulting in either increased or decreased excitability. The interactions between lidocaine and both phases of LPC are also shown. The diagram illustrates the fact that lidocaine's predominant action depended on the characteristics of the matrix altered by LPC. The matrical approach also accommodates the observation that a drug action may change in time despite a constant concentration and that this change in time depends on the match between the arrhythmogenic influence and the antiarrhythmic drug, the net effect reflecting the final shape of the electrophysiologic matrix.

There have been a few attempts to use pacing and pharmacologic probes to elucidate drug mechanisms. Two are of particular interest in terms of our matrical

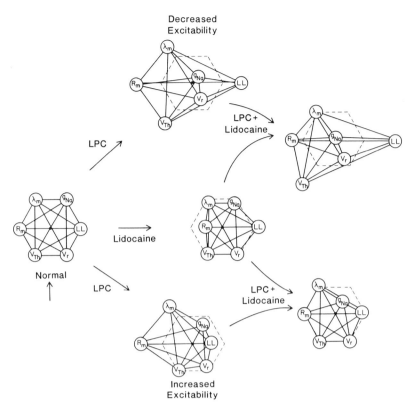

FIG. 39. A simple matrix perturbed first by an arrhythmogenic influence and subsequently by an antiarrhythmic drug. The conventions are the same as in Fig. 36. In the lower pathway, LPC increases excitability in normal tissue by a decrease in the liminal-length requirement, as indicated by a shift in LL toward the center of the hexagon. An LPC-induced increase in excitability is due primarily to increased R_m and λ_m, despite small changes in V_r and V_{th} and an actual decrease in g_{Na}. With the matrix altered into this configuration by LPC, lidocaine decreases excitability and returns LL toward a normal value by decreasing R_m and λ_m, by making V_r less positive despite some decrease in g_{Na}. Note that the effects on passive properties are primarily responsible for the partial normalization of the matrix. In the upper pathway, LPC decreases excitability, as indicated by LL shifting away from the center of the hexagon. Decreased excitability results primarily from a decreased g_{Na} due to direct effects and a less negative V_r and from more positive V_{th}, despite persistently increased R_m and λ_m. With the matrix altered into this configuration by LPC, lidocaine decreases excitability primarily by further depressing g_{Na} and making V_{th} less negative, rather than by affecting passive properties. Note that the effect on active membrane properties further deforms the normal matrix.

approach. Ilvento et al. (108) created complete heart block in dogs and observed both fast and slow idioventricular rhythms that responded differently to pacemaker overdrive. The rate of the fast idioventricular rhythm was slowed by ethmozin, but not by verapamil or lidocaine, and the recovery-cycle length was prolonged by ethmozin and verapamil, but not by lidocaine. The rate of the fast idioventricular rhythm was decreased by lidocaine, was increased by verapamil, and was unaffected by ethmozin; the recovery-cycle length was prolonged by lidocaine, unaltered by ethmozin, and decreased by verapamil. The interpretation was that the fast idioventricular rhythm resulted from an abnormal automatic mechanism at a low membrane potential that was not overdrive-suppressed; the slow rhythm resulted from normal automaticity at a high level of membrane potential and could be overdrive-suppressed. They used the term "matrix" in a different sense in that they created a 3 × 3 table of the responses of normal automaticity, abnormal automaticity, and delayed afterdepolarizations as functions of lidocaine, verapamil, and ethmozin, and they suggested that using pacing and pharmacologic probes might be useful in differentiating the mechanisms of arrhythmias *in vivo*. Sung et al. (177) have used a similar approach of pacing and pharmacologic testing in man in an attempt to differentiate ventricular tachycardia due to reentry, automaticity, and triggered activity. We could reinterpret these data in terms of the normal matrix of electrophysiologic determinants of excitability altered in different ways to produce abnormal and

triggered automaticities that in turn interact differently and perhaps uniquely with specific antiarrhythmic drugs.

Matrix Versus Hierarchy

We believe that our current knowledge favors a matrical approach over a hierarchical approach to drug action. The matrical approach considers multiple changes that occur with arrhythmogenic influences and antiarrhythmic drugs. Even in the qualitative approach used in this chapter, the matrical approach unifies many otherwise isolated observations into a conceptual whole. Perhaps most important, the matrical approach permits development of a quantitative model. The concept of the matrix provides a useful intellectual concept for the necessary experimental and clinical tasks of recognizing and describing sets of interacting electrophysiologic variables.

Clinical Implications

The clinical implications of the matrical approach are several. It allows a link between basic science and clinical science. A number of years ago, we proposed that excitability must be abnormal for premature ventricular beats and even more complex forms to initiate dangerous ventricular arrhythmias, and we termed this the hypothesis of altered excitability (5). Restated at the more basic level of this chapter, the matrix must be altered to produce abnormal excitability and arrhythmias. A major clinical problem is the definition of abnormal excitability with high predictive accuracy.

Electrophysiologic programmed stimulation (EPS) and other provocative techniques are useful when the matrix is deformed and the arrhythmia is triggered in a manner similar to that occurring spontaneously. The response to a provocation should be most predictable, and therapy based on the inhibition of a response most predictably successful, when the matrix remains *fixed* in an arrhythmogenic configuration, such as in reentrant supraventricular tachycardia, particularly those utilizing an accessory atrioventricular bypass connection. With regard to ventricular arrhythmias, the results of provocation and therapy based on the provocation should be most predictable in hemodynamically stable ventricular tachycardia that results from physiologically and anatomically stable pathways, such as in a ventricular aneurysm. Provocative techniques should be least reproducible, and therapy based on the response to provocation less effective, when the matrix is *transiently* deformed into an arrhythmogenic configuration by autonomic surges, ischemia, hypoxia, electrolyte imbalance, pH abnormalities, abnormal myocardial function, drug toxicity, and the like. In this situation, provocative techniques should be used to transiently deform the matrix in the same manner as occurs spontaneously.

Antiarrhythmic interventions should alter the matrix to prevent the arrhythmogenic configuration. On the other hand, there is the risk that a drug may create an arrhythmogenic matrical configuration and produce arrhythmias (156). It is necessary, then, not only to give an antiarrhythmic drug but also to have a rational approach to testing the arrhythmogenic potential of the matrix.

Finally, the antiarrhythmic matrical configuration must be maintained during follow-up. Patient compliance and monitoring of therapy can be assisted by "smart" drug-infusion pumps. Implanted programmable pacemakers that can mimic the protocols used in the invasive electrophysiologic laboratory may be used in the outpatient department to test the continuing efficacy of antiarrhythmic drugs. The use of implantable defibrillators increasingly will complement the use of antiarrhythmic drugs. Drugs will be improved. Knowledge of physicochemical and other characteristics will perhaps allow the design of drugs that can specifically affect portions of the matrix.

ACKNOWLEDGMENTS

Supported in part by USPHS NHLBI grant R01 HL-21788 to Dr. Arnsdorf, as well as by a New Investigator Research Award, USPHS NHLBI HL-30725, and a grant-in-aid from the American Heart Association to Dr. Wasserstrom.

REFERENCES

1. Antzelevitch, C., and Moe, G. K. (1981): Electrotonically mediated delayed conduction and reentry in relation to "slow responses" in mammalian and ventricular conducting tissue. *Cir. Res.*, 49:1129–1139.
2. Arnsdorf, M. F. (1976): Electophysiologic properties of antidysrhythmic drugs as a rational basis for therapy. *Med. Clin. North Am.*, 60:213–232.
3. Arnsdorf, M. F. (1977): Membrane factors in arrhythmogenesis: Concepts and definitions. *Prog. Cardiovasc. Dis.*, 19:413–429.
4. Arnsdorf, M. F. (1977): The effect of antiarrhythmic drugs on sustained rhythmic activity in cardiac Purkinje fibers. *J. Pharmacol. Exp. Ther.*, 201:689–700.
5. Arnsdorf, M. F. (1984): Cable properties and conduction of the action potential: Excitability, sources, and sinks. In: *Physiology and Pathology of the Heart*, edited by N. Sperelakis, pp. 109–140. Martinus Nijhoff, Boston.
6. Arnsdorf, M. F. (1984): Basic understanding of the electrophysiologic actions of antiarrhythmic drugs: Sources, sinks and matrices of information. *Med. Clin. North Am.*, 68:1247–1880.
7. Arnsdorf, M. F. (1986): Electrophysiology and biophysics of cardiac excitation. In: *Cardiovascular Physiology*, edited by O. Garfein, (*in press*). Academic Press, Orlando.
8. Arnsdorf, M. F., and Bigger, J. T., Jr. (1972): Effect of lidocaine hydrochloride on membrane conductance in mammalian cardiac Purkinje fibers. *J. Clin. Invest.*, 51:2252–2263.
9. Arnsdorf, M. F., and Bigger, J. T., Jr. (1975): The effect of lidocaine on components of excitability in long mammalian cardiac Purkinje fibers. *J. Pharmacol. Exp. Ther.*, 195:206–215.
10. Arnsdorf, M. F., and Bigger, J. T., Jr. (1976): The effect of procaine amide on components of excitability in long mammalian cardiac Purkinje fibers. *Circ. Res.*, 38:115–122.
11. Arnsdorf, M. F., and Friedlander, I. (1976): The electrophysiologic effects of tolamolol (UK-6558-01) on the passive membrane properties of mammalian cardiac Purkinje fibers. *J. Pharmacol. Exp. Ther.*, 199:601–610.
12. Arnsdorf, M. F., and Hsieh, Y. (1978): Antiarrhythmic agents. In: *The Heart*, edited by R. W. Hurst, R. B. Logue, R. C. Schlant, et al. pp. 1943–1963. McGraw-Hill, New York.
13. Arnsdorf, M. F., and Mehlman, D. J. (1977): Observations on the effects of selected antiarrhythmic drugs on mammalian cardiac Purkinje fibers with two levels of steady-state potential: Influences of lidocaine, phenytoin, propranolol, disopyramide, and procainamide on repolarization, action potential shape and conduction. *J. Pharmacol. Exp. Ther.*, 207:983–991.
14. Arnsdorf, M. F., and Sawicki, G. J. (1981): The effects of lysophosphatidylcholine, a toxic metabolite of ischemia, on the components of cardiac excitability in sheep Purkinje fibers. *Circ. Res.*, 49:16–30.
15. Arnsdorf, M. F., Schmidt, G. A., and Sawicki, G. J. (1985): Effects of encainide on the determinants of cardiac excitability in sheep Purkinje fibers. *J. Pharmacol. Exp. Ther.*, 232:40–48.
16. Aronson, R. S., Gelles, J. M., and Hoffman, B. F. (1974): Effect of ouabain on the current underlying spontaneous diastolic depolarization in cardiac Purkinje fibers. *Nature* [*New Biol.*], 245:118–120.
17. Ashraf, M., and Halverson, C. (1978): Ultrastructural modifications of nexuses (gap junctions) during early myocardial ischemia. *J. Mol. Cell. Cardiol.*, 10:263–269.
18. Attwell, D., Cohen, I., Eisner, D., Ohba, M., and Ojeda, C. (1979): The steady-state TTX-sensitive ("window") sodium current in cardiac Purkinje fibers. *Pfluegers Arch.*, 379:137–142.
19. Baldwin, K. M. (1977): The fine structure of healing over in mammalian cardiac muscle. *J. Mol. Cell. Cardiol.*, 9:959–966.
20. Baumann, K. (1976): On the actions of nifedipine under conditions of variable stimulation patterns and $[Ca^{++}]_0$ in guinea-pig atrium. *Naunyn Schmiedebergs Arch. Pharmacol.*, 294:161–168.
21. Bayer, R., and Ehara, T. (1978): Comparative studies on calcium antagonists. *Prog. Pharmacol.*, 2:31–37.
22. Bayer, R., Hennekes, R., Kaufmann, R., et al. (1975): Inotropic and electrophysiological actions of verapamil and D-600 in mammalian myocardium. I. Pattern of inotropic effects of the

racemic compounds. *Naunyn Schmiedebergs Arch. Pharmacol.*, 290:49–68.

23. Bayer, R., Kaufmann, R., and Mannhold, R. (1975): Inotropic and electrophysiologic actions of verapamil and D-600 in mammalian myocardium. II. Patterns of inotropic effects of the optical isomers. *Naunyn Schmiedebergs Arch. Pharmacol.*, 290:69–80.

24. Bayer, R., Rodenkirchen, R., Kaufmann, R., Lee, J. H., et al. (1977): The effects of nifedipine on contraction and monophasic action potentials of isolated cat myocardium. *Naunyn Schmiedebergs Arch. Pharmacol.*, 30:29–37.

25. Bean, B. P., Cohen, C. J., and Tsien, R. W. (1983): Lidocaine block of cardiac sodium channels. *J. Gen. Physiol.*, 81:613–642.

26. Beneski, D. A., and Catterall, W. A. (1980): Covalent labeling of protein components of the sodium channel with a photoactivatable derivative of scorpion toxin. *Proc. Natl. Acad. Sci. USA*, 77:639–643.

27. Bianchi, C. P., and Bolton, T. C. (1967): Action of local anesthetics on coupling systems in muscle. *J. Pharmacol. Exp. Ther.*, 157:388–405.

28. Bigger, J. T., Jr., and Jaffee, C. C. (1971): The effect of bretylium tosylate on the electrophysiologic properties of ventricular muscle and Purkinje fiber. *Am. J. Cardiol.*, 27:82–91.

29. Bigger, J. T., Jr., and Mandel, W. J. (1970): Effect of lidocaine on the electrophysiological properties of ventricular muscle and Purkinje fibers. *J. Clin. Invest.*, 49:63–77.

30. Bigger, J. T., Jr., and Mandel, W. J. (1970): The effect of lidocaine on conduction in canine Purkinje fibers and at the ventricular muscle-Purkinje fiber junction. *J. Pharmacol. Exp. Ther.*, 172:239–254.

31. Bodewei, R., Hering, S., Lemke, B., Rosenshtraukh, L. V., Undrovinas, A. I., and Wollenberg, A. (1982): Characterization of the fast sodium current in isolated rat myocardial cells: Simulation of the clamped membrane potential. *J. Physiol. (Lond.)*, 325:301–315.

32. Brown, A. M., Lee, K. S., and Powell, T. (1981): Voltage clamp and internal perfusion of single rat heart muscle cells. *J. Physiol. (Lond.)*, 318:455–477.

33. Brown, A. M., Lee, K. S., and Powell, T. (1981): Sodium currents in single rat heart muscle cells. *J. Physiol. (Lond.)*, 318:479–500.

34. Brown, H., and DiFrancesco, D. (1980): Voltage-clamp investigations of membrane currents underlying the pace-maker activity in rabbit sinoatrial node. *J. Physiol. (Lond.)*, 308:331–351.

35. Bustamante, J. O., and MacDonald, T. F. (1983): Sodium currents in segments of human heart cells. *Science*, 220:320–321.

36. Cachelin, A. B., de Peyer, J. E., Kokubun, S., and Reuter, H. (1983): Sodium channels in cultured cardiac cells. *J. Physiol. (Lond.)*, 340:389–402.

37. Campbell, T. J. (1983): Resting and rate-dependent depression of maximum rate of depolarization ($\dot{V}_{max}$) in guinea pig ventricular action potentials by mexiletine, disopyramide, and encainide. *J. Cardiovasc. Pharmacol.*, 5:291–296.

38. Cardinal, R., and Sasyniuk, B. (1978): Electrophysiologic effects of bretylium tosylate on subendocardial Purkinje fibers from infarcted canine hearts. *J. Pharmacol. Exp. Ther.*, 204:159–174.

39. Carmeliet, E., and Saikawa, T. (1982): Shortening of the action potential and reduction of pacemaker activity by lidocaine, quinidine and procainamide in sheep cardiac Purkinje fibers—an effect on Na or K currents? *Circ. Res.*, 60:257–272.

40. Chen, C.-M., Gettes, L. S., and Katzung, B. G. (1975): Effect of lidocaine and quinidine on steady-state characteristics and recovery kinetics of dV/dt_{max} in guinea pig ventricular myocardium. *Circ. Res.*, 37:20–29.

41. Clarkson, C. W., and Hondeghem, L. M. (1985): Evidence for a specific receptor site for lidocaine, quinidine, and bupivacaine associated with cardiac sodium channels in guinea pig ventricular muscle. *Circ. Res.*, 56:496–506.

42. Clerc, L. (1976): Directional differences of impulse spread in trabecular muscle from mammalian heart. *J. Physiol. (Lond.)*, 255:335–346.

43. Cohen, I. R., Falk, R. P., and Kline, R. P. (1981): Membrane currents following activity in canine cardiac Purkinje fibers. *Biophys. J.*, 33:281–288.

44. Colatsky, T. J. (1980): Voltage clamp measurements of sodium channel properties in rabbit cardiac Purkinje fibres. *J. Physiol. (Lond.)*, 305:215–243.

45. Colatsky, T. J. (1982): Mechanisms of action of lidocaine and quinidine on action potential duration in rabbit cardiac Purkinje fibers—an effect on steady state sodium currents? *Circ. Res.*, 50:17–27.

46. Colatsky, T. J. (1982): Quinidine block of cardiac sodium channels is rate and voltage dependent. *Biophys. J.*, 37:343a.

47. Colatsky, T. J., and Tsien, R. W. (1979): Sodium channels in rabbit cardiac Purkinje fibers. *Nature*, 278:261–268.

48. Cooley, J. W., and Dodge, F. A., Jr. (1966): Digital computer solutions for excitation and propagation of the nerve impulse. *Biophys. J.*, 6:583–599.

49. Coraboeuf, E., Deroubaix, E., and Coulombe, A. (1979): The effect of tetrodotoxin on action potentials of the conducting system in the dog heart. *Am. J. Physiol.*, 236:H561–567.

50. Coromilas, H., Weld, F. M., Bigger, J. T., Jr., and Rottman, J. N. (1983): Mechanism of frequency-dependent depression of maximum upstroke velocity by quinidine in ovine cardiac Purkinje fibers. *Clin. Res.*, 30:180a.

51. Coronado, R., and Latorre, R. (1982): Detection of K^+ and Cl^- channels from calf cardiac sarcolemma in planer lipid bilayer membranes. *Nature (Lond.)*, 298:849–852.

52. Corr, P. R., Gross, R. W., and Sobel, B. E. (1985): Amphipathic metabolites and membrane dysfunction in ischemic myocardium. *Circ. Res.*, 55:135–154.

53. Costa, M. R. C., Casnellie, J. E., and Catterall, W. A. (1982): Selective phosphorylation of the alpha subunit of the sodium channel by cAMP-dependent protein kinase. *J. Biol. Chem.*, 257:7918–7921.

54. Courtney, K. R. (1980): Interval dependent effects of small antiarrhythmic drugs on excitability of guinea pig myocardium. *J. Mol. Cell. Cardiol.*, 12:1273–1286.

55. Cranefield, P. F. (1975): *The Conduction of the Cardiac Impulse.* Futura Publishing, Mount Kisco, N.Y.

56. Dahl, G., and Isenberg, G. (1980): Decoupling of heart muscle cells: Correlation with increased cytoplasmic calcium activity and with changes of nexus ultrastructure. *J. Membr. Biol.*, 53:63–75.

57. Davis, L. D., and Temte, J. V. (1969): Electrophysiologic actions of lidocaine on canine ventricular muscle and Purkinje fibers. *Circ. Res.*, 24:639–655.

58. Deitmer, J., and Ellis, D. (1980): The intracellular sodium activity of sheep heart Purkinje fibers: Effects of local anesthetics and tetrodotoxin. *J. Physiol. (Lond.)*, 300:269–282.

59. Deleze, J. (1970): The recovery of resting potential and input resistance in sheep heart injured by knife or laser. *J. Physiol. (Lond.)*, 208:547–562.

60. DeMello, W. C. (1977): *Intercellular Communication.* Plenum Press, New York.

61. DeMello, W. C., and Dexter, D. (1970): Increased rate of sealing in beating heart muscle of the toad. *Circ. Res.*, 26:481–489.

62. DeMello, W. C., Motta, G. E., and Chapeau, M. (1969): A study of the healing-over of myocardial cells of toads. *Circ. Res.*, 24:475–487.

63. Dhalla, N. S., Ziegelhoffer, A., and Hazzow, J. A. (1977): Regulatory role of membrane systems in heart function. *Can. J. Physiol. Pharmacol.*, 55:1211–1234.

64. DiFrancesco, D. (1981): A new interpretation of the pace-maker current in calf Purkinje fibers. *J. Physiol. (Lond.)*, 314:359–376.

65. DiFrancesco, D. (1981): A study of the ionic nature of the pace-maker current in calf Purkinje fibers. *J. Physiol. (Lond.)*, 314:377–393.

66. DiFrancesco, D., and Ojeda, C. (1980): Properties of the current i_f in the sinoatrial node of the rabbit as compared with those of the current i_{K_2} in Purkinje fibres. *J. Physiol. (Lond.)*, 308:353–367.

67. Dominguez, G., and Fozzard, H. A. (1970): Influence of extracellular K^+ concentration on cable properties and excitability of sheep cardiac Purkinje fibers. *Circ. Res.*, 26:565–574.

68. Ebihara, L., Shigeto, N., Lieberman, M., and Johnson, E. A. (1980): The initial inward current in spherical clusters of chick embryonic heart cells. *J. Gen. Physiol.*, 75:437–456.

69. Ebihara, L., Shigeto, N., Lieberman, M., and Johnson, E. A. (1983): A note on the reactivation of the fast sodium current in spherical clusters of embryonic chick heart cells. *Biophys. J.*, 42:191–194.

70. Ebihara, L., and Johnson, E. A. (1980): Fast sodium current in

cardiac muscle. A quantitative description. *Biophys. J.*, 32:779–790.

71. Ehara, T., and Daufmann, T. (1978): The voltage- and time-dependent effects of (−)verapamil on slow-inward current in isolated cat ventricular myocardium. *J. Pharmacol. Exp. Ther.*, 207:49–55.

72. Ehring, G. R., Moyer, J. W., and Hondeghem, L. M. (1982): Implications from electrophysiological differences resulting from small structural changes in antiarrhythmic drugs. *Proc. West. Pharmacol. Soc.*, 25:65–67.

73. Eisenberg, R. S. (1980): Structural complexity, circuit models and ion accumulation. *Fed. Proc.*, 39:1540–1543.

74. Eisner, D. A., Lederer, W. J., and Sheu, S.-S. (1983): Characterization of the electrogenic sodium pump in cardiac Purkinje fibers. *J. Physiol. (Lond.)*, 340:239–358.

75. El-Sherif, N., and Lazzara, R. (1979): Reentrant ventricular arrhythmias in the late myocardial infarction period. 7. Effect of verapamil and D-600 and the role of the "slow channel." *Circulation*, 60:605–615.

76. El-Sherif, N., Scherlag, B. J., Lazzara, R., and Hope, R. P. (1977): Reentrant ventricular arrhythmias in the late myocardial infarction period. 4. Mechanism of action of lidocaine. *Circulation*, 56:395–402.

76a.Ferrier, G. R., and Moe, G. K. (1973): Effect of calcium on acetylstrophan thidin-induced transient depolarizations in canine Purkinje tissue. *Circ. Res.*, 33:508–515.

77. Ferrier, G. R., Saunders, J. H., and Mendez, C. (1973): A cellular mechanism for the generation of ventricular arrhythmias by acetylstrophanthidin. *Circ. Res.*, 32:600–609.

78. Fleckenstein A. (1983): History of calcium antagonists. *Circ. Res. [Suppl. I]*, 52:3–16.

79. Forbes, M. S., and Sperelakis, N. (1984): Ultrastructure of mammalian cardiac muscle. In: *Function of the Heart in Normal and Pathological States*, edited by N. Sperelakis, pp. 1–42. Martinus Nijhoff, Boston.

80. Fozzard, H. A. (1977): Cardiac muscle: Excitability and passive electrical properties. *Prog. Cardiovasc. Dis.*, 9:343–359.

81. Fozzard, H. A. (1979): Conduction of the action potential. In: *The Handbook of Physiology, Vol. 1, The Cardiovascular System*, edited by R. M. Berne, pp. 335–356. Williams & Wilkins, Baltimore.

82. Fozzard, H. A., and Beeler, G. W., Jr. (1975): The voltage clamp and cardiac electrophysiology. *Circ. Res.*, 37:403–413.

83. Fozzard, H. A., Friedlander, I., January, C. T., Makielski, J. C., and Sheets, M. F. (1984): Second order kinetics of Na$^+$ channel inactivation in internally dialysed canine cardiac Purkinje cells. *J. Physiol. (Lond.)*, 353(Abstr.):72.

84. Fozzard, H. A., January, C. T., and Makielski, J. C. (1985): New studies of the excitatory sodium currents in heart failure. *Circ. Res.*, 56:475–485.

85. Fozzard, H. A., and Schoenberg, M. (1972): Strength-duration curves in cardiac Purkinje fibres: Effects of liminal length and charge distribution. *J. Physiol. (Lond.)*, 226:593–618.

86. Fozzard, H. A., and Wasserstrom, J. A. (1984): Voltage dependence of intracellular sodium and control of contraction. In: *Cardiac Electrophysiology and Arrhythmias*, edited by D. P. Zipes and J. Jalife, pp. 51–57. Grune & Stratton, Orlando.

87. Gintant, G. A., Datyner, N. B., and Cohen, I. S. (1984): Slow inactivation of a tetrodotoxin-sensitive current in canine cardiac Purkinje fibers. *Biophys. J.*, 45:509–512.

88. Golden, S. M., Rhoden, V., and Hess, E. J. (1980): Molecular characterization, reconstitution, and "transport-specific fractionation" of the saxitoxin binding protein/Na$^+$ gate of mammalian brain. *Proc. Natl. Acad. Sci. USA*, 77:6884–6888.

89. Grant, A. O., Starmer, C. F., and Strauss, H. C. (1983): Unitary sodium channels in isolated cardiac myocytes of rabbit. *Circ. Res.*, 53:823–829.

90. Grant, A. O., Trantham, J. L., Brown, K. K., and Strauss, H. C. (1982): pH-dependent effects of quinidine on the kinetics of dV/dt_{max} in guinea pig ventricular myocardium. *Circ. Res.*, 50:210–217.

91. Hamill, O. P., Marty, A., Neher, E., Sakmann, B., and Sigworth, F. J. (1981): Improved patch-clamp techniques for high-resolution current recording from cells and cell-free membrane patches. *Pfluegers Arch.*, 391:85–100.

92. Hanke, W., Boheim, G., Barhanin, J., Pauron, D., and Lazdunski, M. (1984): Reconstitution of highly purified saxitoxin-sensitive Na$^+$-channels into planar lipid bilayers. *EMBO J.*, 3:509–515.

93. Hess, P., and Tsien, R. W. (1984): Mechanism of ion permeation through calcium channels. *Nature (Lond.)*, 309:453–456.

94. Hille, B. (1977): Local anesthetics: Hydrophilic and hydrophobic pathways for the drug-receptor reaction. *J. Gen. Physiol.*, 69:497–515.

95. Hille, B. (1984): *Ionic Channels of Excitable Membranes*. Sinauer Associates, Sunderland, Mass.

96. Hodgkin, A. L. (1975): The optimum density of sodium channels in an unmyelinated nerve. *Philos. Trans. R. Soc. Lond. [Biol.]*, 270:297–300.

97. Hodgkin, A. L., and Huxley, A. F. (1952): A quantitative description of membrane current and its application to conduction and excitation in nerve. *J. Physiol. (Lond.)*, 117:500–544.

98. Hodgkin, A. L., and Rushton, W. A. H. (1946): The electrical constants of a crustacean nerve fibre. *Proc. R. Soc. Lond. [Biol.]*, 133:444–479.

99. Hoffman, B. F. (1957): The action of quinidine and procainamide on single fibers of dog ventricle and specialized conducting system. *An. Acad. Bras. Cienc.*, 29:365–368.

100. Hoffman, B. F., and Bigger, J. T., Jr. (1971): Antiarrhythmic drugs. In: *Drill's Pharmacology in Medicine*, edited by J. R. Di Palma, McGraw-Hill, New York.

101. Holland, R. P., and Arnsdorf, M. F. (1981): Nonspatial determinants of electrograms in guinea pig ventricle. *Am. J. Physiol. (Cell Physiol. 9)*, 240:C148–C160.

102. Hondeghem, L., Grant, A. O., and Jensen, R. A. (1974): Antiarrhythmic drug action: Selective depression of hypoxic cardiac cells. *Am. Heart J.*, 87:602–605.

103. Hondeghem, L., and Katzung, B. G. (1977): Time- and voltage-dependent interaction of antiarrhythmic drugs with cardiac sodium channels. *Biochim. Biophys. Acta*, 472:373–398.

104. Hondeghem, L. E., and Katzung, B. G. (1984): Mechanism of action of antiarrhythmic drugs. In: *Function of the Heart in Normal and Pathological States*, edited by N. Sperelakis, pp. 459–476. Martinus Nijhoff, Boston.

105. Hope, R. R., Williams, D., El-Sherif, N., Lazzara, R., and Scherlag, B. J. (1974): The efficacy of antiarrhythmic agents during acute myocardial ischemia and the role of heart rate. *Circulation*, 50:507–514.

106. Hume, J. R., and Giles, W. (1981): Active and passive electrical properties of single bullfrog atrial cells. *J. Gen. Physiol.*, 78:19–42.

107. Hunter, P. J., McNaughton, P. A., and Noble, D. (1975): Analytical models of propagation in excitable cells. *Prog. Biophys. Mol. Biol.*, 30:99–144.

108. Ilvento, J. P., Provet, J., Danilo, P., Jr., and Rosen, M. R. (1982): Fast and slow idioventricular rhythms in the canine heart: A study of their mechanism using antiarrhythmic drugs and electrophysiologic testing. *Am. J. Cardiol.*, 49:1909–1916.

109. Irisawa, H. (1978): Comparative physiology of the cardiac pacemaker mechanism. *Physiol. Rev.*, 58:461–498.

110. Irisawa, H., Noma, A., Kokubun, S., and Kurachi, Y. (1984): Electrogenesis of pacemaker potential as revealed by AV nodal experiments. In: *Function of the Heart in Normal and Pathological States*, edited by N. Sperelakis, pp. 97–107. Martinus Nijhoff, Boston.

111. Isenberg, G., and Trautwein, W. (1974): The effect of dihydroouabain and lithium ions on the outward current in cardiac Purkinje fibers. *Pfluegers Arch.*, 350:41–54.

112. Jack, J. J. B., Noble, D., and Tsien, R. W. (1975): *Electric Current Flow in Excitable Cells*. Clarendon Press, Oxford.

113. Janse, M. J., and Van Capelle, F. J. L. (1982): Electrotonic interactions across an inexcitable region as a cause of ectopic activity in acute regional myocardial ischemia: A study in intact porcine and canine hearts and computer models. *Circ. Res.*, 50:527–537.

114. January, C. T., and Fozzard, H. A. (1984): The effects of membrane potential, extracellular potassium, and tetrodotoxin on the intracellular sodium ion activity of sheep cardiac muscle. *Circ. Res.*, 54:652–665.

115. Jensen, R. A., and Katzung, B. G. (1970): Electrophysiological action of diphenylhydantoin on rabbit atria: Dependence on

stimulation frequency, potassium, and sodium. *Circ. Res.*, 26: 17–27.

116. Johnson, E. A. (1956): The effects of quinidine, procainamide, and pyrilamine on the membrane resting and action potential of guinea pig ventricular muscle fibers. *J. Pharmacol. Exp. Ther.*, 117:237–244.

117. Johnson, E. A., and McKinnon, M. G. (1957): Differential effect of quinidine and pyridamine on the myocardial action potential at various rates of stimulation. *J. Pharmacol. Exp. Ther.*, 120: 460–465.

118. Jones, L. R., Maddock, S. W., and Besch, H. R., Jr. (1980): Unmasking effect of alamethicine on the (Na+-K+)-ATPase beta-adrenergic receptor-coupled adenylate cyclase and cAMP-dependent protein kinase activities of cardiac sarcolemmal vesicles. *J. Biol. Chem.*, 255:9971–9980.

119. Kabela, E. (1973): The effect of lidocaine on potassium efflux from various tissues of dog heart. *J. Pharmacol. Exp. Ther.*, 184: 611–618.

120. Kanaya, S., Arlock, P., Katzung, B. G., and Hondeghem, L. M. (1983): Diltiazem and verapamil preferentially block inactivated calcium channels. *J. Mol. Cell. Cardiol.*, 15:145–148.

121. Kensler, R. W., and Goodenough, D. A. (1980): Isolation of mouse myocardial gap junctions. *J. Cell Biol.*, 86:755–764.

122. Kohlhardt, M., and Fleckenstein, A. (1977): Inhibition of the slow inward current by nifedipine in mammalian ventricular myocardium. *Naunyn Schmiedebergs Arch. Pharmacol.*, 298: 267–272.

123. Kohlhardt, M., and Mnich, Z. (1978): Studies on the inhibitory effect of verapamil on the slow inward current in mammalian ventricular myocardium. *J. Mol. Cell. Cardiol.*, 10:1037–1052.

124. Kostyuk, P. G. (1984): Intracellular perfusion of nerve cells and its effects on membrane currents. *Physiol. Rev.*, 64:435–454.

125. Kostyuk, P. G., Mironov, S. L., and Shuba, Y. M. (1983): Two ion-selecting filters in the calcium channel of the somatic membrane of mollusc neurons. *J. Membr. Biol.*, 76:83–93.

126. Krueger, B. R., Worly, J. F., III, and French, R. J. (1983): Single sodium channels from rat brain incorporated into planar bilayer membranes. *Nature (Lond.)*, 303:172–175.

127. Kunze, D. L., and Brown, A. M. (1982): Unitary sodium currents in mammalian ventricular cells. *Physiologist*, 25:300.

128. Lapicque, L. (1970): Recherches quantitative sur l'excitation electriques des nerfs traitee comme un poplarisation. *J. Physiol. (Paris)*, 9:620–635.

129. Lederer, W. J., and Tsien, R. W. (1976): Transient inward current underlying arrhythmogenic effects of cardiotonic steroids in Purkinje fibers. *J. Physiol. (Lond.)*, 263:73–100.

130. Lee, C. O. (1981): Ionic activities in cardiac muscle cells and application of ion-selective microelectrodes. *Am. J. Physiol. (Heart Circ. Physiol.* 10), 241:459–478.

131. Lee, C. O., and Fozzard, H. A. (1975): Activities of potassium and sodium in rabbit heart muscle. *J. Gen. Physiol.*, 65:694–708.

132. Lee, C. O., and Fozzard, H. A. (1976): Influence of changes in external potassium and chloride ions on membrane potential and intracellular potassium ions in rabbit ventricular cells. *J. Physiol. (Lond.)*, 256:663–689.

133. Lee, C. O., and Vassalle, M. (1983): Modulation of intracellular Na+ activity and cardiac force by norepinephrine and Ca++. *Am. J. Physiol.*, 244:c110–c114.

134. Lee, K. S., Weeks, T. A., Kao, R. L., Akaike, N., and Brown, A. M. (1979): Sodium current in single heart muscle cells. *Nature (Lond.)*, 278:269–270.

135. Levinson, S. R., and Meves, H. (1975): The binding of tritiated tetrodotoxin to squid giant axons. *Philos. Trans. R. Soc. Lond. [Biol.]*, 270:349–352.

136. Lieberman, M. M., Kootsey, M., Johnson, E. A., and Sawonobari, T. (1973): Slow conduction in cardiac muscle. *Biophys. J.*, 13: 37–55.

137. Linden, J., and Brooker, G. (1980): The influence of resting membrane potential on the effect of verapamil on atria. *J. Mol. Cell. Cardiol.*, 12:325–331.

138. Lowenstein, W. R. (1981): Junctional intercellular communication: The cell-to-cell membrane channel. *Physiol. Rev.*, 61:829–913.

139. McAllister, R. E., Noble, D., and Tsien, R. W. (1975): Reconstruction of the electrical activity of cardiac Purkinje fibers. *J. Physiol. (Lond.)*, 251:1–58.

140. McDonald, T. F., Pelzer, D., and Trautwein, W. (1980): On the mechanism of slow calcium channel block in heart. *Pfluegers Arch.*, 385:175–179.

141. Makielski, J. C., January, C. T., Sheets, M. F., and Undrovinas, A. I. (1983): Single cardiac Purkinje cells for internal perfusion and voltage clamp. *Biophys. J.*, 41:404a.

142. Man, R. Y. K., and Dressel, P. E. (1979): A specific effect of lidocaine and tocainide on ventricular conduction of mid-range extra systoles. *J. Cardiovasc. Pharm.*, 1:329–342.

143. Miller, C., and Racker, E. (1976): Ca induced fusion of fragmented sarcoplasmic reticulum with artificial planar bilayers. *J. Membr. Biol.*, 30:283–300.

144. Moyer, J., and Hondeghem, L. M. (1983): Characterization of activation and inactivation block in a series of aprindine derivatives using voltage clamp technique. *Fed. Proc.*, 42:634.

145. Nakajima, H., Hoshiyama, M., Yamashita, K., et al. (1975): Effect of diltiazem on electrical and mechanical activity of isolated cardiac ventricular muscle on guinea pig. *Jpn. J. Pharmacol.*, 25:383–392.

146. Nayler, W. G., and Grinwald, P. (1981): Calcium entry blockers and myocardial function. *Fed. Proc.*, 40:2855–2861.

147. Noble, D. (1962): Modification of the Hodgkin-Huxley equations applicable to Purkinje fibre action and pacemaker potentials. *J. Physiol. (Lond.)*, 160:317–352.

148. Noble, D., and Stein, R. B. (1966): The threshold conditions for initiation of action potentials by excitable cells. *J. Physiol. (Lond.)*, 187:129–162.

149. Page, E., and Fozzard, H. (1973): Capacitive, resistive, and syncytial properties of heart muscle—ultrastructural and physiological considerations. In: *The Structure and Function of Muscle, Vol. II, Structure, Part 2*, edited by J. Bourne, pp. 91–158. Academic Press, New York.

150. Page, E., and Shibata, Y. (1981): Permeable junctions between cardiac cells. *Annu. Rev. Physiol.*, 43:431–441.

151. Papp, J. G., and Vaughan Williams, E. M. (1969): The effect of bretylium on intracellular cardiac action potentials in relation to its antiarrhythmic and local anesthetic action. *Br. J. Pharmacol.*, 37:380–390.

152. Patlak, J. (1984): Two components of single Na channel inactivation in patch recordings from dissociated cells. *Biophys. J.*, 45: 185a.

153. Raschak, M. (1975): Relationship of antiarrhythmic to inotropic activity and antiarrhythmic qualities of the optical isomers of verapamil. *Naunyn Schmiedebergs Arch. Pharmacol.*, 294:285–291.

154. Reuter, H., and Scholz, H. (1977): A study of the ion selectivity and the kinetic properties of the calcium dependent slow inward current in mammalian cardiac muscle. *J. Physiol. (Lond.)*, 264: 17–47.

155. Reuter, H., Stevens, C. F., Tsien, R. W., and Yellen, G. (1982): Properties of single calcium channels in cardiac cell culture. *Nature*, 297:501–504.

156. Roden, D. M., and Hoffman, B. F. (1985): Action potential prolongation and induction of abnormal automaticity by low quinidine concentrations in cardiac Purkinje fibers. *Circ. Res.*, 56:857–867.

157. Rosen, M. R., Gelband, H., and Hoffman, B. F. (1972): Canine electrocardiographic and cardiac electrophysiologic changes induced by procainamide. *Circulation*, 46:528–536.

158. Rushton, W. A. (1937): Initiation of the propagated disturbance. *Proc. R. Soc. Lond. [Biol.]*, 124:210–243.

159. Sanchez-Chapula, J., and Josephson, I. R. (1983): Effects of phenytoin on the sodium current in isolated rat ventricular cells. *J. Mol. Cell. Cardiol.*, 15:515–522.

160. Sanguinetti, M. C., and Kass, R. S. (1984): Voltage-dependent block of calcium channel current in the calf cardiac Purkinje fiber by dihydropyridine calcium channel antagonists. *Circ. Res.*, 55:336–348.

161. Sano, T. N., Takayama, N., and Shimamoto, T. (1959): Directional difference of conduction velocity in cardiac ventricular syncytium studied by microelectrodes. *Circ. Res.*, 7:262–267.

162. Sawicki, G. J., and Arnsdorf, M. F. (1985): The effects of lidocaine on the electrophysiologic properties of cardiac Purkinje fibers exposed to lysophosphatidylcholine, a toxic metabolite of ischemia. *J. Pharmacol. Exp. Ther.*, 235:829–838.

163. Sheu, S.-S., Korth, M., Lathrop, D. A., and Fozzard, H. A. (1980): Intra- and extracellular K$^+$ and Na$^+$ activities and resting membrane potential in sheep cardiac Purkinje strands. *Circ. Res.,* 47:692–700.

164. Singer, S. J., and Nicholson, G. L. (1972): The fluid mosaic model of the structure of membranes. *Science,* 175:720–731.

165. Singer, D. H., Lazzara, R., and Hoffman, B. F. (1967): Interrelationships between automaticity and conduction in Purkinje fibers. *Circ. Res.,* 21:537–558.

166. Singh, B. N., and Vaughan Williams, E. M. (1971): Effect of altering potassium concentration on the action of lidocaine and diphenylhydantoin on rabbit and ventricular muscle. *Circ. Res.,* 29:286.

167. Sjöstrand, F. S., and Andersson, E. (1954): Electron microscopy of the intercalated discs of cardiac muscle tissue. *Experientia,* 10: 369–372.

168. Sommer, J. R., and Dolber, P. C. (1987): Cardiac muscle: The ultrastructure of its cells and bundles. In: *Normal and Abnormal Conduction of the Heart Beat,* edited by A. Paes de Carvalho, B. F. Hoffman, and M. Lieberman. Futura Publishing, Mt. Kisco, N.Y. (*in press*).

169. Sommer, J. R., and Johnson, E. A. (1979): Ultrastructure of cardiac muscle. In: *Handbook of Physiology, Vol. 1, The Cardiovascular System, Chapter 5, The Heart,* edited by R. M. Berne, N. Sperelakis, and S. R. Geiger, pp. 113–186. Williams & Wilkins, Baltimore.

170. Spach, M. S., Miller, W. T., Dolber, P. C., Kootsey, J. M., Sommer, J. R., and Mosher, C. E., Jr. (1982): The functional role of structural complexities in the propagation of depolarization in the atrium of the dog. Cardiac conduction disturbances due to discontinuities of effective axial resistivity. *Circ. Res.,* 50:175–191.

171. Spach, M. S., Miller, W. T., Geselowitz, D. B., Barr, R. C., Kootsey, J. M., and Johnson, E. A. (1981): The discontinuous nature of propagation in normal canine cardiac muscle. Evidence for recurrent discontinuities of intracellular resistance that affect membrane currents. *Circ. Res.,* 48:39–54.

172. Sperelakis, N. (1979): Origin of the cardiac resting potential. In: *Handbook of Physiology, Vol. 1, The Cardiovascular System,* edited by R. M. Berne, N. Sperelakis, and S. R. Geiger, pp. 187–267. Williams & Wilkins, Baltimore.

173. Sperelakis, N. (1984): The slow action potential and properties of the myocardial slow channels. In: *Function of the Heart in Normal and Pathological States,* edited by N. Sperelakis, pp. 159–186. Martinus Nijhoff, Boston.

174. Staehlin, L. A., and Hull, B. E. (1978): Junctions between living cells. *Sci. Am.,* 238:140–152.

175. Starmer, C. F., Grant, A. O., and Strauss, H. (1984): Mechanisms of use-dependent block of sodium channels in excitable membranes by local anesthetics. *Biophys. J.,* 46:15–27.

176. Strauss, H. C., Bigger, J. T., Thomas, J., Bassett, A. L., and Hoffman, B. F. (1968): Actions of diphenylhydantoin on the electrical properties of isolated rabbit and canine atria. *Circ. Res.,* 23:463–477.

177. Sung, R. J., Shen, E. N., DiCarlo, L., et al. (1983): Beta-adrenergic blockade in the treatment of ventricular tachycardia: Effects on reentry, automaticity, and triggered activity. *Clin. Res.,* 31:220A.

178. Tanaka, J. C., Eccleston, J. F., and Barchi, R. L. (1983): Cation selectivity characteristics of the reconstituted voltage-dependent sodium channel purified from rat skeletal muscle sarcolemma. *J. Biol. Chem.,* 258:7519–7526.

179. Tasaki, I., and Hagiwara, S. (1957): Capacity of muscle fiber membrane. *Am. J. Physiol.,* 188:423–429.

180. Ten Eick, R., Matsuki, N., Quandt, F., and Yeh, J. (1982): Na channels in cultured embryonic chick ventricle: Single channel conductance and open time: Effect of TTX. *Physiologist,* 25:198.

181. Trautwein, W. (1973): Membrane currents in cardiac muscle fibers. *Physiol. Rev.,* 53:793–835.

182. Trautwein, W., Pelzer, D., and McDonald, T. F. (1983): Interval and voltage-dependent effects of the calcium channel blocking agents D-600 and AQA39 on mammalian ventricular muscle. *Circ. Res.,* 52:I-68.

183. Tsien, R. W. (1983): Calcium channels in excitable cell membranes. *Annu. Rev. Physiol.,* 45:341–358.

184. Vassalle, M., and Lee, C. O. (1984): The relationship among intracellular sodium activity, calcium, and strophanthidin inotropy in canine cardiac Purkinje fibers. *J. Gen. Physiol.,* 83:287–307.

185. Vaughan Williams, E. M. (1970): Classification of antiarrhythmic drugs. In: *Symposium on Cardiac Arrhythmias,* edited by E. Sandoe, E. Flensted-Jensen, and K. H. Olesen, pp. 449–472. Astra, Sodertalje, Sweden.

186. Wasserstrom, J. A., and Ferrier, G. R. (1982): Effects of phenytoin and quinidine on digitalis-induced oscillatory afterpotentials, aftercontractions, and inotropy in canine ventricular tissues. *J. Mol. Cell. Cardiol.,* 14:725–736.

187. Wasserstrom, J. A., Sawicki, G. J., and Arnsdorf, M. F. (1982): Effects of tetrodotoxin (TTX), encainide and propranolol on intracellular sodium ion activity, twitch tension and action potentials in sheep cardiac Purkinje fibers. *Circulation [Suppl. II],* 66:II-292.

188. Wasserstrom, J. A., Schwartz, D. J., and Fozzard, H. A. (1984): Relation between intracellular sodium and twitch tension in sheep cardiac Purkinje strands exposed to cardiac glycosides. *Circ. Res.,* 52:697–705.

189. Wasserstrom, J. A., Scanley, B. E., and Fozzard, H. A. (1983): Effects of isoproterenol, phenytoin and quinidine on digitalis-inhibited Na pump in sheep cardiac Purkinje fibers. *Circulation,* 68(Abstr.):II-297.

190. Weidmann, S. (1952): The electrical constants of Purkinje fibres. *J. Physiol. (Lond.),* 118:348–360.

191. Weidmann, S. L. (1955): Effects of calcium ions and local anesthetics on electrical properties of Purkinje fibers. *J. Physiol. (Lond.),* 129:568–582.

192. Weidmann, S. (1966): The diffusion of radiopotassium across intercalated disks of mammalian cardiac muscle. *J. Physiol. (Lond.),* 187:323–342.

193. Weidmann, S. L. (1970): Electrical constants of trabecular muscle from mammalian heart. *J. Physiol. (Lond.),* 210:1041–1053.

194. Wit, A. L., Steiner, C., and Damato, A. N. (1970): Electrophysiologic effects of bretylium tosylate on single fibers of the canine specialized conducting system and ventricle. *J. Pharmacol. Exp. Ther.,* 173:344–356.

195. Wyndham, C. R. C., Arnsdorf, M. F., Levitsky, S., Smith, T. C., Dhingra, R. C., Denes, P., and Rosen, K. (1980): Successful surgical excision of focal paroxysmal atrial tachycardia. Observations in vivo and in vitro. *Circulation,* 62:1365–1372.

The Heart and Cardiovascular System,
edited by H. A. Fozzard et al.
Raven Press, New York © 1986.

CHAPTER 57

Effect of Ischemia on Cardiac Electrophysiology

Leonard S. Gettes

Study of the electrophysiological changes induced by acute ischemia has occupied the efforts of basic and clinical electrophysiologists for many years. The use of microelectrodes, plunge wire electrodes, and intracardiac electrodes has established the phenomenology of the electrical changes associated with acute ischemia. These studies have shown that acute ischemia causes depolarization of the resting membrane, a decrease in the rate of rise and overshoot of the action potential upstroke, and a decrease in action potential duration (64,136,199,214). Conduction speeds transiently (67,112) and then slows until it becomes fractionated or blocked (23,134,251,266). The refractory period in the ischemic zone first shortens (26,68,238) and then lengthens (64,68,213), and the dispersion of the recovery of excitability increases (9,68,98,167,213). A border zone can be demonstrated at the lateral margin of the ischemic area (68,104,125), and injury currents across this border have been measured (3,126,148,186,216). Ventricular premature beats occur commonly and frequently initiate ventricular tachycardia and/or ventricular fibrillation (85,100,101,103,135,220,266,268).

These electrical abnormalities result from the metabolic, ionic, and neurohumoral changes that occur when coronary flow is abruptly interrupted. Thus, an understanding of these electrical changes requires an appreci-

ation of the metabolic, ionic, and neurohumoral events, their effects on membrane structure and function, the translation of the membrane changes into the observed changes in action potential of single cells and fibers, the relationship between these action potential changes and the more global electrophysiological changes seen in the intact heart, and the mechanism whereby these more global changes result in disturbances of cardiac rhythm. Each of these topics will be discussed in this chapter.

METABOLIC, IONIC, AND NEUROHUMORAL CHANGES

Acute ischemia is composed of three essential components: (a) abrupt deprivation of oxygen and metabolic substrates, (b) absence of inflow and outflow, leading to accumulation of the metabolic end products of anaerobic metabolism in the extracellular space, and (c) activation of autonomic reflexes.

The abrupt interruption of coronary flow rapidly lowers the PO_2 in the involved tissue to close to 0 mm Hg (219). Anaerobic glycolysis occurs but is unable to maintain the supply of high-energy phosphates. Within the first 5 min of coronary occlusion, 80% of creatine phosphate is lost (24), and within 15 min the ATP level has decreased by 80% (21,129,203). Intracellular acido-

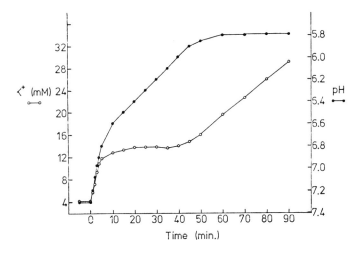

FIG. 1. Simultaneous changes in extracellular potassium and pH from the center of the ischemic zone recorded by ion-selective electrodes following ligation of the left anterior descending coronary artery in the pig.

sis occurs primarily as a result of ATP hydrolysis (90) and is estimated to exceed one pH unit within 30 min (91,195). The level of PCO_2 rises in the extracellular space (34,146,190), extracellular pH falls (45,73,82,107,255), and lactate, phosphate, potassium, free fatty acids, fatty acid esters, phospholipids, and adenosine accumulate in the extracellular space (35,37,48,105,140,149,150,173,180,192,203,262). The recent use of ion-sensitive electrodes has permitted precise characterization of the changes in potassium and pH that occur in the extracellular space following coronary occlusion. The change in potassium consists of three phases (105,149,262) (Fig. 1). The initial phase begins within 30 sec of onset of acute ischemia and lasts from 5 to 15 min. During this period, potassium rises rapidly, achieving levels as high as 15 mM (105,149,264). This is followed by a 10- to 15-min period during which potassium does not change or may actually decline slightly. Weiss and Shine (262) have attributed this plateau to activation of the sodium-potassium pump, because it is prevented by application of acetyl strophanthidin in doses adequate to suppress sodium-potassium ATPase activity.

Following the plateau phase, potassium again begins to rise, but at a slower rate than in the initial phase. This third phase, or slowly rising phase, is thought to mark the period of irreversibility or cell death. It corresponds to the point at which ATP becomes irreversibly depleted (129) and at which extracellular pH decreases to approximately 6.0 (Fig. 1). Weiss and Shine (262,263) have shown that the rate of potassium efflux is slowed and its magnitude diminished by lowering extracellular calcium and by lowering temperature. In their study, the change in potassium was also rate-dependent. However, in other studies (105,149) the potassium rise was independent of the change in heart rate, at least within the physiological range. Kleber (150) has postulated that the increase in extracellular potassium is due to increased potassium efflux that is related to intracellular formation of weak acids during aerobic metabolism, increased permeability of the membrane to lactate and phosphate ions, and secondary redistribution of potassium. Mather and Case (173) studied the changes in coronary sinus potassium, phosphate, and lactate during low-flow ischemia and showed that the molar ratio of lactate to potassium to phosphate was 5:2:1.

The rise in extracellular potassium is accompanied by a fall in extracellular pH, but the characteristics of the changes in potassium and pH differ. The pH level falls continuously and without a plateau until the maximum level of approximately 6.0 is reached (Fig. 1). Thereafter, pH remains relatively constant as the change in extracellular potassium enters its third, or slowly rising, phase.

Reflexly mediated changes in the autonomic nervous system occur following coronary occlusion. Brown (28) and Malliani et al. (170) have reported that occlusion of the left anterior descending coronary artery in cats results in an increased discharge rate in preganglionic fibers of the thoracic sympathetic ganglia. Similar results have been observed by others (168,239). Uchida and Murao have reported that potassium, acidosis, and bradykinins are each capable of stimulating the sympathetic afferents (240–242). Endogenous myocardial catecholamines are released, leading to a decrease in myocardial catecholamine stores (107) and an increase in

TABLE 1. *Effects of some of the constituents of ischemia on action potential characteristics, conduction, and refractoriness*

	RmP	$\dot{V}_{max}$	AP duration	Recovery of $\dot{V}_{max}$	Conduction velocity	Refractoriness
Hypoxia	↓	↓	↓	↑ (in K-depolarized fibers)	↓	Variable
↑ K$_+$	↓	↓	↓	↑	Variable	Variable
↓ Ph	↓	↓	Variable	← →	↓	← →
β-adrenergic agonists	← →	May ↑	Variable	?	May ↑	Variable
α-adrenergic agonists	← →	?	↑	?	?	May lengthen
Acetylcholine	↓	?	↓	?	May ↓	↓
Lysophospholipids	↓	↓	↓	?	↓	?

↑ increases or prolongs; ↓ decreases or shortens; ← → no change; ? not reported.

catecholamines in the coronary sinus (158). There are also increases in circulating epinephrine and norepinephrine following coronary ligation (36,215). Parasympathetic reflexes are also activated by acute coronary occlusion (170).

These metabolic, ionic, and neurohumoral changes induce a variety of action potential changes (Table 1). However, the changes are not uniform across the ischemic area, and multiple border zones are formed (65,105,159,255). Injury currents are generated, changes in impulse formation and propagation occur, and abnormal beats and rhythms emerge (67,84,85,127,182, 224,262,266,268).

EFFECTS OF INDIVIDUAL COMPONENTS OF ISCHEMIA ON ELECTROPHYSIOLOGICAL CHARACTERISTICS OF SINGLE FIBERS

Hypoxia

The dominant effect of hypoxia is to shorten the action potential duration in all cardiac cell types (114,174,182,234). This effect, which is potentiated by lowering extracellular glucose and is prevented by increasing extracellular glucose (174), has been linked to a decrease in glycolytically generated ATP. It is mediated by an increase in the time-independent potassium outward currents (248,249), leading to increased potassium efflux from the cell (201,212,248). This mechanism probably explains a decrease in resting membrane potential that ranges from 5 to 15 mV in normal cells (114,174,182,212) and may be more pronounced in cells depolarized by increasing extracellular potassium (182). In normal fibers, hypoxia causes no change or only a slight decrease in the maximum rate of rise of the action potential upstroke ($\dot{V}_{max}$) even in the presence of a reduced glucose concentration (79,152,212,217). This effect of hypoxia is more pronounced in potassium-depolarized fibers (152). Kodama et al. (152) have also shown that hypoxia has no effect on the recovery of $\dot{V}_{max}$ when potassium is 5.4 mM, as determined in progressively earlier premature responses, but it accentuates the prolongation of the recovery of $\dot{V}_{max}$ that occurs when extracellular potassium is increased (88) (Fig. 2). In contrast to the effect of hypoxia on the action potential upstroke in premature beats, its effects on the action potential duration in premature responses and the time course of the restitution of the action potential duration have not been determined. It is possible that the increased potassium efflux in the non-premature response may alter these characteristics.

It has been suggested that hypoxia decreases the magnitude of the slow, calcium-sensitive inward current (212). However, Vleugels et al. (249) found no such decrease in voltage-clamped papillary muscles.

The combined effects of hypoxia on an action potential

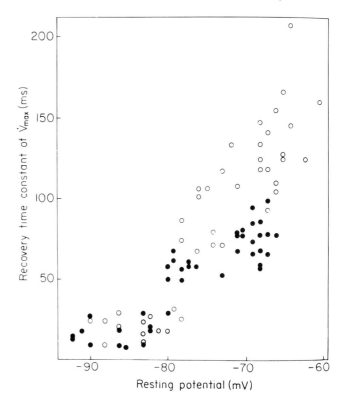

FIG. 2. Resting membrane potential and time constant of recovery of $\dot{V}_{max}$ in guinea pig papillary muscle recorded when potassium was 5, 10, and 12 mM in the absence (*filled circles*) and presence (*open circles*) of hypoxia. Note that the decrease in resting potential induced by hypoxia was more pronounced in the potassium-depolarized cells and that hypoxia prolonged the recovery of $\dot{V}_{max}$ only at the higher potassium levels when resting potential was less negative than −75 mV. (From ref. 152, with permission.)

duration and on the recovery of $\dot{V}_{max}$ probably account for the shortening of the refractory period that occurs when extracellular potassium is 5.4 mM or less and the unchanged or lengthened refractory period that occurs when hypoxia is introduced at higher levels of extracellular potassium (117).

Wojtczak (274) reported that the combination of hypoxia and a decreased concentration of extracellular glucose increased internal longitudinal resistance in cow trabeculae. He postulated that this resistance increase is mediated by an increase in cytoplasmic calcium. Ikeda and Hiraoka (118) demonstrated a hypoxia-induced increase in internal longitudinal resistance even in the absence of glucose. Furata et al. (79) attributed the hypoxia-induced slowing of conduction in rabbit papillary muscles that occurred in the absence of a decrease in $\dot{V}_{max}$ to this effect. It should be noted, however, that Gettes et al. (86) were unable to demonstrate an increase in internal longitudinal resistance in guinea pig papillary muscles perfused with hypoxic glucose-containing solution when potassium was 5.4 mM, although slight increases in longitudinal resistance did occur at higher levels of extracellular potassium. The differences in the results of the various studies concerning the effects of hypoxia on resting membrane potential, $\dot{V}_{max}$, and longitudinal resistance observed in apparently similar experimental models may be due to the differences in PO_2 at the cell surface. In those studies in which PO_2 in the bath was measured, values from less than 5 to more than 40 mm Hg were reported. If the effects of hypoxia are mediated by changes in cellular metabolism, the actual value of PO_2 at the cell surface will be critically important. However, the critical level of PO_2 at which these changes occur has not been determined.

Potassium

An increase in extracellular potassium activity depolarizes the resting membrane, reduces the maximum rate of rise of the action potential upstroke ($\dot{V}_{max}$), lowers the action potential amplitude and plateau potential, accelerates the slope of rapid repolarization, and, in Purkinje fibers, decreases the rate of spontaneous diastolic depolarization (89,109,232,257,259). The change in resting membrane potential associated is due primarily to the change in the potassium equilibrium potential (E_K) (109,260), and the change in $\dot{V}_{max}$ can be attributed primarily to inactivation of the rapid sodium inward current that is dependent on the membrane potential at the onset of depolarization (88,257). However, the precise relationship between sodium channel availability and $\dot{V}_{max}$ of the action potential upstroke has not been uniformly agreed on, although it is probably nonlinear (47). Moreover, Kishida et al. (147) have shown in guinea pig papillary muscles that increasing the extracellular potassium concentration above 11.5 mM causes changes in $\dot{V}_{max}$ that are partially independent of the change in resting membrane potential. They attributed the membrane-potential-independent effect to an increase in potassium conductance resulting in an increase in the background outward current. The decrease in sodium inward current induced by the change in resting potential is responsible for the decrease in action potential overshoot, while the shortening of the action potential duration and suppression of spontaneous depolarization can be attributed to an increase in potassium conductance (259).

An increase in extracellular potassium also prolongs the recovery of $\dot{V}_{max}$ following a preceding depolarization (88) (Fig. 3). This prolongation is voltage-dependent, i.e., the more depolarized the membrane, the longer the time constant of the recovery of $\dot{V}_{max}$. The effect of this phenomenon is to prolong the recovery of excitability beyond the end of the action potential and thereby to dissociate action potential duration and refractoriness (*vide infra*).

Increasing extracellular potassium exerts a biphasic effect on excitability and conduction, first increasing these parameters and then, as potassium is further

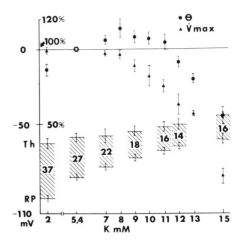

FIG. 3. Effects of changing extracellular potassium from 5.4 to 2.0 mM and from 5.4 to 15.0 mM on changes in conduction velocity (*circles*), $\dot{V}_{max}$ (*triangles*), resting potential (RP), threshold potential (TP), and the mV difference between the two (*shaded area*) in guinea pig papillary muscle. Note that conduction slowed when potassium was decreased from 5.4 to 2.0 mM, in spite of no change in $\dot{V}_{max}$, and note that conduction was speeded when potassium was increased from 5.4 to 10 mM, in spite of a decrease in $\dot{V}_{max}$. These changes were attributed to an increase in the mV difference between RP and TP when potassium was lowered and a decrease in the mV difference when potassium was raised. Above K = 10 mM, the difference between RP and TP remained constant, and conduction slowed as $\dot{V}_{max}$ was further decreased. (From ref. 86, with permission.)

raised, causing a decrease in excitability and a slowing of conduction. This biphasic effect has been observed in Purkinje fibers (63), papillary muscles (31,86), and intact hearts (8,68,97) and can be explained by the effects of increasing extracellular potassium on resting potential threshold potential and $\dot{V}_{max}$. Dominguez and Fozzard (63) reported that increasing extracellular potassium decreased threshold as well as resting potential. However, below a potassium of 7 mM in sheep Purkinje fibers and approximately 9 mM in guinea pig papillary muscle (31,86), the changes in resting potential were of greater magnitude than the change in threshold potential. Thus, the mV difference between the two decreased and was apparently a more critical determinant of conduction velocity and excitability than the decrease in $\dot{V}_{max}$. At higher levels of potassium, the changes in threshold potential parallel the changes in resting potential, and the slowing of $\dot{V}_{max}$ secondary to inactivation of the sodium current becomes dominant, resulting in a decrease in excitability and a slowing of conduction (Fig. 3).

Increasing extracellular potassium does not increase internal longitudinal resistance (63,86), and the slowing of conduction can be attributed entirely to the decrease in $\dot{V}_{max}$. The relationship between $\dot{V}_{max}$ and conduction velocity conforms to that expressed by the cable equation for a one-dimensional model (85) (Fig. 4). This predicts

A

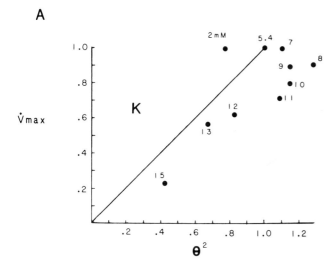

B

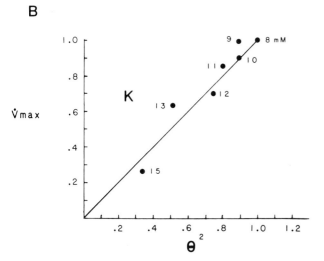

FIG. 4. Relationship between changes in $\dot{V}_{max}$ and changes in Θ^2 (Θ = conduction velocity) as potassium was lowered from 5.4 to 2 mM and raised from 5.4 to 15 mM. The values are taken from Fig. 2. The *solid line* indicates the theoretical relationship predicted from the cable equation assuming no change in other parameters. The values in panel B are replotted from panel A, but referenced against the values at K = 8.0 mM, the level at which the speeding of conduction was maximal. Note that above K = 8.0 mM, the relationship changes in the manner predicted by the theoretical equation. (From ref. 86, with permission.)

that the change in conduction velocity should be linearly related to the square root of the change in $\dot{V}_{max}$ (31,115).

The relationships among the changes in sodium inward current, $\dot{V}_{max}$, and conduction velocity induced by increasing extracellular potassium are complex. The nonlinearity between changes in sodium current and $\dot{V}_{max}$, and the squared relationship between $\dot{V}_{max}$ and conduction velocity, indicate that approximately 90% of the sodium channels must be inactivated or blocked to cause a 25% decrease in conduction velocity. This slowing of conduction will be partially offset by the conduction-speeding effects of an increase in extracellular

potassium. An example of this is seen when extracellular potassium is doubled. Assuming that the resting membrane behaves as a potassium electrode when extracellular potassium is above approximately 3 mM (260), an increase in extracellular potassium from 5.4 to 10.8 mM will cause a 19-mV change in resting potential, i.e., from −85 to −66 mV. According to Cohen et al. (47), this should result in inactivation of approximately 90% of the sodium channels. However, this change in resting potential causes a decrease in $\dot{V}_{max}$ of only 50% (88). Although cable theory predicts that the 50% reduction in $\dot{V}_{max}$ should result in a decrease in conduction velocity of approximately 25%, the effect of the increase in extracellular potassium on threshold potential will counteract some of this conduction slowing, and a decrease in conduction velocity of only 10% will occur (31,86) (Figs. 3 and 4).

The effect of increasing extracellular potassium on refractoriness is also complex, because refractoriness depends on the relationship between the duration of the action potential and the time constant of the recovery from inactivation of $\dot{V}_{max}$. For this reason, a decreased, unchanged, or prolonged refractory period may occur as extracellular potassium is raised.

Acidosis

The effects of acidosis induced either by an increase in PCO_2 (respiratory acidosis) or by replacing bicarbonate with chloride or with weak acids (metabolic acidosis) have been studied in a variety of myocardial tissues (78,130,133,172,182,231,244). Most of these studies have shown that acidosis causes a decrease in conduction velocity, and most (22,85,89,93,95,96,133,172,187,244), but not all (95,130), have reported that acidosis causes a decrease in $\dot{V}_{max}$. Two mechanisms have been postulated to account for a decrease in $\dot{V}_{max}$. One is a decrease in resting potential, with its secondary effect on $\dot{V}_{max}$ (257). The second is a direct effect of acidosis on the relationship between resting potential and $\dot{V}_{max}$. Several investigators (29,30,85,89,93,94,96,98,133,172,187,231, 244) have shown that decreasing pH to the range of 6.5 either by increasing PCO_2 or by decreasing bicarbonate causes a 2- to 5-mV decrease in resting potential, most likely reflecting loss of intracellular potassium (225). Davis et al. (56) reported that reducing pH from 7.2 to 6.0 or 5.2 induced only a slight depolarization of the resting membrane in canine papillary muscle, but caused a progressive depolarization of the resting potential and a progressive decrease in $\dot{V}_{max}$ in false tendons, with eventual development of slow-channel-dependent responses. Kagiyama et al. (133) showed that the effect of respiratory acidosis was greater than that of metabolic acidosis. They attributed this to a greater effect of raising extracellular PCO_2 on intracellular acidosis than that induced by lowering HCO_3^- (196).

Van Bogaert and Carmeliet (22) studied the effects of acidosis induced by lowering HCO_3^- on the relationship between resting potential and $\dot{V}_{max}$ in cow Purkinje fibers and described a shift in this relationship along the voltage axis in the depolarizing direction. A similar shift was described by Kagiyama et al. (133) in guinea pig papillary muscle when pH was lowered from 7.4 to 6.5 by increasing PCO_2 (Fig. 5). This shift was similar to that induced by a fourfold increase in extracellular calcium concentration (15,258,267). Hille (106) noted that acidosis and calcium induced similar shifts in the steady-state voltage dependence of the sodium channel conductance variables. Brown and Noble (30) attributed these changes in conductance variables to the effects of hydrogen and calcium ions on fixed surface charges.

Grant et al. (95) and Kodama et al. (152) studied the effect of decreasing pH to 6.8 on the recovery of $\dot{V}_{max}$. They reported that acidosis did not exert significant effect on this parameter even at potassium levels as high as 12 mM (152). However, these studies did not exclude the possibility that more profound degrees of acidosis might exert an effect similar to that reported when extracellular calcium is raised (88).

Increasing PCO_2 or decreasing bicarbonate in the perfusate has been reported to prolong action potential duration (133,231). Spitzer and Hogan (231) reported that the lengthening of action potential duration induced by lowering bicarbonate was independent of the change in pH. Kagiyama et al. (133) reported that increasing PCO_2 in the extracellular space caused only a transient prolongation of action potential duration but did not significantly alter action potential duration when steady-state conditions were reached.

Acidosis decreases the influx and efflux of calcium (189,197). Davis et al. (56) reported that acidosis induced slow channel responses. Others have reported that acidosis decreases the magnitude of the slow inward current and slows the time constant of activation and inactivation without altering its steady-state characteristics

(38,110,111,154,247,250). The roles of these changes in the electrophysiological effects of ischemia remain to be determined.

Acidosis increases internal longitudinal resistance and by this mechanism decreases cell-to-cell coupling. De Mello (57) reported that intracellular injection of HCl caused a marked increase in intracellular longitudinal resistance in canine Purkinje fibers. Reber and Weingart (202) reported similar results in Purkinje fibers exposed to high PCO_2. Oshita et al. (86,193) studied the effects of acidosis alone and in the presence of high potassium and hypoxia in guinea pig papillary muscle and reported that acidosis to the range of 6.0 caused an increase in internal longitudinal resistance of approximately 20% that was independent of changes in extracellular potassium concentration between 5 and 13 mM. Lowering PO_2 in the presence of high potassium and acidosis resulted in a significantly greater degree of cellular uncoupling. Weiss and Shine (263) showed that the slowing of conduction induced in isolated rabbit septa by high potassium alone was accentuated by concomitant production of extracellular acidosis.

These various effects of acidosis can be attributed to both extracellularly and intracellularly mediated events. The shift in the curve relating $\dot{V}_{max}$ to resting potential and the shift in threshold potential to more positive potentials may be attributed to the effects of extracellular acidosis. The intracellularly mediated effects include leakage of potassium from the intracellular to the interstitial space, which would explain the reduction in resting potential, and an increase in longitudinal resistance leading to cellular uncoupling. It is possible that some of the effects of acidosis may be attributed to changes in calcium activity. However, it should be noted that in the studies of Kagiyama et al. (133), the change in calcium activity induced by acidosis was less than the change in calcium activity required to induce a similar degree of conduction slowing.

The slowing of conduction induced by acidosis cannot

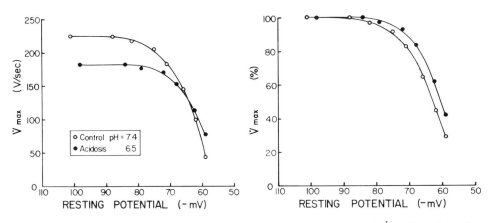

FIG. 5. Effect of acidosis on the steady-state relationship between resting potential and $\dot{V}_{max}$. The data shown in the panel on the left are normalized in the panel on the right and illustrate the shift in the relationship along the voltage axis in a depolarizing direction. (From ref. 133, with permission.)

be attributed entirely to the change in $\dot{V}_{max}$, because the relationship between the changes in conduction velocity and $\dot{V}_{max}$ is greater than that predicted by the equation for a one-dimensional cable (Fig. 6). It is most likely that changes in cell-to-cell uncoupling and/or changes in threshold potential are responsible for this enhanced slowing of conduction.

Sympathetic Agonists

The effects of catecholamines on myocardial fibers depend on whether α-adrenergic and β-adrenergic agonists are studied, whether the fiber is normal or depressed, and whether the depressed fiber is dependent on the rapid sodium-dependent inward current or the slow calcium-dependent inward current. The β-adrenergic agonists increase spontaneous depolarization in both rapid-channel- and slow-channel-dependent fibers (52, 138), increase the rate of rise in slow-channel-dependent action potentials (52,116,117,270,271), hyperpolarize the resting potential of depressed fibers (111), and increase action potential overshoot and plateau voltage in both slow- and rapid-channel-dependent cells (52,205,206,245) (Fig. 7). The β-adrenergic agonists have variously been reported to increase and to decrease action potential duration (14,109,183). These various effects can be attributed to a primary increase in the slow calcium-dependent inward current that is mediated by a catecholamine-induced increase in cyclic AMP (206,237) and to secondary effects of the increase in intracellular calcium and the maximum plateau voltage on the time-dependent and -independent outward currents (13,121,237).

The ability of catecholamines to increase the magnitude of the slow inward current has been demonstrated

in a variety of voltage-clamped fibers (205,206,245) and confirmed in isolated myocytes (122). Moreover, studies using aequorin have demonstrated an increase in free intracellular calcium following exposure to β agonists (1). Evidence has been presented to indicate that the β agonists act by increasing the number of calcium channels without changing their kinetic characteristics (206,207).

Windisch and Tritthart (267) and Arita et al. (5,6) reported that in potassium-depressed fibers having a dual-component upstroke, isoproterenol decreased the $\dot{V}_{max}$ of that component due to the depressed rapid sodium-dependent inward current, while increasing the $\dot{V}_{max}$ of that component due to the slow calcium-dependent inward current.

The increase in the magnitude of the slow inward current explains the increases in action potential amplitude and plateau voltage in rapid- and slow-channel-dependent action potentials and the increases in the rate of spontaneous depolarization and the maximum upstroke velocity of slow-channel-dependent responses, but does not explain the variable effect of the β agonists on the action potential duration. This variable effect can be explained by the interaction of the primary effect on the calcium inward current, which should lengthen action potential duration, and by an increase in the potassium outward current, which should shorten action potential duration. The increase in outward current is caused by the increase in intracellular calcium concentration and the increase in plateau voltage (121,137,205). Several investigators (25,183,200,211) have shown that the effects of the β agonists on action potential duration may be biphasic and may be dependent on the extracellular calcium concentration. When extracellular calcium was less than 1.8 mM, isoproterenol caused tran-

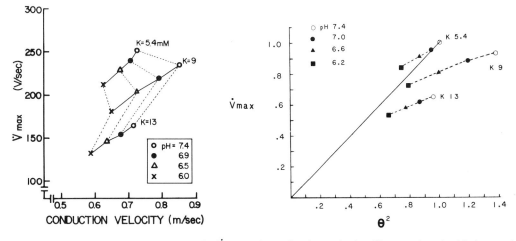

FIG. 6. The panel on the left shows the changes in $\dot{V}_{max}$ and conduction velocity (Θ) associated with increasing potassium from 5.4 to 13 mM (*dotted lines*) and decreasing pH from 7.4 to 6.0 (*solid lines*). Increasing potassium first increases and then decreases Θ in spite of a progressive decrease in $\dot{V}_{max}$. At each level of potassium, acidosis causes decreases in both $\dot{V}_{max}$ and Θ. In the panel on the right, the data are replotted and compared with those predicted by cable theory, assuming no change in any parameter other than $\dot{V}_{max}$ (*solid line*). Note that at each level of potassium, the change in Θ^2 is greater than that predicted by the change in $\dot{V}_{max}$. (From ref. 86, with permission.)

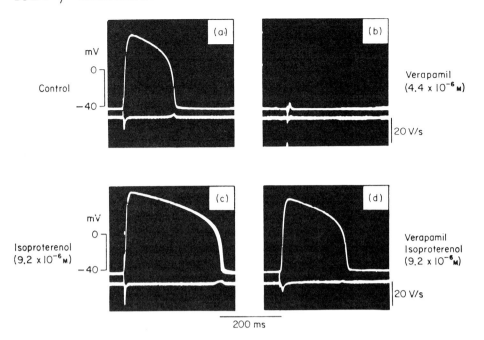

FIG. 7. Effects of verapamil and isoproterenol on slow-channel-dependent action potentials from guinea pig papillary muscle. In each panel the fiber is depolarized to −40 mV by extracellular current injection. The differentiated upstroke is shown in the lower trace of each panel. After exposure to verapamil (panel **b**), the fiber is excitable. Isoproterenol (panel **c**) increases the maximum rate of rise of the upstroke and increases the amplitude and duration of the action potential. Following exposure to verapamil, isoproterenol partially restores the action potential (panel **d**). (From ref. 153, with permission.)

sient lengthening of action potential duration, followed by shortening. When the extracellular calcium concentration was 3.6 mM, isoproterenol caused only shortening of the action potential duration.

The β-adrenergic agonists also cause a transient increase in the dispersion of the recovery of excitability. This is followed by a decrease in dispersion (99). The initial increase may be related to the variable nonsteady-state effects of the β agonists on action potential duration.

The β-adrenergic agonists speed conduction in fibers depolarized by high concentrations of potassium (263).

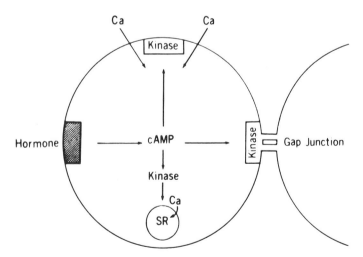

FIG. 8. Different effects of cyclic AMP, including possible activation of a kinase specifically related to the phosphorylation of gap junction proteins. This effect would be expected to improve cell-to-cell coupling by increasing conductance at the gap junction. (From ref. 58, with permission.)

Three possible mechanisms may explain this effect. The first is the hyperpolarization of the resting membrane potential and the associated increases in sodium inward current and $\dot{V}_{max}$ (111). The second is an increase in the magnitude of the slow inward current such that it exceeds the magnitude of the depressed rapid current and becomes responsible for the propagating response (5). The third is an improvement in cell-to-cell coupling (58–60). This latter effect cannot be explained by the increase in intracellular calcium induced by the catecholamines (1), because this would be expected to uncouple cells (61). It has been postulated (60) that the increase in free intracellular calcium may not be able to reach the gap junction because of a low diffusion coefficient in the myoplasm and that the catecholamine-induced rise in cyclic AMP, the mechanism proposed to explain the increase in number of functioning calcium channels, might also increase junctional conductance through activation of specific protein kinases (59,60) (Fig. 8).

The α-adrenergic agonists tend to have effects opposite to those of β-adrenergic agonists. In Purkinje and muscle fibers with normal resting membrane potentials, α-adrenergic stimulation decreases the plateau height slightly and prolongs the action potential duration (94). In addition, the α-adrenergic agonists decrease the spontaneous rate of depolarization in Purkinje fibers (198,210).

Parasympathetic Agonists and Adenosine

The predominant effects of acetylcholine are to shorten action potential duration in all cardiac fiber types and to decrease the rate of spontaneous depolarization (10,55,80,236). These effects result from an increase in potassium conductance during all phases of the action potential (33,80). Acetylcholine is also an inhibitor of the slow calcium-dependent inward current (206,208,233), an effect attributed to inhibition of cyclic AMP activity and possibly to an increase in cyclic GMP (11,254). In many important ways, the cholinergic effects antagonize the effects of β-adrenergic stimulation (165,166,255). Although the precise role of parasympathetic agonists in the electrophysiological changes induced in ventricular and Purkinje fibers by ischemia is not fully understood, it is possible that modulation of adrenergic effects may be important. It has been shown (11) that the shortening of the action potential and the induction of slow channel responses induced by isoproterenol are antagonized by acetylcholine and that the inhibitory effects of cholinergic stimulation on the slow calcium-dependent inward current are particularly pronounced following adrenergic stimulation (19).

Adenosine causes many of the same electrophysiological changes that are induced by acetylcholine (16), particularly the ability to inhibit or modulate the effects of isoproterenol on the slow calcium-dependent inward current (17). Belardenelli and Isenberg (17) have postulated that an ischemia-induced increase in adenosine might prevent the effects of calcium overload induced by β-adrenergic stimulation (180,192).

Fatty Acids

It is clear that acute ischemia induces major changes in fatty acid metabolism that have profound effects on membrane integrity and function (48,140). Although several investigators have suggested a causal relationship between the changes in free fatty acids and their metabolites and the electrophysiological abnormalities induced by ischemia (91,157), the precise role remains an area of active study and discussion. Katz and Messineo (140) proposed three possible mechanisms whereby fatty acids might exert their effects. These include: (a) an increase in free fatty acids, (b) hydrolysis of membrane phospholipids, and (c) intracellular accumulation of long-chain fatty acids. Corr et al. (49) and Cowan and Vaughan Williams (51) found that an increase in free fatty acids failed to induce significant changes in action potential characteristics when glucose was available as a substrate, but did exaggerate the shortening of the action potential duration induced by ischemia. Corr et al. (50) reported that fatty acid esters and lysophospholipids caused changes in action potential characteristics similar to those associated with acute ischemia. Particularly noted were decreases in resting potential, $\dot{V}_{max}$, and action potential duration. These changes were enhanced when pH was lowered to 6.7 (50). Corr and associates have

argued persuasively that these effects are primary causes of the early electrophysiological abnormalities that occur in the setting of acute reversible ischemia. The studies of Arnsdorf and Sawicki (7) in Purkinje fibers and Clarkson and Ten Eick (40) in papillary muscle indicate that the lysophospholipids increase membrane resistance and internal longitudinal resistance and depress the rapid sodium-dependent inward current, the slow calcium-sensitive inward current, and the potassium-sensitive outward currents. These studies have also shown that the low concentrations of lysophospholipids cause an increase in excitability, whereas high concentrations decrease excitability and slow conduction. Thus, in many ways, the effects of lysophospholipids mimic the effect of increasing extracellular potassium while inducing rather nonselective depressant effects on all measured membrane currents. There is continuing discussion whether or not the lysophospholipids contribute in a major way to the early and reversible electrophysiological effects of acute ischemia, particularly because most of the effects of ischemia can be duplicated by models in which ischemia is simulated by changing potassium, PO_2, glucose, pH, and catecholamines in the perfusate. In addition, questions persist whether or not the conditions employed to study the effects of fatty acids and their metabolites *in vitro* duplicate the *in vivo* situation (140). It seems reasonable to conclude that lipid abnormalities are important in the genesis of the structural and functional membrane changes induced by ischemia, but further work will be required to establish their precise contributions to the early electrophysiological abnormalities that characterize acute, reversible ischemia.

Whereas the electrophysiological changes that occur in the setting of acute ischemia can be mimicked by the individual and combined effects of the various recognized components that compose the ischemic process, the relative contribution of each to the changes in the action potential and the changes in the more global electrophysiological properties is not clear. Kleber (149) showed that changes in resting membrane potential associated with acute ischemia could be attributed almost entirely to the increase in extracellular potassium concentration (Fig. 9). Morena et al. (182) showed that action potentials having a configuration similar to those seen during ischemia in the isolated perfused pig heart could be obtained by perfusing the left anterior descending coronary artery with hypoxic, glucose-free solutions in which the potassium was 10 mM and pH was 6.8. They noted that when the coronary artery was perfused with this solution, there was a phase of spontaneous improvement in electrical activity similar to that seen during the acute ischemic process. They attributed this phenomenon to release of catecholamines from cardiac stores, but they were unable to test this hypothesis. The changes in ATP, phosphate, and lactate induced by

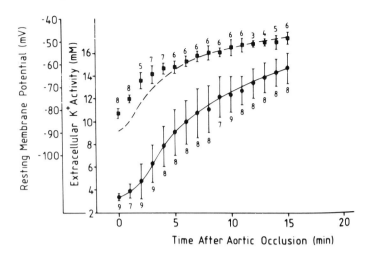

FIG. 9. Time courses of changes in resting membrane potential (*circles*) and extracellular potassium activity (*squares*) during the first 15 min following aortic occlusion in isolated perfused guinea pig heart. The dotted line corresponds to the change in E_K calculated from the values of extracellular K shown, and an assumed intracellular potassium activity of 100 mM. The numbers of observations at each minute are shown. (From ref. 149, with permission.)

ischemia could be reproduced by perfusion of the coronary artery with hypoxic, glucose-free solution alone and did not require an increase in potassium or a lowering in pH. They noted, however, that the changes in T-Q potential in the central area of the ischemic zone were more homogeneous during perfusion of the coronary artery with solutions modified to simulate ischemia than during ischemia induced by occluding the vessel.

Weiss and Shine (263) were able to reproduce most of the ischemia-induced electrophysiological changes induced in the isolated perfused rabbit septum by raising the potassium in the perfusing solution to equal that determined by ion-selective electrodes during ischemia. The pH was lowered to the range of 6.2 to 6.5 by increasing the P_{CO_2} or by adding hydrochloric acid, oxygen was replaced with nitrogen, and norepinephrine was added in concentrations of 10.7 to 10.5 M. Addition of epinephrine caused effects similar to those for norepinephrine. The changes in resting potential, action potential duration, and action potential amplitude were largely reproduced by the combination of increased extracellular potassium and acidosis. However, this combination always caused a greater slowing of conduction than that caused by ischemia. Addition of norepinephrine or epinephrine lessened the conduction slowing, thereby more closely simulating the ischemia-induced change.

These studies, taken together, suggest that the depletion of energy stores is caused by lack of oxygen and lack of glucose. These changes lead to accumulation of potassium, phosphate, lactate, and CO_2 in the extracellular space and to lowering of extracellular pH. The combination of hypoxia, potassium, acidosis, and lack of glucose causes most of the changes in the action potential characteristics, while the increase in local catecholamines may contribute to the transient spontaneous restoration of electrical activity and conduction that has been noted to occur in the setting of acute myocardial ischemia (64,73,105).

RELATIONSHIP OF ELECTROPHYSIOLOGICAL CHANGES IN SINGLE FIBERS TO ELECTROPHYSIOLOGICAL CHANGES IN INTACT HEART

Three types of changes will be considered: (a) changes in excitability and conduction, (b) changes in refractoriness, and (c) inhomogeneities of the changes in conduction and refractoriness and the creation of injury currents.

Changes in Excitability and Conduction

The initial effect of acute ischemia is to render the myocardium slightly more excitable. This is manifest by a decrease in the threshold current and/or stimulus duration required to induce a propagated response (26,68,266). The most likely cause of this effect is the early change in extracellular potassium. Spear and Moore (229) demonstrated a period of supernormal excitability in Purkinje papillary muscle preparations after elevating extracellular potassium. Dominguez and Fozzard (63) noted a shift in the strength–duration curve and a fall in rheobasic current in sheep Purkinje fibers when potassium was raised from 2.7 to 4.0 mM. It has been postulated that this increase in excitability is related to the narrowing of the mV difference between the resting and threshold potentials that occurs as potassium begins to rise. Excitability then decreases as extracellular potassium continues to rise while P_{O_2} and pH fall.

These changes in excitability are paralleled by changes in conduction. Within the first 2 to 3 min of acute coronary ligation, conduction becomes faster (68,112) and then slows progressively. This is frequently followed by spontaneous restoration of conduction (64,105), after which conduction again slows progressively, until, ultimately, impulse propagation is blocked or inhibited (Fig. 10). This latter stage of conduction slowing is rate-

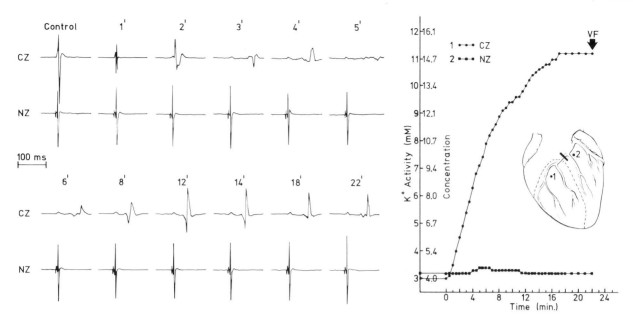

FIG. 10. The bipolar electrograms (**left**) were recorded from the center of the ischemic zone (CZ, position 1 on the diagram of the heart) and from the nonischemic zone (NZ, position 2). The changes in extracellular potassium were recorded from the same positions by potassium-sensitive electrodes. Activation becomes progressively prolonged within 5 min of acute ligation of the left anterior descending coronary artery. This slowing occurs as potassium rises from 4.0 to approximately 8.0 mM. Between 5 and 12 min there is spontaneous restoration of activation while potassium continues to rise, reaching approximately 13.5 mM at 12 min. Thereafter, activation is again delayed as potassium plateaus at a level of approximately 15 mM. (From ref. 105, with permission.)

dependent; i.e., it becomes more pronounced as the heart rate increases (113).

Conduction of the cardiac impulse through the myocardium is a complicated event that depends on interaction between active membrane properties, such as the characteristics of the various ionic currents and the action potential itself, and on passive membrane properties such as membrane resistance and the coupling between Purkinje fibers, between Purkinje and muscle fibers, and between ventricular muscle fibers (74, 91,132,181,183,246). Conduction also depends on fiber orientation and geometry (41,131,227,228). Our understanding of these interactions in the normal myocardium is incomplete and is an area of active ongoing investigation. For this reason, our ability to interpret the changes induced by ischemia is limited.

The initial speeding of conduction that occurs in the setting of ischemia can most likely be attributed to the early increase in extracellular potassium. The subsequent slowing is more pronounced than would be anticipated on the basis of the further increase in potassium (105,182), which by itself should slow conduction in proportion to the square root of changes in upstroke velocity (31,86). The effects of acidosis, hypoxia, and lack of glucose on threshold potential, and cell-to-cell coupling in Purkinje fibers (59,60), at Purkinje-muscle junctions (91,176), and at the gap junctions of the ventricular fibers (86), contribute to this greater degree of conduction slowing. It is also possible that changes

in activation sequence occur that alter the direction of activation and give the appearance of slow conduction.

Conduction frequently improves after the initial period of slowing, despite a continuous increase in extracellular potassium (Fig. 10) and a continued decrease in pH (64,73,105). Morena et al. (182) and Weiss and Shine (262,263) attributed this transient spontaneous improvement in conduction to the effects of endogenously released catecholamine. This hypothesis is supported by the observation of Gilmour et al. (92), who noted that bilateral sympathectomy exacerbated the activation delay induced by acute ischemia in dogs, and by Fleet et al. (73), who reported that the phase of spontaneous improvement progressively diminished when repeated short occlusions were performed, even though the changes in potassium were similar on all occlusions and the fall in pH was slightly less pronounced. They suggested that repetitive occlusions caused a progressive loss of catecholamines from myocardial stores that resulted in the observed changes in activation. However, they did not test this hypothesis.

Following the brief phase of spontaneous improvement, conduction again slows until activation is fractionated or blocked. This phase of conduction slowing is associated with a further rise in extracellular potassium (Fig. 10) and a further fall in pH. It is possible that during this phase, the membrane-potential-independent effects of increasing extracellular potassium on $\dot{V}_{max}$ (147), slowly propagating slow-channel-dependent responses (5,6,52), and greater degrees of cellular uncoupling become important.

Conduction velocities as low as 2 cm/sec have been recorded in single strands (53,272). However, in the intact heart, conduction velocities prior to onset of complete conduction block of less than 12 cm/sec have yet to be recorded (127,148).

Changes in Refractoriness

The refractory period may be defined as the minimum time required for a cell to recover its ability to depolarize after a preceding depolarization. In normal cells of the Purkinje and ventricular muscle fibers, the refractory period is determined principally by the duration of the action potential plateau, because this is the major determinant of the time required for the transmembrane voltage to return to the level at which the inward depolarizing currents and $\dot{V}_{max}$ can be reactivated. Factors that alter the duration of the plateau and/or the reactivation of $\dot{V}_{max}$ of the action potential upstroke can be expected to alter refractoriness. Increased extracellular potassium, hypoxia, and absence of glucose, which are all components of acute ischemia, shorten the action potential duration. The action potential duration is lengthened by extracellular lactate and lowered temperature (109), also components of acute ischemia, and is further influenced by neurotransmitters.

Electrotonic influences from adjacent cells are also important modifiers of the action potential duration and the refractory period. When impulse transmission is blocked, the action potential distal to the area block shortens (176,218). Electrotonically transmitted activity might also increase the action potential duration, and it has been shown to modify the slopes of pacemaker potentials (4,123,124,143,206–209). These electrotonic influences were demonstrated in a variety of models in which active propagation of the action potential was prevented by depolarizing a segment of the preparation or by placing the fiber in a sucrose gap.

In normal fibers, the time constant of reactivation of $\dot{V}_{max}$ is very short (10–20 msec) (88). However, the reactivation time constant of $\dot{V}_{max}$ is voltage-dependent and lengthens as the membrane potential becomes less negative (88) (Fig. 2). For this reason, the refractory period of fibers with lowered resting potentials will exceed the action potential duration, a phenomenon referred to as postrepolarization refractoriness (70,163).

As discussed earlier, the recovery of $\dot{V}_{max}$ is prolonged by high levels of potassium alone as a result of its depolarizing effect on the resting membrane (88). The combination of high potassium and hypoxia has an even greater effect (152). These are the only constituents of ischemia that have thus far been shown to influence this parameter. It should be noted, however, that not all of the constituents have been studied.

The interactions between the changes in action potential duration, the changes in the recovery of $\dot{V}_{max}$, and the effects of electrotonic influences, all of which occur in the setting of ischemia, contribute to the variable changes in refractory period that occur following coronary occlusion (67,68).

The effects of the various factors on the action potential duration and refractoriness have been determined primarily in the nonpremature responses. Their effects in the premature response have not been fully characterized. The duration of the early premature action potential reflects not only the steady-state conductances of the various ionic currents responsible for the plateau but also the background presence of the slowly deactivated outward currents, generated during the preceding nonpremature response, and the effects of ions that accumulate in the extracellular clefts (46,151). The latter two effects will influence the conductance variables of the plateau currents during an early premature response. The influences of these factors on premature responses in Purkinje and ventricular fibers differ (87). In ventricular fibers, the duration of the premature action potential does not shorten until the preceding diastolic interval, i.e., the interval from the end of the preceding repolarization to the depolarization of the premature response has decreased to less than approximately 100 msec (Fig. 11).

In Purkinje fibers, the action potential duration of a late premature response shortens to a value equal to that associated with a steady-state response having the same cycle length. When the diastolic interval shortens to less than approximately 100 msec, the duration of the premature action potential may become shorter than that of the corresponding steady-state cycle length (Fig. 11). Thus, the effects of prematurity on the refractory period of Purkinje and ventricular muscle fibers should differ even under normal conditions. No studies have been performed to characterize the effects of ischemia or the constituents of ischemia on action potential duration or refractoriness in premature beats in either tissue. Nonetheless, studies in normal fibers illustrate that it is the proximity of the onset of the premature response to the repolarization phases of the nonpremature response (i.e., the diastolic interval), rather than the interval between the onsets of the two responses (the coupling interval), that governs the characteristics of the premature response. These studies also suggest that the changes in the characteristics of the premature response induced by ischemia may not be predictable from the changes in the characteristics of the nonpremature response.

Inhomogeneities

Uniform slowing of conduction velocity and shortening of the refractory period would not cause reentry.

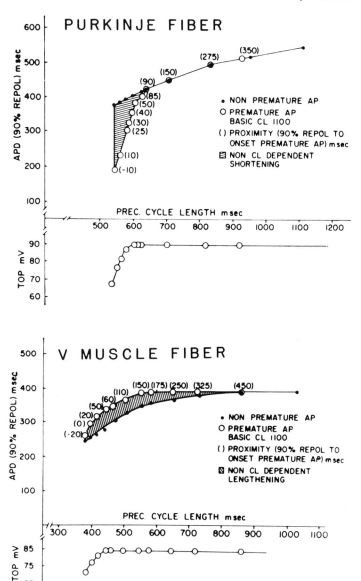

FIG. 11. Durations of premature and nonpremature action potentials having comparable preceding cycle lengths recorded from the right bundle branch (Purkinje fiber) in ventricular (v) muscle of the perfused pig moderator band. In the lower portion of each panel is plotted the membrane potential at the onset of depolarization of the premature action potential (TOP). The closed circles represent the nonpremature action potentials and show the steady-state rate-dependent effects. The open circles represent the premature action potentials. The *shaded area* shows the noncycle-length-(CL)-dependent action potential duration shortening in Purkinje fibers, and the noncycle-length-dependent action potential duration lengthening in the ventricular myocardial fibers. (From ref. 87, with permission.)

Inhomogeneities in these properties are necessary to enable the creation of unidirectional conduction block and the establishment of reentry circuits. Mendez and Moe (175) established that the presence of inhomogeneities in the electrical properties of AV nodal fibers enabled reentry after a properly timed premature response. Han et al. (98,99) showed that lowering the electrical threshold for ventricular fibrillation induced by ischemia, hypoxia, hypothermia, unilateral sympathetic stimulation, and cardioactive drugs correlated with an increase in the inhomogeneities of the recovery of excitability in both nonpremature and premature beats. These results are supported by the observations of others (83,177).

Wallace and Mignone (252) observed repetitive activity after cooling the epicardial surface of the dog ventricle when the refractory period of the cooled epicardium was approximately 150 to 250 msec longer than the refractory period of the noncooled area. Kuo et al. (155) showed that induction of ventricular fibrillation by a single premature stimulus in hearts made inhomogeneous by thermal lesion required that the action potential durations in the cooled and noncooled portions of the myocardium differ by approximately 100 msec.

The changes in extracellular potassium and pH induced by acute ischemia are more marked in the center than in the margin, and more marked in the subendocardium than in the subepicardium (105,255) (Fig. 12). Indeed, differences in potassium of up to 5 mM and in pH of up to 0.5 unit have been observed between subendocardium and subepicardium in the center of the ischemic zone (50,105). Inhomogeneities in extracellular potassium are even recorded by electrodes placed close together at the same myocardial depth (105) (Fig. 12). These inhomogeneities may contribute to the formation of multiple border zones, the most obvious of which is

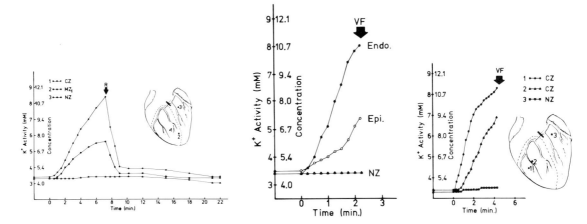

FIG. 12. Inhomogeneities in extracellular potassium recorded from the center (CZ) and margin (MZ) of the ischemic zone (**left panel**), from the endocardium (endo) and epicardium (epi) in the center of the ischemic zone (**middle panel**), and from two closely spaced locations in the mid-myocardium in the center of the ischemic zone (**right panel**) by potassium-sensitive electrodes. In each panel, NZ represents the values in the nonischemic myocardium, and time 0 marks the time at which the left anterior descending coronary artery was occluded. (From ref. 105, with permission.)

at the lateral margin of the ischemic zone. A second discrete border has been recognized between the endocardial fibers and the subendocardial fibers over a distance of approximately 2 mm (71,76,196). There is also a border between the epicardial and subepicardial fibers (204). At the lateral and subendocardial regions, the changes in extracellular potassium and pH that occur during the initial phase may be partially reversed, most likely because of diffusion into the ventricular chamber or into the nonischemic zone (Fig. 13). Differences in lactate, creatine phosphate, and ATP have also been found in these various regions of the ischemic myocardium (125,194) (Fig. 14).

The effects of acute ischemia on sympathetic and parasympathetic discharges are also nonuniform (159) and depend in part on the region involved in the ischemic process. Sympathetic involvement dominates in anterior ischemia, whereas posterior ischemia causes a greater increase in parasympathetic effects (171). A further cause of inhomogeneities is the nonuniform response of Purkinje, subendocardial, and subepicardial fibers to the ionic changes associated with ischemia (93).

The nonuniform changes in resting potential, action potential amplitude, and action potential duration resulting from the various inhomogeneities may be expected to produce inhomogeneous changes in action potential characteristics that are likely to result in inhomogeneous changes in excitability, conduction, and refractoriness and thereby facilitate reentry. Indeed, significant differences in excitability at closely spaced sites within the center of the ischemic zone have been demonstrated (64) (Fig. 15). The inhomogeneous action potential changes are also responsible for generation of injury currents whose magnitudes and directions of flow

vary depending on the location of the more negative potentials. Janse et al. (126) have estimated the magnitudes and directions of injury currents generated at the

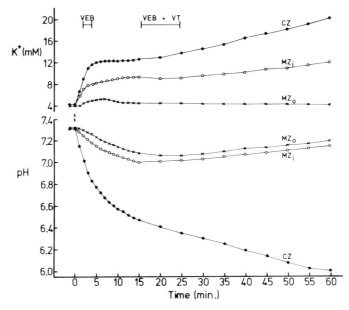

FIG. 13. Changes in extracellular K and pH recorded in the center of the ischemic zone (CZ), on the ischemic side of the lateral margin (MZ_i), and in the prenormal myocardium within 5 mm of the lateral margin (MZ_o) following occlusion of the left anterior descending coronary artery in the open-chest anesthetized pig. Note that in the center (CZ), K rises in three phases as pH progressively falls. On the ischemic side of the lateral margin (MZ_i), there is a slight, transient fall in K after the initial rising phase, while pH progressively increases after its initial decrease. On the normal side of the ischemic margin (MZ_o) there is a progressive decline in K and increase in pH after the initial change. VEB = ventricular extra beats; VT = ventricular tachycardia.

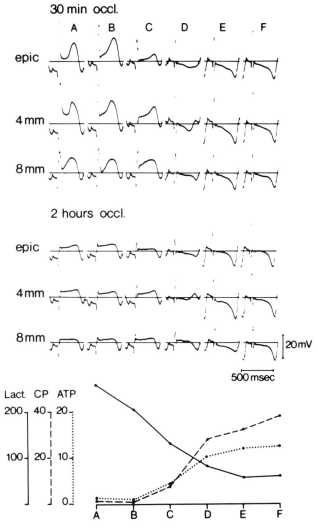

30 min occl.

epic

4 mm

8 mm

2 hours occl.

epic

4 mm

8 mm

|20 mV

500 msec

Lact. CP ATP

200 40 20

100 20 10

0

A B C D E F

FIG. 14. Epicardial and intramural DC electrograms 30 min and 2 hr after occlusion of the left anterior descending coronary artery in the isolated perfused pig heart. Electrodes A–F were in one row separated by 4 mm, extending from the anterior wall of the left ventricular (electrode A), which was in the center of the ischemic zone, to the lateral wall (F), which was in the nonischemic zone. The values of lactate (Lact) creatine phosphate (CP), and ATP shown at the bottom of the figure were obtained 2 hr after occlusion. The figure demonstrates the border zone located between electrodes B and D over a distance of approximately 1.2 cm. (From ref. 125, with permission.)

lateral margin of the ischemic zone by these membrane potential differences throughout the different phases of the cardiac cycle (148) assuming a tissue resistivity of 400 ohms/cm. In diastole, the resting potential is more negative in the normal area than in the ischemic area, and current flows through the intracellular component from ischemic cells to normal cells. The direction of current flow reverses when the cells are excited, because action potential amplitude and plateau voltage are more negative in the ischemic area than in the nonischemic area. The largest flow of injury currents occurs when activation is delayed in the ischemic area (Fig. 16). These investigators estimated current sources on the normal side of the border to be of the order of 2 μA/mm^3 within 15 min of coronary ligation in the isolated perfused pig heart. Current sources calculated during propagation in normal myocardium just ahead of the approaching wave front were on the order of 5 μA/mm^3. Anderson et al. (3) measured injury current in dogs using a uniform resistance of 100 ohms. They reported maximum currents of 1 μA during the T-Q segment, 2 to 3 μA during the S-T segment, and 2 to 5 μA during the T wave. These currents developed within 15 to 30 sec of onset of ischemic and persisted for up to 120 min. These investigators pointed out that the assumption of a uniform resistance did not take into account the anisotropy of resistivity, which depends on fiber direction and orientation and the effect of cellular uncoupling. They attributed an unexpected increase in current 2 hr after occlusion to cellular uncoupling. Other factors might also influence the magnitude of the injury currents generated by the potential differences. For instance, the currents themselves might exert a feedback effect that would influence the magnitude of the potential differences. It may also be speculated that the injury currents will act as a physiological voltage clamp and influence the voltage-dependent conductances of the ionic currents, thereby having an impact on the inhomogeneity of the changes within the ischemic area. These various considerations raise the possibility that the relationship between the ionic changes and the differences in membrane potential and the flow of injury currents might vary with time.

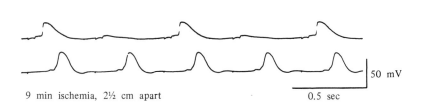

9 min ischemia, 2½ cm apart   0.5 sec

50 mV

FIG. 15. Transmembrane action potentials recorded with microelectrodes from the epicardial surface of the pig heart 9 min after coronary occlusion. The action potentials are recorded from the center of the ischemic zone by microelectrodes placed 2.5 cm apart. The upper panel shows a 2:1 response to an applied stimulus, while the lower panel shows a 1:1 response. (From ref. 64, with permission.)

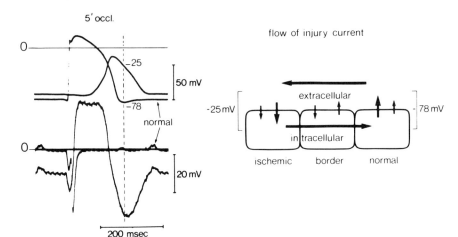

5' occl.

0

—25

50 mV

—78

normal

0

20 mV

200 msec

flow of injury current

extracellular

-25 mV

intracellular

ischemic   border   normal

78 mV

FIG. 16. Left: Transmembrane potentials (**above**) and DC extracellular potentials (**below**) recorded from *in situ* dog heart. The potentials recorded 5 min after occlusion of the left anterior descending coronary artery are superimposed. Note that following occlusion, the membrane potential occurs at the time the normal cells are already repolarized. **Right:** The flow of injury current at the moment indicated by the dotted line is schematically depicted. The injury current produces current sources at the nonischemic side of the border and current sinks on the ischemic side. (From ref. 127, with permission.)

RELATIONSHIP OF PREMATURE BEATS AND RHYTHMS TO ELECTROPHYSIOLOGICAL CHANGES

The electrophysiological changes induced by acute ischemia are capable of inducing abnormalities in impulse formation that might result in premature beats (85,110). Such abnormalities include enhancement of normal pacemaker capability in fully repolarized cells of the specialized conduction system and induction of automaticity in specialized and working myocardial cells with lowered resting potentials. Delayed after potentials and triggered activity are examples of this type of activity (3,5,52,110). The factors associated with ischemia which might enhance spontaneous activity in normal Purkinje fibers include the beta sympathetic catecholamines, myocardial fiber stretch (144) and depolarizing injury currents (235). These factors are also capable of inducing spontaneous activity in Purkinje and myocardial fibers whose resting potential has been lowered by the increase in extracellular potassium. Katzung (141,142) and Imanishi and Surawicz (120) demonstrated that depolarizing ventricular fibers to approximately −40 mV by injecting current induced repetitive activity that could be prevented by blockers of the slow calcium inward current system (119) (Fig. 17). Katzung and Morgenstern (143) were also able to induce spontaneous activity in guinea pig papillary muscle with current generated electrotonically across a sucrose gap. Electrotonically transmitted current has also been shown to alter pacemaker activity in Purkinje fibers mounted in a sucrose gap (4,123,124). These studies demonstrated not only that pacemaker activity in the distal end of the preparation was influenced by the electrotonic spread of current but also that in appropriate circumstances this current could reflect back to excite the proximal end.

Janse and van Capelle (128) used computer simulation to show that electrotonic spread of current through inexcitable tissue was capable of causing latent pacemakers to reach threshold and induce a propagated

response. This suggested that spontaneous impulse generation could be induced by electrotonic-mediated events that might alter the slope of spontaneous depolarizing fibers to allow achievement of the threshold voltage or to bring a subthreshold depolarization to threshold and induce a single response or triggered activity.

Classic reentry has also been suggested as a mechanism for the premature beat. Waldo and Kaiser (251) correlated the occurrence of spontaneous ventricular premature beats following acute coronary ligation in the dog

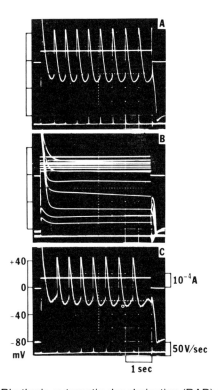

+40
0
-40
-80
mV

10⁻⁴A

50V/sec

1 sec

FIG. 17. Rhythmic automatic depolarization (RAD) produced in guinea pig papillary muscle fiber by depolarizing the membrane to approximately −40 mV by current injection. The **middle trace** shows the effect of Mn^{2+} on the RADs. Panel **C** shows the return to the control solution without Mn^{2+}. (From ref. 120, with permission.)

to the presence of continuous electrical activity on the epicardial surface and concluded that reentry was the underlying mechanism. Similar observations have been made by others studying activation characteristics during development of arrhythmias following coronary occlusion (23,134,266). Reflection may be viewed as a form of reentry in a linear bundle due either to microreentry circuits or to electrotonic transmission of current across an inexcitable segment. Such responses have been observed in Purkinje fiber preparations in which a portion of the fiber has been depolarized by high potassium (53,272), as well as in isolated Purkinje fibers placed in a sucrose gap (4,123,124).

These several mechanisms are also capable of inducing a sustained ventricular arrhythmia, provided the initiating mechanism produces a series of repetitive responses and the responses are capable of propagating out of the ischemic area to excite the entire ventricle. Wiggers (265) reported that following coronary occlusion, there were areas of local reentry that failed to propagate to the intact heart and that this phenomenon preceded the development of ventricular fibrillation.

One of the factors that may influence whether or not the single premature response produces a sustained arrhythmia is the site or origin of the premature response. Burgess et al. (32) examined the influence of the stimulation site on the ventricular fibrillation threshold in dogs following coronary occlusion or regional heating and cooling. They noted that in general, the lowest ventricular fibrillation threshold occurred when the stimulation site was located near the ischemic area or the area with altered temperature. Kuo et al. (155) studied the influence of stimulation site in models employing thermal lesions and observed that a single stimulus induced ventricular fibrillation when it was applied to the noncooled areas with short refractory periods, but not when it was applied to the cooled areas with long refractory periods. Harris and Rojas (103) noted that the ectopic impulse that occurred spontaneously a few minutes after a coronary occlusion in the dog originated at the border of the ischemic area. Janse et al. (126) and Ideker et al. (116) studied spontaneously occurring arrhythmias following coronary artery occlusion with and without reperfusion in porcine and canine models. They found that the initiating beat occurred in the normal myocardium immediately adjacent to the ischemic border. These various results would support the hypothesis linking the initiating premature beat to the flow of injury currents across the lateral border of the ischemic zone, but this does not exclude other factors.

The factors specifically responsible for the transition of ventricular tachycardia to ventricular fibrillation have not been completely explained. It is reasonable to attribute this transition to changes in impulse propagation and refractoriness appropriate to permit reentry, and to

the presence of inhomogeneities that will create the unidirectional block essential to creation of the reentry circuit. These factors are discussed elsewhere by Janse (see Chapter 54). However, it is appropriate to point out that Moe et al. (181) were able to generate reentry circuits in the absence of an anatomical obstacle by increasing the dispersion of atrial refractoriness in their computer model. Allessie et al. (2,215) also showed that an anatomical obstacle was not necessary to produce periods of sustained circus movement in small segments of rabbit atrium following premature stimuli. They showed that a disparity in refractoriness of only 11 to 16 msec among the individual adjacent elements resulted in local conduction block of a properly timed premature impulse. van Capelle and Durrer (243) and Janse and van Capelle (128) reported that reentrant ventricular arrhythmias and fibrillation could be simulated in a computer model even without introducing differences in refractory periods of the individual elements or an obstacle to conduction. In their model, some elements were assigned latent or overt pacemaker characteristics, and inhomogeneities were induced by changing the coupling of the individual elements to simulate ischemia. In this way they were able to induce automatic activity, subthreshold oscillations, and circus movement of activation wave fronts.

CHRONIC ISCHEMIA

An extensive literature exists describing the electrophysiological characteristics of tissues hours to years following myocardial infarction in experimental animals and man. These studies have described abnormalities in action potential configuration (75–77,160,161,185,230) and abnormalities in conduction and refractoriness (70,163,164,209) that contribute to the formation of reentry pathways and abnormal cardiac rhythms. However, these studies have been largely descriptive, and little is known concerning the changes in membrane structure and function or the changes in the characteristics of the ionic currents that underlie the electrophysiological abnormalities.

These studies have shown that the subendocardial Purkinje fibers usually survive the infarction but frequently have abnormal action potentials that demonstrate spontaneous diastolic depolarization. Several layers of subendocardial muscle fibers may also survive, but with abnormal action potentials. The abnormalities appear to be most pronounced within the first several hours of the acute infarction and then to decrease with time. The resting membrane potential is decreased. The action potential amplitude and the rate of rise of the upstroke are decreased, and its duration is frequently prolonged (76) (Fig. 18). Some of these action potentials may be suppressed with verapamil (230), suggesting dependence on the slow calcium-sensitive inward current

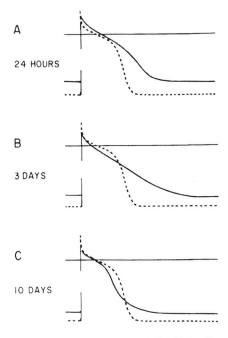

A
24 HOURS

B
3 DAYS

C
10 DAYS

FIG. 18. Surviving subendocardial Purkinje fibers in the infarcted region at the base of the anterior papillary muscle in the dog 24 hr (**A**), 3 days (**B**), and 10 days (**C**) after coronary artery occlusion. The horizontal trace denotes the zero potential. The solid lines show the action potential recorded from a surviving subendocardial Purkinje fiber in the infarct, superimposed on an action potential recorded from a normal subendocardial Purkinje fiber at a comparable site in a noninfarcted preparation (*broken lines*). (From ref. 75, with permission.)

(Fig. 19), whereas others are suppressed with tetrodotoxin (164), suggesting greater dependence on the depressed sodium-dependent, rapid inward current. Adjacent cells often exhibit different action potential characteristics (118,184), indicating significant inhomogeneities in elec-

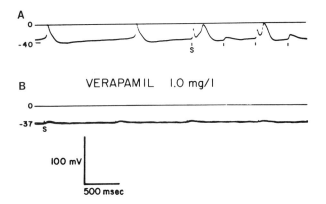

A
0
-40
s

B   VERAPAMIL   1.0 mg/l
0
-37 s

100 mV

500 msec

FIG. 19. Effects of verapamil on spontaneous and paced action potentials recorded from a subendocardial cell in a ventricular aneurysm from a human heart. The recording was made from a region containing tissue that histologically appeared to be ventricular myocardium. Verapamil abolished both stimulated and spontaneous responses. (From ref. 230, with permission.)

trophysiological properties. The infarcted tissue is characterized anatomically by ingrowth of fibrous tissue, creating anatomical and electrical obstacles to impulse propagation (75,76,178,230). Intracellular lipid deposits have been described in the Purkinje fiber cytoplasm within 24 hr of an acute infarction, but usually they are not present several weeks later when the action potentials have become less abnormal (71,75).

Conduction is slowed and fractionated, and the refractory period is longer than anticipated on the basis of the changes in action potential duration (163, 209,222,223,226,230). Losses in sympathetic and parasympathetic effects have been observed not only in the infarcted area but also in regions distal to the infarction (12). The site of the focus initiating premature beats and rhythm is thought to be adjacent to the area of infarction. This conclusion is supported by simulation studies in animals within 1 month of infarction (231) and in man at the time of ventricular aneurysm resection (102,273).

It is clear that major electrophysiological abnormalities persist for an extended period, perhaps indefinitely, following myocardial infarction and that these abnormalities are responsible for serious ventricular arrhythmias. Understanding the fundamental changes responsible for the observed abnormalities remains an area for future investigations.

CONCLUSIONS

This review has attempted to summarize the current understanding of the electrophysiological events that occur in the setting of myocardial ischemia. It is reasonable to conclude that many of the metabolic, ionic, and neurohumoral events have been characterized and that many of the electrophysiological consequences of these events have been described. Yet, there are many important unresolved issues and unanswered questions. A more precise understanding of the roles of fatty acids and their metabolites in the early electrical changes induced by ischemia is one such issue. The effect of ischemia on the electrophysiology of premature beats represents another area of significant clinical relevance that has received little attention. The inhomogeneous nature of the metabolic and ionic events associated with the acute ischemic process suggests that the inhomogeneities themselves may be an independent parameter critical to the development of reentry circuits and the genesis of ventricular fibrillation. Thus, it represents a hypothesis deserving testing. The causes of the changes in the action potential that persist long after myocardial infarction have not been defined and may provide valuable clues to the effect of ischemia on ionic channels, and perhaps their ability to regenerate following an acute ischemic event.

An important role for the autonomic nervous system in the electrophysiological changes during acute ischemia has been suggested by the studies referred to in this chapter and by a variety of other studies of the effects of sympathetic stimulation (156,168,222), sympathetic ablation, and blockade (102,156,223) on monophasic action potential characteristics and susceptibility to ventricular fibrillation, the ability of β-adrenergic blocking agents to prevent sudden death following myocardial infarction (18,108), and the differences in susceptibility to ventricular fibrillation following coronary occlusion in psychologically stressed and unstressed animals (62,169,226). It has recently been reported (20,221) that animals at risk for ventricular fibrillation following recovery from myocardial infarction can be identified on the basis of the cardiac response to baroreceptor testing. These various studies not only illustrate the important role of the autonomic nervous system in the electrophysiology of ischemia but also serve to emphasize the need for continued investigations.

An important role for the slow calcium current and changes in intracellular calcium in the sequence of electrical events that follow coronary occlusion is clearly implied by the studies concerning the electrophysiological effects of the β-adrenergic agonists discussed earlier and by an increasing number of studies showing that the calcium channel blocking agents influence the metabolic, ionic, and electrical events that characterize acute ischemia (27,39,43,66,72,139,145,188,261) (Fig. 20). Yet, our understanding of the role of calcium is incomplete and conjectural (42,43) and represents an area where further studies will undoubtedly reveal important information having significant clinical relevance.

Our understanding of the causes of the abnormalities in conduction and refractoriness that result from the metabolic, ionic, and neurohumoral consequences of ischemia is fragmentary, particularly in the context of its expression in the three-dimensional heart. Further progress in this, as in the other areas mentioned above, will require the application of available and new techniques, sophisticated recording and data processing and computer modeling. Broadening the conceptual framework on which our knowledge is based will permit us to solve some of the unresolved questions outlined earlier and to seek answers to questions that have not yet been formulated.

ACKNOWLEDGMENTS

The author gratefully acknowledges the contributions of the following associates: J. Buchanan, W. Fleet, T. Fugino, C. Grabener, J. Hill, T. Johnson, T. Kagiyamia, S. Oshita, and T. Saito. Without them, much of the work of our laboratory would have been impossible. The author also acknowledges the secretarial and editorial assistance of Elizabeth Otwell.

Some of the studies reported in this chapter were supported by project grant 5-P01-HC-27430-04 from NHLBI.

REFERENCES

1. Allen, D. E., and Blinks, J. R. (1978): Calcium transients in aquorin-injected frog cardiac muscle. *Nature (Lond.)*, 273:509–513.
2. Allessie, M. A., Bonke, F. I. M., and Schopman, F. J. G. (1977): Circus movement in rabbit atrial muscle as a mechanism of tachycardia. III. The "leading circle" concept: A new model of circus movement in cardiac tissue without the involvement of an anatomical obstacle. *Circ. Res.*, 41:9–18.
3. Anderson, G., Reiser, J., Gough, W., and Nydegger, C. (1983): Intramyocardial current flow in acute coronary occlusion in the canine heart. *J. Am. Coll. Cardiol.*, 2:436–443.
4. Antzelevitch, C., Jalife, J., and Moe, G. K. (1980): Characteristics of reflection as a mechanism of reentrant arrhythmias and its relationship to parasystole. *Circulation*, 61:182–191.
5. Arita, M., and Kiyosue, T. (1983): Modification of "depressed fast channel slow conduction" by lidocaine and verapamil in the presence of catecholamines. Evidence for alteration of preferential ionic channels for slow conduction. *Jpn. Circ. J.*, 47:68–81.
6. Arita, M., Kiyosue, T., Aomine, M., and Imanishi, S. (1983): Nature of "residual fast channel" dependent action potentials and slow conduction in guinea pig ventricular muscle and its modification by isoproterenol. *Am. J. Cardiol.*, 51:1433–1440.
7. Arnsdorf, M. F., and Sawicki, G. J. (1981): The effects of lysophosphatidylcholine, a toxic metabolite of ischemia, on the components of cardiac excitability in sheep Purkinje fibers. *Circ. Res.*, 49:16–30.
8. Arnsdorf, M. F., Schreiner, E., Gambetta, M., Friedlander, I., and Childers, R. W. (1977): Electrophysiologic changes in the canine atrium and ventricle during progressive hyperkalemia: Electrocardiographical correlates and the in vivo validation of in vitro predictions. *Cardiovasc. Res.*, 11:409–418.

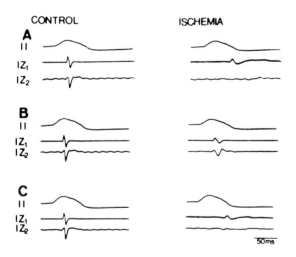

FIG. 20. Effects of verapamil on ischemia-induced conduction delay. IZ_1 and IZ_2 are two epicardial bipolar electrograms obtained from the ischemic zone during pacing at a cycle length of 500 msec. The left and right panels were obtained before (**left**) and 5 min after (**right**) coronary occlusion. The upper panels (**A**) were recorded before administration of verapamil, the middle panels (**B**) were recorded 11 min after preocclusion administration of verapamil (0.2 mg/kg), and the lower panels (**C**) were recorded 47 min after verapamil. Note that the ischemia-induced conduction delays recorded at both areas, 11 min after verapamil (**B**), are less than those recorded either before (**A**) or 47 min after (**C**) verapamil administration. (From ref. 66, with permission.)

9. Avitall, B. S., Naimi, A. H., Brilla, A. H., and Levine, H. J. (1974): A computerized system for measuring dispersion of repolarization in the intact heart. *J. Appl. Physiol.*, 37:456–458.

10. Bailey, J. C., Greenspan, K., Elizari, M. V., Anderson, G. J., and Fisch, C. (1972): Effects of acetylcholine on automaticity and conduction in the proximal portion of the His-Purkinje system in the dog. *Circ. Res.*, 30:210–216.

11. Bailey, J. C., Watanabe, A. M., Besch, H. R., and Lathrop, D. A. (1979): Acetylcholine antagonism of the electrophysiological effects of isoproterenol on canine cardiac Purkinje fibers. *Circ. Res.*, 44:378–383.

12. Barber, M. J., Mueller, T. M., Henry, D. P., Felton, S. Y., and Zipes, D. P. (1983): Transmural myocardial infarction in the dog produces sympathectomy in noninfarcted myocardium. *Circulation*, 67:787–796.

13. Bassingthwaighte, J. B., Fry, C. H., and McGuigan, J. A. S. (1976): Relationship between internal calcium and outward current in mammalian ventricular muscle: A mechanism for the control of the action potential duration? *J. Physiol. (Lond.)*, 262:15–37.

14. Becker, E., Ingebretsen, W. R., and Mayer, S. E. (1977): Electrophysiologic responses of cardiac muscle to isoproterenol covalently linked to glass beads. *Circ. Res.*, 41:653–660.

15. Beeler, G. W., and Reuter, H. (1970): Membrane calcium current in ventricular myocardium fibers. *J. Physiol. (Lond.)*, 207:191–209.

16. Belardinelli, L., and Isenberg, G. (1983): Increase in potassium conductance in isolated guinea pig atrial myocytes by adenosine and acetylcholine. *Am. J. Physiol.*, 244 (*Heart Circ. Physiol.*, 14):H734–H737.

17. Belardinelli, L., and Isenberg, G. (1983): Actions of adenosine and isoproterenol on isolated mammalian ventricular myocytes. *Circ. Res.*, 53:287–297.

18. Beta Blocker Heart Attack Trial Research Group (1982): A randomized trial of propanolol in patients with acute myocardial infarction. *J.A.M.A.*, 247:1707–1712.

19. Biegon, R. L., Epstein, P. M., and Pappano, A. J. (1980): Muscarinic antagonism of the effects of a phosphodiesterase inhibitor (methylisobutylxanthine) in embryonic chick ventricle. *J. Pharmacol. Exp. Ther.*, 215:348–355.

20. Billman, G. E., Schwartz, P. S., and Stone, H. L. (1982): Baroreceptor reflex control of heart rate: A prediction in sudden death. *Circulation*, 66:784–791.

21. Bing, R. J. (1965): Cardiac metabolism. *Physiol. Rev.*, 45:171–213.

22. Van Bogaert, P. P., and Carmeliet, E. (1982): Sodium inactivation and pH in cardiac Purkinje-fibers. *Arch. Int. Physiol. Biochem.*, 80:833–835 (abstract).

23. Boineau, J., and Cox, J. (1973): Slow ventricular activation in acute myocardial infarction. *Circulation*, 47:702–713.

24. Braasch, W., Gudjarnason, S., Puri, P. S., Ravens, K. G., and Bing, R. J. (1968): Early changes in energy metabolism in the myocardium following acute coronary artery occlusion in anesthetized dogs. *Circ. Res.*, 23:429–438.

25. Braveny, P., Simurdova, M., and Sumbera, J. (1974): Effect of epinephrine on duration of action potential of papillary muscles. *Experientia*, 30:166–167.

26. Brooks, C. M., Gilbert, J. L., Greenspan, M. E., Lange, G., and Mazzella, H. M. (1960): Excitability and electrical response of ischemic heart muscle. *Am. J. Physiol.*, 198:1143–1147.

27. Brooks, W. W., Verrier, R. L., and Lown, B. (1980): Protective effect of verapamil on vulnerability to ventricular fibrillation during myocardial ischaemia and reperfusion. *Cardiovasc. Res.*, 14:295–302.

28. Brown, A. M. (1967): Excitation of afferent cardiac sympathetic nerve fibres during myocardial ischaemia. *J. Physiol. (Lond.)*, 190:35–53.

29. Brown, R. H., Cohen, I., and Noble, D. (1978): The interactions of protons, calcium, and potassium ions on cardiac Purkinje fibres. *J. Physiol. (Lond.)*, 282:345–352.

30. Brown, R. H., and Noble, D. (1978): Displacement of activation thresholds in cardiac muscle by protons and calcium ions. *J. Physiol. (Lond.)*, 282:333–343.

31. Buchanan, J. W., Jr., Saito, T., and Gettes, L. S. (1985): The effects of antiarrhythmic drugs, stimulation frequency and potassium-induced resting potential changes on dV/dt max in guinea pig myocardium. *Circ. Res.*, 56:696–703.

32. Burgess, M. J., Williams, D., and Ershler, P. (1977): Influence of test site on ventricular fibrillation threshold. *Am. Heart J.*, 94:55–61.

33. Carmeliet, E., and Ramon, J. (1980): Electrophysiological effects of acetylcholine in sheep cardiac Purkinje fibers. *Pfluegers Arch.*, 383:197–205.

34. Case, R., Felix, A., and Castellana, F. S. (1979): Rate of rise of myocardial P_{CO_2} during early myocardial ischemia in the dog. *Circ. Res.*, 45:324–330.

35. Case, R. B. (1971/72): Ion alterations during myocardial ischemia. *Cardiology*, 56:245–262.

36. Ceremuzynski, L., Staszewska-Barczak, J., and Heroaczynska-Cedro, K. (1969): Cardiac rhythm disturbances and the release of catecholamines after acute coronary occlusion in dogs. *Cardiovasc. Res.*, 3:190–195.

37. Cherbakoff, A., Toyama, S., and Hamilton, W. F. (1957): Relation between coronary sinus plasma potassium and cardiac arrhythmia. *Circ. Res.*, 5:517–521.

38. Chesnais, J. M., Coraboeuf, E., and Suvait, M. P. (1975): Sensitivity to H, Li and Mg ions of the slow inward sodium current in from atrial fibres. *J. Mol. Cell. Cardiol.*, 7:627–642.

39. Clark, R. E., Ferguson, T. B., West, P. N., Schuchleib, R., and Henry, P. D. (1977): Pharmacological preservation of the ischemic heart. *Ann. Thorac. Surg.*, 24:307–314.

40. Clarkson, C. W., and Ten Eick, R. E. (1983): On the mechanism of lysophosphatidylcholine-induced depolarization of cat ventricular myocardium. *Circ. Res.*, 52:543–556.

41. Clerc, L. (1976): Directional differences of impulse spread in trabecular muscle from mammalian heart. *J. Physiol. (Lond.)*, 255:335–346.

42. Clusin, W. T., Bristow, M. R., Baim, D. S., Schroeder, J. S., Jaillon, P., Brett, P., and Harrison, D. C. (1982): The effects of diltazem and reduced serum ionized calcium on ischemic ventricular fibrillation in the dog. *Circ. Res.*, 50:518–526.

43. Clusin, W. T., Buchbinder, M., Ellis, A. K., Kernoff, R. S., Giacomini, J. C., and Harrison, D. C. (1984): Reduction of ischemic depolarization by the calcium channel blocker diltiazem: Correlation with improvements of ventricular conduction and early arrhythmias in the dog. *Circ. Res.*, 54:10–20.

44. Clusin, W. T., Bristow, M. R., Karageuzuan, H. R., Katzung, B. S., and Schroeder, J. S. (1982): Do calcium-dependent ionic currents mediate ischemic ventricular fibrillation? *Am. J. Cardiol.*, 49:606–612.

45. Cobbe, S. M., and Poole-Wilson, P. A. (1980): The time of onset and severity of acidosis in myocardial ischaemia. *J. Mol. Cell. Cardiol.*, 12:745–760.

46. Cohen, L., and Kline, R. P. (1982): K⁺ fluctuations in the extracellular spaces of cardiac muscle: Evidence from the voltage clamp and K⁺ selective extracellular microelectrodes. *Circ. Res.*, 50:1–16.

47. Cohen, C. J., Bean, B. P., and Tsien, R. W. (1984): Maximal upstroke velocity as an index of available sodium conductance: Comparison of maximal upstroke velocity and voltage clamp measurements of sodium current in rabbit Purkinje fibers. *Circ. Res.*, 54:636–651.

48. Corr, P., Gross, R., and Sobel, B. (1984): Amphipathic metabolites and membrane dysfunction in ischemic myocardium. *Circ. Res.*, 55:135–154.

49. Corr, P. B., Cain, M. E., Witkowski, F. X., Price, D. A., and Sobel, B. E. (1979): Potential arrhythmogenic electrophysiological derangements in canine Purkinje fibers induced by lysophosphoglycerides. *Circ. Res.*, 44:822–832.

50. Corr, P. B., et al. (1981): Electrophysiological effects of amphiphiles on canine Purkinje fibers: Implications for dysrhythmia secondary to ischemia. *Circ. Res.*, 49:354–363.

51. Cowan, J. C., and Vaughan Williams, E. M. (1980): The effects of various fatty acids on action potential shortening during sequential periods of ischaemia and reperfusion. *J. Mol. Cell. Cardiol.*, 12:347–369.

52. Cranefield, P. F. (1975): *Conduction of the Cardiac Impulse.* Futura, Mt. Kisco, N.Y.

53. Cranefield, P. F., Wit, A. L., and Hoffman, B. F. (1972):

Conduction of the cardiac impulse. III. Characteristics of very slow conduction. *J. Gen. Physiol.*, 59:227–246.

54. Cranefield, P. F. (1977): Action potentials, after potentials and arrhythmias. *Circ. Res.*, 41:415–423.

55. Danilo, P., Jr., Rosen, M. R., and Hordof, A. J. (1978): Effects of acetylcholine on the ventricular specialized conducting system of neonatal and adult dogs. *Circ. Res.*, 43:777–784.

56. Davis, L. D., Helmer, P. R., and Ballantyne, F., III (1976): Production of slow responses in canine cardiac Purkinje fibers exposed to reduced pH. *J. Mol. Cell. Cardiol.*, 8:61–76.

57. De Mello, W. C. (1980): Influence of intracellular injection of H^+ on the electrical coupling in cardiac Purkinje fibres. *Cell. Biol. Int. Rep.*, 4:51–58.

58. De Mello, W. C. (1983): The role of cAMP and Ca on the modulation of junctional conductance: An integrated hypothesis. *Cell. Biol. Int. Rep.*, 7:1033–1040.

59. De Mello, W. C. (1982): Cell-cell communication in heart and other tissues. *Prog. Biophys. Molec. Biol.*, 39:147–182.

60. De Mello, W. C. (1984): Modulation of junctional permeability. *Fed. Proc.*, 43:2692–2696.

61. De Mello, W. C. (1975): Effects of intracellular injections of calcium and strontium on cell communication in the heart. *J. Physiol. (Lond.)*, 250:231–245.

62. De Silva, R. A. (1982): Central nervous system risk factors for sudden cardiac death. *Ann. N.Y. Acad. Sci.*, 382:143–161.

63. Dominguez, G., and Fozzard, H. (1970): Influence of extracellular K^+ concentration on cable properties and excitability of sheep cardiac Purkinje fibers. *Circ. Res.*, 26:565–574.

64. Downar, E., Janse, M. J., and Durrer, D. (1977): The effect of acute coronary artery occlusion on subepicardial transmembrane potentials in the intact porcine heart. *Circulation*, 56:217–224.

65. Dunn, R. B., and Griggs, D. M. (1975): Transmural gradients in ventricular tissue metabolites produced by stopping coronary blood flow in the dog. *Circ. Res.*, 37:438–445.

66. Elharrar, V., Gaum, W. E., and Zipes, D. P. (1977): Effects of drugs on conduction delay and incidence of ventricular arrhythmias induced by acute coronary occlusion in dogs. *Am. J. Cardiol.*, 39:544–549.

67. Elharrar, V., and Zipes, D. P. (1977): Cardiac electrophysiologic alterations during myocardial ischemia. *Am. J. Physiol.*, 233(*Heart Circ. Physiol.*, 2):H329–H345.

68. Elharrar, V., Foster, P. R., Jirak, T. L., Gaum, W. E., and Zipes, D. P. (1977): Alterations in canine myocardial excitability during ischemia. *Circ. Res.* 40:98–105.

69. El-Sherif, N., Smith, R. A., and Evans, K. (1981): Canine ventricular arrhythmias in the late myocardial infarction period. 8. Epicardial mapping of reentrant circuits. *Circ. Res.*, 49:255.

70. El-Sherif, N., Scherlag, B. J., Lazzara, R., and Samet, P. (1974): Pathophysiology of tachycardia- and bradycardia-dependent block in the canine proximal His-Purkinje system after acute myocardial ischemia. *Am. J. Cardiol.*, 33:529–540.

71. Fenoglio, J. J., Karagueuzian, H. S., Friedman, P. L., Albala, A., and Wit, A. L. (1979): Time course of infarct growth toward the endocardium after coronary occlusion. *Am. J. Physiol.*, 236(*Heart Circ. Physiol.*, 5):H256–H370.

72. Fleet, W. F., Johnson, T. A., Graebner, C., Engle, C. D., and Gettes, L. S. (1984): Verapamil decreases ionic, pH, and activation changes during myocardial ischemia. *Circulation*, 70:II125 (abstract).

73. Fleet, W. F., Johnson, T. A., Graebner, C., and Gettes, L. S. (1985): Effect of serial brief ischemic episodes on extracellular K^+, pH and activation in the pig. *Circulation*, 72:922–932.

74. Fozzard, H. A. (1979): Conduction of the action potential. In: *Handbook of Physiology*, Vol. 1, edited by R. M. Berne, pp. 335–356. American Physiological Society, Bethesda.

75. Friedman, P. L., Fenoglio, J. J., and Wit, A. L. (1975): Time course for reversal of electrophysiological and ultrastructural abnormalities in subendocardial Purkinje fibers surviving extensive myocardial infarction in dogs. *Circ. Res.*, 36:127–144.

76. Friedman, P. L., Stewart, J. R., Fenoglio, J. J., and Wit, A. L. (1973): Survival of subendocardial Purkinje fibers after extensive myocardial infarction in dogs. In vitro and in vivo correlations. *Circ. Res.*, 33:597–611.

77. Friedman, P. L., Stewart, J. R., and Wit, A. L. (1973): Spontaneous

78. Frye, C. H., and Poole-Wilson, P. A. (1979): Electrochemical effects of pH in guinea-pig cardiac ventricular muscle. *J. Physiol. (Lond.)*, 293:74–75.

79. Furuta, T., Kodama, I., Shimuzu, T., Toyama, J., and Yamada, K. (1983): Effects of hypoxia on conduction velocity of ventricular muscle. *Jpn. Heart J.*, 24:417–425.

80. Gadsby, D. C., Wit, A. L., and Cranefield, P. F. (1978): The effects of acetylcholine on the electrical activity of canine cardiac Purkinje fibers. *Circ. Res.*, 43:29–35.

81. Garlick, P. B., Radda, G. K., and Seeley, P. J. (1979): Studies of acidosis in the ischaemic heart by phosphorus nuclear magnetic resonance. *Biochem. J.*, 185:547–554.

82. Gebert, G., Benzig, H., and Strohm, M. (1971): Changes in the interstitial pH of dog myocardium in response to local ischemia, hypoxia, hyper- and hypocapnia, measured continuously by means of glass microelectrodes. *Pfluegers Arch*, 329:72–81.

83. Geddes, J., Burgess, M. J., Millar, K., and Abildskov, J. A. (1974): Accelerated repolarization as a factor in re-entry stimulation of the electrophysiology of acute myocardial infarction. *Am. Heart J.*, 88:61–68.

84. Gettes, L. S. (1974): Electrophysiologic basis of arrhythmias in acute myocardial ischemia. In: *Modern Trends in Cardiology*, edited by M. F. Oliver, pp. 219–246. Butterworth, London.

85. Gettes, L. S. (1984): Ventricular fibrillation. In: *Tachycardias*, edited by B. Surawicz, C. P. Reddy, and E. N. Prystowsky, pp. 37–54. Martinus Nijhoff, Boston.

86. Gettes, L. S., Buchanan, J. W., Saito, T., Kagiyama, Y., Oshita, S., and Fujino, T. (1985): Studies concerned with slow conduction. In: *Cardiac Electrophysiology and Arrhythmias*, edited by D. P. Zipes and J. Jalife, pp. 81–87. Grune & Stratton, Orlando.

87. Gettes, L. S., Morehouse, N., and Surawicz, B. (1972): Effect of premature depolarization on the duration of action potentials in Purkinje and ventricular fibers of the moderator band of the pig heart: Role of proximity and the duration of the preceding action potential. *Circ. Res.*, 30:66.

88. Gettes, L. S., and Reuter, H. (1974): Slow recovery from inactivation of inward currents in mammalian myocardial fibers. *J. Physiol. (Lond.)*, 240:703–724.

89. Gettes, L. S., Surawicz, B., and Shiue, J. C. (1963): Effect of high K, low K, and quinidine on QRS duration and ventricular action potential. *J. Physiol. (Lond.)*, 203:1135–1140.

90. Gevers, W. (1977): Generation of protons by metabolic processes in heart cells. *J. Mol. Cell. Cardiol.*, 9:867–874.

91. Gilmour, R. F., Evans, J. J., and Zipes, D. P. (1984): Purkinje-muscle coupling and endocardial response to hyperkalemia, hypoxia, and acidosis. *Am. J. Physiol.*, 246(*Heart Circ. Physiol.*, 16):H303–H311.

92. Gilmour, R. F., Morrical, D. G., Ertel, P. J., Marsaka, J. F., and Zipes, D. P. (1984): Depressant effects of fast sodium channel blockade on the electrical activity of ischemic canine ventricle: Mediation by the sympathetic nervous system. *Cardiovasc. Res.*, 18:405–413.

93. Gilmour, R. F., and Zipes, D. P. (1980): Different electrophysiologic responses of canine endocardium and epicardium to combined hyperkalemia, hypoxia, and acidosis. *Circ. Res.*, 46:814–825.

94. Giotti, A., Ledda, F., and Mannaioni, P. F. (1968): Electrophysiological effects of alpha and beta-receptor agonists and antagonists on Purkinje fibers of sheep heart. *Br. J. Pharmacol.*, 34:695P–696P.

95. Grant, A. O., Strauss, L. J., and Strauss, H. C. (1980): The influence of pH on the electrophysiological effects of lidocaine in guinea pig ventricular myocardium. *Circ. Res.*, 47:542–550.

96. Griggs, D. M., Jr. (1979): Blood flow and metabolism in different layers of the left ventricle. *Physiologist*, 22:36–40.

97. Han, J., Malozzi, A. M., and Moe, G. K. (1967): Transient ventricular conduction disturbances produced by intra-atrial injection of single doses of KCl. *Circ. Res.*, 21:308.

98. Han, J., and Moe, G. K. (1964): Nonuniform recovery of excitability in ventricular muscle. *Circ. Res.*, 14:44–60.

99. Han, J., Garcia de Jalon, P. D., and Moe, G. K. (1964):

Adrenergic effects on ventricular vulnerability. *Circ. Res.*, 14: 516–524.

100. Harris, A. S. (1950): Delayed development of ventricular ectopic rhythms following experimental coronary occlusion. *Circulation*, 1:1318–1325.

101. Harris, A. S., Bisteni, A., Russell, R. A., Brigham, J. C., and Firestone, J. E. (1954): Excitatory factors in ventricular tachycardia resulting from myocardial ischemia. *Science*, 119:200–202.

102. Harris, A. S., Estandia, A., and Tillotson, R. F. (1951): Ventricular ectopic rhythm and ventricular fibrillation following cardiac sympathectomy and coronary occlusion. *Am. J. Physiol.*, 165: 505–512.

103. Harris, A. S., and Rojas, G. A. (1943): Initiation of ventricular fibrillation due to coronary occlusion. *Exp. Med. Surg.*, 1:105–122.

104. Hearse, D. J., Opie, L. H., Katzeff, I. E., Lubbe, W. F., Van der Werff, T. J., Peisach, M., and Boulle, G. (1977): Characterization of the "border zone" in acute regional ischemia in the dog. *Am. J. Cardiol.*, 40:716–726.

105. Hill, J. L., and Gettes, L. S. (1980): Effect of acute coronary artery occlusion on local myocardial extracellular K^+ activity in swine. *Circulation*, 61:768–777.

106. Hille, B. (1970): Ionic channels in nerve membranes. *Prog. Biophys.*, 21:1–32.

107. Hirche, H. J., Franz, C., Bos, F. L., Bissig, R., Lang, R., and Schramm, M. (1980): Myocardial extracellular K^+ and H^+ increase and noradrenaline release as possible cause of early arrhythmias following acute coronary artery occlusion in pigs. *J. Mol. Cell. Cardiol.*, 12:579–593.

108. Hjalmarson, A., Elmfeldt, D., and Herlitz, J. (1981): Effect on mortality of metoprolol in acute myocardial infarction. *Lancet*, 2:823–827.

109. Hoffman, B. F., and Cranefield, P. F. (1960): *Electrophysiology of the Heart.* McGraw-Hill, New York.

110. Hoffman, B. F., and Rosen, M. R. (1981): Cellular mechanisms for cardiac arrhythmias. *Circ. Res.*, 49:1–15.

111. Hoffman, B. F., and Singer, D. (1967): Appraisal of the effects of catecholamines on cardiac electrical activity. *Ann. N.Y. Acad. Sci.*, 193:914–924.

112. Holland, R., and Brooks, H. (1976): The QRS complex during myocardial ischemia: An experimental analysis in the porcine heart. *J. Clin. Invest.*, 57:541–550.

113. Hope, R. R., Williams, D. O., El-Sherif, N., Lazzara, K., and Schlerlag, B. J. (1974): The efficacy of antiarrhythmic agents during acute myocardial ischemia and the role of heart rate. *Circulation*, 50:507–514.

114. Horio, Y., Okumura, K., Nishi, K., and Tokuomi, H. (1982): Electrophysiological characteristics of ischemia cardiac cells in hypoxia and hyperkalemic conditions. *Jpn. Circ. J.*, 46:980–993.

115. Hunter, P. F., McNaughton, P. A., and Noble, D. (1975): Analytical models of propagation in excitable cells. *Prog. Biophys. Mol. Biol.*, 30:99–144.

116. Ideker, R. E., Klein, G. J., Harrison, L., Smith, W. M., Kasell, J., Reimer, K. A., Wallace, A. G., and Gallagher, J. J. (1981): The transition to ventricular fibrillation induced by reperfusion after acute ischemia in the dog: A period of organized epicardial activation. *Circulation*, 63:1371–1379.

117. Iinuma, H., and Kato, K. (1978): The effect of hypoxia on the refractoriness of the canine ventricular muscle. *J. Electrocardiol.*, 1:15–22.

118. Ikeda, K., and Hiraoka, M. (1982): Effects of hypoxia on passive electrical properties of canine ventricular muscle. *Pfluegers Arch.*, 393:45–50.

119. Imanishi, S., McAllister, R. G., and Surawicz, B. (1978): The effects of verapamil and lidocaine on the automatic depolarization in guinea-pig ventricular myocardium. *J. Pharmacol. Exp. Ther.*, 207:294–303.

120. Imanishi, S., and Surawicz, B. (1976): Automatic activity in depolarized guinea ventricular myocardium. Characteristics and mechanisms. *Circ. Res.*, 39:751–759.

121. Isenberg, G. (1977): Cardiac Purkinje fibers. (Ca^{2+}) controls the potassium permeable via the conductance components gk_1 and gk_2. *Pfluegers Arch.*, 371:7–85.

122. Isenberg, G., and Klockner, U. (1982): Calcium currents of isolated bovine ventricular myocytes are fast of large amplitude. *Pfluegers Arch.*, 395:30–41.

123. Jalife, J., and Moe, G. K. (1976): Effect of electrotonic potentials on pacemaker activity of canine Purkinje fibers in relation to parasystole. *Circ. Res.*, 39:801–809.

124. Jalife, J., and Moe, G. K. (1981): Excitation, conduction, and reflection of impulses in isolated bovine and canine cardiac Purkinje fibers. *Circ. Res.*, 49:233–247.

125. Janse, M. J., et al. (1979): The "border zone" in myocardial ischemia: An electrophysiological, metabolic, and histochemical correlation in the pig heart. *Circ. Res.*, 44:576–583.

126. Janse, M. J., et al. (1980): Flow of "injury current" and patterns of excitation during early ventricular arrhythmias in acute regional myocardial ischemia in isolated porcine and canine hearts: Evidence for two different arrhythmogenic mechanisms. *Circ. Res.*, 47:151.

127. Janse, M. J., and Kleber, A. G. (1981): Electrophysiological changes and ventricular arrhythmias in the early phase of regional myocardial ischemia. *Circ. Res.*, 49:1078–1081.

128. Janse, M. J., and van Capelle, F. J. L. (1982): Electrotonic interactions across an inexcitable region as a cause of ectopic activity in acute regional myocardial ischemia: A study in intact porcine and canine hearts and computer models. *Circ. Res.*, 50: 527.

129. Jennings, R. B., Reimer, K. A., Hill, M. L., and Mayer, S. E. (1981): Total ischemia in dog hearts, in vitro. 1. Comparison of high energy phosphate production, utilization, and depletion, and of adenine nucleotide catabolism in total ischemia in vitro vs. severe ischemia in vivo. *Circ. Res.*, 49:892–900.

130. Johannson, M., and Nilsson, E. (1975): Acid-base changes and excitation-contraction coupling in rabbit myocardium. II. Effects on resting membrane potential, action potential characteristics and propagation velocity. *Acta Physiol. Scand.*, 93:310–317.

131. Joyner, R. W. (1982): Effects of the discrete pattern of electrical coupling on propagation through an electrical syncytium. *Circ. Res.*, 50:192–200.

132. Joyner, R. W., Veenstra, R., Rawling, D., and Chorro, A. (1984): Propagation through electrically coupled cells: Effects of a resistive barrier. *Biophys. J.*, 45:1017–1025.

133. Kagiyama, Y., Hill, J. L., and Gettes, L. S. (1982): Interaction of acidosis and increased extracellular potassium on action potential characteristics and conduction in guinea pig ventricular muscle. *Circ. Res.*, 51:614–623.

134. Kaplinsky, E., Ogawa, S., Balke, W., and Dreifus, L. S. (1979): Role of endocardial activation in malignant ventricular arrhythmias associated with acute ischemia. *J. Electrocardiol.*, 12:299–306.

135. Kaplinsky, E., Ogawa, S., Balke, W., and Dreifus, L. S. (1979): Two periods of early ventricular arrhythmia in the canine acute myocardial infarction model. *Circulation*, 60:397–403.

136. Kardesch, M., Hogancamp, C. E., and Bing, R. J. (1958): The effect of complete ischemia on the intracellular electrical activity of the whole mammalian heart. *Circ. Res.*, 6:715–720.

137. Kass, R. S., and Tsien, R. W. (1976): Control of action potential duration by calcium ions in cardiac Purkinje fibers. *J. Gen. Physiol.*, 67:599–617.

138. Kassebaum, D. G., and Van Dyke, A. R. (1966): Electrophysiological effects of isoproterenol on Purkinje fibers of the heart. *Circ. Res.*, 19:940–946.

139. Katz, A. M., and Reuter, H. (1979): Cellular calcium and cardiac cell death. *Am. J. Cardiol.*, 44:188–190.

140. Katz, A. M., and Messineo, F. C. (1981): Lipid-membrane interactions and the pathogenesis of ischemic damage in the myocardium. *Circ. Res.*, 48:1–16.

141. Katzung, B. G. (1974): Electrically induced automaticity in ventricular myocardium. *Life Sci.*, 14:1133.

142. Katzung, B. G. (1975): Effects of extracellular calcium and sodium on depolarization-induced automaticity in guinea pig papillary muscles. *Circ. Res.*, 37:118–127.

143. Katzung, B. G., and Morgenstern, J. A. (1977): Effects of extracellular potassium on ventricular automaticity and evidence for a pacemaker current in mammalian ventricular myocardium. *Circ. Res.*, 40:105–111.

144. Kaufmann, R., and Theophile, U. (1967): Automatie-fordernde

Dehnungseffekte an Purkinje-faden, Papillarmuskein und Vorhoftrabekeln von Rhesus-Affen. *Pfluegers Arch.*, 297:174–180.

145. Kaumann, A. J., and Aramendia, P. (1968): Prevention of ventricular fibrillation induced by coronary ligation. *J. Pharmacol. Exp. Ther.*, 164:326–332.

146. Khuri, S. F., et al. (1975): Changes in intramyocardial ST segment voltage and gas tensions with regional myocardial ischemia in the dog. *Circ. Res.*, 37:455–463.

147. Kishida, H., Surawicz, B., and Tai Fu, L. (1979): Effects of K^+ and K^+-induced polarization on $(dV/dt)_{max}$, threshold potential, and membrane input resistance in guinea pig and cat ventricular myocardium. *Circ. Res.*, 44:800–814.

148. Kleber, A. G., Janse, M. J., Van Capelle, F. J. L., and Durrer, D. (1978): Mechanism and time course of S-T and T-Q segment changes during acute regional myocardial ischemia in the pig's heart determined by extracellular and intracellular recordings. *Circ. Res.*, 42:603–613.

149. Kleber, A. G. (1983): Resting membrane potential, extracellular potassium activity, and intracellular sodium activity during acute global ischemia in isolated perfused guinea pig hearts. *Circ. Res.*, 52:442–450.

150. Kleber, A. G. (1984): Extracellular potassium accumulation in acute myocardial ischemia. *J. Mol. Cell. Cardiol.*, 16:389–394.

151. Kline, R. P., and Morad, M. (1978): Potassium efflux in heart muscle during activity: Extracellular accumulation and its implications. *J. Physiol. (Lond.)*, 132:537–558.

152. Kodama, I., Wilde, A., Janse, M. J., Durrer, D., and Yamada, K. (1984): Combined effects of hypoxia, hyperkalemia and acidosis on membrane action potential and excitability of guinea-pig ventricular muscle. *J. Mol. Cell. Cardiol.*, 16:247–259.

153. Kohlhardt, M., and Mnich, Z. (1978): Studies on the inhibitory effect on the slow inward current in mammalian ventricular myocardium. *J. Mol. Cell. Cardiol.*, 10:1037–1052.

154. Kohlhardt, M., Haap, K., and Figulla, H. R. (1976): Influence of low extracellular pH upon the Ca inward current and isometric contractile force in mammalian ventricular myocardium. *Pfluegers Arch.*, 366:31–38.

155. Kuo, C. S., Munakata, K., Reddy, C. P., and Surawicz, B. (1983): Characteristics and possible mechanism of ventricular arrhythmias dependent on the dispersion of action potential duration. *Circulation*, 67:1356–1367.

156. Kuo, C. S., and Surawicz, B. (1976): Ventricular monophasic action potential changes associated with neurogenic T wave abnormalities and isoproterenol administration in dogs. *Am. J. Cardiol.*, 38:170–177.

157. Kurien, V. A., Yates, P. A., and Oliver, M. F. (1971): The role of free fatty acids in the production of ventricular arrhythmias after acute coronary artery occlusion. *Eur. J. Clin. Invest.*, 1:225–241.

158. Lammerant, J., De Herdt, P., and De Schryver, C. (1966): Direct release of myocardial catecholamines into the left heart chambers: The enhancing effect of acute coronary occlusion. *Arch. Int. Pharmacodyn.*, 163:219–226.

159. Lathers, C. M., Kelleher, G. J., Roberts, J., and Beasley, A. B. (1978): Nonuniform cardiac sympathetic nerve discharge. Mechanism for coronary occlusion and digitalis-induced arrhythmia. *Circulation*, 57:1058–1065.

160. Lazzara, R., El-Sherif, N., and Scherlag, B. G. (1974): Early and late effects of coronary artery occlusion on canine Purkinje fibers. *Circ. Res.*, 35:391–399.

161. Lazzara, R., El-Sherif, N., and Scherlag, B. J. (1973): Electrophysiological properties of canine Purkinje cells in one day old myocardial infarction. *Circ. Res.*, 33:722–734.

162. Lazzara, R., El-Sherif, N., and Scherlag, B. J. (1975): Disorders of cellular electrophysiology produced by ischemia of the canine His bundle. *Circ. Res.*, 36:444–454.

163. Lazzara, R., El-Sherif, N., Hope, R. R., and Scherlag, B. J. (1978): Ventricular arrhythmias and electrophysiological consequences of myocardial ischemia and infarction. *Circ. Res.*, 42:740–749.

164. Lazzara, R., and Scherlag, B. J. (1980): Role of the slow current in the generation of arrhythmias in ischemic myocardium. In: *The Slow Inward Current and Cardiac Arrhythmias*, edited by

165. Levy, M. N. (1971): Sympathetic-parasympathetic interactions in the heart. *Circ. Res.*, 29:437–445.

166. Levy, M. N., and Martin, P. J. (1979): Neural control of the heart. In: *Handbook of Physiology*, Vol. 1, edited by R. M. Berne, pp. 581–620. American Physiological Society, Bethesda.

167. Levites, R., Banka, V. S., and Helfant, R. H. (1975): Electrophysiologic effects of coronary occlusion and reperfusion: Observations of dispersion of refractoriness and ventricular automaticity. *Circulation*, 52:760–765.

168. Lombardi, F., Verrier, R. L., and Lown, B. (1983): Relationship between sympathetic neural activity, coronary dynamics, and vulnerability to ventricular fibrillation during myocardial ischemia and reperfusion. *Am. Heart J.*, 105:958–965.

169. Lown, B., and Verrier, R. L. (1976): Neural activity and ventricular fibrillation. *N. Engl. J. Med.*, 294:1165–1170.

170. Malliani, A., Schwartz, P. J., and Zanchetti, A. (1969): Sympathetic reflex elicited by experimental coronary occlusion. *J. Physiol. (Lond.)*, 217:703–709.

171. Malliani, A., Schwartz, P. J., and Zanchetti, A. (1980): Neural mechanisms in life-threatening arrhythmias. *Am. Heart J.*, 100:705–715.

172. Marrannes, R., de Hemptinne, A., and Leusen, I. (1979): Influence of lactate and other organic ions on conduction velocity in mammalian heart fibers depressed by "metabolic" acidosis. *J. Mol. Cell. Cardiol.*, 11:359–374.

173. Mather, P. P., and Case, R. B. (1973): Phosphate loss during reversible myocardial ischemia. *J. Mol. Cell. Cardiol.*, 5:375–393.

174. McDonald, T. F., and MacLeod, D. P. (1973): Metabolism and the electrical activity of anoxic ventricular muscle. *J. Physiol. (Lond.)*, 229:559–582.

175. Mendez, C., and Moe, G. K. (1966): Demonstration of a dual A-V nodal conduction system in the isolated rabbit heart. *Circ. Res.*, 19:378–393.

176. Mendez, C., Mueller, W. J., Meredith, J., and Moe, G. K. (1969): Interaction of transmembrane potentials in canine Purkinje fibers and at Purkinje fiber-muscle junctions. *Circ. Res.*, 25:361–373.

177. Merx, W., Yoon, M. S., and Han, J. (1977): The role of local disparity in conduction and recovery time of ventricular vulnerability to fibrillation. *Am. Heart J.*, 94:603–610.

178. Michelson, E. L., Spear, J. F., and Moore, E. N. (1980): Electrophysiologic and anatomic correlates of sustained ventricular tachyarrhythmias in a model of chronic myocardial infarction. *Am. J. Cardiol.*, 45:583–585.

179. Michelson, E. L., Spear, J. F., and Moore, E. N. (1981): Initiation of sustained ventricular tachyarrhythmias in a canine model of chronic myocardial infarction: Importance of the site of stimulation. *Circulation*, 63:776–784.

180. Miller, W. L., Belardinelli, L., Bacch, A., Foley, D., Rubine, R., and Berne, R. M. (1979): Canine myocardial adenosine and lactate production, oxygen consumption and coronary blood flow during stellate ganglion stimulation. *Circ. Res.*, 45:708–718.

181. Moe, G. K., Rheinbold, W. C., and Abildskov, J. A. (1964): A computer model of atrial fibrillation. *Am. Heart J.*, 67:200–207.

182. Morena, H., et al. (1980): Comparison of the effects of regional ischemia, hypoxia, hyperkalemia, and acidosis on intracellular and extracellular potentials and metabolism in the isolated porcine heart. *Circ. Res.*, 46:634–646.

183. Munakata, K., Dominic, J. A., and Surawicz, B. (1982): Variable effects of isoproterenol on action potential duration in guinea-pig papillary muscle: Differences between nonsteady and steady state; role of extracellular calcium concentration. *J. Pharmacol. Exp. Ther.*, 221:806–814.

184. Myerburg, R. J., et al. (1977): Long-term electrophysiological abnormalities resulting from experimental myocardial infarction in cats. *Circ. Res.*, 41:73–80.

185. Myerburg, R. J., et al. (1982): Cellular electrophysiology in acute and healed experimental myocardial infarction. *Ann. N.Y. Acad. Sci.*, 382:90–113.

186. Nahum, L. H., Hamilton, W. F., and Hoff, H. E. (1943): The injury current in the electrocardiogram. *Am. J. Physiol.*, 139:202–207.

187. Nattel, S., Elharrar, V., Zipes, D. P., and Bailey, J. C. (1981): pH-dependent electrophysiological effects of quinidine and lidocaine on canine cardiac Purkinje fibers. *Circ. Res.*, 48:55–61.

188. Nayler, W. G. (1982): Calcium antagonism: A new approach. *Clin. Exp. Pharmacol. Physiol.*, 6:3–13.

189. Nayler, W. G., Poole-Wilson, P. A., and Williams, A. (1979): Hypoxia and calcium. *J. Mol. Cell. Cardiol.*, 11:683–706.

190. Neely, J. R., Whitmer, J. T., and Rovetto, M. J. (1975): Subendocardial distribution of coronary blood flow and the effect of antianginal drugs. *Circ. Res.*, 30:621–627.

191. Oliver, M. F., Kurien, V. A., and Greenwood, T. W. (1968): Relation between serum-free fatty acids and arrhythmias and death after acute myocardial infarction. *Lancet*, 1:710–715.

192. Olsson, R. A. (1970): Changes in content of purine nucleoside in canine myocardium during coronary occlusion. *Circ. Res.*, 26: 301–306.

193. Oshita, S., Buchanan, J., and Gettes, L. (1982): A method for studying internal longitudinal resistance in guinea pig papillary muscles. *Circulation*, 66:II233 (abstract).

194. Patterson, R. E., and Kirk, E. S. (1983): Analysis of coronary collateral structure, function and ischemic border zones in pigs. *Am. J. Physiol.*, 244(*Heart Circ. Physiol.*, 13):H23–H31.

195. Peiper, G. M., et al. (1980): Attenuation of myocardial acidosis by propranolol during ischaemic arrest and reperfusion: Evidence with ^{31}P nuclear magnetic resonance. *Cardiovasc. Res.*, 14:646–653.

196. Poole-Wilson, P. A., and Cameron, I. R. (1975): Intracellular pH and K$^+$ of cardiac and skeletal muscle in acidosis and alkalosis. *Am. J. Physiol.*, 229:1305–1310.

197. Poole-Wilson, P. A., and Langer, G. A. (1975): Effect of pH on ionic exchange and function in rat and rabbit myocardium. *Am. J. Physiol.*, 229:570–581.

198. Posner, P., Farrar, E. L., and Lambert, C. R. (1976): Inhibitory effects of catecholamines in canine Purkinje fibers. *Am. J. Physiol.*, 231:1415–1920.

199. Prinzmetal, M., Toyoshima, H., Ekmekci, A., Mizuno, Y., and Nagaya, T. (1961): Nature of ischemic electrocardiographic patterns in mammalian ventricles as determined by intracellular electrographic and metabolic changes. *Am. J. Cardiol.*, 8:493–503.

200. Quadbeck, J., and Reiter, M. (1975): Cardiac action potential and inotropic effects of noradrenaline and calcium. *Naunyn Schmiedebergs Arch. Pharmacol.*, 228:337–351.

201. Rau, E. E., and Langer, G. A. (1978): Dissociation of energetic state and potassium loss from anoxic myocardium. *Am. J. Physiol.*, 235(*Heart Circ. Physiol.*, 4):H537–H543.

202. Reber, W. R., and Weingart, R. (1982): Ungulate cardiac Purkinje fibres: The influence of intracellular pH on the electrical cell-to-cell coupling. *J. Physiol. (Lond.)*, 328:87–104.

203. Reimer, K. A., Jennings, R. B., and Hill, M. A. (1981): Total ischemia in dog hearts, in vitro. 2. High energy phosphate depletion and associated defects in energy metabolism, cell volume regulation, and sarcolemmal integrity. *Circ. Res.* 49:901–911.

204. Reimer, K. A., Lowe, J. E., Rasmussen, M. M., and Jennings, R. B. (1977): The wavefront phenomenon of ischemic cell death. I. Myocardial infarct size vs. duration of coronary occlusion in dogs. *Circulation*, 56:786–794.

205. Reuter, H. (1979): Properties of two inward membrane currents in the heart. *Annu. Rev. Physiol.*, 41:413–424.

206. Reuter, H. (1983): Calcium channel modulation by neurotransmitters, enzymes and drugs. *Nature*, 301:569–574.

207. Reuter, H. (1984): Ion channels in cardiac cell membranes. *Annu. Rev. Physiol.*, 46:473–474.

208. Reuter, H. (1980): Effects of neurotransmitters on the slow inward current. In: *The Slow Inward Current and Cardiac Arrhythmias*, edited by D. P. Zipes, J. C. Bailey, and V. Elharrar, pp. 205–219. Martinus Nijhoff, The Hague.

209. Richards, D. A., Blake, G. J., Spear, J. F., and Moore, E. N. (1984): Electrophysiologic substrate for ventricular tachycardia: Correlation of properties in vivo and in vitro. *Circulation*, 69:369–381.

210. Rosen, M. R., Hordof, A. J., Ilvento, J. P., and Danilo, P., Jr. (1977): Effects of adrenergic amines on electrophysiological prop-

211. Robinson, R. B., and Sleator, W. W. (1977): Effects of Ca^{2+} and catecholamines on guinea pig atrium action potential plateau. *Am. J. Physiol.*, 233(*Heart Circ. Physiol.*, 2):H203.

212. Ruiz-Ceretti, E., Ragault, P., Leblanc, N., and Zumino, A. Z. P. (1983): Effects of hypoxia and altered K$_0$ on the membrane potential of rabbit ventricle. *J. Mol. Cell. Cardiol.*, 15:845–854.

213. Russell, D. C., and Oliver, M. F. (1978): Ventricular refractoriness during acute myocardial ischaemia and its relationship to ventricular fibrillation. *Cardiovasc. Res.*, 12:221–227.

214. Russell, D. C., Smith, H. J., and Oliver, M. F. (1979): Transmembrane potential changes and ventricular fibrillation during repetitive myocardial ischaemia in the dog. *Br. Heart J.*, 42:88–96.

215. Sakai, K., and Abiko, Y. (1981): Acute changes of myocardial norepinephrine and glycogen phosphorylase in ischemic and nonischemic areas after coronary ligation in dogs. *Jpn. Circ. J.*, 45:1250–1255.

216. Samson, W. E., and Scher, A. M. (1960): Mechanism of S-T segment alteration during acute myocardial injury. *Circ. Res.*, 8:780–787.

217. Sano, T., Horoaka, M., and Sawanobori, T. (1978): Effects of anoxia and metabolic inhibitors on reactivation of the fast sodium system. In: *Recent Advances in Studies on Cardiac Structure and Metabolism*, Vol. 11. *Heart Function and Metabolism*, edited by T. Kobayashi, T. Sano, and N. S. Dhalla, pp. 79–83. University Press, Baltimore.

218. Sasynuck, B. I., and Mendez, C. (1971): A mechanism for reentry in canine ventricular tissue. *Circ. Res.*, 28:3–12.

219. Sayen, J. J., Pierce, G., Katcher, A. H., and Sheldon, W. F. (1961): Correlation of intramyocardial electrocardiograms with polarographic oxygen and contractility in the non-ischemic and regionally ischemic left ventricle. *Circ. Res.*, 9:1268–1279.

220. Scherlag, B. J., El-Sherif, N., Hope, R., and Lazzara, R. (1974): Characterization and localization of ventricular arrhythmias resulting from myocardial ischemia and infarction. *Circ. Res.*, 35:372–383.

221. Schwartz, P. J., Billman, G. E., and Stone, H. L. (1984): Autonomic mechanisms in ventricular fibrillation induced by myocardial ischemia during exercise in dogs with health myocardial infarction. *Circulation*, 69:790–798.

222. Schwartz, P. J., and Stone, H. L. (1982): The role of the autonomic nervous system in sudden coronary death. *Ann. N.Y. Acad. Sci.*, 382:162–180.

223. Schwartz, P. J., Stone, H. L., and Brown, A. M. (1976): Effects of unilateral stellate ganglion blockade on the arrhythmias associated with coronary occlusion. *Am. Heart J.*, 92:589–599.

224. Senges, J., Brachmann, J., Pelzer, D., Mizutani, T., and Keubler, W. (1979): Effects of some components of ischemia on electrical activity and reentry in the canine ventricular conduction system. *Circ. Res.* 44:864–872.

225. Skinner, R. B., Jr., and Kunze, D. L. (1976): Changes in extracellular potassium activity in response to decreased pH in rabbit atrial muscle. *Circ. Res.*, 39:678–683.

226. Skinner, J. E., Lie, J. T., and Entman, M. L. (1975): Modification of ventricular fibrillation latency following coronary artery occlusion in the conscious pig: The effects of psychological stress and beta-adrenergic blockade. *Circulation*, 51:656–667.

227. Spach, M. S., and Kootsey, J. M. (1983): The nature of electrical propagation in cardiac muscle. *Am. J. Physiol.*, 244(*Heart Circ. Physiol.*, 13):H3–H22.

228. Spach, M. S., et al. (1981): The discontinuous nature of propagation in normal canine cardiac muscle. Evidence for recurrent discontinuities of intracellular resistance that affect membrane currents. *Circ. Res.*, 48:39–54.

229. Spear, J. F., and Moore, E. N. (1974): Supernormal excitability and conduction in the His-Purkinje system of the dog. *Circ. Res.*, 35:732–792.

230. Spear, J. F., Horowitz, L. N., Hodess, A. B., MacVaugh, H., and Moore, E. N. (1979): Cellular electrophysiology of human myocardial infarction. *Circulation*, 59:247–256.

231. Spitzer, K. W., and Hogan, P. M., (1979): The effects of acidosis

and bicarbonate on action potential repolarization in canine cardiac Purkinje fibers. *J. Gen. Physiol.*, 73:199–218.

232. Surawicz, B., and Gettes, L. S. (1971): Effect of electrolyte abnormalities on the heart and circulation. In: *Cardiac and Vascular Diseases*, edited by H. L. Conn and O. Horowitz, pp. 539–576. Lea & Febiger, Philadelphia.

233. Ten Eick, R., Nawrath, H., and Trautwein, W. (1976): On the mechanism of the negative inotropic effect of acetylcholine. *Pfluegers Arch.*, 361:207–213.

234. Trautwein, W., and Dudel, J. (1956): Aktionspotential und Kontraktion des Herzmuskels in Sauerstoffmangel. *Pfluegers Arch.*, 263:23–32.

235. Trautwein, W., and Kassebaum, D. C. (1961): On the mechanism of spontaneous impulse generation in the pacemaker of the heart. *J. Gen. Physiol.*, 45:317.

236. Tse, W. W., Han, J., and Yoon, M. S. (1976): Effect of acetylcholine on automaticity of canine Purkinje fibers. *Am. J. Physiol.*, 230:116–119.

237. Tsien, R. W., Filwa, Q., and Greengard, P. (1972): Cyclic AMP mediates the effect of adrenaline on cardiac Purkinje fibers. *Nature [New Biol.]*, 240:181–183.

238. Tsuchida, T. (1965): Experimental studies on the excitability of ventricular musculature in infarcted region. *Jpn. Heart J.*, 65:152–164.

239. Uchida, Y., and Murao, S. (1974): Excitation of afferent cardiac symptomatic nerve fibers during coronary occlusion. *Am. J. Physiol.*, 226:1094–1099.

240. Uchida, Y., and Murao, S. (1974): Potassium-induced excitation of afferent cardiac sympathetic nerve fibers. *Am. J. Physiol.*, 226:603–607.

241. Uchida, Y., and Murao, S. (1975): Acid-induced excitation of afferent cardiac symptomatic nerve fibers. *Am. J. Physiol.*, 228:27–33.

242. Uchida, Y., and Murao, S. (1974): Bradykinin induced excitation of afferent cardiac symptomatic nerve fibers. *Jpn. Heart J.*, 15:84–91.

243. Van Capelle, F. J. L., and Durrer, D. (1980): Computer simulation of arrhythmias in a network of coupled elements. *Circ. Res.*, 47:454–466.

244. Vaughan Williams, E. M., and Whyte, J. M. (1967): Chemosensitivity of cardiac muscle. *J. Physiol. (Lond.)*, 189:119–137.

245. Vassort, G., et al. (1969): Effects of adrenaline on membrane inward currents during the cardiac action potential. *Pfluegers Arch.*, 309:70–81.

246. Veenstra, R. D., Joyner, R. W., and Rawling, D. A. (1984): Purkinje and ventricular activation sequences of canine papillary muscle: Effects of quinidine and calcium on the Purkinje-ventricular conduction delay. *Circ. Res.*, 54:500–515.

247. Vogel, S., and Speralakis, N. (1977): Blockade of myocardial slow inward current at low pH. *Am. J. Physiol.*, 233:C99–103.

248. Vleugels, A., and Carmeliet, E. E. (1976): Hypoxia increases potassium efflux from mammalian myocardium. *Experientia*, 32:483–484.

249. Vleugels, A., Vereecke, J., and Carmeliet, E. E. (1980): Ionic currents during hypoxia in voltage clamped cat ventricular muscle. *Circ. Res.*, 47:501–508.

250. Wada, F., and Goto, Y. (1975): Effects of pH on the processes of excitation-contraction coupling of bullfrog atrium. *Jpn. J. Physiol.*, 25:605–620.

251. Waldo, A. L., and Kaiser, G. A. (1973): A study of ventricular arrhythmias associated with acute myocardial infarction in the canine heart. *Circulation*, 47:1222–1228.

252. Wallace, A. G., and Mignone, R. J. (1966): Physiologic evidence concerning the re-entry hypothesis for ectopic beats. *Am. Heart J.*, 72:60.

253. Walton, M. K., and Fozzard, H. A. (1983): The conducted action potential: Models and comparison to experiments. *Biophys. J.*, 44:9–26.

254. Watanabe, A. M., and Besch, H. R., Jr. (1975): Interaction between cyclic adenosine monophosphate and cyclic guanosine monophosphate in guinea pig ventricular myocardium. *Circ. Res.*, 37:309–317.

255. Watanabe, A. M. (1983): Cholinergic agonists and antagonists: In: *Cardiac Therapy*, edited by M. R. Rosen and B. F. Hoffman, pp. 95–144. Martinus Nijhoff, Boston.

256. Watson, R. M., et al. (1984): Transmural pH gradient in canine myocardial ischemia. *Am. J. Physiol.*, 246(*Heart Circ. Physiol.*, 15):H232–H238.

257. Weidmann, S. (1955): The effect of cardiac membrane potential on the rapid availability of the sodium-carrying system. *J. Physiol. (Lond.)*, 127:213–228.

258. Weidmann, S. (1955): Effects of calcium ions and local anaesthetics on electrical properties of Purkinje fibers. *J. Physiol. (Lond.)*, 129:568–582.

259. Weidmann, S. (1956): Shortening of the action potential due to brief injections of KCl following the onset of activity. *J. Physiol. (Lond.)*, 132:156–163.

260. Weidmann, S. (1956): *Elektrophysiologie der Herzmuskelfaser.* Huber, Stuttgart.

261. Weishaar, R., and Bing, R. J. (1979): The effect of diltiazem, a calcium-antagonist on myocardial ischemia. *Am. J. Cardiol.*, 43:1137–1143.

262. Weiss, J., and Shine, K. I. (1982): [K$^+$]$_o$ accumulation and electrophysiological alterations during early myocardial ischemia. *Am. J. Physiol.* 243(*Heart Circ. Physiol.*, 12):H318–H327.

263. Weiss, J., and Shine, K. I. (1982): Extracellular K$^+$ accumulation during myocardial ischemia in isolated rabbit heart. *Am. J. Physiol.*, 242(*Heart Circ. Physiol.*, 11)H619–H628.

264. Wiegand, V., Guggi, M., Meesmann, W., Kessler, M., and Greitschus, F. (1979): Extracellular potassium activity changes in the canine myocardium after acute coronary occlusion and the influence of beta-blockade. *Cardiovasc. Res.*, 13:297–304.

265. Wiggers, C. J. (1940): The mechanism and nature of ventricular fibrillation. *Am. Heart J.*, 20:399–404.

266. Williams, D. O., Scherlag, B. J., Hope, R. R., El-Sherif, N., and Lazzara, R. (1974): The pathophysiology of malignant ventricular arrhythmias during acute myocardial ischemia. *Circulation*, 50:1163–1172.

267. Windisch, H., and Tritthart, H. A. (1981): Calcium ion effects on the rising phases of action potentials obtained from guinea-pig papillary muscles at different potassium concentrations. *J. Mol. Cell. Cardiol.*, 13:457–469.

268. Windisch, H., and Tritthart, H. A. (1982): Isoproterenol, norepinephrine and phosphodiesterase inhibitors are blockers of the depressed fast Na$^+$-system in ventricular muscle fibers. *J. Mol. Cell. Cardiol.*, 14:431–434.

269. Wit, A. L., and Bigger, J. T. (1975): The electrophysiology of lethal arrhythmias: Possible electrophysiological mechanisms for lethal arrhythmias accompanying myocardial ischemia and infarction. *Circulation [Suppl. 3]*, 51/52:96–115.

270. Wit, A. L., and Cranefield, P. F. (1979): Triggered and automatic activity in the canine coronary sinus. *Circ. Res.*, 41:435–445.

271. Wit, A. L., Cranefield, P. F., and Gadsby, D. C. (1980): Triggered activity. In: *The Slow Inward Current and Cardiac Arrhythmias,* edited by D. P. Zipes, J. C. Bailey, and V. Elharrar, pp. 437–454. Martinus Nijhoff, The Hague.

272. Wit, A. L., Hoffman, B. F., and Cranefield, P. F. (1972): Slow conduction and reentry in the ventricular conducting system. I. Return extrasystole in canine Purkinje fibers. *Circ. Res.*, 30:1–10.

273. Wittig, J. H., and Boineau, J. P. (1975): Surgical treatment of ventricular arrhythmias using epicardial, transmural, and endocardial mapping. *Ann. Thorac. Surg.*, 20:117–126.

274. Wojtczak, J. (1979): Contractures and increase in internal longitudinal resistance of cow ventricular muscle induced by hypoxia. *Circ. Res.*, 44:88–95.

The Heart and Cardiovascular System,
edited by H. A. Fozzard et al.
Raven Press, New York © 1986.

CHAPTER 58

Mechanisms Controlling Cardiac Autonomic Function and Their Relation to Arrhythmogenesis

Peter B. Corr, Kathryn A. Yamada, and Francis X. Witkowski

The sympathetic and parasympathetic nervous systems can, under certain conditions, profoundly influence the electrophysiological properties of the heart and thereby the evolution of both supraventricular and ventricular arrhythmias. In this review, the influence of the autonomic nervous system on arrhythmogenesis is considered from several different levels of complexity, including both *in vitro* and *in vivo* studies in animals and clinical correlates to the experimental findings. Our aim is to present the current state of knowledge and, when appropriate, to define areas where this knowledge is inadequate to arrive at definitive conclusions. This approach should define the framework to stimulate investigations into several areas that appear to be most promising for developing improved interventions for prophylaxis and treatment of malignant ventricular arrhythmias. Prior to considering the cardiac electrophysiologic effects of autonomic input, a brief review of autonomic innervation will be presented.

AUTONOMIC INNERVATION OF THE HEART

The detailed autonomic innervation of the myocardium varies substantially among species, and in many reports the anatomical characteristics have not been correlated with functional indices. The dog is the most extensively studied species relative to detailed cardiac innervation, and although similar to the human, the dog differs in several important respects. In the dog, the two vagi or parasympathetic nerves have their cell bodies in the nodose ganglia and become intermingled with sympathetic fibers between the superior and middle cervical ganglia, each thereby becoming a mixed vagosympathetic nerve. Thus, stimulation of the cervical vagal nerve distal to the middle cervical ganglion results in a mixed sympathetic-parasympathetic response (569). In contrast, in the human, the vagi innervate the heart in nerves distinct from the sympathetic innervation, with little or no interconnections between the vagi emanating from the nodose ganglion and the sympathetic fibers emanating from the cervical or stellate sympathetic ganglia.

In the dog, the middle cervical ganglion on the right side gives off two ansae to the stellate ganglion, from which arises the right stellate nerve. Preganglionic neurons from C-7 to T-5 in the spinal cord synapse in or pass through the stellate ganglion (773). The right stellate nerve originates from either the stellate ganglion per se or the ventral ansa and thus may have cell bodies in both the middle cervical ganglion and stellate ganglion (23). The right stellate nerve, which is also termed the right interganglionic nerve, innervates the right atrial surface and sinoatrial (SA) node and mediates a positive inotropic effect in the atria and a positive chronotropic effect in the SA node (570). Afferent fibers from the

atria also are present in the right stellate nerve (22). Also on the right side in the dog is the recurrent cardiac nerve, a branch of the recurrent laryngeal nerve with primary cell bodies in the caudal cervical ganglion. This nerve also contains input from the middle cervical ganglion through the caudal pole nerve. The right recurrent cardiac nerve contains not only efferents but also afferents from both the atria and ventricles (22). The vagal innervation on the right side in the dog occurs through two major branches below the ansae subclavia, the craniovagal and caudovagal nerves (481). Both nerves contain sympathetic and parasympathetic fibers with both afferent and efferent functions to the right atria (22). Although the sympathetic chain runs caudal to the stellate ganglia, there appears to be little or no functional input to the heart in the dog below the stellate ganglia (24,479), although this point is controversial in that others have demonstrated that cardiac nerves can emanate from the sympathetic chain caudal to the stellate ganglion (103,468). Randall has suggested that these caudal projections in the dog do not influence cardiac function and are not true neural structures.

On the left side in the dog, a number of distinct sympathetic nerves can be found that are not present on the right side. For example, the innominate nerve and the ventromedial nerve emanate from the caudal cervical ganglion as well as from the vagus nerve and thus have both parasympathetic and sympathetic influences with both afferent and efferent functions (22,24,570). The dorsal cardiac nerve is primarily an afferent nerve from aortic receptors with no efferent cardiac neural input but whose cell bodies are in the caudal cervical ganglion (22,480). The ventrolateral cardiac nerve also receives its major input from the caudal cervical ganglion, with additional input from the ansa subclavia and the vagus and recurrent laryngeal nerves, and thus contains both sympathetic and parasympathetic fibers that impinge on the left atrium and left ventricle, including the atrioventricular node (570). The final nerve on the left side in the dog is the left stellate cardiac nerve, which is primarily afferent in nature from the left atrium (22).

It appears that stimulation of discrete cardiac nerves can result in alterations in very specific regions, as demonstrated by Randall (567), and that if control is sufficiently discrete at the central neural level, alterations in very specific regions can occur that may influence not only regional contractility and specific pacemakers but also discrete regional propagation of the cardiac impulse. This differential activation of efferent sympathetic nerves to the heart appears to occur in experimental animals during early myocardial ischemia, evidenced by both an increase and a decrease in neural activity in closely adjacent nerves (*vide infra*).

Evidence also suggests that efferent vagal input to different regions of the heart may be controlled by different central neural structures. Geis and Wurster (234a) have shown that the nucleus ambiguus controls the sinus heart rate whereas the dorsal motor nucleus appears to control vagal input to the ventricle without a change in sinus rate. Since the neurotransmitter at the nucleus ambiguus is γ-aminobutyric acid (GABA) and there is evidence that the transmitter at the dorsal motor nucleus of the vagus may be oxytocin, this may provide a means to control vagal input to the ventricle without altering sinus rate. Future studies should be directed at similar approaches to selectively control central neural autonomic outflow for potential therapeutic advantages.

In the human, the sympathetic and parasympathetic components to the heart are discrete and separate structures. On the right side, the middle cervical ganglion gives off two distinct branches of sympathetic nerves to the right side of the heart, the right dorsomedial and dorsolateral cardiac nerves. The right stellate cardiac nerve originates either from the right stellate ganglion or, in part, from the ventral ansa subclavia. The vagal fibers on the right side in the human originate exclusively from the nodose ganglion and enter the heart through three structures, the recurrent cardiac nerve, the thoracic craniovagal cardiac nerve, and the thoracic caudovagal cardiac nerve. In contrast, on the left side, the left stellate cardiac nerve is large, and the stellate ganglion, a fusion of the inferior cervical ganglion and the first thoracic ganglion, is connected to the middle cervical ganglion by a small ventral ansa subclavia and usually two large dorsal ansae. Most of the cardiac sympathetic innervation in the human emanates from this middle cervical ganglion through four major nerves, the ventral lateral cardiac nerve, the dorsomedial cardiac nerve, the dorsointermedial cardiac nerve, and the left thoracic dorsolateral cardiac nerve, which innervates the atrioventricular node. In addition to these four major nerves from the middle cervical ganglion, there are interconnections to both the vertebral and thyroid ganglia. In some cases, sympathetic fibers course directly from the thyroid and vertebral ganglia to the heart without passing through the middle cervical ganglion.

In summary, autonomic innervation of the heart occurs through complex yet discrete pathways that vary substantially between species. Most important, stimulation of sympathetic structures can result in enhanced parasympathetic input as well, necessitating the use of pharmacological blockade of one component to allow adequate assessment of the other branch of the autonomic nervous system. Likewise, because of the intermingling of both afferent and efferent nerves in most cardiac branches, it is essential to decentralize the structure prior to efferent neural stimulation studies to prevent either ipsilateral effects through other nerves or contralateral influences through spinal or central neural pathways. Because of the discrete nature of efferent responses in the heart (567), multiple simultaneous cardiac mea-

surements are required to adequately assess the influence of neural stimulation. Finally, the magnitude and frequency of neural stimulation used in experimental studies may be excessive compared with the frequency and magnitude of endogenous neural stimulation under physiological or pathophysiological conditions.

ELECTROPHYSIOLOGY OF AUTONOMIC NEUROTRANSMITTERS

In the following section the electrophysiological effects of catecholamines and acetylcholine will be considered separately. Because of disparate effects on different regions of the heart, each region will also be considered separately.

Effects of Catecholamines on the Sinus Node

Information concerning the distribution of both sympathetic and parasympathetic nerves to the SA node remains incomplete (567). Using fluorescence histochemistry to define catecholamine-containing structures and obtain a qualitative assessment of the relative density of adrenergic fibers, a dense network of fluorescent fibers has been described in the area of the SA node in both dogs and rabbits (19,154). These adrenergic fibers appear to innervate most of the SA cells (154). Using isolated atrial preparations with attached and functional sympathetic postganglionic fibers, the influences of both sympathetic nerve stimulation and catecholamine superfusion can be assessed while avoiding the reflex autonomic effects present in situ. Likewise, these procedures permit direct recording of transmembrane action potentials from sinus node cells (723). The frequency of pacemaker discharge is dependent on at least three factors: (a) the slope of phase-4 depolarization, (b) the resting membrane potential (V_m), and (c) the level of the threshold potential (V_{th}). Action potentials recorded from sinus node pacemaker cells reveal several distinct morphological characteristics, including slow depolarization during phase 4, V_m of −50 to −65 mV, and a slow phase-0 depolarization. Using an isolated rabbit SA node preparation, the most prominent effect of sympathetic nerve stimulation is an increase in the slope of phase-4 diastolic depolarization, with threshold level not being altered (723), accounting for an increase in pacemaker firing. The action potential duration measured at 90% repolarization is slightly shortened by sympathetic stimulation, whereas the maximum diastolic potential is unaltered (723). Frequently, sympathetic stimulation is found to convert a true pacemaker fiber, characterized by a smooth transition from the diastolic depolarization to the action potential upstroke, into a latent one (723), which morphologically corresponds to a shift of the pacemaker origin. Likewise, superfusion with norepinephrine induces alterations in the SA node similar to sympathetic nerve stimulation, including an increase in the slope of phase-4 diastolic depolarization as well as a pacemaker shift within the node. These findings imply quantitative differences in receptor density, sensitivity, or coupling to intracellular mediators at each site composing the pacemaker region of the SA node, assuming equal availability of all sites to the superfused neurotransmitter. Similar observations of a complex pacemaker origin with extensive redundancy and multiple levels of functional response have been observed *in situ* with detailed atrial epicardial activation sequence maps and unipolar potential distribution maps (70). Of note, these more recent approaches have revealed a system of possible dominant atrial pacemakers that is considerably more extensive than the sinus node (67). However, in the absence of microelectrode studies of atrial epicardial areas to verify the pacemaker sites, the observations may simply reflect epicardial breakthrough from a single SA node that has a complex tridimensional structure.

Stimulation studies of the stellate ganglia have revealed "sidedness" to the sympathetic innervation of the SA node. Right stellate ganglion stimulation produces sinus tachycardia without discernible shift in P-wave morphology, as grossly determined by a body surface electrocardiogram (568). In contrast, left stellate ganglion stimulation results in less marked increases in heart rate, but is frequently accompanied by a shift in P-wave morphology indicative of a shift from the sinus pacemaker to an ectopic atrial site (568). When more detailed P-wave morphological studies are correlated with accurate sinus node mapping, subtle changes in P-wave morphology are seen, with spontaneous beat-to-beat changes in cycle length (67). In addition, isoproterenol-induced changes in the rate of the SA node are also accompanied by small changes in P-wave morphology (67). Thus, right stellate ganglion stimulation might be expected to produce some, albeit more subtle, changes in pacemaker origin, with resultant alterations of the atrial activation pattern reflected in the P-wave morphology.

In situ electrophysiological procedures used to assess sinus node function in the clinical setting involve assessment of both sinus node automaticity and SA conduction. Refractory period measurements are hampered by the inability to record the effect of premature stimuli directly both proximal and distal to the sinus node, even if sinus node electrogram catheter recording techniques are employed (578). Assessment of the automaticity of the sinus node *in situ* is most frequently achieved by the response of the sinus node to overdrive suppression, where the degree of prolongation of the postdrive cycle length in excess of the control cycle length is assumed to reflect the extent of depression in sinus node automaticity and is termed the sinus node recovery time (446,593). The importance of the release of neurotransmitters rather than the direct excitation of

the sinus node cells in the genesis of some of the effects of overdrive suppression with electrical stimulation has also been investigated (751). The overdrive suppression and the subsequent acceleration of the pacemaker depend on the rate and duration of the driving stimulus and can spontaneously occur after rapid supraventricular tachycardias (386,433). The overdrive suppression is greatest when the driving electrode is placed on the sinus node. Sympathetic nerve stimulation during the last part of the electrical drive sequence shortens the duration of overdrive suppression, and a similar response is obtained with norepinephrine, cocaine, and atropine (386). Thus, at least three factors will influence the response of a normal sinus node complex to electrical overdrive suppression: (a) the proximity of the electrode to the sinus node complex, (b) the relative extent of release of local autonomic neurotransmitters, and (c) the conduction time into and out of the SA node (695). The last factor is likely to be dominant at faster driving rates when the driving stimulus encounters entrance block into the SA node. This finding could be an explanation for the fact that the poststimulus pause is commonly shorter for driving rates in excess of 150 beats/min than at a slower driving rate (446).

Because of the intimate relationship between the autonomic nervous system and intrinsic sinus node electrophysiological properties, autonomic blockade using the procedures of Jose (340) has been invoked to determine the "intrinsic" sinus node function (10). However, these procedures involve the use of pharmacological agents that may result in alteration of the hemodynamic status, competitive antagonism that may be incomplete, and β-adrenergic blocking agents that may possess direct membrane effects. To overcome these inherent difficulties, human transplanted hearts have been studied wherein each patient has two sinus nodes, with the recipient sinus node driving only the atrial remnants and the donor sinus node driving the donor atria and ventricles. The transplanted donor heart appears to remain both anatomically and functionally denervated (399,690,691). Detailed studies of sinus node recovery function in such denervated sinus nodes *in situ* indicate SA node recovery times that increase in a predictable and organized manner with increasing pacing rates in patients without overt donor sinus node dysfunction (55,455). These studies also demonstrate a relatively high incidence of abnormalities of donor SA conduction, as well as SA node automaticity. Patients can be clearly separated into two groups, those with normal sinus node function tests and those with abnormal sinus node function (55), with little overlap between the two groups. In contrast, in patients with sinus node dysfunction with an intact autonomic nervous system, the two groups are not as easily discernible (150,267). The sinus node dysfunction in donor hearts of transplant recipients may contribute to the increased incidence of sudden death and may be related to direct injury of the sinus node.

Effects of Catecholamines on Atrial Tissue

Atrial muscle cells are variable in diameter, with frequent branchings as they traverse atrial walls and the interatrial septum en route to the atrioventricular node or to their insertion into the annulus fibrosus. Whether or not electrical depolarization propagates over preferential conducting pathways is still a debated issue, and the pertinent anatomic, physiological, and clinical evidence that either discredits or supports the existence of such specialized interatrial pathways has been reviewed (191,302,320,323,327,675,726). The weight of evidence does not support the presence of specialized interatrial pathways that resemble the bundle branches in the ventricle. However, rapid conduction between the SA and atrioventricular nodes probably does exist in some parts of the atrium because of wave front initiation, fiber orientation, size, geometry, or factors other than specific specialized tracts.

The distribution of sympathetic fibers to the atria, as assessed by norepinephrine concentrations, is higher in the atria on the right side of the heart than the left in both rabbit and dog (19), with the highest concentration present in the sinus node. The typical transmembrane action potential from contractile atrial tissue is characterized by a resting membrane potential of −80 to −90 mV, a stable level of membrane potential during phase 4, an abrupt onset of rapid depolarization, with rates of depolarization of at least 80 V/sec, and a slow return of repolarization during the terminal phase of the action potential (303). Atrial cells that differ electrophysiologically and anatomically have been described in rabbit, dog, and man. At the venous border of the crista terminalis, fibers usually demonstrate slow depolarization during phase 4, with a prominent rapid phase-0 depolarization and a definitive plateau phase, and are termed plateau fibers or specialized atrial fibers (306). An important functional significance of these fibers is their capacity, as latent pacemakers, to take over as the dominant atrial pacemaker. The embryological derivation of the sinus node is the sinus venosus, and remnants of this embryonic structure have been identified in several areas of the mammalian heart besides the proximal sulcus terminalis, including the musculature of the superior vena cava, coronary sinus, and venous valves.

Excision of the SA node results in residual pacemaker activity arising within the right atrium (233,638) that is responsive to both exercise and autonomic blockade, indicating the presence of sympathetic regulation of functionally dominant subsidiary atrial pacemakers (572). This functional extension of the SA node may correlate to the epicardial breakthrough sites observed using detailed atrial mapping procedures (67). In a conscious dog in which the SA node has been surgically excised, the response to isoproterenol indicates that the subsidiary atrial pacemakers are not capable of a maximum heart rate comparable to that in a control animal with an

intact sinus node subjected to direct β-adrenergic stimulation (571). Interestingly, the "sidedness" is preserved after SA node excision, with both right and left stellate ganglia stimulation causing rate acceleration of subsidiary pacemakers. The response to right stellate stimulation remains greater than that to left stellate stimulation in animals demonstrating subsidiary atrial pacemakers, although shifts in P-wave morphology again occur only with left stellate stimulation (571).

The effects of catecholamines on the electrophysiological properties of atrial muscle cells are minimal compared with effects elicited in pacemaker tissue. Sympathetic stimulation during recordings of the transmembrane potential in atrial muscle elicits little consistent change in the resting membrane potential, the velocity of phase-0 depolarization, or the amplitude of the reversal potential (303). The direct effects of catecholamines on the functional refractory period, as determined by the extrastimulus technique in isolated atrial tissue, has demonstrated a β-adrenergic-mediated decrease in functional refractory period (259). In contrast, an increase in the functional refractory period is seen mediated through α-adrenergic receptor stimulation (259).

Effects of Catecholamines on the Atrioventricular Node

The density of adrenergic innervation in the dog heart in the area of the atrioventricular (AV) node is regarded as high (154), but in both the dog and the rabbit the concentration of norepinephrine in the AV nodal region is not higher than in surrounding tissue (19). Knowledge of the complex cellular composition and precise morphology and architecture of the AV node and its adjacent junctional areas is still incomplete. Morphological counterparts are present for the three classic zones of the AV node: (a) the AN zone located proximal to the zone of Wenckebach block induced by rapid stimulation, (b) the N zone, where the typical increments in conduction time and block occur during rapid stimulation, and (c) the NH zone distal to the zone of block during rapid atrial stimulation. Neither the action potential configuration nor the functional behavior of the tissue in each of the three zones appears to be determined exclusively by cellular morphology (329). Nodal architecture, as well as cellular morphology, plays a significant role in the net electrophysiological properties of the three zones of the AV node (329).

In situ, either right or left stellate ganglion stimulation for only 100 msec in the dog with heart rate fixed by pacing results in acceleration of AV conduction with a latency of 1 to 1.5 sec, a peak response by 6 to 8 sec, and a total duration of action of 13 to 21 sec (676). The acceleration of AV conduction occurs with no effect on atrial, His-Purkinje, or ventricular conduction. Furthermore, there is no discernible difference in responses to AV conduction between right and left stellate ganglion stimulations. Brief bursts of stellate stimulation also have greater effects on AV junctional pacemakers than on ectopic atrial pacemakers, resulting in emergence of transient junctional pacemaker dominance (676).

Most patients (~75%) with AV nodal reentrant supraventricular tachycardia exhibit dual AV nodal pathways in response to atrial stimulation, as identified by a discontinuous response to progressively more premature atrial stimuli (594). Microelectrode recordings in isolated rabbit hearts suggest that the functional discontinuity into dual pathways occurs in the proximal portion of the AV node (472), as derived from atrial extrastimulus studies. A true assessment of slow-pathway refractory properties can be obtained only if the sinus or driven atrial beats are conducted via the slow pathway, which is rarely the case in human studies. The jump from the fast pathway to the slow pathway is typically determined by a rapid increase of at least 50 msec in the A-H interval of the His-bundle electrogram. The demonstration of a dual pathway suggests marked inhomogeneity of conduction and refractoriness in the AV node. β-Adrenergic blockade with propranolol has been shown to increase the refractory period similarly in both the fast and slow pathways, suggesting that the effects of catecholamines on the two pathways are similar (792).

Effects of Catecholamines on Accessory Pathways

In patients with the Wolff-Parkinson-White (WPW) syndrome (789), one limb of the macro-reentry loop that sustains the tachycardia is commonly the accessory AV pathway (226), with the remainder of the loop composed of the atria, the specialized cardiac conduction system, and the ventricles. These pathways may be functional in the antegrade (atrioventricular) and retrograde (ventriculoatrial) directions, although evidence of preexcitation on the electrocardiogram is evident only when functional antegrade conduction exists in sinus rhythm or when manifested during a rapid ventricular response during an episode of atrial fibrillation or flutter.

There is a wide range of antegrade effective refractory periods measured in patients with WPW accessory pathways, with a short antegrade effective refractory period being an important determinant of the ventricular rate occurring during atrial fibrillation (109,775). Furthermore, episodes of supraventricular tachycardia can be induced by ventricular pacing utilizing the bypass tract in a retrograde fashion when the antegrade refractory period of the bypass tract exceeds that of the AV node. This allows premature beats that occur in the interval between these two refractory periods to utilize the AV node antegrade when the accessory pathway is refractory. Such premature timing effectively dissociates the two pathways, allowing the accessory pathway to conduct retrograde when the AV node is then refractory, thus completing the reentrant loop.

An accessory pathway with antegrade conduction that became apparent only with increased sympathetic tone elicited by exercise or isoproterenol infusion was first described in 1979 (772). Subsequently, patients have been reported with documented antegrade ventricular preexcitation during isoproterenol infusion. The antegrade refractory period elicited by isoproterenol is longer than that reported in a large series of patients with spontaneous antegrade accessory pathway conduction (559). Likewise, in patients with functional antegrade accessory pathways, isoproterenol has been shown to shorten the antegrade refractory period of the accessory pathway, with the greatest amount of shortening occurring in patients with the longest initial values of antegrade refractory period (776). The clinical implication of this finding is that states leading to increased adrenergic stimulation may result in shortening of the antegrade refractory period, leading to increased ventricular rates during atrial fibrillation. Furthermore, although isoproterenol induces significant changes in the antegrade refractory characteristics of the accessory pathway, it has little effect on the refractory period of either the atrium or ventricle (776). This suggests that the accessory pathways have different β-adrenergic responsivities and may not be composed of ordinary atrial or ventricular muscle cells (776). No pharmacological studies specifically addressing the relative α- and β-adrenergic receptivities of the accessory pathway have been published, and little is known about the intrinsic adrenergic innervation of the accessory pathway.

Effects of Catecholamines on the Ventricular Conduction System and Ventricular Muscle

The adrenergic innervation of the ventricles is somewhat greater in the left ventricle than in the right in all experimental mammals studied (19), and in the dog, the content of norepinephrine in the ventricle is approximately half that found in the atria (19,154). The adrenergic innervation of the Purkinje cells seen subendocardially both at the bases of the papillary muscles and in the false tendons is also reported to be sparse (154).

Catecholamines elicit changes in action potential parameters in Purkinje fibers mediated through stimulation of both α- and β-adrenergic receptors. In Purkinje cells, β-adrenergic stimulation results in action potential shortening independent of changes in rate, as well as an increase in the rate of spontaneous diastolic depolarization (252,596). The response to α-adrenergic stimulation includes action potential lengthening and a decrease in the spontaneous rate of diastolic depolarization (596). Although α-adrenergic blockade appears to have little effect alone on action potential parameters, α-adrenergic stimulation appears to induce an inhibitory effect on the β-mediated response, because significant enhancement of the β-adrenergic response occurs in the presence of α-adrenergic blockade (596). In normal Purkinje tissue, β-adrenergic receptor stimulation does not alter the membrane response relationship or the conduction velocity of basic or premature impulses. Likewise, catecholamines exert little effect on normal ventricular muscle resting membrane potentials, maximum rate of phase-0 depolarization, action potential amplitude, or conduction velocity (303,788), with variable effects on repolarization (303,583).

In humans, isoproterenol appears to have no effect on the His-Purkinje conduction time at dosages of 1 to 2 μg/min (576,742,776). In patients with the WPW syndrome, no change in right ventricular effective refractory period is induced by isoproterenol (776). However, a significant reduction in right ventricular effective refractory period occurs in response to isoproterenol in patients with recurrent ventricular tachycardia (576). This response is presumably due to inherent abnormalities in ventricular electrophysiological properties. Testing of responses to catecholamines *in vivo* is complicated by the reflex responses to changes in heart rate, blood pressure, ventricular afterload, and ventricular volume.

Effects of Acetylcholine on the Sinus Node

Several lines of evidence are used to determine the extent of parasympathetic innervation to any region of the heart: (a) demonstration of a system of nerves associated with intramyocardial ganglia, (b) measurement of tissue acetylcholine content (89), (c) distribution of the catabolic enzyme acetylcholinesterase (324,362), and (d) distribution of the synthetic enzyme for acetylcholine, choline acetyltransferase (619). Abundant parasympathetic innervation is present in the SA node and is conspicuously more abundant than at any other site in the heart (324). In decreasing order, lower densities of the synthetic and catabolic enzymes for acetylcholine are found in the AV node, right atrium, left atrium, papillary muscles, right ventricular free wall, and left ventricular free wall.

Direct application of acetylcholine to the SA node produces slowing of the spontaneous rate of phase-4 depolarization, likely mediated by an increase in potassium conductance (303). Application of acetylcholine, through a micropipette, directly to the SA node can result in a rapid shift in the pacemaker site (303,779), but direct effects on the resting membrane potential, activation threshold, and action potential duration are inconsistent (303,779). The slight hyperpolarization induced by acetylcholine on SA node cells may be dependent on the diastolic potential prior to acetylcholine administration. Cells with normal diastolic potentials demonstrate only a slight hyperpolarization, but in depolarized cells, acetylcholine induces a marked hyperpolarization (512).

The chronotropic response of the SA node to brief vagal stimuli has been extensively investigated. It was initially observed in the cat that the time course of the changes in basic cycle length following a single vagal stimulation volley exhibited two inhibitory peaks separated by a transient period of acceleration in which the spontaneous rate could exceed the rate prior to vagal stimulation (85). These observations have been confirmed by others in both dogs and rabbits (312,319,413,676,677). This apparent paradox has been resolved using potassium-sensitive extracellular electrodes and multiple transmembrane action potential recordings from SA node cells in an isolated rabbit atrial preparation (677). Stimulation of intramural vagal fibers in this preparation demonstrates the previously described bimodal inhibitory curve. The initial atrial slowing that appears after a latent period of 170 to 300 msec is due to slowing of conduction or a change in the exit pathway out of the sinus node, without an appreciable change in the rate of pacemaker spontaneous diastolic depolarization (Fig. 1). Thus, the initial response reflected a dromotropic response, not a chronotropic response, to vagal stimulation. The initial dromotropic effect was demonstrated not to be secondary to a shift in the pacemaker site using submaximal stimulus intensities; the majority of the delay was within the pacemaker area of the SA node. After the initial phase of deceleration secondary to the dromotropic change, a true slowing of the pacemaker rate was observed associated with a decrease in the rate of phase-4 depolarization, as well as a hyperpolarization of the maximum diastolic potential (677). These changes can be ascribed to a direct action of neurally released acetylcholine on membrane potassium conductance, with no significant accumulation of extracellular potassium activity (677). The subsequent brief acceleratory component in the response to vagal nerve stimulation, when present, is likely due to depolarization of the maximum diastolic potential. This results in early attainment of the threshold, possibly explained by an increased membrane conductance for sodium or secondary to an increase in extracellular potassium (677). The secondary slowing present 1 to 3.5 sec after cessation of vagal stimulation was temporally associated with a rise in extracellular potassium activity that may have contributed to the slowing of the rate of diastolic depolarization.

The initial direct hyperpolarization seen with vagal stimulation in the SA node has been shown to be significantly phase-dependent with respect to when the vagal stimulation is introduced relative to the spontaneous cycle length. If the vagal stimulus is given less than 200 msec in advance of the next expected pacemaker action potential, the initial membrane hyperpolarization does not occur (319). The explanation postulated is that acetylcholine released late in the phase of diastole cannot modulate the inward current responsible for the phase-0 depolarization that becomes activated about 100 msec before the upstroke of the action potential (87).

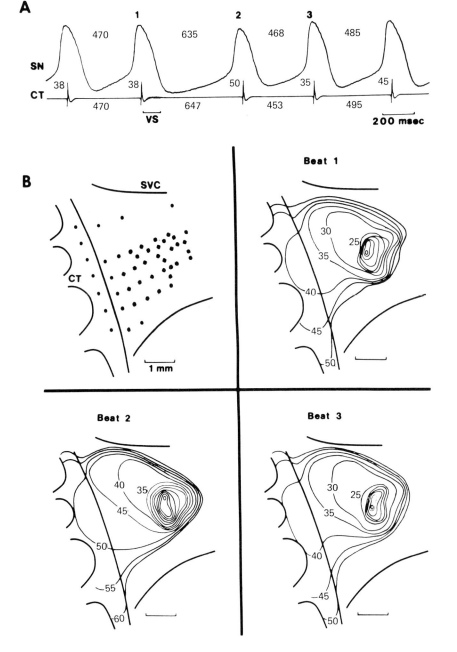

FIG. 1. Effect of vagal stimulation (VS) on the sequence of activation and on the transmembrane action potential recording of the earliest activation in the primary pacemaker area of the isolated rabbit atrium. A: Action potential recordings from the primary pacemaker site (SN) and electrogram recording from the crista terminalis (CT), with VS indicating the time of vagal stimulation. B: Recording sites used in the activation map are indicated by the filled circles, with the stippled area indicating the region from which sinus node action potentials were recorded. The 1, 2, and 3 in A indicate the beats for which activation sequence maps are depicted in B. As can be seen for beat 2, the site of earliest activity has shifted 200–300 μM superiorly, with a prominent slowing of conduction out of the pacemaker site, as compared with the pre-stimulation site (beat 1). (From ref. 677, with permission of the American Heart Association.)

Effects of Acetylcholine in Atrial Tissue

The parasympathetic distribution to the atria is greater on the right than on the left side. It is well known that acetylcholine produces a marked shortening of the action potential duration and absolute refractory period in atrial muscle (303,304). If the initial value of the resting potential is low, acetylcholine or vagal stimulation results in a marked hyperpolarization, but in normal tissue at normal V_m, little effect is seen (303). Importantly, the effects of vagal stimulation and acetylcholine infusion produce an increased dispersion of atrial refractory periods (482,725), which can contribute to the induction and maintenance of atrial fibrillation (277) and atrial flutter (14) in experimental animals.

The effect of acetylcholine on atrial specialized fibers is similar to that in atrial muscle tissue, because it induces a decrease in duration of the action potential, a minimal hyperpolarization, and a marked attenuation of the plateau phase at dosages as low as 0.5 μg/ml (305). Studies in patients investigating the effects of heightened vagal tone on atrial refractoriness have confirmed the abbreviation of the atrial refractory period (558).

Effects of Acetylcholine on the AV Node

Most evidence indicates that the left vagal innervation to the AV node dominates over the right vagal influence (269,315,452). The distribution of cholinergic terminals is more dense in the region of the AV node than in either atrial or ventricular tissue (324,362). The parasympathetic ganglia are not contained within the node itself but at its posterior margin, between the AV node and the anterior wall of the coronary sinus (321).

Studies involving the effects of the parasympathetic nervous system on the AV node are complicated by the concomitant indirect changes on conduction properties produced by cardiac rate, pacemaker location, and atrial activation patterns. AV block produced by acetylcholine superfusion in the isolated rabbit heart was initially described as a failure of transmission occurring at the atrial margin of the AV node (303), with the effect exaggerated at higher pacing rates. However, others, using similar preparations, have localized the area of block to the middle area of the AV node rather than at the AN junction (778), with no effect of acetylcholine on conduction in the His bundle region of the node.

Studies assessing the effects of vagal stimulation on the AV node are impossible to interpret if the effects of heart rate are not controlled. The magnitude of subsequent beat-to-beat changes in AV nodal conduction are critically dependent on the phase in the cardiac cycle at which the vagal stimulus is introduced, similar to the response seen in the SA node. The effects of a single burst of vagal activity have been shown to be rapid in onset (0.5 sec) and transient (<2 sec), permitting modulation of AV node conduction on a beat-to-beat basis (413,676). Concomitant with the conduction delay, the effective refractory period is prolonged by vagal stimulation, and the effect of a given vagal stimulus is more profound at higher heart rates.

In patients, studies have documented the positive dromotropic effects of atropine on AV conduction (9,557). However, in contrast to the predominant parasympathetic effect on sinus node automaticity, in the AV node, conduction appears to be influenced equally, but in opposite directions, by vagal tone and adrenergic tone (557).

Effects of Acetylcholine on Accessory Pathways

Tachycardias involving an accessory bypass tract are modified by vagal tone primarily at the AV node, not at the bypass tract (768). Atropine does not affect either the antegrade effective refractory period or the conduction velocity of the accessory pathway (774). This lack of effect of atropine and the rarity of Wenckebach types of conduction delay in the accessory pathway suggest a different morphologic structure of the accessory pathway as compared with the AV node (774).

Effects of Acetylcholine on the Ventricular Conduction System and Ventricular Muscle

The cholinergic innervation identified by specific histochemical stains for acetylcholinesterase demonstrates a sparse parasympathetic distribution to the ventricular myocardium in both canine and human hearts, with a more richly supplied cholinergic supply to the ventricular conduction system (362). In addition to acetylcholinesterase, choline acetyltransferase, the biosynthetic enzyme (317,598), and muscarinic cholinergic receptors (210) have been demonstrated to be present throughout the ventricular myocardium.

The direct effects of acetylcholine on isolated ventricular muscle and Purkinje fibers in vitro are species-dependent; most notable, however, is the negative chronotropic effect (303,574). The effects of acetylcholine are greatly enhanced in the presence of simultaneous adrenergic stimulation, as discussed in detail in a later section.

Vagal stimulation or acetylcholine administration in intact animals can slow the spontaneous rate of discharge of automatic ventricular foci (157). The effects on ventricular repolarization are more complex. The effects of vagal stimulation to prolong the effective refractory period of the ventricle have been demonstrated to be eliminated by propranolol (375,453) and atropine (453) and to be augmented by simultaneous sympathetic activation (31,453). Thus, vagal stimulation, in the absence of sympathetic stimulation, appears to have little or no significant effect on ventricular repolarization (Fig. 2).

In patients undergoing programmed stimulation for evaluation of a variety of supraventricular and ventricular arrhythmias, the effects of pharmacological blockade with atropine or with atropine plus propranolol have been evaluated on right ventricular endocardium at fixed pacing cycle lengths (557). An effect different from that obtained in experimental preparations (31,375,453)

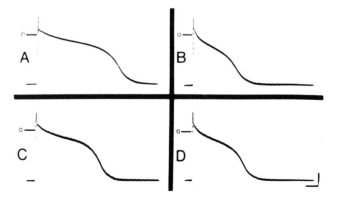

FIG. 2. Effects of acetylcholine on action potential shortening produced by isoproterenol. **A:** Control canine cardiac Purkinje fiber action potential. **B:** Isoproterenol (10^{-7} M) induced action potential shortening. **C:** Acetylcholine (10^{-6} M) in addition to isoproterenol (10^{-7} M) partially reversing the isoproterenol-induced shortening. **D:** Atropine (10^{-6} M) attenuating the effects of acetylcholine. Zero potential indicated in each panel. Calibrations: horizontal bar = 50 msec; vertical bar = 25 mV. (From ref. 31, with permission of the American Heart Association.)

was observed; namely, atropine produced a shortening of refractory period even after β-adrenergic blockade (557). However, the effectiveness of β-adrenergic blockade was assessed in only 2 patients, and all the patients studied demonstrated rhythm or conduction disturbances, suggesting a response that may differ from that seen in normal myocardium.

INTERACTIONS BETWEEN SYMPATHETIC AND PARASYMPATHETIC COMPONENTS

One general but simplistic view of the interaction of the two branches of the autonomic nervous system is that although both systems are involved in the control of cardiac rhythm, activation of the sympathetic nervous system may be deleterious to cardiac rhythm (374,613,630,633), whereas activation of the parasympathetic nervous system may afford protection (363,497). Actually, the overall net influence of the autonomic nervous system on cardiac rhythm represents the complex integration of several factors, including (a) the anatomic region and the extent of neural innervation, (b) the level of central autonomic outflow, (c) the extent of neural activity originating from peripheral afferent sites, (d) the degree of activation of peripheral efferent nerves, and (e) the extent of reflex activity impinging either on central autonomic outflow or directly on peripheral neural activity.

The molecular basis for this integration and the ultimate postsynaptic response depend on the release of neurotransmitter from the presynaptic autonomic nerve terminal or from the adrenal medulla and the binding of the transmitter substances to postsynaptic receptors, with subsequent transduction of that binding to a variety of cellular responses. Modulation of these two major events occurs through chemical, ionic, hormonal, or electrical interactions (765,784). The present discussion will concentrate on presynaptic and transsynaptic mechanisms of autonomic neurotransmitter modulation. For consideration of electrical and ionic mechanisms, the reader is referred to previous reviews (195,740). The mechanisms responsible for the interaction between sympathetic and parasympathetic components have been investigated peripherally (43,541) as well as centrally (44,752).

Modulation of neurotransmission involves both limbs of the autonomic nervous system, as well as other neurotransmitters, modulators, peptides, and hormones. Different mechanisms that have been postulated include (a) those involving presynaptic receptors and (b) transsynaptic mechanisms that involve release of a modulator from the postsynaptic effector cell that then crosses the synapse to modulate activity at the presynaptic terminal, or, alternatively, nonsynaptic mechanisms that involve release of a modulator from one set of neurons that may influence the activity at another set of neurons.

Presynaptic-Receptor-Mediated Modulation

The first suggestion of α-adrenergic-induced alterations in norepinephrine overflow elicited by sympathetic nerve stimulation was reported by Brown and Gillespie, although they did not suggest a presynaptic mechanism for regulation of neurotransmitter release (86). Fifteen years later, six different groups of investigators published data supporting the hypothesis that noradrenergic (204,370,389,681), cholinergic (550), and γ-aminobutyric-acid-ergic (GABAergic) (336) nerve terminals contained presynaptic receptors that could mediate inhibition of neurotransmitter release. Of the presynaptic receptors that serve a regulatory function in feedback inhibition and facilitation of neurotransmitter release, the α_2-adrenoreceptors are the best characterized (240, 387,540,682,683,740,753) (Fig. 3).

Activation of presynaptic α_2-receptors by norepinephrine has been shown to inhibit further norepinephrine release, and blockade of presynaptic α_2-receptors facilitates norepinephrine release. Prejunctional modulation has most often been studied in isolated tissue preparations, where agonists inhibit and antagonists facilitate depolarization-evoked transmitter release. The enhanced release does not appear to depend on the presence of postsynaptic receptors, because enhanced release of norepinephrine after α_2-adrenergic blockade occurs in cultured rat superior cervical ganglion cells, a preparation devoid of postsynaptic receptor sites (775). Furthermore, chemical sympathectomy using 6-hydroxydopamine, which destroys sympathetic nerve terminals, reduces the number of specific α_2 binding sites in the rat ventricle (694), although the denervation may induce a change in postsynaptic α_1 receptors as well as α_2 receptors. Other studies have failed to demonstrate a decrease in α-adrenergic receptors after selective lesioning of noradrenergic neurons. This apparent discrepancy may be explained by the phenomenon of denervation supersensitivity, in which an increase in postsynaptic receptor sites would mask a decrease in presynaptic receptors.

The phenomenon of presynaptic inhibition has been observed across a wide range of species and different tissues. However, there is little direct evidence that the receptors that are activated or blocked are confined to the vicinity of the prejunctional membrane or that the receptors are indeed active during normal physiological conditions *in vivo*. Kalsner (348,349) has raised several objections to the existence of presynaptic receptors modulating norepinephrine release, including the lack of correlation between enhancement of transmitter release by α_2 antagonists and stimulation-induced efflux of the transmitter or the actual magnitude of the postsynaptic response. Other investigators have attempted to resolve the controversy by suggesting modifications of the original theory (54,369). Despite these reservations, presynaptic modulation of transmitter release remains a

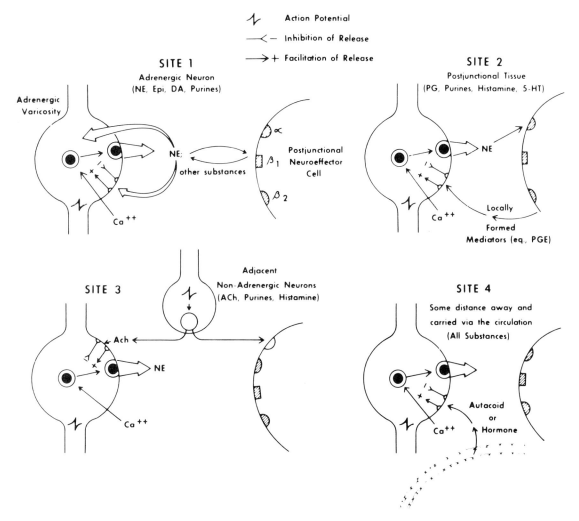

FIG. 3. Sites of origin for the various neuromodulators that influence release of norepinephrine from the adrenergic nerve terminal varicosity. Site 1 represents the presynaptic terminal, from which norepinephrine is released for interaction with presynaptic α_2 or β_2 autoreceptors to feed back and inhibit or enhance, respectively, further release of norepinephrine. This site may be the origin of other catecholaminergic modulators such as epinephrine and dopamine, or of ATP, which may be released with norepinephrine on nerve terminal depolarization. Site 2 represents the postjunctional effector tissue from which mediators, such as prostaglandins or adenosine, are released to traverse the synapse for subsequent transsynaptic modulation of norepinephrine release. Other postjunctional modulator products may include histamine and serotonin. Site 3 represents adjacent nonadrenergic neurons that may produce a variety of nonsynaptic modulators such as acetylcholine, enkephalins, or GABA. These substances diffuse to the adrenergic synapse, where they may influence norepinephrine release. Site 4 represents a distant production site for any of the previously mentioned mediators, as well as for hormones and peptides such as angiotensin. These substances are exposed to the adrenergic synapse from the circulation. (From ref. 781, with permission of the Federation of American Societies for Experimental Biology.)

popular concept. In addition to presynaptic α-adrenergic receptors, the presence of presynaptic β-adrenergic receptors has also been postulated. In contrast to the inhibitory effect of α_2 presynaptic stimulation, stimulation of presynaptic β_2 receptors appears to facilitate the release of norepinephrine (6,796). This mechanism may be of importance in augmenting the cardiac norepinephrine release induced by circulating epinephrine released from the adrenal medulla and may be one of several mechanisms responsible for the effectiveness of β blockade during myocardial ischemia and infarction (*vide infra*).

Transsynaptic and Nonsynaptic Modulation

In addition to the presynaptic effects of catecholamines, several other agents have been reported to affect norepinephrine release. Acetylcholine may inhibit norepinephrine release via activation of presynaptic muscarinic receptors (424,493). Because the heart has a relatively low level of acetylcholinesterase activity, this neuromodulator may be particularly important in cardiac tissue. Although large concentrations of acetylcholine may actually augment the release of norepinephrine through stimulation of nicotinic receptors (780), this mechanism probably is not important *in vivo* because of the high concentrations of acetylcholine required.

Both adenosine and ATP have been shown to inhibit norepinephrine and acetylcholine release from their respective nerve terminals (219,280,693,754). The mechanism for the inhibitory effect of adenosine has been postulated as involving a transsynaptic mechanism (220), because adenosine is released from effector cells (221), adenosine directly inhibits norepinephrine release (280), and adenosine antagonists, although not totally specific and selective for adenosine (655), enhance norepinephrine release (220,279). Although the critical experiments required to prove that the transsynaptic modulatory role of adenosine is physiologically important are lacking, it seems reasonable that adenosine may play a key role in modulating norepinephrine release and hence arrhythmogenesis in several pathophysiological states. For example, hypoxia and ischemia stimulate adenosine production, which may be critical in the autoregulation of blood flow (52) as well as in transsynaptic modulation and inhibition of norepinephrine release and thereby arrhythmogenesis. In contrast to adenosine, ATP as a neuromodulator arises primarily from the presynaptic nerve terminal. ATP coexists with norepinephrine in the nerve terminal vesicles (391) and is released with norepinephrine during depolarization of the nerve terminal.

Angiotensin II has been shown by a number of investigators (102,684,799) to cause facilitation of norepinephrine release, notably in the rabbit heart, where angiotensin II produced up to a fourfold increase in [^{3}H]norepinephrine release, a phenomenon that may be mediated by prostaglandins (68,390). This mechanism may be particularly important in arrhythmogenesis in the ischemic heart, because increased plasma catecholamines can augment renin release directly, thereby resulting in a positive-feedback mechanism to augment further the intramyocardial release of catecholamines (*vide infra*). Dopamine (388), enkephalins and morphine (179,287), histamine (466,467), and serotonin (467) have all been reported to inhibit norepinephrine release, whereas GABA has been shown to enhance the release of norepinephrine (21). Finally, the prostaglandins (PGs) have also been implicated in contributing to transsynaptic modulation of norepinephrine release, with PGs of the E series inhibiting (281) and $PGF_{2\alpha}$ enhancing norepinephrine release (346,553).

Analogous to what has been reported for sympathetic neurons, both adenosine and ATP inhibit acetylcholine release from cholinergic neurons (754). Likewise, both norepinephrine and epinephrine in some systems inhibit acetylcholine release via stimulation of α_2-adrenergic receptors (541,783). Thus, locally released or circulating norepinephrine may regulate the release of either norepinephrine or acetylcholine, and vice versa. Regardless of the extent to which these mechanisms are operative under normal physiological conditions, these processes may become more relevant under pathophysiological conditions, such as myocardial ischemia or infarction, and thereby indirectly contribute to arrhythmogenesis, is discussed in detail in a later section.

Subcellular Mechanisms Responsible for Presynaptic Neural Modulation

The precise mechanisms responsible for presynaptic receptor modulation of neurotransmitter release are for the most part unknown. One important factor appears to be modulation of Ca^{2+} entry into the presynaptic terminal, because only Ca^{2+}-dependent modes of release appear to be modulated by presynaptic receptor mechanisms. Thus, presynaptic inhibitory mechanisms may occur via uncoupling of neuronal depolarization and neurotransmitter release (692). Ultrastructural preparations of noradrenergic nerve terminals stimulated in the presence of phentolamine appear to have more vesicles in close association with terminal membranes (721). Thus, activation of α_2 receptors may interfere with positioning of the transmitter vesicles close to the nerve terminal and might thereby diminish transmitter release. One mechanism for this interference might be an α_2-mediated decrease in the affinity of Ca^{2+} for the tubules, vesicles, or other components of the terminal secretory system. Voltage-dependent influx of Ca^{2+} is critical not only for depolarization-secretion coupling in the neuron but also for impulse conduction. Therefore, α_2-mediated autoinhibition of transmitter release could occur via prevention of neural impulses propagating to the terminal varicosity (692). The mechanism for this could be restricted Ca^{2+} influx or enhanced K^+ efflux, with subsequent hyperpolarization and conduction block in the neuron.

In summary, a vast amount of experimental evidence suggests important interactions among neurotransmitters, hormones, and peptides within the peripheral and central nervous systems. Neurotransmitters may regulate their own activity or the activities of other neuronal systems. However, little is known relative to the effects of this neuromodulation on the generation of supraventricular or ventricular arrhythmias. Many of the studies examining the effects of modulators on norepinephrine and acetylcholine release were assessed in peripheral tissues other than the heart and will require confirmation in cardiac tissues *in vitro* and *in vivo*. Despite these reservations, these findings should provide a framework for designing new approaches to manipulate the release of neurotransmitters and hence their cardiac electrophysiological effects.

CENTRAL NEURAL CONTROL OF CARDIAC FUNCTION: MECHANISMS CONTRIBUTING TO AFFERENT AND EFFERENT ACTIVATION

At least five factors contribute to modulation of the influence of the autonomic nervous system on the heart and thereby arrhythmogenesis. The first factor, presynaptic and transsynaptic modulation, was discussed in the preceding section. The four additional factors, peripheral afferent input, central autonomic outflow, activation of peripheral efferent nerves, and reflex activity, will be discussed in this section. Several excellent reviews of these subjects are available, and the reader is referred to these for added insights and additional references (65,82,126,178,268,378,445,532,678).

Sensory Receptors and Fibers Responsible for Afferent Activation

Three types of receptors reside in the reflexogenic areas of the cardiovascular system: baroreceptors, chemoreceptors, and mechanoreceptors. These receptors, dispersed widely throughout the heart and vasculature, are sensory transducers that transform mechanical or chemical stimuli into electrical signals that are then communicated to the central nervous system through afferent fibers.

Baroreceptors and Chemoreceptors

Baroreceptors are concentrated at the carotid sinus and aortic arch, as well as at various sites along the common carotid artery, in the vessels of the kidney, and in the chambers of the heart itself. The patterns of activity recorded from baroreceptor afferents are well characterized (18,385). However, the mechanism of the transduction from the deformation of the receptor to generation of the afferent nerve action potential is largely unknown, because the nerve endings themselves are so small that it is very difficult to record generator potentials from single baroreceptors. To our knowledge, only one such study has ever been successfully accomplished (458). Based on analogy and extrapolation from studies on crayfish stretch receptors, hypotheses describing mechanoelectrical transduction appear to involve nonselective ion permeability changes (201,382,503,504).

In contrast to the tonic regulatory activity of the baroreceptors (178), chemoreceptors are relatively inactive under normal conditions (126). Information from baroreceptors and chemoreceptors is relayed to the central nervous system via the carotid sinus and aortic depressor nerves. These nerves are composed of both myelinated A fibers with larger diameters and faster conduction velocities and unmyelinated C fibers with smaller diameters and slower conduction velocities (209,532). As is the case with other sensory receptors and fibers, a given functional receptor type is not subserved by a single fiber type. In fact, the bulk of the A fibers in the carotid sinus nerve subserve chemoreceptor function, and most of the C fibers subserve baroreceptor function (209). In contrast, the A fibers in the aortic depressor nerve subserve primarily baroreceptor function, while the C fibers subserve primarily chemoreceptor function (532). Consequently, activation of the two nerves assumes slightly different characteristics in response to baroreceptor or chemoreceptor stimulation (155,160,361,545). The two nerves also have different maximum frequency responses (84). C fibers have higher-pressure thresholds and lower maximum asymptotic discharges and have two different types of discharge patterns, whereas A fibers discharge only regularly (720). It appears, however, that differences in the responses of the carotid sinus and aortic depressor nerves cannot be totally explained by differences in fiber types, but that there is also a central neural component that distinguishes between the carotid and aortic reflex systems (117,149). Furthermore, stimulations of the carotid sinus nerve and the aortic depressor nerve result in quantitatively different effects on the cardiovascular reflex responses. For example, the aortic depressor nerve appears to play a larger role in vagally mediated decreases in heart rate (361).

Mechanoreceptors

The receptors responsible for initiating cardiac reflexes (82) are located in all four chambers of the heart, as well as in the coronary vasculature. These receptors are subserved by both myelinated and unmyelinated vagal and sympathetic afferents, with some afferent fiber types appearing to be more important than others. For example, receptors with myelinated vagal afferents in the atria and ventricles are sparsely distributed, as compared with the more dense distribution for receptors with C-fiber afferents. Cardiac vagal afferents have their cell bodies in the nodose ganglia and project to the medulla via the tenth cranial nerve. These reflexes are generally considered to be inhibitory (27,156,604). Cardiac sympathetic afferents have their cell bodies in the dorsal root ganglia of the T-1 to T-6 segments of the spinal cord and synapse in the dorsal horn. These reflexes are generally considered to be excitatory (83,439,440,547). However, both spinal and supraspinal reflex arcs are involved in responses initiated by the activation of cardiac afferents (609).

Reflexes activated by cardiac mechanoreceptors have often been identified using unnatural and invasive means, including inflation of small and large balloons, puncturing the muscle with needles, and mechanical probing. Characterization of the fibers from which recordings are obtained is difficult because afferent and efferent fibers are intertwined and vagal axons may be present in sympathetic nerve bundles. Even the classification of myelinated and unmyelinated fibers is somewhat arbitrary, because the distinction is usually based largely on conduction velocities.

Atrial receptors subserved by myelinated vagal afferents are either type A, which discharge during atrial contraction, or type B, which are activated by pulsatile increases in atrial volume during filling (25,529,530,575). Activation of the afferent limb of this reflex, also called the Bainbridge reflex (32), results in a sympathetically mediated increase in heart rate (401). In contrast to the myelinated vagal afferents, atrial receptors subserved by unmyelinated vagal afferents, first described by Coleridge and colleagues (124), are relatively quiescent during normal resting conditions (717). During physiological increases in atrial volume, these C fibers discharge with cardiac rhythmicity at the V wave of the atrial pressure pulse wave. Although exclusive activation of C fibers has not been experimentally verified, the reflex response they initiate is transient bradycardia and hypotension (28,185).

Ventricular receptors with large myelinated vagal afferents have been described as discharging during systole, but they are not well characterized and are not thought to play an important physiological role (123). Receptors associated with the coronary arteries are also subserved by myelinated vagal afferents (80). Ventricular receptors with unmyelinated vagal afferents, activated during systole (718), appear to play an important role in pathological conditions such as myocardial ischemia or hemorrhage (516,719) and may be particularly important in arrhythmogenesis. The reflex response seen with activation of these receptors is also bradycardia and hypotension.

Activation of atrial and ventricular receptors subserved by sympathetic afferent fibers produces increased efferent sympathetic outflow (439,440,547,736) and decreases efferent vagal activity (631c). This sympathosympathetic excitatory reflex may play an important role in mediating cardiac pain, particularly pain associated with myocardial ischemia (81,83,442). Foreman has suggested that sympathetic afferents may synapse on spinothalamic cells that receive their primary somatic afferent input from muscle and deep structures and may be the basis for referred pain during angina pectoris and acute myocardial infarction (212).

Sympathetic afferents originating in atrial tissue have been reported as being myelinated and unmyelinated, with the unmyelinated fibers exhibiting less spontaneous activity (441,732). Analogous to the firing patterns of vagal afferents, sympathetic afferent fibers have been identified that discharge synchronously with the A, C, and V waves of the atrial pressure wave (441,732). The atrial receptors appear, therefore, to be excited by atrial contraction and stretch, and by chemical substances as well (733,735).

Myelinated sympathetic afferents arising from ventricular tissue exhibit spontaneous activity, not always coincidental with ventricular contractions (736). These receptors do seem to be excited by increases in ventricular

pressure (441,736), as well as by bradykinin (733) and veratridine (440). Unmyelinated sympathetic afferents from ventricular receptors also appear to be sensitive to both ventricular contraction and distension (108). Although various firing patterns have been observed, activity of the unmyelinated sympathetic afferents most often is associated with ventricular fibrillation (108). Both myelinated and unmyelinated sympathetic afferent fibers discharge in response to interruptions in coronary flow (734), likely resulting in an increase in efferent sympathetic outflow to the heart. In addition to these reflex studies in acute preparations, several different studies of chronic preparations in cats and dogs have demonstrated that cardiac sympathetic afferents are activated in intact, unanesthetized animals, resulting in reflex excitation of efferent sympathetic outflow (64,526). Whether the ventricular receptors are purely mechanosensitive or chemosensitive and whether or not a given receptor subserves both stimuli remain points of contention (65). Most of the data support a dual role for these receptors. Likewise, it appears that cardiac nociception is conveyed via intensified tonic discharges in sympathetic afferents rather than via recruitment of nociceptive-specific fibers (438).

Aside from cardiac receptors that mediate the reflexes just described, there are pulmonary and cardiopulmonary chemoreceptors that when activated result in dramatic depressor responses (444,511,649). Pulmonary stretch receptors subserved by unmyelinated vagal afferents mediate the classic Hering-Breuer respiratory reflex (175), and pulmonary J receptors, when activated by hyperinflation or by increases in interstitial pressure or volume, initiate discharges in unmyelinated vagal fibers that cause reflex hypotension and bradycardia via efferent vagal activation and sympathetic inhibition (175,531). Other cardiopulmonary receptors activated by specific chemical substances, including veratrum alkaloids, phenyl diguanide, capsaicin, nicotine, lobeline, bradykinin, and prostaglandins (65,125,126), mediate efferent vagal activation and sympathetic inhibition through the classic Bezold-Jarisch cardiac chemoreflex (56,331). The afferent neural discharges for this cardiac chemoreflex are carried by unmyelinated vagal fibers. Chemical receptors sensitive to veratridine, serotonin, bradykinin, and cyanide (510,705), subserved by sympathetic afferents, inhibit efferent vagal outflow and may mediate pain perception during myocardial ischemia.

Reflex Pathways Through the Central Nervous System

In the following section the neural pathways in the central nervous system responsible for the net effects of autonomic neural outflow to the heart and vasculature will be discussed (Fig. 4). This information should provide additional avenues for possible future investigations to alter the net autonomic neural outflow in an

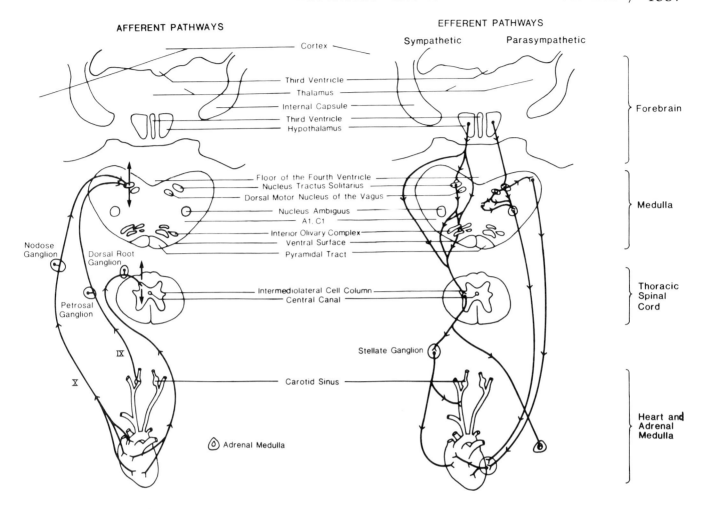

FIG. 4. Schematic diagram of cardiovascular reflex pathways through the central nervous system. **Left:** Afferent limb of the supraspinal and spinal reflex arcs originating from the sensory receptors of the heart and vasculature. The site of the first synapse in the supraspinal arc is at the NTS. **Right:** Efferent sympathetic (*left side of diagram*) and parasympathetic (*right side*) pathways. The sympathetic pathway between NTS and the intermediolateral cell column of the spinal cord, which contains the cell bodies of the preganglionic sympathetic efferent fibers, may include synapses at a variety of medullary sites not specifically delineated in this figure, but discussed in the text. The medulla depicted here is a composite diagram, as all of the structures, as drawn here, do not exist together in any one given section of the brainstem. The parasympathetic pathway between NTS and nucleus ambiguus, which contains the cell bodies of the preganglionic parasympathetic efferent fibers, may include synapses at a variety of sites, including the dorsal motor nucleus of the vagus, the midline raphe nuclei, or the external cuneate nucleus. Forebrain areas, such as the hypothalamus, may influence autonomic outflow, as discussed in the text.

attempt to influence the evolution of malignant cardiac arrhythmias.

Nucleus Tractus Solitarius: The First Synapse of Afferent Input

Numerous reports verify that the first synapse in the cardiovascular reflex pathways occurs at the nucleus tractus solitarius (NTS). The NTS is a longitudinal collection of neurons situated dorsomedially in the medulla oblongata. The caudal two-thirds of the nucleus serves as a vital relay involved in the regulation of cardiovascular, respiratory and other general visceral functions (45). This part of the NTS receives primary

afferent input from baroreceptors and chemoreceptors and from the heart and lungs. Nine distinct subnuclei of the NTS have been identified, most of which receive input from the cardiovascular afferents (347a,347b,422).

Experimental findings indicating that the NTS is the first synapse in cardiovascular reflex pathways include the initial studies tracing degeneration of axons after cutting the rootlets of the ninth and tenth cranial nerves, resulting in terminal degeneration in the NTS (145). Other anatomic techniques such as retrograde transport of horseradish peroxidase from the cut central end of the carotid sinus nerve to the NTS corroborated these results (51). Using electrophysiological techniques, stimulation of fibers in the NTS produced antidromic evoked responses in both the carotid sinus and aortic depressor nerves (149). Several lines of evidence suggest that the evoked potentials were recorded from primary afferent fibers: (a) the ability to follow high-frequency stimulation; (b) 2 min of anoxia or high doses of barbiturates did not change the amplitude of the evoked potentials; (c) short latencies for the responses. Evoked potentials, as well as single-unit recordings in the medulla, can be elicited by stimulation of the afferent nerves (62,63,310, 383,417,490). These units respond, as one would expect, to physiological stimuli and reflexes. However, pulse-synchronous activity recorded from single units in the brainstem is rare (310,462,606,697) and indicates the complexity of connections and interactions at the NTS.

Central Connections Between Afferent and Efferent Limbs: Vagal and Sympathetic Pathways

On the basis of advances in neuroanatomic tract tracing methods, connections from the NTS to other parts of the central nervous system, including the spinal cord, can now be delineated. Microinjections of tritiated amino acids into the NTS, followed by subsequent anterograde transport of the radiolabel, allow for auto-radiographic analysis of NTS connections to nucleus ambiguus, raphe nuclei, Kölliker-Fuse and parabrachial nuclei, and the spinal cord, among other sites (422,585). In direct corroboration, microinjection of horseradish peroxidase into a variety of sites, including the ventro-lateral reticular formation, nucleus ambiguus, ventral medullary surface, spinal cord, and several forebrain structures, resulted in retrograde transport of the per-oxidase to the NTS (194,422,585). Denervation studies performed by lesioning specific areas of the NTS have also been used to determine axonal connections from the NTS to sites such as the dorsal motor nucleus of the vagus and nucleus ambiguus (146,484). Similar anatomic techniques have been used to determine the neuroanatomy of the efferent autonomic pathways (99,234,698,724).

Given the plethora of potential pathways that were found, the next challenge was to determine which were relevant to central cardiovascular control. Electrophysi-ological studies have revealed that the nucleus ambiguus or the dorsal motor nucleus of the vagus may be the site of origin of efferent vagal activity to the heart (118,460,714). Afferents entering the CNS synapse first at the NTS and then project to the nucleus ambiguus, either directly or via the dorsal motor nucleus of the vagus (347a,347b), and possibly via the midline raphe structure (402). The cell bodies for vagal efferents to the heart are located in the nucleus ambiguus. However, the experimentally measured central delay is much longer than a simple disynapse in the NTS and nucleus ambiguus, suggesting that other synapses, presently un-known, may be important in modulating efferent vagal outflow to the heart (461).

With regard to the sympathetic pathways, the connec-tions between the first synapse at the NTS and the cell bodies of the preganglionic sympathetic efferents in the intermediolateral cell column of the spinal cord to the heart have not yet been resolved. The interconnections may involve sites such as the ventral surface of the medulla (16,795), the A1 or C1 catecholaminergic cell groups (65a,421,582,598a,598b) or the inferior olivary complex (660), nucleus gigantocellularis lateralis (84a), the lateral reticular nucleus, or the medullary raphe (16a). In several of these studies, horseradish peroxidase was injected into the intermediolateral cell column to determine the areas contributing to sympathetic outflow (16,16a,421,598a). Although a direct connection from the NTS to the intermediolateral cell column is included in the bulbospinal projections, the cumulative data cited above demonstrate the significance of a vasomotor center, localized to the ventrolateral medulla, in the regulation of autonomic outflow. Specifically lacking, however, are further electrophysiological and neurophysiological studies of bulbospinal neurons (84a), which are needed to characterize the functional significance of anatomically defined pathways influencing autonomic outflow.

Finally, both sympathetic and vagal pathways prob-ably receive important input from the hypothalamus and other forebrain areas. The hypothalamus is an exceedingly complex organ comprising many different areas including the paraventricular nucleus and the dorsal, medial, lateral, anterior, and posterior regions, many of which are involved in cardiovascular control (119,264,297,713). Direct anatomic connections be-tween the hypothalamus have been documented (607), and electrophysiological studies support the role of the hypothalamus in cardiovascular reflexes (272,305,600,731,733).

Central Neurotransmission

In addition to the anatomic data, the nature of neurotransmission along these pathways is now being elucidated. This information is likely to be critical to future approaches to more specifically influence central autonomic outflow by pharmacological means. New techniques in immunohistochemistry have allowed for visualization of neurotransmitters and neuropeptides that often coexist (112) within cell bodies and terminals of these central structures. The identity of the transmitter for primary baroreceptor afferents is controversial, be-cause evidence exists to support a role for glutamate (581) as well as substance P (247). The role of noradren-ergic projections to the spinal cord intermediolateral cell column was first reported 20 years ago (153), but the medullary source of the cell bodies of these projections is still in question. Positive identification of some trans-mitter systems has been made (243). They include epinephrine (598a,598b), GABA (247a), and substance P (281a). Unfortunately, the transmitter systems for most of the anatomically identified pathways remain unknown. Transmitter agonists or antagonists are found to have specific effects on cardiovascular function; yet the site of drug action or anatomic pathway involved is rarely resolved. Thus, future investigations will be required to identify the pathways with respect to the specific neurotransmitters involved as well as the functions they subserve.

Origin of Autonomic Tone

Dittmar was the first to put forth the notion of a vasomotor center, a singular structure that had ultimate control over cardiovascular function and that regulated normal function (169). Subsequent investigators merely modified the boundaries of the center, but the concept remained the same (12). More recently, the complexity of the central nervous system, with the multiple structures and related interconnections involved in cardiovascular function, has indicated that autonomic control is mediated through a number of different "circuits" (793). However, the reported anatomic basis for a number of these circuits does not necessarily imply their functional importance. In order to gain insight into the functional significance of some of these circuits, physiologists have recently studied the individual components of the tonic regulatory and reflex pathways.

Gebber and colleagues (231) have focused on the basic 2- to 6-cycles/sec rhythm inherent in the sympathetic nerve discharges of the cat under both baroreceptor-denervated and innervated conditions. A working model of the brainstem sympathetic generator has been proposed as a hierarchy of independent circuits composed of units with characteristic discharges synchronized to specific points of the sympathetic nerve discharge. The oscillators, located in both the brainstem and the spinal cord, receive input from baroreceptor fibers and forebrain sites such as the hypothalamus (231). Thus, sympathetic outflow appears to be controlled by neuronal oscillators at the bulbar and spinal levels.

Our traditional conception of the spinal cord as a conduit between higher centers and the periphery has also changed. The complexity of connections within the spinal cord is not surprising, because (a) reflex responses in sympathetic nerves may occur in the absence of bulbospinal interactions (609), (b) the spinal cord can maintain normal sympathetic tone and some cardiovascular reflexes in the absence of central neural input, as demonstrated in chronic spinal animals (77) and man (794), and (c) spinal neuronal elements themselves are capable of background neural activation (42,447). In addition, several investigators have demonstrated a spinal component of baroreceptor-induced sympathetic neural inhibition (131,232). Thus, far from being a simple relay station between higher neural structures in the brain and peripheral organs, including the heart, the spinal cord itself is an important site for integration of ascending

and descending pathways and can influence the ultimate magnitude and pattern of sympathetic nerve discharge (39).

Forebrain Sites Influencing Efferent Activation

Many of the initial observations arising from studies of central autonomic control emphasized the independence of brainstem mechanisms in regulating autonomic outflow. However, more recent evidence suggests that forebrain areas such as the hypothalamus are critically involved in modulating autonomic neural control under a wide range of physiological and pathophysiological conditions. The hypothalamus has been known to play an integral role in the expression of emotional behavior since the classic studies by Bard (38). This initial series of neural transections localized the center of integration for the sham-rage response to the diencephalon. More recently, Hilton and colleagues (296) have studied the integral functioning of the hypothalamus, midbrain, pons, and medulla in the defense reaction, a complex response with somatic and autonomic manifestations of profound sympathetic discharge. Furthermore, they and others have demonstrated that the anterior hypothalamus is one link in a bulbo-forebrain loop of the baroreceptor reflex arc (297). Barman and Gebber have also concluded that hypothalamic activity contributes to basal sympathetic nerve discharge and that some units are under baroreceptor control (40).

Most of our basic understanding of cardiovascular regulatory mechanisms has been obtained using anesthetized and often paralyzed laboratory animals. Just as exercise and emotion will yield a given physiological condition, so will altered states of consciousness and varying levels of exogenous anesthetic agents bias the data collected under these conditions. Anesthetics have profound and varied effects on reflex activity and nerve conduction in general. They suppress the brainstem reticular formation and, with it, higher brain function (449). To circumvent these problems, Smith and colleagues have assessed the extent of hypothalamic control of the cardiovascular responses accompanying emotional behavior of conscious baboons (661,659). These investigators found that a specific site in the hypothalamus is responsible for controlling the entire cardiovascular response associated with emotional behavior using classic conditioning. Discrete lesions of this area completely prevented the cardiovascular responses normally seen with the conditioned emotional response, without affecting the somatic response or the cardiovascular response to exercise. These data suggest that there exists within the hypothalamus one specific area that regulates cardiovascular responses associated with one specific behavior, emotion. Whether or not other discrete central neural sites are responsible for specific functional responses remains to be elucidated.

Associations with Arrhythmogenesis

Using classic conditioning, other investigators have also provided links between emotion and cardiovascular responses. Corley found that stressful situations induced electrocardiographic alterations and myocardial abnormalities in squirrel monkeys (135), and others used behavioral paradigms to determine that increases in both sympathetic and parasympathetic tone were required to exacerbate premature ventricular contractions in monkeys previously subjected to myocardial ischemia (565).

These studies raise the question of combined risk factors such as stress in the setting of acute ischemia contributing to the genesis of malignant cardiac arrhythmias. Corbalan and colleagues (132) reported that dogs with evolving myocardial infarction, when stressed, developed ventricular arrhythmias, and Verrier and Lown (744) found that both classic aversive conditioning and inducing angerlike states lowered the threshold for stimulation-induced repetitive extrasystoles. In addition, myocardial ischemia induced in an aversive environment increased the incidence of ventricular fibrillation compared with a nonaversive setting (744). Likewise, Skinner and colleagues (654) demonstrated that in pigs subjected to myocardial ischemia in an unfamiliar environment, the onset to ventricular fibrillation was accelerated, as compared with animals subjected to ischemia in a familiar environment. In addition, in the same experimental preparation, cryoblockade of a corticobulbar pathway prevented ventricular fibrillation associated with ischemia (653). Others have shown that arrhythmias are evoked or enhanced by stimulation of the hypothalamus (379,608).

These experimental studies provide a cogent argument for stress contributing to the genesis of malignant arrhythmias, particularly during acute myocardial ischemia and infarction (745). Proving that stress is a prominent risk factor for ventricular fibrillation and sudden cardiac death in man, however, is more difficult. Although the reports in man suggesting an association between psychological stressors and sudden death are in large part anecdotal, it is likely that psychological factors make a distinctive contribution to arrhythmogenesis in man (165,431). An exciting fund of knowledge is developing around the role of the autonomic nervous system in arrhythmogenesis associated with myocardial ischemia (*see below*). However, our knowledge of the central anatomical and neurophysiological substrates underlying these and other arrhythmias is strikingly deficient.

AUTONOMIC NEURAL INFLUENCES ON ARRHYTHMIAS ASSOCIATED WITH MYOCARDIAL ISCHEMIA

Evidence for Neural Activation During Ischemia

Several lines of evidence indicate that both afferent and efferent autonomic nerves are activated immediately with myocardial ischemia. For example, occlusion of either the left anterior descending (LAD) or circumflex coronary artery in cats enhances efferent sympathetic neural activity from the T-3 ramus coincident with alterations in the ST segment and T wave of the surface electrocardiogram (442,443). Likewise, increased preganglionic efferent sympathetic activity occurs in cats subjected to main left coronary occlusion, associated with the development of malignant ventricular arrhythmias (242). In contrast, Costantin (129) demonstrated that LAD coronary occlusion actually resulted in a decrease in neural activity in the inferior cardiac nerve. Others have reported that although ischemia results in an increase in sympathetic neural discharge, subsequent reperfusion does not (427). This apparent paradox may best be explained by the fact that ischemia results in simultaneous disparate responses in overall cardiac sympathetic neural discharge, with both increases and decreases in activity in different nerve fibers (397). This disparate or asynchronous activation may be particularly arrhythmogenic because of nonuniform effects on excitability, refractoriness, and conduction (270). Although the disparate responses of efferent sympathetic neural activation may be due to discrete control at the central neural level, Malliani and colleagues (442,443) have described a cardiocardiac reflex initiated by coronary occlusion in the cat. This reflex travels in the afferent sympathetic nerves to the stellate ganglia and then returns to the heart through the postganglionic sympathetic nerves. Thus, the reflex is not interrupted by high spinal cord section (442). On the other hand, in the dog, the presence of this cardiocardiac reflex may not be operative, because no increased efferent sympathetic neural activity was seen with coronary occlusion despite vagal nerve section (206). However, in this latter study (206), increased efferent sympathetic neural activity was manifest after spinal cord sectioning, suggesting the presence of tonic inhibition by medullary centers on the cardiocardiac spinal reflexes in the dog. Despite this finding, Schwartz and colleagues have reported that sectioning the dorsal root reduces arrhythmias associated with coronary artery occlusion in cats and dogs, suggesting that fibers running through the dorsal root contribute to the afferent limb of the sympathetic cardiocardiac reflex (631b). Thus, the relevance of this reflex during acute myocardial ischemia remains controversial.

Myocardial ischemia results in activation of vagal afferents (716) as well as sympathetic afferent fibers (730). The activation of afferent neural reflexes during myocardial ischemia may result from a number of factors. For example, myocardial ischemia may excite sensory mechanoreceptors in the ischemic region because of regional dyskinesis (730) or because of stimulation of chemoreceptors by serotonin (326), bradykinin (426,579), acidosis (736), hyperkalemia (731), and prostaglandins (687). Because of a rapid depression in ventricular function, afferent reflexes may also be elicited from the atria, pulmonary region, and systemic baroreceptors (175). When afferent vagal fibers, predominantly C fibers (716), are activated, bradycardia and hypotension result, not only because of increased efferent vagal activity but also because of a decrease in efferent sympathetic activity to the heart and vasculature (517). In the dog, activation of vagal afferents may be more prominent in the inferior wall of the left ventricle, resulting in more pronounced bradycardia and hypotension in inferior as opposed to anterior myocardial ischemia (709). These findings in dogs correlate with findings in humans with acute myocardial ischemia demonstrating more marked activation of the parasympathetic nervous system in patients with inferior as opposed to anterior left ventricular wall involvement (770).

Although activation of the autonomic nervous system during ischemia can occur as a result of activation of cardiopulmonary afferents, several other mechanisms may also be operative. Because of a decrease in arterial pressure coincident with a fall in stroke volume, systemic arterial baroreceptors are activated, resulting in increased efferent sympathetic tone and decreased efferent parasympathetic tone. However, during early ischemia, if vagal afferents are activated, this response may override the baroreceptor input, resulting in a net decrease in efferent sympathetic outflow.

In the absence of increased neural activity, norepinephrine may be released directly within the ischemic zone (1,182,299,384,643,790), even in the presence of ganglionic blockade (1). However, a number of other studies have presented evidence that catecholamines are not released into the local coronary venous effluent during myocardial ischemia (451,465,539,589,590), even in the presence of partial blockade of neuronal reuptake of norepinephrine (588). This apparent lack of an increase in norepinephrine early after ischemia is not due to alterations in neuronal reuptake, because this appears to be normal (555), nor to increased metabolism of norepinephrine, because even in studies using neuronal prelabeling with [^{3}H]-norepinephrine, increased release of metabolites of norepinephrine was not found (588, 589,622). This apparent paradox may be related to the fact that measurement in the local venous effluent may primarily reflect contributions from normal regions during ischemia due to collateral flow, with little or no flow from the ischemic bed. Because release of norepinephrine into the venous effluent is not evident during coronary occlusion but increases markedly with reperfusion (587), this may reflect washout of norepinephrine that accumulated during the antecedent ischemic interval. Despite these methodological considerations, the increase in norepinephrine release during early ischemia does not appear to be large, resulting in only a 5 to 10% loss of tissue catecholamines within the first hour (456,641). Recent catecholamine fluorescence studies of noradrenergic nerve terminals indicate a decrease in fluorescence by 30 min of ischemia, with a more marked loss by 2.5 to 5 hr of ischemia (2). Thus, within the first few

minutes after ischemia there does not appear to be a marked increase in catecholamine release. This conclusion does not preclude the fact that during early ischemia, continued release resulting in postsynaptic receptor stimulation and subsequent neuronal reuptake is likely to occur with little or no net change in venous effluent levels.

There are several factors that may contribute to the release of catecholamines, independent of neural stimulation, during short as well as prolonged ischemia. For example, increases in extracellular K^+ occur within minutes of ischemia (50,71,216,237,238,273,293,294, 299,300,782). Although increases in extracellular K^+ below levels of 15 mM can inhibit the release of norepinephrine from sympathetic nerve terminals, above this level, norepinephrine release is enhanced (429). Because local myocardial concentrations in vivo can exceed 15 mM, as assessed using K^+-sensitive electrodes (238), this mechanism is likely, particularly during prolonged ischemia. Although a reduction in pH to levels that occur during ischemia in vivo has been shown to inhibit norepinephrine release (560), acidosis can also inhibit neuronal reuptake (353) and alter binding and storage of norepinephrine within the nerve terminal (542). Thus, the net effect of acidosis on norepinephrine release may be variable. Increased plasma free fatty acids during ischemia have also been implicated in norepinephrine release (166), possibly because of enhanced neuronal uptake of calcium (680). After prolonged ischemia, reductions in ATP content within the neuron per se may also contribute to the loss of norepinephrine (759), a finding that may explain the loss of contractile response to sympathetic stimulation in the ischemic zone by 30 min, despite maintained responsiveness to injected catecholamines (454).

Regardless of the specific mechanism responsible for increased catecholamines within the myocardium or in the peripheral circulation during myocardial ischemia, numerous clinical studies have presented evidence that plasma and urinary catecholamines are increased during acute myocardial infarction in man (213,230,254, 463,507,586,747,748). Because both epinephrine and norepinephrine are increased, this would suggest release from the adrenal medulla, as well as peripheral nerve terminals. Experimentally, myocardial ischemia results in release of adrenal catecholamines (360,686), which may be secondary to activation of cardiac afferent vagal fibers initiating a centrally mediated increase in efferent splanchnic nerve discharge (685). Despite the associated increase in plasma and urinary catecholamines, the temporal association to arrhythmogenesis remains obscure. Although several studies have reported a temporal relationship between catecholamine release and ventricular arrhythmias in experimental animals, adrenal vein ligation does not alter the pattern of ventricular arrhythmias but does partially attenuate the incidence of ventricular fibrillation during myocardial ischemia (360). However, the fact that chemical sympathectomy with

6-hydroxydopamine, which increases rather than decreases plasma catecholamines (228), is antiarrhythmic during ischemia (650) argues against a major role for adrenal catecholamines. Likewise, increases in plasma catecholamines in patients during the first 48 hr after myocardial infarction fail to correlate with arrhythmogenesis (748), a finding that also occurs in the dog after acute myocardial infarction (586). This apparent paradox and lack of correlation may be due to the insensitivity of plasma catecholamine measurements to reflect specific, and likely heterogeneous, changes in myocardial catecholamine release. Alternatively, plasma catecholamine levels would reflect a relatively homogeneous effect on myocardial electrical properties and would be far less arrhythmogenic than discrete asynchronous neural activation to the heart (270). Thus, little is likely to be gained by assessing the relationship between plasma catecholamines and arrhythmogenesis during ischemia.

Adrenergic Influences During Myocardial Ischemia: Relation to Arrhythmogenesis

In the following sections, the results of studies related to the effects of the sympathetic nervous system during ischemia will be presented in three distinct categories: (a) neural stimulation studies; (b) surgical intervention studies; and (c) pharmacological intervention studies.

Neural Stimulation Studies

Several lines of experimental evidence suggest that stimulation of sympathetic neurons to the heart during ischemia enhances the development of malignant ventricular arrhythmias. For example, psychological stress in experimental animals may contribute to arrhythmogenesis during ischemia (vide supra). Likewise, enhanced neural input through the left stellate ganglion may be particularly arrhythmogenic. Stimulation of the left stellate ganglion during early ischemia enhances the induction of spontaneous ventricular tachycardia and fibrillation as well (630). Despite these findings, there are multiple problems with neural stimulation experiments, because the procedures usually involve stimulation of an entire nerve bundle rather than discrete nerve fibers as occurs under physiological or pathophysiological conditions. In several species, including the dog, sympathetic neural activation can result in simultaneous activation of vagal afferents and efferents. Likewise, in the absence of decentralization of the nerve bundle, stimulation can result in activation or inhibition of contralateral neural inputs due to simultaneous afferent neural activation. Finally, failure to demonstrate intact neural activity after isolation and before decentralization, to rule out neural damage, is critical to the interpretation of subsequent neural stimulation procedures. Because of these inherent problems in stimulation experiments, investigators have focused on the use of surgical and pharmacological denervation procedures.

Surgical Intervention Studies

The results of denervation experiments have corroborated the findings suggesting that enhanced left stellate ganglion stimulation is arrhythmogenic in the ischemic heart. For example, in 1974 Schwartz and colleagues demonstrated that blockade of the left stellate ganglion was antiarrhythmic during ischemia, whereas blockade of the right stellate resulted in an arrhythmogenic effect (634,635). Similar results have been reported by others (533). The protective effect of left stellectomy has also been demonstrated in a conscious canine preparation during acute circumflex occlusion in the presence of a previous 1-month-old anterior myocardial infarction (629). Similar findings have also been demonstrated using ventricular fibrillation threshold (VFT) as the index of vulnerability wherein left stellate ganglion ablation increases the VFT (374,633) and right stellate ganglion ablation decreases the VFT (633). Although others have failed to demonstrate a decrease in VFT with right stellectomy (78), this may be due to a relatively low prevailing level of sympathetic tone reflected as a lower sinus heart rate. Thus, a substantial body of evidence suggests that left stellate ganglion stimulation is arrhythmogenic in the ischemic heart. This is also reflected in the nonischemic heart, wherein right stellectomy increases the incidence of exercise-induced arrhythmias in the dog (628) and in man (26a).

In contrast, the results of bilateral denervation experiments are less conclusive. In 1936, Cox and Robertson (147) reported that acute bilateral stellate ganglionectomy attenuated the incidence of ventricular fibrillation, although evaluation of the data suggests that this difference did not achieve statistical significance. Other reports indicate that bilateral stellate ganglionectomy combined with bilateral removal of the chain ganglia does not influence the incidence of spontaneous ventricular fibrillation during coronary occlusion when adequately rigorous statistical evaluation is employed (183,184,215,272,475,613). However, this acute intervention does apparently reduce the incidence of premature ventricular complexes during ischemia (215,272,613) and attenuates the ischemic-induced fall in VFT (374). In contrast, bilateral stellectomy combined with bilateral removal of the sympathetic chain either 24 hr or 3 weeks prior to myocardial ischemia significantly attenuates the incidence of ventricular fibrillation (464,652). This apparent paradox might be explained by the finding that acute cardiac neural ablation or chronic bilateral stellate ganglionectomy failed to reduce the incidence of ventricular fibrillation associated with ischemia, whereas chronic cardiac neural ablation did (183,184). Because the chronic cardiac neural ablation technique resulted in near total depletion of myocardial catecholamines, whereas acute neural ablation or chronic bilateral stellate ganglionectomy did not (183,184), intramyocardial catecholamine stores, released in response to ischemia, may be critical in the genesis of ventricular fibrillation.

In concert, the foregoing findings would suggest that enhanced sympathetic neural activity has both beneficial and detrimental effects in the ischemic heart. These differential effects may cancel each other under conditions of totally intact innervation or bilateral denervation and only become apparent when innervation or activation is asymmetric. Asymmetry of sympathetic input would be expected to exert disparate effects on refractoriness, conduction, repolarization, and automaticity across the ventricle, potentially providing the milieu for malignant ventricular arrhythmias. Indeed, the finding that perineural inflammation exists at autopsy in some patients who succumb to sudden cardiac death may relate to the induction of asymmetric sympathetic innervation (599). Likewise, recent evidence from Barber and colleagues indicates that myocardial infarction per se can also result in sympathetic denervation, not only to the infarcted region but also to normal regions distal to the infarct (36), raising the possibility that the distal normal zones may have an asymmetric innervation that may potentiate the development of malignant ventricular arrhythmias during a subsequent ischemic episode. Because reinnervation may occur during the subsequent months after myocardial infarction because of the postganglionic nature of the denervation, these findings may explain, at least in part, the relatively high incidence of sudden cardiac death during the first year after infarction. This takes on added significance in patients with anterior myocardial infarction, which would likely have greater denervation of fibers from the right stellate ganglion, leaving a net imbalance, with enhanced left stellate ganglion input. This may also explain the fact that an increased QT interval resulting from increased left stellate ganglion input is an important predictor of sudden cardiac death in man post myocardial infarction (631), with similar results in experimental animals (629).

Several conclusions can be drawn from the multiple denervation studies. First, asymmetry of sympathetic input can be a critical factor in arrhythmogenesis in the ischemic heart. Second, residual catecholamines remaining even after acute or chronic denervation contribute to the development of malignant arrhythmias due to intramyocardial release, independent of neural activation. Third, the fact that several studies have failed to demonstrate a reduction in mortality with denervation may be also be related to an absence of significant endogenous sympathetic tone prior to denervation. Fourth, the majority of experimental studies support the concept that adrenal medullary release of catecholamines is not a primary factor in the development of malignant ventricular arrhythmias during ischemia.

The potential mechanisms responsible for the antiarrhythmic effect of denervation in the ischemic heart are likely to be multiple. For example, adrenergic stimulation will increase myocardial oxygen demand and thereby potentially increase the degree of myocardial damage that is likely to influence arrhythmogenesis. However, if ischemia, with or without previous infarction, is associated with global ventricular failure and ventricular dilation, adrenergic stimulation will increase contractility, thereby decreasing systolic wall tension and the end-diastolic diameter of the ventricle. This sequence of events is likely to decrease rather than increase oxygen demand.

As early as 1931, Leriche and Fontaine (403) reported that stellate ganglionectomy attenuated the degree of necrosis associated with coronary occlusion in the dog. More recent studies have indicated that the effect on necrosis is related to the duration of the denervation prior to coronary occlusion (35,37,338). For example, with acute sympathetic denervation, the degree of necrosis was reduced 25%, versus 90% with chronic denervation (338). Likewise, selective chronic denervation of the ventricle with intact atrial innervation also resulted in a dramatic decrease in the extent of necrosis after coronary occlusion (337). However, others, using necrosis of the papillary muscle as the endpoint, reported that chronic cardiac denervation simply delayed the onset of ischemic injury (190). Indeed, Thomas and colleagues (712) have reported that chronic, but not acute, denervation partially attenuates the reduction in contractile force in the epicardium of the ischemic zone. In contrast, others have reported that chronic denervation does not alter the depression in global ventricular function associated with ischemia (566). Thus, it is likely that adrenergic input may alter the degree of regional necrosis, although the extent of ischemic damage and the prevailing level of sympathetic tone in control hearts are likely to influence the overall global effect of the denervation. Likewise, the fact that acute denervation is less effective than chronic denervation suggests that residual catecholamines, released in the ischemic region, may contribute substantially to the ultimate extent of the necrosis.

Several factors may contribute to the antiischemic effects of chronic denervation and thereby indirectly to the antiarrhythmic effectiveness. For example, chronic denervation results in a 30% reduction in myocardial blood flow, presumably related to a decrease in oxygen demand (37,180,337), because both oxygen consumption and blood flow are reduced concomitantly by chronic denervation, regardless of peripheral hemodynamics (263). However, during regional ischemia, blood flow in the ischemic bed is actually increased with chronic sympathectomy (180,337). The increased blood flow primarily occurs in the periphery of the ischemic zone, possibly related to a decrease in α-adrenergic vasoconstriction or, alternatively, to an increase in collateral flow in the margins of the ischemic zone (180,337,339).

Although chronic sympathetic denervation appears to

substantially alter the degree of necrosis and the incidence of malignant arrhythmias in the ischemic heart, the fact that acute left stellectomy protects against malignant arrhythmias requires other explanations. Left stellectomy increases coronary blood flow and reduces coronary resistance even during exercise (627,628), an effect that leads to a reduction in ischemic damage after 8 hr of coronary occlusion in cats (741). Thus, a portion of the protection effect of left stellectomy is likely to involve an increase in coronary flow to the ischemic region. However, left stellectomy also shifts the strength interval curve to the right, increasing the ventricular refractory period, whereas right stellectomy shifts the curve to the left (637). In contrast, after left stellectomy, removal of the right stellate ganglion further shifts the curve to the right, indicating that the shift after right stellectomy depends on an intact left stellate input (Fig. 5). Thus, the dominant effect of left stellate input is a shortening in the ventricular refractory period, a phenomenon that is likely to enhance the propagation of ventricular arrhythmias dependent on a reentrant mechanism. More recent preliminary evidence indicates that left stellectomy attenuates the decrease in T-Q depression recorded by DC electrograms within ischemic tissue *in vivo,* suggesting an attenuation of the decrease in resting membrane potential; right stellectomy had the opposite effect (328). This apparent paradox might be explained by the fact that the left stellate ganglion is dominant to the left ventricle. Thus, removal of the right stellate ganglion may remove inhibitory afferents through the inferior cardiac nerve, which impinges on the left stellate, resulting in an overall heterogeneous increase in sympa-

thetic tone through the left stellate. However, removal of the dominant left stellate ganglion also results in an increase in right stellate outflow, but the overall net effect is a decrease in sympathetic tone to the left ventricle.

In summary, although cardiac sympathetic denervation can lead to attenuation of malignant arrhythmias in the ischemic heart, the precise mechanisms are unknown. It appears that a portion of the protective influence is mediated by a reduction in the extent of ischemic damage, but the attenuation of the direct electrophysiological effects of catecholamines appears important. Finally, asymmetry of the sympathetic input is crucial, and studies should be directed at detailed analysis of electrophysiological alterations induced by sympathetic activation and denervation in the ischemic heart using both isovoltaic and isochronic mapping procedures.

Pharmacological Intervention Studies

Several different pharmacological approaches have been utilized to inhibit adrenergic influences to the heart during myocardial ischemia. Depletion of myocardial catecholamines with reserpine prior to ischemia does not appear to alter the incidence of ventricular arrhythmias, including fibrillation (184,436,470,674), and may augment their occurrence (470). In contrast, depletion of catecholamines with 6-hydroxydopamine dramatically reduces the incidence of ventricular fibrillation associated with both coronary occlusion and reperfusion (642,650). This apparent paradox is likely to be related to addi-

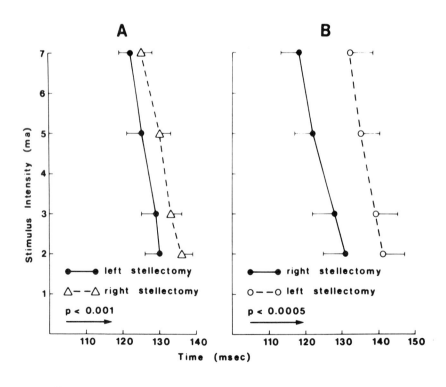

FIG. 5. Effects of right and left stellectomy after contralateral stellate ganglion removal. **A:** Effect of right stellectomy after removal of the left stellate ganglion. In this case, right stellectomy shifted the strength-interval curve 3–6 msec later (panel A). This is in contrast to the leftward shift after right stellectomy in the presence of an intact left stellate ganglion. **B:** Left stellectomy in animals with previous removal of the right stellate ganglion shifted the strength-interval curve 10–14 msec later, an effect similar to that seen in animals with an intact right stellate ganglion. Thus, the effect of right stellectomy is dependent on the presence of intact left stellate ganglion input. (From ref. 637, with permission of the American Heart Association.)

tional postsynaptic effects of reserpine (350) and postsynaptic supersensitivity to remaining adrenal catecholamines (347).

Several findings suggest that β-adrenergic blockade with propranolol at doses from 0.08 to 0.31 mg/kg attenuates the incidence of ventricular arrhythmias and fibrillation associated with ischemia (205,365,366, 546,642), although at higher doses several studies report a lack of significant influence on mortality (137,365,366). In contrast, even at higher doses, practolol significantly attenuates the incidence of ventricular fibrillation during myocardial ischemia (360,544,642), suggesting that intrinsic differences between the two agents may be responsible. Because K^+ release from myocardial cells during ischemia may play an important role in the electrophysiological derangements and thereby arrhythmogenesis (see *Chapter* 57), the differential effects of propranolol and practolol on K^+ uptake may be critical. Through stimulation of β_2 receptors, catecholamines decrease potassium release from myocardial and skeletal muscle (419), an effect blocked by propranolol but not practolol (419). In addition, propranolol actually decreases, whereas practolol increases, the duration of the diastolic period for subendocardial perfusion (450). Finally, propranolol, but not practolol, because of its β_2 blocking properties, may unmask α-adrenergic receptor coronary vasoconstriction, thereby potentially enhancing the degree of ischemic damage (450). Thus, intrinsic differences exist between different β-adrenergic blocking agents, a fact that may contribute to the variable experimental results. Likewise, at higher doses, far in excess of those used clinically and required for blockade of β-adrenergic receptors, most of the agents exhibit direct effects on membranes analogous to those seen with quinidine. It has also been reported that only with these excessive doses is the agent antiarrhythmic in the ischemic rat heart (710). Thus, although β-adrenergic blockade increased the VFT during ischemia in some studies (66,133), others have reported no effect (13). In contrast, there is uniform agreement that β-adrenergic blockade is not antiarrhythmic during reperfusion of ischemic tissue (79,352,650).

To circumvent problems associated with β-adrenergic blocking agents, bretylium has been extensively evaluated. The agent has been shown to attenuate the incidence of ventricular fibrillation associated with ischemia (260), increase the VFT during ischemia (29), and decrease the duration of ventricular arrhythmias (138). Because bretylium has an initial sympathomimetic effect, followed by a sympatholytic effect, the latter is likely to contribute to the antiarrhythmic effects. However, bretylium also has potent membrane effects in cardiac tissue *in vivo,* including an increase in the refractory period of ventricular cells, a phenomenon that is exaggerated in damaged tissue (104). Thus, the precise mechanism responsible for the protective effects of bre-

tylium in the ischemic heart are unknown and are likely to be multiple.

In summary, although most studies have demonstrated a significant reduction in the frequency of premature ventricular complexes after ischemia in the presence of β-adrenergic blockade (143), the influence of β-receptor blockade on the incidence of ventricular fibrillation remains controversial (143). These differences may relate to the dose or agent used, the time of administration, and/or the presence or absence of direct membrane effects independent of β-adrenergic blockade. Likewise, β-adrenergic blockade may decrease the degree of ischemic damage (94,257,580,648), an effect that is likely to be variable, and thereby contribute to its antiarrhythmic effectiveness. On the other hand, multiple clinical studies have demonstrated the effectiveness of β-adrenergic blockade in reducing the incidence of sudden cardiac death in patients with previous myocardial infarction (*vide infra*). Thus, the reduction in mortality is associated with secondary prevention. Indeed, experimental evidence indicates that acute left sympathectomy does reduce the incidence of ventricular fibrillation associated with ischemia in an animal with a previous myocardial infarction (629). The question whether or not β-adrenergic blockade would be effective clinically in primary prevention in patients without previous myocardial infarction remains unanswered.

Because the antiarrhythmic effects of β-adrenergic blockade are variable during ischemia, whereas denervation procedures, particularly those that result in near total depletion of myocardial catecholamines, appear to be far more effective, the role of α-adrenergic stimulation has recently been evaluated. The influence of α-adrenergic stimulation on inotropy in cardiac tissue has recently been reviewed in detail (621), with a positive inotropic effect seen even in human atrial tissue (623). Under normal physiological conditions, α-adrenergic stimulation can affect both the chronotropic and inotropic states of the heart. In this regard, α-adrenergic stimulation results in a negative chronotropic effect in the SA node (325) and in isolated Purkinje fibers (552,596), the latter possibly due to inhibition of ^{42}K uptake (552). However, others have failed to demonstrate any significant chronotropic effect of α-receptor stimulation (757,758). Additional electrophysiological influences of α-adrenergic stimulation include increases in atrial (47,259) and ventricular (400) refractory periods, with associated increases in action potential duration in both atrial (535) and ventricular tissue (251,400,596). Thus, α-adrenergic stimulation in the normal heart exerts small but potentially significant effects on electrophysiological properties, most of which would likely lead to an antiarrhythmic rather than an arrhythmogenic effect.

Assessment of the electrophysiological effects of α-adrenergic receptor stimulation and blockade *in vivo* is complicated by the fact that changes in coronary blood flow and in peripheral and cardiac hemodynamics occur, as well as nonspecific influences of the α-adrenergic blocking agents. Powell and Feigl have demonstrated that a large reduction in pressure in the carotid sinus in dogs of nearly 100 mm Hg induces a 20% increase in coronary resistance mediated primarily by α-adrenergic vasoconstriction (554). Despite the fact that the change in coronary blood flow is small, if the effect were heterogeneous or confined to regions with limited coronary reserve, the effect might induce electrophysiological alterations coincident with regional ischemia. Likewise, the effect of α-adrenergic receptor stimulation or blockade on peripheral hemodynamics may also indirectly alter electrophysiological parameters secondary to changes in regional autonomic tone and coronary blood flow. An additional problem concerns the fact that agents such as phentolamine also block cholinergic actions on isolated smooth muscle (73), inhibit the action of tyramine, and potentiate the action of norepinephrine on isolated guinea pig atrial tissue (46) and at higher doses exhibit quinidine-like membrane depressant effects on canine Purkinje fibers (595). Phenoxybenzamine also can directly reduce the rate of depolarization in isolated atrial tissue, as well as lengthen the refractory period and decrease excitability (700,701).

Even with these concerns, recent experimental evidence indicates that under certain pathophysiological conditions, the effect of α-adrenergic stimulation may be enhanced. For example, central neural stimulation with picrotoxin results in ventricular arrhythmias that are mediated through stimulation of cardiac α-adrenergic mechanisms, as assessed from the protective effects of phentolamine, tolazoline, and denervation and the ineffectiveness of β-adrenergic blockade (167). Both α- and β-adrenergic mechanisms appear to contribute to the evolution of ventricular fibrillation in animals treated with probucol (188). Others reported that in dogs with regional ischemia, either epinephrine or stellate nerve stimulation induced a positive inotropic response mediated through stimulation of β-adrenergic receptors in the normal myocardium but through α-adrenergic receptor stimulation in the ischemic myocardium (344). More recently, α_1-adrenergic blockade has been shown to induce potent antiarrhythmic effects during both coronary occlusion and reperfusion in the cat, independent of hemodynamic alterations or changes in regional myocardial blood flow (650). Likewise, the beneficial antiarrhythmic effects of α_1-adrenergic blockade with prazosin (50 μg/kg) in the cat have been confirmed (159), and in the dog, systemic administration of phentolamine (0.2 mg/kg) is antiarrhythmic during reperfusion and blocks the associated increase in effective refractory period (689). Similar findings during ischemia and reperfusion have been reported in the dog with prazosin, although the effectiveness in the pig is less

pronounced (48). Likewise, intracoronary phentolamine in the dog at the time of reperfusion completely attenuates the incidence of ventricular fibrillation (786). More recent evidence using left stellate ganglion stimulation within a brief 2-min ischemic interval indicates that α_1-adrenergic blockade with prazosin (100 μg/kg) reduces the incidence of ventricular complexes but is less effective in reducing the occurrence of ventricular fibrillation (636,741). Several studies in the rat also indicate that α-adrenergic blockade is antiarrhythmic during both coronary occlusion and reperfusion (352,710). In contrast, one report in the dog indicates that neither prazosin (1 mg/kg) nor phentolamine (5 mg/kg) significantly alters the incidence of ventricular fibrillation associated with reperfusion (69). This apparent discrepancy may be due to the relatively high doses of α-adrenergic blocking agents for the dog used in this latter study.

One explanation for the enhanced α-adrenergic responsivity seen *in vivo* during reperfusion (650) may be related to the twofold increase in α_1-adrenergic receptor density confined to the ischemic region, with no alteration in receptor affinity (142). The increase in α_1 receptors returns to control values with sustained reperfusion with a time course that corresponds to the decrease in α-adrenergic responsivity (142). In the dog, both α_1-adrenergic (492) and β-adrenergic receptor numbers (491) increase in ischemic myocardium. The increase in β-receptor number does not occur until 1 hr and is associated with increased tissue production of cyclic AMP and phosphorylase kinase activity in response to isoproterenol. Although the precise mechanisms responsible for the change in adrenergic receptors during ischemia are unknown, preliminary evidence in cultured myocytes suggest that lysophosphatides, which accumulate in ischemic regions *in vivo* (for review see ref. 140), can expose latent α_1-adrenergic receptors (645). However, it is unknown whether or not these newly exposed receptors are coupled intracellularly and whether or not they mediate important electrophysiological effects, analogous to what occurs *in vivo*. That α-adrenergic receptors can be altered by changes in the phospholipid environment has been suggested previously (425). Likewise, in frog erythrocytes, phospholipase A_2, which can result in the production of lysophosphatides, decreases ^{3}H-dihydroalprenolol binding to β receptors and isoproterenol-stimulated adenylate cyclase activity (416), although effects on the α_1-adrenergic receptor have not been assessed. Methylation of membrane phospholipids also alters receptor number, apparently because of differential uncovering of receptors in a more fluid membrane environment (696). Thus, changes in adrenergic receptors in the ischemic heart may alter the responsivity to α- versus β-adrenergic stimulation and may explain, at least in part, the enhanced α_1-adrenergic responsivity and associated effectiveness of α-adrenergic blockade on arrhythmogenesis. It should be emphasized, however, that some of the protective effects of α-adrenergic blockade may be mediated directly by the pharmacological agent used independent of blockade of the α-adrenergic receptor (710).

Electrophysiological Effects of α- and β-Adrenergic Stimulation

Under physiological conditions, the effects of sympathetic stimulation in the heart are mediated primarily through β-receptors. These effects include an acceleration of sinus node rate (723), an increase in AV node conduction velocity (760), decreases in AV junctional and His-bundle refractoriness, with shortening of Purkinje fiber and ventricular muscle action potential durations, and increases in excitability and automaticity in the His-Purkinje network (252,308). The reduction in refractory period may contribute to arrhythmogenesis, particularly in the ischemic heart. Over the past several years, interest has also focused on the role of β-adrenergic receptor stimulation in maintaining very slow conduction through activation of the slow inward current (I_{si}). During myocardial ischemia, depolarization of the tissue may inactivate the fast sodium channel, with the result that depolarization and conduction may then be exclusively dependent on the I_{si}. Catecholamines can increase the magnitude of the I_{si} and decrease its threshold for excitation, which apparently occurs through stimulation of β-adrenergic receptors and is mediated by increases in intracellular cyclic AMP (414). However, findings suggest that the slow inward current does not maintain depolarization in the ischemic heart (372), although there is disagreement (122). However, to date there are no detailed data available to indicate the precise electrophysiological effects of β-adrenergic stimulation in the ischemic heart *in vivo*. Until this information is available, the precise mechanisms responsible for the beneficial effects of β-adrenergic blockade *in vivo* will remain speculative.

Under normal physiological conditions, α-adrenergic stimulation results in effects that would be expected to be primarily antiarrhythmic, including a decrease in automaticity in the sinus node and latent ventricular pacemakers, lengthening of the refractory period, and an increase in the VFT. However, in depressed tissue the arrhythmogenic effects of α-adrenergic stimulation may become manifest. For example, in rabbit papillary muscle depolarized by high $[K^+]_0$, α-adrenergic mechanisms appear to increase the I_{si} and maintain depolarization (478). *In vivo*, the augmentation of contractility in response to stellate nerve stimulation may be mediated through α-adrenergic receptors in the ischemic region, but by β-adrenergic receptors in the normal zone (344). Potentially, both of these effects may involve modulation of intracellular calcium. Likewise, *in vivo* in the cat,

reperfusion after coronary occlusion results in an increased idioventricular rate that can be abolished by α-adrenergic blockade or catecholamine depletion with 6-hydroxydopamine, but not by β-adrenergic blockade (650). Likewise, the idioventricular rate can be enhanced during reperfusion by regional infusion of methoxamine, an α agonist, into the reperfused zone (650). This finding is in contrast to the β-mediated effects on idioventricular rate in nonischemic animals (Fig. 6). Thus, evidence would suggest that α_1-adrenergic stimulation may result in electrophysiological derangements peculiar to ischemia and reperfusion and not evident in normal tissue. Recent work also suggests that α-adrenergic mechanisms may mediate a large portion of the increase in intracellular calcium during reperfusion (646). In untreated animals subjected to 35 min of coronary occlusion followed by reperfusion, there was a twofold increase in total tissue calcium, and using measurements of vascular space and the interstitium, the increase was confirmed to be largely intracellular (646). This was confirmed by pyroantimonate precipitation of the calcium and X-ray microprobe analysis. α-Adrenergic blockade even 2 min prior to reperfusion completely prevented the increase in intracellular calcium. This calcium accumulation during reperfusion in *reversibly* injured tissue is not a passive process but appears to be modulated by α-adrenergic stimulation (Fig. 7). This increase in intracellular calcium may be important not only in the progression of cellular damage but also in arrhythmogenesis. Recently, using microelectrodes and membrane patches derived from cultured myocytes, an inward current has been characterized that is activated by increased cytosolic calcium (127). *In vivo*, during ischemia or reperfusion, α-adrenergic stimulation may enhance this inward current by increasing cytosolic calcium. This inward current may contribute to depolarization, which is likely to be slow, and may also contribute to the development of delayed afterdepolarizations and triggered activity (see *Chapter 60*). This type of response may be involved in the accelerated idioventricular rates seen during reperfusion in both animals (650) and man (253).

There is a substantial amount of evidence to suggest that α-adrenergic stimulation in tissues other than the heart can lead to increased calcium influx (139). In ischemic tissue *in vivo*, exposure of α-adrenergic receptors may lead to a receptor-coupled increase in intracellular calcium. A potential mechanism may involve phospholipid inositol turnover, leading to an increase in intracellular calcium (749).

Parasympathetic Influences During Myocardial Ischemia: Relation to Arrhythmogenesis

There is a substantial amount of evidence to suggest that manipulation of vagal influences to the myocardium during ischemia will affect arrhythmogenesis. However,

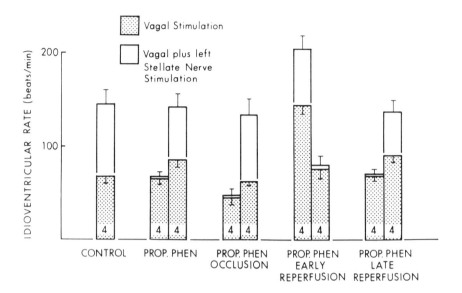

FIG. 6. Effects of left stellate nerve stimulation on the idioventricular rate determined by intense vagal nerve stimulation in the cat. Intrinsic idioventricular rates are shown in the stippled bars under control, coronary occlusion, early reperfusion, and late reperfusion conditions in the presence of either β-adrenergic blockade with propranolol (PROP) or α-adrenergic blockade with phentolamine (PHEN). Responses induced by left stellate nerve stimulation are shown by open bars. The increase in idioventricular rate induced by left stellate nerve stimulation was blocked by propranolol, but not phentolamine, during control and ischemic conditions. In contrast, during early reperfusion, there was an intrinsic increase in idioventricular rate that was further increased by stellate nerve stimulation, despite β-adrenergic blockade with propranolol, but was blocked by phentolamine, indicating an α-adrenergic-mediated response. During late reperfusion, the response reverted back to a normal β-mediated effect. Values are means ± SEM, and numbers within histograms indicate numbers of animals in the groups. (From ref. 650, with permission of the Journal of Clinical Investigation.)

there is controversy regarding whether excessive vagal tone is antiarrhythmic due to a direct electrophysiological effect in the ventricle or whether it is arrhythmogenic due to excessive bradycardia. The experimental findings during early ischemia are in many ways inconsistent with clinical findings in patients with acute myocardial infarction, probably because the time after the initial ischemic insult varies, as does the apparent mechanism responsible for the arrhythmia. As pointed out by Greenberg (261), vagally mediated bradycardia associated

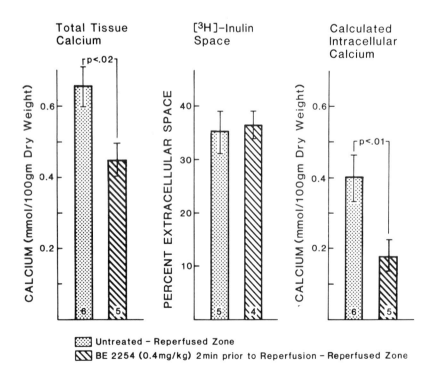

FIG. 7. Effects of α₁-adrenergic blockade with BE-2254 given intravenously 2 min prior to reperfusion after a 35-min ischemic interval on the total tissue calcium (left), the ³H-inulin space (middle), and the calculated intracellular calcium (right). Values represent means ± SEM in the reperfused zone in either untreated control animals or animals with α₁-adrenergic blockade. Although total tissue calcium was reduced by α₁-adrenergic blockade, it was still elevated over that seen in control tissue (0.3 mmole/100 g dry weight). The increase in total tissue calcium in the presence of α₁-adrenergic blockade was due to a maintained increase in inulin space that was 24% in control, nonischemic tissue and likely reflects movement into irreversibly injured cells. However, α₁-adrenergic blockade with BE-2254 completely prevented the increase in intracellular calcium. These results were verified with pyroantimonate precipitation of calcium and electron microscopic X-ray microprobe analysis. (From ref. 646, with permission of the Journal of Clinical Investigation.)

with inferior wall infarction in man is quite different from bradyasystolic cardiac arrest. In the former, the bradycardia response is reversible by atropine, a pacemaker, or catecholamines. In contrast, the latter is likely attributable to several mechanisms (261), including: (a) complete heart block associated with acute anterior infarction due to ischemia or infarction involving the His bundle and bundle branches, usually unresponsive to pharmacological therapy; (b) myocardial rupture during evolving infarction; (c) drug-induced bradycardic death due to agents that depress conduction and/or automaticity and include digitalis, antiarrhythmic agents, and β-adrenergic blocking agents; (d) bradycardia-induced ventricular tachycardia or fibrillation secondary to a decrease in coronary perfusion pressure with associated ischemia; and (e) bradycardic asystolic death, which may involve, in part, a Bezold-Jarisch-type reflex but appears not to be responsive to medical intervention. Thus, the following sections on the influence of parasympathetic tone during ischemia and infarction will be restricted to the effects associated with infarction, but not those associated with bradyasystolic cardiac arrest. As in the case of adrenergic neural influences, the following section will be divided into three categories: (a) neural stimulation studies, (b) surgical denervation studies, and (c) pharmacological intervention studies.

Neural Stimulation Studies

The results derived from animal studies appear to depend in part on the time interval after the ischemic insult. Within the first hour after coronary occlusion in the dog, vagal nerve stimulation suppresses or abolishes ventricular arrhythmias (617), increases the VFT (363), reduces the incidence of malignant arrhythmias, defined as those with a coupling interval less than 0.43 sec (255), increases the rate of rise of the ischemic zone electrogram (309,616), decreases the incidence of spontaneous ventricular fibrillation (497), and delays the onset of malignant ventricular arrhythmias (137,497). Likewise, use of the cholinesterase inhibitor edrophonium to enhance the effect of parasympathetic tone in the dog also increases the VFT, an effect abolished by atropine (274). Physostigmine also dramatically reduces the incidence of spontaneous ventricular fibrillation associated with ischemia (158). However, with preexisting vagal tone, stimulation does not appear to enhance the protection (137).

In contrast to the protective effects of vagal tone during early ischemia, at 1 day after myocardial infarction, vagal stimulation enhances ventricular arrhythmias, possibly because of an unmasking of enhanced ventricular automaticity (616). Even at 5 hr after coronary occlusion, vagal stimulation appears to exacerbate ventricular arrhythmias, although the incidence of ventricular tachycardia and fibrillation is not increased (364),

a finding that agrees with clinical results wherein edrophonium fails to alter, and may actually increase, the incidence of arrhythmias in patients following the first 24 hr after acute myocardial infarction (521). Thus, any protective influence of increased vagal tone is likely to be confined to the early ischemic interval, analogous to the prehospital phase of acute myocardial infarction. Unfortunately, clinical data related to the effectiveness of vagal tone during this early time interval are lacking.

Surgical Denervation Studies

Studies in the conscious dog would suggest that bilateral vagotomy has no effect on the incidence of ventricular fibrillation after LAD coronary occlusion (184). In contrast, in the cat, bilateral vagotomy results in a highly significant increase in the incidence of ventricular fibrillation, independent of changes in sinus rate (136,173). These results are consistent, because the conscious dog exhibits a tachycardia in response to an anterior ischemic insult, with no increase in efferent vagal tone (548). On the other hand, the cat exhibits an increase in vagal tone and associated bradycardia in response to an anterior ischemic insult (136). Thus, vagotomy will be expected to exert only a deleterious influence in the cat under identical experimental conditions, because of a preexisting level of vagal tone.

Pharmacological Intervention Studies

Several experimental investigations have assessed the influence of atropine on arrhythmogenesis during ischemia. It appears that the effect is critically dependent on the site of coronary occlusion. For example, atropine administration does not appear to alter the incidence of malignant arrhythmias after circumflex coronary occlusion in the conscious or anesthetized dog (404). In contrast, after anterior myocardial ischemia induced by LAD coronary occlusion, atropine significantly increases the incidence of ventricular fibrillation, independent of changes in sinus rate (136). Likewise, in the same experimental preparation, malignant arrhythmias associated with inferior myocardial ischemia were not influenced by atropine (141). In addition, the protective influences of enhanced vagal stimulation detailed earlier were all demonstrated in animals with anterior myocardial ischemia. Several additional findings indicate that atropine has detrimental influences on rhythm during acute anterior ischemia, including exacerbation of arrhythmias 10 min after ischemia (255) and enhancement of the incidence of ventricular fibrillation (136). In contrast, atropine is actually antiarrhythmic 24 hr after coronary occlusion (435), presumably related to overdrive suppression of enhanced ventricular automaticity, and appears to obliterate arrhythmias associated with a relatively long (0.43-sec) coupling interval (192). Thus, the detrimental influence of atropine on rhythm appears to be dependent on the time after the ischemic insult as well as the region of the myocardium affected by the insult.

Clinical results in patients with acute myocardial infarction appear to support these experimental conclusions. For example, in most clinical studies, atropine is used to improve hemodynamics in patients with acute myocardial infarction with associated bradycardia, hypotension, and/or heart block. Most of these patients have inferior myocardial infarction and would be expected to respond favorably to atropine. In clinical studies performed to determine whether or not atropine resulted in detrimental effects on rhythm during acute myocardial infarction (111,615), most of the patients had inferior infarction and were studied 5 to 7 hr after onset of symptoms. Likewise, in patients given atropine within the first hour after onset of symptoms, the majority of patients had inferior infarction (763). Thus, each of these clinical studies (111,615,763) failed to demonstrate an adverse effect of atropine on the evolution of arrhythmias. In contrast, in patients seen early after myocardial infarction, edrophonium may reduce the incidence of ventricular tachycardia (476). However, despite the fact that patients seen within the first hour, even with anterior infarction, have a relatively high incidence of bradycardia (770), the potential deleterious effect of atropine has not been assessed. Possibly, based on experimental findings, enhancement of vagal tone in this population may be protective relative to arrhythmogenesis if hemodynamics are not compromised.

Potential Electrophysiological Mechanisms

Although the influence of the parasympathetic nervous system on electrophysiological properties of the SA and AV nodes and atrial tissue is unequivocal, controversy continues regarding whether or not similar influences are exerted in the ventricle. Although parasympathetic innervation to the ventricle has been verified by histologic analysis of the His bundle and bundle branches in both the dog and man (362), the enzyme responsible for synthesis of acetylcholine, choline acetyltransferase, is prominent in ventricular muscle as well (317,598). Likewise, both acetylcholine (89) and a high density of muscarinic cholinergic receptors (210) are found throughout both ventricles. Thus, it is apparent that the capacity for direct parasympathetic effects on ventricular electrophysiological properties exists.

Although early *in vitro* studies failed to demonstrate an effect of acetylcholine on action potentials derived from Purkinje fibers or ventricular muscle (304,335), more recent evidence indicates several important alterations. For example, in both canine Purkinje fibers and the His bundle *in vitro,* acetylcholine induces a dose-dependent decrease in automaticity (30,225,728). In contrast, in sheep Purkinje fibers, the rate of diastolic

depolarization is enhanced by acetylcholine (107), likely because of a depolarization shift of the activation curve for the pacemaker current (105). In the dog (225), guinea pig (518), and chick heart (536), acetylcholine shortens the action potential duration, secondary to a decrease in the slow inward current, with no change in the outward (i_x) or background (i_{K_1}) potassium currents (298,518). In direct contrast, in the sheep, acetylcholine increases the action potential duration in the ventricle, associated with a shift in the plateau phase to a more positive direction (107), because of a reduction in the background outward current carried by potassium (105,106). Thus, it is apparent that under some conditions, acetylcholine can alter the electrophysiological properties of ventricular tissue *in vitro,* which may mediate some of the antiarrhythmic effects seen in the ischemic heart *in vivo.*

In vivo, vagal stimulation can directly decrease the idioventricular rate (49,189,256,743) even after removal of the sympathetic ganglia (256), suggesting that the negative chronotropic effect is evidenced *in vivo* and appears to be independent of inhibition of catecholamine release. As early as 1934 it was reported that the negative chronotropic effect of vagal stimulation was increased in the presence of an enhanced sympathetic drive (597), a phenomenon later termed accentuated antagonism by Levy (411). Thus, a relatively strong sympathetic input can be overcome by a relatively weak parasympathetic response. Most studies addressing the electrophysiological effects of acetylcholine do not take into account the presence of tissue catecholamines, suggesting that some of the "direct" effects may be due to either presynaptic or postsynaptic inhibition of the effects of catecholamines (*vide supra*). For example, acetylcholine reverses the isoproterenol-induced decrease in action potential duration, but not the decrease in action potential duration induced by elevation of extracellular calcium (31), indicating that the response is due exclusively to the antiadrenergic effect of acetylcholine. In ventricular muscle from the embryonic chick heart, calcium-dependent action potentials are suppressed by acetylcholine only when isoproterenol is used to augment the I_{si}. However, in 5-day-old chick heart, the suppression of I_{si} in depolarized tissue is mediated not only through an antiadrenergic effect but also through a direct effect on the I_{si} (59,536). Likewise, in both sheep (107) and guinea pig (298), the electrophysiological effects of acetylcholine appear to be direct, independent of adrenergic neural input. Thus, during myocardial ischemia, the protective effect of vagal tone is likely to result primarily from an antiadrenergic effect as well as a potential direct effect.

The antiadrenergic effect of parasympathetic input is likely to be mediated by several mechanisms. First, acetylcholine or vagal nerve stimulation inhibits norepinephrine outflow from the isolated perfused rabbit heart (424) and coronary sinus norepinephrine overflow *in vivo* (398,412), an effect likely mediated through stimulation of presynaptic muscarinic receptors on the sympathetic nerve endings (494). Second, a postsynaptic antiadrenergic effect is also likely, because acetylcholine will antagonize the effects of norepinephrine infusion (162,307). Third, muscarinic-cholinergic stimulation directly attenuates the β-adrenergic-induced increase in cyclic AMP (88,227) and thereby the electrophysiological effects of catecholamines. Fourth, muscarinic-cholinergic stimulation induces increases in cyclic GMP and thereby inhibition of cyclic AMP (236,766), although there is substantial evidence to indicate that the electrophysiological effects of acetylcholine can occur independent of changes in cyclic GMP (477). Thus, the antiadrenergic effects of acetylcholine occur at both presynaptic and postsynaptic sites.

The antiarrhythmic effect of vagal tone *in vivo* also appears to be mediated, at least in part, by an antiadrenergic effect. For example, vagal stimulation will increase both the ventricular fibrillation threshold and the repetitive extrasystole threshold *in vivo* only in the presence of an elevated sympathetic tone (224,376, 562,798). Likewise, the increase in ventricular effective refractory periods *in vivo* induced by vagal stimulation also depends exclusively on the presence of sympathetic tone (453), although conflicting results on changes in the monophasic action potential have also been reported (17).

In summary, the protective influence of vagal tone during ischemia may be in part mediated through a decrease in heart rate independent of any electrophysiologic effects. Alternatively, it may be related to direct effects to decrease the rate of ventricular pacemakers and thereby ventricular automaticity, depress or abolish the I_{si} and hence potentially interfere with slowed conduction in ischemic regions, and lengthen the effective refractory period, changes that would be expected to interrupt a reentrant circuit. However, the inhibition of the I_{si} may not be critical in the ischemic heart, because slowed conduction appears to depend on depressed fast-response action potentials. Additionally, vagal stimulation, by inhibiting either the release or postsynaptic effect of intramyocardial catecholamines in the ischemic heart, may improve the marked disparities in repolarization between the ischemic region and normal region, a phenomenon linked to initiation of malignant ventricular arrhythmias in the ischemic heart (330).

CLINICAL FINDINGS RELATED TO THE AUTONOMIC NERVOUS SYSTEM IN SUDDEN CARDIAC DEATH

Sudden death associated with coronary artery disease is primarily a result of disturbances in cardiac rhythm, culminating in ventricular fibrillation (134). Coronary disease is one of the principal causes of death in the Western world, and more than half of these patients die suddenly because of abnormalities in cardiac rhythm (187,430). Among the many causes of sudden cardiac

death, in addition to ischemic heart disease, are lethal rhythm disorders associated with mitral valve prolapse, cardiomyopathy, myocarditis, WPW syndrome, metabolic and electrolyte disturbances, acquired and congenital valvular lesions and other malformations, infiltration or degeneration of the cardiac conduction system, cardiac sensitivity to drugs such as quinidine, digitalis, phenothiazines, and tricyclic antidepressants, and the long-QT syndrome. In the following section we shall briefly review the clinical findings implicating the autonomic nervous system in sudden death associated with coronary artery disease.

Clinical evidence implicating the autonomic nervous system in the genesis of sudden cardiac death associated with coronary artery disease takes two forms: (a) cardiovascular observations in patients during acute myocardial ischemia and infarction; (b) pharmacological intervention studies in the same population.

Evidence that the Autonomic Nervous System Is Activated in Patients During Acute Myocardial Ischemia and Infarction

Pantridge and colleagues (5,534,770) have evaluated the incidence of autonomic disturbances present within 1 hr of onset of symptoms in patients suffering acute myocardial infarction who had not experienced ventricular tachycardia, ventricular fibrillation, supraventricular arrhythmias, or prior therapy with digitalis or β-adrenergic blocking agents. Sympathetic overactivity was assessed by the presence of sinus tachycardia and transient hypertension; parasympathetic overactivity was indicated by sinus bradycardia, AV block, or transient hypotension. The vast majority of patients had signs of autonomic imbalance within the first 30 min, with signs of excessive sympathetic activity more common in patients with anterior ischemic insult, whereas signs of vagal overactivity were more frequent in patients with inferior ischemic insult. Furthermore, sympathetic and parasympathetic overactivities may coexist, because correction of vagal overactivity by atropine usually gives rise to tachycardia and transient hypertension (534).

The plasma norepinephrine level is considered an indicator of global sympathetic tone, reflecting release from sympathetic postganglionic nerve endings. Measurements of plasma catecholamines in the setting of acute myocardial infarction by several investigators have all demonstrated increases (213,230,254,463,507,586, 747,748). The extent of the myocardial infarction has correlated directly with the plasma norepinephrine level, and, not surprisingly, the presence of shock or a course complicated by congestive heart failure has contributed to higher levels, as compared with patients with an uncomplicated course. The norepinephrine elevation, while rapid in its initial rise, usually persists for at least 2 days in patients undergoing myocardial infarction. The elevation in plasma catecholamines probably also

TABLE 1. *Summary of results of trials assessing effectiveness of β-adrenergic blockade for secondary prevention*

Study	Ref.	No. of patients	Definition of sudden death	Drug
Wilhelmsson, 1974	785	230	<24 hr	Alprenolol
Ahlmark, 1976	7	162	<24 hr	Alprenolol
European multicenter, 1975, 1977	314, 577	3,038	<2 hr	Practolol
Norwegian multicenter study group, 1981	514	1,884	≤24 hr	Timolol
β-blocker heart attack trial, 1982	53	3,837	<1 hr	Propranolol
Hansteen, 1982	271	560	<12 hr	Propranolol
Julian, 1982	345	1,456	<24 hr	Sotalol

reflects reflex adrenal epinephrine release (437). However, the relationship between arrhythmias and plasma catecholamines is not definitive, likely because of the nonspecificity of the measurement compared with the more important alterations in intramyocardial catecholamines (*vide supra*).

Summary of Results from Trials Evaluating the Effectiveness of β-Adrenergic Blockade

A clearly defined group at significant risk of sudden cardiac death are the survivors of acute infarction, with patients under 70 years of age having 10% mortality during the first year and subsequent 5% annual mortality (459). Almost half of these deaths are sudden. Since 1974, seven double-blind randomized trials of β-adrenergic blockade in postinfarction patients have been performed, with the definition of sudden death being variable (Table 1). Pooled data reveal that treatment led to a 28% reduction in mortality, with a 33% reduction in sudden cardiac death and a 20% reduction in non-sudden cardiac death (223), which suggests a primary antiarrhythmic effect to explain the beneficial actions of β-adrenergic blockade. These findings in chronic survivors of myocardial infarction are the first reports that a pharmacological intervention has enhanced survival in

TABLE 2. *Summary of acute intervention trials with β-adrenergic blockade*

Study	Ref.	No. of patients	Drug	Route of administration
Balcon, 1966	33	114	Propranolol 20 mg q. 6 hr	Oral
Clausen, 1966	121	130	Propranolol 10 mg q.i.d.	Oral
Norris, 1968	513	536	Propranolol 10 mg q.i.d.	Oral
Barber, 1975	34	298	Practolol 300 mg q. 12 hr	Oral
Evemy, 1978	200	94	Practolol 15 mg i.v., 200 mg q. 12 hr	Initial dose i.v., then oral
Johansson, 1980	334	85	Practolol 20 mg i.v. then Atenolol 50 mg b.i.d.	Initial dose i.v., then oral
Hjalmarson, 1981, and Ryden, 1983	301 601	1,395	Metoprolol 15 mg i.v., 100 mg b.i.d.	Initial dose i.v., then oral
International collaborative study group, 1984	711	144	Timolol i.v. × 24 hr, 10 mg b.i.d.	First 24 hr i.v., then oral

Relative β_1 selective activity	Intrinsic sympathomimetic activity	Membrane-stabilizing activity	Sudden deaths		p, significance
			β blockade	Placebo	
0	+	+	3	11	<0.05
0	+	+	1	9	<0.05
+	+	0	48	78	<0.01
0	0	0	47	95	<0.001
0	0	++	64	89	<0.05
0	0	++	11	23	<0.038
0	0	0	4.6%	4.7%	N.S.

the period after infarction (459) and suggest that increased sympathetic activity contributes to mortality associated with coronary artery disease. Although the precise mechanisms responsible for the reduction in cardiovascular mortality with chronic β-adrenergic blockade are unknown, the mechanisms likely include reduction in the extent of myocardial ischemia, a direct antiarrhythmic effect, and improvement in left ventricular dysfunction. The observed beneficial effects are likely related to the β-adrenergic blocking properties of the drugs rather than to some other property of the compounds, because the beneficial effects have been noted with several different agents possessing inherently

different properties (Table 1). The fact that sotalol, a nonselective agent, failed to significantly reduce mortality despite a spectrum of activity similar to that of timolol suggests that sotalol may have additional properties that offset its beneficial β blocking property. Sotalol differs importantly in possessing a class-3 antiarrhythmic effect that may account for the apparent differences.

The influence of β-adrenergic blockade as an acute intervention during myocardial infarction is less definitive (223). The results from the nine double-blind, placebo-controlled, randomly assigned acute intervention trials for evaluating β-adrenergic blockade are conflicting (Table 2) (33,34,121,200,301,334,513,601,711). These stud-

Relative β_1 selectivity	Intrinsic sympathomimetic activity	Membrane-stabilizing activity	Patients with VT and/or VF		p, significance
			β blockade	Placebo	
0	0	++	2	2	N.S.
0	0	++	3	2	N.S.
0	0	++	3	4	N.S.
+	+	0	—	—	N.S.
+	+	0	5	7	N.S.
+	+	0	5	2	
+	0	0			
+	0	0	6 (VF)	17 (VF)	<0.05
0	0	0	2	4	

ies differed in regard to route of administration, β-adrenergic blocking agent used, and dosage regimen. With the exception of the large-scale metoprolol study, which demonstrated a statistically significant reduction in the incidence of fatal arrhythmias (301,601), each of the other trials failed to demonstrate a significant difference between placebo and β-adrenergic blockade (Table 2). Thus, it appears that β-adrenergic blockade may be useful as an acute intervention to decrease the incidence of sudden cardiac death associated with myocardial infarction, but the response may be peculiar to the specific agent employed.

The efficacy of α-adrenergic blockade in primary or secondary prevention has not as yet been evaluated in controlled randomized studies. Although experimental results indicate that α-adrenergic blockade may prove beneficial in primary prevention, there are no experimental data to indicate that this mode of therapy will be useful in secondary prevention.

AUTONOMIC NEURAL INFLUENCES ON SUPRAVENTRICULAR TACHYCARDIAS, ATRIAL FLUTTER, AND ATRIAL FIBRILLATION

The effects of both parasympathetic and sympathetic neurotransmitters on cardiac impulse formation and conduction were discussed earlier. In this section, the effects of autonomic neural modulation on the initiation, perpetuation, and termination of supraventricular rhythm disturbances will be examined.

AV Node Reentry

The electrophysiology inhomogeneity of the AV node provides the substrate for this reentrant rhythm, which

is the most common cause of paroxysmal supraventricular tachycardia (342,343), with no predilection for age, sex, or preexisting heart disease. Most patients with AV nodal reentrant supraventricular tachycardia will demonstrate dual AV node pathways in response to progressively more premature atrial stimulation, with conduction proceeding down the fast (β) pathway initially. However, because of the relatively longer refractory period of the β pathway, earlier coupled atrial premature beats block in the β pathway, but will then conduct antegrade in the slower α pathway (Fig. 8). Demonstration of inhomogeneity of conduction and refractoriness in the AV node is not a prerequisite for either the presence or absence of clinical supraventricular tachycardia (164). This inability to demonstrate dual AV nodal pathways may reflect inability to elicit the inhomogeneity because of the limitations of atrial prematurity due to the functional refractory period of the atrium, the similarity of refractory periods under basal conditions, or variations in the heterogeneity between the fast (β) and slow (α) pathways of conduction and refractoriness both antegrade and retrograde in the AV node. Thus, the occurrence of supraventricular tachycardia in a particular patient depends on a critical relationship between the refractory period and conduction velocity within the AV node, both factors that are profoundly regulated by the autonomic nervous system. Neither the atria nor the ventricles are necessary to maintain AV nodal supraventricular tachycardia, as demonstrated by the ability to depolarize either the atria (341) or the ventricles (343) from multiple sites without affecting the tachycardia and by its maintenance in the presence of AV node dissociation (341).

AV nodal reentrant tachycardia is usually initiated by either spontaneous or artificially induced atrial premature depolarizations (342,343,769). For spontaneous AV nodal reentry to occur, both critically timed atrial pre-

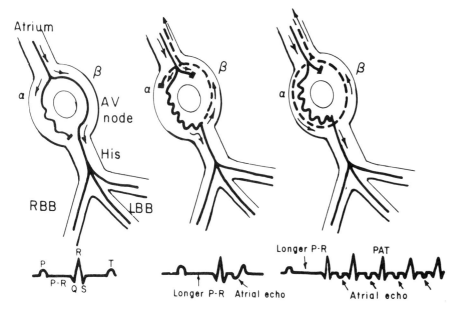

FIG. 8. Pictorial representation of dual AV nodal pathways and mechanism of AV nodal reentrant tachycardia. The AV node is depicted as divided into a slow (α) pathway and a fast (β) pathway. In the center is the response to a single atrial premature beat that is blocked in the fast (β) pathway but can propagate slowly down the α pathway. However, the return beat, as demonstrated by the atrial echo, finds the α pathway refractory. In the right panel, a critically timed atrial premature beat fulfills the requirements for initiating a sustained reentrant circuit, and a paroxysmal atrial tachycardia ensues. (From ref. 342, with permission of *Annals of Internal Medicine*.)

mature depolarizations and the correct balance between AV node refractoriness and conduction velocity must occur. Augmentation of sympathetic tone with exercise or isoproterenol infusion may evoke an atrial premature depolarization and thus initiate this type of supraventricular tachycardia (768). In a series of 14 patients with dual AV nodal pathways and spontaneously recurrent paroxysms of supraventricular tachycardia, 7 patients failed to induce or sustain the rhythm with programmed stimulation because of a long refractory period in the retrograde fast (β) pathway (791). However, atropine, by shortening the refractory period retrograde, resulted in induction of the supraventricular tachycardia in all patients (791). In contrast, atropine may enhance both retrograde fast (β) pathway and antegrade slow (α) pathway conduction and decrease the effective refractory period in the fast pathway. Thus, the retrograde impulse could arrive prior to atrial recovery of excitability and thereby might actually prevent induction of the supraventricular tachycardia (791). The actions of β-adrenergic blockade with propranolol are more complex, with increases in the effective and functional refractory periods of both the slow and fast pathways (792). However, the effects vary in both pathways, with the net result being either depression or facilitation of the initiation of supraventricular tachycardia (792). This variation is likely the result of not only differences in sympathetic innervation to regions of the AV node but also differences in the degree of adrenergic tone prior to β-adrenergic blockade.

The cycle length of the AV nodal reentrant tachycardia is significantly shortened by parasympathetic neural blockade with atropine, reflecting the increases in both antegrade slow pathway and retrograde fast pathway conduction velocities (791). In contrast, minimal lengthening of the tachycardia cycle length with β-adrenergic blockade has been reported (792). Because of the interactions between the sympathetic and parasympathetic nervous systems detailed earlier, the effect of isoproterenol on acceleration of the rate of supraventricular tachycardia is attenuated by edrophonium and exacerbated by atropine (769).

Termination of AV node reentrant supraventricular tachycardia involves intervening in the critical relationship between conduction velocity and refractory periods in the AV node. The most frequently employed methods are those that further slow AV nodal conduction, with the only requirement for termination being that the refractory period of the reentrant circuit exceed the conduction time (343). Vagal-stimulation-induced termination is preceded by slowing because of depression of the AV node conduction velocity, and the level of vagal tone required to terminate the tachycardia is modulated by the concomitant background sympathetic tone. Augmentation of sympathetic tone through reflex mechanisms increases vagal tone, and it is this reflex

parasympathetic augmentation that is responsible for termination, because termination is prevented by adrenergic stimulation in the presence of muscarinic-cholinergic receptor blockade (769).

Supraventricular Tachycardia Associated with an Accessory Bypass Tract

This form of reentrant tachycardia is the second most common cause of supraventricular tachycardia and represents a true anatomically definable dual-pathway mechanism. In patients with the WPW syndrome, an accessory pathway connects the atria and the ventricles, providing an additional parallel conduction pathway to the normal AV node conduction. The conduction velocity of the accessory pathway is usually faster than that of the AV node, but its refractory period is longer. Thus, a premature atrial depolarization may block in the accessory pathway, propagate via the AV node to the ventricles, and retrogradely conduct via the accessory pathway to initiate a macro-reentrant loop. In contrast to AV node reentry, where only the AV node is essential to continuation of the supraventricular tachycardia, the atria, ventricles, AV node, and accessory pathway are all necessary components of the reentrant loop. When some degree of antegrade excitation is present via the accessory pathway during sinus rhythm, a preexcitation, or delta wave, is apparent, but when antegrade accessory conduction is not apparent, the bypass tract is referred to as concealed. Although the reentrant circuit can propagate in either direction, antegrade AV node conduction with retrograde conduction through the bypass tract is more common, but retrograde AV node conduction and antegrade accessory pathway propagation can also occur.

Initiation of the more common form of supraventricular tachycardia utilizing an accessory pathway is via a premature beat, either from the atrium, producing unidirectional block in the accessory pathway, or from the ventricle, producing unidirectional block in the normal AV nodal pathway (181,699). The inducibility of the tachycardia is correlated to the presence of rapid antegrade normal pathway conduction, as well as rapid retrograde conduction through the accessory pathway (163). Vagal stimulation, via carotid sinus massage, has been shown to allow antegrade accessory pathway conduction to become manifest, presumably on the basis of prolonging the cycle length beyond the refractory period of the accessory pathway (559). Similarly, isoproterenol infusion can reinstitute antegrade conduction over a concealed accessory pathway (559) and shorten the antegrade refractory period of the accessory pathway (776), but the inducibility of the tachycardia has not been specifically addressed relative to these effects on the accessory pathway. The rate of the tachycardia utilizing an accessory bypass tract is significantly affected by changes in autonomic tone to the AV node (768). Termination of the reentrant tachycardia associated with an accessory pathway can occur at multiple possible points in the loop. For example, isoproterenol can accelerate the AV nodal conduction velocity, which can lead to encroachment of the retrograde impulse on the refractory period of the bypass tract and can thereby terminate the tachycardia (768).

Supraventricular Tachycardia Associated with SA Node Reentry

This form of supraventricular tachycardia is usually initiated by an atrial premature depolarization (505,771) and represents one of the more rare forms of supraventricular tachycardia (343). The inhomogeneity of conduction and refractory periods is presumably in the sinus node, with variation in these parameters resulting in abolition or facilitation of the tachycardia (505), probably because of the varied effects of vagal stimulation on these indices. The effects of vagal stimulation include lengthening of the sinus node refractory period, shortening of the atrial refractory period, and, during sinus node reentry, lengthening of the echo circuit time (114). Because the reentrant circuit principally involves the sinus node and the SA perinodal tissues, the ventricles, AV node, and most of the atria are not required for tachycardia initiation or maintenance. The role of sympathetic stimulation or blockade in SA node reentry has not been studied systematically relative to initiation, perpetuation, or termination.

Atrial Flutter and Atrial Fibrillation

Atrial fibrillation is a common arrhythmia in patients both with and without organic heart disease and can be initiated by atrial premature depolarizations. This type of atrial arrhythmia can be induced in approximately 5% of normal patients using atrial stimulation, although in this case it is usually self-terminating (343). In contrast, initiation of atrial flutter is uncommon in patients without spontaneous atrial flutter. Atrial flutter is frequently associated with intraatrial conduction delays and can be most reliably initiated by rapid atrial pacing (343). Cholinergic stimulation has been known for years to be associated with the induction and maintenance of atrial fibrillation, with similar effects produced by blockade of cholinesterase (93), application or administration of methacholine (502) or acetylcholine (92,428,499), or efferent vagus nerve stimulation (428). Although the effects of vagal stimulation on atrial fibrillation are blocked by atropine, the mechanism of the induction of atrial fibrillation is not completely understood. The effects have been attributed to a nonuniform shortening of the atrial refractory period by vagal stimulation (11),

as well as intraatrial conduction delays (677), which would, of course, predispose the atria to a reentrant arrhythmia. Similar approaches have been used in conjunction with detailed mapping procedures in which the reentrant nature of the atrial flutter has been clearly demonstrated (14).

Modulation of the ventricular response rate to atrial fibrillation and flutter is significantly affected by autonomic tone. Either exercise or passive tilt to induce augmentation of sympathetic tone can increase the AV nodal conduction velocity and thus the ventricular response rate, an effect blocked by propranolol (768). Although enhancement of vagal tone frequently slows the ventricular response rate to both atrial flutter or fibrillation, rarely is this procedure effective in reestablishing sinus rhythm, based on the foregoing discussion demonstrating initiation of the arrhythmia with vagomimetic interventions.

AUTONOMIC NEURAL CONTRIBUTIONS TO DIGITALIS-INDUCED ARRHYTHMIAS

Digitalis possesses unique properties that enable it to have profound direct effects on the heart, involving myocardial contractility as well as electrophysiological alterations in the atria and ventricles (662,663). The mechanism responsible for these direct effects of digitalis is primarily due to inhibition of Na^+–K^+ ATPase (664). Although digitalis is used widely as a positive inotropic and antiarrhythmic agent, it is also one of the most powerful arrhythmogenic agents, with a narrow therapeutic index often leading to significant and deleterious side effects. As stated by Smith and Haber (665), "cardiac toxicity manifest by [digitalis-induced] arrhythmias can take the form of essentially every known rhythm disturbance." Experimentally, the most common endpoints studied with respect to digitalis-induced arrhythmias are ventricular arrhythmias, including premature ventricular contractions and ventricular tachycardia, and fibrillation.

Although referred to as a cardiac glycoside, Gillis and Quest (244) suggested that digitalis may just as accurately be referred to as a "neural glycoside." Direct and indirect effects on nerves, neural centers, reflexes, and neurotransmitter mechanisms contribute to the complex profile of digitalis (244,393). The primary experimental evidence implicating the neural contributions to digitalis-induced arrhythmias is threefold: (a) surgical denervation of sympathetic nerves and/or ganglia increases the toxic dose of digitalis; (b) enhanced neural activity occurs during digitalis intoxication; (c) pharmacological modulation of the autonomic nervous system during digitalis intoxication influences arrhythmogensis. The discussion will initially involve the contributions of the sympathetic nervous system to digitalis-induced arrhythmias, followed by the contributions of the parasympathetic and serotonergic systems.

Sympathetic Contributions to Digitalis-Induced Arrhythmias

Denervation Studies

Numerous levels of surgical denervation have been employed, ranging from cardiac denervation and spinal cord transection to central neural lesions and adrenalectomy. The majority of results from these studies indicate that the sympathetic nervous system contributes to the arrhythmogenic effect of digitalis. Cardiac denervation has been accomplished in both acute (96,473) and chronic (30,668,761) preparations. Both types of preparations demonstrate that larger doses of digitalis are required to elicit the same degree of intoxication in denervated animals, whether the endpoint is benign ventricular arrhythmias, ventricular fibrillation, or death. As early as 1913, Rothberger and Winterberg (600) demonstrated that acute removal of the thoracic sympathetic chains increased the dose of digitalis required to produce arrhythmias. However, others have found either no effect (486) or even a greater sensitivity to ouabain after denervation (235). The disparate results may be due to several differences, including (a) the animal model, including the anesthetic and background level of sympathetic tone, (b) the actual extent of cardiac denervation, and whether or not in addition to stellate ganglionectomy the upper four thoracic ganglia were also removed, (c) the dose of digitalis used, and (d) the actual arrhythmogenic endpoint measured.

Chronic denervation studies support the consensus that denervation protects animals from digitalis-induced arrhythmias (668,761). However, in addition to the one study mentioned previously (486), two other studies using autotransplantation as a means of cardiac denervation found no effect on ouabain-induced ventricular arrhythmias (658,787). A more recent study (395) also concluded that chronic sympathetic denervation did not protect against digitalis-induced arrhythmias and that the adrenergic nerve terminal "is an important factor in providing the proper milieu for the protection afforded by sympathectomy." In an interesting study by Cavoto and Kelliher (110), even isolated Purkinje fibers from chronically denervated hearts showed greater protection against ouabain-induced electrophysiological alterations than fibers obtained from control nondenervated hearts. This study suggests that isolated Purkinje fibers from denervated hearts are less sensitive to the arrhythmogenic effects of ouabain. The mechanism for the protection is unknown, but may be related to decreased norepinephrine stores, altered Na^+-K^+ ATPase activity, or altered binding of ouabain due to local changes induced by denervation.

Spinal cord transection is another technique used to interrupt neural outflow to the heart. As early as 1930, Macdonald and Schlapp (434) reported higher lethal doses of digitalis in spinal-cord-transected animals, which

has since been confirmed by several groups of investigators (97,249,408,563,673). Although a portion of the protection after spinal transection may be a direct result of reduced systemic arterial pressures and heart rates, lowering blood pressure pharmacologically does not alter the arrhythmogenic effects of digitalis (193,669). Interestingly, digitalis distributes within the heart in transected animals at even higher levels, despite reduced sensitivity to the arrhythmogenic effects (97,408,409). However, the reduction in heart rate may contribute to reducing the sensitivity to digitalis, because pacing the hearts of transected animals partially reverses the protective effect of the transection (98).

Finally, in an effort to localize the central neural component of the sympathetic pathway involved in digitalis toxicity, midcollicular decerebrations were performed by two groups in anesthetized animals. In one study, decerebration provided protection (286), whereas in the other, the procedure did not alter the dose required to produce lethal ventricular arrhythmias (670). Different anesthetics used may partially account for the differences in effects seen. An unanesthetized, decerebrate model would be more appropriate to test for forebrain involvement in digitalis-induced arrhythmias. In summary, from these studies alone, no conclusion can be reached concerning whether or not digitalis may act at forebrain sites to produce its toxic effect on cardiac rhythm. There is some evidence that cortical input into the hypothalamus may mediate part of the arrhythmogenic properties of digitalis (161). Because there is some evidence demonstrating that spinal, and possibly central, neural sites may be activated by toxic levels of digitalis, the potential role of enhanced release of adrenal catecholamines has also been evaluated (116,278,289,373,524). It appears that although adrenalectomy alone does not provide significant protection, when it is combined with other treatments that inhibit the sympathetic nervous system, there is enhanced protection (116,289,373).

Digitalis-Induced Alterations in Neural Activity

Functioning sympathetic neural pathways appear to be important for the arrhythmogenic effects of digitalis, as assessed by monitoring the activity in preganglionic and postganglionic sympathetic nerves during digitalis intoxication. Digitalis alters activity in both preganglionic and postganglionic nerves, which has been correlated with the onset of ventricular arrhythmias (241,249,469,524). Lathers and colleagues have shown that nonuniform changes in cardiac sympathetic nerve discharge may be responsible for digitalis-induced arrhythmias (397), and activation (199) or inhibition (241,246,248,250) of sympathetic neural discharges in the presence of digitalis enhances or abolishes, respectively, the associated cardiac arrhythmias.

Pharmacological Modulation of the Autonomic Nervous System During Digitalis Intoxications

The interaction between digitalis and pharmacological methods of modulating the autonomic nervous system has provided additional evidence for the importance of sympathetic influences on the arrhythmias associated with digitalis toxicity. Clonidine, an agent known to depress central sympathetic outflow, has been shown to antagonize the digitalis-induced ventricular arrhythmias associated with increases in cardiac sympathetic nerve activity (246,524). Likewise, depletion of catecholamines by reserpine (72,116,171,407), 6-hydroxydopamine (498,603), or guanethidine (564) increases the dose of digitalis required to produce ventricular arrhythmias. The sites of action of the protective effects of these agents are most likely peripheral cardiac stores of norepinephrine (396). Because several of these agents can also act by first producing a sympathomimetic effect prior to depletion of norepinephrine stores or blockade of transmitter release, they are also capable of exacerbating digitalis toxicity (432). These effects have been observed with acute administration of bretylium (584) or with administration of bretylium to digitalis-intoxicated animals (245,418).

β-Adrenergic blockade has also been shown clinically (26,239,707,729) and experimentally (198,358,392) to protect against arrhythmias due to digitalis toxicity. Various β-adrenergic antagonists, including stereospecific isomers (41,172,357), have been evaluated, and the conclusion is that the protection is mediated by blockade of β-adrenergic receptors rather than by a nonspecific effect of the agents. α-Adrenergic blockade has also been demonstrated as being antiarrhythmic against digitalis-induced arrhythmias in cats, dogs, and man (15,197,258). Whether this antiarrhythmic effect is due to specific α blockade, nonspecific local anesthetic effects of the agents, or effects secondary to increased coronary flow is unknown. Presumably, α- as well as β-adrenergic receptors may be activated during digitalis intoxication as a result of increased sympathetic neural activity. In addition, subtoxic doses of digitalis enhance the arrhythmogenic effects of adrenergic agonists (543,639), and exogenously administered catecholamines exacerbate digitalis toxicity (485,573,584,727).

Potential Mechanisms Responsible for the Sympathetic Component of Digitalis Toxicity

The sites of action of the neuroexcitatory effects of digitalis range from afferent systems to the central nervous system to the efferent systems, including peripheral sensory receptors and autonomic ganglia. This wide spectrum of potential sites complicates precise determination of the area contributing to exacerbation of digitalis toxicity, but it is likely that digitalis acts via a few common mechanisms at a wide variety of sites. Digitalis has been shown by several groups to sensitize baroreceptors (561), activate chemoreceptors (620), and stimulate mechanoreceptors (515,708) in the heart. A large part of these effects may be explained by the ability of digitalis to inhibit the electrogenic sodium pump. Inhibition of the pump by digitalis may lead to prevention of postexcitatory depression in baroreceptor preparations (610), a reduction in the resting membrane potential of sensory neurons leading to spontaneous discharge of the neuron (667), and other effects depending on where the targeted pump is located.

Interactions with Neurotransmitters at Central Neural Sites

Digitalis has been shown to have salient interactions with neurotransmitter systems and may interact with adrenergic receptors per se. These interactions have been shown to take place in the central nervous system, as well as in the periphery (*vide infra*). Although digitalis produces a biphasic effect on norepinephrine release (405) and inhibits norepinephrine uptake *in vitro* (722), the concentrations used in these *in vitro* studies are well in excess of the toxic doses of digitalis. Indeed, Helke and colleagues have reported that lethal doses of digitalis had no effect on norepinephrine uptake in several central neural areas (284). Other central neural effects of digitalis on noradrenergic systems include inhibition of the catabolic enzyme monoamine oxidase (551), possible reduction in norepinephrine content (20), and elevation of the norepinephrine metabolite 3-methoxy-4-hydroxyphenethylene glycol in the hypothalamus (286), which is not consistent with inhibition of monoamine oxidase. Additional lines of evidence exist for hypothalamic involvement in digitalis-induced increases in sympathetic outflow and associated ventricular arrhythmias (611), and stimulation of certain areas of the hypothalamus may protect against digitalis-induced arrhythmias (115,523).

The area postrema, a hindbrain structure devoid of the blood-brain barrier, is another area implicated in enhanced central sympathetic outflow in response to digitalis (670). Polar digitalis glycosides that do not cross the blood-brain barrier were found to have the same therapeutic index as less polar compounds (672). The fact that the centrally acting polar glycosides were not found in the cerebral spinal fluid supports the area postrema as a possible site of action. High concentrations of digoxin were found in the area postrema after intravenous infusions of ^{3}H-digoxin that produced ventricular arrhythmias (217).

The other CNS neurotransmitter system that may contribute to the increase in sympathetic outflow produced by digitalis is dopamine. Digitalis has been reported to increase the dopamine content in the hypothalamus. Other lines of evidence suggest that digitalis reduces dopaminergic function in the central nervous system (170,282). Specifically, intracerebroventricular administration of apomorphine, a specific dopamine agonist, increases the dose of deslanoside required to produce ventricular arrhythmias. Conversely, administration of haloperidol, a specific dopamine antagonist, counteracts the protective effects obtained with apomorphine (282).

Interactions with Neurotransmitters at Peripheral Sites

The effects of digitalis on peripheral adrenergic neurotransmission have also been evaluated. Ouabain and acetylstrophanthidin both enhance stimulation-induced or potassium-evoked norepinephrine release from isolated cardiac (354) and splenic (371) tissue. However, at very high nonclinical doses (10^{-4}–10^{-3} M), digitalis appears to inhibit stimulation-induced norepinephrine release, possibly secondary to blockade of axonal conduction. The effect of digitalis on neuronal reuptake has also been studied both *in vitro* and *in vivo*. In both cases, the majority of studies agree that digitalis inhibits uptake of norepinephrine, probably due to inhibition of Na^+-K^+ ATPase (186,284,647), an effect that appears to correlate with [^{3}H]ouabain binding (647). The effect, if any, of digitalis on peripheral adrenergic receptors has not been well characterized. There have been reports that digitalis both augments (76) and blocks β-adrenergic receptors (473). Although radioligand binding assays have been performed to study digitalis receptors, to our knowledge, interactions between digitalis and β- or α-adrenergic receptors have not been documented.

In summary, these combined data provide a compelling argument for the sympathetic nervous system mediating a significant contribution to the malignant arrhythmias associated with digitalis toxicity. Reduction of sympathetic neural activity anywhere between the central origins of sympathetic outflow and the adrenergic receptors located postsynaptically in the heart appears to dramatically alter the dose required to induce the arrhythmogenic response to digitalis. Although digitalis will directly induce delayed afterdepolarizations and triggered activity in isolated cardiac tissue in the absence of catecholamines, the delayed afterdepolarizations are exacerbated by catecholamines, an effect attenuated by β-adrenergic blockade (292) (see *Chapter* 60 for further details).

Parasympathetic Contributions to Digitalis-Induced Arrhythmias

Although the sympathetic nervous system appears to contribute, at least in part, to the arrhythmogenic effects of digitalis, the parasympathetic nervous system appears to impart protection. The role of the parasympathetic

system is not minor, because toxic doses of digitalis will activate both sympathetic and vagal nerves to the heart (249). Despite sparse cholinergic innervation of the ventricles, the protective effect of vagal activation appears to be antagonism of sympathetic effects on the ventricles via increased efferent vagal tone (525). Because of the combined effects of cholinergic activation at the SA node and the sparse cholinergic innervation of the ventricles, it is not surprising that reports variously indicating a protective influence and no effect of parasympathetic tone have been published. With respect to the former case, bilateral vagotomy or atropine pretreatment lowers the dose of digitalis required to produce ventricular arrhythmias (410). With respect to the lack of protection, activation of cholinergic neural pathways may not be able to compete with the more profound sympathetic activation. Furthermore, during vagal stimulation, particularly in the presence of digitalis, the SA node may be suppressed, subsequently unmasking ectopic ventricular pacemakers (381), augmented by both the direct effects of digitalis and the enhanced sympathetic tone to the ventricle.

Serotonergic Contributions to Digitalis-Induced Arrhythmias

One other peripheral neurotransmitter system has been implicated as playing a significant role in digitalis-induced arrhythmias: the serotonergic system. Administration of serotonin receptor antagonists increases the dose of digitalis required to produce ventricular arrhythmias (285). Conversely, exogenously administered serotonin enhances the arrhythmogenicity of digitalis (283). The mechanism for this enhanced arrhythmogenic effect of digitalis by serotonin may involve enhanced inhibition of cardiac Na^+-K^+ ATPase or an interaction between serotonin and the peripheral sympathetic nervous system.

Role of Neurotransmitter Modulation

Sympathetic mechanisms involved in digitalis-induced arrhythmias appear to dominate over all other neural mechanisms. Sympathetic involvement occurs at multiple levels of the nervous system, spanning central to peripheral sites. Other components such as cholinergic or serotonergic elements may contribute to the overall profile of digitalis intoxication. Although they are not of primary consideration, these elements most likely operate in modulating sympathetic mechanisms, possibly via interactions between presynaptic and postsynaptic constituents as discussed earlier.

It is interesting to note that endogenous prostaglandins may also impart protection against digitalis-induced arrhythmias (356). It is debatable whether or not part of this action is independent of an action on sympathetic neural influences (359). More likely is the hypothesis that prostaglandins are acting via neurotransmitter modulation, as discussed earlier. Although the source of the prostaglandins has not been clarified, there is indirect evidence that prostaglandins may be located presynaptically (359). Most studies, however, agree that prostaglandins from a postsynaptic site inhibit norepinephrine release through a transsynaptic mechanism (279).

Angiotensin II and histamine, on the other hand, are thought to enhance ouabain-induced cardiotoxicity. Angiotensin II exacerbates the lethal ventricular arrhythmias due to ouabain in dogs (211). This arrhythmogenic effect was initially thought to be via a central neural mechanism mediated by increased sympathetic neural activity, although a peripheral effect of angiotensin II to facilitate norepinephrine release is possible. Tackett and Holl (702) concluded that ouabain may activate histaminergic neurons via H_2 receptor activation, which in turn activates sympathetic outflow from fibers originating in the hypothalamus. In addition, the data published by Somberg and colleagues (671) suggest that H_1 antagonists block the direct effects of ouabain on the heart and that H_2 antagonists block a neural component of ouabain. The latter neural H_2-receptor-mediated effect is abolished by spinal cord transection (671).

Additional Considerations

Unfortunately, to date the neural contributions to the arrhythmogenic effects of digitalis have not been properly evaluated in experimental settings that would simulate the various disease states in which digitalis is used clinically. The response to digitalis and its arrhythmogenic influences may depend, to a large extent, on preexisting heart disease or autonomic dysfunction. Myocardial ischemia, for example, has been shown to predispose the heart to the arrhythmogenic actions of digitalis (488). The mechanism for this decreased tolerance may be due to local metabolic alterations associated with ischemia (368). However, very little is known regarding the pathological conditions that might alter, exacerbate, or modulate the interaction between the autonomic nervous system and digitalis in the genesis of malignant arrhythmias.

ADRENERGIC NEURAL FACTORS IN ARRHYTHMOGENESIS ASSOCIATED WITH THE IDIOPATHIC LONG-QT SYNDROME

Background

Substantial evidence indicates that prolongation of the QT interval of the electrocardiogram is associated with ventricular arrhythmias and sudden death (333, 367,489,591,632,666,750,762). The delay in repolarization has been categorized as either primary or idiopathic, with or without inheritable features (333,591,632,

750,762). In addition, acquired forms of the long-QT syndrome have also been described (367,489,666) due to such diverse causes as cardiac effects of pharmacological agents (168,214,509,612,640), electrolyte disturbances (152,351,420), cerebral insults (265,756), liquid protein diets (316), and patients recovering from myocardial infarction (8,176,631). The heritable prolonged-QT-interval syndrome associated with deafness and exhibiting syncopal episodes and sudden death was first described in 1957 as autosomal recessive and is referred to as the Jervell and Lange-Nielsen syndrome (333). The autosomal dominant form, which is not associated with congenital deafness, was described in 1963 by Romano and Ward (591,762). More recently, patients have also been described with idiopathic QT prolongation associated with life-threatening arrhythmias and sudden death, but without the heritable features of either the Jervell and Lange-Nielsen syndrome or the Romano and Ward syndrome (487).

Transient symptomatic episodes, with or without unconsciousness, are the major clinical features of the long-QT syndrome. The episodes usually begin in early life, although onset has been reported late in the second and third decades (750). Precipitating factors for these often lethal syncopal episodes include exercise, anxiety, fear, and sudden noises, each of which is commonly associated with a sudden increase in sympathetic neural activity. Alternation of the T wave characteristically occur and may often presage or follow ventricular fibrillation (632). The QT prolongation also may vary in a given patient, sometimes prolonged only with exercise (549) or in the upright position (355). The episodes of recurrent syncope have been documented to be due to transient ventricular fibrillation (591,762) or, less often, ventricular asystole (520). The frequency of attacks is variable, from many times per day to once in several years, and there is a tendency for the frequency of the attacks to decrease with increasing age. Milder attacks, without syncope, may also occur, with transient palpitations, visual blurring, dizziness, numbness, and anginal-type chest pain. The mortality among untreated patients from the largest series was 77% (626).

Pathology

In patients with the long-QT syndrome, routine gross and microscopic examination of the heart and other organs is usually unremarkable (406,750,762). Although no distinctive findings are present in all cases, findings have included thickening of the tunica media of the intranodal portion of the sinus node artery, hemorrhage at the junction of the sinus node and right atrium, hemorrhage of parasympathetic ganglia near both the sinus node and AV node (218,322), and focal sclerosis and degeneration of the AV bundle (457,549). However, there have been no abnormalities of the ventricular conduction system or its blood supply reported to date (406,762). Electron microscopy of cardiac tissue in one case has demonstrated rounded dense bodies in mitochondria (483), but no specific ion-probe analysis was performed to clarify their composition.

Electrophysiological Findings in Patients with the Long-QT Syndrome

A prolonged QT interval with a normal activation sequence could be caused by two conditions: (a) homogeneous prolongation of repolarization throughout both ventricles associated with a stable T-wave morphology; (b) heterogeneous prolongation of repolarization resulting in increased dispersion of refractory periods across the ventricle. Using suction electrodes, monophasic action potential recordings have been obtained from the endocardial surface of the right ventricle in patients with the long-QT syndrome (70,229). Monophasic action potentials obtained from normals do not differ in duration by more than 40 msec when recorded from several areas of the right ventricular endocardial surface at fixed cycle lengths (70). In contrast, recordings in the 4 patients reported to date with long-QT syndrome demonstrate differences in action potential duration of 105 to 190 msec (70,229), reflecting a marked dispersion of ventricular repolarization and likely a similar dispersion in ventricular refractory periods. Similar studies have not been performed in the left ventricle, nor has any transmural information been obtained. Although the results suggest that dispersion of refractory periods may contribute to lethal arrhythmias in this syndrome, the small sample size of patients studied precludes definitive conclusions.

A second important alteration observed with the monophasic action potential recordings is the heterogeneous presence of transient afterdepolarizations that are not attributable to movement artifacts and progressively disappear with very early premature stimulation (70,229). Although afterdepolarizations in normal patients rarely exceed 10% of the monophasic action potential amplitude, in patients with the long-QT syndrome the amplitudes can range from 25 to 55% of total action potential amplitude. Interestingly, no afterdepolarizations were noted, but evidence of dispersions of repolarization was observed in two cases of prolonged QT interval due to hypothyroidism (222). Afterdepolarizations were also recorded from both the right and left ventricles in a single case of the long-QT syndrome; they increased in magnitude in response to epinephrine (614). Afterdepolarizations induced by acetylstrophanthidin appear to depend on an inward calcium current, and the amplitude is enhanced by an increase in the driving rate, as well as by premature stimulation (208). In contrast, the afterdepolarizations in patients with the long-QT syn-

drome decrease in amplitude when the ventricular rate is increased or a premature stimulus is introduced (70). Interestingly, the afterdepolarizations induced by cesium chloride are also decreased with increases in pacing rate and are blocked by tetrodotoxin, suggesting that the depolarization is due to an inward current carried through the sodium channel (74). In general, in cells that do demonstrate delayed afterdepolarizations, the amplitude as well as the ease of triggering a tachycardia are enhanced by catecholamines (148), suggesting that adrenergic factors may contribute to initiating the malignant tachycardias associated with this syndrome.

Invasive programmed stimulation of the heart is a valuable adjunct for evaluation of antiarrhythmic therapy as well as elucidation of potential electrophysiological mechanisms. However, in patients with the long-QT syndrome, the incidence of inducibility is low (58,276,277), despite simultaneous infusion of isoproterenol (58). Thus, with the limited information available, it appears that programmed electrical stimulation for evaluation of patients with the long-QT syndrome is of little therapeutic or prognostic significance. This finding may be secondary to the transient nature of the sympathetic imbalance that characteristically initiates the tachycardia in these patients or to the possibility that the factors responsible for the tachycardias are not dependent on a reentrant mechanism. The fact that intravenous infusion of isoproterenol does not initiate the tachycardias (58) does not indicate that the sympathetic neural component failed to contribute, because it is likely that sympathetic imbalance rather than homogeneous sympathetic stimulation is an initiating factor.

Potential Influence of the Adrenergic Nervous System

Sympathetic imbalance refers to any condition that results in cardiac sympathetic neural influences to the ventricle in quantities or ratios different from the normal right and left contributions of cardiac sympathetic innervation. A role for the adrenergic nervous system in the pathogenesis of the long-QT syndrome was initially suggested by the associated clinical findings of syncope and malignant ventricular arrhythmias with states commonly associated with increased sympathetic neural activity (632,750). Experimentally, an increased dispersion of refractory periods across the ventricle is observed with unilateral left stellate stimulation (270), and an increase in the ventricular fibrillation threshold is seen with left stellate ablation (633), findings that suggest an arrhythmogenic influence associated with augmentation of left-sided sympathetic neural input. Conversely, right stellectomy, leaving the left sympathetic input unopposed, results in a decrease in the ventricular fibrillation threshold (633). As indicated earlier, these findings could be due to the fact that left sympathetic input is usually dominant to the left ventricle and that removal of the left input, although resulting in removal of inhibitory afferent input to the right stellate, results in an overall net decrease in sympathetic tone. Conversely, removal of the right stellate ganglion also results in ablation of afferent inhibitory input to the left stellate ganglion, resulting in a net overall increase in sympathetic tone to the ventricle. The fact that unilateral sympathetic stimulation increases the disparities in repolarization across the ventricle (797) may be a major contributing mechanism, because this may result in nonhomogeneous depolarization and repolarization and provide the substrate for initiation of these rapid ventricular tachyarrhythmias, particularly in patients with the long-QT syndrome. This suggestion is supported in part by experimental findings indicating that the effect of unilateral right stellectomy on ventricular refractory periods is critically dependent on the presence of an intact left stellate ganglion (637). Others have reported that sympathetic stimulation does not alter refractory periods measured at the endocardium and epicardium of the anterior left ventricle (453). However, repolarization across the ventricular wall cannot be deduced by interpolation of the end of systole at only endocardial and epicardial sites, because the intramural layers may be more repolarized than either the outer or inner layers (739). Thus, transmural repolarization information at multiple depths at several simultaneous left and right ventricular sites is required to adequately address the effects of unilateral augmentation of sympathetic tone.

Results of Therapeutic Trials

Evaluating therapeutic efficacy is complicated in patients with the long-QT syndrome because of the inherent temporal fluctuations of symptoms and the low prevalence of the long-QT syndrome. The largest experience accumulated to date is that of Schwartz who has reported data from more than 750 patients with the long-QT syndrome (625,626). If left untreated, the long-QT syndrome results in 71% mortality (625,626). With treatment that does not include β-adrenergic blockade, mortality remains high at 35%, but this is markedly reduced to 7% with β blockade (626). Based on experimental findings suggesting a role for left stellectomy, in patients with the long-QT syndrome the electrophysiological responses to left sympathetic blockade or ablation include (a) shortening of the QT interval, with amelioration of symptoms and only 6% mortality (626), (b) no shortening of the QT interval, but symptoms are ameliorated (626), (c) no shortening of the QT interval and no therapeutic efficacy (276), and (d) shortening of the QT interval without change in symptoms (58). Thus, the endogenous sympathetic nerve imbalance may function in only some of the patients with the long-QT syndrome, with amelioration of either the dispersion in refractory periods or depression in the initial triggering rhythm. It is of

interest that in those patients reported initially resistant to therapy with β-adrenergic blocking agents who underwent left cervicothoracic sympathectomy and subsequently required additional therapy for ventricular arrhythmias, in several cases β-adrenergic blockade was then efficacious (58). Finally, the adequacy of the denervation is critical, because in the human, left sympathetic input may occur through the first four to five thoracic ganglia independent of the left stellate ganglia.

ARRHYTHMOGENIC ASSOCIATIONS WITH CENTRAL NEURAL DISORDERS AND PERIPHERAL NEURAL DISEASE

Although a transplanted, denervated heart may allow the recipient to resume normal functioning under limited environmental and physiological conditions, the importance of central neural influences should not be underestimated. These influences allow anticipation and response to a host of physical, psychological, and emotional demands. The arrhythmogenic associations with central and peripheral neural dysfunction are numerous; yet our understanding of the mechanisms of these associations is limited. Most of the disorders discussed in this section have both peripheral and central components. Because of the close association between the central nervous system and the heart, it is often difficult to ascertain whether the arrhythmogenic influences are due primarily to peripheral neural dysfunction or to disorders within central neural structures. However, for the sake of organization, and realizing the inaccuracy, we shall discuss central disorders, followed by peripheral disorders.

Central Disorders

Subarachnoid Hemorrhage and Cerebrovascular Accidents

Abnormalities in the electrocardiogram, cardiac arrhythmias, and sudden cardiac death have been associated with a variety of conditions in which patients have had no history or clinical indication of heart disease. Almost 40 years ago, Byer and colleagues (95) published the first report of abnormalities in the electrocardiogram associated with subarachnoid hemorrhage. Since then, characteristic alterations in the electrocardiogram have been reported by a number of investigators in association with subarachnoid hemorrhage (151,527,651,679), intracranial bleeding (151,380), cerebrovascular accidents (90,207,275,474,764), stroke (496), head injuries (290), brain tumors (377), and lesions and infections involving the central nervous system (174,291). The most common manifestations of these abnormalities deceptively mimic the electrocardiographic changes resulting from myocardial infarction and include disturbances in repolarization: large, wide upright or deeply inverted T waves, prolonged QT intervals, prominent U waves, and displacement of the ST segment. In fact, incidents have been reported in which myocardial infarction has been diagnosed on the basis of electrocardiographic abnormalities, when in fact the primary cause of the alterations has been subarachnoid hemorrhage (151,679). Indeed, T-wave and ST-segment deflections seen with subarachnoid hemorrhage and cerebrovascular accidents may be identical with those seen with myocardial ischemia, although T waves usually are not as wide during ischemia. QT prolongation and sustained bradycardia are also more pronounced with a cerebrovascular accident or subarachnoid hemorrhage than during ischemia, suggesting that intense vagal stimulation may occur with both forms of cerebral disease.

Arrhythmias associated with these central disorders have not been as well documented as the electrocardiographic changes, but include atrial arrhythmias, premature ventricular contractions, AV block, and ventricular tachycardia and fibrillation (496,538,651), both in experimental animals (318,519) and in man (196,537,656). Parizel (538) has suggested that more than one mechanism is responsible for the arrhythmias associated with a subarachnoid hemorrhage, because of the variety of arrhythmias evoked.

Various mechanisms have been proposed for the electrocardiographic changes as well, because both sympathetic and parasympathetic activations can occur. Structural changes within the myocardium have been reported in patients who have died of subarachnoid hemorrhage (128,508) and in experimental animals subjected to intracranial hemorrhage (91,311). The myocardial lesions appear to be mediated by excessive release of catecholamines with an associated cardiomyopathy, because they are prevented by β-adrenergic blockade (311). Likewise, acute stroke may also increase sympathetic outflow, resulting in electrocardiographic abnormalities and myocardial cell necrosis (495). Although there appears to be a much higher incidence of arrhythmias in stroke patients versus controls, there does not appear to be an association between high sympathetic activity and arrhythmias (495). However, elevated plasma norepinephrine levels are associated with high serum creatine kinase values, which may indicate an association between high sympathetic activity and myocardial damage. These findings are supported by experimental results demonstrating that stimulation of selected brain regions produces cardiac arrhythmias (471). Indeed, Chen and colleagues have demonstrated both cardiac arrhythmias and myocardial damage with stimulation of the hypothalamus, midbrain, pons, and medulla, and they suggest that the effects are similar to those obtained by other investigators studying catecholamine-induced cardiomyopathy (113). Several investigators have suggested that cortical involvement is important in the electrocar-

diographic changes associated with a cerebral vascular accident or subarachnoid hemorrhage. Area 13 of the frontal lobe, the main cortical representation of the parasympathetic nervous system, appears to be very sensitive to stimulation (151), although release of adrenal catecholamines and electrolyte status may also be important. The primary stimulus for the electrocardiographic alterations and cardiac arrhythmias in these patients has been questioned. For example, changes were more common in patients with cerebral hemorrhage than in patients with primary cerebral infarctions (207) and more pronounced with subarachnoid hemorrhage than with cerebral hemorrhage (90). Finally, there is evidence to suggest that the electrocardiographic abnormalities are the direct result of increases in intracranial pressure rather than the specific size of the lesion (496,657).

An important point is that a large percentage of patients suffering from central neural lesions do not demonstrate any electrocardiographic abnormalities. This may be due to the variability of the site of the hemorrhagic lesion, or more probably due to the reversibility of the cardiac changes over time (207,275,651). A large part of the literature on central neural lesions and cardiac rhythm disturbances consists of case reports. The nature of the patient populations and their different lesions, procedures, treatments, laboratory tests, monitoring of vital signs, and postmortem examinations preclude a systematic investigation of the cause-and-effect relationships. It appears that systematic, carefully controlled laboratory experimentation is warranted in order to determine which exact brain sites are susceptible to which specific stimuli and to determine the contribution of sympathetic versus parasympathetic influences, the role of circulating catecholamines, and the incidences of different types of arrhythmias and how they might be associated with electrolyte disturbances, catecholamine levels, and autonomic tone. Such experimental work would provide extremely valuable information given the high mortality among patients with these types of central neural lesions. Although massive cerebral damage may be the cause of death in some patients suffering from subarachnoid hemorrhage, there is often little or no evidence of focal brain damage in patients dying from this disorder, suggesting that prevention of malignant cardiac arrhythmias by interfering with autonomic neural outflow may be beneficial (538).

Epilepsy

Electrocardiographic abnormalities, cardiac arrhythmias, and sudden cardiac death are associated with another central neural disease, epilepsy (332), likely a result of enhanced cardiac sympathetic neural activity (738). Recently, correlations between enhanced sympathetic and parasympathetic neural discharge and atrial and ventricular arrhythmias in an experimental model of epilepsy have been made (394). Interestingly, the enhanced neural discharges occurred during subconvulsive interictal activity and preceded the rhythm alterations (394). Thus, autonomic imbalance may be an arrhythmogenic factor responsible for sudden death in epileptics.

Sudden Infant Death Syndrome

A clinically important condition in which autonomic dysfunction may be responsible for producing lethal cardiac arrhythmias during sleep is the sudden infant death syndrome (SIDS). SIDS has been considered as being primarily a problem of apnea produced by upper airway obstruction (688). However, additional data suggest that central mechanisms involving respiratory control areas may also be important in the pathogenesis of SIDS (618,703). Indeed, SIDS may be associated with various pathological findings indicative of chronic or recurrent hypoxia (75,500,501,704).

Other sources, however, suggest that abnormalities in autonomic regulation of cardiovascular activity may be of primary importance in SIDS (144,448,605,624). Although brainstem gliosis and astroglial proliferation at the NTS, nucleus ambiguus, and dorsal motor nucleus of the vagus, the key regulatory sites for autonomic control of cardiac function, have been observed in patients with SIDS (501,703,704), consistent histological abnormalities in the central nervous system specific to SIDS have not been reported.

Abnormal vagal activation may be a major contributing factor in SIDS (144). In approximately 50% of potential SIDS babies who experienced apneic episodes, transient bradycardia is observed prior to apnea (144), and enhanced vagal activity may also be responsible for the gastroesophageal reflux seen in SIDS patients. Furthermore, Manoach and colleagues have suggested that acetylcholine-induced ventricular fibrillation may contribute to SIDS (448).

The peak occurrence of SIDS is within the first 12 months after birth, coincident with development of the autonomic nervous system. Because the mechanisms responsible for autonomic control of the heart may be unstable even in normal infants, it is difficult to determine the primary defect in SIDS. Additional mechanisms that may contribute to SIDS include (a) cardiac conduction disorders, (b) infections, (c) allergies, and (d) other environmental factors (644,737).

Similar to the patients with central neural lesions discussed earlier, a large percentage of SIDS victims have no premonitory arrhythmias. However, in the infant with an underdeveloped autonomic nervous system that may produce paroxysmal vagal or sympathetic activation, this autonomic imbalance may lead to cardiac arrhythmias and sudden death. Vagal activation may lead to asystole or respiratory arrest secondary to reduced cardiac output, poor perfusion, and hypoxia. Heterogeneous activation in an underdeveloped sympathetic nervous system may lead to lethal ventricular arrhythmias via a mechanism similar to or identical with that responsible for lethal arrhythmias occurring in patients with the long-QT syndrome. Thus, depending on the specific mechanism underlying a given case of SIDS, pharmacological prevention of SIDS may consist of atropine or β-adrenergic blockade, although no definitive data are yet available.

Peripheral Disorders

Thus far, we have considered disorders in which the primary abnormalities are mediated largely via central neural sites. Both the Guillain-Barré syndrome and diabetic neuropathy are associated with primarily peripheral autonomic neuropathy.

Guillain-Barré Syndrome

This relatively rare disorder is sometimes classified as polyradiculitis, indicating inflammation of nerve roots (4). Pathologically the disease is characterized by discrete focal inflammation throughout the peripheral nervous system, especially at plexuses, spinal nerves, and dorsal root ganglia (556). The pathogenesis appears to be a result of a cell-mediated immunologic response directed against peripheral myelin (3,4,556,602) and may be of viral origin (177), and it results in demyelination and subsequent nerve degeneration.

Motor paralysis and areflexia are common (506) but are often reversible (266,423,522). However, extensive autonomic dysfunction may lead to excessive or reduced activity in sympathetic or parasympathetic nerves. Cardiac alterations evoked by the imbalance in autonomic activity include bradyarrhythmias, including AV block, and supraventricular or ventricular tachyarrhythmias (262). Electrocardiographic abnormalities, including inverted T waves and, less frequently, ST-segment depression and QT prolongation, were observed in 64% of patients in the study reported by Lichtenfeld (415). Although increases in peroneal sympathetic nerve activity in patients during the acute phase of Guillain-Barré syndrome have been demonstrated, no attempts have been made to correlate the sympathetic hyperactivity with arrhythmogenesis (203).

Death among patients with the Guillain-Barré syndrome has, in the past, been attributed to respiratory failure. However, with improved means of administering supportive care, arrhythmias and sudden death, secondary to increased sympathetic activity, may account for the majority of fatalities (415). Because of the widespread abnormalities associated with the Guillain-Barré syndrome, including involvement in peripheral nerves (556), brainstem nuclei (592), and the spinal cord (60), the site and mechanism responsible for autonomic dysfunction have not yet been delineated. Lesions in afferent nerve fibers, central regulatory nuclei, or efferent sites in the spinal cord or ganglia, singly or in combination, may result in abnormal reflexes as well as altered autonomic tone to the heart and vasculature. Finally, although sudden death in patients with the Guillain-Barré syndrome has been reported, Greenland and Griggs (262) observed that none of their four fatalities were cardiac in origin, suggesting that cardiac arrhythmias may not be a common cause of unexplained death. The contribution of the autonomic nervous system in the generation of arrhythmias in the Guillain-Barré syndrome and the contributions of catecholamines or peptides, myocardial lesions, and the functioning of cardiovascular reflexes during the acute stages of the disease have not yet been elucidated.

Diabetic Neuropathy

This is an insidious and variable complication of long-term insulin-dependent diabetes. Demyelination and degeneration of autonomic nerves result in sympathetic and parasympathetic denervation of several peripheral organs. The abnormalities of diabetic neuropathy are highly variable, which has contributed to the controversy as to the primary site and nature of the lesion. The morphology of diabetic neuropathy, as reviewed by Bischoff (61), involves both demyelination, with secondary Wallerian degeneration of the nerve fiber, and primary axonal degeneration. Inclusion bodies and hyperplasia of the basement membrane are other characteristic ultrastructural observations that have been reported.

The clinical manifestations of diabetic autonomic neuropathy involve the cardiovascular, gastrointestinal, and genitourinary systems, as well as pupillary and sudomotor abnormalities (101). The cardiovascular derangements are indicative of sympathetic and parasympathetic deterioration. Usually the vagal neuropathy is manifest initially, although in some patients sympathetic defects may develop in parallel with parasympathetic defects (295,767).

Painless or "silent" myocardial infarction has been associated with diabetic neuropathy (202) and has been suggested as the cause of sudden death in diabetic patients. However, painful myocardial infarction has also been documented in patients with diabetic neuropathy and abnormal cardiovascular reflex tests (100). In addition, one study reported a reduced proportion of deaths due to myocardial infarction among patients with diabetic neuropathy (120). It has been postulated that abnormal autonomic reflexes associated with respiratory control may lead to cardiorespiratory arrest and

"sudden" death in patients with severe diabetic autonomic neuropathy (528). However, studies investigating the incidence of cardiac arrhythmias associated with diabetic neuropathy are lacking. It appears that diabetic neuropathy, associated with abnormal cardiovascular function tests, produces a high mortality of 50% over 5 years (120). Although there appears to be a significant proportion of sudden deaths in this patient group, the influence of autonomic nervous system dysfunction and the potential correlation with arrhythmogenesis have not yet been adequately addressed.

ACKNOWLEDGMENTS

The authors would like to thank Ms. Ava Ysaguirre for superb secretarial assistance and Ms. Ysaguirre and Ms. Evelyn Kanter for preparation of the manuscript throughout this project.

Research from the authors' laboratory was supported by National Institutes of Health grants HL-17646, SCOR in Ischemic Heart Disease, and HL-28995, and by grant RR00396 from the Division of Research Resources. This work was done during the tenure of an Established Investigatorship (Dr. Corr) of the American Heart Association and with funds contributed in part by the Missouri Heart Affiliate. Dr. Yamada is the recipient of a Research Fellowship of the American Heart Association, Missouri Affiliate.

REFERENCES

1. Abrahamsson, T., Almgren, O., and Holmgren, S. (1982): Effects of ganglionic blockade on noradrenaline release and cell injury in the acutely ischemic rat myocardium. *J. Cardiovasc. Pharm.,* 4:584–591.
2. Abrahamsson, T., Holmgren, S., and Almgren, O. (1982): Noradrenaline release in acute myocardial ischaemia, a fluorescence-histochemical and biochemical study. In: *Early Arrhythmias Resulting from Myocardial Ischaemia. Mechanisms and Prevention by Drugs,* edited by J. R. Parrott, pp. 153–169. Macmillan, London.
3. Abramsky, O., Teitelbaum, D., and Arnon, R. (1977): Experimental allergic neuritis induced by a basic neuritogenic protein (P₁L) of human peripheral nerve origin. *Eur. J. Immunol.,* 7:213–217.
4. Adams, R. D., and Victor, M. (editors) (1981): *Principles of Neurology,* ed. 2, pp. 894–899. McGraw-Hill, New York.
5. Adgey, A. A. J., Allen, J. D., Geddes, J. S., James, R. G. G., Webb, S. W., Zaidi, S. A., and Pantridge, J. F. (1971): Acute phase of myocardial infarction. *Lancet,* 2:501–504.
6. Adler-Graschinsky, E., and Langer, S. Z. (1975): Possible role of a β-adrenoceptor in the regulation of noradrenaline release by nerve stimulation through a positive feed-back mechanism. *Br. J. Pharmacol.,* 53:43–50.
7. Ahlmark, G., and Saetre, H. (1976): Long-term treatment with β-blockers after myocardial infarction. *Eur. J. Clin. Pharmacol.,* 10:77–83.
8. Ahnve, S., Helmers, C., and Lundman, T. (1980): QTc intervals at discharge after acute myocardial infarction and long-term prognosis. *Acta Med. Scand.,* 208:55–60.
9. Akhtar, M., Damato, A. N., Caracta, A. R., Batsford, W. P., Josephson, M. E., and Lau, S. H. (1974): Electrophysiologic effects of atropine on atrioventricular conduction studied by His bundle electrogram. *Am. J. Cardiol.,* 33:333–343.

10. Alboni, P., Malcarne, C., Pedroni, P., Masoni, A., and Narula, O. S. (1982): Electrophysiology of normal sinus node with and without autonomic blockade. *Circulation*, 65:1236–1242.

11. Alessi, R., Nusynowitz, M., Abildskov, J. A., and Moe, G. K. (1958): Nonuniform distribution of vagal effects on the atrial refractory period. *Am. J. Physiol.*, 194:406–410.

12. Alexander, R. S. (1946): Toxic and reflex functions of medullary sympathetic cardiovascular centers. *J. Neurophysiol.*, 9:205–217.

13. Allen, J. D., Shanks, R. G., and Zaidi, S. A. (1971): Effects of lignocaine and propranolol on experimental cardiac arrhythmias. *Br. J. Pharmacol.*, 42:1–12.

14. Allessie, M. A., Lammers, W. J. E. P., Bonke, I. M., and Hollen, J. (1984): Intra-atrial reentry as a mechanism for atrial flutter induced by acetylcholine and rapid pacing in the dog. *Circulation*, 70:123–135.

15. Alps, B. J., Hill, M., Fidler, K., Johnson, E. S., and Wilson, A. B. (1971): The reversal of experimental cardiac arrhythmias by indoramine (Wy 21901). *J. Pharm. Pharmacol.*, 23:678–686.

16. Amendt, K., Czachurski, J., Dembowsky, K., and Seller, H. (1978): Neurones within the "chemosensitive area" on the ventral surface of the brainstem which project to the intermediolateral column. *Pfluegers Arch.*, 375:289–292.

16a. Amendt, K., Czachurski, J., Dembowsky, K., and Seller, H. (1979): Bulbospinal projections to the intermediolateral cell column; a neuroanatomical study. *J. Auton. Nerv. Syst.*, 1:103–117.

17. Amlie, J. P., and Refsum, H. (1981): Vagus-induced changes in ventricular electrophysiology of the dog heart with and without β-blockade. *J. Cardiovasc. Pharmacol.*, 3:1203–1210.

18. Angell-James, J. E., and Daly, M. de B. (1970): Comparison of the reflex vasomotor responses to separate and combined stimulation of the carotid sinus and aortic arch baroreceptors by pulsatile and non-pulsatile pressures in the dog. *J. Physiol. (Lond.)*, 209:257–293.

19. Angelakos, E. T., King, M. P., and Millard, R. W. (1969): Regional distribution of catecholamines in the hearts of various species. *Ann. N.Y. Acad. Sci.*, 156:219–240.

20. Angelucci, L., Lorentz, G., and Baldieri, M. (1966): The relation between noradrenaline content of rabbit heart muscle and the amount of k-strophanthin needed to produce arrhythmias. *J. Pharm. Pharmacol.*, 18:775–782.

21. Arbilla, S., and Langer, S. Z. (1979): Facilitation by GABA of the potassium-evoked release of ^{3}H-noradrenaline from the rat occipital cortex. *Naunyn Schmiedebergs Arch. Pharmacol.*, 306:161–168.

22. Armour, J. A. (1973): Physiological behavior of thoracic cardiovascular receptors. *Am. J. Physiol.*, 225:177–185.

23. Armour, J. A., and Hopkins, D. A. (1981): Localization of sympathetic postganglionic neurons of physiologically identified cardiac nerves in the dog. *J. Comp. Neurol.*, 202:169–184.

24. Armour, J. A., and Randall, W. C. (1975): Functional anatomy of canine cardiac nerves. *Acta Anat.*, 91:510–528.

25. Arndt, J. O., Brambring, P., Hindorf, K., and Rohnelt, M. (1971): The afferent impulses traffic from atrial A-type receptors in cats. *Pfluegers Arch.*, 326:300–315.

26. Aronow, W. S., and Uyeyama, R. R. (1972): Treatment of arrhythmias with pindolol. *Clin. Pharmacol. Ther.*, 13:15–22.

26a. Austoni, P., Rosati, R., Gregorini, L., Bianchi, E., Bortolani, E., and Schwartz, P. J. (1979): Stellectomy and exercise in man. *Am. J. Cardiol.*, 43:399.

27. Aviado, D. M., Jr., and Schmidt, C. F. (1955): Reflexes from stretch receptors in blood vessels, heart and lungs. *Physiol. Rev.*, 35:247–300.

28. Aviado, P. M., Jr., Li, T. H., Kalow, W., Schmidt, C. F., Turnbull, G. L., Peskin, G. W., Hess, M. E., and Weiss, A. J. (1951): Respiratory and circulatory reflexes from the perfused heart and pulmonary circulation of the dog. *Am. J. Physiol.*, 165:261–277.

29. Bacaner, M. B., and Schrienemachers, D. (1968): Bretylium tosylate for suppression of ventricular fibrillation after experimental myocardial infarction. *Nature*, 220:294–296.

30. Bailey, J. C., Greenspan, K., Elizari, M. V., Anderson, G. J., and Fisch, C. (1972): Effects of acetylcholine on automaticity and conduction in the proximal portion of the His-Purkinje specialized conduction system of the dog. *Circ. Res.*, 30:210–216.

31. Bailey, J. C., Watanabe, A. M., Besch, H. R., Jr., and Lathrop, D. A. (1979): Acetylcholine antagonism of the electrophysiological effects of isoproterenol on canine cardiac Purkinje fibers. *Circ. Res.*, 44:378–383.

32. Bainbridge, F. A. (1915): The influence of venous filling upon the rate of the heart. *J. Physiol. (Lond.)*, 50:65–84.

33. Balcon, R., Jewitt, D. E., Davies, J. P. H., and Oram, S. (1966): A controlled trial of propranolol in acute myocardial infarction. *Lancet*, 2:917–920.

34. Barber, J. M., Boyle, D. M., Chaturvedi, N. C., Singh, N., and Walsh, M. J. (1976): Practolol in acute myocardial infarction. *Acta Med. Scand. [Suppl.]*, 587:213–219.

35. Barber, M. J., Euler, D. E., Thomas, J. X., Jr., and Randall, W. C. (1980): Changes in blood flow and S-T segment during coronary arterial occlusion in denervated and nondenervated canine hearts. *Am. J. Cardiol.*, 45:973–978.

36. Barber, M. J., Mueller, T. M., Henry, D. P., Felten, S. Y., and Zipes, D. P. (1983): Transmural myocardial infarction in the dog produces sympathectomy in noninfarcted myocardium. *Circulation*, 67:787–796.

37. Barber, M. J., Thomas, J. X., Jr., Jones, S. B., and Randall, W. C. (1982): Effect of sympathetic nerve stimulation and cardiac denervation on myocardial blood flow during coronary artery occlusion. *Am. J. Physiol.*, 243:H566–H574.

38. Bard, P. (1928): A diencephalic mechanism for the expression of rage with special reference to the sympathetic nervous system. *Am. J. Physiol.*, 84:490–515.

39. Barman, S. M. (1984): Spinal cord control of the cardiovascular system. In: *Nervous Control of Cardiovascular Function*, edited by W. C. Randall, pp. 321–345. Oxford University Press, New York.

40. Barman, S. M., and Gebber, G. L. (1982): Hypothalamic neurons with activity patterns related to sympathetic nerve discharge. *Am. J. Physiol.*, 242:R34–R43.

41. Barrett, A. M., and Cullen, V. A. (1968): The biological properties of the optical isomers of propranolol and their effects on cardiac arrhythmias. *Br. J. Pharmacol.*, 34:43–55.

42. Beacham, W. S., and Perl, E. R. (1964): Background and reflex discharge of sympathetic preganglionic neurons in the spinal cat. *J. Physiol. (Lond.)*, 173:400–416.

43. Beani, L., Bianchi, C., and Crema, A. (1969): The effect of catecholamines and sympathetic stimulation on the release of acetylcholine from the guinea-pig colon. *Br. J. Pharmacol.*, 36:1–17.

44. Beani, L., Bianchi, C., Giacomelli, A., and Tamberi, F. (1978): Noradrenaline inhibition of acetylcholine release from guinea-pig brain. *Eur. J. Pharmacol.*, 48:179–193.

45. Beckstead, R. M., and Norgren, R. (1979): An autoradiographic examination of the central distribution of the trigeminal, facial, glossopharyngeal, and vagus nerves in the monkey. *J. Comp. Neurol.*, 184:455–472.

46. Benfey, B. G., and Greeff, K. (1961): Interactions of sympathomimetic drugs and their antagonists on the isolated atrium. *Br. J. Pharmacol. Chemother.*, 17:232–235.

47. Benfey, B. G., and Varma, D. R. (1967): Interactions of sympathomimetic drugs, propranolol and phentolamine, on atrial refractory period and contractility. *Br. J. Pharmacol. Chemother.*, 30:603–611.

48. Benfey, B. G., Elfellah, M. S., Ogilvie, R. I., and Varma, D. R. (1984): Anti-arrhythmic effects of prazosin and propranolol during coronary artery occlusion and re-perfusion in dogs and pigs. *Br. J. Pharmacol.*, 82:717–725.

49. Benforado, J. M. (1958): A depressant effect of acetylcholine on the idioventricular pacemaker of the isolated perfused rabbit heart. *Br. J. Pharmacol. Chemother.*, 13:415–418.

50. Benzing, H., Strohm, M., and Gebert, G. (1972): The effect of local ischaemia on the ionic activity of dog myocardial interstitium. In: *Vascular Smooth Muscle*, edited by E. Betz, pp. 172–174. Springer-Verlag, Berlin.

51. Berger, A. J. (1979): Distribution of carotid sinus nerve afferent fibers to solitary tract nuclei of the cat using transganglionic transport of horseradish peroxidase. *Neurosci. Lett.*, 14:153–158.

52. Berne, R. M., and Rubio, R. (1978): Role of adenosine, adenosine triphosphate and inorganic phosphate in resistance vessel vaso-

dilatation. In: *Mechanisms of Vasodilatation,* edited by P. M. Vanhoutte and I. Leusen, pp. 214–221. S. Karger, Basel.

53. β-Blocker Heart Attack Trial Research Group (1982): A randomized trial of propranolol in patients with acute myocardial infarction. I. Mortality results. *J.A.M.A.,* 247:1707–1714.

54. Bevan, J. A., Tayo, F. M., Rowan, R. A., and Bevan, R. D. (1984): Presynaptic α-receptor control of adrenergic transmitter release in blood vessels. *Fed. Proc.,* 43:1365–1370.

55. Bexton, R. S., Nathan, A. W., Hellestrand, K. J., Cory-Pearce, R., Spurrell, R. A. J., English, T. A. H., and Camm, A. J. (1984): Sinoatrial function after cardiac transplantation. *J. Am. Coll. Cardiol.,* 3:712–723.

56. Bezold, A. von, and Hirt, L. (1867): Über die physiologischen Wirkungen des essigsauren Veratrins. *Physiol. Lab. Wurzburg Untersuchungen,* 1:75–156.

57. Bhandari, A. K., Morady, F., Shen, E. N., Schwartz, A., Mason, J., and Scheinman, M. (1983): Is left cervicothoracic sympathectomy effective treatment for patients with the prolonged QT syndrome. *Circulation [Suppl. III],* 68:427.

58. Bhandari, A. K., Shapiro, W. A., Evans-Bell, T., Morady, F., Mason, J., and Scheinman, M. (1983): Electrophysiologic studies in patients with the long QT syndrome. *Circulation [Suppl. III],* 68:426.

59. Biegon, R. L., and Pappano, A. J. (1980): Dual mechanism for inhibition of calcium dependent action potentials by acetylcholine in avian ventricular muscle: Relationship to cyclic AMP. *Circ. Res.,* 46:353–362.

60. Birchfield, R. I., and Shaw, C. M. (1964): Postural hypotension in the Guillain-Barré syndrome. *Arch. Neurol.,* 10:149–157.

61. Bischoff, A. (1980): Morphology of diabetic neuropathy. *Horm. Metab. Res. [Suppl.],* 9:18–28.

62. Biscoe, T. J., and Sampson, S. R. (1970): Field potentials evoked in the brainstem of the cat by stimulation of the carotid sinus, glossopharyngeal, aortic and superior laryngeal nerves. *J. Physiol. (Lond.),* 209:341–358.

63. Biscoe, T. J., and Sampson, S. R. (1970): Responses of cells in the brainstem of the cat to stimulation of the sinus, glossopharyngeal, aortic and superior laryngeal nerves. *J. Physiol. (Lond.),* 209:359–373.

64. Bishop, V. S., Lombardi, F., Malliani, A., Pagani, M., and Recordati, G. (1976): Reflex sympathetic tachycardia during intravenous infusions in chronic spinal cats. *Am. J. Physiol.,* 230:25–29.

65. Bishop, V. S., Malliani, A., and Thorén, P. (1983): Cardiac mechanoreceptors. In: *Handbook of Physiology,* Vol. III, edited by J. T. Shepherd and F. M. Abboud, pp. 497–555. American Physiological Society, Bethesda.

65a. Blessing, W. W., and Reis, D. J. (1982): Inhibitory cardiovascular function of neurons in the caudal ventrolateral medulla of the rabbit: relationship to the area containing A1 noradrenergic cells. *Brain Res.,* 253:161–171.

66. Bloor, C. M., Ehsani, A., and White, F. C. (1975): Ventricular fibrillation threshold in acute myocardial infarction and its relation to myocardial infarct size. *Cardiovasc. Res.,* 9:468–472.

67. Boineau, J. P., Miller, C. B., Schuessler, R. B., Roeske, W. R., Autry, L. J., Wylds, A. C., and Hill, D. A. (1984): Activation sequence and potential distribution maps demonstrating multicentric atrial impulse origin in dogs. *Circ. Res.,* 54:332–347.

68. Böke, T., and Malik, K. U. (1983): Enhancement by locally generated angiotension II of release of the adrenergic transmitter in the isolated rat kidney. *J. Pharmacol. Exp. Ther.,* 226:900–907.

69. Bolli, R., Brandon, T. A., Fisher, D. J., Taylor, A. A., and Miller, R. R. (1982): Alpha-adrenergic blockade does not prevent arrhythmias during coronary occlusion and reperfusion in the dog. *Clin. Res.,* 30:173A.

70. Bonatti, V., Rolli, A., and Botti, G. (1983): Recording of monophasic action potentials of the right ventricle in long QT syndromes complicated by severe ventricular arrhythmias. *Eur. Heart J.,* 4:168–179.

71. Bös, L., Franz, C., and Hirche, H. (1978): Cardiac arrhythmia and increase of local myocardial extracellular K⁺ activity in pigs. *J. Physiol. (Lond.),* 284:88P.

72. Boyajy, L. D., and Nash, C. B. (1965): Influence of reserpine on arrhythmias, inotropic effects and myocardial potassium balance induced by digitalis materials. *J. Pharmacol. Exp. Ther.,* 148:193–201.

73. Boyd, H. G., Burnstock, G., Campbell, G., Jowett, A., O'Shea, J., and Wood, M. (1963): The cholinergic blocking action of adrenergic blocking agents in the pharmacological analysis of autonomic innervation. *Br. J. Pharmacol. Chemother.,* 20:418–435.

74. Brachmann, J., Scherlag, B. J., Rosenshtraukh, L. V., and Lazzara, R. (1983): Bradycardia-dependent, triggered activity: Relevance to drug-induced multiform ventricular tachycardia. *Circulation,* 68:846–856.

75. Brand, M. M., and Bignami, A. (1969): The effects of chronic hypoxia on the neonatal and infantile brain. A neuropathological study of five premature infants with the respiratory distress syndrome treated by prolonged artificial ventilation. *Brain,* 92:233–254.

76. Broekaert, A., and Godfraind, T. (1973): The actions of ouabain on isolated arteries. *Arch. Int. Pharmacodyn. Ther.,* 203:393–395.

77. Brooks, C. M. (1935): The reaction of chronic spinal animals to hemorrhage. *Am. J. Physiol.,* 114:30–39.

78. Brooks, W. W., Verrier, R. L., and Lown, B. (1978): Influence of vagal tone on stellectomy-induced changes in ventricular electrical stability. *Am. J. Physiol.,* 234:H503–H507.

79. Brooks, W. W., Verrier, R. L., and Lown, B. (1980): Protective effect of verapamil on vulnerability to ventricular fibrillation during myocardial ischemia and reperfusion. *Cardiovasc. Res.,* 14:295–302.

80. Brown, A. M. (1965): Mechanoreceptors in or near the coronary arteries. *J. Physiol. (Lond.),* 177:203–214.

81. Brown, A. M. (1968): Excitation of afferent cardiac sympathetic nerve fibers during myocardial ischaemia. *J. Physiol. (Lond.),* 190:35–53.

82. Brown, A. M. (1979): Cardiac reflexes. In: *Handbook of Physiology,* Vol. I, edited by R. M. Berne, pp. 677–689. American Physiological Society, Bethesda.

83. Brown, A. M., and Malliani, A. (1971): Spinal sympathetic reflexes initiated by coronary receptors. *J. Physiol. (Lond.),* 212:685–705.

84. Brown, A. M., Saum, W. R., and Yasui, S. (1978): Baroreceptor dynamics and their relationship to afferent fiber type and hypertension. *Circ. Res.,* 42:694–702.

84a. Brown, D. L., and Guyenet, P. G. (1984): Cardiovascular neurons of brain stem with projections to spinal cord. *Am. J. Physiol.,* 247:R1009–R1016.

85. Brown, G. L., and Eccles, J. C. (1934): The action of a single vagal volley on the rhythm of the heart beat. *J. Physiol. (Lond.),* 82:211–240.

86. Brown, G. L., and Gillespie, J. S. (1957): The output of sympathetic transmitter from the spleen of the cat. *J. Physiol. (Lond.),* 138:81–102.

87. Brown, H. F., Giles, W., and Noble, S. J. (1977): Membrane currents underlying activity in frog sinus venosus. *J. Physiol. (Lond.),* 271:783–816.

88. Brown, J. H. (1979): Depolarization-induced inhibition of cyclic AMP accumulation: Cholinergic-adrenergic antagonism in murine atria. *Mol. Pharmacol.,* 16:841–850.

89. Brown, O. M. (1976): Cat heart acetylcholine: Structural proof and distribution. *Am. J. Physiol.,* 231:781–785.

90. Burch, G. E., Meyers, K., and Abildskov, J. A. (1954): A new electrocardiographic pattern observed in cerebrovascular accidents. *Circulation,* 9:719–723.

91. Burch, G. E., Sun, S. C., Calcolough, H. L., DePasquale, N. P., and Sohal, R. S. (1967): Acute myocardial lesions following experimentally-induced intracranial hemorrhage in mice: A histological and histochemical study. *Arch. Pathol.,* 84:517–521.

92. Burn, J. H., Vaughan Williams, E. M., and Walker, J. M. (1955): The effects of acetylcholine in the heart-lung preparation including the production of auricular fibrillation. *J. Physiol. (Lond.),* 128:277–293.

93. Burn, J. H., Vaughan Williams, E. M., and Walker, J. M. (1955): The production of block and auricular fibrillation in the heart-lung preparation by inhibitors of cholinesterase. *Br. Heart J.,* 17:431–447.

94. Bush, L. R., Haack, D. W., Shlafer, M., and Lucchesi, B. R. (1980): Protective effects of β-adrenergic blockade in isolated ischemic hearts. *Eur. J. Pharmacol.,* 67:209–217.
95. Byer, E., Ashman, R., and Toth, L. A. (1947): Electrocardiogram with large upright T waves and long Q-T intervals. *Am. Heart J.,* 33:796–806.
96. Cagin, N., Freeman, E., Somberg, J., Bounous, H., Mittag, T., Raines, A., and Levitt, B. (1974): A comparison of the *in vivo* and *in vitro* actions of ouabain to produce cardiac arrhythmia. *Arch. Int. Pharmacodyn. Ther.,* 207:162–169.
97. Cagin, N. A., Somberg, J., Bounous, H., Mittag, T., Raines, A., and Levitt, B. (1974): The influence of spinal cord transection on the capacity of digitoxin to induce cardiotoxicity. *Arch. Int. Pharmacodyn. Ther.,* 207:340–347.
98. Cagin, N. A., Somberg, J., Freeman, E., Bounous, H., Raines, A., and Levitt, B. (1978): The influence of heart rate on ouabain cardiotoxicity in cats with spinal cord transection. *Eur. J. Pharmacol.,* 50:69–74.
99. Calaresu, F. R., and Cottle, M. K. (1965): Origin of cardiomotor fibres in the dorsal nucleus of the vagus in the cat: A histological study. *J. Physiol. (Lond.),* 176:252–260.
100. Campbell, I. W., Ewing, D. J., and Clarke, B. F. (1978): Painful myocardial infarction in severe diabetic autonomic neuropathy. *Acta Diabetologica Latina,* 15:201–204.
101. Campbell, I. W., Ewing, D. J., and Clarke, B. F. (1980): Tests of cardiovascular reflex function in diabetic autonomic neuropathy. *Horm. Metab. Res. [Suppl.],* 9:61–68.
102. Campbell, W. B., and Jackson, E. K. (1979): Modulation of adrenergic transmission by angiotensins in the perfused rat mesentery. *Am. J. Physiol.,* 236:211–217.
103. Cannon, W. B., Lewis, J. T., and Britton, S. W. (1926): Studies on the conditions of activity in endocrine glands. XVII. A lasting preparation of the denervated heart for detecting internal secretion, with evidence for accessory accelerator fibers from the thoracic sympathetic chain. *Am. J. Physiol.,* 77:326–352.
104. Cardinal, R., and Sasyniuk, B. I. (1978): Electrophysiological effects of bretylium tosylate on subendocardial Purkinje fibers from infarcted canine hearts. *J. Pharmacol. Exp. Ther.,* 204:159–174.
105. Carmeliet, E., and Ramon, J. (1980): Effects of acetylcholine on time-dependent currents in sheep cardiac Purkinje fibers. *Pfluegers Arch.,* 387:217–223.
106. Carmeliet, E., and Ramon, J. (1980): Effects of acetylcholine on the time-independent currents in sheep cardiac Purkinje fibers. *Pfluegers Arch.,* 387:207–216.
107. Carmeliet, E., and Ramon, J. (1980): Electrophysiological effects of acetylcholine in sheep cardiac Purkinje fibers. *Pfluegers Arch.,* 387:197–205.
108. Casati, R., Lombardi, F., and Malliani, A. (1979): Afferent sympathetic unmyelinated fibers with left ventricular endings in cats. *J. Physiol. (Lond.),* 292:135–148.
109. Castellanos, A., Jr., Myerburg, R. J., Craparo, K., Befeler, B., and Agha, A. S. (1973): Factors regulating ventricular rates during atrial flutter and fibrillation in pre-excitation (Wolff-Parkinson-White) syndrome. *Br. Heart. J.,* 35:811–816.
110. Cavoto, F. B., and Kelliher, G. J. (1974): Protection by cardiac denervation of the arrhythmogenic effects of ouabain in isolated cat Purkinje fibers. *Fed. Proc.,* 33:476.
111. Chadda, K. D., Lichstein, E., Gupta, P. K., and Choy, R. (1975): Bradycardia-hypotension syndrome in acute myocardial infarction. *Am. J. Med.,* 59:158–164.
112. Chan-Palay, V., Jonsson, G., and Palay, S. L. (1978): Serotonin and substance P coexist in neurons of the rat's central nervous system. *Proc. Natl. Acad. Sci. U.S.A.,* 75:1582–1586.
113. Chen, H. I., Sun, S. C., Chai, C. Y., Kau, S. L., and Kou, C. (1974): Encephalogenic cardiomyopathy after stimulation of the brainstem in monkeys. *Am. J. Cardiol.,* 33:845–852.
114. Childers, R. W., Arnsdorf, M. F., de la Fuente, D. J., Gambetta, M., and Svenson, R. (1973): Sinus nodal echos: Clinical case report and canine studies. *Am. J. Cardiol.,* 31:220–231.
115. Chinn, C., and Natelson, B. H. (1984): Termination of ouabain-induced cardiac arrhythmias by anterior hypothalamic stimulation. *Res. Commun. Chem. Pathol. Pharmacol.,* 43:203–208.
116. Ciofalo, F., Levitt, B., and Roberts, J. (1967): Some factors affecting ouabain-induced arrhythmias in the reserpine-treated cat. *Br. J. Pharmacol.,* 30:143–154.
117. Ciriello, J., and Calaresu, F. R. (1979): Separate medullary pathways mediating reflex vagal bradycardia to stimulation of buffer nerves in the cat. *J. Autonom. Nerv. Syst.,* 1:13–32.
118. Ciriello, J., and Calaresu, F. R. (1980): Distribution of vagal cardioinhibitory neurons in the medulla of the cat. *Am. J. Physiol.,* 238:R57–R64.
119. Ciriello, J., and Calaresu, F. R. (1980): Role of paraventricular and supraoptic nuclei in central cardiovascular regulation in the cat. *Am. J. Physiol.,* 239:R137–R142.
120. Clarke, B. F., Campbell, I. W., and Ewing, D. J. (1980): Prognosis in diabetic autonomic neuropathy. *Horm. Metab. Res. [Suppl.],* 9:101–104.
121. Clausen, J., Felsby, M., Jørgensen, F. S., Nielsen, B. L., Roin, J., and Strange, B. (1966): Absence of prophylactic effect of propranolol in myocardial infarction. *Lancet,* 2:920–924.
122. Clusin, W. T., Buchbinder, M., Bristow, M. R., and Harrison, D. C. (1984): Evidence for a role of calcium in the genesis of early ischemic cardiac arrhythmias. In: *Calcium Antagonists and Cardiovascular Disease,* edited by L. H. Opie, pp. 293–302. Raven Press, New York.
122a.Cohen, M. I. (1979): Neurogenesis of respiratory rhythm in the mammal. *Physiol. Rev.,* 59:1105–1173.
123. Coleridge, H. M., and Coleridge, J. C. G. (1972): Cardiovascular receptors. In: *Modern Trends in Physiology,* edited by C. B. B. Downman, pp. 245–267. Appleton-Century-Crofts, New York.
124. Coleridge, H. M., Coleridge, J. C. G., Dangel, A., Kidd, C., Luck, J. C., and Sleight, P. (1973): Impulses in slowly conducting vagal fibers from afferent endings in the veins, atria and arteries of dogs and cats. *Circ. Res.,* 33:87–97.
125. Coleridge, H. M., Coleridge, J. C. G., Ginzel, K. H., Baker, D. G., Banzett, R. B., and Morrison, M. A. (1976): Stimulation of "irritant" receptors and afferent C-fibers in the lungs by prostaglandins. *Nature,* 264:451–453.
126. Coleridge, J. C. G., and Coleridge, H. (1979): Chemoreflex regulation of the heart. In: *Handbook of Physiology,* Vol. I, edited by R. M. Berne, pp. 653–676. American Physiological Society, Bethesda.
127. Colquhoun, D., Neher, E., Reuter, H., and Stevens, C. F. (1981): Inward current channels activated by intracellular Ca in cultured cardiac cells. *Nature,* 294:752–754.
128. Connor, R. C. R. (1970): Fuchsinophilic degeneration of myocardium in patients with intracranial lesions. *Br. Heart J.,* 32:81–84.
129. Costantin, L. (1963): Extracardiac factors contributing to hypotension during coronary occlusion. *Am. J. Cardiol.,* 11:205–217.
130. Cooper, T., Gilbert, J. W., Bloodwell, R. D., and Crout, R. J. (1961): Chronic extrinsic cardiac denervation by regional neural ablation. *Circ. Res.,* 9:275–281.
131. Coote, J. H., and Macleod, V. H. (1974): Evidence for the involvement in the baroreceptor reflex of a descending inhibitory pathway. *J. Physiol. (Lond.),* 241:477–496.
132. Corbalan, R., Verrier, R. L., and Lown, B. (1974): Psychologic stress and ventricular arrhythmias during myocardial infarction in the conscious dog. *Am. J. Cardiol.,* 34:692–696.
133. Corbalan, R., Verrier, R. L., and Lown, B. (1976): Differing mechanisms for ventricular vulnerability during coronary occlusion and release. *Am. Heart J.,* 92:223–230.
134. Corday, E. (1977): Symposium on identification and management of the candidate of sudden cardiac death: Introduction. *Am. J. Cardiol.,* 39:813–815.
135. Corley, K. C., Shiel, F. O., Mauck, H. P., Clark, L. S., and Barber, J. H. (1977): Myocardial degeneration and cardiac arrest in squirrel monkey: physiological and psychological correlates. *Psychophysiology,* 14:322–328.
136. Corr, P. B., and Gillis, R. A. (1974): Role of the vagus nerves in the cardiovascular changes induced by coronary occlusion. *Circulation,* 49:86–97.
137. Corr, P. B., and Gillis, R. A. (1975): Effect of autonomic neural influences on the cardiovascular changes induced by coronary occlusion. *Am. Heart J.,* 89:766–774.
138. Corr, P. B., and Gillis, R. A. (1975): Effect of bretylium on cardiovascular changes induced by coronary occlusion in the cat. *Eur. J. Pharmacol.,* 33:401–404.

139. Corr, P. B., and Sharma, A. D. (1984): α-Adrenergic-mediated effects on myocardial calcium. In: *Calcium Antagonists and Cardiovascular Disease*, edited by L. H. Opie, pp. 193–204. Raven Press, New York.

140. Corr, P. B., Gross, R. G., and Sobel, B. E. (1984): Amphipathic metabolites and membrane dysfunction in ischemic myocardium. *Circ. Res.*, 55:135–154.

141. Corr, P. B., Pearle, D. L., and Gillis, R. A. (1976): Coronary occlusion site as a determinant of the cardiac rhythm effects of atropine and vagotomy. *Am. Heart J.*, 92:741–749.

142. Corr, P. B., Shayman, J. A., Kramer, J. B., and Kipnis, R. J. (1981): Increased α-adrenergic receptors in ischemic cat myocardium: A potential mediator of electrophysiological derangements. *J. Clin. Invest.*, 67:1232–1236.

143. Corr, P. B., Witkowski, F. X., and Sobel, B. E. (1978): Mechanisms contributing to malignant dysrhythmias induced by ischemia in the cat. *J. Clin. Invest.*, 61:109–119.

144. Coryllos, E. (1982): Vagal dysfunction and sudden infant death syndrome. *N.Y. State J. Med.*, 82:731–734.

145. Cottle, M. K. (1964): Degeneration studies of primary afferents of IXth and Xth cranial nerves in the cat. *J. Comp. Neurol.*, 122: 329–343.

146. Cottle, M. K. W., and Calaresu, F. R. (1975): Projections from the nucleus and tractus solitarius in the cat. *J. Comp. Neurol.*, 161:143–158.

147. Cox, V. W., and Robertson, H. F. (1936): The effect of stellate ganglionectomy on the cardiac function of intact dogs, and its effect on the extent of myocardial infarction and on cardiac function following coronary artery occlusion. *Am. Heart J.*, 12: 285–300.

148. Cranefield, P. (1977): Action potentials, afterpotentials, and arrhythmias. *Circ. Res.*, 41:415–423.

149. Crill, W. E., and Reis, D. J. (1968): Distribution of carotid sinus and depressor nerves in cat brain stem. *Am. J. Physiol.*, 214: 269–276.

150. Crook, B., Kitson, D., McComish, M., and Jewitt, D. (1979): Indirect measurement of sinoatrial conduction time in patients with sinoatrial disease and in controls. *Br. Heart J.*, 39:771–777.

151. Cropp, G. J., and Manning, G. W. (1960): Electrocardiographic changes simulating myocardial ischemia and infarction association with spontaneous intracranial hemorrhage. *Circulation*, 22:25–38.

152. Curry, P., Fitchett, D., Stubbs, W., and Krikler, D. (1976): Ventricular arrhythmias and hypokalaemia. *Lancet*, 2:231–233.

153. Dahlström, A., and Fuxe, K. (1964): Evidence for the existence of monoamine-containing neurons in the central nervous system. I. Demonstration of monoamines in cell bodies of brainstem neurons. *Acta Physiol. Scand. [Suppl. 232]*, 62:1–53.

154. Dahlström, A., Fuxe, K., Mya-Tu, M., and Zetterström, B. E. M. (1965): Observations on adrenergic innervation of dog heart. *Am. J. Physiol.*, 209:689–692.

155. Daly, M. de B., and Unger, A. (1966): Comparison of the reflex responses elicited by stimulation of the separately perfused carotid and aortic chemoreceptors in the dog. *J. Physiol. (Lond.)*, 182: 379–403.

156. Daly, M. de B., and Verney, E. B. (1926): Cardiovascular reflexes. *J. Physiol. (Lond.)*, 61:268–274.

157. Danilo, P., Jr., Rosen, M. R., and Hordof, A. J. (1978): Effects of acetylcholine on the ventricular specialized conducting system of neonatal and adult dogs. *Circ. Res.*, 43:777–784.

158. Das, P. K., and Bhattacharya, S. K. (1972): Studies on the effect of physostigmine on experimental cardiac arrhythmias in dogs. *Br. J. Pharmacol.*, 44:397–403.

159. Davey, M. J. (1980): Relevant features of the pharmacology of prazosin. *J. Cardiovasc. Pharmacol.*, 2:S287–S301.

160. DeGroat, W. C., and Lalley, P. M. (1974): Reflex sympathetic firing in response to electrical stimulation of the carotid sinus nerve in the cat. *Brain Res.*, 80:17–40.

161. DeLuca, B., Cerciello, A., and Monda, M. (1982): Cortical control of neurally-mediated arrhythmogenic properties of desacetyl lanatoside C: The role of the posterior hypothalamus. *Neuropharmacology*, 21:1211–1214.

162. Dempsey, P. J., and Cooper, T. (1969): Ventricular cholinergic receptor systems: Interaction with adrenergic systems. *J. Pharmacol. Exp. Ther.*, 167:282–290.

163. Denes, P., Wu, D., Amat-y-Leon, F., Dhingra, R., Wyndham, C., Kehoe, R., Ayres, B. F., and Rosen, K. M. (1979): Paroxysmal supraventricular tachycardia induction in patients with Wolff-Parkinson-White syndrome. *Ann. Intern. Med.*, 90:153–157.

164. Denes, P., Wu, D., Dhingra, R., Amat-y-Leon, F., Wyndham, C., and Rosen, K. M. (1975): Dual atrioventricular nodal pathways. A common electrophysical response. *Br. Heart J.*, 37:1069–1076.

165. DeSilva, R. A. (1982): Central nervous system risk factors for sudden cardiac death. *Ann. N.Y. Acad. Sci.*, 382:143–161.

166. Didier, J. P., Moreau, D., and Opie, L. H. (1980): Effects of glucose and of fatty acids on rhythm, enzyme release and oxygen uptake in isolated perfused working rat heart with coronary artery ligation. *J. Mol. Cell. Cardiol.*, 12:1191–1206.

167. DiMicco, J. A., Prestel, T., Pearle, D. L., and Gillis, R. A. (1977): Mechanism of cardiovascular changes produced in cats by activation of the central nervous system with picrotoxin. *Circ. Res.*, 41:446–451.

168. DiSegni, E., Klein, H. O., David, D., Libhaber, C., and Kaplinsky, E. (1980): Overdrive pacing in quinidine syncope and other long QT-interval syndrome. *Arch. Intern. Med.*, 140:1036–1040.

169. Dittmar, C. (1873): Über die Lage des sogenannten Gefässcentrums in der Medulla Oblongata. *Ber. Verh. Sächs. Ges. Wiss. Leipzig. Math. Phys. Kl.*, 25:449–469.

170. Doggett, N. S. (1973): Possible involvement of a dopaminergic pathway in the depressant effects of ouabain on the central nervous system. *Neuropharmacology*, 12:213–220.

171. Doggett, N. S., and Case, G. (1975): Some observations on the interaction between cardiac glycosides and reserpine in the heart and central nervous system. *Toxicol. Appl. Pharmacol.*, 33:87–93.

172. Dohadwalla, A. N., Freedberg, A. S., and Vaughan Williams, E. M. (1969): The relevance of β-receptor blockade to ouabain-induced cardiac arrhythmias. *Br. J. Pharmacol.*, 36:257–267.

173. Dokukin, A. V. (1964): Blood pressure and pulse changes in normal and vagotomized animals during acute myocardial ischemia. *Fed. Proc.*, 23:T583–T586.

174. Dolgopol, V. B., and Cragan, M. B. (1948): Myocardial changes in poliomyelitis. *Arch. Pathol.*, 46:202–211.

175. Donald, D. E., and Shepherd, J. T. (1978): Reflexes from the heart and lungs: Physiological curiosities or important regulatory mechanisms. *Cardiovasc. Res.*, 12:449–469.

176. Doroghazi, R. M., and Childers, R. (1978): Time-related changes in the Q-T interval in acute myocardial infarction: Possible relation to local hypocalcemia. *Am. J. Cardiol.*, 41:684–688.

177. Dowling, P. C., and Cook, S. D. (1981): Role of infection in Guillain-Barré syndrome: Laboratory confirmation of herpes viruses in 41 cases. *Ann. Neurol. [Suppl.]*, 9:45–55.

178. Downing, S. E. (1979): Baroreceptor regulation of the heart. In: *Handbook of Physiology*, Vol. I, edited by R. M. Berne, pp. 621–652. American Physiological Society, Bethesda.

179. Dubocovich, M. L., and Langer, S. Z. (1980): Pharmacological differentiation of presynaptic inhibitory alpha-adrenoceptors and opiate receptors in the cat nictitating membrane. *Br. J. Pharmacol.*, 70:383–393.

180. DuPont, E., Jones, C. E., Luedecke, R. A., and Smith, E. E. (1979): Chronic ventricular sympathectomy: Effect on myocardial perfusion after ligation of the circumflex artery in dogs. *Circ. Shock*, 6:324–331.

181. Durrer, D., Schoo, L., Schuilenburg, R. M., and Wellens, H. J. J. (1967): The role of premature beats in the initiation and termination of supraventricular tachycardia in the Wolff-Parkinson-White syndrome. *Circulation*, 36:644–662.

182. Dutta, S. N., and Booker, W. M. (1970): Possible myocardial adaptation to acute coronary occlusion: Relation to catecholamines. *Arch. Int. Pharmacodyn. Ther.*, 185:5–12.

183. Ebert, P. A., Allgood, R. J., and Sabiston, D. C. (1968): The antiarrhythmic effects of cardiac denervation. *Ann. Surg.*, 168: 728–735.

184. Ebert, P. A., Vanderbeek, R. B., Allgood, R. J., and Sabiston, D. C. (1970): Effect of chronic cardiac denervation on arrhythmias after coronary artery ligation. *Cardiovasc. Res.*, 4:141–147.

185. Edis, A. J., Donald, D. E., and Shepherd, J. T. (1970): Cardiovascular reflexes from stretch of pulmonary vein-atrial junctions in the dog. *Circ. Res.*, 27:1091–1100.

186. Eikenburg, D. C., and Stickney, J. L. (1977): Inhibition of

sympathetic neuronal transport and ouabain-induced cardiac arrhythmias. *Res. Commun. Chem. Pathol. Pharmacol.,* 18:587–599.

187. Eisenberg, M. S., Hallstrom, A., and Bergner, L. (1982): Long-term survival after out-of-hospital cardiac arrest. *N. Engl. J. Med.,* 306:1340–1343.

188. Elharrar, V., Watanabe, A. M., Molello, J., Besch, H. R., Jr., and Zipes, D. P. (1979): Adrenergically mediated ventricular fibrillation in probucol-treated dogs: Roles of alpha and beta adrenergic receptors. *P.A.C.E.,* 2:435–443.

189. Eliakim, M., Bellet, S., Elias, T., and Muller, O. (1961): Effect of vagal stimulation and acetylcholine on the ventricle. *Circ. Res.,* 9:1372–1379.

190. Elson, J. L., Ten Eick, R. E., and Singer, D. H. (1981): Autonomic nervous system and cellular injury from circumflex ligation in dogs. *Am. J. Physiol.,* 240:H738–H745.

191. Emberson, J. W., and Challice, C. E. (1970): Studies on the impulse conducting pathways in the atrium of the mammalian heart. *Am. Heart J.,* 79:653–667.

192. Epstein, S. E., Berser, G. D., Rosing, D. R., Tolano, J. V., and Karsh, R. B. (1973): Experimental acute myocardial infarction: Characterization and treatment of the malignant premature ventricular contraction. *Circulation,* 47:446–454.

193. Erlij, D., and Mendez, R. (1964): The modification of digitalis intoxication by excluding adrenergic influences on the heart. *J. Pharmacol. Exp. Ther.,* 144:97–103.

194. Errington, M. L., and Dashwood, M. R. (1979): Projections to the ventral surface of the cat brain stem demonstrated by horseradish peroxidase. *Neurosci. Lett.,* 12:153–158.

195. Erulkar, S. D. (1983): The modulation of neurotransmitter release at synaptic junctions. *Rev. Physiol. Biochem. Pharmacol.,* 98:63–175.

196. Estanol, B. V., and Marin, O. S. (1975): Cardiac arrhythmias and sudden death in subarachnoid hemorrhage. *Stroke,* 8:382–386.

197. Ettinger, S., Gould, L., Carmichael, J. A., and Tashjian, R. J. (1969): Phentolamine: Use in digitalis-induced arrhythmias. *Am. Heart J.,* 77:636–640.

198. Evans, D. B., Peschka, M. T., Lee, R. J., and Laffan, R. J. (1976): Antiarrhythmic action of nadolol, a β-adrenergic receptor blocking agent. *Eur. J. Pharmacol.,* 35:17–27.

199. Evans, D. E., and Gillis, R. A. (1974): Effect of diphenylhydantoin and lidocaine on cardiac arrhythmias induced by hypothalamic stimulation. *J. Pharmacol. Exp. Ther.,* 191:506–517.

200. Evemy, K. L., and Pentecost, B. L. (1978): Intravenous and oral practolol in the acute stages of myocardial infarction. *Eur. J. Cardiol.,* 7:391–398.

201. Eyzaguirre, C., and Kuffler, S. W. (1955): Further study of soma, dendrite, and axon excitation in single neurons. *J. Gen. Physiol.,* 39:121–153.

202. Faerman, I., Faccio, E., Milei, J., Nunez, R., Jadzinsky, M., Fox, D., and Rapaport, M. (1977): Autonomic neuropathy and painless myocardial infarction in diabetic patients: Histological evidence of their relationship. *Diabetes,* 26:1147–1158.

203. Fagius, J., and Wallin, G. (1983): Microneurographic evidence of excessive sympathetic outflow in the Guillain-Barré syndrome. *Brain,* 106:589–600.

204. Farnebo, L. O., and Hamberger, B. (1971): Drug induced changes in the release of ³H-noradrenaline from field stimulated rat iris. *Br. J. Pharmacol.,* 43:97–106.

205. Fearon, R. E. (1967): Propranolol in the prevention of ventricular fibrillation due to experimental coronary artery occlusion. *Am. J. Cardiol.,* 20:222–228.

206. Felder, R. B., and Thames, M. D. (1981): The cardiocardiac sympathetic reflex during coronary occlusion in anesthetized dogs. *Circ. Res.,* 48:685–692.

207. Fentz, V., and Gormsen, J. (1962): Electrocardiographic patterns in patients with cerebrovascular accidents. *Circulation,* 25:22–28.

208. Ferrier, G. R., and Moe, G. K. (1973): Effect of calcium on acetylstrophanthidin-induced transient depolarizations in canine Purkinje tissue. *Circ. Res.,* 33:508–515.

209. Fidone, S. J., and Sato, A. A. (1969): A study of chemoreceptor and baroreceptor A and C fibers in the carotid sinus nerve. *J. Physiol. (Lond.),* 205:527–548.

210. Fields, J. Z., Roeske, W. R., Morkin, E., and Yamamura, H. I. (1978): Cardiac muscarinic cholinergic receptors: Biochemical identification and characterization. *J. Biol. Chem.,* 253:3251–3258.

211. Fleming, J. T., and Holl, J. R. (1982): Centrally mediated enhancement of ouabain cardiotoxicity by angiotensin II in dogs. *Eur. J. Pharmacol.,* 85:259–268.

212. Foreman, R. D. (1984): Mechanisms of cardiac pain: Processing of cardiac afferent information in ascending spinal pathways. In: *Nervous Control of Cardiovascular Function,* edited by W. C. Randall, pp. 369–390. Oxford University Press, New York.

213. Forssman, O., Hansson, G., and Jensen, C. (1952): The adrenal function in coronary thrombosis. *Acta Med. Scand.,* 142:441–449.

214. Fowler, N. O., McCall, D., Chou, T., Holmes, J. C., and Hanenson, I. B. (1976): Electrocardiographic changes and cardiac arrhythmias in patients receiving psychotropic drugs. *Am. J. Cardiol.,* 37:223–230.

215. Fowlis, R. A. F., Sang, C. T. M., Lundy, P. M., Ahuja, S. P., and Calhoun, H. (1974): Experimental coronary artery ligation in conscious dogs six months after bilateral cardiac sympathectomy. *Am. Heart J.,* 88:748–757.

216. Franz, C., Lang, R., Bös, L., Schramm, M., Bissig, R., and Hirche, H. (1978): The release of K⁺ and noradrenaline as cause of arrhythmia and ventricular fibrillation following myocardial ischemia in pigs. *Pfluegers Arch.,* 377:R3.

217. Frazer, G., and Binnion, P. (1981): ³H-digoxin distribution in the nervous system in ventricular tachycardia. *J. Cardiovasc. Pharmacol.,* 3:1296–1305.

218. Frazer, G. R., Froggatt, P., and James, T. N. (1964): Congenital deafness associated with electrocardiographic abnormalities, fainting attacks and sudden death. *Q. J. Med.,* 33:361–385.

219. Fredholm, B. B. (1974): Vascular and metabolic effects of theophylline, dibutyryl cyclic AMP and dibutyryl cyclic GMP in canine subcutaneous adipose *in situ. Acta Physiol. Scand.,* 90:226–236.

220. Fredholm, B. B. (1981): Trans-synaptic modulation of transmitter release—with special reference to adenosine. In: *Chemical Neurotransmission 75 Years,* edited by L. Stjärne, P. Hedqvist, H. Lagercrantz, and Å. Wennmalm, pp. 211–222. Academic Press, London.

221. Fredholm, B. B., and Sollevi, A. (1981): The release of adenosine and inosine from canine subcutaneous adipose tissue by nerve stimulation and noradrenaline. *J. Physiol. (Lond.),* 313:351–367.

222. Fredlund, B. O., and Olsson, S. B. (1983): Long QT interval and ventricular tachycardia of "Torsade de Pointes" type in hypothyroidism. *Acta Med. Scand.,* 213:231–235.

223. Frishman, W. H., Furberg, C. D., and Friedewald, W. T. (1984): β-Adrenergic blockade for survivors of acute myocardial infarction. *N. Engl. J. Med.,* 310:830–837.

223a. Froggatt, P., and James, T. N. (1973): Sudden unexpected death infants. Evidence on a lethal cardiac arrhythmia. *Ulster Med. J.,* 42:136–152.

224. Furey, S. A., III, and Levy, M. N. (1983): The interactions among heart rate, autonomic activity, and arterial pressure upon the multiple repetitive extrasystole threshold in the dog. *Am. Heart J.,* 106:1112–1120.

225. Gadsby, D. C., Wit, A. L., and Cranefield, P. F. (1978): The effects of acetylcholine on the electrical activity of canine cardiac Purkinje fibers. *Circ. Res.,* 43:29–35.

226. Gallagher, J. J., Gibbert, M., Svenson, R. H., Sealy, W. C., Kasell, J., and Wallace, A. G. (1975): Wolff-Parkinson-White syndrome: The problem, evaluation, and surgical correction. *Circulation,* 51:767–785.

227. Gardner, R. M., and Allen, D. O. (1977): The relationship between cyclic nucleotide levels and glycogen phosphorylase activity in isolated rat hearts perfused with epinephrine and acetylcholine. *J. Pharmacol. Exp. Ther.,* 202:346–353.

228. Gauthier, P., Nadeau, R., and de Champlain, J. (1972): Acute and chronic cardiovascular effects of 6-hydroxydopamine in dogs. *Circ. Res.,* 31:207–217.

229. Gavrilescu, S., and Luca, C. (1978): Right ventricular monophasic action potentials in patients with long QT syndrome. *Br. Heart J.,* 40:1014–1018.

230. Gazes, P. C., Richardson, J. A., and Woods, E. F. (1959): Plasma catecholamine concentrations in myocardial infarction and angina pectoris. *Circulation*, 19:657–661.

231. Gebber, G. L. (1984): Brainstem systems involved in cardiovascular regulation. In: *Nervous Control of Cardiovascular Function*, edited by W. C. Randall, pp. 346–368. Oxford University Press, New York.

232. Gebber, G. L., Taylor, D. G., and Weaver, L. C. (1973): Electrophysiological studies on organization of central vasopressor pathways. *Am. J. Physiol.*, 224:470–481.

233. Geesbreght, J. M., Randall, W. C., and Brynjolfsson, G. (1970): Area localization of supraventricular pacemaker activity before and after SA node excision. *Physiologist*, 13:202.

234. Geis, G. S., and Wurster, R. D. (1980): Horseradish peroxidase localization of cardiac vagal preganglionic somata. *Brain Res.*, 181:19–30.

234a.Geis, G. S., and Wurster, R. D. (1980): Cardiac responses during stimulation of the dorsal motor nucleus and nucleus ambiguus in the cat. *Circ. Res.*, 46:606–611.

235. George, A., Spear, J. F., and Moore, E. N. (1974): The effects of digitalis glycosides on the ventricular fibrillation threshold in innervated and denervated canine hearts. *Circulation*, 50:353–359.

236. George, W. J., Polson, J. B., O'Toole, A. G., and Goldberg, N. D. (1970): Elevation of guanosine 3'5'-cyclic phosphate in rat heart after perfusion with acetylcholine. *Proc. Natl. Acad. Sci. U.S.A.*, 66:398–403.

237. Gettes, L. S. (1974): Electrophysiologic basis of arrhythmias in acute myocardial ischemia. In: *Modern Trends in Cardiology*, Vol. 3, edited by M. F. Oliver, pp. 219–246. Butterworth, London.

238. Gettes, L. S., and Hill, J. L. (1981): The use of K^+ sensitive electrodes to gain an understanding of myocardial ischemia. In: *Progress in Enzyme and Ion-Selective Electrodes*, edited by D. W. Lübbers, H. Acker, R. P. Buck, G. Eisenmann, M. Kessler, and W. Simon, pp. 171–178. Springer-Verlag, Berlin.

239. Gianelly, R., Griffen, J. R., and Harrison, D. C. (1967): Propranolol in the treatment and prevention of cardiac arrhythmias. *Ann. Intern. Med.*, 66:667–676.

240. Gillespie, J. (1980): Presynaptic receptors in the autonomic nervous system. *Handb. Exp. Pharmacol.*, 54:169–205.

241. Gillis, R. A. (1969): Cardiac sympathetic nerve activity: Changes induced by ouabain and propranolol. *Science*, 166:508–510.

242. Gillis, R. A. (1971): Role of the nervous system in the arrhythmias produced by coronary occlusion in the cat. *Am. Heart J.*, 81:677–684.

243. Gillis, R. A. (1982): Neurotransmitters involved in the central nervous system control of cardiovascular function. In: *Circulation, Neurobiology, and Behavior*, edited by O. A. Smith, R. A. Gialosy, and S. M. Weiss, pp. 41–53. Elsevier, New York.

244. Gillis, R. A., and Quest, J. A. (1980): The role of the nervous system in the cardiovascular effects of digitalis. *Pharmacol. Rev.*, 31:19–97.

245. Gillis, R. A., Clancy, M. M., and Anderson, R. J. (1973): Deleterious effects of bretylium in cats with digitalis-induced ventricular tachycardia. *Circulation*, 47:974–983.

246. Gillis, R. A., Dionne, R. A., and Standaert, F. G. (1972): Suppression by clonidine (St-155) of cardiac arrhythmias induced by digitalis. *J. Pharmacol. Exp. Ther.*, 182:218–226.

247. Gillis, R. A., Helke, C. J., Hamilton, B. L., Norman, W. P., and Jacobowitz, D. M. (1980): Evidence that substance P is a neurotransmitter of baro- and chemoreceptor afferents in nucleus tractus solitarius. *Brain Res.*, 181:476–481.

247a.Gillis, R. A., Quest, J. A., and DiMicco, J. A. (1986): Central regulation of autonomic function by GABA receptors. In: *GABA and Benzodiazepine Receptors*, edited by R. F. Squires. CRC Press, Boca Raton (*in press*).

248. Gillis, R. A., McClellan, J. R., Sauer, T. S., and Standaert, F. G. (1971): Depression of cardiac sympathetic nerve activity by diphenylhydantoin. *J. Pharmacol. Exp. Ther.*, 179:599–610.

249. Gillis, R. A., Raines, A., Sohn, Y. T., Levitt, B., and Standaert, F. G. (1972): Neuroexcitatory effects of digitalis and their role in the development of cardiac arrhythmias. *J. Pharmacol. Exp. Ther.*, 183:154–168.

250. Gillis, R. A., Thibodeaux, H., and Barr, L. (1974): Antiarrhythmic properties of chlordiazepoxide. *Circulation*, 49:272–282.

251. Giotti, A., Ledda, F., and Mannaioni, P. F. (1968): Electrophysiological effects of alpha- and beta-receptor agonists and antagonists on Purkinje fibres of sheep heart. *Br. J. Pharmacol.*, 34:695P–696P.

252. Giotti, A., Ledda, F., and Mannaioni, P. F. (1973): Effects of noradrenaline and isoprenaline, in combination with α- and β-receptor blocking substances, on the action potential of cardiac Purkinje fibers. *J. Physiol. (Lond.)*, 229:99–113.

253. Goldberg, S., Greenspon, A. J., Urban, P. L., Muza, B., Berger, B., Walinsky, P., and Maroko, P. R. (1983): Reperfusion arrhythmias: A marker of restoration of antegrade flow during intracoronary thrombolysis for acute myocardial infarction. *Am. Heart J.*, 105:26–32.

254. Goldstein, D. S. (1981): Plasma norepinephrine as an indicator of sympathetic neural activity in clinical cardiology. *Am. J. Cardiol.*, 48:1147–1154.

255. Goldstein, R. E., Karsh, R. B., Smith, E. R., Orlando, M., Norman, D., Farnham, M., Redwood, D. R., and Epstein, S. E. (1973): Influence of atropine and of vagally mediated bradycardia on the recurrence of ventricular arrhythmias following acute coronary occlusion in closed chest dogs. *Circulation*, 47:1180–1190.

256. Gonzáles-Serrato, H., and Alanís, J. (1962): La accion de los nervios cardiacos y de la acetilcolina sobre el automatismo del corazon. *Acta Physiology Latinoamerica*, 12:139–152.

257. Goodlett, M., Dowling, K., Eddy, L. J., and Downey, J. M. (1980): Direct metabolic effects of isoproterenol and propranolol in ischemic myocardium of the dog. *Am. J. Physiol.*, 239:H469–H476.

258. Gould L., Zahir, M., Shariff, M., and Guiliani, M. G. (1969): Treatment of cardiac arrhythmias with phentolamine. *Am. Heart J.*, 78:189–193.

259. Govier, W. C., Mosal, N. C., Whittington, P., and Broom, A. H. (1966): Myocardial alpha and beta adrenergic receptors as demonstrated by atrial functional refractory-period changes. *J. Pharmacol. Exp. Ther.*, 154:255–263.

260. Grayson, J., and Lapin, B. A. (1966): Observations on the mechanisms of infarction in the dog after experimental occlusion of the coronary artery. *Lancet*, 1:1284–1288.

261. Greenberg, H. M. (1984): Bradycardia at onset of sudden death: Potential mechanisms. *Ann. N.Y. Acad. Sci.*, 427:241–251.

262. Greenland, P., and Griggs, R. C. (1980): Arrhythmic complications in the Guillain-Barré syndrome. *Arch. Intern. Med.*, 140:1053–1055.

263. Gregg, D. E., Khouri, E. M., Donald, D. E., Lowensohn, H. A., and Pasyk, S. (1972): Coronary circulation in the conscious dog with cardiac neural ablation. *Circ. Res.*, 31:129–144.

264. Grizzle, W. E., Johnson, R. N., Schramm, L. P., and Gann, D. S. (1975): Hypothalamic cells in an area mediating ACTH release respond to right atrial stretch. *Am. J. Physiol.*, 228:1039–1045.

265. Grossman, M. A. (1976): Cardiac arrhythmias in acute central nervous system disease: Successful management with stellate ganglion block. *Arch. Intern. Med.*, 136:203–207.

266. Guillain, G., Barré, J. A., and Strohl, A. (1916): Sur un syndrome de radiculonévrite avec hyperalbuminose du liquide céphalorachidien sans réaction cellulaire. *Bull. Soc. Med. Hop. Paris*, 40:1462–1470.

267. Gupta, P. K., Lichstein, E., Chadda, K. D., and Badui, E. (1977): Appraisal of sinus nodal recovery time in patients with sick sinus syndrome. *Am. J. Cardiol.*, 34:265–270.

268. Hainsworth, R., Kidd, C., and Linden, R. J. (editors) (1979): *Cardiac Receptors*. Cambridge University Press, Cambridge, U.K.

269. Hamlin, R. L., and Smith, C. R. (1968): Effects of vagal stimulation on S-A and A-V nodes. *Am. J. Physiol.*, 215:560–568.

270. Han, J., and Moe, G. K. (1964): Nonuniform recovery of excitability in ventricular muscle. *Circ. Res.*, 14:44–60.

271. Hansteen, V., Møinichen, E., Lorentsen, E., Andersen, A., Strøm, O., Søiland, K., Dyrbekk, D., Refsum, A.-M., Tromsdal, A., Knudsen, K., Eika, C., Bakkenjun, J., Smith, P., and Hoff, P.I. (1982): One year's treatment with propranolol after myocardial

infarction: Preliminary report of Norwegian multicentre trial. *Br. Med. J.*, 284:155–160.

272. Harris, A. S., Estandia, A., and Tillotson, R. F. (1951): Ventricular ectopic rhythms and ventricular fibrillation following cardiac sympathectomy and coronary occlusion. *Am. J. Physiol.*, 65:505–512.

273. Harris, A. S., Toth, L. A., and Hoey, T. E. (1958): Arrhythmic and antiarrhythmic effects of sodium, potassium and calcium salts and of glucose injected into coronary arteries of infarcted and normal hearts. *Circ. Res.*, 6:570–579.

274. Harrison, L. A., Harrison, L. H., Kent, K. M., and Epstein, S. E. (1974): Enhancement of electrical stability of acutely ischemic myocardium by edrophonium. *Circulation*, 50:99–102.

275. Harrison, M. T., and Gibb, B. H. (1964): Electrocardiographic changes associated with a cerebrovascular accident. *Lancet*, 2:429–430.

276. Hartzler, G. O., and Osborn, M. J. (1981): Invasive electrophysiological study in the Jervell and Lange-Nielsen syndrome. *Br. Heart J.*, 45:225–229.

277. Hashimoto, K., Chiba, S., Tanaka, S., Hirata, M., and Suzuki, Y. (1968): Adrenergic mechanism participating in induction of atrial fibrillation by ACh. *Am. J. Physiol.*, 215:1183–1191.

278. Hashimoto, K., Kimura, T., and Kubota, K. (1973): Study of the therapeutic and toxic effects of ouabain by simultaneous observations on the excised and blood-perfused sinoatrial node and papillary muscle preparations and the in situ heart of dogs. *J. Pharmacol. Exp. Ther.*, 186:463–471.

279. Hedqvist, P. (1981): Trans-synaptic modulation versus α-autoinhibition of norepinephrine secretion. In: *Chemical Neurotransmission 75 Years*, edited by L. Stjärne, P. Hedqvist, H. Lagercrantz, and Å. Wennmalm, pp. 223–233. Academic Press, London.

280. Hedqvist, P., and Fredholm, B. B. (1976): Effects of adenosine on adrenergic neurotransmission: Prejunctional inhibition and postjunctional enhancement. *Naunyn Schmiedebergs Arch. Pharmacol.*, 293:217–223.

281. Hedqvist, P., Stjärne, L., and Wennmalm, Å. (1970): Inhibition by prostaglandin E₂ of sympathetic neurotransmission in the rabbit heart. *Acta Physiol. Scand.*, 79:139–141.

281a. Helke, C. J. (1982): Neuroanatomical localization of substance P: Implications for central cardiovascular control. *Peptides*, 3:479–483.

282. Helke, C. J., and Gillis, R. A. (1978): Centrally mediated protective effects of dopamine agonists on digitalis-induced ventricular arrhythmias. *J. Pharmacol. Exp. Ther.*, 207:263–270.

283. Helke, C. J., Dias Souza, J., and Gillis, R. A. (1978): Interaction of serotonin and deslanoside on cardiac rhythm in the cat. *Eur. J. Pharmacol.*, 51:167–177.

284. Helke, C. J., Kellar, K. J., and Gillis, R. A. (1978): Effect of arrhythmogenic doses of deslanoside on the uptake of monoamines in brain tissue and in cardiac tissue. *Eur. J. Pharmacol.*, 52:47–55.

285. Helke, C. J., Quest, J. A., and Gillis, R. A. (1978): Effects of serotonin antagonists on digitalis-induced ventricular arrhythmias. *Eur. J. Pharmacol.*, 47:443–449.

286. Helke, C. J., Zavadil, A. P., III, and Gillis, R. A. (1979): Forebrain noradrenergic mechanisms and digitalis-induced ventricular arrhythmias. *J. Pharmacol. Exp. Ther.*, 208:57–62.

287. Henderson, G., and Hughes, J. (1976): The effects of morphine on the release of noradrenaline from the mouse vas deferens. *Br. J. Pharmacol.*, 57:551–557.

288. Reference deleted in proof.

289. Hermansen, K. (1970): Evidence for adrenergic mediation of ouabain induced arrhythmias in the guinea pig. *Acta Pharmacol. Toxicol.*, 28:57–86.

290. Hersch, C. (1961): Electrocardiographic changes in head injuries. *Circulation*, 23:853–866.

291. Hersch, C. (1964): Electrocardiographic changes in subarachnoid haemorrhage, meningitis, and intracranial space-occupying lesions. *Br. Heart J.*, 26:785–793.

292. Hewett, K. W., and Rosen, M. R. (1984): Alpha and beta adrenergic interactions with ouabain-induced delayed afterdepolarizations. *J. Pharmacol. Exp. Ther.*, 229:188–192.

293. Hill, J. L., and Gettes, L. S. (1980): Effect of acute coronary artery occlusion on local myocardial extracellular K⁺ activity in swine. *Circulation*, 61:768–778.

294. Hill, J. L., Gettes, L. S., Lynch, M. R., and Hebert, N. C. (1978): Flexible valinomycin electrodes for on-line determination of intravascular and myocardial K⁺. *Am. J. Physiol.*, 235:H455–H459.

295. Hilsted, J. (1982): Pathophysiology in diabetic autonomic neuropathy: Cardiovascular, hormonal, and metabolic studies. *Diabetes*, 31:730–737.

296. Hilton, S. M. (1979): The defense reaction as a paradigm for cardiovascular control. In: *Integral Function of the Autonomic Nervous System*, edited by C. M. Brooks, K. Koizumi, and A. Sato, pp. 443–449. Elsevier/North-Holland, Amsterdam.

297. Hilton, S. M., and Spyer, K. M. (1971): Participation of the anterior hypothalamus in the baroreceptor reflex. *J. Physiol. (Lond.)*, 218:271–293.

298. Hino, N., and Ochi, R. (1979): Effect of acetylcholine on membrane currents in guinea-pig papillary muscle. *J. Physiol. (Lond.)*, 307:183–197.

299. Hirche, H., Addicks, K., Deutsch, H. J., Friedrich, R. Griebenow, R., McDonald, F. M., and Zylka, V. (1981): The effect of lignocaine on the release of K⁺ and of noradrenaline from ischemic pig heart. *Pfluegers Arch.*, 389:R5.

300. Hirche, H., Gaehtgens, P., Hagemann, H., Kebbel, U., Kleine, H.-J., Schramm, M., and Schumacher, E. (1976): Untersuchungen über die Acidose im ischämischen Hundemyokard mit H⁺-sensitiven Minielektroden. *Verh. Dtsch. Ges. Kreislaufforsch.*, 42:311–315.

301. Hjalmarson, Å., Elmfeldt, D., Herlitz, J. Holmberg, S., Málek, I., Nyberg, G., Rydén, L., Swedberg, K., Vedin, A., Waagstein, F., Waldenström, A., Waldenström, J., Wedel, H., Wilhelmsen, L., and Wilhelmsson, C. (1981): Effect on mortality of metoprolol in acute myocardial infarction: A double-blind randomised trial. *Lancet*, 2:823–827.

302. Hoffman, B. F. (1979): Fine structure of internodal pathways. *Am. J. Cardiol.*, 44:385–386.

303. Hoffman, B. F., and Cranefield, P. F. (1960): *Electrophysiology of the Heart.* McGraw-Hill, New York.

304. Hoffman, B. F., and Suckling, E. E. (1953): Cardiac cellular potentials: Effect of vagal stimulation and acetylcholine. *Am. J. Physiol.*, 173:312–320.

305. Hogan, P. M., and Davis, L. D. (1968): Evidence for specialized fibers in the canine right atrium. *Circ. Res.*, 23:387–396.

306. Hogan, P. M., and Davis, L. D. (1971): Electrophysiological characteristics of canine atrial plateau fibers. *Circ. Res.*, 28:62–73.

307. Hollenberg, M., Carrierie, S., and Barger, A. C. (1965): Biphasic action of acetylcholine on ventricular myocardium. *Circ. Res.*, 16:527–536.

308. Hordof, A. J., Rose, E., Danilo, P., Jr., and Rosen, M. R. (1982): α- and β-adrenergic effects of epinephrine on ventricular pacemakers in dogs. *Am. J. Physiol.*, 242:677–682.

309. Hoskins, E. J., Priola, D. V., and Weiss, G. K. (1976): Postischemic vagal stabilization of the canine ventricle. *Physiologist*, 19:231.

310. Humphrey, D. R. (1967): Neuronal activity in the medulla oblongata of the cat evoked by stimulation of the carotid sinus nerve. In: *Baroreceptors and Hypertension*, edited by P. Kezdi, pp. 131–168. Pergamon Press, Oxford.

311. Hunt, D., and Gore, L. (1972): Myocardial lesions following experimental intracranial hemorrhage: Prevention with propranolol. *Am. Heart J.*, 83:232–236.

312. Iano, T. L., Levy, M. N., and Lee, M. H. (1973): An acceleratory component of the parasympathetic control of heart rate. *Am. J. Physiol.*, 224:997–1005.

313. Reference deleted in proof.

314. (1975): Improvement in prognosis of myocardial infarction by long-term beta-adrenoceptor blockade using practolol: A multicentre international study. *Br. Med. J.*, 3:735–740.

315. Irisawa, H., Caldwell, W. M., and Wilson, M. F. (1971): Neural regulation of atrioventricular conduction. *Jpn. J. Physiol.*, 21:15–25.

316. Isner, J. M., Sours, H. E., Paris, A. L., Ferrans, V. J., and Roberts, W. C. (1979): Sudden, unexpected death in avid dieters using the liquid-protein-modified-fast diet: Observations in 17 patients and the role of the prolonged QT interval. *Circulation*, 60:1401–1412.

317. Jacobowitz, D., Cooper, T., and Barner, H. B. (1967): Histochemical and chemical studies of the localization of adrenergic and cholinergic nerves in normal and denervated cat hearts. *Circ. Res.,* 20:289–298.

318. Jacobson, S. A., and Danufsky, P. (1954): Marked electrocardiographic changes produced by experimental head trauma. *J. Neuropath. Exp. Neurol.,* 13:462–466.

319. Jalife, J., and Moe, G. K. (1979): Phasic effects of vagal stimulation on pacemaker activity of the isolated sinus node of the young cat. *Circ. Res.,* 45:595–608.

320. James, T. N. (1963): The connecting pathways between the sinus node and the A-V node and between the right and the left atrium in the human heart. *Am. Heart J.,* 66:498–508.

321. James, T. N. (1967): Cardiac innervation: Anatomic and pharmacologic relations. *Bull. N.Y. Acad. Med.,* 43:1041–1086.

322. James, T. N. (1967): Congenital deafness and cardiac arrhythmias. *Am. J. Cardiol.,* 19:627–643.

323. James, T. N., and Sherf, I. (1971): Specialized tissues and preferential conduction in the atria of the heart. *Am. J. Cardiol.,* 28:414–427.

324. James, T. N., and Spence, C. A. (1966): Distribution of cholinesterase within the sinus node and AV node of the human heart. *Anat. Rec.,* 155:151–162.

325. James, T. N., Bear, E. S., Lang, K. F., and Green, E. W. (1968): Evidence for adrenergic alpha receptor depressant activity in the heart. *Am. J. Physiol.,* 215:1366–1375.

326. James, T. N., Isobe, J. H., and Urthaler, F. (1975): Analysis of components in a hypertensive cardiogenic chemoreflex. *Circulation,* 52:179–192.

327. Janse, M. J., and Anderson, R. H. (1974): Specialized internodal atrial pathways—fact or fiction? *Eur. J. Cardiol.,* 2:117–136.

328. Janse, M. J., and Schwartz, P. J. (1983): Effect of cardiac sympathetic nerves on electrophysiologic changes induced by acute myocardial ischemia in dogs. *Eur. Heart J. [Suppl. E],* 4: 38.

329. Janse, M. J., Van Capelle, F. J. L., Anderson, R. H., Touboul, P., and Billette, J. (1976): Electrophysiology and structure of the atrioventricular node of the isolated rabbit heart. In: *The Conduction System of the Heart, Structure, Function and Clinical Implications,* edited by H. J. J. Wellens, K. I. Lie, and M. J. Janse, pp. 296–315. Lea & Febiger, Philadelphia.

330. Janse, M. J., Van Capelle, F. J. L., Morsink, H., Kleber, A. G., Wilms-Schopman, F., Cardinal, R., D'Alnoncourt, C. H., and Durrer, D. (1980): Flow of "injury" current and patterns of excitation during early ventricular arrhythmias in acute regional myocardial ischemia in isolated porcine and canine hearts. Evidence for two different arrhythmogenic mechanisms. *Circ. Res.,* 47:151–165.

331. Jarisch, A., and Richter, H. (1939): Die afferenten Bahnen des Veratrineffektes in den Herznerven. *Arch. Exp. Pathol. Pharmakol.,* 193:355–371.

332. Jay, G. W., and Leestma, J. E. (1981): Sudden death in epilepsy. A comprehensive review of the literature and proposed mechanisms. *Acta Neurol. Scand. [Suppl. 82],* 63:1–66.

333. Jervell, A., and Lange-Nielsen, F. (1957): Congenital deaf-mutism, functional heart disease with prolongation of the Q-T interval, and sudden death. *Am. Heart J.,* 54:59–68.

334. Johansson, B. W. (1980): A comparative study of cardioselective β-blockade and diazepam in patients with acute myocardial infarction and tachycardia. *Acta Med. Scand.,* 207:47–53.

335. Johnson, E. A., and McKinnon, M. G. (1956): Effect of acetylcholine and adenosine on cardiac cellular potentials. *Nature,* 178: 1174–1175.

336. Johnston, G. A. R., and Mitchell, J. F. (1971): The effect of bicuculline, metrazol, picrotoxin and strychnine on the release of [³H]GABA from rat brain slices. *J. Neurochem.,* 18:2441–2446.

337. Jones, C. E., Beck, L. Y., DuPont, E., and Barnes, G. E. (1978): Effects of coronary ligation on the chronically sympathectomized ventricle. *Am. J. Physiol.,* 235:H429–H434.

338. Jones, C. E., Devous, M. D., Thomas, J. X., Jr., and DuPont, E. (1978): The effect of chronic cardiac denervation on infarct size following acute coronary occlusion. *Am. Heart J.,* 95:738–746.

339. Jones, C. E., Hurst, T. W., and Randall, W. C. (1982): Reduced oxygen and blood flow demands in the chronically sympathectomized heart. *Circ. Shock,* 9:469–480.

340. Jose, A. D. (1966): Effect of combined sympathetic and parasympathetic blockade on heart rate and cardiac function in man. *Am. J. Cardiol.,* 18:476–478.

341. Josephson, M. E., and Kastor, J. A. (1976): Paroxysmal supraventricular tachycardia: Is the atrium a necessary link? *Circulation,* 54:430–435.

342. Josephson, M. E., and Kastor, J. A. (1977): Supraventricular tachycardia: Mechanisms and management. *Ann. Intern. Med.,* 87:346–358.

343. Josephson, M. E., and Seides, S. F. (1979): Supraventricular tachycardias. In: *Clinical Cardiac Electrophysiology Techniques and Interpretations,* pp. 147–190. Lea & Febiger, Philadelphia.

344. Juhasz-Nagy, A., and Aviado, D. M. (1976): Increased role of alpha-adrenoceptors in ischemic myocardial zones. *Physiologist,* 19:245.

345. Julian, D. G., Prescott, R. J., Jackson, F. S., and Szekely, P. (1982): Controlled trial of sotalol for one year after myocardial infarction. *Lancet,* 1:1142–1147.

346. Kadowitz, P. J., Sweet, C. S., and Brody, M. J. (1972): Enhancement of sympathetic neurotransmission by prostaglandin F₂α in the cutaneous vascular bed of the dog. *Eur. J. Pharmacol.,* 18: 189–194.

347. Kaiman, M., and Shibata, S. (1975): Sensitivity of guinea pig aorta to norepinephrine, phenylephrine, methoxamine and potassium: Effect of reserpine, 6-hydroxydopamine, and cocaine. *Proc. Western Pharmacol. Soc.,* 18:93–94.

347a. Kalia, M., and Mesulam, M.-M. (1980): Brain stem projections of sensory and motor components of the vagus complex in the cat: I. The cervical vagus and nodose ganglion. *J. Comp. Neurol.,* 193:435–465.

347b. Kalia, M., and Mesulam, M.-M. (1980): Brain stem projections of sensory and motor components of the vagus complex in the cat: II. Laryngeal, tracheobronchial, pulmonary, cardiac, and gastrointestinal branches. *J. Comp. Neurol.,* 193:467–508.

348. Kalsner, S. (1984): Limitations of presynaptic theory: No support for feedback control of autonomic effectors. *Fed. Proc.,* 43:1358–1364.

349. Kalsner, S. (1984): The noradrenergic presynaptic receptor controversy. *Fed. Proc.,* 43:1351.

350. Kalsner, S., and Nickerson, M. (1969): Effect of reserpine on the disposition of sympathomimetic amines in vascular tissue. *Br. J. Pharmacol.,* 35:394–405.

351. Kambara, H., Iteld, B. J., and Phillips, J. (1977): Hypocalcemia and intractable ventricular fibrillation. *Ann. Intern. Med.,* 86: 583–584.

352. Kane, K. A., Parratt, J. R., and Williams, F. M. (1984): An investigation into the characteristics of reperfusion-induced arrhythmias in the anaesthetized rat and their susceptibility to antiarrhythmic agents. *Br. J. Pharmacol.,* 82:349–357.

353. Karpati, P., Preda, I., and Endroczi, E. (1974): Effect of acidosis and noradrenaline infusion on ¹⁴C-noradrenaline uptake by the rat myocardium. *Acta Physiol. Hung.,* 45:109–114.

354. Katz, R. I., and Kopin, I. J. (1969): Electrical field-stimulated release of norepinephrine-H³ from rat atrium. *J. Pharmacol. Exp. Ther.,* 169:229–236.

355. Kay, G. N., Plumb, V. J., Arciniegas, J. G., Henthorn, R. W., and Waldo, A. L. (1983): Torsade de Pointes: The long-short initiating sequence and other clinical features: Observations in 32 patients. *J. Am. Coll. Cardiol.,* 2:806–817.

356. Kelliher, G. J., and Glenn, T. M. (1983): Effect of prostaglandin E₁ on ouabain-induced arrhythmia. *Eur. J. Pharmacol.,* 24:410–414.

357. Kelliher, G. J., and Roberts, J. (1972): The effect of *d*(+)- and *l*(−)-practolol on ouabain-induced arrhythmia. *Eur. J. Pharmacol.,* 20:243–247.

358. Kelliher, G. J., and Roberts, J. (1974): A study of the antiarrhythmic action of certain beta-blocking agents. *Am. Heart J.,* 87:458–467.

359. Kelliher, G. J., Jurkiewicz, N., and Soifer, B. (1981): Effect of prostaglandin synthesis inhibition and sympathectomy on ouabain-induced arrhythmia in cats. *J. Cardiovasc. Pharmacol.,* 3:1278–1286.

360. Kelliher, G. J., Widmar, C., and Roberts, J. (1975): Influence of adrenal medulla on cardiac rhythm disturbances following acute coronary artery occlusion. In: *Recent Advances in Cardiac Structure and Metabolism,* Vol. 10, edited by P. E. Roy and G. Rona, pp. 387–400. University Park Press, Baltimore.

361. Kendrick, J. E., and Matson, G. L. (1973): A comparison of the cardiovascular responses to stimulation of the aortic and carotid sinus nerves of the dog. *Proc. Soc. Exp. Biol. Med.,* 144:404–411.

362. Kent, K. M., Epstein, S. E., Cooper, T., and Jacobowitz, D. M. (1974): Cholinergic innervation of the canine and human ventricular conducting system, anatomic and electrophysiologic correlations. *Circulation,* 50:948–955.

363. Kent, K. M., Smith, E. R., Redwood, D. R., and Epstein, S. E. (1973): Electrical stability of acutely ischemic myocardium: Influences of heart rate and vagal stimulation. *Circulation,* 47:291–298.

364. Kerzner, J., Wolf, M., Kosowsky, B. K., and Lown, B. (1973): Ventricular ectopic rhythms following vagal stimulation in dogs with acute myocardial infarction. *Circulation,* 47:44–50.

365. Khan, M. I., Hamilton, J. T., and Manning, G. W. (1972): Protective effect of beta adrenoreceptor blockade in experimental coronary occlusion in conscious dogs. *Am. J. Cardiol.,* 30:832–837.

366. Khan, M. I., Hamilton, J. T., and Manning, G. W. (1973): Early arrhythmias following experimental coronary occlusion in conscious dogs and their modification by beta adrenoceptor blocking drugs. *Am. Heart J.,* 86:347–358.

367. Khan, M. M., Logan, K. R., McComb, J. M., and Adgey, A. A. J. (1981): Management of recurrent ventricular tachyarrhythmias associated with Q-T prolongation. *Am. J. Cardiol.,* 47: 1301–1308.

368. Kim, D., Akera, T., and Weaver, L. C. (1984): Role of sympathetic nervous system in ischemia-induced reduction of digoxin tolerance in anesthetized cats. *J. Pharmacol. Exp. Ther.,* 228:537–544.

369. Kirpekar, S. M. (1984): Support for a role for feedback regulation of norepinephrine release. *Fed. Proc.,* 43:1375–1378.

370. Kirpekar, S. M., and Puig, M. (1971): Effect of flow stop on noradrenaline release from normal spleens treated with cocaine, phentolamine or phenoxybenzamine. *Br. J. Pharmacol.,* 43:359–369.

371. Kirpekar, S. M., Prat, J. C., and Yamamoto, H. (1970): Effects of metabolic inhibitors on norepinephrine release from the perfused spleen of the cat. *J. Pharmacol. Exp. Ther.,* 172:342–350.

372. Kléber, A. G., Janse, M. J., Van Capelle, F. J. L., and Durrer, D. (1978): Mechanism and time course of S-T and T-Q segment changes during acute regional myocardial ischemia in the pig heart determined by extracellular and intracellular recordings. *Circ. Res.,* 42:603–613.

373. Klepser, M., Kelliher, G. J., and Roberts, J. (1973): Modification of the cardiotoxic action of digoxin by 6-hydroxydopamine and adrenalectomy. *Clin. Res.,* 21:949.

374. Kliks, B. R., Burgess, M. J., and Abildskov, J. A. (1975): Influence of sympathetic tone on ventricular fibrillation threshold during experimental coronary occlusion. *Am. J. Cardiol.,* 36:45–49.

375. Kolman, B. S., Verrier, R. L., and Lown, B. (1976): Effect of vagus nerve stimulation upon excitability of the canine ventricle. *Am. J. Cardiol.,* 37:1041–1045.

376. Kolman, B. S., Verrier, R. L., and Lown, B. (1976): The effect of vagus nerve stimulation upon vulnerability of the canine ventricle: Role of the sympathetic parasympathetic interactions. *Circulation,* 52:578–585.

377. Korczyn, H. D., Spitzer, S., Kott, E., and Bornstein, B. (1971): Electrocardiographic abnormalities in patients with brain-stem tumor. *Confin. Neurol.,* 33:304–308.

378. Korner, P. I. (1979): Central nervous control of autonomic cardiovascular function. In: *Handbook of Physiology,* Vol. I, edited by R. M. Berne, pp. 691–739. American Physiological Society, Bethesda.

379. Korteweg, G. C. J., Boeles, T. J., and Tencate, J. (1957): Influence of stimulation of some subcortical areas on electrocardiogram. *J. Neurophysiol.,* 20:100–107.

380. Koskelo, P., Punsar, S., and Sipilä, W. (1964): Subendocardial hemorrhage and ECG changes in intracranial bleeding. *Br. Med. J.,* 1:1479–1480.

381. Kreuger, E., and Unna, K. (1942): Comparative studies on the toxic effects of digitoxin and ouabain in cats. *J. Pharmacol. Exp. Ther.,* 76:282–294.

382. Kuffler, S. W., and Eyzaguirre, C. (1955): Processes of excitation in the dendrites and in the soma of single isolated sensory nerve cells of the lobster and crayfish. *J. Gen. Physiol.,* 39:87–119.

383. Kumada, M., and Nakajima, H. (1972): Field potentials evoked in rabbit brainstem by stimulation of the aortic nerve. *Am. J. Physiol.,* 223:575–582.

383a. Lagercrantz, H. (1976): On the composition and function of large dense cored vesicles in sympathetic nerves. *Neuroscience,* 1:81–92.

384. Lammerant, J., Delterdt, P., and DeSchryver, C. (1966): Direct release of myocardial catecholamines into the left heart chambers; the enhancing effect of acute coronary occlusion. *Arch. Int. Pharmacodyn. Ther.,* 163:219–226.

385. Landgren, S. (1952): On the excitation mechanism of the carotid baroreceptors. *Acta Physiol. Scand.,* 26:1–34.

386. Lange, G. (1965): Action of driving stimuli from intrinsic and extrinsic sources on in situ cardiac pacemaker tissues. *Circ. Res.,* 17:449–459.

387. Langer, S. Z. (1981): Presynaptic regulation of the release of catecholamines. *Pharmacol. Rev.,* 32:337–362.

388. Langer, S. Z., and Dubocovich, M. L. (1979): Physiological and pharmacological role of the regulation of noradrenaline release by presynaptic dopamine receptors. In: *Peripheral Dopaminergic Receptors,* edited by J. L. Imbs, and J. Schwartz, pp. 233–245. Pergamon Press, Oxford.

389. Langer, S. Z., Adler, E., Enero, M. A., and Stefano, F. J. E. (1971): The role of the alpha-receptor in regulating noradrenaline overflow by nerve stimulation. In: *Proceedings of the International Union of the Physiological Sciences,* Vol. IX, p. 335.

390. Lanier, S. M., and Malik, K. U. (1983): Facilitation of adrenergic transmission in the canine heart by intracoronary infusion of angiotensin II: Effect of prostaglandin synthesis inhibition. *J. Pharmacol. Exp. Ther.,* 227:676–682.

391. Reference deleted in proof.

392. Lathers, C. M. (1980): Effect of timolol on autonomic neural discharge associated with ouabain-induced arrhythmia. *Eur. J. Pharmacol.,* 64:95–106.

393. Lathers, C. M., and Roberts, J. (1980): Digitalis cardiotoxicity revisited. *Life Sci.,* 27:1713–1733.

394. Lathers, C. M., and Schraeder, P. L. (1982): Autonomic dysfunction in epilepsy: Characterization of autonomic cardiac neural discharge associated with pentylenetetrazol-induced epileptogenic activity. *Epilepsia,* 23:633–647.

395. Lathers, C. M., Gerard-Ciminera, J. L., Baskin, S. I., Krusz, J. C., Kelliher, G. J., Goldberg, P. B., and Roberts, J. (1982): Role of the adrenergic terminal in digitalis-induced cardiac toxicity: A study of the effects of pharmacological and surgical denervation. *J. Cardiovasc. Pharmacol.,* 4:91–98.

396. Lathers, C. M., Gerard-Ciminera, J. L., Baskin, S. I., Krusz, J. C., Kelliher, G. J., and Roberts, J. (1981): The action of reserpine, 6-hydroxydopamine, and bretylium on digitalis-induced cardiotoxicity. *Eur. J. Pharmacol.,* 76:371–379.

397. Lathers, C. M., Kelliher, G. J., Roberts, J., and Beasley, A. B. (1978): Nonuniform cardiac sympathetic nerve discharge: Mechanism for coronary occlusion and digitalis induced arrhythmia. *Circulation,* 57:1058–1065.

398. Lavallée, M., de Champlain, J., Nadeau, R. A., and Yamaguchi, N. (1978): Muscarinic inhibition of endogenous myocardial catecholamine liberation in the dog. *Can. J. Physiol. Pharmacol.,* 56:642–649.

399. Leachman, R. D., Cokkinos, D. V. P., Zamalloa, O., and Alvarez, A. (1969): Electrocardiographic behavior of recipient and donor atria after human heart transplantation. *Am. J. Cardiol.,* 24:49–53.

400. Ledda, F., Marchetti, P., and Manni, A. (1971): Influence of phenylephrine on transmembrane potentials and effective refractory period of single Purkinje fibers of sheep heart. *Pharmacol. Res. Commun.,* 3:195–205.

401. Ledsome, J. R., and Linden, R. J. (1964): A reflex increase in heart rate from distension of the pulmonary-vein-arterial junctions. *J. Physiol. (Lond.),* 170:456–473.

402. Lee, T. M., Kuo, J. S., and Chai, C. Y. (1972): Central integrating

mechanism of the Bezold-Jarish and baroreceptor reflexes. *Am. J. Physiol.*, 222:713–720.

403. Leriche, R., and Fontaine, R. (1931): Les resultats actuels du traitement chirurgical de l'angine de poitrine. *J. Chir. (Paris)*, 38:785–815.

404. LeRoy, G. V., Fenn, G. K., and Gilbert, N. C. (1942): The influence of xanthine drugs and atropine on the mortality rate after experimental occlusion of a coronary artery. *Am. Heart J.*, 23:637–643.

405. Levi, G., Roberts, P. J., and Raiteri, M. (1976): Release and exchange of neurotransmitters in synaptosomes: Effects of the ionophore A 23187 and of ouabain. *Neurochem. Res.*, 1:409–416.

406. Levine, S. A., and Woodworth, C. R. (1958): Congenital deaf-mutism, prolonged QT interval, syncopal attacks and sudden death. *N. Engl. J. Med.*, 259:412–417.

407. Levitt, B., and Roberts, J. (1967): The capacity of different digitalis materials to induce ventricular rhythm disturbances in the reserpine-pretreated cat. *J. Pharmacol. Exp. Ther.*, 156:159–165.

408. Levitt, B., Cagin, N. A., Somberg, J., Bounous, H., Mittag, T., and Raines, A. (1973): Alteration of the effects and distribution of ouabain by spinal cord transection in the cat. *J. Pharmacol. Exp. Ther.*, 185:24–28.

409. Levitt, B., Cagin, N. A., Somberg, J. C., and Kleid, J. J. (1976): Neural basis for the genesis and control of digitalis arrhythmias. *Cardiology*, 61:50–60.

410. Levitt, B., Gillis, R. A., Roberts, J., and Raines, A. (1970): Influence of the cardiac vagus nerves on the cardiotoxicity of acetylstrophanthidin (AcS), ouabain (O), and digitoxin (D). *Pharmacologist*, 12:304.

411. Levy, M. N. (1971): Sympathetic-parasympathetic interactions in the heart. *Circ. Res.*, 29:437–445.

412. Levy, M. N., and Blattberg, B. (1976): Effect of vagal stimulation on the overflow of norepinephrine into the coronary sinus during cardiac sympathetic nerve stimulation in the dog. *Circ. Res.*, 38:81–85.

413. Levy, M. N., Martin, P. J., Iano, T., and Zieske, H. (1970): Effects of single vagal stimuli on heart rate and atrioventricular conduction. *Am. J. Physiol.*, 218:1256–1262.

414. Li, T., and Sperelakis, N. (1983): Stimulation of slow action potentials in guinea pig papillary muscle cells by intracellular injection of cAMP, Gpp(NH)$_p$, and cholera toxin. *Circ. Res.*, 52:111–117.

415. Lictenfeld, P. (1971): Autonomic dysfunction in the Guillain-Barré syndrome. *Am. J. Med.*, 50:772–780.

416. Limbird, L. E., and Lefkowitz, R. J. (1976): Adenylate cyclase-coupled beta adrenergic receptors: Effect of membrane lipid-perturbing agents on receptor binding and enzyme stimulation by catecholamines. *Mol. Pharmacol.*, 12:559–567.

417. Lipski, J., McAllen, R. M., and Spyer, K. M. (1975): The sinus nerve and baroreceptor input to the medulla of the cat. *J. Physiol. (Lond.)*, 251:61–78.

418. Lipski, J. I., Donoso, E., and Friedberg, C. K. (1972): The effect of bretylium tosylate on the normal and digitalis-sensitized dog heart. *Am. Heart J.*, 83:769–776.

419. Lockwood, R. H., and Lum, B. K. B. (1974): Effects of adrenergic agonists and antagonists on potassium metabolism. *J. Pharmacol. Exp. Ther.*, 189:119–129.

420. Loeb, H. S., Pietras, R. J., Gunnar, R. M., and Tobin, J. R., Jr. (1968): Paroxysmal ventricular fibrillation in two patients with hypomagnesemia. Treatment by transvenous pacing. *Circulation*, 37:210–215.

421. Loewy, A. D. (1981): Descending pathways to sympathetic and parasympathetic preganglionic neurons. *J. Autonom. Nerv. Syst.*, 3:265–275.

422. Loewy, A. D., and Burton, H. (1978): Nuclei of the solitary tract. Efferent projections to the lower brainstem and spinal cord of the cat. *J. Comp. Neurol.*, 181:421–450.

423. Löffel, N. B., Rossi, L. N., Mumenthaler, M., Lütschg, J., and Ludin, H.-P. (1977): The Landry-Guillain-Barré syndrome. *J. Neurol. Sci.*, 33:71–79.

424. Löffelholz, K., and Muscholl, E. (1969): A muscarinic inhibition of the noradrenaline release evoked by postganglionic sympathetic nerve stimulation. *Naunyn Schmiedebergs Arch. Pharmacol.*, 265:1–15.

425. Loh, H. H., and Law, P. Y. (1980): The role of membrane lipids in receptor mechanisms. *Annu. Rev. Pharmacol. Toxicol.*, 20:201–234.

426. Lombardi, F., Patton, C. P., Bella, P. D., Pagani, M., and Malliani, A. (1982): Cardiovascular and sympathetic responses reflexly elicited through the excitation with bradykinin of sympathetic and vagal cardiac sensory endings in the cat. *Cardiovasc. Res.*, 16:57–65.

427. Lombardi, F., Verrier, R. L., and Lown, B. (1983): Relationship between sympathetic neural activity, coronary dynamics, and vulnerability to ventricular fibrillation during myocardial ischemia and reperfusion. *Am. Heart J.*, 105:958–965.

428. Loomis, T. A., and Krop, S. (1955): Auricular fibrillation induced and maintained by acetylcholine or vagal stimulation. *Circ. Res.*, 3:390–396.

429. Lorenz, R. R., and Vanhoutte, P. M. (1975): Inhibition of adrenergic neurotransmission in isolated veins of the dog by potassium ions. *J. Physiol. (Lond.)*, 246:479–500.

430. Lown, B. (1979): Sudden cardiac death: The major challenge confronting contemporary cardiology. *Am. J. Cardiol*, 43:313–328.

431. Lown, B., DeSilva, R. A., Reich, P., and Murawski, B. J. (1980): Psychophysiologic factors in sudden cardiac death. *Am. J. Psychiatry*, 137:1325–1335.

432. Lown, B., Ehrlich, L., Lipschultz, B., and Blake, J. (1961): Effect of digitalis in patients receiving reserpine. *Circulation*, 24:1184–1191.

433. Lu, H. H., Lange, G., and Brooks, C. M. (1965): Factors controlling pacemaker action in cells of the sinoatrial node. *Circ. Res.*, 17:460–471.

434. Macdonald, A. D., and Schlapp, W. (1930): The assay of digitalis by the cat method. *Q. J. Pharm. Pharmacol.*, 3:450–454.

435. Madan, B. R., and Gupta, R. S. (1969): Acetylcholine and atropine in ventricular arrhythmias following coronary occlusion in the dog. *Arch. Int. Pharmacodyn.*, 178:43–52.

436. Maling, H. M., Cohn, V. H., and Highman, B. (1959): The effects of coronary occlusion in dogs treated with reserpine and in dogs treated with phenoxybenzamine. *J. Pharmacol. Exp. Ther.*, 127:229–235.

437. Malliani, A., and Lombardi, F. (1978): Neural reflexes associated with myocardial ischemia. In: *Neural Mechanisms in Cardiac Arrhythmias*, edited by P. J. Schwartz, A. M. Brown, A. Malliani, and A. Zanchetti, pp. 209–219. Raven Press, New York.

438. Malliani, A., and Lombardi, F. (1982): Consideration of the fundamental mechanisms eliciting cardiac pain. *Am. Heart J.*, 103:575–578.

439. Malliani, A., Parks, M., Tuckett, R. P., and Brown, A. M. (1973): Reflex increases in heart rate elicited by stimulation of afferent cardiac sympathetic nerve fibers in the cat. *Circ. Res.*, 32:9–14.

440. Malliani, A., Peterson, D. F., Bishop, V. S., and Brown, A. M. (1972): Spinal sympathetic cardiocardiac reflexes. *Circ. Res.*, 30:158–166.

441. Malliani, A., Recordati, G., and Schwartz, P. J. (1973): Nervous activity of afferent cardiac sympathetic fibers with atrial and ventricular endings. *J. Physiol. (Lond.)*, 29:457–469.

442. Malliani, A., Schwartz, P. J., and Zanchetti, A. (1969): A sympathetic reflex elicited by experimental coronary occlusion. *Am. J. Physiol.*, 217:703–709.

443. Reference deleted in proof.

444. Mancia, G., and Donald, D. E. (1975): Demonstration that the atria, ventricles and lungs each are responsible for a tonic inhibition of the vasomotor center in the dog. *Circ. Res.*, 36:310–318.

445. Mancia, G., and Zanchetti, A. (1981): Hypothalamic control of autonomic functions. In: *Handbook of Hypothalamus*, edited by P. J. Pankseep and J. Morgane, pp. 147–202. Marcel Dekker, New York.

446. Mandel, W., Hayakawa, H., Danzig, R., and Marcus, H. S. (1971): Evaluation of sino-atrial node function in man by overdrive suppression. *Circulation*, 44:59–66.

447. Mannard, A., and Polosa, C. (1973): Analysis of background firing of single sympathetic preganglionic neurons of cat cervical nerve. *J. Neurophysiol.*, 36:398–408.

448. Manoach, M., Amitzur, G., Netz, H., Weinstock, M., and Gitter, S. (1982): Acetylcholine induced ventricular fibrillation in mammals: Possible model for sudden infant death. *Jpn. Heart J.* [*Suppl. 1*], 23:142–144.

449. Marshall, B. E., and Wollman, H. (1980): General anesthetics. In: *The Pharmacological Basis of Therapeutics*, ed. 6, edited by G. A. Gilman, L. S. Goodman, and A. Gilman, p. 292. Macmillan, New York.

450. Marshall, R. J., and Parratt, J. R. (1976): Comparative effects of propronolol and practolol in the early stages of experimental canine myocardial infarction. *Br. J. Pharmacol.*, 57:295–303.

451. Marshall, R. J., and Parratt, J. R. (1980): The early consequences of myocardial ischaemia and their modification. *J. Physiol. (Paris)*, 76:699–715.

452. Martin, P. (1977): The influence of the parasympathetic nervous system on atrioventricular conduction. *Circ. Res.*, 41:593–599.

453. Martins, J. B., and Zipes, D. P. (1980): Effects of sympathetic and vagal nerves on recovery properties of the endocardium and epicardium of the canine left ventricle. *Circ. Res.*, 46:100–110.

454. Martins, J. B., Kerber, R. E., Marcus, M. L., Laughlin, D. L., and Levy, D. M. (1980): Inhibition of adrenergic neurotransmission in ischaemic regions of the canine left ventricle. *Cardiovasc. Res.*, 14:116–124.

455. Mason, J. W. (1980): Overdrive suppression in the transplanted heart: Effect of the autonomic nervous system on human sinus node recovery. *Circulation*, 62:688–696.

456. Mathes, P., and Gubjarnason, S. (1971): Changes in norepinephrine stores in the canine heart following experimental myocardial infarction. *Am. Heart J.*, 81:211–219.

457. Mathews, E. C., Blount, A. W., Jr., and Townsend, J. I. (1972): Q-T prolongation and ventricular arrhythmias, with and without deafness, in the same family. *Am. J. Cardiol.*, 29:702–711.

458. Matsuura, S. (1973): Depolarization of sensory nerve endings and impulse initiation in common carotid baroreceptors. *J. Physiol. (Lond.)*, 235:31–56.

459. May, G. S., Eberlein, K. A., Furberg, C. D., Passamani, E. R., and DeMets, D. L. (1982): Secondary prevention after myocardial infarction: A review of long-term trials. *Prog. Cardiovasc. Dis.*, 24:331–352.

460. McAllen, R. M., and Spyer, K. M. (1976): The location of cardiac vagal preganglionic motoneurones in the medullar of the cat. *J. Physiol. (Lond.)*, 258:187–204.

461. McAllen, R. M., and Spyer, K. M. (1978): The baroreceptor input to cardiac vagal motorneurones. *J. Physiol. (Lond.)*, 282:365–374.

462. McCall, R. B., Gebber, G. L., and Barman, S. M. (1977): Spinal interneurons in the baroreceptor reflex arc. *Am. J. Physiol.*, 232:H657–H665.

463. McDonald, L., Baker, C., Bray, C., McDonald, A., and Restieaux, N. (1969): Plasma-catecholamines after cardiac infarction. *Lancet*, 2:1021–1023.

464. McEachern, C. G., Manning, G. W., and Hall, G. E. (1940): Sudden occlusion of coronary arteries following removal of cardiosensory pathways. *Arch. Intern. Med.*, 65:661–670.

465. McGrath, B. P., Lim, S. P., Leversha, L., and Shanahan, A. (1981): Myocardial and peripheral catecholamine responses to acute coronary artery constriction before and after propranolol treatment in the anaesthetized dog. *Cardiovasc. Res.*, 15:28–34.

466. McGrath, M. A., and Shepherd, J. T. (1976): Inhibition of adrenergic neurotransmission in canine vascular smooth muscle by histamine. Mediation by H_2-receptors. *Circ. Res.*, 39:566–573.

467. McGrath, M. A., and Shepherd, J. T. (1978): Histamine and 5-hydroxytryptamine inhibition of transmitter release mediated by H_2 and 5-hydroxytryptamine receptors. *Fed. Proc.*, 37:195–198.

468. McKibben, J. S., and Getty, R. (1968): A comparative morphologic study of the cardiac innervation of domestic animals. I. The canine. *Am. J. Anat.*, 122:533–544.

469. McLain, P. L. (1969): Effects of cardiac glycosides on spontaneous efferent activity in vagus and sympathetic nerves of cats. *Int. J. Neuropharmacol.*, 8:379–387.

470. Melville, K. I., and Varma, D. R. (1962): The combined effects of reserpine and various coronary dilator drugs: An experimental study. *Can. Med. Assoc. J.*, 86:1014–1019.

471. Melville, K. I., Blum, B., Shister, H. E., and Silver, M. D. (1963): Cardiac ischemic changes and arrhythmias induced by hypothalamic stimulation. *Am. J. Cardiol.*, 12:781–791.

472. Mendez, C., and Moe, G. K. (1966): Demonstration of a dual A-V nodal conduction system in the isolated rabbit heart. *Circ. Res.*, 19:378–393.

473. Mendez, C., Aceves, J., and Mendez, R. (1961): Inhibition of adrenergic cardiac acceleration by cardiac glycosides. *J. Pharmacol. Exp. Ther.*, 131:191–198.

474. Mikolich, J. R., Jacobs, W. C., and Fletcher, G. F. (1981): Cardiac arrhythmias in patients with acute cerebrovascular accidents. *J.A.M.A.*, 246:1314–1317.

475. Milch, E., Zimdahl, W. T., Egan, R. W., Hsia, T. W., Anderson, A. A., and David, J. (1955): Experimental prevention of sudden death from acute coronary artery occlusion in the dog. *Am. Heart J.*, 50:483–491.

476. Miller, R. R., Olson, H. G., Vera, Z., Demaria, A. N., Amsterdam, E. A., and Mason, D. T. (1977): Clinical evaluation of the enhancement of vagal tone in acute myocardial infarction by edrophonium chloride: Effects on ventricular arrhythmias, His bundle electrocardiography and left ventricular function. *Am. Heart J.*, 93:222–228.

477. Mirro, M. J., Bailey, J. C., and Watanabe, A. M. (1979): Dissociation between the electrophysiological properties and total tissue cyclic guanosine monophosphate content of guinea pig atria. *Circ. Res.*, 45:225–233.

477a.Miura, M., and Reis, D. J. (1969): Termination and secondary projections of the carotid sinus nerve in the cat brainstem. *Am. J. Physiol.*, 217:142–153.

478. Miura, Y., Inui, J., and Imamura, H. (1978): Alpha-adrenoceptor-mediated restoration of calcium dependent potentials in the partially depolarized rabbit papillary muscle. *Naunyn Schmiedebergs Arch. Pharmacol.*, 301:201–205.

479. Mizeres, N. J. (1955): The anatomy of the autonomic nervous system in the dog. *Am. J. Anat.*, 96:285–318.

480. Mizeres, N. J. (1957): The course of the left cardioinhibitory fibers in the dog. *Anat. Rec.*, 127:109–116.

481. Mizeres, N. J. (1958): The origin and cause of the cardioaccelerator fibers in the dog. *Anat. Rec.*, 132:261–279.

482. Moe, G. K., and Abildskov, J. A. (1959): Atrial fibrillation as a self-sustaining arrhythmia independent of focal discharge. *Am. Heart J.*, 58:59–70.

483. Moothart, R. W., Pryor, R., Hawley, R. L., Clifford, N. J., and Blount, S. G. (1976): The heritable syndrome of prolonged Q-T interval, syncope, and sudden death. Electron microscopic observations. *Chest*, 70:263–266.

484. Morest, P. K. (1967): Experimental study of the projections of the nucleus of the tractus solitarius and the area postrema in the cat. *J. Comp. Neurol.*, 130:277–293.

485. Morrow, D. H. (1967): Anesthesia and digitalis toxicity. II. Effect of norepinephrine infusion on ouabain tolerance. *Anesth. Analg. Curr. Res.*, 46:319–323.

486. Morrow, D. H., Gaffney, T. E., and Braunwald, E. (1963): Studies on digitalis. VIII. Effect of autonomic innervation and of myocardial catecholamine stores upon the cardiac action of ouabain. *J. Pharmacol. Exp. Ther.*, 140:236–242.

487. Moss, A. J., and Schwartz, P. J. (1982): Delayed repolarization (GT or GTU prolongation) and malignant ventricular arrhythmias. *Mod. Concepts Cardiovasc. Dis.*, 51:85–90.

488. Moss, A. J., Davis, H. T., Conard, D. L., DeCamilla, J. J., and Odoroff, C. L. (1981): Digitalis-associated cardiac mortality after myocardial infarction. *Circulation*, 64:1150–1156.

488a.Moss, A. J., Schwartz, P. J., Crampton, R. S., Locati, E., and Carleen, E. (1985): The long QT syndrome: a prospective international study. *Circulation*, 71:17–21.

489. Motté, G., Coumel, P. H., Abitol, G., Dessertenne, F., and Slama, R. (1970): Le syndrome QT long et syncopes par "torsades de pointe." *Arch. Mal. Coeur*, 63:831–853.

490. Muira, M., and Reis, D. J. (1969): Termination and secondary projections of the carotid sinus nerve in the cat brainstem. *Am. J. Physiol.*, 217:142–153.

491. Mukherjee, A., Bush, L. R., McCoy, K. E., Duke, R. J., Hagler, H., Buja, L. M., and Willerson, J. T. (1982): Relationship between β-adrenergic receptor numbers and physiological responses

during experimental canine myocardial ischemia. *Circ. Res.,* 50: 735–741.

492. Mukherjee, A., Hogan, M., McCoy, K., Buja, L. M., and Willerson, J. T. (1980): Influence of experimental myocardial ischemia on alpha₁-adrenergic receptors. *Circulation [Suppl. III],* 64:149.

493. Muscholl, E. (1979): Presynaptic muscarine receptors and inhibition of release. In: *The Release of Catecholamine from Adrenergic Neruons,* edited by D. M. Paton, pp. 87–110. Pergamon Press, Oxford.

494. Muscholl, E. (1980): Peripheral muscarinic control of norepinephrine release in the cardiovascular system. *Am. J. Physiol.,* 239:H713–H720.

495. Myers, M. G., Norris, J. W., Hachinski, V. C., and Sole, M. J. (1981): Plasma norepinephrine in stroke. *Stroke,* 12:200–204.

496. Myers, M. G., Norris, J. W., Hachinski, V. C., Weingert, M. E., and Sole, M. J. (1982): Cardiac sequelae of acute stroke. *Stroke,* 13:838–842.

497. Myers, R. W., Pearlman, A. S., Hyman, R. M., Goldstein, R. A., Kent, K. M., Goldstein, R. E., and Epstein, S. E. (1974): Beneficial effects of vagal stimulation and bradycardia during experimental acute myocardial ischemia. *Circulation,* 49:943–947.

498. Nadeau, R., and deChamplain, J. (1973): Comparative effects of 6-hydroxydopamine and of reserpine on ouabain toxicity. *Life Sci.,* 13:1753–1761.

499. Nadeau, R. A., Roberge, F. A., and Billette, J. (1970): Role of the sinus node in the mechanism of cholinergic atrial fibrillation. *Circ. Res.,* 27:129–138.

500. Naeye, R. L. (1973): Pulmonary arterial abnormalities in the sudden-infant-death syndrome. *N. Engl. J. Med.,* 289:1167–1170.

501. Naeye, R. L. (1976): Brain-stem and adrenal abnormalities in the sudden-infant-death syndrome. *Am. J. Clin. Pathol.,* 66:526–530.

502. Nahum, L. H., and Hoff, H. E. (1940): Production of auricular fibrillation by application of acetyl-β methylcholine chloride to localized regions of the auricular surface. *Am. J. Physiol.,* 129: P428–P429.

503. Nakajima, S., and Onodera, K. (1969): Membrane properties of the stretch receptor neurones of crayfish with particular reference to mechanisms of sensory adaptation. *J. Physiol. (Lond.),* 200: 161–185.

504. Nakajima, S., and Onodera, K. (1969): Adaptation of the generator potential in the crayfish stretch receptors under constant length and constant tension. *J. Physiol. (Lond.),* 200:187–204.

505. Narula, O. S. (1974): Sinus node reentry. *Circulation,* 50:1114–1128.

506. National Institute of Neurologic and Communicative Disorders and Stroke (1978): Criteria for diagnosis of Guillain-Barré syndrome. *Ann. Neurol.,* 3:565–566.

507. Nazum, F. R., and Bischoff, F. (1953): The urinary output of catechol derivatives including adrenaline in normal individuals in essential hypertension and in myocardial infarction. *Circulation,* 7:96–101.

508. Neil-Dwyer, G., Walter, P., Cruickshank, J. M., Doshi, B., and O'Gorman, P. (1978): Effect of propranolol and phentolamine on myocardial necrosis after subarachnoid hemorrhage. *Br. Med. J.,* 2:990–992.

509. Nicholson, W. J., Martin, C. E., Gracey, J. G., and Knoch, H. R. (1979): Disopyramide-induced ventricular fibrillation. *Am. J. Cardiol.,* 43:1053–1055.

510. Nishi, K., and Takenaka, F. (1973): Chemosensitive afferent fibers in the cardiac sympathetic nerve of the cat. *Brain Res.,* 55: 214–218.

511. Nishi, K., Sakanashi, M., and Takenaka, F. (1974): Afferent fibres from pulmonary arterial baroreceptors in the left cardiac sympathetic nerve of the cat. *J. Physiol. (Lond.),* 240:53–66.

512. Nishi, K., Yoshikawa, Y., Takenaka, F., and Akaiki, N. (1977): Electrical activity of sinoatrial node cells of the rabbit surviving a long exposure to cold Tyrode's solution. *Circ. Res.,* 41:242–247.

513. Norris, R. M., Caughey, D. E., and Scott, P. J. (1968): Trial of propranolol in acute myocardial infarction. *Br. Med. J.,* 2:398–400.

514. Norwegian Multicenter Study Groups (1981): Timolol-induced

515. Öberg, B., and Thorén, P. (1972): Studies on left ventricular receptors, signalling in non-medullated vagal afferents. *Acta Physiol. Scand.,* 85:145–163.

516. Öberg, B., and Thorén, P. (1972): Increased activity in left ventricular receptors during hemmorrhage or occlusion of caval veins in the cat. A possible cause of the vaso-vagal reaction. *Acta Physiol. Scand.,* 85:164–173.

517. Öberg, B., and Thorén, P. (1973): Circulatory responses to stimulation of medullated and non-medullated afferents in the cardiac nerve in the cat. *Acta Physiol. Scand.,* 87:121–132.

518. Ochi, R., and Hino, N. (1978): Depression of slow inward current by acetylcholine in mammalian ventricular muscle. *Proc. Japan. Acad.,* 54:474–477.

519. Offerhaus, I., and Van Gool, J. (1969): Electrocardiographic changes and tissue catecholamines in experimental subarachnoid hemorrhage. *Cardiovasc. Res.,* 3:433–440.

520. Olley, P. M., and Fowler, R. S. (1970): The surdo-cardiac syndrome and therapeutic observations. *Br. Heart J.,* 32:467–471.

521. Olson, H. G., Milla, R. R., DaSilva, O., Amsterdam, E. A., and Mason, D. T. (1974): Vagal stimulation in patients with acute myocardial infarction: Antiarrhythmic and hemodynamic effects of edrophonium. *Circulation [Suppl. III],* 50:33.

522. Osler, L. D., and Sidell, A. D. (1960): The Guillain-Barré syndrome. The need for exact diagnostic criteria. *N. Engl. J. Med.,* 262:964–969.

523. Otsuka, K., Kaba, H., Saito, H., Seto, K., and Yanaga, T. (1982): The hypothalamus and digitalis cardiotoxicity. *Am. Heart J.,* 104:649–651.

524. Pace, D. G., and Gillis, R. A. (1976): Neuroexcitatory effects of digoxin in the cat. *J. Pharmacol. Exp. Ther.,* 199:583–600.

525. Pace, D. G., and Martin, P. (1978): Interactions between digoxin and brief vagal bursts influencing atrioventricular conduction. *J. Pharmacol. Exp. Ther.,* 205:657–665.

526. Pagani, M., Pizzinelli, P., Bergamaschi, M., and Malliani, A. (1982): A positive feedback sympathetic pressor reflex during stretch of the thoracic aorta in conscious dogs. *Circ. Res.,* 50: 125–132.

527. Page, A., Boulard, G., and Guérin, J. (1983): Anomalies, électrocardiographiques an cours des hémorragies sous-arachnoidiennes. *Arch. Mal. Coeur,* 76:1031–1037.

528. Page, M. M., and Watkins, P. J. (1978): Cardiorespiratory arrest and diabetic autonomic neuropathy. *Lancet,* 1:14–16.

529. Paintal, A. S. (1953): A study of right and left atrial receptors. *J. Physiol. (Lond.),* 120:596–610.

530. Paintal, A. S. (1963): Natural stimulation of type B atrial receptors. *J. Physiol. (Lond.),* 169:116–136.

531. Paintal, A. S. (1969): Mechanism of stimulation of type J pulmonary receptors. *J. Physiol. (Lond.),* 203:511–532.

532. Paintal, A. S. (1972): Cardiovascular receptors. In: *Handbook of Sensory Physiology,* Vol. 3, edited by E. Neil, pp. 1–45. Springer-Verlag, Berlin.

533. Pandey, R. C., Srivastava, R. D., and Bathnagar, V. N. (1979): Effect of unilateral stellate ganglion blockade and stimulation on experimental arrhythmias. *Int. J. Physiol. Pharmacol.,* 23:305–314.

534. Pantridge, J. F. (1978): Autonomic disturbance at the onset of acute myocardial infarction. In: *Neural Mechanisms in Cardiac Arrhythmias,* edited by P. J. Schartz, A. M. Brown, A. Malliani, and D. Zanchetti, pp. 7–17. Raven Press, New York.

535. Pappano, A. J. (1971): Propranolol-insensitive effects of epinephrine on action potential repolarization in electrically driven atria of the guinea pig. *J. Pharmacol. Exp. Ther.,* 177:85–95.

536. Pappano, A. J., and Inoue, D. (1984): Development of different electrophysiological mechanisms for muscarinic inhibition of atria and ventricles. *Fed. Proc.,* 43:2607–2612.

537. Parizel, G. (1973): Life threatening arrhythmias in subarachnoid hemorrhage. *Angiology,* 24:17–21.

538. Parizel, G. (1979): On the mechanism of sudden death with subarachnoid hemorrhage. *J. Neurol.,* 220:71–76.

539. Parratt, J. R. (1980): Beta-adrenoceptor blockade and early postinfarction dysrhythmias. In: *The Clinical Impact of Beta-*

reduction in mortality and reinfarction in patients surviving acute myocardial infarction. *N. Engl. J. Med.,* 304:801–807.

Adrenoceptor Blockade, edited by D. M. Burley and G. F. B. Birdwood, pp. 29–49. Ciba, Horsham, Surrey.

540. Paton, D. M. (editor) (1979): *The Release of Catecholamine from Adrenergic Neurons.* Pergamon Press, Oxford.

541. Paton, W. D. M., and Vizi, E. S. (1969): The inhibitory action of noradrenaline and adrenaline on acetylcholine output by guinea-pig ileum longitudinal muscle strip. *Br. J. Pharmacol.,* 35:10–28.

542. Peach, M. J., Ford, G. D., Azzaro, A. J., and Fleming, W. W. (1970): The effects of acidosis on chronotropic responses, norepinephrine storage and release in isolated guinea-pig atria. *J. Pharmacol. Exp. Ther.,* 172:289–296.

543. Pearle, D. L., and Gillis, R. A. (1974): Effect of digitalis on response of the ventricular pacemaker to sympathetic neural stimulation and to isoproterenol. *Am. J. Cardiol.,* 34:704–710.

544. Pearle, D. L., Williford, D., and Gillis, R. A. (1978): Superiority of practolol versus propranolol in protection against ventricular fibrillation induced by coronary occlusion. *Am. J. Cardiol.,* 42:960–964.

545. Pelletier, C. L., Clement, D. L., and Shepherd, J. T. (1972): Comparison of afferent activity of canine aortic and sinus nerves. *Circ. Res.,* 31:557–568.

546. Pentecost, B. L., and Austen, W. G. (1966): Beta-adrenergic blockade in experimental myocardial infarction. *Am. Heart J.,* 72:790–796.

547. Peterson, D. F., and Brown, A. M. (1971): Pressor reflexes produced by stimulation of afferent fibers in the cardiac sympathetic nerves of the cat. *Circ. Res.,* 28:605–610.

548. Peterson, D. F., Kasper, R. L., and Bishop, V. S. (1973): Reflex tachycardia due to temporary coronary occlusion in the conscious dog. *Circ. Res.,* 32:652–659.

549. Phillips, J., and Ichinose, H. (1970): Clinical and pathologic studies in the hereditary syndrome of a long QT interval, syncopal spells and sudden death. *Chest,* 58:236–243.

550. Polak, R. L. (1971): Stimulating action of atropine on the release of acetylcholine by rat cerebral cortex in vitro. *Br. J. Pharmcol.,* 41:600–606.

551. Popov, N., and Forster, W. (1966): Über den Einfluss verschiedener Digitaliskörper auf die monoaminoxydase Aktivität im Ratten, Meerschweinchen und Katzengehirn. *Acta Biol. Med. Ger.,* 17:221–231.

552. Posner, P., Farrar, E. L., and Lambert, C. R. (1976): Inhibitory effects of catecholamines in canine cardiac Purkinje fibers. *Am. J. Physiol.,* 231:1415–1420.

553. Powell, J. R., and Brody, M. J. (1973): Peripheral facilitation of reflex vasoconstriction by prostaglandin $F_{2\alpha}$. *J. Pharmacol. Exp. Ther.,* 187:495–500.

554. Powell, J. R., and Feigl, E. O. (1979): Carotid sinus reflex coronary vasoconstriction during controlled myocardial oxygen metabolism in the dog. *Circ. Res.,* 44:44–51.

555. Preda, I., Karpati, P., and Endsoczi, E. (1975): Myocardial noradrenaline uptake after coronary occlusion in the rat. *Acta Physiol. Hung.,* 46:99–106.

556. Prineas, J. W. (1981): Pathology of the Guillain-Barré syndrome. *Ann. Neurol. [Suppl.],* 9:6–19.

557. Prystowsky, E. N., Jackman, W. M., Rinkenberger, R. L., Heger, J. J., and Zipes, D. P. (1981): Effect of autonomic blockade on ventricular refractoriness and atrioventricular nodal conduction in humans. Evidence supporting a direct cholinergic action on ventricular muscle refractoriness. *Circ. Res.* 49:511–518.

558. Prystowsky, E. N., Naccarelli, G. V., Jackman, W. M., Rinkenberger, R. L., Heger, J. J., and Zipes, D. P. (1983): Enhanced parasympathetic tone shortens atrial refractoriness in man. *Am. J. Cardiol.,* 51:96–100.

559. Przybylski, J., Chiale, P. A., Halpern, M. S., Nau, G. J., Elizari, M. V., and Rosenbaum, M. G. (1980): Unmasking of ventricular preexcitation by vagal stimulation or isoproterenol infusion. *Circulation,* 61:1030–1037.

560. Puig, M., and Kirpekar, S. M. (1971): Inhibitory effects of low pH on norepinephrine release. *J. Pharmacol. Exp. Ther.,* 176:134–138.

561. Quest, J. A., and Gillis, R. A. (1974): Effect of digitalis on carotid sinus baroreceptor activity. *Circ. Res.,* 35:247–255.

562. Rabinowitz, S. H., Verrier, R. L., and Lown, B. (1976): Muscarinic effects of vagosympathetic trunk stimulation on the repetitive extrasystole (RE) threshold. *Circulation,* 53:622–627.

563. Raines, A., Levitt, B., and Standaert, F. G. (1967): The effect of spinal section on ventricular rhythm disorders induced by ouabain. *Arch. Int. Pharmacodyn. Ther.,* 170:485–490.

564. Raines, A., Moros, D., and Levitt, B. (1968): The effect of guanethidine on ouabain-induced ventricular arrhythmia in the cat. *Arch. Int. Pharmacodyn. Ther.,* 174:373–377.

565. Randall, D. C., and Hasson, D. M. (1981): Cardiac arrhythmias in the monkey during classically conditioned fear and excitement. *Pavlovian J. Biol. Sci.,* 16:97–107.

566. Randall, D. C., Evans, J. M., Billman, G. E., Ordway, G. A., and Knapp, C. F. (1981): Neural, hormonal and intrinsic mechanisms of cardiac control during acute coronary occlusion in the intact dog. *J. Autonom. Nerv. Syst.,* 3:87–99.

567. Randall, W. C. (editor) (1977): *Neural Regulation of the Heart.* Oxford University Press, New York.

568. Randall, W. C. (1984): Selective autonomic innervation of the heart. In: *Nervous Control of Cardiovascular Function,* edited by W. C. Randall, pp. 46–67. Oxford University Press, New York.

569. Randall, W. C., and Armour, J. A. (1974): Regional vagosympathetic control of the heart. *Am. J. Physiol.,* 227:444–452.

570. Randall, W. C., Armour, J. A., Geis, W. P., and Lippincott, D. B. (1972): Regional cardiac distribution of the sympathetic nerves. *Fed. Proc.,* 31:1119–1208.

571. Randall, W. C., Jones, S. B., Lipsius, S. L., and Rozanski, G. J. (1984): Subsidiary atrial pacemakers and their neural control. In: *Nervous Control of Cardiovascular Function,* edited by W. C. Randall, pp. 199–224. Oxford University Press, New York.

572. Randall, W. C., Talano, J., Kaye, M. P., Euler, D., Jones, S., and Brynjolfsson, G. (1978): Cardiac pacemakers in absence of the SA node: Responses to exercise and autonomic blockade. *Am. J. Physiol.,* 234:H465–H470.

573. Raper, C., and Wale, J. (1969): Cardiac arrhythmias produced by interaction of ouabain and beta-receptor stimulation. *Eur. J. Pharmacol.,* 6:223–234.

574. Rardon, D. P., and Bailey, J. C. (1983): Direct effects of cholinergic stimulation on ventricular automaticity in guinea pig myocardium. *Circ. Res.,* 52:105–110.

575. Recordati, G., Lombardi, F., Bishop, V. S., and Malliani, A. (1976): Mechanical stimuli exciting type A atrial vagal receptors in the cat. *J. Appl. Physiol.,* 38:397–403.

575a. Recordati, G., Schwartz, P. J., Pagani, M., Maliani, A., and Brown, A. M. (1971): Activation of cardiac vagal receptors during myocardial ischemia. *Experientia,* 27:1423–1424.

576. Reddy, C. P., and Gettes, L. S. (1979): Use of isoproterenol as an aid to electric induction of chronic recurrent ventricular tachycardia. *Am. J. Cardiol.,* 44:705–713.

577. (1977): Reduction in mortality after myocardial infarction with long-term beta-adrenoceptor blockade: Multicentre international study: Supplementary report. *Br. Med. J.,* 2:419–421.

578. Reiffel, J. A., Gang, E., Gliklich, J., Weiss, M. B., Davis, J. C., Patton, J. N., and Bigger, J. T., Jr. (1980): The human sinus node electrogram: A transvenous catheter technique, and a comparison of directly measured and indirectly estimated sinoatrial conduction time in adults. *Circulation,* 62:1324–1334.

579. Reimann, K. A., and Weaver, L. C. (1980): Contrasting reflexes evoked by chemical activation of cardiac afferent nerves. *Am. J. Physiol.,* 239:316–325.

580. Reimer, K. A., Rasmussen, M. M., and Jennings, R. B. (1976): On the nature of protection by propranolol against myocardial necrosis after temporary coronary occlusion in dogs. *Am. J. Cardiol.,* 37:520–527.

581. Reis, D. J., Granata, A. R., Perrone, M. H., and Talman, W. T. (1981): Evidence that glutamic acid is the neurotransmitter of baroreceptor afferents terminating in the nucleus tractus solitarius (NTS). *J. Autonom. Nerv. Syst.,* 3:321–334.

582. Reis, D. J., Ross, C. A., Ruggiero, D. A., Granata, A. R., and Joh, T. H. (1984): Role of adrenaline neurons of ventrolateral medulla (the C1 group) in the tonic and phasic control of arterial pressure. *Clin. Exp. Hyper. Theory and Practice [A],* 6:221–241.

583. Reuter, H. (1974): Localization of beta adrenergic receptors, and effects of noradrenaline and cyclic nucleotides on action potentials,

ionic currents and tension in mammalian cardiac muscle. *J. Physiol. (Lond.),* 242:429–451.

584. Reynolds, A. K., and Horne, M. L. (1969): Studies on the cardiotoxicity of ouabain. *Can. J. Physiol. Pharmacol.,* 47:165–170.

585. Ricardo, J. A., and Koh, E. T. (1978): Anatomical evidence of direct projections from the nucleus of the solitary tract to the hypothalamus, amygdala and other forebrain structures in the rat. *Brain Res.,* 153:1–26.

586. Richardson, J. A. (1963): Circulating levels of catecholamines in acute myocardial infarction and angina pectoris. *Prog. Cardiovasc. Dis.,* 6:56–62.

587. Riemersma, R. A. (1982): Myocardial catecholamine release in acute myocardial ischaemia: Relationship to cardiac arrhythmias. In: *Early Arrhythmias Resulting from Myocardial Ischaemia. Mechanisms and Prevention by Drugs,* edited by J. R. Parratt, pp. 125–138. Macmillan, London.

588. Riemersma, R. A., and Forfar, J. C. (1981): Myocardial norepinephrine release during acute coronary occlusion. *Fed. Proc.,* 40:646.

589. Rochette, L., Didier, J.-P., Moreau, D., and Bralet, J. (1980): Effect of substrate on release of myocardial norepinephrine and ventricular arrhythmias following reperfusion of the ischaemic isolated working rat heart. *J. Cardiovasc. Pharmacol.,* 2:267–279.

589a.Rogers, R. C., and Nelson, D. O. (1984): Neurons of the vagal division of the solitary nucleus activated by the paraventricular nucleus of the hypothalamus. *J. Auton. Nerv. Syst.,* 10:193–197.

590. Rogg, H., and Bucher, U. M. (1979): Effects of an isolated myocardial ischaemia in dogs on plasma catecholamines in the systemic and local coronary venous blood. *Naunyn Schmiedebergs Arch. Pharmacol.,* 307:R42.

591. Romano, C., Gemme, G., and Pongiglione, R. (1963): Aritimie cardiache rare dell'eta pediatrica. II. Accessi sincopali per fibrillazione ventricolare parossistica. (Pesentazione del primo caso della letteratura pediatrica Italiana.) *Clin. Pediatr. (Bologna),* 45:656–683.

592. Roseman, E., and Aring, C. D. (1941): Infectious polyneuritis. *Medicine (Baltimore),* 20:463–494.

593. Rosen, K. M., Loeb, H. S., Sinno, M. Z., Rahimtoola, S. H., and Gunnar, R. M. (1971): Cardiac conduction in patients with symptomatic sinus node disease. *Circulation,* 43:836–844.

594. Rosen, K. M., Mehta, A., and Miller, R. A. (1974): Demonstration of dual atrioventricular nodal pathways in man. *Am. J. Cardiol.,* 33:291–294.

595. Rosen, M. R., Gelband, H., and Hoffman, B. F. (1971): Effects of phentolamine on electrophysiologic properties of isolated canine Purkinje fibers. *J. Pharmacol. Exp. Ther.,* 179:586–593.

596. Rosen, M. R., Hordof, A. J., Ilvento, J. P., and Danilo, P., Jr. (1977): Effects of adrenergic amines on electrophysiological properties and automaticity of neonatal and adult canine Purkinje fibers. Evidence for α- and β-adrenergic actions. *Circ. Res.,* 40:390–400.

597. Rosenblueth, A., and Simeone, F. A. (1934): Interrelationships of vagal and accelerator effects on the cardiac rate. *Am. J. Physiol.,* 110:42–55.

598. Roskoski, R., Jr., Schmid, P. G., Mayer, H. E., and Abboud, F. M. (1975): *In vitro* acetylcholine biosynthesis in normal and failing guinea pig hearts. *Circ. Res.,* 36:547–552.

598a.Ross, C. A., Ruggiero, D. A., Joh, R. H., Park, D. H., and Reis, D. J. (1984): Rostral ventrolateral medulla: Selective projections to the thoracic autonomic cell column from the region containing C1 adrenaline neurons. *J. Comp. Neurol.,* 228:168–185.

598b.Ross, C. A., Ruggiero, D. A., Park, D. H., Joh,T. H., Sved, A. F., Fernandez-Pardal, J., Saavedra, J. M., and Reis, D. J. (1984): Tonic vasomotor control by the roastral ventrolateral medulla: Effect of electrical or chemical stimulation of the area containing C1 adrenaline neurons on arterial pressure, heart rate, and plasma catecholamines and vasopressin. *J. Neurosci.,* 4:474–494.

599. Rossi, L. (1979): *Histopathology of Cardiac Arrhythmias,* ed. 2. Casa Editrice Ambrosiana, Milan.

600. Rothberger, C. J., and Winterberg, H. (1913): Über den Einfluss von Strophanthin auf die Rerzbildungfahigkeit der automatischen Zentren des Herzens. *Pfluegers Arch.,* 150:217–242.

601. Rydén, L., Ariniego, R., Arnman, K., Herlitz, J., Hjalmarson, Å., Holmberg, S., Reyes, C., Smedgård, P., Svedberg, K., Vedin, A., Waagstein, F., Waldenström, A., Wilhemsson, C., Wedel, H., and Yamamoto, M. (1983): A double-blind trial of metoprolol in acute myocardial infarction: Effects on ventricular tachyarrhythmias. *N. Engl. J. Med.,* 308:614–618.

602. Saida, T., Saida, K., Dorfman, S. H., Silberberg, D. H., Sumner, A. J., Manning, M. C., Lisak, R. P., and Brown, M. J. (1979): Experimental allergic neuritis induced by sensitization with galactocerebroside. *Science,* 204:1103–1106.

603. Saito, H., Otani, T., Shudo, I., and Tanabe, T. (1974): Effect of 6-hydroxydopamine on cardiotoxicity of ouabain in guinea pigs. *Jpn. J. Pharmacol.,* 24:923–925.

604. Salisbury, P. F., Cross, C. E., and Rieben, D. A. (1960): Reflex effects of left ventricular distension. *Circ. Res.,* 8:530–534.

605. Salk, L., Grellong, B. A., and Dietrich, J. (1974): Sudden infant death. Normal cardiac habituation and poor autonomic control. *N. Engl. J. Med.,* 291:219–222.

606. Salmoiraghi, G. C. (1962): "Cardiovascular" neurones in the brainstem of cat. *J. Neurophysiol.,* 25:182–197.

607. Saper, C., Loewy, A. D., Swanson, L. W., and Cowan, W. M. (1976): Direct hypothalamo-autonomic connections. *Brain Res.,* 117:305–312.

608. Satinsky, J., Kosowsky, B., and Lown, B. (1971): Ventricular fibrillation induced by hypothalamic stimulation during coronary occlusion. *Circulation [Suppl. II],* 44:60.

609. Sato, A., and Schmidt, R. F. (1973): Somatosympathetic reflexes: Afferent fibers, central pathways, discharge characteristics. *Physiol. Rev.,* 53:916–947.

610. Saum, W. R., Brown, A. M., and Tuley, F. H. (1976): An electrogenic sodium pump and baroreceptor function in normotensive and spontaneously hypertensive rats. *Circ. Res.,* 39:497–505.

610a.Sawchenko, P. E., and Swanson, L. W. (1982): The organization of noradrenergic pathways from the brainstem to the paraventricular and supraoptic nuclei in the rat. *Brain Res. Rev.,* 4:275–325.

611. Saxena, P. R., and Bhargava, K. P. (1975): The importance of central adrenergic mechanism in the cardiovascular responses to ouabain. *Eur. J. Pharmacol.,* 31:332–346.

612. Scagliotti, D., Strasberg, B., Hai, H. A., Kehoe, R., and Rosen, K. (1982): Aprindine-induced polymorphous ventricular tachycardia. *Am. J. Cardiol.,* 49:1297–1300.

613. Schaal, S. F., Wallace, A. G., and Sealy, W. C. (1969): Protective influence of cardiac denervation against arrhythmias of myocardial infarction. *Cardiovasc. Res.,* 3:241–244.

614. Schechter, E., Freeman, C. C., and Lazzara, R. (1984): Afterdepolarizations as a mechanism for the long QT syndrome: Electrophysiologic studies of a case. *J. Am. Coll. Cardiol.,* 3:1556–1561.

615. Scheinman, M. M., Thorburn, D., and Abbott, J. A. (1975): Use of atropine in patients with acute myocardial infarction and sinus bradycardia. *Circulation,* 52:627–633.

616. Scherlag, B. J., El-Sherif, N., Hope, R., and Lazzara, R. (1974): Characterization of ventricular arrhythmias resulting from myocardial ischemia and infarction. *Circ. Res.,* 35:372–383.

617. Scherlag, B. J., Helfant, R. H., Haft, J. I., and Damato, A. N. (1970): Electrophysiology underlying ventricular arrhythmias due to coronary ligation. *Am. J. Physiol.,* 291:1665–1671.

618. Schlaefke, M. E. (1981): Central chemosensitivity: A respiratory drive. *Rev. Physiol. Biochem. Pharmacol.,* 90:171–244.

619. Schmid, P. G., Grief, B. G., Lund, D. D., and Roskoski, R., Jr. (1978): Regional choline acetyltransferase activity in the guinea pig heart. *Circ. Res.,* 42:657–660.

620. Schmitt, G., Müller-Limmroth, H. W., and Guth, V. (1958): Über die Bedeutung der Chemoreceptoren der Carotis und Aorta für die toxische Digitalis bradykardie bei der Katze. *Z. Gesamte Exp. Med.,* 130:190–202.

621. Scholz, H. (1980): Effects of beta- and alpha-adrenoceptor activators and adrenergic transmitter releasing agents on the mechanical activity of the heart. In: *Handbook of Experimental Pharmacology,* Vol. 54, edited by L. Szekeres, pp. 651–733. Springer-Verlag, Berlin.

622. Schömig, A., Dietz, R., Rascher, W., Stasser, R., and Kübler, W.

(1980): Noradrenaline release from the ischaemic myocardium. *Circulation,* 61:669.

623. Schumann, H. J., Wagner, J., Knorr, A., Reidmeister, J. C., Sadony, V., and Schramm, G. (1978): Demonstration in human atrial preparations of α-adrenoceptors mediating positive inotropic effects. *Naunyn Schmiedebergs Arch. Pharmacol.,* 302:333–336.

624. Schwartz, P. J. (1976): Cardiac sympathetic innervation and the sudden infant death syndrome: A possible pathogenetic link. *Am. J. Med.,* 60:167–172.

624a.Schwartz, P. J. (1983): Autonomic nervous system, ventricular fibrillation, and SIDS. In: *Sudden Infant Death Syndrome,* edited by J. T. Tildon, L. M. Roeder, and A. Steinschneider, pp. 319–339. Academic Press, New York.

625. Schwartz, P. J. (1984): Sympathetic imbalance and cardiac arrhythmias. In: *Nervous Control of Cardiovascular Function,* edited by W. C. Randall, pp. 225–252. Oxford University Press, New York.

626. Schwartz, P. J. (1985): Idiopathic long QT syndrome: Progress and questions. *Am. Heart J.,* 109:399–410.

627. Schwartz, P. J., and Stone, H. L. (1977): Tonic influence of the sympathetic nervous system on myocardial reactive hyperemia and on coronary blood flow distribution. *Circ. Res.,* 41:51–58.

628. Schwartz, P. J., and Stone, H. L. (1979): Effects of unilateral stellectomy upon cardiac performance during exercise in dogs. *Circ. Res.,* 44:637–645.

629. Schwartz, P. J., and Stone, H. L. (1980): Left stellectomy in the prevention of ventricular fibrillation caused by acute myocardial ischemia in conscious dogs with anterior myocardial infarction. *Circulation,* 62:1256–1265.

630. Schwartz, P. J., and Vanoli, E. (1981): Cardiac arrhythmias elicited by interaction between acute myocardial ischemia and sympathetic hyperactivity: A new experimental model for the study of antiarrhythmic drugs. *J. Cardiovasc. Pharmacol.,* 3:1251–1259.

631. Schwartz, P. J., and Wolf, S. (1978): QT interval prolongation as predictor of sudden death in patients with myocardial infarction. *Circulation,* 57:1074–1077.

631a.Schwartz, P. J., Billman, G. E., and Stone, H. L. (1984): Autonomic mechanisms in ventricular fibrillation induced by myocardial ischemia during exercise in dogs with healed myocardial infarction. *Circulation,* 69:790–800.

631b.Schwartz, P. J., Foreman, R. D., Stone, H. L., and Brown, A. M. (1976): Effect of dorsal root section on the arrhythmias associated with coronary occlusion. *Am. J. Physiol.,* 231:923–928.

631c.Schwartz, P. J., Pagani, M., Lombardi, F., Malliani, A., and Brown, A. M. (1973): A cardiocardiac sympathovagal reflex in the cat. *Circ. Res.,* 32:215–220.

632. Schwartz, P. J., Periti, M., and Malliani, A. (1975): The long Q-T syndrome. *Am. Heart J.,* 89:378–390.

633. Schwartz, P. J., Snebold, N. G., and Brown, A. M. (1976): Effects of unilateral cardiac sympathetic denervation on the ventricular fibrillation threshold. *Am. J. Cardiol.,* 37:1034–1040.

634. Schwartz, P. J., Stone, H. L., and Brown, A. M. (1974): Effects of unilateral cardiac sympathetic denervation on arrhythmias induced by coronary occlusion. *Circulation [Suppl. III],* 50:204.

635. Schwartz, P. J., Stone, H. L., and Brown, A. M. (1976): Effects of unilateral stellate ganglion blockade on the arrhythmias associated with coronary occlusion. *Am. Heart J.,* 92:589–599.

636. Schwartz, P. J., Vanoli, E., Zaza, A., and Zuanetti, G. (1985): The effect of antiarrhythmic drugs on life-threatening arrhythmias induced by the interaction between acute myocardial ischemia and sympathetic hyperactivity. (*Submitted for publication*).

637. Schwartz, P. J., Verrier, R. L., and Lown, B. (1977): Effect of stellectomy and vagotomy on ventricular refractoriness in dogs. *Circ. Res.,* 40:536–540.

638. Sealy, W. C., Bache, R. J., Seaber, A. V., and Bhattacharga, S. K. (1973): The atrial pacemaking site after surgical exclusion of the sinoatrial node. *J. Thorac. Cardiovasc. Surg.,* 65:841–850.

639. Seevers, M. H., and Meek, W. J. (1935): The cardiac irregularities produced by ephedrine after digitalis. *J. Pharmacol. Exp. Ther.,* 53:295–303.

640. Selzer, A., and Wray, H. W. (1964): Quinidine syncope: Paroxysmal ventricular fibrillation occurring during treatment of chronic atrial arrhythmias. *Circulation,* 30:17–26.

641. Serrano, P. A., Chavaz-Lara, B., Bisteni, A., and Sodi-Pallares, D. (1971): Effect of propranolol on catecholamine content of injured cardiac tissue. *J. Mol. Cell. Cardiol.,* 2:91–97.

642. Sethi, V., Haider, B., Ahmed, S., Oldewurtel, H. A., and Regan, T. J. (1973): Influence of beta blockade and chemical sympathectomy on myocardial function and arrhythmias in acute ischaemia. *Cardiovasc. Res.,* 7:740–747.

643. Shahab, L., Wollenberger, A., Hause, M., and Schiller, U. (1969): Noradrenalineabgabe aus dem Hundenherzen nach vorubergehender Okklusion einer Koronararterie. *Acta Biol. Med. Ger.,* 22:135–143.

644. Shannon, D. C., and Kelly, D. H. (1982): SIDS and near-SIDS. *N. Engl. J. Med.,* 306:959–965.

645. Sharma, A. D., Ahumada, G. G., Sobel, B. E., and Corr, P. B. (1983): Lysophosphatide-induced increases in α-adrenergic receptor number in intact myocytes. *Circulation [Suppl. III],* 68:57.

646. Sharma, A. D., Saffitz, J. E., Lee, B. I., Sobel, B. E., and Corr, P. B. (1983): Alpha adrenergic-mediated accumulation of calcium in reperfused myocardium. *J. Clin. Invest.,* 72:802–818.

647. Sharma, V. K., and Banerjee, S. P. (1977): Inhibition of [^{3}H]norepinephrine uptake in peripheral organs of some mammalian species by ouabain. *Eur. J. Pharmacol.,* 41:417–429.

648. Shatney, C. H., MacCarter, D. J., and Lillehei, R. C. (1976): Effects of allopurinol, propranolol and methylprednisolone on infarct size in experimental myocardial infarction. *Am. J. Cardiol.,* 37:572–580.

649. Shepherd, J. T. (1981): The lungs as receptor sites for cardiovascular regulation. *Circulation,* 63:1–10.

650. Sheridan, D. J., Penkoske, P. A., Sobel, B. E., and Corr, P. B. (1980): Alpha-adrenergic contributions to dysrhythmia during myocardial ischemia and reperfusion in cats. *J. Clin. Invest.,* 65:161–171.

651. Shuster, S. (1960): The electrocardiogram in subarachnoid haemorrhage. *Br. Heart J.,* 22:316–320.

652. Skelton, R. B., Gergely, N., Manning, G. W., and Coles, J. C. (1962): Mortality studies in experimental coronary occlusion. *J. Thorac. Cardiovasc. Surg.,* 44:90–96.

653. Skinner, J. E., and Reed, J. C. (1981): Blockade of frontocortical-brainstem pathway prevents ventricular fibrillation of ischemic heart. *Am. J. Physiol.,* 240:H156–H163.

654. Skinner, J. E., Lie, J. T., and Entman, M. L. (1975): Modification of ventricular fibrillation latency following coronary artery occlusion in the conscious pig: The effects of psychological stress and beta-adrenergic blockade. *Circulation,* 51:656–667.

655. Smellie, F. W., Davis, C. W., Daly, J. W., and Wells, J. N. (1979): Alkylxanthines: Inhibition of adenosine-elicited accumulation of cyclic AMP in brain slices and of brain phosphodiesterase activity. *Life Sci.,* 24:2475–2482.

656. Smith, M. (1972): Ventricular bigeminy and quadrigeminy occurring in a case of subarachnoid hemorrhage. *J. Electrocardiol.,* 5:78–85.

657. Smith, M., and Ray, C. T. (1972): Cardiac arrhythmias, increased intracranial pressure, and the autonomic nervous system. *Chest,* 61:125–133.

658. Smith, N. T., Gerschwin, M. E., and Hurley, E. J. (1968): Hemodynamic effects of ouabain on the surgically denervated, autotransplanted dog heart. *Arch. Int. Pharmacodyn. Ther.,* 173:95–114.

659. Smith, O. A., and DeVito, J. L. (1984): Central neural integration for the control of autonomic responses associated with emotion. *Annu. Rev. Neurosci.,* 7:43–65.

660. Smith, O. A., Jr., and Nathan, M. A. (1966): Inhibition of the carotid sinus reflex by stimulation of the inferior olive. *Science,* 154:674–675.

661. Smith, O. A., Astley, C. A., DeVito, J. L., Stein, J. M., and Walsh, K. E. (1980): Functional analysis of hypothalamic control of the cardiovascular responses accompanying emotional behavior. *Fed. Proc.,* 39:2487–2494.

662. Smith, T. W., and Haber, E. (1973): Digitalis. *N. Engl. J. Med.,* 289:945–952.

663. Smith, T. W., and Haber, E. (1973): Digitalis. *N. Engl. J. Med.,* 289:1010–1015.

664. Smith, T. W., and Haber, E. (1973): Digitalis. *N. Engl. J. Med.,* 289:1063–1072.

665. Smith, T. W., and Haber, E. (1973): Digitalis. *N. Engl. J. Med.*, 289:1125–1129.
666. Smith, W. M., and Gallagher, J. J. (1980): "Les torsade de pointes": An unusual ventricular arrhythmia. *Ann. Intern. Med.*, 93:578–584.
667. Sokolove, P. G., and Cooke, I. M. (1971): Inhibition of impulse activity in a sensory neuron by an electrogenic pump. *J. Gen. Physiol.*, 57:125–163.
668. Solti, F., Iskum, M., and Nagy, J. (1965): Studies on the acute cardiac action of strophanthin in the dog by means of cardiac denervation. *Acta Physiol. Acad. Sci. Hung.*, 26:377–385.
669. Somani, P., and Lum, B. K. B. (1965): The antiarrhythmic actions of beta adrenergic blocking agents. *J. Pharmacol. Exp. Ther.*, 147:194–204.
670. Somberg, J. C., and Smith, T. W. (1979): Localization of the neurally mediated arrhythmogenic properties of digitalis. *Science*, 204:321–323.
671. Somberg, J. C., Bounous, H., Cagin, N., and Levitt, B. (1980): Histamine antagonists as antiarrhythmic agents in ouabain cardiotoxicity in the cat. *J. Pharmacol. Exp. Ther.*, 214:375–380.
672. Somberg, J. C., Mudge, G. H., Risler, T., and Smith, T. W. (1980): Neurally mediated augmentation of arrhythmogenic properties of highly polar cardiac glycosides. *Am. J. Physiol.*, 238:H202–H208.
673. Somberg, J. C., Risler, T., and Smith, T. W. (1978): Neural factors in digitalis toxicity: Protective effect of C-1 spinal cord transection. *Am. J. Physiol.*, 235:H531–H536.
674. Sommers, H. M., and Jennings, R. B. (1972): Ventricular fibrillation and myocardial necrosis after transient ischemia: Effect of treatment with oxygen, procainamide, reserpine and propranolol. *Arch. Intern. Med.*, 129:780–789.
675. Spach, M. S., Lieberman, M., Scott, J. G., Barr, R. C., Johnson, E. A., and Kootsey, J. M. (1971): Excitation sequences of the atrial septum and the AV node in isolated hearts of the dog and rabbit. *Circ. Res.*, 29:156–172.
676. Spear, J. F., and Moore, E. N. (1973): Influence of brief vagal and stellate nerve stimulation on pacemaker activity and conduction within the atrioventricular conduction system of the dog. *Circ. Res.*, 32:27–41.
677. Spear, J. F., Kronhaus, K. D., Moore, E. N., and Kline, R. P. (1979): The effect of brief vagal stimulation on the isolated rabbit sinus node. *Circ. Res.*, 44:75–88.
678. Spyer, K. M. (1981): Neural organisation and control of the baroreceptor reflex. *Rev. Physiol. Biochem. Pharmacol.*, 88:23–124.
679. Srivastava, S. C., and Robson, A. O. (1964): Electrocardiographic abnormalities associated with subarachnoid haemorrhage. *Lancet*, 2:431–433.
680. Stamm, H., and Hulsmann, W. C. (1978): The role of endogenous catecholamines in the depressive effects of free fatty acids on isolated, perfused rat hearts. *Basic Res. Cardiol.*, 73:208–219.
681. Starke, K. (1971): Influence of α-receptor stimulants on noradrenaline release. *Naturwissenschaften*, 58:420.
682. Starke, K. (1977): Regulation of noradrenaline release by presynaptic receptor systems. *Rev. Physiol. Biochem. Pharmacol.*, 77:1–124.
683. Starke, K. (1981): Presynaptic receptors. *Annu. Rev. Pharmacol. Toxicol.*, 21:7–30.
684. Starke, K., Werner, U., Hellerforth, R., and Schümann, H. J. (1970): Influence of peptides on the output of noradrenaline from isolated rabbit hearts. *Eur. J. Pharmacol.*, 9:136–140.
685. Staszewska-Barczak, J. (1971): The reflex stimulation of catecholamine secretion during the acute stage of myocardial infarction in the dog. *Clin. Sci.*, 41:419–439.
686. Staszewska-Barczak, J., and Ceremuzynski, L. (1968): The continuous estimation of catecholamine release in the early stages of myocardial infarction in the dog. *Clin. Sci.*, 34:531–539.
687. Staszewska-Barczak, J., Ferreira, S. H., and Vane, J. R. (1976): An excitatory nocioceptive cardiac reflex elicited by bradykinin and potentiated by prostaglandins and myocardial ischaemia. *Cardiovasc. Res.*, 10:314–327.
688. Steinschneider, A. (1972): Prolonged apnea and the sudden infant death syndrome: Clinical and laboratory observations. *Pediatrics*, 50:646–654.
689. Stewart, J. R., Burmeister, W. E., Burmeister, J., and Lucchesi,

B. R. (1980): Electrophysiologic and antiarrhythmic effects of phentolamine in experimental coronary artery occlusion and reperfusion in the dog. *J. Cardiovasc. Pharmacol.*, 2:77–91.
690. Stinson, E. B., Griepp, R. B., Schroeder, J. S., Dong, E., Jr., and Shumway, N. E. (1972): Hemodynamic observations one and two years after cardiac transplantation in man. *Circulation*, 45:1183–1194.
691. Stinson, E. B., Schroeder, J. S., Griepp, R. B., Shumway, N. E., and Dong, E., Jr. (1972): Observations on the behavior of recipient atria after cardiac transplantation in man. *Am. J. Cardiol.*, 30:615–622.
692. Stjärne, L. (1981): On sites and mechanisms of presynaptic control of noradrenaline secretion. In: *Chemical Neurotransmission 75 Years*, edited by L. Stjärne, P. Hedqvist, H. Lagercrantz, and Å. Wennmalm, pp. 257–272. Academic Press, London.
693. Stone, T. W. (1981): Physiological roles for adenosine and adenosine 5'-triphosphate in the nervous system. *Neuroscience*, 6:523–555.
694. Story, D. K., Brileg, M. S., and Langer, S. Z. (1979): The effects of chemical sympathectomy with 6-hydroxydopamine on α-adrenoceptor and muscarinic cholinoceptor binding in rat heart ventricle. *Eur. J. Pharmacol.*, 57:423–426.
695. Strauss, H. C., Saroff, A. L., Bigger, J. T., Jr., and Giardina, E. G. V. (1973): Premature atrial stimulation as a key to the understanding of sinoatrial conduction in man; presentation of data and critical review of the literature. *Circulation*, 47:86–93.
696. Strittmatter, W. J., Hirata, F., and Axelrod, J. (1979): Phospholipid methylation unmasks cryptic β-adrenergic receptors in rat reticulocytes. *Science*, 204:1205–1207.
697. Stroh-Werz, M., Langhorst, P., and Camerer, H. (1977): Neuronal activity with cardiac rhythm in the nucleus of the solitary tract in cats and dogs. I. Differential discharge patterns related to the cardiac cycle. *Brain Res.*, 133:65–80.
698. Sugimoto, T., Itoh, K., Mizuno, N., Nomura, S., and Konishi, A. (1979): The site of origin of cardiac preganglionic fibers of the vagus nerve: An HRP study in the cat. *Neurosci. Lett.*, 12:53–58.
699. Sung, R. J., Castellanos, A., Mallon, S. M., Gelband, H., Mendoza, I., and Myerburg, R. J. (1977): Mode of initiation of reciprocating tachycardia during programmed ventricular stimulation in the Wolff-Parkinson-White syndrome. *Am. J. Cardiol.*, 40:24–31.
700. Szekeres, L., and Papp, G. J. (1971): *Experimental Cardiac Arrhythmias and Antiarrhythmic Drugs*. Akademiai Kiado, Budapest.
701. Szekeres, L., and Vaughan Williams, E. M. (1962): Antifibrillatory action. *J. Physiol. (Lond.)*, 160:470–482.
702. Tackett, R. L., and Holl, J. E. (1980): Histaminergic mechanisms involved in the centrally mediated effects of ouabain. *J. Pharmacol. Exp. Ther.*, 215:552–556.
703. Takashima, S., Armstrong, D., Becker, L., and Bryan, C. (1978): Cerebral hypoperfusion in the sudden infant death syndrome? Brainstem gliosis and vasculature. *Ann. Neurol.*, 4:257–262.
704. Takashima, S., Armstrong, D., Becker, L. E., and Huber, J. (1978): Cerebral white matter lesions in sudden infant death syndrome. *Pediatrics*, 62:155–159.
705. Takenaka, F., Nishi, K., and Sakanashi, M. (1975): A pharmacological study of sympathetic afferent discharges originating from the cardiac region. *Proc. Western Pharmacol. Soc.*, 18:1–4.
706. Taylor, G. J., Crampton, R. S., Gibson, R. S., Stebbins, P. T., Waldman, M. T. G., and Beller, G. A. (1981): Prolonged Q-T interval at onset of acute myocardial infarction in predicting early phase ventricular tachycardia. *Am. Heart J.*, 102:16–24.
707. Taylor, R. R., Johnston, C. I., and Jose, A. D. (1964): Reversal of digitalis intoxication by beta-adrenergic blockade with pronethalol. *N. Engl. J. Med.*, 271:877–882.
708. Thames, M. D. (1979): Acetyl strophanthidin-induced reflex inhibition of canine renal sympathetic nerve activity mediated by cardiac receptors with vagal afferents. *Circ. Res.*, 44:8–15.
709. Thames, M. D., Klopfenstein, H. S., Abboud, F. M., Mark, A. L., and Walker, J. L. (1978): Preferential distribution of inhibitory cardiac receptors with vagal afferents to the inferoposterior wall of the left ventricle activated during coronary occlusion in the dog. *Circ. Res.*, 43:512–519.
710. Thandroyen, F. T., Worthington, M. G., Higginson, L. M., and

Opie, L. H. (1983): The effect of alpha- and beta-adrenoceptor antagonist agents on reperfusion ventricular fibrillation and metabolic status in the isolated perfused rat heart. *J. Am. Coll. Cardiol.,* 14:1056–1066.

711. The International Collaborative Study Group (1984): Reduction of infarct size with the early use of timolol in acute myocardial infarction. *N. Engl. J. Med.,* 310:9–15.

712. Thomas, J. X., Jr., Randall, W. C., and Jones, C. E. (1981): Protective effect of chronic versus acute cardiac denervation on contractile force during coronary occlusion. *Am. Heart J.,* 102:157–161.

713. Thomas, M. R., and Calaresu, F. R. (1972): Responses of single units in the medial hypothalamus to electrical stimulation of the carotid sinus nerve in the cat. *Brain Res.,* 44:49–62.

714. Thomas, M. R., and Calaresu, F. R. (1974): Localization and function of medullary sites mediating vagus bradycardia. *Am. J. Physiol.,* 226:1344–1349.

715. Thomas, M. R., and Calaresu, F. R. (1974): Medullary sites involved in hypothalamic inhibition of reflex vagal bradycardia in the cat. *Brain Res.,* 80:1–16.

716. Thoren, P. N. (1976): Activation of left ventricular receptors with non-medullated vagal afferent fibers during occlusion of a coronary artery in the cat. *Am. J. Cardiol.,* 37:1046–1051.

717. Thorén, P. N. (1976): Atrial receptors with nonmedullated vagal afferents in the cat: discharge frequency and pattern in relation to atrial pressure. *Circ. Res.,* 381:357–362.

718. Thorén, P. (1977): Characteristics of left ventricular receptors with nonmedullated vagal afferents in cats. *Circ. Res.,* 40:415–421.

719. Thorén, P. (1978): Vagal depressor reflexes elicited by left ventricular C-fibers during myocardial ischemia in cats. In: *Neural Mechanisms in Cardiac Arrhythmias,* edited by P. J. Schwartz, A. M. Brown, A. Malliani, and A. Zanchetti, pp. 179–190. Raven Press, New York.

720. Thorén, P., Saum, W. R., and Brown, A. M. (1977): Characteristics of rat aortic baroreceptors with nonmedullated afferent nerve fibers. *Circ. Res.,* 40:231–237.

721. Thureson-Klein, Å, and Stjärne, L. (1981): Dense-cored vesicles inactively secreting noradrenergic neurons. In: *Chemical Neurotransmission 75 Years,* edited by L. Stjärne, P. Hedqvist, H. Lagercrantz, and Å. Wennmalm, pp. 153–164. Academic Press, London.

722. Tissari, A. H., and Bogdanski, D. F. (1971): Biogenic amine transport. VI. Comparison of effects of ouabain and K$^+$ deficiency on the transport of 5-hydroxytryptamine and norepinephrine by synaptosomes. *Pharmacology,* 5:225–234.

723. Toda, N., and Shimamoto, K. (1968): The influence of sympathetic stimulation on transmembrane potentials in the SA node. *J. Pharmacol. Exp. Ther.,* 159:298–305.

724. Todo, K., Yamamoto, T., Satomi, H., Ise, H., Takata, H., and Takahashi, I. (1977): Origins of vagal preganglionic fibers to the sino-atrial and atrio-ventricular node regions in the cat heart as studied by the horseradish peroxidase method. *Brain Res.,* 130:545–550.

725. Trautwein, W. (1963): Generation and conduction of impulses in the heart as affected by drugs. *Pharmacol. Rev.,* 15:277–332.

726. Truex, R. C. (1976): The sinoatrial node and its connections with the atrial tissues. In: *The Conduction System of the Heart, Structure, Function and Clinical Implications,* edited by H. J. J. Wellens, K. I. Lie, and M. J. Janse, pp. 209–226. Lea & Febiger, Philadelphia.

727. Tse, W. W., and Han, J. (1974): Interaction of epinephrine and ouabain on automaticity of canine Purkinje fibers. *Circ. Res.,* 34:777–782.

728. Tse, W. W., Han, J., and Yoon, M. (1976): Effect of acetylcholine on automaticity of canine Purkinje fibers. *Am. J. Physiol.,* 230:116–119.

729. Turner, J. R. B. (1966): Propranolol in the treatment of digitalis-induced and digitalis-resistant tachycardia. *Am. J. Cardiol.,* 18:450–455.

730. Uchida, Y., and Murao, S. (1973): Excitation of afferent cardiac sympathetic nerve fibers during coronary occlusion. *Am. J. Physiol.,* 226:1094–1099.

731. Uchida, Y., and Murao, S. (1973): Potassium-induced excitation of afferent cardiac sympathetic nerve fibers. *Am. J. Physiol.,* 226:603–607.

732. Uchida, Y., and Murao, S. (1974): Afferent sympathetic nerve fibers originating in left atrial wall. *Am. J. Physiol.,* 227:753–758.

733. Uchida, Y., and Murao, S. (1974): Bradykinin-induced excitation of afferent cardiac sympathetic nerve fibers. *Jpn. Heart J.,* 15:84–91.

734. Uchida, Y., and Murao, S. (1974): Excitation of afferent cardiac sympathetic nerve fibers during coronary occlusion. *Am. J. Physiol.,* 226:1094–1099.

735. Uchida, Y., and Murao, S. (1975): Acid-induced excitation of afferent cardiac sympathetic nerve fibers. *Am. J. Physiol.,* 228:27–33.

736. Ueda, H., Uchida, Y., and Kamisaka, K. (1969): Distribution and responses of the cardiac sympathetic receptors to mechanically induced circulatory changes. *Jpn. Heart J.,* 10:70–80.

737. Valdés-Dapena, M. A. (1980): Sudden infant death syndrome: A review of the medical literature. 1974–1979. *Pediatrics,* 66:597–614.

738. Van Buren, J. M., and Ajmone-Marsan, C. (1960): Correlations of autonomic and EEG components in temporal lobe epilepsy. *Arch. Neurol.,* 3:683–703.

739. Van Dam, R. T., and Durrer, D. (1961): Experimental study of the intramural distribution of the excitability cycle and on the form of the epicardial T wave in the dog heart in situ. *Am. Heart J.,* 61:537–542.

740. Vanhoutte, P. M., Verbeuren, T. J., and Webb, R. C. (1981): Local modulation of adrenergic neuroeffector interaction in the blood vessel wall. *Physiol. Rev.,* 61:151–247.

741. Vanoli, E., Zaza, A., Zuanetti, G., Pappalettera, M., and Schwartz, P. J. (1982): Reduction in infarct size produced by left stellectomy. *9th World Congress of Cardiology (Moscow),* 2:1312.

742. Vargas, G., Akhtar, M., and Damato, A. N. (1975): Electrophysiologic effects of isoproterenol on cardiac conduction system in man. *Am. Heart J.,* 90:25–34.

743. Vassalle, M., Carlos, D. L., and Slovin, A. J. (1967): On the cause of ventricular asystole during vagal stimulation. *Circ. Res.,* 20:228–241.

744. Verrier, R. L., and Lown, B. (1982): Experimental studies of psychophysiological factors in sudden cardiac death. *Acta Med. Scand. [Suppl.],* 660:57–68.

745. Verrier, R. L., and Lown, B. (1984): Behavior stress and cardiac arrhythmias. *Annu. Rev. Physiol.,* 46:155–176.

746. Reference deleted in proof.

747. Vetter, N. J., Strange, R. C., Adams, W., and Oliver, M. F. (1974): Initial metabolic and hormonal response to acute myocardial infarction. *Lancet,* 1:284–289.

748. Videbaek, J., Christensen, N. J., and Sterndorff, B. (1972): Serial determination of plasma catecholamines in myocardial infarction. *Circulation,* 46:846–855.

749. Villalobos-Molina, R., Mirna, U. C., Hong, E., and García-Sáinz, J. A. (1982): Correlation between phosphatidylinositol labeling and contraction in rabbit aorta: Effect of alpha-1 adrenergic activation. *J. Pharmacol. Exp. Ther.,* 222:258–261.

750. Vincent, G. M., Abildskov, J. A., and Burgess, M. J. (1974): Q-T interval syndrome. *Prog. Cardiovasc. Dis.,* 16:523–530.

751. Vincenzi, F. F., and West, T. C. (1963): Release of autonomic mediators in cardiac tissue by direct subthreshold electrical stimulation. *J. Pharmacol. Exp. Ther.,* 141:185–194.

752. Vizi, E. S. (1972): Stimulation, by inhibition of (Na$^+$-K$^+$-Mg^{2+})-activated ATPase, of acetylcholine release in cortical slices from rat brain. *J. Physiol. (Lond.),* 226:95–117.

753. Vizi, E. S. (1979): Presynaptic modulation of neurochemical transmission. *Prog. Neurobiol.,* 12:181–290.

754. Vizi, E. S., and Knoll, J. (1976): The inhibitory effect of adenosine and related nucleotides on the release of acetylcholine. *Neuroscience,* 1:391–396.

755. Vogel, S. A., Silberstein, S. D., Berv, K. R., and Kopin, I. J. (1972): Stimulation-induced release of norepinephrine from rat superior cervical ganglion in vitro. *Eur. J. Pharmacol.,* 20:308–311.

756. Vourc'h, G., and Tannières, M. L. (1978): Cardiac arrhythmia induced by pneumoencephalography. *Br. J. Anaesth.,* 50:833–839.

757. Wagner, J., and Brodde, O.-E. (1978): On the presence and distribution of α-adrenoceptors in the heart of various mammalian species. *Naunyn Schmiedebergs Arch. Pharmacol.,* 302:239–254.

758. Wagner, J., and Reinhardt, D. (1974): Characterisation of the

adrenoceptors mediating the positive ino- and chronotropic effect of phenylephrine on isolated atria from guinea pigs and rabbits by means of adrenolytic drugs. *Naunyn Schmiedebergs Arch. Pharmacol.*, 282:295–306.

759. Wakade, A. R., and Furchgott, R. F. (1968): Metabolic requirements for the uptake and storage of norepinephrine by the isolated left atrium of the guinea pig. *J. Pharmacol. Exp. Ther.*, 163:123–135.

760. Wallace, A. G., and Sarnoff, S. J. (1964): Effects of sympathetic nerve stimulation on conduction in the heart. *Circ. Res.*, 14:86–92.

761. Wallace, A. G., Schaal, S., Tauneaki, S., Rozear, M., and Alexander, J. A. (1967): The electrophysiologic effects of beta-adrenergic blockade and cardiac denervation. *Bull. N.Y. Acad. Med.*, 43:1119–1137.

762. Ward, O. C. (1964): A new familial cardiac syndrome in children. *J. Ir. Med. Assoc.*, 54:103–106.

763. Warren, J. V., and Lewis, R. P. (1976): Beneficial effects of atropine in the prehospital phase of coronary care. *Am. J. Cardiol.*, 37:68–72.

764. Wasserman, F., Choquette, G., Cassinelli, R., and Bellet, S. (1956): Electrocardiographic observations in patients with cerebrovascular accidents. *Am. J. Med. Sci.*, 231:502–510.

765. Watanabe, A. M. (1984): Cellular mechanisms of muscarinic regulation of cardiac function. In: *Nervous Control of Cardiovascular Function*, edited by W. C. Randall, pp. 130–164. Oxford University Press, New York.

766. Watanabe, A. M., and Besch, H. R., Jr. (1975): Interaction between cyclic adenosine monophosphate and cyclic guanosine monophosphate in guinea pig ventricular myocardium. *Circ. Res.*, 37:309–317.

767. Watkins, P. J., and Edmonds, M. E. (1983): Sympathetic nerve failure in diabetes. *Diabetologia*, 25:73–77.

768. Waxman, M. B., Wald, R. W., and Cameron, D. (1983): Interactions between the autonomic nervous system and tachycardias in man. *Cardiology Clinics*, 1:143–185.

769. Waxman, M. B., Wald, R. W., Sharma, A. D., Huerta, F., and Cameron, D. A. (1980): Vagal techniques for termination of paroxysmal supraventricular tachycardia. *Am. J. Cardiol.*, 46:655–664.

770. Webb, S. W., Adgey, A. A. J., and Pantridge, J. F. (1972): Autonomic disturbance at onset of acute myocardial infarction. *Br. Med. J.*, 3:89–92.

771. Weisfogel, G. M., Batsford, W. P., Paulay, K. L., Josephson, M. E., Ogunkelu, J. B., Akhtar, M., Seides, S. F., and Damato, A. N. (1975): Sinus node re-entrant tachycardia in man. *Am. Heart J.*, 90:295–304.

772. Weisfogel, G. M., Stein, R. A., Fernaine, A., and Krasnow, N. (1979): Increasing pre-excitation during exercise and isoproterenol infusion. Evidence for a catecholamine sensitive bypass tract. *J. Electrocardiol.*, 12:315–320.

773. Weisman, G. G., Jones, D. S., and Randall, W. C. (1966): Sympathetic outflows from cervical spinal cord in the dog. *Science*, 152:381–382.

774. Wellens, H. J. J. (1976): The electrophysiologic properties of the accessory pathway in the Wolff-Parkinson-White syndrome. In: *The Conduction System of the Heart, Structure, Function and Clinical Implications*, edited by H. J. J. Wellens, K. I. Lie, and M. J. Janse, pp. 567–612. Lea & Febiger, Philadelphia.

775. Wellens, H. J. J., and Durrer, D. (1974): Relation between refractory period of the accessory pathway and ventricular frequency during atrial fibrillation in patients with Wolff-Parkinson-White syndrome. *Am. J. Cardiol.*, 33:178.

776. Wellens, H. J. J., Brugada, P., Roy, D., Weiss, J., and Bär, F. W. (1982): Effect of isoproterenol on the antegrade refractory period of the accessory pathway in patients with the Wolff-Parkinson-White syndrome. *Am. J. Cardiol.*, 50:180–184.

777. Wellens, H. J. J., Farré, J., Brugada, P., and Bär, F. W. H. M. (1982): The method of programmed stimulation in the study of ventricular tachycardia. In: *Ventricular Tachycardia—Mechanisms and Management*, edited by M. E. Josephson, pp. 237–283. Futura Publishing, Mt. Kisco, N.Y.

778. West, T. C., and Toda, N. (1967): Response of the A-V node of the rabbit to stimulation of intracardiac cholinergic nerves. *Circ. Res.*, 20:18–31.

779. West, T. C., Falk, G., and Cervoni, P. (1956): Drug alteration of transmembrane potentials in atrial pacemaker cells. *J. Pharmacol. Exp. Ther.*, 117:245–252.

780. Westfall, T. C. (1977): Local regulation of adrenergic neurotransmission. *Physiol. Rev.*, 57:659–728.

781. Westfall, T. C. (1984): Evidence that noradrenergic transmitter release is regulated by presynaptic receptors. *Fed. Proc.*, 43:1352–1357.

782. Wiegand, V., Güggi, M., Meesmann, W., Kessler, M., and Greitschus, F. (1979): Extracellular potassium activity changes in the canine myocardium after acute coronary occlusion and the influence of β-blockade. *Cardiovasc. Res.*, 13:297–302.

783. Wikberg, J. (1978): Pharmacological classification of adrenergic α receptors in the guinea pig. *Nature*, 273:164–166.

784. Wikberg, J. E. S., and Lefkowitz, R. J. (1984): Adrenergic receptors in the heart: Pre- and postsynaptic mechanisms. In: *Nervous Control of Cardiovascular Function*, edited by W. C. Randall, pp. 95–129. Oxford University Press, New York.

785. Wilhelmsson, C., Vedin, J. A., Wilhelmsen, L., Tibblin, G., and Werkö, L. (1974): Reduction of sudden deaths after myocardial infarction by treatment with alprenolol: Preliminary results. *Lancet*, 2:1157–1160.

786. Williams, L. T., Guerrero, J. L., and Leinbach, R. C. (1982): Prevention of reperfusion dysrhythmia by selective coronary alpha-adrenergic blockade. *Am. J. Cardiol.*, 49:1046.

787. Willman, V. L., Cooper, T., Kaiser, G. C., and Hanlon, C. R. (1965): Cardiovascular response after cardiac autotransplant in primate. *Arch. Surg.*, 91:805–806.

788. Wit, A. L., Hoffman, B. F., and Rosen, M. R. (1975): Electrophysiology and pharmacology of cardiac arrhythmias. IX. Cardiac electrophysiologic effects of beta adrenergic receptor stimulation and blockade. *Am. Heart J.*, 90:521–533.

789. Wolff, L., Parkinson, J., and White, P. D. (1930): Bundle-branch block with short P-R interval in healthy young people prone to paroxysmal tachycardia. *Am. Heart J.*, 5:685–704.

790. Wollenberger, A., and Shahab, L. (1965): Anoxia-induced release of noradrenaline from the isolated perfused heart. *Nature*, 207:88–89.

791. Wu, D., Denes, P., Bauernfeind, R., Dhingra, R. C., Wyndham, C., and Rosen, K. M. (1979): Effects of atropine on induction and maintenance of atrioventricular nodal reentrant tachycardia. *Circulation*, 59:779–788.

792. Wu, D., Denes, P., Dhingra, R., Khan, A., and Rosen, K. M. (1974): The effects of propranolol on induction of A-V nodal reentrant paroxysmal tachycardia. *Circulation*, 50:665–677.

793. Wurster, R. D. (1984): Central nervous system regulation of the heart: An overview. In: *Nervous Control of Cardiovascular Function*, edited by W. C. Randall, pp. 307–320. Oxford University Press, New York.

794. Wurster, R. D., and Randall, W. C. (1979): Cardiovascular responses to bladder distension in patients with spinal transection. *Am. J. Physiol.*, 228:1288–1292.

795. Yamada, K. A., McAllen, R. M., and Loewy, A. D. (1984): GABA antagonists applied to the ventral surface of the medulla oblongata block the baroreceptor reflex. *Brain Res.*, 297:175–180.

796. Yamaguchi, N., DeChamplain, J., and Nadeau, R. A. (1977): Regulation of norepinephrine release from cardiac sympathetic fibers in the dog by presynaptic alpha- and beta-receptors. *Circ. Res.*, 41:108–117.

797. Yanowitz, F., Preston, J. B., and Abildskov, J. A. (1966): Functional distribution of right and left stellate innervation to the ventricles: Production of neurogenic electrocardiographic changes by unilateral alteration of sympathetic tone. *Circ. Res.*, 18:416–428.

798. Yoon, M. S., Han, J., Tse, W. W., and Rogers, R. (1977): Effect of vagal stimulation, atropine and propranolol on fibrillation threshold of normal and ischaemic ventricles. *Am. Heart J.*, 93:60–65.

799. Zimmerman, B. G., and Whitmore, L. (1967): Effect of angiotensin and phenoxybenzamine on release of norepinephrine in vessels during sympathetic nerve stimulation. *Int. J. Neuropharmacol.*, 6:27–38.

The Heart and Cardiovascular System,
edited by H. A. Fozzard et al.
Raven Press, New York © 1986.

CHAPTER 59

Epidemiology of Ventricular Arrhythmias and Clinical Trials with Antiarrhythmic Drugs

J. Thomas Bigger, Jr., Linda M. Rolnitzky, and Jacques Merab

It is our objective in this chapter to discuss the prevalence and significance of ventricular arrhythmias in apparently normal persons and in patients with heart disease. We shall discuss the methods currently used to detect and quantify ventricular arrhythmias and the methods used to classify them. We shall discuss the prevalence and significance of ventricular arrhythmias in normal subjects as a function of age and sex and in patients with various etiologic forms of heart disease. We shall discuss the relationship between sporadic ventricular arrhythmias and symptomatic, sustained ventricular arrhythmias and mortality. Also, we shall consider how ventricular arrhythmias relate to the severity of left ventricular dysfunction in patients with cardiac disease. Spontaneous variabilities in the frequency and complexity of ventricular arrhythmias will be discussed as they relate to the possibility of misclassification of patients or as they relate to the conclusions drawn about the effect of therapy. Finally, we shall discuss the conduct of trials to determine the effects of drugs proposed for control of ventricular arrhythmias. Although many electrophysiologic mechanisms have been shown to be capable of producing ventricular arrhythmias, clinical epidemiologic studies have not attempted, to any significant extent, to relate the mechanisms of ventricular arrhythmias to outcomes such as death or the occurrence of symptomatic, sustained ventricular arrhythmias. This type of investigation remains for the future.

DETECTION AND QUANTIFICATION OF VENTRICULAR ARRHYTHMIAS

Ventricular arrhythmias arise in the ventricles, i.e., in an "ectopic location." These events are often asymptomatic and for more than 70 years have been detected by their characteristically wide QRS complex, along with other features. Because ventricular arrhythmias often occur sporadically, reasonably long samples of EKGs are required to obtain an accurate estimate of the frequency and character of ventricular arrhythmias in an individual.

Holter EKG Recordings

The invention of the Holter technique was a critical step forward for study of the epidemiology of cardiac arrhythmias. This technique permits 24- to 48-hr continuous two-lead EKG recordings to sample normal cardiac rhythm and arrhythmias. Modern computer methods permit accurate and reproducible analysis of the massive amount of data essential for obtaining sufficient EKG data to correlate with other predictor or outcome variables.

Continuous Recorders

There are now more than a dozen portable reel-to-reel or cassette recorders available for recording ambulatory EKGs. Modern continuous EKG recorders are light in weight (0.3–0.9 kg) and are worn on shoulder straps or belts (11,123). Most record two channels of EKG data and are powered by disposable alkaline batteries or rechargeable nickel/cadmium batteries. Also, modern recorders permit patients to insert a high-frequency signal into one of the recorded leads when symptoms occur. These markers permit careful analysis of the relationship between symptoms and corresponding arrhythmic events. Some recorders have a clock display that can be used by the patient in conjunction with the event marker to note the time of symptoms.

Reel-to-reel recorders use two-track heads to record the EKG on 6.4-mm-wide magnetic tape coated with ferric oxide or chromium dioxide (123). Cassette recorders use four-track heads to record signals on 3.2-mm-wide magnetic tape coated with ferric oxide. The third track of the cassette recorder is used as a timing track to modulate playback speed and correct for deviations that occur in recording rate (usually up to 20%). This is particularly important, because cassette monitors tend to have less precise tape-transport mechanisms than their reel-to-reel counterparts. Because cassette recorders record four tracks of information on a 3.2-mm-wide tape and reel-to-reel recorders record two tracks of information on 6.4-mm-wide tape, cassette recordings tend to be noisier than reel-to-reel recordings (11).

Virtually all recorder manufacturers indicate that their recorders have a frequency response of 0.05 to 100 Hz (−3 db), the frequency response recommended by the American Heart Association for diagnostic-quality, di-

rect-writing EKG machines. However, Bragg-Remschel et al. (26) evaluated eight recorders and found that none had the frequency response recommended by the American Heart Association. Most recorders have adequate bandwidth for ventricular arrhythmia detection, but their accuracy for quantitative S-T-segment analysis requires further investigation (11,26,190).

Analysis of Holter EKG Recordings

AVSEP. Audiovisual superimposed EKG presentation (AVSEP) is a technique developed in 1961 by Holter and associates for rapid analysis of recorded long-term EKGs (64,78). This technique was used to analyze recordings from the first epidemiologic studies. Tapes were played back at a speed of 7.5 inches per second, which was 60 times faster than the recorded speed of 7.5 inches per minute. Later, units that play recordings back at 120 or 240 times real time were developed. The AVSEP system playing back the tape at 60 to 240 times real time (recording speed) presents the EKG signals on an oscilloscope, with each QRS superimposed on the preceding QRS complex. If the morphology and R-R cycle lengths are unchanged, this procedure results in a stable and unchanging EKG signal on the oscilloscope screen. The EKG signal also is translated to an audio signal with a pitch that varies with the R-R interval. The system loudspeaker produces a steady hum when both rate and QRS-T patterns remain unchanged. Ventricular premature depolarizations (VPDs) are identified by seeing the characteristic VPD morphology on screen and hearing a simultaneous drop in tone on the audio output. Holter (78) also developed an arrhythmiograph that converted each R-R interval to a vertical line, with height proportional to R-R interval to permit graphic display of cycle length changes that might be missed on the EKG display. AVSEP scanners are prone to miss short runs of ventricular tachycardia (13).

Computerized analysis of Holter EKG recordings. State-of-the-art analysis of Holter EKG recordings involves the use of digital computers to perform high-speed analysis of 24-hr EKG recordings to take advantage of certain computer attributes: speed, tirelessness, and reproducibility (51,133). Figure 1 indicates the typical steps in computer analysis of a 24-hr EKG recording. Many analysis systems do substantial analog preprocessing prior to or during digitization of the EKG signals, e.g., analog filtering, QRS or pacemaker pulse detection. The first step in computer analysis is detection of the QRS. After the QRS is detected, its beginning and end are delineated, and certain features of the QRS complex are measured and used to classify QRS morphology. Alternatively, the QRS or QRS-T can be matched to the template of a QRS complex that has been called normal by the operator during setup. Feature-extraction and correlation-template methods can be used separately

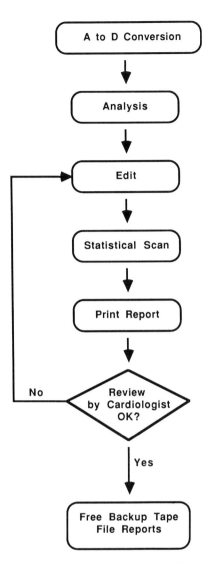

FIG. 1. Holter processing flow chart. Steps in 24-hr continuous EKG analysis by a typical computerized arrhythmia detector.

data and stored in a computerized research data base. For epidemiologic research, it is important to use a computerized system with known reproducibility and accuracy to analyze Holter EKG recordings. Reproducibility can be evaluated by reprocessing EKG recordings in a blinded fashion. Accuracy is much harder to evaluate, because it requires validation on data bases of EKG recordings in which every QRS complex has been labeled and reviewed by a panel of experts.

Only recently have two data bases of validated, labeled QRS complexes become available: the American Heart Association (AHA) data base of ventricular arrhythmias and the Massachusetts Institute of Technology–Beth Israel Hospital (MIT/BIH) data base of ventricular and supraventricular arrhythmias. The AHA data base has a learning set of 80 tapes and a test set of 80 tapes (72). Each tape consists of 3 hr of two-channel EKG data, with the last 30 min containing validated, labeled QRS complexes. The MIT/BIH data base consists of 48 two-channel Holter EKG recordings, each 30 min in length (104). There are two series of tapes in the MIT/BIH annotated data set. The 100 series consists of 23 tapes randomly selected from a library of 4,000 tapes. The 200 series consists of 25 tapes selected for events of clinical interest. Every QRS complex in both series of the MIT/BIH set is annotated. After a set of annotated tapes has been analyzed, sensitivity and positive predictive accuracy are used to summarize the performance of the computerized analysis system. These are defined as follows:

$$\text{sensitivity} = \frac{\text{true positives}}{\text{true positives} + \text{false negatives}}$$

$$\frac{\text{positive}}{\text{predictive accuracy}} = \frac{\text{true positives}}{\text{true positives} + \text{false positives}}$$

On many recordings, automatic arrhythmia detectors achieve over 99% sensitivity and 97% predictive accuracy for ventricular ectopy activity (21).

Duration of Holter recordings. The duration of EKG recording used in epidemiologic studies of cardiac arrhythmias varies with the objective of the study and with the cost and practicality of making the recordings. Bigger et al. (12) examined the relationship between the probability of detecting VPD and the duration of recording in a set of 200 24-hr ambulatory EKG recordings made 2 weeks after acute myocardial infarction. All 200 patients included in the study were hospitalized, and their activities were reasonably standardized with respect to exercise, meals, and visiting hours. The 24-hr EKG recordings were analyzed by the computer program Columbia IV, using strict quality-control measures (21). Table 1 gives the expected VPD rates (middle column) needed to detect VPDs in records 1 min and 1, 6, and 24 hr in duration. The expectation given is based on

or combined in order to classify QRS morphology. QRS shape information, along with R-R interval and perhaps context information, can be used to label each QRS as follows: normal, supraventricular premature complex, ventricular premature complex, ventricular escape complex, or unknown. As the analysis proceeds, a file accumulates that indicates the label of each QRS and the time since the previous QRS, along with other information that may be useful in editing the results. After the automated analysis is complete, the results are edited. Modern editing programs permit propagation of certain decisions to all members of a class or family of QRS complexes. When editing is complete, the results are documented by printing the important EKG events that occurred during the 24-hr EKG recording. Then the results are reviewed by a cardiologist. The information from Holter EKG analysis can be merged with demographic and historical information and laboratory

the assumption that VPD frequency is spread evenly throughout the 24-hr period. For example, if VPDs were equally likely to occur in each hour of the day, an average daily frequency of about 50 per hour would be required in order for a VPD to be detected in an EKG recording of 40- to 50-sec duration. The right column in Table 1 gives the actual proportion of patients in the sample who had the theoretical VPD rates listed in the middle column. A 1-hr recording should detect patients who have one or more VPDs per hour; 47% of the study patients had a frequency of one or more VPDs per hour. These considerations suggest that the 1-hr daytime EKG recording employed by the HIP study gives a reasonable estimate of the proportion of patients who have VPD frequencies of one per hour or greater (152,153). To examine further the ability of 1-hr EKG recordings to classify VPD frequency, Bigger et al. (12) classified their 200 patients using the first hour of a 24-hr EKG recording and compared the result with the findings in the remaining 23 hr. Table 2 shows the association between the VPD count in the first hour and the average VPD count in the remaining 23 hr. The overall χ^2 is large, indicating a significant lack of correspondence between the two variables (Stuart-Maxwell $\chi^2 = 73.9$). Inspection of Table 2 shows that counts above zero in the first hour correspond reasonably well with the average VPD frequency in the last 23 hr. Most of the large χ^2 is caused by the 75 patients who had no VPD in the first hour but had 1 to 230 VPDs in the remainder of the tape. This was formally evaluated by collapsing the 3 × 3 table shown in Table 2 into two 2 × 2 tables, one partitioned as presence versus absence of VPDs (McNemar $\chi^2 = 72.1$) and another for VPDs fewer than 10 versus 10 or more (McNemar $\chi^2 = 0.8$). Thus, a 1-hr recording performs very well in detecting persons with moderately frequent or frequent VPDs; it will produce many false negatives in the group with a low frequency of VPDs.

Next, the ability of EKG recordings of various lengths to identify patients with certain complex VPD features was examined (12). Figure 2 shows the cumulative frequency of paired VPDs, ventricular tachycardia (three or more consecutive VPDs), R-on-T, and complex VPDs (defined as any combination of the aforementioned

TABLE 1. Relationship among duration of EKG recording, VPD frequency, and probability of detecting VPDs

Duration of recordings	Average VPDs per hour needed for detection (expected)	% With VPDs present (observed)
1 min	50.00	11
1 hr	1.00	47
6 hr	0.17	66
24 hr	0.04	84

TABLE 2. Relationship between VPD count in the first hour and average VPD frequency in the last 23 hr of a 24-hr EKG recording[a]

| VPD count, first hour | Average no. of VPDs, last 23 hr | | | Total |
	0	>0–<10	≥10	
0	35	75	2	112
1–9	1	41	6	48
≥10	0	4	36	40
Total	36	120	44	200

[a] Stuart-Maxwell $\chi^2 = 73.9$; d.f. = 4.

characteristics) as a function of EKG duration for a 24-hr period. As shown in Fig. 2, detection of these VPD features increases nonlinearly as a function of recording duration. For all features except ventricular tachycardia, the rate of rise in incidence was much greater in the first 6 to 12 hr than in the latter portion of the recording. In contrast, ventricular tachycardia incidence accumulates almost linearly over the entire 24-hr recording period. The steeper initial slope found for most features may be attributable to the fact that the waking hours were always in the first half of the EKG recording. The almost linear rise in detection of ventricular tachycardia over 24 hr suggests that longer recordings will significantly improve the detection of persons with this arrhythmia. The cumulative percentages of complex VPDs, R-on-T, paired VPDs, and ventricular tachycardia each were calculated as a function of the recording duration; 100% was taken as the total number of persons who had a given feature in the entire 24-hr record. In the first hour, about 30% of the persons who had R-on-T VPDs at any time during the 24-hr EKG were detected. However, only 20% of those with ventricular tachycardia were detected in the first hour. By the sixth hour of recording, about 40 to 60% of persons with any given complex VPD feature were detected. For individual characteristics such as R-on-T or paired VPDs or ventricular tachycardia, the greater the proportion of persons with the characteristic, the more were identified in a relatively brief monitoring period. Detection in the first 6 hr of about half the patients with a complex VPD feature may be due to the fact that recordings were started during the morning, i.e., frequent, complex VPDs are more likely to occur during the day. Certainly by the 12th hour of the recording a substantial fraction of the patients with one or more complex features had been identified.

Also, the interaction of VPD frequency with complexity was examined, searching for a way to predict rare events from brief recordings. Only one strong relationship emerged from this analysis. Ten or more VPDs in the first hour identified 12 of the 18 persons (67%) who had ventricular tachycardia on a 24-hr

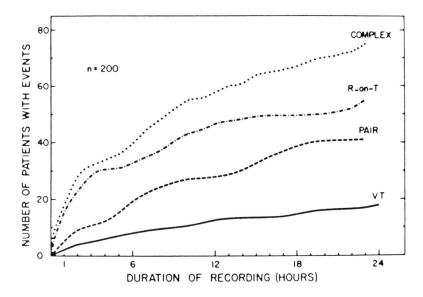

FIG. 2. Detection of complex ventricular arrhythmias as a function of the duration of the recording.

recording, even though only 3 actually had an episode of ventricular tachycardia in the first hour. Twelve of the 40 persons (30%) who had 10 or more VPDs in the first hour had ventricular tachycardia on a 24-hr recording.

Winkle et al. (189) also studied the relationship between the duration of continuous EKG recordings and the likelihood of detecting ventricular tachycardia. They recorded EKGs for 72 consecutive hours in 57 patients 8 to 11 days after myocardial infarction. One 24-hr recording performed very well with respect to detection of VPD frequency of 10 or more per hour. Also, there was more than 90% day-to-day concordance on this level of frequency. The detection of ventricular tachycardia was quite different. Of the 12 patients ultimately found to have ventricular tachycardia, none was detected in the first 6 hr of recording; only 5 patients (42%) were detected in the first 24 hr, and 7 patients (58%) in the first 48 hr. Winkle et al. (189) commented that long recording periods may be required to detect ventricular tachycardia. However, using long recordings may obligate the investigator to use the frequency of ventricular tachycardia events to classify patients, rather than just presence or absence.

So many factors bear on the decision about how many hours of EKG to record and analyze for observational studies that conclusions must be individualized for each study. If complex VPD features are to be fully accounted for, 12 to 24 hr of EKG recording would seem to be a minimum requirement when doing observational studies in patients with recent acute myocardial infarction.

Other Methods for Quantifying Spontaneous Ventricular Arrhythmias

The Holter technique of continuously recording the EKG for 1 to 72 hr has been used most commonly for studies of the epidemiology of cardiac arrhythmias. However, new technology is available that could be adapted for future studies (11,123). Two important new devices with potential for epidemiologic research are the intermittent recorders and the real-time recorders.

Intermittent EKG Recorders

Intermittent recorders have been used primarily to study symptoms that suggest arrhythmias but occur too infrequently to be recorded using a 24-hr continuous EKG recording. A large array of recording devices have been marketed, each with a slightly different concept for documenting the cardiac rhythm at the time of symptoms. Some units are attached via EKG skin electrodes all the time, whereas with other units, electrodes are applied by the patient when symptoms occur. Recorders also may have on-board memory that can store EKG recordings for telephone transmission or for recording on a tape recorder. Intermittent recorders are usually activated by the patient when symptoms occur, by pushing a button or switch. Passive recorders will lose the onset of symptomatic arrhythmias, but those with memory can document the onset of the arrhythmia if the recorder is activated within a minute or so of its onset. For some epidemiologic investigations, patient-activated intermittent recorders could be useful for identifying the cause of occasional arrhythmic symptoms and relating them to outcomes of interest. Also, intermittent recorders are available that take samples at predefined times over many days. This type of recorder could be used to implement innovative sampling strategies for epidemiologic research in cardiac arrhythmias. Also, transtelephonic systems can provide immediate feedback and could be used to conduct trials with experimental treatments. When a symptom is experienced, the patient can phone in and verify the presence of the qualifying arrhythmia by transmitting a recording. Then the patient can take the trial medication, e.g., active drug or placebo, and the results can be documented at an appropriate time by another EKG transmission. This type of system permits control and documentation of the arrhythmia and treatment. Also, appropriate safeguards can be instituted; thus, transtelephonic monitoring systems can increase the range of ethical investigation of potentially malignant or malignant cardiac arrhythmias.

Real-Time EKG Monitoring

Another technique with significant potential for epidemiologic research in cardiac arrhythmias is real-time EKG monitoring, a technique that incorporates the EKG acquisition and analysis phases of the Holter concept. A computer programmed with arrhythmia-detection algorithms is worn by the patient and analyzes the EKG in real time, storing digital results. The device worn by the patient is ready to produce a report of the heart rate and rhythm when the patient returns after the monitoring interval. Some computer/recorders provide feedback to enlist the patient's help in the monitoring or documentation processes. These devices may indicate loose electrodes, battery failure, or arrhythmic events. Currently available devices usually communicate via signal lights. In the future, we expect that real-time monitoring devices will use voice synthesizers for communication. In addition to warnings, real-time monitoring equipment can ask about activities and symptoms or give protocol instructions when programmed, individualized conditions are satisfied. There are many problems to solve before the potential of real-time monitoring for cardiac arrhythmia detection can be fully realized. The current generation of real-time monitoring equipment will require additional development and testing of arrhythmia-detection algorithms before achieving acceptance as accurate and reliable tools for epidemiologic research. To date, most real-time recorders have incorporated or adapted algorithms from CCU computerized arrhythmia detectors or, more often, from high-speed computerized arrhythmia detectors in Holter scanning systems. Adapting algorithms from these two environments has caused serious problems and probably will never bring real-time monitoring to its full potential. For future generations of real-time monitoring systems, new algorithms should be developed that will address the unique problems of this mode of monitoring. The real-time monitoring systems can take advantage of the fact that they have 60 to 480 times as much time to process the EKG data as does a high-speed computerized Holter EKG analysis system. This provides the opportunity to use signal-processing techniques, e.g., EKG transforms and digital filters, that would be unthinkably slow for Holter analysis systems. Herein lies the oppor-

tunity to develop the sophisticated algorithms that will be required in the future to translate the concepts of real-time monitoring for the needs of epidemiologic research on cardiac arrhythmias. When real-time arrhythmia-detection algorithms have been developed and tested adequately, these devices will significantly extend the capabilities for observational and experimental epidemiologic studies.

Exercise Testing

A number of studies have evaluated exercise testing as a method for detecting cardiac arrhythmias for epidemiologic research. The general conclusion has been that exercise is much less sensitive than 24-hr continuous EKG recordings for detecting arrhythmias. A few studies have surveyed ventricular arrhythmias during exercise testing in populations of coronary heart disease patients and related these to subsequent mortality (9,35,96,132, 157,177,182,185). For the most part, those studies that have focused on arrhythmias detected during exercise testing early (less than 30 days) after myocardial infarction have shown that they are associated with subsequent mortality (96,185). The positive studies were careful to record the EKG continuously during the exercise test session so that VPDs could be quantified precisely (185). Comparing exercise arrhythmias with those detected by 24-hr continuous recordings in the same patients reveals that the exercise test is less sensitive overall but is more sensitive per unit time, i.e., the rate of detection is higher with exercise testing (185). It may be that previous studies did not use methods that were accurate enough for detecting ventricular arrhythmias, and thus exercise should be reevaluated as an efficient means for evaluating ventricular arrhythmias in epidemiologic studies. Exercise is likely to be more valuable for establishing risk than for evaluating the effects of antiarrhythmic therapy, because exercise ventricular arrhythmias show even more day-to-day variability than 24-hr continuous EKG recordings (167).

Electrophysiologic Studies

There has been great difficulty in diagnosis and treatment of malignant sustained ventricular arrhythmias, i.e., sustained ventricular tachycardia and ventricular fibrillation. Because the clinical presentation of these arrhythmias is often so dramatic, they usually are not documented adequately, i.e., patients often are treated with cardioversion or defibrillation without first having a 12-lead EKG. Lack of documentation causes severe limitations in arrhythmia research and management. When patients are found in ventricular fibrillation, it is not possible to know how the rhythm began, e.g., as a result of primary ventricular tachycardia or as a result of an ischemic attack. Continuous 24-hr EKG recording was the first method used to study ventricular arrhythmias in patients who presented with sustained ventricular tachycardia. This method was used to evaluate spontaneous unsustained ventricular arrhythmias in patients who presented with sustained ventricular arrhythmias and to guide therapy with antiarrhythmic drugs. One of the problems with this approach is that it assumes that spontaneous arrhythmias and their responses to treatment reflect the responses of sustained arrhythmias. Also, about 20 to 25% of patients will have very few spontaneous ventricular arrhythmias in a 24-hr EKG recorded soon after an episode of sustained ventricular arrhythmia. The frequency of recurrence of sustained ventricular tachycardia and ventricular fibrillation in patients who have presented with clinical episodes is variable, but often low. A period of telemetry in hospital or several 24-hr Holter EKG recordings nearly always fail to document the onset of sustained ventricular arrhythmias. Based on principles learned in the study of supraventricular tachycardia, programmed ventricular stimulation has been used to provoke sustained ventricular arrhythmias. By pacing the ventricles and applying premature stimuli, sustained ventricular tachycardia usually can be provoked in a patient who has experienced a clinical episode of malignant ventricular arrhythmia. Many questions have been raised about this technique. Are the sustained ventricular arrhythmias evoked by programmed ventricular stimulation the same as those that occurred spontaneously? What are the sensitivity, specificity, and reproducibility of the technique? Which stimulation protocol should be used? Does the sensitivity or specificity depend on the presence of or type of heart disease?

Substantial data exist on the comparability of spontaneous ventricular tachycardia and the ventricular tachycardia that is induced by programmed ventricular stimulation. In patients with recurrent sustained ventricular tachycardia, an arrhythmia that is similar in rate and morphology can be induced in the majority of cases, depending on the intensity of the stimulation protocol. Additional arrhythmias, i.e., ventricular tachycardia with a different morphology or ventricular fibrillation, are occasionally induced, particularly with intense programmed ventricular stimulation. Currently, induction of sustained uniform ventricular tachycardia in patients with spontaneous sustained ventricular tachycardia is thought to represent a true-positive response. To support this point of view, more and more cases are accumulating in which a "nonclinical" tachycardia occurs spontaneously during follow-up. Conversely, the current concept is that ventricular fibrillation induced during V1V2V3V4 stimulation, i.e., with three premature stimuli, is a false-positive response in patients who have recurrent, sustained uniform ventricular tachycardia clinically.

With respect to programmed ventricular stimulation, sensitivity is the probability of inducing sustained ventricular tachycardia in patients with spontaneous sustained ventricular tachycardia. Substantial data exist on the sensitivity of programmed ventricular stimulation as a function of the intensity of stimulation in patients with recurrent, sustained ventricular tachycardia. Table 3 shows that sensitivity increases from about 30% to 90% as the number of premature stimuli increases from one to three (32,53,100,107,180). In addition to intensity of stimulation, several other factors substantially influence the sensitivity of programmed ventricular stimulation: presence and type of heart disease; arrhythmia history; the definition of a positive response, e.g., sustained ventricular tachycardia versus ventricular fibrillation; adjunctive maneuvers used during programmed ventricular stimulation, e.g., isoproterenol infusion. If one restricts attention to patients who have sustained ventricular tachycardia clinically, the sensitivity of programmed ventricular stimulation seems to vary with the type of cardiac disease. It is often said that programmed ventricular stimulation has greater sensitivity in patients with coronary heart disease than in patients with cardiomyopathy, mitral valve prolapse, or no detectable heart disease. The experience of Prystowsky et al. (143) with the sensitivity of programmed ventricular stimulation in patients who had clinical episodes of sustained ventricular tachycardia but no coronary heart disease runs counter to this view (143). They found that programmed ventricular stimulation had excellent sensitivity (83%) in patients who had no apparent heart disease. Sensitivity was lower (60%) in cardiomyopathy. The number of patients with mitral valve prolapse was too small to give a reliable estimate of sensitivity, but 6 of 7 patients (86%) were inducible. Other groups have found sensitivity to be lower in patients with mitral valve prolapse (30). The probability of detecting ventricular tachycardia is greater in patients with clinically documented sustained ventricular tachycardia (31,150,155) and less in patients who are resuscitated after cardiac arrest (120,150,155). Sustained ventricular arrhythmias are induced with programmed ventricular stimulation in 40 to 70% of cardiac arrest survivors. This low probability can be attributed to the varied pathophysiologies that can initiate ventric-

TABLE 3. Sensitivity and specificity of programmed ventricular stimulation[a]

Number of premature stimuli	Sensitivity (%)	Specificity (%)
1	30–40	100
2	60–70	100
3	80–90	100

[a] Specificity defined as the induction of sustained, uniform ventricular tachycardia.

ular fibrillation. Some episodes occur in patients with scarred ventricles and are initiated by a run of sustained ventricular tachycardia; these are likely to have inducible sustained ventricular tachycardia. Other episodes of ventricular fibrillation are induced by a period of intense ischemia; these are unlikely to have inducible sustained ventricular tachycardia.

Specificity is the probability of a negative test response among patients free of the condition of interest. If sustained ventricular tachycardia is taken as the endpoint, then the specificity of programmed ventricular stimulation is 100% even when three premature stimuli are used (20,29,53,100,180). However, three premature stimuli elicited unsustained ventricular tachycardia in about 25% and ventricular fibrillation in about 5% of the patients studied (29,121).

There is still relatively little information available on the day-to-day reproducibility of programmed ventricular stimulation. Recently, Bigger et al. (20) reported a prospective study to determine the between-day reproducibility of inducible ventricular tachycardia in terms of being sustained or nonsustained and, secondarily, to determine if inducible ventricular tachycardia was reproducible in terms of morphology and rate. Of the 181 patients who had ventricular tachycardia induced, 52 (29%) were studied on two days, drug-free and with identical stimulation protocols. The mean age for these 52 patients was 57 years; 85% of them were male, and 60% had ischemic heart disease. The indication for electrophysiologic study was documentation of sustained ventricular tachycardia or cardiac arrest in 85% and syncope in 15%. Testing was conducted drug-free, i.e., without class I, II, or III antiarrhythmic drugs. The stimulation protocol used in each study included three premature stimuli at two basic pacing rates (100 and 150 per minute) and at two right ventricular sites and burst pacing. Of 47 patients who had sustained ventricular tachycardia induced at the first study, 87% were induced during the second study. In 32 of the 41 patients (78%), the stimulation mode that was required was the same for the two studies, whereas for 13 patients (32%) a different mode of stimulation was needed. In terms of being sustained or unsustained, ventricular tachycardia was reproducible in 85% of the patients, ventricular tachycardia morphology was reproducible in 85%, and ventricular tachycardia rate was reproducible in 91%. Ventricular tachycardia was reproducible for duration, morphology, and rate in 75% of the patients. Schoenfeld et al. (163) studied the long-term reproducibility of programmed ventricular stimulation in 17 patients with ventricular arrhythmias: 10 patients with sustained ventricular tachycardia, 5 patients with unsustained ventricular tachycardia, and 2 patients with ventricular fibrillation. Heart disease was present in 14 patients, 11 of whom had coronary heart disease. The interval between the two tests averaged 18 months. All 11 patients with

coronary heart disease had ventricular tachycardia inducible at both studies, compared with only 1 of 6 patients who did not have coronary heart disease. These two small studies of day-to-day reproducibility of programmed ventricular stimulation suggest that reproducibility is good when studies are repeated after long intervals, as well as after short intervals. The data also suggest that reproducibility is a function of underlying heart disease, just as sensitivity is. With respect to reproducibility, programmed ventricular stimulation compares very favorably with the other techniques available for evaluation of patients with malignant ventricular arrhythmias, e.g., Holter EKG recording or exercise testing.

CLASSIFICATION OF VENTRICULAR ARRHYTHMIAS

It has been found that the mere presence of ventricular arrhythmias is not very specific for outcomes of interest in patients with ventricular arrhythmias, e.g., mortality from all causes, sudden cardiac death, arrhythmic death, or sustained ventricular arrhythmias. This problem has led to attempts to classify arrhythmias on some ordinal or quantitative scale that has prognostic significance (17,101,103,130).

Lown Grading System

In 1971, Lown and Wolf (103) proposed a system for grading ventricular arrhythmias in the coronary care unit. They classified arrhythmias into one of seven mutually exclusive grades. Their hypothesis was that the higher the arrhythmia grade, the more likely it is that sudden cardiac death or sustained ventricular arrhythmias will occur. The Lown grading system uses three levels of VPD frequency (0, >0 but <30, ≥30 VPDs per hour) and four complex features of VPD (multiform, paired VPD, ventricular tachycardia, and R-on-T VPD) to classify a given 24-hr continuous EKG recording into one of seven grades (Table 4). The system is mutually exclusive and hierarchical. For example, if R-on-T VPDs are present, the arrhythmia is called grade 5, regardless of VPD frequency or any other complex feature. Given the three VPD frequency categories and four complex VPD features, 33 possible arrhythmia categories can be enumerated ($2^5 + 1$). However, many of these individual categories are aggregated into single Lown grades. The Lown arrhythmia grades are assumed to be ranked in order of prognostic significance, i.e., the higher arrhythmia grade, the more likely it is that arrhythmic death or sustained ventricular arrhythmias will occur.

Bigger and Weld (18) tested three of the critical assumptions of the Lown arrhythmia grading system in a group of 400 patients who had had recent myocardial infarctions. They analyzed 24-hr, two-channel continuous

TABLE 4. *Lown arrhythmia grade and mortality for 400 patients with recent myocardial infarction*

Lown grade	Definition	No. of patients	No. of subgroups	Medium VPDs/hr	Mortality (%)
0	No VPD[a]	64	1	0.0	14
1	<30 VPDs per hour	85	1	0.1	11
2	≥30 VPDs per hour	2	1	300.0	0
3	Multiform VPDs	68	2	1.5	15
4A	Paired VPDs	44	4	5.0	20
4B	≥3 consecutive VPDs	21	8	20.0	33
5	R-on-T VPDs (R − V/QT < 1.0)	116	16	8.0	29
	All patients	400	33	1.0	20

[a] VPD = ventricular premature depolarization.
From ref. 18, with permission.

recordings made between 10 and 20 days after myocardial infarction using a digital-computer program with high sensitivity and specificity for VPD detection (21).

First, the assumption that high VPD frequency exerts negligible additional risk in patients who have complex VPD was tested. That assumption was incorrect. Frequent VPDs (10 or more per hour) doubled or tripled the risk for subsequent cardiac death in each of the four highest Lown grades, i.e., those that are assigned on the basis of complex features. Interestingly, much of the mortality gradient that is attributed to the hierarchy of complex features is attributable to a tendency for VPD frequency to increase as the Lown grade increases (Table 4). Note also in Table 4 that high VPD frequency cannot be evaluated in the Lown grading system. Only 2 of the 56 patients who had a VPD frequency of 30 or more lacked complex features and remained in Lown grade 2. The other 54 patients are scattered throughout Lown grades 3 to 5.

Second, the assumption that the Lown arrhythmia grades are ranked in order of increasing mortality risk was tested. That was not the case. Lown grade 4B has higher mortality after myocardial infarction than Lown grade 5 (Table 4). Like VPD frequency, ventricular tachycardia is not accounted for in the Lown grading system; cases of ventricular tachycardia are divided approximately equally between grades 4B and 5.

Third, the assumption that any given Lown grade is homogeneous with respect to likelihood of dying during follow-up was tested. That assumption was not true either. A lack of homogeneity was found in the Lown grades that aggregate subgroups. We have already mentioned the striking influence of VPD frequency on mortality within Lown grades 3 to 5. Additional examples of heterogeneity can be found in grade 5, a grade that contains 16 subgroups (18). In the 400 patients, the mortality in grade 5 subgroups ranged from 0 to 75%; statistically significant differences in mortality were found among the subgroups. Two *a priori* contrasts were made in Lown grade 5. First, the 22 patients who had only R-on-T VPDs without high VPD frequency or any other

complex VPD feature were compared with the 17 patients who had not only R-on-T VPDs but also high VPD frequency and all other complex features. The mortality in the former group was 9%, compared with 59% in the latter group, a difference that was statistically significant ($p < 0.001$). The second contrast was between the 58 patients in grade 5 who had repetitive VPDs and the 58 patients who did not. Those with repetitive VPDs had a mortality of 48%, compared with 10% for those who did not have repetitive VPDs, another highly significant difference ($p < 0.001$). Obviously, there is very significant heterogeneity in Lown grade 5, and the high- and low-risk subsets can be easily identified using the usual VPD characteristics that are quantified in a 24-hr continuous EKG recording. The presence or absence of high VPD frequency and the presence or absence of repetitive VPDs are the most important features for this purpose. The fundamental cause for the poor performance of the Lown grading system in observational studies of coronary heart disease was that insufficient emphasis was given to VPD frequency and to repetitive forms of VPDs.

In 1975, Lown et al. (101) extended their grading system to include an "arrhythmia equation" that enumerates the number of hours spent in each arrhythmia grade and provides details about the ventricular arrhythmias in a 24-hr EKG recording. Bigger and Weld have demonstrated the awkwardness of the arrhythmia equation (17).

Multivariate Classification

It has been shown that frequency and certain other characteristics of ventricular arrhythmias, e.g., repetitiveness, multiformity, or prematurity, can have prognostic significance. In coronary heart disease and cardiomyopathy, the most impressive associations have been between mortality and VPD frequency or repetitiveness (10,57). Also, it has been shown that VPD frequency and repetitiveness are independently associated with mortality in coronary heart disease (10,13). Therefore, the prognostic information from long-term EKG recordings can best be extracted by enumerating the VPD frequency and other characteristics and using these directly in statistical models to predict mortality or other endpoints, e.g., occurrence of sustained ventricular arrhythmias. The ventricular arrhythmia variables can be grouped on some ordinal scale or as measured. For example, VPD frequency can simply be dichotomized, to divide the study into subgroups with low and high frequencies, e.g., <10 or ≥10 VPDs per hour. Or the average VPD frequency or total VPD count during the recording period can be entered directly, e.g., log(VPD count +1). Similarly, the presence or absence of other VPD characteristics can be entered as absent or present, on an ordinal scale or as measured. For example, ventricular tachycardia can be dichotomized as absent or present, trichotomized as <5, 5 to 9, or ≥10 episodes per recording period, or used as continuous data, i.e., the average number of episodes per hour. It should be noted that using the categories absent/present or counts per recording period, patients will be classified differently depending on the duration of the recording period. Especially for rare events such as ventricular tachycardia, the likelihood of detecting an event will increase strikingly as a function of recording duration. Up to 72 to 96 hr, the probability of detecting ventricular tachycardia increases with the duration of the recording (11,176). In long continuous EKG recordings, the significance of ventricular tachycardia may vary in accordance with the number of events per unit time, analogous to average VPD frequency.

INCIDENCE AND SIGNIFICANCE OF VENTRICULAR ARRHYTHMIAS

In this section we shall discuss the prevalence and significance of ventricular arrhythmias in normal subjects and in patients who have heart disease. Such information is useful in interpreting the results of 24-hr EKG recordings and for making therapeutic decisions. Individual case studies often have the objective of correlating symptoms with arrhythmic events. However, epidemiologic studies usually test hypotheses about associations between arrhythmias and mortality or symptomatic arrhythmias during follow-up.

There have been more studies of the incidence of ventricular arrhythmias in subjects or patients with heart disease than studies to evaluate the significance of ventricular arrhythmias by following the patients for a relatively long period of time. It is almost impossible to attribute causality to an association such as one between unsustained ventricular arrhythmias and subsequent death. It is always possible that other variables that are associated with ventricular arrhythmias are causing the deaths. If these factors are not known and accounted for, an erroneous conclusion can be drawn about the association between ventricular arrhythmias and death.

One important issue that is not entirely settled concerns the relationships among ventricular arrhythmias, left ventricular dysfunction, and mortality.

Ventricular Arrhythmias in Normal Persons

To accurately estimate the incidence and significance of ventricular arrhythmias in the normal population, stringent criteria for normalcy must be fulfilled, and the group under study must be a random sample of the normal population. However, application of the full cardiac diagnostic armamentarium (including catheterization and angiography) is not practical in large epidemiologic trials. Furthermore, normalcy is constantly being redefined by the advent of new diagnostic modalities such as echocardiography, endomyocardial biopsy, and positron-emitting tomography. Most studies to date have used selected samples, e.g., volunteers (28,41,168) or referred patients (75,93,165), rather than random samples of the normal population.

Incidence of VPDs

In 1960, Hiss, Averill, and Lamb (5,75) studied the incidence of ventricular ectopy on standard EKGs (48 sec in duration) for 67,375 asymptomatic men on flying status with the U.S. Air Force (75): 90% of these subjects were between 20 and 40 years of age. Only 437 men (0.65%) had one or more VPDs in a recording that lasted less than 1 min. One pilot had multiform VPDs, and one had unsustained ventricular tachycardia (three complexes).

Several studies summarized in Table 5 have described the incidences of ventricular ectopy in apparently normal populations using 24-hr EKG recordings (28,93,145, 149,165,168). Ventricular ectopy (≥1 VPD/day) was found in about 30 to 55% of subjects, depending on the study. The incidences of ventricular ectopy increased somewhat with age (28,65,93,149,165,182) and did not differ significantly between the sexes (28,168). There were conflicting reports whether or not the incidence of VPD is subject to diurnal variation (149).

VPD frequency greater than 10 per hour did not occur in any of the normal young men (average age 25) studied by Brodsky et al. (28) and occurred in 2% of the normal young women (average age 25) studied by Sobotka et al. (168). Kostis et al. (93) studied 101 middle-aged men and women (average age 49) and found that only 1% had a VPD frequency greater than 10 per hour. Romhilt et al. (149) studied a random sample of 101 women who were employed by a metal company, with an age range of 20 to 60 years, and found that only 1% had more than 10 VPDs per hour and that VPD frequency increased somewhat with age.

All studies concur that complex ventricular arrhythmias are rare in normal individuals. It should be noted

TABLE 5. *Incidences of spontaneous ventricular arrhythmias in apparently normal persons*

	Scott (165)	Brodsky (28)	Sobotka (168)	Romhilt (149)	Kostis (93)	Raftery (145)	Clarke (41)	Fleg (55)	Bjerregaard (22)
No. studied	131	50	50	101	101	53	86	98	260
Age range	10–13	23–27	22–28	20–60	16–68	20–70+	16–65	60–85	40–79
Mean age	12	25	25	40	49	47	—	70	56
Male/female	131M	50M	50F	101F	51M/50F	29M/24F	41M/45F	69M/29F	170M/90F
Hours of recording	24	24	24	24	24	24	48	24	24
VPD characteristics (%)									
Any present	26	50	54	34	39	17	73	78	69
Frequency (>10 VPDs/hr)	0	0	2	1	1	2	7	—	8
Multiform	—	12	10	9	4	1	15	35	23
R-on-T	—	6	4	0	2	—	2	1	1
Paired VPDs	—	0	2	0	3	0	2	0	11
Ventricular tachycardia	0	2	2	1	0	0	2	4	2

that there is more interobserver variance in assigning the diagnoses of multiform and R-on-T than in assigning the diagnoses of paired VPDs or ventricular tachycardia (40). Brodsky et al. (28) found multiform VPDs in 12% of 50 healthy men and 10% of 50 healthy women in 24-hr continuous EKG recordings. With 48-hr EKG recordings, Clarke et al. (41) found multiform VPDs in 15% of 86 subjects. Between 23 and 35% of apparently normal old persons had multiform VPDs (22,55). Repetitive VPDs, paired VPDs, and ventricular tachycardia were rare in all but the oldest group of patients (22,55). Up to age 60 or so, paired VPDs occurred in 0 to 3% and ventricular tachycardia in 0 to 2% of about 500 patients studied in all the series (Table 5). In the group of normal persons of average age 70 years studied by Fleg and Kennedy (55), 11% had paired VPDs, and 4% had ventricular tachycardia.

Of interest, Kostis et al. (93) recorded continuous ambulatory EKGs for two additional 24-hr periods in 30 persons randomly selected from their original 101 subjects. The percentage of subjects who did not have any VPDs during the 72-hr recording decreased to 17%, compared with 61% in the initial 24-hr recording. The occurrence of VPDs varied considerably among the three successive 24-hr recordings within patients. Also, Clarke et al. (41) obtained 48-hr continuous EKG recordings in 86 normal subjects and found a higher incidence (73%) of ventricular ectopy in apparently healthy subjects than did Brodsky and others who used 24-hr EKG recordings. Kostis et al. (93) found that the detection of complex forms did not increase substantially with 72 hr versus 24 hr of recording. Multiform VPDs were noted in only 4 subjects, and bigeminy in 3 subjects. No patients had paired VPDs or ventricular tachycardia during the 72 hr. This finding by Kostis et al. (93) in middle-aged normal subjects contrasts strikingly with that of Winkle et al. (189), who found that the incidence of repetitive VPDs increased almost linearly with increasing duration of recording time in middle-

aged patients who had had previous myocardial infarctions.

Subtle Heart Disease in Apparently Normal Persons with VPDs

Persons who present with VPDs and appear to be normal by routine clinical and laboratory examinations may be found to have heart disease when studied more intensively.

Left ventricular dysfunction. From another perspective, several studies have identified subtle subclinical abnormalities of left ventricular performance in apparently healthy individuals with frequent VPDs (84,171,172). Kennedy et al. (84) examined hemodynamic and angiographic data in 18 patients with VPDs and normal results on coronary angiography and left ventriculography. They found an elevated left ventricular systolic volume index in 10 patients (56%) and an elevated left ventricular end-diastolic volume index in 11 (61%). A decreased mean velocity of circumferential fiber shortening was also noted in 10 persons (56%). This study suggests that clinically inapparent primary myocardial disease is often present when frequent and repetitive VPDs occur in apparently healthy individuals.

Left ventricular false tendons. Suwa et al. (172) performed two prospective echocardiographic studies of the association between left ventricular false tendons and VPDs. First, they studied 1,055 consecutive patients referred to their echocardiographic laboratory for routine diagnostic echocardiograms in order to estimate the incidence of left ventricular false tendons and their association with ventricular arrhythmias. Age, sex, and health status for these 1,055 patients were not given. Of the 1,055 patients in the study, 36 (3%) had left ventricular false tendons detected by two-dimensional echocardiograms. Of the 36 patients with false tendons, 10 had organic heart disease excluded noninvasively, and 2 of these (20%) had VPDs. In addition, Suwa et al. (172)

performed a second study to determine the incidence of left ventricular false tendons in normal persons who had frequent VPDs. They identified 62 patients with VPDs detected by a standard EKG or a 24-hr continuous EKG recording but no evidence of heart disease by noninvasive evaluation, i.e., physical examination, 12-lead EKG, chest X-ray, exercise test, and echocardiograms. Among the 62 patients with VPDs, 35 (56%) had false tendons demonstrated by two-dimensional echocardiography. These investigators concluded that there is a reasonably strong association between VPDs and left ventricular false tendons and speculated that false tendons might be the source of the VPDs. False tendons contain Purkinje fibers, and the automaticity of these specialized fibers is increased, and their conductivity is decreased, by stretching. Suwa et al. (172) noted a diastolic figure-eight pattern of false tendons in some patients with VPDs, suggesting that during diastole the false tendon was under considerable tension, perhaps enough to cause functional abnormalities. VPD frequency decreased in persons with left ventricular false tendons, a finding they attributed to a decrease in diastolic stretch of the false tendon due to decreased diastolic filling at higher heart rates. Interestingly, Suwa et al. (172) found that persons with VPDs and left ventricular false tendons were more resistant to antiarrhythmic drug treatment than normal persons with frequent VPDs but no false tendons demonstrated by two-dimensional echocardiography.

Heart biopsy abnormalities. Strain et al. (171) performed right endomyocardial biopsy in 18 patients with symptomatic ventricular tachycardia or fibrillation and no other evidence of cardiac disease by invasive and noninvasive studies, including exercise testing, echocardiography, cardiac catheterization, and coronary angiography. Abnormal biopsy results were found in 16 of 18 subjects (89%); 9 (50%) had nonspecific cardiomyopathy; 3 (17%) had myocarditis; 2 (11%) had intramyocardial vascular abnormalities; 2 (11%) had adipose infiltration consistent with arrhythmogenic right ventricular dysplasia. One subject with a normal biopsy had Wolff-Parkinson-White syndrome; the other had mitral valve prolapse (as shown on echocardiography, but not ventriculography). This study suggests that ventricular arrhythmias may be the first and only clinically apparent manifestation of primary myocardial disease, especially myocarditis.

Significance of VPDs in Normal Subjects

Several longitudinal studies have examined the prognostic significance of ventricular ectopy in apparently normal individuals (53,67,73,74,85,88,142,144,146,148). For normal subjects with ventricular ectopy on a 12-lead EKG, the risk of death is not clearly increased. However, there seems to be an increased risk of devel-

oping coronary heart disease, especially of experiencing sudden death as a first manifestation of coronary heart disease.

Rabkin et al. (144) prospectively followed 401 men in apparent good health who had VPDs in a standard 12-lead EKG. These men were drawn from a cohort of 3,983 Canadian pilots who had 12-lead EKGs recorded at the time of medical examination for licensing. The duration of follow-up was 10.8 ± 0.5 years. The endpoint was the appearance of clinical coronary heart disease, as manifested by angina, myocardial infarction, or sudden death. Rabkin showed that in men 40 to 59 years of age, but not in men younger than 40 years or older than 60 years, the age-specific incidence of coronary heart disease was increased for those who had VPDs on the 12-lead EKG, as compared with men who did not have VPDs. However, Rabkin's conclusion is weakened by his use of *post hoc* age stratification. Furthermore, he did not state whether or not the incidences of coronary risk factors were equal in the subjects with and without VPDs. Therefore, no conclusion can be drawn from his study about the ability of VPDs to predict coronary heart disease independent of standard coronary risk factors.

In the Tecumseh study (39), 5,129 randomly selected members of the Tecumseh community had standard 12-lead EKGs and were followed prospectively to assess the occurrence of coronary heart disease and sudden cardiac death. The incidence of VPDs in the Tecumseh population was 1.5%. Over a 6-year follow-up, 98 deaths from coronary disease were recorded; 45 of these deaths were sudden. Among persons over 30 years of age, the incidence of coronary disease was higher in persons with VPDs than in persons without them. Furthermore, the incidence of sudden death in persons with VPDs was higher than in persons without VPDs. Diastolic and systolic blood pressures, cholesterol, weight, glucose tolerance, and smoking habits among patients with VPDs did not significantly differ from the expected values for the upper quintile of the age- and sex-specific distribution. These authors concluded that VPDs predict sudden death independent of known coronary risk factors. However, in their analysis, Chiang et al. (38,39) did not specifically address the prognostic significance of VPDs in apparently healthy individuals.

There is no VPD characteristic, such as frequency, configuration, or coupling interval, that predicts which subjects will develop coronary heart disease. In the Canton study, the presence of EKG abnormalities other than VPDs in standard 12-lead EKG recordings, e.g., nonspecific T-wave abnormalities and left axis deviation, carried the same increased risk of sudden death (52).

With the advent of Holter EKG recording, it became possible to address the roles of VPD frequency and complexity in a more quantitative manner. However, no longitudinal studies of the significance of VPDs in apparently normal individuals have been done in un-biased samples of the population. So far, studies have been done in patients who presented for evaluation of symptomatic VPDs or evaluation of VPDs detected in the course of some form of health survey.

Kennedy et al. (83) followed 73 subjects referred for evaluation of ventricular ectopy. These subjects were asymptomatic and had been evaluated extensively by noninvasive means to exclude cardiac abnormalities. Cardiac catheterization and angiography were performed in a subset of 31 subjects, and serious (>50%) coronary artery narrowing was found in 6 subjects. Subjects with any coronary narrowing (13 patients) were given beta-blocker therapy and continued in the study. The mean age was 46 at the time of entry into the study. The mean VPD frequency was 566 per hour (range 78–1,994); 63% had multiform VPDs, 60% had paired VPDs, and 25% had ventricular tachycardia. Of the original cohort, 70 subjects were followed for a mean of 6.5 years (range 3–9.5 years). There were two deaths, one from cancer and one sudden death. Using Monson's U.S. white and nonwhite death-rate data (118), the survival rate was comparable to that for the healthy population. When compared with survival for patients with coronary heart disease of moderate severity based on data from Proudfit's study (142), or with the survival of men with silent myocardial infarction based on data from the Framingham study (82), the prognosis was clearly superior in Kennedy's subjects. However, Kennedy's study suffered from lack of concurrent controls and a relatively small sample size. No endomyocardial biopsies were performed to exclude subclinical myocardial disease. Inclusion in the study of subjects with coronary disease and subjects on beta-blocker therapy may have confounded the relationship between VPDs and outcome. Because Kennedy's patients were highly selected, some had had ventricular ectopy for years before entering the study. Therefore, it is possible that similar subjects with ventricular ectopy might have died before coming to medical attention.

Kennedy's observations concur with and extend the findings of Montague et al. (119), who studied 45 subjects 2 weeks to 62 years of age (mean age 25) who had been referred for frequent VPDs but were otherwise in good health (with normal results on physical examination, echocardiogram, and EKG, except 2 subjects with nonspecific ST-T changes). Mean VPD frequency was 444 ± 454 VPDs per hour; 16% of the patients had multiform VPDs, 24% had ventricular couplets, and 7% had ventricular tachycardia (119). All 27 subjects who were available for follow-up (including an examination and 24-hr EKG recording) remained well 8 months later. Of the 18 subjects available for follow-up at 22 months, 16 remained well, and two experienced arrhythmic events. One was an infant who died of sudden crib death, and one was an adult who developed sustained ventricular tachycardia. The latter subject had normal results on cardiac catheterization and coronary angiography; ventricular tachycardia could not be induced during an electrophysiologic study. Of interest, in the 27 subjects who had repeat Holter recordings at 8 months after entry into the study, Montague found that despite marked individual variability of VPD frequency in that subgroup, there was no significant change in group mean values. There was also a high linear correlation of VPD frequencies at initial and follow-up studies.

Kennedy and Underhill (85) observed that in apparently healthy subjects, VPDs are more often of a morphology suggesting a right ventricular origin. Buxton et al. (30) recently reported a series of 30 patients without evidence of myocardial disease and with ventricular tachycardia of left bundle branch block morphology and inferior axis. These patients had a relatively high frequency of exercise-induced ventricular tachycardia (14/23) or isoproterenol-facilitated induction (13/23) of ventricular tachycardia, as well as relatively high rates of response to both beta-blocking and class 1 antiarrhythmic agents. In 10 patients in whom endocardial activation mapping was performed, the earliest site of ventricular activation during the tachycardia occurred at the right ventricular outflow tract on the interventricular septum. During a mean follow-up of 30 months, no deaths occurred, and no further evidence of cardiac disease appeared in patients with right ventricular outflow tract tachycardia.

Exercise

Several studies have examined the incidence and significance of exercise-induced VPDs and their reproducibility (35,110,111). Using treadmill testing, McHenry et al. (110) examined 561 Indiana state policemen between 25 and 54 years of age without evidence of cardiovascular disease. The overall incidence of VPDs was 32% (183 subjects). The incidence of frequent VPDs (defined as more than six VPDs per minute) was 10%. Complex ectopy was rare, with an incidence of 2% for multiform VPDs, 3.5% for paired VPDs, and 1% for ventricular tachycardia. These figures are in the ranges described by others (23,47,56,58). The incidence of VPDs during exercise increases with age (50,110). Ekblom et al. (47) noted that at any given decade of age, the incidence of exercise-induced VPDs was lower in women than in men.

Blackburn et al. (23) studied 196 men between 40 and 59 years of age. Their group consisted of apparently healthy men at high risk for coronary heart disease (by standard coronary risk factors). These men were drawn from a random sample of Minneapolis households and from faculty members at Pennsylvania State University. When subjected to treadmill testing, the proportion of men who had VPDs increased from 3% in a preexercise rest period to 50% when maximal oxygen consumption was achieved. At submaximal-exercise heart rates, the frequency of VPDs during exercise was not related to heart rate. However, with maximal exercise, the likelihood of VPDs increased with the external work load imposed.

Kennedy and Underhill (85) observed the exercise responses of 23 subjects in apparent good health who had been referred for frequent and complex ectopy. These subjects had a mean VPD frequency of 559 VPDs per hour. In 21 of the 23 subjects, the ventricular ectopy resolved during the last stage of maximal exercise. In 21 subjects, grade 3 or higher ventricular ectopy appeared during the postexercise recovery period. Similar findings were reported by Montague. In Montague's study, there were 45 patients in apparent good health (by invasive testing) with frequent complex ectopy on 24-hr continuous EKG recordings (119). The average VPD frequency was 444 VPDs per hour, and 18 of 45 patients had complex VPDs (defined by the investigators as multiform, repetitive, or R-on-T). Of 37 subjects who had VPDs during the preexercise rest period, only 11 had VPDs at peak exercise; VPDs reappeared during the recovery period in all.

Kennedy and others have noted that a marked decrease in frequency of VPDs during exercise is not specific for healthy individuals, because this response also is seen in patients with angiographically documented significant coronary artery disease.

Using three different exercise protocols (gymnasium exercise, bicycle ergometry, and arm ergometry), Ekblom et al. (47) found that the incidences of exercise-induced ectopy were the same for subjects who achieved similar heart rates during the three types of exercise. Pantano and Oriel (135) recorded the EKG continuously in 60 well-conditioned runners during both a distance run and a maximal treadmill test. Although the subjects were able to maintain submaximal heart rates during the distance run, the maximal treadmill test significantly underestimated both the incidence and grade of ventricular ectopy. These investigators suggested that the difference was related to the duration of the distance run and its effect on the total work load.

On repeating the exercise testing both within 2 weeks (47) and at a 2- to 3-year interval (110), the incidence of exercise-induced ectopy was reproducible for the subjects tested as a group, but there was marked variability in the incidence of exercise-induced ectopy in individuals. However, in patients with a negative first test, Ekblom found that the repeat exercise test was almost always negative, i.e., free of ventricular ectopy.

In their longitudinal study, Froelicher et al. (58) followed 710 apparently healthy men with a mean age of 37 years for a period of 6 years after exercise testing. These men were aircrewmen referred for evaluation of their flying status. The investigators found that, except

when associated with an abnormal ST-segment response, exercise-induced ventricular ectopy had very low sensitivity, predictive value, and risk ratio as an indicator of risk for development of coronary heart disease.

Fleg and Lakatta studied the incidence and prognosis in exercise-induced ventricular tachycardia in 922 community volunteers from the Baltimore Longitudinal Study on Aging (56). Ten subjects (1% of the group) had exercise-induced ventricular tachycardia, and 9 subjects were 65 years of age or older. Thus, exercise-induced ventricular tachycardia occurred almost exclusively in the elderly, and it usually consisted of short asymptomatic runs (three to six QRS complexes) and was not associated with increased risk for cardiac morbidity or mortality during a 2-year follow-up.

Spontaneous Ventricular Arrhythmias in Coronary Heart Disease

Incidence of ventricular arrhythmias early after myocardial infarction. There have been several studies to characterize ventricular arrhythmias at about the time of discharge from hospital after myocardial infarction (10,18,90,126,127,129,134,179). This time has been selected because recordings done at this time are convenient for patients and physicians and because of the high mortality early after discharge. The incidence of VPDs at the time of discharge is summarized in Table 6. About 15% have no VPDs at all in a 24-hr continuous EKG recording, 50% average less than 1 VPD per hour, and 20% have more than 10 VPDs per hour. Also, at the time of discharge, about 50% of patients with myocardial infarction will have multiform VPDs, 25% will have R-on-T VPDs, 20% will have paired VPDs, and 10% will have ventricular tachycardia.

Time course of ventricular arrhythmias after myocardial infarction. Although most studies of ventricular arrhythmias have been done at about the time of hospital discharge, i.e., 2 to 3 weeks after infarction, VPD frequency is quite variable over the first few weeks after myocardial infarction (8). During the first 48 hr after myocardial infarction, almost 90% of patients will have VPDs, and 40% will have ventricular tachycardia. Three to five days after infarction, VPD frequency is at a minimum; only about 10% of patients have ≥ 10 VPDs per hour, and only 5% have ventricular tachycardia at this time. VPD frequency continues to rise to reach a maximum at 6 to 12 weeks after infarction (99).

Significance of ventricular arrhythmias after myocardial infarction. Mortality is an S-shaped function of VPD frequency recorded at the time of discharge (Fig. 3). Below 1 VPD per hour, the 2-year mortality is very low (10). Above 1 VPD per hour, mortality rises steeply, and about half of the VPD-associated mortality increase is reached at a frequency of 3 VPDs per hour. The 2-year mortality rate approaches a plateau of about 20%

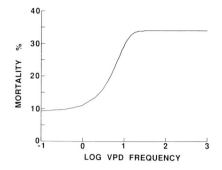

FIG. 3. Two-year mortality as a function of average VPD frequency in a 24-hr continuous EKG recording made 11 ± 3 days after myocardial infarction. The y axis is the 2-year mortality, and the x axis is the common logarithm of the 24-hr average VPD frequency. These data come from the Multicenter Post-Infarction Program (10).

between 10 and 30 VPDs per hour. In conventional clinical practice, treatment with an antiarrhythmic drug is not seriously considered until VPD frequency is greater than 60 to 100 VPDs per hour. It is interesting that the VPD frequency at which the maximum mortality effect is expressed is considerably lower than the conventional clinical criterion for treatment. Recently, controlled clinical antiarrhythmic drug trials, such as the Cardiac Arrhythmia Pilot Study or the Timolol, Encainide, Sotalol Trial, have used a criterion of 10 VPDs per hour as an enrollment criterion (7). In terms of predicting mortality, repetitiveness is the most significant complex VPD feature found in predischarge 24-hr continuous EKG recordings after myocardial infarction. As shown in Table 6, about 25% of patients will have repetitive VPDs, and about 10% will have unsustained ventricular tachycardia. Nearly every large study has found that ventricular tachycardia has the strongest association with subsequent mortality of any ventricular arrhythmia variable. Table 7 provides base-line and follow-up data from four studies of unsustained ventricular tachycardia after myocardial infarction (3,10,14,90). The incidence of ventricular tachycardia at the time of hospital discharge depends importantly on the duration of EKG recording, the age and degree of illness of the patient population studied, the definition of ventricular tachycardia, and the sensitivity of the analysis method. When 24-hr continuous EKG recordings were made in a representative sample of the postinfarction population in the United States and analyzed by sensitive and specific digital-computer programs that used three or more consecutive VPDs at any rate as the definition of ventricular tachycardia, the incidence of ventricular tachycardia was slightly greater than 10% (10). The four studies displayed in Table 7 all showed a strong association between ventricular tachycardia recorded at the time of hospital discharge and mortality over the next several years. The odds of dying were about 2.5 to 3.5

times greater for patients with ventricular tachycardia than for patients without ventricular tachycardia in each of these studies. This strong association between unsustained ventricular tachycardia and long-term mortality is a little surprising considering the fact that ventricular tachycardia episodes tend to be infrequent, brief, and asymptomatic 2 to 3 weeks after myocardial infarction. Half of patients who have ventricular tachycardia will have only three VPDs in the longest run, and 30% will have only one episode of ventricular tachycardia in the entire 24-hr recording. So far, no relationship has been found between the number of ventricular tachycardia episodes, the length of the episodes, or the rate of ventricular tachycardia and subsequent mortality (3,14,90). However, the relationship of these features of ventricular tachycardia to mortality could bear further examination, because the studies to date have been relatively small and have not had much power to detect an association between these features of ventricular tachycardia and mortality. Two studies have shown that repetitive VPDs are associated with mortality independent of VPD frequency (8,10). Despite a moderately strong association between VPD frequency and repetitive VPDs, there is a substantial and statistically significant association between repetitive ventricular arrhythmias and mortality after adjusting for VPD frequency.

Relationships among ventricular arrhythmias, left ventricular dysfunction, and mortality. Strategies for secondary prevention of arrhythmic death after myocardial infarction depend importantly on the relationships among ventricular arrhythmias, left ventricular dysfunction, and mortality. Until quite recently, many investigators believed that the ventricular arrhythmias that occur after myocardial infarction were so strongly related to left ventricular dysfunction that they had no important independent association with mortality. One retrospective study in chronic coronary heart disease suggested that this view was correct (34). However, many patients in

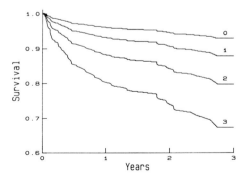

FIG. 4. Relationship between 2-year mortality and repetitive VPDs detected in 820 24-hr continuous EKG recordings made 11 ± 3 days after myocardial infarction. The percentages of patients in the categories are as follows: 0 = no VPD at all, 14%; 1 = only single VPD, 58%; 2 = paired VPDs, 17%; 3 = runs of VPDs, 11%.

TABLE 6. *Frequency and characteristics of ventricular arrhythmias 2 weeks after acute myocardial infarction*

Institution	Duration of recording (hr)	No. of patients	Frequency of VPDs (%)			VPD characteristics (%)			
			0	≥1/hr	≥10/hr	Multi-form	Pairs	VT[a]	R-on-T
Stanford University	10	95	24	76	30	43	16	17	—
University of Rochester	6	500	47	—	5	10	3	1	10[b]
University of Ghent	6–8	150	41	58	23	24	24	15	2[c]
Washington University	10	238	26	43	17	45	15	2	18[b]
Columbia University	24	616	16	50	25	54	31	12	27[b]
MPIP	24	819	14	41	20	64	17	11	24[b]
MILIS	24	533	16	—	15	66	26	11	10[b]

[a] Ventricular tachycardia.
[b] $R - V/QT < 1.00$.
[c] $R - V/QT < 0.85$.

the study by Califf et al. (34) had not had previous myocardial infarction. The four studies that have addressed the question of the independence of ventricular arrhythmias as a risk predictor after myocardial infarction are summarized in Table 8. Ruberman et al. (152) and Moss et al. (126) evaluated the relationship between "complex" ventricular arrhythmias and mortality after myocardial infarction using the clinical diagnosis of heart failure to adjust for left ventricular dysfunction. Both of these studies were large, enrolling 1,739 and 940 patients, respectively. Both used relatively short continuous EKG recordings, 1 and 6 hr, respectively, to detect the ventricular arrhythmias. Both studies concluded that ventricular arrhythmias were significantly associated with total mortality and with sudden cardiac death during 3 or 4 years of follow-up after adjusting for clinical heart failure. These two studies could have underadjusted for left ventricular dysfunction by using the clinical diagnosis of heart failure as the measure for this important covariate. It is known that multivariate

techniques, such as the Cox regression or log-linear models, tend to underadjust when an important covariate is measured imprecisely and then used in the adjustment procedures. Shulze et al. (164) studied 81 patients with radionuclide ventriculograms and 24-hr EKG recordings, but too few deaths (eight) were observed in follow-up to permit any conclusions. More recently, two multicenter studies have addressed this problem. The Multicenter Investigation of the Limitation of Infarct Size (MILIS) analyzed their data two different ways to address the question of the independence of the relationship between ventricular arrhythmias and mortality after myocardial infarction (128,129). In the first analysis, MILIS used radionuclide ejection fraction dichotomized at 40% to adjust for left ventricular dysfunction and repetitive VPDs detected in a 24-hr continuous EKG recording as the arrhythmia variable to relate to 1-year mortality among 388 patients (128). They found that repetitive ventricular arrhythmias were significantly associated with 1-year mortality after adjusting for left ventricular dys-

TABLE 7. *Studies of unsustained ventricular tachycardia (VT) recorded about 2 weeks after myocardial infarction*

	Anderson (3)	Bigger (14)	Kleiger (90)	Bigger (10)
No. of patients	915	430	289	819
Age limit	<66	<76	<71	<70
One-year mortality	4%	13%	9%	9%
Duration of EKG recording (hr)	6	24	10	24
Definition of VT				
Number of VPDs	≥3	≥3	≥3	≥3
Rate	≥100/min	Any	Any	Any
Incidence of VT	1%	12%	3%	12%
Follow-up time (months)	48	36	12	24
Mortality				
With VT	25%	38%	14%	25%
Without VT	13%	12%	7%	9%
Odds ratio	4.8	4.7	2.1	3.0

TABLE 8. *Independent relationship between ventricular arrhythmias or left ventricular dysfunction and mortality in coronary heart disease*

	Ruberman (152)	Moss (126)	MILIS (129)	MPIP (10)
No. of patients	1,739	940	533	766
Time of enrollment (weeks after infarction)	12	2–3	1–2	1–2
Measure of left ventricular dysfunction	Clinical	Clinical	RNEF	RNEF
Duration of EKG recording (hr)	1	6	24	24
Ventricular arrhythmia variable	Complex VPDs	Complex VPDs	Frequent VPDs	Frequent or repetitive VPDs
Duration of follow-up (years)	3	4	1.5	2
No. of deaths	208	115	66	101
Mortality effect of ventricular arrhythmias independent of left ventricular dysfunction	Yes	Yes	Yes	Yes

Note: Complex ventricular arrhythmias = R-on-T VPDs, ≥2 consecutive VPDs, multiform VPDs, or bigeminy. Frequent VPDs = ≥10 per hour. Repetitive VPDs = ≥2 consecutive VPDs. RNEF = radionuclide ejection fraction.

function using left ventricular ejection fraction. Later, the MILIS investigators evaluated the same relationships in a larger sample (533 patients). In the second analysis, they used VPD frequency dichotomized at 10 per hour as the arrhythmia variable to relate to mortality after adjusting for left ventricular dysfunction using left ventricular ejection fraction dichotomized at 40% (129). This analysis also showed a relationship between ventricular arrhythmias and mortality independent of left ventricular dysfunction. The Multicenter Post-Infarction Program (MPIP) performed similar analyses in a group of 766 patients. First, the MPIP group evaluated the relationship between VPD frequency dichotomized at 10 per hour and 2-year mortality, adjusting for left ventricular dysfunction using left ventricular ejection fraction dichotomized at 40%. Ventricular arrhythmias were significantly and independently associated with mortality in this analysis (174). Analyses done later showed that frequent and repetitive VPDs were each independently associated with 2-year mortality after adjusting for ejection fraction divided into four groups (10) or as measured (19). Thus, it seems well established that spontaneous ventricular arrhythmias are an independent risk predictor after myocardial infarction. The independent risk represented by ventricular arrhythmias recorded after myocardial infarction provides a strong rationale for clinical trials to test the effects of antiarrhythmic drug treatment in the years immediately after infarction.

Exercise Ventricular Arrhythmias After Myocardial Infarction

There has been little work done to evaluate the incidence and significance of ventricular arrhythmias that occur during or after exercise testing early after myocardial infarction. Ericsson et al. (49) were among the first investigators to demonstrate the safety and potential utility of exercise testing before discharge after acute myocardial infarction. They studied 100 patients with a treadmill exercise test 3 weeks after myocardial infarction. The test started with a load of 16 or 33 watts and was advanced every 4 to 6 min by 16 watts. The treadmill test was discontinued for (a) angina pectoris or dyspnea, (b) frequent VPDs, or (c) heart rate >140 per minute. Seventy-five percent of the patients stopped exercise at 50 watts of effort or less. Before the test, 3% of the patients had VPDs, and during the test 19% had VPDs. Later, the same group (69) studied the incidence and prognostic significance of ventricular arrhythmias after myocardial infarction in 205 patients. There were 183 men and 22 women, with a mean age of 59 ± 9 years. The same treadmill test as used by Ericsson was used at 3 and 9 weeks after acute myocardial infarction, and patients were followed for as long as 5 years. During the treadmill exercise test 3 weeks after acute myocardial infarction, ventricular arrhythmias were seen in 34 patients (17%). During an average follow-up of over 2 years, 16 of the 34 patients with exercise-induced ventricular arrhythmias (47%) died, compared with 41 of 171 of those without ventricular arrhythmias (24%). This difference is statistically significant ($p < 0.05$). The odds of dying during follow-up were 2.8 times greater for those who had exercise-induced ventricular arrhythmias than for those who did not. At 9 weeks after myocardial infarction, exercise tests were performed in 174 of the patients, and 40 of them (23%) had ventricular arrhythmias. During follow-up, 16 of the 40 patients with ventricular arrhythmias died (40%), compared with 25 of the 134 patients without ventricular arrhythmias (19%). This difference is statistically significant. The odds of dying for patients with exercise ventricular arrhythmias in the 9-week exercise test were 2.9 times greater than for those who did not have ventricular arrhythmias.

Weld et al. (185) evaluated exercise ventricular arrhythmias in 250 patients who performed a low-level exercise test just before hospital discharge. This study was different from several other early studies of exercise testing before discharge after myocardial infarction in that it enrolled consecutive patients who had had myocardial infarction and who were under age 70 years. Patients with complicated myocardial infarction were not excluded if they were able to walk 100 feet in the hallway. A 9-min exercise protocol was designed to finish at an energy expenditure comparable to that required for activities of ordinary daily living, approximately 4 MET. The final 3-min stage was identical with stage I of the standard Bruce exercise protocol. The exercise test was performed 1 or 2 days before anticipated hospital discharge. Patients with unstable angina pectoris, those with orthostatic systolic blood pressure less than 90 mm Hg, or those with an unsteady gait were not exercised even though they were enrolled. In order to evaluate arrhythmias, the EKG was recorded continuously for 9 min prior to exercise, during exercise, and for 10 min after exercise was completed. VPD frequency was calculated by dividing the number of VPDs recorded by the duration of the recording interval. The study group consisted of 200 men and 50 women, mean age 57 ± 9 years. The average interval between hospitalization for myocardial infarction and exercise testing was 16 ± 4 days. Of the 236 patients who were able to perform the exercise test, 102 (43%) had one or more VPDs during exercise or the 10 min after exercise. VPD frequency was at least 10 per hour in 56 patients (24%); 50 patients (22%) had complex VPDs (i.e., multiform VPDs, R-on-T VPDs, VPD pairs, or ventricular tachycardia). To determine if ventricular arrhythmias were associated with left ventricular dysfunction, exercise-test VPDs were associated with clinical variables reflecting left ventricular failure. There was no significant association between exercise-test VPDs and left ventricular failure in the CCU, left ventricular failure at the time of exercise, cardiomegaly or pulmonary congestion in

the discharge chest X-ray, or exercise duration less than 10 min. VPDs were significantly associated with digoxin treatment at the time of the exercise test. As shown in Table 9, VPD frequency of 10 or more per hour or paired VPDs or ventricular tachycardia showed a reasonably strong association with cardiovascular death within a year of the infarct. Also, in a multiple logistic regression analysis using 1-year cardiovascular mortality as the endpoint, ventricular arrhythmias during exercise test were significantly and independently associated with mortality, simultaneously adjusting for age, previous myocardial infarction, cardiomegaly on chest X-ray, pulmonary vascular congestion on chest X-ray, exercise ST depression, and exercise duration. These results indicate that ventricular arrhythmias are relatively common after myocardial infarction, have a weak association with left ventricular dysfunction, and contribute independently to the prediction of 1-year cardiovascular mortality when adjusting for several important clinical variables and other exercise variables that indicate left ventricular dysfunction and myocardial ischemia.

Another important exercise study was performed by the MPIP group (96). This was a natural-history study that enrolled patients under 70 years who were discharged from CCU after acute myocardial infarction; it involved nine hospitals in four cities: New York City, Tucson, Arizona, Rochester, New York, and St. Louis, Missouri. Of the 867 patients enrolled in the study, 667 patients took the low-level treadmill exercise test. The MPIP used the same treadmill exercise test protocol as described by Weld et al. (185). A total of 187 patients (28%) were taking digoxin, and 207 patients (31%) were taking a beta blocker at the time of the test. Patients were not taken off either of these drugs systematically before the test. The presence of VPDs or couplets before, during, or after the exercise test was associated with increased cardiac mortality in the first year. To evaluate the possible effects of treatment on the relationship between ventricular arrhythmias during or after an exercise test and cardiac mortality, the subgroups who took or did not take beta blockers or digitalis were analyzed separately. When patients taking beta blockers were analyzed separately, the relationship of VPDs to cardiac mortality

TABLE 9. *Relationship between exercise ventricular arrhythmias and 1-year cardiac mortality after myocardial infarction*

	CPMC (N = 236)			MPIP (N = 667)		
	Incidence (%)	p value	Odds ratio	Incidence (%)	p value	Odds ratio
Any VPD	43	0.01	4.3	43	0.05	2.4
VPDs ≥10 per hour	24	0.001	6.3	—	—	—
Paired VPDs	8	0.001	9.2	7	0.05	3.9

Note: CPMC = Columbia-Presbyterian Medical Center; MPIP = Multicenter Post-Infarction Program.

was seen only in the patients not taking beta blockers. There was no relationship between VPDs at the time of the exercise test and cardiac mortality in those taking beta blockers. This finding could be related to the increased survival of postinfarction patients with arrhythmias when treated with beta blockers (15,60). The opposite relationship was seen in patients who were taking digitalis at the time of the exercise test. Patients who were taking digitalis had a higher incidence of death when VPDs also were present. However, patients not taking digitalis showed no such relationship. These results are difficult to interpret, because patients were not randomly but rather selectively treated with beta blockers or digitalis, and thus many other variables aside from treatment were likely to have been different between those persons taking drugs and those not taking drugs. In a stepwise logistic regression model, paired VPDs contributed significantly to the prediction of mortality when simultaneously adjusting for other clinical and exercise-derived variables, e.g., pulmonary congestion on chest X-ray, heart rate greater than or equal to 90 per minute, systolic blood pressure less than 110 mm Hg. Thus, in this study also, exercise-related VPDs were significantly related to mortality as univariates and after adjusting for a variety of clinical and other exercise variables. This indicates the significant independent value of exercise-induced ventricular arrhythmias in predicting cardiac mortality in the year after myocardial infarction. This finding has been corroborated in more chronic phases of coronary heart disease (35).

Electrophysiologic Studies After Myocardial Infarction

Electrophysiologic studies have become a standard method for evaluating patients who have spontaneous episodes of sustained ventricular arrhythmias. These studies are useful for characterizing the type and severity of ventricular arrhythmias and for evaluating therapy. Programmed ventricular stimulation has excellent sensitivity, specificity, and reproducibility for sustained

ventricular tachycardia (20). Also, the response of ventricular arrhythmias induced by programmed ventricular stimulation to drug therapy or surgery has excellent predictive accuracy for death and recurrence of symptomatic arrhythmias in patients with spontaneous sustained ventricular arrhythmias (79,108,138,173,191). Because programmed ventricular stimulation is an invasive study, its ability to detect arrhythmic potential after myocardial infarction in patients who have not yet manifested clinical arrhythmias has not been studied extensively. The potential of electrophysiologic studies to detect the substrate for malignant arrhythmias after acute myocardial infarction is an ongoing area of clinical research at the present time. Since 1981, at least eight studies of programmed ventricular stimulation have been reported that have included patients with complicated and those with uncomplicated myocardial infarction (Table 10). Most of the studies done thus far have been small and have involved biased samples, and therefore are difficult to interpret. Three groups have reported studies that included more than 100 patients (27,46,147,151). These studies provide a reasonable estimate of the incidence and significance of inducible ventricular arrhythmias after myocardial infarction.

Incidence of inducible ventricular tachycardia. Studies of the incidence of unsustained ventricular tachycardia or sustained ventricular tachycardia after acute myocardial infarction are summarized in Table 11 (27,46,70,71, 105,147,151,159). These results vary with the selection of patients, the time after infarction when the studies were done, and the stimulation protocols that were used. In 1981, Haerten et al. (70) reported 64 patients who were studied an average of 25 days after acute myocardial infarction. Programmed ventricular stimulation consisted of four basic ventricular pacing rates (120, 140, 160, and 180 per minute) and one or two premature stimuli delivered via bipolar catheter electrodes placed under fluoroscopy in the right ventricular apex. These workers found that 30% of the patients had unsustained ventricular tachycardia, i.e., four complexes

TABLE 10. *Studies of programmed ventricular stimulation after acute myocardial infarction*

Author	Year	No. of patients studied	No. of ventricular pacing rates	No. of sites stimulated	Stimulus No.	Stimulus Amplitude (mA)	Response (%) VT-U	Response (%) VT-S	Response (%) VF
Haerten (70)	1981	64	4	1	2	<2	30	←20→	
Hamer (71)	1982	70	2	2	2	<2	15	11	NA
Richards (147)	1983	165	1	2	2	<2, 20	—	←23→	
Marchlinski (105)	1983	46	2	1	2	<2	11	11	NA
Santarelli (159)	1983	38	2	2	2	<2	18	26	NA
Breithardt (27)	1985	132	4	2	2	<2	25	←20→	
Roy (151)	1985	150	2	2	2	<2	11	11	1
Denniss (46)	1985	306	1	2	2	<2, 20	—	20	—

Note: NA = not available; VT-U = unsustained ventricular tachycardia; VT-S = sustained ventricular tachycardia; VF = ventricular fibrillation.

TABLE 11. *Significance of programmed ventricular stimulation early after myocardial infarction*

	Breithardt (27)	Roy (151)	Denniss (46)
Year of study	1985	1985	1985
No. of patients	132	150	306
Average time from MI to EPS (days)	22	12	10
Stimulus width (msec)	1.8	1.5	2
Stimulus amplitude (mA)	<2	<1.5	<2, 20
Follow-up (months)	15 ± 11	10 ± 5	10 ± 6
No. of deaths	8	5	23
Occurrences of spontaneous VT-S	9	2	6
Incidence of inducible VT-S	21%	11%	20%
Mortality			
With inducible VT-S	3%	3%	21%
Without inducible VT-S	8%	4%	4%
Spontaneous VT-S during follow-up			
With inducible VT-S	25%	3%	8%
Without inducible VT-S	2%	1%	0.4%

Note: EPS = electrophysiologic study; MI = myocardial infarction; VT-S = sustained ventricular tachycardia.

to 30 sec of consecutive VPDs, and 20% had sustained ventricular tachycardia or ventricular fibrillation. Hamer et al. (71) studied 70 patients whose acute myocardial infarction was complicated by arrhythmias or left ventricular failure. In each patient, continuous 24-hr EKG recordings and electrophysiologic studies were done while patients were off antiarrhythmic medications. The electrophysiologic evaluation included two basic ventricular pacing rates (120 and 150 per minute) and one premature stimulus delivered to the right ventricular apex in all 70 patients, a high current (20 mA) and two premature stimuli in 33 patients, and stimulation at a second right ventricular site in 50 patients. Of the 37 patients who underwent the entire protocol, 8 had sustained ventricular tachycardia (22%), and 4 had unsustained ventricular tachycardia (11%) of more than five consecutive complexes.

Richards et al. (147) performed electrophysiologic studies in 165 patients 6 to 28 days after uncomplicated myocardial infarction. All patients were off all cardioactive medications at the time of study. Programmed ventricular stimulation consisted of ventricular pacing at a rate of 100 per minute, with one and two premature stimuli applied to the right ventricular apex and outflow tract at both low (twice threshold) and high (20 mA) current amplitudes. Of the 165 patients, 38 (23%) had inducible ventricular tachycardia that lasted more than 10 sec or ventricular fibrillation. In a 1985 abstract, the group from Westmead, Australia, gave a current status report showing that 62 of 306 patients (20%) had inducible sustained ventricular arrhythmias when studied within the month after myocardial infarction (46). In 1985, Breithardt et al. (27) reported 132 patients studied an average of 22 days after myocardial infarction. Pro-

grammed stimulation included four ventricular pacing rates (120, 140, 160, and 180 per minute) and one and two premature stimuli delivered at the right ventricular apex or right ventricular outflow tract. When four or more ventricular echo complexes occurred, stimulation was stopped. In this study, 25% of the patients had four repetitive responses to 30 sec of unsustained ventricular tachycardia, and 20% had sustained ventricular tachycardia or ventricular fibrillation. In 1985, Roy et al. (151) reported a group of patients studied 12 ± 2 days after myocardial infarction with ventricular pacing at two rates (100 and 150 per minute), one and two premature stimuli, and two sites of stimulation; 11% had unsustained ventricular tachycardia, 11% had sustained ventricular tachycardia, and 1% had ventricular fibrillation. Thus, studies to date indicate that about 15 to 20% of patients have inducible, sustained ventricular tachycardia soon after myocardial infarction. Interestingly, the proportion who had inducible ventricular arrhythmias as a response to programmed ventricular stimulation soon after uncomplicated myocardial infarction seems to be about the same as after complicated infarction.

Time course of inducible ventricular tachycardia. The time course of inducible tachyarrhythmias after myocardial infarction has not been clarified. Klein et al. (91) studied 70 patients 3 to 4 weeks after myocardial infarction with programmed ventricular stimulation and found that 16% had sustained ventricular tachycardia or ventricular fibrillation as a response. Subsequent studies done at 6 months in 40 patients and at 12 months in 35 patients showed no significant difference in the proportion who responded to programmed ventricular stimulation with sustained ventricular arrhythmia. Costard et al. (44) studied 18 patients on days 6 and 24 after infarction with programmed ventricular stimulation (up to three premature stimuli). They found that 2 patients (11%) had inducible ventricular tachycardia or fibrillation on day 6, and 9 (50%) on day 24. Given the disparate results of these two small studies, conclusions cannot be reached concerning changes in the incidence of inducible ventricular tachycardia as a function of time after myocardial infarction.

Infarct size and incidence of inducible ventricular tachycardia early after acute myocardial infarction. Richards et al. (147) found a trend for inducible patients to have a higher incidence of diagnostic Q waves in EKGs and lower left ventricular ejection fractions. These findings suggest that the patients who had inducible ventricular tachycardia also had larger infarcts than the noninducible patients. On the other hand, Costard et al. (44) found no relationship between the inducibility of sustained ventricular arrhythmias and the peak creatine kinase, the left ventricular ejection fraction, the area of wall-motion abnormality on left ventriculograms, or the left ventricular end-diastolic pressure. The lack of correlation of inducible sustained arrhythmias with indices of infarct size early after infarction in the latter study conflicts with data from patients with chronic coronary heart disease and from animal models. Patients with chronic coronary heart disease and large scars, particularly those with ventricular aneurysms and/or significant ventricular arrhythmias detected by 24-hr EKG recordings, appear more likely to have sustained ventricular tachycardia induced during electrophysiologic studies. Spielman et al. (169) studied a group of patients with coronary heart disease and previous myocardial infarction who had both 10 or more VPDs per hour and left ventricular ejection fraction less than 50%. In this group, about 50% had inducible sustained ventricular tachycardia, a much higher rate than those found in studies of unselected patients. These human data agree with animal data showing that about 40% of dogs with subacute myocardial infarction will have inducible sustained ventricular arrhythmias (43,62). In dogs with experimental myocardial infarction, the probability of having sustained ventricular tachycardia as a response to programmed ventricular stimulation is very strongly related to infarct size. More than two-thirds of animals with ≥20% of the left ventricle infarcted have inducible sustained ventricular arrhythmias (43,62). In humans, the relationship between infarct size and the likelihood of inducing sustained ventricular tachycardia with programmed ventricular stimulation early after myocardial infarction has not yet been defined. It is reasonably clear from the studies of Breithardt et al. (27) and Roy et al. (151) that there is no significant relationship between the extent of coronary artery disease, as judged by coronary angiography, and the incidence of inducible ventricular tachycardia.

Prediction of mortality by programmed ventricular stimulation. The data on prediction of mortality by programmed ventricular stimulation are scanty at the present time. Data on the significance of ventricular tachycardia induced by programmed ventricular stimulation early after myocardial infarction are summarized in Table 11; only studies with more than 100 patients are included. In the study of Hamer et al. (71), 5 of the 12 patients (42%) with inducible sustained or unsustained ventricular tachycardia died within 12 months, compared with only 1 of 25 (4%) without ventricular tachycardia. Of the 12 patients with inducible ventricular tachycardia, only 5 had spontaneous ventricular arrhythmias in their 24-hr EKG recordings that "suggested a need for treatment." In the Westmead Hospital study (46,147), patients with 10 sec or more of ventricular tachycardia or ventricular fibrillation had a 1-year mortality of 26%, contrasted with 6% for patients who did not have one of these arrhythmias induced ($p < 0.001$). In inducible patients, 80% of the deaths were instantaneous, and ventricular tachyarrhythmias were documented in 63%, whereas none of the uninducible patients died instantaneously. A more recent report by the same group indicated a 21% mortality for inducible patients, compared with 4% in the uninducible group (Fig. 5) (46). Also, Denniss et al. (46) reported that whereas sustained ventricular tachycardia induced by programmed ventricular stimulation had a strong relationship with subsequent mortality, ventricular fibrillation did not. This finding is congruent with the experience with programmed ventricular stimulation in chronic coronary heart disease patients with spontaneous sustained uniform ventricular tachycardia, in whom ventricular fibrillation induced with three premature stimuli also is

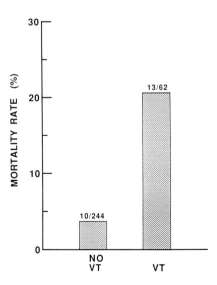

FIG. 5. Relationship between mortality and response to programmed ventricular stimulation early after myocardial infarction. The odds of dying are increased sixfold in the 306 patients who were inducible.

a nonspecific response. This finding may account for some of the variability in results from many small studies of programmed ventricular stimulation early after myocardial infarction, in which ventricular tachycardia and fibrillation have been used as joint endpoints because of small numbers. Denniss et al. (46,147) reported that the results of programmed ventricular stimulation done within a month of myocardial infarction predicted the future occurrence of symptomatic sustained ventricular arrhythmias as well. The numbers of deaths in the studies by Breithardt (27) and Roy (151) are too small to permit meaningful assessment of the relationship between inducible ventricular tachycardia and total mortality or sudden cardiac death. Breithardt reported that predischarge programmed ventricular stimulation after myocardial infarction did have high predictive accuracy for future occurrences of sustained ventricular tachycardia during follow-up. Seven of 28 patients (25%) with sustained ventricular tachycardia had spontaneous sustained ventricular tachycardia during follow-up, compared with 2% of 104 patients who did not have inducible ventricular tachycardia. Thus, the odds of having spontaneous sustained ventricular tachycardia during follow-up were increased 14-fold in patients who had sustained ventricular tachycardia induced by programmed ventricular stimulation before discharge after myocardial infarction. In the study of Roy et al. (151), only 2 patients with sustained ventricular tachycardia were detected during follow-up. In Spielman's study of patients with chronic coronary heart disease with frequent ventricular arrhythmias and reduced left ventricular ejection fraction, about 50% had inducible sustained ventricular tachycardia, and the mortality was substantially higher in inducible patients (169). Such patients have a mortality of about 50% in 2 years. Gomes et al. (66) reported similar findings.

Although much remains to be learned about the utility of programmed ventricular stimulation as a screening test for subsequent arrhythmic events after myocardial infarction, we can say with confidence that 15 to 20% of patients will have sustained ventricular tachycardia inducible after myocardial infarction. Inducible ventricular tachycardia is clearly independent of the extent of coronary atherosclerosis, but its relationships to infarct size and spontaneous ectopy are yet to be defined. Preliminary results suggest that despite a relationship to both infarct size and spontaneous ectopy, ventricular tachycardia inducible by programmed ventricular stimulation has independent prognostic significance. The incidence of sustained ventricular tachycardia in the year after myocardial infarction is low, about 3%. Nearly all of the patients with spontaneous sustained ventricular tachycardia occurring during follow-up had ventricular tachycardia induced prior to discharge from hospital; the odds of having ventricular tachycardia during follow-up are increased more than 10-fold in

inducible patients. The time course of inducible ventricular tachycardia and its significance in terms of total or arrhythmic mortality are yet to be clarified. The preliminary results on mortality suggest that programmed ventricular stimulation predicts total death to some extent and predicts arrhythmic death even better. It is very rare indeed for spontaneous sustained ventricular tachycardia to occur in patients who are not inducible at the time of hospital discharge.

Ventricular Arrhythmias in Variant Angina Pectoris

In 1959, Prinzmetal described variant angina pectoris, a syndrome that differs strikingly from Herberden's classic form of effort angina (140,141). Variant angina pectoris occurs at rest without relationship to emotion; it lasts longer and often is more severe than classic angina pectoris. The attacks may recur at the same time of day and have been attributed to coronary artery spasm, usually at the site of an atherosclerotic lesion (6,86). The hallmark of variant angina pectoris is ST elevation during the attack that is thought to represent severe transmural ischemia (48,89,184). ST-segment elevation often is accompanied by an increase in R-wave amplitude in the same leads (87). Various rhythm or conduction disturbances have been described in variant angina pectoris: ventricular tachycardia, ventricular fibrillation (98), frequent VPDs (162), A-V block (24,86), and asystole (116). The incidence of arrhythmias is between 40 and 50% (87,116), with about half of the patients with arrhythmias having ventricular arrhythmias and half having either A-V block or sinus bradycardia/asystole. Arrhythmias tend to occur near the peak of the ST-segment elevation or as the ST segments are returning toward base line, suggesting intense ischemia or reperfusion as a contributing mechanism (176). Kerin et al. (87) studied 26 patients to evaluate the relationship between the development of arrhythmias and the degree of ST elevation and R-wave amplitude. In this study, 46% had significant ventricular arrhythmias: 6 had ventricular tachycardia (4) or ventricular fibrillation (2), 3 had frequent VPDs (>60 per hour), and 3 had A-V block. The degree of ST-segment change had a strong influence on the probability of having significant arrhythmias during angina. The conditional probability of having an arrhythmia when the ST-segment increase was ≥0.4 mV was 100% in this sample, versus a probability of 0% when the ST-segment increase was <0.4 mV. Also, the R-wave amplitude increased significantly more in the patients who developed arrhythmias. There was no relationship between the likelihood of developing arrhythmias and the extent of coronary atherosclerosis or left ventricular dysfunction (86). A relationship was suggested between the ischemic segment of left ventricular wall and the type of arrhythmia. Patients with ventricular arrhythmias were more likely to have anterior-wall ischemia, whereas patients with A-V block were more likely to have inferior-wall ischemia. R-on-T VPDs started many episodes of ventricular tachycardia, suggesting that the arrhythmia had an ischemic cause.

Miller et al. (116) followed 114 patients with variant angina pectoris for an average of 26 months (6 died, and 13 experienced cardiac arrest, with successful resuscitation). Each of the patients had at least 3 days of continuous EKG monitoring in hospital to search for the maximum ST-segment elevation and to quantify their arrhythmias. Coronary angiography was performed in 110 patients, and if a lesion was seen, angiography was repeated after nitroglycerin administration. Ergonovine was not given during angiography. About half of the 114 patients (49%) had a significant arrhythmia during the monitoring period, and half (51%) did not. The group with arrhythmias was similar to the nonarrhythmia group with respect to age, sex, incidence of multivessel coronary artery disease, and left ventricular dysfunction (Table 12). However, on the average, ST-segment elevation was much greater in the patients who had arrhythmias. Also, sudden death (<1 hr) or cardiac arrest was more common in the arrhythmia group (29% versus 5%). Classified by outcome, the patients who experienced sudden cardiac death or cardiac arrest were significantly more likely to have had ventricular tachycardia or ventricular fibrillation, second- or third-degree A-V block, or asystole.

Incidence and Significance of Ventricular Arrhythmias in Effort Angina Pectoris

The only large study of ventricular arrhythmias in patients who had angina of effort without prior acute myocardial infarction was conducted by the Health Insurance Plan of Greater New York investigators (154). Between March 1972 and December 1975, 416 men with angina of effort, but no previous myocardial in-

TABLE 12. *Features of patients with ventricular arrhythmias during attacks of variant angina pectoris*

	Ventricular arrhythmias in 3 days of monitoring	
	Yes (N = 56)	No (N = 58)
Mean age	51	53
Male sex	71%	72%
Multivessel disease	30%	36%
Abnormal ventriculogram	20%	36%
Maximum ST elevation (mm)	7.4 ± 5.7	3.3 ± 2.3[a]
Death/cardiac arrest	29%	5%[a]

[a] $p < 0.05$.
From ref. 116, with permission.

farction, were recruited from a group of 120,000 men between ages 35 and 74 years. At base line, all patients had standardized interviews, physical and laboratory examinations, and 1-hr single-lead EKG recordings that were analyzed by digital computer. Patients were followed for an average of 3.5 years (range 2–5.5 years), and 62 deaths occurred during follow-up. Comparisons were made between the angina cohort and a group of patients who had previously had myocardial infarction recruited from the same population of insured men (Table 13). The angina group was older and had a longer history of heart disease, but had fewer abnormalities in the 12-lead EKG and less congestive heart failure than the previous-myocardial-infarction group. Table 13 lists the frequency and complex features of ventricular arrhythmias determined by analyzing the 1-hr base-line EKG recordings. VPD frequency was significantly higher in the patients with previous myocardial infarction than in the angina-only patients. Men with effort angina were divided into two subgroups based on the presence or absence of VPDs in the 1-hr EKG recording and were compared for long-term mortality. The 143 angina patients (34%) who had VPDs had a cumulative 5-year mortality of over 25%, compared with 10% mortality for the 273 patients without VPDs ($p < 0.001$). Cox's regression model was used to evaluate the prognostic significance of VPDs when up to 11 clinical variables were taken into account. Variables that did not improve the fit of the model were successively eliminated. The best fit to survivorship over 5 years of follow-up was given by a three-variable model that included age dichotomized at 65 years (relative risk = 2.3), presence or absence of VPDs (relative risk = 2.1), and ST-segment depression in the 12-lead EKG (relative risk = 2.9). VPDs increase the risk of dying twofold over the 5-year follow-up period independent of the other risk indicators. Because the three indicators are independently associated with mortality, they are multiplied to estimate risk. For example, a group of patients with angina pectoris over age 65 with VPDs and ST depression has 5-year mortality more than 13 times that for a group with angina but none of these three risk indicators.

This important study from the HIP investigators suggests that VPDs are significantly less prevalent in patients with angina of effort who have not experienced previous myocardial infarction, even though the angina group is significantly older, and VPDs tend to increase somewhat with age. However, the presence of VPDs has about the same significance in patients with angina pectoris as in patients with previous myocardial infarction. Adjusted for age and a number of other clinical risk variables, the presence of VPDs increases mortality at least twofold. It should be noted that VPDs are excellent predictors of mortality in coronary heart disease in subgroups (e.g., angina only) in which congestive heart failure is rare (6%), as well as in groups (e.g., prior

TABLE 13. *Health Insurance Plan of New York angina study: comparison of patients with angina but no previous myocardial infarction to patients with previous infarction*

	Angina only (%) (N = 416)	Previous AMI (%) (N = 1,739)	Z score[a]
Clinical features			
Age ≥65 years	39	29	3.91
Heart disease ≥1 year	81	42	14.24
ST-segment depression	19	39	7.62
T-wave abnormality	29	62	12.12
Congestive heart failure	6	34	11.29
No. of VPDs in 1-hr EKG			
0	66	49	6.18
1–9	19	25	2.52
≥10	15	26	4.86
Complex VPDs in 1-hr EKG			
Multiform	13	21	3.63
R-on-T	3	5	1.62
Bigeminy	6	12	3.45
>2 consecutive	5	10	3.10

[a] Z score ≥ 1.96; $p < 0.05$.
From ref. 154, with permission.

myocardial infarction) in which congestive heart failure is common (34%).

Ventricular Arrhythmias in Dilated Cardiomyopathy

Incidence. Although the numbers of patients in individual studies of ventricular arrhythmias in cardiomyopathy have been small, the number of studies is sufficient to give a clear picture. On the average, more than 80% of patients with dilated cardiomyopathy and congestive heart failure will have VPDs, and about 50% will have unsustained ventricular tachycardia (Table 14). Meinertz et al. (114) reported the incidence and prognostic significance of VPDs in 74 patients with idiopathic dilated cardiomyopathy. These patients were classified on the basis of the clinical criteria of Fuster et al. (61), and all patients underwent cardiac catheterization and angiography. Continuous 24-hr EKG recordings performed at entry into the study revealed that 96% of the patients had VPDs: 35% had frequent VPDs (defined as more than 1,000 VPDs per 24 hr), 20% had paired unsustained ventricular tachycardia, and 49% had ventricular tachycardia. Von Olshausen et al. (183) studied 60 patients with idiopathic dilated cardiomyopathy and found that 100% of the patients had VPDs during a 24-hr EKG recording; 42% had frequent VPDs (more than 1,000 per 24 hr), 78% had paired VPDs, and 42% had ventricular tachycardia. Studies by Meinertz, von Olshausen, and others suggest that the incidence of VPDs, including complex forms, is greater in dilated cardiomyopathy than in hypertrophic cardiomyopathy or coronary disease.

Relation of ventricular arrhythmias to left ventricular dysfunction. Meinertz et al. (114) found that the incidence of frequent VPDs varied inversely with left ventricular ejection fraction. Patients with frequent VPDs were

TABLE 14. *Incidence and significance of ventricular arrhythmias in patients with congestive heart failure*

Author	N	Unsustained ventricular tachycardia (VT) (%)	Average follow-up (months)	Mortality (%) VT present	Mortality (%) VT absent
Huang (80)	35	60	34	14	7
Wilson (186)	77	51	12	64	50
Meinertz (114)	74	49	11	39	13
Von Olshausen (183)	60	80	12	20	6
Holmes (77)	31	39	14	59	11
Chakko (37)	43	51	16	36	13
Unverferth (178)	69	22	12	60	28

highly likely to have higher Lown grades of ectopy, although the converse was not true. There was a significant association between the number of ventricular pairs and the number of episodes of unsustained ventricular tachycardia. However, no clinical or hemodynamic findings were identified in this study that distinguished patients who had unsustained ventricular tachycardia from those who did not. This finding is in agreement with a retrospective study of 35 patients with idiopathic dilated cardiomyopathy conducted by Huang et al. (80). In contrast, von Olshausen et al. (183) found highly significant differences in indices of diastolic and systolic left ventricular function (cardiac index, diastolic pressure, and left ventricular ejection fraction) between patients who had unsustained ventricular tachycardia and patients without it. Despite its statistical significance, the association between left ventricular ejection fraction and ventricular tachycardia was weak, just as it is in coronary heart disease (10).

Prognostic significance of ventricular arrhythmias. There have been conflicting reports on the prognostic significance of ventricular arrhythmias in dilated cardiomyopathy. In general, patients with significant ventricular arrhythmias experience mortality rates at least twice as great as that for comparable patients without VPDs (Table 14). Von Olshausen et al. (183) followed their patients for a mean of 12 months. The annual rate of death from all causes was 12%, and that for sudden death was 5%. Severe impairment of left ventricular function was predictive of death, but ambulatory EKG findings and hemodynamic parameters did not significantly differ between patients who died of congestive heart failure and those who died suddenly. However, there were only seven deaths in this study. Wilson et al. (186) prospectively followed 77 patients with New York Heart Association functional class III or IV heart failure for an average of 11 months; 40 of 77 patients had cardiomyopathy. The mortality was 48% and was equally divided between sudden death and congestive heart failure. Using multivariate analysis, only functional class was an independent prognostic indicator; ventricular arrhythmia frequency and repetitiveness detected by 24-hr EKG recordings provided no additional predictive power. Wilson's study was limited by its small size and by the fact that all patients were severely symptomatic and had been referred for vasodilator therapy of worsening congestive heart failure. Holmes et al. (77) examined the prognostic significance of VPDs classified by the Lown grading system in 31 patients who had been referred for vasodilator therapy; 16 had ischemic and 15 had nonischemic dilated cardiomyopathy. Fourteen patients died during 1 year of follow-up (49%), and 12 of the 14 died suddenly. Patients with simple ventricular arrhythmias (Lown grades 1 to 3) experienced mortality of 11% (1 of 9), compared with 59% (13 of

22) for patients with complex VPDs (Lown grades 4 or 5). The difference in mortality between the two subgroups could not be attributed to differences in hemodynamic parameters alone, suggesting that repetitive or early cycle VPDs were independent predictors of death. In Meinertz's study (114), at 11 months of follow-up, the incidence of all-cause mortality was 26%, and that for sudden cardiac death was 16%. The incidence of paired VPDs and ventricular tachycardia was significantly higher in patients who died suddenly than in survivors or patients who died from congestive heart failure. Using a linear stepwise discriminant-function analysis, Meinertz found that the combination of two hemodynamic (left ventricular ejection fraction, cardiac index) and two arrhythmic variables (number of episodes of ventricular tachycardia, number of VPD pairs per 24 hr) allowed a separation between survivors and patients who died. Left ventricular ejection fractions of $\leq 40\%$, with >20 VPD pairs or >20 episodes of ventricular tachycardia, constituted the best predictors of sudden death. In their 60 patients with nonischemic dilated cardiomyopathy, Unverferth et al. (178) performed univariate and multivariate analyses using 30 variables (from history, physical examination, echocardiography, catheterization, and endomyocardial biopsy) in order to identify prognostic factors. The 1-year mortality was 35%. Univariate analysis showed that ventricular arrhythmia was the third most powerful predictor of death ($p = 0.007$), after left ventricular conduction delay ($p = 0.003$) and pulmonary capillary wedge pressure ($p = 0.005$). Using stepwise logistic regression, the combination of left intraventricular conduction delay, right atrial pressure, and ventricular arrhythmia was the best independent predictor of death.

Ventricular arrhythmias, ventricular dysfunction, and mortality. The available evidence on the prognostic significance of ventricular arrhythmias in dilated cardiomyopathy suggests that frequent and repetitive VPDs predict all-cause mortality and sudden cardiac death, just as they do after myocardial infarction. However, dilated cardiomyopathy has not been studied sufficiently to define clearly the relationship between left ventricular dysfunction and ventricular arrhythmias. McKenna et al. (112) have pointed out that in the small population of patients with isolated right ventricular cardiomyopathy, including right ventricular dysplasia, prognosis depends more on the development of ventricular arrhythmias than on right ventricular dysfunction. The latter is often severe but asymptomatic. Fitchett et al. (54) studied 14 patients with right-sided dilated cardiomyopathy, 10 of whom presented with symptoms suggestive of arrhythmias. Six patients had syncope due to sustained ventricular tachycardia. Of the 12 patients followed for an average of 4.1 years, 11 died, 5 suddenly. The fact that patients with class III or IV congestive heart failure and ventricular arrhythmias experience higher mortality than patients with class III or IV congestive heart failure and no significant ventricular arrhythmias suggests an independent role for ventricular arrhythmias.

Programmed ventricular stimulation in dilated cardiomyopathy. Only a few small series have used programmed ventricular stimulation to evaluate and manage ventricular arrhythmias in dilated cardiomyopathy. Poll et al. (139) studied 9 patients with spontaneous uniform sustained ventricular tachycardia with programmed stimulation in the drug-free state. Sustained ventricular tachycardia was induced in 8 patients. The patient whose ventricular tachycardia was not induced was not tested with triple premature stimuli. Ventricular tachycardia was induced by two premature stimuli in 3 patients (one by left ventricular stimulation only), by three premature stimuli in 4 patients, and by rapid pacing of the left ventricle in 1 patient. Leclercq et al. (97) studied 12 patients with programmed stimulation, but details of the stimulation protocol were not given. Ventricular tachycardia was induced in only 4 patients (33%). Leclercq et al. (97) made the observation that inducible ventricular tachycardia often started late in diastole or after an interpolated sinus beat, following the last premature stimulus. Other published studies on electrophysiologic testing in patients who had spontaneous sustained ventricular tachycardia unrelated to coronary disease either had very few cases of dilated cardiomyopathy or did not identify them clearly.

Exercise ventricular arrhythmias. There is practically no information on exercise-induced ventricular arrhythmias in dilated cardiomyopathy. Considering the functional status of most patients with this condition, this is no surprise.

Effect of treatment on survival. Chakko and Gheorghiade (37) tried to answer the difficult question whether or not antiarrhythmic therapy improves survival for patients with dilated cardiomyopathy. Forty-three patients (28 with ischemic and 15 with idiopathic dilated cardiomyopathy) had 24-hr EKG recordings classified by a hierarchical grading system: 9% had fewer than 30 VPDs per hour and no complex features, 12% had greater than 30 VPDs per hour or multiform VPDs, and 65% had VPD pairs or unsustained ventricular tachycardia. Of the 43 patients, 20 were not given antiarrhythmic therapy; 20 were given procainamide, and 3 quinidine. Before treatment, the two groups were similar for clinical variables, left ventricular ejection fraction, and ventricular ectopy. The method of assigning patients to antiarrhythmic agents was not disclosed. Results were analyzed only for those patients who had "therapeutic" plasma concentrations of antiarrhythmic drugs. At a mean follow-up of 16 months, the all-cause mortality was 37%, and the sudden death rate was 23%. There was no significant difference in incidences of sudden death attributable to drug treatment. However,

this study had major limitations. The study was retrospective; the effect of "antiarrhythmic plasma concentrations" on the arrhythmia was not assessed; and proarrhythmic effects of the antiarrhythmic drugs were not sought. Recently, Parmley and Chatterjee (136) presented preliminary results suggesting that antiarrhythmic drug treatment may have decreased mortality among 78 patients with severe congestive heart failure, most of whom were New York Heart Association (NYHA) class IV. The 6-month mortality in this group was 64%, and about one-third of these deaths were sudden. Twenty-six patients with complex ventricular arrhythmias were treated either with class I antiarrhythmic drugs (13 patients treated with quinidine or procainamide) or with amiodarone (13 patients). The sudden death rate was reduced substantially in the patients who were treated with antiarrhythmic drugs. This study also was retrospective, with treatment initiated on a patient-by-patient basis. These two studies were much too small to detect a treatment effect. Assuming the observed death rate to be the real rate, about 1,000 patients would be required to detect a 25 to 30% difference in mortality due to antiarrhythmic treatment. Thus, it remains for the future to determine if antiarrhythmic drug treatment will improve outcome in patients with severe heart failure due to dilated cardiomyopathy and significant ventricular arrhythmias.

Hypertrophic Cardiomyopathy

The incidence and significance of ventricular arrhythmias also have been studied in patients with hypertrophic cardiomyopathy (25,160). The NIH group (106,160) studied the incidence of VPDs using continuous 24-hr EKG recordings in a large number of patients with hypertrophic cardiomyopathy. These patients had a mean age of 38 years (range of 12–64) and were selected on the basis of history (syncope, family history of sudden death or cardiomyopathy) and EKG findings (sinus rhythm, atrial fibrillation). The 24-hr EKG recordings showed that 83% of the patients had VPDs; 28% had more than 100 VPDs per 24 hr; 60% had multiform VPDs; 32% had paired VPDs; and 19% had ventricular tachycardia. McKenna et al. (112) recorded continuous 24-hr EKGs in 86 unselected patients with hypertrophic cardiomyopathy: 77% had had less than 30 VPDs per hour; 23% had more than 30 VPDs per hour; 17% had multiform VPDs; 37% had paired VPDs; and 30% had ventricular tachycardia. Thus, in both these studies, there were higher incidences of frequent and repetitive VPDs than in the normal or postinfarction populations, but fewer than in patients with congestive cardiomyopathy in NYHA functional class III or IV.

Extent of hypertrophy and ventricular arrhythmias. Savage et al. (160) found no correlation between left ventricular outflow gradient and the presence or severity of VPDs. There was no linear relation between ventricular septal thickness and the VPD grade, but patients with septal thickness greater than 20 mm had a higher incidence of high-grade VPDs. Patients with unsustained ventricular tachycardia had significantly greater mean septal thicknesses and total 24-hr VPD counts than those who did not have ventricular tachycardia. Of interest, symptoms of lightheadedness correlated with either atrial or ventricular arrhythmias detected with 24-hr EKG recordings in only 2 of the 19 patients who had this symptom during a recording.

Mechanisms of sudden death. Several mechanisms have been proposed to account for sudden death in hypertrophic cardiomyopathy. These include outflow obstruction, diastolic dysfunction, myocardial infarction, and arrhythmias. Although unsustained ventricular tachycardia is often asymptomatic in patients with hypertrophic cardiomyopathy, it appears to have prognostic significance. In Savage's series, the possibility of death or a sustained ventricular arrhythmia during a mean 3-year follow-up was 24% in patients with unsustained ventricular tachycardia, contrasted with 3% in patients without ventricular tachycardia (160). In McKenna's series, the combination of multiform and paired VPDs also was associated with sudden death (113).

Exercise tests. Both Savage (160) and McKenna (112) noted that continuous 24-hr EKG recording was superior to exercise testing for detecting ventricular arrhythmias. Exercise tests underestimated VPD grade in 57% of patients with greater than grade 3 VPDs on Holter in Savage's series. None of the patients with high-grade VPDs on exercise went undetected by Holter.

Programmed ventricular stimulation. There is little information on electrophysiologic testing in patients with hypertrophic cardiomyopathy. Anderson et al. (4) performed programmed stimulation on 17 patients in the operating room at the time of myectomy and induced ventricular tachycardia or ventricular fibrillation in 14 patients. None of 5 control patients with coronary disease and normal ventricular function had inducible sustained ventricular arrhythmias, and the difference between the two groups was statistically significant. Only 6 of the 17 patients with hypertrophic cardiomyopathy had a previous history of cardiac arrest or syncope. However, the performance of electrophysiologic testing at the time of surgery and the requirement of three ventricular premature stimuli for induction of ventricular tachycardia or ventricular fibrillation in 4 patients raise questions about the significance of the findings. More recently, Kowey et al. (94) studied 7 patients with hypertrophic cardiomyopathy referred for cardiac arrest or syncope. Ventricular tachycardia was inducible in 3, and ventricular fibrillation in 1 patient. At a mean of 17 months of follow-up, with antiarrhythmic drugs

predicted to be effective based on the electrophysiologic testing, no patient had a recurrence of symptoms. While promising, these results are inconclusive and controversial. One of the major issues raised by these data is the significance of polymorphic ventricular tachycardia or ventricular fibrillation induced by programmed ventricular stimulation. Some consider these responses to be false-positive findings without prognostic significance. Others believe that polymorphic ventricular tachycardia and ventricular fibrillation are common in hypertrophic cardiomyopathy because premature activation of the disordered whorls of hypertrophic muscle during programmed stimulation is likely to result in fragmented propagation. The latter hypothesis leads to the view that polymorphic ventricular tachycardia and ventricular fibrillation may have prognostic significance.

Mitral Valve Prolapse

Mitral valve prolapse has been thought to be associated with increased probabilities of ventricular arrhythmias and of sudden death (81,137). More recently, these concepts have been challenged and have become controversial (2). There are three areas of controversy: (a) the echocardiographic criteria for a diagnosis of prolapse, (b) the association between mitral valve prolapse and ventricular arrhythmias, and (c) the relationship between mitral valve prolapse and sudden death.

Population-based studies. Savage et al. (161) examined the incidence of VPDs in mitral valve prolapse in a large sample of offspring of the original Framingham cohort. A total of 1,370 men and 1,470 women, mean age 44 years, were studied. To determine the incidence of VPDs, resting 12-lead EKGs of 15 sec duration were obtained in 156 subjects with mitral valve prolapse and 1,801 control subjects; treadmill exercise tests were obtained in 192 subjects with mitral valve prolapse and 2,455 controls; and 24-hr continuous EKG recordings were obtained in 61 subjects with mitral valve prolapse and 179 age-matched controls. On the 12-lead EKG, VPDs occurred in none of the subjects who had mitral valve prolapse and 1% of the control subjects. During treadmill exercise, VPDs occurred in 10% of subjects with mitral valve prolapse and 13% of the control group. In the 24-hr continuous EKG recording, at least one VPD occurred in 89% of subjects with mitral valve prolapse and in 68% of the control group. Of the 61 persons with mitral valve prolapse, 49% had complex or frequent VPDs in their Holter recordings, and 20% had VPD pairs or runs. Of 179 control subjects, 40% had complex or frequent VPDs; 12% had VPD pairs or runs. None of the differences in VPD incidence between subjects with mitral valve prolapse and the control group reached statistical significance. The Framingham study did not exclude the possibility that specific subgroups of patients with mitral valve prolapse might have had an excess incidence of VPDs. Because Jeresaty (81) had suggested that middle-aged women with mitral valve prolapse have a high risk for sudden death, Savage et al. (161) examined the Framingham black and white populations of women ≥40 years of age and found that 16 of 22 women (73%) with mitral valve prolapse had Lown grade 2 or higher VPDs, compared with 24 of 52 women (46%) without mitral valve prolapse. The difference was statistically significant ($p < 0.05$).

Ventricular arrhythmias in symptomatic patients. Winkle et al. (188) found that mitral valve prolapse subjects with auscultatory findings or unexplained chest pain had a high incidence of VPDs. They studied 24 such patients (5 men, 19 women) who had been referred for cardiologic evaluation but were unselected with respect to presence or absence of arrhythmias. Their mean age was 45 years. Each patient had a 12-lead EKG, a maximal treadmill exercise test, and a 24-hr continuous EKG recording. VPDs were present in 75% of the 24-hr EKG recordings; frequent VPDs (defined as >425 VPDs per 24 hr) occurred in 50%, multiform VPDs in 41%, paired VPDs in 50%, and unsustained ventricular tachycardia in 21%. There was a striking separation of patients into groups with low- and high-frequency VPDs. There was a strong correlation between complex and frequent VPDs. There was poor correlation between symptoms and arrhythmias detected in 24-hr EKG recordings. In particular, 2 patients had syncopal attacks at a time when they had normal blood pressure and only occasional VPDs in the EKG recording. In Winkle's study, Holter EKG recordings were more sensitive than treadmill exercise tests for detecting arrhythmias. Although there were no control subjects in Winkle's study, his findings are supported by those of DeMaria et al. (45) in a group of 31 patients with mitral valve prolapse, 28 of whom had abnormal auscultatory findings. The results of 24-hr EKG recordings and treadmill exercise tests for the 31 mitral valve prolapse patients were compared with those for 40 patients evaluated for atypical chest pain and documented to be free of heart disease or mitral valve prolapse by cardiac catheterization and coronary angiography. None of their 40 control patients had any abnormality in the resting 12-lead EKG. Fourteen (45%) of the 31 patients with mitral valve prolapse had rhythm disturbances in the 12-lead EKG, and 14 (45%) had inferior or lateral ST-T abnormalities. During 24-hr continuous EKG recordings, the mitral valve prolapse patients had a 52% incidence of frequent or complex VPDs, compared with 10% in the control group. Supraventricular arrhythmias were recorded in 35% of the mitral valve prolapse group, compared with 10% in the control group. Bradyarrhythmias occurred in 29% of the mitral valve prolapse group, compared with 5% of the control group.

Clinical predictors of ventricular arrhythmias. In an attempt to identify clinical predictors of ventricular arrhythmias in mitral valve prolapse patients, DeMaria et al. (45) related their Holter data according to sex, age (greater or less than 40 years), severity of prolapse, ST-T-wave abnormalities, QT intervals, and auscultatory findings. No statistically significant correlation was found between any clinical factor and cardiac arrhythmias detected by Holter recordings. Campbell et al. (36) studied 20 patients with midsystolic click and/or late systolic murmur. Echocardiography confirmed the presence of mitral valve prolapse in 17. Twenty-four-hour EKG recordings showed that 3 patients had ventricular tachycardia, and 1 had spontaneously terminating ventricular fibrillation. Eight patients had nonspecific ST-T-wave changes in the inferolateral leads of their resting 12-lead EKGs. All 4 patients with ventricular tachycardia or ventricular fibrillation were in the group with inferolateral ST and T-wave abnormalities. Campbell concluded that the "auscultatory-electrocardiographic variant of the balloon mitral valve syndrome" constituted a group at risk for arrhythmic death (36).

Kramer et al. (95) have recently disputed Winkle's and DeMaria's observations. In an effort to assess the contribution of selection bias, Kramer compared 24-hr EKG recordings in 63 mitral valve prolapse patients with those for 28 symptom-matched control subjects. He found no statistically significant difference in VPD incidence between the two groups.

Mitral valve prolapse and sudden death. An association between mitral valve prolapse and sudden death has been proposed by Jeresaty (in 25 documented cases) and others. Jeresaty (81) concluded that risk factors for sudden death in mitral valve prolapse were as follows: female sex, age greater than 40, a history of syncope or presyncope, a late systolic murmur preceded by a click or a pansystolic murmur with late systolic accentuation, inferolateral ST and T-wave changes, frequent VPDs, and severe mitral valve prolapse on ventriculography. However, the significance of the association of mitral valve prolapse with sudden death remains unclear, because cases of sudden death usually have been collected retrospectively, and despite dramatic case histories, the incidence appears to be low despite the high incidence of mitral valve prolapse. Furthermore, the specificity of the risk factors outlined by Jeresaty has been questioned on the basis of case reports of sudden death in patients with mitral valve prolapse who lacked auscultatory abnormalities or EKG changes.

Follow-up studies in mitral valve prolapse. From another prospective, longitudinal studies have examined the prognostic significance of mitral valve prolapse and associated auscultatory abnormalities. Allen et al. (1) identified 62 patients with isolated late systolic murmurs from the phonocardiographic records of their hospitals. Thirty-three patients had been referred because of palpitations and VPDs. Fifty-eight patients were followed for a mean of 14 years (range 9–22), with a murmur known for a mean of 27 years (range 13–51). Mechanical and infectious mitral valvular complications occurred in 7 patients (bacterial endocarditis in 5, ruptured chordae in 1, progressive mitral regurgitation in 1), and atrial fibrillation occurred in 10 patients. No primary lethal ventricular arrhythmias occurred during long-term follow-up. However, Allen et al. (1) excluded patients with electrocardiographic abnormalities, and no echocardiograms were performed. Koch and Hancock (92) followed 40 patients with the midsystolic-click/late-systolic-murmur syndrome for 10 years, 90% of whom had an abnormal EKG. No bacterial endocarditis occurred, but 5 patients died suddenly. Mills et al. (117) followed 53 patients with midsystolic click or late systolic murmur a mean of 14 years; 33 of 53 (62%) patients had normal EKGs. During follow-up, 9 deaths occurred; 1 died of acute chordal rupture during an episode of bacterial endocarditis, 1 died suddenly during quinidine treatment, and 7 died of causes unrelated to mitral valve prolapse.

In summary, although the "auscultatory-electrocardiographic" variant of mitral valve prolapse may constitute a subgroup at risk for arrhythmic death, the available data do not conclusively support this hypothesis, because of the methods used to select these cases and the small numbers of patients in the available studies.

Programmed ventricular stimulation. Morady et al. (122) have reported recently on the results of electro-physiologic testing in 36 patients with echocardiographically documented mitral valve prolapse. Despite an aggressive stimulation protocol (with three ventricular premature stimuli), no ventricular tachycardia or ventricular fibrillation was inducible in 11 patients without syncope, even among those who had complex ventricular ectopy on Holter recordings. At a mean follow-up of 23 months, these patients remained well. Among 20 patients with syncope or presyncope and documented unsustained ventricular tachycardia, multiform unsustained ventricular tachycardia was induced in 8, uniform sustained ventricular tachycardia was induced in 2, and ventricular fibrillation in 3. Two patients with syncope but no documented ectopy were not inducible. All 3 patients with documented spontaneous sustained ventricular tachycardia or ventricular fibrillation had inducible uniform ventricular tachycardia. Naccarelli et al. (131) studied patients with mitral valve prolapse. Three of 5 (60%) with a history of sustained ventricular tachycardia had sustained ventricular tachycardia induced by programmed ventricular stimulation. Among 13 patients with unsustained ventricular tachycardia detected by 12-lead or 24-hr continuous EKG, no sustained ventricular tachycardia was induced. Thus, in both of these studies, a history of sustained ventricular arrhythmia was the best predictor of inducible sustained ventricular tachycardia.

EVALUATION OF ANTIARRHYTHMIC DRUGS

The task of evaluating the effects of antiarrhythmic drugs on ventricular arrhythmias presents many difficult and complex problems. The most elemental aspect of assessing drug effect is to determine if an antiarrhythmic drug significantly reduces the frequency of VPDs or of repetitive VPDs. This is far from a simple issue because of the substantial spontaneous hour-to-hour and day-to-day variability in VPD rates. A number of statistical techniques have been proposed to determine when a drug-induced change in VPD rate is beyond the limits of spontaneous variability. These methods will be critically evaluated in this section.

Patterns of Occurrence of VPDs

The advent of the Holter recorder and the development of sophisticated computerized systems for analyzing long-term EKG recordings have enabled researchers to study cardiac rhythms over prolonged periods of time. Studies in patients with frequent VPDs have shown that there is substantial variability in ventricular arrhythmias from hour to hour and from day to day. Several investigators have noted decreases in the frequencies of VPDs and of repetitive VPDs during sleep (102,170). It is not surprising that there is diurnal variation in VPD frequency during sleep, considering the overall decreases in heart rate and sympathetic tone during sleep. What is surprising is the substantial variability from day to day in the frequency of VPDs and of repetitive VPDs. This variability was noted by a number of investigators using 24-hr EKG recordings to develop criteria for determining antiarrhythmic drug efficacy. Morganroth et al. (124) selected 15 patients from an antiarrhythmic drug study who had VPD rates of at least 30 per hour on a 24-hr continuous EKG screening recording. After enrollment, the patients were monitored for 3 successive days prior to antiarrhythmic drug therapy in order to evaluate the variability of ventricular arrhythmias. There was as much variance in the average hourly VPD rates between daily monitoring periods as there was between patients. In one-third of the patients there was at least a fourfold difference in the average hourly VPD rates among the three daily records; in one-half of the patients there was a twofold difference. Sami et al. (158) studied 21 patients who had average hourly VPD counts of 6 or more on 24-hr continuous EKG recordings. Each of these patients had a second drug-free 24-hr EKG recording 2 weeks later. The patients studied by Sami showed less day-to-day variability than did those of Morganroth. However, the extent of variability is still impressive; 9 of the 19 patients showed at least a 50% change in average hourly VPD rates between the two recordings.

Hour-to-Hour Variability

The ranges of hour-to-hour variability in VPD rates and rates of occurrence of repetitive VPDs are considerable. Morganroth et al. (124) found that in their population of 15 patients, for an individual patient, hour-to-hour variability accounted for 48% of total variability. Winkle (187) published 20 examples of marked spontaneous variability recorded during 5.5-hr time periods selected from 24-hr EKG recordings of patients referred to the Stanford University Medical Center for cardiac arrhythmias. All patients had average VPD rates of 60 or more per hour. The objective of the study was to determine if hour-to-hour variability in VPD frequency might invalidate the technique of acute drug testing. In acute drug testing, a 30-min control period was compared with the 5.5 hr after a single large dose of antiarrhythmic drug (63). Winkle noted that, when compared with the first half-hour period, the variation in VPD rate for subsequent half-hour periods ranged from a 99% decline to an 1,100% increase (187). Winkle's examples mimicked antiarrhythmic drug success in 65% of the cases.

Interpatient Variability

Unfortunately, there have been only a few studies concerning the distribution of average hourly VPD rates occurring over 24-hr periods in the general population. In several studies, continuous EKGs were recorded in patients who had sustained myocardial infarction, and information is available on the average hourly VPD distribution in this population. Figure 6 shows the distribution of hourly VPD frequencies for 733 patients admitted to Columbia-Presbyterian Medical Center with myocardial infarction over the past 5 years. The distribution is highly skewed to the left. Approximately one-half the patients had less than 1 VPD per hour over the 24-hr period. At frequencies greater than 10 to 20 VPDs per hour, the distribution remains relatively constant. This is an interesting phenomenon: In this population, there were as many patients with very high VPD rates as with moderately high VPD rates.

Figure 7 shows the logarithmic transformation of the distribution in Figure 6. Many investigators use the logarithmic transformation of average hourly VPD frequency in statistical analyses to conform to a normal distribution and to stabilize the variance. As is shown in Fig. 7, the log-transformed distribution is still highly skewed, indicating that the transformation fails to normalize the distribution.

Modeling the Occurrence of VPDs

Ruttimann et al. (156) searched for a mathematical model to describe the occurrence of VPDs. Twenty-

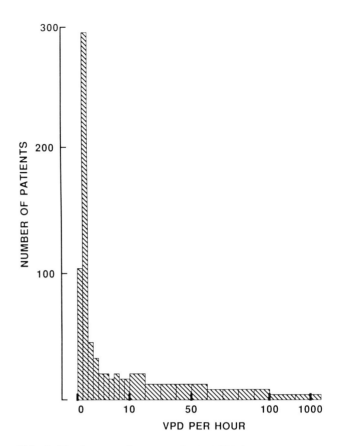

FIG. 6. Distribution of average 24-hr VPD frequency (VPDs per hour) 10 ± 4 days after myocardial infarction. These data were obtained from 733 patients treated at the Columbia-Presbyterian Medical Center.

four-hour continuous EKG recordings for 21 patients in the George Washington University Hospital CCU were analyzed. Ruttimann found that the occurrence of VPDs could be described as a "renewal process" in 18 of the 21 patients. In a renewal process, the expected number of events observed in a given time interval depends solely on the underlying "true" event rate and is unrelated to the previous sequence of events. In other words, there appears to be no regular pattern to the occurrence of these events. During episodes of bigeminy and ventricular tachycardia, there is a regularity in the occurrence of VPDs, so that the occurrence of a VPD is related to the pattern of occurrence of previous VPDs. Nevertheless, unless sustained bigeminy or ventricular tachycardia occurs frequently in a record, the occurrence of VPDs can be adequately described as a renewal process.

A Poisson process is a special case of a renewal process. In addition to the general characteristics of a renewal process given earlier, the intervals between events in a Poisson process are distributed exponentially. Ruttimann found that in 52% of his cases, the occurrence of VPDs showed a good fit with a Poisson process. An important characteristic of a Poisson process is that the

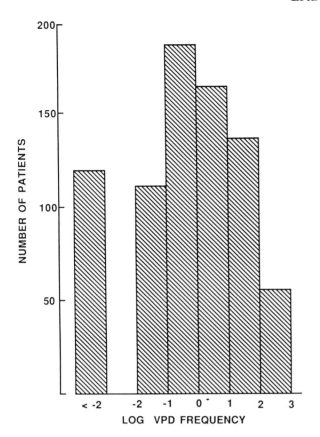

FIG. 7. The same data shown in Fig. 6 are presented with VPD frequency plotted on a logarithmic scale.

variability of intervals between events is equal to the mean interevent time. In the case of VPD occurrence, this means that 24-hr continuous EKG recordings with a higher average hourly VPD rate will show less variability than recordings with a lower average hourly VPD rate. Ruttimann found that, not only in the records fitting the Poisson model but also in 81% of his cases, the variability of interectopic intervals was approximately equal to the mean interectopic interval. That is, for the vast majority of his cases, Ruttimann found that as the VPD rate increased, the variability of the interectopic intervals decreased. This fact has been of concern to investigators in choosing an arbitrary enrollment criterion for patients in antiarrhythmic drug studies. In many studies, high VPD rates on predrug EKG recordings are required for enrollment, on the rationale that records with high VPD rates also will have relatively low variability in VPD rates, making it easier to recognize a drug effect. The necessity and desirability of using such stringent entry criteria will be discussed later.

Estimates of Limits of Spontaneous Variability

A number of investigators have developed criteria for determining when the effect of an antiarrhythmic drug is greater than that due to spontaneous variability of

VPD rate, or of repetitive VPD rate. The data used to develop these criteria were indeed limited. Most analyses involved data from 15 to 20 patients with high VPD rates, although results were assumed to be valid for a more diverse population. For example, Ruttimann analyzed records of CCU patients, presumably patients who had experienced myocardial infarction, and assumed that his results with the acute phase of infarction could be applied to patients being tested for antiarrhythmic drug efficacy.

Heuristic approach. In his evaluation of the utility of acute drug testing, discussed previously, Winkle (187) analyzed continuous 24-hr EKG recordings for 20 patients with an average hourly VPD frequency of at least 60 VPDs per hour. Winkle concluded that in order for the Lown 6-hr acute drug testing protocol to yield correct results, the effect of an antiarrhythmic drug cannot be considered significant unless there is 100% suppression of VPDs for a half-hour period or a 90% reduction in VPDs in two or three consecutive half-hour periods following drug administration. He decided that these stringent criteria were necessary because 19 of his 20 patients exhibited less than this degree of reduction spontaneously. This, in effect, established a method with an alpha level near 0.05. That is, assuming that his patients were representative of patients with high VPD rates, Winkle's criteria for drug efficacy would incorrectly indicate that there is a significant drug effect about 5% of the time.

Winkle examined the criteria proposed for acute drug tests in the light of his findings (187). In their acute drug testing studies, Gaughan et al. (63) used as criteria for significant drug effect a 50% reduction in VPD rate or abolition of repetitive VPDs in a 30-min period within 1 to 3 hr after administration of a test drug, as compared with a 30-min control period. Winkle observed that if these criteria were applied to his data, 14 of the 20 patients would be classified as responders, solely because of spontaneous variability of ventricular ectopic events. Even if an 80% reduction criterion were used, 7 of the 20 patients would be classified as responders. Winkle concluded that the criteria used by Gaughan were not stringent enough to distinguish between drug response and spontaneous variability. His paper made the important contribution of alerting researchers to the need to use carefully developed criteria when dealing with events in which there is considerable spontaneous variability.

Winkle's direct, heuristic approach has the appeal of a nonparametric statistic: No assumptions need be made about the underlying distribution of VPD rates. However, the inclusion of only 20 patients in this study seems less than adequate; if only 1 patient had demonstrated a different pattern in the occurrence of VPDs, Winkle might have proposed different criteria.

Analysis-of-variance approach. Using the data cited

previously from three successive 24-hr EKG recordings for each of 15 patients, Morganroth et al. (124) used classic analysis-of-variance procedures to evaluate antiarrhythmic drug efficacy. They used a logarithmic transformation of the VPD data attempting to normalize the distribution and to ensure homogeneous variance.

A four-way nested analysis-of-variance design was used to compute the minimal percentage VPD reduction values required to prove significant antiarrhythmic drug effect (Table 15). The minimal percentage VPD reduction is a function of the duration of EKG recording and the numbers of control and test days. The magnitude of VPD reduction required to declare efficacy is greatest for short durations of recording and few recording periods: For one 8-hr control record and one 8-hr test record, a 90% reduction is needed. Note that this criterion is similar to Winkle's. The criterion value for one 24-hr control record and one 24-hr test record is an 83% reduction in VPD frequency.

Total variation in VPD frequency was partitioned into its components: variation between patients, between daily records for each patient, between 8-hr periods within a 24-hr recording, and between hourly VPD counts within an 8-hr period (Table 16).

Morganroth et al. (124) analyzed the EKG recordings in 8-hr units, making the statistical assumption that there was no difference in VPD rates at different times of the day. However, Morganroth noted a tendency toward decreased arrhythmic frequency during sleep. The findings in this study suggest that the most valid comparisons for drug effect are made using 24-hr records. If records shorter than 24 hr are used for between-day drug comparisons, they should be recorded during the same time interval each day.

Analysis-of-variance approach for variability of repetitive VPDs. Michelson and Morganroth (115) applied the analysis-of-variance procedure to examine the spontaneous variability of repetitive VPDs. For this analysis they used 96 hr of consecutive ambulatory EKG record-

TABLE 15. *Percentage reductions in mean hourly frequency of total VPD, VPD pairs, and ventricular tachycardia required to demonstrate drug efficacy*

No. of days[a]		Percentage reduction		
Control	Test	Total VPD	Pairs	VT
1	1	83	75	65
1	2	79	70	60
1	3	77	68	57
2	1	79	70	60
2	2	72	63	52
3	3	65	55	45
7	7	49	41	33

[a] Number of 24-hr EKG recordings.
From ref. 16, with permission.

TABLE 16. *Sources of variance in mean hourly frequencies of total VPDs, VPD pairs, and ventricular tachycardia*

Source	Percentage variance from each source		
	Total VPDs	VPD pairs	VT
Pooled data			
Between patients	66	65	46
Between days	8	4	7
Between 8-hr periods	10	8	9
Between hours	16	23	38
Total	100	100	100
Data from individual patients			
Between days	23	12	12
Between 8-hr periods	29	24	17
Between hours	48	64	71
Total	100	100	100

From ref. 16, with permission.

ings from 21 patients with various cardiac disorders. As before, they related the percentage reduction required to declare a significant reduction of repetitive VPDs to the duration of recording (Table 15). Surprisingly, efficacy criteria for repetitive VPDs were found to be less stringent than for total VPD frequency. The percentage reduction needed to assert that an antiarrhythmic drug exerts a significant effect on paired VPDs was 75% using two 24-hr recordings, and 86% using two 8-hr recordings. For ventricular tachycardia, the corresponding reductions were 65% and 80%. A decrease in repetitive ventricular arrhythmias was noted during sleep. As with their earlier paper, the group performed a components-of-variance analysis for paired VPDs and ventricular tachycardia (Table 16). In this study, variance between days for mean hourly frequency for repetitive VPDs made up a smaller proportion of total variance than daily variance in total VPD frequency. The proportion of intrapatient variability attributable to day-to-day variability is half as great for repetitive VPDs (12%) as for nonrepetitive VPDs (23%). Hourly variability made up a larger proportion of variability for repetitive VPDs than for VPD frequency. It accounted for 64% of intrapatient variability for paired VPDs and 71% for ventricular tachycardia, compared with 48% for total VPD frequency. It remains to be seen if this finding holds for many different samples.

Linear-regression techniques. Sami et al. (158) used linear regression to develop criteria for drug efficacy. Twenty-one patients who had an average of 6 or more VPDs per hour on a 24-hr EKG recording were studied. For each patient, an initial 24-hr continuous EKG recording was obtained. Each patient was treated with placebo for 2 weeks, and then a second 24-hr EKG was recorded. The VPD rate during placebo treatment was regressed on the pretreatment VPD rate, and 95% and 99% confidence intervals were calculated to account for spontaneous variability. Sami et al. (158) estimated the minimum percentage reduction in VPD frequency required to establish drug efficacy as a function of the initial VPD rate. For rates below 2.2 VPDs per hour, this regression method cannot be used. For rates from 2.2 to 3 VPDs per hour, the critical value in Sami's sample was a 90% reduction in VPD rate. For an initial VPD rate of 30 or more VPDs per hour, the critical value was a 65% reduction in VPD rate.

Comparison of analysis-of-variance and regression methods. There is a considerable difference in the one criterion value that can be compared in the Morganroth and Sami studies, i.e., the minimum percentage reduction in VPD frequency required to prove antiarrhythmic drug efficacy using two 24-hr EKG recordings in patients with 30 or more VPDs per hour in the initial record. Morganroth et al. (124) proposed an 83% reduction for this analysis; Sami et al. (158) proposed a 65% reduction. In an attempt to reconcile these differences, Shapiro et al. (166) applied both Morganroth's and Sami's methods to a much more extensive data set. The data set consisted of three 24-hr ambulatory EKG recordings, obtained within a 14-day period, for 162 patients with severe ventricular arrhythmias. Each recording averaged at least 30 VPDs per hour.

Shapiro et al. (166) obtained very similar results using both Morganroth's analysis-of-variance approach and Sami's regression method. They obtained separate results for each pairwise comparison of the three records obtained for each patient. The percentage reduction needed to declare antiarrhythmic drug effect varied from 74% (record 1 versus record 2) to 83% (record 1 versus record 3) with an analysis-of-variance approach similar to that of Morganroth et al. (124). With regression techniques, the percentage reduction needed to declare antiarrhythmic drug effect varied from 72% (record 1 versus record 3) to 84% (record 1 versus record 3). The similarity of results is reassuring, but not expected, because these analysis-of-variance and regression models are not equivalent. As an example of the disparity between the two methods, Morganroth's method analyzed EKG data in 8-hr units, whereas Sami used data averaged over a 24-hr period. Shapiro more closely aligned the two methods by using a one-tailed nested analysis of variance. This differs from Morganroth's two-tailed analyses and is equivalent to Sami's one-tailed approach. Shapiro attributed the discrepancy between Sami's results and those of Morganroth and himself to a smaller day-to-day variance of the VPDs in the Sami sample.

It is somewhat surprising that Sami's data demonstrated less daily variability than Morganroth's, because Morganroth's data consisted of sets of recordings made on consecutive days, whereas Sami's recordings were made 2 weeks apart. Also, Sami's second record for each patient included any effect on arrhythmia due to placebo treatment. The discrepancy in the two data sets is probably best explained by the fact that they were both very small, too small to confidently represent the population of patients with high VPD rates. Shapiro's study points out the need to use data sets large enough to represent adequately the population to which results will be applied.

Poisson model. Thomas and Miller (175) used the Poisson model to derive a set of criteria that can be used easily in a clinical research setting. They used the variance of a Poisson process to estimate between-day variability, and they combined this with estimates of day-to-day intrapatient variability to derive criteria for assessing antiarrhythmic drug efficacy. The estimate of between-day intrapatient variability was obtained from results of an unpublished drug trial in which six 24-hr continuous EKG recordings were made for each of 20 patients, consisting of two control recordings, two placebo recordings, and two postdrug recordings per patient. Although Ruttimann et al. (156) found that only half of the EKG records they examined fit the Poisson model, they did find that the variance of intervals between VPDs was close to the variance of a Poisson process in 81% of the cases. Therefore, it seems justified to use the Poisson variance in this analysis.

Figure 8, taken from Thomas and Miller (175), shows the 95% confidence limits for spontaneous variability of ventricular arrhythmias. This approach indicates that the percentage reduction required to show significant antiarrhythmic drug efficacy varies with VPD frequency in the predrug ambulatory EKG recording. For initial EKG recordings with 30 or more VPDs in 24 hr, an 84% reduction in frequency is required to demonstrate antiarrhythmic drug efficacy. This value is essentially identical with Morganroth's value of 83%. For predrug 24-hr EKG recordings with less than 20 ventricular events per day, Thomas and Miller required a 95% reduction to show significant antiarrhythmic drug effect. They stated that this criterion might be used when investigating the effect of an antiarrhythmic drug on relatively rare events such as VPD pairs. For even rarer events, such as ventricular tachycardia, the confidence limits would become even wider. The results of Thomas and Miller (175) concerning VPD pairs differ sharply from those of Michelson and Morganroth (115). Michelson and Morganroth found that a smaller percentage reduction in frequency of VPD pairs was needed to show significant drug effect than for VPDs occurring singly. These divergent results were in part due to the fact that Michelson and Morganroth used different variance estimates for simple and for repetitive ventricular episodes. Morganroth's variance estimates for simple ventricular ectopic events were calculated from the records of only 15 patients; the variance estimates for

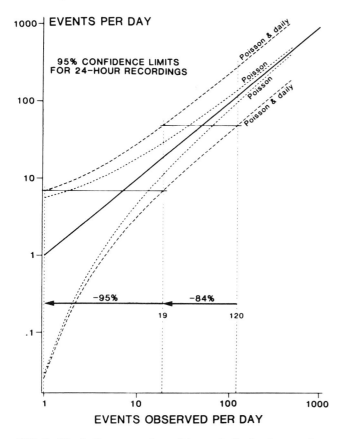

FIG. 8. Ninety-five percent confidence limits for the number of VPDs observed in a 24-hr continuous recording (on a log-log scale). Confidence limits are shown for Poisson counting statistics alone, as well as for Poisson counting statistics plus between-day variation. (From ref. 175, with permission.)

repetitive ventricular ectopic events were obtained from the records of only 20 patients. Substantiation of variance estimates for paired VPDs or ventricular tachycardia with a larger data set is needed to settle the issue whether or not components of variance differ for simple and repetitive ventricular events.

Enrolling Criteria for Antiarrhythmic Studies

In many antiarrhythmic drug studies, an average hourly VPD rate of 30 or more on a 24-hr continuous EKG recording has been used as an arbitrary enrolling criterion. The usual argument for using a value as high as 30 VPDs per hour is that it simplifies judgments about antiarrhythmic drug efficacy. However, the use of an enrolling criterion of this magnitude presents a number of problems. For one, it is more difficult to obtain subjects for antiarrhythmic drug therapy when the enrolling criterion is set this high. For example, 10 days after myocardial infarction, only 8% will have 30 or more VPDs per hour in a 24-hr EKG. Also, it would be more informative to conduct antiarrhythmic drug testing on the full range of patients who might use them,

because the effects of antiarrhythmic drugs may be different for patients with differing VPD rates. Recent data have shown that in the population who have experienced recent myocardial infarction, mortality rises rapidly as the average hourly VPD rate increases from 1 to 10. However, mortality remains relatively constant for patients with average hourly VPD rates of 10 or greater (Fig. 3). Therefore, in our current state of knowledge, it would be as appropriate to treat a patient with an average VPD rate of 10 per hour after myocardial infarction with antiarrhythmic drugs as to treat a patient with an average VPD rate of 30 or more per hour.

Researchers have been concerned that a possible pitfall in extending the enrolling criterion to include patients with an average VPD frequency of, say, 10 per hour is that the statistical power to detect antiarrhythmic drug efficacy may be decreased. That is, as the qualifying VPD frequency is lowered, the ability to detect a significant reduction in VPD frequency due to treatment will be appreciably diminished. Dr. Bruce Levin (*personal communication*) has argued that power is not compromised substantially by reducing the enrollment criterion from 30 VPDs per hour to 10 VPDs per hour. By his calculations, the reduction in power will be no more than 5%.

Levin used the following assumptions in his analysis: (a) the occurrence of VPDs in both the predrug and postdrug 24-hr EKG recordings can be described by a Poisson process (175), and (b) the logarithmic transformation of the average hourly VPD rate is distributed uniformly in the range between 5 and 1,000 VPDs per hour. This second assumption accurately reflects empirical findings in postinfarction populations. Also, in his calculations he used a 70% reduction to define a drug success. This is lower than the critical values suggested in the publications of Winkle, Morganroth, Sami, and Miller (124, 158, 175, 187), but it is in accord with the Cardiac Arrhythmic Pilot Study criterion for drug efficacy (33). This value was used because clinical experience indicates that a 70% reduction is sufficient to indicate an antiarrhythmic drug effect and because researchers have been wary of using the critical values for drug efficacy obtained from studies involving small sample sizes. This disparity between theoretical results based on small sample sizes and criteria based on clinical practicality underscores the need for further studies involving larger samples to estimate the limits of spontaneous variability of VPD frequency.

Levin (*personal communication*) calculated the probabilities of declaring antiarrhythmic drug efficacy as a function of the VPD rate used as an enrolling criterion, the true (not the manifest) predrug base-line VPD rate, and the true "reduction fraction" achieved during antiarrhythmic drug therapy. He did this in order to compare these probabilities for the two entry criteria: an average rate of 10 VPDs per hour and an average rate of 30 VPDs per hour. The "reduction fraction" expresses the posttreatment VPD rate as a fraction of the predrug VPD rate. For example, if the predrug VPD occurrence rate is 100 VPDs per hour and the postdrug rate is 30 VPDs per hour, the reduction fraction is 0.30, indicating a 70% reduction in VPD rate. The true reduction fraction is the underlying reduction fraction, which can be estimated only from long-term EKG recordings. Similarly, the true predrug base-line VPD rate is the underlying base-line rate, which can be estimated only from long-term EKG recording. It is the observed, not the true, reduction fraction that is used to make the decision whether or not an antiarrhythmic drug is effective.

Levin plotted the probability of declaring antiarrhythmic drug success against the logarithmic transform of the true predrug VPD rate for each of a set of true reduction fractions and for each of the two enrolling criteria, 10 and 30 VPDs per hour. Figure 9 shows the probabilities of declaring antiarrhythmic drug success based on the results of a postdrug 24-hr EKG recording if the eligibility criterion is 30 or more VPDs per hour on a predrug 48-hr continuous EKG recording. This figure displays curves for reduction fractions of 0.25 to 0.30 for the true drug effect. In this figure, the y axis represents the probability of recognizing a true drug effect. Figure 10 shows similar curves assuming an eligibility criterion of 10 or more VPDs per hour. These two figures differ in the area bounded by the x axis values of 1 to 1.5, representing an underlying base-line VPD rate of 10 VPDs per hour to 30 VPDs per hour. The reason is as follows: Figure 9 assumes an enrolling criterion of 30 VPDs per hour, so that the probability of defining a drug success remains near 1 until a VPD rate of around 30 VPDs per hour is reached. With this

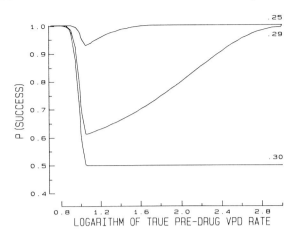

FIG. 10. The probability of declaring a drug success as a function of the true predrug VPD rate and the true reduction fraction. This figure differs from Fig. 9 in that an enrolling criterion of 10 VPDs per hour is assumed.

enrolling criterion, some patients whose true predrug rates are less than 30 per hour will be enrolled, and these patients will have a substantial chance of manifesting a false-positive test result. Similarly, in Fig. 10, the probability of defining a drug success remains near 1 until a VPD rate of around 10 VPDs per hour is reached. The effect of the enrolling criterion on the probability of declaring a drug efficacious is known as selection bias.

By comparing the curves in Figs. 9 and 10, one can see that lowering the eligibility criterion from 30 to 10 VPDs per hour does not substantially affect the probability of declaring a successful outcome when considering all patients entering an antiarrhythmic drug trial.

To estimate the difference in power for two common enrolling criteria, 10 and 30 VPDs per hour, Levin (*personal communication*) calculated the probabilities of declaring drug efficacy among all patients entering an antiarrhythmic drug trial for a set of true reduction fractions and for each of the two enrolling criteria. Levin assumed that the logarithmic transform of the VPD rate in the patient population was uniform in the range between 5 and 1,000 VPDs per hour. Figure 11 presents these results. Note that in the previous figures, values were calculated for different predrug VPD rates, but in this figure the distribution of VPD rates in the population is used to obtain an integrated probability of success for the population in general. There are two sets of probabilities shown in this figure; the squares indicate the probabilities if the enrolling criterion is 30 VPDs per hour, and the circles indicate these probabilities for the enrolling criterion of 10 VPDs per hour. Note that in most cases, for the same true-reduction criterion, the probabilities associated with the different enrolling criteria differ by 5 percentage points or less. Thus, given the assumptions used in this analysis, power is not

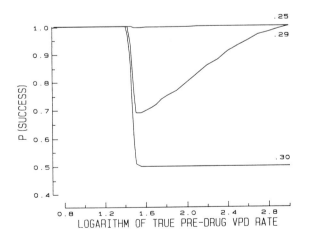

FIG. 9. The probability of declaring a drug success as a function of the true predrug VPD rate and the true reduction fraction. Drug success is defined as an observed reduction fraction of 0.30. One curve is shown for each of three true reduction fractions: 0.25, 0.29, and 0.30. An enrolling criterion of 30 VPDs per hour is assumed.

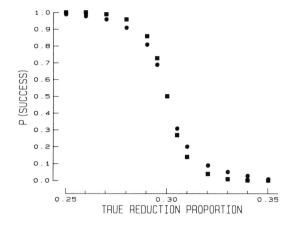

FIG. 11. The probability of declaring a drug success as a function of the enrollment criterion used (10 or 30 VPDs per hour) and of the true reduction fraction. These values represent the average rate of positive results among a hypothetical set of patients entering a drug trial. *Squares:* Values associated with an enrollment criterion of 30 VPDs per hour. *Circles:* Values associated with an enrollment criterion of 10 VPDs per hour. Note that the two sets of values never differ by more than about 5 percentage points.

sacrificed by more than 5 percentage points by using the enrolling criterion of 10 VPDs per hour instead of 30 VPDs per hour.

Note that if a reduction criterion of 70% is used to signify antiarrhythmic drug effect, and if a patient has a true reduction of exactly 70% (i.e., a reduction fraction of 0.30), then there is a 50% chance of not detecting this effect and failing to declare a drug success! In this case, the power to detect a true drug effect is low, i.e., there is only a 50% chance of recognizing a true drug effect. The power curve is steep in this region, for if the true reduction is 71%, the power to detect the drug effect is around 80%. These power considerations suggest that special procedures may be required for dealing with patients whose on-drug arrhythmia reduction is very close to the efficacy criterion value.

It should be kept in mind that Levin's work is theoretical and needs to be confirmed using real data.

Secondary Prevention Trials for Potentially Malignant Ventricular Arrhythmias

With recent studies clearly showing that potentially malignant ventricular arrhythmias are independent predictors of mortality, the next question arises: Will reducing potentially malignant ventricular arrhythmias significantly reduce mortality? Clearly, we do not know the answer to this question. Several small retrospective and uncontrolled studies have been encouraging in that they have shown that patients whose spontaneous ventricular arrhythmias are controlled by antiarrhythmic drugs fare better than those who are poorly controlled

(68,76). But there really have been no controlled trials that have addressed this question. Recently, May et al. (109) and Furberg (59) reviewed the short-term and long-term postinfarction secondary-prevention trials with antiarrhythmic drugs. Studies were selected based on three criteria: (a) total sample size of at least 100, (b) random assignment to either a treatment group or control group, and (c) reporting of all-cause mortality. Trials reported up to March 1, 1983, were included in their reviews. There were 14 acute-phase trials (follow-up 1 hr to 6 weeks) and 6 long-term trials (follow-up 3 to 24 months) that met the criteria for review. Four different antiarrhythmic drugs were evaluated in 14 short-term trials: disopyramide, lidocaine, procainamide, and quinidine. In addition, four drugs were evaluated in 6 long-term trials: aprindine, mexiletine, phenytoin, and tocainide. Altogether, more than 4,500 patients were enrolled in these trials. However, none of these studies adequately tested the hypothesis that reducing ventricular arrhythmias by drug treatment after myocardial infarction will reduce mortality. Instead, most tested the hypothesis that treatment with a fixed dose of a single antiarrhythmic drug would show a beneficial trend in mortality. Most studies did not require the presence of ventricular arrhythmias for enrollment. No study permitted a change in drug, and only one study permitted dosage adjustment based on the effect of treatment on ventricular arrhythmia reflected in serial 24-hr EKG recordings (59). Most important, none of the previous long-term studies was large enough to detect a drug-related reduction in mortality even as large as 50%. No trial enrolled enough participants to have any reasonable chance of finding a statistically significant difference between active treatment and placebo. Therefore, these studies can all be regarded as feasibility studies at best.

Table 17 lists some of the features that are important to consider in secondary-prevention trials to evaluate the effects of antiarrhythmic drugs on mortality. For a trial that uses mortality as an endpoint, a sample size

TABLE 17. *Requirements for clinical trials to study the effect of antiarrhythmic drugs*

Adequate sample size

Patients selected for arrhythmias

Flexible dosing strategies

Adequate drug plasma concentration

Evaluation of antiarrhythmic effect

Search for proarrhythmic effects

Evaluation of other drug adverse effects, e.g., aggravation of myocardial failure or ischemia

Analysis of mortality

of about 4,000 to 5,000 patients will be required. If one considers that not only arrhythmias but also heart failure and ischemic events contribute to mortality, then even larger sample sizes may be necessary. There is no reason to expect that a drug that is a potent antiarrhythmic but has no beneficial effect on left ventricular dysfunction or ischemia will prevent deaths from nonarrhythmic causes. Thus, expectations concerning arrhythmic death should be considered in sample-size calculations as well as total mortality. Patients who have potentially malignant ventricular arrhythmias should be selected for secondary-prevention trials with antiarrhythmic drugs. Unfortunately, many previous studies have treated all postinfarction patients, i.e., have not required an arrhythmia to qualify patients for enrollment. If the question being addressed is whether or not reducing potentially malignant ventricular arrhythmias will reduce mortality, then the antiarrhythmic effect of treatment must be documented carefully. Also, adjustment of dosage should be permitted in order to reach the level of arrhythmia control defined as effective by the trial. Unless the drug used in the trial is extremely potent, it is desirable to permit a change in drug if the first drug used is not effective even after dose ranging. Because there is a great deal of day-to-day variability in the frequency of isolated ventricular premature depolarizations and even more for repetitive ventricular arrhythmias, it may be desirable to require some minimum plasma concentration of drug as well as arrhythmia control, as judged by analysis of 24-hr EKG recordings. Because antiarrhythmic drugs can produce proarrhythmic effects (125,181), an effort should be made to detect patients who have this undesirable response and to change the patients who experience proarrhythmic effects to another drug. In the same vein, some attempt should be made to detect the adverse effect of antiarrhythmic drug treatment on left ventricular dysfunction or myocardial ischemia. If an effective antiarrhythmic drug causes deaths due to heart failure or ischemic events, it will be more difficult to detect an overall benefit of treatment. To minimize the dropouts, drug changes should be permitted for patients who experience intolerable adverse effects from the first drug in a trial.

Finally, the deaths should be analyzed carefully. A potent antiarrhythmic drug with a single action should affect only arrhythmic deaths. Unfortunately, our ability to classify death into functional categories, e.g., due to arrhythmia, ischemia, or heart failure, is poor at best. Also, it is common for more than one of these three mechanisms to operate in the terminal event for coronary heart disease patients. This is an area in which we need substantial progress. Until we are able to classify death by functional category, we shall continue to experience considerable difficulty in the interpretation of trial results. For example, let us assume that deaths in the 2 years after myocardial infarction are partitioned as follows:

arrhythmic 40%, ischemic 40%, and heart failure 20%. If we had an extraordinary antiarrhythmic drug that achieved arrhythmia control in 80% of patients and reduced mortality by 80% in patients who were controlled, total mortality would be reduced by only 26% in a clinical trial, assuming that the drug did not change the mortality due to ischemic events or heart failure.

Cardiac Arrhythmia Pilot Study

Because so many design features for secondary-prevention trials with antiarrhythmic drugs were not established by field trials, the Cardiac Arrhythmia Pilot Study (CAPS), a 10-center study, was sponsored by the National Heart, Lung, and Blood Institute to determine the feasibility of conducting a full-scale trial to test the hypothesis that reducing ventricular arrhythmias after acute myocardial infarction would decrease mortality (31). The overall decision flow in the CAPS is shown in Fig. 12. Patients less than 75 years of age with myocardial infarction are screened with a 24-hr Holter EKG recording 6 to 60 days after myocardial infarction. For a patient to qualify for the CAPS, the 24-hr EKG recording has to contain an average of ≥ 10 VPDs per hour or ≥ 5 runs of 3 to 9 consecutive VPDs regardless of total frequency. Patients who do not qualify on the first 24-hr EKG recording can be screened again up to 60 days after myocardial infarction.

Patients with qualifying arrhythmias have a series of base-line tests to search for conditions that will exclude patients who cannot safely participate in the study. A series of behavioral studies is done to evaluate the relationship between behavioral factors and ventricular arrhythmias or the responses to drugs and to test physiologic reactivity.

Enrolled patients are randomized to one of the five treatment "tracks," 100 patients to each track. One track is placebo treatment to provide a comparison with other treatment strategies and to control for spontaneous VPD variability. The four active drug treatments were selected on the basis of potential efficacy, safety, and prospect of developing new information for planning a full-scale trial. "Standard" antiarrhythmic drugs were not selected, because the information about them was considered adequate to determine their relative worth for a full-scale trial. Unapproved drugs were chosen for their efficacy, convenience of use, lack of known adverse effects, and likelihood of being marketed before the beginning of a full-scale trial. Based on these considerations, encainide, ethmozine, flecainide, and imipramine were selected for the CAPS. All of these drugs were judged to be at least as effective as quinidine or procainamide but more convenient to use or less likely to cause serious adverse effects.

Each of the four active treatment tracks permits up to three doses of the first drug to be evaluated using 24-

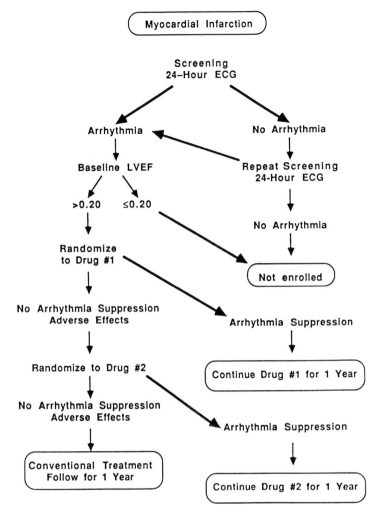

FIG. 12. Diagram of the protocol decision flow in Cardiac Arrhythmia Pilot Study.

hr EKG recordings. The CAPS efficacy criterion, 70% reduction in VPDs, was chosen to provide a balance between substantial reduction in frequency and a low rate of adverse effects. If efficacy is achieved on the first drug in a treatment track, the patient is treated on that drug and dosage for 1 year (Fig. 12). If the first drug fails to achieve efficacy or causes intolerable adverse effects, the patient is crossed over to the second drug in the track by random assignment to one of two possible drugs. Then, dose ranging resumes. Should the highest dose of drug 2 not meet the efficacy criterion, the patient is left on the dosage of drug 2 that gave the best VPD suppression, unless some dosage of drug 1 gave 50% better VPD suppression; in that case the patient is treated with the best dosage of drug 1 for the remainder of the trial.

Follow-up. Once an effective drug and dosage are found, patients are followed for a year. At 3, 6, 9, and 12 months after myocardial infarction, clinical and laboratory tests and a 24-hr EKG are done. At 3, 6, and 12 months the behavioral tests are repeated.

End of study. After 12 months of treatment, a 24-hr EKG is recorded to evaluate treatment, and then the CAPS drug is stopped. One week later, a final 24-hr EKG is recorded, and the patient's follow-up is completed. The results of the last two EKG recordings are discussed with the patient's personal physician, who takes one of the following actions: (a) use no antiarrhythmic drugs, (b) use a conventional antiarrhythmic drug, or (c) use the CAPS drug on a compassionate-use basis.

The CAPS data are expected to contribute substantially to the planning of a definitive secondary-prevention trial with antiarrhythmic drugs. Some of the important planning topics are described briefly in the following paragraphs.

Qualifying arrhythmia. A key feature of secondary-prevention trials with antiarrhythmic drugs after myocardial infarction is selection of patients with suitable arrhythmias. The CAPS study is gathering data on when and how to screen for qualifying arrhythmias. Earlier studies have shown that arrhythmias occurring in the CCU phase of myocardial infarction have a weak association with long-term mortality (13). This finding virtually eliminates screening for arrhythmias in the CCU phase of infarction. Also, the incidence of ventricular arrhythmias increases substantially from 3 to 5 days to 6 weeks after myocardial infarction (13,42,99). The increase in ventricular ectopic activity during the first 6 weeks complicates screening and enrollment procedures in antiarrhythmic secondary-prevention trials. We expect the proportion of patients with qualifying ventricular arrhythmias to increase by about twofold between 6 and 60 days. Thus, a late screening Holter recording would detect more patients with arrhythmias. However, pre-discharge enrollment is preferable in terms of convenience and the potential for protection against early arrhythmic death. CAPS screens with 24-hr continuous EKG recordings over a 60-day enrollment window. Analysis of these data may suggest more effective ways of screening for qualifying arrhythmias. Ten or more VPDs per hour are required for eligibility in CAPS, a value chosen on the basis of the relationship between VPD frequency and mortality (10,19).

Treatment effect. To test the ventricular arrhythmia hypothesis, VPD reduction must be substantial, and a large percentage of participants must have arrhythmia control. Based on judgment and practicality, a 70% reduction in VPD frequency was chosen for the CAPS efficacy criterion (16,175). Also, it is hoped that 75% of the population treated will achieve the 70% reduction. Given the variability in the relationships among dosages, plasma drug concentrations, and antiarrhythmic effects in a human population, the CAPS efficacy goals probably cannot be achieved without dosage adjustment. Also, given a substantial incidence of adverse effects with any single antiarrhythmic drug, an option to change drugs is desirable. The CAPS will provide information on drug and dosage changes that should help in designing the dosing strategy of a full-scale trial.

VPD suppression over time. To test the ventricular arrhythmia hypothesis adequately, the drug effect must be maintained for at least 1 year. Thus, ventricular arrhythmias will have to be quantified during the course of the trial. The current CAPS protocol does not permit dosage changes after the initial dose ranging to find the effective drug and dosage. Because ventricular arrhythmias tend to increase in frequency and repetitiveness during the first 3 months after myocardial infarction (13,99), late dosage adjustment may be desirable in future trials. To evaluate safety, all CAPS drugs are started in the hospital under EKG surveillance. Depending on the incidence and character of adverse drug effects, this precaution may or may not need to be used in a full-scale trial. This decision has important implications in terms of convenience and cost.

Sample size. In most trials, sample-size calculations are based on observed mortality in reference populations. CAPS will provide reasonably precise estimates of mortality and treatment effects in the population that will be enrolled in a subsequent full-scale trial, permitting accurate sample sizes to be calculated.

Cause-specific mortality. CAPS is carefully documenting each death, cardiac arrest, or episode of sustained ventricular tachycardia so that arrhythmic endpoints can be defined before a full-scale trial.

Proarrhythmic effects. During the past 5 years, the proarrhythmic effects of antiarrhythmic drugs have caused growing concern (181). In a secondary-prevention trial, undetected drug proarrhythmic effects could nullify some of the benefit of arrhythmia control. The CAPS will produce vital information on proarrhythmic effects. There are 24-hr EKG recordings during dosage determinations and routinely at 3, 6, 9, and 12 months. Additional recordings are done when patients report symptoms suggesting cardiac arrhythmias, e.g., palpitations or lightheadedness. When the CAPS proarrhythmia criteria are met, patients are admitted to hospital, and drug washout is done to determine if the increase in arrhythmic activity is due to the CAPS drug or to a spontaneous increase in arrhythmia. The placebo group will provide the first information on false-positive rates in the diagnosis of proarrhythmia.

Cardiac Arrhythmia Treatment Study

The first patient was randomized to CAPS on July 25, 1983, and enrollment ended on July 25, 1985. Follow-up will end for the last patient in the summer of 1986, and the drug code can be broken and final analyses done. CAPS should answer its primary question: Can any of the treatment strategies reduce VPD frequency by 70% in 75% of the patients for a 1-year period? Also, it should provide information on many issues that are vital for the planning and conduct of a full-scale trial (Table 18), e.g., information on the time course of arrhythmias in the first year after myocardial infarction, the tolerance to antiarrhythmic drugs early after myocardial infarction, the relationship of behavioral characteristics to ventricular arrhythmias, etc. These

TABLE 18. *Trial-design questions that are being answered in the Cardiac Arrhythmia Pilot Study*

What is the best time and method to screen for qualifying arrhythmias?

Can the qualifying arrhythmia be suppressed in the majority of patients?

What are the problems of dosage and drug changes in a placebo-controlled, double-blind study?

Can suppression of qualifying ventricular arrhythmias be sustained for a year?

How frequently will proarrhythmic effects be encountered?

What is the best management for proarrhythmic effects?

Are behavioral factors related to ventricular arrhythmias after myocardial infarction?

results will be pivotal in designing a full-scale trial. Meanwhile, planning is proceeding for a definitive trial, the Cardiac Arrhythmia Treatment Study (CATS), which is scheduled to begin in 1987. CATS will be a 25-center, 4,500-patient study to determine whether or not reducing ventricular arrhythmias after myocardial infarction will result in a significant reduction in mortality.

REFERENCES

1. Allen, H., Harris, A., and Leatham, A. (1974): Significance and prognosis of an isolated late systolic murmur: A 9 to 22 year follow-up. *Br. Heart J.,* 36:525–532.
2. Alpert, J. S. (1984): Association between arrhythmias and mitral valve prolapse. *Arch. Intern. Med.,* 144:2333–2334 (editorial).
3. Anderson, K. P., DeCamilla, J., and Moss, A. J. (1978): Clinical significance of ventricular tachycardia (3 beats or longer) detected during ambulatory monitoring after myocardial infarction. *Circulation,* 57:890–897.
4. Anderson, K. P., Stinson, E. B., Derby, G. C., Oyer, P. E., and Mason, J. W. (1983): Vulnerability of patients with obstructive hypertrophic cardiomyopathy to ventricular arrhythmia induction in the operating room. Analysis of 17 patients. *Am. J. Cardiol.,* 51:811–816.
5. Averill, K., and Lamb, L. (1960): Electrocardiographic findings in 67,375 asymptomatic subjects. I. Incidence of abnormalities. *Am. J. Cardiol.,* 6:76–83.
6. Betriu, A., Solignac, A., and Bourassa, M. G. (1974): The variant form of angina: Diagnostic and therapeutic implications. *Am. Heart J.,* 87:272–278.
7. Bigger, J. T. (1984): Identification of patients at high risk for sudden death. *Am. J. Cardiol.,* 54:3D–8D.
8. Bigger, J. T., Jr., Coromilas, J., Weld, F. M., Reiffel, J. A., and Rolnitzky, L. M. (1985): Identification of high-risk patients after myocardial infarction: Pointers for management. In: *Sudden Cardiac Death,* edited by J. Morganroth and L. N. Horowitz, pp. 109–146. Grune & Stratton, Orlando.
9. Bigger, J. T., Jr., Dresdale, R. J., Heissenbuttel, R. H., Weld, F. M., and Wit, A. L. (1977): Ventricular arrhythmias in ischemic heart disease: Mechanism, prevalence, significance, and management. *Prog. Cardiovasc. Dis.,* 19:255–283.
10. Bigger, J. T., Jr., Fleiss, J. L., Kleiger, R., Miller, J. P., Rolnitzky, L. M., and Multicenter Post-Infarction Research Group (1984): The relationships among ventricular arrhythmias, left ventricular dysfunction, and mortality in the 2 years after myocardial infarction. *Circulation,* 69:250–258.
11. Bigger, J. T., Jr., Reiffel, J. A., and Coromilas, J. (1986): Ambulatory electrocardiography. In: *Cardiac Arrhythmias: Non-Pharmacologic Management,* edited by E. V. Platia, (in press). Lippincott, Philadelphia.
12. Bigger, J. T., Jr., Rolnitzky, L. M., Leahey, E. B., Jr., and La-Pook, J. (1981): Ambulatory ECG recording: Duration of recording and activity protocol. In: *Ambulatory Electrocardiographic Recording,* edited by N. K. Wenger, M. B. Mock, and I. Ringqvist, pp. 87–102. Year Book, Chicago.
13. Bigger, J. T., Jr., Weld, F. M., Coromilas, J., Rolnitzky, L. M., and DeTurk, W. E. (1983): Prevalence and significance of arrhythmias in 24-hour ECG recordings made within one month of acute myocardial infarction. In: *The First Year After a Myocardial Infarction,* edited by H. E. Kulbertus and H. J. J. Wellens, pp. 161–175. Futura, Mt. Kisco, N.Y.
14. Bigger, J. T., Jr., Weld, F. M., and Rolnitzky, L. M. (1981): Prevalence, characteristics and significance of ventricular tachycardia (three or more complexes) detected with ambulatory electrocardiographic recording in the late hospital phase of acute myocardial infarction. *Am. J. Cardiol.,* 48:815–823.
15. Bigger, J. T., Jr., and Coromilas, J. (1984): How do beta-blockers protect after myocardial infarction? *Ann. Intern. Med.,* 101:256–258.
16. Bigger, J. T., Jr., and Rolnitzky, L. M. (1985): The evaluation of antiarrhythmic drug efficacy. In: *Mechanism and Treatment of Cardiac Arrhythmias: Relevance of Basic Studies to Clinical*

Management, edited by H. J. Reiser and L. N. Horowitz, pp. 117–135. Urban & Schwarzenberg, Baltimore.
17. Bigger, J. T., Jr., and Weld, F. M. (1980): Shortcomings of the Lown grading system for observational or experimental studies in ischemic heart disease. *Am. Heart J.,* 100:1081–1088.
18. Bigger, J. T., Jr., and Weld, F. M. (1981): Analysis of prognostic significance of ventricular arrhythmias after myocardial infarction. Shortcomings of Lown grading system. *Br. Heart J.,* 45:717–724.
19. Bigger, J. T., Jr. (1985): Risk stratification after myocardial infarction. *Z. Kardiol.* [*Suppl. 4*], 74:141–152.
20. Bigger, J. T., Jr., Reiffel, J. A., Livelli, F. D., Jr., and Wang, P. J. (1986): Sensitivity, specificity, and reproducibility of programmed ventricular stimulation. *Circulation,* [Suppl. II] 73: II73–II79.
21. Birman, K. P., Rolnitzky, L. M., and Bigger, J. T., Jr. (1978): A shape oriented system for automated Holter ECG analysis. In: *Computers in Cardiology,* pp. 217–220. IEEE Computer Society, Long Beach, Calif.
22. Bjerregaard, P. (1982): Premature beats in healthy subjects 40–79 years of age. *Eur. Heart J.,* 3:493–503.
23. Blackburn, H., Taylor, H., Harrell, B., Buskirk, E., Nicholas, W., and Thorsen, R. (1973): Premature ventricular complexes induced by stress testing. *Am. J. Cardiol.,* 31:441–449.
24. Botti, R. E. (1966): A variant form of angina pectoris with recurrent transient complete heart block. *Am. J. Cardiol.,* 17: 443–446.
25. Bourmayan, C. I., Nouhaud, M., Fournier, C. I., Bouajina, A., Desnos, M., Gay, J., and Gerbaux, A. (1983): Arythmies ventriculaires de la myocardiopathie hypertrophique obstructive. Etude par enregistrement electrocardiographique continu. *La Presse Medicale,* 12:2089–2092.
26. Bragg-Remschel, D. A., Anderson, C. M., and Winkle, R. A. (1982): Frequency response characteristics of ambulatory ECG monitoring systems and their implications for ST segment analysis. *Am. Heart J.,* 103:20–31.
27. Breithardt, G., Borggrefe, M., and Haerten, K. (1985): Role of programmed ventricular stimulation and noninvasive recording of ventricular late potentials for the identification of patients at risk of ventricular tachyarrhythmias after acute myocardial infarction. In: *Cardiac Electrophysiology and Arrhythmias,* edited by D. P. Zipes, and J. Jalife, pp. 553–561. Grune & Stratton, New York.
28. Brodsky, M., Wu, D., Denes, P., Kanakis, C., and Rosen, K. (1977): Arrhythmias documented by 24-hour continuous electrocardiographic monitoring in 50 male medical students without apparent heart disease. *Am. J. Cardiol.,* 39:390–395.
29. Brugada, P., Green, M., Abdollah, H., and Wellens, H. J. J. (1984): Significance of ventricular arrhythmias initiated by programmed ventricular stimulation: The importance of the type of ventricular arrhythmia induced and the number of premature stimuli required. *Circulation,* 69:87–92.
30. Buxton, A. E., Marchlinski, F., Doherty, J. U., Cassidy, D. M., Vassalo, J. A., Flores, B. T., and Josephson, M. E. (1984): Repetitive, monomorphic ventricular tachycardia: Clinical and electrophysiological characteristics in patients with and patients without organic heart disease. *Am. J. Cardiol.,* 54:997–1002.
31. Buxton, A. E., Waxman, H. L., Marchlinski, F. E., Simson, M. B., Cassidy, D. M., and Josephson, M. E. (1983): Right ventricular tachycardia: Clinical and electrophysiologic characteristics. *Circulation,* 5:917–927.
32. Buxton, A. E., Waxman, H. L., Marchlinski, F. E., Untereker, W. J., Waspe, L. E., and Josephson, M. E. (1984): Role of triple extrastimuli during electrophysiologic study of patients with documented sustained ventricular tachyarrhythmias. *Circulation,* 69:532–540.
33. CAPS investigators (1986): The Cardiac Arrhythmia Pilot Study. *Am. J. Cardiol.,* 57:91–95.
34. Califf, R., Burks, J., Behar, V., Margolis, J., and Wagner, G. (1978): Relationships among ventricular arrhythmias, coronary artery disease, and angiographic and electrocardiographic indicators of myocardial fibrosis. *Circulation,* 57:725–732.
35. Califf, R., McKinnis, R., McNeer, F., Harrell, F., Jr., Lee, K., Pryor, D., Waugh, R., Harris, P., Rosati, R., and Wagner, G. (1983): Prognostic value of ventricular arrhythmias associated with treadmill exercise testing in patients studied with cardiac

catheterization for suspected ischemic heart disease. *J. Am. Coll. Cardiol.,* 2:1060–1067.

36. Campbell, R. W., Godman, M. G., Fiddler, G. I., Marquis, R. M., and Julian, D. G. (1976): Ventricular arrhythmias in syndrome of balloon deformity of mitral valve. Definition of possible high risk group. *Br. Heart J.,* 38:1053–1057.

37. Chakko, C. S., and Gheorghiade, M. (1985): Ventricular arrhythmias in severe heart failure: Incidence, significance, and effectiveness of antiarrhythmic therapy. *Am. Heart J.,* 109:497–504.

38. Chiang, B., Perlman, L., Fulton, M., Ostrander, L., Jr., and Epstein, F. (1970): Predisposing factors in sudden cardiac death in Tecumseh, Michigan. A prospective study. *Circulation,* 46:31–37.

39. Chiang, B., Perlman, L., and Ostrander, L., Jr. (1969): Relationship of premature systoles to coronary heart disease and sudden death in the Tecumseh epidemiologic study. *Ann. Intern. Med.,* 6:1159–1166.

40. Clark, K. W., Rolnitzky, L. M., Miller, J. P., DeCamilla, J. J., Kleiger, R. E., Thanavaro, S., Bigger, J. T., Jr., and other MPIP participants (1981): Ambulatory ECG analysis shared by two independent computer labs in the multicenter post-infarction program (MPIP). In: *Computers in Cardiology,* pp. 271–275. IEEE Computer Society, Long Beach, Calif.

41. Clarke, J. M., Hamer, J., Shelton, J. R., Taylor, S., and Venning, G. R. (1976): The rhythm of the normal human heart. *Lancet,* 2:508–512.

42. Coromilas, J., and Bigger, J. T., Jr. (1983): The prevalence of VPD in the post CCU and late hospital phases of acute myocardial infarction (abstr.). *Circulation [Suppl. III],* 68:412.

43. Coromilas, J., Bigger, J. T., Jr., Gang, E. S., and Zimmerman, J. M. (1985): Relationship between infarct size and ventricular arrhythmias. In: *Cardiac Electrophysiology and Arrhythmias,* edited by D. P. Zipes and J. Jalife, pp. 523–530. Grune & Stratton, Orlando.

44. Costard, A., Schluter, M., and Geiger, M. (1985): Inducibility of ventricular arrhythmias after myocardial infarction. Influence of time on stimulation results and prognostic significance. *Circulation,* 72:477.

45. DeMaria, A. N., Amsterdam, E. A., Vismara, L. A., Neumann, A., and Mason, D. T. (1976): Arrhythmias in the mitral valve prolapse syndrome. Prevalence, nature, and frequency. *Ann. Intern. Med.,* 84:656–660.

46. Denniss, A. R., Richards, D. A., Cody, D. V., Russell, P. A., Young, A. A., Ross, D. L., and Uther, J. B. (1985): Comparable prognostic significance of delayed potentials and inducible ventricular tachycardia after myocardial infarction. *Circulation,* 72:359.

47. Ekblom, B., Hartley, L., and Day, W. (1979): Occurrence and reproducibility of exercise-induced ventricular ectopy in normal subjects. *Am. J. Cardiol.,* 43:35–40.

48. Ekmekci, A., Toyoshima, H., Kwoczynski, J. K., Nagaya, T., and Prinzmetal, M. (1961): Angina pectoris. IV. Clinical and experimental differences between ischemia with S-T elevation and with S-T depression. *Am. J. Cardiol.,* 7:413–420.

49. Ericsson, M., Granath, A., Ohlsen, P., Sodermark, T., and Volpe, U. (1973): Arrhythmias and symptoms during treadmill testing three weeks after myocardial infarction in 100 patients. *Br. Heart J.,* 35:787–790.

50. Faris, J., McHenry, P., Jordan, J., and Morris, S. (1976): Prevalence and reproducibility of exercise-induced ventricular arrhythmias during maximal exercise testing in normal men. *Am. J. Cardiol.,* 37:617–622.

51. Feldman, C. L. (1981): How should Holter monitoring analysis be performed? In: *The Evaluation of New Antiarrhythmic Drugs,* edited by J. Morganroth, E. N. Moore, L. S. Dreifus, and E. L. Michelson, pp. 87–102. Martinus Nijhoff, The Hague.

52. Fisher, F., and Tyroler, H. (1973): Relationship between ventricular premature contractions on routine electrocardiography and subsequent sudden death from coronary heart disease. *Circulation,* 47:712–719.

53. Fisher, J. D., Cohen, H. L., Mehra, R., Altschuler, H., Escher, D. J. W., and Furman, S. (1977): Cardiac pacing and pacemakers. II. Serial electrophysiologic-pharmacologic testing for control of recurrent tachyarrhythmias. *Am. Heart J.,* 93:658–668.

54. Fitchett, D. H., Sugrue, D. D., MacArthur, C. G., and Oakley, C. M. (1984): Right ventricular dilated cardiomyopathy. *Br. Heart J.,* 41:25–29.

55. Fleg, J. L., and Kennedy, H. L. (1982): Cardiac arrhythmias in a healthy elderly population: Detection by 24-hour ambulatory monitoring. *Chest,* 81:302–307.

56. Fleg, J., and Lakatta, E. (1984): Prevalence and prognosis of exercise-induced nonsustained ventricular tachycardia in apparently healthy volunteers. *Am. J. Cardiol.,* 54:762–764.

57. Follansbee, W. P., Michelson, E. L., and Morganroth, J. (1980): Nonsustained ventricular tachycardia in ambulatory patients: Characteristics and association with sudden cardiac death. *Ann. Intern. Med.,* 92:741–747.

58. Froelicher, V., Jr., Thomas, M., Pillow, C., and Lancaster, M. (1974): Epidemiologic study of asymptomatic men screened by maximal treadmill testing for latent coronary artery disease. *Am. J. Cardiol.,* 34:770–776.

59. Furberg, C. D. (1983): Effect of antiarrhythmic drugs on mortality after myocardial infarction. *Am. J. Cardiol.,* 52:32C–36C.

60. Furberg, C. D., Hawkins, C. M., Lichstein, E., and the Beta-Blocker Heart Attack Trial study group (1984): Effect of propranolol in postinfarction patients with mechanical or electrical complications. *Circulation,* 69:761–765.

61. Fuster, V., Gersh, B. J., Giuliani, E. R., Tajik, A. J., Brandenburg, R. O., and Frye, R. L. (1981): The natural history of idiopathic dilated cardiomyopathy. *Am. J. Cardiol.,* 47:525–531.

62. Gang, E. S., Bigger, J. T., Jr., and Livelli, F. D., Jr. (1982): A model of chronic ischemic arrhythmias: The relationships among electrically inducible ventricular tachycardia, ventricular fibrillation threshold and myocardial infarct size. *Am. J. Cardiol.,* 50:469–477.

63. Gaughan, C. E., Lown, B., Lanigan, J., Voukydis, P., and Besser, H. (1976): Acute oral drug testing for determining antiarrhythmic drug efficacy. 1. Quinidine. *Am. J. Cardiol.,* 38:677–684.

64. Gilson, J. S., Holter, N. J., and Glasscock, W. R. (1964): Clinical observations using the electrocardiorecorder: AVSEP continuous electrocardiographic system: Tentative standards and typical patterns. *Am. J. Cardiol.,* 14:204–217.

65. Glasser, S., Clark, P., and Applebaum, H. (1979): Occurrence of frequent complex arrhythmias detected by ambulatory monitoring. Findings in an apparently healthy asymptomatic elderly population. *Chest,* 5:565–568.

66. Gomes, J. A. C., Harriman, R. I., Kang, P. S., El-Sherif, N., Chowdhry, I., and Lyons, J. (1984): Programmed electrical stimulation in patients with high-grade ventricular ectopy: Electrophysiologic findings and prognosis for survival. *Circulation,* 1:43–51.

67. Gordon, J. B., Evans, L. C., Beckwith, G. H., McCall, M. M., Simpson, R. J., and Foster, J. R. (1979): Follow-up of complex ventricular arrhythmias in healthy young adults and children. *Clin. Res.,* 27:170A (abstract).

68. Graboys, T. B., Lown, B., Podrid, P. J., and DeSilva, R. (1982): Long-term survival of patients with malignant ventricular arrhythmia treated with antiarrhythmic drugs. *Am. J. Cardiol.,* 50:437–443.

69. Granath, A., Sodermark, T., Winge, T., Volpe, U., and Zetterqvist, S. (1977): Early work load tests for evaluation of long-term prognosis of myocardial infarction. *Br. Heart J.,* 39:758–763.

70. Haerten, K., Abendroth, R. R., Breithardt, G., et al. (1981): Programmierte Stimulation zur Prufung der Vulnerabilitat der Kammern in der Postinfarktphase. *Z. Kardiol.,* 70:325.

71. Hamer, A., Vohra, J., Hunt, D., and Sloman, G. (1982): Prediction of sudden death by electrophysiologic studies in high risk patients surviving acute myocardial infarction. *Am. J. Cardiol.,* 50:223–229.

72. Hermes, R. E., and Oliver, G. C. (1981): Use of the American Heart Association data base. In: *Ambulatory Electrocardiographic Recording,* edited by N. K. Wenger, M. B. Mock, and I. Ringqvist, pp. 165–181. Year Book, Chicago.

73. Hinkle, L., Carver, S., and Argyros, D. C. (1974): The prognostic significance of ventricular premature contractions in healthy people and in people with coronary heart disease. *Acta Cardiol.,* 18:5–32.

74. Hinkle, L., Carver, S., and Stevens, M. (1969): The frequency of asymptomatic disturbances of cardiac rhythm and conduction in middle-aged men. *Am. J. Cardiol.,* 24:629–650.

75. Hiss, R., Averill, K., and Lamb, L. (1960): Electrocardiographic findings in 67,375 asymptomatic subjects. III. Ventricular rhythms. *Am. J. Cardiol.,* 6:96–107.

76. Hoffman, A., Buhler, F. R., and Burckhardt, D.: High-grade ventricular ectopic activity and 4-year survival in patients with chronic heart disease and in healthy subjects. *Cardiology,* 170:82–87.

77. Holmes, J., Kubo, S. H., and Cody, R. J. (1984): Ventricular arrhythmia analysis and mortality risk stratification in congestive cardiomyopathy. *J. Am. Coll. Cardiol.,* 3:548 (abstract).

78. Holter, N. J. (1961): New methods for heart studies: Continuous electrocardiography of active subjects over long periods of time is now practical. *Science,* 134:1214–1220.

79. Horowitz, L., Josephson, M., Farshidi, A., Spielman, S., Michelson, E., and Greenspan, A. (1978): Recurrent sustained ventricular tachycardia. 3. Role of the electrophysiologic study in selection of antiarrhythmic regimens. *Circulation,* 58:986–997.

80. Huang, S. K., Messer, J. V., and Denes, P. (1983): Significance of ventricular tachycardia in idiopathic dilated cardiomyopathy: Observations in 35 patients. *Am. J. Cardiol.,* 51:507–511.

81. Jeresaty, R. M. (1976): Sudden death in the mitral valve prolapse click syndrome. *Am. J. Cardiol.,* 37:317–318.

82. Kannel, W. B., Sorlie, P., and McNamara, P. M. (1979): Prognosis after initial myocardial infarction: The Framingham study. *Am. J. Cardiol.,* 44:53–59.

83. Kennedy, H. L., Whitlock, J. A., Sprague, M. K., Kennedy, L. J., Buckingham, T. A., and Goldberg, R. J. (1985): Long-term follow-up of asymptomatic healthy subjects with frequent and complex ventricular ectopy. *N. Engl. J. Med.,* 312:193–197.

84. Kennedy, H., Pescarmona, J., Bouchard, J., Goldberg, R., and Caralis, D. (1982): Objective evidence of occult myocardial dysfunction in patients with frequent ventricular ectopy without clinically apparent heart disease. *Am. Heart J.,* 104:57–65.

85. Kennedy, H., and Underhill, S. (1976): Frequent or complex ventricular ectopy in apparently healthy subjects. A clinical study of 25 cases. *Am. J. Cardiol.,* 38:141–148.

86. Kerin, N., and MacLeod, C. A. (1974): Coronary artery spasm associated with variant angina pectoris. *Br. Heart J.,* 36:224–227.

87. Kerin, N. Z., Rubenfire, M., Naini, M., Wajszczuk, W. J., Pamatmat, A., and Cascade, P. N. (1979): Arrhythmias in variant angina pectoris. Relationship of arrhythmias to ST-segment elevation and R-wave changes. *Circulation,* 60:1343–1350.

88. Kirkland, J. L., Lye, M., Faragher, E. B., and dos Santos, A. G. R. (1983): A longitudinal study of the prognostic significance of ventricular ectopic beats in the elderly. *Gerontology,* 29:199–201.

89. Kjekshus, J. K., Maroko, P. R., and Sobel, B. E. (1972): Distribution of myocardial injury and its relation to epicardial ST-segment changes after coronary artery occlusion in the dog. *Cardiovasc. Res.,* 6:490–499.

90. Kleiger, R. E., Miller, J. P., Thanavaro, S., Martin, T. F., Province, M. A., and Oliver, G. C. (1981): Relationship between clinical features of acute myocardial infarction and ventricular runs two weeks to one year following infarction. *Circulation,* 63:64–69.

91. Klein, H., Trappe, H. J., Hartwig, C. A., Kuhn, E., and Juppner, L. (1985): Repeated programmed stimulation within the first year after myocardial infarction. *Circulation,* 72:359.

92. Koch, F. M., and Hancock, W. E. (1976): Ten year follow-up of 40 patients with the midsystolic click/late systolic murmur syndrome. *Am. J. Cardiol.,* 37:149 (abstract).

93. Kostis, J. B., McCrone, K., Moreyra, A. E., Gotzoyannis, S., Aglitz, N. M., Natarajan, N., and Kuo, P. T. (1981): Premature ventricular complexes in the absence of identifiable heart disease. *Circulation,* 63:1351–1356.

94. Kowey, P. R., Eisenberg, R., and Engel, T. R. (1984): Sustained arrhythmias in hypertrophic obstructive cardiomyopathy. *N. Engl. J. Med.,* 24:1566–1569.

95. Kramer, H. M., Kligfield, P., Devereux, R. B., Savage, D. D., and Kramer-Fox, R. (1984): Arrhythmias in mitral valve prolapse. *Arch. Intern. Med.,* 144:2360–2364.

96. Krone, R. J., Gillespie, J. A., Weld, F. M., Miller, J. P., Moss, A. J., and the Multicenter Post-Infarction Research Group (1985): Low-level exercise testing after myocardial infarction: Usefulness in enhancing clinical risk stratification. *Circulation,* 71:80–89.

97. Leclercq, J. F., Maison, B. P., Cauchemez, B., Attuel, P., and Coumel, P. (1984): Ventricular rhythm disorders in congestive cardiomyopathy. *Arch. Mal. Coeur,* 77:937–945.

98. Levi, G. F., and Proto, C. (1973): Ventricular fibrillation in the course of Prinzmetal's angina pectoris. *Br. Heart J.,* 35:601–603.

99. Lichstein, E., Morganroth, J., Harrist, R., Hubble, E., and BHAT Study Group (1983): Effect of propranolol on ventricular arrhythmias. The Beta-Blocker Heart Attack Trial experience. *Circulation* [*Suppl. I*], 67:1–5.

100. Livelli, F. D., Jr., Bigger, J. T., Jr., Reiffel, J., Gang, E., Patton, J. N., Noethling, P., Rolnitzky, L., and Gliklich, J. (1982): Response to programmed ventricular stimulation: Sensitivity, specificity and relation to heart disease. *Am. J. Cardiol.,* 50:452–458.

101. Lown, B., Calvert, A. F., Armington, R., and Ryan, M. (1975): Monitoring for serious arrhythmias and high risk of sudden death. *Circulation* [*Suppl. III*], 51–52:189–198.

102. Lown, B., Tykocinski, A., Garfein, M., and Brooks, P. (1973): Sleep and ventricular premature beats. *Circulation,* 48:691–701.

103. Lown, B., and Wolf, M. (1971): Approaches to sudden death from coronary heart disease. *Circulation,* 44:130–142.

104. MIT-BIH Arrhythmia Data Base (1980): *Tape Directory and Format Specification.* Technical report no. 010, Vol. 5, pp. 391–399. Biomedical Engineering Center for Clinical Instrumentation. MIT, Cambridge.

105. Marchlinski, F. E., Buxton, A. E., Waxman, H. L., and Josephson, M. E. (1983): Identifying patients at risk of sudden death after myocardial infarction: Value of the response to programmed stimulation, degree of ventricular ectopic activity and severity of left ventricular dysfunction. *Am. J. Cardiol.,* 52:1190–1196.

106. Maron, B. J., Savage, D. D., Wolfson, J., and Epstein, S. E. (1981): Prognostic significance of 24-hour ambulatory electrocardiographic monitoring in patients with hypertrophic cardiomyopathy. A prospective study. *Am. J. Cardiol.,* 48:252–257.

107. Mason, J. W., Swerdlow, C. D., Winkle, R. A., Ross, D. L., Echt, D. S., Anderson, K. P., Mitchell, L. B., and Clusin, W. T. (1984): Ventricular tachyarrhythmia induction for drug selection: Experience with 311 patients. In: *Clinical Pharmacology of Antiarrhythmic Therapy,* edited by B. R. Lucchesi, J. V. Dingell, and R. P. Schwarz, Jr., pp. 229–239. Raven Press, New York.

108. Mason, J. W., and Winkle, R. A. (1978): Electrode-catheter arrhythmia induction in the selection and assessment of antiarrhythmic drug therapy for recurrent ventricular tachycardia. *Circulation,* 58:971–985.

109. May, G. S., Eberlein, K. A., Furberg, C. D., Passamani, E. R., and DeMets, D. L. (1982): Secondary prevention after myocardial infarction: A review of long-term trials. *Prog. Cardiovasc. Dis.,* 24:331–352.

110. McHenry, P., Fisch, C., Jordan, J., and Corya, B. (1972): Cardiac arrhythmias observed during maximal treadmill exercise testing in clinically normal men. *Am. J. Cardiol.,* 29:331–336.

111. McHenry, P., Morris, S., Kavalier, M., and Jordan, J. (1976): Comparative study of exercise-induced ventricular arrhythmias in normal subjects and patients with documented coronary artery disease. *Am. J. Cardiol.,* 37:609–616.

112. McKenna, W. J., Chetty, S., Oakley, C. M., and Goodwin, J. F. (1980): Arrhythmia in hypertrophic cardiomyopathy: Exercise and 48-hour ambulatory electrocardiographic assessment with and without beta adrenergic blocking therapy. *Am. J. Cardiol.,* 45:1–5.

113. McKenna, W. J., England, D., Doi, Y. L., Deanfield, J. E., Oakley, C., and Goodwin, J. F. (1981): Arrhythmia in hypertrophic cardiomyopathy. I. Influence on prognosis. *Br. Heart J.,* 46:168–172.

114. Meinertz, T., Hofmann, T., Kasper, W., Treese, N., Bechtold, H., Stienen, U., Pop, T., Leitner, E.-R. V., Andresen, D., and Meyer, J. (1984): Significance of ventricular arrhythmias in idiopathic dilated cardiomyopathy. *Am. J. Cardiol.,* 53:902–907.

115. Michelson, E. L., and Morganroth, J. (1980): Spontaneous variability of complex ventricular arrhythmias detected by long-term electrocardiographic recording. *Circulation,* 61:690–695.

116. Miller, D. D., Waters, D. D., Szlachcic, J., and Theroux, P. (1982): Clinical characteristics associated with sudden death in patients with variant angina. *Circulation,* 66:588–592.

117. Mills, P., Rose, J., Hollingsworth, J., Amara, I., and Craige, E.

(1977): Long-term prognosis of mitral-valve prolapse. *N. Engl. J. Med.*, 297:13–18.

118. Monson, R. R. (1974): Analysis of relative survival and proportional mortality. *Comput. Biomed. Res.*, 7:325–332.

119. Montague, T., McPherson, D., MacKenzie, B., Spencer, C., Nanton, M., and Horacek, B. (1983): Frequent ventricular ectopic activity without underlying cardiac disease: Analysis of 45 subjects. *Am. J. Cardiol.*, 52:980–984.

120. Morady, F., Scheinman, M. M., Hess, D. S., Sung, R. J., Shen, E., and Shapiro, W. (1983): Electrophysiologic testing in the management of survivors of out-of-hospital cardiac arrest. *Am. J. Cardiol.*, 51:85–89.

121. Morady, F., Shapiro, W., Shen, E., Sung, R. J., and Scheinman, M. M. (1984): Programmed ventricular stimulation in patients without spontaneous ventricular tachycardia. *Am. Heart J.*, 107:875–882.

122. Morady, F., Shen, E., Bhandari, A., Schwartz, A., and Scheinman, M. M. (1984): Programmed ventricular stimulation in mitral valve prolapse: Analysis of 36 patients. *Am. J. Cardiol.*, 53:135–138.

123. Morganroth, J. (1985): Ambulatory Holter electrocardiography: Choice of technologies and clinical uses. *Ann. Intern. Med.*, 102:73–81.

124. Morganroth, J., Michelson, E. L., Horowitz, L. N., Josephson, M. E., Pearlman, A. S., and Dunkman, W. B. (1978): Limitations of routine long-term monitoring to assess ventricular ectopic frequency. *Circulation*, 58:408–414.

125. Morganroth, J., and Horowitz, L. N. (1984): Flecainide: Its proarrhythmic effect and expected changes on the surface electrocardiogram. *Am. J. Cardiol.*, 53:89B–94B.

126. Moss, A. J., Davis, H. T., DeCamilla, J., and Bayer, L. W. (1978): Ventricular ectopic beats and their relation to sudden and nonsudden cardiac death after myocardial infarction. *Circulation*, 60:998–1003.

127. Moss, A. J., DeCamilla, J. J., Davis, H. P., and Bayer, L. (1977): Clinical significance of ventricular ectopic beats in the early posthospital phase of myocardial infarction. *Am. J. Cardiol.*, 39:635–640.

128. Mukharji, J., Rude, R. E., Poole, K., Croft, C., Thomas, L. J., Jr., Strauss, H. W., Roberts, R., Raabe, D. S., Jr., Braunwald, E., Willerson, J. T., and cooperating investigators Multicenter Investigation of the Limitation of Infarct Size (MILIS) (1982): Late sudden death following acute myocardial infarction, importance of combined presence of repetitive ventricular ectopy and left ventricular dysfunction. *Clin. Res.*, 30:108A.

129. Mukharji, J., Rude, R. E., Poole, W. K., Gustafson, N., Thomas, L. J., Jr., Strauss, H. W., Jaffe, A. S., Muller, J. E., Roberts, R., Raabe, D. S., Jr., Croft, C. H., Passamani, E., Braunwald, E., Willerson, J. T., and the MILIS study group (1984): Risk factors for sudden death after acute myocardial infarction: Two-year follow-up. *Am. J. Cardiol.*, 54:31–36.

130. Myerburg, R. J., Kessler, K. M., Luceri, R. M., Zaman, L., Trohman, G., Estes, E., and Castellanos, A. (1984): Classification of ventricular arrhythmias based on parallel hierarchies of frequency and form. *Am. J. Cardiol.*, 54:1355–1357.

131. Naccarelli, G. V., Prystowsky, E. N., Jackman, W. M., Heger, J. J., Rahilly, G. T., and Zipes, D. P. (1982): Role of electrophysiologic testing in managing patients who have ventricular tachycardia unrelated to coronary artery disease. *Am. J. Cardiol.*, 50:165–171.

132. Nair, C., Thomson, W., Aronow, W., Pagano, T., Ryschon, K., and Sketch, M. (1984): Prognostic significance of exercise-induced complex ventricular arrhythmias in coronary artery disease with normal and abnormal left ventricular ejection fraction. *Am. J. Cardiol.*, 54:1136–1138.

133. Oliver, G. C., Ripley, K. L., and Miller, J. P. (1977): A critical review of computer arrhythmia detection. In: *Computer Electrocardiography: Current Status and Criteria*, edited by L. Pordy, pp. 319–348. Futura, Mt. Kisco, N.Y.

134. Olson, H. G., Lyons, K. P., Troop, P., Butman, S. M., and Piters, K. M. (1984): Prognostic implications of complicated ventricular arrhythmias early after hospital discharge in acute myocardial infarction: A serial ambulatory electrocardiography study. *Am. Heart J.*, 108:1221–1228.

135. Pantano, J., and Oriel, R. (1982): Prevalence and nature of

cardiac arrhythmias in apparently normal well-trained runners. *Am. Heart J.*, 104:762–768.

136. Parmley, W. W., and Chatterjee, K. (1986): Congestive heart failure and arrhythmias: An overview. *Am. J. Cardiol.*, 57:34B–37B.

137. Pocock, W. A., Bosman, C. K., Chesler, E., Barlow, J. B., and Edwards, J. E. (1984): Sudden death in primary mitral valve prolapse. *Am. Heart J.*, 107:378–382.

138. Podrid, P. J., Schoeneberger, A., Lown, B., Lampert, S., Matos, J., Porterfield, J., Raeder, E., and Corrigan, E. (1983): Use of nonsustained ventricular tachycardia as a guide to antiarrhythmic drug therapy in patients with malignant ventricular arrhythmia. *Am. Heart J.*, 105:181–188.

139. Poll, D. S., Marchlinski, F. E., Buxton, A. E., Doherty, J. U., Waxman, H. L., and Josephson, M. (1984): Sustained ventricular tachycardia in patients with idiopathic dilated cardiomyopathy: Electrophysiologic testing and lack of response to antiarrhythmic drug therapy. *Circulation*, 70:451–456.

140. Prinzmetal, M., Kennamer, R., Merliss, R., Wada, T., and Bor, N. (1959): Angina pectoris. 1. A variant form of angina pectoris; preliminary report. *Am. J. Med.*, 27:375–388.

141. Prinzmetal, M., Ekmekci, A., Kennamer, R., Kwoczynski, J., Shubin, H., and Toyoshima, H. (1960): Variant form of angina pectoris. Previously undelineated syndrome. *J.A.M.A.*, 174:1794–800.

142. Proudfit, W. L., Bruschke, A. V. G., and Sones, F. M., Jr. (1980): Clinical course of patients with normal or slightly or moderately abnormal coronary angiograms: 10 year follow-up of 521 patients. *Circulation*, 62:712–717.

143. Prystowsky, E. N., Heger, J. J., Lloyd, E. A., and Zipes, D. P. (1983): Clinical electrophysiology of ventricular tachycardia. *Cardiology Clinics*, 1:253.

144. Rabkin, S., Mathewson, F., and Tate, R. (1981): Relationship of ventricular ectopy in men without apparent heart disease to occurrence of ischemic heart disease and sudden death. *Am. Heart J.*, 2:135–141.

145. Raftery, E., and Cashman, P. (1976): Long-term recording of the electrocardiogram in a normal population. *Postgrad. Med. J.*, [Suppl. 7], 52:32–37.

146. Rahilly, G. T., Prystowsky, E. N., Zipes, D. P., Naccarelli, G. V., Jackman, W. M., and Heger, J. J. (1982): Clinical and electrophysiologic findings in patients with repetitive monomorphic ventricular tachycardia and otherwise normal electrocardiogram. *Am. J. Cardiol.*, 50:459–468.

147. Richards, D. A., Cody, D. V., Denniss, A. R., Russell, P. A., Young, A. A., and Uther, J. B. (1983): Ventricular electrical instability: A predictor of death after myocardial infarction. *Am. J. Cardiol.*, 51:75–80.

148. Rodstein, M., Wolloch, L., and Gubner, R. (1971): Mortality study of the significance of extrasystoles in an insured population. *Circulation*, 44:617–625.

149. Romhilt, D., Chaffin, C., Choi, S., and Claiborne Irby, E. (1984): Arrhythmias on ambulatory electrocardiographic monitoring in women without apparent heart disease. *Am. J. Cardiol.*, 54:582–586.

150. Roy, D., Waxman, H. L., Kienzle, M. G., Buxton, A. E., Marchlinski, F. E., and Josephson, M. E. (1983): Clinical characteristics and long-term follow-up in 119 survivors of cardiac arrest: Relation to inducibility at electrophysiologic testing. *Am. J. Cardiol.*, 52:969–974.

151. Roy, D., Marchand, E., Theroux, P., Waters, D. D., Pelletier, G. B., and Bourassa, M. G. (1985): Programmed ventricular stimulation in survivors of an acute myocardial infarction. *Circulation*, 72:487–494.

152. Ruberman, W., Weinblatt, E., Goldberg, J. D., Frank, C. W., and Shapiro, S. (1977): Ventricular premature beats and mortality after myocardial infarction. *N. Engl. J. Med.*, 297:750–757.

153. Ruberman, W., Weinblatt, E., Goldberg, J. D., Frank, C. W., Chaudhary, B. S., and Shapiro, S. (1981): Ventricular premature complexes and sudden death after myocardial infarction. *Circulation*, 64:297–305.

154. Ruberman, W., Weinblatt, E., Goldberg, J. D., Frank, C. W., Shapiro, S., Chaudhary, B. S. (1980): Ventricular premature complexes in prognosis of angina. *Circulation*, 61:1172–1178.

155. Ruskin, J. N., DiMarco, J. P., and Garan, H. (1980): Out-of-

hospital cardiac arrest: Electrophysiologic observations and selection of long-term antiarrhythmic therapy. *N. Engl. J. Med.*, 303: 607–613.

156. Ruttimann, U. E., Bassir, R., and Yamamoto, W. S. (1972): A statistical description of the occurrence of premature ventricular contractions based on the Poisson process. *Comput. Biomed. Eng.*, 10:431–442.

157. Sami, M., Chaitman, B., Fisher, L., Holmes, D., Fray, D., and Alderman, E. (1984): Significance of exercise-induced ventricular arrhythmia in stable coronary artery disease: A coronary artery surgery study project. *Am. J. Cardiol.*, 54:1182–1187.

158. Sami, M., Kraemer, H., Harrison, D. C., Houston, N., Chimasaki, S., and DeBusk, R. F. (1980): A new method for evaluating antiarrhythmic drug efficacy. *Circulation*, 62:1172–1179.

159. Santarelli, P., Bellocci, F., Loperfido, F., Mazzari, M., Mongiardo, R., and Denes, P. (1983): Ventricular electrical instability in acute myocardial infarction: Clinical, angiographic and electrophysiologic correlations. *Circulation [suppl. III]*, 68:108.

160. Savage, D. D., Seides, S. F., Maron, B. J., Myers, D. J., and Epstein, S. E. (1979): Prevalence of arrhythmias during 24-hour electrocardiographic monitoring and exercise testing in patients with obstructive and nonobstructive hypertrophic cardiomyopathy. *Circulation*, 59:866–875.

161. Savage, D. D., Levy, D., Garrison, R. J., Castelli, W. P., Kligfield, P., Devereux, R. B., Anderson, S. J., Kannel, W. B., and Feinleib, M. (1983): Mitral valve prolapse in the general population. 3. Dysrhythmias: The Framingham study. *Am. Heart J.*, 106:582–586.

162. Schamroth, L., and Levenstein, J. H. (1974): Variant (Prinzmetal's) form of angina pectoris manifesting in complicating ventricular extrasystoles. *S. Afr. Med. J.*, 48:1146–1149.

163. Schoenfeld, M. H., McGovern, B., Garan, H., and Ruskin, J. N. (1984): Long-term reproducibility of responses to programmed cardiac stimulation in spontaneous ventricular tachyarrhythmias. *Am. J. Cardiol.*, 54:564–568.

164. Schulze, R. A., Humphries, J. O., Griffith, L. S. C., Ducci, H., Achuff, S., Baird, M. G., Mellits, E. D., and Pitt, B. (1977): Left ventricular and coronary angiographic anatomy. Relationship to ventricular irritability in the late hospital phase of acute myocardial infarction. *Circulation*, 55:839–843.

165. Scott, O., Williams, G., and Fiddler, G. (1980): Results of 24-hour ambulatory monitoring of electrocardiogram in 131 healthy boys aged 10 to 13 years. *Br. Heart J.*, 44:304–308.

166. Shapiro, W., Canada, W. B., Lee, G., DeMaria, A. N., Low, R. I., Mason, D. T., and Laddu, A. (1982): Comparison of two methods of analyzing frequency of ventricular arrhythmias. *Am. Heart J.*, 104:874–883.

167. Sheps, D., Ernst, J., Briese, F., Lopez, L., Conde, C., Castellanos, A., and Myerburg, R. (1977): Decreased frequency of exercise-induced ventricular ectopic activity in the second of two consecutive treadmill tests. *Circulation*, 55:892–895.

168. Sobotka, P., Mayer, J., Bauernfeind, R., Kanakis, C., Jr., and Rosen, K. (1981): Arrhythmias documented by 24-hour continuous ambulatory electrocardiographic monitoring in young women without apparent heart disease. *Am. Heart J.*, 101:753–758.

169. Spielman, S. R., Greenspan, A. M., Kay, H. R., Disigil, K. F., Webb, C. R., Sokoloff, N. M., Rai, A. P., Morganroth, J., and Horowitz, L. N. (1985): Electrophysiologic testing in patients at high risk to sudden death. Nonsustained ventricular tachycardia and abnormal ventricular function. *J. Am. Coll. Cardiol.*, 6:31–40.

170. Steinback, K., Goldar, D., Weber, H., Joskowicz, G., and Kaindl, F. (1982): Frequency and variability of ventricular premature contractions the influence of heart rate and circadian rhythms. *Pace*, 5:38–51.

171. Strain, J., Grose, R., Factor, S., and Fisher, J. (1983): Results of endomyocardial biopsy in patients with spontaneous ventricular tachycardia but without apparent structural heart disease. *Circulation*, 6:1171–1181.

172. Suwa, M., Hirota, Y., Nagao, H., Kino, M., and Kawamura, K. (1984): Incidence of the coexistence of left ventricular false tendons and premature ventricular contractions in apparently healthy subjects. *Circulation*, 5:793–798.

173. Swerdlow, C. D., Winkle, R. A., and Mason, J. W. (1983): Prognostic significance of the number of induced ventricular complexes during assessment of therapy for ventricular tachyarrhythmias. *Circulation*, 68:400–405.

174. The Multicenter Post-Infarction Research Group (1983): Risk stratification and survival after myocardial infarction. *N. Engl. J. Med.*, 309:331–336.

175. Thomas, L. J., and Miller, J. P. (1984): Long-term ambulatory ECG recording in the determination of antidysrhythmic drug efficacy. In: *The Clinical Pharmacology of Antiarrhythmic Drugs*, edited by B. R. Lucchesi, J. V. Dingell, and R. P. Schwartz, Jr., pp. 249–265. Raven Press, New York.

176. Tzivoni, D., Keren, A., Granot, H., Gottlied, S., Benhorin, J., and Stern, S. (1983): Ventricular fibrillation caused by myocardial reperfusion in Prinzmetal's angina. *Am. Heart J.*, 105:323–325.

177. Udall, J., and Ellestad, M. (1977): Predictive implications of ventricular premature contractions associated with treadmill stress testing. *Circulation*, 56:985–989.

178. Unverferth, D. V., Magorien, R. D., Moeschberger, M. L., Baker, P. B., Fetters, J. K., and Leier, C. V. (1984): Factors influencing the one-year mortality of dilated cardiomyopathy. *Am. J. Cardiol.*, 54:147–152.

179. Van Durme, J. P., and Pannier, R. H. (1976): Prognostic significance of ventricular dysrhythmias one year after myocardial infarction. *Am. J. Cardiol.*, 37:178 (abstract).

180. Vandepol, C., Farshidi, A., Spielman, S., Greenspan, A., Horowitz, L., and Josephson, M. (1980): Incidence and clinical significance of induced ventricular tachycardia. *Am. J. Cardiol.*, 45:725–731.

181. Velebit, B., Podrid, P., Lown, B., Cohen, B. H., and Graboys, T. B. (1982): Aggravation and provocation of ventricular arrhythmias by antiarrhythmic drugs. *Circulation*, 65:886–894.

182. Vlay, S., and Reid, P. (1982): Ventricular ectopy: Etiology, evaluation, and therapy. *Am. J. Med.*, 73:899–913.

183. Von Olshausen, K., Schafer, A., Mehmel, H. C., Schwarz Sengles, J., and Kubler, W. (1984): Ventricular arrhythmias in idiopathic dilated cardiomyopathy. *Br. Heart J.*, 51:195–201.

184. Wegria, R., Segers, M., Keating, R. P., and Ward, H. P. (1949): Relationship between the reduction in coronary flow and the appearance of electrocardiographic changes. *Am. Heart J.*, 38:90–96.

185. Weld, F. M., Chu, K.-L., Bigger, J. T., Jr., and Rolnitzky, L. M. (1981): Risk stratification with low level exercise testing two weeks after acute myocardial infarction. *Circulation*, 64:306–314.

186. Wilson, J. R., Schwartz, J. S., St. John Sutton, M., Ferraro, N., Horowitz, L., Reichek, N., and Josephson, M. (1983): Prognosis in heart failure: Relation to hemodynamic measurements and ventricular ectopic activity. *J. Am. Coll. Cardiol.*, 2:403–410.

187. Winkle, R. A. (1978): Antiarrhythmic drug effect mimicked by spontaneous variability of ventricular ectopy. *Circulation*, 57:1116–1121.

188. Winkle, R. A., Lopes, M. G., Fitzgerald, J. W., Goodman, D. J., Schroeder, J. S., and Harrison, D. H. (1975): Arrhythmias in patients with mitral valve prolapse. *Circulation*, 52:73–81.

189. Winkle, R. A., Peters, F., and Hall, R. (1981): Characterization of ventricular tachyarrhythmias on ambulatory ECG recordings in postmyocardial infarction patients: Arrhythmia detection and duration of recording, relationship between arrhythmia frequency and complexity, and day-to-day reproducibility. *Am. Heart J.*, 102:162–169.

190. Winkle, R. A., Rodriguez, I., and Bragg-Remschel, D. A. (1984): Technological status and problems of ambulatory electrocardiographic monitoring. *Ann. N.Y. Acad. Sci.*, 432:108–116.

191. Zipes, D. P., Prystowsky, E. N., and Heger, J. J. (1982): Electrophysiologic testing of antiarrhythmic agents. *Am. Heart J.*, 103: 610–614.

The Heart and Cardiovascular System,
edited by H. A. Fozzard et al.
Raven Press, New York © 1986.

CHAPTER **60**

Afterdepolarizations and Triggered Activity

Andrew L. Wit and Michael R. Rosen

"Triggered activity" is the term used to describe impulse initiation in cardiac fibers that is dependent on afterdepolarizations (73,75). It is separate and distinct from automaticity, which results from the spontaneous diastolic depolarization caused by the pacemaker current (85). Afterdepolarizations are oscillations in membrane potential that follow the upstroke of an action potential. They may occur early, that is, during repolarization of the action potential (early afterdepolarizations), or they may be delayed until repolarization is complete or nearly complete (delayed afterdepolarizations). When afterdepolarizations are large enough to reach the threshold potential for activation of a regenerative inward current, the resultant action potentials are referred to as "triggered." It is therefore apparent that for triggered activity to occur, at least one action potential must precede it (the trigger).

The concept of triggered activity is not new, although it has been called by different names. Oscillations or afterdepolarizations have long been a known cause of rhythmic firing in neural tissue (13,124). Also, afterpotentials were originally given strong endorsement as a mechanism for cardiac arrhythmias by Scherf as early as 1926 (for review, see ref. 253). He classified "true

extrasystoles" as being *precipitated by the preceding beat* and distinguished this mechanism from ectopic arrhythmias, in which two or more independent centers of impulse formation exist, "the activity of neither deriving from that of the other." Wenckebach and Winterberg (309) interpreted this behavior as indicative of circus movement, because it is also characteristic of reentry. However, Scherf objected to the circus-movement theory as an explanation of extrasystoles and believed that "negative afterpotentials" like those shown by neurophysiologists were the causes of extrasystoles in the heart (253).

Phenomena resembling triggered activity also were identified by other investigators. In 1936, Goldenberg and Rothberger (131) showed discharges arising from prolonged negative afterpotentials in canine Purkinje fibers exposed to veratrine. They emphasized the resemblance of the grouped discharges caused by the afterpotential to attacks of paroxysmal tachycardia in patients.

In 1941, Segers showed early and delayed afterdepolarizations in frog ventricle by recording monophasic action potentials (73). He pointed out that extrasystoles in intact hearts can be caused by the same agents that enhance afterdepolarizations, such as Ba^{2+}, elevated

$[Ca^{2+}]_o$, aconitine, veratrine, adrenaline, and cardiac glycosides. He suggested that the phenomenon we call triggered activity be called "self-sustained beating" (*batement auto-entretenu*) and clearly differentiated this form of impulse initiation from automaticity (255). Bozler (29), in experiments on turtle ventricle in 1943, also described afterpotentials in which an afterhyperpolarization was followed by an afterdepolarization that could reach threshold (delayed afterdepolarization). The amplitude of the delayed afterdepolarizations was enhanced by increasing $[Ca^{2+}]_o$ or by adding epinephrine. "Afterdischarges," i.e., triggered activity, were noted under conditions where the afterpotentials were largest, such as following a short series of driven responses. Bozler (29) commented that "oscillatory afterpotentials . . . provide a simple explanation for coupled extrasystoles and paroxysmal tachycardia."

Many of these important observations made before 1945 were almost forgotten during the subsequent 30 years. Although Trautwein (270) stressed the possible importance of early afterdepolarizations as a cause of arrhythmias, other discussions of arrhythmia mechanisms did not emphasize or even include this cause. Studies on the electrophysiological effects of digitalis in the early 1970s that suggested a possible role for afterdepolarizations as a cause of digitalis-toxic arrhythmias revived interest in this concept of an arrhythmogenic mechanism (111,115,245,246).

DELAYED AFTERDEPOLARIZATIONS AND TRIGGERED ACTIVITY

Delayed afterdepolarizations are oscillations in membrane potential that occur after repolarization of an action potential and that are caused by that action potential. As shown in Fig. 1A, a delayed afterdepolarization may be preceded by an afterhyperpolarization, in which case the membrane potential transiently becomes more negative after the action potential than it was just before it. The transient nature of the afterdepolarization clearly distinguishes it from normal spontaneous diastolic (pacemaker) depolarization, during which the membrane potential declines monotonically until the next action potential occurs. All oscillations in membrane potential that occur during phase 4 are not delayed afterdepolarizations, because some oscillations may not be caused by the action potential, but may occur at random.

A triggered impulse is initiated when a delayed afterdepolarization reaches the threshold potential for activation of the inward current responsible for the upstroke of the action potential (Fig. 1B). Afterdepolarizations do not always reach threshold, so that triggerable fibers may sometimes be stimulated regularly without becoming

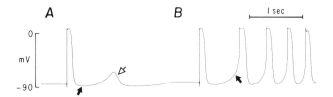

FIG. 1. An example of a delayed afterdepolarization in an atrial fiber from the canine coronary sinus. **A:** An action potential that was elicited by a stimulus. The delayed afterdepolarization is a transient depolarization that follows the action potential (*open arrow*) and is preceded by an afterhyperpolarization (*black arrow*). **B:** Only the first action potential was stimulated. Triggered action potentials then occurred because the afterdepolarization following the stimulated action potential (*arrow*) reached threshold potential (part of the plateau of the first three triggered action potentials is off the scale of the pen recorder).

rhythmically active. The conditions under which they can reach threshold vary in different types of cardiac fibers and will be discussed later.

A triggered action potential is also followed by an afterdepolarization that may or may not reach threshold. Quite often the first triggered action potential is followed by a short or long "train" of additional triggered action potentials, each arising from the afterdepolarization caused by the previous action potential (Fig. 1B). The merging of the rising phase of the afterdepolarization with the upstroke of the action potential may be smooth, and the fiber may show phase-4 depolarization during triggered activity that is indistinguishable from the phase-4 depolarization seen during automatic activity.

Causes of Delayed Afterdepolarizations and Triggered Activity

Delayed afterdepolarizations usually occur under a variety of conditions in which there appears to be a large increase in Ca in the myoplasm and the sarcoplasmic reticulum (sometimes referred to as "Ca overload"). Abnormalities in the sequestration and release of Ca by the sarcoplasmic reticulum also may contribute to their occurrence. However, there are also several examples of delayed afterdepolarizations occurring in presumably normal fibers (*vide infra*). The proposed mechanisms by which intracellular Ca may cause delayed afterdepolarizations will be discussed in detail later. Before that discussion, we shall outline the conditions and kinds of cardiac fibers in which delayed afterdepolarizations have been observed. All these data on triggered activity have been derived from studies with microelectrodes on isolated, superfused preparations of cardiac tissue. Later we shall describe attempts to demonstrate triggered activity in the *in situ* heart, a necessary prerequisite to proving that this mechanism causes arrhythmias.

Triggered Activity Caused by Digitalis Toxicity

Triggered activity caused by cardiac glycosides was first studied in detail in isolated cardiac tissues in the early 1970s (9,83,113,115,141,155,245,246). It was found that toxic concentrations of ouabain or acetylstrophanthidin could induce one or more oscillations in membrane potential following stimulated action potentials in Purkinje fibers, ventricular muscle, and atrial muscle (Fig. 2). These oscillations increase in amplitude with an increase in extracellular Ca. The oscillations (delayed afterdepolarizations) are cycle-length dependent; that is, as drive rate is increased, they increase in amplitude; as a result, increases in drive rate are associated with an increased incidence of arrhythmias. Not only do the delayed afterdepolarizations cause arrhythmias, but they also can lead to abnormalities of impulse conduction; action potentials arising from delayed afterdepolarizations that do not reach threshold conduct slowly because of partial inactivation of the Na channel at the reduced level of membrane potential (245,251).

Cardiac glycosides cause delayed afterdepolarizations by inhibiting the Na-K pump. In toxic amounts, this effect results in a measurable increase in intracellular Na (84,194). Interventions that lead to an increase in Na_i may, in turn, cause an increase in Ca_i (195,206,292); when Na_i is increased, the driving force for Na across the sarcolemma is decreased, which, in turn, diminishes Ca extrusion from the cell by Na-Ca exchange. Hence, there is a net inward Ca movement (4,171,221,222,239). Other pharmacological agents that increase Na_i either by inhibiting Na extrusion (e.g., see effects of zero potassium, *infra*) or by increasing Na entry into cells

(33) may also lead to increases in Ca_i and delayed afterdepolarizations for a similar reason.

Triggered Activity in Embryonic Heart Cells

Some pacemaker activity in embryonic chick heart cells can be attributed to delayed afterdepolarizations (261). Sustained rhythmic activity in embryonic heart cells sometimes ends abruptly with a delayed afterdepolarization following the last action potential. At times, the cycle length of rhythmic activity fluctuates with abrupt changes from rapid to slow rates and then a return to rapid rates. At the slow rates, action-potential repolarization may be followed by an afterhyperpolarization and then a delayed afterdepolarization. Following the delayed afterdepolarization, phase-4 depolarization causes the next action potential to occur spontaneously. The rate abruptly increases when the delayed afterdepolarization appears to reach threshold, causing rapid triggered activity. Thus, it appears that both automaticity and triggering occur in the same cells. Digitalis can also cause delayed afterdepolarizations in embryonic hearts (183).

Triggered Activity in the Sinus Node

The sinus node has always been regarded as a prime example of automatic activity. However, Cranefield (74) has pointed out that phase-4 depolarization during triggered activity appears virtually identical with phase-4 depolarization during automatic activity. There is little in the characteristics of phase 4 to suggest that a rhythm

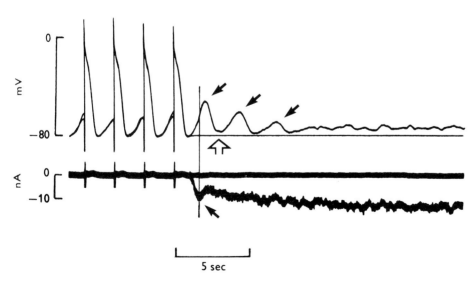

FIG. 2. Delayed afterdepolarization and transient inward (TI) current. **Top:** Two superimposed records of membrane potentials from a Purkinje fiber intoxicated with 1 μM strophanthidin and driven at a cycle length of 2 sec. During the first sequence of recordings, external stimulation was discontinued, and three delayed afterdepolarizations occurred in succession (*black arrows*). The Purkinje fiber was then stimulated again, but following the last stimulated action potential the membrane potential was clamped at its maximum diastolic potential (*open arrow*). **Bottom:** Membrane current recorded during the clamp. A TI current (*arrow*) is shown superimposed on the decaying pacemaker potential. The vertical bar runs through the peak of the TI and shows its relationship to the afterdepolarization. The magnitude of the TI is 10 nA. (From ref. 193, with permission.)

1452 / CHAPTER 60

is triggered unless the rhythm stops. If it stops, a delayed afterdepolarization should be seen. Because the sinus node normally does not stop initiating impulses, it therefore is difficult to determine if afterdepolarizations are occurring. However, under certain experimental conditions, rhythmic activity in the sinus node does cease, and activity then can be triggered from delayed afterdepolarizations. When Na$^+$ in the perfusing solution is decreased to 20% of normal, no action potentials occur in sinus fibers; only subthreshold oscillations are seen. If calcium is also decreased to 50% of normal and isoproterenol is added to the perfusate, action potentials can be elicited by electrical stimulation, and these action potentials are followed by afterhyperpolarizations and delayed afterdepolarizations that can reach threshold to cause triggered impulses (310). Also, after the sinus node is divided in two, the inferior part is often quiescent, while rhythmic activity continues in the superior part. The inferior part can then be triggered into sustained rhythmic activity by a stimulus (32).

Thus, triggered activity can be demonstrated in sinus node fibers under unusual experimental conditions. This suggests the possibility that sustained rhythmic activity of the sinus node might sometimes be caused by delayed afterdepolarizations.

Triggered Activity in Atrial Fibers

AV valve leaflets. Triggerable fibers in mammalian atria were first demonstrated in the simian anterior mitral valve leaflet (314) and the human mitral valve leaflet (319) in the presence of exogenous catecholamines. The catecholamines may cause the increase in intracellular Ca necessary for the afterdepolarizations to occur (238) by increasing the slow inward (Ca) current (237). Catecholamines may also cause the appearance of delayed afterdepolarizations in other atrial and ventricular tissues (*vide infra*) (77,192,225).

Muscle fibers in the mitral valves have relatively low resting potentials of −60 to −70 mV, and their action potentials are slow responses (72). These myocardial cells have the ultrastructure of typical atrial muscle, which suggests that cells that can be triggered need not have a specialized structure.

Coronary sinus. Atrial fibers lining the coronary sinus in the canine heart can be triggered, but as in mitral valve fibers, catecholamines usually are needed (315). When stimulated at rates of about 100/min *in vitro*, these fibers may have a high level of maximum diastolic potential (−80 to −90 mV) and action potentials with fast upstrokes. Action-potential repolarization is followed by a small afterhyperpolarization, but no afterdepolarization. Superfusion with catecholamines under these conditions often causes only small afterdepolarizations, and triggering may not occur. After a period of stimu-

lation at a slow rate (< about 60/min) or after a period with no stimulation, resting potential often decreases to between −50 and −65 mV, a level at which the fibers do not initiate action potentials in response to electrical stimuli. When fibers at this low level of membrane potential are exposed to low concentrations of norepinephrine, resting potential increases rapidly (25), and the fibers become excitable, generating action potentials followed by large afterdepolarizations that may reach threshold, resulting in triggered activity.

Although the mechanism for this increase in afterdepolarization amplitude has not been investigated, we can offer a hypothesis that might explain these observations. Depolarization has been shown to increase Ca entry into squid axon (223,224) and cardiac muscle (3,52). This response to depolarization is greatly increased by elevating extracellular Na and occurs when intracellular Na is elevated (96). The elevation in Ca$_i$ has been proposed to be caused by a voltage-dependent Na-Ca exchange (94). If a similar mechanism exists in the atrial cells, depolarization prior to catecholamine administration will be expected to increase intracellular Ca. Furthermore, Na$_i$ may be elevated because of the large Na leak in these cardiac fibers, enhancing the net influx of Ca (26). Once the tissue is exposed to catecholamines and hyperpolarization occurs, a decrease in Ca$_i$ can be expected. However, catecholamines can also cause uptake of Ca by the sarcoplasmic reticulum (219), and thus much of the increased intracellular Ca may remain in the cells. In addition, catecholamines may cause a further increase in Ca by increasing the slow inward current (238).

Pectinate muscle. Triggerable fibers in the upper pectinate muscles bordering the crista terminalis in the rabbit heart may be located in branches of the sinoatrial ring bundle or in transitional fibers between the ring bundle and ordinary pectinate muscle (249). They have relatively high resting potentials ($\geq$ −70 mV), and afterdepolarizations arise from this high membrane potential in the absence of exogenous catecholamines. The afterdepolarizations do not appear to follow afterhyperpolarizations, but rather occur just prior to complete repolarization of the action potentials.

Human atria. Apparently normal fibers in human atrial myocardium (resting potentials of −70 to −75 mV) can have delayed afterdepolarizations and can be triggered (208). Resting membrane potential decreases to around −60 mV when stimulation is discontinued, much like the decline that occurs when coronary sinus fibers are not stimulated. The atrial fibers, unlike coronary sinus fibers, become automatic at relatively slow rates because of spontaneous diastolic depolarization. Delayed afterdepolarizations in these spontaneously active fibers are superimposed on the spontaneous diastolic depolarization that causes the automatic activity. When a delayed afterdepolarization reaches threshold, it triggers a more rapid rhythm.

Spontaneous diastolic depolarization, delayed afterdepolarizations, and triggered activity also are evident in human atrial fibers with very low membrane potentials (−60 mV) and slow-response action potentials (156,208,269). Such preparations are obtained from atria that are dilated as a result of cardiac disease. Catecholamines are sometimes necessary for the afterdepolarizations to occur. Similar phenomena also occur in atria from feline hearts with cardiomyopathy (27).

Triggered Activity in Purkinje Fibers and Ventricular Muscle

Overdrive excitation in Purkinje fibers. The usual effect of overdrive stimulation on Purkinje fibers is to suppress spontaneous diastolic depolarization and automaticity by increasing the electrogenic Na-K pump current (279). Increasing extracellular Ca over the range of 2 to 10 mM also decreases automaticity by shifting the threshold potential toward more positive levels (302). In addition to these suppressive effects, both overdrive and elevated Ca interact to cause a phenomenon in Purkinje fibers that Vassalle (282,286,295) called overdrive excitation, which is probably the same as triggered activity. When superfused with Tyrode solution containing elevated Ca (8.1 mM), Purkinje fibers are quiescent, but develop what appears to be spontaneous diastolic depolarization during a period of stimulation (267), followed by persistent rhythmic activity after stimulation is stopped (276,277). The rate of the rhythmic activity is fastest immediately after drive and then progressively slows, accompanied by a decrease in the slope of the diastolic depolarization. The period of overdrive excitation is longer after faster drive rates (276). A similar phenomenon occurs in the presence of norepinephrine, which normally inhibits overdrive suppression (286). Although during rhythmic activity delayed afterdepolarizations are not apparent, an oscillatory potential can be recognized after the last beat. The combination of high Ca (8.1 mM) and norepinephrine is even more effective in causing overdrive excitation and increases the amplitude of the oscillatory potentials (276). Overdrive excitation is most likely a result of delayed afterdepolarizations that cause the steepening of the diastolic depolarization during and after a period of drive. The combination of a period of drive (189), norepinephrine (238), and elevated extracellular Ca (236,277) brings about an increase in Ca influx and the increase in intracellular Ca necessary to cause the appearance of delayed afterdepolarizations.

Hypertrophied and diabetic ventricular muscle. Delayed afterdepolarizations and triggered activity may occur in rat ventricular muscle that is hypertrophic secondary to

renovascular hypertension, particularly if Ca_o is moderately elevated (7.2–12.0 mM) (8). Afterdepolarizations also appear in the presence of 10 to 30 mM tetraethylammonium ion (8), which decreases outward currents (177). Afterdepolarizations do not occur under these conditions in normal ventricular muscle. The occurrence of delayed afterdepolarizations may be related to abnormalities in membrane Ca currents or in sarcoplasmic reticulum uptake and release of Ca that occur concomitantly with hypertrophy, as discussed by Aronson (8). Ventricular myocardium from diabetic rats is also more prone to develop delayed afterdepolarizations under conditions believed to cause myoplasmic Ca overload, such as the presence of ouabain and increased Ca_o (227).

Altered ionic environment. Cranefield and Aronson (75) first described delayed afterdepolarizations and triggered activity in Purkinje fibers exposed to Na^+-free and Ca^{2+}-rich solutions. Purkinje fibers exhibit two stable levels of resting membrane potentials in these solutions (311) and can be triggered only at the low level of membrane potential.

Delayed afterdepolarizations and triggered activity also occur in ventricular muscle superfused with a K^+-free solution containing normal or elevated Ca^{2+} (92,150–152). Superfusates lacking K^+ cause delayed afterdepolarizations by inhibiting the Na-K pump (92,93). When the pump is inhibited, Na_i increases (84). Simultaneously, twitch tension increases, and aftercontractions appear, indicating an increase in Ca_i (92).

When bovine or ovine Purkinje fibers are exposed to a superfusate containing high (16 mM) K^+, resting potential is reduced, and the fibers are inexcitable. Addition of catecholamines to the superfusing solution restores excitability to the inexcitable fibers, causing action potentials with slow upstrokes and long durations (47). In the presence of normal levels of extracellular Ca, no afterdepolarizations occur, but when Ca^{2+} is increased to 16 mM, delayed afterdepolarizations appear; single or trains of triggered impulses may arise from the afterdepolarizations. Caffeine added to the superfusate has effects very similar to those of the catecholamines (47). However, delayed afterdepolarizations do not occur in canine Purkinje fibers in the presence of high K^+ and catecholamines (318).

Purkinje fibers in myocardial infarcts. Purkinje fibers survive on the endocardial surfaces of transmural infarcts in the canine heart, probably because they are nourished by blood within the left ventricular cavity. By 24 hr after the coronary occlusion, maximum diastolic potential is reduced, as are the action-potential upstroke velocity and amplitude. Action-potential duration is prolonged, and spontaneous diastolic depolarization is evident (118,191). Automaticity in these surviving Purkinje fibers causes ventricular arrhythmias 1 day after coronary artery ligation. In addition to the spontaneous diastolic depolarization, delayed afterdepolarizations occur (99) and might be related to the increase in intracellular Ca thought to be caused by ischemia. Their role in the genesis of the ventricular arrhythmias is unclear. The occurrence of delayed afterdepolarizations (198) appears to be dependent on (a) the size of the infarct, (b) the membrane potential of the Purkinje fibers, and (c) the temperature of the superfusate. Membrane potential, in turn, is related to the extent of infarction and the time of superfusion in the tissue chamber. Membrane potential is lower in more extensive infarcts, being lowest toward the apex, where damage is usually more severe. Membrane potential also increases during the period of superfusion and may improve by as much as 30 mV over a period of 2 to 3 hr (191). Delayed afterdepolarizations are not usually seen when membrane potential is very low (< −65 mV) in the extensive infarcts, but are more common in Purkinje fibers with membrane potentials in the range of −70 mV in smaller infarcts. Two to three days after an infarct, membrane potentials are higher than at 24 hr. Automatic rhythms usually are not seen here, but delayed afterdepolarizations and triggered rhythms can be induced by pacing (198). The appearance of delayed afterdepolarizations in Purkinje fibers overlying infarcts is also dependent on the temperature of the superfusate. At temperatures of 35 to 36°C, delayed afterdepolarizations may predominate in infarcted tissues that nonetheless demonstrate automatic rhythms when the superfusate is maintained at 38 to 39°C (normal canine body temperature). The mechanism for this temperature effect is unknown.

Some ventricular arrhythmias that occur after reperfusion of a previously ischemic area might also be caused by delayed afterdepolarizations. When Purkinje fibers superfused *in vitro* are subjected to an ischemic-like environment (hypoxia, acidosis, elevated lactate, zero substrate), they depolarize to low levels of membrane potential. If they are then reperfused with a normally oxygenated solution, membrane potential rapidly repolarizes, depolarizes, and then once again repolarizes. The action potentials occurring during the second phase of depolarization are followed by delayed afterdepolarizations (114).

Isolated myocytes. Single myocytes can be isolated from mammalian ventricle by enzymatic dissociation (88,129). Sometimes such myocytes can have delayed afterdepolarizations even when resting and action potentials are normal (16,210). Delayed afterdepolarizations have not been recorded from muscle cells in intact tissues in the absence of pharmacological interventions. Delayed afterdepolarizations can also be induced in myocytes by low concentrations of isoproterenol (1–10 μM) (16), unlike the situation in intact ventricular muscle, in which much larger concentrations are required (192). The reason that delayed afterdepolarizations appear so readily in isolated myocytes is unknown, but we can offer two suggestions. First, isolation of cells may increase intracellular Ca to the extent necessary to cause afterdepolarizations, perhaps by increasing the permeability of the membrane to Ca. Second, uncoupling of cells and removal of the electrotonic load may enhance the ability of the weak transient inward current to depolarize the membrane.

Triggered Activity Caused by Electrotonic Interactions Between Pacemaker and Nonpacemaker Cells

In the next section we discuss the specific membrane current to which delayed afterdepolarizations are usually attributed. However, oscillations in membrane potential occurring after an action potential and resembling delayed afterdepolarizations caused by this current might also result from passive interactions among cells in a syncytial sheet having different kinds of action potentials, according to Van Capelle and Durrer (278). They simulated these interactions in a computer model using a sheet of excitable elements coupled together by passive resistances that could be set to different values. Transmembrane potentials and currents flowing between elements were included in the simulation. When cells with spontaneous diastolic depolarization and pacemaker activity are coupled to nonpacemaker cells by a critically low resistance in this model, the repetitive activity of the pacemaker cells is completely inhibited. A single stimulus then can evoke an action potential and start sustained rhythmic activity. The rhythmic activity can also be stopped by a single stimulus. If the coupling resistance is lowered a bit more, the action potential evoked by the stimulus is followed by oscillatory activity resembling afterdepolarizations. These apparent afterdepolarizations result from the electrotonic effect of the nonpacemaker cell on the pacemaker cell. The diastolic membrane potential of the pacemaker cells begins to depolarize, but then may be returned to the maximum diastolic level before reaching threshold because of current flow from the nonpacemaker cell. If threshold potential is reached, repolarization of the triggered action potential will be followed by spontaneous diastolic depolarization to threshold if coupling resistance between the two kinds of cells is not low enough to prevent it (278).

Ionic Mechanisms Responsible for Delayed Afterdepolarizations

Transient Inward Current

Delayed afterdepolarizations and triggered activity are caused by an oscillatory membrane current that is distinct from both the pacemaker current and other membrane currents occurring during the course of the action potential (11,12,149,193). This membrane current was called the transient inward (TI) current by Lederer and Tsien (193), who were among the first to characterize it in digitalis-toxic Purkinje fibers using the two-micro-electrode voltage-clamp technique. Similar experimental approaches have since been extended to other preparations and conditions in which afterdepolarizations occur to define the properties of the membrane current(s) that cause them. These include ventricular muscle exposed to digitalis (170), Purkinje fibers in normal or high Ca (203,293) or low K^+ (92,93), and catecholamine-induced afterdepolarizations in atrial fibers (273). A TI current with properties similar to those of the one originally identified in digitalis-toxic Purkinje fibers causes the afterdepolarizations under this variety of experimental conditions.

Characteristics of Transient Inward Current

As described earlier, delayed afterdepolarizations develop when driven Purkinje fibers are exposed to toxic concentrations of digitalis. If the membrane potential is clamped at the maximum diastolic level following a series of driven beats, and the membrane currents following the last stimulated action potential are measured, an inward current transient occurs, superimposed on the decaying pacemaker potential (Fig. 2) (193). This current has the appropriate time course and magnitude to be a cause of the delayed afterdepolarizations. The TI current is also recorded after a depolarizing voltage-clamp pulse in the form of a square wave that mimics to some extent the action potential (depolarization for 200–500 msec, followed by repolarization). The current appears after the repolarizing step (Fig. 3). The procedure of using a square-wave depolarizing clamp step has also been used in voltage-clamp studies on afterdepolarizations in other preparations and under other conditions (vide infra). The magnitude of the membrane depolarization, the duration of the depolarization, and the level of repolarization can all be varied and all influence the kinetics and amplitude of the current.

Effects of membrane depolarization. The TI current can be elicited on repolarization after a depolarizing pulse (Fig. 3). The holding potential that has been used for studies of the TI current under different conditions has ranged from around −80 mV (293) to −20 mV (193) and has mainly been varied to distinguish the TI current from other membrane currents such as the fast inward current and the pacemaker current, both of which can be eliminated by selecting a particular holding potential. At holding potentials (and repolarization potentials) less negative than about −60 mV, the pacemaker current is not seen, but a large TI current may occur

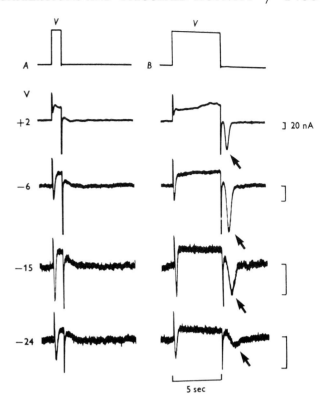

FIG. 3. Effects of depolarizing voltage-clamp pulse duration and magnitude on the amplitude of the TI current in calf Purkinje fiber exposed to 1 μM strophanthidin (two-micro-electrode voltage-clamp technique). From a holding potential of −41 mV, depolarizing voltage-clamp pulses were imposed for either 1 sec (**A**) or 4 sec (**B**), as shown in the top traces. The range of depolarization was from −24 to +2 mV, as indicated on the left-hand side of the figure. Note the variation in scale of the different current records (vertical bars at the right of each trace are 20 nA). At the same pulse duration, the TI current is larger as depolarizations become more positive [compare records in B, where TI current (*arrows*) is most prominent]. At comparable depolarizations, the TI current becomes larger as the pulse duration is increased (compare records in A with those in B). (From ref. 193, with permission.)

(193). Similarly, the TI current can be elicited after the fast inward current is first inactivated by voltage-clamp steps to potentials less negative than −60 to −50 mV (193,293).

The threshold of depolarization required to elicit the TI current ranges widely from −60 mV in atrial muscle from the coronary sinus (273) to −13 mV in ferret papillary muscle exposed to toxic amounts of digitalis (170). We shall describe in detail later the hypothesis that the TI current is caused by Ca overload in the cell interior and that under certain conditions the magnitude of the current is related to the level of myoplasmic or sarcoplasmic reticulum Ca. The threshold level of depolarization probably also depends to some extent on the intracellular Ca levels. Raising Ca_o (and thereby Ca_i) shifts the level of depolarization necessary to elicit the

TI current in a negative direction (293). Intracellular Ca levels have probably been different under the variety of experimental conditions in which the TI current has been studied, explaining, to some extent, the variability in the threshold potentials.

Different physiological properties of different kinds of myocardial fibers may also play roles in determining the threshold for activation of the TI current, in particular, the handling of intracellular Ca. Histological studies show that mammalian atrial cells have a better-developed sarcoplasmic reticulum than mammalian ventricular muscle or Purkinje fibers (107). The Ca level required for Ca-triggered Ca release from the sarcoplasmic reticulum is lower in atrial cells than in ventricular cells or Purkinje fibers (102). These tissue variations might contribute to the observations that in atrial fibers of the coronary sinus the depolarizing clamp pulse voltage is lower (and duration is shorter) for inducing the transient inward current than in ventricular muscle or Purkinje fibers.

Increasing the magnitude of the depolarization enhances the amplitude of the TI current and causes it to develop more rapidly (Fig. 4) (170,193,273,293). The relationship between the amplitude and time course of the TI current and the amplitude of the activating clamp pulse has been studied in detail in ventricular muscle in the presence of ouabain (Fig. 4) (170); in that tissue, this relationship is sigmoid, with the amplitude of the TI current increasing slowly after depolarizations from about −20 to 0 mV and rapidly after depolarizations from 0 to +20 mV. The descending limb of the curve (decreasing TI current with increasing depolarization) occurs between +20 and +40 mV. The negative limb of the curve was considered by Karagueuzian and Katzung (170) to result either from accumulation of K in the extracellular space with more positive clamps (increased K can depress the TI current) (92,293) or from intracellular accumulation of the TI-current charge carrier, causing a decrease in the current's reversal potential and a parallel decrease in driving force. In atrial fibers exposed to catecholamines, the relationship between TI-current magnitude and activation clamp pulse amplitude is also sigmoid, but the steepest slope occurs between −20 and 0 mV (273).

The effects of the amplitude of the depolarizing clamp pulse on the TI current may depend on the effects of the depolarizing pulses on intracellular Ca. Ca influx via the slow inward current might play some role. The steep part of the curve relating TI current to the level of depolarization occurs over a range of membrane potentials at which the slow inward current is activated and increases in amplitude (59). Increasing the level of external Ca increases the TI current (171,175,293). An increase in Ca_o may increase intracellular Ca by increasing the magnitude of the slow inward current (236). However, depolarizing clamp steps that do not activate the slow inward current may also activate the TI current (see ref. 293 for details), and the slope factor for the TI current may be more positive and steeper than the activation curve for the slow inward current (170). Therefore, other mechanisms such as membrane-potential-dependent Na-Ca exchange (94) or release of Ca from internal stores may also play a role in causing the increasing TI current that follows depolarizing steps of increasing amplitude.

Effects of duration of depolarization. The minimal duration of membrane depolarization required for appearance of the TI current also varies markedly, de-

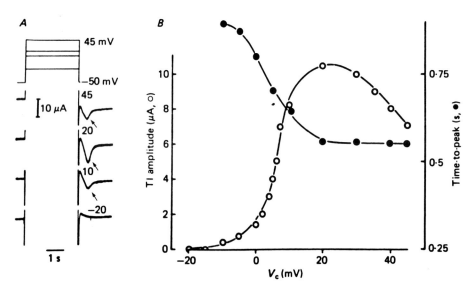

FIG. 4. Dependence of TI amplitude and kinetics in ferret papillary muscle on activating voltage (sucrose-gap voltage-clamp technique). The preparation was superfused with 1.8 μM ouabain. **A:** Chart records showing (*top*) the superimposed voltage-clamp pulses and (*below*) the current records at high sensitivity. The TI current is indicated by the *arrows*. The activating clamp voltage level (V_c) is shown at the right margin of each record. Currents flowing during the depolarizing steps were off scale. **B:** Plot of a complete series of clamps in the same preparation. Inward ("negative") current is plotted upward. Note the sigmoid relationship of TI current amplitude (*open circles*) to activating clamp voltage level. The time to peak (*solid circles*) of the TI current increases at voltage levels from −20 to +20 mV. (From ref. 170, with permission.)

pending on the conditions of the experiments and the preparations used. As with the variation in depolarization threshold, the differences among experiments are likely to be dependent both on intracellular Ca levels and on the functional properties of the sarcoplasmic reticulum. In atrial fibers from the coronary sinus, pulses as short as 100 msec sometimes elicit a TI current (273), whereas in digitalis-toxic Purkinje fibers, pulses 5 sec in duration may be required for a clear TI current at the weakest depolarization level (193). At fixed levels of depolarization, increasing the duration of the voltage-clamp pulse (and membrane depolarization) increases the amplitude of the TI current and accelerates the time course at which it achieves maximum amplitude (Fig. 3) (170,193,273,293). The increase in the TI-current amplitude has a sigmoid relation to the clamp pulse duration in digitalis-toxic Purkinje fibers (193) and in atrial fibers of the coronary sinus (273); TI amplitude and time to peak eventually reach a plateau or decline as pulse duration is increased.

The prolongation of the clamp pulse and the duration of membrane depolarization might also increase intracellular Ca by increasing the flow of slow inward current (59,173). However, during prolonged pulses from 100 msec to 3 or 5 sec, the slow inward current may become inactivated to a large extent (172); yet the TI current may increase over this range of pulse durations. Therefore, intracellular Ca may increase by another mechanism that has not yet been defined.

Effects of successive depolarizations. The relationship between the duration of the depolarizing clamp pulse and the amplitude of the TI current described earlier shows that increasing the amount of time the membrane is maintained in the depolarized state can enhance the TI current. For the same reason, it has been found that the amplitude of the TI current increases after repeated clamp pulses and is inversely related to the interval between pulses and directly related to the number of pulses (193,293). The repetitive depolarizations can increase intracellular Ca because of repeated activation of the slow inward current. Repetitive clamp pulses to low potentials that do not activate the slow inward current can also lead to an increase in the TI current, and therefore there may be an additional mechanism for increasing Ca_i (293). If the fast inward current is activated by repetitive clamp pulses, intracellular Ca might also rise secondary to an increase in intracellular Na (164). An increase in Ca_i is indicated by the positive staircase effect on contraction of repetitive stimulation (127).

Effects of level of repolarization. Current–voltage relationships for the TI current have been established with a clamp protocol in which a fixed depolarization step is used to elicit the current and the level of repolarization (membrane potential at which the current is measured) is varied over a wide range (Fig. 5). As the level of repolarization is decreased from about −60 mV toward

0, the amplitude of the TI current decreases, and its time to peak increases. A decrease also occurs as the level of repolarization is increased from −60 mV toward more negative potentials, and no current may be observed at −90 to −100 mV (6,170,175,293). This experimental procedure has also been used to determine the reversal potential of the TI current, and the difference in the data from different laboratories provides the source of an important controversy as to whether or not the TI current flows through gated membrane channels. In their studies on digitalis-toxic Purkinje fibers, Kass et al. (175) found a reversal potential for the TI current of around −5 mV (at repolarization to −5 mV after clamps well into the positive range of membrane potentials, the TI current was zero, and at more positive repolarization levels the TI current was outward) (Fig. 5). The reversal potential was shifted in a negative direction when Na in the superfusate was decreased (Na is the charge carrier for the current, as will be described later). However, in other studies on the TI current in digitalis-toxic ventricular muscle fibers (6,170), a reversal potential was not apparent: The TI current became smaller at more positive potentials and approached zero current or a finite inward current in a curvilinear fashion between −40 and +10 mV. An outward TI current was never seen even when the Na in the superfusate was replaced by choline chloride or sucrose. Also, a clear reversal potential was not seen in studies on the TI current in embryonic rat ventricular muscle cell aggregates (294), rabbit sinus node (34) and atrial fibers exposed to catecholamines (273). The absence of a reversal potential has been interpreted to suggest that the TI current does not flow through gated membrane channels but rather results from electrogenic Na-Ca exchange (6), as will be discussed later.

In experiments on the current–voltage relationship of the TI current it usually has been assumed that the repolarization level of membrane potential influences the membrane conductance and hence the magnitude of the TI current. However, this level might affect not only the membrane channels or "system" mediating the TI current but also Ca movements inside the cells that in turn influence the magnitude of the TI current. At membrane potentials positive to −20 or −30 mV, there may be a continuous high free Ca level in the cytoplasm, as indicated by increases in tonic tension over this voltage range (218). The sarcoplasmic reticulum may not be able to take up and release as much Ca because of the high-free-Ca level at the positive level of membrane potential, and the myoplasmic Ca oscillations necessary to induce the TI current may be small. The TI current may be diminished, and there may be only low-amplitude current oscillations. At membrane potentials negative to −20 mV, the sarcoplasmic reticulum uptake function may be improved: a larger amount of Ca being released from and taken up by the sarcoplasmic reticulum,

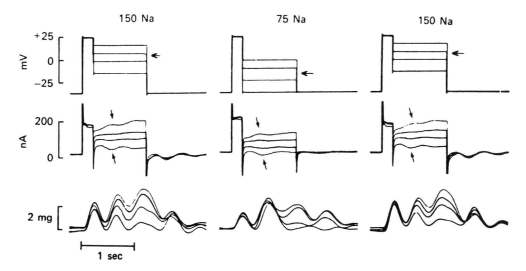

FIG. 5. A: Experiment demonstrating reversal potential in calf Purkinje fibers superfused with strophanthidin and the effects of reducing Na on TI reversal. In each column, step repolarizations to varying potentials are superimposed (*top*). Membrane current (*middle*) and contractile force (*bottom*) follow the same vertical sequence as the voltage traces. Horizontal *arrows* in the voltage trace (*top*) indicate reversal potential values obtained by graphic analysis of data. *Arrows* in current trace indicate TI current. **Left:** Control run in 150 mM Na. **Center:** Records taken 3 to 5 min after changing external solution to 75 mM Na (choline). **Right:** Records taken 19 to 21 min after readmitting 150 mM Na. (From ref. 175, with permission.)

resulting in sizable free intracellular Ca oscillations and a large TI current. At still more negative potentials, the sarcoplasmic reticulum release mechanism may decrease, resulting in less Ca release and a smaller TI current. If the time to peak of the TI current can be taken as an indicator of the efficiency of the Ca release mechanism of the sarcoplasmic reticulum, the monotonic increase in time to peak of the current as the repolarization level becomes more negative can be explained by less efficient Ca release from the sarcoplasmic reticulum at more negative voltages. That aftercontractions are influenced by the repolarization level in a similar way as the TI current (175) supports the supposition that this membrane potential affects intracellular Ca release (amplitude and time course of aftercontractions reflect the level and time course of intracellular Ca changes). Therefore, the results of Kass et al. (175) indicate that voltage-dependent Ca movements between the myoplasm and sarcoplasmic reticulum may play an important role in determining the current–voltage relationship of the TI current.

Creep Current

Sodium-pump blockade with K-free superfusates or with digitalis may also cause a time-dependent increase in a nonoscillatory inward current during long voltage-clamp steps, called the "creep current" by Eisner and Lederer (92). The appearance of this current parallels the development of voltage-dependent tonic tension (Fig. 6). After returning to the holding potential, the oscillatory TI current that develops is superimposed on a gradual decrease in net inward current. The creep current has some similarities to the TI current and may

be related to it. Both are decreased by manipulations that decrease Ca entry into the cell (92). The oscillatory TI current is due to the oscillatory release and uptake of Ca from the sarcoplasmic reticulum (*vide infra*), whereas the tail currents have been proposed to result from nonoscillatory extrusion of Ca from the cell (see ref. 282 for more details).

Subcellular Mechanism of Delayed Afterdepolarizations

Overview.

Based on the results of their voltage-clamp studies on digitalis toxic Purkinje fibers, Tsien et al. (274) proposed a hypothesis to explain the subcellular mechanism that causes membrane oscillations and delayed afterdepolarizations. We shall first summarize this hypothesis and then describe some of the experimental data pertinent to its formulation.

The occurrence of delayed afterdepolarizations is usually associated with a situation in which intracellular Ca levels are elevated. An elevation of cytoplasmic Ca may lead to an elevation in the calcium contained in the sarcoplasmic reticulum. Calcium is normally released from the sarcoplasmic reticulum during the plateau of the action potential to activate the contractile machinery and is taken up by the sarcoplasmic reticulum during repolarization, resulting in relaxation. When the sarcoplasmic reticulum is overloaded with calcium, the reuptake of Ca that results in relaxation is followed by a secondary release of Ca from the sarcoplasmic reticulum *following* repolarization. It is this secondary release of Ca that leads to the transient increases in membrane

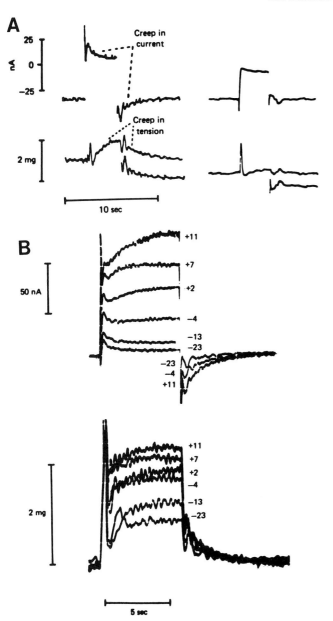

FIG. 6. A: Effects of prolonged exposure to K-free superfusate in voltage-clamped sheep Purkinje fibers: current (*top*), tension (*bottom*). Holding potential −60 mV. A 3-sec depolarizing pulse to −40 mV is shown. **A:** The right-hand panel was obtained 3 min after changing from 4 mM K_o to the K-free solution. The left-hand panel was obtained after 32 min in K-free solution. The creep current that appears during depolarization and after returning to the holding potential is indicated. A creep in tension also occurs. In both panels, the current tail after the depolarizing pulse has been inverted and delayed by 100 msec and placed below the tension trace. **B:** Reversal of creep current: current (*top*), tension (*bottom*). The records were obtained after 20-min exposure to K-free solution. Six-second depolarizing pulses were applied from a holding potential of −50 mV to the potentials shown. To improve the amplification of the records, the instantaneous current jump on depolarization has been reduced by moving the traces nearer to the base line. Current tails are shown only from pulses to −23, −4, and +11 mV. Part of the twitch is off scale at this gain for all but the weakest depolarizing pulses. (From ref. 92, with permission.)

conductance and inward current that cause the afterdepolarization.

Relationships of delayed afterdepolarizations to contractions and aftercontractions.

Much of the evidence that led to the hypothesis described earlier has come from studies in which tension has been measured simultaneously with membrane potential or transmembrane current. Interventions that cause delayed afterdepolarizations also cause an increase in twitch tension and the appearance of aftercontractions that follow the TI current (110,112,170,171,175,203). A large body of evidence relates the occurrence of aftercontractions to elevated intracellular Ca. This suggests that the afterdepolarizations also occur because of the increased intracellular calcium. Furthermore, a strong relationship between the TI current and aftercontractions can be seen from the results of voltage-clamp studies. Clamp protocols that affect the TI current also affect aftercontractions in a similar way. The amplitudes of both the TI current and the aftercontractions increase with a sigmoid time course as the duration of the depolarizing clamp pulse is increased; increasing the strength of depolarization produces parallel increases in current and aftercontraction. The TI current and aftercontractions have similar dependences on the level of repolarization; repeated depolarizations cause increases in both TI current and aftercontractions (171,175). The clamp protocols that increase the aftercontractions and afterdepolarizations probably cause an increase in intracellular Ca, as was previously discussed. Furthermore, experimental evidence suggests that both afterdepolarizations and aftercontractions are caused by a common mechanism (oscillatory release and reuptake of Ca by the sarcoplasmic reticulum), rather than the afterdepolarizations causing the aftercontractions (92,93,175,274). In support of this statement is the demonstration that the TI current can be dissociated from the aftercontraction. As described earlier, as the level of repolarization after a depolarizing clamp pulse is made more and more positive, the magnitude of the TI current decreases and may approach zero, or even reverse. Despite the absence of the TI current, the aftercontraction remains (171,175). A similar dissociation between the TI current and aftercontractions occurs initially after removing Na from the external environment; the TI current disappears because Na is the charge carrier, but the aftercontractions may not disappear (175).

Increases in tonic tension also occur under conditions that cause delayed afterdepolarizations (92,93,170, 171,175). The relationship between the occurrence of delayed afterdepolarizations and the development of tonic tension provides additional evidence that links afterdepolarizations to an increase in Ca_i, because the tonic tension developed is probably dependent on the level of Ca_i (96,170). The TI current in Purkinje fibers in a normal physiologic solution requires depolarization of the membrane to about -20 mV and subsequent repolarization to -40 mV (293). Coincidentally, -20 mV is the threshold for appearance of voltage-dependent tonic tension (126). The TI current occurs on repolarization after the depolarizing clamp step. Vassalle and Mugelli (293) have pointed out that this repolarization also coincides with relaxation of the tonic contraction. It therefore seems that the occurrence of the TI current actually coincides with removal of Ca from the myofilaments. This may, in fact, lead to release of Ca from the sarcoplasmic reticulum by, for example, Ca-induced release of Ca (103).

In the presence of digitalis or in the absence of external K, the TI current appears simultaneously with an increase in tonic tension at more negative holding potentials (92,93,170). Tonic tension also becomes voltage-dependent after pump inhibition, whereas it is not usually voltage-dependent; there is an increase in tonic tension during the clamp pulses used to activate the TI current, and the increase is dependent on the magnitude of the clamp pulse (92,93,170). The voltage-dependent tonic tension may reflect an increase in myoplasmic Ca during depolarization and thus a voltage dependence of factors regulating Ca_i (92,93). Eisner and Lederer (92,93) have considered the possibility that it indicates either voltage-dependent Ca movement across the plasma membrane or voltage-dependent Ca flux from intracellular stores into the cytoplasm. Removal of external Ca decreases augmented tonic tension along with the aftercontraction and TI current (92,93).

Therefore, the evidence shows a strong relationship between afterdepolarizations or TI current, on the one hand, and indices of contractile activity that reflect intracellular Ca levels, on the other.

Relationship of delayed afterdepolarizations to oscillatory Ca movements.

The TI current is a manifestation of what Tsien et al. (274) have called an internal oscillator. This is an oscillatory control loop contained within the cell that for the most part excludes the membrane potential across the sarcolemma. The oscillations in the membrane potential that are sometimes manifested as delayed afterdepolarizations occur as a secondary consequence of this oscillatory mechanism. Changes in membrane potential, although not essential for the oscillations, can modify their characteristics (174). The experimental evidence suggests that the internal oscillator is the sarcoplasmic reticulum and that it is responsible for oscillations in the myoplasmic Ca levels that occur when Ca_i is elevated. Thus, under conditions of elevated intracellular Ca in unstimulated cells, fluctuations in tension (43,130,184), membrane potential, and current occur (92,93,174,210) simultaneously with fluctuations in myoplasmic Ca levels (2,190,229,303). Such oscilla-

tions can increase in amplitude and frequency after interventions that further increase intracellular Ca, such as digitalis (174), absence of external K (92,93), or low Na (2,3,210). Lowering external Ca or intracellular injection of EGTA, which are expected to lower myoplasmic free Ca, cause the disappearance of spontaneous voltage and current fluctuations (174,210).

The oscillatory changes in myoplasmic Ca levels are believed to result from an oscillatory release and uptake of Ca from the sarcoplasmic reticulum, perhaps by Ca-induced Ca release (103). The evidence for this statement includes the following: (a) Increasing Ca around mechanically skinned cardiac muscle has been shown to produce cyclic contractions (106). (b) Cyclic contractions are abolished in skinned cardiac muscle after Ca is buffered with EGTA or the sarcoplasmic reticulum is destroyed (106). (c) Oscillatory Ca release has also been shown from isolated sarcoplasmic reticulum loaded with Ca (230). (d) Oscillations in membrane potential (210), tension, and myoplasmic Ca_i in tissues or isolated cells are inhibited by caffeine or ryanodine, two agents that inhibit the function of the sarcoplasmic reticulum (2,262). (e) The high frequency of the oscillations (around 0.8 Hz) makes it unlikely that they are due to Ca uptake and release by mitochondria, a process that is much slower.

A relationship is thought to exist between spontaneous oscillations in membrane current, voltage, tension, and myoplasmic Ca levels, on the one hand, and the TI current, afterdepolarizations, and aftercontractions, on the other, because they have similar properties and are affected in the same ways by a variety of interventions. The similar properties are as follows: (a) The power spectrum of spontaneous oscillations in Ca-loaded Purkinje fibers is similar to that of the TI current evoked in the same preparation (174). (b) The period of oscillations of myoplasmic Ca levels measured by aequorin in nonstimulated, Ca-loaded ferret papillary muscle is similar to the period of the oscillatory increase and decrease of myoplasmic Ca after a stimulated twitch in the same preparation (aftercontraction) (Fig. 7) (2). (c) Ca-dependent spontaneous current fluctuations have the same frequency as the larger oscillatory TI current (174). (d) Interventions that affect the spontaneous oscillations in myoplasmic Ca and membrane current have similar effects on the TI current, afterdepolarizations, and aftercontractions. For example, increasing intracellular Ca_i increases the frequency and amplitude of aequorin-measured spontaneous oscillations in myoplasmic Ca and the oscillations in myoplasmic Ca following a stimulated twitch (2). The spontaneous oscillations in membrane current and voltage, as well as the TI current, also increase (174,210). Repetitive stimulation increases the magnitude and frequency of both spontaneous oscillations in myoplasmic Ca and the oscillations following a stimulated twitch (2). EGTA inhibits spontaneous

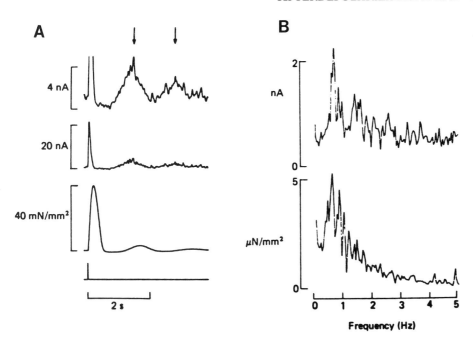

FIG. 7. Comparison of stimulated and spontaneous oscillations of aequorin light and tension. **A:** Stimulated oscillations. Traces show averaged (N = 4) records of aequorin light (high gain) (**top**), aequorin light (low gain) (**middle**), and tension (**bottom**). The stimulus marker is shown below. The *arrows* in the **top trace** show the period of oscillations of light accompanying an aftercontraction (**bottom trace**). The muscle was stimulated at 0.03 Hz in a solution containing Ca^{2+} (8 mmol/liter) and strophanthidin (10 µmol/liter). All solutions were buffered with HCO_3^-/CO_2. **B:** Spontaneous oscillations. Traces show Fourier amplitude spectra of aequorin light (**top**) and tension (**bottom**). The spectra were obtained in the same solutions as in A, and the muscle was not stimulated. (From ref. 2, with permission.)

oscillations in both membrane current and TI current (174). Caffeine and ryanodine also inhibit spontaneous myoplasmic Ca oscillations and spontaneous oscillations in membrane current (262), as well as oscillations following an action potential (delayed afterdepolarizations) or a depolarizing voltage-clamp pulse (10,288).

The voltage changes in the membrane potential are not an essential part of the oscillatory loop between sarcoplasmic reticulum and myoplasm and can be eliminated (e.g., by clamping the membrane at a constant voltage) without altering the intracellular oscillatory process. However, changes in membrane potential can exert influences on the magnitude, frequency, and coherence of the subcellular oscillations (Fig. 8). This was shown by Kass and Tsien (174), who measured spontaneous current fluctuations induced by strophanthidin in Purkinje fibers at a series of membrane potentials ranging from 0 to −80 mV (extracellular Na of 37 mM). The amplitude of the voltage fluctuations decreased at more negative potentials between −2 and −40 mV, and the minimum fluctuation in potentials was found at −40 mV. This falls within the range of reversal potentials at similar Na_o for the TI current (175). The amplitude of the oscillations increased from −40 to −80 mV. The oscillatory frequency also showed voltage dependence: Frequency increased over a range of potentials from −80 to −20 mV. This is similar to the acceleratory effect of decreasing membrane potential on the TI current.

If the spontaneous oscillations in myoplasmic Ca and membrane current in unstimulated cells are related to the oscillations following activity, it then seems that the spontaneous oscillations must somehow be synchronized by the occurrence of an action potential (174,210,262).

In the absence of a stimulated action potential, different cells may not oscillate in synchrony, and even within a cell, different regions may oscillate out of phase with each other (43). When an action potential occurs, release and uptake of Ca by the sarcoplasmic reticulum are synchronized (210). On depolarization of the membrane, the intracellular free Ca is increased by Ca influx through

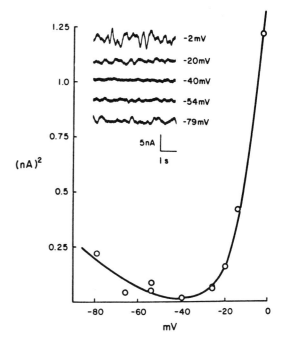

FIG. 8. Voltage dependence of noise variance. **Inset:** Representative traces showing current fluctuations at various holding potentials. **Graph:** Noise variance calculated from these records and others from same experiments. Smooth curve drawn by eye. (From ref. 174, with permission.)

the slow channel. Initially the rapid rate of change of intracellular Ca triggers Ca release from the sarcoplasmic reticulum, which causes a further rise in intracellular free Ca (104). Repolarization then induces a synchronous Ca uptake by the whole population of sarcoplasmic reticulum in the cell. If intracellular Ca is very high or if catecholamines or cyclic AMP are present, the Ca in the sarcoplasmic reticulum may rise to a critical level at which a secondary spontaneous and synchronous release of Ca from the sarcoplasmic reticulum occurs (106). This secondary release of Ca generates the TI current and the afterdepolarization (possible mechanisms are discussed in the next section). After one or several afterdepolarizations, myoplasmic Ca may decrease because of Na-Ca exchange.

Inward current during delayed afterdepolarizations.

The exact mechanism by which the secondary rise in myoplasmic Ca causes the TI current is unclear and is a source of controversy. At least two possibilities are being actively considered: (a) the rise in calcium increases membrane conductance to ions (mainly Na), which flow through gated channels down a concentration gradient. (b) The rise in calcium causes an inward current through an electrogenic exchange of Ca for Na.

The charge carrier for the inward TI current that causes delayed afterdepolarizations appears to be mainly Na^+. This has been elucidated by changing the concentrations of ions in the extracellular fluid. Removal of Na leads to decreases in the afterdepolarizations and TI current (6,170,175). However, the effects of Na removal may be complex. In digitalis-toxic Purkinje fibers, Na removal leads first to increases in afterdepolarization amplitude and TI current, accompanied by an increase in twitch tension and an aftercontraction. This is followed by decreases in afterdepolarization amplitude and TI current while the increased aftercontraction is maintained (175,284). When Na_o is lowered, there is a net increase in intracellular Ca via Na-Ca exchange that causes the initial increases in tension, aftercontraction (18,51), TI current, and afterdepolarization amplitude (175). Subsequently the TI current decreases because the charge carrier is decreased, but the effects of the increased intracellular Ca on the aftercontraction may persist.

The studies of Kass et al. (175) on digitalis-toxic Purkinje fibers led to the proposal that the TI current flows through gated channels, down an ion concentration gradient. This conclusion was reached because the TI current was shown to have a reversal potential (−5 mV) as predicted for a membrane current caused by passive ion flux through channels. The reversal potential was shifted by approximately 15 mV (to −15 to −20 mV) when nonpermeant anions were substituted for 75% of the Na in the superfusate (Fig. 5). This shift is to be

expected if the TI current is caused by a transient conductance change to Na in the presence of a driving force ($E − E_{rev}$); changes in E_{rev} would be expected to result from changes in Na_o. The reversal potential did not change when Ca_o was reduced, and therefore Ca does not appear to act as a charge carrier. However, the results also indicate that the TI current cannot be a Na-specific current, because E_{Na} is normally about +70 mV. The reversal potential of the TI current does not correspond specifically to the equilibrium potential of any major ion, being less negative than E_{Na} and more positive than E_K or E_{Cl}. Therefore, other ions with more negative equilibrium potentials, such as K or Cl, were also proposed to act as charge carriers, and it was suggested that the TI channel was a nonselective leak channel (175). Nonselective membrane channels similar to those proposed by Kass et al. (175) were identified in experiments using the patch-clamp technique on cultured cardiac cells (58). However, a shift in E_{rev} was not seen when the concentrations of these other ions in the perfusate were altered or when K currents were blocked by cesium (175).

Other investigators did not find a reversal potential in their studies on the TI current, although the studies were not performed on digitalis-toxic Purkinje fibers. A major difficulty in establishing a reversal potential arises because the TI current is oscillatory. Brown et al. (34) suggested that the apparent reversal potential that they and Kass et al. (175) described may be attributable to a phase shift in the oscillation, so that the most negative rather than most positive current excursion was considered to be a measurement of the TI current. Eisner and Lederer (94) believe that this possibility was excluded in the studies of Kass et al. (175) on digitalis-toxic Purkinje fibers, because force oscillations were measured simultaneously with membrane current. At the reversal potential, the aftercontractions maintained the same phase delay to the peak of TI current, suggesting that the reversal of the current cannot be accounted for by a phase shift (Fig. 5) (94).

Kass et al. (175) also considered the alternative hypothesis that an electrogenic Na-Ca exchange might cause the TI current. According to this hypothesis, the transient rise in myoplasmic Ca released from the sarcoplasmic reticulum after the action potential is expected to result in Ca efflux across the sarcolemma. Such an efflux is coupled to a Na influx by the Na-Ca exchanger, and if more than 2 Na enter for each Ca, a net inward current occurs. However, if the TI current is caused by electrogenic Na-Ca exchange, theory predicts that the current will not have a reversal potential, because an increase in the free internal Ca will always lead to a net inward current (6,221,222,226). Because of the reversal potential found in their studies, Kass et al. (175) rejected the Na-Ca exchange hypothesis. However, the finding of a reversal potential does not eliminate entirely a contribution of electrogenic Na-Ca exchange to the TI current (94).

The concept of a Na-Ca exchange mechanism causing the TI current is favored by Katzung and associates (6,170). A reversal potential was not found in their sucrose-gap experiments on digitalis-toxic ventricular muscle. Replacement of Na by either choline or sucrose caused a reduction in the TI current at potentials in the steep part of the current–voltage relationship (−40 to −10 mV) and sometimes a shift of the maximum inward TI current to more negative potentials, but no outward current was detected as in the study of Kass et al. (175). Arlock and Katzung (6) have suggested that the results may indicate that at more positive voltages there is an additional current, perhaps a Ca-activated outward current (98), that follows the time course of intracellular Ca oscillations and masks or exceeds the TI current, thereby causing the decrease in the inward current measured at more depolarized levels of membrane potential.

Characteristic Properties of Delayed Afterdepolarizations and Triggered Activity

Many of the properties and characteristics of delayed afterdepolarizations and triggered activity induced in different tissues and under different experimental conditions are quite similar. These similarities probably result from the similar properties of the TI current under the different conditions. However, differences also exist. The most prominent (and most thoroughly studied) differences can be found between properties of afterdepolarizations and triggered activity caused by digitalis and those caused by calcium overload not related to blockade of the Na-K pump.

Dependence of Delayed Afterdepolarizations on Rate and Rhythm

The amplitude of a delayed afterdepolarization and the coupling interval to the previous action potential are dependent on the cycle length at which action potentials are occurring. Digitalis-induced delayed afterdepolarizations occur singly or as two or more "damped" oscillations following the action potential (115,245). When two or more afterdepolarizations are present, their relationship to the drive-cycle length is complex (Fig. 9). As drive-cycle length is decreased, the amplitude of the first afterdepolarization increases, reaching a peak at a cycle length of about 500 msec. At shorter drive-cycle lengths, the magnitude of this afterdepolarization decreases if triggered activity has not occurred by that time. However, the second delayed afterdepolarization

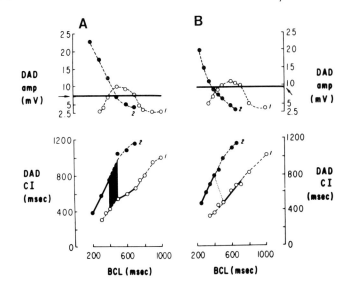

FIG. 9. Relationship between amplitude (DAD amp) and coupling intervals (CL) of delayed afterdepolarizations in digitalis-toxic Purkinje fibers and drive-cycle length (BCL). The first delayed afterdepolarization (DAD 1) is indicated by the *open circles*, the second afterdepolarization (DAD 2) by the *filled circles*. **A** and **B** show data from two different experiments. The coupling intervals for both afterdepolarizations decrease with a decrease in BCL (**bottom panels**). The amplitude of DAD 1 begins to increase at longer BCL than DAD 2 and reaches threshold first (indicated by *solid horizontal line*) to cause triggered activity (BCL about 650 msec). As BCL is decreased further, the amplitude of DAD 1 decreases, but DAD 2 increases to threshold and causes triggered activity. (From ref. 248, with permission.)

continues to increase in magnitude as drive-cycle length shortens further and may reach threshold and induce triggered activity. The drive-cycle length at which triggered activity occurs varies markedly in different preparations and may be partly related to the extent of digitalis toxicity.

In other experimental situations (catecholamines, ischemic Purkinje fibers, hypertrophy), usually only one afterdepolarization occurs, although occasionally there may be several. When one afterdepolarization is present, its amplitude increases as the drive-cycle length decreases, and that can result in triggered activity (8,99,227, 249,314,315). A decline in amplitude with a decrease in cycle length below a critical point has not been directly demonstrated under these conditions, as it has been for digitalis. However, in Purkinje fibers exposed to high concentrations of Ca and catecholamines, triggered activity can be initiated by decreasing the drive-cycle length to a critical level, below which triggering does not occur (276). The afterdepolarization may, therefore, decrease at the shorter drive-cycle lengths, perhaps because of an increase in outward pump current. In human atrial fibers and embryonic heart cells that have both automaticity and subthreshold delayed afterdepolarizations, a spontaneous increase in the rate of automatic activity can cause increases in afterdepolarization amplitude and triggering in the same way as increasing the extrinsic drive rate (208,261).

Decreasing the drive-cycle length also tends to decrease the coupling interval of both digitalis-induced and other kinds of delayed afterdepolarizations measured to the action-potential upstroke or terminal phase of repolarization (Fig. 9). In general, the rate of depolarization of the afterdepolarization also increases (115,245,249,315).

A decrease in the length of even a single drive cycle (i.e., a premature impulse) tends to result in an increase in the amplitude of the delayed afterdepolarization that follows the curtailed cycle. Because the premature impulse occurs earlier after the previous impulse, the amplitude of the afterdepolarization that follows the premature impulse increases and may reach threshold, initiating triggered activity (Fig. 10) (216,249,315). For digitalis-toxic Purkinje fibers, the premature coupling interval at which triggered activity occurs is also dependent on the basic drive-cycle length. As the drive-cycle length decreases, the premature coupling interval needed to induce triggered activity may increase (216).

The amplitude of delayed afterdepolarizations is dependent on the number of action potentials that precede them. That is, after a period of quiescence, the initiation of a single action potential may be followed by either no afterdepolarization or only a small one. With continued stimulation, the afterdepolarizations increase in amplitude (8,115,144,245,314,315). In digitalis-toxic Purkinje fibers, usually five to eight successive action potentials are needed for the delayed afterdepolarizations to attain their peak magnitude (115,245). On occasion, however, afterdepolarizations in atrial fibers of the mitral valve or coronary sinus exposed to catecholamines are large enough to cause triggered activity after a single stimulated action potential (166,314).

The tendency for afterdepolarization amplitude to increase and coupling interval to decrease with increased activity is consistent with the results of the voltage-clamp studies described in an earlier section; the increased time during which the membrane is in the depolarized state increases Ca in the myoplasm and the sarcoplasmic reticulum and increases the TI current. As the number of action potentials is increased or the rate of stimulation is increased, a rate-related shortening of action-potential duration might be expected to offset part of this effect (28). However, in atrial fibers of the coronary sinus in the presence of catecholamines, action-potential duration sometimes *increases* with increased activity, possibly increasing Ca influx further (144). Whether or not this also occurs under other conditions in which afterdepolarizations are found has not been described. Other factors may also contribute to the increase in afterdepolarization amplitude following a period of activity. Rapid stimulation of atrial fibers in the canine coronary sinus (182), pectinate fibers in the rabbit (249), hypertrophied ventricular muscle (8), and Purkinje fibers exposed to high Ca and catecholamines (276) may cause a decline in the maximum diastolic potential that is associated with the increase in afterdepolarization amplitude. Depolarization of the atrial fibers in the coronary sinus coincides with, and is probably caused by, an accumulation of K in the extracellular space resulting from the rapid drive (180,182). Although an increase in K_o has been described to decrease the TI current in some experiments (293), the enhancing effects of depolarization on the amplitude of the TI current and afterdepolarization (142,299) may sometimes predominate (the effects of the level of repolarization were discussed in an earlier section). In addition, the decrease in maximum diastolic potential may bring the afterdepolarization closer to threshold.

There is also an additional mechanism that might cause depolarization during rapid drive. As mentioned earlier, under conditions of calcium overload, the rela-

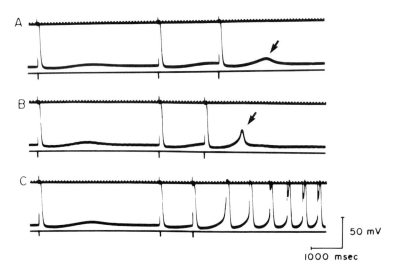

FIG. 10. Effects of premature stimulation on afterdepolarization amplitude and triggering. Transmembrane potentials are recorded from an atrial fiber in canine coronary sinus superfused with Tyrode solution containing norepinephrine. *Bottom trace* marks time of stimulus. Each panel shows the last two impulses of a series of 10 impulses driven at a cycle length of 4,000 msec. A premature impulse was then induced at progressively shorter coupling intervals. The afterdepolarization of the premature impulse is larger in **B** than in **A** (*arrows*) because the premature coupling interval is shorter. In **C**, at a still shorter coupling interval, the premature impulse induces triggered activity. (From ref. 315, with permission of the American Heart Association.)

50 mV

1000 msec

tively brief oscillatory TI current may be superimposed on a slowly decaying inward current called the creep current (92,93). Valenzuela and Vassalle (277) have suggested that the creep current may be maximal at the end of a period of drive and could shift the maximum diastolic potential toward less negative values and the threshold potential to more negative values.

Dependence of Delayed Afterdepolarizations on Action-Potential Characteristics

Delayed afterdepolarizations are influenced by the level of membrane potential at which the action potentials occur. In the digitalis-toxic Purkinje system, a "window" of membrane voltage has been identified (approximately −75 to −80 mV) at which the amplitude of delayed afterdepolarizations tends to be greatest (109,299). When delayed afterdepolarizations are occurring at membrane potentials that are optimal for their peak amplitude, any intervention that hyperpolarizes or depolarizes the membrane (such as rapid pacing, a spontaneous change in rate, or intracellular application of hyperpolarizing or depolarizing current) will tend to reduce their magnitude and to suppress any rhythms the afterdepolarizations might induce. Similarly, in instances in which a preparation shows no delayed afterdepolarizations in the presence of digitalis and is at a membrane voltage less than or greater than the "window," the use of the same interventions to bring them into this voltage range often will induce delayed afterdepolarizations. A similar dependence on membrane potential has been shown for atrial fibers of the coronary sinus (142) and Purkinje fibers from infarcts (198). This effect of membrane potential may be exerted in several different ways, either because of voltage dependence of the TI current (vide supra) or because of changes in membrane resistance that accompany changes in membrane potential (89).

Delayed afterdepolarizations are also influenced by the action-potential duration. Given the same exposure to digitalis, the amplitude of delayed afterdepolarizations at the area of maximum action-potential duration in the Purkinje system tends to be greater than at sites more proximal or distal, where action-potential duration is shorter (M. R. Rosen, unpublished observations). In atrial fibers of the coronary sinus exposed to catecholamines, prolonging the action-potential duration with depolarizing current pulses, applied during repolarization, increases afterdepolarization amplitude and decreases their coupling interval, whereas shortening the action-potential duration with repolarizing current pulses has the opposite effect (Fig. 11) (144). The effects of action potential duration on afterdepolarizations are most likely related to its effects on Ca entering the cell either via

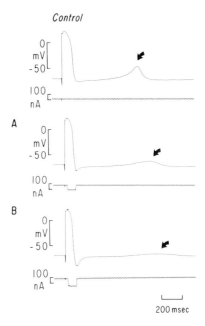

FIG. 11. Effects of action-potential duration on the amplitude of a delayed afterdepolarization in an atrial fiber of canine coronary sinus superfused with norepinephrine. The **top trace** in each panel is the transmembrane voltage recording; the **bottom trace** in each panel shows the current passed through a second microelectrode positioned close to the recording electrode. The **top panel** (control) shows the action potential and afterdepolarization (*arrow*) during regular stimulation. The records in **A** and **B** were taken while action potential repolarization was accelerated by passing current in the repolarizing direction. Decreasing action-potential duration caused the amplitude of the delayed afterdepolarization to decrease (*arrows*). (Record kindly provided by Dr. Berthold Henning.)

the slow inward current or by other mechanisms (*vide supra*).

Rate of Triggered Activity

The increase in amplitude of delayed afterdepolarizations with increasing activity, described previously, is probably largely responsible for the perpetuation of triggered activity, once the first nondriven (triggered) action potential has occurred. If the first nondriven action potential arises from the peak of the delayed afterdepolarization, then the coupling interval (cycle length) between the upstroke of the first nondriven action potential and the last driven one often is shorter than the drive-cycle length. Hence, the afterdepolarization following the first nondriven action potential will be even larger than the afterdepolarization from which it arose, and a second nondriven action potential will occur at a short coupling interval. The continuation of triggered activity is then dependent on the delayed afterdepolarization after each triggered action potential reaching threshold.

In Purkinje fibers made toxic with digitalis, the rate of triggered activity is dependent on the preceding drive-cycle length: As the drive-cycle length decreases, the rate tends to increase (216). This increase in rate is best seen during the first few beats. The rate may remain constant thereafter or may increase still further or decrease. The stimulus rate may also influence the rate of triggered activity of Purkinje fibers surviving in infarcts (198) and Purkinje fibers exposed to elevated Ca and catecholamines (276,277) in the same way that it influences digitalis-induced triggered activity. In atrial fibers exposed to catecholamines, only the first triggered beat shows this cycle-length dependence (shorter cycle length at faster drive rates), but the fastest rate attained is not related to the cycle length of the basic drive (166). Data from other experimental preparations are not available.

When Purkinje fibers, toxic from digitalis, have sub-threshold delayed afterdepolarizations that are brought to threshold by stimulated premature depolarizations or periods of rapid drive, the rhythms that are triggered tend not to be sustained. In a study by Moak and Rosen (216), only 21 to 28% of such fibers showed persistence of triggered activity for more than 25 beats. Termination of triggered activity in this situation may either be abrupt or may occur after a period of slowing or acceleration in rate. During the course of triggered activity, maximum diastolic potential may decrease, and there may be further depolarization as the rhythm stops. Membrane potential then drifts to its more negative initial level (241).

Catecholamine-induced triggered activity in atrial fibers (315), as well as some other kinds of triggering not dependent on digitalis, may have different characteristics than that associated with digitalis toxicity. The differences in the characteristics of triggered activity after digitalis and after catecholamines may be related to the function of the Na-K pump, partly or mostly inhibited during the former but still active during the latter. Catechol-amine-induced triggered activity in atrial fibers can be subdivided into several well-defined phases (181,182,317) (Fig. 12): an initial phase of 5 to 10 sec during which there is a marked increase in rate that is sometimes associated with membrane depolarization; a second phase during which the rate accelerates more gradually and that is associated with membrane depolarization; a third phase during which maximum diastolic potential hyper-polarizes, the rate slows, and triggered activity eventually terminates; a final phase following termination during which maximum diastolic potential hyperpolarizes rel-ative to the maximum diastolic potential prior to trig-gering and then returns to the control value.

The mechanism for the initial rapid increase in rate occurring with the first few triggered beats is the same as we described at the beginning of this section—it results from the influence of the short cycle length of the first triggered beats on afterdepolarization amplitude and rate of depolarization. After triggered activity is initiated, there is an increase in K_o that begins during the first few beats (Fig. 12) (181,182). It most likely results from K efflux during the action potential and the inability of diffusion out of the extracellular space and the Na-K pump to balance this efflux (180). After the first 5 to 10 beats, as K_o continues to increase, the maximum diastolic potential declines simultaneously. Subsequent to the first few triggered impulses, the rest of the increase in rate during triggered activity parallels the progressive rise in K_o and depolarization of the maximum diastolic potential (181). The rise in K_o and

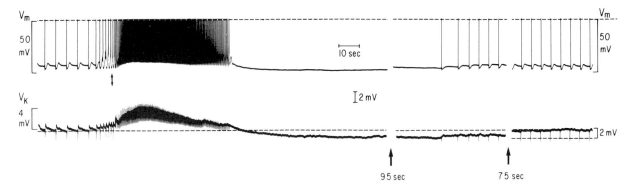

FIG. 12. Changes in membrane potential and extracellular K during triggered activity in an atrial fiber of canine coronary sinus. The **top trace** is the transmembrane voltage recording. The top of the record has been cut off so that 0 potential is not shown. Maximum diastolic potential is −80 mV. The preparation was first stimulated at a long cycle length (**left**). Stimulus cycle length was then abruptly decreased, and triggered activity began at the *arrow*. The subsequent changes in maximum diastolic potential, as described in the text, are shown. Triggered activity terminated spontaneously, and after a period of quiescence (95 sec between the **left** and **middle panels**) stimulation was resumed (**right**). The **bottom trace** is a record of extracellular K activity simultaneously recorded with a K^+-selective microelectrode inserted into the extracellular space of the triggered fibers (180). The 4-mV voltage scale is equivalent to 2 mM K^+. Note the K_o accumulation and subsequent depletion during and after triggered activity. (Record kindly provided by Dr. R. P. Kline.)

decrease in maximum diastolic potential may therefore contribute to the further increase in rate, because the rate of triggered activity is related to the membrane potential (181). The decrease in membrane potential may accelerate the rate either by enhancing the rate of development of the TI current (*vide supra*) or by shifting the maximum diastolic potential closer to threshold potential. In addition, it is predicted that with each beat, Na and Ca enter and K leaves the cells, resulting in increases in Na_i, Ca_i (56,164,189), and K_o (180). The net effect of these three ionic changes should be to initially speed the triggering rate.

Soon after depolarization of the maximum diastolic potential reaches a maximum, it slowly starts to hyperpolarize (Fig. 12), in a manner similar to the hyperpolarization that occurs during prolonged rapid stimulation (35,279). K_o begins to decrease after hyperpolarization begins. Activation of an outward current from the electrogenic Na-K pump (activated as Na_i continues to accumulate during triggered activity) is expected to contribute to the hyperpolarization and the decrease in K_o (120,121). The increase in maximum diastolic potential and the outward electrogenic current both probably play roles in slowing and eventually stopping triggered activity (317).

After an episode of triggered activity there is further hyperpolarization of the maximum diastolic potential to levels usually negative to those prior to triggering (Fig. 12). Both hyperpolarization and further K_o depletion are interpreted to be associated with enhanced Na pumping driven by intracellular Na accumulated during rapid activity (35,180,186,279). Currents associated with Na pumping hyperpolarize the membrane, which may be further hyperpolarized by the direct action of reduced K_o. The return of membrane potential and K_o to control levels is then due to return of the pump rate to its original base-line value as extrusion of intracellular Na is completed.

After termination of triggered activity in atrial fibers of the canine coronary sinus and rabbit pectinate muscle, the stimulated action potentials at the hyperpolarized membrane potential are followed by afterdepolarizations of reduced amplitude, and triggering is more difficult to induce (181,249). Several possible reasons for these observations include (a) a decrease in transient inward current at hyperpolarized membrane potentials (175), (b) decreases in Na_i and Ca_i following a period of rapid activity (56,189), (c) the direct opposing effect of increased outward electrogenic pump current on the afterdepolarization, and (d) a decrease in action-potential duration caused by enhanced electrogenic pump current (121,122), which in turn decreases afterdepolarization amplitude (144).

The changes in maximum diastolic potential and rate during triggered activity caused by high Ca and catecholamines in Purkinje fibers (overdrive excitation) are different from those in atrial fibers (276). Purkinje fibers show progressive slowing after overdrive without the initial acceleration. After a fast rate of drive, the first triggered impulse occurs at a cycle length longer than the drive-cycle length because of the long time needed for the afterdepolarization to reach threshold. The afterdepolarization following the triggered action potential is somewhat smaller because of the long cycle length and takes even longer to reach threshold. Slowing of the triggered rate occurs gradually because of the decreasing oscillatory potential (276). In addition, activation of an outward current due to electrogenic sodium extrusion may contribute to cessation of activity.

Effects of Electrical Stimulation on Established Triggered Activity

We have discussed how triggered activity is initiated by stimulation. These characteristics may be of use in identifying triggered activity in the *in situ* heart (*vide infra*). Also of importance in identifying triggered arrhythmias *in situ* are the effects of electrical stimulation on established triggered activity.

In general, triggered activity is markedly influenced by overdrive stimulation (stimulation at a rate faster than the triggered rate). The effects of overdrive have been studied in only a few experimental situations: triggered activity caused by catecholamines in atrial fibers, and digitalis or myocardial infarction in Purkinje fibers. The effects of overdrive on triggered activity in the atrial fibers of the canine coronary sinus are dependent on both the rate and duration of overdrive (166,317). During a short period of overdrive at a rate only moderately faster than the triggered rate, there is a decrease in the maximum diastolic potential; following the period of overdrive the rate of triggered activity may be faster than it was before overdrive (overdrive acceleration), perhaps because of the decrease in the maximum diastolic potential (Fig. 13). The decrease in maximum diastolic potential may result, at least partly, from additional K_o accumulation during overdrive (R. P. Kline and A. L. Wit, *unpublished observations*). The postoverdrive acceleration may last for several seconds, and then the rate of triggered activity gradually slows and maximum diastolic potential increases until preoverdrive values are attained. If either the rate of overdrive or the duration of overdrive is increased to a critical degree, the decline in maximum diastolic potential during overdrive is greater, as is the postoverdrive acceleration. The rate then gradually decreases and maximum diastolic potential increases until the fiber becomes quiescent (Fig. 13). When triggered activity stops after a period of overdrive at a moderate rate, some 10 to 50 impulses may occur after termination of

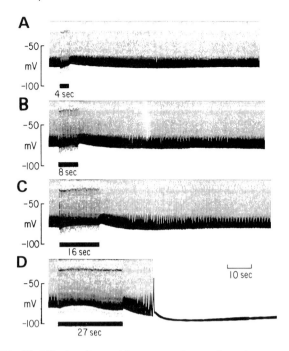

FIG. 13. Effects of overdrive on maximum diastolic potential of an atrial fiber in canine coronary sinus superfused with Tyrode solution containing catecholamines. The records are displayed at high amplification to emphasize the changes in maximum diastolic potential; hence, the tops of the action potentials are not shown. The cycle length of this burst of triggered activity stabilized at 400 msec after about 900 sec. The *horizontal bars* below each panel indicate the periods of overdrive at a cycle length of 300 msec. The periods of overdrive lasted 4, 8, 16, and 27 sec. After each period of overdrive there was a decrease in maximum diastolic potential associated with postoverdrive acceleration, followed by an increase in membrane potential and postoverdrive suppression. Following the 27-sec period of overdrive, the burst of activity stopped after a period of membrane hyperpolarization. (From ref. 317, with permission of the American Heart Association.)

the overdrive before termination of the triggered activity. The increase in maximum diastolic potential and the slowing and termination of triggered activity following a period of overdrive probably are caused by enhanced activity of the electrogenic sodium pump (317). During the period of overdrive there is probably a transient increase in intracellular Na, because of the increased number of action potentials, that stimulate the pump (35,56,120,121,279). When the rate at which coronary sinus fibers are overdriven is very fast, triggered activity may stop immediately on termination without the prior increase in maximum diastolic potential or gradual slowing (313). In the experiments of Saito et al. (249), triggered activity in rabbit pectinate muscle was not terminated by overdrive stimulation, although maximum diastolic potential did increase following overdrive, and the rate of triggered activity slowed. It is possible that more rapid rates or longer periods of overdrive than

used in that study would have terminated the triggered activity.

In digitalis-toxic Purkinje fibers, overdrive stimulation can also terminate triggered activity; termination occurs more frequently at more rapid overdrive rates (216). Termination may not be caused by increased Na-K pump activity, because the pump is partially inhibited by digitalis. Instead, it might result from accumulation of Na or Ca during overdrive.

Premature stimuli may also terminate triggered rhythms in digitalis-toxic Purkinje fibers (216) or atrial fibers (166,314), although much less frequently than overdrive. Whether or not the premature impulse must occur at a critical point in the cycle length of triggered activity has not been demonstrated, although in studies of digitalis, such a critical cycle length has been sought (216). In a study on triggering in the mitral valve, it was shown that a premature impulse that terminates triggered activity may be followed by an increased afterhyperpolarization that, in turn, is followed by an afterdepolarization that does not reach threshold, perhaps because it arises from the more negative membrane potential of the preceding afterhyperpolarization (314). Whether or not this mechanism applies to other kinds of triggered activity is not known. Triggered activity could not be terminated by a single premature stimulus in rabbit pectinate muscle (249).

Pharmacology of Triggered Activity

The effects of pharmacological agents on delayed afterdepolarizations and triggered activity are of interest for at least two reasons. First, drugs have provided insights into possible mechanisms causing afterdepolarizations and triggered activity. Second, because triggered activity is increasingly thought of as an arrhythmogenic mechanism, the effects of neurohumors and antiarrhythmic agents are of clinical importance.

There are several possible mechanisms of action by which drugs may act on delayed afterdepolarizations. Effects might be exerted through alterations in the action potential and the membrane currents that cause the action potential. Changes in the time course of repolarization, for example, markedly affect afterdepolarizations, because this influences Ca release from the sarcoplasmic reticulum or intracellular Ca levels (144,258). A drug might therefore modify inward Na or Ca currents or outward K currents during repolarization or modify the possible contribution of an electrogenic Na-Ca exchange mechanism to repolarization to influence the action potential duration and thereby the amplitude of delayed afterdepolarizations. Changes in the upstroke of an action potential caused by a drug might influence the afterdepolarization if Na_i is altered, because Na_i influences Ca_i (95,257,258). Drugs might also directly modify the function of the membrane channels through which the TI current passes. Changes in the maximum diastolic potential, caused by a drug, might also affect the afterdepolarization, because the membrane voltage influences the TI current (*vide supra*). Drugs might also influence delayed afterdepolarizations by acting during diastole or during periods of quiescence to influence intracellular Ca levels (a) by modifying resting membrane conductances, decreasing Na or Ca leak conductances, for example, (b) by changing the activity of the Na-K pump, thereby increasing or decreasing Na_i (92,93), or (c) by influencing Na-Ca exchange. Finally, drugs might influence the function of the sarcoplasmic reticulum and either enhance or suppress oscillatory movements of Ca between the sarcoplasmic reticulum and myoplasm.

Autonomic Neurohumors

We have already indicated that catecholamines cause afterdepolarizations to occur in mitral valve fibers (313,314), atrial fibers in the coronary sinus (315), some fibers from diseased human (208) and animal atria (27), and in Purkinje fibers (77,282) and ventricular muscle (192,225). They also increase the magnitude of digitalis- or ischemia-induced delayed afterdepolarizations in Purkinje fibers and may cause subthreshold afterdepolarizations to attain threshold (147). Catecholamines may exert this effect by increasing the slow inward current and intracellular Ca through beta-receptor stimulation (237). Catecholamines thereby increase the TI current and the range of repolarization levels at which the current appears (273,293). This effect on delayed afterdepolarizations is antagonized by beta-blocking concentrations of propranolol (147). Beta-receptor blockade in the absence of exogenously administered catecholamines does not prevent digitalis-induced delayed afterdepolarizations (169). Alpha-adrenergic agonists appear to have more variable effects than beta agonists. Although one study showed them to have no significant effect on digitalis-toxic Purkinje fibers (147), in another study on feline Purkinje fibers in the presence of high external Ca, concentrations of alpha agonists that may have induced Ca loading increased the magnitude of afterdepolarizations (178).

Histamine, another natural substance found in the heart, can also cause delayed afterdepolarizations, possibly by increasing the slow inward current. This effect is mediated through stimulation of H_2 receptors (200).

Acetylcholine reduces the amplitude of afterdepolarizations in atrial fibers that are not caused by digitalis, while at the same time increasing maximum diastolic potential (208,315). In the presence of acetylcholine, therefore, triggering can occur only at high rates of drive or very short premature coupling intervals. Addition of acetylcholine during triggered activity lowers the rate of

that activity and often stops it. Acetylcholine can also suppress delayed afterdepolarizations caused by digitalis toxicity in the atria (141). Both its known effects to increase membrane K^+ conductance (158) and to reduce slow inward Ca current (128,268) may play roles in acetylcholine's actions.

Fast-Channel-Blocking Drugs

Tetrodotoxin (TTX) blocks the fast Na^+ channel (55) and the Na window current (14). In concentrations that cause marked decreases in action-potential amplitude and upstroke velocity of fibers in the anterior atrial wall, it does not alter the amplitude of the slow-response action potentials in the mitral valve muscle and does not have any effect on catecholamine-induced delayed afterdepolarizations (314). Sustained rhythmic activity can be triggered at the same rate in the presence of TTX as in its absence. Similarly, TTX has little effect on catecholamine-dependent delayed afterdepolarizations in human atrial fibers, which also may generate slow responses (208). However, TTX does depress delayed afterdepolarizations in coronary sinus atrial fibers exposed to catecholamines (143) and in digitalis-toxic Purkinje fibers (242). In the atrial fibers, part of the suppression is a result of the decrease in duration of the plateau phase of the action potential and an increase in the maximum diastolic potential. In Purkinje fibers, there also appears to be a relationship between depression of the afterdepolarization and changes in the action potential plateau. TTX also decreases the TI current in Purkinje fibers after inhibition of the Na-K pump in K-free solution. The decrease in this TI current parallels a decrease in Na_i that results from Na-channel blockade. It has been proposed that the decrease in Na_i in turn causes a decrease in Ca_i and therefore diminishes the TI current (95).

Although TTX decreases afterdepolarization amplitude and may inhibit induction of triggered activity normally caused by changes in rate and rhythm in atrial fibers of the coronary sinus, TTX applied to fibers that are already triggered has no effect on triggered activity (G. N. Tseng and A. L. Wit, *unpublished observations*). Triggering in these atrial fibers may be accompanied by a significant decrease in maximum diastolic potential and a change in action-potential configuration to resemble a slow response (313). Under these conditions the fast Na channel may already be inactivated. This triggered activity is blocked by the slow-channel-blocking drugs D600 and verapamil (A. L. Wit, *unpublished observations*).

Antiarrhythmic drugs that block Na channels also depress delayed afterdepolarizations and prevent induction of triggered activity in digitalis-toxic Purkinje fibers. Drugs that have been shown to have this effect are lidocaine (169,258,242), aprindine (100), procainamide, quinidine, ethmozin (80,146), phenytoin (243,300), mexiletine (304), and propranolol in high concentrations (147). Lidocaine's effects have been correlated with a decrease in Na_i resulting from blockade of Na channels. The concentration of lidocaine used in these experiments was higher than the therapeutic level, and it is uncertain whether or not a decrease in Na_i can explain the antiarrhythmic effect at lower doses, where abolition of triggered activity may sometimes occur much more rapidly than a decrease in Na_i. This rapid effect may result from the decrease in action-potential duration (258). In human atrial fibers, lidocaine does not have an effect on delayed afterdepolarizations (208). In atrial fibers of the canine coronary sinus, quinidine also does not depress afterdepolarizations, but actually makes them larger and causes triggered activity (272). Part of this effect results from a prolongation of the action-potential duration.

Slow Channel Blocking Drugs

Pharmacological blockade of the slow channel with inorganic Mn^{2+} or organic blockers (e.g., verapamil, D600, nifedipine) causes a decrease in TI current, afterdepolarizations, and aftercontractions (Fig. 14) (78,113, 135,136,169,171,208,247,315). The time course for this decrease lags behind the time course for diminution of the slow inward current (171). When blockade with Mn^{2+} is reversed in digitalis-toxic Purkinje fibers by washing it out with Mn^{2+}-free solution, the slow current reappears *before* the reappearance of the TI current. These observations are compatible with the interpretation that slow-channel blockade leads to a decrease in intra-

cellular Ca stores by decreasing the slow inward current, and the decrease in intracellular Ca then causes a decrease in the TI current (171).

Drugs that Alter Sarcoplasmic Reticulum Function

In addition to increasing the slow inward current, catecholamines enhance uptake of Ca^{2+} by the sarcoplasmic reticulum, leading to release of an increased amount of Ca from the sarcoplasmic reticulum during the twitch (105,107,219). The increased Ca in the sarcoplasmic reticulum induced by catecholamines also may trigger the secondary Ca release after relaxation that causes afterdepolarizations.

The pharmacological agents caffeine and ryanodine, which influence the release of Ca from the sarcoplasmic reticulum, as well as its uptake, also have marked effects on delayed afterdepolarizations. Caffeine has a biphasic effect, causing Ca release in low concentrations and preventing Ca uptake in higher concentrations, eventually depleting the sarcoplasmic reticulum of Ca (22,101,301; cf. 145). Low concentrations of caffeine increase the amplitudes of the TI current and delayed afterdepolarizations and cause triggered activity in digitalis-toxic Purkinje fibers, and in atrial fibers in the presence of catecholamines (Fig. 15) (10,232). Caffeine also induces a TI current in cultured cardiac cells (54). Higher concentrations cause afterdepolarizations to occur earlier during the repolarization phase of the action potential, then to decrease in size and eventually disappear (Fig. 15). The TI current is also inhibited (10,288,289). These changes in afterdepolarizations probably are due to changes in myoplasmic Ca resulting from the effects of caffeine on the sarcoplasmic reticulum (SR). According

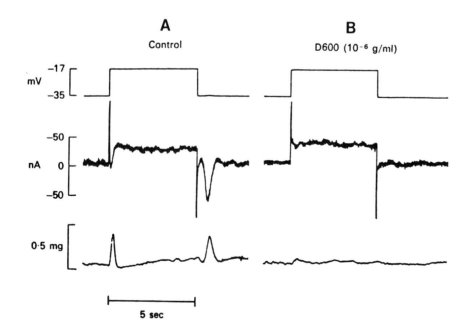

FIG. 14. Inhibition of the TI current and aftercontraction with the organic calcium-channel blocker D600 in a sheep Purkinje fiber superfused with 1 μM strophanthidin. **A:** A depolarizing step from −35 to −17 mV (**upper trace**) evokes a surge of slow inward current (**middle trace**) and a twitch (**bottom trace**). The pulse is terminated, and the TI current and an aftercontraction occur on repolarization. **B:** The slow inward current and TI are almost completely abolished by exposure to D600 (10^{-6} g/ml) for 13 min. The tension trace is virtually flat. (From ref. 171, with permission.)

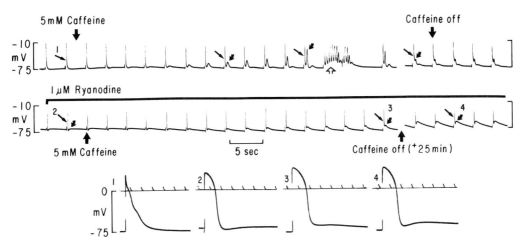

FIG. 15. Effects of caffeine and caffeine after treatment with ryanodine on afterdepolarizations and action potentials in an atrial fiber of the canine coronary sinus. Norepinephrine was present throughout the experiment. *Broad black arrows* indicate when caffeine-containing solution was started and stopped; *small straight black arrows* indicate the terminal phase of repolarization of the action potential; *black curved arrows* indicate the peak of the delayed afterdepolarizations; the *open broad arrow* indicates triggered activity. The numbers indicate when the corresponding action potentials at the bottom of the figure were recorded; time marks, 100 msec. **A:** Exposure to caffeine in **top trace** initially caused an increase in afterdepolarization amplitude and triggered activity. Following the period of triggered activity and just prior to removal of caffeine, afterdepolarization amplitude and coupling interval were decreased. **B:** Exposure to caffeine shortly after treatment with ryanodine (*horizontal bar*) caused only a small increase in the afterdepolarization amplitude. Caffeine and Ryanodine both increased the action potential plateau. (From ref. 10, with permission.)

to one hypothesis (10), the biphasic effect of caffeine on delayed afterdepolarizations is explained as follows: The phasic rise in calcium in the myoplasm during the action-potential plateau causes Ca release from the SR at a threshold level of myoplasmic Ca (104). The release of Ca from the SR might then be followed by a secondary release if the SR is overloaded. If early sequestration of Ca by the SR is impaired by low concentrations of caffeine leading to a rise in myoplasmic Ca, then myoplasmic Ca might reach the level needed to induce Ca release earlier in the cardiac cycle, thus causing the delayed afterdepolarization to occur earlier. Afterdepolarizations initially have increased amplitudes if increased amounts of Ca are released. The eventual decrease in the amplitude of the delayed afterdepolarization results from eventual depletion of Ca from the SR.

Ryanodine decreases delayed afterdepolarization amplitude and inhibits triggered activity without causing the initial increase that caffeine does. Ryanodine may either block release of Ca from the SR (266) or induce a leak of Ca from the SR, causing depletion (148,157). Blockade of Ca-induced Ca release could explain the findings that ryanodine abolishes the delayed afterdepolarizations seen in the presence of digitalis toxicity (207,275) and catecholamines and after low concentrations of caffeine (10).

Doxorubicin

The anthracycline antibiotic doxorubicin also suppresses digitalis-induced delayed afterdepolarizations in

Purkinje fibers (21). This occurs at concentrations that have no other effect on the action potential than to prolong its duration slightly. The basis for this action of doxorubicin is uncertain, although some studies have suggested it acts through suppression of the Na-Ca exchange mechanism (48). Such an effect might decrease intracellular Ca. Alternatively, doxorubicin might act more directly via an effect on the TI current itself.

Delayed Afterdepolarizations and Triggered Activity as a Cause of Arrhythmias

Identifying Triggered Activity in the In Situ Heart

It has yet to be established that triggered activity causes arrhythmias in the *in situ* human heart. Triggered activity can readily be induced in both normal and diseased isolated cardiac tissue preparations when exposed to an environment not unlike that expected to exist *in situ* (catecholamines, ischemia, digitalis toxicity). Therefore, because there is reasonable evidence that isolation and superfusion of cardiac tissue *in vitro* do not drastically change its basic electrophysiological properties, we see every reason to believe that triggered activity should occur *in situ*. Although identification of delayed afterdepolarizations in cardiac fibers of the arrhythmic heart would provide an irrefutable proof that they constitute an arrhythmogenic mechanism, Bozler (29), after concluding in 1943 that extrasystoles and tachycardias might be caused by oscillatory afterpotentials, went on to say that "unfortunately, the study of these weak and localized potentials in the heart *in situ* presents great technical difficulties." This statement still holds true today.

Extracellular recordings.

It may now be possible to make extracellular recordings of afterdepolarizations in the heart by means of catheter electrodes. Cramer et al. (71) have developed a technique for recording the extracellular currents that occur during spontaneous diastolic depolarization in automatic foci using unipolar recordings with high amplification. The extracellular records from *in vitro* rabbit sinus node show a slow diastolic potential change in regions where pacemaker depolarization is prominent in microelectrode recordings. Extracellular recordings have also been made of afterdepolarizations in isolated preparations of canine coronary sinus; a transient extracellular current flows at the same time that the afterdepolarization appears in the intracellular records (Fig. 16) (313).

This technique for recording extracellular potentials has been used in *in situ* canine and human hearts to record spontaneous diastolic depolarization from the sinus node (139,140,235) and the region of the atrioventricular (AV) junction (137,138). It seems possible, therefore, that afterdepolarizations might similarly be detected by the same technique. A major problem will be discriminating the voltage deflections induced by motion of the heart from potential changes that are in fact the result of afterdepolarizations. A second important problem is the difficulty in locating focal sites at which triggered activity may be originating, using a catheter electrode. Nevertheless, catheter electrodes have been used to demonstrate what appear to be delayed afterdepolarizations occurring in the *in situ* heart (202).

Because the direct recording techniques have major

difficulties at present, an effort has been made to determine the responses of experimental models of triggered activity and afterdepolarizations to interventions such as drugs or pacing-induced changes in rate and rhythm. These studies are intended to find unique characteristics that might be used to identify triggered activity *in situ* and differentiate it from other arrhythmogenic mechanisms such as reentry or automaticity, as described next.

Use of pacing techniques to initiate triggered arrhythmias.

Many clinically occurring tachycardias can be initiated by an increase in heart rate or by premature depolarizations, as reviewed elsewhere (1,36,40,41,167,307). These arrhythmias cannot be caused by automatic pacemakers, because automaticity is not initiated characteristically by prior activity. The evidence that some of these tachycardias are caused by reentry is convincing. For example, the onset of tachycardias presumed to be caused by AV nodal reentry can be precisely correlated with a critical amount of slowed conduction in the AV node of the initiating premature or basic impulse (132). There is often a reciprocal (inverse) relationship between the coupling interval of premature impulses that initiate reentry and the intervals between the premature impulses and the first reentrant beat (19). Because the premature impulse occurs earlier in the cycle (shorter coupling interval), it conducts more slowly through the reentrant circuit, resulting in a longer time before occurrence of the reentrant beat (longer coupling interval). (See *Chapter 54* for a detailed discussion of the causes and characteristics of reentry.) Slowed conduction of premature impulses has also been shown to result in this reciprocal relationship during initiation of some ventricular tachyarrhythmias (305,308) Assigning a reentrant mechanism

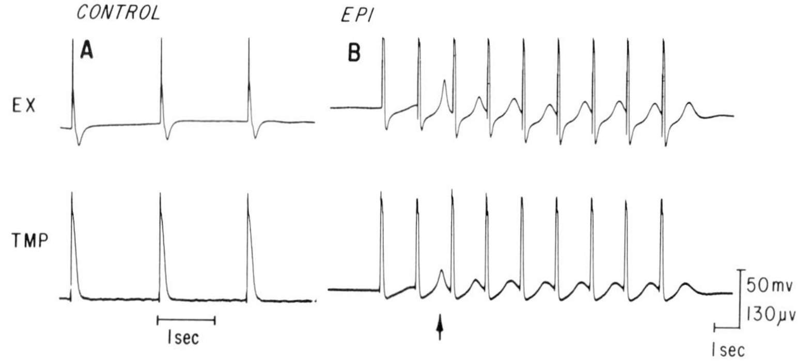

FIG. 16. Comparison of extracellular recordings of coronary sinus electrical activity with intracellular recording of electrical activity using the recording technique of Cramer et al. (71). The **top trace** in each panel is extracellular potential recording (EX), and the bottom trace is the transmembrane potential recording (TMP). **A:** Control records during superfusion with normal Tyrode solution. **B:** Records obtained when epinephrine (EPI) (0.5 μg/ml) was added to the perfusate. The preparation was stimulated at the same rate in all panels; the time scale in **B** is shorter than in **A**. Note the appearance of afterdepolarizations (*arrow*) in both the intracellular and extracellular records (the transmembrane potential recording in **B** is not from the same fiber as in **A**, explaining why maximum diastolic potential in **B** is less than in **A**). Amplitude calibration in millivolts at lower right is for transmembrane potential record, and calibration in microvolts is for extracellular record. (From ref. 313, with permission.)

to other atrial and ventricular tachycardias is solely based on observations that they can be started (and stopped) by premature impulses or a train of stimulated impulses with shorter cycle lengths than the sinus rate, particularly when a region of slow conduction cannot be identified (296,322). Arrhythmias caused by triggered activity, however, are also predicted to follow an increase in the heart rate or a premature impulse.

If both reentrant and triggered rhythms can be induced by prior activity (premature or rapid stimulation), are there any characteristics that might indicate a distinction between the two? An attempt to distinguish between the two mechanisms is further complicated by experimental results suggesting that triggering resulting from different causes might also have different characteristics (*vide supra*). The following guidelines have been proposed to assist in distinguishing delayed afterdepolarization-induced triggered activity from other causes of arrhythmias, particularly reentrant excitation (244,248). The guidelines are based to a large extent on the characteristics of triggered activity determined from the *in vitro* studies described earlier:

1. Arrhythmias caused by delayed afterdepolarizations should be more easily induced by rapid drive or a series of premature stimuli than by a single premature stimulus. Also, they should be more easily induced by premature stimuli superimposed on a rapid drive than a slow one. In contrast, some reentrant rhythms are more easily and reproducibly induced by single premature impulses (1,305,307), although others require a number of premature impulses (37). In some instances, single premature impulses may be more effective in inducing reentry at slow drive cycles (168). Triggered arrhythmias often cannot be initiated in a reproducible manner by the same stimulus protocol (216), whereas reentrant tachycardias are often reproducibly initiated by the same stimulus protocol.

2. A propensity for an arrhythmia to occur more frequently when the preceding cardiac rhythm shows a short rather than a long cycle length (and in the case of digitalis toxicity, with peak occurrence following a rhythm with a 500–700-msec cycle length) is consistent with delayed afterdepolarizations (244).

3. Premature beats or the first beat of tachycardias caused by delayed afterdepolarizations are predicted to occur late in the cardiac cycle (244). This proposal is based on experimental data from studies of isolated tissue showing that delayed afterdepolarizations rarely reach their peak amplitude at less than 50% of the cardiac cycle when the drive-cycle length is less than 1,000 msec. In contrast, reentrant beats may occur very early in the cycle (312).

4. One would expect a direct relationship between the coupling interval of the first beat of tachycardia and the premature coupling interval or drive-cycle length,

because at short cycle lengths the coupling interval of the afterdepolarizations to the preceding action potential decreases (*vide supra*). In the case of digitalis, this relationship is sometimes complicated by the presence of two afterdepolarizations and the possibility of a triggered impulse arising from either one (*vide supra*) (Fig. 9).

5. The demonstration that the cycle length of an arrhythmia diminishes when the cycle length of the basic rhythm that induces it is decreased is characteristic of digitalis-induced delayed afterdepolarizations (*vide supra*). However, as discussed under guideline 4, this relationship can be complicated by the presence of two afterdepolarizations. The steady-state cycle length of triggered rhythms resulting from causes other than digitalis has not been shown to have this relationship to the cycle length of the inducing rhythm (166). The cycle length of the initiating impulses should not influence the cycle length of reentry in an anatomical circuit. The effects on functional reentry are, at this time, unknown.

Characteristics of triggered arrhythmias.

Several studies of triggering in atrial fibers have shown a gradual increase in the rate after the initiation of triggered activity (27,317). However, a gradual increase in rate does not always occur in diseased human atrial fibers (208) or Purkinje or ventricular muscle fibers (276), or in the presence of digitalis toxicity (115, 245,246), and is therefore not diagnostic of triggered activity. *In vitro*, triggered activity often terminates spontaneously. Triggered arrhythmias might therefore occur in bursts. Although termination of triggered activity in some atrial and Purkinje fibers is preceded by a slowing of the rate, this is not characteristic of triggering in all fibers. Triggering caused by digitalis can terminate abruptly (*vide supra*).

Use of pacing techniques to terminate triggered arrhythmias.

We can now continue the guidelines for identifying triggered rhythms based on their responses to stimulation during the triggered rhythm (244,248).

1. Single premature impulses may terminate triggered arrhythmias, but termination is predicted to be infrequent and usually is not reproducible at the same critical premature cycle length (*vide supra*). In contrast, single premature impulses often (but not always) terminate reentrant arrhythmias in a reproducible manner and over a consistent range of premature cycle lengths in any one individual (1,167,305,307). Premature impulses usually do not terminate automatic arrhythmias.

2. Overdrive stimulation either should have no effect on arrhythmias caused by abnormal automaticity (automaticity at reduced levels of membrane potential) or should transiently accelerate them (81), whereas this

procedure should transiently suppress arrhythmias caused by normal automaticity (automaticity at normal levels of membrane potential) without terminating them (279). On the other hand, overdrive stimulation should terminate most triggered arrhythmias if the rate and duration of overdrive are sufficient (166,216,317). Overdrive stimulation may cause acceleration of triggered arrhythmias, followed by gradual slowing and termination, or rapid overdrive may cause abrupt termination (*vide supra*). Overdrive stimulation may also terminate reentrant arrhythmias or accelerate them (297). However, a gradual slowing of the rate prior to termination might not be expected.

It is therefore apparent that although the response of triggered arrhythmias to stimulation can be predicted from the experimental studies, there is no single feature that will positively enable a triggered rhythm to be distinguished from reentry. Because the characteristics of initiation and termination of triggered rhythms by stimulation are very different from the characteristics of automatic rhythms, it should be easier to distinguish between these mechanisms by pacing techniques. However, this differentiation may be made more difficult when an arrhythmia is persistent and the initiation cannot be studied. Also, entrance block of stimulated impulses into arrhythmogenic foci, whether automatic or triggered, may negate the use of pacing techniques to distinguish between these mechanisms.

Use of pharmacological agents to differentiate triggered activity from reentry and automaticity.

Because pacing techniques alone are inadequate to differentiate triggered activity from other arrhythmogenic events, attempts have been made to identify drugs that have different effects on the different arrhythmogenic mechanisms. In particular, drugs have been sought that might suppress arrhythmias caused by one mechanism, such as delayed afterdepolarizations, and not other mechanisms, such as automaticity or reentry. One example of this approach was provided using ethmozin and lidocaine to distinguish among arrhythmias that might be caused by normal automaticity, abnormal automaticity, or triggered activity (160). The rationale for using these drugs was provided by studies on isolated tissues. Lidocaine, in therapeutic concentrations, suppresses delayed afterdepolarizations (242,258) and normal automaticity (20), but has little or no effect on abnormal automaticity (5,161,198). Therapeutic concentrations of ethmozin suppress delayed afterdepolarizations (80,146) but have little effect on normal automaticity, while suppressing abnormal automaticity (80). Hence, the effects of these two drugs provide a matrix whereby an arrhythmia responding to lidocaine alone might be normally automatic, one responding to eth-

mozin alone might be abnormally automatic, and one responding to both drugs might be triggered. This matrix was used to study three kinds of arrhythmias in conscious dogs: accelerated idioventricular arrhythmias occurring about 24 hr following experimental induction of heart block, slow idioventricular rhythms occurring days to weeks after heart block, and ventricular tachycardia induced by experimental myocardial infarction (160,198). (Because of their electrocardiographic characteristics, these arrhythmias were not thought to result from reentry.) The first and third of these models responded only to ethmozin, and the second only to lidocaine. These results suggested that both the accelerated idioventricular rhythm and the infarct-induced ventricular tachycardia were abnormally automatic and that the slow idioventricular rhythm resulted from normal automaticity.

Addition of another drug, doxorubicin, to the matrix has permitted further study of triggering as a mechanism in the infarct, as well as in digitalis-toxic, arrhythmias. In isolated tissue studies, doxorubicin has been shown to have a specific depressant effect on delayed afterdepolarizations in concentrations that have no effect on normal or abnormal automaticity or on fast- and slow-response action potentials (21,197) (*vide supra*). When administered to dogs having ventricular tachycardia, 24 hr after occlusion of the left anterior descending coronary artery, doxorubicin had no effect on the arrhythmia (197). In contrast, doxorubicin abolished digitalis-induced ventricular tachycardias in dogs treated with ouabain (197). Hence, it appears that doxorubicin shows the same selectivity in intact animal studies that was predicted in studies of isolated tissues. Although the likelihood that doxorubicin might find clinical application for diagnosis of arrhythmias is small, given its cumulative cardiac and bone marrow toxicity (64,196), other drugs having similar selectivity can be sought in an effort to improve our attempts at diagnosis. No experimental studies have yet been reported using drugs in an attempt to differentiate between triggered activity and reentrant excitation.

Experimental Animal Models of Triggered Arrhythmias

Triggered rhythms induced by digitalis.

The characteristics of ventricular arrhythmias caused by digitalis toxicity in the canine heart have been thoroughly studied, and there is little doubt that some of these arrhythmias are caused by triggered activity. Ventricular arrhythmias (repetitive responses) caused by digitalis can be initiated by pacing the heart. As toxicity progresses, the duration of these trains of repetitive responses increases. Pacing can also induce arrhythmias in the digitalis-toxic human heart (50,204,205). There is also a direct relationship between the coupling interval of premature impulses that initiate ventricular arrhythmias and the first beat of the arrhythmia—as premature stimuli are induced with shorter and shorter coupling intervals, the duration of the return cycle following the stimulated premature impulse also decreases (133,134). The rates of ventricular tachycardias induced by pacing in canine hearts with digitalis toxicity are also dependent on the pacing rate (134,321,324). As the stimulus rate is increased, so is the rate of the resultant tachycardia. Digitalis-induced tachyarrhythmias can be abolished by caffeine, a drug that inhibits afterdepolarizations (86,87).

Triggered rhythms induced by myocardial infarction.

Delayed afterdepolarizations can be recorded from isolated preparations of Purkinje fibers that survive on the endocardial surfaces of myocardial infarcts 1 to 3 days after coronary artery ligation (99). However, the evidence from studies on *in situ* ventricular arrhythmias 1 to 3 days after coronary occlusion suggests that most are caused by abnormal automaticity, although triggered tachycardias sometimes may occur (197,198). Overdrive pacing of spontaneous ventricular tachycardia at cycle lengths of 300 to 500 msec in dogs with 1-day-old infarcts usually either has no effect or causes some degree of overdrive suppression (82,197,198). In only a small number of experiments (82) did overdrive acceleration occur as might be expected with triggered activity. The effects of the antiarrhythmic drugs ethmozin and lidocaine and of the anthracycline antibiotic doxorubicin on the infarction-related arrhythmias are also more consistent with abnormal automaticity than with triggered activity (*vide supra*). Most dogs with 2- to 3-day-old infarcts are in sinus rhythm. In these dogs, ventricular premature beats or tachycardia can sometimes be induced by overdrive pacing. The coupling interval between the ventricular premature beat and the last paced beat is directly related to the pacing cycle length, as is expected of triggered activity (198). The occurrence of triggered activity at 2 to 3 days may be related to the fact that with time after infarction, Purkinje fibers

hyperpolarize and attain the range of membrane potentials at which afterdepolarizations occur more readily (*vide supra*).

Idioventricular arrhythmias and overdrive acceleration.

After acute AV block, application of single stimuli to the ventricle can initiate nonstimulated repetitive activity. During slow stimulation rates, the nonstimulated beats appear coupled to the drive beats. Fast drive rates induce rhythmic activity that persists when the drive is discontinued (overdrive excitation) (Fig. 17) (287,290,291). In general, the combination of decreasing the duration of diastole during drive and increasing the number of drive beats (both to a maximum point beyond which suppression occurs) enhances the occurrence of the induced rhythmic activity (Fig. 17). This induced rhythm persists for a variable period of time and then slows down before stopping (290,287). Similarly, fast idioventricular rhythms can be induced by spontaneously occurring premature impulses. These characteristics of induction and termination of rhythmic activity are identical with those of overdrive excitation (276,286) or triggered activity (315) in cardiac fibers exposed to catecholamines (*vide supra*). In fact, the overdrive excitation may result from the increased catecholamine levels found acutely after surgery causing AV block. Sympathetic stimulation or norepinephrine administration and Ca infusions enhance overdrive excitation, making the induced rhythms faster and longer lasting (291). Overdrive excitation is not seen after chronic AV block (160,285).

Studies of Clinical Cardiac Arrhythmias

Two different approaches have been used to determine whether or not clinical arrhythmias are caused by delayed afterdepolarization-induced triggered activity. One has utilized analysis of the ECG characteristics of arrhythmias to determine if their spontaneous behavior is consistent with the predicted behavior of triggered activity. In the second, invasive electrophysiologic techniques have been used to change the heart rate and rhythm.

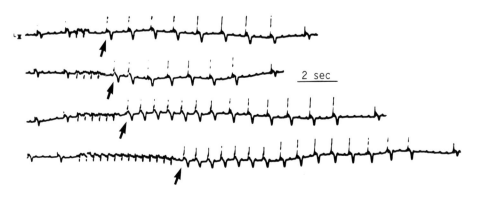

FIG. 17. Rhythm induced by overdrive pacing in canine heart with heart block. Each trace is a lead II ECG. At the **left** is one cycle (two beats) of the idioventricular rhythm prior to overdrive. The duration of the driven beats (small complexes with prominent S waves) was progressively increased from 0.33 sec (**first strip**) to 5 sec (**fourth strip**). Drive is followed in each case by an induced tachycardia (*arrows* and prominent R waves). The duration and rate of the tachycardia are related to the duration of the drive. (From ref. 287, with permission.)

2 sec

The ECG characteristics of accelerated AV junctional escape rhythms are consistent with those expected of a triggered mechanism (244). These arrhythmias occur predominantly as a result of digitalis toxicity or myocardial infarction and obey many of the rules presented earlier. There is a consistent relationship between the occurrence of the junctional escape beats and previous sinus cycle lengths, so that junctional beats occur more frequently after shorter preceding cycle lengths. The first junctional escape beat also occurs late in the cycle. As the dominant cardiac cycle length shortens, so does the interval between the last sinus beat and the junctional beat and that between the first junctional beat and subsequent junctional impulses. There also is a tendency for the rate of the junctional rhythm to accelerate over several successive cycles (244).

Clinical electrophysiological studies utilizing stimulation of the heart have led to the conclusion that only a small percentage of atrial and ventricular tachycardias are caused by triggered activity (38). In these studies, a crucial aspect has been to determine if there is a direct relationship between the coupling interval of stimulated premature beats and the first beat of tachycardia. About 10% of patients with ventricular tachycardias of diverse causes, as well as patients with mitral valve prolapse and with atrial tachyarrhythmias, have shown the characteristics expected of triggered activity.

It must be recognized, however, that there are subgroups of arrhythmias in which the primary cause may be triggered activity. One of the best candidates appears to be exercise-related ventricular tachycardia in patients with normal coronary arteries and no overt evidence of heart disease (17,40,67–69,209,234, 265,298). These tachycardias can often be initiated and terminated by programmed stimulation or rapid pacing, even from the atrium (125,306,325). Tachycardias also can be initiated by isoproterenol infusion (117) and follow an acceleration in the sinus rhythm (68,69). The spontaneous onset of such tachycardias is also dependent on the sinus rate increasing to some threshold level. At an upper level of rate, the arrhythmia disappears (68,69). The first beat of the tachycardia occurs late in the cycle length, and the coupling interval to the last sinus beat is directly related to the sinus cycle (199,324). The second beat of the tachycardia has a shorter cycle length, and the cycle length may then increase until the arrhythmia terminates (68,69). The tachycardia can be slowed or terminated by verapamil (17,209,265,298) or beta-adrenergic blockade (42,68,69,231,323). In addition to these features, which are consistent with the characteristics that we expect of triggered activity dependent on delayed afterdepolarizations [but see Coumel et al. (68,69) for a different interpretation], this kind of ventricular tachycardia can be terminated by intravenous adenosine, and this response has been proposed to be specific for a delayed afterdepolarization mechanism (199).

EARLY AFTERDEPOLARIZATIONS AND TRIGGERED ACTIVITY

Early afterdepolarizations are oscillations of membrane potential that occur during repolarization of an action potential that usually has been initiated from a high level of membrane potential (between −75 and −90 mV) (Fig. 18). They may appear as oscillations at the plateau level of membrane potential or later during phase 3 of repolarization. Under certain conditions these oscillations can lead to "second upstrokes" (72,73) or action potentials; when an oscillation is large enough, the decrease in membrane potential leads to an increase in net inward (depolarizing) current, and a second action potential occurs prior to complete repolarization of the first (Fig. 18). The second action potential occurring during repolarization is triggered in the sense that it is evoked by an early afterdepolarization, which in turn is induced by the preceding action potential. The second action potential may also be followed by other action potentials, all occurring at the low level of membrane potential characteristic of the plateau or phase 3. The sustained rhythmic activity may continue for a variable number of impulses and terminates when repolarization of the initiating action potential returns membrane potential to a high level (Fig. 19). Sometimes repolarization to the high level of membrane potential may not occur, and membrane potential may remain at the plateau level or at a level intermediate between the plateau level and the resting potential (Fig. 18). The sustained rhythmic activity may then continue at the reduced level of membrane potential.

Cranefield (73) has pointed out a terminological and conceptual difficulty associated with triggered activity caused by early afterdepolarizations: "If an action potential arising from a high resting potential is followed by a second upstroke that interrupts repolarization, that

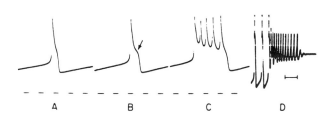

FIG. 18. Early afterdepolarization and triggered activity. Action potentials are from a rhythmically active canine Purkinje fiber exposed to normal Tyrode solution. **A:** Normal action potential. **B:** An early afterdepolarization is seen (*arrow*). **C:** Four nondriven action potentials occur at a membrane potential corresponding to that of the early afterdepolarization. **D:** Record obtained from a different fiber shows a series of three normal action potentials followed by a train of activity at a low membrane potential followed in turn by quiescence at a low level of membrane potential. (From ref. 73, with permission of the American Heart Association.)

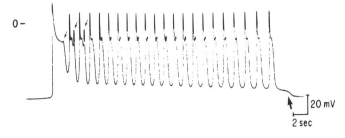

FIG. 19. Example of a self-terminating triggered rhythm resulting from a cesium-induced early afterdepolarization. After 80 min of exposure to cesium chloride (5 mM) and 2 mM potassium, stimulation was discontinued. After 18 sec of quiescence, a single spontaneous action potential arose at a membrane potential of −76 mV. This was followed by a triggered rhythm initiated before full repolarization. As the activation voltage of the rhythm increased, the rhythm slowed and terminated with a subthreshold early afterdepolarization (arrow). Also, note the presence of low-membrane-potential early afterdepolarizations associated with the precipitating action potential and the triggered action potentials (arrows). (From ref. 76, with permission of the American Heart Association.)

second upstroke can be said to be triggered. But what if a series of action potentials arise before the cell finally repolarizes to the high resting potential? Are the later action potentials in the series triggered or has the loss of resting potential merely shifted the membrane potential into a region in which automatic activity occurs?" (72,161,176) Certainly, based on the response of the early afterdepolarization-induced sustained rhythm to pacing (vide infra), it is not readily differentiated from abnormal automaticity occurring at low membrane potentials. In fact, the major differentiation between triggered and abnormally automatic rhythms may be that the former results from interruption of repolarization by an oscillation, and the latter from steady depolarization of the membrane to the same range of potentials. This being the case, it is reasonable to think of "triggered activity" as an appropriate generic term to incorporate all rhythms that require a trigger or impulse to initiate them. The sustained rhythmic activity that is triggered by an early afterdepolarization may well be triggered in its mechanism of onset but automatic in its sustained form. With this in mind, the term "triggered automaticity," which has often been misused as a synonym for "triggered activity," probably is a good description of that sustained rhythm that is triggered only by an early afterdepolarization.

Another possibility suggested by Cranefield (73) is that, once triggered, the rhythmic activity is a result of delayed afterdepolarizations, because the TI current can be activated at these low levels of membrane potential. In support of this suggestion is the observation that when triggered activity initiated by an early afterdepo-

larization terminates at the plateau level, it is often followed by a delayed afterdepolarization (Fig. 18D).

Causes of Early Afterdepolarizations and Triggered Activity

Early afterdepolarizations and triggered activity have been produced in studies on isolated heart muscle under a variety of experimental conditions.

Triggered Activity Caused by Changes in Ionic Environment

In potassium-free solutions, Purkinje fibers depolarize to approximately −50 mV of resting potential. The loss mainly reflects a decrease in K permeability, although there also may be a contribution from the reduced Na-K-pump current (44,72,119). There is a tendency for oscillatory activity during repolarization of action potentials in this situation, and this is enhanced by substituting acetyl glycinate for Cl⁻ in the superfusate (159).

Triggered Activity Caused by Hypoxia, pH, Catecholamines

Lowering the oxygen in the perfusate causes single action potentials or repetitive activity to arise from the plateau of Purkinje fiber action potentials (at membrane potentials of −50 to −30 mV) (271). In the presence of hypoxia clinically, alterations in Purkinje fiber action potentials similar to those shown in the in vitro studies might be expected in situ. It has also been shown that in the extracellular space of cardiac muscle made ischemic by coronary occlusion, the CO₂ tension increases (49). This increased CO₂ content might also cause early afterdepolarizations and triggered arrhythmias, because increasing CO₂ in Tyrode solution to 20% causes early afterdepolarizations in Purkinje fibers (60,62,63). After prolonged exposure to elevated CO₂, the membrane potential following the upstroke of an action potential initiated at a high membrane potential can remain somewhere between the plateau level and the original maximum diastolic potential, and rhythmic activity can persist at this low level of membrane potential. Catecholamines also may be released from nerve endings in ischemic and infarcting regions of the ventricles (153). High concentrations of catecholamines have been shown to cause early afterdepolarizations and triggered activity in Purkinje fibers in vitro (31,154). Therefore, the extracellular environment of cardiac fibers in an ischemic or infarcting region appears to be conducive to triggered activity caused by early afterdepolarizations (259). Whether or not this is a mechanism for the ischemic arrhythmias that occur soon after coronary occlusion requires more study.

Pharmacological Agents

Aconitine, veratridine, cesium.

Aconitine reduces membrane potential and induces early afterdepolarizations and triggered activity (212,254). Reduction of Na_o suppresses the aconitine-induced arrhythmias, but not the early afterdepolarization (254). It was suggested by Peper and Trautwein (233) that aconitine increases Na^+ permeability and that this is the cause of both the early afterdepolarizations and the triggered activity (*vide infra*). Observations similar to those with aconitine have been made with veratridine (211).

In contrast to agents like aconitine, which appear to act by increasing inward current, cesium causes early afterdepolarizations and triggered activity (30,76) by inhibiting outward K^+ current (i_{K_1}) (162). Here, the superimposition of normally occurring inward current can account for the early afterdepolarizations.

Antiarrhythmic drugs.

Antiarrhythmic drugs that prolong the duration of the action potential of Purkinje fibers [e.g., sotalol (46,264), *N*-acetyl procainamide (79), and quinidine (240)] can cause early afterdepolarizations and triggered activity. This may be the mechanism by which toxic concentrations of these drugs cause cardiac arrhythmias (*vide infra*).

Both the *d* and the *l* (beta-blocking) forms of sotalol prolong the action-potential duration by inhibiting i_K. This blocking effect is not accompanied by a change in activation kinetics or in reversal potential but is due entirely to a decrease in the fully activated conductance (46).

Quinidine is particularly effective in prolonging Purkinje fiber action-potential duration when the stimulus cycle length is long and K_o^+ is lower than normal (2.7 mM) (240). The prolongation of the action potential may be related to quinidine's blocking effect on I_X (57) and is not related to quinidine's well-known effect to block the Na channel. In fact, $\dot{V}_{max}$ is unchanged at the low concentrations (1 μM) of quinidine that can cause early afterdepolarizations (240). The lack of blockade of Na channels at low concentrations of quinidine may favor the development of early afterdepolarizations, because the inward Na window current may be important (*vide infra*). Under these conditions, repolarization is often arrested at the second level of resting potential (119) at which rhythmic activity occurs. Interventions that increase outward current (raising K_o) or decrease inward current (TTX) restore a normal level of resting potential and abolish triggered activity caused by quinidine (240).

Injury

Early afterdepolarizations and triggered activity occasionally occur in Purkinje fibers superfused with a normal Tyrode solution soon after dissection from the heart (7,316,320). They may disappear after the fiber is stimulated at a reasonably rapid rate (about 100/min). This triggered activity may be related to stretch (91) or damage during the dissection and suggests the interesting possibility that mechanical injury or stretch of Purkinje fibers *in situ* might cause similar triggering. Under certain conditions, stretch might also cause delayed afterdepolarizations and triggered activity; see Lab (187,188) for details. Stretch of the ventricles might occur during acute heart failure or in a ventricular aneurysm.

A similar phenomenon often is seen in cardiac muscle and Purkinje cells subjected to enzymatic and mechanical disaggregation. In the presence of normal K_o^+, the membrane sometimes fails to repolarize after stimulation of the fiber; rather, membrane potential persists in the plateau range (119), and early afterdepolarizations and triggered activity can occur (P. A. Boyden, *unpublished observations*). Elevation of the K_o to 6 or 8 mM immediately repolarizes the cells to higher levels of membrane potential and terminates this activity.

Electrotonic Interactions

Sano and Sawanobori (250) described initiation of prolonged repolarization and early afterdepolarizations as the result of electrotonic effects on Purkinje fibers. They bathed one end of a Purkinje fiber bundle in Tyrode solution containing Ca, and the other in Ca-free Tyrode. Repolarization was prolonged markedly in the Ca-free superfusate, and this resulted in a delay in repolarization and the occurrence of early afterdepolarizations at the end of the fiber bundle in the normal superfusate. Hence, in situations in which there is disparity of repolarization, that part of the fiber bundle that remains at positive membrane potentials can induce a secondary depolarization of the other end of the fiber bundle.

Ionic and Membrane Mechanisms for Early Afterdepolarizations

Little is known about the ionic mechanisms that cause early afterdepolarizations, although they are likely to result from abnormalities in the repolarizing membrane currents. During the plateau phase of the action potential, net membrane current is outward throughout the range of membrane potentials between zero and the resting potential. The net repolarizing current results from an imbalance between inward and outward membrane currents (281). Inward current components include a background Na current (119), Na current flowing through incompletely inactivated Na channels (61,90), and the slow inward current (45,59). One of the outwardly directed membrane currents is probably a potassium current flowing in a gated channel whose permeability is both time- and voltage-dependent (214). Other contributions to outward membrane current in the plateau range may be a time-independent K current that is small because of inward rectification (89) and the current generated by the electrogenic Na-K pump (121,122,163). Normally the net outward membrane current shifts membrane potential progressively in a negative direction, and the final rapid phase of action-potential repolarization takes place. An early afterdepolarization might occur if there were a shift in the current–voltage relationship resulting in a region of net inward current during the plateau range of membrane potentials (270). This would retard or prevent repolarization and might lead to a secondary depolarization during the plateau or phase 3 if a regenerative inward current were activated.

The ionic current responsible for the upstrokes of the action potentials during triggered activity is determined by the level of membrane potential at which the action potentials occur. Triggered action potentials occurring during the plateau phase and early during phase 3, at a time when most fast Na channels are still inactivated, will most likely have upstrokes caused by the slow inward current (72,320). At higher membrane potentials, where there is partial reactivation of the fast Na channels, fast responses should predominate. Current flowing through both slow channels and partially reactivated fast channels may be involved over intermediate ranges of membrane potential.

The ionic mechanism causing early afterdepolarizations and triggered activity has been investigated in greatest detail in Purkinje fibers exposed to a slightly acid medium (pH reduced to 6.9 by increasing CO_2 partial pressure or by changing the buffer system) (62,66). These early afterdepolarizations start from a membrane potential of -60 mV or greater, a level at which the fast Na channel is partly reactivated. The triggered action potentials have a fast rising phase. The early afterdepolarizations are decreased by reduction of external Na or by TTX. The TTX effect occurs concomitantly with a decrease in action-potential duration (61). During washout of TTX, early afterdepolarizations reappear before the action-potential duration returns to control level. Thus, the early afterdepolarizations appear to result at least partly from a Na current flowing through TTX-sensitive channels. This current may be the Na window

current that occurs in a potential range more negative than approximately -50 mV (14). The Na current that flows throughout the plateau range in the noninactivating or slowly inactivating channels may not participate, because the TTX effect on early afterdepolarizations can be separated from the TTX effect on the plateau (66).

Coulombe et al. (65,66) simulated early afterdepolariations caused by acidosis by modifying the equations in the Purkinje fiber action-potential model of McAllister et al. (213). In the presence of a normal Na conductance, a modification of the i_{K_1}–E_m relationship (increasing i_{K_1} at membrane potentials more positive than approximately -45 mV, and decreasing it at more negative membrane potentials) simulated the change in repolarization caused by acidosis but did not result in early afterdepolarizations. The initial part of phase 3 was accelerated, and the terminal part delayed. Under these conditions, an increase in current entering the cell through the Na window (by increasing the overlap between activation and inactivation curves) generated early afterdepolarizations and, when increased sufficiently, single or multiple reexcitations. When early afterdepolarizations reached a noticeable size as a result of the simultaneous changes in i_{K_1} and the Na window current, they became very sensitive to further changes in i_{K_1}; a small additional decrease in inward-going rectification triggered premature action potentials. A reduction in the delayed repolarizing current, I_X, which occurs mainly during the late plateau phase, also increased early afterdepolarization amplitude and caused repetitive activity. In this model, a decrease in maximum sodium conductance (g_{Na}) reduced early afterdepolarizations without affecting action-potential duration. The partial inhibition of another population of Na channels without an inactivation mechanism mimics the action-potential-shortening effect of TTX. Inhibition of the pacemaker current, I_f, either by experiments using low concentrations of Cs or in the computer model, did not depress early afterdepolarization amplitude, probably because I_f increases slowly during diastole after the occurrence of the early afterdepolarization (65,66).

An increase in the Na window current may not explain the occurrence of early afterdepolarizations at membrane potentials less negative than about -50 mV. These are suppressed by slow channel blockade, suggesting that the slow inward current may be involved in their genesis (320).

Other outward and inward currents may also be involved in the control of early afterdepolarizations, for example, the inward current channels responsible for delayed afterdepolarizations that are also activated during the plateau phase (65,66). Electrogenic Na-Ca exchange might also induce oscillations at the plateau level (116).

Characteristic Properties of Early Afterdepolarizations and Triggered Activity

Early afterdepolarizations show a cycle length dependence; they are markedly influenced by the rate at which the triggering action potentials occur (76). At a "physiological range" of cycle lengths (a range that encompasses the normal sinus rhythm of the adult human heart, 1,000–700 msec), early afterdepolarizations rarely occur. As cycle length is increased and repolarization prolongs early afterdepolarizations occur, and their amplitude increases (Fig. 20). In studies of cesium-induced early afterdepolarizations in Purkinje fibers, the early afterdepolarization amplitude increased to achieve a peak as drive-cycle length increased, and then, as cycle length was prolonged still further, they again decreased in magnitude (76). Therefore, there appears to be a range of cycle lengths at which these oscillations have a maximal amplitude, and above or below this range the balance of inward and outward currents is less favorable for their occurrence.

Once early afterdepolarizations have achieved a steady-state magnitude at a constant drive-cycle length, any event that even transiently shortens the drive-cycle length tends to reduce their amplitude (76). Hence, initiation of a single premature depolarization, which is associated with an acceleration of repolarization, will reduce the magnitude of the early afterdepolarizations that follow the premature impulse.

As drive-cycle length is prolonged, the level of membrane potential at which the early afterdepolarization occurs tends to become more positive, and the interval

between the primary action-potential upstroke and the early afterdepolarization or triggered action potential tends to decrease. Thus, there is a tendency—with increasing bradycardia—for the coupling interval of the afterdepolarization-induced ectopic impulse to decrease. The triggered impulse also conducts more slowly and aberrantly (a reflection of the more positive membrane potential). The result is a bradycardia-induced tachycardia in which there is a tendency for very slow conduction (76).

The ectopic impulses generated by early afterdepolarizations tend to have consistent (fixed) coupling to the impulses that induce them, if the cycle length is constant. For some time it was thought that such fixed coupling, or bigeminy, was characteristic mainly of reentrant impulses. More recently, we have learned that with automatic rhythms in the setting of parasystole, this same bigeminal pattern may be observed (217). It is apparent that with early afterdepolarizations, too, the pattern of fixed coupling is to be expected.

Another important characteristic is that the longer the basic drive-cycle length, the greater the number of ectopic impulses that are triggered by early afterdepolarizations (Fig. 20). Once a triggered rhythm is induced, it may be sustained or it may slow gradually and then terminate with a subthreshold early afterdepolarization.

Overdrive pacing and premature stimulation protocols have been used to characterize these triggered rhythms in Purkinje fibers superfused with Tyrode solution containing cesium (76). The likelihood of termination of prolonged periods of triggered activity by stimulation depends largely on the membrane potential at which the rhythm is occurring. A single premature depolarization can terminate triggered rhythms occurring at membrane potentials greater than about −65 mV. The basis for termination is the hyperpolarization of the membrane and acceleration of repolarization that follow the premature impulse. Premature stimuli usually are unable to terminate rhythms caused by early afterdepolarization-induced triggered activity at membrane potentials less than −50 to −55 mV, and tend only to reset them.

Whereas relatively short periods of overdrive have no effect on the membrane potential or the triggered rate following stimulation (unlike the effects on normal automaticity) (279,280), longer periods of overdrive hyperpolarize the membrane and cause some transient overdrive suppression, similar to that which occurs after long periods of overdrive of a focus with abnormal automaticity (81). The more positive the maximum diastolic potential of the triggered rhythm, the more difficult it is to overdrive-suppress it.

A mechanism for the effects of overdrive can be proposed based on what is known concerning the basis for overdrive suppression of automatic rhythms (81,279). At low levels of membrane potential, the fast inward current is largely inactivated. Overdrive for a short

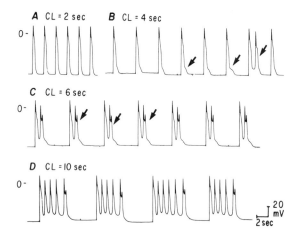

FIG. 20. Effects of basic drive-cycle length (CL) on early afterdepolarizations caused by cesium chloride in canine Purkinje fiber. A: At a CL of 2 sec, early afterdepolarizations are not apparent. B: They appear after CL was increased to 4 sec (*arrows*), and one triggered action potential occurs. C: A triggered action potential occurs after every driven action potential at a CL of 6 sec (*arrows*). D: At a CL of 10 sec, a triggered burst of four impulses follows every stimulated action potential. (From ref. 76, with permission of the American Heart Association.)

period of time probably causes little additional Na accumulation in the cells and no appreciable increase in activity of the electrogenic Na-K pump (108). With an increased duration of overdrive, the amount of Na that enters the cells presumably increases, stimulating activity of the electrogenic Na-K pump and causing hyperpolarization. The triggered rhythm slows both because of the increased outward current that opposes the net inward current causing diastolic depolarization and because of the increase in membrane potential. Triggered activity may terminate if membrane potential increases to a stable high level after the overdrive.

Pharmacology of Triggered Activity Induced by Early Afterdepolarizations

Cranefield (72) has described the means whereby drugs theoretically could abolish triggered activity caused by early afterdepolarizations. These include (a) facilitating or accelerating repolarization to a high level of resting potential (repolarization from a low level of membrane potential at which the sustained rhythmic activity occurs in Purkinje fibers to a high level of membrane potential at which it does not occur can be facilitated by increasing the outward repolarizing K current or by decreasing the steady background Na current), (b) reducing the inward current responsible for the depolarization phase of the triggered action potentials, or shifting the threshold potential of the slow upstroke toward zero, and (c) decreasing phase-4 depolarization of the triggered action potentials either by reduction of the inward current or by an increase in repolarizing current.

Small increases in K_o or acetylcholine increase the steady-state outward current during the plateau or low level of membrane potential and accelerate repolarization. This suppresses triggered activity (119,123). Lidocaine can terminate the triggered activity induced by early afterdepolarizations by repolarizing the membrane to higher potential levels at which the oscillatory activity ceases (7). Lidocaine decreases the inward window current carried by Na. This favors a shortening of the plateau and diminution of the magnitude of early afterdepolarizations (57). Procainamide also suppresses early afterdepolarization-induced triggered activity (7). Its actions are attributed to the reduction of inward Na current during the plateau. The beta-blocker tolamolol has a similar effect, although the mechanism is uncertain (7).

The upstrokes of the action potentials occurring during triggered activity at membrane potentials positive to −60 mV are probably caused by the slow inward current. Verapamil, by blocking slow channels, can decrease both the amplitude and the cycle length of this activity, and in sufficient concentrations can abolish it (320). However, early afterdepolarizations and triggered

activity may sometimes occur at membrane potentials negative to −60 mV. Verapamil and Mn have little or no effect, probably because the depolarization causing triggered activity occurs via a fast-channel mechanism. Procainamide decreases Na conductance and has been reported to stop such triggered activity (7).

Early Afterdepolarizations and Triggered Activity as a Cause of Arrhythmias

Identifying Triggered Activity in In Situ Heart

The studies on early afterdepolarizations and the triggered activity that they cause were done in isolated tissues, in some cases under conditions that might never exist *in situ*. It remains to be determined whether or not similar triggered activity occurs in the *in situ* heart. Furthermore, it is uncertain whether or not triggered activity that occurs at very low levels of resting potential and that is associated with action potentials of low upstroke velocity can excite normal myocardial fibers, as must occur if it is to cause arrhythmias (215). Early afterdepolarizations also occur at very long cycle lengths that might not arise in the *in situ* heart in the absence of protection of the site generating the early afterdepolarizations by entry block.

The approach to identification of early afterdepolarization-induced triggered activity *in situ* is similar to that which we described for identification of delayed afterdepolarization-induced triggered activity. It involves extracellular recordings, predictions concerning the electrocardiographic characteristics of the arrhythmias, and the response of the arrhythmias to pacing and drugs based on studies of isolated tissues.

Extracellular recordings. Extracellular recordings of early afterdepolarization-induced triggered activity can be obtained from Purkinje fibers *in vitro* using unipolar electrodes (79,201). This technique might therefore be useful to identify triggered arrhythmias *in situ*. We have already discussed the difficulties that might arise.

Characteristics of triggered activity. If, in fact, early afterdepolarizations do cause arrhythmias, some of their characteristics might be predicted from the results of *in vitro* studies and from Scherf's studies on the *in situ* heart with aconitine (253). The extrasystoles that are caused by early afterdepolarizations should appear as the heart rate decreases, rather than increases as described for delayed afterdepolarizations. They also should have a relatively fixed coupling to a preceding beat, because they tend to occur at the same time during repolarization of the action potential that induces them. Bigeminal rhythms may occur if only one action potential is triggered; polygeminal rhythms or tachycardia may also occur. The rate of bursts of nonsustained tachycardia should gradually slow prior to termination. That a single beat is necessary to initiate the extrasystoles or tachycardia can be shown by inhibiting the initiating beat, for example, by stimulating the vagus to inhibit the sinus node if the extrasystoles follow sinus impulses; triggered extrasystoles should then disappear. Some of these characteristics can also be predicted for reentrant beats, so they cannot distinguish triggered activity caused by early afterdepolarizations from reentry.

Use of pacing techniques to differentiate early after-depolarization-induced triggered activity from other arrhythmogenic mechanisms. Arrhythmias caused by early afterdepolarizations should not be inducible by overdrive pacing or programmed-stimulation protocols, unlike arrhythmias caused by delayed afterdepolarizations or reentry. As mentioned earlier, the appearance of early afterdepolarization-induced triggered activity is facilitated by slowing the basic heart rate. This characteristic does not distinguish them from automatic rhythms, which are also facilitated by slowing the heart rate. However, once the heart rate is slowed, the triggered rhythms may occur in bursts, with a gradual slowing of the triggered rate prior to termination, whereas automatic rhythms may gradually speed up because of removal of over-drive suppression and then persist at a constant cycle length (285).

If a polygeminal rhythm or short, repeated bursts of tachycardia are caused by afterdepolarizations, pacing the heart at faster rates than the basic, underlying rhythm is predicted to cause disappearance of the periods of tachycardia. Increasing the basic heart rate shortens the action-potential duration and thereby suppresses early afterdepolarizations. When the pacing is stopped, arrhythmias should reappear as the action potential returns to its original duration. In contrast, triggered arrhythmias caused by delayed afterdepolarizations may become more frequent as heart rate increases (244). The effects of increasing the heart rate on extrasystoles caused by reentry may be variable; reentry might be exacerbated, or it might stop (318). Increasing the basic heart rate may also cause disappearance of automatic rhythms during the periods of pacing.

Triggered arrhythmias caused by early afterpolarizations might also be sustained. When sustained, their response to single premature stimuli or overdrive pacing can be predicted on the basis of the results of the *in vitro* studies described earlier. Some arrhythmias might be terminated by premature stimuli, and others not, depending on the maximum diastolic potential. Some arrhythmias also might be terminated by overdrive pacing, and others not (*vide supra*). This variability of response may not be of much help in determining the mechanism, because arrhythmias caused by delayed afterdepolarizations and reentry might also be terminated by premature impulses or overdrive. When termination occurs, it is expected to immediately follow the overdrive, whereas termination of triggered activity caused by delayed afterdepolarizations may sometimes be preceded

by up to 10 triggered "afterbeats" (216,317). Reentrant arrhythmias may also terminate immediately after over-drive. When termination does not occur, overdrive is not expected to cause significant postoverdrive suppression; the response should be more similar to an arrhythmia caused by abnormal automaticity (81), rather than normal automaticity, which is readily overdrive-suppressed (279).

Therefore, as with the triggered arrhythmias caused by delayed afterdepolarizations, there is no single feature that will positively enable an early afterdepolarization-induced triggered rhythm to be distinguished from other arrhythmogenic mechanisms. Early afterdepolarization-induced rhythms usually can be differentiated by pacing from rhythms induced by delayed afterdepolarizations or automaticity at high membrane potentials, and sometimes from reentry, but their response to pacing is often indistinguishable from abnormal automaticity at low membrane potentials.

Experimental Animal Models of Early Afterdepolarization-Induced Arrhythmias

One of the first models of early afterdepolarization-induced rhythms was provided by Scherf in his studies of aconitine (253). Administration of aconitine to dogs induced extrasystoles (usually bigeminal) occurring during the T wave. Direct application of aconitine to the atrial or ventricular epicardium resulted in rapid tachycardias that—in the ventricles—had the characteristics of so-called ventricular flutter. Inhibition of the sinus rhythm with vagal stimulation prevented occurrence of the arrhythmias. Brachmann et al. (30) induced pleomorphic ventricular tachycardias that sometimes resembled torsades de pointes (*vide infra*) by infusing dogs with cesium. Moreover, the tachycardia was preceded by Q-T-interval prolongation, and the initial beat of the tachycardia often occurred during repolarization. In a study of cesium-induced ventricular tachycardia, phenomena resembling early afterdepolarizations and triggered activity were seen in monophasic action potentials recorded from the epicardial surface of the heart during repolarization (201).

Clinical Arrhythmias

Brugada and Wellens (39) recently have considered the role of early afterdepolarizations in clinical arrhythmias. While stressing that lack of direct evidence leaves the role of oscillations largely open to conjecture, they do suggest that early afterdepolarizations at low membrane potential might induce "bizarre, unusual forms of conduction block and . . . prolonged repolarization-dependent reexcitation."

Long Q-T interval. Hereditary prolongation of the Q-T interval of the electrocardiogram may be accompanied by syncopal episodes and sudden death due to paroxysmal ventricular arrhythmias (165). Although the mechanism for the prolongation is uncertain, it probably reflects a prolonged time course for repolarization of ventricular muscle. Because prolongation of action-potential duration can lead to early afterdepolarizations, some of these arrhythmias may be triggered. Phenomena similar to early afterdepolarizations have been recorded with monophasic action-potential techniques in patients with prolonged Q-T intervals and ventricular arrhythmias (24).

Torsades de pointes. "Torsades de pointes" is a term used to describe a rapid and often self-terminating ventricular tachycardia during which the peaks of the QRS complex gradually twist around the isoelectric line. The coupling interval of the first beat of the torsade is usually in the range of 500 to 800 msec (long-coupled), and subsequent beat-to-beat intervals are generally more rapid and irregular. The onset of torsades often follows periods of bradycardia and may sometimes be prevented by pacing the heart (see ref. 70 for review).

Abnormalities of repolarization of the ventricles are part of the definition of torsades de pointes. They may take the form of the congenital prolonged-Q-T-interval syndrome mentioned in the previous section or prolonged Q-T interval caused by electrolyte imbalance (most frequently potassium deficiency) or by antiarrhythmic drugs (70) that prolong the action-potential duration. Quinidine is a prime example (15,260). Interestingly, the arrhythmia may occur at low plasma quinidine concentrations that do not cause QRS widening (256). Hypokalemia and bradycardia both predispose to the occurrence of quinidine-induced torsades de pointes (260). Torsades has also been associated with *N*-acetyl procainamide (53,228,263) and sotalol (185).

It is reasonable to suggest that early afterdepolarization-induced triggered activities occurring at two sites in the heart might influence one another such that the characteristic QRS morphology of torsades is seen. The long-coupled interval of the first beat, its occurrence after bradycardia, and the relationship of the arrhythmia to prolonged repolarization provide further supportive evidence. It should be emphasized, however, that any pathological event in which two disparate foci are initiating impulses could give rise to the phenomenon of torsades de pointes. Reentrant excitation with different exit points from the reentrant circuit could give rise to a similar phenomenon. Hence, to attribute torsades uniquely to early afterdepolarizations is certainly premature and may turn out to be inappropriate as well.

ACKNOWLEDGMENTS

Supported by the following grants from the National Heart, Lung, and Blood Institute: HL 28958, 28223, 33727, and 30557. Andrew L. Wit was on leave in the Department of Physiology, Rijksuniversitat Maastricht, The Netherlands, and was supported by the Stichting voor Fundamental Geneeskundig Onderzoek (Fungo) while this chapter was being written.

REFERENCES

1. Akhtar, M. (1984): Supraventricular tachycardias. Electrophysiologic mechanisms, diagnosis, and pharmacologic therapy. In: *Tachycardias: Mechanisms, Diagnosis, Treatment,* edited by M. E. Josephson and H. J. J. Wellens, pp. 137–169. Lea & Febiger, Philadelphia.
2. Allen, D. G., Eisner, D. A., and Orchard, C. H. (1984): Characterization of oscillations of intracellular calcium concentration in ferret ventricular muscle. *J. Physiol. (Lond.),* 352:113–128.
3. Allen, D. G., Eisner, D. A., and Orchard, C. H. (1984): Factors influencing free intracellular calcium concentration in quiescent ferret ventricular muscle. *J. Physiol. (Lond.),* 350:615–630.
4. Allen, D. G., and Orchard, C. H. (1984): Measurements of intracellular calcium concentration in heart muscle: The effects of inotropic interventions and hypoxia. *J. Mol. Cell. Cardiol.,* 16:117–128.
5. Allen, J. D., Brennan, F. J., and Wit, A. L. (1978): Actions of lidocaine on transmembrane potentials of subendocardial fibers surviving in infarcted canine heart. *Circ. Res.,* 43:470–481.
6. Arlock, P., and Katzung, B. G. (1985): Effects of sodium substitutes on transient inward current and tension in guinea-pig and ferret papillary muscle. *J. Physiol. (Lond.),* 360:105–120.
7. Arnsdorf, M. F. (1977): The effect of antiarrhythmic drugs on triggered sustained rhythmic activity in cardiac Purkinje fibers. *J. Pharmacol. Exp. Ther.,* 201:689–700.
8. Aronson, R. S. (1981): Afterpotentials and triggered activity in hypertrophied myocardium from rats with renal-hypertension. *Circ. Res.,* 48:720–727.
9. Aronson, R. S., and Cranefield, P. F. (1974): The effect of resting potential on the electrical activity of canine cardiac Purkinje fibers exposed to Na-free solution or to ouabain. *Pfluegers. Arch.,* 347:101–116.
10. Aronson, R. S., Cranefield, P. F., and Wit, A. L. (1985): The effects of caffeine and ryanodine on the electrical activity of the canine coronary sinus. *J. Physiol. (Lond.),* 368:593–610.
11. Aronson, R. S., and Gelles, J. M. (1977): The effect ouabain, dinitrophenol and lithium on the pacemaker current in sheep cardiac Purkinje fibers. *Circ. Res.,* 40:517–524.
12. Aronson, R. S., Gelles, J. M., and Hoffman, B. F. (1973): Effect of ouabain on the current underlying spontaneous diastolic depolarization in cardiac Purkinje fibers. *Nature (New Biol.),* 245:118–120.
13. Arvanitaki, A. (1940): Reactions electriques declenchees par le passage de l'influx en un point differencie de l'axons qui le conduit. *C. R. Soc. Biol. (Paris),* 113:36–45.
14. Atwell, D., Cohen, I., Eisner, D., Ohba, M., and Ojeda, C. (1979): The steady-state TTX-sensitive (window) sodium current in cardiac Purkinje fibers. *Pfluegers Arch.,* 379:137–142.
15. Bauman, J. L., Bauernfeind, R. A., Hoff, J. V., Strasberg, B., Swiryn, S., and Rosen, K. M. (1984): Torsade de pointes due to quinidine: Observations in 31 patients. *Am. Heart J.,* 107:425–430.
16. Belardinelli, L., and Isenberg, G. (1983): Actions of adenosine and isoproterenol on isolated mammalian ventricular myocytes. *Circ. Res.,* 53:287–297.
17. Belhassen, B., Shapira, I., Pelleg, A., Copperman, I., Kauli, N., and Laniado, S. (1984): Idiopathic recurrent sustained ventricular tachycardia responsive to verapamil: An ECG-electrophysiologic entity. *Am. Heart J.,* 108:1034–1037.
18. Bers, D. M., and Ellis, D. (1982): Intracellular calcium and sodium activity in sheep heart Purkinje fibers. Effect of changes of external sodium and intracellular pH. *Pfluegers Arch.,* 393:171–178.
19. Bigger, J. T., Jr., and Goldreyer, B. N. (1970): The mechanisms of supraventricular tachycardia. *Circulation,* 42:673–688.
20. Bigger, J. T., Jr., and Mandel, W. J. (1970): Effect of lidocaine

on transmembrane potentials of ventricular muscle and Purkinje fibers. *J. Clin. Invest.*, 49:63–77.

21. Binah, O., Cohen, I. S., and Rosen, M. R. (1983): The effects of adriamycin on normal and ouabain-toxic canine Purkinje and ventricular muscle fibers. *Circ. Res.*, 53:655–662.

22. Blinks, J. R., Olson, C. B., Jewell, B. R., and Braveny, P. (1972): Influence of caffeine and other methylxanthines on mechanical properties of isolated mammalian heart muscle. Evidence for a dual mechanism of action. *Circ. Res.*, 30:367–392.

23. Bonatti, V., Finardi, A., and Botti, G. (1979): Enregistrements des potentiels d'action monophasiques du ventricule droit dans un cas QT long et alternance isolee de l'onde. *Arch. Mal. Coeur*, 72:1180–1186.

24. Bonatti, V., Rolli, A., and Botti, G. (1983): Recording of mono-phasic action potentials of the right ventricle in the long QT syndrome complicated by severe ventricular arrhythmias. *Eur. Heart J.*, 4:168–172.

25. Boyden, P. A., Cranefield, P. F., and Gadsby, D. C. (1983): Noradrenalin hyperpolarizes cells of the canine coronary sinus by increasing their permeability to potassium ions. *J. Physiol. (Lond.)*, 339:185–206.

26. Boyden, P. A., Cranefield, P. F., Gadsby, D. C., and Wit, A. L. (1983): The basis for the membrane potential of quiescent cells of the canine coronary sinus. *J. Physiol. (Lond.)*, 339:161–183.

27. Boyden, P. A., Tilley, L. P., Albala, A., Liu, S. K., Fenoglio, J. J., Jr., and Wit, A. L. (1984): Mechanisms for atrial arrhythmias associated with cardiomyopathy: A study of feline hearts with primary myocardial disease. *Circulation*, 69:1036–1047.

28. Boyett, M. R., and Jewell, B. R. (1980): Analyses of the effects of changes in rate of rhythm upon electrical activity in the heart. *Prog. Biophys. Mol. Biol.*, 36:1–52.

29. Bozler, E. (1943): The initiation of impulses in cardiac muscle. *Am. J. Physiol.*, 138:273–282.

30. Brachmann, J., Scherlag, B. J., Rosenshtraukh, L. V., and Lazzara, R. (1983): Bradycardia-dependent triggered activity: Relevance to drug-induced multiform ventricular tachycardia. *Circulation*, 68:846–856.

31. Brooks, C. M., Hoffman, B. F., Suckling, E. E., and Orias, O. (1955): *Excitability of the Heart.* Grune & Stratton, New York.

32. Brooks, C. M., and Lu, H.-H. (1972): *The Sinoatrial Pacemaker of the Heart.* Charles C Thomas, Springfield, Ill.

33. Brown, B. S., Akera, T., and Brody, T. M. (1981): Mechanism of grayanotoxin-III-induced afterpotentials in feline cardiac Purkinje fibers. *Eur. J. Pharmacol.*, 75:271–281.

34. Brown, H. F. F., Noble, D., Noble, S., and Taupignon, A. (1984): Transient inward current and its relation to the very slow inward current in the rabbit sinoatrial node. *J. Physiol. (Lond.)*, 349:47 P.

35. Browning, D. J., Tiedman, T. S., Stagg, A. L., Benditt, D. G., Scheinman, N. N., and Strauss, H. C. (1979): Aspects of rate-related hyperpolarization in feline Purkinje fibers. *Circ. Res.*, 44:612–624.

36. Brugada, P., and Wellens, H. J. J. (1984): Electrophysiology, mechanisms, diagnosis and treatment of paroxysmal recurrent atrioventricular nodal reentrant tachycardia. In: *Tachycardias*, edited by B. Surawicz, C. R. Reddy, and E. N. Prystowsky, pp. 131–157. Martinus Nijhoff, The Hague.

37. Brugada, P., and Wellens, H. J. J. (1984): Programmed electrical stimulation of the human heart: General principles. In: *Tachy-cardias: Mechanisms, Diagnosis, Treatment*, edited by M. E. Josephson and H. J. J. Wellens, pp. 61–89. Lea & Febiger, Philadelphia.

38. Brugada, P., and Wellens, H. J. J. (1984): The role of triggered activity in clinical ventricular arrhythmias. *Pace*, 7:260–271.

39. Brugada, P., and Wellens, H. J. J. (1985): Early afterdepolarizations: Role in conduction block, prolonged repolarization dependent reexcitation, and tachyarrhythmias in the human heart. *Pace*, 8:889–896.

40. Buxton, A. E., Marchlinski, F. E., Doherty, J. U., Cassidy, D. M., Vassallo, J. A., Flores, B. T., and Josephson, M. E. (1984): Repetitive, monomorphic ventricular tachycardia: Clinical and electrophysiologic characteristics in patients with and patients without organic heart disease. *Am. J. Cardiol.*, 54:997–1002.

41. Buxton, A. E., Waxman, H. L., Marchlinski, F. E., and Josephson, M. E. (1984): Electrophysiologic characterization of nonsustained

42. Buxton, A. E., Waxman, H. L., Marchlinski, F. E., Simson, M. B., Cassidy, D., and Josephson, M. E. (1983): Right ventricular tachycardia: Clinical and electrophysiologic characteristics. *Circulation*, 68:917–927.

43. Capogrossi, M. C., and Lakatta, E. G. (1985): Frequency modu-lation and synchronization of spontaneous oscillations in cardiac cells. *Am. J. Physiol.*, 248:H412–418.

44. Carmeliet, E. (1961): Chloride ions and the membrane potential of Purkinje fibers. *J. Physiol. (Lond.)*, 156:375–388.

45. Carmeliet, E. (1980): The slow inward current: Non-voltage-clamp studies. In: *The Slow Inward Current and Cardiac Arrhyth-mias*, edited by D. P. Zipes, J. C. Bailey, and V. Elharrar, pp. 97–110. Martinus Nijhoff, The Hague.

46. Carmeliet, E. (1985): Electrophysiologic and voltage clamp analyses of the effects of sotalol on isolated cardiac muscle and Purkinje fibers. *J. Pharmacol. Exp. Ther.*, 232:817–825.

47. Carmeliet, E., and Vereecke, J. (1969): Adrenaline and the plateau phase of the cardiac action potential. *Pfluegers Arch*, 313:300–315.

48. Caroni, P., Villani, E., and Carafoli, E. (1981): The cardiotoxic antibiotic doxorubicin inhibits Na/Ca exchange of dog heart sarcolemmal vesicles. *FEBS Lett.*, 30:184–186.

49. Case, R. B., Felix, A., and Castellana, F. S. (1979): Rate of rise of myocardial pCO_2 during early myocardial ischemia in the dog. *Circ. Res.*, 45:324–330.

50. Castellanos, A., Lemberg, L., Centruion, M. J., and Berkovits, B. V. (1967): Concealed digitalis induced arrhythmias unmasked by electrical stimulation of the heart. *Am. Heart J.*, 73:484–490.

51. Chapman, R. A., Coray, A., and McGuigan, J. A. S. (1983): Sodium/calcium exchange in mammalian ventricular muscle: A study with sodium-sensitive microelectrodes. *J. Physiol.*, 343:253–276.

52. Chapman, R. A., and Tunstall, J. (1981): The tension-depolar-ization relationship of frog atrial trabeculae as determined by potassium contractures. *J. Physiol. (Lond.)*, 310:97–115.

53. Chow, M. J., Piergies, A. A., Bowsker, D. J., Murphy, J. J., Kushner, W., Ruo, T. I., Asada, A., Talano, J. Y., and Atkinson, A. J. (1984): Torsades de pointes induced by N-acetylprocainamide. *J. Am. Coll. Cardiol.*, 4:621–624.

54. Clusin, W. T. (1983): Caffeine induces a transient inward current in cultured cardiac cells. *Nature*, 301:248–250.

55. Cohen, C. J., Bean, B. P., Colatsky, T. J., and Tsien, R. W. (1981): Tetrodotoxin block of sodium channels in rabbit Purkinje fibers: Interaction between toxin binding and channel gating. *J. Gen. Physiol.*, 78:383–411.

56. Cohen, C. J., Fozzard, H. A., and Sheu, S. (1982): Increase in intracellular sodium ion activity during stimulation in mammalian cardiac muscle. *Circ. Res.*, 50:651–662.

57. Colatsky, T. (1982): Mechanisms of action of lidocaine and quinidine on action potential duration in rabbit cardiac Purkinje fibers: An effect on steady-state sodium currents. *Circ. Res.*, 50:17–27.

58. Colquhoun, D., Neher, E., Reuter, H., and Stevens, C. F. (1981): Inward current channels activated by intracellular Ca in cultured cardiac cells. *Nature*, 294:752–754.

59. Coraboeuf, E. (1980): Voltage clamp studies of the slow inward current. In: *The Slow Inward Current and Cardiac Arrhythmias*, edited by D. P. Zipes, J. C. Bailey, and V. Elharrar, pp. 25–96. Martinus Nijhoff, The Hague.

60. Coraboeuf, E., and Boistel, J. (1953): L'action des taux eleves de gaz carbonique sur le tissu cardiaque etudiee a Paide de micro-electrodes intracellulaires. *C. R. Soc. Biol. (Paris)*, 147:654–658.

61. Coraboeuf, E., Deroubaix, E., and Coulombe, A. (1979): Effect of tetrodotoxin on action potentials of the conducting system in the dog heart. *Am. J. Physiol.*, 236:561–567.

62. Coraboeuf, E., Deroubaix, E., and Coulombe, A. (1980): Acidosis-induced abnormal repolarization and repetitive activity in isolated dog Purkinje fibers. *J. Physiol. (Paris)*, 76:97–106.

63. Coraboeuf, E., Deroubaix, E., and Hoerter, J. (1976): Control of ionic permeabilities in normal and ischemic heart. *Circ. Res. [Suppl. I]*, 38:92–98.

64. Cortes, E. P., Lutman, G., and Wanka, J. (1975): Adriamycin (NSC-123127) cardiotoxicity: A clinicopathologic correlation. *Cancer Chemother. Rep.*, 6:215–225.

65. Coulombe, A., Coraboeuf, E., and Deroubaix, E. (1980): Computer simulation of acidosis-induced abnormal repolarization and repetitive activity in dog Purkinje fibers. *J. Physiol. (Paris)*, 76: 107–112.

66. Coulombe, A., Coraboeuf, E., Malecot, C., and Deroubaix, E. (1984): Role of the Na window current and other ionic currents in triggering early afterdepolarizations and resulting reexcitations in Purkinje fibers. In: *Cardiac Electrophysiology and Arrhythmias*, edited by D. P. Zipes and J. Jalife, pp. 43–50. Grune & Stratton, New York.

67. Coumel, P., and Attuel, P. (1983): Which arrhythmias are specifically susceptible to calcium antagonists? In: *Frontiers of Cardiac Electrophysiology*, edited by M. B. Rosenbaum and M. V. Elizari, pp. 341–348. Martinus Nijhoff, The Hague.

68. Coumel, P., Attuel, P., and Leclercq, J. F. (1980): The role of calcium antagonists in ventricular arrhythmias. In: *Calcium Antagonism in Cardiovascular Therapy: Experience with Verapamil*, edited by A. Zanchetti and D. M. Krikler, pp. 373–387. Excerpta Medica, Amsterdam.

69. Coumel, P., Leclercq, J. F., Attuel, P., Rosengarten, M. E., Milosevic, D., Slama, R., and Bouvrain, Y. (1980): Tachycardies ventriculaires en salves. Etude electrophysiologique et therapeutique. *Arch. Mal. Coeur*, 73:153–164.

70. Coumel, P., Leclercq, J., and Dessertenne, F. (1984): Torsades de pointes. In: *Tachycardias: Mechanisms, Diagnosis, Treatment*, edited by M. E. Josephson and H. J. J. Wellens, pp. 325–351. Lea & Febiger, Philadelphia.

71. Cramer, M., Siegal, M., Bigger, J. T., Jr., and Hoffman, B. F. (1977): Characteristics of extracellular potentials recorded from the sinoatrial pacemaker of the rabbit. *Circ. Res.*, 41:292–300.

72. Cranefield, P. F. (1975): *The Conduction of the Cardiac Impulse: The Slow Response and Cardiac Arrhythmias*. Futura Publishing, Mt. Kisco, N.Y.

73. Cranefield, P. F. (1977): Action potentials, afterpotentials and arrhythmias. *Circ. Res.*, 41:415–423.

74. Cranefield, P. F. (1978): Does spontaneous activity arise from phase 4 depolarization or from triggering? In: *The Sinus Node: Structure, Function and Clinical Relevance*, edited by F. I. M. Bonke, pp. 348–356. Martinus Nijhoff, The Hague.

75. Cranefield, P. F., and Aronson, R. S. (1974): Initiation of sustained rhythmic activity by single propagated action potentials in canine cardiac Purkinje fibers exposed to sodium free solution or to ouabain. *Circ. Res.*, 34:477–481.

76. Damiano, B. P., and Rosen, M. (1984): Effects of pacing on triggered activity induced by early afterdepolarizations. *Circulation*, 69:1013–1025.

77. Dangman, K. H., Danilo, P., Hordof, A. J., Mary-Rabine, L., Reder, R. F., and Rosen, M. R. (1982): Electrophysiologic characteristics of human ventricular and Purkinje fibers. *Circulation*, 65:362–368.

78. Dangman, K. H., and Hoffman, B. F. (1980): Effects of nifedipine on electrical activity of cardiac cells. *Am. J. Cardiol.*, 46:1059–1067.

79. Dangman, K. H., and Hoffman, B. F. (1981): In vivo and in vitro antiarrhythmic and arrhythmogenic effects of *N*-acetyl procainamide. *J. Pharmacol. Exp. Ther.*, 217:851–862.

80. Dangman, K. H., and Hoffman, B. F. (1983): Antiarrhythmic effects of ethmozin in cardiac Purkinje fibers: Suppression of automaticity and abolition of triggering. *J. Pharmacol. Exp. Ther.*, 227:578–586.

81. Dangman, K. H., and Hoffman, B. F. (1983): Studies on overdrive stimulation of canine cardiac Purkinje fibers: Maximal diastolic potential as a determinant of the response. *J. Am. Coll. Cardiol.*, 2:1183–1190.

82. Davis, J., Glassman, R., and Wit, A. L. (1982): Method for evaluating the effects of antiarrhythmic drugs on ventricular tachycardias with different electrophysiologic characteristics and different mechanisms in the infarcted canine heart. *Am. J. Cardiol.*, 49:1176–1184.

83. Davis, L. D. (1973): Effects of changes in cycle length on diastolic depolarization produced by ouabain in canine Purkinje fibers. *Circ. Res.*, 32:206–214.

84. Deitmar, J. W., and Ellis, D. (1978): The intracellular sodium activity of cardiac Purkinje fibers during inhibition and reactivation of the Na-K pump. *J. Physiol. (Lond.)*, 284:241–259.

85. DiFrancesco, D. (1981): A new interpretation of the pacemaker current in calf Purkinje fibers. *J. Physiol. (Lond.)*, 314:359–376.

86. DiGennaro, M., Carbonin, P., and Vassalle, M. (1984): On the mechanism by which caffeine abolishes the fast rhythms induced by cardiotonic steroids. *J. Mol. Cell. Cardiol.*, 16:851–862.

87. DiGennaro, M., Valle, R., Pakor, M., and Carbonin, P. (1983): Abolition of digitalis tachyarrhythmias by caffeine. *Am. J. Physiol.*, 244:H215–H222.

88. Dow, J. W., Harding, N. G. L., and Powell, T. (1981): Isolated cardiac myocytes. II. Functional aspects of mature cells. *Cardiovasc. Res.*, 15:549–579.

89. Dudel, J., Peper, K., Rudel, R., and Trautwein, W. (1967): The potassium component of membrane current in Purkinje fibers. *Pfluegers Arch.*, 296:308–327.

90. Dudel, J., Peper, K., Rudel, R., and Trautwein, W. (1967): The effect of tetrodotoxin on the membrane current in cardiac muscle (Purkinje fibers). *Pfluegers Arch.*, 295:213–226.

91. Dudel, J., and Trautwein, W. (1954): Das Aktionspotential und Mechanogramm des Herzmuskels unter dem Einfluss der Dehnung. *Cardiologia*, 25:344–362.

92. Eisner, D. A., and Lederer, W. J. (1979): Inotropic and arrhythmogenic effects of potassium depleted solutions on mammalian cardiac muscle. *J. Physiol. (Lond.)*, 294:255–277.

93. Eisner, D. A., and Lederer, W. J. (1979): The role of the sodium pump in the effects of potassium depleted solutions on mammalian cardiac muscle. *J. Physiol. (Lond.)*, 294:279–301.

94. Eisner, D. A., and Lederer, W. J. (1985): Na-Ca exchange: Stoichiometry and electrogenicity. *Am. J. Physiol. (Cell. Physiol.*, 17), 248:189–202.

95. Eisner, D. A., Lederer, W. J., and Sheu, S. S. (1983): The role of intracellular Na activity in the antiarrhythmic action of local anesthetics in sheep Purkinje fibers. *J. Physiol. (Lond.)*, 340:239–257.

96. Eisner, D. A., Lederer, W. J., and Vaughan Jones, R. D. (1983): The control of tonic tension by membrane potential and intracellular sodium activity in the sheep cardiac Purkinje fiber. *J. Physiol. (Lond.)*, 335:723–743.

97. Eisner, D. A., Orchard, C. H., and Allen, D. G. (1984): Control of intracellular ionized calcium concentration by sarcolemmal and intracellular mechanisms. *J. Mol. Cell. Cardiol.*, 16:137–146.

98. Eisner, D. A., and Vaughan Jones, R. D. (1983): Do calcium-activated potassium channels exist in the heart? *Cell Calcium*, 4: 371–386.

99. El-Sherif, N., Gough, W. B., Zeiler, R. H., and Mehra, R. (1983): Triggered ventricular rhythms in one-day-old myocardial infarction in the dog. *Circ. Res.*, 52:566–579.

100. Elharrar, V., Bailey, J. C., Lathrop, D. A., and Zipes, D. P. (1978): Effects of aprindine on slow channel action potentials and transient depolarizations in canine Purkinje fibers. *J. Pharmacol. Exp. Ther.*, 205:410–417.

101. Endo, M. (1977): Calcium release from the sarcoplasmic reticulum. *Physiol. Rev.*, 57:71–108.

102. Fabiato, A. (1982): Calcium release in skinned cardiac cells: Variations with species, tissues and development. *Fed. Proc.*, 41: 2238–2244.

103. Fabiato, A. (1983): Calcium-induced release of calcium from the cardiac sarcoplasmic reticulum. *Am. J. Physiol.*, 245:C1–C14.

104. Fabiato, A. (1985): Simulated calcium current can both cause calcium loading in and trigger calcium release from the sarcoplasmic reticulum of a skinned canine cardiac Purkinje cell. *J. Gen. Physiol.*, 85:291–320.

105. Fabiato, A., and Fabiato, F. (1973): Activation of skinned cardiac cells. Subcellular effects of cardioactive drugs. *Eur. J. Cardiol.*, 1:143–155.

106. Fabiato, A., and Fabiato, F. (1975): Contraction induced by a calcium-triggered release of calcium from the sarcoplasmic reticulum of single skinned cardiac cells. *J. Physiol. (Lond.)*, 249: 469–495.

107. Fabiato, A., and Fabiato, F. (1977): Calcium release from the sarcoplasmic reticulum. *Circ. Res.*, 40:119–129.

108. Falk, R. T., and Cohen, I. S. (1984): Membrane current following

activity in canine cardiac Purkinje fibers. *J. Gen. Physiol.*, 83: 771–799.

109. Ferrier, G. R. (1981): Effects of transmembrane potential on oscillatory afterpotentials induced by acetylstrophanthidin in canine ventricular tissues. *J. Pharmacol. Exp. Ther.*, 215:332–341.

110. Ferrier, G. R. (1976): The effects of tension on acetylstrophanthidin-induced transient depolarizations and aftercontractions in canine myocardial and Purkinje tissue. *Circ. Res.*, 38:156–162.

111. Ferrier, G. R. (1977): Digitalis arrhythmias: Role oscillatory afterpotentials. *Prog. Cardiovasc. Dis.*, 19:459–474.

112. Ferrier, G. R. (1977): Relationship between acetylstrophanthidin-induced aftercontractions and the strength of contraction of canine ventricular myocardium. *Circ. Res.*, 41:622–629.

113. Ferrier, G. R., and Moe, G. K. (1973): Effect of calcium on acetylstrophanthidin-induced transient depolarizations in canine Purkinje tissue. *Circ. Res.*, 33:508–515.

114. Ferrier, G. R., Moffat, M. P., and Lukas, A. (1985): Possible mechanisms of ventricular arrhythmias elicited by ischemia followed by reperfusion: Studies on isolated canine ventricular tissues. *Circ. Res.*, 56:184–194.

115. Ferrier, G. R., Saunders, J. H., and Mendez, C. (1973): A cellular mechanism for the generation of ventricular arrhythmias by acetylstrophanthidin. *Circ. Res.*, 32:600–609.

116. Fischmeister, R., and Vassort, G. (1981): The electrogenic Na-Ca exchange and cardiac electrical activity. I. Stimulation on Purkinje fibre action potential. *J. Physiol. (Paris)*, 77:705–709.

117. Freedman, R. A., Sherdlow, C. D., Echt, D. S., Winkle, R. A., Soderholm-Difatte, V., and Mason, J. W. (1984): Facilitation of ventricular tachyarrhythmic induction by isoproterenol. *Am. J. Cardiol.*, 54:765–770.

118. Friedman, P. L., Fenoglio, J. J., Jr., and Wit, A. L. (1975): Time course for reversal of electrophysiological and ultrastructural abnormalities in subendocardial Purkinje fibers surviving extensive myocardial infarction in dogs. *Circ. Res.*, 36:127–144.

119. Gadsby, D. C., and Cranefield, P. F. (1977): Two levels of resting potential in cardiac Purkinje fibers. *J. Gen. Physiol.*, 70:725–746.

120. Gadsby, D. C., and Cranefield, P. F. (1979): Direct measurement of changes in sodium pump current in canine cardiac Purkinje fibers. *Proc. Natl. Acad. Sci. (USA)*, 76:1783–1787.

121. Gadsby, D. C., and Cranefield, P. F. (1979): Electrogenic sodium extrusion in cardiac Purkinje fibers. *J. Gen. Physiol.*, 73:819–837.

122. Gadsby, D. C., and Cranefield, P. F. (1982): Effects of electrogenic sodium extrusion on the membrane potential of cardiac Purkinje fibers. In: *Normal and Abnormal Conduction in the Heart*, edited by A. Paes de Carvalho, B. F. Hoffman, and M. Lieberman, pp. 225–248. Futura Publishing, Mt. Kisco, N.Y.

123. Gadsby, D. C., Wit, A. L., and Cranefield, P. F. (1978): The effects of acetylcholine on the electrical activity of canine cardiac Purkinje fibers. *Circ. Res.*, 43:29–35.

124. Gasser, H. S., and Grundfest, H. (1936): Action and excitability in mammalian A fibers. *Am. J. Physiol.*, 117:113–133.

125. German, L. D., Packer, D. L., Bardy, G. H., and Gallagher, J. J. (1983): Ventricular tachycardia induced by atrial stimulation in patients without symptomatic cardiac disease. *Am. J. Cardiol.*, 52:1202–1207.

126. Gibbons, W. R., and Fozzard, H. A. (1971): Voltage dependence and time dependence of contraction in sheep cardiac Purkinje fibers. *Circ. Res.*, 28:446–460.

127. Gibbons, W. R., and Fozzard, H. A. (1975): Relationships between voltage and tension in sheep cardiac Purkinje fibers. *J. Gen. Physiol.*, 65:345–365.

128. Giles, W., and Noble, S. J. (1976): Changes in membrane currents in bullfrog atrium produced by acetylcholine. *J. Physiol. (Lond.)*, 261:103–123.

129. Glick, M. R., Burns, A. H., and Reddy, W. J. (1974): Dispersion isolation of beating cells from adult rat heart. *Anal. Biochem.*, 61:32–42.

130. Glitsch, H. G., and Pott, L. (1975): Spontaneous tension oscillations in guinea pig atrial trabeculae. *Pfluegers Arch.*, 358:11–25.

131. Goldenberg, M., and Rothberger, C. J. (1936): Über die Werkung von Veratrin auf den Purkinje-Faden. *Pfluegers Arch.*, 238:137–152.

132. Goldreyer, B. N., and Damato, A. N. (1971): The essential role of atrioventricular conduction delay in the initiation of paroxysmal supraventricular tachycardia. *Circulation*, 43:679–687.

133. Gorgels, A. P. M., Beekman, H. D. M., Brugada, P., Dassen, W. R. M., Richards, D. A. B., and Wellens, H. J. J. (1983): Extrastimulus related shortening of the first postpacing interval in digitalis induced ventricular tachycardia. *J. Am. Coll. Cardiol.*, 1:840–857.

134. Gorgels, A. P. M., De Wit, B., Beekman, H. D. M., Dassen, W. R. M., and Wellens, H. J. J. (1986): Triggered activity induced by pacing during digitalis intoxication. *Pace (in press)*.

135. Gough, W. B., Zeiler, R. H., and El-Sherif, N. (1984): Effects of diltiazem on triggered activity in canine 1-day-old infarction. *Cardiovasc. Res.*, 18:339–343.

136. Gough, W. B., Zeiler, R. H., and El-Sherif, N. (1984): Effects of nifedipine on triggered activity in 1-day-old MI in dogs. *Am. J. Cardiol.*, 53:303–306.

137. Hariman, R. J., and Chen, C. (1983): Recording of diastolic slope from the junctional area in dogs with junctional rhythm. *Circulation*, 68:636–643.

138. Hariman, R. J., Gomes, J. A. C., and El-Sherif, N. (1984): Recording of diastolic slope with catheters during junctional rhythm in humans. *Circulation*, 69:485–491.

139. Hariman, R. J., Hoffman, B. F., and Naylor, R. E. (1980): Electrical activity from the sinus node region in conscious dogs. *Circ. Res.*, 47:775–791.

140. Hariman, R. J., Krongrad, E., Boxer, R. A., Bowman, F. O., Jr., Malm, J. R., and Hoffman, B. F. (1980): Methods for recording electrograms of the sinoatrial node during cardiac surgery in man. *Circulation*, 61:1024–1029.

141. Hashimoto, K., and Moe, G. K. (1973): Transient depolarizations induced by acetylstrophanthidin in specialized tissue of dog atrium and ventricle. *Circ. Res.*, 32:618–624.

142. Henning, B., and Wit, A. L. (1981): Action potential characteristics control afterdepolarization amplitude and triggered activity in canine coronary sinus. *Circulation*, 64:50.

143. Henning, B., and Wit, A. L. (1982): Multiple mechanisms for antiarrhythmic drug action on delayed afterdepolarizations and triggered activity in canine coronary sinus. *Am. J. Cardiol.*, 49:921 (abstract).

144. Henning, B., and Wit, A. L. (1984): The time course of action potential repolarization effects delayed afterdepolarization amplitude in atrial fibers of the canine coronary sinus. *Circ. Res.*, 55:110–115.

145. Hess, P., and Wier, W. G. (1984): Excitation-contraction coupling in cardiac Purkinje fibers. Effects of caffeine on the intracellular Ca^{2+} transient, membrane currents, and contraction. *J. Gen. Physiol.*, 83:417–433.

146. Hewitt, K., Gessman, L., and Rosen, M. R. (1983): Effects of procaineamide, quinidine and ethmozin on delayed afterdepolarizations. *Eur. J. Pharmacol.*, 96:21–28.

147. Hewitt, K. W., and Rosen, M. R. (1984): Alpha and beta adrenergic interactions with ouabain-induced delayed afterdepolarizations. *J. Pharmacol. Exp. Ther.*, 229:188–192.

148. Hilgemann, D. W., Delay, M. J., and Langer, G. A. (1983): Activation-dependent cumulative depletions of extracellular free calcium in guinea pig atrium measured with antipyrylazo III and tetramethylmurexide. *Circ. Res.*, 53:779–793.

149. Hiraoka, M. (1977): Membrane current changes induced by acetylstrophanthidin in cardiac Purkinje fibers. *Jpn. Heart J.*, 18:851–859.

150. Hiraoka, M., and Kawano, S. (1984): Regulation of delayed afterdepolarization and aftercontractions in dog ventricular muscle fibres. *J. Mol. Cell. Cardiol.*, 16:285–289.

151. Hiraoka, M., Okamoto, Y., and Sano, T. (1979): Effects of Ca^+ and K^+ on oscillatory afterpotentials in dog ventricular muscle-fibers. *J. Mol. Cell. Cardiol.*, 11:999–1015.

152. Hiraoka, M., Okamoto, Y., and Sano, T. (1981): Oscillatory afterpotentials in dog ventricular muscle fibers. *Circ. Res.*, 48:510–518.

153. Hirsche, H. J., Franz, C., Bos, L., Bissig, R., and Schramm, M. (1980): Myocardial extracellular K^+ and H^+ increase and noradrenaline release as a possible cause of early arrhythmias following acute coronary artery occlusion in pigs. *J. Mol. Cell. Cardiol.*, 12:579–593.

154. Hoffman, B. F., and Cranefield, P. F. (1960): *Electrophysiology of the Heart.* McGraw-Hill, New York.
155. Hogan, P. M., Wittenberg, S. M., and Klocke, F. J. (1973): Relationship of stimulation frequency to automaticity in the canine Purkinje fiber during ouabain administration. *Circ. Res.,* 32:377–383.
156. Hordof, A. J., Edie, R., Malm, J. R., Hoffman, B. F., and Rosen, M. R. (1976): Electrophysiologic properties and response to pharmacologic agents of fibers from diseased human atria. *Circulation,* 54:774–779.
157. Hunter, D. R., Haworth, R. A., and Berkoff, H. A. (1983): Modulation of cellular calcium stores in the perfused rat heart by isoproterenol and ryanodine. *Circ. Res.,* 53:703–712.
158. Hutter, O. F. (1964): The action of the vagus, of acetylcholine and other parasympathetic drugs on the heart. In: *Second International Pharmacological Meeting, Vol. 5, Pharmacology of Cardiac Function,* edited by O. Krayer and A. Kovarikova, pp. 87–94. Pergamon Press, Oxford.
159. Hutter, O. F., and Noble, D. (1961): Anion conductance of cardiac muscle. *J. Physiol. (Lond.),* 157:335–350.
160. Ilvento, J. P., Provet, J., Danilo, P., and Rosen, M. R. (1982): Fast and slow idioventricular rhythms in the canine heart; a study of their mechanism using antiarrhythmic drugs and electrophysiologic testing. *Am. J. Cardiol.,* 49:1909–1916.
161. Imanishi, S., McAllister, R. G., Jr., and Surawicz, B. (1978): The effects of verapamil and lidocaine on the automatic depolarizations in guinea-pig ventricular myocardium. *J. Pharmacol. Exp. Ther.,* 207:294–303.
162. Isenberg, G. (1976): Cardiac Purkinje fibers: Cesium as a tool to block inward rectifying potassium currents. *Pfluegers Arch.,* 365:99–106.
163. Isenberg, G., and Trautwein, W. (1974): The effect of dihydroouabain and lithium-ions on the outward current in cardiac Purkinje fibers. *Pfluegers Arch.,* 350:41–54.
164. January, T., and Fozzard, H. A. (1984): The effects of membrane potential, extracellular potassium, and tetrodotoxin on the intracellular sodium ion activity of sheep cardiac muscle. *Circ. Res.,* 54:652–665.
165. Jervell, A., and Lange-Nielsen, F. (1957): Congenital deaf mutism functional heart disease with prolongation of Q-T interval and sudden death. *Am. Heart J.,* 54:59–68.
166. Johnson, N., Danilo, P., Wit, A., and Rosen, M. (1985): Response to pacing of triggered activity occurring in catecholamine-treated canine coronary sinus. *Circulation,* 72:III–381.
167. Josephson, M. E., Marchlinski, F. E., Buxton, A. E., Waxman, H. L., Doherty, J. U., Kiengle, M. G., and Falcone, R. (1984): Electrophysiologic basis for sustained ventricular tachycardia—role of reentry. In: *Tachycardias: Mechanisms, Diagnosis, Treatment,* edited by M. E. Josephson and H. J. J. Wellens, pp. 305–324. Lea & Febiger, Philadelphia.
168. Karagueuzian, H. S., Fenoglio, J. J., Jr., Weiss, M. B., and Wit, A. L. (1979): Protracted ventricular tachycardia induced by premature stimulation of the canine heart after coronary occlusion and reperfusion. *Circ. Res.,* 44:833–846.
169. Karagueuzian, H. S., and Katzung, B. G. (1981): Relative inotropic and arrhythmogenic effects of 5 cardiac steroids in ventricular myocardium: Oscillatory afterpotentials and the role of endogenous catecholamines. *J. Pharmacol. Exp. Ther.,* 218:348–356.
170. Karagueuzian, H. S., and Katzung, B. G. (1982): Voltage clamp studies of transient inward current and mechanical oscillations induced by ouabain in ferret papillary muscle. *J. Physiol. (Lond.),* 327:255–271.
171. Kass, R. S., Lederer, W. J., Tsien, R. W., and Weingart, R. (1978): Role of calcium ions in transient inward currents and aftercontractions induced by strophanthidin in cardiac Purkinje fibers. *J. Physiol. (Lond.),* 281:187–208.
172. Kass, R. S., and Sanguinetti, M. C. (1984): Inactivation of calcium channel current in the calf cardiac Purkinje fiber—evidence for voltage-mediated and calcium-mediated mechanisms. *J. Gen. Physiol.,* 84:705–726.
173. Kass, R. S., and Scheuer, T. (1982): Slow inactivation of calcium channels in the cardiac Purkinje fiber. *J. Mol. Cell. Cardiol.,* 14:615–618.
174. Kass, R. S., and Tsien, R. W. (1982): Fluctuations in membrane current driven by intracellular calcium in cardiac Purkinje fibers. *Biophys. J.,* 38:259–269.
175. Kass, R. S., Tsien, R. W., and Weingart, R. (1978): Ionic basis of transient inward current induced by strophanthidin in cardiac Purkinje fibers. *J. Physiol. (Lond.),* 281:209–226.
176. Katzung, B. O., and Morgenstern, J. A. (1977): Effects of extracellular potassium on ventricular automaticity and evidence for a pacemaker current in mammalian ventricular myocardium. *Circ. Res.,* 40:105–111.
177. Kenyon, J. L., and Gibbons, W. R. (1979): Influence of chloride, potassium and tetraethylammonium on the early outward current of sheep cardiac Purkinje fibers. *J. Gen. Physiol.,* 73:117–138.
178. Kimura, S., Cameron, J. S., Kozlovsky, P. L., Bassett, A. L., and Meyerberg, R. J. (1984): Delayed afterdepolarizations and triggered activity induced in feline Purkinje fibers by alpha-adrenergic stimulation in the presence of elevated calcium levels. *Circulation,* 70:1074–1082.
179. Kimura, S., Hazamia, S., Fujii, T., Nakaya, H., and Kanno, M. (1984): Delayed afterdepolarizations and triggered activity in canine Purkinje fibers treated with neuroaminidase. *Cardiovasc. Res.,* 18:294–301.
180. Kline, R. P., and Kupersmith, J. (1982): Effects of extracellular potassium accumulation and sodium pump activation on automatic canine Purkinje fibers. *J. Physiol. (Lond.),* 324:507–533.
181. Kline, R. P., Siegal, M. S., Henning, B., and Wit, A. L. (1986): Triggered activity in atrial fibers of the canine coronary sinus. The role of extracellular K^+ accumulation and depletion. *J. Physiol. (Lond.), (in press).*
182. Kline, R. P., Siegal, M. S., Kupersmith, J., and Wit, A. L. (1982): Effects of strophanthidin on changes in extracellular potassium during triggered activity in the arrhythmic canine coronary sinus. *Circulation [Suppl. II],* 66:356.
183. Kojima, M., and Sperelakis, N. (1984): Properties of oscillatory afterpotentials in young embryonic chick hearts. *Circ. Res.,* 55:497–503.
184. Kort, A. A., and Lakatta, E. G. (1984): Calcium-dependent mechanical oscillations occur spontaneously in unstimulated mammalian cardiac tissues. *Circ. Res.,* 54:396–404.
185. Kuck, K. H., Kunze, K. P., Roewer, N., and Bleifeld, W. (1984): Sotalol-induced torsade de pointes. *Am. Heart J.,* 107:179–180.
186. Kunze, D. L. (1977): Rate dependent changes in extracellular potassium in the rabbit atrium. *Circ. Res.,* 41:122–127.
187. Lab, M. J. (1978): Mechanically dependent changes in action potentials recorded from the intact frog ventricle. *Circ. Res.,* 42:519–528.
188. Lab, M. J. (1980): Transient depolarization and action potential alterations following mechanical changes in isolated myocardium. *Cardiovasc. Res.,* 14:624–637.
189. Lado, M. G., Sheu, S. S., and Fozzard, H. A. (1982): Changes in intracellular Ca^{2+} activity with stimulation in sheep cardiac Purkinje strands. *Am. J. Physiol.,* 243:H133–H137.
190. Lakatta, E. G., and Lappe, D. L. (1981): Diastolic scattered light fluctuation, resting force and twitch force in mammalian cardiac muscle. *J. Physiol. (Lond.),* 315:369–394.
191. Lazzara, R., El-Sherif, N., and Scherlag, B. J. (1973): Electrophysiological properties of canine Purkinje cells in one-day-old myocardial infarction. *Circ. Res.,* 33:722–734.
192. Lazzara, R., Hope, R. R., and Leh, B. K. (1978): Implication of CAMP and calcium as mediators of automaticity induced in working myocardium. *Am. J. Cardiol.,* 41:417.
193. Lederer, W. J., and Tsien, R. W. (1976): Transient inward current underlying arrhythmogenic effects of cardiotonic steroids in Purkinje fibers. *J. Physiol. (Lond.),* 263:73–100.
194. Lee, C. O., and D'Agostino, M. (1982): Effect of strophanthidin on intracellular Na ion activity and twitch tension of constantly driven canine cardiac Purkinje fibers. *Biophys. J.,* 40:185–198.
195. Lee, C. O., Kang, D. H., Sokol, J. H., and Lee, K. S. (1980): Relation between intracellular Na ion activity and tension of sheep cardiac Purkinje fibers exposed to dihydro-ouabain. *Biophys. J.,* 29:315–330.
196. Lefrak, E. A., Pitha, J., Rosenheim, S., and Gottlieb, J. A. (1973): A clinicopathologic analysis of adriamycin cardiotoxicity. *Cancer,* 32:302–314.
197. LeMarec, H., Spinelli, W., and Rosen, M. R. (1985): Effects of

doxorubicin on ventricular tachycardia in conscious dogs. *Circulation*, 72:226.

198. LeMarec, H., Dangman, K. H., Danilo, P., and Rosen, M. R. (1985): An evaluation of automaticity and triggered activity in the canine heart one to 4 days after myocardial infarction. *Circulation*, 71:1224–1236.

199. Lerman, B. B., Belardinelli, L., West, G. A., Berne, R. M., and DiMarco, J. P. (1986): Adenosine sensitive ventricular tachycardia: Evidence suggesting cyclic AMP triggered activity. *Circulation*, (*in press*).

200. Levi, R., Malm, J. R., Bowman, F. O., and Rosen, M. R. (1981): The arrhythmogenic actions of histamine on human atrial fibers. *Circ. Res.*, 49:545–550.

201. Levine, J. H., Spear, J. F., Guarnier, T., Weisfeldt, M., DeLangen, C. D. J., Becker, L. C., and Moore, E. N. (1985): Cesium chloride-induced long QT syndrome: Demonstration of afterdepolarizations and triggered activity in vivo. *Circulation*, 72:1092–1104.

202. Levine, J. H., Weisfeldt, M. L., Burkhoff, D., Franz, M. R., and Guarnieri, T. (1984): Delayed afterdepolarization in monophasic action potentials in vivo. *Circulation*, 70:222.

203. Lipsius, S. L., and Gibbons, W. R. (1982): Membrane currents, contractions and aftercontractions in cardiac Purkinje fibers. *Am. J. Physiol.*, 243:H77–H86.

204. Lown, B. (1968): Electrical stimulation to estimate the degree of digitalization. *Am. J. Cardiol.*, 22:251–259.

205. Lown, B., Cannon, R. L., and Rossi, M. A. (1967): Electrical stimulation and digitalis drugs: Repetitive response in diastole. *Proc. Soc. Exp. Biol. Med.*, 126:628–701.

206. Marban, E., and Tsien, R. W. (1982): Enhancement of calcium current during digitalis inotropy in mammalian heart: Positive feedback regulation by intracellular Ca? *J. Physiol.*, 329:589–614.

207. Marban, E., and Weir, W. G. (1985): Ryanodine suppresses drug-induced triggered arrhythmias in isolated ferret ventricular muscle. *Circulation*, 72:III–380.

208. Mary-Rabine, L., Hordof, A. J., Danilo, P., Malm, J. R., and Rosen, M. R. (1980): Mechanisms for impulse initiation in isolated human atrial fibers. *Circ. Res.*, 47:267–277.

209. Mason, J. W., Swerdlow, C. D., and Mitchell, L. B. (1983): Efficacy of verapamil in chronic, recurrent ventricular tachycardia. *Am. J. Cardiol.*, 51:1614–1617.

210. Matsuda, H., Noma, A., Kurachi, Y., and Irisawa, H. (1982): Transient depolarization and spontaneous voltage fluctuations in isolated single cells from guinea-pig ventricles: Calcium-mediated membrane potential fluctuations. *Circ. Res.*, 51:142–151.

211. Matsuda, K., Hoffman, B. F., Ellner, C. N., Katz, M., and Brooks, C. M. (1953): Veratridine-induced prolongation of repolarization in the mammalian heart. In: *Nineteenth International Physiological Congress*, pp. 596–597. American Physiological Society.

212. Matsuda, K., Hoshi, T., and Kameyama, S. (1959): Effects of aconitine on the cardiac membrane potential of the dog. *Jpn. J. Physiol.*, 9:419–429.

213. McAllister, R. E., Noble, D., and Tsien, R. W. (1975): Reconstruction of the electrical activity of cardiac Purkinje fibers. *J. Physiol. (Lond.)*, 251:1–59.

214. McAllister, R. E., and Noble, D. (1966): The time and voltage dependence of the slow outward current in cardiac Purkinje fibers. *J. Physiol. (Lond.)*, 186:632–662.

215. Mendez, C., and Delmar, M. (1984): Triggered activity: Its possible role in cardiac arrhythmias. In: *Cardiac Electrophysiology and Arrhythmias*, edited by D. P. Zipes and J. Jalife, pp. 311–314. Grune & Stratton, New York.

216. Moak, J. P., and Rosen, M. R. (1984): Induction and termination of triggered activity by pacing in isolated canine Purkinje fibers. *Circulation*, 69:149–162.

217. Moe, G. K., Jalife, J., Mueller, W. J., and Moe, B. (1977): A mathematical model of parasystole and its application to clinical arrhythmias. *Circulation*, 56:968–979.

218. Morad, M., and Goldman, Y. (1973): Excitation-contraction coupling in heart muscle: Membrane control of development of tension. *Prog. Biophys. Mol. Biol.*, 27:259–316.

219. Morad, M., and Rolett, E. (1972): Relaxing effect of catecholamine on mammalian heart. *J. Physiol. (Lond.)*, 224:537–558.

220. Mugelli, A. (1982): Separation of the oscillatory current from

other currents in cardiac Purkinje fibers. *Cardiovasc. Res.*, 16:637–645.

221. Mullins, L. J. (1979): The generation of electrical currents in cardiac fibers by Na/Ca exchange. *Am. J. Physiol.*, 236:C103–C110.

222. Mullins, L. J. (1981): *Ion Transport in Heart*. Raven Press, New York.

223. Mullins, L. J., and Requena, J. (1981): The "late" Ca channel in squid axons. *J. Gen. Physiol.*, 78:683–700.

224. Mullins, L. J., Tiffert, T., Vassort, G., and Wittemby, J. (1983): Effects of internal sodium and hydrogen ions and of external calcium ions and membrane potential on calcium entry in squid axons. *J. Physiol. (Lond.)*, 338:295–319.

225. Nathan, D., and Beeler, G. W. (1975): Electrophysiologic correlates of the inotropic effects of isoproterenol in canine myocardium. *J. Mol. Cell. Cardiol.*, 7:1–15.

226. Noble, D. (1984): The surprising heart: A review of recent progress in cardiac electrophysiology. *J. Physiol. (Lond.)*, 353:1–50.

227. Nordin, C., Gilat, E., and Aronson, R. S. (1985): Delayed afterdepolarizations and triggered activity in ventricular muscle from rats with streptozotocin-induced diabetes. *Circ. Res.*, 57:28–34.

228. Olshansky, B., Martins, J., and Hunt, S. (1982): *N*-acetylprocainamide causing torsades de pointes. *Am. J. Cardiol.*, 50:1439–1441.

229. Orchard, C. H., Eisner, D. A., and Allen, D. G. (1983): Oscillations of intracellular Ca^{2+} in mammalian cardiac muscle. *Nature*, 304:735–738.

230. Palade, P., Mitchell, R. D., and Fleisher, S. (1983): Spontaneous calcium release from sarcoplasmic reticulum. General description and effects of calcium. *J. Biol. Chem.*, 258:8098–8107.

231. Palileo, E. V., Ashley, W. W., Swiryn, S., Bauernfeind, R. A., Strasberg, B., Petropoulos, A. T., and Rosen, K. M. (1982): Exercise-provocable right ventricular outflow tract tachycardia. *Am. Heart J.*, 104:185–193.

232. Paspa, P., and Vassalle, M. (1984): Mechanism of caffeine-induced arrhythmias in cardiac Purkinje fibers. *Am. J. Cardiol.*, 53:313–319.

233. Peper, K., and Trautwein, W. (1966): Über den Mechanismus der Extrasystolen des Aconitin-vergifteten Herzmuskels. *Pfluegers Arch.*, 291:R16.

234. Rahilly, G. T., Prystowsky, E. N., Zipes, D. P., Naccarelli, G. V., Jackman, W. M., and Heger, J. J. (1982): Clinical and electrophysiologic findings in patients with repetitive monomorphic ventricular tachycardia and otherwise normal electrocardiogram. *Am. J. Cardiol.*, 50:459–468.

235. Reiffel, J. A., Gang, E., Gliklich, J., Weiss, M. B., Davis, J. C., Patton, J. N., and Bigger, J. T., Jr. (1980): The human sinus node electrogram: A transvenous catheter technique and a comparison of directly measured and indirectly estimated sinoatrial conduction time in adults. *Circulation*, 62:1324–1334.

236. Reuter, H. (1973): Divalent cations as charge carriers in excitable membranes. *Prog. Biophys. Mol. Biol.*, 26:1–43.

237. Reuter, H. (1974): Localization of beta adrenergic receptors and effects of noradrenaline and cyclic nucleotides on action potentials, ionic currents and tension in mammalian cardiac muscle. *J. Physiol. (Lond.)*, 242:429–451.

238. Reuter, H., and Scholz, H. (1977): The regulation of the calcium conductance of cardiac muscle by adrenaline. *J. Physiol. (Lond.)*, 264:49–62.

239. Reuter, H., and Seitz, N. (1968): The dependence of calcium efflux from cardiac muscle on temperature and external ion composition. *J. Physiol. (Lond.)*, 195:451–470.

240. Roden, D. M., and Hoffman, B. F. (1985): Action potential prolongation and induction of abnormal automaticity by low quinidine concentrations in canine Purkinje fibers. Relationship to potassium and cycle length. *Circ. Res.*, 56:857–867.

241. Rosen, M. R., and Danilo, P. (1980): Digitalis-induced delayed afterdepolarizations. In: *The Slow Inward Current and Cardiac Arrhythmias*, edited by D. P. Zipes, J. C. Bailey, and V. Elharrar, pp. 417–436. Martinus Nijhoff, The Hague.

242. Rosen, M. R., and Danilo, P. (1980): Effects of tetrodotoxin, lidocaine, verapamil and AHR-2666 on ouabain-induced delayed afterdepolarizations in canine Purkinje fibers. *Circ. Res.*, 46:117–124.

243. Rosen, M. R., Danilo, P., Alonso, M. B., and Pippenger, C. E. (1974): Effects of therapeutic concentrations of diphenylhydantoin on transmembrane potentials of normal and depressed Purkinje fibers. *J. Pharmacol. Exp. Ther.*, 197:594–604.

244. Rosen, M. R., Fisch, C., Hoffman, B. F., Danilo, P., Lovelace, D. E., and Knoebel, S. B. (1980): Can accelerated AV junctional escape rhythms be explained by delayed afterdepolarization? *Am. J. Cardiol.*, 45:1272–1282.

245. Rosen, M. R., Gelband, H. B., Merker, C., and Hoffman, B. F. (1973): Mechanics of digitalis toxicity. Effects of ouabain on phase 4 of canine Purkinje fiber transmembrane potentials. *Circulation*, 47:681–689.

246. Rosen, M. R., Gelband, H. B., and Hoffman, B. F. (1973): Correlation between effects of ouabain on the canine electrocardiogram and transmembrane potentials of isolated Purkinje fibers. *Circulation*, 47:65–72.

247. Rosen, M. R., Ilvento, J. P., Gelband, H., and Merker, C. (1974): Effect of verapamil on electrophysiologic properties of canine cardiac Purkinje fibers. *J. Pharmacol. Exp. Ther.*, 189:414–422.

248. Rosen, M. R., and Reder, R. F. (1981): Does triggered activity have a role in the genesis of cardiac arrhythmias? *Ann. Intern. Med.*, 94:794–801.

249. Saito, T., Otoguro, M., and Matsubara, T. (1978): Electrophysiological studies on the mechanism of electrically induced sustained rhythmic activity in the rabbit right atrium. *Circ. Res.*, 42:199–206.

250. Sano, T., and Sawanobori, T. (1972): Abnormal automaticity in canine Purkinje fibers focally subjected to low external concentrations of calcium. *Circ. Res.*, 16:423–430.

251. Saunders, J. H., Ferrier, G. R., and Moe, G. K. (1973): Conduction block associated with transient depolarizations induced by acetylstrophanthidin in isolated canine Purkinje fibers. *Circ. Res.*, 32:610–617.

252. Schechter, E., Freeman, C. C., Lazzara, R. (1984): Afterdepolarizations as a mechanism for the long QT syndrome: Electrophysiologic studies of a case. *J. Am. Coll. Cardiol.*, 3:1556–1562.

253. Scherf, D., and Schott, A. (1973): *Extrasystoles and Allied Arrhythmias.* Heinemann, Chicago.

254. Schmidt, R. F. (1960): Versuche mit Aconitin zum Problem der spontanen Erregungsbildung im Herzen. *Pfluegers Arch.*, 271:526–536.

255. Segers, M. (1947): Le battement auto-entretenu du coeur. *Arch. Int. Pharmacodyn.*, 75:144–156.

256. Selzer, A., and Wray, H. W. (1964): Quinidine syncope. Paroxysmal ventricular fibrillation occurring during treatment of chronic atrial arrhythmias. *Circulation*, 30:17–26.

257. Sheu, S. S., and Fozzard, H. A. (1982): Transmembrane Na$^+$ and Ca^{2+} electrochemical gradients in cardiac muscle and their relationship to force development. *J. Gen. Physiol.*, 80:325–351.

258. Sheu, S. S., and Lederer, W. J. (1985): Lidocaine's negative inotropic and antiarrhythmic actions: Dependence on shortening of action potential duration and reduction of intracellular sodium activity. *Circ. Res.*, 57:578–590.

259. Singer, D. H., Baumgarten, C. M., and Ten Eick, R. E. (1981): Cellular electrophysiology of ventricular and other dysrhythmias: Studies on diseased and ischemic heart. *Prog. Cardiovasc. Dis.*, 24:97–156.

260. Smith, W. M., and Gallagher, J. J. (1980): Les torsades de pointes. An unusual ventricular arrhythmia. *Ann. Intern. Med.*, 93:578–584.

261. Sperelakis, N. (1972): Electrical properties of embryonic heart cells. In: *Electrical Phenomena in the Heart*, edited by W. C. DeMello, pp. 1–62. Academic Press, New York.

262. Stern, M. D., Kort, A. A., Bhatnagar, G., and Lakatta, E. G. (1983): Scattered-light intensity fluctuations in diastolic rat cardiac muscle caused by spontaneous Ca^{++}-dependent cellular mechanical oscillations. *J. Gen. Physiol.*, 82:119–153.

263. Stratmann, H. G., Walter, K. E., and Kennedy, H. L. (1985): Torsade de pointes associated with elevated N-acetylprocainamide. *Am. Heart J.*, 109:375–377.

264. Strauss, H. C., Bigger, J. R., and Hoffman, B. F. (1970): Electrophysiological and beta-blocking effects of MJ-1999 on dog and rabbit cardiac tissue. *Circ. Res.*, 26:661–678.

265. Sung, R. J., Shapiro, W. A., Shen, E. N., Morady, F., and Davis, J. (1983): Effects of verapamil on ventricular tachycardias possibly caused by reentry, automaticity, and triggered activity. *J. Clin. Invest.*, 72:350–360.

266. Sutko, J. L., and Kenyon, J. L. (1983): Ryanodine modification of cardiac muscle responses to potassium-free solutions. Evidence for inhibition of sarcoplasmic reticulum calcium release. *J. Gen. Physiol.*, 82:385–404.

267. Temte, J. V., and Davis, L. D. (1967): Effect of calcium concentration on the transmembrane potentials of Purkinje fibers. *Circ. Res.*, 20:32–44.

268. Ten Eick, R., Nawrath, H., McDonald, T. F., and Trautwein, W. (1976): On the mechanism of the negative inotropic effect of acetylcholine. *Pfluegers Arch.*, 361:207–213.

269. Ten Eick, R. E., and Singer, D. H. (1979): Electrophysiological properties of diseased human atrium: I. Low diastolic potential and altered cellular response to potassium. *Circ. Res.*, 44:545–557.

270. Trautwein, W. (1970): Mechanisms of tachyarrhythmias and extrasystoles. In: *Symposium on Cardiac Arrhythmias*, edited by E. Sandoe, E. Flenstad-Jensen, and K. Olesen, pp. 53–66. Ab Astra, Sodertalje, Sweden.

271. Trautwein, W., Gottstein, U., and Dudel, J. (1954): Der Aktionsstrom der myokard Faser im Sauerstoffmangel. *Pfluegers Arch.*, 260:40–60.

272. Tseng, G., and Wit, A. L. (1985): Arrhythmogenic effects of quinidine on triggered activity in atrial muscle. *Circulation*, 72:III-380.

273. Tseng, G. N., and Wit, A. L. (1984): Characteristics of a transient inward current causing catecholamine-induced triggered atrial tachycardia. *Circulation*, 70:221.

274. Tsien, R. W., Kass, R. S., and Weingart, R. (1979): Cellular and subcellular mechanisms of cardiac pacemaker oscillations. *J. Exp. Biol.*, 81:205–215.

275. Valdeolmillos, M., and Eisner, D. A. (1985): The effects of ryanodine on calcium-overloaded sheep cardiac Purkinje fibers. *Circ. Res.*, 56:452–456.

276. Valenzuela, F., and Vassalle, M. (1983): Interaction between overdrive excitation and overdrive suppression in canine Purkinje fibers. *Cardiovasc. Res.*, 17:608–619.

277. Valenzuela, F., and Vassalle, M. (1985): Overdrive excitation and cellular calcium load in canine cardiac Purkinje fibers. *J. Electrocardiol.*, 18:21–29.

278. Van Capelle, F. J. L., and Durrer, D. (1980): Computer simulation of arrhythmias in a network of coupled excitable elements. *Circ. Res.*, 47:454–466.

279. Vassalle, M. (1970): Electrogenic suppression of automaticity in sheep and dog Purkinje fibers. *Circ. Res.*, 27:361–377.

280. Vassalle, M. (1977): The relationship among cardiac pacemakers: Overdrive suppression. *Circ. Res.*, 41:268–277.

281. Vassalle, M. (1979): Electrogenesis of the plateau and pacemaker potential. *Annu. Rev. Physiol.*, 41:425–440.

282. Vassalle, M. (1985): Overdrive excitation: The onset of spontaneous activity following a fast drive. In: *Cardiac Electrophysiology and Arrhythmias*, edited by D. P. Zipes and J. Jalife, pp. 97–107. Grune & Stratton, Orlando.

283. Vassalle, M., and Bhattacharyya, M. (1981): Interactions of norepinephrine and strophanthidin in cardiac Purkinje fibers. *Int. J. Cardiol.*, 1:179.

284. Vassalle, M., and Bhattacharyya, M. T. (1978): Role of sodium in strophanthidin toxicity in cardiac Purkinje fibers. *Am. J. Physiol.*, 243:H477–H486.

285. Vassalle, M., Caress, D. L., Slovin, A. J., and Stuckey, J. H. (1967): On the cause of ventricular asystole during vagal stimulation. *Circ. Res.*, 20:228–241.

286. Vassalle, M., and Carpentier, R. (1972): Overdrive excitation: Onset of activity following fast drive in cardiac Purkinje fibers exposed to norepinephrine. *Pfluegers Arch.*, 332:198–205.

287. Vassalle, M., Cummins, M., Castro, C., and Stuckey, J. H. (1976): The relationship between overdrive suppression and overdrive excitation in ventricular pacemakers in dogs. *Circ. Res.*, 38:367–374.

288. Vassalle, M., and DiGennaro, M. (1983): Caffeine eliminates the oscillatory current in cardiac Purkinje fibers. *Eur. J. Pharmacol.*, 94:361–362.

289. Vassalle, M., and DiGennaro, M. D. (1985): Caffeine actions on

currents induced by calcium overload in Purkinje fibers. *Eur. J. Pharmacology,* 106:121–131.

290. Vassalle, M., Knob, R. E., Cummins, M., Lara, G. A., Castro, C., and Stuckey, J. H. (1977): An analysis of fast idioventricular rhythm in the dog. *Circ. Res.,* 41:218–226.

291. Vassalle, M., Knob, R. E., Lara, G. A., and Stuckey, J. H. (1976): The effect of adrenergic enhancement on overdrive excitation. *J. Electrocardiol.,* 9:335–343.

292. Vassalle, M., and Lee, C. O. (1984): The relationship among intracellular sodium activity, calcium, and strophanthidin inotropy in canine cardiac Purkinje fibers. *J. Gen. Physiol.,* 83:287–307.

293. Vassalle, M., and Mugelli, A. (1981): An oscillatory current in sheep cardiac Purkinje fibers. *Circ. Res.,* 48:618–631.

294. Van Ginnehen, A. (1983): Oscillatory currents in aggregates of neonatal rat heart cells. *Biophys. J.,* 41:176.

295. Wald, R. W., and Waxman, M. B. (1981): Pacing-induced automaticity in sheep Purkinje fibers. *Circ. Res.,* 48:531–538.

296. Waldo, A. L., Cooper, T. B., and MacLean, W. A. H. (1977): Need for additional criteria for the diagnosis of sinus node reentrant tachycardias. *J. Electrocardiol.,* 10:103–104.

297. Waldo, A. L., Cooper, T. B., and MacLean, W. A. H. (1978): Overdrive pacing for supraventricular tachycardia: A review of theoretical implications and therapeutic techniques. *Pace,* 1:196.

298. Ward, D. E., Nathan, A. W., and Camm, A. J. (1984): Fascicular tachycardia sensitive to calcium antagonists. *Eur. Heart J.,* 5:896–905.

299. Wasserstrom, J. A., and Ferrier, G. R. (1981): Voltage dependence of digitalis afterpotentials, aftercontractions, and inotropy. *Am. J. Physiol.,* 241:H646–H653.

300. Wasserstrom, J. A., and Ferrier, G. R. (1982): Effects of phenytoin and quinidine on digitalis-induced oscillatory afterpotentials, aftercontractions and inotropy in canine ventricular tissues. *J. Mol. Cell. Cardiol.,* 14:725–736.

301. Weber, A., and Herz, R. (1968): The relationship between caffeine contracture of intact muscle and the effect of caffeine on reticulum. *J. Gen. Physiol.,* 52:750–759.

302. Weidmann, S. (1955): Effects of calcium ions and local anesthetics on electrical properties of Purkinje fibers. *J. Physiol.,* 129:568–582.

303. Weir, W. G., Kort, A. A., Stern, M. D., Lakatta, E. G., and Marban, E. (1983): Cellular calcium fluctuations in mammalian heart: Direct evidence from noise analysis of aequorin signals in Purkinje fibers. *Proc. Natl. Acad. Sci. (USA),* 80:7367–7371.

304. Weld, F. M., Bigger, J. T., Swistel, D., Bordiuk, J., and Lau, Y. H. (1979): Electrophysiological effects of mexiletine (K-1173) on ovine cardiac Purkinje fibers. *J. Pharmacol. Exp. Ther.,* 210:222–228.

305. Wellens, H. J. J. (1978): Value and limitations of programmed electrical stimulation of the heart in the study and treatment of tachycardia. *Circulation,* 57:845–853.

306. Wellens, H. J. J., Bar, F. W., Farre, J., Ross, D. L., Weiner, I., and Vanagt, E. J. (1980): Initiation and termination of ventricular tachycardia by supraventricular stimuli: Incidence and electrophysiologic determinants as observed during programmed stimulation of the heart. *Am. J. Cardiol.,* 46:576–580.

307. Wellens, H. J. J., and Brugada, P. (1984): Value of programmed stimulation of the heart in patients with the Wolff-Parkinson-White syndrome. In: *Tachycardias: Mechanisms, Diagnosis, Treatment,* edited by M. E. Josephson and H. J. J. Wellens, pp. 199–221. Lea & Febiger, Philadelphia.

308. Wellens, H. J. J., Schuilenburg, R. M., and Durrer, D. (1972): Electrical stimulation of the heart in patients with ventricular tachycardia. *Circulation,* 46:216–226.

309. Wenckebach, K. F., and Winterberg, H. (1927): *Die unregelmassige Herztatigkeit.* Engelmann, Leipzig.

310. West, T. C. (1961): Effects of chronotropic influences on subthreshold oscillations in the sino-atrial node. In: *The Specialized Tissues of the Heart,* edited by A. Paes de Carvalho, W. C. DeMello, and B. F. Hoffman, pp. 81–94. Elsevier, New York.

311. Wiggins, J. R., and Cranefield, P. F. (1976): Two levels of resting potential in canine cardiac Purkinje fibers exposed to sodium-free solutions. *Circ. Res.,* 39:466–474.

312. Wit, A. L., Allessie, M. A., Bonke, F. I. M., Lammers, W., Smeets, J., and Fenoglio, J. J., Jr. (1982): Electrophysiologic mapping to determine the mechanism of experimental ventricular tachycardia initiated by premature impulses: Experimental approach and initial results demonstrating reentrant excitation. *Am. J. Cardiol.,* 49:166–185.

313. Wit, A. L., Boyden, P. A., Gadsby, D. C., and Cranefield, P. F. (1979): Triggered activity as a cause of atrial arrhythmias. In: *Cardiac Arrhythmias: Electrophysiology, Diagnosis and Management,* edited by O. S. Narula, pp. 14–31. Williams & Wilkins, Baltimore.

314. Wit, A. L., and Cranefield, P. F. (1976): Triggered activity in cardiac muscle fibers of the simian mitral valve. *Circ. Res.,* 38:85–98.

315. Wit, A. L., and Cranefield, P. F. (1977): Triggered and automatic activity in the canine coronary sinus. *Circ. Res.,* 41:435–445.

316. Wit, A. L., Cranefield, P. F., and Gadsby, D. C. (1980): Triggered activity. In: *The Slow Inward Current and Cardiac Arrhythmias,* edited by D. P. Zipes, J. C. Bailey, and V. Elharrar, pp. 437–454. Martinus Nijhoff, The Hague.

317. Wit, A. L., Cranefield, P. F., and Gadsby, D. C. (1981): Electrogenic sodium extrusion can stop triggered activity in the canine coronary sinus. *Circ. Res.,* 49:1029–1042.

318. Wit, A. L., Cranefield, P. F., and Hoffman, B. F. (1972): Slow conduction and reentry in the ventricular conducting system. II. Single and sustained circus movement in networks of canine and bovine Purkinje fibers. *Circ. Res.,* 30:11–22.

319. Wit, A. L., Fenoglio, J. J., Jr., Hordof, A. J., and Reemtsma, K. (1979): Ultrastructure and transmembrane potentials of cardiac muscle in the human anterior mitral valve leaflet. *Circulation,* 59:1284–1292.

320. Wit, A. L., Wiggins, J. R., and Cranefield, P. F. (1976): The effects of electrical stimulation on impulse initiation in cardiac fibers; its relevance for the determination of the mechanisms of clinical cardiac arrhythmias. In: *The Conduction System of the Heart: Structure, Function, and Clinical Implications,* edited by H. J. J. Wellens, K. I. Lie, and M. J. Janse, pp. 163–181. Stenfert Kroese, Leiden.

321. Wittenberg, S. M., Streuli, F., and Klocke, F. J. (1970): Acceleration of ventricular pacemakers by transient increases in heart rate in dogs during ouabain administration. *Circ. Res.,* 26:705–716.

322. Wu, D., Amat-Y-Leon, F., Denes, P., Dhingra, R. C., Pietras, R. J., and Rosen, K. M. (1975): Demonstration of sustained sinus and atrial reentry as a mechanism of paroxysmal supraventricular tachycardia. *Circulation,* 51:234–243.

323. Wu, D., Kou, H. C., and Hung, J. S. (1981): Exercise-triggered paroxysmal ventricular tachycardia: A repetitive rhythmic activity possibly related to afterdepolarization. *Ann. Intern. Med.,* 95:410–414.

324. Zipes, D. P., Arbel, E., Knope, R. F., and Moe, G. K. (1974): Accelerated cardiac escape rhythms caused by ouabain intoxication. *Am. J. Cardiol.,* 33:248–253.

325. Zipes, D. P., Foster, P. R., Troup, P. J., and Pendersen, D. H. (1979): Atrial induction of ventricular tachycardia: Reentry vs. triggered automaticity. *Am. J. Cardiol.,* 44:1–7.

326. Zipes, D. P., Foster, P. R., Troup, P. J., and Pendersen, D. H. (1979): Atrial induction of ventricular tachycardia: Reentry vs. triggered automaticity. *Am. J. Cardiol.,* 44:1–7.

The Heart and Cardiovascular System,
edited by H. A. Fozzard et al.
Raven Press, New York © 1986.

CHAPTER 61

Biological Mechanisms of Hypertrophy

Lawrence Bugaisky and Radovan Zak

Cardiac muscle growth can be envisioned to be regulated by two sets of factors: those that during normal growth maintain the proper allometric ratio of heart to body size, and those that are responsible for matching the heart size to the functional load during adaptation to altered hemodynamic requirements. It must be realized, however, that often this distinction is merely hypothetical, because normal growth can be accompanied by altered function. This is best demonstrated by the dramatic changes in the growth of the two ventricles of the heart following parturition. Such growth becomes primarily influenced by the increased peripheral resistance, which is superimposed on the inverted exponential growth curve, typical of the same period. Despite the lack of a clear distinction in the foregoing example between normal growth and that due to altered function, experimental delineation of time- and function-dependent factors holds the key to an eventual understanding of the nature of adaptive cardiac growth.

Early biochemical studies of cardiac growth centered on the descriptive approaches, such as evaluation of protein composition and metabolic and biosynthetic pathways (2). These types of studies provided a considerable amount of information that suggested the dynamic nature of the heart. When appropriately challenged, the heart can sustain a considerable workload. At the same time, it can become an efficient protein-synthetic machine, with output similar to very active cells (e.g. hemoglobin-reproducing reticulocytes). Conversely, when the load of the heart decreases, the degradation of the constituent proteins is highly stimulated, and the heart's size ultimately diminishes.

During growth, the activation of the biosynthetic pathways is manifested by rapid changes in cardiac RNAs (149). Evidence of this can be found in the increased DNA-dependent RNA polymerase activity, labelling of nascent RNA with tracers, and in the amount of total RNA, which all provide an accurate index for the biosynthetic state of the organ. Increased protein-synthesizing capacity in the heart (and other eucaryotic cells) is thus not carried out by simply increasing the level of mRNA, as in bacteria, but by a proportional increase of all species of RNA.

Recent impressive progress in recombinant DNA technology has yielded experimental tools, with which cardiac hypertrophy can be examined at the molecular level. Thus, rather than measuring the products of multiple genes, the activity of specific genes will be accessible for investigation. Once a gene's anatomy, including it's regulatory domain, is defined, the quest for growth-controlling factors will be on much more solid ground than it is at present.

NORMAL DEVELOPMENT OF THE HEART

Cytodifferentiation of Cardiac Myocytes

A general description of the earliest stages of muscle differentiation can be formulated that applies to both mammals and birds (71). The majority of experimental work, however, has been undertaken in chicken because of ease of developmental staging.

Myogenesis in the heart bears a resemblance to that observed in skeletal muscle, but significant differences exist in several critical features (148). In both skeletal and cardiac muscle, the first stage of differentiation consists of proliferation of nondifferentiated precursor cells, referred to as presumptive myoblasts or premyoblasts (92). These myoblastic cells, which are derived from precardiac splanchnic mesoderm, possess no apparent identifiable characteristics to distinguish them from other types of proliferating cells.

In the next stage of differentiation, which can be considered "overt myogenesis" (i.e., the cells can be definitively identified as muscle cells by particular cellular constituents), the presumptive myoblasts begin to elongate, and some initiate synthesis of muscle-specific proteins. The synthesis of these contractile proteins culminates in the appearance of cross-striations and spontaneous contractions. Such cells can be referred to as developing myocytes (92).

Because cytodifferentiation in the heart is not synchronized, the presumptive myoblasts and developing myocytes initially coexist. Eventually, however, more and more cells initiate synthesis of cell-specific proteins, and all the cells acquire myofibrils. With the accumulation of myofibrillar mass, the developing myocytes are gradually transformed to fully functioning adult myocytes. Myofibrillar acquisition by all cardiac cells contrasts with that in skeletal muscle, in which a sizable population of myogenic precursor cells (satellite cells) remain even in the adult muscle (147). At present, differentiated myogenic cells have not been identified in the heart, although micrographs have shown that cells that bear a resemblance to satellite cells have been observed to bind tightly to myocytes in adult rat ventricles (35).

Even at the advanced stages of cytodifferentiation in cardiac cells described earlier, mitosis and cellular division still occur (91). This duality of heart-specific protein expression and DNA synthesis stands in opposition to the situation in skeletal muscle, where only the myoblasts are able to proliferate during myogenesis. In skeletal myogenesis, once the multinucleated myotube formation and synthesis of muscle-specific proteins begin, DNA synthesis in the incorporated myoblast nucleus is repressed. These multinucleated myotubes eventually become multinucleated "structural" syncytia, known as myofibers. Cardiac tissue, on the other hand, will form a "functional" syncytium because of tight, low-resistance junctions between the mostly (greater than 90%) binucleated myocytes.

Because cardiac myogenesis takes place prior to any apparent physiological influence from the undeveloped circulatory system, it may be safe to assume that the previously described events are governed by a time-dependent developmental program. This is further illustrated by the fact that the basic events leading to cardiomyogenesis can be reproduced in primary cultures of cardiac cells obtained from embryonic hearts of rats and chickens. Such in vitro experiments have confirmed that, first of all, there is "an in vivo shift of myoblasts to myocytes in the muscle cell population as the rat ages" (98). Second, cells containing myofibrils can both beat and divide (75,77,94).

Cardiac Morphogenesis

Heart formation in the chick begins with the inward movement of two folds of precardiac mesoderm, which eventually fuse to form a tubular heart rudiment (71). During the next stage, the tubular heart becomes asymmetric through its bending and rotation to the right, a process referred to as "looping." This transformation coincides with the first contractile activity, but appears to be independent of it (93). When the beating of the heart is blocked, the progression of looping is not altered from that seen in functioning hearts. When sarcomere assembly or protein synthesis is prevented, however, no looping takes place. Thus, the first morphological transformation of the heart depends on a critical mass of myofilaments.

When cardiac morphogenesis begins, each region of the primitive heart tube consists of a homogeneous myocardial layer, only several cells thick, and the endocardial portion, which is separated from the myocardium by the extracellular matrix of cardiac jelly. Only myocytes are present; there are no fibroblasts, coronary vessels, or differentiated conduction tissue (92).

After looping, cardiac morphogenesis becomes progressively more complex, with a variety of nonmuscle cells invading the myocardium. This results in the heart's gradual conversion to an organ containing a heterogeneous cell population. In general, the nonmuscle cells have greater mitotic activity, so that eventually they outnumber myocytes by a ratio of 3 to 1. Some of the cell types found in this population of nonmuscle cells include fibroblasts, endothelial cells, nerve cells, and phagocytes (Fig. 1). The importance of these nonmuscle cells can be illustrated by several recent in vitro experiments.

By using time-lapse cinematography, Gross (65) demonstrated frequent interactions between fibroblasts and myocytes during cardiomyogenesis in culture. Several different phenomena were observed in this study, including fibroblast-monocyte contact, myocyte movement with the fibroblasts, and accelerated formation of polarized myocytes, with resulting beating. Additionally, the joining of myocytes in a fibroblast-free area of a culture was an extremely rare event. Gross hypothesized that, as a rule, myocytes do not unite in culture to form their syncytial beating masses without the aid of fibroblasts. Precisely how strict this relationship is in vivo is still unknown, although we do know that the earliest stages of cardiomyogenesis occur in a homogeneous myocyte population.

HEART CELL PEDIGREES

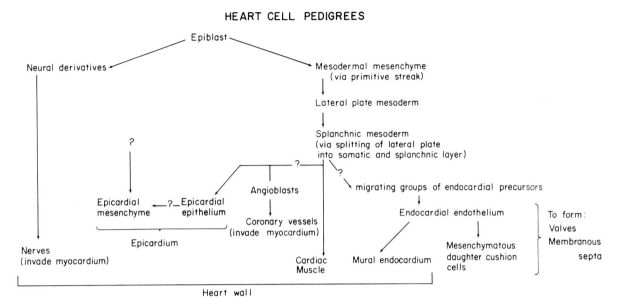

FIG. 1. Splanchnic mesoderm layers of the developing embryo give rise, directly or indirectly, to most of the cell types that form the heart. These include myocardium, endocardium, valves, membranous septa, and epicardium. Each cell type has a distinct lineage that becomes segregated early in cardiac development. The autonomic nerves invade the myocardium later in embryonic development. A question mark indicates that tissue origin is not certain (Courtesy of F. J. Manesek).

Furthermore, it has been demonstrated that the metabolic interactions between myocytes and fibroblasts constitute more than a mere additive effect. In fact, the two cell populations "coexist in a metabolically functional synergism" (124). This is based on a series of observations demonstrating that *mixed cultures* utilize glucose more rapidly than enriched cultures of either myocytes or fibroblasts and that they are insulin-sensitive (whereas enriched cultures of myocytes are not) and are more resistant to starvation.

Finally, a striking example of the importance of myocyte-nonmyocyte interaction can be observed in the *in vivo* work of Borg and Caulfield (14). When neonatal rats were treated with a drug (BAPN) that prevented cross-linking of collagen, a major product of connective tissue cells, the hearts did not attain their normal ellipsoid shape. Instead, they appeared globular and presented evidence of ventricular aneurysms. Thus, the lack of production of a nonmyocyte synthetic product results in structural instability in the heart.

After looping, the heart morphologically and functionally separates into atrial, ventricular, and conotruncal regions by the development of endocardial cushions (71). The atrium differentiates into thin-walled, venous receptacles, and the ventricular myocardium thickens through trabeculation. From the onset of myocardial contractility, each region of the heart has its own intrinsic rate of contraction (142). These observed differences in contraction rates are not associated with any currently identifiable markers in gross morphology, stages of cytodifferentiation, or functional demands placed on ventricular, atrial, or sinus venosus primordia. [We have

also observed this intrinsic difference in tissue cultures made from atrium or ventricle (19).] Moreover, the membrane specializations and ion transport systems appear to be primitive at this stage, although some regional differences are already noticeable (135).

Certainly, the distinction between endogenous developmental programs and the influence of circulation on cardiac morphogenesis is difficult to determine at this point, because both heart and circulation develop simultaneously. It seems, however, that hemodynamic factors do influence the progression of morphogenesis. For example, occlusion of the atrioventricular canal was shown to result in an abnormally small left atrium and ventricle and concurrent enlargement of the right heart chamber (26).

Other factors that should be considered when discussing the cytodifferentiation and morphogenesis of the heart are the roles of the nervous and neurohumoral systems.

During embryogenesis in the rat, the heart begins to beat about 9.6 days after conception (63). Adrenergic and cholinergic responses have been reported in the heart at 10 and 10.5 days, respectively (115). By 14 to 16 days, the fetal heart can respond to a wide variety of stimuli, including uterine contraction, hypoxia, hypercapnia, needle prick, and norepinephrine (1). Because nerves do not invade the sinus pacemaker until about 16 days *in utero* (61), these early responses may be either self-regulated or dependent on neurohumoral influences. Also, functional sympathetic innervation (i.e., response to reflex stimulation) does not appear in most rats until 6 to 8 days of postnatal age (7). This time course can, however, be accelerated to as early as 2 days after birth by triiodothyronine administration (82).

Several investigators have suggested that sympathetic innervation of cardiac muscle is involved in the control of myocyte proliferation and differentiation (7,28,41). Alternatively, it has been suggested that such innervation may in fact not be "obligatory" to the normal development of the heart (6). Further complicating this situation is the fact that despite the lack of functional neurotransmission, receptors are already present in the early neonate (41). In this way, when examining the early role of nervous influences in the heart, two different effects must be considered: first, the actual nervous transmission, and second, the humoral influences. The isolated cardiac myocyte in tissue culture is a potentially rich source of information regarding both nervous and neurohumoral effectors and the role of sympathetic innervation, or the lack thereof, on cardiac myocyte development and function.

Experiments in tissue culture have already produced evidence to suggest that *in vitro* nervous tissue can influence contractile protein expression in both skeletal and cardiac muscle (50,141). Co-culturing of cardiac myocytes from embryonic chick with motor or sympathetic neurons, or in medium containing nerve extract, produced immunologic staining specific for adult cardiac troponin. In the absence of nerves, the myocytes stained with both skeletal and cardiac troponin antibodies, similar to the embryo *in vivo*. Ecob et al. (50) have used immunofluorescence in mouse cultures to show that newly formed myofibers in skeletal muscle react with antibodies to adult fast myosin. This "maturation" occurs only after dendrites from dorsal root ganglia contact the muscle. In an electrophysiological study (57), microcultures of cardiac cells from newborn rats in culture responded differently, depending on whether there was interaction with adrenergic or cholinergic co-cultured nerves. In yet another study, it has been proposed that cell proliferation may be controlled by adrenergic innervation, using norepinephrine and cAMP as chemical mediators (28). These experiments clearly demonstrate that both biochemical and physiological characteristics of myocytes in culture can be modified by nervous influences.

Although it is clear that the nervous system is one of the factors that control cell proliferation, the ultimate mechanism responsible for the decline in the mitotic activity of the cardiac myocyte is unknown. Several hypotheses have been proposed, but as with other cell types, none of them is entirely satisfactory (11).

According to one, the accumulating muscle-specific structures present a hindrance to mitotic division. A few lines of evidence support this theory. First, the cell cycle becomes longer as the myofibrillar mass increases. Second, the myofibrils in dividing myocytes become disorganized, and after nuclear division, they reassemble

again. Third, the number of binucleated myocytes increases with development, possibly resulting from inability of the cells to undergo cytokinesis. Still, there are data to contradict the mass-hindrance hypothesis. For example, cultured cells derived from hearts of neonatal rats were shown to undergo cytokinesis while they continued to beat. Moreover, atrial myocytes, which have a similar relative cellular content of myofibrils to ventricular cells, respond to organ injury by resumed mitotic activity (116).

Postnatal Cardiac Development

In contrast to skeletal muscle, myocytes of the heart continue to possess mitotic activity at birth (60). Nevertheless, the trend of decreasing cellular divisions, already seen during the embryonic period, persists, or even accelerates, after birth. As a result, only about 2% of rat myocytes are still dividing at birth, compared with 15% of hepatocytes (149). In addition to the declining mitotic activity, nuclear division frequently leads to binucleation. Consequently, the population of cells containing more than one nucleus increases during the neonatal period (79) and amounts to greater than 80% of the myocyte population in the rat by 3 weeks. Despite the decreased cellular division, the number of myocytes in the heart doubles during the first 3 to 4 weeks of life.

As myocytes lose their ability to proliferate, greater heart growth is accomplished through enlargement of existing cells. The diameter of a myocyte increases from about 5 μm at birth to 14 to 18 μm in the adult (149). In contrast to the embryonic period, cell death is rarely seen, if at all, in the healthy heart (92). The myocytes, therefore, must have the same life span as the entire organism.

The number of divisions that each myocyte undergoes after birth does not appear to be genetically programmed. For example, experiments manipulating litter size have shown that decreasing the size of the litter results in an increased growth rate for the newborn rat pups, which is accompanied by enhanced proliferation of myocytes (114).

The importance of hemodynamic factors in the regulation of cardiac growth following birth is clearly established, with the best example being the increased left ventricular growth after the postnatal increase in peripheral resistance. Another example is abnormal growth of the heart due to congenital errors in the circulatory system.

WORK-INDUCED ENLARGEMENT OF THE HEART

The hemodynamic load has been definitively identified as the key epigenetic factor that regulates the growth of the heart. Any change in the demands placed on the heart, either because of physiological activity or because of pathological alterations in the cardiovascular system, eventually leads to heart:body weight ratios that differ from those typical in the normal animal. The observed enlargement or reduction in heart size is referred to in both clinical and experimental studies as hypertrophy or atrophy, respectively.

It should be realized that these terms refer strictly to cardiac size, as opposed to the mode of cellular growth; cardiac hypertrophy can occur by cell proliferation (hyperplasia) and/or enlargement (hypertrophy) of the individual cells. Furthermore, it should be noted that cardiac hypertrophy may not even include an increase in the heart's mass, as is seen in cardiac dilation.

Models of Cardiac Hypertrophy

Many models of cardiac hypertrophy have been used in the past, each with its own limitations. As far as applicability to human disease is concerned, an investigator might choose models that approximate either valvular insufficiency or stenosis (Table 1). The characteristics of the growth responses vary widely, depending on experimental conditions. Commonly recognized variables are the severity, duration, and type of overload (i.e., pressure versus volume), the rate of overload application (i.e., acute versus gradual), and the age and species of the animal.

A major complication in the study of in vivo models of hypertrophy is the growth in body weight of the animal. Normal growth can be affected by any of the following: surgical trauma, nutritional anemia, thyrotoxicosis, or carbon monoxide poisoning. In such cases, to evaluate the degree of hypertrophy, one must rely not on the size of the heart but on its ratio to body size. The possible fallacy of this approach is that during the starvation of animals, the decrement in heart size is less than that in the entire body. Thus ensues a false index of hypertrophy. The second complication arises when the overload is accompanied by necrotic changes in the heart. This might lead to myofibrillar disorganization and mitochondrial damage or to proliferation of connective-tissue cells, with consequent accumulation of collagen, or both of these (11).

A possible way to bypass some of these complications may be to simulate cardiac hypertrophy in tissue culture. The use of tissue culture permits analysis of the effects of specific variables directly at the cellular level, instead of complicated systemic interactions that usually affect the interpretation of in vivo experiments. Three potential tissue-culture models that could be used are the monolayer, the reaggregate, and the synthetic cardiac strand.

Cardiac myocytes in culture undergo both hypertrophy and hyperplasia. In this way their behavior differs from that of myocytes in vivo in the adult animal. In the fully mature adult mammal, myocyte division apparently does not occur (147), and it is solely by myocyte hypertrophy that the adult heart enlarges in response to growth stimuli.

Depending on the type of myocyte growth in culture, it is necessary to view most of the reported experiments with isolated cells as not representing adult hypertrophy. We should instead consider the cells as representing either (a) myocytes, similar to those in the neonatal heart immediately after parturition, that undergo a "natural" developmental hypertrophy accompanied by cell division or (b) myocytes, similar to cardiac cells in the weanling heart, that respond to a hypertrophic stimulus by both hyperplasia and hypertrophy (18,46).

A major question, which it is hoped can be answered by the use of tissue-culture systems, concerns what factors governing myocyte growth are intrinsic to the cell itself. At least two reports concerning training effects in utero (13,21) have presented evidence for intrinsic changes in the growth behavior of isolated cells. Bonner et al. (13) observed that beating cardiac cells prepared from neonatal rats whose mothers had participated in an exercise regimen possessed a slower beating rate.

TABLE 1. *Various models of experimental cardiac hypertrophy*[a]

Pressure overload	Volume overload	Overload due to multiple factors
Aortic stenosis	Arteriovenous fistula (rat) (38)	Hyperthyrodism (rat) (8), (rabbit) (24)
Ascending (rat) (34)	Aortic insufficiency (rat) (67)	CO exposure (rat) (108)
Abdominal (rat) (9)	Sideropenic anemia (rat) (8)	Hypoxia, simulated high altitude
Pulmonary artery stenosis (cat) (32), (rat) (73)	Bradycardia (dog) (17)	(rat) (8)
Hypertension		Catecholamines (rat) (8)
Renal ischemia (rat) (59)		Exercise
Nephrectomy (rat) (64)		Running (rat) (68)
Nephrectomy + DOCA + salt (rat) (8)		Swimming (rat) (118)
Aldosterone + salt (rat) (58)		Cardiomyopathy (hamster) (4)
Spontaneous SHR (rat) (105)		Embryonic development at low
Spontaneous, Dahl, salt-sensitive (rat) (109)		temperature (chicken) (83)

[a] Only representative references are given, disregarding the date when the procedure was originally introduced. Additional models can be found in the work of Bishop (10).

Additionally, after 2 days in culture, they were 20% larger than their respective controls. These are characteristics that might be used to describe a trained heart *in vivo*. Changes that may have occurred to the cells during the training regimen seem to have carried over to the culture dish. Furthermore, Butler et al. (21) have demonstrated differences in beating responses to verapamil, isoproterenol, and propranolol between cells isolated from "trained" and "untrained" hearts. From these results, they hypothesize that the training effects produced *in utero* may affect the Ca^{2+} dynamics (i.e., uptake and binding) in the neonatal hearts. Thus, evidence is accumulating that characteristics of the myocytes gained *in vivo* may be carried over to culture.

Other studies have attempted to examine the growth characteristics of the myocytes once they are removed from all *in vivo* influences. When grown in culture, cells from neonatal rat hearts show about a 21% increase in cell diameter between days 0 and 6 (99). Such an increase could be comparable to the growth of the heart that occurs during the first week after birth. An increase in myocyte size during time spent in culture has also been reported by Simpson et al. (132). This latter work is a more extensive examination of the growth question, and it demonstrates increases not only in cell volume but also in protein and surface area of the myocyte with time spent in culture. Furthermore, it shows that catecholamines, which are known to produce hypertrophy *in vivo* (133), have a similar effect *in vitro*. However, no effect of epinephrine on protein synthesis has been reported using cultures obtained from canine heart (144).

Another interesting and potentially important question regarding the suitability of cells in culture as a model for hypertrophy is raised by Simpson et al. (132). It has been believed for many years that a major cause of hypertrophy *in vivo* is an increase in the work load of the heart. In tissue culture, however, cellular hypertrophy occurs without the "required" apparent increase in work load. Thus, certain intrinsic factors may play roles in determining the size of a cardiac cell in culture.

Another possible model for *in vitro* study of cardiac hypertrophy is the adult cardiac myocyte in culture. Several groups (30,72,102) have been able to maintain these cells in culture for several weeks. Unfortunately, these cells undergo a period of "dedifferentiation." During this period of dedifferentiation, the myocytes synthesize DNA, an atypical characteristic of adult myocytes *in vivo* (29).

An alternative preparation that may more closely resemble the *in vivo* heart is that of Piper et al. (110). Cells in this preparation maintain their *in vivo* geometry and do not appear to go through dedifferentiation. It has yet to be determined if such cells also synthesize DNA when in culture. Although a thorough examination of both these types of preparations is just beginning, many interesting results have already been reported (111).

The growth of dissociated heart cells in monolayers is the most commonly used and extensively investigated technique for study of cardiac myocytes *in vitro*. However, the limitation of this technique is the loss of three-dimensional relationships between various cell types that might regulate DNA or protein synthesis and general physiological functioning. In attempts to avoid this shortcoming, several other systems have been devised. The two major examples are synthetic cardiac strands (84,110) and spherical reaggregates (55).

Synthetic cardiac strands are grown in a groove scraped into a agar-coated Petri dish. In such a preparation, a cell bundle can be grown from dissociated chick heart cells that is 1 to 30 mm in length and 250 to 400 μm in width. These strands are spontaneously active and contract uniformly for as long as 3 weeks when grown in a conditioned medium (84). Furthermore, it has been observed that these strands consist of an inner core of well-differentiated muscle cells surrounded by what appears to be an epimysium (113). Between the muscle cells there is observed a region of close fiber apposition with well-differentiated nexi, fascia, and macula adherents. As an electrophysiological preparation, the synthetic strand behaves like a simple one-dimensional cell. This may be a useful model to study membrane permeability and active transport and to correlate morphological and biochemical information.

The second major alternative to monolayer culture was used by Fischman and Moscona (55). In this model, embryonic hearts were enzymatically dissociated and then allowed to reaggregate on a gyratory shaker at low speed. There was evidence of cellular sorting of myogenic from nonmyogenic cells. The nonmyogenic cells migrate to the periphery of the aggregate and form a layer of squamous-like epithelium that encloses a central core of myocytes. There is also a formation of tight junctions (gap junction and adherent junctions), and synchronous contractility resumes within 2 to 3 hr (130). The resumption of contractility can occur either with or without *de novo* protein synthesis (131).

Electrophysiologically, the aggregates behave differently than cell monolayers in that they develop tetrodotoxin sensitivity. DeHaan and Fozzard (39) concluded that the individual cells in an aggregate are tightly coupled electrically and behave as an isopotential system; i.e., there is virtually no distance-dependent delay in the spread of an injected current. Thus, their passive electrical properties are similar to those of the intact myocardium (40). If aggregate cultures are made using cardiac myocytes and sympathetic neurons, a positive chronotropy mediated by the nerves is apparent (33). Another aspect of cardiac myocyte biology that has been examined in the reaggregates is DNA synthesis. In a comparison of monolayers and reaggregates from embryonic chick hearts, Fischman et al. (56) found a lower level of ^{3}H-thymidine incorporation over time into the aggregates. Similar differences between monolayers and reaggregates were shown for cultures made from embryonic rat ventricles (103).

Fischman et al. (56) also demonstrated that the difference in ^{3}H-thymidine incorporation was not simply a diffusion problem, because cells in the core of the aggregate were observed to label equally as well as those on the exterior of the aggregate. When these already formed reaggregates were dissociated into single cells, the new monolayers presented more that a twofold increase in ^{3}H-Tdr incorporation. Hence, the three-dimensional relationships in the reaggregates result in declining DNA synthesis, similar to that seen in the living heart.

Finally, a logical extension of the aggregate work has recently come from Bkaily et al. (12). They kept aggregates of adult cardiac cells from rabbits for up to a month. These aggregates remained quiescent, but were responsive to electrical stimulation.

Cellular Features of Cardiac Enlargement

Organ growth can occur as a result of either cell division (hyperplasia) or cell enlargement (hypertrophy), or a combination of both processes (147). In practice, distinguishing between these possibilities is a rather difficult task. The most widely used indication of cell proliferation is measurement of ^{3}H-thymidine incorporation into DNA. Unfortunately, this technique, particularly when applied to the heart, has several limitations, which are often overlooked. First, DNA synthesis does not necessarily result in nuclear or cellular division. It is possible to increase either the DNA content per nucleus (ploidy) or the number of nuclei per cell without increasing the number of cells. Second, the possibility of DNA repair synthesis must be considered, though work done by Lampidis and Schaiberger (80) suggests that this type of DNA synthesis is turned off in isolated adult cells.

An alternative to measuring DNA synthesis is to estimate the total number of cells prior to and after induction of a growth stimulus to the heart. This cannot, however, be done on a single animal. Another major limitation is that the derivation of cell volume, which is implicit in this type of calculation, involves both technical and conceptual difficulties.

Despite these limitations, it appears that the cellular basis of cardiac enlargement, for at least several weeks after birth, depends on the ability of the myocytes to synthesize DNA. In young rats, in which nuclear DNA synthesis still takes place (though at a very low level), the heart enlargement accompanying nutritional anemia (79) and pressure overload due to aortic constriction (46) is followed by activation of DNA synthesis. This activated synthesis of DNA has been proved by the incorporation of ^{3}H-thymidine into the muscle cell nuclei and by the increase in DNA polymerase α. An *in vitro* DNA stimulator has been demonstrated in cytoplasmic extracts (18a).

Because no change has been established either in the frequency of multinucleated cells or in cell ploidy, nuclear activity appears to be followed by cytokinesis. Measurements of cell volume indicate that cellular hypertrophy is also involved (18). The compensatory enlargement of the heart in young animals consists of the same modes that are observed during normal postnatal growth of animals, namely, a combination of hypertrophy and hyperplasia.

When an overload similar to that in young animals is used in adults, in which DNA synthesis is already repressed, there is no activation of DNA synthesis. The growth of the heart therefore occurs solely through the hypertrophy of existing myocytes (147). Under these circumstances, cellular proliferation has been detected only in the population of nonmyocytes. However, the capacity to synthesize DNA by muscle nuclei is not necessarily lost. Studies of nuclear ploidy in hearts of some animal species, notably primates (including man), indicate that a large proportion of myocyte nuclei endoreplicate their DNA complement, increasing the number of nuclei with more than one set of chromosomes (polyploidy) (147). The significance and consequences of this DNA endoreplication are still unknown.

Mitosis in an enlarging adult heart has never been seen in myocytes. Nevertheless, cytometric studies using stereological techniques support the original Linzbach idea that addition of a new cell takes place when cardiac enlargement exceeds a certain "critical" size (147).

Ultrastructure of Hypertrophied Heart

The question whether the relative contents of cellular constituents in the heart change or remain constant is of considerable importance to our understanding and evaluation of compensatory cardiac growth. Growth accompanied by coordinated accumulation of organelles and their respective proteins might be expected to maintain unaltered cellular function. It would mean that the heart would be better suited to cope with functional overload. In contrast, decreases in some components might lead to impairment of cellular functioning, resulting in cardiac failure.

The available data suggest (11,54) that cellular symmetry is maintained to a large degree in some models of cardiac hypertrophy, although a disproportionality has been found, especially as far as mitochondria are concerned. Both quantitative ultrastructural investigations and biochemical analyses indicate that the relative mass of mitochondria is moderately increased in the early stage of hypertrophy. The relationship between plasma membrane volume and cell volume remains unchanged in the left ventricles of hearts enlarged secondary to aortic constriction and thyrotoxicosis. The same is true for the ratio of sarcotubular membrane to myofibrillar volume. The preferential accumulation of mitochondria and their constituent cytochromes and respiratory enzymes is only a transitory event. After the early phase of overload, myofibrils accumulate more rapidly than mitochondria. Subsequently there is a progressive decline in the fraction of mitochondria per unit of myocardial mass. This sequence of initially increased and then decreased mitochondrial mass does not take place in other models of hypertrophy, such as volume or gradual pressure overload. A more in-depth description of the ultrastructure of the hypertrophic heart can be found in reviews by Bishop (10) and Ferrans (54).

REDUCTION OF CARDIAC MASS

Models

Although both cardiac hypertrophy and atrophy are interesting to the clinician and researcher, it is the clinician who has studied atrophy more closely. As a result, few animal models of cardiac atrophy are found in the literature. Loss of cardiac mass occurs whenever the hemodynamic load of the heart decreases below that level normally maintained by a given animal. In practice, this can be observed in two distinct situations: the unloading of the healthy heart, such as during prolonged bed rest or disease states, and the regression of hypertrophy after the removal of work overload. Several examples of reduced hemodynamic load include restrictive pericardial disease, chronic reduction of mean arterial pressure, Addison's disease, and decreased body mass during starvation. Experimental studies, such as the unloading of papillary muscles by section of their chordae tendineae or the beating empty heart, also result in cardiac atrophy.

The second major area of study involves regression of acquired hypertrophy. This has been demonstrated in a variety of models, such as the correction of coarcted abdominal (34) or ascending aorta (9), cessation of a hyperthyroid state (9) or nutritional anemia (9), removal of DOCA-salt overload of a single kidney (9), and the antihypertensive treatment of spontaneously hypertensive rats (126,127).

Unloading the Heart

Most descriptions of cardiac atrophy associated with decreased hemodynamic load concern clinical observations. Although it is frequently mentioned that cardiac atrophy accompanies aging, in a systematic study of a large number of patients the incidence of senile atrophy was not confirmed (149).

Commonly observed in studies of cardiac atrophy due to unloading of an otherwise normal heart is a loss in mass accompanied by a decrease in the diameter of muscle cells and an increase in nuclear density. Presently, little is known about the functional characteristics of the unloaded heart. In addition to mechanical unloading, other factors (e.g., hormones) undoubtedly contribute to cardiac changes in at least some of the cases mentioned earlier, e.g., Addison's disease or starvation.

Experimental studies in which the unloading has been accomplished without complicating factors have been few. In two such studies, the right ventricular papillary muscles of a cat were examined after transection of the chordae tendineae (138,140). The operation was followed by a rapid loss of cardiac mass and a corresponding decrease in the size of the muscle cells. Accumulation of collagen, partial disorientation of myofilaments, and infiltration with fibroblasts and macrophages were observed. The mechanical properties of these muscles also deteriorated. Furthermore, the force–velocity curve and force–shortening relationship shifted with a reduction in maximal developed tension (31). Oxygen consumption by these muscles did not change. Thus, some aspects of cardiac atrophy in this case appeared similar to those of a degenerative process.

Another potentially useful model of unloading is the heterotopically isotransplanted empty beating heart (139). In this model, coronary flow was preserved, but preload and afterload were substantially reduced, and a loss of cardiac mass ensued.

Regression of Cardiac Hypertrophy

Rapid regression of cardiac hypertrophy resulting in a ratio of heart to body weight expected for control animals has been described in the models listed earlier. In these hearts, the concentration of RNA and the incorporation of radiolabeled lysine into total proteins return to normal values. Quantitative morphometric data also indicate that the cellular ratio of mitochondria to myofibrils returns to normal in the ferret myocardium after 14 days of hypertrophy, followed by 6 weeks of regression (16).

In contrast to the unequivocal regression of acquired hypertrophy seen in experimental studies, the results of corrective heart surgery are less conclusive (149). In some reports, such as those that dealt with repair of ventricular septal defects in children, regression of left ventricular (LV) volume was achieved. In other studies, regression was not noted. This discrepancy is undoubtedly related to the different characteristics of the hypertrophic heart prior to corrective surgery. This was demonstrated in a study in which the courses of regression differed depending on the length of the preceding overload of the heart (34). Whereas LV weight and RNA content declined following removal of stress in hearts overloaded for 10 and 28 days, the rate of decline in the first group of rats was faster than in the 28-day group. The collagen and DNA contents remained elevated in both groups of debanded animals, even though a declining trend was noticed in the short-banded group. The elevated content of collagen in the heart, coupled with a decrease in cardiac mass, increased the collagen concentration. A similar accumulation of collagen was noticed after antihypertensive therapy in spontaneously hypertensive rats (126). In these cases, alterations of mechanical properties of the heart, such as resting tension or resistance to passive stretching, can be anticipated. However, regression of hypertrophy does not necessarily lead to altered contractility, as indicated by a study of the right ventricle in pressure-overloaded cat heart, in which cardiac function returned to normal (31).

As far as the biochemical pathways leading to loss of cardiac mass are concerned, it is interesting that the activity of cathepsin D was found to increase during regression of thyroxine-induced hypertrophy (146).

WORK LOAD AS A DETERMINANT OF CARDIAC GROWTH

A change in the functional load of the heart has two consequences that involve the growth process: changes in organ mass and composition. The latter response includes both the relative amounts and the properties of intracellular proteins. Therefore, the work load not only affects the overall rate of gene transcription but also selectively regulates the expression of specific genes. The need to differentiate between the responses of individual genes became apparent when numerous studies pointed out that many muscle proteins demonstrate extensive polymorphism. In other words, proteins are members of large gene families whose members have corresponding overall structures and functions, but they are products of different genes. As a result of the slight differences in amino acid sequences, called microheterogeneity, properties vary between members of a given family. Thus far, molecular polymorphism has been detected not only in enzymes (isozymes) but also in some sarcoplasmic and contractile proteins. There is no reason not to expect diversity among other cellular constituents, such as sarcoplasmic reticulum and mitochondria. Assorted terms are used to indicate the molecular variants: isoforms, isoproteins, or, more specifically, isomyosin, isoactin, etc. As discussed in *Chapter 45*, the genes for some isoforms of muscle proteins are being identified and characterized. This, in turn, allows for the construction and application of probes for specific genes. This undoubtedly will lead to a more thorough analysis of the factors that control cardiac growth.

Control of Gene Expression in the Heart

Early analyses of the contractile properties of functionally overloaded heart led to detailed examinations of myosin ATPase that indicated subtle changes in its molecule. These pioneering studies of Alpert and Morkin and their associates (5,137) were later refined when it was realized that cardiac myosin, like its skeletal muscle counterpart, has multiple forms. So far, two types of myosin have been detected in the heart: ventricular and atrial. The two classes can be further subdivided into isomyosins: V_1, V_2, and V_3 in the ventricle, and A_1 and A_2 in the atrium. This classification is based on electrophoretic mobility in the native state, in which the migration rate reflects the combined properties of both the heavy chains (HC) and light chains (LC).

The multiplicity of ventricular isomyosin arises from an association between $HC\alpha$ and $HC\beta$ that forms homodimers α_2 and β_2 (V_1 and V_3, respectively) and one heterodimer, V_2. The primary structures of $HC\alpha$ and $HC\beta$ differ, as seen in analyses of amino acid sequences, in the cDNA correspondence to their respective messages, and in the genes themselves. In contrast to the HCs, the LC complement of ventricular isomyosin represents identical proteins (70).

The unraveling of myosin complexity in the heart was greatly aided by the use of electrophoresis under nondenaturing conditions, developed independently by D'Albis et al. (36) and Hoh et al. (69). This method readily detects isomyosins in some animal species, notably mouse, rat, rabbit, and hamster. In other species, however, microheterogeneity results in smaller charge differences than in the foregoing cases. Consequently, the isomyosins do not separate readily according to their migration rates under ordinary conditions (e.g., guinea pig, pig, and human) (27). In this case, improved resolution of electrophoresis is required (121), or additional procedures, such as immunochemical analysis or peptide mapping, must be used (27).

As for the atrial class of isomyosin, its study has thus far attracted less attention than has the ventricular class (145). Nevertheless, it is known that atrial LCs differ from those of the ventricle. The predominant HCs, on the other hand, are indistinguishable, both by amino acid sequence (23) and by cDNA analysis (89,134), from ventricular $HC\alpha$. The differences in electrophoretic behaviors of ventricular and atrial isomyosins thus must reside in the properties of their LCs. This was proved by an exchange of the LCs present in atrial isomyosins with those in the ventricle (24). The cross-hybridized atrial isomyosins migrate as a single band only, with mobility identical with that for V_1 isomyosin. The difference in the mobilities of A_1 and A_2 isomyosins, however, is still obscure at this time.

In published studies, both classes of HCs have been detected in ventricles and atria of all mammals. The relative proportions of the two HCs differ between animal species and seem to be related to body size and pattern of physical activity and hence to basal metabolic rate. In small animals, such as mice, $HC\alpha$ dominates in both heart chambers throughout the entire life. In middle-sized animals, such as rats (88), hamsters (121), and rabbits (52), both the HCs are expressed in the ventricles, and all three isomyosins (V_1–V_3) appear. Even among these species, some gradations can be seen. The ventricles of young adult rats contain predominantly V_1 isomyosin, and the other two isoforms are detectable only in neonates or in very old animals (88,125). In contrast, the ventricle in young adult rabbit contains mostly V_3 isomyosin, and V_1 and V_2 are seen only in neonates and adolescent animals. In the atria of middle-sized animals, HCα predominates. Animals of large body size have ventricles in which HCβ is predominantly expressed (15,101). It also appears substantially in the atria (15), although HCα still remains the main form there.

The functional consequences of different myosin phenotypes have not yet been unfolded with all their details. Nevertheless, it is clear that the high beating heart rates seen in small animals require a high shortening velocity and hence a fast cross-bridge cycling rate and a corresponding high ATPase activity. These postulates have received full support from studies of isolated isomyosin, as well as studies of intact heart preparations containing one or the other isoform of myosin. Thus, the actin-activated ATPase of purified V_1 isomyosin is about three times that of the V_3, whereas the V_2 isoforms have activities analogous to the average of V_1 and V_3 (112). Similarly, the shortening velocity for skinned fibers and papillary muscle (107) correlates with the isomyosin phenotype. Measurements of tension-dependent heat production and isometric twitch tension indicate that the efficiency of contraction varies depending on the type of myosin present (3). So a shift toward predominance of the V_3 isoform is associated with a decreased rate of cross-bridge cycling and an increased "on" time of the individual cross-bridges, resulting in increased economy of force production (see also *Chapter 62*).

One aspect of myosin phenotype that has not yet been explained satisfactorily is the cellular heterogeneity in isomyosin distribution. In a ground-breaking study, Schiaffino and associates showed a checkerboard pattern in a ventricle stained with isomyosin-specific antibodies (123). Most interesting was that adjacent cells expressed different classes of myosin HCs. Moreover, myocytes isolated from enzymatically dispersed adult rat heart (122) revealed three populations of cells after immunofluorescence staining. Half of the cells were stained exclusively with anti-V_1 antibody, 10% were stained with anti-V_3, and the remaining 40% reacted with both.

When an entire free left ventricular wall was examined by immunofluorescence and histochemical staining for Ca^{2+}-ATPase, a striking transmural gradient became apparent (51). In the outer epicardial region, V_1-containing myocytes predominated, whereas the midwall and endocardial portions showed a checkerboard pattern, with a minimum of V_1-reacting cells in the middle third

of the wall. The functional consequences of such isomyosin distributions are unknown. Other transmural gradients (Table 2) in the heart are also known, as discussed by Eisenberg et al. (51). For example, the length of the action potential in epicardial myocytes is longer than that in endocardial myocytes, the effect being that force is generated first in endocardial myocytes, and the epicardial layers have the shortest contractions. During the normal cycle, the endocardial cells are believed to do more work than the epicardial cells, but after a while the epicardial layers are recruited. Sarcomere length also varies with anatomical location, the greatest length being in the midwall, and the shortest close to the epicardium. No regional differences in cell organization are readily seen in normal myocardium; with hypertrophy, however, some differences become obvious. Namely, the degree of cell enlargement in the overloaded heart is greater in the epicardial than in the endocardial portion, and the mitochondria/myofibril ratio and the density of the T system change disproportionately in different regions of the wall.

Insofar as functional effects of the transmural isomyosin gradient are involved, any explanation must take into account the fact that such organization is not always apparent. In young rabbits (51) and hypothyroid rabbits (143), the heart contains only one type of myosin: V_1 and V_3, respectively. Moreover, the fact that adjacent myocytes, connected via an intercalated disc and having similar electrical and mechanical properties, can differ in isomyosin content indicates that the functional load cannot be the sole determinant of myosin phenotype. Because the cellular microenvironment is not known to vary over a short distance of two myocytes, one must consider the possibility that the expression of myosin HC genes is programmed and in some way is related to the number of mitoses experienced by each cell. Support

TABLE 2[a]

	Portion of the wall	
Property	Epicardial	Endocardial
Phylogenetic origin	New	Old
Predominant myocytes	V_1	V_3
Electrical: length of AP	Short	Long
Mechanical:		
Length of contraction	Short	Long
Onset of force generation	Late	Early
Morphological:		
Sarcomere length	Short	Long
Cellular hypertrophy (pressure overload)	Large	Small
Metabolic: onset of ischemia (decreased pH)	Late	Early

[a] The documentation for this table can be found in ref. 51.

for this belief comes from the demonstration that in developing avian atria, changes in mitotic activity (136) and in the expression of HCs (62) appear to be connected. Thus, the cellular heterogeneity of isomyosin might reflect the uncoordinated nature of mitotic activity in the heart.

One of the most fascinating aspects of cardiac myosin phenotype is that although it is typical of a given animal species, it changes during normal development and can change because of a variety of experimental interventions and possibly because of disease states (Table 3). Thus, the reference to adult myocytes as "terminally" differentiated requires revision.

In normal development, which thus far has been systematically examined only in the rat (25,125) and rabbit (52,88), all three isomyosins are present in the ventricles of the late fetus, with V_3 predominant. Soon after birth, however, the myosin profile begins to change, so that at about 2 weeks after birth the V_1 becomes the main isomyosin present. Such preferential synthesis of $HC\alpha$ coincides very closely with the rapid postnatal increase in the blood level of thyroid hormone (52). In the period that follows, the close correlation between circulating thyroid hormone and myosin phenotype gradually disappears. This is especially true for the rabbit, in which the trend in myosin expression reverses itself at the time the thyroid hormone is stabilized at the adult level (52). Consequently, in mature and old animals, the "embryonic" V_3 form predominates again. The same is true in the rat (125), except that the reappearance of V_3 isomyosin occurs later than in the rabbit.

Many experimental manipulations and abnormal situations have been shown to be accompanied by changes in the isomyosin composition of the heart. Of those interventions examined, thyroid hormone is by far the most potent. The hyperthyroid state favors expression of $HC\alpha$ at the expense of $HC\beta$, and the opposite is true

for hypothyroidism (23,70,86,95). These reciprocal changes in gene activities can be seen in animals previously made thyroid-deficient and in euthyroid animals at the age when both HCs are normally present. In either case, the activation of $HC\alpha$ is quite rapid, with the mRNA rising at 2 hr (53,89) and apparent changes in the isomyosin profile noticeable at day 2 of thyroid treatment (95). The dependence of HC expression on the thyroid state has been shown in rat adults, neonates, and late embryos (25). In the atrium, the response to thyroid hormone is considerably less than that in the ventricle; nevertheless, a small increase in $HC\beta$ message in thyroidectomized animals was detected (90). One of the reasons for this difference between the two chambers might be that the metabolic consequence of hypothyroidism in the atrium is different from that in the ventricle, as disclosed in a study of enzymes of catecholamine metabolism by Bukhari and Rupp (20).

The second condition that has been examined intensively is the response of the ventricular isomyosin profile to hemodynamic overload. Various procedures, such as aortic constriction (86,87,100) and renal- and aldosterone-induced hypertension (97,117), as well as hypertension in spontaneously hypertensive rats (SHR) (118), are known to result in myosin redistribution toward the V_3 isoform. However, the observed changes are less dramatic than those seen in hypothyroidism, in which case there is complete disappearance of the V_1 isoform after about 3 weeks of treatment. Pressure overload has been shown only to decrease the relative proportion of V_1, never to completely eliminate it. In contrast to the pathological situation, an increase in the hemodynamic load during exercise by experimental animals (106,117,118), both normal and hypertensive (118,119), results in the opposite change: a shift toward the V_1 isoform. However, the redistribution has been demonstrated only after swimming, not after running (121). This is interesting, because both forms of exercise result

TABLE 3. *Some determinants of ventricular complements of isomyosins[a]*

	Situations favoring V_1 isomyosin	Situations favoring V_3 isomyosin
Development	Neonates[b]	Fetal life, maturation, and aging[f]
Hormones	Thyroid hormone, steroid hormones[c]	Hypothyroid state, diabetes[f]
Function	Swimming exercise	Hemodynamic overload,[g] sympathectomy
Nutrition	High-fructose diet,[d] inhibition of fatty-acid oxidation,[e] perinatal overnourishment	Semistarvation,[g] perinatal undernourishment

[a] The information compiled in this table is based on studies of rat and rabbit. In other species, only a few studies have been done. For references, see text.
[b] Correlates with high plasma level of thyroid hormone.
[c] Hydrocorticosteroid treatment of adrenalectomized animals.
[d] Especially pronounced in diabetic animals.
[e] Done in diabetic animals.
[f] Independent of plasma thyroid hormone.
[g] In some, but not all, instances, the plasma level of thyroid hormone was decreased by the treatment.

in normalization of pressure in SHR. Therefore, the change in HC expression seen during exercise is not necessarily related to normalization of blood pressure.

Among other factors examined for their influence on myosin phenotype in the heart, the alteration of metabolic pathways is quite interesting. Based on the available information, a generalization emerges: The decreased glycolytic flux and the corresponding increase in the relative contribution of fatty-acid oxidation to energy production, as seen in the case of diabetes, favor synthesis of the V_3 isomyosin. Replacement of insulin (42), feeding a high-fructose diet (44), or administration of methyl palmixirate (45) (an inhibitor of carnitine-dependent transport of long-chain fatty acids into the mitochondria) to an animal previously made diabetic by streptozotocin results in increased glycolytic flux and a shift to the synthesis of V_1 isomyosin. This shift was also noticed after feeding a high-fructose diet to hypophysectomized rats (129).

Redistributions of ventricular isomyosins have also been shown to be influenced by glucocorticosteroids and overall nutrition. Thus, adrenalectomy in euthyroid rats increases the expression of V_3 isomyosin and consequently reduces the V_1 form (129). Intermittent starvation (43), as well as perinatal undernutrition (47) (achieved by increasing the number of rat pups per mother), favors the V_3 isomyosin. Decreasing the litter size, on the other hand, increases the rate of V_3-to-V_1 conversion normally seen in newly born animals (47).

Finally, the adrenergic system has recently been implicated (mainly in studies conducted by Rupp and Jacob) in modulation of the isomyosin composition of the heart. Peripheral sympathectomy by 6-OH-dopamine and β-blockage by atenolol induce synthesis of V_3 and decrease ATPase in myosin (119). Isoproterenol, when administered at 0.1 to 1.0 mg/kg, favors the V_1 isomyosin, but doses of 5 mg/kg have the opposite effect (121). Experimental stress induced by electrical stimulation of rats in pairs, with a resulting increase in aggression, did not change the myosin profile in normotensive Wistar rats, but in SHR it enhanced the normally occurring trend toward synthesis of V_3 isomyosin (120,121). Notably, the change in myosin profile produced by stress was prevented when the electrostimulation was followed by swimming.

β-Adrenergic stimulation with isoproterenol and blockade with propranolol, however, have been also reported not to have any effect on the isomyosin profile of the heart (129).

To understand the determinants of cardiac myosin phenotype, it is important to keep in mind that an interplay of multiple factors likely occurs. For example, semistarvation (43) and aortic constriction of weanling rats (47), but not adult rats, exhibited an association with a decreased level of thyroid hormone. In contrast, perinatal nutritional modification of the isomyosin profile

(47) and the effects of diabetes (42) was found to be independent of thyroid status. Swimming resulted not only in increased and possibly altered patterns of energy utilization but also in alterations of the activities of several key enzymes of catecholamine metabolism (120). Moreover, the close relationship between the adrenergic system and thyroid hormone is well-documented. For example, the functional ontogeny of efferent sympathetic pathways is accelerated by an increased level of thyroid hormone (82). In the adult, catecholamine metabolism (81) and adrenergic responsiveness correlate (22) with the thyroid state of the animal, with hypothyroidism generally damping the effects of the adrenergic system. In addition, the action of thyroid hormone on the heart undoubtedly has a peripheral component due to the increased overall oxygen utilization. However, it is of interest that myocytes isolated from rat fetal ventricles respond to the thyroid hormone level in defined growth medium in a manner similar to that in cells of intact hearts (104).

Resolving the complex nature of phenotype determinants, as described here briefly, will certainly demand detailed delineation of myosin gene structure, including elucidation of the receptor mechanisms for gene-regulating molecules.

Search for Stimuli to Control Cardiac Growth

Numerous ingenious theories of growth regulation in the heart by its functional load have been advanced in the past. Still, none of them is entirely satisfactory. One of the reasons that this important topic in cardiac functioning is so elusive is that up to now, no probes for specific genes have been available. Consequently, the investigator has had to rely on studies of overall growth response. Recently, however, application of recombinant DNA technology to cardiovascular research has led to the cloning of cDNA probes for several myofibrillar proteins, including those for myosin HCs. The latter probes have allowed us to analyze the level of gene regulation in the heart by thyroid hormone. As a logical first step, the amount of myosin-specific mRNA was compared with the rate of HC synthesis in euthyroid rabbits, as well as after induction of HCα synthesis by administration of thyroid hormone (53). In both situations, a close relationship was found between HC synthesis and the level of its mRNA, which strongly suggests that thyroid hormone regulates expression of the myosin gene in one of the steps that precedes translation. This could include gene transcription, storage, or masking and degradation of cytoplasmic mRNA. In order to further define gene regulation, the rates of α and β HC gene transcription were measured within nuclei isolated from rabbit ventricles after manipulation of the thyroid state of the animal (37). The nascent gene transcripts were quantitated by hybridization to probes consisting of highly divergent 5' noncoding sequences of β and α HC genes. The transcription rates of these two genes correlated with the relative ratios of the respective mRNAs. This indicates, in this model of cardiac growth, that transcription is the primary target of the regulating signal. These experiments, however, are just one example of gene regulation in the heart. It might well be that when growth is induced by other stimuli, another level of regulation might supplement gene transcription.

In addition to the thyroid hormone triggering growth, two other mechanisms have recently been examined: the effects of mechanical stretch (148) and the humoral factors produced by an overloaded heart. It has been known for some time that passive stretch applied to skeletal muscle produces rapid enlargement. After denervation of one hemidiaphragm, for example, the muscle becomes rhythmically stretched by the functioning half, and in about a week it is enlarged by 40%. When the stretch of the paralyzed hemidiaphragm is eliminated, there is no enlargement. This is analogous to the anterior musculus latissimus dorsi when a weight-induced stretch not only results in enlargement of the muscle but also profoundly affects the type of myosin expressed (74). That stretch plays a role in regulating the growth of the heart was suggested by studies in which the stretch of the ventricular wall, as a consequence of increased aortic pressure, increased the rate of protein synthesis (discussed in *Chapter* 45).

The roles of humoral factors are hinted at by the frequent reports that both chambers of the heart respond when only one is overloaded (96). These puzzling results can be explained by reports describing the presence of substances produced by the enlarging heart that are able to promote protein synthesis. In one report (66), the extract from a pressure-overloaded heart, when introduced into the perfusion medium, increased cell-free protein synthesis, directed by cytoplasmic RNA that was extracted from a perfused normal heart. Two other examples of soluble factors that regulate protein synthesis have been described. One study reported that incorporation of labeled amino acid into sliced normal heart was increased by addition of postribosomal supernatant obtained from a hypertrophic heart (78). In another study (128), a protein fraction, isolated from 1,500 $\times$ g supernatant of heart homogenate from SHR, increased protein synthesis when added to the medium used to incubate myocytes isolated from the hearts of normotensive rats.

Regarding the factors that control the development of cardiac hypertrophy, particularly interesting is the demonstration by Sen et al. (126) that in the SHR model of hypertension, a close correlation between blood pressure and degree of hypertrophy does not always exist. Some drugs, such as hydralazine, lower blood pressure to a normotensive level but have no effect on cardiac hypertrophy. Administration of minox-

idil even increases the degree of hypertrophy while lowering the pressure overload (127). These models offer an excellent chance to clarify the processes that trigger compensatory growth of the heart.

ACKNOWLEDGMENTS

This investigation was supported in part by the United States Public Health Service grants HL16637 and HL20592 from the National Heart, Lung, and Blood Institute and by a grant from the Muscular Dystrophy Association of America.

We would like to thank Dr. Gabrielle Bugaisky for her helpful comments concerning this manuscript.

REFERENCES

1. Adolph, E. F. (1965): Capacities of regulation of heart rate in fetal, infant and adult rats. *Am. J. Physiol.,* 209:1095–1105.
2. Alpert, N. (1971): *Cardiac Hypertrophy.* Academic Press, New York.
3. Alpert, N. R., and Mulieri, L. A. (1982): Heat, mechanics, and myosin ATPase in normal and hypertrophied heart muscle. *Fed. Proc.,* 41:192–198.
4. Bajusz, E., Baker, J. R., Nixon, C. W., and Homburger, F. (1969): Spontaneous hereditary myocardial degeneration and congestive heart failure in a strain of Syrian hamster. *Ann. N.Y. Acad. Sci.,* 156:105–129.
5. Banerjee, S. K., Kabbas, E. G., and Morkin, E. (1977): Enzymatic properties of the heavy meromyosin subfragment of cardiac myosin from normal and thyrotoxic rabbits. *J. Biol. Chem.,* 252: 6925–6929.
6. Bareis, D. L., Morgan, R. E., Lau, C., and Slotkin, T. A. (1981): Maturation of sympathetic neurotransmission in the rat heart. IV. Effects of guanethidine-induced sympathectomy in neonatal development of synaptic vesicles, synaptic terminal function and heart growth. *Dev. Neurosciences,* 4:15–24.
7. Bareis, D. L., and Slotkin, T. A. (1978): Responses of the heart ornithine decarboxylase and adrenal catecholamines to methadone and sympathetic stimulants in developing and adult rats. *J. Pharmacol. Exp. Ther.,* 205:164–174.
8. Bartsova, D., Chvapil, M., Korecky, B., Poupa, O., Rakusan, K., Turek, Z., and Vizek, M. (1969): The growth of the muscular and collagenous parts of the rat heart in various forms of cardiomegaly. *J. Physiol. (Lond.),* 200:285–295.
9. Beznak, R., Korecky, B., and Thomas, G. (1969): Regression of cardiac hypertrophies of various origin. *Can. J. Physiol. Pharmacol.,* 47:579–586.
10. Bishop, S. P. (1982): Animal models. In: *Congestive Heart Failure,* edited by E. Braunwald, M. B. Mock, and J. T. Watson, pp. 125–149. Grune & Stratton, New York.
11. Bishop, S. P. (1983): Ultrastructure of the myocardium in physiologic and pathologic hypertrophy in experimental animals. *Perspect. Cardiovasc. Res.,* 7:127–147.
12. Bkaily, G., Sperelakis, N., and Doane, J. (1984): A new method for preparation of isolated single adult cells. *Am. J. Physiol.,* 247: H1018–1026.
13. Bonner, H. W., Buffington, C. K., Newman, J. J., Farrar, R. P., and Acosta, D. (1978): Contractile activity of neonatal heart cells in culture derived from offspring of exercised pregnant rats. *Eur. J. Appl. Physiol.,* 39:1–6.
14. Borg, T. K., and Caulfield, J. B. (1979): Collagen in the heart. *Tex. Rep. Biol. Med.,* 39:321–333.
15. Bouvagnet, P., Leger, J., Pons, F., Dechesne, C., and Leger, J. J. (1984): Fiber types and myosin types in human atrial and ventricular myocardium. Anatomical description. *Circ. Res.,* 55: 794–804.

16. Breisch, E. A., Bove, A. A., and Phillips, S. J. (1980): Myocardial morphometrics in pressure overload left ventricular hypertrophy and regression. *Cardiovasc. Res.*, 14:161–168.
17. Brockman, S. K. (1965): Cardiodynamics of complete heart block. *Am. J. Cardiol.*, 16:72–83.
18. Bugaisky, L., and Zak, R. (1979): Cellular growth of cardiac muscle after birth. *Tex. Rep. Biol. Med.*, 39:123–138.
18a. Bugaiski, L., Rabinowitz, M., and Zak, R. (1985): Nuclear-cytoplasmic interactions affecting DNA synthesis during induced cardiac muscle growth in the rat. *Cardiovasc. Res.*, 19:89–94.
19. Bugaisky, L., and Zak, R. (1985): *In vitro* development of ventricular and atrial myocytes from fetal rabbit and rat. *J. Cell. Biochem.*, 9B:83.
20. Bukhari, A. R., and Rupp, H. (1983): Differential effect of thyroid hormone on catecholamine enzymes and myosin isoenzymes in ventricles and atria of rat heart. In: *Cardiac Adaptation to Hemodynamic Overload, Training and Stress*, edited by R. Jacob, R. W. Gulch, and G. Kissling, pp. 59–64. Steinkopff Verlag, Tubingen.
21. Butler, A. W., Farrar, R. P., and Acosta, D. (1984): Effects of cardioactive drugs on the beating activity of myocardial cell cultures isolated from offspring of trained and untrained pregnant rats. *In Vitro*, 20:629–634.
22. Chang, H. Y., and Kunos, G. (1981): Short term effects of triiodothyronine on rat heart adrenoceptors. *Biochem. Biophys. Res. Commun.*, 100:313–320.
23. Chizzonite, R. A., Everett, A. W., Clark, W. A., Jakovcic, S., Rabinowitz, M., and Zak, R. (1982): Isolation and characterization of two molecular variants of myosin heavy chains from rabbit ventricle: Change in their content during normal growth and after treatment with thyroid hormone. *J. Biol. Chem.*, 257:2056–2065.
24. Chizzonite, R. A., Everett, A. W., Prior, G., and Zak, R. (1984): Comparison of myosin heavy chains in atria and ventricles from hyperthyroid, hypothyroid, and euthyroid rabbits. *J. Biol. Chem.*, 259:15564–15571.
25. Chizzonite, R. A., and Zak, R. (1984): Regulation of myosin isoenzyme composition in fetal and neonatal rat ventricle by endogenous thyroid hormone. *J. Biol. Chem.*, 259:12628–12632.
26. Clark, E. B. (1984): Functional aspects of cardiac development. In: *Growth of the Heart in Health and Disease*, edited by R. Zak, pp. 81–103. Raven Press, New York.
27. Clark, W. A., Chizzonite, R. A., Everett, A. W., Rabinowitz, M., and Zak, R. (1982): Species correlations between cardiac isomyosins. *J. Biol. Chem.*, 257:5449–5454.
28. Claycomb, W. C. (1976): Biochemical aspects of cardiac muscle differentiation: Possible control of deoxyribonucleic acid synthesis and cell differentiation by adrenergic innervation and cyclic adenosine 3':5'-monophosphate. *J. Biol. Chem.*, 251:6082–6089.
29. Claycomb, W. C., and Bradshaw, B. D. (1980): Acquisition of multiple nuclei and the activity of DNA polymerase-α and reinitiation of DNA replication in terminally differentiated adult cardiac muscle cells in culture. *Dev. Biol.*, 99:331–337.
30. Claycomb, W. C., and Palazzo, M. C. (1980): Culture of the terminally differentiated adult cardiac muscle cell: A light and scanning electron microscope study. *Dev. Biol.*, 80:466–482.
31. Cooper, G., Satava, R. M., Harrison, C. E., and Coleman, H. N. (1974): Normal myocardial function and energetics after reversing pressure-overload hypertrophy. *Am. J. Physiol.*, 226:1158–1165.
32. Cooper, G., Tomanek, R. J., Ehrhardt, J. C., and Marcus, M. L. (1981): Chronic progressive pressure-overload of the cat right ventricle. *Circ. Res.*, 48:488–497.
33. Culver, N. (1977): Sympathetic innervation of the embryonic chick heart. PhD thesis, University of Chicago.
34. Cutilletta, A. F., Dowell, R. T., Rudnik, M., Arcilla, R. A., and Zak, R. (1975): Regression of myocardial hypertrophy. I. Experimental model, changes in heart weight, nucleic acids and collagen. *J. Mol. Cell. Cardiol.*, 7:767–780.
35. Cutilleta, A. F., Aumont, M.-C., Nag, A. C., and Zak, R. (1977): Separation of muscle and non-muscle cells from adult rat myocardium: An application to the study of RNA polymerase. *J. Mol. Cell. Cardiol.*, 9:399–407.
36. D'Albis, A., Pantaloni, C., Bechet, J.-J. (1979): An electrophoretic study of native myosin isoenzymes and of their subunit content. *Eur. J. Biochem.*, 99:261–272.
37. Darling, D. S., Kennedy, J. M., DeGroot, L. J., Jakovcic, S.,

Zak, R., and Umeda, P. K. (1985): Transcriptional regulation of cardiac myosin heavy chain expression by thyroid hormone. *Circulation*, 72:III–25.
38. Dart, C. H., and Holloszy, J. O. (1969): Hypertrophied non-failing rat heart: Partial biochemical characterization. *Circ. Res.*, 25:245–253.
39. DeHaan, R. L., and Fozzard, H. A. (1975): Membrane response to current pulses in spheroidal aggregates of embryonic heart cells. *J. Gen. Physiol.*, 65:207–222.
40. DeHaan, R. L., McDonald, T. F., and Sachs, H. G. (1975): Development of tetrodotoxin sensitivity of embryonic chick heart cells in vitro. In: *Developmental and Physiological Correlates of Cardiac Muscle*, edited by M. Lieberman and T. Sano, pp. 155–68. Raven Press, New York.
41. Deskin, R., Mills, E., Whitmore, W. L., Seidler, F. J., and Slotkin, T. A. (1980): Maturation of the sympathetic neurotransmission in the rat heart. VI. The effect of neonatal central catecholaminergic lesions. *J. Pharmacol. Exp. Ther.*, 215:342–347.
42. Dillman, W. H. (1982): Influence of thyroid hormone administration on myosin ATPase activity and myosin isoenzyme distribution in the hearts of diabetic rats. *Metabolism*, 31:199–204.
43. Dillman, W. H., Berry, S., and Alexander, N. M. (1983): A physiological dose of triiodothyronine normalizes cardiac myosin adenosine triphosphatase activity and changes myosin isoenzyme distribution in semistarved rats. *Endocrinology*, 112:2081–2087.
44. Dillman, W. H. (1984): Fructose feeding increases Ca^{++}-activated myosin ATPase activity and changes myosin isoenzyme distribution in the diabetic rat heart. *Endocrinology*, 114:1678–1685.
45. Dillman, W. H. (1985): Methyl palmoxirate increases Ca^{2+}-myosin ATPase activity and changes myosin isoenzymes distribution in the diabetic rat heart. *Am. J. Physiol.*, 248:E602–606.
46. Dowell, R. T., and McManus, R. E. (1978): Pressure induced cardiac enlargement in neonatal and adult rats: Left ventricular functional characteristics and evidence of cardiac cell proliferation in the neonate. *Circ. Res.*, 42:303–310.
47. Dowell, R. T., Haithcoat, J. L., Thirkill, H. M., and Palmer, W. K. (1984): Heart cyclic nucleotide responses to sustained aortic constriction in neonatal and adult rat. *Am. J. Physiol.*, 246:H197–206.
48. Dowell, R. T., and Martin, A. F. (1984): Perinatal nutritional modification of weanling rat heart contractile protein. *Am. J. Physiol.*, 247:H967–972.
49. Ebrecht, G., Rupp, H., and Jacob, R. (1982): Alterations of mechanical parameters in chemically skinned preparations of rat myocardium as a function of isoenzyme pattern of myosin. *Basic Res. Cardiol.*, 77:220–234.
50. Ecob, M. S., Butler-Browne, G. S., and Whalen, R. G. (1983): The adult fast isoenzyme of myosin is present in tissue culture system. *Differentiation*, 25:84–87.
51. Eisenberg, B. R., Edwards, J. A., and Zak, R. (1985): Transmural distribution of isomyosin in rabbit ventricle during maturation examined by immunofluorescence and staining for calcium-activated adenosine triphosphatase. *Circ. Res.*, 56:548–555.
52. Everett, A. W., Clark, W. A., Chizzonite, R. A., and Zak, R. (1983): Change in synthesis rates of alpha- and beta-myosin heavy chains in rabbit heart after treatment with thyroid hormone. *J. Biol. Chem.*, 258:2421–2425.
53. Everett, A. W., Sinha, A. M., Umeda, P. K., Jakovcic, S., Rabinowitz, M., and Zak, R. (1984): Regulation of myosin synthesis by thyroid hormone: Relative change in the α- and β-myosin heavy chain mRNA levels in rabbit heart. *Biochemistry*, 23:1596–1599.
54. Ferrans, V. J. (1984): Cardiac hypertrophy: Morphological aspects. In: *Growth of the Heart in Health and Disease*, edited by R. Zak, pp. 187–239. Raven Press, New York.
55. Fischman, D. A., and Moscona, A. A. (1971): Reconstruction of heart tissue from suspensions of embryonic myocardial cells: Ultrastructural studies on disposed and reaggregated cells. In: *Cardiac Hypertrophy*, edited by N. R. Alpert, pp. 125–139. Academic Press, New York.
56. Fischman, D. A., Doyle, C. M., and Zak, R. (1975): DNA synthesis in chick cardiac muscle: Comparative observations of *in vivo* and *in vitro* growth. In: *Developmental and Physiological Correlates of Cardiac Muscle*, edited by M. Lieberman and T. Sano, pp. 67–79. Raven Press, New York.

57. Furshspan, E. J., MacLeish, P. R., O'Lague, P. H., and Potter, D. D. (1976): Chemical transmission between rat sympathetic neurons and cardiac myocytes developing in microcultures: Evidence for cholinergic, adrenergic and dual function neurons. *Proc. Natl. Acad. Sci. USA,* 73:4225–4229.

58. Garwitz, E. T., and Jones, A. W. (1982): Aldosterone infusion into the rat and dose-dependent changes in blood pressure and arterial ionic transport. *Hypertension,* 4:374–381.

59. Goldblatt, H., Lynch, J., Hanzal, R. F., and Summerville, W. W. (1934): Studies of experimental hypertension; I. production of persistent elevation of systolic blood pressure by means of renal ischemia. *J. Exp. Med.,* 59:347–379.

60. Goldstein, M. A., Claycomb, W. C., and Schwartz, A. (1974): DNA synthesis and mitosis in well-differentiated mammalian cardiocytes. *Science,* 183:212–213.

61. Gomez, H. (1958): The development of the innervation of the heart in the rat embryo. *Anat. Rec.,* 130:53–71.

62. Gonzales-Sanchez, A., and Bader, D. (1984): Immunochemical analysis of myosin heavy chains in the developing chicken heart. *Dev. Biol.,* 103:151–158.

63. Goss, C. M. (1938): The first contractions of the heart in rat embryos. *Anat. Rec.,* 70:505–524.

64. Grollman, A. (1944): A simplified procedure for inducing chronic renal hypertension in the mammal. *Proc. Soc. Exp. Biol.,* 57:102.

65. Gross, W. O. (1982): Fibroblast-myocyte interactions in in vitro cardiomyogenesis. *Exp. Cell. Res.,* 142:341–356.

66. Hammond, G. L., Lai, Y. K., and Market, C. L. (1982): The molecules that initiate cardiac hypertrophy are not species specific. *Science,* 216:529–531.

67. Hatt, P. Y., Berjal, G., Moravec, J., and Swynghedauw, B. (1970): Heart failure: An electron microscopic study of the left ventricular capillary muscle in aortic insufficiency in the rabbit. *J. Mol. Cell. Cardiol.,* 1:235–247.

68. Hickson, R. C., Hammons, G. T., and Holloszy, J. O. (1979): Development and regression of exercise-induced hypertrophy in the rat. *Am. J. Physiol.,* 236:H268–272.

69. Hoh, J. F. Y., McGrath, P. A., and White, R. I. (1976): Electrophoretic analysis of multiple forms of myosin in fast-twitch and slow-twitch muscles of the chick. *Biochem. J.,* 157:87–95.

70. Hoh, J. F. Y., McGrath, P. A., and Hale, P. T. (1978): Electrophoretic analysis of multiple forms of cardiac myosin: Effect of hypophysectomy and thyroxine replacement. *J. Mol. Cell. Cardiol.,* 10:1053–1076.

71. Icardo, J. M. (1984): The growing heart: An anatomical perspective. In: *Growth of the Heart in Health and Disease,* edited by R. Zak, pp. 41–79. Raven Press, New York.

72. Jacobson, S. L. (1977): Culture of spontaneously contracting myocardial cells from adult rats. *Cell Struct. Func.,* 2:1–9.

73. Julian, F. J., Morgan, D. L., Moss, R. L., Gonzales, M., and Dwivedi, P. (1981): Myocyte growth without physiological impairment in gradually induced rat cardiac hypertrophy. *Circ. Res.,* 49:1300–1310.

74. Kamel, S., Kennedy, J., Vrbova, G., and Zak, R. (1985): Changes in myosin isozymes during normal and stretch induced growth in chicken skeletal muscles. *Fed. Proc.,* 44:1373.

75. Kasten, F. H. (1972): Rat myocardial cells in vitro: Mitosis and differentiated properties. *In Vitro,* 8:128–150.

76. Katzberg, A. A., Farmer, B. B., and Harris, R. A. (1977): The predominance of binucleation in isolated rat heart myocytes. *Am. J. Anat.,* 149:489–499.

77. Kelly, A. M., and Chacko, S. (1976): Myofibril organization and mitosis in cultured cardiac muscle cells. *Dev. Biol.,* 48:421–430.

78. Kolbel, F., and Schreiber, V. (1983): Biochemical regulators in cardiac hypertrophy. *Basic Res. Cardiol.,* 78:351–363.

79. Korecky, B., Sweet, S., and Rakusan, K. (1979): Number of nuclei in mammalian cardiac myocytes. *Can. J. Physiol. Pharmacol.,* 57:1122–1129.

80. Lampidis, T. J., and Schaiberger, G. E. (1975): Age related loss of DNA repair synthesis in isolated mammalian cells. *Exp. Cell Res.,* 96:412–416.

81. Landsberg, L., and Axelrod, J. (1968): Influence of pituitary, thyroid, and adrenal hormones on norepinephrine turnover and metabolism in the rat heart. *Circ. Res.,* 22:559–571.

82. Lau, C., and Slotkin, T. A. (1979): Accelerated development of rat sympathetic neurotransmission caused by neonatal triiodothyronine administration. *J. Pharmacol. Exp. Ther.,* 208:485–490.

83. Leighton, J., Merkow, L., and Locker, M. (1964): Alteration in the size of the heart of late chick embryo after incubation at varied temperatures. *Nature,* 201:198–199.

84. Lieberman, M., Roggeveen, A. E., Purdy, J. E., and Johnson, E. A. (1972): Synthetic strands of cardiac muscle: Growth and physiological implications. *Science,* 175:909–911.

85. Lieberman, M., Sawanoburi, T., Kootsey, J. M., and Johnson, E. A. (1975): A synthetic strand of cardiac muscle. Its passive electrical properties. *J. Gen. Physiol.,* 65:527–550.

86. Litten, R. Z., Martin, B. J., Low, R. B., and Alpert, N. R. (1982): Altered myosin isozyme pattern from pressure-overloaded and thyrotoxic hypertrophied rabbit hearts. *Circ. Res.,* 50:856–864.

87. Lompre, A. M., Schwartz, K., D'Albis, A., Lacombe, G., Van Thiem, N., and Swynghedauw, B. (1979): Myosin isoenzyme redistribution in chronic heart overload. *Nature,* 282:105–107.

88. Lompre, A. M., Mercadier, J. J., Wisnewsky, C., Bouveret, P., Pantaloni, C., D'Albis, A., and Schwartz, K. (1981): Species- and age-dependent changes in the relative amounts of cardiac myosin isoenzymes in mammals. *Dev. Biol.,* 84:286–290.

89. Lompre, A. M., Nadal-Ginard, B., and Mahdavi, V. (1984): Expression of the cardiac ventricular α- and β-myosin heavy chain genes is developmentally and hormonally regulated. *J. Biol. Chem.,* 259:6437–6446.

90. Mahdavi, V., Strehler, E. E., Periasamy, M., Wieczorek, D., Izumo, S., Grund, S., Chambers, A. P., Strehler, M. A., and Nadal-Ginard, B. (1985): Sarcomeric myosin heavy chain gene family organization and pattern of expression. *J. Cell. Biochem.* [Suppl.], 9B:57.

91. Manasek, F. J. (1968): Mitosis in developing cardiac muscle. *J. Cell Biol.,* 37:191–196.

92. Manasek, F. J. (1970): Histogenesis of the embryonic myocardium. *Am. J. Cardiol.,* 25:149–168.

93. Manasek, F. J., Kulikowski, R. R., Nakamura, A., Nguyenphuc, Q., and Lacktis, J. W. (1984): Early heart development: A new model of cardiac morphogenesis. In: *Growth of the Heart in Health and Disease,* edited by R. Zak, pp. 105–130. Raven Press, New York.

94. Mark, G. E., and Strasser, F. F. (1966): Pacemaker activity and mitosis in cultures of newborn rat heart ventricle cells. *Exp. Cell Res.,* 44:217–233.

95. Martin, A. F., Pagani, E. D., and Solaro, R. J. (1982): Thyroxine-induced redistribution of isoenzymes of rabbit ventricular myosin. *Circ. Res.,* 50:117–124.

96. Martin, A. F., Robinson, D. C., and Dowell, R. T. (1985): Isomyosin and thyroid hormone level in pressure-overloaded weanling and adult rat hearts. *Am. J. Physiol.,* 248:H305–310.

97. Martin, A. F., Paul, R. J., and McMahon, E. G. (1986): Isomyosin transitions in ventricles of aldosterone-salt hypertensive rats. *Hypertension,* 8:128–132.

98. Masse, M. J. O., and Harary, I. (1981): The use of fluorescent antimyosin and DNA labelling for the estimation of the myoblast and myocyte population of primary rat heart cell cultures. *J. Cell. Physiol.,* 106:165–172.

99. McCarl, R. L., Hartzell, C. R., Schroedl, N., Kunze, E., and Ross, P. D. (1980): Mammalian heart cells in culture. In: *Hearts and Heartlike Organs,* Vol. 3, edited by G. H. Bourne, pp. 1–44. Academic Press, New York.

100. Mercadier, J. J., Lompre, A. M., Wisnewsky, C., Samuel, J. L., Bercovici, J., Swynghedauw, B., and Schwartz, K. (1981): Myosin isoenzymic changes in several models of rat cardiac hypertrophy. *Circ. Res.,* 49:525–532.

101. Mercadier, J. J., Bouveret, P., Gorza, L., Schiaffino, S., Clark, W. A., Zak, R., Swynghedauw, B., and Schwartz, K. (1983): Myosin isoenzymes in normal and hypertrophied human ventricular myocardium. *Circ. Res.,* 53:52–62.

102. Nag, A. C., Cheng, M., Fischman, D. A., and Zak, R. (1983): Long-term cell culture of adult mammalian cardiac myocytes: Electron microscopic and immunofluorescent analyses of myofibrillar structure. *J. Mol. Cell. Cardiol.,* 15:301–317.

103. Nag, A. C., and Cheng, M. (1983): DNA synthesis in mammalian heart cells: Comparative studies of monolayer and aggregate cultures. *Cell. Mol. Biol.,* 29:451–459.

104. Nag, A. C., Cheng, M., and Zak, R. (1985): Distribution of isomyosin in cultured cardiac myocytes as determined by mono-

clonal antibodies and adenosine triphosphatase activity. *Exp. Cell Res.*, 158:53–62.

105. Okamoto, K. (1969): Spontaneous hypertension in rats. *Int. Rev. Exp. Pathol.*, 7:227–270.

106. Pagani, E. D., and Solaro, R. J. (1983): Swimming exercise, thyroid state, and the distribution of myosin isoenzyme in rat heart. *Am. J. Physiol.*, 245:713–720.

107. Pagani, E. D., and Julian, F. J. (1984): Rabbit papillary muscle myosin isozymes and the velocity of papillary muscle shortening. *Circ. Res.*, 54:586–594.

108. Penney, D. G. (1984): Carbon monoxide induced cardiac hypertrophy. In: *Growth of the Heart in Health and Disease*, edited by R. Zak, pp. 337–362. Raven Press, New York.

109. Pfeffer, M. A., Pfeffer, J., Mirsky, I., and Iwai, J. (1984): Cardiac hypertrophy and performance of Dahl hypertensive rats on graded salt diets. *Hypertension*, 6:475–481.

110. Piper, H. M., Probst, I., Schwartz, P., Hutter, F. J., and Spieckerman, P. G. (1982): Culturing of calcium stable adult cardiac myocytes. *J. Mol. Cell. Cardiol.*, 14:397–412.

111. Piper, H. M., and Spieckerman, P. G. (1985): Isolation, properties and applications. In: *Adult Heart Muscle Cells: Isolation, Properties and Application*. Springer-Verlag, New York.

112. Pope, B., Hoh, J. F. Y., and Weeds, A. (1980): The ATPase activities of rat cardiac myosin isoenzymes. *FEBS Lett.*, 118:205–208.

113. Purdy, J. E., Lieberman, M., Roggeveen, A. E., and Kirk, R. G. (1972): Synthetic strands of cardiac muscle: Formation and ultrastructure. *J. Cell Biol.*, 55:563–578.

114. Rakusan, K., Raman, S., Layberry, R., and Korecky, B. (1978): The influence of aging and growth on the postnatal development of cardiac muscle in rats. *Circ. Res.*, 42:212–218.

115. Robkin, M. A., Shepard, T. H., Dyer, D. C., and Guntheroth, W. G. (1976): Autonomic receptors of the early rat embryo heart: Growth and development. *Proc. Soc. Exp. Biol. Med.*, 151:799–803.

116. Rumyantsev, P. P. (1977): Interrelations of the proliferation and differentiation processes during cardiac myogenesis and regeneration. *Int. Rev. Cytol.*, 51:187–273.

117. Rupp, H. (1981): The adaptive changes in the isoenzyme pattern of myosin from hypertrophied rat myocardium as a result of pressure overload and physical training. *Basic Res. Cardiol.*, 76:79–88.

118. Rupp, H., and Jacob, R. (1982): Response of blood pressure and cardiac myosin polymorphism to swimming training in the spontaneously hypertensive rat. *Can. J. Physiol. Pharmacol.*, 60:1098–1103.

119. Rupp, H., Bukhari, A. R., and Jacob, R. (1983): Regulation of cardiac myosin isoenzymes: The interrelationship with catecholamine metabolism. *J. Mol. Cell. Cardiol. [Suppl. I]*, 15:317.

120. Rupp, H., Felbier, H.-R., Bukhari, A. R., and Jacob, R. (1984): Modulation of myosin isoenzyme populations and activities of monoamine oxidase and phenylethanolamine-N-methyltransferase in pressure loaded and normal rat heart swimming exercise and stress arising from electrostimulation in pairs. *Can. J. Physiol. Pharmacol.*, 62:1209–1218.

121. Rupp, H., and Jacob, R. (1984): Ventricular myocardium as a fast- or slow-type muscle. The influence of stressors and the preventative action of intensive exercise. In: *Pathogenesis of Stress-Induced Heart Disease*, edited by R. E. Beamish, V. Panagia, and N. S. Dhalla, pp. 147–158. Kluwer Academic, Boston.

122. Samuel, J. L., Rappaport, L., Mercadier, J. J., Lompre, A. M., Sartore, S., Triban, C., Schiaffino, S., and Schwartz, K. (1983): Distribution of myosin isoenzymes within single cardiac cells: An immunohistochemical study. *Circ. Res.*, 52:200–209.

123. Sartore, S., Gorza, L., Bormioli, S. P., Libera, L. D., and Schiaffino, S. (1981): Myosin types and fiber types in cardiac muscle. *J. Cell Biol.*, 88:226–233.

124. Schroedl, N. A., and Hartzell, C. R. (1983): Myocytes and fibroblasts exhibit functional synergism in mixed cultures of neonatal rat heart cells. *J. Cell. Physiol.*, 117:326–332.

125. Schwartz, K., Lompre, A. M., Bouveret, P., Wisnewsky, C., and Whalen, R. G. (1982): Comparison of cardiac myosins at fetal stages, in young animals and in hypothyroid adults. *J. Biol. Chem.*, 257:14412–14418.

126. Sen, S., Tarazi, R. C., and Bumpus, F. M. (1976): Biochemical

changes associated with development and reversal of cardiac hypertrophy in spontaneously hypertensive rats. *Cardiovasc. Res.*, 10:254–261.

127. Sen, S., Tarazi, R. C., and Bumpus, F. M. (1977): Cardiac hypertrophy and antihypertensive therapy. *Cardiovasc. Res.*, 11:427–433.

128. Sen, S., and Hollinger, C. (1983): A factor that may initiate myocardial hypertrophy in hypertension. *Circulation [Suppl. III]*, 68:224.

129. Sheer, D., and Morkin, E. (1984): Myosin isoenzyme expression in rat ventricle: Effects of thyroid hormone analogs, cathecholamines, glucocorticoids, and high carbohydrate diet. *J. Pharmacol. Exp. Ther.*, 229:872–879.

130. Shimada, Y., Moscona, A. A., and Fischman, D. A. (1974): Scanning electron microscopy of cell aggregation: Cardiac and mixed retina-cardiac cell suspension. *Dev. Biol.*, 36:428–446.

131. Shimada, Y., and Fischman, D. A. (1975): Cardiac cell aggregation by scanning electron microscopy. In: *Developmental and Physiological Correlates of Cardiac Muscle*, edited by M. Lieberman and T. Sano, pp. 81–101. Raven Press, New York.

132. Simpson, P., McGrath, A., and Savion, S. (1982): Myocyte hypertrophy in neonatal rat heart cultures and its regulation by serum and by catecholamines. *Circ. Res.*, 51:787–801.

133. Simpson, P., and Savion, S. (1982): Differentiation of rat myocytes in single cell cultures with and without proliferating non-myocardial cells: Cross-striation, ultrastructures and chronotropic response to isoproteronol. *Circ. Res.*, 50:101–116.

134. Sinha, A. M., Friedman, D. J., Nigro, J. M., Jakovcic, S., Rabinowitz, M., and Umeda, P. K. (1984): Expression of rat ventricular α-myosin heavy chain messenger RNA sequences in atrial muscle. *J. Biol. Chem.*, 259:6674–6680.

135. Sperelakis, N. (1979): Origin of the cardiac resting potential. In: *Handbook of Physiology*, pp. 187–267. American Physiological Society, Bethesda.

136. Stalsberg, H. (1969): Regional mitotic activity in the precardiac mesoderm and differentiating heart tube in the chick embryo. *Dev. Biol.*, 20:18–45.

137. Thomas, L. L., and Alpert, N. R. (1977): Functional integrity of the SH1 site in myosin from hypertrophied myocardium. *Biochim. Biophys. Acta*, 481:680–688.

138. Thompson, E. W., Marino, T. A., Uboh, C. E., Kent, R. L., and Cooper, G. (1984): Atrophy reversal and cardiocyte redifferentiation in reloaded cat myocardium. *Circ. Res.*, 54:367–377.

139. Tolnai, S., and Korecky, B. (1980): Lysosomal hydrolases in the heterotopically isotransplanted heart undergoing atrophy. *J. Mol. Cell. Cardiol.*, 12:869–890.

140. Tomanek, R. J., and Cooper, G. (1981): Morphological changes in the mechanically unloaded myocardial cell. *Anat. Rec.*, 200:271–280.

141. Toyota, N., and Shimada, Y. (1983): Isoform variants of troponin in skeletal and cardiac muscle cells cultured with and without nerves. *Cell*, 33:297–304.

142. Van Mierop, L. H. S. (1967): Location of pacemaker in chick embryo heart at the time of initiation of heartbeat. *Am. J. Physiol.*, 212:407–415.

143. Weisberg, A., Winegrad, A., Tucker, M., and McClellan, G. (1982): Histochemical detection of specific isozymes of myosin in rat ventricular cells. *Circ. Res.*, 51:802–809.

144. Wikman-Coffelt, J., Fenner, C., and Mason, D. T. (1978): Synthesis and phosphorylation of canine cardiac myosin in tissue culture, assessment of hypertrophying factors. In: *Recent Advances in Studies on Cardiac Structure and Function*, 12:677–682, edited by T. K. Kobayashi, Y. Ito, and G. Rona. University Park Press, Baltimore.

145. Wikman-Coffelt, J., and Srivastava, S. (1979): Differences in atrial and ventricular myosin light chains. *FEBS Lett.*, 106:207–212.

146. Wildenthal, K., and Mueller, E. A. (1974): Increased myocardial catheptic activity during regression of thyrotoxic cardiac hypertrophy. *Nature*, 249:478–479.

147. Zak, R. (1974): Development and proliferation capacity of cardiac muscle cells. *Circ. Res. [Suppl. II]*, 34-35:17–26.

148. Zak, R. (1984): Factors controlling cardiac growth. In: *Growth of the Heart in Health and Disease*, edited by R. Zak, pp. 165–185. Raven Press, New York.

149. Zak, R. (1984): Cardiac hypertrophy and atrophy. In: *The Heart*, edited by L. H. Opie, pp. 198–209. Grune & Stratton, London.

The Heart and Cardiovascular System,
edited by H. A. Fozzard et al.
Raven Press, New York © 1986.

CHAPTER 62

Cellular Basis of the Mechanical Properties of Hypertrophied Myocardium

Burt B. Hamrell and Norman R. Alpert

A sustained increase in external work of either cardiac ventricle results in enlargement of the muscle fibers in the ventricular wall (12,13,24,74,104,115,122,139,140, 193) and proliferation of connective tissue (20,28,31–33). Although there is a relationship between the extent of increase in ventricular work with the amount of hypertrophy (62), the specific cellular mechanism or mechanisms that transform a sustained increase in external work into myocardial fiber enlargement and connective tissue proliferation are unknown. Identification of the mechanisms involved in the transformation is a problem of general importance, because in addition to the increase in muscle mass during hypertrophic growth there are fundamental changes from normal in excitation-contraction coupling (16,37,55,64,77,106,110,167,184, 189,191), force development (2,71), active shortening (71), and resting muscle properties (2). The accretion of cellular elements during hypertrophic growth results not only in more tissue but also in tissue that is structurally and mechanically different from normal.

Studies of the quantitative and qualitative changes that occur during the development of hypertrophy provide unique opportunities for learning more about the fundamental mechanical properties of muscle. The documented alterations from normal in morphology, excitation-contraction coupling, and mechanics are derived

from interrelated changes in protein metabolism that culminate in hypertrophic growth. For example, changes from normal in the contractile proteins result in abnormalities in muscle biochemistry that are the basis of altered muscle mechanics (2) and energetics (8). During hypertrophic growth, sarcomeres are added within each muscle cell, and the amount of sarcomere shortening during contraction is less than normal (73,74), a finding that may be important for understanding excitation-contraction coupling, mechanics, and energetics in hypertrophy. The following is a discussion of the mechanical properties of hypertrophied heart muscle from perspectives that relate to all of the previously mentioned areas and that we have attempted to relate to each other.

MODELS OF VENTRICULAR HYPERTROPHY

There are several methods used to produce experimental hypertrophy. Pressure overload of a ventricle induced by acute partial obstruction of one of the great vessels (14,23,59,61,71,94,96,198), systemic hypertension (13,16,18,22,44,64,70,76–78,92,96,101,102,111,115, 129,132,134,136,143,144,166,192,193,196), or pulmonary (107,126) hypertension will result in hypertrophy. A nonconstricting but snug band applied to a great vessel of a young animal or a nonconstricting band composed of ameroid, which absorbs moisture and swells, will result in slow onset of ventricular hypertrophy. Gradual-onset pressure-overload hypertrophy also can be induced with intravenous infusions of silica, monocrotaline (107), or Sephadex (126). Another model involves the induction of volume overload of the ventricle by means of an arteriovenous fistula (186) or an atrial septal defect (38). Chronic endurance exercise also is used to induce ventricular hypertrophy (18,131,161) and may prove to be another type of volume overload.

The characteristics of hypertrophy in response to these mechanical stresses are, in part, dependent on levels of circulating hormones (154). In addition, hypertrophy can be induced by administration of hormones. For instance, a combination of systolic systemic high blood pressure and high cardiac output occurs with the increased metabolic load of hyperthyroidism (128). Hypertrophic growth is affected by growth hormone (21) or administration of a β agonist (47,105) or adrenocorticoids (21). A number of stresses, including cold acclimatization (137), viral infection (119), and bacterial endocarditis (46), have been shown to result in myocardial hypertrophy. Coronary artery ligation results in loss of function and scarring of the ischemic portion of the ventricular wall, with hypertrophy of the remaining muscle of that ventricle (125). In aged heart muscle there is hypertrophy with changes in mechanical function that are similar to the alterations from normal in pressure-overload hypertrophy; shortening and force development are reduced as compared with those in ventricular myocardium isolated from younger hearts (198).

The discussions of myocardial function that follow concern several types of hypertrophy, including the entire spectrum from slow contracting pressure overload to fast thyrotoxic hypertrophy.

CELLULAR PATHOPHYSIOLOGY UNDERLYING THE MECHANICAL CHANGES IN HYPERTROPHY

Morphological Alterations Important for Mechanical Function During Hypertrophic Growth

After the early neonatal period there is limited capacity for myocardial cell hyperplasia (147,148). The structural response to a sustained increase in ventricular work is myocardial cell enlargement and, under some conditions, connective tissue hyperplasia and accretion. The myocardial cell organelles are not much changed in appearance, but there is a greater than proportionate increase above normal in the number of parallel myofibrils in hypertrophied myocardial cells (139,140), and sarcomeres are added in series to the myofibrils (75,104) (Table 1). The ratio of surface area to volume of hypertrophied myocardial cells is less than normal (97), but the surface

areas of membranous structures such as mitochondria and sarcoplasmic reticulum increase in proportion with myocyte enlargement (140) (Table 1). The increase in muscle mass in hypertrophy in the absence of heart failure apparently is proportionate to the increase in ventricular work (52,62).

Page et al. (139) used microchemical determinations of trace metals to quantitate the proportion of specific cellular structures within normal myocardial cells and within cells in hearts subjected to various types of chronic stress. The results of microchemical techniques correlate highly with those from stereological analyses, and both indicate that there is a proportionate decrease in mitochondrial volume (Table 1) and an increase in myofibrillar volume in myocardial cells in the left ventricle in rats with aortic constriction. Anversa et al. (12–14) reported results similar to the foregoing, as did Kamereit and Jacob (96) in progressive aortic stenosis in rabbits (Table 1). In thyroidectomized rats treated with thyroxine (140), the proportion of myocardial cell volume consisting of myofibrils is unchanged, but the relative amounts of mitochondrial cristae and T system both increase. Therefore, sarcolemma-plus-T-system surface area increases in proportion with the increase in myocardial cell volume that occurs with hypertrophic growth secondary to pressure overload of a ventricle or thyroid hormone administration. There is a greater increase in myofibrillar volume than in cell volume in pressure-overload hypertrophic growth, but the mitochondrial mass and cristae surface area increase less than cell volume (Table 1).

In hypertrophy with heart failure, longitudinal splitting of myofibrils may occur, there is contortion of the intercalated discs, and the Z lines are more out of register (24). When heart failure is present, the ratio of myofibrillar to mitochondrial mass is decreased to levels

TABLE 1. *Morphometric changes from normal in hypertrophy*

| Myocardial cell | Pressure overload | | Thyrotoxicosis |
	Sudden	Gradual	
Number of parallel myofibrils	+↑	↑	↑
Number of series sarcomeres	↑	↑	
Surface area/volume	↓		↓
Membranous surface area (mitochondria and sarcoplasmic reticulum)	+↑		+↑
Mitochondrial volume	↓	↓	

The direction of an arrow indicates the change from normal, and a plus sign denotes that the change is greater than proportionate with cell enlargement.

less than in hypertrophy without heart failure (24), but the ratio of mitochondria surface area to mitochondria volume and the number of mitochondria per unit cross-sectional area are increased (24). In future studies we need to learn whether or not larger numbers of smaller mitochondria with less than normal total mitochondrial volume relative to myocardial cell volume are adequate for the greater than normal contractile mass in the hypertrophied cell. There is the possibility that the reduced ratio of mitochondrial volume to myocardial cell volume may indicate a mismatch of myofibrillar mass with the energy-producing capacity of the cell (123,124).

In pressure-overload and thyrotoxic hypertrophy the Z lines are widened and have been proposed as a site of sarcomerogenesis (58,108,160). Stretch of the ventricular wall appears to be the mechanical factor that is most related to an increase in protein synthesis in hearts from rats with aortic constriction or with thyrotoxicosis (127). Consequently, if the Z lines are sites that are important in sarcomerogenesis, they are optimally located for transformation of muscle stretch into the addition of series sarcomeres (75,95,104).

In rats studied 8 days after constriction of the aorta below the diaphragm, the increase in myofibrillar volume above normal is in proportion with the enlargement of myocardial cell volume (14). There is significant longitudinal myocardial cell growth from an average of 49.1 ± 7.1 μm in sham-operated controls to 65.6 ± 3.7 μm (±SEM) in the hypertrophied group (14). In dogs with pulmonary artery constriction (right ventricular pressure 50–80 mm Hg) for 2 to 7 weeks, the length of right ventricular cells increases from a normal mean of 85.3 μm to 101.5 μm, and sarcomere length in the hypertrophied myocardial cells is 1.96 μm and 2.25 μm in the normals (104). In the normals there are 38 sarcomeres in series per fiber, and 52 in the hypertrophied right ventricles (104). In young rats with slowly progressive pulmonary artery narrowing, the mean length of myocytes obtained with enzymatic dispersion is 135.2 μm, as compared with 113.3 μm in normal rats, and sarcomere length is 1.7 μm in both groups (95); there are 79 sarcomeres in series per myocardial cell in the hypertrophied rat hearts and 67 in the normals. The increase above normal in the number of sarcomeres in series per myocardial cell in hypertrophy is consistent with a site of sarcomerogenesis being present in series (58,108,160) with the sarcomeres and sensitive to stretch (127). Apparently the proliferation of series sarcomeres is an important facet of the structural alterations that characterize hypertrophic growth in animals (74) and humans (17). Specific sites where myofibrils are added in parallel are not as evident. However, it is clear that myofibrils added in parallel are essential in pressure-overload hypertrophic growth in order to maintain active ventricular wall stress at normal levels (62).

The foregoing data suggest that resting sarcomere length in hypertrophied hearts should be less than normal at any given diastolic ventricular volume. In rabbit left ventricles hypertrophied due to aortic constriction, Anversa et al. (11) fixed the ventricles at known diastolic pressures and documented sarcomere lengths at several sites through the thickness of the ventricular wall. When sarcomere lengths in normal hearts over a resting pressure range are compared with those at comparable sites and pressures in hypertrophied hearts, the sarcomere lengths are shorter than normal in hypertrophy (11).

In addition to the number of sarcomeres in series, the diastolic properties of the hypertrophied ventricle must be considered when analyzing the relationship between resting ventricular pressure and sarcomere length. For instance, a decrease in passive ventricular compliance (2,133,190) during hypertrophic growth would result in greater than normal filling pressures at a particular sarcomere length. Hydroxyproline content is greater than normal in pressure-overload hypertrophy (31,176), and there is an increase in the DNA content in hypertrophy related to proliferation of cells other than muscle cells, i.e., connective tissue cells (25,63,199). There is more than normal connective tissue in pressure-overload hypertrophy (97), but myocardial hydroxyproline content and compliance are normal in thyrotoxicosis (85). The amount of connective tissue proliferation may be related to the nature of the stimulus for hypertrophic growth (20,113). Focal connective tissue proliferation is present in sudden-onset pressure-overload hypertrophy in cats with constriction of the pulmonary artery and in rabbits with aortic constriction (25); the connective tissue foci may result from transient focal ischemia due to a demand for coronary flow that exceeds flow capacity when a great vessel is constricted.

As myocardial cells increase in cross-sectional area, the number of capillaries per muscle cell remains constant (146,151,169); thus, the mean diffusion distance from intracellular sites to capillaries is greater than normal in hypertrophy (85). The capillary density of the endocardium in cats with severe constriction of the aorta is less than normal, and with adenosine in the coronary perfusate to induce maximal coronary blood flow there is a smaller than normal ratio of endocardial to epicardial blood flow in the chronically stressed left ventricle (29). Without adenosine perfusion, the aforementioned ratio in the hypertrophied left ventricles is the same as normal; the increase in coronary blood flow resulting from addition of adenosine to the perfusate is less than normal in hypertrophy, a finding that is consistent with a reduction in coronary blood flow reserve (29). Rembert et al. (149) reported findings similar to the foregoing except for a less than normal ratio of endocardial to epicardial blood flow at rest as well as with maximal blood flow following ischemia.

Marcus et al. (118) also noted a reduction of the previously mentioned ratio and cited earlier experiments of others that were consistent with an abnormal distribution of coronary blood flow in left ventricular hypertrophy.

The coronary circulation is normal in hypertrophy secondary to volume overload related to increased ventricular filling in the presence of complete heart block in dogs (54). Gascho et al. (54) proposed that with constriction of the aorta the high coronary blood pressure may lead to abnormalities in the coronary vasculature, with a consequent increase in coronary vascular resistance in experimental left ventricular hypertrophy. However, in hypertrophy secondary to volume overload induced by complete heart block (54) or to sudden-onset pressure overload due to pulmonary artery constriction, coronary perfusion pressure remains close to normal.

Excitation-Contraction Coupling

In papillary muscles isolated from pressure-overloaded hypertrophied hearts, the time from onset of an isometric twitch to the twitch peak (time to peak tension, TPT) is increased (2,38,66,71,94), whereas the maximum rate of relaxation is less than normal (94). In hyperthyroidism, TPT is 47% shorter than normal (9). It is likely that the foregoing changes from normal in the time course of the isometric twitch in hypertrophy involve the sarcolemma, the T tubular system, and the sarcoplasmic reticulum. The plateau phase of the transmembrane potential in pressure-overload hypertrophy is longer and slightly less positive than normal (16,64,77,167,191); Ten Eick (189) reported similar findings and possible changes in ionic currents. The time for initial repolarization to -20 to -40 mV is shorter than normal in hypertrophy secondary to thyrotoxicosis (167).

In thyrotoxicosis, the plateau of the action potential is longer than normal at slow stimulation rates and is shorter than normal at fast rates of stimulation (167). Concomitant with the cascade of events that begin with depolarization of the sarcolemma and release of trigger calcium, the release, storage, and uptake of calcium by the sarcoplasmic reticulum are of critical importance in the contractile process. There may be an increase above normal in calcium uptake, and the coupling to ATPase remains intact in more mild forms of pressure overload (110). In severe pressure overload, the uptake of calcium by the sarcoplasmic reticulum is less than normal, and calcium uptake is uncoupled from ATPase activity (55,106,184). Uptake of calcium by the sarcoplasmic reticulum is accelerated in thyrotoxic hypertrophy (37).

The force-velocity relationship is depressed below normal in papillary muscles isolated from hypertrophied right ventricles and studied in solutions containing 2.5 mM Ca^{2+} and a normal Na^+ concentration (2,23,71,175).

When the solution Ca^{2+} concentration is increased to 11 mM and the Na^+ concentration is reduced, there is less depression of the force-velocity relationship below normal than in the 2.5 mM Ca^{2+}-containing solution (97). Kaufmann et al. (97) suggested that in pressure-overload hypertrophy, activation may be compromised because of a reduction in the ratio of surface area to volume in the hypertrophied myocardial cells (Table 1). Although isolated myocardial cells are not circular (26) and may be close to elliptical in cross section, they can be approximated by a right circular cylinder; with an increase in cross-sectional area of a cylinder, the ratio of surface area to volume decreases (3). However, based on stereological analyses of electron micrographs, mentioned earlier in the discussion of cell structure, the surface area of the sarcolemma plus the T system relative to myocardial cell volume is increased above normal in hypertrophy (122,140); apparently there is proliferation of the T system and its plasma membrane (Table 1). Consequently, the greater than normal mechanical response of hypertrophied cardiac muscle to increased external calcium is not due simply to a larger ratio of surface area to volume, and it may be related to the abnormalities in intracellular Ca^{2+} translocation discussed earlier. Another possibility is that high activator Ca^{2+} levels may reduce a higher than normal proportion of attached but noncycling cross-bridges in the hypertrophied preparations. Measurement of cross-bridge dynamics will be discussed in a later section.

Contractile System: Contractile Proteins

We have observed a consistent decrease below normal in myosin ATPase activity in hypertrophy due to pressure overload (2,6,48,112). However, there have been conflicting reports of an increase or no change in myosin ATPase activity, and we attribute the differences from one laboratory to another to the unexpected sensitivity of the adaptive responses of the contractile system to the precise details of the applied chronic stress. Consequently, the duration, intensity, and time course of the stress and the status of the animal at the time of application of the stress (162) determine whether a sustained increase in ventricular pressure development results in an increase, decrease, or no change in myosin ATPase activity and determine the rate of isometric active tension development and the velocity of shortening. Myosin ATPase activity (19,37,60,197) is greater than normal in hypertrophy secondary to thyrotoxicosis, as is the velocity of muscle shortening and the rate of isometric force development (65,171,181).

With reference to the foregoing variations among laboratories and animal models, it is important to note that there are several isoenzymic forms of myosin present in a number of heart preparations used in the study of hypertrophy. In ventricular myocardium there are at least three isoenzymes of myosin: (a) a high-ATPase (V_1) isoenzyme consisting of two α heavy chains; (b) a low-ATPase (V_3) isoenzyme made up of two β heavy chains; (c) a heterodimer (V_2) with intermediate ATPase activity and consisting of an α heavy chain and a β heavy chain. With the use of monoclonal antibodies, at least four regions of antigenic differences have been identified in the V_1 as compared with the V_3 myosin isoenzyme (36). When tryptic digests from the two types of enzymes are compared, there are at least three major differences in peptide maps (109,112,128) and two areas of difference in alkylation studies (112). There is a direct correlation of the rate of force development and the velocity of shortening with the myocardial V_1/V_3 iso-enzyme ratio and with the level of myosin ATPase activity (1,138,164,185), whereas the economy of iso-metric active force maintenance (*vide infra*) is inversely related to the V_1/V_3 isoenzyme ratio (9).

There is an increase in V_1 isoenzyme concentration in myocardium hypertrophied because of thyrotoxicosis, volume overload, or exercise (112,117,163,164,200), whereas in pressure-overload hypertrophy it is the activity of the V_3 isoenzyme that is increased. The extent and direction of changes in isoenzyme activity are very sensitive to the age, species, and hormonal status of the animals and the intensity of the stress applied to the ventricle (112,165,200). Also, it is important to note that in normal hearts studied with immunofluorescent microscopic techniques, the V_1 isoenzyme is more abundant in the right ventricle and in the epicardial layers, and V_3 is more abundant in the left ventricle and in endocardial layers (163).

MECHANICAL PROPERTIES OF HYPERTROPHIED MYOCARDIUM

Muscle Preparations

Thin long trabeculae and papillary muscles are especially suited for quantitative study of myocardial mechanical properties because they can be isolated from the heart and remain functionally stable for long periods in oxygenated, buffered saline and can be linked to devices to measure and control force and shortening. Although such preparations are particularly well suited for measurements of discrete mechanical properties, it is important to know if they are representative of ventricular myocardial function. In order to compare papillary muscle function with ventricular wall mechanical properties, Cronin et al. (43) attached strain gauges through a left atriotomy along the longitudinal aspect of an anterior or posterior left ventricular papillary muscle in dogs, the epicardium adjacent to the papillary muscle, and the interventricular septum. In response to positive inotropic interventions and volume loading, the

force development in the papillary muscle is similar to that of the ventricular wall. Consequently, force development of the left ventricular wall appears to be well represented in measurements from papillary muscles. Also, isolated myocardial preparations participate in hypertrophic growth in response to a sustained pressure overload. In right ventricular septal papillary muscles from cats with hypertrophy due to pulmonary artery constriction, fiber length (97) and width (97,175) are increased above normal levels. In left ventricular anterior papillary muscles of the rat there are no changes in fiber length, but fiber width is increased above control levels in response to aortic constriction (15). In rabbits with pulmonary artery constriction, enzymatically dissociated myocytes from subvalvular right ventricular free wall trabeculae are longer and wider than normal (75). Therefore, with respect to both structure and function, isolated myocardial preparations respond to perturbations that alter a ventricle.

Isometric Force Development

In papillary muscles from the left ventricle in rats with constriction of the ascending aorta, the active tension per unit dry muscle weight is increased, as compared with normal controls at comparable preloads; heart weight varies from 8 to 80% above control levels, and the active tension per unit dry muscle weight is related directly to the extent of hypertrophy (100). In rats with chronic subdiaphragmatic aortic constriction, the active and passive tensions per unit wet weight of columnae carneae are the same as normal; the weight of the hypertrophied left ventricle varies from 8.5 to 42.6% above control values (61). In these two studies, the use of dry (100) and wet (61) weights as denominators in the normalization of force measurements may account for some of the differences in the results, particularly if edema was present (percentage water was not presented in either study). The extent of active force development is related to the number of interacting sites on the thin filaments with the thick filaments; therefore, the total amount of active isometric force development is related to the number of parallel force-generating units. Consequently, in all the experiments to be discussed later, force is expressed as tension, defined as force per unit cross-sectional area.[1]

In rats studied 28 days after aortic constriction (left ventricular weight 40% greater than normal), the level of peak active isometric tension development in left ventricular columnae carneae muscles is not different

---

[1] Tension is more correctly defined as force per unit length, and stress is force per unit cross-sectional area; however, here we are presenting the generally used definition of tension in muscle physiology, which is identical with that for stress.

from normal and sham-operated control levels. TPT (time to peak tension; time from onset of a twitch to its peak) at L_{max} (muscle length where peak active twitch tension amplitude, P_{max}, is maximal) is prolonged (23).

In cats with sustained reduction of pulmonary artery external diameter to 80% of normal and no evidence of heart failure, the mean peak active isometric tension levels are the same as normal in papillary muscles from hypertrophied right ventricles studied at lengths from 45% below to 3% above L_{max} and at 1 to 90 days postoperatively. The ratio of right ventricular weight to body weight (RV/BW) is 90% above control levels. In papillary muscles from hypertrophied right ventricles from cats with heart failure induced by a 90% reduction of pulmonary artery external diameter, peak active isometric twitch tension is significantly less than normal; the RV/BW ratio is 142% above control levels (175).

TPT can be the same as normal in papillary muscles from hypertrophied or failed right ventricles (175) or prolonged in papillary muscles from cats with right ventricular hypertrophy without failure (38,66). Whether or not TPT is prolonged may depend on subtle differences in the effects of chronic stress on the excitation-contraction coupling mechanism. The maximum rate of isometric active twitch tension development, $(dP/dt)_{max}$, is significantly less than normal in cats with hypertrophy or with hypertrophy and heart failure (175).

In papillary muscles from rabbits with constriction of the pulmonary artery for 2 weeks, TPT is longer than normal (2,71). P_{max} is the same as normal in hypertrophied rabbit papillary muscles (2,71). There have been other reports of a decrease (35,38,80) or no change (65,66) in P_{max} and a decrease in $(dP/dt)_{max}$ (23,35,65,66) in hypertrophy as compared with normal.

A summary of the foregoing mechanical studies suggests that P_{max} is not substantially changed from normal in pressure-overload hypertrophy, whereas $(dP/dt)_{max}$ is reduced to less than normal, and TPT is prolonged. Because the extent of isometric force development is dependent in part on the balance of factors that determine TPT and dP/dt, it is not surprising that there is a range of values of P_{max} in hypertrophy in the several species studied over a range of ages and in the presence of a variety of experimental conditions.

Isotonic Shortening

In rats with aortic constriction for up to 28 days, postoperatively columnae carneae muscles from the left ventricle manifest less than normal muscle shortening velocity "at the lightest possible preload . . . at a slightly shorter muscle length [than L_{max}]" (23).

At up to 85 days after pulmonary artery constriction in cats, there is a significant depression to less than normal levels of the isotonic afterloaded force-velocity relationship in right ventricular papillary muscles at an initial external length determined by a 0.5 g/mm² pre-load;[2] the force-velocity relationship is depressed further in the presence of heart failure (175). Kaufmann et al. (97) found a similar depression of the force-velocity relationship in cats with pulmonary constriction, right ventricular hypertrophy, and no evidence for congestive heart failure. At a superfusate calcium concentration of 11.0 mM with reduced sodium-ion concentration, the force-velocity relationship is higher than in 2.5 mM calcium in normal and hypertrophied cat right ventricular papillary muscles (97). However, as was discussed earlier in relation to excitation-contraction coupling in hypertrophy, the shift in the hypertrophied muscles is greater than normal.

In the foregoing studies, afterloaded isotonic twitches were used to study muscle shortening. In an afterloaded contraction, shortening begins at a time in the isometric twitch that is inversely related to the total load; the muscle shortens with light loads earlier in the twitch than with heavier loads. Therefore, the amount of auxotonic sarcomere shortening (73,103) and the extent of intracellular release and uptake of calcium are dependent variables, as well as the velocity of muscle shortening. If the muscle is released at a selected instant in the isometric twitch and then shortens with a range of constant loads, one can measure the instantaneous force-velocity relationship with isotonic afterloaded quick releases. When force and shortening are measured with quick releases at the conclusion of the first third of TPT, the force-velocity relationship is depressed below normal in the hypertrophied muscles (2,71). V_{max}, the estimated shortening velocity at zero load, is independent of resting muscle length in normal and hypertrophied muscles and is depressed in hypertrophy (71). In the presence of substantial myocardial hypertrophy due to pressure overload, all laboratories report depression of isotonic shortening velocity (35,38,65,66).

V_{max}, measured with quick releases early in the twitch over a range of temperatures, is directly linearly related to calcium-activated myosin ATPase activity in rabbit and marmot myocardium when the biochemical measures are obtained from the same hearts and at the same temperatures as the mechanical measurements (72). The values for calcium-activated myosin ATPase activity (2) and V_{max} in right ventricular myocardium from rabbits with pulmonary artery constriction and normal rabbits fall along the foregoing linear relationship.

In contrast to the above studies involving substantial amounts of hypertrophy, in an experiment in which a modest amount of pulmonary artery constriction (pulmonary artery external diameter reduced to 35–40% of normal) was induced in cats, there was no change from normal isometric and isotonic mechanical properties

---

[2] Approximately 90% L_{max} based on our estimate from the graph of muscle length versus resting tension.

(141). The degree of pulmonary artery constriction used by Pannier (141) was less than that reported by Spann et al. (175) or Kaufmann et al. (97).

Transient Mechanical Responses to Pressure Overload

In some instances there are initial changes from normal in the mechanical properties of pressure-overloaded ventricles, but with the return of some of these changes to normal in the presence of persistent high pressure (94,195). When 200- to 250-g Wistar rats with abdominal aortic constriction were compared with normal and sham-operated controls at 5 to 28 days after surgery, there were initial decreases in P_{max}, $(dP/dt)_{max}$, and maximal muscle shortening velocity at the lightest total load in the hypertrophied muscles (94). However, the depressed values returned to close to control levels by 28 days postoperatively (94). The ventricular wet weight was 30% to 40% above control levels, and the muscle measurements were obtained at 5, 8, 15, and 28 days postoperatively. At 8 days after surgery, TPT was significantly prolonged, and this persisted throughout the 28 days of the study; in some of the rats the aortic constriction was removed at 5, 8, or 15 days, and the prolonged TPT persisted, but the other changes from normal mechanical function noted earlier returned to control or greater than control levels. The maximal rate of isometric twitch relaxation at L_{max} was less than control levels at 5, 8, and 15 days after surgery, and when the constriction was removed, it returned to control levels in the hypertrophy muscles.

There is an inverse relationship between active isometric twitch tension and stimulus frequency in rat myocardium, i.e., there is a negative rate treppe. Papillary muscles from the hypertrophied rat ventricles described above developed more than normal P_{max} levels as stimulus frequency was increased from 0.1 to 1.0 Hz, and the inverse relation of developed tension with stimulation frequency was shifted to the right as a result of hypertrophy (94). After removal of the constriction, the force–frequency curves returned to normal (94).

In cats with pulmonary artery constriction for 6 to 24 weeks, which resulted in a 70% increase above normal right ventricular weight, there was a symmetrical depression below normal of the length–active-tension relationship at 6 weeks, but by 24 weeks P_{max} returned to normal levels (195). The pattern of depression at 6 weeks, with return to control levels at 24 weeks, also was noted for the isotonic afterloaded force-velocity relationship and $(dP/dt)_{max}$ at L_{max} with paired stimulation and with norepinephrine in the superfusate (195). The length–resting-tension relationship did not change over the 24 weeks.

Changes from normal in ventricular function in the presence of pressure overload are consistent with the transient changes in isolated muscle function described earlier. In conscious, instrumented dogs, left ventricular dimensions and pressure are used to assess function over time after the onset of sustained aortic constriction with an encircling cuff inflated to an extent that is determined by the magnitude of increase in left ventricular systolic and end-diastolic pressures (159). Left ventricular wall thickness, internal diameter at a minor axis, and intraventricular pressure are measured with implanted sensors prior to the constriction, when left ventricular dilatation is maximal, during stable hypertrophy, immediately following the release of the stenosis, and finally 24 hr after release. The extent and rate of left ventricular shortening decrease immediately after constriction and then gradually return to normal as the constriction is maintained and hypertrophy progresses. Peak left ventricular wall stress per unit cross-sectional area initially increases and then returns toward normal. At an average of 9 days after onset of constriction, high left ventricular wall stress and maximal dilatation are present; wall stress is close to normal, end-diastolic internal diameter is at control levels, and there is normal circumferential shortening at 2 weeks after constriction; ventricular dimensions and ejection return to normal, and wall stress decreases to less than normal levels. In some dogs, 6 to 7 days after release of the cuff constriction there is a decrease in left ventricular wall thickness to 7% above control levels.

From all of the foregoing studies of muscle shortening in the presence of substantial pressure-overload hypertrophy it is apparent that the force-velocity relationship is depressed below normal levels, although the depression may be transient in some experiments in some species. Meerson (124) has proposed that the ventricle responds to pressure overload in stages: (a) stage of damage: increased oxygen consumption per unit mass of myocardium, anaerobic glycolysis, and decreases in P_{max} and $(dP/dt)_{max}$; (b) stage of compensation: force per unit tissue dimension and overall ventricular performance return to normal because of hypertrophic growth; and (c) stage of exhaustion and heart failure: depletion of myocardial norepinephrine, scar tissue appears, and atrophy, depressed ATPase activity, ATP depletion, and depressed mitochondrial activity appear (124).

Gradual-Onset Pressure-Overload Hypertrophy

As we noted earlier, focal fibrotic reactions may occur following the imposition of a sudden pressure overload (25). Gradual pressure overload can be induced by applying a snug but not constricting band to the great vessel of a young animal, and as the animal grows the relative stenosis becomes more severe; when this is done in kittens, eventually there is a substantial increase above normal in right ventricular pressure and mass (Table 2), but cardiac output and ejection fraction remain normal (40). There are no important differences

TABLE 2. *Slow as compared with sudden-onset right ventricular hypertrophy*

	RV weight	RV pressure (mm Hg)		Septal papillary muscle				
		S	ED	P_{max}	P_{rest}	$(dP/dt)_{max}$	TPT	dL/dt
Slow	52%↑	50	3–4	↓	↓	↓	↑	↓
Sudden	65%↑	40	3	—	—	↓	↑	↓

Slow-onset hypertrophy data are from Cooper et al. (40), and data are from Alpert et al. (2) and Hamrell and Alpert (71) for sudden onset. RV is right ventricular, and S and ED refer to systolic and end-diastolic intraluminal pressures, respectively. P_{rest} is the resting tension at L_{max}, and dL/dt is the rate of muscle shortening as the lowest load measured in each study. The arrows indicate an increase or decrease as compared with normal; a dash indicates no change from normal.

in mechanical properties when the sudden-onset pressure-overload model is compared with the gradual-onset model (Table 2). The several types of cardiac hypertrophy models condense what may take years to develop in human heart disease into several weeks or months; the presence or absence of focal connective tissue does not appear to complicate analysis of the functional characteristics of the various pressure-overload models.

Thyrotoxic Hypertrophy

In animals given repeated injections of L-thyroxine, the rate of active tension development is greater than in muscle isolated from normal controls (60,172,181,187). In some studies, the extent of active tension development is greater in heart muscle preparations from hyperthyroid animals than from controls (187), but usually it is unchanged from normal (172,181–183). The combination of the rate of force development with TPT determines the amount of active force development. During the initial 3 weeks of treatment of guinea pigs with L-thyroxine, $(dP/dt)_{max}$ increases, TPT is reduced, and peak tension is greater than normal (60,172). Active peak isometric twitch force levels from hypothyroid rat left ventricular papillary muscles normalized to muscle weight are less than normal (194). Smitherman et al. (173) reported less than normal active isometric twitch tension, $(dP/dt)_{max}$ and TPT in thyrotoxicosis in rabbits, which they attributed to abnormally arrayed thick filaments and focal areas of contracture.

There is faster than normal release and/or uptake of calcium by the sacroplasmic reticulum in hyperthyroidism (135), which is consistent with the aforementioned changes in TPT and $(dP/dt)_{max}$. It is also important to note that differences based on comparisons of isometric twitches from hyperthyroid animals with those from normals are most apparent at a slow stimulus rate (0.2 Hz) and may be absent at faster rates (60,187).

Mechanical Properties at the Sarcomere Level

Thin isolated myocardial preparations can be studied with an optical system suitable for imaging the diffraction

patterns that result when a laser beam is focused on the muscle (73,103). The myofibrils, which consist of sarcomeres in series, constitute a repeating array of alternating bands of refractive index levels that diffract light (158). A diffraction pattern can be imaged by a suitable optical system when the coherent light beam of a laser is focused onto a trabeculum with a diameter less than approximately 200 μm (73,103). The modal sarcomere length in the region of the muscle illuminated by the laser beam is inversely proportional to the distance from the center of distribution of the zeroth order to that of one of the first orders. Sarcomere length determined with diffraction is highly correlated with sarcomere length determined from photomicrographs of the same region of the muscle illuminated by the laser beam (r = 0.91) (73); the diffraction patterns and photomicrographs include data from normal and hypertrophied muscles (rabbit right ventricular free wall trabeculae) at rest and at the peak of the twitch (73).

Resting sarcomere length at L_{max} is less than normal (2.32 ± 0.02 μm; ±SEM) in pressure-overload hypertrophy (2.24 ± 0.01 μm) (73,74). There is less than normal auxotonic sarcomere shortening during isometric active tension development in pressure-overload hypertrophied myocardium (73,74,86). Myocytes have been enzymatically dispersed from right ventricular free wall trabeculae in the same region of the heart as those used for the diffraction studies (75). The average length of the myocytes from the hypertrophied ventricles is 109.8 ± 1.0 μm, as compared with 102.9 ± 0.9 μm (±SEM; $p <$ 0.05) in the normals, and the respective values for myocyte width are 20.0 ± 0.2 μm and 15.4 ± 0.2 μm (75). Hamrell et al. (73–75,86) hypothesized that the greater than normal number of sarcomeres in series per myocyte in hypertrophy in part accounts for the reduced auxotonic sarcomere shortening during active tension development in hypertrophied myocardium. Series compliance is the same as normal in hypertrophy (71,94,95,142). Therefore, during isometric active force development to a particular force level, as the myocytes shorten auxotonically and stretch the series compliant elements, the absolute amount of fiber shortening should be the same as normal in hypertrophy, whereas fiber shortening relative to initial fiber length will be reduced. Consequently, the amount of shortening per sarcomere in the longer hypertrophied myocytes is less than normal (73,74,86). There also is less than normal sarcomere shortening for a given amount of isotonic muscle shortening in hypertrophy (74), which is consistent with the foregoing auxotonic data.

Consequently, there is less work than normal per sarcomere during the contraction of hypertrophied cardiac muscle. Also, because there is less sarcomere shortening than normal during hypertrophied muscle shortening, there may be less shortening deactivation (93). Less susceptibility to shortening-related deactivation and less sarcomere work may be important aspects of compensation in hypertrophy that are important to explore. In the hypertrophied ventricle, if there is less than normal sarcomere shortening to produce a particular ejection fraction, that could be important for maintaining a given level of ventricular function.

MYOCARDIAL ENERGY MEASUREMENTS

Energy measurements provide the thermodynamic envelope within which all of the mechanical and biochemical events during systole and diastole must fit. Thus, under appropriate conditions, energy measurements can be used to shed light on the molecular events taking place during contraction, relaxation, and recovery. The major methods available to the investigator for evaluating the energy fluxes of the heart are thermal, chemical, and the measurement of oxygen consumption or nuclear magnetic resonance (NMR). Myothermal measurements offer the advantage of speed, and under steady-state conditions, in conjunction with mechanical information, they provide a total picture of the energy fluxes. Rapid thermal measurements are limited to isolated preparations such as the papillary muscle. For measurements on the entire organ, thermal measurements are slow and therefore have the same temporal limitations as do measurements of oxygen consumption. Quantification of oxygen consumption and lactate production provides an overall index of aerobic and anaerobic metabolism and can be applied to whole organs as well as isolated preparations; however, the measurements, although inclusive, suffer from an intrinisic lack of speed. NMR measurements are noninvasive and can provide repeated measurements in the same tissue of CrP, ATP, P_i, and H^+ levels. Although the rate constants for some reactions have been measured, the instantaneous levels of the high-energy compounds during contraction and relaxation have not been satisfactorily assessed. NMR studies require substantial amounts of tissue and are difficult to carry out on simple systems such as very thin muscle bundles or papillary muscles, a problem that can be addressed if measurements are carried out on an array of muscle bundles organized so as to permit simultaneous mechanical and NMR mea-

surements. Finally, detailed chemical analyses of tissues can be used to provide the time course of energy fluxes, but they are time-consuming and require multiple preparations.

Mitochondria

The ADP/O ratio and state-3 respiration of mitochondria from pressure- or volume-overloaded hypertrophied hearts are normal (38,86,152,174). Similar data were obtained from thyrotoxic hypertrophied hearts (179). Recovery heat production (discussed in detail later) provides information concerning the efficiency with which ATP is resynthesized from ADP during the recovery period. For a given quantity of ADP presented to the mitochondria (assessed by measurements of initial heat), the recovery heat production is normal in pressure overload and is decreased in thyrotoxic hypertrophied hearts (9).

Energetics

Hill (83) pioneered the use of heat measurements in skeletal muscle to analyze the relationship between mechanical performance and energy consumption. The key to making those measurements was the development of a low-resistance, sensitive planar thermopile that permitted simultaneous assessment of muscle heat output with force or work. The first comparable thermometric measurements on isolated heart papillary muscles were made using high-resistance, plated wire thermopiles (150). There is broad agreement regarding the energetics of papillary muscles or intact perfused hearts based on measurements of oxygen consumption, NMR, or heat output (42,53,89,116,155). Gibbs et al. (56,57) developed the approach used to analyze heat data from thin trabeculae or small papillary muscles from the left or right ventricle of hearts in a manner that generally followed the outline developed by Hill for skeletal muscle (83). The heat production (and accordingly the muscle temperature above ambient) (Fig. 1) can be divided into a resting component and an activity-related component. The activity-related heat (T_A) is partitioned into the initial (I) and recovery (R) phases. The initial heat is made up of tension-dependent (TDH) and tension-independent (TIH) portions.

A muscle at rest produces a steady quantity of heat that results from all of the energy-consuming processes involved in maintaining the integrity of the resting cell (from the energetic viewpoint it is equivalent to the resting oxygen consumption). There have been no reported differences from normal in the resting heat of hearts hypertrophied secondary to pressure overload or thyrotoxicosis.

When heart muscle is stimulated repetitively and steady-state conditions prevail, the total activity-related

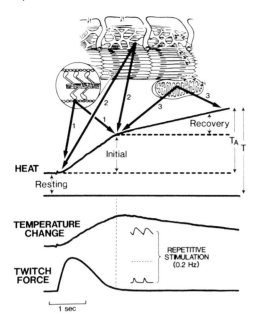

FIG. 1. Components of muscle heat and the time course of their liberation. Presented from the bottom upward are the isometric twitch force, the muscle temperature change, the muscle heat production, and the muscle components responsible for the heat production. The uncorrected temperature change observed following repetitive steady-state stimulation oscillates around a mean above the base temperature (**inset, lower right**). The mean value above the baseline and the height of the oscillation depend on the rate and quantity of heat production, the thermal capacity of the muscle and temperature-measuring system, and the heat loss characteristics of the system. In the upper portion of this diagram is a corrected heat record and the sources of that heat. The total heat (T) is made up of resting heat and total activity-related heat (T_A). The initial heat portion of the T_A arises from the cross-bridge cycling heat (TDH) (arrows labeled 1) and the calcium cycling heat (TIH) (arrows labeled 2). The recovery portion of the T_A arises from the mitochondria and is believed to be associated with the resynthesis of ATP from ADP.

heat is a reflection of all the energy-producing processes associated with excitation, contraction, relaxation (initial heat), and recovery heat (Fig. 1). In pressure-overload hypertrophy in rabbit right ventricles, the ratio of recovery heat to initial heat (R/I) is normal (4,6–9). In contrast, when the rabbit heart is hypertrophied following thyroxine administration, the R/I ratio is significantly less than normal (6,8,9), an observation that suggests that the recovery processes (resynthesis of ATP by mitochondria) are more efficient in the thyrotoxic hypertrophied hearts. The unidirectional reaction rate constants for both the forward and reverse creatine kinase reactions are reported to be depressed in pressure-overload hypertrophied heart preparations (27,90). Comparable measurements have not been made under thyrotoxic conditions.

In isometric contractions under steady-state conditions, the initial heat per tension-time integral is less than normal for pressure-overload hypertrophied hearts and

greater than normal for thyrotoxic hypertrophied hearts (6,8). The tension-dependent portion of the initial heat (TDH) is associated with myosin cross-bridge cycling. TDH, normalized for the isometric tension-time integral (TDH/∫Pdt), is low in pressure-overload and high in thyrotoxic hypertrophied hearts (6,8). TDH/∫Pdt varies directly with the actomyosin ATPase activity and the percentage V_1 myosin isoenzyme from those hearts (6,8). Thus, isometric force development is more economical (economy = ∫Pdt/TDH) in pressure-overload hearts with a low myosin ATPase activity and less economical in thyrotoxic hearts with a high ATPase activity; these results can be interpreted in terms of a kinetic analysis of myosin cross-bridge head cycling (Fig. 2) (49). There are several features of this analysis: (a) In

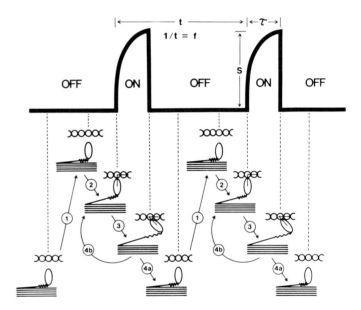

FIG. 2. Interpretation of myothermal data in terms of a kinetic analysis of myosin cross-bridge head cycling (6,8). In the upper part of the diagram the cross-bridge head cycle is presented in a sequence of states that do not produce force (OFF) and force-producing states (ON). Thus, force development can be analyzed in terms of the tension-time integral, τ, and the frequency of cross-bridge cycling, f. In terms of an enzyme kinetic view, the cross-bridge cycle can be analyzed in terms of steps 1 through 4 in the lower portion of the diagram. In step 1, actin and myosin are dissociated and undergo a transformation from the refractory M**ADP-P_i state to the nonrefractory M^{++}ADP-P_i state. At this stage in the cycle the myosin can combine with actin, yielding AM^{++}ADP-P_i (step 2). In step 3 there is an obligatory rotation of the cross-bridge head (AM-ADP-P_i) that stretches the compliant filaments and produces force. In step 4a, ADP and P_i are liberated, ATP combines with actomyosin, causing dissociation of actin and myosin, and the cycle then repeats itself starting with M**ADP-P_i. An alternative pathway is indicated by step 4b, where ADP and P_i are liberated, with a new molecule of ATP binding to the system, but total dissociation does not occur; the actomyosin oscillates from a force-producing step to a step that does not produce force, with the molecule of ATP being hydrolyzed for each cycle. (Adapted from ref. 49.)

developing force, the myosin cross-bridge head attaches to actin, rotates from a 90° position to a 45° position, and stretches the compliant links, and (b) following the development of force, the myosin cross-bridge head detaches from the actin to repeat the cycle. For each cycle, one ATP is hydrolyzed, producing heat at 11 kcal/mole. Consequently, the force development in each of the preparations can be analyzed from the myothermal and mechanical data in terms of the cycling rate and the tension-time integral for each cross-bridge (6,8).

In pressure-overloaded hypertrophied hearts (P), the cross-bridge cycling rate is decreased, while the tension-time integral is increased, findings that are associated with a decreased myosin ATPase activity and an increase in the V_3/V_1 myosin isoenzyme ratio. Conversely, in thyrotoxic hypertrophied hearts (T), the cross-bridge cycling rate is increased, and the tension-time integral is decreased; in these hearts, myosin ATPase activity is increased, and the V_3/V_1 myosin isoenzyme ratio is decreased. The ratios of myosin cross-bridge cycling rates and tension-time integrals for hypertrophied versus control (C) hearts are presented in Table 3.

In the pressure-overloaded preparation, the tension-independent heat is low and is liberated more slowly than normal, a finding that can be interpreted in terms of less calcium cycled with each stimulus and slower sequestration of the calcium that is liberated (4,41), and this is consistent with the increase above normal in TPT and decreased $(dP/dt)_{max}$ observed in these preparations (2,8,71). Furthermore, isolated sarcoplasmic reticular (SR) preparations from similarly hypertrophied hearts sequester calcium at a slower rate than normal (30,91,152,174). Tension-independent heat is liberated more rapidly than normal in thyrotoxic hearts; consequently, the SR from these hearts has the capability of taking up calcium from the cytoplasm more rapidly than the normal SR.

From the thermal data on pressure-overload hypertrophied hearts, one would expect that oxygen consumption would also be depressed, and in a number of experiments this was observed to be the case (30,40). However, a number of studies indicated that resting and

TABLE 3. *Cross-bridge cycling frequency and tension-time integral in pressure-overload (P) and thyrotoxic (T) hypertrophied hearts as compared with controls (C)*

Preparation	f	s_T	V_3/V_1	$E = \int Pdt/TDH$
P/C	0.65	1.54	↑	↑
T/C	1.56	0.47	↓	↓

f = cross-bridge cycling frequency; s_T = cross-bridge tension-time integral; V_3 and V_1 refer to the myosin isoenzymes, with V_3 being the β homodimer with low ATPase activity and V_1 representing the α homodimer with high ATPase activity; E = economy of isometric force development.

tension-related oxygen consumptions for pressure-overloaded hypertrophied hearts were greater than normal (38,39,66,170,180). Although there is no simple explanation for the contrast between these results and the observations of decreased energy output per tension-time integral discussed previously, there are at least two possibilities. The experiments for the hypertrophied group may have been carried out at lengths slightly above L_{max}, where activity-related energy production is greater than at shorter lengths (130). A second possibility is that the experimental groups might have had a higher V_1/V_3 isoenzyme ratio prior to initiation of the stress than the control rabbits; if this was so, then even after the stress the ratio might still have been higher than control levels and yielded a higher than normal oxygen consumption for those preparations. In light of the extraordinary sensitivity of the V_1/V_3 myosin isoenzyme ratios to the age of the animals and the substantial variation known to exist at a given age within a group, the foregoing possibility exists. Thus, it is wise to know the isoenzyme composition of the preparations used. If that is not possible, then great care must be given to randomizing the experiments. In thyrotoxic hypertrophy, myothermal and oxygen consumption measurements agree in that there is an augmentation of energy dissipation per tension-time integral in both (5,67,130).

FUTURE DIRECTIONS

A model that relates overall cross-bridge cycling rate and tension-time integral with biochemical and thermodynamic data from normal and hypertrophied myocardial preparations has been presented (Fig. 2, Table 3). Programmed mechanical perturbations have been used to assess the relative number of attached cross-bridges and to derive rate constants for cross-bridge turnover in single skeletal muscle fibers. Similar perturbations have been used to study normal heart muscle, but the complex geometry of heart muscle complicates interpretation of the data. A model of cardiac muscle mechanics that attempts to account for the relationship between mechanical work and energy consumption eventually must be tested with quantitative measures of cross-bridge dynamics.

By applying small (<0.5% of muscle length) length perturbations at the ends of an intact skeletal muscle fiber and then analyzing the relationship between length change and the resulting force change, a stiffness can be calculated that bears a direct relationship to active tension development (88). The slope of the linear relationship of the ratio of the force level (T_1, Fig. 3) at the end of phase 1 (Fig. 3) to the active force level (T_0, Fig. 3) with relative length change is positive, and the magnitude of the slope is proportional to active tension and the amount of overlap of actin with myosin filaments on the descending limb of the length–active-tension

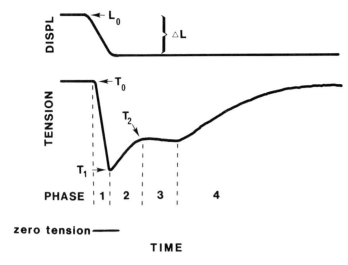

FIG. 3. Tension response to a rapid length transient. L_0 is the muscle length prior to onset of a shortening transient at the arrow next to L_0; ΔL is the length change during the transient. DISPL is displacement. T_0 is the active tension level at the moment of onset of the transient. The rest of the tension transient characteristics are discussed in the text. The time scale depends on the type of preparation and the conditions of the experiment.

relationship (81). The amount of active tension developed in skinned skeletal muscle fibers exposed to submaximal activating levels of calcium is proportional to active stiffness, determined as described above (81). Consequently, the stiffness described may be a reflection of the relative number of force-generating cross-bridges during contraction.

During contraction, cross-bridge cycling occurs as biochemical energy stores are converted to muscular work (51). Consequently, if these stiffness measurements are to reflect the number of attached cross-bridges at any given instant, the length perturbation and force response must be completed rapidly. When a sufficiently rapid length transient is used (complete within 0.2 msec in skeletal muscle), the relationship between force and length during the transient is linear (68). With large length changes and a long phase 1 tension redevelopment begins during the transient. As a result, the level of T_1 is higher than expected at the large length changes, and the relationship between force and length during phase 1 and the plot of T_1 versus length change will be nonlinear.

The initial rapid force change is followed by a phase of rapid recovery of force (88) toward the level that pertained prior to the length transient (phase 2, Fig. 3). The rapid recovery phase could be related to a rapid change in the number of force-generating cross-bridges (145) or to a change in configuration (88) or state (50) of existing attached cross-bridges. Guth et al. (69) and Cecchi et al. (34) concluded that phase 2 reflects the behavior of existing attached cross-bridges rather than

the attachment of additional cross-bridges, because stiffness was only slightly reduced during phase 2.

Following the rapid recovery phase, there is a phase of reduced rate of tension recovery or reversal of tension recovery (phase 3, Fig. 3) (88) that is thought to be due to cross-bridge detachment or attachment (80). Finally, in skeletal muscle, the remainder of tension recovery (phase 4, Fig. 3) is believed to be related to cross-bridges cycling and reaching a new equilibrium at the isometric force level following the length change (88).

Force transients similar to the foregoing have been observed in actively contracting heart muscle (80, 153,156,177). However, in cardiac muscle studies, only three distinct phases have been identified: (a) a change in force concurrent with the length change, analogous to phase 1; (b) a rapid recovery of force toward the level before the length change, similar to phase 2; (c) a subsequent slowing down or a reversal of force recovery, a phase that may be a combination of phases 3 and 4. In cardiac muscle, the rate constant of the most rapid recovery phase (phase 2) following a rapid length change is dependent on the amplitude of the length change for a stretch but is independent of the extent of length change for releases (177).

Because the rapid and then slower phases of force recovery that are present in contracting muscle are absent from length transient studies of relaxed cardiac muscle or cardiac muscle in contracture, Saeki et al. (156) argued that the recovery phases are related to the kinetics of cycling cross-bridges. The proposition that the rapid and then slower force recovery phases are associated with the behavior of cycling cross-bridges in myocardial preparations is consistent with the dependence of the amplitude and/or rate constant of the force recovery phases on the rapidity, direction (stretch or release), and amplitude of the length change (156,177), on the degree of activation of the muscle (80,177), on the level of substrate concentration (Mg-ATP) (153), and on the extent of phosphorylation of the myosin light chains (153).

Active muscle stiffness is greater than normal in septal papillary muscles from the right ventricles of rabbits with pulmonary artery constriction (87), although P_{max} is unchanged. An increase in active muscle stiffness could mean that the number of cross-bridges attached at a given active force level might be greater than normal in hypertrophy or that the stiffness per cross-bridge might be increased, or a combination of these two possibilities might be present. The decreased resting compliance of hypertrophied cardiac muscle (2) is a potential confounding variable in such an interpretation. Another variable difficult to control in stiffness measurements in cardiac muscle is series compliance, which resides predominantly at the ends of a myocardial preparation damaged during attachment to the measuring apparatus (103). However, it is important to note that series compliance, measured in muscle preparations from the same rabbit model as for the stiffness measurements, is the same as normal in hypertrophy (71).

Problems of interpretation of myocardial stiffness presented by the presence of end compliance could be solved by resolving cardiac muscle length perturbations at the level of the sarcomere by using laser diffraction. However, the level of resolution of sarcomere length by diffraction in cardiac muscle may not be high enough to be applied consistently for this purpose (45).

Sinusoidal length perturbations have been used to investigate the characteristics of cardiac muscle (114, 157,178,188). Exponential rate processes within the cross-bridge cycle can be assessed by analyzing the force response to small-amplitude sinusoidal length perturbations applied to an isometrically contracting muscle. In theory, the response to cyclic perturbations is not different than that to length transients described earlier; Kawai and Brandt (98) described the correspondence of the exponential rate processes resolved by sinusoidal analysis with phases 2, 3, and 4 of the force transient response to rapid small-amplitude length changes of skeletal muscle fibers (88).

Although stiffness attributable to attached cross-bridge number is difficult to measure in cardiac muscle preparations, the study of rate constants that can be derived from analyses of tension responses to sinusoidal length perturbations is fruitful. Because the frequency of the length perturbations is known, the frequency of the force response is known, and therefore one can use powerful signal processing techniques, e.g., fast Fourier transforms, to enhance the signal-to-noise ratio. Consequently, interpretable force change measurements can be obtained with small-amplitude length perturbations. Also, the sinusoidal technique is well-suited to distinguishing among exponential processes with similar rate constants (99).

Small sinusoidal length perturbations at frequencies from 0.05 to 50 Hz were applied to right ventricular papillary muscles from normal rabbits and rabbits treated with thyroxine in order to assess dynamic myocardial stiffness (168). Stable contracture was induced in the muscles by incubation in a solution containing barium (168). In a plot of dynamic stiffness versus frequency there is a minimum at 1.2 and 2.6 Hz for the normal and thyrotoxic muscles, respectively. Such minima are interpreted as an index of cross-bridge cycling rate. The higher frequency at which the minimum occurs for the thyrotoxic muscles is consistent with an expected higher than normal cross-bridge cycling frequency related to the increase in V_1/V_3 isoenzyme ratio in muscles from rabbits treated with thyroid (112). The ratio of thyrotoxic to normal rabbit myocardial cross-bridge cycling rate calculated from the sinusoidal perturbation measurements was 2.2, as compared with 1.6 from the thermal measurements (Table 3), a difference that in part may

be attributed to differences in methodology (including any possible effects of barium on cycling rate). Also, the V_1/V_3 isoenzyme ratio decreases with age. Starting with older rabbits with a lower V_1/V_3 ratio and cross-bridge cycling rate would result in a higher ratio of the findings in thyrotoxicosis to those in normals.

Pseudo-random-noise length perturbations were applied to rat papillary muscles with a high V_1 myosin isoenzyme electrophoretic profile and compared with muscles with a low profile (83). Contracture was induced with barium. With a perturbation analysis similar to that described earlier, the calculated cycling rate for the high-profile muscles was 2.1, as compared with 1.1 for the low-profile preparations. In contrast, myothermal analysis of absolute cross-bridge cycling rate of rat heart papillary muscles tetanized in a solution containing high calcium and caffeine was 6.5 Hz for the high-V_1 hearts and 2.7 Hz for the low-V_1 muscles (10). In these experiments the high- and low-V_1 rats were similar to those used by Hoh (83). The absolute difference found when the results of pseudo-random-noise experiments are compared with the myothermal results may be a result of the effects of the incubation medium on cross-bridge cycling or may involve intrinsic differences in the methodology.

Another approach to the study of normal and hypertrophied cardiac muscle is to "skin" small bundles of cardiac fibers by exposing them to a detergent (Brij-58, 0.5% wt/vol) (121). The bundles of cells are obtained from the right ventricular free wall of normal and hypertrophied rabbit hearts by briefly grinding the tissue in relaxing solution (120,121). Once affixed to an apparatus that permits the measurement of force and shortening, contraction can be induced by exposing the bundle of skinned cells to solutions containing calcium (120,121). In a comparison of such preparations from normal rabbits, rabbits with pressure-overload hypertrophy, and thyrotoxic rabbits, there was no significant variation from one curve relating muscle force to pCa^{2+} for the three groups (121). Consequently, there is no evidence for an alteration from normal of calcium sensitivity of the contractile system of ventricles hypertrophied due to pressure overload or thyrotoxicosis; the implication is that the regulatory proteins function normally in hypertrophy. The force-velocity relation of skinned fibers is above normal levels in thyrotoxicosis and is below normal in pressure-overload hypertrophy (121). Consequently, there is a change in shortening speed intrinsic to the contractile system concomitant with hypertrophic growth and changes in the level of myosin ATPase activity (121). The latter findings of a reduced rate of muscle shortening in these muscle fragments from throughout the free wall of hypertrophied right ventricles are in accord with the extent of reduction of shortening velocity in septal papillary muscles from the same model (2,71). There are future directions, such as applying one of the aforementioned perturbation techniques to skinned fibers, that are important to explore.

CONCLUSIONS

In the process of adapting to stress, fundamental changes occur in the structural and functional characteristics of the contractile apparatus and membrane system of myocardial cells. Study of the functional changes from normal in hypertrophied heart muscle has yielded valuable clues to fundamental aspects of myocardial mechanics and the relationship between structure and function. Observations in normal and hypertrophied myocardium have revealed basic aspects of adaptation to stress by the contractile proteins and broadened our understanding of the processes by which chemical energy is converted into mechanical work. Consequently, the study of myocardial hypertrophy has emerged as an important tool with which one can investigate the fundamental behavior of muscle and, as a consequence, learn more about the basic aspects of heart disease.

ACKNOWLEDGMENTS

The authors wish to express their sincere appreciation to Dr. Michael R. Berman for his helpful suggestions as regards the material on length perturbations of muscles. However, we accept all responsibility for any inaccuracies. Dr. Hamrell's research was supported in part by grants P01-28001, R01-HL21182, R01-HL31260, and PHS-5429-23-14, and by grants-in-aid from the Vermont Affiliate of the American Heart Association. Support for Dr. Alpert's research was derived in part from USPHS grants R01-HL34179-01 and P01-HL28001-04A1

REFERENCES

1. Alpert, N. R., Gale, H. H., and Taylor, N. (1967): The effect of age on contractile protein ATPase activity and the velocity of shortening. In: *Factors Influencing Myocardial Contractility*, edited by R. D. Tanz, F. Kavaler, and J. Roberts, pp. 127–133. Academic Press, New York.
2. Alpert, N. R., Hamrell, B. B., and Halpern, W. (1974): Mechanical and biochemical correlates of cardiac hypertrophy. *Circ. Res.* [*Suppl. II*], 34:71–82.
3. Alpert, N. R., and Hamrell, B. B. (1975): Cardiac hypertrophy: A compensatory and anticompensatory response to stress. In: *Cardiac Physiology for the Clinician*, edited by M. Vassalle, pp. 173–201. Academic Press, New York.
4. Alpert, N. R., and Mulieri, L. A. (1977): The partitioning of altered mechanics in hypertrophied heart muscle between the sarcoplasmic reticulum and the contractile apparatus by means of myothermal measurements. *Basic. Res. Cardiol.*, 72:153–159.
5. Alpert, N. R., Litten, R. Z., and Mulieri, L. A. (1978): Myothermal vs enzymatic changes in thyrotoxic hypertrophy. *Physiologist*, 21:2.
6. Alpert, N. R., Mulieri, L. A., and Litten, R. Z. (1979): Functional significance of altered myosin adenosine triphosphatase activity in enlarged hearts. *Am. J. Cardiol.*, 44:947–953.
7. Alpert, N. R., and Mulieri, L. A. (1981): Increased myothermal economy of isometric force generation in compensated hypertrophy induced by pulmonary artery constriction in the rabbit. A characterization of heat liberation in normal and hypertrophied right ventricular papillary muscles. *Circ. Res.*, 50:491–500.
8. Alpert, N. R., and Mulieri, L. A. (1982): Heat, mechanics and myosin ATPase activity in normal and hypertrophied heart muscle. *Fed. Proc.*, 41:192–198.
9. Alpert, N. R., and Mulieri, L. A. (1983): Thermomechanical economy of hypertrophied hearts. In: *Myocardial Hypertrophy and Failure*, edited by N. R. Alpert, pp. 619–630. Raven Press, New York.
10. Alpert, N. R., Mulieri, L. A., Litten, R. Z., and Holubarsch, C. (1984): A myothermal analysis of the myosin crossbridge cycling rate during isometric tetanus in normal and hypothyroid rat hearts. *Eur. Heart J.* [*Suppl. F*], 5:3–11.
11. Anversa, P., Vitali-Mazza, L., Odoardo, V., and Marchetti, G. (1971): Experimental cardiac hypertrophy: A quantitative ultrastructural study in the compensatory stage. *J. Mol. Cell. Cardiol.*, 3:213–227.
12. Anversa, P., Loud, A. V., and Vitali-Mazza, L. (1976): Morphometry and autoradiography of early hypertrophic changes in the ventricular myocardium of adult rat: An electronic microscopic study. *Lab. Invest.*, 35:475–483.
13. Anversa, P., Loud, A. V., Giacomelli, F., and Weiner, J. (1978): Absolute morphometric study of myocardial hypertrophy in experimental hypertension. II. Ultrastructure of myocytes and interstitium. *Lab. Invest.*, 38:597–609.
14. Anversa, P., Olivetti, G., Melissari, M., and Loud, A. V. (1979): Morphometric study of myocardial hypertrophy induced by abdominal aortic stenosis. *Lab. Invest.*, 40:341–349.
15. Anversa, P., Olivetti, G., Melissari, M., and Loud, A. V. (1980): Stereological measurement of cellular and subcellular hypertrophy and hyperplasia in the papillary muscle of adult rat. *J. Mol. Cell. Cardiol.*, 12:781–795.
16. Aronson, R. S. (1980): Characteristics of action potentials of hypertrophied myocardium from rats with renal hypertension. *Circ. Res.*, 47:443–454.
17. Astorri, E., Bolognesi, R., Colla, B., Chizzola, A., and Visioli, O. (1977): Left ventricular hypertrophy: A cytometric study on 42 human hearts. *J. Mol. Cell. Cardiol.*, 9:763–775.
18. Bache, R. J., and Vrobel, T. R. (1979): Effects of exercise on blood flow in hypertrophied heart. *Am. J. Cardiol.*, 44:1029–1033.
19. Banerjee, S. K., Kabbas, E. G., and Morkin, E. (1977): Enzymatic properties of the heavy meromyosin subfragment of cardiac myosin from normal and thyrotoxic rabbits. *J. Biol. Chem.*, 252:6925–6929.
20. Bartosova, D., Chvapil, M., Korecky, B., Poupa, O., Rakusan, K., Turek, Z., and Vizek, M. (1969): The growth of the muscular and collagenous parts of the rat heart in various forms of cardiomegaly. *J. Physiol. (Lond.)*, 200:285–295.
21. Beznak, M. (1952): The effect of the pituitary and growth hormone on the blood pressure and on the ability of the heart to hypertrophy. *J. Physiol. (Lond.)*, 116:74–83.
22. Beznak, M., Korecky, B., and Thomas, G. (1969): Regression of cardiac hypertrophies of various origin. *Can. J. Physiol. Pharmacol.*, 47:579–586.
23. Bing, O. H. L., Matshushita, S., Fanburg, B. L., and Levine, H. J. (1973): Mechanical properties of rat cardiac muscle during experimental hypertrophy. *Circ. Res.*, 28:234–245.
24. Bishop, S. P., and Cole, C. R. (1969): Ultrastructural changes in the canine myocardium with right ventricular hypertrophy and congestive heart failure. *Lab. Invest.*, 20:219–229.
25. Bishop, S. P., and Melsen, L. R. (1976): Myocardial necrosis, fibrosis, and DNA synthesis in experimental cardiac hypertrophy induced by sudden pressure overload. *Circ. Res.*, 39:238–245.
26. Bishop, S. P., Oparil, S. Reynolds, R. H., and Drummond, J. L. (1979): Regional myocyte size in normotensive and spontaneously hypertensive rats. *Hypertension*, 1:378–383.
27. Bittl, J. A., and Ingwall, J. S. (1985): Reaction rates of creatine kinase and ATP synthesis in isolated rat heart: A ^{31}P NMR magnetization transfer study. *J. Biol. Chem.*, 260:3512–3517.
28. Bonnin, C. M., Sparrow, M. P., and Taylor, R. R. (1981): Collagen synthesis and content in right ventricular hypertrophy in the dog. *Am. J. Physiol.*, 241:708–713.

29. Breisch, E. A., Houser, S. R., Carey, R. A., Spann, J. F., and Bove, A. A. (1980): Myocardial blood flow and capillary density in chronic pressure overload of the feline left ventricle. *Cardiovasc. Res.,* 14:469–475.

30. Breisch, E. A., Houser, S. R., and Coulson, R. L. (1983): Reduced heat production in compensated pressure-overload hypertrophy of the left ventricle of the cat. In: *Myocardial Hypertrophy and Failure,* edited by N. R. Alpert, pp. 587–599. Raven Press, New York.

31. Buccino, R. A., Harris, E., Spann, J. F., Jr., and Sonnenblick, E. H. (1969): Response of myocardial connective tissue to development of experimental hypertrophy. *Am. J. Physiol.,* 216: 425–428.

32. Carey, R. A., Natarjan, G., Bove, A. A., Santamore, W. P., and Spann, J. F. (1980): Elevated collagen content in volume overload induced cardiac hypertrophy. *J. Mol. Cell. Cardiol.,* 12:929–936.

33. Caulfield, J. B. (1983): Morphologic alterations of the collagen matrix with cardiac hypertrophy. In: *Myocardial Hypertrophy and Failure,* edited by N. R. Alpert, pp. 167–175. Raven Press, New York.

34. Cecchi, G., Griffiths, P. J., and Taylor, S. (1982): Muscular contraction: Kinetics of crossbridge attachment studied by high-frequency stiffness measurements. *Science,* 217:70–72.

35. Chandler, B. M., Sonnenblick, E. H., Spann, J. F., Jr., and Pool, P. (1967): Association of depressed myofibrillar adenosine triphosphatase and reduced contractility in experimental heart failure. *Circ. Res.,* 21:717–725.

36. Chizzonite, R. A., Everett, A. W., Clark, W. A., and Zak, R. (1983): Molecular variants of cardiac myosin: Identification, isolation, quantitation and measurement of synthesis rates. In: *Myocardial Hypertrophy and Failure,* edited by N. R. Alpert, pp. 477–496. Raven Press, New York.

37. Conway, G., Heazlitt, R. A., Fowler, N. O., Gabel, M., and Green, S. (1976): The effect of hyperthyroidism on the sarcoplasmic reticulum and myosin ATPase of dog hearts. *J. Mol. Cell. Cardiol.,* 8:39–51.

38. Cooper, G., Satava, R. M., Harrison, C. E., and Coleman, H. N. (1973): Mechanisms for abnormal energetics of pressure-induced hypertrophy of the cat myocardium. *Circ. Res.,* 33:213–223.

39. Cooper, G., Puga, F. J., Zujko, K. J., Harrison, C. E., and Coleman, H. N. (1973): Normal myocardial function and energetics in volume overload hypertrophy in the cat. *Circ. Res.,* 32: 140–148.

40. Cooper, G., Tomanek, R. J., Ehrhardt, J. C., and Marcus, M. L. (1981): Chronic progressive pressure overload of the cat right ventricle. *Circ. Res.,* 48:488–497.

41. Coughlin, P., and Gibbs, C. L. (1981): Cardiac energetics in short and long term hypertrophy induced by aortic coarctation. *Cardiovasc. Res.,* 15:623–631.

42. Coulson, R. L. (1976): Energetics of isovolumic contractions of the isolated rabbit heart. *J. Physiol. (Lond.),* 260:45–53.

43. Cronin, R., Armour, J. A., and Randall, W. C. (1969): Function of the in-situ papillary muscle in the canine left ventricle. *Circ. Res.,* 25:57–75.

44. De Champlain, J., Mueller, R. A., and Axelrod, J. (1969): Turnover and synthesis of norepinephrine in experimental hypertension in rats. *Circ. Res.,* 25:285–291.

45. Dealy, M. J., Vassallo, D. V., Iwazumi, T., and Pollack, G. H. (1979): Fast response of cardiac muscle to quick length changes. In: *Crossbridge Mechanism in Muscle Contraction,* edited by H. Sugi and G. H. Pollack, pp. 71–83. University Park Press, Baltimore.

46. Dhalla, N. S., Ziegelhoffer, A., Singal, P. K., Panagia, V., and Dhillon, K. S. (1980): Subcellular changes during cardiac hypertrophy and heart failure due to bacterial endocarditis. *Basic. Res. Cardiol.,* 75:81–91.

47. Dhalla, N. S., Dzurba, A., Pierce, G. N., Tregaskis, M. G., Panagia, V., and Beamish, R. E. (1983): Membrane changes in myocardium during catecholamine-induced pathological hypertrophy. In: *Myocardial Hypertrophy and Failure,* edited by N. R. Alpert, pp. 527–534. Raven Press, New York.

48. Draper, M., Taylor, N., and Alpert, N. R. (1971): Alteration in the contractile protein in hypertrophied guinea pig hearts. In: *Cardiac Hypertrophy,* edited by N. R. Alpert, pp. 315–331. Academic Press, New York.

49. Eisenberg, E., and Hill, T. L. (1978): A crossbridge model of muscle contraction. *Prog. Biophys. Mol. Biol.,* 33:55–82.

50. Eisenberg, E., Hill, T. L., and Chen, Y. (1980): Cross-bridge model of muscle contraction—quantitative analysis. *Biophys. J.,* 29:195–227

51. Eisenberg, E., and Hill, T. L. (1985): Muscle contraction and free energy transduction in biological systems. *Science,* 227:999–1006.

52. Ford, L. (1976): Heart size. *Circ. Res.,* 39:297–303.

53. Fossel, E. T., Morgan, H. E., and Ingwall, J. S. (1980): Measurement of changes in high-energy phosphates in the cardiac cycle using gated P-31 NMR. *Proc. Natl. Acad. Sci. U.S.A.,* 77:3654–3658.

54. Gascho, J. A., Mueller, T. N., Eastham, C., and Marcus, M. L. (1982): Effect of volume-overload hypertrophy on the coronary circulation in awake dogs. *Cardiovasc. Res.,* 16:288–292.

55. Gertz, E. W., Hess, J. L., Lain, R. F., and Briggs, F. N. (1967): Activity of the vesicular calcium pump in the spontaneously failing heart-lung preparation. *Circ. Res.,* 20:477–484.

56. Gibbs, C. L., Ricchiuti, N. V., and Mommaerts, W. F. H. M. (1967): Energetics of cardiac contractions. *J. Physiol. (Lond.),* 191:25–46.

57. Gibbs, C. L., and Chapman, J. B. (1979): Cardiac heat production. *Annu. Rev. Physiol.,* 41:507–519.

58. Goldstein, M. A., Sordahl, L. A., and Schwartz, A. (1974): Ultrastructural analysis of left ventricular hypertrophy in rabbits. *J. Mol. Cell. Cardiol.,* 6:265–273.

59. Gonzalez, N. C., Wemken, H., and Heisler, N. (1979): Intracellular pH regulation of normal and hypertrophic rat myocardium. *J. Appl. Physiol.,* 47:651–656.

60. Goodkind, M. J., Damback, G. E., Thyrum, P. T., and Luchi, R. J. (1974): Effect of thyroxine on ventricular myocardial contractility and ATPase activity in guinea pigs. *Am. J. Physiol.,* 226:66–72.

61. Grimm, A. F., Kubota, R., and Whitehorn, W. V. (1963): Properties of the myocardium in cardiomegaly. *Circ. Res.,* 12: 118–124.

62. Grossman, W. (1980): Cardiac hypertrophy: Useful adaptation or pathologic process? *Am. J. Med.,* 69:576–584.

63. Grove, D., Zak, R., Nair, K. G., and Aschenbrunner, V. (1969): Biochemical correlates of cardiac hypertrophy: IV. Observations on the cellular organization of growth during myocardial hypertrophy in the rat. *Circ. Res.,* 25:473–485.

64. Gulch, R. W., Baumann, R., and Jacob, R. (1979): Analysis of myocardial action potential in left ventricular hypertrophy of Goldblatt rats. *Basic Res. Cardiol.,* 74:69–82.

65. Gunning, J. F., and Coleman, H. N. (1972): The effects of hypertrophy on myocardial energy utilization. In: *Recent Advances in Studies on Cardiac Structure and Metabolism.* Vol. I. *Myocardiology,* edited by E. Bajusz and E. Rona, pp. 190–199. University Park Press, Baltimore.

66. Gunning, J. F., Cooper, G., Harrison, C. E., and Coleman, H. N. (1973): Myocardial oxygen consumption in experimental hypertrophy and congestive heart failure due to pressure overload. *Am. J. Cardiol.,* 32:427–436.

67. Gunning, J. F., Harrison, C. E., and Coleman, N. H. (1974): Myocardial contractility and energetics following treatment with d-thyroxine. *Am. J. Physiol.,* 226:1166–1171.

68. Guth, K., Kuhn, H. J., Drexler, B., Berberich, W., and Ruegg, J. C. (1979): Stiffness and tension during and after sudden length changes of glycerinated single insect fibrillar muscle fibres. *Biophys. Struct. Mech.,* 5:255–276.

69. Guth, K., Kuhn, H. J., Tsuchiya, T., and Ruegg, J. C. (1981): Length dependent state of activation—length change dependent kinetics of cross bridges in skinned insect flight muscle. *Biophys. Struct. Mech.,* 7:139–169.

70. Hall, O., Hall, C. E., and Ogden, E. (1953): Cardiac hypertrophy in experimental hypertension and its regression following reestablishment of normal blood pressure. *Am. J. Physiol.,* 174:175–178.

71. Hamrell, B. B., and Alpert, N. R. (1977): The mechanical characteristics of hypertrophied rabbit cardiac muscle in the absence of congestive heart failure: The contractile and series elastic elements. *Circ. Res.,* 40:20–25.

72. Hamrell, B. B., and Low, R. B. (1978): The relationship of

mechanical V_{max} to myosin ATPase activity in rabbit and marmot ventricular muscle. *Pfluegers Arch.*, 377:119–124.

73. Hamrell, B. B., Hultgren, P. B., and Dale, L. (1983): Reduced auxotonic sarcomere shortening in pressure-overload cardiac hypertrophy: Subcellular cardiac compensation. In: *Myocardial Hypertrophy and Failure*, edited by N. R. Alpert, pp. 311–322. Raven Press, New York.

74. Hamrell, B. B., and Hultgren, P. B. (1985): Sarcomere shortening in pressure overload hypertrophy. *Fed. Proc.*, (*in press*).

75. Hamrell, B. B., Roberts, E. T., Carkin, J. A., and Delaney, C. L. (1986): Myocyte morphology of free wall trabeculae in right ventricular pressure overload hypertrophy in rabbits. *J. Mol. Cell. Cardiol.*, 18:127–138.

76. Hawthorne, E. W., Hinds, J. E., Crawford, W. J., and Tearney, R. J. (1974): Left ventricular myocardial contractility during the first week of renal hypertension in conscious instrumented dogs. *Circ. Res. [Suppl. I]*, 34:223–234.

77. Heller, L. J., and Stauffer, E. K. (1981): Membrane potentials and contractile events of hypertrophied rat cardiac muscle. *Proc. Soc. Exp. Biol. Med.*, 166:141–147.

78. Henning, M. (1969): Noradrenaline turnover in renal hypertensive rats. *J. Pharm. Pharmacol.*, 21:61–63.

79. Henry, P. D., Ahumada, G. G., Friedman, W. F., and Sobel, B. E. (1972): Simultaneously measured isometric tension and ATP hydrolysis in glycerinated fibers from normal and hypertrophied rabbit heart. *Circ. Res.*, 31:740–749.

80. Herzig, J. W., and Ruegg, J. C. (1977): Myocardial cross-bridge activity and its regulation by Ca^{2+}, phosphate and stretch. In: *Myocardial Failure*, edited by G. Riecker, A. Weber, and J. Goodwin, pp. 41–51. Springer-Verlag, Berlin.

81. Herzig, J. W., Yamamoto, T., and Ruegg, J. C. (1981): Dependence of force and immediate stiffness on sarcomere length and Ca^{2+} activation in frog skinned muscle fibres. *Pfluegers Arch.*, 389:97–103.

82. Hill, A. V. (1965): *Trails and Trials in Physiology*. Williams & Wilkins, Baltimore.

83. Hoh, J. F. Y., and Rossmanith, G. H. (1983): Crossbridge dynamics in rat papillary muscle containing V1 and V3 isomyosins: Effect of adrenaline. *J. Mol. Cell. Cardiol. [Suppl. 2]*, 15:65.

84. Holubarsch, C., Holubarsch, T., Jacob, R., Medugorac, I., and Thiedemann, K. (1983): Passive elastic properties of myocardium in different models and stages of hypertrophy: A study comparing mechanical, chemical, and morphometric parameters. In: *Myocardial Hypertrophy and Failure*, edited by N. R. Alpert, pp. 323–336. Raven Press, New York.

85. Honig, C. R., and Bourdean-Martini, J. (1974): Extravascular component of oxygen transport in normal and hypertrophied hearts with special reference to oxygen therapy. *Circ. Res. [Suppl. II]*, 34–35:97–103.

86. Hultgren, P. B., and Hamrell, B. B. (1985): Reduced auxotomic sarcomere shortening in pressure overload hypertrophy in rabbits. *Am. J. Physiol.*, 249:820–826.

87. Hultgren, P. B., and Hamrell, B. B. (1986): Increased active elastic stiffness in tetanized rabbit papillary muscles. *Basic Res. Cardiol.* (*in press*).

88. Huxley, A. F., and Simmons, R. M. (1972): Mechanical transients and the origin of muscular force. *Cold Spring Harbor Symp. Quant. Biol.*, 37:669–680.

89. Ingwall, J. (1982): Phosphorus nuclear magnetic resonance spectroscopy of cardiac and skeletal muscles. *Am. J. Physiol.*, 242:729–744.

90. Ingwall, J. S., and Fossel, E. T. (1983): Changes in the creatine kinase system in the hypertrophied myocardium of the dog and rat. In: *Myocardial Hypertrophy and Failure*, edited by N. R. Alpert, pp. 601–617. Raven Press, New York.

91. Ito, Y., Suko, J., and Chidsey, C. A. (1974): Intracellular calcium and myocardial contractility. V. Calcium uptake of sarcoplasmic reticulum fractions in hypertrophied and failing rabbit hearts. *J. Mol. Cell. Cardiol.*, 6:237–247.

92. Jacob, R., Ebrecht, G., Kammereit, A., Medugorac, I., and Wendt-Gallitelli, M. F. (1977): Myocardial function in different models of cardiac hypertrophy. An attempt at correlating mechanical, biochemical, and morphological parameters. *Basic. Res. Cardiol.*, 72:160–167.

93. Jewell, B. R. (1977): A reexamination of the influence of muscle length on myocardial performance. *Circ. Res.*, 40:221–230.

94. Jouannot, P., and Hatt, P. Y. (1975): Rat myocardial mechanics during pressure-induced hypertrophy development and reversal. *Am. J. Physiol.*, 229:355–364.

95. Julian, F. J., Morgan, D. L., Moss, R. L., Gonzalez, M., and Dwivedi, P. (1981): Myocyte growth without physiological impairment in gradually induced rat cardiac hypertrophy. *Circ. Res.*, 49:1300–1310.

96. Kamereit, A., and Jacob, R. (1979): Alterations in rat myocardial mechanics under Goldblatt hypertension and experimental aortic stenosis. *Basic Res. Cardiol.*, 74:389–405.

97. Kaufmann, R. L., Homburger, H., and Wirth, H. (1971): Disorders in excitation-contraction coupling of cardiac muscle from cats with experimentally produced right ventricular hypertrophy. *Circ. Res.*, 28:346–357.

98. Kawai, M., and Brandt, P. W. (1980): Sinusoidal analysis: A high resolution method for correlating biochemical reactions with physiological processes in activated skeletal muscles of rabbit, frog and crayfish. *J. Muscle Res. Cell. Motil.*, 1:279–303.

99. Kawai, M., Cox, R. N., and Brandt, P. W. (1981): Effect of Ca^{2+} ion concentration on cross-bridge kinetics in rabbit psoas fibers. Evidence for the presence of two Ca^{2+}-activated states of thin filament. *Biophys. J.*, 35:375–384.

100. Kerr, A., Winterburger, A. R., and Giambattista, M. (1961): Tension developed by papillary muscles from hypertrophied cat hearts. *Circ. Res.*, 9:103–105.

101. Keung, E. C. H., and Aronson, R. S. (1981): Non-uniform electrophysiological properties and electrotonic interaction in hypertrophied rat myocardium. *Circ. Res.*, 49:150–158.

102. Kissling, G., Gassenmaier, T., Wendt-Gallitelli, M. F., and Jacob, R. (1977): Pressure volume relations, elastic modulus and contractile behaviour of the hypertrophied left ventricle of rats with Goldblatt II hypertension. *Pfluegers Arch.*, 369:213–221.

103. Krueger, J. W., and Pollack, G. H. (1975): Myocardial sarcomere dynamics during isometric contractions. *J. Physiol. (Lond.)*, 251:627–643.

104. Laks, M. M., Morady, F., Garner, D., and Swan, H. J. L. (1974): Temporal changes in canine right ventricular volume, mass, cell size, and sarcomere length after banding the pulmonary artery. *Cardiovasc. Res.*, 8:106–111.

105. Laks, M. M. (1977): Norepinephrine, the producer of myocardial cellular hypertrophy and/or necrosis and/or fibrosis. *Am. Heart J.*, 94:394–399.

106. Lamers, J. M. M., and Stinis, J. T. (1979): Defective calcium pump in the sarcoplasmic reticulum of the hypertrophied rabbit heart. *Life Sci.*, 18:2313–2319.

107. Larson, D. F., Womble, J. R., Copeland, J. G., and Russell, D. H. (1982): Concurrent left and right ventricular hypertophy in dog models of right ventricular overload. *J. Thorac. Cardiovasc. Surg.*, 84:543–547.

108. Legato, M. J. (1970): Sarcomerogenesis in human myocardium. *J. Mol. Cell. Cardiol.*, 1:425–437.

109. Leger, J., Klotz, C., and Leger, J. J. (1983): Cardiac myosin heavy chains and tropomyosin in mechanical heart overloading and aging. In: *Myocardial Hypertrophy and Failure*, edited by N. R. Alpert, pp. 385–392. Raven Press, New York.

110. Limas, C. J., Spier, S. S., and Kahlon, J. (1980): Enhanced calcium transport by sarcoplasmic reticulum in mild cardiac hypertrophy. *J. Mol. Cell. Cardiol.*, 12:1103–1116.

111. Limas, C. J. (1982): Enhanced myocardial RNA synthesis in spontaneously hypertensive rats. Possible role of high-mobility group non-histone proteins. *Biochim. Biophys. Acta*, 696:37–43.

112. Litten, R. Z., Martin, B. J., Low, R. B., and Alpert, N. R. (1982): Altered myosin isoenzyme patterns from pressure-overloaded and thyrotoxic hypertrophied rabbit hearts. *Circ. Res.*, 50:856–864.

113. Ljungqvist, A., and Unge, G. (1973): The proliferative activity of the myocardial tissue in various forms of experimental cardiac hypertrophy. *Acta Pathol. Microbiol. Scand.*, A81:233–240.

114. Loeffler, L., and Sagawa, K. (1975): A one-dimensional viscoelastic model of cat heart muscle studied by small length perturbations during isometric contraction. *Circ. Res.*, 36:498–512.

115. Loud, A. V., Anversa, P., Giancomelli, F., and Wiener, J. (1978): Absolute morphometric study of myocardial hypertrophy in

experimental hypertension. I. Determination of myocyte size. *Lab. Invest.,* 38:586–596.

116. MacDonald, R. H. (1971): Myocardial heat production: Its relationship to tension development. *Am. J. Physiol.,* 220:894–900.

117. Malhotra, A., Pempargkul, T. F., Schaible, T. F., and Scheuer, J. (1981): Contractile proteins and sarcoplasmic reticulum in physiologic cardiac hypertrophy. *Am. J. Physiol.,* 241:263–267.

118. Marcus, M. L., Mueller, T. M., Gascho, J. A., and Kerber, R. E. (1979): Effects of cardiac hypertrophy secondary to hypertension on the coronary circulation. *Am. J. Cardiol.,* 44:1023–1028.

119. Matsumori, A., and Kawai, C. (1982): An animal model of congestive (dilated) cardiomyopathy: Dilatation and hypertrophy of the heart in the chronic stage in DBA/2 mice with myocarditis caused by encephalomyocarditis virus. *Circulation,* 66:355–360.

120. Maughan, D., Low, E., Litten, R., and Alpert, N. (1979): Calcium-activated muscle from hypertrophied rabbit hearts: Mechanical and correlated biochemical changes. *Circ. Res.,* 44:279–287.

121. Maughan, D. (1983): Use of functionally skinned tissue in studying altered contractility in hypertrophied myocardium. In: *Myocardial Hypertrophy and Failure,* edited by N. R. Alpert, pp. 337–343. Raven Press, New York.

122. McCallister, L. P., and Page, E. (1973): Effects of thyroxin on ultrastructure of rat myocardial cells: A stereological study. *J. Ultrastruct. Res.,* 42:136–155.

123. Meerson, F. Z., Zaletayeve, T. A., Lagutchev, S. S., and Pshennikova, M. G. (1964): Structure and mass of mitochondria in the process of compensatory hyperfunction and hypertrophy of the heart. *Exp. Cell Res.,* 36:568–578.

124. Meerson, F. Z. (1969): The myocardium in hyperfunction, hypertrophy and heart failure. *Circ. Res. [Suppl. II],* 25:1–163.

125. Meerson, F. Z. (1983): *The Failing Heart: Adaptation and Deadaptation,* edited by A. M. Katz, pp. 51–52. Raven Press, New York.

126. Matsuhashi, T., Arai, R., and Sawa, H. (1980): Right ventricular hypertrophy following chronic pulmonary embolism induced by repeated administration of Sephadex particles. *Tohoku J. Exp. Med.,* 131:143–150.

127. Morgan, H. E., Gordon, E. E., Kira, Y., Siehl, D. L., Watson, P. A., and Chua, B. H. L. (1985): Biochemical correlates of myocardial hypertrophy. *Physiologist,* 28:18–27.

128. Morkin, E., Flink, I. L., and Goldman, S. (1983): Biochemical and physiologic effects of thyroid hormone on cardiac performance. *Prog. Cardiovasc. Dis.,* 25:435–464.

129. Mueller, T. M., Marcus, M. L., Kerber, R. E., Young, J. A., Barnes, R. W., and Abboud, F. M. (1978): Effect of renal hypertension and left ventricular hypertrophy on the coronary circulation in dogs. *Circ. Res.,* 42:543–549.

130. Mulieri, L. A., and Alpert, N. R. (1977): Length dependence of initial heat in cardiac muscles. *Biophys. J.,* 17:161A.

131. Muntz, K. H., Gonyea, W. J., and Mitchell, J. H. (1981): Cardiac hypertrophy in response to an isometric training program in the cat. *Circ. Res.,* 49:1092–1101.

132. Nakamura, K., Gerold, M., and Thoenen, H. (1971): Experimental hypertension of the rat: Reciprocal changes of norepinephrine turnover in heart and brain-stem. *Naunyn Schmiedebergs Arch. Pharmacol.,* 268:125–139.

133. Natarajan, G., Bove, A. A., Coulson, R. L., Carey, R. A., and Spann, J. F. (1979): Increased passive stiffness of short-term pressure-overload hypertrophied myocardium in cat. *Am. J. Physiol.,* 237:676–680.

134. Nishiyama, K., Nishiyama, A., and Frohlich, E. D. (1976): Regional blood flow in normotensive spontaneously hypertensive rats. *Am. J. Physiol.,* 230:691–698.

135. Nwoye, L., Mommaerts, W. F. H. M., Simpson, D. R., Seraydarian, K., and Marusich, M. (1982): Evidence for a direct action of thyroid hormone in specifying muscle properties. *Am. J. Physiol.,* 242:401–408.

136. Okamoto, K., and Aoki, K. (1963): Development of a strain of spontaneously hypertensive rats. *Jpn. Circ. J.,* 21:282–293.

137. Oliviero, A., and Stjarne, L. (1965): Acceleration of noradrenaline turnover in the mouse heart by cold exposure. *Life Sci.,* 4:2339–2343.

138. Pagani, E. D., and Julian, F. J. (1984): Rabbit papillary muscle isozymes and the velocity of muscle shortening. *Circ. Res.,* 54:586–594.

139. Page, E., Polimeni, P. I., Zak, R., Earley, J., and Johnson, M. (1972): Myofibrillar mass in rat and rabbit heart muscle: Correlation of microchemical and stereological measurements in normal and hypertrophied. *Circ. Res.,* 30:430–439.

140. Page, E., and McCallister, L. P. (1973): Quantitative electron microscopic description of heart muscle cells: Application to normal, hypertrophied and thyroxin-stimulated hearts. *Am. J. Cardiol.,* 31:172–181.

141. Pannier, J. L. (1971): Contractile state of papillary muscles obtained from cats with moderate right ventricular hypertrophy. *Arch. Int. Physiol.,* 79:743–752.

142. Parmley, W. W., Spann, J. F., Jr., Taylor, R. R., and Sonnenblick, E. H. (1968): The series elasticity of cardiac muscle in hyperthyroidism, ventricular hypertrophy and heart failure. *Proc. Soc. Exp. Biol. Med.,* 127:606–609.

143. Pfeffer, M. A., Pfeffer, J. M., and Frohlich, E. D. (1976): Pumping ability of the hypertrophying left ventricle of the spontaneously hypertensive rat. *Circ. Res.,* 38:423–429.

144. Piesche, L., Hilse, H., and Skcheer, E. (1971): Verhalten des endogenen Noradrenalin-Spiegels und Gehirn sowie des ³H-Noradrenalin-Umsatzes wahrend Entwicklung und Ausbildung einer experimentellen Hypertonie bei Ratten. *Acta Biol. Med. Ger.,* 27:949–960.

145. Podolsky, R. J., and Nolan, A. C. (1972): Muscle contraction transients, cross-bridge kinetics, and the Fenn effect. *Cold Spring Harbor Symp. Quant. Biol.,* 37:661–668.

146. Rakusan, K. (1971): Quantitative morphology of capillaries of the heart. Number of capillaries in animal and human hearts under normal and pathological conditions. *Methods Achiev. Exp. Pathol.,* 5:272–286.

147. Rakusan, K., Korecky, B., and Mezl, V. (1983): Cardiac hypertrophy and/or hyperplasia. In: *Myocardial Hypertrophy and Failure,* edited by N. R. Alpert, pp. 103–109. Raven Press, New York.

148. Rakusan, K. (1984): Cardiac growth, maturation and aging. In: *Growth of the Heart in Health and Disease,* edited by R. Zak, pp. 131–164. Raven Press, New York.

149. Rembert, J. C., Kleinman, L. H., Fedor, J. M., Wechsler, A. S., and Greenfield, J. C., Jr. (1978): Myocardial blood flow distribution in concentric left ventricular hypertrophy. *J. Clin. Invest.,* 62:379–386.

150. Ricchiuti, N. V., and Mommaerts, W. F. H. M. (1965): Techniques for myothermic measurements. *Physiologist,* 8:259.

151. Roberts, J. T., and Wearn, J. T. (1941): Quantitative changes in the capillary-muscle relationship in human hearts during normal growth and hypertrophy. *Am. Heart J.,* 2:617–633.

152. Rouslin, W., Cubicciotti, R. S., Edwards, W. D., Matlib, M. A., Wilson, D. R. Hamrell, B. B., and Schwartz, A. (1979): Phosphorylative respiratory activity of mitochondria isolated from left and right ventricles of rabbit hearts following partial pulmonary trunk occlusion. *J. Mol. Cell. Cardiol.,* 11:91–99.

153. Ruegg, J. C., Kuhn, H. J., Guth, K., Pfitzer, G., and Hofman, F. (1984): Tension transients in skinned muscle fibres of insect flight muscle and mammalian cardiac muscle: Effect of substrate concentration and treatment with myosin light chain kinase. In: *Contractile Mechanisms in Muscle,* edited by G. H. Pollack and H. Sugi, pp. 605–615. Plenum Press, New York.

154. Rupp, H., Kissling, G., and Jacob, R. (1983): Hormonal and hemodynamic determinants of polymorphic myosin. In: *Myocardial Hypertrophy and Failure,* edited by N. R. Alpert, pp. 373–383. Raven Press, New York.

155. Rusy, B. F., and Coulson, R. L. (1973): Energy consumption in the isolated rabbit heart. *Anaesthesiology,* 39:428–454.

156. Saeki, Y., Sagawa, K., and Suga, H. (1980): Transient tension responses of heart muscle in Ba²⁺ contracture to step length changes. *Am. J. Physiol.,* 238:340–347.

157. Sagawa, K., Saeki, Y., Loeffler, L., and Nakayama, K. (1979): Dynamic stiffness of heart muscle in twitch and contracture. In: *Cross-bridge Mechanism in Muscle Contraction,* edited by H. Sugi and G. H. Pollack, pp. 171–190. University Park Press, Baltimore.

158. Sandow, A. (1936): Diffraction patterns of the frog sartorius

and sarcomere behavior under stretch. *J. Cell. Comp. Physiol.*, 9:37–54.

159. Sasayama, S., Ross, J., Jr., Franklin, D., Bloor, C., Bishop, S., and Dilly, R. B. (1976): Adaptations of the left ventricle to chronic pressure overload. *Circ. Res.*, 38:172–178.

160. Schaper, J., Thiedemann, K. U., Flameng, W., and Schaper, W. (1974): The ultrastructure of sarcomeres in hypertrophied canine myocardium in spontaneous subaortic stenosis. *Basic. Res. Cardiol.*, 69:509–515.

161. Scheuer, J., and Tipton, C. M. (1977): Cardiovascular adaptations to physical training. *Annu. Rev. Physiol.*, 39:221–251.

162. Scheuer, J., and Bhan, A. K. (1979): Cardiac contractile proteins: Adenosine triphosphatase activity and physiological function. *Circ. Res.*, 45:1–12.

163. Schiaffino, S., Gorza, L., and Sartore, S. (1983): Distribution of myosin types in normal and hypertrophied hearts: An immunocytochemical approach. In: *Myocardial Hypertrophy and Failure*, edited by N. R. Alpert, pp. 149–166. Raven Press, New York.

164. Schwartz, K., Lecarpentier, Y., Martin, J. L., Lompre, A. M., Mercadier, J. J., and Swynghedauw, B. (1981): Myosin isoenzymic distribution correlates with speed of myocardial contraction. *J. Mol. Cell. Cardiol.*, 13:1071–1075.

165. Schwartz, K., Lompre, A. M., Lacombe, G., Bouveret, P., Wisnewsky, C., Whalen, R. G., D'Albis, A., and Swynghedauw, B. (1983): Cardiac myosin isoenzymic transitions in mammals. In: *Myocardial Hypertrophy and Failure*, edited by N. R. Alpert, pp. 345–358. Raven Press, New York.

166. Sen, S., Tarazi, R. C., Khairallah, P. A., and Bumpus, F. M. (1974): Cardiac hypertrophy in spontaneously hypertensive rats. *Circ. Res.*, 35:775–781.

167. Sharp, N. A., and Parsons, R. L. (1983): Alterations in ventricular action potentials in pressure-overload and thyroxine-induced hypertrophy. In: *Myocardial Hypertrophy and Failure*, edited by N. R. Alpert, pp. 211–220. Raven Press, New York.

168. Shibata, T., Hunter, W. C., and Sagawa, K. (1985): Thyroxine treatment of rabbit shifts frequency spectrum of myocardial dynamic stiffness to higher region. *Biophys. J.*, 47:287a.

169. Shipley, R. A., Shipley, L. J., and Wearn, J. T. (1937): Capillary supply in normal and hypertrophied hearts of rabbits. *J. Exp. Med.*, 65:29–42.

170. Skelton, C. L., Coleman, H. N., Wildenthal, K., and Braunwald, E. (1970): Augmentation of myocardial oxygen consumption in hypertrophied cat hearts. *Circ. Res.*, 27:301–309.

171. Skelton, C. L., and Sonnenblick, E. H. (1974): Heterogeneity of contractile function in cardiac hypertrophy. *Circ. Res. [Suppl. II]*, 34:83–96.

172. Skelton, C. L., Su, J. Y., and Pool, P. E. (1976): Influence of hyperthyroidism on glycerol-extracted cardiac muscle from rabbits. *Cardiovasc. Res.*, 10:380–384.

173. Smitherman, T. C., Johnson, R. S., Taubert, K., Decker, R. S., Wildenthal, K., Shapiro, W., Butsch, R., and Richards, E. G. (1979): Acute thyrotoxicosis in the rabbit: Changes in cardiac myosin, contractility and ultrastructure. *Biochem. Med.*, 21:277–298.

174. Sordahl, L. A., McCollum, W. B., Wood, W. G., and Schwartz, A. (1973): Mitochondria and sarcoplasmic reticulum function in cardiac hypertrophy and failure. *Am. J. Physiol.*, 224:497–502.

175. Spann, J. F., Buccino, R. A., Sonnenblick, E. H., and Braunwald, E. (1967): Contractile state of cardiac muscle obtained from cats with experimentally produced ventricular hypertrophy and heart failure. *Circ. Res.*, 21:341–345.

176. Spann, J. F., Sonnenblick, E. H., Harris, E. D., and Buccino, R. A. (1971): Connective tissue of the hypertrophied heart. In: *Cardiac Hypertrophy*, edited by N. R. Alpert, pp. 141–145. Academic Press, New York.

177. Steiger, G. J. (1977): Tension transients in extracted rabbit heart muscle preparations. *J. Mol. Cell. Cardiol.*, 9:671–685.

178. Steiger, G. J., Brady, A. J., and Tan, S. T. (1978): Intrinsic regulatory properties of contractility in the myocardium. *Circ. Res.*, 42:349–360.

179. Stoner, C. D., Ressalat, M. M., and Sirak, H. D. (1968): Oxidative phosphorylation in mitochondria isolated from chronically stressed dog hearts. *Circ. Res.*, 23:87–97.

180. Strauer, B. E., and Tauchert, M. (1973): Evidence for inefficient

energy utilization in cardiac hypertrophy. Studies on isolated human ventricular myocardium. *Klin. Wochenschr.*, 51:322–326.

181. Strauer, B. E., and Scherpe, A. (1975): Experimental hyperthyroidism. II: Mechanics of contraction and relaxation of isolated ventricular myocardium. *Basic. Res. Cardiol.*, 70:130–141.

182. Strauer, B. E., and Scherpe, A. (1975): Experimental hyperthyroidism. IV: Myocardial muscle mechanics and oxygen consumption in eu- and hyperthyroidism. *Basic. Res. Cardiol.*, 70:246–255.

183. Strauer, B. E., and Scherpe, A. (1975): Experimental hyperthyroidism. I: Hemodynamics and contractility in situ. *Basic Res. Cardiol.*, 70:115–129.

184. Suko, J., Vogel, H. K., and Chidsey, C. A. (1970): Intracellular calcium and myocardial contractility. III. Reduced calcium uptake and ATPase of sarcoplasmic reticular fraction prepared from chronically failing calf hearts. *Circ. Res.*, 27:235–247.

185. Swynghedauw, B., Moalic, J. M., Lecarpentier, Y., Rey, A., Mercadier, J. J., Aumont, M. C., and Schwarts, K. (1983): Adaptational changes in contractile proteins in chronic cardiac overloading: Structure and rate of synthesis. In: *Myocardial Hypertrophy and Failure*, edited by N. R. Alpert, pp. 465–476. Raven Press, New York.

186. Taylor, R. R., Covell, J. W., and Ross, J., Jr. (1968): Left ventricular function in experimental aorta-caval fistula with circulatory congestion and fluid retention. *J. Clin. Invest.*, 47:1333–1342.

187. Taylor, R. R. (1970): Contractile properties of cardiac muscle in hyperthyroidism: Analysis of behavior of hyperthyroid cat papillary muscle in vitro relevant to thyrotoxic heart disease. *Circ. Res.*, 27:539–549.

188. Templeton, G. H., Donald, T. C., III, Mitchell, J. H., and Hefner, L. L. (1973): Dynamic stiffness of papillary muscle during contraction and relaxation. *Am. J. Physiol.*, 224:692–698.

189. Ten Eick, R. E., Bassett, A. L., and Robertson, L. L. (1983): Possible electrophysiological basis for decreased contractility associated with myocardial hypertrophy in the cat: A voltage clamp approach. In: *Myocardial Hypertrophy and Failure*, edited by N. R. Alpert, pp. 245–259. Raven Press, New York.

190. Thiedemann, K. U., Holubarsch, C., Medugorac, I., and Jacob, R. (1983): Connective tissue content and myocardial stiffness in pressure overload hypertrophy. A combined study of morphologic, morphometric, biochemical, and mechanical parameters. *Basic Res. Cardiol.*, 78:140–155.

191. Tritthart, H., Luedcke, H., Bayer, R., Stierle, H., and Kaufmann, R. (1975): Right ventricular hypertrophy in the cat. An electrophysiological and anatomical study. *J. Mol. Cell. Cardiol.*, 7:163–174.

192. Weiss, L., and Lundgren, Y. (1978): Left ventricular hypertrophy and its reversibility in young spontaneously hypertensive rats. *Cardiovasc. Res.*, 12:635–638.

193. Wendt-Gallitelli, M. F., Ebrecht, G., and Jacob, R. (1979): Morphological alterations and their functional interpretation in the hypertrophied myocardium of Goldblatt hypertensive rats. *J. Mol. Cell. Cardiol.*, 11:275–287.

194. Whitehorn, W. V., Ullrick, W. C., and Andersen, B. R. (1959): Properties of hyperthyroid rat myocardium. *Circ. Res.*, 7:250–255.

195. Williams, J. F., and Potter, R. D. (1974): Normal contractile state of hypertrophied myocardium after pulmonary artery constriction. *J. Clin. Invest.*, 54:1266–1272.

196. Yamori, Y. (1974): Contribution of cardiovascular factors to the development of hypertension in spontaneously hypertensive rats. *Jpn. Heart. J.*, 15:194–196.

197. Yazaki, Y., and Raben, M. S. (1975): Effect of thyroid state on the enzymatic characteristics of cardiac myosin: A difference in behavior of rat and rabbit cardiac myosin. *Circ. Res.*, 36:208–215.

198. Yin, F. P., Spurgeon, H. A., Weisfeldt, M. L., and Lakatta, E. G. (1980): Mechanical properties of myocardium from hypertrophied rat hearts. A comparison between hypertrophy induced by senescence and by aortic banding. *Circ. Res.*, 46:292–300.

199. Zak, R. (1973): Cell proliferation during cardiac growth. *Am. J. Cardiol.*, 31:211–219.

200. Zak, R. (1984): Factors controlling cardiac growth. In: *Growth of the Heart in Health and Disease*, edited by R. Zak, pp. 165–185. Raven Press, New York.

The Heart and Cardiovascular System,
edited by H. A. Fozzard et al.
Raven Press, New York © 1986.

CHAPTER 63

Cardiac Consequences of Vasomotor Changes in the Periphery: Impedance and Preload

Jay N. Cohn

The peripheral circulation plays a vital role in the control of left ventricular performance. In considering the pump function of the left ventricle, the heart, the arterial resistance vessels, and the venous capacitance vessels all must be viewed as an integrated unit. The roles of these resistance and capacitance functions in influencing cardiac performance are importantly dependent on the intrinsic contractile strength of the ventricular myocardium. Therefore, comprehensive consideration of the influence of peripheral vascular changes on ventricular function must include the effects in both normal and abnormal cardiac states.

INTERACTION OF LEFT VENTRICLE WITH PERIPHERAL CIRCULATION

Aortic Input Impedance

Factors Contributing to Impedance

The downstream resistance faced by blood as it leaves the left ventricle is determined by inertial and viscous factors as well as by the compliance and resistance imposed by the arterial vasculature (Table 1). These factors have a direct influence on left ventricular emp-tying during systole when the aortic valve is open. During diastole, these factors play a major role in determining the rate of aortic runoff and the residual aortic pressure at the time of the next systole (end-diastolic aortic pressure). Thus, they also influence the duration of systole by affecting the time of aortic valve opening and closing (40).

The terms used to describe these peripheral factors that influence left ventricular ejection have been somewhat controversial, but definition of terms is important so that measurements can be used in a precise way. Some of the terms applied are as follows:

Systemic vascular resistance. The ratio of pressure drop across the arterial bed to cardiac output. This is a mean resistance that is calculated from mean flow and mean pressures. The site of this resistance is predominantly in the small arteries and arterioles, and there is marked systemic heterogeneity of resistance. The total resistance therefore represents the sum of resistances in multiple parallel circuits that represent the regional vascular beds. Because flow and pressure are pulsatile, use of an integrated pressure and an integrated flow over time to calculate a mean resistance provides a value that has no true biological equivalent in an intact circulation (38).

TABLE 1. *Factors that may contribute to impedance to left ventricular ejection*

1. Aortic valve (negligible except in stenosis)
2. Aortic compliance
3. Muscular artery compliance
4. Blood viscosity
5. Inertia
6. Small artery caliber (resistance)
7. Arteriolar caliber (resistance)
8. Capillary and venous pressure (negligible)

Arterial compliance. The rato of change in volume of the arterial bed to change in pressure. This dynamic relationship between pressure and volume is a determinant of the storage capacity of the arteries during systole (13). Although arterial compliance is comparatively low, changes in this compliance induced by drugs, physiologic responses, aging, or disease may have a striking impact on dynamic aortic inflow resistance.

Impedance. The total opposition to flow consisting of inertial, viscosity, resistance, and compliance components. Impedance changes dynamically during systole as there are continual changes in pressure, compliance, inertia, and apparent viscosity. Impedance can be measured at any point in the vasculature. In the root of the aorta it is representative of total systemic impedance (aortic input impedance), whereas in regional vascular beds it may represent localized impedance. The traditional means of assessing impedance has been by Fourier analysis of high-fidelity pressure and flow wave signals (43).

Afterload. A measure of cardiac load best defined as the stress or tension on the ventricular wall during ejection. Afterload is importantly determined by impedance, but it is also affected by ventricular volume and shortening fraction, because these latter factors influence ventricular chamber diameter during ejection and thus wall tension and stress, by the Laplace relationship (41). The term *afterload* therefore is most appropriate for isolated heart muscle preparations in which the muscle tension during shortening is directly related to the weight the muscle is asked to lift.

Responses to Changes in Aortic Input Impedance

Changes in impedance will influence the left ventricle by altering stroke volume, left ventricular systolic pressure, left ventricular volume during ejection, and left ventricular wall tension and stress. If the contractile force of the left ventricular myocardium is unchanged, a reduction in impedance allows ejection of blood into the aorta at a lower generated pressure; ventricular emptying is enhanced by a longer systole because of earlier opening and delayed closure of the aortic valve as a result of the lower aortic pressure. An increase in impedance will have the opposite effect by shortening

the systolic ejection time and reducing stroke volume. These impedance-related changes in stroke volume are inversely related to changes in wall tension. Because wall tension is a product of both instantaneous intraventricular pressure and chamber diameter (6), a higher stroke volume is associated with a greater systolic reduction in chamber size and a lower mean systolic wall tension. Conversely, the smaller stroke volume associated with a high aortic impedance is accompanied by a higher left ventricular wall tension. Because the oxygen consumption of the myocardium is directly related to wall tension during ejection (53), the increased stroke volume and cardiac output that accompany a reduced aortic impedance are not oxygen-consuming, but actually may be accomplished with a lowered oxygen consumption.

Although these responses to pure changes in aortic impedance would be anticipated in a model system in which pump performance was maintained at a constant level, the response in the intact organism appears to be more complex. At least two factors appear to play roles in altering the simple relationship between aortic impedance and stroke volume described above:

1. An increase in stroke volume, by decreasing end-systolic volume, may result in some reduction in end-diastolic volume in the next beat and a resultant reduction in contractile force (Frank-Starling mechanism) that may counterbalance the effect of a lowered impedance (44). Similarly, an increase in end-systolic volume may result in augmentation of the subsequent end-diastolic volume and an increase in contractile force that may counteract the increased impedance. Modest changes in preload may therefore obscure a simple relationship between aortic input impedance and stroke volume.

2. A mechanism that may adjust myocardial contractility in response to a change in impedance has been postulated (48). The magnitude of this autoregulatory mechanism, as compared with the changes in loading that also have been described, remains controversial. Nonetheless, it is clear that the myocardium does have the capacity for acute change in contractility that may be important in setting cardiac performance to match peripheral demands when the heart is normal. It appears likely that this autoregulatory mechanism is blunted in the presence of myocardial disease (6), as is the response to preload changes (46).

Mechanisms Controlling Aortic Input Impedance

Changes in caliber or tone of the arterial vasculature can have profound effects on total systemic impedance. These vessels are under neural and humoral control as well as under the influence of local structural factors that may influence both compliance and resistance. The major variables that can influence resistance and compliance include the sympathetic nervous system through locally released and circulating norepinephrine, the renin-angiotensin system through circulating angiotensin II and possibly local vascular levels of angiotensin II, and the antidiuretic hormone system through circulating vasopressin levels (10). Activation of any of these systems with pressor levels of hormone can result in an increase in aortic input impedance. Autoregulation of the vasculature also appears to play a role in the control of resistance. At least two forms of autoregulation may be involved in this process. The traditional autoregulatory mechanism is a local mechanical or metabolic factor that adjusts resistance in the vasculature to maintain a constant flow in the face of changes in perfusion pressure (31). This form of autoregulation is a prompt adjustment of the vasculature. A more slowly developing autoregulation has been described by Guyton and his colleagues, who theorize that this process is a generalized systemic response designed to keep flow constant at the expense of changes in resistance and in perfusion pressure (28). The sites in the vasculature at which these two autoregulatory mechanisms act have not been entirely clarified.

In summary, aortic input impedance is composed of a variety of factors that influence resistance and compliance of the vasculature. The vasomotor component of these impedance changes is under the influence of neural and humoral factors that can be activated by a variety of physiologic and pathologic stresses. The normal ventricle can use intrinsic mechanisms to adjust to changes in impedance and thus to lessen the impact of these impedance changes on the performance of the heart. In the presence of myocardial disease, however, these regulatory mechanisms are blunted, and cardiac pump function becomes more intimately related to the vascular resistance and compliance.

Ventricular Filling (Preload)

End-diastolic filling of the right and left ventricles is an important determinant of ventricular performance, based on the Frank-Starling mechanism. Changes in ventricular filling may occur abruptly by virtue of acute shifts in intravascular volume or more chronically by virtue of total changes in intravascular volume. Major factors include the following:

Systemic venous capacitance. Because the majority of intravascular blood is contained in the venous vessels, these vessels exert considerable capacitance function. An acute increase in tone of these capacitance vessels will result in translocation of blood volume from the systemic venous bed into the right ventricle (14). This augmentation of right ventricular filling should in the normal circulation lead to comparable augmentation of left ventricular filling and thus an increase in left ventricular preload.

Pulmonary vascular capacitance. Filling of the left ventricle also is dependent on the capacitance function of the pulmonary circulation. Capacitance is markedly affected by changes in lung volume and in pleural pressures during the respiratory cycle (9). Pulmonary vascular capacitance also can be influenced by physiologic and pharmacologic interventions.

Ventricular compliance. The pressure-volume relationship of the right and left ventricles during diastole may have a profound effect on the magnitude of ventricular volume increments in response to changes in filling pressure. The right ventricle is more compliant than the left and thus may serve as a volume reservoir (37). The left ventricular pressure-volume relationship is so steep that considerable changes in pressure may be observed with very small alterations in chamber size (22).

Role of right ventricle. The primary circulatory role of the right ventricle in the normal individual appears to be as a booster pump to help support left ventricular filling while maintaining pulmonary flow at an adequate level. It is clear that normal resting left ventricular filling can be maintained adequately in the absence of a functioning right ventricle when the pulmonary vascular resistance is low (55). Under these circumstances the left ventricle fills passively through a low-impedance pulmonary vasculature utilizing the systemic venous pressure as a driving force. When the pulmonary vascular resistance rises, however, or when left ventricular compliance is decreased and therefore a higher filling pressure is demanded, the right ventricle becomes exceedingly important in maintaining an adequate pulmonary artery pressure to sustain left ventricular filling (8). The function of the right ventricle also becomes intimately involved with the intraventricular septum, a structure shared by both the left and right ventricles. Shifts of this intraventricular septum toward and away from the left ventricle can influence the compliance characteristics of the left ventricle and thus its preload (7). The position of the system during diastole may be determined, at least in part, by the transeptal pressure gradient. The effectiveness of the septum in contributing to right or left ventricular ejection during systole may be critically dependent on its position at the end of diastole.

Intravascular volume. Vasomotor changes can influence the plasma volume by altering the rate of filtration at the capillary level (34). In general terms, an increase in arteriolar resistance will reduce capillary pressure and thus slow the rate of capillary filtration and expand the intravascular plasma volume. Conversely, a decrease in arteriolar resistance can lead to increases in capillary pressure and transcapillary filtration (4). Even more important may be changes in venous resistance. An increase in postcapillary venous resistance should augment capillary pressure and lead to a depletion of intravascular volume (4).

In summary, left ventricular preload may be under considerable influence from vasomotor change of the peripheral vasculature. In the normal heart, changes in ventricular preload can have profound effects on the performance of the ventricle. In abnormal cardiac states in which the Frank-Starling curve of ventricular function is flattened and shifted to the right, changes in preload may be less important in controlling cardiac performance. Indeed, the sensitivity of the ventricle to changes in impedance in the setting of left ventricular dysfunction may in large part reflect attenuation of the negative feedback preload mechanism.

MEASUREMENT OF CHANGES IN AORTIC INPUT IMPEDANCE

Vasomotor changes can produce, at most, only a small change in hematocrit (23), and therefore viscosity changes will not be considered in the following discussion. Force is required to set the flow in motion in the root of the aorta at the onset of systole; because this force also is essentially unaltered by vasomotor changes, it also will be disregarded. Inertial forces at the end of systole can be importantly influenced by the velocity of flow achieved during systolic ejection. The greater the velocity of flow, the more likely it is that flow will continue at the end of systole against a pressure gradient (54). Although vasomotor change may have some influence on flow velocity, the inertial component of total systemic impedance also will be disregarded in the following discussion.

Arterial Compliance

The most direct means of assessing the compliance of large arteries is to measure simultaneously the pulsatile pressure and pulsatile diameter of the artery. This approach is of limited value, however, because caliber changes of *in vivo* arteries are difficult to measure, and the results may apply only to the specific artery under study. Measurements of caliber changes in large arteries have been attempted by use of angiographic and echocardiographic techniques (1) and with ultrasonic crystals (56).

Simultaneous recording of high-fidelity pressure and flow signals allows assessment of impedance in the frequency domain (23). Fourier analysis of these signals provides data on resistance at a series of frequencies. The average of the resistance moduli at frequencies

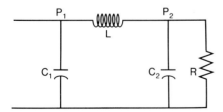

FIG. 1. Modified Windkessel model of the vasculature used to analyze compliance of the peripheral vascular bed. (Reprinted from ref. 19, with permission.)

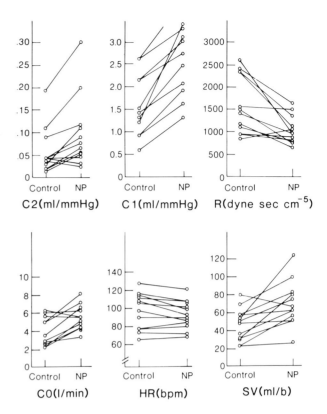

FIG. 2. Response to nitroprusside infusion in patients with heart failure. Proximal (C1) and distal (C2) compliance increases in response to the drug. The hemodynamic changes induced by the drug [fall in resistance (R), rises in cardiac output (CO) and stroke volume (SV), with no change in heart rate (HR)] are typical of the responses to vasodilators in heart failure.

from approximately 2 to 12 cycles per second often is used to calculate the characteristic impedance, which is defined ideally as the impedance in a system without reflected waves. This value should be inversely related to arterial compliance (20).

Measurements in the time domain consist of various analyses of the arterial pulse wave. One approach has been to measure the pulse wave velocity by assessing the timing of the pulse wave measured at various sites in the arterial tree using an external pulse wave pickup. The pulse wave velocity is inversely related to the arterial compliance, resulting in increasing pulse wave velocity with aging (32).

A second approach has been to analyze the contour of the arterial pulse wave. The simplest approach to this analysis has been to measure the height of the dicrotic wave, which is directly related to stiffness of the vascular tree (42). Another approach has been to describe the slope of arterial pressure decay during diastole. In its simplest form, this pressure decay can be viewed as a first-order equation, and this slope, when related to the stroke volume, can provide a direct measure of diastolic compliance.

A more complex analysis uses a Windkessel model of the circulation that incorporates proximal and distal compliance elements in the model (Fig. 1). The proximal compliance is viewed as characteristic of the aorta and large vessels proximal to the site of pressure measurement. The distal compliance is taken as representative of the arterial vascular bed distal to the pressure measurement, which usually is in the brachial or femoral artery. Data from several laboratories (19,50,57) have confirmed that the distal compliance is strikingly altered in the presence of hypertension or congestive heart failure, thus suggesting stiffening of the distal vascular segment. Changes in distal compliance have also been demonstrated in response to vasoconstrictor and vasodilator drugs in both human and animal experimentation (61) (Fig. 2). These data suggest that this analysis may provide a sensitive means for assessing the compliance of the vascular bed as a lumped parameter. Because these parameters have no distinct anatomic equivalence, the measurements are weakened by the inability to precisely localize the site of the changes. On the other hand, this lumped parameter model provides a functionally important measurement that appears to be of physiologic significance.

Small Artery Resistance

Calculation of total systemic vascular resistance as the ratio of the pressure drop across the circulation and the flow (cardiac output) has classically served as a guide to the state of the arteriolar vascular caliber. Although this crude measurement has provided useful data that have been widely used in both pharmacologic and physiologic assessments of the circulation, it clearly has limitations in its ability to define the location or the mechanism of vascular resistance changes. A more sensitive technique involves assessment of regional changes in vascular resistance. Measurement of organ blood flow by use of electromagnetic flow probes enables one to assess the resistance in a regional vascular bed. By measuring the blood flow in multiple regional beds, it is possible to assess the effects of various physiologic, pharmacologic, and pathologic interventions on vascular resistance in specific beds. Similar data can be obtained in animals by use of microspheres for measurement of regional blood flow.

Drug effects can be assessed either by systemic administration or more precisely by regional administration. Local arterial infusion of a drug at a dose insufficient to affect systemic hemodynamics allows measurement of direct changes in vascular resistance that reflect the direct vasomotor changes induced by the drug (3). Similar experiments can be carried out in regionally perfused beds, with flow being held constant, and the effects of changes in resistance in response to a drug are reflected by changes in perfusion pressure in the vascular

bed under study. None of these regional flow techniques allows assessment of the exact locations of the vascular changes in question, but it is generally considered that the changes occur in the smaller terminal arteries and in arterioles approximately 20 to 100 μm in diameter.

MEASUREMENT OF CHANGES IN CAPACITANCE

Systemic Venous Capacitance

The capacitance of the systemic venous bed is an important determinant of venous return to the heart. Basically, this capacitance can be viewed as the pressure-volume relationship of the venous bed. Venous return curves were popularized by Guyton and his colleagues, who used the rapidly equilibrating pressure when the heart was arrested, a pressure they termed the mean circulatory pressure, as a guide to the capacitance of the system (29). The higher this mean circulatory pressure, or the lesser the compliance of the system, the more the system will encourage venous return to the heart. Drugs or interventions that increase the mean circulatory pressure therefore should augment venous return (27).

A more direct measurement of venous return can be carried out in open-chest animals in which venous blood is drained into a reservoir from which it can be pumped at a constant rate either into the right ventricle or into the pulmonary artery, or, by means of an oxygenator, into the left side of the heart (45). When output from the pump and the reservoir level are held constant, changes in reservoir volume can be viewed as indicative of changes in the capacitance of the systemic bed. In such studies it has been possible to demonstrate that venoconstrictor drugs augment the reservoir volume, suggesting mobilization of blood from venous capacitance vessels, whereas drugs that have a venodilator effect may actually deplete the reservoir of blood.

A less invasive way to assess the capacitance of the systemic bed has been measurement of the ratio of central blood volume to total blood volume (11). Measurements of central blood volume in most experiments have used indicator dilution curves for measuring the transit time of the indicator from a central injection site to a sampling site. Because cardiac output can be computed from the indicator dilution curve, it is possible to use the mean transit time to determine a volume that represents all blood contained between the injection site and sampling site and temporally equidistant points (39). If total blood volume is measured by using the equilibration concentration of a plasma or red cell label, it is possible to calculate the central blood volume as a fraction of the total blood volume. Venoconstrictor interventions that tend to reduce the compliance of the venous bed force a larger percentage of the total volume centrally and thus increase the ratio of central blood volume to total blood volume. Venodilator interventions have an opposite effect.

Because these systemic measurements are either highly invasive or relatively nonspecific, efforts have been made to carry out capacitance studies in more isolated vascular beds. The forearm vascular bed has been employed commonly in man. Venous responses in this bed can be assessed by several techniques. Venous tone can be measured by plethysmography using simultaneous measurements of forearm blood flow and the rate of pressure rise in a superficial vein during venous occlusion (49). The ratio of the slope of pressure rise to the simultaneously measured forearm blood flow is a measurement of venous tone. Because these measurements can vary when made in different forearm veins, and because the dynamic pressure changes in veins can be influenced by stress-relaxation, the venous capacitance of the entire forearm bed has been assessed at steady state by recording arm girth increments at various venous distending pressures (59). If the arm girth is allowed to stabilize while venous occluding pressure is progressively increased, the equilibrium point at increasing venous occluding pressures describes a slope that represents the increment in volume at small increments in venous occluding pressure. The more compliant the venous bed, the larger the volume increment will be recorded as the venous pressure is progressively increased. These measurements are extremely sensitive to the initial starting points of venous pressure and venous volume, because the venous pressure-volume curve is not linear (16).

A third technique that has been used in the forearm vascular bed in both animals and man is measurement of the pressure gradient between the small veins and large veins (30). Small venous pressure can be measured directly by advancing a small catheter distally in a hand vein until it wedges in a venule. The pressure gradient from this wedged position to the large free venous pressure, when factored by blood flow, allows measurement of the venous resistance. In previous experiments in our laboratory this venous resistance appeared to be directly related to venous tone and inversely related to venous capacitance, thus suggesting that these various techniques for assessing the venous bed have appropriate relationships with one another (4).

Pulmonary Vascular Capacitance

Venous return to the left ventricle is dependent not only on systemic venous return to the right ventricle and on right ventricular function but also on the capacitance function of the pulmonary bed. In man, the pulmonary vascular bed may serve as a reservoir to augment left ventricular filling under some circumstances (51). The pulmonary blood volume is closely dependent on the respiratory cycle. An increase in volume during inspiration more than compensates for an increased right ventricular output during inspiration, thus leading to a modest fall in left ventricular filling during inspiration (12). Expiration mobilizes blood from the pulmonary bed to augment left ventricular filling and increase left ventricular stroke volume at the onset of expiration (15).

The volume of blood in the central circulation is measured most frequently by indicator dilution techniques. As previously noted, the mean transit time between a central injection site and a central sampling site, when factored by the cardiac output, provides a measure of the volume contained between these two sites. Transit time can be measured by direct injection and withdrawal using an intravascular label such as indocyanine green dye (35) or by radioisotope techniques, including external probe methods, in which arrivals of blood in the right ventricle and in the left ventricle can be timed separately after bolus injection (24). The relationship between transmural pressure and volume contained in the pulmonary vascular bed varies under certain clinical situations, thus suggesting the likelihood that changes in compliance of the pulmonary vascular bed could play an important role in hemodynamics (60).

MEASUREMENT OF INDUCED CHANGES IN LEFT VENTRICULAR PERFORMANCE

In order to assess the effects on left ventricular function of vasomotor changes in the periphery, it is necessary to have techniques that can accurately quantitate changes in both systolic and diastolic performance. Furthermore, changes in cardiac output necessarily result in changes in regional blood flow, and it is these organ-specific flows that can impact on organ function.

Systolic Left Ventricular Function

The effect of preload changes on the left ventricle should be reflected in changes in stroke volume, cardiac output, and stroke work or cardiac work. Frank-Starling curves relating the left ventricular filling pressure or preload to output from the heart have similar relationships whether the filling pressure is plotted against stroke volume, cardiac output, or a measure of cardiac work (47). For these purposes, cardiac output can be measured either on the basis of the Fick principle or by indicator dilution techniques. Both of these methods require invasive studies. Indicator dilution techniques using indocyanine green can be performed peripherally with the venous injection cannula inserted well into an antecubital vein and a cannula in a peripheral artery for sampling blood through a cuvette densitometer. Thermodilution techniques have become popular in recent years and can be performed through a single catheter with a proximal injection site and a distal thermistor positioned in the pulmonary artery (18). Noninvasive techniques also have been used to monitor changes in cardiac output. These are less reliable than the well-established invasive techniques, but under some circumstances they provide adequate data for analysis. The most popular noninvasive technique is the carbon dioxide rebreathing method (21), which uses the Fick principle by providing a noninvasive estimation of arterial and mixed venous CO_2 concentrations. The impedance cardiograph technique provides a calculation of stroke volume using measured electrical impedance changes across the chest wall during each cardiac cycle (33).

Less quantitative but often useful indirect methods for measuring cardiac output include radionuclide and echocardiographic techniques. Gated radionuclide studies allow for fairly reproducible measurements of the ejection fraction from the left ventricle. In some laboratories these radionuclide studies are also used to calculate absolute end-diastolic and end-systolic volumes that allow for calculation of an absolute stroke volume (52). These methods, although not always quantitatively reliable from patient to patient, should provide adequate measurements of changes in stroke volume in an individual patient. Valvular regurgitation, however, will invalidate this technique as a measure of forward stroke volume.

Echocardiographic techniques allow for assessment of the wall motion of the left ventricle, including regional abnormalities. Changes in performance of the heart may be reflected in the absolute wall movement from diastole to systole and in the velocity of the wall motion.

Diastolic Left Ventricular Function

Changes in preload of the left ventricle usually are assessed by monitoring changes in the pressure at end-diastole in the left ventricle, left atrium, or pulmonary wedge position. Under normal circumstances these pressures are in equilibrium at the end of diastole, and they should provide comparable values. Discrepancy between these pressures may become prominent in certain circumstances, particularly when there is pulmonary vascular disease or mitral valve disease.

Because preload refers most directly to the end-diastolic myocardial fiber length, diastolic ventricular volume rather than ventricular pressure would seem to be a more appropriate measurement to quantitate diastolic function. However, ventricular volumes are considerably more difficult to measure accurately than pressures, and most investigators have therefore relied on pressure measurements as a guide to preload. However, as volume measurements have become more readily available both for investigational and clinical use, it has become apparent that changes in ventricular volume do not always reflect comparable changes in end-diastolic

fiber length; plastic changes in the ventricle can result in considerable alteration in volume, with little, if any, change in the length of individual fibers (36). Furthermore, the compliance of the ventricle under various physiologic and pathologic states can alter the relationship between changes in pressure and changes in fiber length (25).

Despite the concerns about the reliability and significance of ventricular volume measurements, it is generally held that changes in diastolic volume measured in an individual patient over a short period of intervention should reflect comparable changes in pressure and in preload. In many studies in which acute intervention with a vasodilator drug has led to a striking increase in stroke volume, measured by indicator dilution techniques, measurement of systolic function of the left ventricle, whether by echocardiographic or radionuclide techniques, has not revealed the magnitude of change indicated by cardiac output assessment (17). The reasons for these apparent discrepancies between the noninvasive methods for evaluating ventricular volume changes and the invasive methods for measuring cardiac output have been attributed to the insensitivity of the volume measurement techniques and to changes in the volume of valvular regurgitation. Further analysis of this problem is required.

Regional Distribution of Blood Flow

Changes in cardiac output induced by vasomotor effects on the periphery can lead to striking differences in the regional distributions of flow. The effects on different regional beds depend on the state of the circulation at the time of the intervention, the specific intervention used, and the neurohumoral response to that intervention. For example, if cardiac output is low and the body has responded to this low-flow state with activation of the sympathetic nervous system, renal blood flow may be strikingly reduced. In these circumstances, a drug that increases cardiac output, either by augmenting preload or reducing impedance, might cause relaxation of the heightened sympathetic tone and thus preferential redistribution of the blood to the renal vascular bed, even if the drug employed did not have a direct renal vascular action (26). Therefore, individual responses to a specific drug cannot be predicted merely from an understanding of the pharmacologic action of that drug, but must be based on an understanding of the integrated cardiovascular and neurohumoral effects of that agent in the specific situation in which it is employed.

Blood flow in experimental animals can be measured by electromagnetic flow probes or, in acute terminal experiments, by measurement of the regional distribution of radiolabeled microspheres. Both in experimental animals and in clinical situations it is possible to measure blood flow more indirectly in several vascular beds. The extremity bed can be assessed by plethysmographic techniques. The method most commonly employed at present is to use a mercury-in-rubber Whitney gauge placed around the extremity that is capable of measuring changes in extremity girth, which, during venous occlusion, represent arterial inflow (58). Renal blood flow and hepatic blood flow can be measured by clearance techniques using indicators that are selectively cleared by the kidney and liver, respectively. Renal blood flow studies most frequently employ paraaminohippurate or Hippuran (2). For hepatic flow determination, indocyanine green dye is most popular (5). These indicators can be given either by constant infusion or by bolus injection, with measurement of the peripheral disappearance rate. Clearance of these substances without simultaneous measurement of extraction across the organ in question can provide only an estimate of absolute flow. Changes in flow therefore can be assessed accurately only if one can assume that extraction of the substance is not changed by the intervention.

REFERENCES

1. Arndt, J. O., and Kober, G. (1970): Pressure-diameter relationship of the intact femoral artery in conscious man. *Pfluegers Arch.,* 318:130–146.
2. Beyer, K. H., Mattis, P. A., Patch, E. A., and Russa, H. F. (1945): Para-aminohippuric acid: Its pharmacodynamic actions. *J. Pharmacol. Exp. Ther.,* 84:136–146.
3. Cohn, J. N. (1965): Comparative cardiovascular effects of tyramine, ephedrine and norepinephrine in man. *Circ. Res.,* 16:174–182.
4. Cohn, J. N. (1966): Relationship of plasma volume changes to resistance and capacitance vessels: Effects of sympathomimetic amines and angiotensin in man. *Clin. Sci.,* 30:267–278.
5. Cohn, J. N. (1968): Hemodynamic technics in the study of liver diseases. In: *Laboratory Diagnosis of Liver Diseases,* edited by F. W. Sunderman, Jr., pp. 388–393. Warren H. Green, St. Louis.
6. Cohn, J. N. (1973): Blood pressure and cardiac performance. *Am. J. Med.,* 55:351–361.
7. Cohn, J. N. (1979): Right ventricular infarction revisited. *Am. J. Cardiol.,* 43:666–668.
8. Cohn, J. N., Guiha, N. H., Broder, M. I., and Limas, C. J. (1974): Right ventricular infarction: Clinical and hemodynamics features. *Am. J. Cardiol.,* 33:209–214.
9. Cohn, J. N., and Hamosh, P. (1982): Experimental observations on pulsus paradoxus and hepatojugular reflux. In: *Pericardial Disease,* edited by P. S. Reddy, D. F. Leon, and J. A. Shaver, pp. 7–11. Raven Press, New York.
10. Cohn, J. N., Levine, T. B., Francis, G. S., and Goldsmith, S. (1981): Neurohumoral control mechanisms in congestive heart failure. *Am. Heart J.,* 102:509–514.
11. Cohn, J. N., and Luria, M. H. (1966): Studies in clinical shock and hypotension. IV. Variations in reflex vasoconstriction and cardiac stimulation. *Circulation,* 34:823–832.
12. Cohn, J. N., Pinkerson, A. L., and Tristani, F. E. (1967): Mechanism of pulsus paradoxus in clinical shock. *J. Clin. Invest.,* 46:1744–1755.
13. Dobrin, P. B. (1978): Mechanical properties of arteries. *Physiol. Rev.,* 58:397–460.
14. Drees, J. A., and Rothe, C. F. (1974): Reflex venoconstriction and capacity vessel pressure-volume relationships in dogs. *Circ. Res.,* 34:360–373.
15. DuBois, A., and Marshall, R. (1957): Measurement of pulmonary capillary blood flow and gas exchange throughout the respiratory cycle in man. *J. Clin. Invest.,* 36:1566–1571.
16. Eckstein, J. W., Hamilton, W. K. amd McCammond, J. M. (1958): Pressure-volume changes in the forearm veins of man during hyperventilation. *J. Clin. Invest.,* 37:956–961.
17. Firth, B. G., Dehmer, G. J., Markham, R. V., Willerson, J. T., and Hillis, L. D. (1982): Assessment of vasodilator therapy in patients with severe congestive heart failure: Limitations of measurements of left ventricular ejection fraction and volumes. *Am. J. Cardiol.,* 50:954–959.
18. Forrester, J. S., Ganz, W., Diamond, G., McHugh, T., Chonette, D., and Swan, H. J. C. (1972): Thermodilution cardiac output with a single flow-directed catheter. *Am. Heart J.,* 83:306–311.
19. Finkelstein, S. M., Cohn, J. N., Collins, R. V., Carlyle, P. F., and Shelley, W. (1985): Vascular hemodynamic impedance in congestive heart failure. *Am. J. Cardiol.,* 55:423–427.
20. Finkelstein, S. M., and Collins, V. R. (1982): Vascular hemodynamic impedance measurements. *Prog. Cardiovasc. Dis.,* 24:401–418.
21. Franciosa, J. A., Ragan, D. O., and Rubenstone, S. J. (1976): Validation of the CO_2 rebreathing method for measuring cardiac output in patients with hypertension or heart failure. *J. Lab. Clin. Med.,* 88:672–682.
22. Gaasch, W. H., Alexander, J. K., Cole, J. S., and Quinones, M. A. (1975): Dynamic determinants of left ventricular diastolic pressure-volume relations in man. *Circulation,* 51:317–323.
23. Gabe, I. T., Karnell, J., Porje, I. G., and Rudewald, B. (1964): The measurement of input impedance and apparent phase velocity in the human aorta. *Acta Physiol. Scand.,* 61:73–84.
24. Giuntini, C., Lewis, M. L., SalesLuis, A., and Harvey, R. M. (1963): A study of the pulmonary blood volume in man by quantitative radiocardiography. *J. Clin. Invest.,* 42:1589–1605.
25. Glantz, S. A., and Parmley, W. W. (1978): Factors which affect the diastolic pressure volume curve. *Circ. Res.,* 42:171–180.
26. Guiha, N. H., Cohn, J. N., Mikulic, E., Franciosa, J. A., and Limas, C. J. (1974): Treatment of refractory heart failure with infusion of nitroprusside. *N. Engl. J. Med.,* 291:587–592.
27. Guyton, A. C. (1955): Determination of cardiac output by equating venous return curves with cardiac response curves. *Physiol. Rev.,* 35:123–129.
28. Guyton, A. C., and Coleman, T. G. (1969): Quantitative analysis of the pathophysiology of hypertension. *Circ. Res.,* 24:1–19.
29. Guyton, A. C., Polizo, D., and Armstrong, G. G. (1954): Mean circulatory filling pressure measured immediately after cessation of heart pumping. *Am. J. Physiol.,* 179:261–272.
30. Haddy, F. J., Molnar, J. I., Borden, C. W., and Texter, E. C. (1962): Comparison of direct effects of angiotensin and artery vasoactive agents on small and large blood vessels in several vascular beds. *Circulation,* 25:239–246.
31. Johnson, P. C., and Henrich, H. A. (1975): Metabolic and myogenic factors in local regulation of the microcirculation. *Fed. Proc.,* 34:2020–2024.
32. Jordan, H. (1959): Investigations on the relationship between central pulse velocity and so-called delay time. *Cardiologia,* 35:228–236.
33. Kubicek, W. G., Karnegis, S. N., Patterson, R. P., Witsoe, D. A., and Mattson, R. H. (1966): Development and evaluation of an impedance cardiac output system. *Aerospace Med.,* 37:1208–1212.
34. Landis, E. M. (1934): Capillary pressure and capillary permeability. *Physiol. Rev.,* 14:404–481.
35. Levinson, G. E., Frank, M. J., and Hellems, H. K. (1964): The pulmonary vascular volume in man. Measurement from atrial dilution curves. *Am. Heart J.,* 67:734–741.
36. Linzbach, A. J. (1960): Heart failure from the point of quantitative anatomy. *Am. J. Cardiol.,* 5:370–382.
37. Mashiro, I., Cohn, J. N., Heckel, R., Nelson, R. R., and Franciosa, J. A. (1978): Left and right ventricular dimensions during ventricular fibrillation in the dog. *Am. J. Physiol.,* 235:H231–H236.
38. McDonald, D. A. (1955): The relation of pulsatile pressure to flow in arteries. *J. Physiol. (Lond.),* 127:533–552.
39. Meier, P., and Zierler, K. L. (1954): On the theory of the indicator-dilution method for measurement of blood flow and volume. *J. Appl. Physiol.,* 6:731–744.
40. Milnor, W. R. (1975): Arterial impedance as ventricular afterload. *Circ. Res.,* 36:565–570.
41. Mirsky, I. (1969): Left ventricular stresses in the intact human heart. *Biophys. J.,* 9:189–208.

42. O'Rourke, M. F. (1971): The arterial pulse in health and disease. *Am. Heart J.,* 82:687–702.
43. O'Rourke, M. F., and Taylor, M. G. (1967): Input impedance of the systemic circulation. *Circ. Res.,* 20:365–380.
44. Patterson, W. W., and Starling, E. H. (1914): On mechanical factors which determine output of ventricles. *J. Physiol. (Lond.),* 48:357–379.
45. Rose, J. C., Kot, P. A., Cohn, J. N., Freis, E. D., and Eckert, G. E. (1962): Comparison of effects of angiotensin and norepinephrine on pulmonary circulation, systemic arteries and veins, and systemic vascular capacity in the dog. *Circulation,* 25:247–252.
46. Ross, J., Jr. (1976): Afterload mismatch and preload reserve. A conceptual framework for analysis of ventricular function. *Progr. Cardiovasc. Dis.,* 18:255–264.
47. Sarnoff, S. J., and Berglund, E. (1954): Ventricular function. I. Starling's law of the heart studied by means of simultaneous right and left ventricular function curves in the dog. *Circulation,* 9:706–718.
48. Sarnoff, S. J., Mitchell, J. H., Gilmore, J. P., and Remensnyder, J. P. (1960): Homeometric autoregulation of the heart. *Circ. Res.,* 9:706–718.
49. Sharpey-Schafer, E. P. (1961): Venous tone. *Br. Med. J.,* 2:1589–1595.
50. Simon, A. C., Safar, M. E., Levenson, J. A., London, G. M., Levy, B. I., and Chau, N. P. (1979): An evaluation of large artery compliance in man. *Am. J. Physiol.,* 237:H550–H554.
51. Sjostrand, T. (1953): Volume and distribution of blood and their significance in regulating the circulation. *Physiol. Rev.,* 33:202–228.
52. Slutsky, R., Karliner, J., Ricci, D., Kaiser, R., Pfisteier, M., Gordon, D., Peterson, K., and Ashburn, W. (1979): Left ventricular volumes by gated equilibrium radionuclide angiography: A new method. *Circulation,* 60:556–564.
53. Sonnenblick, E. H., Ross, J., Jr., and Braunwald, E. (1968): Oxygen consumption of the heart. New concept of its multifactorial determination. *Am. J. Cardiol.,* 22:328–336.
54. Spencer, M. P., and Greiss, F. C. (1962): Dynamics of ventricular ejection. *Circ. Res.,* 10:274–279.
55. Starr, I., Jeffers, W. A., and Meade, R. H. (1943): Absence of conspicuous increments of venous pressure after severe damage to the right ventricle of the dog, with a discussion of the relation between clinical congestive failure and heart disease. *Am. Heart J.,* 26:291–301.
56. Vatner, S. F., Hintze, T. H., and Macho, P. (1982): Regulation of large coronary arteries by β-adrenergic mechanisms in the conscious dog. *Circ. Res.,* 51:56–66.
57. Watt, T. B., and Burrus, C. (1976): Arterial pressure contour analysis for estimating human vascular properties. *J. Appl. Physiol.,* 40:171–176.
58. Whitney, R. J. (1953): The measurement of volume changes in the human limb. *J. Physiol. (Lond.),* 121:1.
59. Wood, J. E., and Eckstein, J. W. (1958): A tandem plethysmograph for study of acute responses of the peripheral veins of man; the effect of environmental and local temperature change and the effect of pooling blood in the extremities. *J. Clin. Invest.,* 37:41–50.
60. Yu, P. N., Murphy, G. W., Schneiner, B. F., and James, D. H. (1967): Distensibility characteristics of the human pulmonary vascular bed. Study of pressure-volume response to exercise in patients with and without heart disease. *Circulation,* 35:710–723.
61. Zobel, L. R., Finkelstein, S. M., Carlyle, P. F., and Cohn, J. N. (1980): Pressure pulse contour analysis in determining the effect of vasodilator drugs on vascular hemodynamic impedance characteristics in dogs. *Am. Heart J.,* 100:81–88.

The Heart and Cardiovascular System,
edited by H. A. Fozzard et al.
Raven Press, New York © 1986.

CHAPTER 64

Cardiac Mechanoreceptors

John T. Shepherd

HISTORICAL NOTES

Since the classic experiments of William Harvey in 1628 (49), the way in which the heart operates as a highly efficient pump has dominated the attention of cardiovascular clinicians and scientists. The enunciation of the Fick principle (38) for measurement of cardiac output, Waller's demonstration (154) of the electrical activity of the heart, the advent of the string galvanometer for easy recording of this activity (34), Keith and Flack's discovery (63) of the sinoatrial node, and Otto Loewi's proof (69) of chemical transmission of the nervous impulse formed the basis for the rapid growth of knowledge of the fundamental processes concerned with cardiac excitability, excitation-contraction coupling, and contraction.

Although terms such as "warm-heart, faint-heart" have been in common use for centuries, it was the observations of von Bezold and Hirt (13) that demonstrated the presence in the heart of receptors that affect the cardiovascular system. They observed that injections of veratrine caused a decrease in arterial blood pressure that could not be fully explained by the accompanying bradycardia and that did not occur after bilateral cervical vagotomy. This vasodepressor effect of veratridine was

explained by the stimulation in the heart of sensory nerve endings whose afferent fibers are in the vagus. Several other substances were shown to induce a similar depressor reflex (54,55) that was later named the Bezold-Jarisch reflex (29,68). Daly and Verney (27), using a heart-lung preparation, showed that an increase in perfusion pressure in the left side of the heart caused slowing of the heart; because aortic pressure was kept constant, this provided evidence for mechanoreceptors in the left ventricle. Aviado et al. (8) found that increasing the pressure on the right side of the heart also caused cardiac slowing and a decrease in systemic arterial blood pressure that was prevented by vagotomy (9).

Histological and electrophysiological studies have demonstrated the presence of mechanoreceptors in the atria, ventricles, coronary arteries, and pericardium. The receptors are subserved by either myelinated or unmyelinated afferent nerve fibers that pass either in the vagal nerves to the brainstem or via the sympathetic nerves (the so-called sympathetic or spinal afferents) to the spinal cord (Fig. 1) (16,19,39,51,66,67,95,96,101,102,146,149).

The time-honored approach to analysis of the role of a particular reflex is to isolate the receptors concerned, to eliminate or hold constant other sensory inputs to

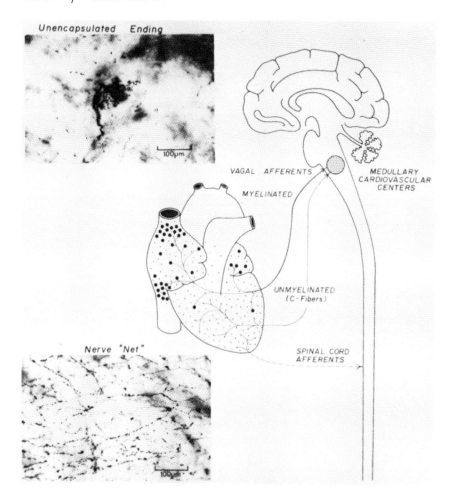

FIG. 1. Mechanoreceptors in the heart and their afferent fibers. Those subserved by the fast-conducting myelinated vagal afferents (8–30 m/sec) are localized to the junctions of (a) the caval veins with the right atrium and (b) the pulmonary veins with the left atrium. Those subserved by the slowly conducting unmyelinated afferents (less than 2.5 m/sec) arise from a widespread nerve net present in all chambers of the heart. Those subserved by the spinal cord afferents (sympathetic afferents, myelinated and unmyelinated) also arise from a diffuse network of fibers throughout the heart. **Insets:** histological appearance (methylene blue stain) of the large unencapsulated endings that are connected to the myelinated vagal afferents and the nerve "net" from which the unmyelinated vagal afferents seem to arise. (From ref. 71, with permission of the American Heart Association Inc.)

the central nervous system, and then to determine the relationship between graded stimulation of the receptors and the response of the cardiovascular system as a whole and the responses of its individual components. In the case of the anatomy at the site of the carotid baroreceptors and chemoreceptors, isolation can be accomplished with relative ease, but in the case of the cardiac receptors, it is difficult to separate the response of the total array of receptors in the heart from the response of those in the lungs, and it is even more difficult to study the contributions of the different receptors in the heart itself. However, many studies in recent years have demonstrated that sensory endings in the heart can be activated mechanically by pressure changes during the cardiac cycle and can participate in reflex regulation of the cardiovascular system. Other important considerations on which attention has been focused include the central terminations of receptor afferents, the differential engagement of the various receptor systems in regulation of the sympathetic outflow to the heart and systemic vascular beds, interactions between the different cardiovascular reflexes, and the influence of anesthesia on reflex responses.

In this chapter, our current knowledge of the cardiac mechanoreceptors is outlined. It is hoped that this will

encourage new approaches to gain answers to the many intriguing questions still to be resolved regarding the role of the heart as a sensory organ. For further details, excellent reviews by Thorén (138), Bishop et al. (16), Mark and Mancia (90), and Abboud and Thames (3) should be consulted.

CARDIAC MECHANORECEPTORS WITH VAGAL AFFERENTS

Myelinated Cardiac Vagal Afferents

The end formations of these afferent nerves appear to be unencapsulated endings (95,96) localized mainly in the atrial endocardium, especially at the junctions of the great veins with the right atrium and the pulmonary veins with the left atrium (20,47,91). They are subserved by myelinated vagal afferents with conduction velocities of 8 to 32 m/sec, are spontaneously active, and discharge with a cardiac rhythmicity at an average frequency of 18 impulses per second. Paintal (101–103) divided the atrial endings into A receptors, which fire during atrial systole, and B receptors, which fire during atrial diastole. There are also many fibers with both A and B discharges that he called intermediate endings (Fig. 2). The question

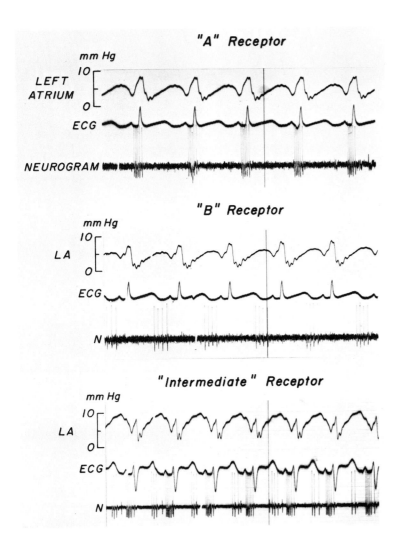

FIG. 2. Single-fiber recordings from left atrial receptors with myelinated vagal afferents. **Top:** Receptor is firing during the A wave of atrial pressure pulse ("A" receptor). **Middle:** Receptor is firing during the V wave ("B" receptor). **Bottom:** Receptor that is activated during both A and V waves ("intermediate" receptor). (Data from P. Thorén, G. Mancia, R. R. Lorenz, and J. T. Shepherd, *unpublished observations.*)

has been raised whether the atrial A and B receptors are two different types or whether they belong to the same group of endings. As far as their excitatory properties are concerned, they seem to belong to a homogeneous population, because the discharge patterns of types A and B behave in the same way during sinusoidal stretch of the receptor area *in situ.* The different patterns of their discharge are due to their arrangement in the atrial wall in relation to the contractile elements (6,7,48). It seems that the A receptors are activated by the tension developed by the atria during their contraction, because they are characterized by a brief high-frequency burst during the atrial A wave. Changes in heart rate do not affect the number of spikes with each atrial contraction. Thus, they provide information on heart rate to the cardiovascular center. In intact animals the endings seem to have reached their saturation point, and an increase in the inotropic state of the atria does not increase their discharge. However, a marked decrease in inotropy may reduce it (6,113,115). In contrast to the A receptors, the discharge of the B receptors is related to atrial filling (V wave). Thus, they are very sensitive to changes in central venous pressure. The frequency of

the B discharge is related not only to the absolute tension but also to the rate of change in tension development (114). Neither A nor B receptors respond to changes in plasma osmolality (43).

There are also endings in the ventricles with myelinated vagal afferents that discharge at the onset of ventricular systole (101,102). However, these are few in number compared with the many unmyelinated vagal afferents, particularly in the left ventricle (24). Other mechanoreceptors with myelinated vagal afferents in or near the coronary arteries are spontaneously active.

Unmyelinated Cardiac Vagal Afferents

The existence of atrial receptors with unmyelinated vagal afferents was first shown by Coleridge et al. (22), and the functional characteristics of this receptor group were studied by Thorén (136). Because the conduction velocity of these afferents is 2.5 m/sec, they are classified as C fibers. In the cat the cardiac vagal branch contains about 2,500 afferents, of which about 75% are unmyelinated (4,16). In contrast to the A and B receptors, the atrial C fiber endings are located throughout the

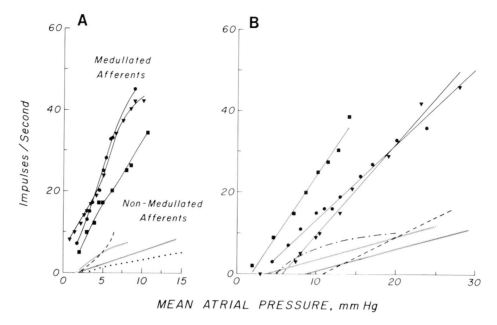

FIG. 3. Relationship between activity in myelinated and unmyelinated vagal afferents from right atrium (**A**) and left atrium (**B**) of cats during increases in atrial pressure caused by graded occlusion of the respective outflow tract. Each set of recordings is from a single fiber. (From ref. 136, with permission of the American Heart Association Inc.)

atria, including the interatrial septum and atrial appendices (136). Under resting conditions, both in artificially ventilated and in naturally breathing cats, these receptors are silent or have no discharge or a low-frequency irregular discharge (mean 1.4 impulses/sec). However, when excited above threshold levels, most receptors discharge with cardiac rhythmicity in phase with either atrial contraction (A wave) or atrial filling (V wave). The threshold for individual receptors is between 2 and 3 mm Hg (mean pressure) in the right atrium and between 5 and 12 mm Hg (mean pressure) in the left atrium (Fig. 3). In spontaneously respiring cats the receptors discharge with cardiac rhythmicity during end inspiration and early expiration when atrial transmural pressure is greatest and are silent for the remainder of the respiratory cycle. This effect is enhanced by augmenting respiration by brief inhalation of CO_2. Thus, these receptors can respond to physiological changes in atrial volume. During blood volume expansion these receptors become active throughout the entire respiratory cycle (Fig. 4) (128).

The existence of left ventricular C fibers was first demonstrated in the dog by Coleridge et al. (21), and they were shown to have a low firing rate with irregular rhythm. They were activated by probing the epicardium or by injections of capsaicin and veratridine. Further studies showed that these epimyocardial receptors could be stimulated by aortic occlusion and usually displayed cardiac rhythmicity. Epinephrine injection induced a more powerful activation of the receptors than aortic

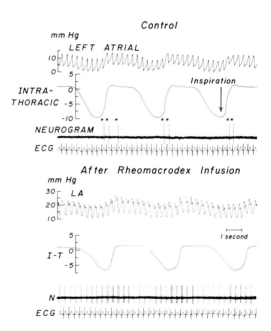

FIG. 4. Influences of respiration and of expansion of blood volume with Rheomacrodex on the rate and pattern of discharge of left atrial receptor with unmyelinated vagal afferent in the closed-chest spontaneously breathing cat. The asterisks indicate the times during the cardiac cycle during which the receptor was activated when the appropriate correction is made for conduction time from receptor to recording electrodes. The receptor's anatomical location was the venoatrial junction draining the left lower lobe. The left atrial pressure tracing is overdamped due to slight wedging of the catheter tip. (From ref. 128, with permission of the American Heart Association Inc.)

occlusion. Carotid occlusion to activate the sympathetic fibers to the heart, or electrical stimulation of these nerves, also activated them, and some were activated by increasing the coronary venous pressure by partial occlusion of the coronary sinus (24,92,93,124). The characteristics of left ventricular epimyocardial C fibers in the cat are similar to those in the dog. When recording from C fibers, which normally have low-frequency activity, the method of selecting the receptors is important, because they include a large number of fibers with heterogeneous characteristics (138). Because it is not possible to find a silent C fiber, every dissected filament must be manipulated to increase the receptor activity. Some are mechanoreceptors capable of signaling changes in the inotropic state of the ventricles, as well as changes in volume. Others are chemosensitive, and their importance may lie in their stimulation by substances produced in the myocardium when metabolic demands on it are high (10,11). Baker et al. (11) suggested that the chemosensitive endings may be concerned with "protective" rather than regulatory reflexes, reducing metabolic demands on the myocardium by slowing heart rate and diminishing afterload. Differences in results between

studies might well be explained by the way fibers are selected. In the cat, ventricular C fiber activity was studied according to their ability to respond to aortic occlusion, so that only mechanoreceptors were examined (138). Although usually activated during systole, in no experimental conditions was an increase in receptor discharge observed wthout a concomitant rise in left ventricular end-diastolic pressure; when systolic pressure alone was raised, the receptors did not increase their rate of discharge (Fig. 5). Thus, there seems to be the paradox that the left ventricular receptors with unmyelinated vagal afferents are activated mainly during systole, although the frequency in discharge correlates well with increase in end-diastolic pressure, i.e., appears to relate to diastolic events (10,23,137). This finding will probably be explained when more information is obtained about the structure of the receptors and the relationship between the endings and the myocardium. The receptors may be some type of branching nerve endings of unmyelinated fibers situated between the myocardial cells throughout the entire myocardium. An increased left ventricular end-diastolic pressure that markedly influences the following systole because of the

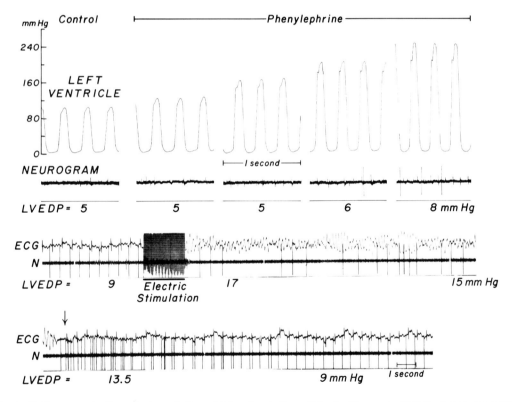

FIG. 5. Activity in C fiber vagal afferents from left ventricle of cat. **Top:** Effect of increase in left ventricular outflow resistance (infusion of phenylephrine) on discharge frequency. Note that left ventricular systolic pressure increased by 60 mm Hg without an increase in left ventricular end-diastolic pressure (LVEDP), during which the receptor remained silent. With the first increase in left ventricular diastolic pressure (6 mm Hg), the receptor discharged. **Lower panels:** Effects of electrically induced fibrillation of ventricle on spontaneous activity of left ventricular afferent fibers. During fibrillation, activity decreased immediately, but after spontaneous defibrillation (arrow), traffic markedly increased before it returned to control. Increases in end-diastolic pressure were not accompanied by increases in receptor discharge until there was a coordinated ventricular contraction. ECG, electrocardiogram; N, neurogram. (From ref. 31, with permission.)

Frank-Starling mechanism and resulting increase in stroke volume may trigger the receptor to fire. On the other hand, this does not explain why purely systolic events, such as an isolated increase in systolic pressure, are relatively weak in activating the receptors. The discharge of ventricular receptors also is augmented by positive inotropic interventions and reduced by negative interventions. Thus, the discharge pattern of ventricular receptors with unmyelinated afferents is influenced by increases in preload and afterload and by changes in cardiac contractility (137). Each of these factors has been shown to influence cardiac contraction by changing the force and speed of shortening of the ventricular myocardium. Thus, the apparent dependence of the rate of discharge of these receptors on the left ventricular end-diastolic pressure can now be viewed as a contribution of this pressure to determination of the mechanical events of ventricular systole. Another peculiarity of these receptors is the fact that recordings of spontaneous activity of left ventricular C fibers often show a period

of increased activity without concomitant changes in cardiac dynamics. The mechanisms behind the odd behavior of the cardiac C fibers remain to be elucidated (16,138).

CARDIAC RECEPTORS WITH SYMPATHETIC (SPINAL) AFFERENTS

Receptors that are widely distributed in each of the cardiac chambers and great vessels and whose afferent fibers course in the cardiac sympathetic nerves to the spinal cord, with cell bodies in the dorsal root ganglia, have been described in the cat, the dog, and the monkey (Fig. 6). From electrophysiological recordings, afferent sympathetic nerve fibers with receptive endings in the heart have been detected in the cardiac sympathetic nerves, the rami communicantes, and the spinal dorsal roots (16,50,80,81). Similarly, innervated receptors also have been described in or near the coronary vessels (19), the aorta (147), the caval and pulmonary veins

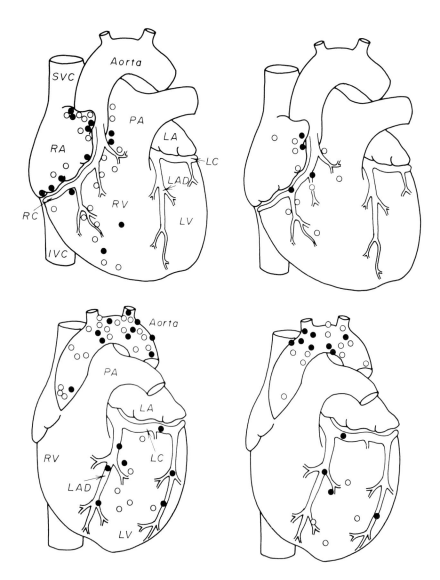

FIG. 6. Distribution in dogs of cardiac mechanoreceptors subserved by myelinated (left) and unmyelinated (right) afferent sympathetic nerve fibers. Open circles, spontaneously firing; filled circles, silent except when stimulated mechanically; SVC, superior vena cava; LC, left circumflex coronary artery; PA, pulmonary artery; LA, left atrium; LV, left ventricle; RA, right atrium; IVC, inferior vena cava; RV, right ventricle; LAD, left anterior descending coronary artery; RC, right coronary artery. (Data from refs. 30 and 146.)

(75,146,149), and extrapulmonic portions of pulmonary artery (66). Electrophysiological studies indicate that the majority of sympathetic afferent fibers are unmyelinated (C fibers). However, the functional importance of the myelinated versus unmyelinated afferents in reflex control of the circulation has still to be determined (119).

Atrial Receptors

Afferent sympathetic nerve fibers from these receptors are myelinated and unmyelinated, as inferred from their conduction velocities. These fibers may discharge in phase with atrial systole (A wave), with bulging of the atrioventricular valves (C wave), and with atrial filling (V wave) (145). Unlike the myelinated afferent vagal fibers from atrial endings that usually yield bursts of impulses, these receptors generate a single impulse during each cardiac cycle. The silent fibers are more numerous among the unmyelinated afferents and can be activated both by mechanical stimuli and by chemical substances

such as potassium chloride or bradykinin applied topically on the epicardial surface (16).

Ventricular Receptors

Ventricular receptors with afferent myelinated nerve fibers are sensitive to mechanical events of the cardiac cycle. The discharge increases during increases in ventricular pressure and decreases during reductions. These ventricular endings are also excited by chemical substances such as bradykinin, veratridine, and acids.

Unlike the discharge of myelinated sympathetic ventricular afferents, cardiac receptors with unmyelinated afferents have an irregular discharge that has no apparent relation to cardiac events (Fig. 7). However, when they are excited by distension of the cardiac chamber in which they are located and corrections are made for the conduction time, most of the spontaneous impulses appear to occur during ventricular systole.

Some receptors with myelinated and unmyelinated

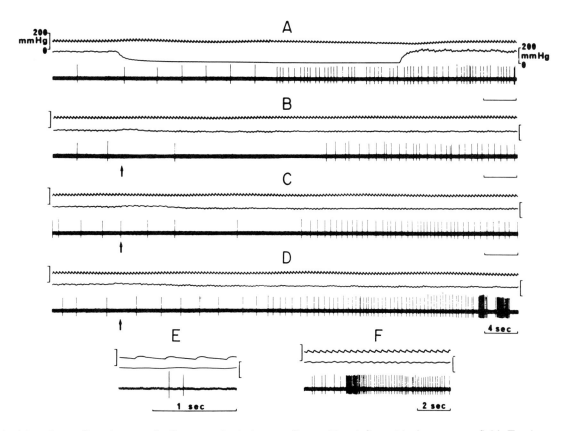

FIG. 7. Activity of an afferent sympathetic unmyelinated nerve fiber with a left ventricular sensory field. Tracings represent, from top to bottom, systemic arterial pressure, coronary perfusion pressure, and nerve impulse activity (cathode-ray oscilloscope recordings). **A:** Interruption of left main coronary artery perfusion. **B:** Intracoronary administration, beginning at the arrow, of bradykinin, 5 ng/kg. **C:** Intracoronary administration of bradykinin, 10 ng/kg. **D:** Intracoronary administration of bradykinin, 30 ng/kg. **E:** Electrical stimulation of left inferior cardiac nerve activating the afferent fiber; the biphasic first deflection is the artifact of the stimulus, and the second biphasic deflection is the action potential of the fiber. The approximate length of the fiber was 8 cm. The conduction velocity calculated for this fiber was 0.45 m/sec. **F:** Mechanical probing, marked by a bar, of an area of the external surface of the left ventricle; notice the afterdischarge, which is typical of unmyelinated afferents. (From ref. 76, with permission of the American Heart Association Inc.)

fibers display properties of "polymodal" receptors, i.e., they are sensitive to both mechanical and chemical stimuli (16,76). Several receptors might be connected to the same afferent fibers, as suggested by the finding of multiterminal afferent fibers from the thoracic viscera in sympathetic rami communicantes of cats and dogs. These receptors are not necessarily from the same anatomical structure (26). Because of the difficulties in distinguishing primarily chemosensitive receptors from polymodal receptors, no definite conclusion can be reached concerning the two populations of receptors: those primarily sensitive to mechanical events and those sensitive to chemical stimuli (16).

Coronary Receptors

Afferent sympathetic nerve fibers can be excited by increases in coronary blood flow and pressure and by occlusion of the coronary sinus. Some of these fibers are also activated during the period of myocardial ischemia caused by temporary interruption of coronary blood flow. It is uncertain whether or not these coronary receptors should be distinguished from ventricular receptors that are also excited by increased coronary blood flow and pressure (19,144).

Cardiac Nociceptors

Spinal (sympathetic) afferent pathways appear to be solely responsible for signaling the pain of myocardial ischemia. In man this pain can be relieved by bilateral stellectomy and excision of T-1 through T-5 thoracic ganglia (157). Chemical substances released by the ischemic myocardium probably activate chemosensitive endings with unmyelinated fibers (144). Bradykinin, a powerful algesic agent, is released by the ischemic heart (64). This substance, in anesthetized cats, excites both chemosensitive and mechanosensitive sympathetic afferent fibers from the heart and great vessels. It is suggested that it is the activity transmitted in the most slowly conducting group of chemosensitive afferent fibers that arouses a sensation of pain (11).

Electrical stimulation of cardiopulmonary sympathetic afferents excites spinothalamic tract neurons in the upper thoracic spinal cord. This is inhibited by stimulation of vagal afferent fibers, as is the activation of sympathetic afferents by bradykinin. This suggests that vagal afferents can modulate the sensation of cardiac pain. These studies provide an explanation for the clinical observations of "silent" myocardial infarction (5).

**FUNCTION OF ATRIAL
RECEPTORS WITH VAGAL AFFERENTS**

In the dog, distension of the vein-atrial junctions with small balloons increases heart rate, augments renal

blood flow by a minimal amount, and has no effect on hindlimb vascular resistance. These effects are abolished by vagotomy. Balloon inflation is accompanied by an increase in impulse activity in both afferent vagal myelinated and unmyelinated fibers and in efferent cardiac sympathetic fibers. There is no concomitant change in the activity of efferent cardiac vagal nerves. The sympathetic fibers that mediate this reflex tachycardia are separate from those involved in other cardiac reflexes (73). Sympathetic nerve activity to the kidney is decreased, while that to the hindlimb and spleen is unaffected. Because the increases in heart rate and urine flow and the reduction in the activity of the renal sympathetic nerves are abolished by cooling the cervical vagi to 8 to 10°C, it has been concluded that these responses are likely to be due to activation of receptors with myelinated vagal afferents (60–62,71,72). The response of the sympathetic nervous system to left atrial receptor activation is thus nonuniform and can be directionally opposite, increasing to the heart and decreasing slightly to the kidney. Balloon inflation does not increase left ventricular contractility, suggesting that the efferent limb of the cardiac reflex is limited to the sympathetic nerves to the sinus node. Thus, stimulation of the area where the endings with vagal myelinated afferents predominate (i.e., the vein-atrial junctions) causes a tachycardia, solely of sympathetic origin, and uses a bundle of efferent neurons separate from those in any other reflex. It has been proposed that this reflex increase in heart rate acts to maintain cardiac volume relatively constant during an increase in venous return (71).

When larger areas of the vein-atrial junctions are stimulated, C fiber afferents that are more widely distributed may also be activated to cause a vasodepressor response (16,33,138). The finding by Karim et al. (61) that a small balloon inflated in the pulmonary vein-atrial junction could induce not only reflex tachycardia but also inhibition of the renal sympathetic traffic might be partly explained by simultaneous stimulation of receptors with both myelinated and unmyelinated vagal afferents. Activation of atrial C fibers is likely to contribute to renal sympathetic nerve withdrawal because of the pronounced inhibitory effect this has on the sympathetic nerve traffic to the kidney even at low levels of activation (74,138). Further support for this hypothesis comes from the studies of Öberg and Thorén (98), which showed that electrical stimulation of the vagal afferents from the heart, with parameters such that only the myelinated fibers were activated, induced an excitatory reflex response. In contrast, electrical activation of the cardiac C fibers induced vasodepressor reflexes. This is consistent with the finding that atrial receptors, presumably those with C fiber afferents, continuously inhibit the vasomotor center (see Fig. 9).

In 1951, Gauer and associates suggested that extracellular fluid volume is regulated through stretch receptors in the intrathoracic circulation. They considered that the atrial receptors were situated advantageously to sense the "fullness of the circulation" and that those receptors with myelinated vagal afferents might serve as volume receptors and act to regulate the circulating level of antidiuretic hormone (vasopressin) (40,41). Balloon distension of the pulmonary vein–atrial junction in dogs results not only in an increase in heart rate but also in an increase in urine flow that can be prevented by cooling the cervical vagi (59,70). There are minor increases in excretions of sodium and potassium. Similar changes are observed when the superior vena cava–right atrial junction or the right atrial appendage is stretched (58). The diuresis still occurs after denervation of the kidneys, and so is due, at least in part, to a blood-borne agent. It seems that stimulation of the unencapsulated endings in the atria with myelinated vagal afferents results in increases in urine flow and sodium excretion as a consequence of changes in the plasma concentration of a humoral agent, affecting only water excretion, and of decreased efferent sympathetic nerve activity to the kidney affecting both water and sodium excretions (72). The cardiopulmonary receptors with afferent vagal fibers exert a tonic inhibitory influence on antidiuretic hormone secretion (3,44,134,135). However, there has been much debate whether the diuresis caused by discrete stimulation of the unencapsulated atrial receptors with small balloons is due to a reduction in the concentration of circulating antidiuretic hormone or to secretion of a diuretic substance (72). In evaluating the various studies it is important to exclude the possibility that the accompanying circulatory changes might be held responsible for an alteration in antidiuretic hormone secretion; for example, Goetz et al. (45) have shown that reduction in atrial transmural pressure by distension of a previously prepared pericardial pouch still causes decreases in urine flow and renal sodium excretion in dogs with acute cardiac denervation. In dogs, after administration of bretylium tosylate, atropine, and atenolol, to prevent any hemodynamic changes accompanying balloon distension of the pulmonary vein–left atrial junctions and the left atrial appendage, there was an increase in urine flow and a decrease in the plasma concentration of vasopressin. It has still to be determined if this decrease is sufficient to explain the increase in urine flow (12).

During space flight, when zero gravity is reached, blood from the legs is displaced centrally. This is manifest by a feeling of fullness in the head and distension of the neck veins. Diuresis follows, the plasma and red cell volume decrease, and the intrathoracic blood volume is restored to normal. However, the total blood volume is decreased, so that on return to earth gravity, the blood is redistributed to the legs, and the central blood volume and the filling pressure of the heart are reduced; as a result, there is a reduced tolerance for standing, and fainting may occur. Presumably these large venoatrial receptors have an important role in causing the diuresis, but this has still to be assessed.

FUNCTION OF VENTRICULAR RECEPTORS WITH VAGAL AFFERENTS

While there is evidence for some mechanoreceptors in the ventricles that discharge into myelinated fibers, there is little evidence for their functional role. Mechanoreceptors in or near the coronary arteries, however, are spontaneously active, like those of the unencapsulated endings at the vein–atrial junctions. Their discharge frequency is directly related to coronary perfusion pressure, most being activated during the systolic phase of the coronary arterial pressure pulse (18). Paintal (102) has suggested that these coronary artery receptors belong to the same group as the ventricular mechanoreceptors

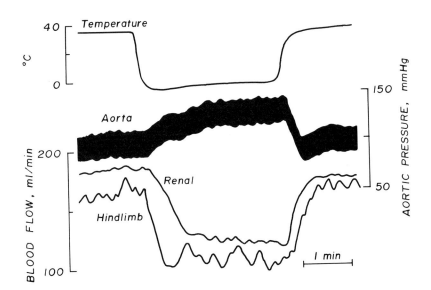

FIG. 8. Vascular responses to vagal cold block in a dog on cardiopulmonary bypass. The arterial baroreceptors were denervated, the lungs were removed, and the heart was left *in situ.* One hindlimb and kidney were perfused at a constant pressure of 120 mm Hg. Cooling the cervical vagi to 0°C caused an increase in aortic blood pressure and decreases in renal and hindlimb blood flow. (Data from ref. 83.)

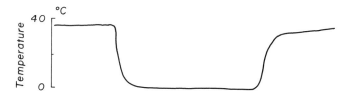

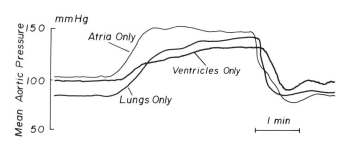

FIG. 9. Evidence that the atria, ventricles, and lungs each contribute to tonic inhibition of the vasomotor center. Dogs on cardiopulmonary bypass; vagi divided below the diaphragm, and arterial baroreceptors denervated. Study 1: Lungs and ventricles removed, leaving the beating atria. Study 2: Lungs removed and atria denervated, leaving the innervated beating ventricles. Study 3: Heart removed, leaving the lungs, which were mechanically ventilated. When the traffic in the vagal afferents from the receptors in each of these structures was interrupted by cooling (**top**), there was an increase in aortic blood pressure due to increased sympathetic outflow to systemic blood vessels. (From ref. 31, with permission.)

and that their different firing pattern is due to their location.

Receptors with unmyelinated afferent fibers are widely distributed throughout the heart, including the interatrial and interventricular septa, and constitute the major part of the afferent innervation of the ventricles. They cannot be associated with any specific nerve endings, although they may be part of the fine network of fibers (39). Some of the C fiber endings appear to be located superficially in or near the epicardium, while others are situated more deeply in the myocardium; hence, they have been described as epicardial, epimyocardial, and myocardial.

The intracardiac route of left ventricular C fibers has been studied by Thorén (137) in the cat. The afferent fibers from the posterior surface of the heart pass along the posterior descending artery into the right atrium to join the right main cardiac nerve; those from the an-

terolateral region pass behind the aorta and the pulmonary trunk. Most of the C fibers seem to exit from the heart at the junction of the superior caval vein and the right atrium in the main cardiac branch of the right vagus, which passes underneath the azygos vein. The depressor effects of veratrum alkaloids are also mediated by the same vagal branch (57,138).

Interruption of all afferent vagal traffic from the heart in atropinized animals with aortic nerves sectioned and carotid sinuses denervated and vascularly isolated results in increases in arterial blood pressure and in renal, mesenteric, and muscle vascular resistance and decreased splanchnic capacitance and tachycardia (30,82,141). These changes are due to an increase in sympathetic adrenergic outflow. The cutaneous veins are not involved. Thus, these vagally innervated cardiac receptors, like the arterial baroreceptors, act to tonically inhibit the vasomotor center (Fig. 8). Further, receptors in the atria,

FIG. 10. Effects of anodal block of myelinated vagal fibers, and subsequent vagal cold block, on aortic blood pressure and renal blood flow in cat. The compound action potentials were recorded before and during the anodal block. Disappearance of the A and Aδ potentials during block demonstrates that conduction in the myelinated fibers has been prevented. The large downward deflection is the stimulus artifact. (From ref. 141, with permission of the American Heart Association Inc.)

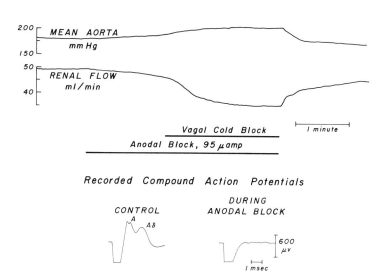

the ventricles, and the lungs each exert tonic inhibition of the center (Fig. 9); although the surgical techniques employed in these experiments make it difficult to compare the relative inhibition exerted by each region, the findings suggest considerable occlusion of the neural input from each organ (83).

To determine if receptors served by myelinated or unmyelinated fibers were responsible for this tonic vasomotor inhibition, techniques of selective stimulation

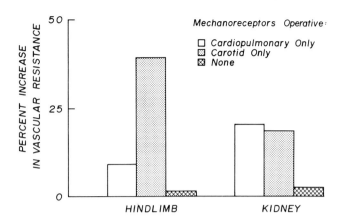

FIG. 12. Roles of cardiopulmonary and carotid mechanoreceptors in circulatory control during 10% hemorrhage in dogs. (From ref. 107.)

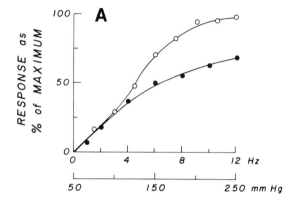

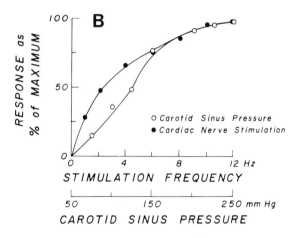

FIG. 11. Changes in muscle (**A**) and renal (**B**) vascular resistance in cats in response to electrical stimulation of right cardiac nerve and to alterations in pressure within the partially isolated carotid sinus. Data plotted as percentage of maximal decrease in resistance at a carotid sinus pressure of 33.3 kPa (250 mm Hg) (1 kPa = 7.5 mm Hg). The stimulus–response curves to changes in activity in the cardiac and carotid sinus nerves have been adjusted so that the threshold and maximal responses of each coincide. As carotid sinus pressure is increased above 20.0 kPa (150 mm Hg), the resultant increase in activity of the carotid baroreceptors reduces muscle resistance more than does the increase in activity in cardiac C fiber vagal afferents; both are similar in their modulation of renal resistance. As carotid sinus pressure increases from 6.7 to 16.0 kPa (50 to 120 mm Hg), the resultant increase in activity of the carotid baroreceptors is less effective in decreasing renal resistance than is an increase in activity of cardiac C fiber vagal afferents; both are similar in their modulation of muscle resistance. (Data from refs. 30 and 74.)

and interruption of nerve activity have been employed. In cats, electrical excitation of the right cardiac nerve with stimuli of appropriate parameters showed that excitation of unmyelinated fibers resulted in arterial hypotension, decreased renal and muscle vascular resistance, and bradycardia (98). Selective cervical vagal cold block in rabbits (140) and anodal block of the same nerve in cats (143) demonstrated that tonic inhibition of the vasomotor center could be ascribed to inhibition of nerve activity in unmyelinated fibers (Fig. 10).

Although the afferent fibers from the arterial and cardiopulmonary mechanoreceptors converge on the same general pool of neurons in the brainstem, and both groups of receptors act to tonically inhibit the vasomotor center, there are important differences in the extents to which the inputs from the two groups regulate the sympathetic outflow to the different vascular beds. As with the carotid and arterial baroreceptors, the effects of the cardiopulmonary receptors on sympathetic adrenergic outflow to different vascular beds are nonuniform. Studies in cats and dogs indicate that at moderate and high levels of stimulation of both receptor systems, muscle vasomotor fibers are less engaged by cardiopulmonary than by carotid baroreceptors (Fig. 11). At low levels of stimulation, sympathetic outflow to muscle vessels appears to be influenced equally by both systems. At low levels of stimulation, the renal vasomotor fibers appear to be more inhibited by the cardiopulmonary than by the carotid baroreceptors, whereas at high levels the responses are similar (30,74,84). This differential engagement of the carotid and cardiopulmonary receptors with the central neuronal pools governing sympathetic outflow to the periphery dictates the role of each system in counteracting various stresses. For example, during a moderate hemorrhage the more powerful control of muscle resistance vessels by the carotid than by the cardiopulmonary baroreceptors is the reason why arterial blood pressure is better sustained by the former (Fig. 12) (107).

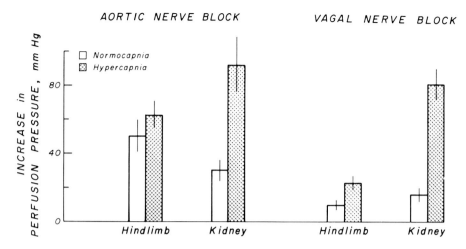

FIG. 13. Effects of hypercapnia on inhibition of hindlimb and renovascular resistance by aortic and cardiopulmonary mechanoreceptors in anesthetized rabbits. **Left panel:** Vagal and carotid sinus nerves were cut before aortic nerve block by cooling (N = 11). **Right panel:** Carotid sinus and aortic nerves were cut before cold block of cervical vagal nerves (N = 19). Note the greater augmentation by hypercapnia of the inhibitory influences of both systems on renal but not on hindlimb vascular resistance. (From ref. 30.)

During hypercapnia, reflex inhibition of renal vasomotor tone exerted by cardiopulmonary and arterial baroreceptors is augmented (Fig. 13). The mechanism is not known, but it permits renal blood flow to be preserved and has its obvious benefits in helping restore the acid-base balance in respiratory acidosis (85,99,100).

REFLEX CONTROL OF RELEASE OF RENIN AND ANTIDIURETIC HORMONE

Excitation of the renal sympathetic nerves causes an increase in renal vascular resistance and a decrease in urinary excretion of sodium. This may activate one or all of the mechanisms that govern the release of renin; these are the intrarenal vascular receptors, the sodium load to the macula densa, and the direct sympathetic innervation of the juxtaglomerular cells. Changes in the activity of arterial and cardiopulmonary mechanoreceptors subserved by vagal afferents, sufficient to cause an increase or decrease in sympathetic nerve traffic to the kidney, result in increases or decreases in renin release, respectively. Also, very weak stimulation of the renal nerves, insufficient to cause an increase in renin release, can potentiate release through local nonneural mechanisms (131). No particular group of cardiac receptors that modulate the release of renin has been identified. Because receptors in the heart and lungs with vagal myelinated and unmyelinated afferents can reflexly alter renal sympathetic nerve activity, it is assumed that all of them can influence renin release. Thus, interruption of afferent inhibitory activity from vagally innervated cardiopulmonary receptors by cold block or nerve section in dogs with sinoaortic denervation results in an increase

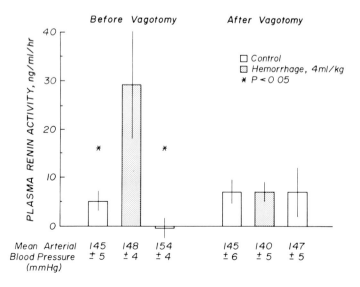

FIG. 14. Increases in plasma renin activity during nonhypotensive hemorrhage (4 cm^3·kg^{-1}) in 10 anesthetized dogs. Mean values (±SE) before, 3 min after completion of hemorrhage, and 15 min after reinfusion of the withdrawn blood. The increase was absent after vagotomy. Because arterial systolic and diastolic and pulse pressures did not change significantly with hemorrhage, these studies imply that cardiopulmonary receptors are more sensitive detectors of small changes in circulating blood volume than are arterial baroreceptors. (Data from refs. 122 and 129, with permission.)

in secretion of renin that is abolished following section of the renal nerves (84). Stimulation of left atrial receptors by outflow obstruction in normal (17) and in salt-depleted dogs (158) and chemical excitation of the left ventricular receptors with cryptenamine in dogs subjected to a moderate hemorrhage act to decrease the release of renin (127). These experiments establish a role for vagally innervated cardiopulmonary receptors in control of renin release and demonstrate that this is exerted by the receptors in the atria and the left ventricle. It is not yet known if receptors in the right ventricle and the lungs also modulate the release of renin. The fact that a very mild hemorrhage can cause an increase in renin release without changing the arterial baroreceptor activity indicates that a tonic inhibition of renin release by vagal cardiopulmonary receptors occurs in the presence of intact arterial baroreceptors and also that the cardiopulmonary receptors can respond to changes in blood volume to which arterial baroreceptors are insensitive (Fig. 14).

CARDIAC RECEPTORS WITH VAGAL AFFERENTS: STUDIES IN CONSCIOUS DOGS

Because general anesthesia alters the cardiovascular reflexes, it is important, as far as possible, to study these reflexes in conscious animals. Bilateral vagal cold block or section has been used to interrupt the afferent traffic. Thus, in interpreting the results, it must be recognized that all vagal afferents from the cardiopulmonary region are interrupted, and thus the roles of different receptor groups cannot be determined. Collectively, these afferents exert a restraining influence on the vasomotor center in the conscious resting dog. This was demonstrated by increases in systemic arterial blood pressure, heart rate, and cardiac output during bilateral cervical vagal cold block. In the absence of functioning arterial baroreflexes, the vagal block caused a significantly greater increase in arterial pressure, while the heart rate response was less, and there was an increase in total systemic vascular resistance (15).

Lability of Arterial Blood Pressure

When the arterial baroreflexes are acutely or chronically interrupted, the variability in systemic arterial blood pressure is increased in dogs both at rest and during exercise. This indicates that the arterial baroreflexes are controlling the moment-to-moment fluctuations in sympathetic outflow. By contrast, the cardiopulmonary reflexes do not appear to be involved in moment-to-moment control of arterial blood pressure, because interruption of these reflexes in dogs whose arterial baroreflexes have been either acutely or chronically interrupted does not increase lability (150,151).

Arterial Blood Pressure During Exercise

During rhythmic exercise there is a locally mediated vasodilatation in the active muscles, a reflex constriction of the splanchnic and renal vascular beds, and an increase in cardiac output, each proportional to the work load. These events permit a modest elevation in mean arterial pressure as the exercise becomes more severe, and this, together with the local vasodilatation, provides for adequate blood flow to the active muscles so that their metabolic requirements are met. Some of this rise in pressure is due to an increase in the set point of the arterial baroreceptors that occurs rapidly when exercise commences (65).

Surprisingly, the cardiopulmonary reflexes appear to have little or no role in the arterial blood pressure response to exercise in dogs either acutely or chronically deprived of their arterial baroreflexes. In dogs exercising following chronic denervation of the aortic arch, and with the carotid baroreflexes acutely interrupted, there is a profound increase in arterial blood pressure as the intensity of the exercise increases, and this increase is maintained in the postexercise period. The heart rate and cardiac output responses are the same as those seen during and after the same exercise prior to interruption of the baroreflexes. Thus, the role of the arterial baroreflexes is to govern total systemic vascular resistance during and after exercise. Heart rate and cardiac output are regulated by different mechanisms. Section of both cervical vagi does not alter the blood pressure response to moderately severe exercise, indicating that the cardiopulmonary receptors do not contribute to maintenance of a normal arterial blood pressure response to exercise after acute removal of the arterial baroreflexes (150,151).

After chronic sinoaortic denervation, the arterial blood pressure is little changed from resting values during graded exercise. Obviously, some adaptation has occurred. To see if this adaptation involved cardiopulmonary receptors, arterial blood pressure, cardiac output, and heart rate responses to graded exercise were examined in chronic sinoaortic-denervated dogs before and after vagotomy. These hemodynamic changes were similar during the exercise before and after vagotomy. However, in the postexercise period, the arterial blood pressure, after vagotomy, increased markedly at a time when the cardiac output and heart rate were decreasing rapidly, just as before vagotomy, to the resting level. This suggests that in these circumstances, the cardiopulmonary reflexes are necessary to restore the arterial blood pressure to normal after exercise by causing relaxation of systemic resistance vessels, presumably those in the splanchnic bed and the kidneys (28,152).

Thus, whereas each of the mechanoreceptor systems, carotid sinus, aortic arch, and cardiopulmonary, contributes to the mean level of arterial blood pressure in the conscious dog by tonic inhibition of the vasomotor center, the cardiopulmonary reflexes are not capable of substantially limiting the rise in pressure when the arterial baroreflexes are acutely abrogated. Possibly the mechanoreceptors in the heart and lungs have a prime role in setting the mean pressure over long periods, while the arterial baroreflexes are more concerned with short-term regulation (150,151).

FUNCTION OF CARDIAC RECEPTORS WITH SYMPATHETIC AFFERENTS

Some of the cardiac receptors have afferent fibers that travel in the sympathetic nerves to the spinal cord. One group of myelinated afferents has a spontaneous discharge at normal cardiac pressures. Another group does not spontaneously discharge, but does so irregularly if coronary occlusion is imposed. Low-frequency electrical stimulation of the myelinated fibers leads to a reduction in arterial blood pressure, due to inhibition of efferent sympathetic nerve activity to the heart and systemic circulation. With high-frequency stimulation to activate the unmyelinated fibers, the opposite occurs. Thus, the cardiovascular sympathetic afferents have the potential to exert an excitatory or inhibitory influence on those neurons that control the sympathetic outflow to the heart and systemic blood vessels, and particularly that to the kidney (112,155). The excitatory effect, which seems to predominate, operates through a spinal reflex and exhibits positive-feedback characteristics (19,78,79,110). However, when the spinal cord is intact, the role of this spinal reflex in control of sympathetic outflow to the heart is attenuated. Thus, in dogs with spinal cords sectioned, cardiac sympathetic nerves exert an excitatory influence on the sympathetic discharge to the heart, but may not with spinal cords intact. It appears that inhibitory bulbospinal pathways minimize the response (37). Because the sympathetic afferents constitute the pathway of the pain response to coronary occlusion (157), conceivably this might lead to tachycardia and hypertension by a supraspinal mechanism. However, to date, the contribution of receptors in the heart and lungs with sympathetic afferents to the normal integrated neural adjustments of the cardiovascular system is not known (14,77,78,148,155).

Central Integration of Cardiac Reflexes

In order to determine the role of a particular reflex in circulatory control, it is necessary to eliminate the participation of other reflexes in the response. This is known as the open-loop approach. However, in the intact organism, a perturbation in one reflex system is often accompanied by or causes changes in other sensory inputs. Thus, the final outcome in terms of the cardiovascular adjustments will depend on the way in which this array of sensory signals is processed by the central nervous system (3).

Central Nervous Structures

The baroreceptor and chemoreceptor afferents that travel in the glossopharyngeal and vagal nerves relay in the cell bodies of the petrosal and nodose ganglia, respectively, and terminate in the nucleus tractus solitarius of the medulla. The cardiac vagal unmyelinated afferents seem to project to the same part of the nucleus tractus solitarius as the myelinated fibers. This nucleus also has inputs from many other sites, including receptors in the skeletal muscles, the trigeminal and vestibular nerves, and hypothalamus and the locus ceruleus. This array of connections makes the nucleus tractus solitarius an important integrating center for reflex control of the cardiovascular system (3,104,105,125).

In the nucleus tractus solitarius, the neurotransmitter(s) released from the nerve terminals that alters the activity in other central pathways regulating cardiovascular reflex activity is not known. While this nucleus is richly supplied with catecholamine-containing varicosities, there is no evidence that norepinephrine is the neurotransmitter. The sensory nerve terminals of the baroreceptor and chemoreceptor afferents have a direct connection with catecholaminergic bodies in this nucleus, and axon terminals containing substance P, a vasoactive undecapeptide, may form synapses with these bodies. Thus, substance P might be a neurotransmitter for the baroreceptor and chemoreceptor afferents. Glutamic acid injection into the nucleus causes hypotension and bradycardia. This substance may also be a mediator of the baroreflexes in the nucleus (126).

The efferent fibers of the nucleus tractus solitarius project to the cardiac vagal nuclei of the medulla (the nucleus ambiguus and the dorsal motor nucleus), to other nuclei in the reticular formation of the brainstem, to the sympathetic preganglionic nuclei in the intermediolateral horns of the spinal cord, and to the hypothalamus and other higher brain centers. Changes in the traffic in these efferent fibers thus can excite or inhibit the vagal cholinergic efferent pathway to the heart and can activate the excitatory or inhibitory bulbospinal pathways, which terminate close to the preganglionic sympathetic neurons in the intermediolateral horn of the thoracic and lumbar segments of the spinal cord. Activation of these bulbospinal pathways cause a release of norepinephrine or 5-hydroxytryptamine and excitation or inhibition, respectively, of the preganglionic sympathetic neurons.

The arterial baroreceptor afferents that control cardiac vagal efferents diverge in the nucleus tractus solitarius from those afferent fibers that influence sympathetic neurons. This permits selective baroreflex control of cardiac vagal and sympathetic motor neurons (111).

Serotoninergic neurons also are located near sites of neural cardiovascular control, and changes in the central serotoninergic system can modulate arterial blood pressure. Stimulation of the fastigial nucleus of the cerebellum causes tachycardia and an increase in arterial blood pressure. It seems that afferent impulses that originate in the vestibular apparatus and pass to the fastigial nucleus assist the arterial and cardiopulmonary mechanoreflexes in achieving circulatory adjustments to the upright posture.

Interaction of Cardiovascular Reflexes

When two or more reflexes are triggered simultaneously, each may activate a discrete pool of neurons in the central nervous system, leading to summation of the separate effects on autonomic outflow to discrete parts of the cardiovascular system. There may also be a facilitative or occlusive interaction leading to enhancement or diminution, respectively, of the separate responses. In view of the complexity of brain centers, such as the nucleus tractus solitarius, it is not surprising that our current understanding is still rudimentary.

Studies in anesthetized dogs have shown that the inhibitory influence of the cardiopulmonary receptors on the vasomotor center varies inversely with that of the arterial baroreceptors. This was shown by performing bilateral vagal cold block at different carotid sinus pressures in dogs with aortic nerves sectioned. When the carotid baroreceptors were activated maximally, there was no vascular response to the vagal block. As the inhibition exerted by the carotid baroreceptors was withdrawn, there was a progressive increase in the response to the block (86). The small reflex increase in blood flow to the kidney from stimulation of the pulmonary vein–atrial junctions, which is attributed to activation of the complex unencapsulated endings with myelinated vagal afferents, also is modulated in the same manner by the carotid sinus baroreceptors (62).

The cardiopulmonary and carotid receptors also interact in control of renin release. Thus, in dogs with aortic nerves cut, when the carotid baroreceptors were free to exert their buffering influence, vagal cold block did not result in increased release of renin, but it did when the carotid sinuses were isolated and maintained at a normal arterial pressure (Fig. 15) (53).

Whereas osmolality of body fluids is an important regulator of antidiuretic hormone secretion, this secretion is also regulated by carotid baroreceptors and cardiopulmonary receptors (120,133). However, a tonic inhibitory influence of the carotid baroreceptors on antidiuretic hormone secretion can be demonstrated only after vagotomy, indicating an interaction between carotid and cardiopulmonary receptors in the release of this hormone from the posterior pituitary (133).

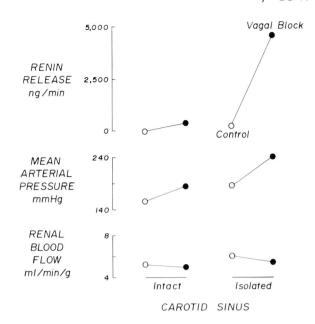

FIG. 15. Suppression by carotid sinus of renin release induced by vagal cold block. Dog with aortic nerves cut. With the carotid sinuses intact, bilateral vagal cold block caused a modest increase in arterial blood pressure, but not in renin release. When the buffering activity of the carotid baroreceptors was prevented by their vascular isolation, there was, with the vagal block, a marked increase in renin release, despite the blood pressure rise. (Data from refs. 121 and 129.)

Stimulation of cardiac receptors with vagal afferents in dogs by intracoronary injection of a veratrum alkaloid caused reflex suppression of vasopressin secretion in dogs with sinoaortic baroreceptor denervation. This response was abolished by vagotomy. When the baroreceptors were present, injection of cryptenamine resulted in profound hypotension. This hypotension would be expected to result in arterial-baroreflex-induced increases in plasma vasopressin. However, this was prevented by activation of the cardiac receptors by the cryptenamine. These data suggest that there is an interaction between cardiac receptors with vagal afferents and arterial baroreceptors in the control of vasopressin secretion. Because the reflex effects of bradycardia and hypotension with injection of veratrum alkaloids may be attributed primarily to activation of left ventricular receptors with vagal afferents, it seems that the suppressive influence of this drug on vasopressin secretion was mediated principally by these receptors (134).

In the conscious dog, each of the mechanoreceptor systems, aortic and carotid sinus and cardiopulmonary, contributes to the mean level of arterial pressure. While the former two receptor groups are equally effective in buffering elevations in arterial blood pressure, the cardiopulmonary are not capable of limiting substantially the rise in pressure when the arterial baroreflexes are acutely abrogated (150,151).

In conscious dogs in which similar reductions in cardiac output and systemic arterial pressure had been caused by hemorrhage and by embolization of the coronary vessels, the former group had marked reductions in renal blood flow and urine production, while in the latter both were maintained (46). With the hemorrhage, combined withdrawal of the inhibition exerted by each receptor group would result in a marked increase in renal sympathetic nerve traffic, whereas the bulging of the ischemic myocardium activated vagal C fiber afferents, and this opposed the reduced input from the carotid sinus, and there was less increase in sympathetic outflow.

Role of Cardiac Afferents in Humans

Obvious restrictions in experimental procedures limit the conclusions that can be drawn about the role of cardiac mechanoreceptors in reflex regulation of the cardiovascular system. However, a body of evidence has accumulated to indicate that receptors in the cardiopulmonary region have a more important role than the arterial baroreflexes in reflex regulation of the muscle blood vessels during gravitational stresses and that they may also have a role in reflex control of renin secretion (1,90,118).

Procedures that increase intrathoracic blood volume, such as raising the legs of a recumbent subject to the vertical position, can cause an increase in forearm blood flow. The increase in flow did not occur following inflation of thigh cuffs to suprasystolic pressure or after blockade of the sympathetic nerves to the forearm blood vessels. Thus, the fall in vascular resistance was mediated reflexly and resulted from translocation of blood to the thorax. Analysis of the oxygen content of venous blood draining skin and muscle showed that the response was confined to the muscle vessels. Failure of atropine to reduce the vasodilatation demonstrated that sympathetic cholinergic fibers were not involved (Fig. 16). Because this maneuver did not cause a change in arterial blood pressure, it was concluded that the reflex originated in intrathoracic low-pressure receptors. Activation of the same receptors also explains the dilatation of the forearm resistance vessels that occurs when the intrathoracic blood volume is increased by negative-pressure breathing (116–118).

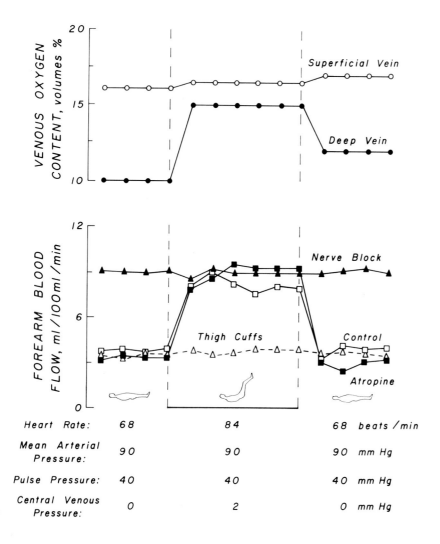

FIG. 16. Effect of passive elevation of the legs of a normal subject on circulation through the forearm. With leg elevation, blood flow in the forearm increases. This is due to an increase in muscle blood flow, because the oxygen content of the blood draining the forearm muscles increases (deep vein), but that of the blood draining the forearm skin (superficial vein) does not. The increased flow was due to reflex dilatation, because it was prevented by blocking the sympathetic nerves to the forearm vessels with a local anesthetic. The dilatation was not affected by atropine, indicating that it was caused by decreased activity of noradrenergic fibers, not by activation of cholinergic fibers. It was caused by displacement of blood from the legs, because it was prevented by inflation of thigh cuffs to suprasystolic pressure before the leg elevation. Because arterial mean and pulse pressures were unchanged, and central venous pressure increased, the reflex dilatation was attributed to excitation of receptors somewhere in the heart and lungs. (From ref. 30, with permission.)

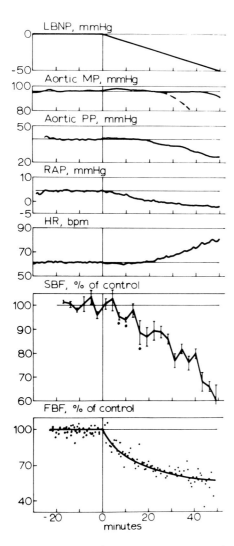

FIG. 17. Average values for responses to ramp lower-body negative pressure (LBNP) in 9 subjects. MP, mean aortic pressure; PP, pulse pressure; RAP, right atrial pressure; HR, heart rate; SBF, splanchnic blood flow; FBF, forearm blood flow. Ramp LBNP applied at −1 mm Hg/min. Bars with entries for SBF indicate SE; values for SE for other variables were too small to be shown. *Asterisks* denote first three significant decrements in SBF below control. At 0–20 mm Hg, LBNP decreased RAP without decreasing aortic MP or PP and without increasing HR. This mild LBNP produced substantial decreases in FBF and slight decreases in SBF. At 20–50 mm Hg, LBNP decreased aortic PP and RAP and produced increases in HR, and further decreases in SBF and FBF. (From ref. 56, with permission of the American Heart Association Inc.)

Conversely, application of negative pressure to the lower body sufficient to cause displacement of blood from the central circulation and a decrease in central venous pressure, but not to significantly alter arterial blood pressure, arterial dP/dt, and heart rate, results in increases in forearm and splanchnic vascular resistances. When translocation of blood to the lower body is greater, as with upright tilting or lower-body negative pressure of 40 mm Hg or greater, the changes include a decrease in mean aortic blood pressure and narrowing of the arterial pressure pulse, an increase in heart rate, and further constriction of the muscle and splanchnic resistance vessels (56,161) (Fig. 17). It is likely that in these latter circumstances both high- and low-pressure baroreceptor systems contribute to the compensatory hemodynamic changes (56). Other procedures that decrease the intrathoracic blood volume, such as tilting to a feet down position, positive-pressure breathing, and the Valsalva maneuver, also cause reflex constriction of the muscle resistance vessels (117).

Activation of receptors in the skeletal muscles by isometric hand-grip exercise reflexly increases sympathetic activity to the heart and circulation. Removal of the inhibitory influence of the cardiopulmonary receptors by pooling blood in the lower extremities enhances this exercise reflex. This indicates an interaction between cardiopulmonary and somatic reflexes in the control of forearm vascular resistance in man (153).

Cardiopulmonary Receptors and Diuresis

When normal subjects are immersed to the neck in water, about 700 ml of blood is redistributed from the peripheral veins to the central circulation, and the right atrial pressure increases from −2 to +16 mm Hg. The arterial blood pressure increases by 10 mm Hg or less. The stroke volume and cardiac output increase, but there is no change or a decrease in heart rate. Diuresis and natriuresis occur, as well as decreases in urinary excretion of antidiuretic hormone, plasma renin activity, and plasma aldosterone level. This can be explained by stimulation of receptors in the heart and lungs, particularly in the easily distensible atria by the increase in intracardiac pressures. In addition to antidiuretic hormone, release of an unidentified diuretic and natriuretic substance adds to the complexity of the mechanisms as yet not understood that maintain the blood volume within narrow limits (35). It has been suggested that in the primate, volumetric control of salt and water homeostasis has shifted from low-pressure to high-pressure receptors and that vagally innervated cardiac receptors are not necessary for the renal response to water immersion, although they may make some contribution to it. It is concluded that the major receptors involved in the control of antidiuretic hormone in the primate, including humans, reside in the high-pressure side of the vascular tree (42).

In man, the relative importances of the arterial and cardiopulmonary receptors for control of renin release are uncertain. Some studies claim that a decrease in thoracic blood volume insufficient to perturb the arterial baroreceptors causes a reflex release of renin. Other studies imply that this does not occur until the decrease in volume is sufficient to reduce the arterial pressure and thus unload the arterial baroreceptors. It may be that decreased activities of both sets of receptors are necessary; when the activity of only one set is reduced, continued restraint of sympathetic outflow by the other prevents release (53).

ROLE OF CARDIAC MECHANORECEPTORS IN ABNORMAL CIRCUMSTANCES

Aortic Stenosis

Patients with aortic stenosis are prone to syncope on exertion. When they undertake supine exercise, the usual reflex constriction of the forearm vessels is inhibited or reversed; this has been attributed to excessive activation of left ventricular receptors (87).

Cardiac Failure

The early hypervolemic phase of heart failure is associated with suppression of the renin-angiotensin aldosterone system, possibly through cardiac distension and enlargement. This phase is followed by one in which there is a chronic decrease in cardiac afferent activity. The evidence for this is that there is a decrease in frequency of discharge of afferent vagal fibers during expansion of blood volume of chronic-heart-failure dogs and humans, with elevations of norepinephrine, renin, angiotensin II, aldosterone, and antidiuretic hormone. The latter may account in part for the retention of sodium and water. The increase in antidiuretic hormone that normally attends nonhypotensive hemorrhage is attenuated in dogs with chronic mitral stenosis. This can be attributed to reduced sensitivity of the cardiac mechanoreceptors and hence decreased tonic inhibition of the vasomotor center. This decreased inhibition can be explained by a decrease in atrial compliance and degenerative changes in receptor endings (159,162). During the relatively mild exercise of which patients in heart failure are capable, there are greater increases in plasma levels of norepinephrine than with similar exercise in normal subjects, and greater reflex constriction of systemic vascular beds outside the active muscles. This also may be due to decreased ability of the cardiac mechanoreceptors to buffer the excitatory reflex from the active muscles. In normal subjects, with a change from supine to upright posture, plasma levels of norepinephrine increase, and forearm vessels constrict. By contrast, in patients with heart failure, levels of norepinephrine do not increase, and forearm vessels dilate. The gravitational shift of blood from the central circulation in these patients may result in a shift to a more favorable position of the ventricular compliance curve; resultant increased activity of the cardiac afferent nerve endings might account for this paradoxical response (2). Digitalis glycosides sensitize the cardiac mechanoreceptors, and this augments the inhibition of efferent sym-

pathetic nerve activity caused by increases in cardiac pressures; this may account in part for their beneficial action in patients with heart failure (135,163).

Hemorrhage

During hemorrhage, combined withdrawal of the inhibition exerted by arterial mechanoreceptors and cardiopulmonary receptors results in a marked increase in renal sympathetic nerve traffic and reductions in renal blood flow and urine production. Syncope may occur during hemorrhage; the sudden decrease in arterial blood pressure may be precipitated by increased activity of left ventricular mechanoreceptors as a consequence of the decrease in stroke volume and the increasing cardiac contractility (97).

Myocardial Ischemia

Coronary occlusion may simultaneously excite a wide variety of receptors that exert different reflex effects on the cardiovascular system. The early hemodynamic changes that accompany acute myocardial infarction in man may result, therefore, not only from cardiac impairment but also from changes in activities of different receptor systems. Among patients seen within 30 min after onset of infarction, only 17% had normal heart rate and blood pressure, 48% had evidence of parasympathetic overactivity manifested by bradyarrhythmia and hypotension, and 35% showed evidence of sympathetic overactivity with sinus tachycardia or elevated blood pressure or both (106). It is likely that these different manifestations are the results of different degrees of activation and interaction between the vagal and sympathetic afferent input from cardiac receptors to the central nervous system and the input from the high-pressure baroreceptors.

Reduction in coronary blood flow in animals activates cardiac receptors with vagal and sympathetic myelinated and nonmyelinated fibers. Left ventricular receptors with unmyelinated vagal afferents situated in the region supplied by the occluded coronary artery increased their activity in concert with systolic bulging of the ischemic myocardium, suggesting that excitation is mechanical rather than chemical (Fig. 18). These inhibitory cardiac receptors have a preferential distribution in the inferoposterior wall of the left ventricle of the dog (129,130). Occlusion of the coronary artery supplying the inferior wall of the heart in man has frequently been observed to result in bradycardia and hypotension (106). During coronary occlusion in cats, the resultant increase in the receptor discharge usually decreases toward control over several minutes. This is in keeping with the clinical observation that the bradycardia and hypotension are transient. Injection of radiographic contrast medium into the coronary artery supplying the posteroinferior

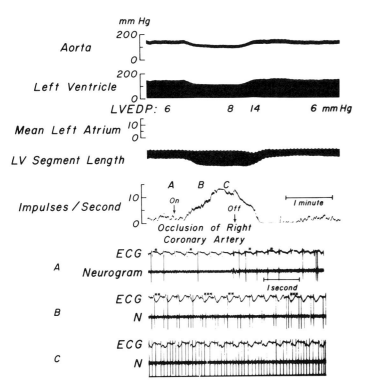

mm Hg

Aorta

Left Ventricle

LVEDP: 6   8 14   6 mm Hg

Mean Left Atrium

LV Segment Length

Impulses / Second

A B C

On   Off

1 minute

Occlusion of Right
Coronary Artery

A   ECG
     Neurogram

1 second

B   ECG
     N

C   ECG
     N

FIG. 18. Left ventricular vagal afferent C fiber activity during occlusion of right coronary artery in the cat. Aortic, left ventricular, left ventricular end-diastolic (LVEDP), and mean left atrial pressures, left ventricular (LV) segment length (downward deflection means increased length), and discharge frequency in a left ventricular receptor are shown before and during occlusion. The electrocardiogram (ECG) and neurograms were recorded at times A, B, and C. The receptor initially (A) had a low rate of discharge that was greatly increased 20 sec after onset of coronary occlusion. At time B, the receptor discharge had a cardiac-modulated rhythmicity, with two or three impulses every cycle. From the total conduction time (220 msec), the receptor was calculated to be activated in systole (asterisks indicate the corrected position in the cardiac cycle of receptor activation, which occurred 220 msec before the recorded spike). At time C, the receptor was firing continuously. The reciprocal S-T segment depression in the electrocardiogram was already obvious at time B. During occlusion, the increased firing occurred together with the bulging of the ischemic area. The time lag between the release of occlusion and the decrease in systolic bulging was probably due to an observed spasm of the coronary artery, which relaxed slowly on release of the ligature. Disappearance of the dyskinesia was accompanied by a rapid decrease in discharge frequency. (From refs. 138 and 142, with permission.)

wall of the heart in man is more often accompanied by bradycardia, vasodilatation, and hypotension than when the contrast medium is injected into the artery supplying the anterior wall (32,108). Such injections also cause reflex dilatation of forearm blood vessels that may be mediated by sympathetic cholinergic fibers, because it is prevented by atropine (160). The hypotension results more from the reflex decrease in systemic vascular resistance than from the bradycardia, because preventing the bradycardia by atrial pacing only slightly reduces the hypotension (31). In the cat, coronary artery occlusion can cause relaxation of the stomach; this is due to activation of vagal noncholinergic relaxatory fibers to the stomach as a consequence of the increased activity in cardiac vagal C fibers (138). In dogs, circumflex coronary artery occlusion, and to a lesser degree occlusion of the anterior descending coronary artery, results in reflex withdrawal of renal sympathetic nerve activity mediated by left ventricular receptors with vagal afferents. Despite the attendent hypotension, this withdrawal can occur even in the presence of functional sinoaortic baroreceptors (132). Although the cardiac receptors do not respond directly to hypoxia and hypercapnia (88), prostaglandins and bradykinin, released by the ischemic heart, may stimulate afferent nerves in the heart and cause circulatory changes. It has been suggested that a local reduction in oxygen tension might activate brady-kinin synthesis, which in turn stimulates local reduction of prostaglandins. Bradykinin- and prostaglandin-acti-vating chemosensitive endings will then contribute to the vagally mediated depressor reflexes observed during

myocardial infarction (25,94). The inhibitory influence exerted by these cardiac receptors with vagal afferents, particularly during inferoposterior ischemia, obviously limits the ability of the arterial baroreceptors to combat the circulatory changes (36).

On the other hand, the hypertension and tachycardia observed in some cases following myocardial ischemia or infarction may be caused by excitatory sympathetic reflexes that are initiated from the heart, and perhaps mainly when the ischemia involves the anterior wall of the left ventricle (Fig. 19). Studies in cats have shown that occlusion of the left anterior descending coronary artery causes reflex excitation of renal nerve activity in cats in which vagi and arterial baroreceptor afferent nerves have been severed. Stimulation of vagal afferents by coronary occlusion consistently produced inhibition of renal nerve activity and marked depressor responses. When both components of cardiac innervation remained intact, increases or decreases in renal nerve activity and blood pressure were elicited by coronary artery occlusion in the presence or absence of arterial baroreceptors (156). The excitation of the sympathetic efferents may be due in part or in whole to local release of chemicals in the ischemic myocardium. Thus, bradykinin and prostaglandins may reinforce each other to stimulate the sensory sympathetic nerves that signal the pain of myocardial ischemia and to elicit reflex tachycardia and hypertension (25,75). Whereas the predominance of vagal and sympathetic endings to different parts of the left ventricle may explain the predominance of vagal or sympathetic reflexes in myocardial infarction, much remains to be understood about their separate and combined roles.

A cardiogenic hypertensive chemoreflex might contribute to bradycardia and hypertension during myocardial ischemia. Chemoreceptors with a blood supply from the initial portion of the left coronary artery may be activated by release of 5-hydroxytryptamine from platelet thrombi (52).

Hypertension

Hypertension also may cause changes in the cardiopulmonary reflexes. Initially, the inhibitory influence of the cardiopulmonary reflexes may increase as that of the arterial baroreceptors is reduced (Fig. 20). Thus, in mildly or moderately hypertensive young men, the vasoconstrictor response in the forearm resulting from deactivation of the cardiopulmonary receptors (by applying lower-body negative pressure) is greater than in normal subjects. This is consistent with the fact that patients with mild hypertension have augmented increases in systemic vascular resistance and plasma renin activity. Later, as cardiac hypertrophy develops, it is possible that the cardiopulmonary reflexes become impaired. At this stage the decreased ability of both arterial and cardiopulmonary mechanoreceptors to inhibit sympathetic outflow, combined with the enhanced constriction of the systemic resistance vessels due to hypertrophy of vascular smooth muscles, leads to perpetuation and enhancement of the high blood pressure (89).

In spontaneously hypertensive rats, the threshold mean left atrial pressure to activate the atrial vagal C fibers was about twice that in normotensive rats. This resetting

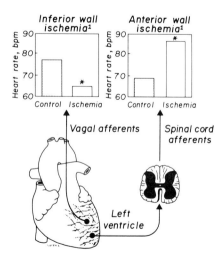

FIG. 19. Afferent innervation of the heart. Changes in heart rate during anterior wall and inferior wall ischemia in patients with coronary spasm and Prinzmetal's angina. Heart rate increased during anterior wall ischemia and decreased during inferior wall ischemia. (Adapted from ref. 109; from ref. 121, with permission.)

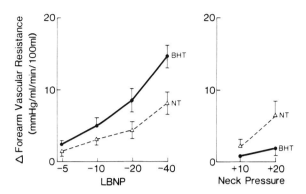

FIG. 20. Forearm vascular responses to lower-body negative pressure (LBNP) and neck pressure in borderline hypertensive and normotensive subjects. Forearm vasoconstrictor responses to LBNP were augmented, whereas forearm vasoconstrictor responses to neck pressure were impaired in borderline hypertensive subjects. This indicates that the cardiopulmonary baroreflexes are augmented but the carotid baroflexes are impaired in young men with borderline hypertension. (From ref. 89, with permission of the American Heart Association Inc.)

of the atrial receptors is probably due to decreased distensibility of the atrium (138).

REFERENCES

1. Abboud, F. M., and Mark, A. L. (1979): Cardiac baroreceptors in circulatory control in humans. In: *Cardiac Receptors*, edited by R. Hainsworth, C. Kidd, and R. J. Linden, pp. 437–461. Cambridge University Press, Cambridge, U.K.
2. Abboud, F. M., Thames, M. D., and Mark, A. L. (1981): Role of cardiac afferent nerves in the regulation of circulation during coronary occlusion and heart failure. In: *Disturbances in Neurogenic Control of the Circulation*, edited by F. M. Abboud, H. A. Fozzard, J. P. Gilmore, and D. J. Reis, pp. 65–86. American Physiological Society, Bethesda.
3. Abboud, F. M., and Thames, M. D. (1983): Interaction of cardiovascular reflexes in circulatory control. In: *Handbook of Physiology: Peripheral Circulation and Organ Blood Flow*, edited by J. T. Shepherd and F. M. Abboud, pp. 675–753. American Physiological Society, Washington, D.C.
4. Agostoni, E., Chinnock, J. E., Daly, M. de Burgh, and Murray, J. G. (1957): Functional and histological studies of the vagus nerve and its branches to the heart, lungs and abdominal viscera in the cat. *J. Physiol. (Lond.)*, 135:182–205.
5. Ammons, W. S., Blair, R. W., and Foreman, R. D. (1983): Vagal afferent inhibition of spinothalamic cell responses to sympathetic afferents and bradykinin in the monkey. *Circ. Res.*, 53:603–612.
6. Arndt, J. O. (1979): Neurophysiological properties of atrial mechanoreceptors. In: *Cardiac Receptors*, edited by R. Hainsworth, C. Kidd, and R. J. Linden, pp. 89–115. Cambridge University Press, Cambridge, U.K.
7. Arndt, J. O., Brambring, P., Hindorf, K., and Rhonelt, M. (1974): The afferent discharge pattern of atrial mechano-receptors in the cat during sinusoidal stretch of atrial strips in situ. *J. Physiol. (Lond.)*, 240:33–52.
8. Aviado, D. M., Jr., Li, T. H., Kalow, W., Schmidt, C. F., Turnbull, G. L., Peskin, G. W., Hess, M. E., and Weiss, A. J. (1951): Respiratory and circulatory reflexes from the perfused heart and pulmonary circulation of the dog. *Am. J. Physiol.*, 165: 261–277.
9. Aviado, D. M., and Schmidt, C. F. (1955): Reflexes from stretch receptors in blood vessels, heart and lungs. *Physiol. Rev.*, 35: 247–300.

10. Baker, D. G., Coleridge, H. M., and Coleridge, J. C. G. (1979): Vagal afferent C-fibers from the ventricles. In: *Cardiac Receptors,* edited by R. Hainsworth, C. Kidd, and R. J. Linden, pp. 117–137. Cambridge University Press, Cambridge, U.K.

11. Baker, D. G., Coleridge, H. M., Coleridge, J. C. G., and Nerdrum, T. (1980): Search for a cardiac nociceptor: Stimulation by bradykinin of sympathetic afferent nerve endings in the heart of cat. *J. Physiol. (Lond.),* 306:519–536.

12. Bennett, K. L., Linden, R. J., and Mary, D. A. S. G. (1983): The effect of stimulation of atrial receptors on the plasma concentration of vasopressin. *Q. J. Exp. Physiol.,* 68:579–589.

13. Bezold, A. von, and Hirt, L. (1867): Über die physiologischen Wirkungen des essigsauren Veratrins. *Untersuchungen aus dem physiologischen Laboratorium Wurzburg,* 1:75–156.

14. Bishop, V. S., Lombard, F., Malliani, A., Pagani, M., and Recordati, G. (1976): Reflex sympathetic tachycardia during intervenous infusions in chronic spinal cats. *Am. J. Physiol.,* 230:25–29.

15. Bishop, V. S., and Barron, K. W. (1980): Contribution of vagal afferents in the regulation of the circulation in conscious dogs. In: *Arterial Baroreceptors in Hypertension,* edited by P. Sleight, pp. 91–97. Oxford University Press, Oxford, U.K.

16. Bishop, V. S., Malliani, A., and Thorén, P. (1983): Cardiac mechanoreceptors. In: *Handbook of Physiology: Peripheral Circulation and Organ Blood Flow,* edited by J. T. Shepherd and F. M. Abboud, pp. 497–555. American Physiological Society, Washington, D.C.

17. Brennan, L. A., Malvin, R. L., Jochim, K. E., and Roberts, D. E. (1971): Influence of right and left atrial receptors on plasma concentration of ADH and renin. *Am. J. Physiol.,* 221:273–278.

18. Brown, A. M. (1965): Mechanoreceptors in or near the coronary arteries. *J. Physiol. (Lond.),* 177:203–214.

19. Brown, A. M., and Malliani, A. (1971): Spinal sympathetic reflexes initiated by coronary receptors. *J. Physiol. (Lond.),* 212:685–705.

20. Coleridge, J. C. G., Hemingway, A., Holmes, R. L., and Linden, R. J. (1957): The location of atrial receptors in the dog: A physiological and histological study. *J. Physiol. (Lond.),* 136:174–197.

21. Coleridge, H. M., Coleridge, J. C. G., and Kidd, C. (1964): Cardiac receptors in the dog, with particular reference to two types of afferent endings in the ventricular wall. *J. Physiol. (Lond.),* 174:323–339.

22. Coleridge, H. M., Coleridge, J. C. G., Dengel, A., Kidd, C., Luck, J. C., and Sleight, P. (1973): Impulses in slowly conducting vagal fibers from afferent endings in the veins, atria and arteries of dogs and cats. *Circ. Res.,* 33:87–97.

23. Coleridge, J. C. G., and Coleridge, H. M. (1977): Afferent C-fibers in cardiorespiratory chemoreflexes. *Am. Rev. Respir. Dis.,* 115:251–260.

24. Coleridge, J. C. G., Coleridge, H. M., and Baker, D. G. (1979): Vagal afferent C-fibers from the ventricle. In: *Cardiac Receptors,* edited by R. Hainsworth, C. Kidd, and R. J. Linden, pp. 117–137. Cambridge University Press, Cambridge, U.K.

25. Coleridge, J. C. G., and Coleridge, H. M. (1979): Chemoreflex regulation of the heart. In: *Handbook of Physiology: The Cardiovascular System. The Heart,* Vol. I, edited by R. M. Berne and M. Sperelakis, pp. 653–676. American Physiological Society, Bethesda.

26. Coleridge, H. M., and Coleridge, J. C. G. (1980): Cardiovascular afferents involved in regulation of peripheral vessels. *Annu. Rev. Physiol.,* 42:413–427.

27. Daly, I. de Burgh, and Verney, E. B. (1927): The localization of receptors involved in the reflex regulation of the heart rate. *J. Physiol. (Lond.),* 62:330–340.

28. Daskalopoulos, D. A., Shepherd, J. T., and Walgenbach, S. C. (1984): Cardiopulmonary reflexes and blood pressure in exercising sinoaortic denervated dogs. *J. Appl. Physiol.,* 57(5):1417–1421.

29. Dawes, G. S., and Comroe, J. H., Jr. (1954): Chemoreflexes from the heart and lungs. *Physiol. Rev.,* 34:167–201.

30. Donald, D. E., and Shepherd, J. T. (1978): Reflexes from the heart and lungs: Physiological curiosities or important regulatory mechanisms? *Cardiovasc. Res.,* 12:449–469.

31. Donald, D. E., and Shepherd, J. T. (1979): Cardiac receptors: normal and disturbed function. *Am. J. Cardiol.,* 44:873–878.

32. Eckberg, D. L., White, C. W., Kioschos, J. M., and Abboud, F. M. (1974): Mechanisms mediating bradycardia during coronary arteriography. *J. Clin. Invest.,* 54:1445–1461.

33. Edis, A. J., Donald, D. E., and Shepherd, J. T. (1970): Cardiovascular reflexes from stretch of pulmonary vein–atrial junctions in the dog. *Circ. Res.,* 27:1091–1100.

34. Einthoven, W. (1909): Die Konstruktion des Saitengalvanometers. *Pfluegers Arch.,* 130:287.

35. Epstein, M. (1976): Cardiovascular and renal effects of head-out water immersion in man: Application of the model in the assessment of volume homeostasis. *Circ. Res.,* 39:619–628.

36. Felder, R. B., and Thames, M. D. (1979): Interaction between cardiac receptors and sinoaortic baroreceptors in the control of efferent sympathetic nerve activity during myocardial ischemia in dogs. *Circ. Res.,* 45:728–736.

37. Felder, R. B., and Thames, M. D. (1981): The cardiocardiac sympathetic reflex coronary occlusion in anesthetized dogs. *Circ. Res.,* 48:685–692.

38. Fick, A. (1870): Über die Messung des Blutquantums in den Herzventrikeln. *Sitzungsber. Phys.-Med. Ges. Wurzburg,* July 9.

39. Floyd, K. (1979): Light microscopy of nerve endings in the atrial endocardium. In: *Cardiac Receptors,* edited by R. Hainsworth, C. Kidd, and R. J. Linden, pp. 3–26. Cambridge University Press, Cambridge, U.K.

40. Gauer, O. H., and Henry, J. P. (1963): Circulatory basis of fluid volume control. *Physiol. Rev.,* 43:423–481.

41. Gauer, O. H., and Henry, J. P. (1976): Neurohumoral control of plasma volume. In: *International Review of Physiology, Cardiovascular Physiology II,* Vol. 19, edited by A. C. Guyton and A. W. Cowley, pp. 145–190. University Park Press, Baltimore.

42. Gilmore, J. P. (1983): Neural control of extracellular volume in the human and non-human primate. In: *Handbook of Physiology: Peripheral Circulation and Organ Blood Flow,* edited by J. T. Shepherd and F. M. Abboud, pp. 885–915. American Physiological Society, Washington, D.C.

43. Gilmore, J. P., and Zucker, I. H. (1974): Failure of the type B atrial receptors to respond to increase in plasma osmolality in the dog. *Am. J. Physiol.,* 227:1005–1007.

44. Goetz, K. L., Bond, G. C., and Bloxham, D. D. (1975): Atrial receptors and renal function. *Physiol. Rev.,* 55:157–205.

45. Goetz, K. L., Bloxham, D. D., Bond, G. C., and Sharma, J. M. (1976): Persistence of the renal response to atrial tamponade after cardiac denervation. *Proc. Soc. Exp. Biol. Med.,* 152:423–427.

46. Gorfinkel, H. J., Szidon, J. P., Hirsch, L. J., and Fishman, A. P. (1972): Renal performance in experimental cardiogenic shock. *Am. J. Physiol.,* 222:1260–1268.

47. Gupta, B. N. (1977): The location and distribution of type A and type B atrial endings in cats. *Pfluegers Arch.,* 367:271–275.

48. Gupta, B. N. (1977): Studies on the adaptation rate and frequency distribution of type A and type B atrial endings in cats. *Pfluegers Arch.,* 367:277–281.

49. Harvey, W. (1628): *Exercitatio anatomica de motu cordis et sanguinis in animalibus.* G. Fitzeri, Francofurti.

50. Hess, G. L., Zuperku, E. J., Coon, R. L., and Kampine, J. P. (1974): Sympathetic afferent nerve activity of left ventricular origin. *Am. J. Physiol.,* 227:543–546.

51. Holmes, R. L. (1957): Structures in the atrial endocardium of the dog which stain with methylene blue and the effects of unilateral vagotomy. *J. Anat.,* 91:259–266.

52. James, T. N., Hageman, G. F., and Urthaler, F. (1979): Anatomic and physiologic consideration of a cardiogenic hypertensive chemoreflex. *Am. J. Cardiol.,* 44:852–859.

53. Jarecki, M., Thorén, P., and Donald, D. E. (1978): Release of renin by the carotid baroreflex in anesthetized dogs. Role of cardiopulmonary vagal afferents and renal arterial pressure. *Circ. Res.,* 42:614–619.

54. Jarisch, A., and Richter, H. (1939): Die Kreislaufwirkung des Veratrins. *Arch. Exp. Pathol. Pharmakol.,* 193:347–354.

55. Jarisch, A., and Richter, H. (1939): Die afferenten Bahnen des Veratrineffektes in den Herznerven. *Arch. Exp. Pathol. Pharmakol.,* 193:355–371.

56. Johnson, J. M., Rowell, L. B., Neiderberger, M., and Eisman, M. M. (1974): Human splanchnic and forearm vasoconstrictor

responses to reductions of right atrial and aortic pressure. *Circ. Res.*, 31:515–524.

57. Jones, J. V. (1953): The afferent pathways of the Bezold-reflex: The right vagal branches in cats. *Br. J. Pharmacol.*, 8:352–355.

58. Kappagoda, C. T., Linden, R. J., and Snow, H. M. (1973): Effect of stimulating right atrial receptors on urine flow in the dog. *J. Physiol. (Lond.)*, 235:493–502.

59. Kappagoda, C. T., Linden, R. J., Snow, H. M., and Whitaker, E. M. (1974): Left atrial receptors and the antidiuretic hormone. *J. Physiol. (Lond.)*, 237:663–683.

60. Kappagoda, C. T., Linden, R. J., and Sivananthan, N. (1979): The nature of the atrial receptors responsible for a reflex increase in heart rate in the dog. *J. Physiol. (Lond.)*, 291:393–412.

61. Karim, F., Kidd, C., Malpus, C. M., and Penna, P. E. (1972): The effect of stimulation of the left atrial receptors on sympathetic efferent nerve activity. *J. Physiol. (Lond.)*, 227:243–260.

62. Karim, F., Mackay, D., and Kappagoda, C. T. (1982): Influence of carotid sinus pressure on atrial receptors and renal blood flow. *Am. J. Physiol.*, 242(*Heart Circ. Physiol.*, 11):H220–H226.

63. Keith, A., and Flack, M. (1907): The form and nature of the muscular connections between the primary divisions of the vertebrate heart. *J. Anat.*, 41:172.

64. Kimura, E., Hashimoto, K., Furukawa, S., and Hayakawa, H. (1973): Changes in bradykinin level in coronary sinus blood after the experimental occlusion of a coronary artery. *Am. Heart J.*, 85:635–647.

65. Korner, P. I. (1979): Central nervous control of autonomic cardiovascular function. In: *Handbook of Physiology: The Cardiovascular System. The Heart*, Vol. I, edited by R. M. Berne and N. Sperelakis, pp. 691–739. American Physiological Society, Bethesda.

66. Kostreva, D. R., Zuperku, E. J., Hess, G. L., Coon, R. L., and Kampine, J. P. (1975): Pulmonary afferent activity recorded from sympathetic nerves. *J. Appl. Physiol.*, 39:37–40.

67. Kostreva, D. R., Zuperku, E. J., Purtock, R. V., Coon, R. L., and Kampine, J. P. (1975): Sympathetic nerve activity of right heart origin. *Am. J. Physiol.*, 229:911–915.

68. Krayer, O. (1961): The history of the Bezold-Jarisch effect. *Naunyn Schmiedebergs Arch. Pharmacol.*, 240:361–368.

69. Loewi, O. (1921): Über humorale Ubertragbarkeit der Herznervenwirkung. I. Mitteilung. *Pfluegers Arch.*, 189:239.

70. Ledsome, J. R., and Linden, R. J. (1968): The role of the left atrial receptors in the diuretic response to left atrial distension. *J. Physiol. (Lond.)*, 198:487–503.

71. Linden, R. J. (1973): Function of cardiac receptors. *Circulation*, 48:463–480.

72. Linden, R. J., and Kappagoda, C. T. (1982): Atrial receptors. Monographs of the Physiological Society, No. 39, Cambridge University Press, Cambridge, U.K.

73. Linden, R. J., Mary, D. A. S. G., and Weatherill, D. (1982): The response in efferent cardiac sympathetic nerves to stimulation of atrial receptors, carotid sinus baroreceptors and carotid chemoreceptors. *Q. J. Exp. Physiol.*, 67:151–163.

74. Little, R., Wennergren, G., and Oberg, B. (1975): Aspects of the central integration of arterial baroreceptor and cardiac ventricular receptor reflexes in the cat. *Acta Physiol. Scand.*, 93:85–96.

75. Lombardi, F., Malliani, A., and Pagani, M. (1976): Nervous activity of afferent sympathetic fibers innervating the pulmonary veins. *Brain Res.*, 113:197–200.

76. Lombardi, F., Della Bella, P., Casati, R., and Malliani, A. (1981): Effects of intracoronary administration of bradykinin on the impulse activity of afferent sympathetic unmyelinated fibers with left ventricular endings in the cat. *Circ. Res.*, 48:69–75.

77. Malliani, A. (1979): Afferent cardiovascular sympathetic nerve fibers and their function in the neural regulation of the circulation. In: *Cardiac Receptors*, edited by R. Hainsworth, C. Kidd, and R. J. Linden, pp. 319–338. Cambridge University Press, Cambridge, U.K.

78. Malliani, A. (1982): Cardiovascular sympathetic afferent fibers. *Rev. Physiol. Biochem. Pharmacol.*, 94:11–74.

79. Malliani, A., Schwartz, P. J., and Zanchetti, A. (1969): A sympathetic reflex elicited by experimental coronary occlusion. *Am. J. Physiol.*, 217:703–709.

80. Malliani, A., Recordati, G., and Schwartz, P. J. (1973): Nervous activity of afferent cardiac sympathetic fibers with atrial and ventricular endings. *J. Physiol. (Lond.)*, 229:457–469.

81. Malliani, A., Lombardi, F., Pagani, M., Recordati, G., and Schwartz, P. J. (1975): Spinal cardiovascular reflexes. *Brain Res.*, 87:239–246.

82. Mancia, G., Donald, D. E., and Shepherd, J. T. (1973): Inhibition of adrenergic outflow to peripheral blood vessels by vagal afferents from the cardiopulmonary region in the dog. *Circ. Res.*, 33:713–721.

83. Mancia, G., and Donald, D. E. (1975): Demonstration that the atria, ventricles, and lungs each are responsible for a tonic inhibition of the vasomotor center in the dog. *Circ. Res.*, 36:310–318.

84. Mancia, G., Romero, J. C., and Shepherd, J. T. (1975): Continuous inhibition of renin release in dogs by vagally innervated receptors in the cardiopulmonary region. *Circ. Res.*, 36:529–535.

85. Mancia, G., Shepherd, J. T., and Donald, D. E. (1975): Role of cardiac, pulmonary and carotid mechanoreceptors in the control of hind-limb and renal circulation in dogs. *Circ. Res.*, 37:200–208.

86. Mancia, G., Shepherd, J. T., and Donald, D. E. (1976): Interplay among carotid sinus, cardiopulmonary, and carotid body reflexes in dogs. *Am. J. Physiol.*, 230:19–24.

87. Mark, A. L., Kioschos, J. M., Abboud, F. M., Heistad, D. D., Schmid, P. G. (1973): Abnormal vascular responses to exercise in patients with aortic stenosis. *J. Clin. Invest.*, 52:1138–1146.

88. Mark, A. L., Abboud, F. M., Heistad, D. D., Schmid, P. G., and Johannsen, U. J. (1974): Evidence against the presence of ventricular chemoreceptors activated by hypoxia and hypercapnia. *Am. J. Physiol.*, 227:178–182.

89. Mark, A. L., and Kerber, R. E. (1982): Augmentation of cardiopulmonary baroreflex control of forearm vascular resistance in borderline hypertension. *Hypertension*, 4:39–46.

90. Mark, A. L., and Mancia, G. (1983): Cardiopulmonary baroreflexes in humans. In: *Handbook of Physiology: The Cardiovascular System. Peripheral Circulation and Organ Blood Flow*, Vol. III, edited by J. T. Shepherd and F. M. Abboud, pp. 795–813. American Physiological Society, Washington, D.C.

91. Miller, M. R., and Kasahara, K. (1964): Studies on the nerve endings in the heart. *Am. J. Anat.*, 115:217–234.

92. Muers, M. F., and Sleight, P. (1972): The reflex cardiovascular depression caused by occlusion of the coronary sinus in the dog. *J. Physiol. (Lond.)*, 221:259–282.

93. Muers, M. F., and Sleight, P. (1972): Action potentials from ventricular mechanoreceptors stimulated by occlusion of the coronary sinus in the dog. *J. Physiol. (Lond.)*, 221:283–309.

94. Needleman, P. (1976): The synthesis and function of prostaglandins in the heart. *Fed. Proc.*, 35:2376–2381.

95. Nonidez, J. F. (1937): Identification of the receptor areas in the venae cavae and pulmonary veins which initiate reflex cardiac acceleration (Bainbridge's reflex). *Am. J. Anat.*, 61:203–231.

96. Nonidez, J. F. (1941): Studies of the innervation of the heart. II. Afferent nerve endings in the large arteries and veins. *Am. J. Anat.*, 68:151–189.

97. Öberg, B., and Thorén, P. (1971): Increased activity in left ventricular receptors during hemorrhage or occlusion of caval veins in the cat. A possible cause of the vasovagal reaction. *Acta Physiol. Scand.*, 85:164–173.

98. Öberg, B., and Thorén, P. (1973): Circulatory responses to stimulation of medullated and non-medullated afferents in the cardiac nerve of the cat. *Acta Physiol. Scand.*, 87:121–132.

99. Ott, N. T., and Shepherd, J. T. (1973): Modifications of the aortic and vagal depressor reflexes by hypercapnia in the rabbit. *Circ. Res.*, 33:160–165.

100. Ott, N. T., and Shepherd, J. T. (1975): Modification of vagal depressor reflex by CO_2 in spontaneously breathing rabbits. *Am. J. Physiol.*, 228:530–535.

101. Paintal, A. S. (1971): Cardiovascular receptors. In: *Handbook of Sensory Physiology. Enteroreceptors*, Vol. III, edited by E. Neil, pp. 1–45. Springer-Verlag, Berlin.

102. Paintal, A. S. (1973): Vagal sensory receptors and their reflex effects. *Physiol. Rev.*, 53:159–227.

103. Paintal, A. S. (1979): Electrophysiology of atrial receptors. In:

Cardiac Receptors, edited by R. Hainsworth, C. Kidd, and R. J. Linden, pp. 73–87. Cambridge University Press, Cambridge, U.K.

104. Palkovits, M. (1980): The anatomy of central cardiovascular neurons. In: *Central Adrenaline Neurons: Basic Aspects and Their Role in Cardiovascular Functions,* edited by K. Fuxe, M. Goldstein, B. Hokfelt, and T. Hokfelt, pp. 3–17. Pergamon Press, Oxford.

105. Palkovits, M. (1981): Neuropeptides and biogenic amines and central cardiovascular control mechanisms. In: *Central Nervous System Mechanisms in Hypertension,* edited by J. P. Buckle and C. M. Ferrario, pp. 73–97. Raven Press, New York.

106. Pantridge, J. F., Adgey, A. A. J., Geddes, J. S., and Webb, S. W. (1975): The acute coronary attack. In: *Clinical Cardiology Monographs,* p. 141. Grune & Stratton, New York.

107. Pelletier, C. L., Edis, A. J., and Shepherd, J. T. (1971): Circulatory reflex from vagal afferents in response to hemorrhage in the dog. *Circ. Res.,* 29:626–634.

108. Perez-Gomez, F., and Garcia-Aguado, A. (1977): Origin of ventricular reflexes caused by coronary arteriography. *Br. Heart J.,* 39:967–973.

109. Perez-Gomez, F., et al. (1979): *Br. Heart J.,* 42:81–87. Prinzmetal's angina: reflex cardiovascular response during episode of pain.

110. Peterson, D. F., and Brown, A. M. (1971): Pressor reflexes produced by stimulation of afferent fibers in cardiac sympathetic nerves of the cat. *Circ. Res.,* 28:605–610.

111. Porazasz, J. T., Barankay, J., Szolcsanzi, J., Gibiszer-Porszasz, K., and Madarasz, K. (1962): Studies of the neural connection between the vasodilator and vasoconstrictor centers in the cat. *Acta Physiol. Acad. Sci. Hung.,* 22:29–41.

112. Purlock, R. V., von Colditz, J. H., Seagard, J. L., Igler, F. O., Zuperku, E. J., and Kampine, J. P. (1977): Reflex effects of thoracic sympathetic afferent nerve stimulation on the kidney. *Am. J. Physiol.,* 233(*Heart Circ. Physiol.,* 2):H580–H586.

113. Recordati, G. (1978): Type A atrial receptors in the cat: Effects of changes in atrial volume and contractility. *J. Physiol. (Lond.),* 280:303–317.

114. Recordati, G., Lombardi, F., Bishop, V. S., and Malliani, A. (1975): Response of type B atrial vagal receptors to changes in wall tension during atrial filling. *Circ. Res.,* 36:682–691.

115. Recordati, G., Lombardi, F., Bishop, V. S., and Malliani, A. (1976): Mechanical stimuli exciting type A atrial vagal receptors in the cat. *Circ. Res.,* 38:397–403.

116. Roddie, I. C., and Shepherd, J. T. (1956): The reflex nervous control of human skeletal muscle blood vessels. *Clin. Sci.,* 15:433–440.

117. Roddie, I. C., Shepherd, J. T., and Whelan, R. F. (1957): Reflex changes in vasoconstrictor tone in human skeletal muscle in response to stimulation of receptors in a low-pressure area of the intrathoracic vascular bed. *J. Physiol. (Lond.),* 139:369–376.

118. Roddie, I. C., and Shepherd, J. T. (1963): Circulation in skeletal muscle. *Br. Med. Bull.,* 19:115–119.

119. Seagard, J. L., and Kampine, J. P. (1980): Electrophysiological investigation of sympathetic cardiac afferent fibers. *Proc. Soc. Exp. Biol. Med.,* 164:93–100.

120. Share, L. (1968): Control of plasma ADH titer in hemorrhage: Role of atrial and arterial receptors. *Am. J. Physiol.,* 215:1384–1389.

121. Shepherd, J. T. (1981): Reflex control of arterial blood pressure. In: *Blood Pressure Measurement and Systemic Hypertension,* edited by A. C. Arntzenius, A. J. Dunning, and H. A. Snellen, p. 321. Medical World Press.

122. Shepherd, J. T. (1982): Regulation of arterial blood pressure. *Cardiovasc. Res.,* 16:357–370.

123. Shepherd, J. T., and Vanhoutte, P. M. (1985): Spasm of the coronary arteries: causes and consequences (the scientist's viewpoint). *Mayo Clin. Proc.,* 60:33–46.

124. Sleight, P., and Widdicombe, J. G. (1965): Action potentials in fibres from receptors in the epicardium and myocardium of the dog's left ventricle. *J. Physiol. (Lond.),* 181:235–258.

125. Spyer, K. M. (1981): The neural organization and control of the baroreflex. *Rev. Physiol. Biochem. Pharmacol.,* 88:24–124.

126. Talman, W. T., Perrone, M. H., and Reis, D. J. (1981): Acute hypertension after the local injection of kainic acid into the nucleus tractus solitarius of rats. *Circ. Res.,* 48:292–298.

127. Thames, M. D. (1977): Reflex suppression of renin release by

ventricular receptors with vagal afferents. *Am. J. Physiol.,* 233(*Heart Circ. Physiol.,* 2):H181–H184.

128. Thames, M. D., Donald, D. E., and Shepherd, J. T. (1977): Behavior of cardiac receptors with non-myelinated vagal afferents during spontaneous respiration in cats. *Circ. Res.,* 41:696–701.

129. Thames, M. D., Jerecki, M., and Donald, D. E. (1978): Neural control of renin secretion in anesthetized dogs. Interaction of cardiopulmonary and carotid baroreflexes. *Circ. Res.,* 42:237–245.

130. Thames, M. D., Kloppenstein, H. S., Abboud, F. M., Mark, A. L., and Walker, J. L. (1978): Preferential distribution of inhibitory cardiac receptors with vagal afferents to the inferoposterior wall of the left ventricle activated during coronary occlusion in the dog. *Circ. Res.,* 43:512–519.

131. Thames, M. D., and Dibona, G. F. (1979): Renal nerves modulate the secretion of renin mediated by non-neural mechanisms. *Circ. Res.,* 44:645–652.

132. Thames, M. D., and Abboud, F. M. (1979): Reflex inhibition of renal sympathetic nerve activity during myocardial ischemia mediated by left ventricular receptors with vagal afferents in dogs. *J. Clin. Invest.,* 63:395–402.

133. Thames, M. D., and Schmid, P. G. (1979): Cardiopulmonary receptors with vagal afferents tonically inhibit ADH release in the dog. *Am. J. Physiol.,* 237(3):H299–H304.

134. Thames, M. D., Peterson, M. G., and Schmid, P. G. (1980): Stimulation of cardiac receptors with veratrum alkaloids inhibits ADH secretion. *Am. J. Physiol.,* 239(*Heart Circ. Physiol.,* 8):H784–H788.

135. Thames, M. D., Waickman, L. A., and Abboud, F. M. (1980): Sensitization of cardiac receptors (vagal afferents) by intracoronary acetylstrophanthidin. *Am. J. Physiol.,* 239:H628–H635.

136. Thorén, P. (1976): Atrial receptors with non-medulated vagal afferents in the cat: Discharge frequency and pattern in relation to atrial pressure. *Circ. Res.,* 38:357–362.

137. Thorén, P. (1977): Characteristics of left ventricular receptors with non-medullated vagal afferents in cats. *Circ. Res.,* 40:415–421.

138. Thorén, P. (1979): Role of cardiac vagal C-fibers in cardiovascular control. *Rev. Physiol. Biochem. Pharmacol.,* 86:1–94.

139. Thorén, P. (1980): Characteristics of right ventricular receptors with non-medullated vagal afferents in the cat. *Acta Physiol. Scand.,* 110:431–434.

140. Thorén, P., Mancia, G., and Shepherd, J. T. (1975): Vasomotor inhibition in rabbits by vagal non-medullated fibers from cardiopulmonary area. *Am. J. Physiol.,* 229:1410–1413.

141. Thorén, P., Donald, D. E., and Shepherd, J. T. (1976): Role of heart and lung receptors with non-medullated vagal afferents in circulatory control. *Circ. Res. [Suppl. II],* 38:2–9.

142. Thorén, P. (1976): Activation of left ventricular receptors with nonmedullated vagal afferents during occlusion of a coronary artery in the cat. *Am. J. Cardiol.,* 37:1046–1051.

143. Thorén, P., Shepherd, J. T., and Donald, D. E. (1977): Anodal block of medullated cardiopulmonary vagal afferents in cats. *J. Appl. Physiol. Respirat. Environ. Exercise Physiol.,* 42:461–465.

144. Uchida, Y., and Murao, S. (1974): Excitation of afferent cardiac sympathetic nerve fibers during coronary occlusion. *Am. J. Physiol.,* 226:1094–1099.

145. Uchida, Y., and Murao, S. (1974): Afferent sympathetic nerve fibers originating in the left atrial wall. *Am. J. Physiol.,* 227:753–758.

146. Uchida, Y. (1975): Afferent sympathetic nerve fibers with mechanoreceptors in the right heart. *Am. J. Physiol.,* 228:223–230.

147. Uchida, Y. (1975): Afferent aortic nerve fibers with their pathways in cardiac sympathetic nerves. *Am. J. Physiol.,* 228:990–995.

148. Uchida, Y. (1979): Mechanisms of excitation of cardiac "sympathetic" afferents. In: *Cardiac Receptors,* edited by R. Hainsworth, C. Kidd, and R. J. Linden, pp. 301–318. Cambridge University Press, Cambridge, U.K.

149. Ueda, H., Uchida, Y., and Kamisaka, K. (1969): Distribution and responses of the cardiac sympathetic receptors to mechanically induced circulatory changes. *Jpn. Heart J.* 10:70–81.

150. Walgenbach, S. C., and Donald, D. E. (1983): Cardiopulmonary reflexes and arterial pressure during rest and exercise in dogs. *Am. J. Physiol.,* 244:H326–H369.

151. Walgenbach, S. C., and Donald, D. E. (1983): Inhibition by carotid baroreflex of exercise-induced increase in arterial pressure. *Circ. Res.,* 52:253–262.
152. Walgenbach, S. C., and Shepherd, J. T. (1984): Role of arterial and cardiopulmonary mechanoreceptors in the regulation of arterial pressure during rest and exercise in conscious dogs. *Mayo Clin. Proc.,* 59:467–475.
153. Walker, J. L., Abboud, F. M., Mark, A. L., and Thames, M. D. (1980): Interaction of cardiopulmonary and somatic reflexes in humans. *J. Clin. Invest.,* 65:1491–1497.
154. Waller, A. D., and Reid, E. W. (1887): On the action of the excised mammalian heart. *Philos. Trans. R. Soc. Lond.* [*Biol.*], 178:215.
155. Weaver, L. C. (1977): Cardiopulmonary sympathetic afferent influences on renal nerve activity. *Am. J. Physiol.,* 233(*Heart Circ. Physiol.,* 2):H592–H599.
156. Weaver, L. C., Danos, L. M., Oehl, R. S., and Meckler, R. L. (1981): Contrasting reflex influences of cardiac afferent nerves during coronary occlusion. *Am. J. Physiol.,* 240(*Heart Circ. Physiol.,* 9):H620–H629.
157. White, J. C. (1957): Cardiac pain. Anatomic pathways and physiologic mechanisms. *Circulation,* 16:644–655.
158. Zehr, J. E., Hasbargen, J. A., and Kurz, K. D. (1976): Reflex suppression of renin secretion during distention of cardiopulmonary receptors in dog. *Circ. Res.,* 38:232–239.
159. Zehr, J. E., Hawe, A., Tsakiris, A. G., Rastelli, G. C., McGoon, D. C., and Segar, W. E. (1971): ADH levels following nonhypotensive hemorrhage in dogs with chronic mitral stenosis. *Am. J. Physiol.,* 221:312–317.
160. Zelis, R., Caudill, C. C., Baggette, K., and Mason, D. T. (1976): Reflex vasodilatation induced by coronary angiography in human subjects. *Circulation,* 53:490–493.
161. Zoller, R. P., Mark, A. L., Abboud, F. M., Schmid, P. G., and Heistad, D. D. (1972): The role of low pressure baroreceptors in reflex vasoconstrictor responses in man. *J. Clin. Invest.,* 51:2967–2972.
162. Zucker, I. H., Earle, A. M., and Gilmore, J. P. (1977): The mechanism of adaptation of the left atrial stretch receptors in dogs with chronic congestive heart failure. *J. Clin. Invest.* 60:323–331.
163. Zucker, I. H., Peterson, T. V., and Gilmore, J. P. (1980): Ouabain increases left atrial stretch receptor discharge in the dog. *J. Pharmacol. Exp. Ther.,* 212:320–324.

The Heart and Cardiovascular System,
edited by H. A. Fozzard et al.
Raven Press, New York © 1986.

CHAPTER 65

Atrial Natriuretic Factor: Biosynthetic Regulation and Role in Circulatory Homeostasis

Robert M. Graham and Jerome B. Zisfein

Atrial natriuretic factor (ANF) is a newly described peptide hormone that is potentially of major importance in volume and pressure homeostasis. It is synthesized in cardiac atria, where it is processed and then stored in membrane-bound secretory granules. An increase in blood volume, presumably leading to augmented atrial stretch, appears to be the major signal for its release. The circulating form of the hormone is a 24–28-amino-acid peptide containing a 17-member disulfide-linked ring that is essential for biological activity. After release into the circulation, ANF produces a variety of hemodynamic effects due to its potent natriuretic, diuretic, and vasorelaxant properties, in addition to influencing other hormonal modulators of blood volume and arterial pressure, such as renin, aldosterone, and antidiuretic hormone. Specific receptor sites that bind the biologically active forms of ANF with high affinity have been identified in a variety of tissues, and evidence has been presented that its cellular action may, in part, involve increased generation of cGMP due to activation of particulate guanylate cyclase. Sensitive and specific assays have been developed for quantitation of ANF in tissue extracts and in plasma. Preliminary findings suggest that alteration in the normal levels of ANF may occur with

changes in fluid and electrolyte balance, as well as in a variety of clinical disorders, such as congestive heart failure, supraventricular tachyarrhythmias, and hypertension. However, the position of ANF in the hierarchy of cardiovascular control systems, its role in the pathogenesis of various disease states, and its potential as a therapeutic agent have only begun to be defined.

BACKGROUND

In addition to a variety of neural, humoral, and structural influences, blood pressure homeostasis is critically dependent on the state of sodium and water balance (54). Sodium output is closely related to extracellular fluid volume: Sodium depletion causes a fall in urinary sodium excretion, whereas sodium loading causes natriuresis. In humans, sodium output changes such that sodium balance is achieved within a few days of an alteration of intake (124). This change in sodium excretion is mediated by changes in renal tubular reabsorption rather than by changes in glomerular filtration rate (16); subtle changes in sodium reabsorption lead to profound alterations in sodium excretion. Of the 1,000 mEq of sodium filtered per hour, less than 10 mEq is excreted in the urine; the remaining 99% is reabsorbed by the renal tubule. Thus, a fall in renal tubular sodium reabsorption from 99% to 98% will cause a doubling of urinary sodium excretion. In the process of reabsorption, sodium-containing fluid moves from the tubular lumen to the peritubular capillaries. Sodium reabsorption can therefore be altered by changes in physical factors—the hydrostatic and protein oncotic pressure gradients across the renal tubule—as well as by changes in cellular transport processes. Renal blood flow is a major determinant of these physical forces, and renal vasodilatation can cause natriuresis by increasing peritubular capillary hydrostatic pressure.

Given these complexities of renal sodium handling and the central role of sodium in modulating blood pressure, it is not surprising that the fine control of renal sodium excretion has been an issue of importance and interest for decades (40). With the isolation of aldosterone, it was assumed that changes in mineralocorticoid activity, balanced by changes in glomerular filtration, were sufficient to preserve sodium balance at a particular level. The experiments of de Wardener and Mills (9,38,91) and others (14,19,68,77) showed that that was not the case, because a sodium load still produced natriuresis when both these influences were removed. Such studies led to the concept of a "third factor" or "natriuretic hormone," and much attention has been focused on the hypothalamus as a site of its synthesis and release (37,76).

While the evidence for such a hypothalamic hormone continues to accumulate (27,57), over the past 5 years atrial peptides have been isolated and characterized (96). In addition to potent natriuretic and diuretic activities, these peptides have vasorelaxant properties and potentially can influence other modulators of volume and blood pressure, such as renin, aldosterone, and antidiuretic hormone.

Indeed, as postulated by Gauer and associates (46,47), the atria, because of their great distensibility and their independence of alterations in systemic pressure, are the prime location for a control mechanism involved in the detection and modulation of intravascular volume. This notion was based on the findings of a number of physiological studies that demonstrated that maneuvers leading to expansion of blood volume, such as atrial distension, negative pressure and carbon dioxide breathing, and total-body water immersion, were associated with an increase in urinary flow. Although a suppression of antidiuretic hormone release was initially postulated to account for some of these findings, Kappagoda et al. (71) more recently provided direct evidence that atrial stretch leads to release of a diuretic substance into plasma.

Nevertheless, the discovery of ANF resulted not from these physiological insights but rather from considerations of the functional morphology of cardiac muscle cells.

Kisch (75) and Jamieson and Palade (66) demonstrated that mammalian atrial cardiocytes, but not ventricular cardiocytes, had morphological features of secretory cells, containing electron-dense, membrane-bound storage granules. Further evidence for the secretory nature of atrial cardiocytes and for the link with volume regulation was the demonstration by de Bold that the kinetics of labeling of atrial granules with [³H]leucine resembled that found in cells producing polypeptide hormones and that the density of the atrial granules varied with changes in volume and electrolyte balance (33). Subsequently, de Bold and his colleagues (34) demonstrated that intravenous administration of atrial extracts caused a marked increase in urinary sodium excretion in rats, and he and others gained evidence for the peptide nature and amino acid content of the atrial material (33).

Numerous studies have confirmed the natriuretic activity of atrial extracts (20,21,72,73,97,104,121,128,129), and evidence for the location of this activity in atrial granules has been presented (33,141). Over the past 3 years, a prodigious amount of work has led to complete isolation, sequencing, and synthesis of ANF in active form. Much has been learned about the physiology, pharmacology, molecular biology, and mechanisms of action of ANF. Quantitative assays for ANF have been developed, and questions concerning its role in various disease states have begun to be addressed.

Because many of these insights have already been discussed in excellent reviews (26,83,86,95,96), they will be considered here only briefly. Rather, this chapter will focus on the more recent advances in our understanding of ANF.

NOMENCLATURE

With the isolation and sequencing of atrial peptides by numerous laboratories, various trivial names, in addition to ANF, have been used to identify the various peptides, which differ not in amino acid sequence but in the lengths of the peptide chains isolated (Fig. 1). It is now clear that these differences in chain length were generally due to artifactual truncation of the peptides that occurred during the isolation procedures.

The numbering system used to identify the amino acids of the ANF peptides has also changed with the elucidation of the prohormone and preprohormone sequences. As shown in Fig. 1, the longest peptide initially isolated contained 33 residues (26), the N-terminal leucine residue being identified as the first amino acid, and the C-terminal tyrosine as the thirty-third amino acid. More recently, the reference amino acid has been changed to either the first amino acid of the prohormone sequence (asparagine) or the first amino acid of the preprohormone (methionine). The former numbering system is preferred by some investigators because the

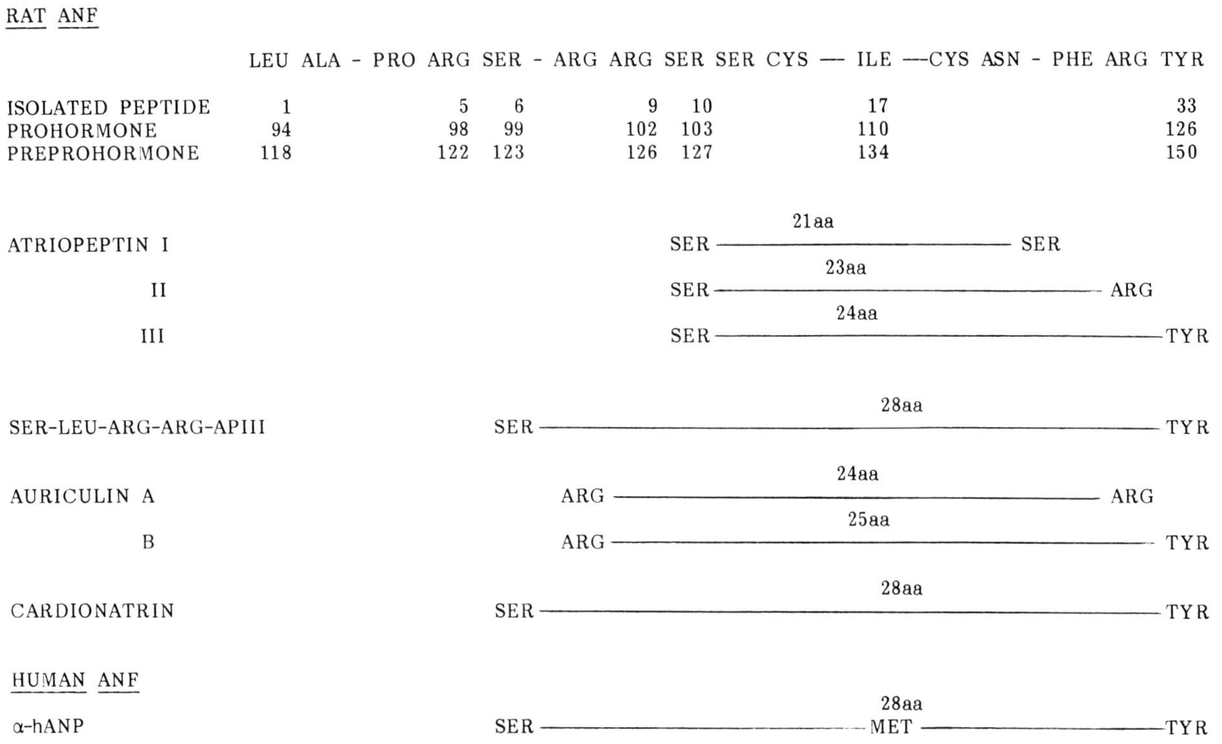

RAT ANF

LEU ALA - PRO ARG SER - ARG ARG SER SER CYS — ILE —CYS ASN - PHE ARG TYR

ISOLATED PEPTIDE	1	5	6	9	10	17	33
PROHORMONE	94	98	99	102	103	110	126
PREPROHORMONE	118	122	123	126	127	134	150

ATRIOPEPTIN I   SER ——————21aa—————— SER

II   SER ——————23aa—————— ARG

III   SER ——————24aa—————— TYR

SER-LEU-ARG-ARG-APIII   SER ——————28aa—————— TYR

AURICULIN A   ARG ——————24aa—————— ARG

B   ARG ——————25aa—————— TYR

CARDIONATRIN   SER ——————28aa—————— TYR

HUMAN ANF

α-hANP   SER ——————28aa—— MET ——————TYR

FIG. 1. Amino acid sequences and trivial names for the various ANF peptides isolated from atria and plasma (26,83,86,96,115,119). Numbering of the amino acids is based on the sequence of the longest peptide initially isolated (leucine-1, tyrosine-33; ANF 1–33), the structure of the prohormone (asparagine-1, leucine-94, tyrosine-126; ANF 94–126), or the structure of the preprohormone (methionine-1, leucine-118, tyrosine-150; ANF 118–150).

length of the prohormone is 126 amino acids in all species, whereas the length of the preprohormone varies because of species differences in the length of the signal peptide, 23 amino acids in the dog, 24 in the rodent, and 25 in the human and rabbit.

MOLECULAR AND CELLULAR BIOLOGY

Biosynthesis

With the availability of amino acid sequence data following the isolation and complete purification of ANF from rat and human atrial tissue (26,83,86,95,96). It has been possible to isolate cDNA and genomic copies of the gene encoding the precursor polypeptide (52,70,88,93,98,101,102,116–118,137). From these studies, the structures of human, rat, mouse, rabbit, and dog ANF (Fig. 2) have been deduced from the determined nucleotide sequences, and much has been learned about the molecular biology of ANF.

It is now apparent that ANF is synthesized as a 150–152-amino-acid precursor, preproANF, containing a 24–25-amino-acid hydrophobic leader sequence. PreproANF is cleaved to a 126-amino-acid prohormone, proANF. The biologically active 24–28-amino-acid "hormone" is located at the carboxyl-terminal end of proANF. The sequence of human and dog ANF differs from the rodent

and rabbit hormone by the substitution of a single isoleucine residue with a methionine.

In all mammalian species examined thus far, the preprohormone is encoded by a single gene that is highly conserved and that contains many features of a typical eukaryotic gene. These include a TATAA box (T, thymidine; A, adenosine), two intervening sequences bounded by splicing signals (GT-AG) (G, guanosine), and an AATAAA polyadenylation addition signal. Initiation of ANF mRNA transcription begins 27 base pairs after the TATAA box (cap site). PreproANF is encoded in three separate exons (coding blocks). Coding block I encodes the first 40–41 amino acids, including the hydrophobic leader sequence and the first 20 amino acid residues of proANF. Coding block II encodes the remainder of proANF except for 1–3 carboxyl-terminal amino acids that are encoded by coding block III.

The rat, mouse, and rabbit ANF gene contains nucleotide sequences that encode two amino acids (Arg-Arg) more at the C terminus than the human and dog ANF gene. This is due to a single nucleotide change (C to T) at the 3' end of the gene that defines a terminating codon in humans and dogs, rather than an arginine in rodents and rabbits. The nucleotide sequences for these terminal arginine residues are present on the rat mRNA, but the Arg-Arg sequence has not been identified on the peptides isolated from rodent atria. This suggests that

FIG. 2. Comparison of complete amino acid sequences for human, rat, mouse, rabbit, and dog preproANF deduced from nucleotide sequence analysis of ANF cDNA clones (70,88,93,98,101,102,118,137). Residues s1–s25 (*bold type*) compose the signal sequence, and residues 1–126 and 1–128 the sequences of the human and dog proANF and rodent and rabbit proANF, respectively. Residues 99–126 and 103–126 (*bold type*) compose the sequences of the biologically active, circulating forms of ANF. Where an amino acid is not shown, its identity is the same as the amino acid indicated immediately above. A dash indicates the absence of an amino acid in that position.

Signal sequence (s1–s25):

	s1									s10										s20					s25
Human	**Met**	**Ser**	**Ser**	**Phe**	**Ser**	**Thr**	**Thr**	**Thr**	**Val**	**Ser**	**Phe**	**Leu**	**Leu**	**Leu**	**Leu**	**Ala**	**Phe**	**Gln**	**Leu**	**Leu**	**Gly**	**Gln**	**Thr**	**Arg**	**Ala-**
Mouse		Gly				---	Ile		Leu	Gly			Phe		Val			Trp		Pro		His	Ile	Gly	
Rat						---			Lys						Phe										
Dog		---	---			Pro	Ala	Ala	Ser						Leu			Val	Gln		Leu		Gln	Thr	
Rabbit		Pro	Phe			Thr	Thr	Val					Phe	Cys				Phe	Trp	His	Pro	Asp		Ile	

Residues 1–25:

	1									10										20					
Human	Asn	Pro	Met	Tyr	Asn	Ala	Val	Ser	Asn	Ala	Asp	Leu	Met	Asp	Phe	Lys	Asn	Leu	Leu	Asp	His	Leu	Glu	Glu	Lys-
Mouse			Val		Ser					Thr															
Rat																									
Dog			Gly	Ser						Ala			Leu							Arg			Asp		
Rabbit			Asn	Ala	Met								Met							His					Arg

Residues 26–50:

					30										40										50
Human	Met	Pro	Leu	Glu	Asp	Glu	Val	Val	Pro	Pro	Gln	Val	Leu	Ser	Asp	Pro	Asn	Glu	Glu	Ala	Gly	Ala	Ala	Leu	Ser-
Mouse			Val					Met				Ala			Glu	Gln	Thr								
Rat																	Asp								
Dog			Leu				Ala	Glu	Ser								Asn	Ala							
Rabbit			Phe					Val	Pro								Ser	Asp							

Residues 51–75:

										60										70					
Human	Pro	Leu	Pro	Glu	Val	Pro	Pro	Trp	Thr	Gly	Glu	Val	Ser	Pro	Ala	Gln	Arg	Asp	Gly	Gly	Ala	Leu	Gly	Arg	Gly-
Mouse	Ser														Asn	Pro	Leu			Ser		Ser	Arg		Ser
Rat		Ser		Ser																					
Dog	Pro														Ser	Ala	Gln			Gly		Leu	Gly		
Rabbit																				Glu					

Residues 76–100:

					80										90										100
Human	Pro	Trp	Asp	Ser	Ser	Asp	Arg	Ser	Ala	Leu	Leu	Lys	Ser	Lys	Leu	Arg	Ala	Leu	Leu	Thr	Ala	Pro	Arg	**Ser**	**Leu-**
Mouse				Pro																Ala	Gly				
Rat																									
Dog				Ser																Ala					
Rabbit	Thr		Glu	Ala		Glu														Thr					

Residues 101–125:

					105					110										120					
Human	**Arg**	**Arg**	**Ser**	**Ser**	**Cys**	**Phe**	**Gly**	**Gly**	**Arg**	**Met**	**Asp**	**Arg**	**Ile**	**Gly**	**Ala**	**Gln**	**Ser**	**Gly**	**Leu**	**Gly**	**Cys**	**Asn**	**Ser**	**Phe**	**Arg-**
Mouse										Ile															
Rat																									
Dog										**Met**															
Rabbit										**Ile**															

Residues 126–128:

	126		
Human	**Tyr**	---	---
Mouse		Arg	Arg
Rat			
Dog		---	---
Rabbit		Arg	Arg

these terminal sequences are cleaved following translation of the rodent mRNA, but the site of this cleavage has not yet been defined.

Northern-blot analysis using ANF cDNA has revealed a single, abundant (1–3% of total atrial mRNA) message of approximately 850 bases in poly(A)$^+$ mRNA from atria. In contrast, no mRNA or mRNA present only in extremely low abundance has been found in liver, ventricle, kidney, aorta, cartoid artery, pituitary, hypothalamus, adrenal, pancreas, testes, or epididymis (117).

Processing

Following the synthesis of preproANF on rough endoplasmic reticulum (rER) microsomes by translation of ANF mRNA, the signal peptide, which may facilitate transduction of the nascent polypeptide across the microsomal membrane into the rER cisternae, is likely cotranslationally cleaved from proANF by a membrane-associated enzyme. ProANF is then packaged and stored in membrane-bound secretory granules that on electron microscopy appear as dense osmophilic structures (250–500 nm) (33). These granules are most abundant in the perinuclear region of atriocytes, often in association with prominent Golgi, from which they likely arise. The granules are present in the atrial but not ventricular cells of all mammalian species, numbering up to 600 per cell (26,33). In nonmammalian species, however, including amphibians, reptiles, birds, teleost fish, and elasmobranchs, such as sharks, granules are present in both ventricular and atrial cardiocytes (33). And it is of interest that ANF has been found to stimulate chloride secretion from the shark rectal gland (120), an organ that plays a primary role in maintenance of water and electrolyte balance in this species.

The finding that the biologically active C-terminal 24–28-amino-acid peptide is the major circulating form in rodents (115) and possibly humans (136), and also the major form detected in perfusates of isolated atria (33), has led to the suggestion that proANF is cleaved before its release into the circulation. Recent evidence from studies of isolated atrial cardiocytes in culture, however, indicates that the 17-kd proANF is stored and released intact and can be cleaved by a serum protease to the 3-kd C-terminal hormone and a 14-kd peptide (17,18,48). The serum protease, responsible for this cleavage has been partially purified and characterized (140), although the factors regulating its activity and thus its role in modulating the availability of the biologically active hormone have not yet been determined.

Intrachain disulfide-bond formation to yield the 17-member ring critical for biological activity must also occur posttranslationally, probably prior to granular packaging, but the site of this processing has not been defined. In this regard, it is of interest that a 56-amino-acid peptide has been isolated from human atrial tissue, which has a unique dimeric structure in which two identical 28-amino-acid carboxyl-terminal peptides are arranged in an antiparallel fashion linked by two sets of interchain disulfide bridges (69). The significance of this structure is unknown.

As indicated earlier, the proANF-cleaving enzyme in serum produces an apparent specific endolytic cleavage of proANF to a product that migrates as a 3-kd band on SDS-gel electrophoresis. Radioactive sequence analysis of this band revealed that it contains both the C-terminal 28- and 24-amino-acid sequences of ANF in a ratio of approximately 3:1 (18). Resolution of these two peptides also proved to be possible by HPLC. This finding is in keeping with the identification of a 3-kd peptide as the major circulating form of ANF in humans and with the identification of both the carboxyl-terminal 28- and 24-amino-acid sequences of ANF, in a ratio of approximately 10:1, as the major circulating forms of ANF in the rat (115). Because the amino acid sequences at the site of proANF cleavage to yield both the 28- and 24-amino-acid peptides are identical (Arg-Ser), it is possible that a single protease is responsible for the production of both peptides. Nevertheless, the existence of an additional arginine-serine dipeptide sequence in proANF (residues 82 and 83) and the inability to detect a C-terminal 43-amino-acid peptide, which would result from cleavage between these residues, suggest that proANF-activating enzyme has relatively specific substrate requirements that permit generation of only the C-terminal 28- and 24-amino-acid peptides. Differences in the relative abundances of the 28- and 24-amino-acid peptides may be due to differences in substrate affinities for the proteolytic enzyme or to differences in clearance rates.

Clearance

Little is known about the fate of ANF following its release into the circulation. Some evidence has been presented to suggest that glandular kallikrein or a similar serine protease may be involved in its catabolism. Pharmacokinetic studies in humans and rats indicate a short half-life of 177 and 26.5 sec, and clearance rates of 1.4 to 1.8 and 0.5 liter/min, respectively, for the 24-amino-acid form of ANF (85,138). In the rat studies, no ANF could be detected in urine (85). This finding and the observation that the plasma half-life is doubled in anephric animals suggest that the kidneys are a major site of elimination by a degradative pathway, presumably involving peptide hydrolysis, rather than by excretion. Because the brush border of the renal proximal tubule is resplendent with proteolytic enzymes, this finding is not unexpected. However, it has yet to be established that ANF is filtered across the glomerular membrane.

Release

The finding that ANF is stored in granules suggests that its release is regulated rather than constitutive (74). In other systems in which release of proteins is regulated, secretion involves application of an appropriate stimulus, leading to an alteration in the level of a cytoplasmic messenger, such as calcium. As a result, the secretory vesicles fuse with the plasma membrane and extrude their contents into the circulation. However, the specific stimulus leading to release or alterations of an appropriate cytoplasmic messenger has not been defined for ANF. Preliminary in vitro investigations suggested that a variety of humoral substances, such as epinephrine, vasopressin, and acetylcholine (122), as well as the calcium ionophore A23187 (108), increase ANF release, whereas dibutyryl cAMP inhibits ANF release (112). Similar findings were reported from in vivo studies in which vasopressin and other pressor agents resulted in ANF release (89). However, because those compounds activated diverse cellular mechanisms and ANF release was not observed with nonpressor analogs, their relevance to physiological control of ANF secretion remains unclear.

At present, the most convincing mechanism suggested for ANF release is an increase in atrial distension, presumably leading to augmented atrial stretch. Evidence for such a mechanism is the finding of enhanced ANF release with increases in the central venous pressure or right atrial pressure of isolated perfused heart or heart-lung preparations (32,39,80). Similarly, volume expansion produced by infusion of fluids (80,136) or by salt loading (62,126) has been demonstrated in animals and humans to result in increased plasma levels of ANF. Finally, increased plasma ANF levels have been reported in a variety of disease states, such as congestive heart failure (119) and supraventricular tachyarrhythmias (135), conditions known to be associated with elevated atrial pressures. By contrast, ANF levels may not be altered in other conditions, such as cirrhosis of the liver, in which atrial pressures are likely to be normal or low (119).

QUANTITATION OF ANF

Initially, quantitation of ANF relied on the use of bioassays, natriuresis and diuresis in whole animals, and relaxation in isolated smooth-muscle preparations (26,96). Although these assays proved invaluable for evaluating biological activity during purification procedures and for qualitative or semiquantitative measurements of ANF in tissue extracts, their sensitivities are low, in the nanogram range for smooth-muscle assays and in the microgram range for the *in vivo* assays.

With the availability of synthetic ANF peptides for immunization and radiotracer synthesis, radioimmunoassays capable of detecting the picogram levels of ANF present in plasma have now been developed. Even with the availability of these assays, quantitation of the low levels of ANF in plasma, which in the basal state are close to the limits of sensitivity of most assays, remains a difficult undertaking. Confounding the analysis of ANF is the fact that substances in plasma interfere with antibody binding, and an initial extraction step is required. This necessitates careful quantitation of recoveries if valid plasma ANF levels are to be obtained. Extraction of ANF from plasma is generally achieved by passing the plasma over octadecasilyl cartridges, which bind ANF by hydrophobic interaction, and then elution with an organic solvent, such as methanol or acetonitrile. These solvents can then be removed by evaporation under N_2 or by lyophilization, which additionally allows the sample to be concentrated before assay.

Most commercially available antisera recognize both the carboxyl-terminal 24- and 28-amino-acid ANF peptides, but not biologically inactive or unrelated peptides. Sensitivity is generally enhanced by performing the assays under nonequilibrium conditions in which the antibody is preincubated with the plasma or unlabeled standards before addition of the radiotracer.

Synthesis of the radioiodinated tracer is generally achieved by standard chloramine-T or iodogen methods, and labeled peptide is purified on an octadecasilyl cartridge, or preferably by HPLC. The latter method results in higher specific radioactivity of the tracer and less contamination by unlabeled or diiodinated peptides or breakdown products.

PHARMACOLOGY AND MECHANISM OF ACTION

In addition to the natriuretic and diuretic effects observed with atrial extracts or synthetic ANF peptides,

relaxation of intestinal and vascular smooth muscle has been identified from *in vitro* studies as a major pharmacological property. These effects of ANF have been used as tools to evaluate the biological activities of isolated and synthetic peptides and to define the structure-activity relationships for a variety of ANF analogs. From such studies it is clear that in addition to the 17-member disulfide-linked ring (30,92), biological activity is dependent on the presence of the C-terminal Phe-Arg residues (Fig. 1) (30,125). The C-terminal Tyr residue probably is not essential for biological activity but is present on the native peptide. By contrast, modifications at the amino terminus appear less crucial for biological activity. Thus, for example, the 24- and 28-amino-acid peptides (Fig. 1) display reasonably similar vasorelaxant and diuretic activities (96).

In *in vitro* systems, half-maximal responses to the most active peptides are generally observed with concentrations in the low nanomolar range. Specific ANF receptor binding sites of high affinity (K_d 10^{-10}–10^{-9} M) have also been identified in radioligand binding studies using membranes prepared from a variety of tissues, including kidney, adrenal, pituitary, platelet, liver, aorta, glomerular mesangial cells, and cultured aortic smooth-muscle and renal epithelial cell lines (11,35,60,61,67,84,94,113,114). In those studies, the radioiodinated forms of the C-terminal 24- and 28-amino-acid peptides were used as radioligands. Specificity was demonstrated by showing appropriate inhibition of ligand binding by a variety of unlabeled ANF analogs, but no inhibition of binding by a variety of unrelated peptide hormones. The structural requirements for ANF binding identified in those studies are similar to the requirements for biological activity, namely, the presence of the 17-member disulfide-linked ring and the C-terminal Phe-Arg residues (11,35,60).

Photolabile radioiodinated analogs of ANF have also been developed and used to identify a 140-kd receptor glycoprotein in renal and liver plasma membranes (139). In those studies, the radioligand was covalently linked to the binding protein by photoactivation and then subjected to subunit size analysis by SDS-polyacrylamide-gel electrophoresis and autoradiography.

Regulation of ANF receptors in response to changes in the endogenous ANF concentration associated with alterations in fluid and electrolyte balance, or to changes in the ANF concentration resulting from exogenous administration of the hormone, have been observed in studies of isolated glomerular and cultured smooth-muscle cells (11,60). In these investigations, reciprocal changes in receptor density were noted with maneuvers that increased the concentration of ANF to which the cells were exposed.

In a variety of tissues, including liver, lung, kidney, aorta, testes, and intestine, ANF activates the membrane-bound form of guanylate cyclase without altering the activity of the soluble form of the enzyme (132). As a result of this enzyme activation, cGMP levels increase. In vascular tissue this effect of ANF is not dependent on the presence of an intact endothelium (134). Increases in urinary and plasma cGMP levels have also been reported with infusion of atrial extracts into rats (44,45,55). Because of the potential role of cGMP in the spasmolytic actions of other vasodilators, such as sodium nitroprusside, it has been suggested that cGMP acts as the intracellular mediator of ANF's vasorelaxant effects (132). Support for this notion is the finding of a strong correlation between the structural requirement for receptor binding by the various ANF peptides, their ability to activate guanylate cyclase, and their ability to produce vasorelaxation (11,60,61,132). Additionally, the spasmolytic effects of ANF can be attenuated by methylene blue, an inhibitor of guanylate cyclase (100). Nevertheless, a discrepancy in this schema that has not yet been reconciled is the finding that the concentration of ANF required to produce a 50% maximal vasodilator response is in the range of 10^{-10} to 10^{-9} M, whereas that required for cGMP accumulation is $\geq 10^{-8}$ M (11). This implies that cGMP accumulation will not occur until a concentration of ANF is achieved that will already have maximally saturated the receptor binding sites. Thus, it is possible that guanylate cyclase activation is linked only indirectly to receptor activation.

It is of interest, nonetheless, that in keeping with the selectivity of low doses of ANF for the renal vascular bed (131), preliminary findings suggest that ANF produces a selective increase in cGMP accumulation in cultured smooth-muscle cells from renal as compared with mesenteric artery (111).

ANF has also been reported to decrease cAMP levels by inhibiting adenylate cyclase activity in preparations of aorta, renal artery, and mesenteric artery, as well as anterior and posterior pituitary (2,3). Both basal and hormone-stimulated adenylate cyclase activities were inhibited dose-dependently in these preparations, with an IC_{50} of 10^{-10} to 10^{-9} M. Because receptor-independent activation of adenylate cyclase by fluoride or forskolin was also attenuated by ANF, it is likely that the effects of ANF occur at the level of the guanine nucleotide binding protein and/or the catalytic subunit of adenylate cyclase. However, the significance of these observations remains unclear, because inhibition of adenylate cyclase activity and alterations in urinary cAMP levels have not been universal findings (55,100,132,134).

SPASMOLYTIC AND HEMODYNAMIC EFFECTS OF ANF

Atrial extracts and synthetic ANF produce potent relaxant effects, particularly when applied in vitro to precontracted isolated smooth-muscle preparations or isolated perfused vascular beds (96). However, significant variability in the sensitivities of different vascular beds has been noted. The renal vasculature and isolated aortic strips respond readily to the spasmolytic actions of ANF, whereas relative insensitivity has been observed with application of ANF to mesenteric, femoral, carotid, coronary, and vertebral arteries (30,31,43,44,65).

The hemodynamic effects of ANF are complex because of confounding reflexogenic influences that tend to counteract the vasodilator effects of ANF, because of its differential actions in various vascular beds, and because of the level of vascular tone at the time of ANF administration. In animals, bolus administration of ANF leads to a reduction in arterial pressure that is due to a fall in peripheral resistance (81). By contrast, with infusions of ANF, the reduction in arterial pressure is due to a fall in cardiac output, and peripheral resistance actually increases (82). The fall in cardiac output may be due to a venodilating action of ANF, leading to a reduction in venous return, rather than to a negative inotropic effect that has been suggested from in vitro studies with an isolated perfused heart preparation (133). The increase in resistance, on the other hand, is most likely the result of a counteracting baroreceptor-mediated increase in sympathetic activity, because it can be prevented by surgical or chemical sympathectomy (82).

A possible venodilating effect of ANF is suggested by the fall in stroke volume that accompanies the fall in cardiac output, and by in vitro evidence that ANF causes dilatation of certain isolated vein preparations (83). A fall in venous return may also account, in part, for the failure of ANF to produce a marked increase in heart rate. Thus, with agents such as hydralazine that selectively reduce resistance but not capacitance vessel tone, venous return is augmented, and heart rate increases markedly. By contrast, with agents such as sodium nitroprusside that produce balanced reductions in both resistance tone and capacitance tone, there is little increase in heart rate. However, the failure of heart rate to increase with ANF may also be due to stimulation of cardiac sensory receptors with vagal afferents (1,90).

RENAL EFFECTS OF ANF

The renal actions of ANF are complex and not completely defined. However, inhibition of Na^+-K^+ ATPase, Na^+-K^+ pump activity, or sodium transport in isolated preparations, such as the toad bladder, is not involved (103,127). In animals and in humans, administration of ANF produces marked increases in renal sodium and water excretions (34,73,79,107,121). These natriuretic and diuretic effects are paralleled by increases in chloride and osmolal excretions and by increased but less marked losses of other solutes such as potassium, calcium, phosphate, and magnesium. These changes in solute excretion, coupled with the fact that most potent natriuretic agents act by depressing renal tubular transport mechanisms, whereas other renal vasodilators, such as acetylcholine and bradykinin, produce less marked or less sustained increases in sodium excretion, have led to the notion that ANF inhibits tubular solute transport. Because inhibition of solute transport in the more proximal segments of the nephron leads to more avid distal reabsorption, a tubular action of ANF would have to involve the thick ascending limb of the loop of Henle or more distal nephron segments to account for the marked solute losses (21,73,121). In support of a tubular action are the findings from clearance studies of increased lithium and phosphate excretions (96), the demonstration of reduced sodium-phosphate cotransport in proximal tubular brush border membrane vesicles prepared from rats pretreated with ANF (56), and the finding that ANF increases cGMP generation in renal papillary collecting tubule cells (6).

Less direct, but nevertheless provocative, evidence for an effect of ANF on solute transport are the finding of ANF receptors and modulation by ANF of amiloride-sensitive sodium transport in a cultured renal epithelial cell line (LLC-PK$_1$) (25,114) and the demonstration that ANF increases chloride excretion by the shark rectal gland (120). This latter action of ANF does not involve a hemodynamic mechanism, but rather appears to be an indirect effect involving release of a neurohormone, vasointestinal polypeptide (F. Epstein and P. Silva, *personal communication*). Whether such an action of ANF is confined to electrolyte homeostasis in lower-order species or has been evolutionarily conserved in mammals is presently unknown.

Evidence against a direct tubular action of ANF is the recent finding from stop-flow experiments that tubular handling of sodium, potassium, and water is not altered by ANF (123). Additionally, the proximal nephron is devoid of ANF receptors (26), and direct effects of ANF on isolated proximal tubules (13) or brush border vesicles (56) are not demonstrable with *in vitro* application of the peptide. Finally, ANF produces marked natriuresis even in the setting of water deprivation (104), in which avid distal tubular reabsorption would likely offset any increase in delivery of sodium from the proximal nephron.

The most striking effect of ANF on renal function in both animals and humans is an increase in filtration fraction, even in the setting of reduced renal blood flow and increased renal vascular resistance. The glomerular filtration rate (GFR) is also generally increased, although enhanced renal sodium excretion occurs even when GFR is unaltered (34,72,97,104,121). In micropuncture studies, single-nephron GFR increases with infusion of ANF, because of afferent arteriolar dilatation and mild efferent constriction that result in augmented glomerular capillary hydraulic pressure (64). The glomerular ultra-filtration coefficient (K_f) is unaltered by ANF. Increased efferent arteriolar resistance is also observed with ad-ministration of ANF to preparations of isolated perfused glomeruli (42).

Like the effects of ANF on systemic vascular resistance, changes in total renal resistance and renal flow are influenced by basal vascular tone at the time of ANF administration and by associated reflexogenic effects. Thus, total renal blood flow has been observed to increase with bolus administration of atrial extracts or synthetic ANF (20,45), particularly in studies of anesthetized animals, in which basal renal vascular tone is likely to be high. In contrast, when basal renal resistance is low, as in studies of conscious animals, infusions of ANF lead to no change (23,63) or a fall in total renal blood flow (81) or only to a selective increase in blood flow to certain regions of the kidney, such as the inner cortex (109). Similarly, in the isolated perfused kidney, ANF increases total vascular resistance. However, if the renal vasculature is initially preconstricted with angiotensin, norepinephrine, or vasopressin, ANF produces a vasodilatory response (83).

It is tempting to speculate from these findings that the increase in GFR is the sole mechanism responsible for the effects of ANF on solute and water excretions. However, as mentioned earlier, ANF produces natriuresis in the absence of an increase in GFR. Also, increases in peritubular capillary oncotic forces resulting from the augmented filtration fraction are likely to favor avid proximal reabsorption and thus to counteract, at least in part, the effect of enhanced delivery of filtered sodium (22). Micropuncture studies indicate a marked increase in sodium delivery to the outer medullary collecting duct, whereas sodium delivery to more proximal nephron segments is increased only slightly (121). Net addition of sodium to distal nephron segments, therefore, has been postulated to play a major role in the natriuretic effects of ANF (121). The most likely site for such an effect is the papillary collecting duct, which is exposed to the high concentrations of sodium in the renal papillary interstitium. Nevertheless, this postulated action of ANF remains speculative, because in the micropuncture studies mentioned earlier, only the proximal segments of superficial nephrons were available for sampling. Increased sodium delivery to papillary collecting ducts could thus also have resulted from the contributions of deeper proximal nephron segments. Additionally, preliminary studies in which the papillae were chemically ablated indicated an unaltered natriuretic response to ANF (59).

It is evident from these considerations that much remains to be learned about the renal actions of ANF. Results of studies using anesthetized animal preparations, such as micropuncture investigations, must be carefully considered. Although detailed insights can be gained from such studies and care is usually taken to ensure adequate hydration, increased basal renal vascular tone may still be present and may alter responses to ANF that would occur under more physiological conditions. It is also likely that the net effect of ANF on renal function is influenced, both chronically and perhaps acutely, by interactions of ANF with other hormonal modulators of renal function, such as renin, aldosterone, and antidiuretic hormone (*vide infra*). Finally, most studies reported to date have evaluated the renal functional effects of ANF after bolus administration or with short-term infusions. The effects of prolonged alterations in ANF levels are thus largely unknown. Indeed, it is of interest that substantially different effects have recently been reported with 45-min as compared with 5-day infusions of ANF in conscious dogs (51). With the former, GFR and renal sodium excretion increased significantly, whereas mean arterial pressure was reduced only slightly. The 5-day infusions, on the other hand, produced greater reductions in arterial pressure, but no long-term effects on GFR or sodium excretion.

ENDOCRINE INTERRELATIONSHIPS

Interactions between ANF and several other hormonal systems involved in volume and blood pressure homeostasis have been identified from both *in vitro* and *in vivo* studies.

Adrenal Steroids

Crude atrial extracts, as well as synthetic ANF, inhibit aldosterone production by isolated rat and bovine adrenal zona glomerulosa cells (96), and specific ANF receptor sites have been identified in adrenal cell membranes (35). In bovine cells, the effect of ANF on basal aldosterone production has been variable, with both inhibition and no change in production being reported (8,49). This may be related to the state of sodium balance at the time the adrenal cells are harvested. For example, elevated basal aldosterone production that is inhibited by ANF is observed in cells prepared from sodium-depleted rats but not sodium-replete rats (24). Inhibitions of angiotensin-II- (AII-), ACTH-, PGE-, cAMP-, K$^+$-, and forskolin-stimulated aldosterone production have also been demonstrated. The inhibitory effect of ANF on AII-stimulated aldosterone production is not due to AII receptor blockade, because ANF does not alter AII binding or AII-induced phosphatidylinositol turnover or changes in Ca^{2+} flux (49). Also, neither AII nor ACTH interferes with ANF receptor binding (36).

The effect of ANF on both basal and AII-stimulated aldosterone production appears to involve the early pathway in steroidogenesis, because pregnenolone accumulation is inhibited (24,49). An inhibitory effect on the late pathway (aldosterone production from exogenous progesterone and exogenous 25-OH cholesterol) has also been observed in studies of rat but not bovine adrenal cells (24,49).

Suppression of aldosterone secretion has been noted with *in vivo* administration of ANF, particularly when basal secretion is high, as in studies of anesthetized animals or animals with severe sodium restriction and ascites due to inferior vena cava constriction. In conscious sodium-replete animals, aldosterone secretion is unaltered with ANF administration (51).

ANF does not alter basal or stimulated corticosterone release *in vitro* or cortisol levels *in vivo* (8,24,87).

Renin

An inhibitory effect of ANF on renin secretion has been documented in animals with high basal renin activity, but not in normal animals (41,51,87). Suppression of renin release from rat renal slices has also been reported (58). This latter finding suggests a direct effect on the renin-producing juxtaglomerular cells, although an action at the macula densa due to an increase in distal delivery of sodium has not been excluded.

Antidiuretic Hormone and Water Homeostasis

Recent evidence suggests a multisite interaction among ANF, antidiuretic hormone (ADH), and water homeostasis. ANF inhibits dehydration- and hemorrhage-induced ADH release in rats and both basal and AII-stimulated ADH release from isolated superfused rat posterior pituitary glands (99,110). Specific high-affinity ANF binding sites have also been identified in pituitary gland membranes (67). In isolated perfused cortical collecting tubules, ANF inhibits ADH-stimulated hydraulic conductivity (an index of osmotic water permeability) (4).

A direct central nervous system interaction between ANF and water homeostasis is suggested by the finding that ANF inhibits dehydration and AII-induced water intake (5) and that certain areas in the brain, such as the hypothalamus, involved in the regulation of fluid balance, contain both ANF and ANF receptors, as determined by immunohistochemical and radioligand binding studies, respectively (96,105).

EFFECTS OF ANF IN HUMANS

There are, as yet, few reports on the effects of ANF administration in humans. The available evidence suggests that bolus administration of synthetic ANF to normal subjects and patients with essential hypertension results in rapid and marked increases in water and solute (sodium, chloride, calcium, phosphorus, and magnesium) excretions, a fall in urine osmolality, and a transient increase in creatinine clearance (79,106,107). These renal effects are accompanied by a small but significant fall in mean arterial pressure and an increase in heart rate, but no significant changes in plasma renin activity, aldosterone, cortisol, norepinephrine, or ADH.

In normal subjects, infusion of the synthetic C-terminal 25-amino-acid rat peptide at a rate of 0.1 μg/kg/min for 1 hr produced diuresis, increases in sodium and free-water clearances, and an increase in filtration fraction (28). GFR and renal blood flow remained unchanged. These effects were accompanied by small but significant reductions in systolic arterial pressure, plasma renin activity, and aldosterone. Similar findings have been reported with more prolonged (4 hr) infusions of the C-terminal 24-amino-acid rat peptide at 0.5 and 5 μg/min, although a fall in mean arterial blood pressure and an increase in heart rate were significant only with the higher dose (15). Renal blood flow was reduced with both doses. Plasma renin activity, AII, and aldosterone were unaltered during peptide infusion, but increased after its administration was discontinued. Again, increases in filtration fraction were noted with both doses, due to the divergence of GFR and renal blood flow.

THERAPEUTIC POTENTIAL AND ROLE IN DISEASE STATES

If ANF is a physiologically relevant hormone, it is likely that a defect in its biosynthesis, release, catabolism, or end-organ effects may play a pathophysiological role or that ANF may have therapeutic potential in any number of disease states. These may include cardiac disorders such as congestive heart failure and supraventricular tachyarrhythmias, hypertensive disorders such as low-renin essential hypertension, preeclampsia, and Gordon's syndrome, disorders of liver function such as cirrhosis and the hepatorenal syndrome, fluid and electrolyte disorders such as Bartter's syndrome and hyporeninemic hypoaldosteronism, and renal disorders such as nephrosis and acute or chronic renal failure.

Evidence for such a role for ANF in animal models of hypertension and congestive heart failure has been sought and discussed in previously published reviews of ANF (26,83,86,95,96). More recently, preliminary evidence from investigations in animals has been presented for a possible role for ANF in the "escape" natriuresis that is characteristic of mineralocorticoid excess (10,53). Additionally, a potential therapeutic role for ANF has been identified in a model of ischemic renal failure (29). Infusion of synthetic ANF in that study resulted in marked and sustained increases in GFR and in urine and sodium excretions, even though renal blood flow remained unaltered. These changes are particularly impressive because an animal with reduced renal mass already has an elevated single-nephron GFR and is excreting near-maximal amounts of sodium per nephron.

Increased plasma ANF levels have recently been demonstrated in patients with marked edema due to congestive heart failure (119) and in patients with biventricular dysfunction (12), but not in patients with cirrhosis and edema (119). This difference may be due to elevations in atrial pressure and stretch in the patients with heart disease, because correlations between plasma ANF levels and right atrial and pulmonary capillary wedge pressures were documented in one of these studies. In contrast, increased atrial pressure is not a common feature of cirrhosis leading to salt retention (119). Increased plasma ANF levels have also been reported in some, but not all, patients with essential hypertension (7). However, the normal control subjects were not carefully matched for age, sex, and weight, and a number of variables likely to influence plasma ANF levels, such as sodium intake and posture, were not defined.

Sodium diuresis has been well described in association with paroxysmal atrial tachyarrhythmias. In several studies, increases in plasma ANF levels were reported in patients who spontaneously developed supraventricular tachycardia, as well as in patients undergoing atrial pacing (78,135). However, the significance of this finding remains unclear, because in neither situation was enhanced solute excretion documented.

Finally, alterations in plasma ANF levels have been observed both basally and with volume expansion in patients with a variety of fluid and electrolyte disorders (130). For example, plasma ANF levels were appropriately raised in patients with primary hyperaldosteronism and fell following removal of an aldosterone-producing tumor, or with dexamethasone suppression of aldosterone overproduction. In contrast, inappropriate elevations in plasma ANF levels were observed in patients with Bartter's syndrome (a disorder characterized by a contracted plasma volume) and rose further with volume expansion. This latter finding is of particular interest because it suggests primary hypersecretion or impaired clearance of ANF in patients with Bartter's syndrome. However, in one informative kindred with Bartter's syndrome, a link between the gene for ANF and the disease has been definitively excluded (50).

FUTURE DIRECTIONS

Fewer than 5 years have elapsed since the pivotal experiment by de Bold (34) first demonstrated a potent natriuretic substance in atrial tissue. Since that time, much has been learned about the structure, biosynthesis, release, and actions of this unique cardiac hormone, and insights have been gained into its potential role as a regulator of cardiovascular homeostasis. There are, however, at every level of study, crucial questions that remain unanswered. Although the ANF gene structure has been elucidated, the stimuli leading to transcription of the gene and the mechanisms involved in its control are unknown. Similarly, the neural, humoral, and mechanical stimuli leading to release of proANF from the atria and the significance of its cleavage in the circulation have not been fully defined. The major renal sites of action and mechanism by which ANF exerts its natriuretic effect are still unknown, and there are seemingly equal bodies of evidence in support of both renal hemodynamic and renal tubular models.

Perhaps the most important question is how ANF fits into the intricate network of neural and humoral checks and balances that effect fluid and electrolyte homeostasis. Although increases in salt and intravascular volume lead to prompt release of ANF from atriocytes, how crucial is its natriuretic action to restoring equilibrium? Similarly, are there pathological conditions, such as those that exist for other peptide hormones, attributable to the absence or overabundance of ANF, or to alterations in receptor-mediated responsiveness?

The diagnostic and therapeutic implications of ANF are potentially exciting. Measurement of plasma ANF levels might be a useful clinical tool for detecting the earliest stages of congestive heart failure and for identification of those most at risk for developing the cardiac sequelae of essential hypertension. Equally promising is potential pharmacological use of synthetic ANF or its analogs in acute or chronic treatment of salt-retaining states, such as cirrhosis and congestive heart failure, as well as conditions of impaired renal function due to either parenchymal or hemodynamic abnormalities.

Whatever the answers to these questions, there is no doubt that the discovery of ANF represents a significant milestone in the study of circulatory physiology. Through continued study of this new hormone, we are sure to gain useful and perhaps unique insights into the factors regulating fluid and electrolyte homeostasis.

ACKNOWLEDGMENTS

We thank Debra Rollins for typing the manuscript, our colleagues Charles Homcy, Kenneth Bloch, Jonathan Seidman, Christine Seidman, Gary Matsueda, Edgar Haber, John Fallon, and Michael Margolies, who participated in the research, and Professor Richard Gordon for sharing unpublished data with us.

Studies reported here were supported in part by NIH grants NS-19583 and HL-35642 and by a grant from the R. J. Reynolds Company. R.M.G. is an Established Investigator of the American Heart Association (82-240).

REFERENCES

1. Ackerman, U., Trizawa, T. G., Milojeric, S., and Sonnenberg, H. (1984): Cardiovascular effects of atrial extracts in anesthetized rats. *Can. J. Physiol. Pharmacol.*, 62:819–826.
2. Anad-Srivastava, M. B., Cantin, M., and Genest, J. (1985): Inhibition of pituitary adenylate cyclase by atrial natriuretic factor. *Life Sci.*, 36:1873–1879.
3. Anad-Srivastava, M. B., Franks, D. J., Cantin, M., and Genest, J. (1984): Atrial natriuretic factor inhibits adenylate cyclase activity. *Biochem. Biophys. Res. Commun.*, 121:855–862.
4. Anderson, R. J., and Dillingham, M. A. (1986): Atrial natriuretic factor inhibition of arginine vasopressin (AVP) action in rabbit cortical collecting tubule. *Kidney Int.*, 29:328A.
5. Antunes-Rodrigues, J., McCann, S. M., Robergs, L. C., and Samson, W. K. (1985): Atrial natriuretic factor inhibits dehydration- and angiotensin II-induced water intake in the conscious, unrestrained rat. *Proc. Natl. Acad. Sci. (USA)*, 82:8720–8723.
6. Appel, R. G., and Dunn, M. J. (1985): Effect of synthetic atrial natriuretic factor (sANF) on cGMP synthesis in rat renal papillary collecting tubule (RPCT) cells. *Clin. Res.*, 33:618A.
7. Arendt, R. M., Stangl, E., and Zahringer, J. (1985): Alpha-atrial natriuretic factor in human plasma: Differences between normotensive and hypertensive patients. *Circulation*, 72:103A.
8. Atrashi, K., Mulrow, P. J., Franco-Saenz, R., Snajdar, R., and Rapp, J. (1984): Inhibition of aldosterone production by an atrial extract. *Science*, 224:992–993.
9. Bahlmann, J., McDonald, S. J., Ventom, M. G., and de Wardener, H. E. (1967): The effect on urinary sodium excretion of blood volume expansion without changing the composition of blood in the dog. *Clin. Sci.*, 32:403–413.
10. Ballerman, B. J., Bloch, K. D., Seidman, J. G., and Brenner, B. M. (1986): Atrial natriuretic peptide (ANP) secretion, biosynthesis and glomerular receptor activity during mineralocorticoid escape. *Kidney Int.*, 29:329A.
11. Ballerman, B. J., Hoover, R. L., Karnovsky, M. J., and Brenner, B. M. (1986): Physiologic regulation of atrial natriuretic peptide receptors in rat renal glomeruli. *J. Clin. Invest.*, 76:2049–2056.
12. Bates, E. R., Shenker, Y., and Grekin, R. J. (1985): Plasma atrial natriuretic factor levels are markedly elevated in humans with biventricular dysfunction. *Circulation*, 72:4111A.
13. Baum, M. (1985): Effect of atrial natriuretic factor on the rabbit proximal convoluted tubule. *Clin. Res.*, 33:477A.
14. Bengele, H. H., Houttuin, E., and Pearce, J. W. (1972): Volume natriuresis without renal nerves and renal vascular pressure rise in the dog. *Am. J. Physiol.*, 223:68–73.
15. Biollaz, J., Nussberger, J., Waeber, B., Brunner-Ferber, F., Gomez, H. J., Otterbein, E. S., and Brunner, H. R. (1985): Four hour infusion of synthetic atrial natriuretic factor in normal volunteers: Metabolic and hormonal effects. *Hypertension*, 7:845A.
16. Black, D. A. K., Platt, R., and Stanbury, S. W. (1950): Regulation of sodium excretion in normal and salt-depleted subjects. *Clin. Sci.*, 9:205–221.
17. Bloch, K. D., Scott, J. A., Zisfein, J. B., Fallon, J. T., Margolies, M. N., Seidman, C. E., Matsueda, G. R., Homcy, C. J., Graham, R. M., and Seidman, J. G. (1985): Biosynthesis and secretion of proatrial natriuretic factor by cultured rat cardiocytes. *Science*, 230:1168–1171.
18. Bloch, K. D., Zisfein, J. B., Margolies, M. N., Homcy, C. J., Graham, R. M., Seidman, J. G. (1986): Atrial natriuretic factor biosynthesis: A serum protease cleaves proANF into a 14-kilodalton peptide and ANF. (*submitted for publication*).
19. Blythe, W. B., D'Avila, D., Gitelman, H. J., and Welt, L. G. (1971): Further evidence for a humoral natriuretic factor. *Circ. Res.*, 28:21–31.
20. Borenstein, H. B., Cupples, W. A., Sonnenberg, H., and Veness, A. T. (1983): The effects of natriuretic atrial extract on renal haemodynamics and urinary excretion in anesthetized rats. *J. Physiol. (Lond).*, 334:133–140.
21. Briggs, J. P., Steipe, B., Schubert, G., and Schnermann, J. (1982): Micropuncture studies of the renal effects of atrial natriuretic substances. *Pfluegers Arch.*, 395:271–276.
22. Burg, M. B. (1981): Renal handling of sodium chloride, water, amino acids, and glucose. In: *The Kidney*, edited by B. M. Brenner and F. C. Rector, Jr., pp. 328–370. W. B. Saunders, Philadelphia.
23. Burnett, J. C., Jr., Granger, J. P., and Opgenorth, T. J. (1984): Effects of synthetic atrial natriuretic factor on renal function and renin release. *Am. J. Physiol.*, 247:F863–F866.
24. Campbell, W. B., and Needleman, P. (1985): Inhibition of aldosterone biosynthesis by atriopeptins in rat adrenal cells. *Circ. Res.*, 57:113–118.
25. Cantiello, H. F., and Ausiello, D. A. (1986): Atrial natriuretic factor and cGMP inhibit amiloride-sensitive Na^+ transport in the cultured renal epithelial cell line, LLC-PK$_1$. *Biochem. Biophys. Res. Commun.*, (*in press*).

26. Cantin, M., and Genest, J. (1985): The heart and the atrial natriuretic factor. *Endocrine Rev.*, 6:107–127.
27. Carilli, C. T., Berne, M., Cantley, L. C., and Haupert, G. T., Jr. (1985): Hypothalamic factor inhibits the (Na,K)ATPase from the extracellular surface. *J. Biol. Chem.*, 260:1027–1031.
28. Cody, R. J., Covit, A. B., Laragh, J. H., and Atlas, S. (1985): Atrial natriuretic factor (ANF) in normal men: Renal hemodynamic/hormonal responses. *Hypertension*, 7:845A.
29. Cole, B. R., Kuhnline, M. A., and Needleman, P. (1986): Atriopeptin III: A potent natriuretic, diuretic and hypotensive agent in rats with chronic renal failure. *J. Clin. Invest., (in press)*.
30. Currie, M. G., Geller, D. M., Cole, B. R., Boylan, J. C., Yu Sheng, W., Holmberg, S. W., and Needleman, P. (1983): Bioactive cardiac substances: Potent vasorelaxant activity in mammalian atria. *Science*, 221:71–73.
31. Currie, M. G., Geller, D. M., Cole, B. R., Siegel, N. R., Fok, K. F., Adams, S. P., Eubanks, S. R., Galluppi, G. R., and Needleman, P. (1984): Purification and sequence analysis of bioactive atrial peptides (atriopeptins). *Science*, 223:67–69.
32. Currie, M. G., Sulkin, D., Geller, D. M., Cole, B. R., and Needleman, P. (1984): Atriopeptin release from the isolated perfused rabbit heart. *Biochem. Biophys. Res. Commun.*, 124:711–717.
33. de Bold, A. J. (1985): Atrial natriuretic factor: A hormone produced by the heart. *Science*, 230:767–770.
34. de Bold, A. J., Borenstein, H. B., Veress, A. T., and Sonnenberg, H. (1981): A rapid and potent natriuretic response to intravenous injection of atrial myocardial extract in rats. *Life Sci.*, 28:89–94.
35. de Lean, A., Gutkowska, J., McNicoll, N., Schiller, P. W., Cantin, M., and Genest, J. (1984): Characterization of specific receptors for atrial natriuretic factor in bovine adrenal zona glomerulosa. *Life Sci.*, 35:2311–2318.
36. de Lean, A., Racz, K., Gutkowska, J., Nguyen, T.-T., Cantin, M., and Genest, J. (1984): Specific receptor-mediated inhibition by synthetic atrial natriuretic factor of hormone-stimulated steroidogenesis in cultured bovine adrenal cells. *Endocrinology*, 115:1636–1638.
37. de Wardener, H. E. (1977): Natriuretic hormone. *Clin. Sci. Mol. Med.*, 53:1–8.
38. de Wardener, H. E., Mills, I. H., Clapham, W. F., and Hayter, C. J. (1961): Studies of the efferent mechanism of the sodium diuresis which follows the administration of intravenous saline in the dog. *Clin. Sci.*, 21:249–258.
39. Dietz, J. R. (1984): Release of natriuretic factor from rat heart-lung preparations by atrial distension. *Am. J. Physiol.*, 247:R1093–R1096.
40. Editor (1977): Natriuretic hormone. *Lancet*, 2:1163–1164.
41. Freeman, R. H., Davis, J. O., and Vari, R. C. (1985): Renal response to atrial natriuretic factor in conscious dogs with caval constriction. *Am. J. Physiol.*, 248:R495–R500.
42. Fried, T. A., McCoy, R. N., Osgood, R. W., Reineck, H. J., and Stein, J. H. (1985): The effect of atrial natriuretic peptide on glomerular hemodynamics. *Clin. Res.*, 33:584A.
43. Garcia, R., Thibault, G., Cantin, M., and Genest, J. (1984): Effect of a purified atrial natriuretic factor on rat and rabbit vascular strips and vascular beds. *Am. J. Physiol.*, 247:R34–R39.
44. Garcia, R., Thibault, G., Gutkowska, J., Cantin, M., and Genest, J. (1985): Changes of regional blood flow induced by atrial natriuretic factor (ANF) in conscious rats. *Life Sci.*, 36:1687–1692.
45. Garcia, R., Thibault, G., Gutkowska, J., Hamet, P., Cantin, M., and Genest, J. (1985): Effect of chronic infusion of synthetic atrial natiuretic factor (ANF 8-33) in conscious two-kidney, one-clip hypertensive rats. *Proc. Soc. Exp. Biol. Med.*, 178:155–159.
46. Gauer, O. H., and Henry, J. P. (1976): Neurohormonal control of plasma volume. In: *International Review of Physiology*, edited by A. C. Guyton and A. W. Cowley, p. 145. University Park Press, Baltimore.
47. Gauer, O. H., Henry, J. P., and Behn, C. (1970): The regulation of extracellular fluid volume. *Annu. Rev. Physiol.*, 32:547–595.
48. Glembotski, C. C., and Gibson, T. R. (1985): Molecular forms of immunoactive atrial natriuretic peptide released from cultured rat atrial myocytes. *Biochem. Biophys. Res. Commun.*, 132:1008–1017.
49. Goodfriend, T. L., Elliott, M. E., and Atlas, S. A. (1984): Actions of synthetic atrial natriuretic factor on bovine adrenal glomerulosa. *Life Sci.*, 35:1675–1682.
50. Graham, R. M., Bloch, K. D., Delaney, V. B., Bourke, E., and Seidman, J. G. (1986): Bartter's syndrome and the atrial natriuretic factor gene. *Hypertension, (in press)*.
51. Granger, J. P., Opgenorth, T. J., Salazar, J., Romero, J. C., and Burnett, J. C., Jr. (1986): Chronic hypotensive and renal effects of atrial natriuretic factor. *Hypertension, (in press)*.
52. Greenberg, B. D., Bencen, G. H., Seilhamer, J. J., Lewicki, J. A., and Fiddes, J. C. (1984): Nucleotide sequence of the gene encoding human atrial natriuretic factor precursor. *Nature*, 312:656–658.
53. Grekin, R. J., Ling, W. D., Shenker, Y., and Bohr, D. F. (1985): Plasma levels of immunoreactive atrial natriuretic factor (IR-ANF) during the developement of DOCA hypertension in pigs. *Hypertension*, 7:839A.
54. Guyton, A. C., Coleman, T. G., Cowley, A. W., Jr., Scheel, K. W., Manning, R. D., Jr., and Norman, R. A., Jr. (1972): Arterial pressure regulation: Overriding dominance of the kidneys in long-term regulation and in hypertension. *Am. J. Med.*, 52:582–589.
55. Hamet, P., Tremblay, J., Pang, S. C., Garcia, R., Thibault, G., Gutkowska, J., Cantin, M., and Genest, J. (1984): Effect of native and synthetic atrial natriuretic factor on cyclic GMP. *Biochem. Biophys. Res. Commun.*, 123:515–527.
56. Hammond, T. G., Yusufi, A. N. K., Knox, F. G., and Dousa, T. P. (1985): Administration of atrial natriuretic factor inhibits sodium-coupled transport in proximal tubules. *J. Clin. Invest.*, 75:1983–1989.
57. Haupert, G. T., Carilli, C. T., and Cantley, L. C. (1984): Hypothalamic sodium-transport inhibitor is a high-affinity reversible inhibitor of Na^+-K^+-ATPase. *Am. J. Physiol.*, 247:F919–F924.
58. Henrich, W., McAllister, L., Smith, P., Needleman, P., and Campbell, W. (1985): Direct effects of atriopeptin (AP) on renin release. *Clin. Res.*, 33:528A.
59. Hildebrandt, D. A., and Banks, R. O. (1986): Atrial natriuretic factor (ANF)- and furosemide-induced natriuresis in rats with papillary necrosis. *Kidney Int.*, 29:298A.
60. Hirata, Y., Tomita, M., Takada, S., and Yoshimi, H. (1985): Vascular receptor binding activities and cyclic GMP responses by synthetic human and rat atrial natriuretic peptides (ANP) and receptor down-regulation by ANP. *Biochem. Biophys. Res. Commun.*, 128:538–546.
61. Hirata, Y., Tomita, M., Yoshimi, H., and Ikeda, M. (1984): Specific receptors for atrial natriuretic factor (ANF) in cultured vascular smooth muscle cells of rat aorta. *Biochem. Biophys. Res. Commun.*, 125:562–568.
62. Hollister, A. S., Tanaka, I., Onrot, J., Biaggioni, I., and Inagami, T. (1985): Modulation of plasma atrial natriuretic factor levels in human subjects by sodium loading and posture change. *Hypertension*, 7:846A.
63. Huang, C.-L., Lewicki, J., Johnson, L. K., and Cogan, M. G. (1985): Renal mechanism of action of rat atrial natriuretic factor. *J. Clin. Invest.*, 75:769–773.
64. Ichikawa, I., Dunn, B. R., Troy, J. L., Maack, T., and Brenner, B. M. (1985): Influence of atrial natriuretic peptide on glomerular microcirculation in vivo. *Clin. Res.*, 33:487A.
65. Ishihara, T., Aisaka, K., Hattori, K., Hamasake, S., Morita, M., Noguchi, T., Kanagawa, K., and Matsuo, H. (1985): Vasodilatory and diuretic actions of alpha-human atrial natriuretic polypeptide (alpha-hANP). *Life Sci.*, 36:1205–1215.
66. Jamieson, J. D., and Palade, G. E. (1984): Specific granules in atrial muscle. *J. Cell Biol.*, 23:151–172.
67. Januszewicz, P., Gutkowska, J., de Lean, A., Thibault, G., Garcia, R., Genest, J., and Cantin, M. (1985): Synthetic atrial natriuretic factor induces release (possibly receptor-mediated) of vasopressin from rat posterior pituitary. *Proc. Soc. Exp. Biol. Med.*, 178:321–325.
68. Kaloyanides, G. J., and Azer, M. (1971): Evidence for a humoral mechanism in volume expansion natriuresis. *J. Clin. Invest.*, 50:1603–1612.
69. Kangawa, K., Fukuda, A., and Matsuo, H. (1985): Structural

identification of β- and α-human atrial natriuretic polypeptides. *Nature,* 313:397–400.

70. Kangawa, K., Tawaragi, T., Oikawa, S., Mizuno, A., Sakuragawa, Y., Nakazato, H., Fukuda, A., Minamino, N., and Matsuo, H. (1984): Identification of rat alpha-atrial natriuretic polypeptide and characterization of the cDNA encoding its precursor. *Nature,* 312:152–155.

71. Kappagoda, C. T., Knapp, M. F., Linden, R. J., Pearson, M. J., and Whitaker, E. M. (1979): Diuresis from left atrial receptors: Effect of plasma on the secretion of the Malpighian tubules of *Rhodnius prolixus. J. Physiol. (Lond.),* 291:381–391.

72. Keeler, R. (1982): Atrial natriuretic factor has a direct, prostaglandin-independent action of kidneys. *Can. J. Physiol. Pharmacol.,* 60:1078–1082.

73. Keeler, R., and Azzarolo, A. M. (1983): Effects of atrial natriuretic factor on renal handling of water and electrolytes in rats. *Can. J. Physiol. Pharmacol.,* 61:996–1002.

74. Kelly, R. B. (1985): Pathways of protein secretion in eukaryotes. *Science,* 230:25–32.

75. Kisch, B. (1956): Electron microscopy of the atrium of the heart. I. Guinea pig. *Exp. Med. Surg.,* 114:99–112.

76. Klahr, S., and Rodriguez, H. J. (1975): Natriuretic hormone. *Nephron,* 15:387–408.

77. Knox, F. G., Howards, S. S., Wright, F. S., Davis, B. B., and Berliner, R. W. (1968): Effect of dilution and expansion of blood volume on proximal sodium reabsorption. *Am. J. Physiol.,* 215:1041–1048.

78. Koller, P. T., Nicklas, J. M., DiCarlo, L. A., Shenker, Y., and Grekin, R. J. (1985): Marked elevation of plasma atrial natriuretic factor during paroxysmal supraventricular tachycardia. *Circulation,* III:102A.

79. Kuribayashi, T., Nakazato, M., Tanaka, M., Nagamine, M., Kurihara, T., Kanagawa, K., and Matsuo, H. (1985): Renal effects of human alpha-atrial natriuretic polypeptide. *N. Engl. J. Med.,* 312:1456–1457.

80. Lang, R. E., Tholken, H., Ganten, D., Luft, F. C., Ruskoaho, H., and Unger, T. (1985): Atrial natriuretic factor—a circulating hormone stimulated by volume loading. *Nature,* 314:264–266.

81. Lappe, R. W., Smits, J. F. M., Todt, J. A., Debets, J. J. M., and Wendt, R. L. (1985): Failure of atriopeptin II to cause arterial vasodilation in the conscious rat. *Circ. Res.,* 56:606–612.

82. Lappe, R. W., Todt, J. A., and Wendt, R. L. (1986): Mechanism of action of the vasoconstrictor responses to atriopeptin II in conscious SHR. *Am. J. Physiol., (in press).*

83. Laragh, J. H. (1985): Atrial natriuretic hormone, the renin-aldosterone axis, and blood pressure-electrolyte homeostasis. *N. Engl. J. Med.,* 313:1330–1339.

84. Leitman, D. C., Waldman, S. A., Kuno, T., and Murad, F. (1985): Specific atrial natriuretic factor receptors mediate increased cyclic GMP accumulation in cultured bovine aortic endothelial and smooth muscle cells. *Clin. Res.,* 33:599A.

85. Luft, F. C., Lang, R. E., Aronoff, G. R., Ruskoaho, H., Toth, M., Ganten, D., Sterzel, R. B., and Unger, T. H. (1986): Atriopeptin III kinetics and dynamics in rats. *Kidney Int.,* 29:340A.

86. Maack, T., Camargo, M. J. F., Kleinert, H. D., Laragh, J. H., and Atlas, S. A. (1985): Atrial natriuretic factor: Structure and functional properties. *Kidney Int.,* 27:607–615.

87. Maack, T., Marion, D. N., Camargo, M. J. F., Kleinart, H. D., Laragh, J. H., Vaughan, E. D., Jr., and Atlas, S. A. (1984): Effects of auriculin (atrial natriuretic factor) on blood pressure, renal function, and the renin-aldosterone system in dogs. *Am. J. Med.,* 77:1069–1075.

88. Maki, M., Takayanagi, R., Misono, K. S., Pandey, K. N., Tibbetts, C., and Inagami, T. (1984): Structure of rat atrial natriuretic factor precursor deduced from cDNA sequence. *Nature,* 309:722–724.

89. Manning, P. T., Schwartz, D., Katsube, N. C., Holmberg, S. W., and Needleman, P. (1985): Vasopressin-stimulated release of atriopeptin: Endocrine antagonists in fluid homeostasis. *Science,* 229:395–397.

90. Mark, A. L., Thoren, P., O'Neill, T. P., Morgan, D., Needleman, P., and Brody, M. J. (1985): Atriopeptins stimulate cardiac sensory receptors with vagal afferents in rats. *Clin. Res.,* 33:596A.

91. Mills, I. H., de Wardener, H. E., Hayter, C. J., and Clapham, W. F. (1961): Studies on the afferent mechanism of the sodium chloride diuresis which follows intravenous saline in the dog. *Clin. Sci.,* 21:259–264.

92. Misono, K. S., Fukumi, H., Grammer, R. T., and Inagami, T. (1984): Rat atrial natriuretic factor: Complete amino acid sequence and disulfide linkage essential for biological activity. *Biochem. Biophys. Res. Commun.,* 119:524–529.

93. Nakayama, K., Ohkubo, H., Hirose, T., Inayama, S., and Nakanishi, S. (1984): mRNA sequence for human cardiodilatin-atrial natriuretic factor precursor and regulation of precursor mRNA in rat atria. *Nature,* 310:699–701.

94. Napier, M. A., Vandlen, R. L., Albers-Schonberg, G., Nutt, R. F., Brady, S., Lyle, T., Winquist, R., Faison, E. P., Heinel, L. A., and Blaine, E. H. (1984): Specific membrane receptors for atrial natriuretic factor in renal and vascular tissue. *Proc. Natl. Acad. Sci. (USA),* 81:5946–5950.

95. Needleman, P., Currie, M. G., Geller, D. M., Cole, B. R., and Adams, S. P. (1984): Atriopeptins: Potential mediators of an endocrine relationship between heart and kidney. *Trends Pharmacol. Sci.,* 5:506–509.

96. Needleman, P., Adams, S. P., Cole, B. R., Currie, M. G., Geller, D. M., Michener, M. L., Saper, C. B., Schwartz, D., and Standaert, D. G. (1985): Atriopeptins as cardiac hormones. *Hypertension,* 7:469–482.

97. Nemeh, M. N., and Gilmore, J. P. (1983): Natriuretic activity of human and monkey atria. *Circ. Res.,* 53:420–423.

98. Nemer, M., Chamberland, M., Sirois, D., Argentin, S., Drouin, J., Dixon, R. A. F., Zivin, R. A., and Condra, J. H. (1984): Gene structure of human cardiac hormone precursor, pronatriodilatin. *Nature,* 312:654–656.

99. Obana, K., Naruse, M., Inagami, T., Brown, A., Naruse, K., Kurimoto, F., Sakurai, H., Demura, H., and Shizume, K. (1985): Atrial natriuretic factor inhibits vasopressin secretion from rat posterior pituitary. *Biochem. Biophys. Res. Commun.,* 132:1088–1094.

100. Ohlstein, E. H., and Berkowitz, B. A. (1985): Cyclic guanosine monophosphate mediates vascular relaxation induced by atrial natriuretic factor. *Hypertension,* 7:306–310.

101. Oikawa, S., Imai, M., Inuzuka, C., Tawaragi, Y., Nakazato, H., and Matsuo, H. (1985): Structure of dog and rabbit precursors of atrial natriuretic polypeptides deduced from nucleotide sequence of cDNA. *Biochem. Biophys. Res. Commun.,* 132:892–899.

102. Oikawa, S., Imai, M., Ueno, A., Tanaka, S., Noguchi, T., Nakazato, H., Kanagawa, K., Fukuda, A., and Matsuo, H. (1984): Cloning and sequence analysis of cDNA encoding a precursor for human atrial natriuretic polypeptide. *Nature,* 309:724–726.

103. Pammani, M. B., Clough, D. L., Chen, J. S., Link, W. T., and Haddy, F. J. (1984): Effect of rat atrial extract on sodium transport and blood pressure in the rat. *Proc. Soc. Exp. Biol. Med.,* 176:123–131.

104. Pollock, D. M., and Banks, R. O. (1983): Effect of atrial extract on renal function in the rat. *Clin. Sci.,* 65:47–55.

105. Quirion, R., Dalpe, M., and Dam, T.-V. (1986): Characterization and distribution of receptors for the atrial natriuretic peptides in mammalian brain. *Proc. Natl. Acad. Sci. (USA),* 83:174–178.

106. Richards, A. M., Nicholls, M. G., Espiner, E. A., Ikram, H., Yandle, T. G., Joyce, S. L., and Cullens, M. M. (1985): Effects of α-human atrial natriuretic peptide in essential hypertension. *Hypertension,* 7:812–817.

107. Richards, A. M., Nicholls, M. G., Ikram, H., Webster, M. W. I., Yandle, T. G., and Espiner, E. A. (1985): Renal, haemodynamic, and hormonal effects of human alpha atrial natriuretic peptide in healthy volunteers. *Lancet,* 1:545–549.

108. Ruskoaho, H., Toth, M., and Lang, R. E. (1985): Atrial natriuretic peptide secretion: Synergistic effect of phorbol ester and A23187. *Biochem. Biophys. Res. Commun.,* 133:581–588.

109. Salazar, J., Fiksen-Olsen, M. J., Opgenorth, T. J., Granger, J. P., Burnett, J. C., Jr., and Romero, J. C. (1985): Renal hemodynamic and prostglandin (PG) effects of atrial natriuretic peptide (ANP). *Circulation [Suppl. IV],* 72:215A.

110. Samson, W. K. (1985): Atrial natriuretic factor inhibits dehydration and hemorrhage-induced vasopressin release. *Neuroendocrinology,* 40:277–279.

111. Sato, M., Abe, K., Takeuchi, K., Yasujima, M., and Yoshinaga, K. (1986): Atrial natriuretic factor and cGMP in vascular smooth muscle cells in culture. *Kidney Int.*, 29:258A.

112. Schiebinger, R. J. (1985): Dibutyryl cAMP inhibits atrial natriuretic factor secretion by rat atria in vitro. *Circulation [Suppl. III]*, 72: 310.

113. Schiffrin, E. L., Chartier, L., Thibault, G., St.-Louis, J., Cantin, M., and Genest, J. (1985): Vascular and adrenal receptors for atrial natriuretic factor in the rat. *Circ. Res.*, 56:801–807.

114. Schiffrin, E. L., Deslongchamps, M., and Thibault, G. (1985): Receptors for atrial natriuretic factor in human platelets: Characterization and effect of sodium. *Hypertension*, 7:838.

115. Schwartz, D., Geller, D. M., Manning, P. T., Siegel, N. R., Fok, K. R., Smith, C. E., and Needleman, P. (1985): Ser-Leu-Arg-Arg-atriopeptin III: The major circulating form of atrial peptide. *Science*, 229:397–400.

116. Seidman, C. E., Bloch, K. D., Klein, K. A., Smith, J. A., and Seidman, J. G. (1984): Nucleotide sequences of the human and mouse atrial natriuretic factor genes. *Science*, 226:1206–1209.

117. Seidman, C. E., Bloch, K. D., Zisfein, J. B., Smith, J. A., Haber, E., Homcy, C. J., Duby, A. D., Choi, E., Graham, R. M., and Seidman, J. G. (1985): Molecular studies of the atrial natriuretic factor gene. *Hypertension*, 7:31–34.

118. Seidman, C. E., Duby, A. D., Choi, E., Graham, R. M., Haber, E., Homcy, C. J., Smith, J. A., and Seidman, J. G. (1984): The structure of rat preproatrial natriuretic factor as defined by a complementary DNA clone. *Science*, 225:324–326.

119. Shenker, Y., Sider, R. S., Ostafin, E. A., and Grekin, R. J. (1985): Plasma levels of immunoreactive atrial natriuretic factor in healthy subjects and in patients with edema. *J. Clin. Invest.*, 76: 1684–1687.

120. Solomon, R., Taylor, M., Dorsey, D., Silva, P., and Epstein, F. H. (1985): Atriopeptin stimulation of rectal gland function in *Squalus acanthias. Am. J. Physiol.*, 249:R348.

121. Sonnenberg, H., Cupples, W. A., de Bold, A. J., and Veress, A. T. (1982): Intrarenal localization of the natriuretic effect of cardiac atrial extracts. *Can. J. Physiol. Pharmacol.*, 60:1149–1152.

122. Sonnenberg, H., and Veress, A. T. (1984): Cellular mechanisms of release of atrial natriuretic factor. *Biochem. Biophys. Res. Commun.*, 124:443–449.

123. Steigerwalt, S., Carretero, O. A., and Beierwaltes, W. H. (1986): Intrarenal effects of atrial natriuretic factor. *Kidney Int.*, 29:408A.

124. Strauss, M. B., Lamdin, E., Smith, W. P., and Bleifer, D. J. (1958): Surfeit and deficit of sodium: A kinetic concept of sodium excretion. *Arch. Intern. Med.*, 102:527–531.

125. Sugiyama, M., Fukume, H., Gammer, R. T., Misono, K. S., Yabe, Y., Morisawa, Y., and Inagami, T. (1984): Synthesis of atrial natriuretic peptides and studies on structural factors in tissue specificity. *Biochem. Biophys. Res. Commun.*, 123:338–344.

126. Tanaka, I., Misono, K. S., and Inagami, T. (1984): Atrial natriuretic factor in rat hypothalamus, atria, and plasma: Determination by specific radioimmunoassay. *Biochem. Biophys. Res. Commun.*, 124:663–668.

127. Thibault, G., Garcia, R., Cantin, M., and Genest, J. (1983): Atrial natriuretic factor: Characterization and partial purification. *Hypertension*, 5:75–80.

128. Trippodo, N. C., MacPhee, A. A., and Cole, F. E. (1983): Partially purified human and rat atrial natriuretic factor. *Hypertension [Suppl. I]*, 5:81–88.

129. Trippodo, N. C., MacPhee, A. A., Cole, F. E., and Blakesley, H. L. (1982): Partial chemical characterization of a natriuretic substance in rat atrial heart tissue. *Proc. Soc. Exp. Biol. Med.*, 170:502–528.

130. Tunny, T. J., Higgins, B. A., and Gordon, R. D. (1986): Atrial natriuretic peptide (ANP) in man in primary aldosteronism, in Gordon's syndrome and in Bartter's syndrome. *Clin. Exp. Pharmacol. Physiol., (in press).*

131. Wakitani, K., Cole, B. R., Geller, D. M., Currie, M. G., Fok, K. F., and Needleman, P. (1985): Atriopeptins: Correlation between renal vasodilation and natriuresis. *Am. J. Physiol.*, 249: F49–F53.

132. Waldman, S. A., Rapoport, R. M., and Murad, F. (1984): Atrial natriuretic factor selectively activates particulate guanylate cyclase and elevates cyclic GMP in rat tissues. *J. Biol. Chem.*, 259: 14332–14334.

133. Wangler, R. D., Breuhaus, B. A., Otero, H. O., Hastings, D. A., Holzman, M. D., Saneii, H. H., Sparks, H. V., Jr., and Chimoskey, J. E. (1985): Coronary vasoconstrictor effects of atriopeptin II. *Science*, 230:558–561.

134. Winquist, R. J., Faison, E. P., Waldman, S. A., Schwartz, K., Murad, F., and Rapoport, R. M. (1984): Atrial natriuretic factor elicits an endothelium-independent relaxation and activates particulate guanylate cyclase in vascular smooth muscle. *Proc. Natl. Acad. Sci. (USA)*, 81:7661–7664.

135. Yamaji, T., Ishibashi, M., Nakaoka, H., Imataka, K., Amono, M., and J. Fujii. (1985): Possible role for atrial natriuretic peptide in polyuria associated with paroxysmal atrial arrhythmias. *Lancet*, 1:1211.

136. Yamaji, T., Ishibashi, M., and Takaku, F. (1985): Atrial natriuretic factor in human blood. *J. Clin. Invest.*, 76:1705–1709.

137. Yamanaka, M., Greenberg, B., Johnson, L., Seilhamer, J., Brewer, M., Friedemann, T., Miller, J., Atlas, S., Laragh, J., Lewicki, J., and Fiddes, J. (1984): Cloning and sequence analysis of the cDNA for the rat atrial natriuretic factor precursor. *Nature*, 309: 719–722.

138. Yandle, T. G., Crozier, I., Espiner, E. A., Ikram, H., and Nicholls, M. G. (1985): Production, plasma levels, and clearance of atrial natriuretic peptide in man. *Hypertension*, 7:838A.

139. Yip, C. C., Laing, L. P., and Flynn, T. G. (1985): Photoaffinity labeling of atrial natriuretic factor receptors of rat kidney cortex plasma membranes. *J. Biol. Chem.*, 260:8229–8232.

140. Zisfein, J. B., Graham, R. M., and Homcy, C. J. (1986): Purification and characterization of the serum protease that cleaves pro-atrial natriuretic factor (PRO-ANF) to ANF. *Clin. Res., (in press).*

141. Zisfein, J. B., Matsueda, G. R., Fallon, J. T., Seidman, C. E., Seidman, J. G., Homcy, C. J., and Graham, R. M. (1985): Immunologic analysis of the structure of rat atrial natriuretic factor. *Clin. Res.*, 33:240A.

The Heart and Cardiovascular System,
edited by H. A. Fozzard et al.
Raven Press, New York © 1986.

CHAPTER 66

Digitalis

Eduardo Marban and Thomas W. Smith

In this chapter we shall consider selected aspects of current research related to fundamental aspects of digitalis glycosides. Clinical pharmacology and use are not covered, nor are hemodynamic and neurally mediated effects; these topics, together with manifestations and treatment of digitalis toxicity, recently have been reviewed elsewhere (211).

EXCITATION-CONTRACTION COUPLING IN MAMMALIAN HEART MUSCLE

Excitation and contraction in heart are linked by a series of events that alter the intracellular calcium activity $[Ca^{2+}]_i$ and its capacity to activate the contractile proteins. Each major structural element of the cardiac cell participates in the regulation of $[Ca^{2+}]_i$, and each must be considered as a potential locus for the effects of cardiotonic agents such as digitalis. Surface-membrane mechanisms control Ca entry into the cell, as well as extrusion of Ca from the cell interior. The sarcoplasmic reticulum (SR) releases and takes up Ca during the cardiac cycle. The contractile proteins sense an increase in $[Ca^{2+}]_i$ and convert this signal into mechanical force, as Ca binds to troponin and disinhibits the interaction of actin and myosin. Despite its primacy, the regulation of $[Ca^{2+}]_i$ is not the sole mechanism for modulation of contractility. The $[Ca^{2+}]$ dependence of contractile-protein activation

is itself subject to modulation, so that myofilament sensitivity must be considered when investigating the inotropic effects of pharmacologic agents.

Surface Membrane: Ionic Channels

The first step leading to cardiac contraction is depolarization of the surface membrane of each cell. Depolarization normally occurs in the form of an action potential, which represents the concerted response of the ionic channels in the surface membrane. Cardiac action potentials are of two general types, fast and slow responses, whose characteristics are reviewed in *Chapter* 31. Both types of action potential are associated with force production in the form of a twitch.

The ionic channels participating in cardiac excitation are of various types, but they share some basic features. All are thought to be integral membrane proteins spanning the surface membrane, with "gates" determining whether or not the channel is open at any given instant, and pores allowing ions to traverse the channel when it is open. Each type of channel is distinctive and can be characterized by three properties: (a) its *permeation* characteristics, including the conductance of a single channel, its selectivity, and the capacity to distinguish among the many ions present in aqueous solution near the mouth of the channel; (b) its *gating* characteristics, i.e., the probability that the channel will be open at any given potential and time; (c) its *pharmacologic sensitivity.*

Ionic channels function in ensemble, with each population of channels giving rise to a macroscopic ionic current. The voltage-clamp technique, which will be reviewed later (see also *Chapter* 32), has been used to identify the various ionic currents present in cardiac cells. The current most important in generating the cardiac contraction is the Ca current, I_{Ca}, which is activated in the plateau range of potentials (above -60 mV) (152,192). This current, carried by Ca channels, underlies plateau depolarization during fast-response action potentials, as well as the upstroke of slow responses. The kinetics are characterized by rapid (<5 msec) activation, followed by a slower multiexponential decline (117). When examined in isolation using the patch voltage-clamp technique (see *Chapter* 31), the single Ca channels composing I_{Ca} have conductances in the range of 15 pico-Siemens (pS) (194), a value similar to that for Ca channels in other tissues. I_{Ca} is blocked by inorganic ions such as cobalt and lanthanum, as well as by various organic molecules, including verapamil and nifedipine. I_{Ca} is augmented by β-adrenergic stimulation and, under certain conditions, by digitalis (*vide infra*) (175,221).

Pharmacologic blockade of Ca channels reduces or totally abolishes cardiac contraction, as does removal of extracellular Ca. On the other hand, agents that are associated with an increase in I_{Ca} generally increase force. Beyond this general correlation, it is still uncertain what fraction of Ca ions activating contraction arrives by direct influx through the Ca channels in the surface membrane [see Marban and Wier (154) for a pharmacologic approach to this question in Purkinje fibers]. Functional evidence in mammalian heart argues for an intimate but indirect link between tension and I_{Ca}, as summarized in *Chapter* 36. This conclusion is supported by a number of studies showing dissociation between tension and I_{Ca} when Ca release from intracellular stores is reduced (162). The positive inotropic effect of agents that act by augmenting I_{Ca} is at least partly explained by an increase in the amount of Ca released by the SR.

Ca channels are modulated by several mechanisms, with cyclic nucleotides and $[Ca^{2+}]_i$ as recognized second messengers. Catecholamines, which augment contraction, increase I_{Ca} by increasing adenylate cyclase activity (40). This, in turn, increases intracellular cAMP concentration, which leads to an increase in the number of functional Ca channels and/or an increase in the probability of channel opening (24,36). Conversely, parasympathetic agonists decrease Ca current and contractile force, effects that may be mediated in part by a rise in cGMP (220) but also involve reduced cAMP levels. Digitalis alters I_{Ca} via changes in $[Ca^{2+}]_i$ (153), which has dual effects on I_{Ca}, as will be discussed at greater length later.

In an approach complementary to electrophysiologic techniques, traditional methods of receptor biochemistry have been applied in an effort to characterize (and, ultimately, to isolate) ionic channels. The highly specific pharmacologic sensitivity of an individual channel type is exploited by radiolabeling agonists or antagonists, exposing them to intact or fragmented cells or tissue, and observing their binding and/or displacement by unlabeled ligand. This approach has already proved fruitful in the characterization of the nitrendipine receptor, which is presumed to be part of the Ca channel. Although initial studies with fragmented tissue reported only very high affinity binding inconsistent with electrophysiologic estimates of channel blockade, Marsh et al. (154a) have identified a second low-affinity binding mode in intact cultured heart cell monolayers. Part of the apparent discrepancy between electrophysiologic and biochemical data may arise from differences in membrane potentials in intact and fragmented tissues, because dihydropyridine Ca channel antagonists and agonists bind preferentially to inactivated channels (21,112).

Although we have spoken of the Ca channel as a single entity, ample evidence is emerging to indicate that there are at least two distinct types of Ca channels in a wide variety of cell types, including heart cells (22). The predominant type, corresponding to the "traditional" Ca current measured from holding potentials of -50 mV and above, is open longer than the second type, which becomes available only at negative holding potentials and inactivates rapidly with depolarization. More experiments will be required to determine the functions of the two Ca channel types in heart cells.

Surface Membrane: Ca-Efflux Pathways

The surface membrane not only allows phasic Ca influx during depolarization but also controls Ca extrusion. Sodium-calcium (Na-Ca) exchange occurs via a carrier mechanism that can use the electrochemical-energy gradient of Na across the surface membrane to drive Ca from the cell, so that Na entry via the carrier is coupled to Ca extrusion (given the normal Na and Ca gradients). The existence of this mechanism helps explain the well-known effects of Na on contraction. For example, removal of Na_o leads to a contracture, usually explained by net Ca influx via Na-Ca exchange. The most widely accepted hypothesis for the positive inotropic effect of digitalis invokes Na-Ca exchange to link a rise in Na_i to increased contractility. Digitalis compounds inhibit the NaK-ATPase enzyme complex that maintains the normal Na gradient across the sarcolemma. If this gradient is reduced, $[Ca^{2+}]_i$ will increase to a new, higher level, leading to increased availability of activator Ca and therefore to increased force. This is commonly known as the Na-pump lag hypothesis and will be discussed subsequently in more detail.

Despite the common assumption that the Na-Ca

carrier functions principally to extrude Ca from the cell, it is still unclear how many Na^+ are countertransported with each Ca^{2+}. Multiple experimental approaches have been used in an attempt to answer this question, with results ranging from 2 to 6 Na^+ per Ca^{2+} (68). Any stoichiometry above 2:1 is expected to produce a net membrane current, i.e., to be electrogenic, and such a stoichiometry appears to be required if the Na gradient is the sole energy source used to maintain $[Ca^{2+}]_i$ at its low resting level. Attempts to measure the current generated by Na-Ca exchange are difficult to interpret because of likely interference from Ca^{2+}- and/or Na^+-activated membrane conductances. Progress has been hampered by the lack of a specific Na-Ca exchange inhibitor.

The existence of Na-Ca exchange explains the importance of $[Na]_i$ as a determinant of myocardial contractility. In general, an increase in $[Na^+]_i$ will lead to an increase in $[Ca^{2+}]_i$. In addition to NaK-ATPase inhibition, which decreases Na efflux, $[Na^+]_i$ can rise as a result of increased influx through voltage-dependent Na channels. These channels underlie the upstroke of fast-response action potentials; the amount of Na entering the cell through these channels parallels the stimulation frequency (52,58). Influx also increases when Na-channel gating is modified chemically by ceveratrum alkaloids or other toxins that increase the open-state probability. Substantial progress has been made in biochemical characterization of Na channels, culminating recently in cloning of the channel gene isolated from eel electric organ (176). Along with receptor-binding and electrophysiologic techniques, the molecular biologic approach will be instrumental in increasing our understanding of Na channels in particular and transmembrane pathways in general.

Na-Ca exchange has generally been assumed to be the major route for Ca removal from the cell, but an ATP-dependent sarcolemmal Ca pump operates in parallel with the exchange (43). This pump appears to be chemically distinct from the Ca^{2+}-ATPase in the SR; studies to date imply that it forms a low-capacity but high-affinity Ca^{2+}-efflux system. The relative contributions of these two systems to Ca extrusion have yet to be determined, but the existence of an alternative pathway may help explain the puzzling observation that Na_o removal does not invariably lead to a large increase in tension or $[Ca^{2+}]_i$ (151) and that increases in tension are transient despite the continuing absence of Na_o.

Sarcoplasmic Reticulum

The SR constitutes another major locus for $[Ca^{2+}]_i$ regulation. Ca release from the SR plays a central role in excitation-contraction (E-C) coupling, and Ca uptake by the SR is important for relaxation of tension. The SR is entirely intracellular, but its terminal cisternae are apposed to the sarcolemma at specialized sites (see *Chapter* 4). In skeletal muscle, where contraction is not markedly dependent on Ca_o, an electrical signal is believed to initiate SR Ca release directly (200). In contrast, cardiac muscle is dependent on Ca influx for contraction; depolarization per se is not sufficient.

In heart, the entering Ca is thought to act as the signal for Ca release by the SR in a process known as Ca-induced Ca release. This mechanism amplifies the small $[Ca^{2+}]_i$ increment directly attributable to entry into a much larger rise in $[Ca^{2+}]_i$. The evidence for this phenomenon comes principally from mechanically skinned cardiac cells in which the sarcolemma is dissected away, leaving only the myofilament space and the SR. In such preparations, a small rapid increase in bathing $[Ca^{2+}]$ triggers tension oscillations attributed to Ca release from the SR (79,80). Ca-induced Ca release can also occur in skinned skeletal muscle fibers, but in that tissue it is suppressed by physiologic Mg concentrations (76). Such Mg levels do not inhibit Ca release in skinned cardiac cells.

Ca-induced Ca release explains many features of E-C coupling, including the dissociation of I_{Ca} and force when SR Ca stores are depleted (164). However, it hinges on observations in skinned cells, in which the SR is swollen and perhaps functionally aberrant. Thus, it is encouraging that certain observations in intact preparations are most readily explained by invoking Ca-induced Ca release. For example, in digitalis-intoxicated Purkinje fibers (or in K_o-depleted solutions, where NaK-ATPase is also inhibited), $[Ca^{2+}]_i$ increases, and this rise is associated with oscillations in tension like those seen in skinned cells (124). Under similar conditions, oscillations in $[Ca^{2+}]_i$ have been documented directly using aequorin (179,231); these oscillations are abolished by the SR Ca-transport inhibitors caffeine and ryanodine (231). Such results provide evidence for Ca-induced Ca release in intact preparations, at least under conditions of increased cellular Ca loading.

Like the other elements in E-C coupling, the SR is subject to modulation. Experiments with SR membrane vesicles have demonstrated an increased rate of Ca uptake after phosphorylation of a specific membrane protein, phospholamban, by cAMP-dependent protein kinase (127) and also by protein kinase C and calmodulin-dependent protein kinase (167). Catecholamines, by increasing intracellular cAMP, enhance Ca uptake by the SR. An increased rate of uptake is presumed to contribute to the relaxant effects of catecholamines on tension, i.e., the increased rate of twitch relaxation and the attenuation of contracture tension (163). Operating in parallel with cAMP, $[Ca^{2+}]_i$ itself leads to phosphorylation of phospholamban, as a consequence of interaction with the regulatory protein calmodulin (149). Such multiple regulatory mechanisms can provide sensitive control over $[Ca^{2+}]$ transport.

Myofilaments

The ultimate level of contractile regulation lies not in the SR or the surface membrane but rather in the myofilaments themselves. In this case the variable is not $[Ca^{2+}]_i$, but rather the *sensitivity* to $[Ca^{2+}]_i$. In skinned fibers, myofilament sensitivity changes can be measured as changes in the steady-state pCa-tension relation, so that a given $[Ca^{2+}]$ results in either an increase or a decrease in contractile activation (234). The biochemical basis for these effects centers around changes in the Ca^{2+} affinity of troponin C.

Various factors that alter the force of contraction may do so by changing myofilament Ca sensitivity. The best known of these factors is an increase in muscle length, which increases the force of contraction over a broad range (the Frank-Starling effect) (see *Chapter* 40). In skinned fibers, an increase in length has been reported to increase myofilament Ca sensitivity, manifested as a shift of the steady-state pCa–tension curve to higher pCa values (a leftward shift in the usual convention for plotting such curves) (113). This observation provides an alternative to the traditional myofilament-overlap explanation for the Frank-Starling effect. Another manifestation of this phenomenon has been observed with rapid length changes in aequorin-injected ventricular muscle, in which shortening is associated with an increment in luminescence (10). The extra luminescence reflects Ca^{2+} release from troponin as a result of decreased Ca^{2+} affinity when the muscle shortens. The detailed molecular mechanisms remain to be determined.

Another variable affecting myofilament Ca sensitivity is pH. Fabiato and Fabiato (79,80) found that a decrease in the pH of a solution bathing skinned fibers depressed myofilament Ca sensitivity. This finding was consistent with Katz and Hecht's hypothesis (126) that such a change might explain early pump failure during ischemia, possibly because of competition between H^+ and Ca^{2+} for binding to an activator site on troponin C. Intracellular acidification also occurs with exposure to high concentrations of digitalis (59).

Hormones and drugs can also act on myofilament sensitivity. McClellan and Winegrad (160), using a hyperpermeable rat ventricular preparation, found that high levels of cAMP reduced myofilament sensitivity, an effect potentiated by phosphodiesterase inhibition. Cyclic GMP had the opposite effect. Catecholamines increase cAMP; the observed reduction in Ca sensitivity seems paradoxical in light of the positive inotropic effect of catecholamines on twitch force. However, catecholamines also shorten the twitch and actually *decrease* contracture tension, effects compatible with a decrease in Ca sensitivity. Although compelling, the evidence available is predominantly from hyperpermeable or myofibrillar preparations, and the physiologic importance of these findings remains to be determined. As will be discussed subsequently, there is no evidence that changes in myofilament sensitivity underlie the positive inotropy of digitalis, although such changes may contribute to the decline in force that occurs in advanced digitalis intoxication.

Until recently it had been impossible to determine the steady-state relationship between $[Ca^{2+}]_i$ and force in intact heart tissue. Such measurements would allow assessment of the physiologic importance of modulatory mechanisms identified in skinned muscles. Yue et al. (235) have recently measured $[Ca^{2+}]_i$ and force at steady state during tetani in intact papillary muscles, an approach that may prove fruitful in future studies of myofilament sensitivity.

Depolarization activates I_{Ca}, allowing entry of Ca ions down their steep concentration gradient, thereby increasing $[Ca^{2+}]_i$. Even a small increase in $[Ca^{2+}]_i$ may act as a signal for Ca release from the SR. Ca ions bind to troponin C and allow actin and myosin to interact, producing force. The amount of force varies with changes in myofilament sensitivity. Relaxation occurs as Ca ions dissociate from troponin and are either sequestered by the SR or extruded from the cell. Using this simplified framework, we can proceed to consider the mechanism of action of digitalis in a cellular context.

EFFECTS OF DIGITALIS

Inotropic Effects of Cardiac Glycosides

By the late 1920s it was evident that digitalis evokes a positive inotropic effect on the intact ventricle, with a consequent increase in the rate of rise of intracavitary pressure during isovolumic systole with heart rate and aortic pressure kept constant (233). Cattell and Gold (46) first demonstrated a direct increase in force generation in isolated cardiac muscle in response to ouabain, and it was soon evident that this effect is manifest in normal as well as failing cardiac muscle. Cardiac glycoside administration causes the ventricular-function (Frank-Starling) curve of the intact heart to shift upward and to the left, so that more stroke work is generated at a given filling pressure. This is true of both right and left ventricles, and of atrial as well as ventricular myocardium. Force–velocity curves for isolated cardiac muscle, as would be expected, are shifted in parallel upward and to the right by cardioactive steroids (215). These effects appear to be sustained during *in vivo* administration of digitalis, at least over periods of weeks to months, without evidence of desensitization or tachyphylaxis (13,146). The time to peak force generation and the relaxation rates are altered little by subtoxic doses or concentrations of cardioactive steroids (188), but the positive inotropic effect observed is highly dependent on contraction frequency (134), declining on either side of an intermediate frequency yielding maximal inotropic response.

It is now generally agreed that digitalis compounds bring about an increase in the availability of activator Ca in heart cells (8,9,166,232). There are two principal questions with regard to the mechanism of digitalis action: (a) Does the increase in $[Ca^{2+}]_i$ suffice to explain the inotropic and arrhythmogenic effects of digitalis? (b) How does the increase in $[Ca^{2+}]_i$ arise? We shall summarize evidence indicating that the increase in $[Ca^{2+}]_i$ is indeed sufficient and that this increase arises from NaK-ATPase inhibition.

The most direct evidence for a rise in $[Ca^{2+}]_i$ during digitalis inotropy comes from studies using the Ca-activated photoprotein aequorin (32). Although several approaches are available for measuring $[Ca^{2+}]_i$ (vide infra), aequorin is the only indicator widely available at present that has rapid responsiveness while not buffering intracellular Ca, thereby yielding useful estimates of the $[Ca^{2+}]_i$ transient during twitch contractions. During the inotropic effect of digitalis, there is a close association between the increase in peak systolic aequorin luminescence (directly related to $[Ca^{2+}]_i$) and the increase in twitch force (232), as illustrated in Fig. 1. Panel A shows the action potential, aequorin luminescence, and twitch under control conditions in a dog Purkinje fiber. After 25 min of exposure to 100-nM ouabain (B), the action potential is not much changed, but systolic aequorin luminescence and the twitch are both markedly augmented.

The issue whether or not *diastolic* $[Ca^{2+}]_i$ rises with digitalis has important mechanistic implications, in that most theories (in their simplest form) predict increases in both diastolic and systolic $[Ca^{2+}]_i$. Unfortunately, there is little evidence to indicate whether or not a rise in diastolic $[Ca^{2+}]_i$ is invariably associated with the positive inotropic effect. Although there is no indication

of a rise in aequorin luminescence during the positive inotropic effect illustrated in Fig. 1B, this may be because aequorin is not a sensitive indicator at low levels of $[Ca^{2+}]_i$. Experiments using other techniques in beating heart tissue [e.g., Ca-sensitive microelectrodes (58), Ca^{45} accumulation (28)] confirm that there is a rise in overall $[Ca^{2+}]_i$ during the positive inotropic effect, but the limited time responsiveness of the measurements precludes further resolution. If there is a rise in diastolic $[Ca^{2+}]_i$ during the early inotropic effect, it is likely to be small [less than 200 nM above diastolic levels before drug, according to Wier and Hess (232)], suggesting that an amplifying mechanism (such as enhanced I_{Ca}) may be required for full expression of the inotropic effect.

During exposure to high concentrations of digitalis, isolated myocardial preparations manifest small unstimulated contractions and depolarizations following action potentials, as illustrated in Fig. 1C after 47 min of exposure to ouabain (see ref. 222 for review). These oscillatory events coincide with the development of digitalis-toxic arrhythmias (such as premature ventricular contractions) in intact animals exposed to the same concentrations of digitalis (196). There is no doubt that systolic and diastolic $[Ca^{2+}]_i$ both increase during the arrhythmogenic effect of digitalis, as manifested by the increased aequorin luminescence accompanying aftercontractions and afterdepolarizations (Fig. 1C). Such an increase in $[Ca^{2+}]_i$ was first inferred from changes in tension (81,123) and led to the idea that intracellular "Ca overload" contributes to the arrhythmogenic effects. In this formulation, $[Ca^{2+}]_i$ increases progressively, until the SR is no longer capable of retaining all the Ca that is taken up with each cycle. Spontaneous cycles of Ca release and reuptake ensue (137,179,231). These cycles are brought into phase by stimulated activity (124,216), resulting in the aftercontraction. The associated afterdepolarization is the result of a Ca-activated transient

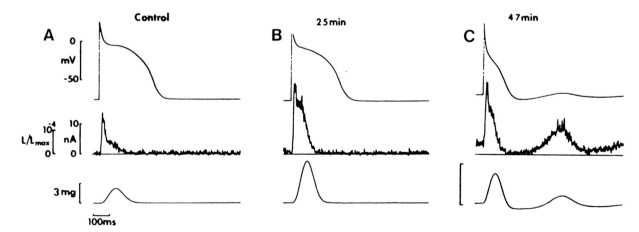

FIG. 1. Calcium transients measured with aequorin during exposure to digitalis. Simultaneous signal-averaged recordings of membrane potential, aequorin luminescence, and tension in a canine cardiac Purkinje fiber before **(A)** and during **(B,** 25 min; **C,** 47 min) exposure to 100-nM ouabain. (From ref. 232, with permission.)

inward current (123) thought to be the macroscopic manifestation of Ca-activated nonspecific cation channels (12,55). The fundamental link is the increase in cellular Ca loading. In this formulation, the inotropic and arrhythmic effects of digitalis constitute a spectrum dependent on the overall level of intracellular Ca loading.

The effects of antiarrhythmic drugs that decrease transient inward current often appear to be attributable to a decrease in cellular Ca loading. For example, the reduction in transient inward current produced by lidocaine is thought to occur because it blocks Na influx and reduces Na loading and, in turn, Ca loading (72,73), thereby decreasing the propensity for oscillatory Ca release. Ca-channel blockers, which reduce digitalis-induced afterdepolarizations (197), may do so indirectly by inhibiting Ca influx and thereby decreasing $[Ca^{2+}]_i$.

Chemistry and Structure-Activity Relationships

The sources and chemistry of the cardiac glycosides are extensively considered in standard texts (103,155). By about 1960, structural determinants required for cardiotonic activity of digitalis glycosides seemed to be evident (218). These included a steroidal 14β-hydroxy skeleton with cis, trans, and cis configurations at the A-B, B-C, and C-D ring junctions, respectively. An unsaturated lactone (γ-lactone or α-pyrone) as a 17β side chain and 3β-oriented oxygen function in the form of an OH group of glycosidic linkage were considered requisite. The distance between the carbonyl group of the lactone and the C_3 oxygen function (electronegative poles) was considered critical. Sugar components were recognized to be important pharmacokinetically, but not to the fundamental pharmacodynamic properties of these drugs. More recent synthesis work has occasioned some modifications of these precepts.

The 3-desoxy derivative of digitoxigenin was synthesized by Saito et al. (198) and found to be nearly as active as the latter compound. A-B trans compounds have been reported to be highly active (181). The C_{14} OH group is not essential, although substitution by -H yields considerably less active derivatives (178). Although certainly an important determinant, the cis β configuration of the C and D rings appears to be less than absolutely necessary, because synthetic derivatives of prednisone and prednisolone have appreciable biological activity despite their 14α-H structures (138). The β orientation of the C_{17} side chain appears to be essential, but the position of attachment of the butenolide ring to the 17β site does not. Thomas et al. (219) have studied the role of the 17β side chain extensively and have demonstrated activity in trans acrylic acid methyl ester and trans acrylonitrile C_{17} derivatives. The distribution of electron density in the 17β side chain does seem to be decisive, and there is evidence suggesting that the

part of the receptor that interacts with the C_{17} side chain lies within a cleft (207). Further insights into the importance of the chemistry of the C_{17} functional group are available from the recent work of From et al. (88).

The ultimate goal of structure-activity studies, apart from insights into the fundamental nature of interactions of cardiac glycosides with NaK-ATPase, is the recognition or discovery of compounds with improved therapeutic ratios. One hopes that this goal will be realized, but studies of several hundred cardiac glycosides and aglycones over many decades have yielded remarkably similar therapeutic ratios, as might be anticipated if toxic manifestations are a consequence of a greater degree of occupancy of the same receptor, i.e., NaK-ATPase, that mediates the therapeutic (inotropic) effects.

Inhibition of NaK-ATPase

All cardioactive steroids share the property of being potent and highly specific inhibitors of transmembrane movement of Na^+ and K^+ mediated by the intrinsic membrane monovalent-cation active-transport protein NaK-ATPase, the enzymatic equivalent of the "sodium pump." This Mg^{2+}- and ATP-dependent, Na^+- and K^+-activated transport enzyme complex consists of two polypeptide subunits, termed α (about 100 kd) and β (a sialoglycoprotein with a mass of approximately 50 kd), that occur in 1:1 stoichiometry. A 12-kd proteolipid component tends to copurify, but is not known to be essential to the activity of the enzyme complex (84). One cardiac glycoside binding site is present per α chain; optimal binding requires Na^+, Mg^{2+}, and ATP (202) and results in complete inhibition of enzymatic and transport functions of each NaK-ATPase site occupied. NaK-ATPase is generally agreed to be the receptor for the biological actions of digitalis glycosides. The term "receptor," as used here, although well established, has a somewhat different connotation from its use in relation to, for example, the β-adrenergic or muscarinic cholinergic receptor. Blinks (*personal communication*) has therefore questioned the term "receptor" for NaK-ATPase in relation to digitalis, likening it to calling a machine the receptor for a monkey wrench.

Earlier evidence supporting a role for NaK-ATPase as a receptor for the inotropic action of digitalis glycosides includes the following:

1. NaK-ATPase is inhibited by cardioactive analogues but not by inactive analogues; a close relationship has been demonstrated between potency for NaK-ATPase inhibition and cardiac activity (83).

2. Cardiac glycoside sensitivity in various species is closely correlated with the ability of glycosides to inhibit myocardial NaK-ATPase of that species. The rat, for

example, is highly resistant to the cardiac actions of digitalis, and the myocardial NaK-ATPase of the rat is about 100 times less sensitive to digitalis glycosides than is NaK-ATPase from sensitive species such as dog or cat (11).

3. The time course of NaK-ATPase inhibition is similar to the time course for inotropic effects in the hearts of species studied, with regard to both onset and offset of inotropic effects (3).

4. Enhancement of the positive inotropic and toxic effects of digitalis glycosides occurs under conditions that increase intracellular Na^+ concentration, including paired stimulation or the presence of drugs that increase Na^+ influx (5). Digitalis-induced inotropy is delayed under conditions that reduce intracellular Na^+ concentration, such as low extracellular Na^+ concentration (5) or tetrodotoxin (227).

5. Several interventions, including low temperature, increased extracellular K^+ concentration, and low pH, all have parallel tendencies to reduce both the inotropic effect and the inhibition of NaK-ATPase by cardiac glycosides (210).

6. An independent intervention that inhibits NaK-ATPase activity, reduction in extracellular K^+ concentration, exerts similar positive inotropic effects, a similar degree of NaK-ATPase inhibition, and similar enhancement of intracellular sodium content (19). In the intact dog, doses of digitalis glycosides producing positive inotropic effects inhibit NaK-ATPase activity in myocardial enzyme preparations from the heart of the same animal (2).

7. Serial myocardial biopsy studies have demonstrated that sustained subtoxic plasma and myocardial cardiac glycoside concentrations producing a positive inotropic effect cause inhibition of myocardial monovalent-cation transport capacity (114,213).

8. Relatively high concentrations of extracellular K^+ slow the rate of cardiac glycoside binding by myocardium and also slow the onset of inotropic effect, as well as the rate of binding of cardiac glycosides to NaK-ATPase (187). The well-known ability of K^+ to suppress clinical digitalis intoxication supports this set of observations.

9. The erythrophleum alkaloids differ chemically from the digitalis glycosides, but they share both the ability to inhibit NaK-ATPase and the ability to produce a positive inotropic effect (33).

10. NaK-ATPase inhibitors, including *N*-ethylmaleimide and parachloromercuribenzoate, produce positive inotropic effects accompanied by inhibition of NaK-ATPase. Monovalent cations such as Rb^+ and Tl^+ that inhibit NaK-ATPase in the presence of Na^+ and K^+ produce sustained positive inotropic effects in isolated cardiac muscle (1). Tl^+ concentrations and digitalis levels that are equieffective in inhibiting the Na^+ pump produce comparable increases in myocardial contractility.

Theories for the Positive Inotropic Effect of Cardiac Glycosides

Sodium-Pump Lag

Having defined a highly specific interaction between digitalis glycosides and NaK-ATPase, it remains to determine the basis for coupling of this interaction with the observed inotropic effects of digitalis on the intact heart. More than 50 years ago, Calhoun and Harrison (41) documented a net K^+ efflux from myocardium after toxic cardiac glycoside doses. Subsequent studies have confirmed decreases in intracellular K^+ and, in some instances, increases in intracellular Na^+ in responses to high, toxic doses or concentrations of digitalis glycosides, whereas results with subtoxic but inotropic doses have been more equivocal (147). The seminal contributions of Repke and colleagues deserve particular credit in the development of the sodium-pump lag hypothesis (189,190).

Studies using isotope-flux and washout techniques supported the view that positive inotropic effects of cardiac glycosides are accompanied by net K^+ loss and a gain in Na^+, accompanied by a net accumulation of intracellular Ca^{2+} (139). Overt toxicity was accompanied by further changes in the same direction, but of greater magnitude. Important direct evidence supporting the presence of cardiac-glycoside-induced increases in intracellular Na^+ is now available from ion-sensitive microelectrode studies (*vide infra*).

How might inhibition of the Na^+ pump, with consequent accumulation of intracellular Na^+, result in a positive inotropic effect? It has been postulated that this might result from exchange of intracellular Na^+ for extracellular Ca^{2+}, as has been observed in the squid giant axon (15), as well as mammalian myocardium (96). The proposed sequence is as follows:

$$\text{cardiac glycoside} \atop {\downarrow \atop \downarrow \text{Na pump}} \xrightarrow{\text{Na-Ca} \atop \text{exchange}} \uparrow[Na^+]_i \rightarrow \uparrow[Ca^{2+}]_i \rightarrow \uparrow\text{contractile force}$$

This mechanism is consistent with the well-known dependence of digitalis-induced inotropy on the number and rate of contractions following drug exposure (134). Transmembrane influx of Na^+ occurring with each action potential, together with reduced outward Na^+ transport, leads to increased Na^+ content in the myocardial cell. At rapid heart rates, Na^+ influx may be of sufficient magnitude to provide the maximum level of intracellular Na^+ that can be utilized, thus accounting for the diminished inotropic effects of digitalis at high frequencies. It is possible, as suggested by Akera and Brody (4), that most or all of the sodium entering the cell during a single beat could be extruded by the end of that beat, but over a longer time period in the presence of digitalis glycosides. This could account for enhanced availability of activator Ca via Na^+-Ca^{2+} exchange without net accumulation of intracellular Na^+, although the hypothesis is not readily testable using current techniques.

Studies using cultured myocardial cells have demonstrated direct correlations between ouabain-induced positive inotropic effects and inhibition of monovalent-cation active transport, as well as enhanced intracellular contents of both Na^+ and Ca^{2+} (28). Further support is provided by studies demonstrating that decreased extracellular K^+ produces positive inotropic effects equivalent to those of cardiac glycosides at similar levels of Na^+-transport inhibition, similar increases in intracellular Na^+, and similar enhancement of Na^+-Ca^{2+} exchange (19).

Displacement of a Labile Ca^{2+} Pool

It has been argued that the positive inotropic effect of digitalis, although dependent on specific binding to NaK-ATPase, does not depend on inhibition of monovalent-cation active transport. It is difficult to exclude the possibility that more direct interactions between NaK-ATPase and release of Ca^{2+} during E-C coupling could be modified by digitalis glycosides, as suggested by Lüllmann and colleagues (93,150). Direct experimental evidence for this interesting theory has been difficult to obtain by available techniques.

Sodium-Pump Stimulation

Evidence from several laboratories suggests that low concentrations of cardiac glycosides may, under some circumstances, produce apparent stimulation of monovalent-cation active transport. This observation has been made most frequently in systems consisting of intact myocardium or Purkinje fibers with their endogenous pools of norepinephrine and acetylcholine. Noble (174) has discussed in detail the evidence that pump stimulation may occur at low but positively inotropic concentrations of cardiac glycosides.

Catecholamine Release

It is well known that high concentrations of cardiac glycosides will stimulate the release, and block the reuptake, of norepinephrine from adrenergic nerve terminals in intact myocardium (203,211). Consequently, these phenomena have been suggested to be causally related to the inotropic effects of cardiac glycosides under some circumstances. We have demonstrated that low concentrations of cardiac glycosides in the nanomolar range stimulate the sodium pump by a mechanism involving the action of endogenous catecholamine stores (114). It seems unlikely, however, that catecholamines are involved in the major positive inotropic effects of cardiac glycosides that are of clinical and pharmacologic interest (133). Nevertheless, these effects may contribute under selected circumstances and can potentially complicate the interpretation of experimental results. Useful approaches include depletion of catecholamine stores from intact myocardium by the use of reserpine or 6-OH-dopamine, as well as the use of specific adrenergic and muscarinic blocking agents (140).

Enhanced Calcium Current

One way in which digitalis compounds could produce an increase in $[Ca^{2+}]_i$ would be by increasing Ca influx through sarcolemmal Ca channels (86,125). Although an increase in the related Ca current (also called "slow inward current") was not found in many early studies (for review, see ref. 153), reexamination of the question by Weingart et al. (228) provided evidence that increased Ca current in fact accompanies digitalis inotropy in Purkinje fibers. Marban and Tsien (153) extended this observation to mammalian ventricle: Figure 2 shows membrane potential, current, and tension during depolarizing voltage-clamp pulses in a ferret papillary muscle before and during exposure to ouabain. The increase in inward current associated with the increase in force was interpreted as an increase in I_{Ca}. This interpretation was confirmed in Purkinje fibers using a new technique for blocking outward currents that had clouded the previous measurements of I_{Ca}. Marban and Tsien also proposed a mechanism for the increase in I_{Ca}: A small increase in $[Ca^{2+}]_i$ (by Na-pump lag or any other mechanism) acts as a positive-feedback signal to increase I_{Ca} ("positive regulation" of Ca channels by $[Ca^{2+}]_i$). This conclusion was based on several lines of evidence, including abolition of the increase in I_{Ca} when $[Ca^{2+}]_i$ was buffered by intracellular EGTA (Fig. 2C). A similar mechanism was proposed by Lederer and Eisner (141) to explain the changes in membrane current they observed during NaK-ATPase inhibition by K_o withdrawal.

The relative contribution of increased I_{Ca} to the inotropic effect of digitalis is still undetermined. One way in which it could be important is in amplifying small changes in diastolic $[Ca^{2+}]_i$ to much larger changes in systolic $[Ca^{2+}]_i$. The increase in I_{Ca} also helps explain the prolongation of the cardiac action potential seen in various tissues on exposure to cardiotonic steroids (for review, see ref. 211). On the other hand, a positive inotropic effect can seemingly occur without an increase in I_{Ca} in frog ventricle (50,100), in mammalian heart when strontium replaces Ca as the cation activating tension (153), and with high concentrations of digitalis (228). In this regard, it should be noted that $[Ca^{2+}]_i$ also

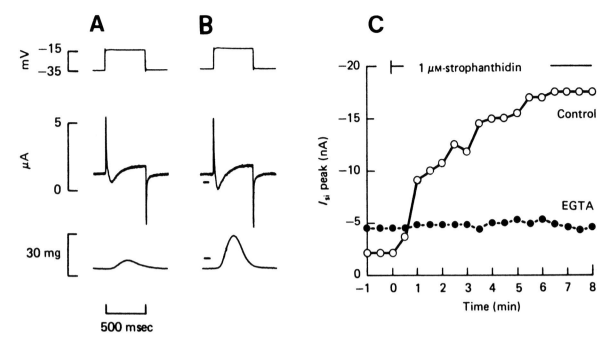

FIG. 2. Calcium currents in mammalian heart during exposure to digitalis. **A:** Membrane potential, Ca current, and force before and during exposure to 1-μM ouabain in a ferret papillary muscle voltage-clamped using the single-sucrose-gap technique. **B:** Peak Ca current before (*open circles*) and after (*filled circles*) EGTA injection in a calf Purkinje fiber, during exposures to 1-μM strophanthidin. (Adapted from ref. 153.)

has negative-feedback effects on I_{Ca}: Ca-channel inactivation is partly Ca-dependent (148; see ref. 65 for review), so that increased $[Ca^{2+}]_i$ may actually lead to a net decrease in I_{Ca} at the high $[Ca^{2+}]_i$ associated with toxic effects of digitalis.

Other Mechanisms

Other mechanisms, including altered intermediary metabolism or altered sensitivity of the contractile element to calcium, have been sought as possible explanations for the positive inotropic effects (PIE) of cardiac glycosides. Although occasional positive correlations have been reported, none has stood the test of time as a reproducible finding. We are not aware of any promising leads in these directions under study at the present time.

Unanswered Questions

There seems little doubt that inhibition of Na^+ transport leading to an increased intracellular Ca^{2+} pool available at the time of E-C coupling is an important mechanism underlying the PIE of cardiac glycosides on the heart. Unanswered, however, is the question whether the dominant mechanism involves enhanced Ca^{2+} entry via Na^+-Ca^{2+} exchange or whether dissipation of the Na^+ gradient results in reduced Ca^{2+} efflux. It is entirely possible that both phenomena may contribute in different circumstances or even in the same preparation. The

absence of a measurable increase in $[Na^+]_i$ in intact preparations noted by some workers (25) may simply reflect the insensitivity of the methods used, but it invites the ingenuity of the experimenter to devise methods to test the hypothesis of Akera and Brody (4) that an enhanced intracellular Na^+ transient might enhance $[Ca^{2+}]_i$ via Na-Ca exchange without measurably increasing steady-state Na levels. Optical indicators of free intracellular Na^+, if available, would provide new directions for further work in this regard.

Also unanswered is the question whether or not other mechanisms also make significant contributions to the PIE. Under selected circumstances, endogenous neuroeffectors appear to modulate the inotropic as well as toxic effects of cardiac glycosides (140). As discussed earlier, the relative importance of enhanced Ca^{2+} entry via the slow Ca channel during the plateau phase of the action potential is an interesting but as yet unresolved issue.

Unanswered questions abound in the clinical sphere (208), but they are beyond the scope of the present discussion. In this context, however, despite the weight of accumulated evidence that the therapeutic ratios of various cardioactive steroids are fundamentally similar, it must be asked again if naturally occurring or synthetic compounds can be found with better separation between therapeutic and toxic effects. Even if myocardial toxicity resulting in arrhythmias is a straightforward extension of the desired inotropic effect (i.e, occupancy of a still greater fraction of NaK-ATPase sites), advantage could be taken (in principle) of the fact that neural mechanisms are important in the mediation of electrophysiologic and most unwanted extracardiac effects of cardiac glycosides (212). Although we were disappointed to learn that highly polar cardiac glycosides that did not cross the blood-brain barrier still exerted typical neurally mediated toxic effects (168,213) (perhaps because of the lack of a blood-brain barrier in the area postrema), the obvious clinical importance of the issue should encourage investigators to continue to seek cardiac glycosides or derivatives thereof with an improved therapeutic ratio over currently used agents.

APPROACHES TO THE STUDY OF INOTROPIC MECHANISMS

Sarcolemma: NaK-ATPase

The interaction of cardiac glycosides with NaK-ATPase has been reviewed in detail recently by Hansen (108). As mentioned earlier, the specific binding site is located facing the outer cell surface on the larger or α subunit of the transport-enzyme complex. Whereas the α- and β-subunit proteins are quite well defined, the enzyme requires a less well defined phospholipid matrix for activity (120).

Enzymatic turnover of NaK-ATPase involves transphosphorylation at a β-aspartyl site of the α subunit, forming an acyl phosphate that is relatively acid-stable but sensitive to hydroxylamine (177). Charnock and Post (49) first suggested that ouabain bound preferentially to the phosphoenzyme, and Matsui and Schwartz (158) confirmed and extended this finding in their early studies with radiolabeled cardiac glycosides. Many details of the conditions favoring reversible ouabain binding to and inhibition of NaK-ATPase have been worked out, including the existence of two major pathways, the more physiologic of which requires the presence of Mg^{2+}, Na^+, and ATP. A second pathway, also capable of supporting high-affinity binding, occurs preferentially at low ionic strength in the absence of monovalent cations and is accelerated by Mg^{2+} and P_i (204). It is now generally agreed that ouabain binds preferentially to the E_2P form of the phosphoenzyme, as designated in the Albers-Post model (7,186), in which E_1 binds ATP and, in the presence of Mg^{2+}, Na^+, and nucleotide, is phosphorylated to E_1P. This undergoes a conformational change to E_2P in the continued presence of Mg^{2+}; E_2P is dephosphorylated by K^+, accounting in part for the well-known ability of K^+ to reduced ouabain binding by NaK-ATPase. ^{31}P nuclear magnetic resonance (NMR) observations by Fossel et al. (85) have demonstrated the phosphoenzyme intermediate in highly purified NaK-ATPase from avian salt gland, as well as skeletal-muscle SR Ca-ATPase.

Nonideality (i.e., inadequate description as a simple bimolecular interaction) of ouabain binding kinetics to various NaK-ATPase preparations has been reported, and proposed explanations for such behavior have included multiple classes of cooperatively interacting sites, multiple independent binding sites, and artifacts. The finding of Sweadner (217) that two distinct molecular forms of NaK-ATPase exist in brain, with different cardiac glycoside binding properties, indicates that assumptions about homogeneity of binding-site affinities are not generally warranted.

There is doubt that each step of the sequential Albers-Post model must be traversed in the hydrolytic cycle of the enzyme, and Plesner et al. (185) have suggested that the main flux does not require an acid-stable phosphoenzyme intermediate. An area of particularly active debate concerns the issue whether the functional enzyme is an $\alpha\beta$ protomer or a dimer ($\alpha_2\beta_2$) (119,120,180). The actual mechanism of enzyme action (and monovalent-cation transport) in the living cell continues to be a focus of active research efforts (97).

Sarcolemma: Electrogenic-Pump Current

When the NaK-ATPase of heart cells is inhibited (e.g., by K withdrawal), intracellular Na accumulates. Reactivation of the pump then results in a transient hyperpolarization of the cell (94,95). Under voltage-clamp conditions, pump reactivation produces a transient outward current that is abolished by strophanthidin (90,92). The amount of charge transported is directly related to the degree of Na loading (69,70). Pump current measurements have failed to substantiate a role for Na-pump stimulation in the positive inotropic effect of strophanthidin (67).

Other less direct methods have been used to assess the activity of the Na pump under voltage-clamp conditions. The restricted space in the intercellular clefts of cardiac Purkinje fibers creates the milieu for profound changes in local extracellular $[K^+]$ in response to changes in Na-pump activity. Based on their measurements of the K-sensitive current i_{K2}, Cohen et al. (54) inferred that the Na pump was stimulated by low concentrations of glycosides. The reversal potential of the current shifted to more negative values during ouabain exposure, consistent with a decrease in $[K^+]_o$. The observed change in reversal potential was taken as evidence for Na-pump stimulation by ouabain. These results have since been questioned for several reasons: (a) i_{K2} has been reinterpreted as an inward current (62), with K sensitivity explicable only on the basis of a model with numerous unproven assumptions (64); (b) the reversal potentials in the original records of Cohen et al. (54) were not always clear-cut; (c) the effects were seen primarily at unphysiologically elevated bulk $[K^+]$ of 6 to 8 mM;

(d) there was no experimental correlation with inotropic effects, although the authors speculated that pump stimulation might underlie the positive inotropic effects of low digitalis concentrations.

Hart et al. (109) reexamined this question using a related approach to deduce Na-pump activity from voltage-clamp measurements in sheep Purkinje fibers, coupled with force measurements. Rather than specifically measuring the i_{K2} reversal potential, these investigators measured steady-state current–voltage relations and tension during exposure to various concentrations of strophanthidin. An outward shift in the current–voltage relation observed with strophanthidin concentrations of 5 to 500 nM was taken as evidence of pump stimulation; however, changes in other pathways (such as the background K current i_{K1}) were not excluded. The outward shift in steady-state current was found to be accompanied by either positive or negative inotropic effects. The results were highly variable, and on balance they do not substantiate a role for Na-pump stimulation in the positive inotropic effects of cardiotonic steroids.

NaK-ATPase: Pharmacology

In contrast to the substantial literature on interactions of ouabain and other cardiac glycosides with purified or partially purified NaK-ATPase in particulate preparations, much less has been published with respect to ouabain interactions with NaK-ATPase in membranes of living cells, particularly sarcolemmal membranes of cardiac cells. Such data are obviously important to the examination of pharmacologic issues, and it would be hazardous indeed to assume that binding properties would be the same in disrupted cell fragments or purified enzyme as compared with intact, functioning cells with normal ion gradients, high-energy phosphate stores, and membrane polarization.

Kim et al. (130) defined the relationships among ^{3}H-ouabain binding, sodium-pump inhibition, and inotropic response in a monolayer preparation of spontaneously beating chick-embryo ventricular cells that was free of appreciable diffusion limitations. Ouabain binding followed pseudo-first-order kinetics, and K_D values derived kinetically and from equilibrium binding data were in good agreement. The Scatchard plot of ouabain binding in K^+-free medium was linear, consistent with the presence of a single class of binding sites ($K_D = 1.3 \times 10^{-7}$ M). In normal (4 mM) $[K^+]_o$, the K_D increased to about 5×10^{-7} M, and 10% of total NaK-ATPase sites were occupied by 10^{-7}-M ouabain, a concentration just below the threshold for a measurable positive inotropic effect or increase in $[Na^+]_i$. At 10^{-6} M, ouabain occupied 38% of NaK-ATPase sites, inhibited active $^{42}K^+$ uptake by 36%, increased steady-state $[Na^+]_i$ by 35%, and produced a 50% mean increase in amplitude of motion of individual cells in the culture. Thus, in this model system, more than 10% of sodium-pump sites must be inhibited to produce an appreciable change in the monovalent-cation active transport rate, in $[Na^+]_i$, or in contractile state. The reserve capacity of the ouabain-sensitive monovalent-cation active transport system in these myocytes is such that the initial rate of $^{42}K^+$ uptake in cells preloaded with Na^+ is four times greater than that observed without Na^+ loading. With 36% of NaK-ATPase sites blocked by ouabain, however, positive inotropy is readily observed and is closely correlated with increased $[Na^+]_i$. The remaining 64% of unblocked sites must cycle more rapidly to maintain the new steady-state level of $[Na^+]_i$, assuming that Na influx undergoes no substantial change.

Regulation of the number of NaK-ATPase sites in myocardial as well as other cells appears to be mediated via a mechanism that maintains surveillance over the intracellular Na^+ concentration. Thus, pharmacologic responsiveness to an agent that acts by inhibition of the Na^+ pump would be expected to change with altered numbers of sarcolemmal pump sites. Kim et al. (131) tested this hypothesis by growing cultured embryonic chick heart cells in low-$[K^+]_o$ medium (1.0 mM), 2-μM ouabain, or 1-μM veratridine, producing 60%, 40%, and 20% increases, respectively, in the total number of NaK-ATPase sites in intact cells, as judged by ^{3}H-ouabain binding. Each of the three interventions caused an acute increase in $[Na^+]_i$, followed by a gradual fall coincident with the emergence of larger numbers of identifiable NaK-ATPase sites over a period of 48 hr. The increased number of Na-pump sites in response to growth in 1.0-mM $[K^+]_o$ produced no change in inotropic responsiveness to isoproterenol, but shifted the ouabain concentration–effect curve to the right (Fig. 3). Shifts in ouabain responsiveness as a consequence of altered numbers of NaK-ATPase sites and $[Na^+]_i$ levels were accompanied by corresponding changes in Na-Ca exchange demonstrated by ^{45}Ca influx in response to a step change to zero $[Na^+]_o$. These findings support the view that elevated $[Na^+]_i$ due to NaK-ATPase inhibition mediates the inotropic response to ouabain, via altered Na-Ca exchange. According to the alternative proposal that binding of digitalis to NaK-ATPase causes altered release of Ca from enzyme-associated sarcolemmal sites (150), and if binding of a cardiac glycoside molecule caused a similar alteration in Ca binding at that locus irrespective of the density of NaK-ATPase sites, one would expect greater Ca mobilization (and a greater positive inotropic effect) in cells with increased numbers of pump sites, contrary to what was observed.

Other physiologic events may well alter pharmacologic responsiveness of the heart to cardiac glycosides through changes in NaK-ATPase. Thyroid hormone, for example, is known to increase the number of Na-pump sites in a number of tissues (66), including heart (57). Kim and Smith (129) examined the effects of thyroid hormone

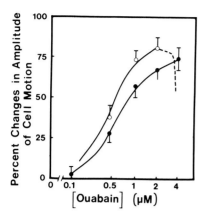

FIG. 3. Effects of growth of cells in medium containing zero or 10^{-8}-M T_3 on the concentration–effect relation for ouabain. Contractile responses of cells to several concentrations of ouabain (0.1–4 μM) were determined using the optical-video system. The response of a single cell to ouabain is expressed as a percentage of the response of that same cell to 3.6-mM Ca^{2+}. *Open circles* and *filled circles* represent responses of cells grown in medium containing 0 and 10^{-8}-M T_3, respectively. *Dotted line* represents the development of toxicity. (From ref. 129, with permission.)

on Na-pump sites, Na content, and contractile responses to ouabain in monolayer cultures of chick ventricular cells in order to gain insight into the well-known resistance of hyperthyroid patients to cardiac glycosides. Cells grown in relatively high concentrations of triiodothyronine (T_3) (10^{-8} M) showed a 60% increase in the number of NaK-ATPase sites per cell, as judged by ^{3}H-ouabain binding; these sites were functional and caused a significant reduction in steady-state $[Na^+]_i$. As in the case of cells with increased numbers of NaK-ATPase sites in response to growth under conditions such as low $[K]_o$, positive inotropic and also toxic effects (as well as $[Na]_i$ levels) were diminished at any given ouabain concentration in cells grown in the presence of high T_3 levels. Although thyroid hormone may alter cardiac responsiveness because of other mechanisms in the intact animal or patient, these findings account, at least in part, for reduced cardiac glycoside sensitivity in the presence of hyperthyroidism.

This discussion has emphasized the use of cultured heart cells as a model system for the study of pharmacologic interactions with sarcolemmal structures such as NaK-ATPase, not because it is perfect for such a purpose but because it tends to have fewer drawbacks than alternative systems. In particular, it affords stability over periods of days, and the lack of diffusion limitations in the monolayer preparation facilitates radioligand binding studies in intact, functioning cells and flux studies where rapid-sequence, unidirectional flux measurements are desirable (14). For studies of cardiac glycoside mechanisms, the absence of endogenous neuroeffectors, as are present in intact tissue preparations, greatly simplifies the interpretation of experimental results.

Studies of NaK-ATPase Structure and Function: New Directions

Specific Antibodies

Several laboratories have raised antibodies to NaK-ATPase for use as probes of its structure and function. McCans et al. (159) showed that antibody populations could be obtained that interacted specifically with catalytic sites or with ouabain binding sites on the enzyme. Our own studies indicated substantial cross-reactivity of NaK-ATPase from various organs and species and indicated that inhibition of monovalent-cation transport occurred only when the antibodies had access to the inner (cytoplasmic) cell surface (209). Highly specific monoclonal antibodies may prove useful as probes of structure and function of sarcolemmal components, including NaK-ATPase. The use of antibodies specific for cardiac glycosides in diagnostic and therapeutic applications has recently been reviewed elsewhere (211).

Digitalis Antagonists

Perhaps the most useful discovery that one might imagine in this field would be a substance that would act as a true cardiac glycoside antagonist, i.e., would compete for and displace cardioactive steroids from the inhibitory site on NaK-ATPase without itself inhibiting the enzyme. Agents acting on this principle have achieved major importance in the modulation of α- and β-adrenergic, muscarinic cholinergic, histaminergic, and opiate receptor functions, to name only a few examples. Regrettably, no molecule has been discovered that competes for the cardiac glycoside binding site without itself inhibiting the enzyme, and we are not aware of any promising leads in this direction.

NMR Studies of Monovalent-Cation Distribution

Pike et al. (183) have described a new approach to discrimination between intracellular and extracellular Na and K in intact, beating Langendorff heart preparations using shift reagents such as Dy(TTHA)$^{3-}$ that permeate extracellular spaces but do not enter intracellular spaces. Such shift reagents can thus be used to discriminate the resonances of ^{23}Na and ^{39}K ions in these spaces. We have observed that interventions, such as addition of ouabain to the perfusate, that inhibit NaK-ATPase cause an increase in the resonance peak corresponding to $[Na^+]_i$. Exclusion of K^+ from the perfusing medium caused a similar enhancement of the $[Na^+]_i$ peak, and this increase was reversed when $[K^+]_o$ perfusing the heart was returned to normal. Further work is needed to determine the details of the relationships between total and NMR-visible Na^+ and K^+ in the beating heart (183).

Endogenous Digitalis-like Factors

The possibility that there are endogenous ligands for the cardiac glycoside binding site on NaK-ATPase has been the source of considerable speculation. The presence of binding sites for digitalis glycosides on NaK-ATPase is analogous to the presence of specific receptors for exogenous opiate compounds *in vivo,* suggesting that there might be an endogenous digitalis, just as there is an endogenous opioid peptide system. If these inhibitors of the Na pump exist, they may be involved in the regulation of blood pressure and Na homeostasis. The early volume-expansion and cross-circulation experiments of de Wardener and colleagues (for review, see ref. 61) and the renal-transplantation experiments of Nizet et al. (173) supported the hypothesis that a separate natriuretic hormone or "third factor" exists. Subsequent work of Buckalew et al. (37) and of Gonick et al. (98) suggested that such a factor might be an inhibitor of NaK-ATPase.

Apart from its role in increasing renal Na excretion, a circulating NaK-ATPase inhibitor could function as a vasoconstrictor hormone, as postulated by Blaustein (29). In this formulation, a rise in $[Na^+]_i$ would cause an increase in $[Ca^{2+}]_i$ via Na-Ca exchange across the vascular smooth-muscle cell membrane, leading in turn to vasoconstriction; the Na-pump inhibitor would be released in response to volume expansion or an increase in dietary salt.

None of these mechanisms has yet been proved to be the means by which either an endogenous NaK-ATPase inhibitor or chronic administration of digitalis glycosides themselves exerts a hypertensive effect. Most of the evidence for the presence of endogenous NaK-ATPase inhibitors has been indirect, based on bioassays for effects on Na-pump activity *in vitro* by samples from plasma or other tissues from humans or experimental animals. Also, the Na-Ca antiport that appears to be important in determining levels of $[Ca^{2+}]_i$ in myocardial cells and vascular tone in the aorta has not been proved to be physiologically important in smooth-muscle cells of peripheral vascular resistance vessels (171).

Bioassay techniques such as ^{22}Na efflux from leukocytes, ^{86}Rb (a K^+ analogue) uptake into erythrocytes, or histochemical techniques thought to reflect NaK-ATPase activity have suggested that there is an endogenous NaK-ATPase inhibitor. Plasma from volume-expanded patients with chronic renal failure and patients with essential hypertension, or from normotensive subjects on a high-Na diet, has been reported to yield positive results in these assays (see ref. 61 for review). Plasma from animals with experimental hypertension also has been shown to contain Na-pump inhibitory activity. This NaK-ATPase inhibitory activity has been described consistently only in the volume-expanded and low-renin models of experimental hypertension, such as in the DOCA-saline model, the reduced-renal-mass model, or the one-kidney, one-clip Goldblatt model of hypertension (105).

Although the origin of putative endogenous Na-pump inhibitors is unknown, there is some evidence that the central nervous system (CNS) may release or regulate the release of such factors. Disruption of neuronal pathways in the preoptic hypothalamic, periventricular tissue of the anteroventral third ventricle (AV3V) can attenuate or prevent many forms of experimental hypertension in the rat, suggesting that this anatomic region may function as a central processing site in control of blood pressure by the sympathetic nervous system. Haddy and associates demonstrated that AV3V-lesioned rats with reduced-renal-mass/saline hypertension failed to develop hypertension as severe as that in control animals and also had significantly higher levels of vascular NaK-ATPase activity (38). AV3V lesions in rats have been reported to be associated with increases in NaK-ATPase activity in vessels and to prevent hypertension in the DOCA-salt-hypertensive rat model (214). AV3V lesions also induce alterations in fluid balance, presumably because of interruption of neural pathways involved in salt and water balance, as well as CNS angiotensin-II- and vasopressin-dependent mechanisms. However, AV3V lesions in rats also are associated with higher levels of NaK-ATPase activity in blood vessels of volume-expanded rats, suggesting that these rats have lower circulating levels of a Na-pump inhibitor. Finally, Bealer and colleagues have reported that lesions in the AV3V area decrease the natriuretic response to acute volume expansion (20).

Reports from several laboratories (6,110,230) have described NaK-ATPase inhibitors from mammalian brain. Halperin et al. reported that there is NaK-ATPase inhibitory activity in human cerebrospinal fluid and that this activity can increase rapidly following intravenous infusion of saline.

Despite evidence that circulating Na-pump inhibitors may be involved in the pathogenesis of hypertension, none of the putative factors has been isolated and characterized. Indeed, it is unknown whether or not they act as high-affinity ligands for the digitalis binding site on NaK-ATPase. Although there are known compounds in mammalian plasma that are NaK-ATPase inhibitors, they do not bind to the glycoside binding site and are not specific for NaK-ATPase. Vanadate, for example, acts as a transition-state phosphate analogue and inhibits NaK-ATPase function by binding to an ATP binding site. Vanadate, like ATP, facilitates cardiac glycoside binding to the enzyme in the presence of sodium and magnesium (108). However, unlike the digitalis glycosides, vanadate inhibits other phosphate-transferring enzymes, including Ca- and myosin-ATPase. Despite this lack of specificity, vanadate is concentrated in a number of mammalian tissues and in certain conditions could conceivably function as a physiologically important Na-pump inhibitor.

A variety of long-chain fatty acids and phospholipids can inhibit NaK-ATPase (199). The inhibitory potential of these lipids is dependent on the net charge and tends to be inversely correlated with the degree of aliphatic-chain saturation. These effects tend to be nonspecific, however, and apply to other membrane-bound ATPases as well as NaK-ATPase (195).

The fact that digitalis glycosides are steroid compounds has led investigators to search for endogenous steroid derivatives with cardiac-glycoside-like properties. There are steroids in amphibian skin and plasma (bufodienolides) that inhibit binding of cardiac glycosides to and activity of NaK-ATPase (132). However, all known mammalian endogenous steroids exist in a relatively planar conformational state and lack the cis A-B and C-D ring-junction structure characteristic of digitalis glycosides.

Nevertheless, evidence has emerged that compounds with at least some structural similarity to the digitalis glycosides do exist in the plasma and tissues of mammals and other species. With a more sensitive radioimmunoassay for digoxin than the standard clinical assay techniques, Gruber et al. (101) reported a low-molecular-weight substance in the plasma of volume-expanded dogs that cross-reacted with anti-digoxin antibodies and inhibited NaK-ATPase. The factor was not found in the plasma of normovolemic dogs. Gruber et al. (102) then described the presence of digoxin-like immunoreactivity in the plasma of several subhuman primate species and found that plasma levels of the substance correlated with the degree of hypertension. Kojima (136) also reported a plasma factor with NaK-ATPase inhibitory activity and digoxin-like immunoreactivity in rats with DOCA-salt hypertension.

The significance of digoxin-like immunoreactivity in plasma remains controversial. Several investigators have reported identifying substances in plasma with NaK-ATPase inhibitory activity that do not have digoxin-like immunoreactivity (51) or have failed to find any relationship between plasma levels of NaK-ATPase activity and digoxin-like immunoreactivity (107). False-positive digoxin radioimmunoassay results, as measured by standard digoxin clinical assays, have been found in patients with chronic renal failure, in the plasma of neonates, and in women in the third trimester of pregnancy (99). Higher levels have been reported to occur in preeclamptic than normotensive pregnant women (104). Despite these intriguing findings, few investigators have examined the factor with more than one antibody or have rigorously defined the radioimmunoassay technique to exclude potential artifacts.

We have recently identified three fractions in desalted, deproteinized plasma from normal humans that contain potent inhibitors of NaK-ATPase (128). The inhibitors in these fractions are low-molecular-weight compounds that are resistant to acid hydrolysis and proteases and that also displace ouabain from NaK-ATPase and cross-react variably with differing populations of polyclonal and monoclonal anti-digoxin antibodies. We have also identified a fourth fraction in plasma that cross-reacts with anti-digoxin antibodies but does not appear to inhibit NaK-ATPase. Despite these immunologic and functional similarities to the digitalis glycosides, the compounds in these plasma fractions differ in some details of the nature of their interactions with NaK-ATPase.

In summary, there is evidence for the existence of endogenous NaK-ATPase inhibitors in plasma of humans. Thus far, the evidence is largely circumstantial and incomplete. Nevertheless, the specific high-affinity binding sites for the digitalis glycosides on NaK-ATPase will continue to engender speculation about the existence of native ligands for these receptors. The potential biological importance of an endogenous Na-pump inhibitor will ensure a continued search for an endogenous digitalis-like hormone.

Sarcolemma: Na Channels and Ca Channels

The techniques available to characterize ionic channels in the heart are described extensively in other chapters in this book and will be described only briefly here, concentrating on Na and Ca channels.

Some properties of ionic channels can be deduced from action potentials. Na-channel activity is reflected predominantly in the maximal upstroke velocity of fast-response action potentials (53,230a). Current flow through Ca channels contributes to the overshoot of the action potential (156) but is most directly manifested in the action-potential plateau amplitude and duration (124).

Direct electrophysiologic measurement of channel activity requires the voltage-clamp technique. Current is applied across the cell membrane to control its potential. Ionic current is determined from the total membrane current by subtraction of the capacitive component. Because the cells of cardiac muscle are connected by low-resistance gap junctions, they form an electrical syncytium, making it possible to control the membrane potential even in multicellular preparations (87). This approach has two advantages: Tissue is studied in its intact state, and force can be measured simultaneously. There are also distinct disadvantages. The narrow intercellular clefts introduce a resistance in series with the cell membrane, making voltage control difficult (if not impossible) during rapid currents. These clefts also constitute a restricted space in which ion concentrations are not easily measured or controlled.

The development of techniques for enzymatic dissociation of adult hearts into single cells, and for maintaining embryonic or neonatal heart cells in culture, has allowed the application of potent new approaches to voltage-clamp studies of single cells (106,144). The techniques permit dialysis of the cell interior with solutions of the desired composition. The patch-clamp method can also be used to measure currents flowing through single channels.

The effects of digitalis on ionic currents have primarily been studied in multicellular preparations, in which force can be measured during voltage clamp (see ref. 153 for review). Recently, Beresewicz et al. (26) have documented an increase in peak Ca current in single guinea pig ventricular myocytes under voltage clamp, confirming the work in Purkinje fibers and ventricular muscle. Fischmeister et al. (82) measured ionic currents in single frog ventricular cells during pump inhibition by digitalis or by activator cation (Cs) depletion. They found that either of these maneuvers alone was associated with a decrease in Ca current; however, when cells were exposed to ouabain or dihydroouabain after the NaK-ATPase had already been inhibited by Cs depletion, an increase in I_{Ca} was observed. The relationship of these observations to the inotropic effect of digitalis is difficult to determine, in that $[Ca^{2+}]_i$ was heavily buffered by internal dialysis with 5-mM EGTA. More experiments in this area are required.

Sarcolemma: Na-Ca Exchange

As outlined previously, Na-Ca exchange has been implicated as a key step in the sequence of events linking occupancy of NaK-ATPase inhibitory sites by cardiac glycosides to their positive inotropic effect. Baker et al. (15) proposed this mechanism of digitalis action based on their studies of Na-Ca exchange in the squid giant axon. Also relevant are the early studies of Reuter and Seitz (193), yielding evidence for a Na-Ca exchange carrier in mammalian myocardium. A general consideration of Na-Ca exchange in cardiac tissue has been provided by Mullins (170).

Although a substantial literature exists describing the phenomenology associated with Na-Ca exchange, details at the molecular level are scant and constitute a fertile area for further exploration. Thus far, no potent and highly specific inhibitors of Na-Ca exchange are known to exist, although some progress has been made in identifying compounds with the ability to block this process (206).

The stoichiometry, capacity, and physiologic role of Na-Ca exchange continue to be subjects of considerable debate. Based on different specific assumptions for the stoichiometry, the carrier has been assigned diverse physiologic roles ranging from Ca extrusion [e.g., Reuter (191), assuming 2 Na per 1 Ca] to voltage-dependent Ca influx [Mullins (169), assuming at least 4 Na per 1 Ca]. The uncertainties arise primarily because of other

pathways acting either in parallel or in series with the exchange.

Three basic approaches have been applied in experimental attempts to characterize the Na-Ca exchange: (a) measurement of counterfluxes of Na and Ca; (b) determination of changes in intracellular ion activities in response to changes in transmembrane gradients of Na or Ca; (c) measurement of membrane potential (or current) changes associated with altered Na or Ca gradients. Each of these approaches will be considered briefly here; the reader is referred to Chapter 26 and to recent reviews (31,68) for more comprehensive treatments.

Counterfluxes of Na and Ca have been measured in a variety of cardiac preparations, including sarcolemmal vesicles (184,226), chick heart cells in culture (17), and whole rabbit hearts (34). Assuming no parallel pathways, the vesicle experiments find flux ratios of 3 Na per 1 Ca. Nevertheless, self-exchange of Ca (Ca-Ca exchange) (142) or Ca-activated Na-conductance changes cannot be excluded. Barry et al. (19) documented Na-dependent Ca influx and found no evidence for (but could not exclude) Ca efflux through Na-Ca exchange. Although these results are consistent with the view that Na-Ca exchange functions physiologically to produce net Ca influx, the results can also be explained if ^{45}Ca is largely extruded via Ca-Ca exchange in the absence of Na. The experiments in whole rabbit hearts measured total cellular Na and Ca, thereby avoiding the complications that Ca-Ca exchange can introduce into radioisotope flux measurements, and also arrived at a stoichiometry of 3 Na per 1 Ca. Because changes in other pathways (such as passive Na influx) were not excluded, the stoichiometry remains in doubt. These examples point out the major uncertainties that plague experiments on Na-Ca exchange.

Another approach has been to measure the changes in $[Na^+]_i$ and $[Ca^{2+}]_i$ (or tonic tension as an indication of $[Ca^{2+}]_i$) during maneuvers such as NaK-ATPase inhibition and Na_o withdrawal (27,72,73,205), then derive a coupling ratio from thermodynamic-equilibrium equations. Using this approach, Sheu and Fozzard argued for a ratio of 2.5; Eisner and associates found a slightly higher ratio. However, these values assume that equilibrium was reached, which, as pointed out by the authors, is not substantiated by experimental evidence. A specific problem with this assumption was pointed out by Wier et al. (231) [see also Kort et al. (137)], who noted that spontaneous Ca fluctuations associated with tonic tension would preclude the attainment of a steady state, a necessary condition for thermodynamic equilibrium.

Any carrier with a ratio other than 2 Na per 1 Ca would be "electrogenic," i.e., would produce a change in membrane current with changes in the Na or Ca gradients. A number of investigators have found that the increase in force produced by Na removal occurs in conjunction with membrane hyperpolarization (56), as would be expected if a transient increase in outward current were produced by exchange-mediated Na efflux. Attempts to measure the Na-Ca exchange current under voltage clamp, including the recent study by Mentrard et al. (161), have failed to exclude Ca-activated changes in membrane conductance (143).

Sarcolemma: Ca-ATPase

Although not directly implicated in current schemes to explain the mechanism of positive inotropic effects of cardiac glycosides, the sarcolemmal Ca^{2+} pump (Ca-ATPase) has a potentially important bearing on the physiologic expression of any intervention that alters cellular Ca handling. A useful review of the general aspects of plasma membrane Ca-ATPase as an active Ca transport system is that of Penniston (182). This transport system is widely distributed in eukaryotic organisms and appears to be regulated by a variety of mechanisms, including protein phosphorylation (hence regulated by kinases and phosphatases), calmodulin, acidic phospholipids, and substrates. Compared with the Na-Ca exchanger, sarcolemmal Ca-ATPase has a higher affinity for Ca but a lower capacity to move Ca across the sarcolemmal membrane at relatively high $[Ca]_i$ levels (182).

Caroni and Carafoli (42) have described in some detail an ATP-dependent Ca^{2+}-pumping system in cardiac sarcolemma, also recognized by Morcos and Drummond (165). Isolated from calf heart sarcolemma by calmodulin affinity chromatography (43,44) as a 140,000-d protein, the purified enzyme has a high affinity for Ca^{2+} (K_m 0.4 μM) in the presence of calmodulin, but shifts to a lower affinity (K_m 20 μM) in its absence (45). Calmodulin was also found to increase V_{max}. The enzyme from cardiac sarcolemma appears to be homologous with that from other sources, as judged by cross-reactivity with antibody raised against erythrocyte Ca-ATPase; under similar conditions, purified SR Ca-ATPase did not react (45).

The presence of an ATP-dependent Ca pump in the sarcolemma is presumed to account for the ability of heart cells to relax after being put into contracture by exposure to medium containing zero $[Na^+]_o$, which produces Ca influx via Na-Ca exchange and effectively precludes Ca extrusion by that pathway (18). The responses of cardiac tissues of various sorts to a given level of cardiac glycoside may be expected, based on the arguments put forward in this chapter, to depend on (among other things) the capacity of sarcolemmal Ca-ATPase to extrude the excess Ca that enters via Na-Ca exchange when Na-pump sites are blocked by the glycoside and $[Na^+]_i$ accumulates.

Full exploration of the physiologic role of the ATP-dependent Ca transport system, like Na-Ca exchange, is hampered by the lack of a potent and specific inhibitor.

Cytoplasm

Thus far we have pursued the premise that digitalis compounds act directly on sarcolemmal pathways and that their intracellular effects are indirect consequences of the increase in cellular Ca loading. Various lines of experimental evidence support the absence of direct effects of digitalis on the contractile proteins or the SR. Fabiato and Fabiato (79) found no effect of digitalis on the pCa–tension relation or on Ca-induced Ca release in mechanically skinned heart cells. Similarly, Hess and Müller (111) exposed the cut ends of bovine ventricular trabeculae to digoxin as a means of introducing the compound into the tissue. The extracellular bathing medium included specific anti-digoxin antibodies to eliminate any possibility that leakage of digoxin into the extracellular space might obscure the results. They saw no change in contractile force, despite evidence for intracellular accumulation of the glycoside.

An intriguing exception to the notion that digitalis has no significant direct intracellular effects comes from the work of Isenberg (116), who injected ouabain, digoxin, or digitoxin into isolated bovine ventricular cells and measured their degree of shortening. He found that injection of the glycosides could more than double the contraction. The effect of intracellularly applied digoxin was not abolished by extracellular anti-digoxin antibody. An increase in cell shortening was observed even under Na-free conditions, suggesting that the degree of Na loading played no role in the intracellular effects. Isenberg interpreted his results as indicating a direct effect of digitalis to potentiate Ca release from the SR. These results are at odds with the findings in skinned cells and in trabeculae; new experiments in those preparations, as well as injection experiments in isolated cells coupled with direct measurements of $[Ca^{2+}]_i$, will be needed to resolve the discrepancies.

A number of techniques have been applied to determine the effects of cardiotonic steroids on intracellular ion concentrations, in particular $[Na^+]_i$ and $[Ca^{2+}]_i$. Although total cellular concentrations of ions have been measured using flame photometry (25) or electron-probe microanalysis (229), the most useful techniques have been those that yield estimates of free-ion concentrations: ion-sensitive microelectrodes and optical indicators. We shall limit our discussion to the application of these methods to measure $[Na^+]_i$ and $[Ca^{2+}]_i$ during exposure to cardiotonic steroids in heart cells; more general reviews are available in *Chapters* 28 and 33.

Ion-Sensitive Microelectrodes

These are made by incorporating a membrane of ion-selective glass or resin at the tip of a siliconized-glass microelectrode. The ion-sensitive electrode measures the sum of the membrane potential and the ion-specific potential difference across the tip, necessitating subtraction of the membrane potential (usually measured with a separate conventional voltage-sensing microelectrode). Although in principle such electrodes can provide explicit values for intracellular ion concentrations, in practice their usefulness is rather limited given the current level of technology. The responses of the electrodes to changes in the relevant ions are often much slower than the physiologically relevant signals; rapid transients can be missed altogether or filtered in misleading ways (because of the nonlinear responses of the electrodes). Furthermore, the high tip resistance of the microelectrodes results in attenuation of the membrane-potential component of the signal. They sample from only one point in one cell, which may not be representative of the preparation as a whole. The tips of ion-sensitive microelectrodes are large compared with conventional microelectrodes, so that impalement-induced damage is always a worry, especially in small cells. It is not surprising that ion-sensitive microelectrodes have been of greatest utility in measuring ion concentrations at rest or during slow changes (on the time scale of minutes).

The first measurements of $[Na^+]_i$ in heart cells by Ellis (75) and Deitmer and Ellis (59) applied recessed-tip glass microelectrodes to sheep Purkinje fibers. These investigators found that $[Na^+]_i$ increased in response to high concentrations (>100 nM) of strophanthidin. Lower concentrations sometimes (but not always) produced a slight decrease in $[Na^+]_i$; such a fall in $[Na^+]_i$ did not occur with dihydroouabain, a cardiotonic steroid not believed capable of producing Na-pump stimulation (174). Deitmer and Ellis made their measurements with the preparations quiescent; this made it easier to obtain the Na-sensitive potential signal, because the membrane potential could be subtracted without filtering the reference microelectrode signal to match the RC characteristics of the high-resistance ion-sensitive electrode. However, the quiescent state fails to mimic the normal conditions in which there is rhythmic voltage-dependent Na influx and a higher baseline level of $[Na^+]_i$ (52,118,144).

Lee and associates were the first to correlate a rise in $[Na^+]_i$ with the positive inotropic effect of cardiotonic steroids; they allowed $[Na^+]_i$ in Purkinje fibers to reach a steady state during exposure to various concentrations of dihydroouabain, then stimulated the preparation to determine twitch tension at that level of $[Na^+]_i$. They found a linear relationship between $[Na^+]_i$ and twitch tension; twitch tension doubled with each 8-mM increase in $[Na^+]_i$. A linear relationship between $[Na^+]_i$ and force during exposure to cardiotonic steroids has been confirmed, although other studies have found a fourfold to eightfold steeper dependence of twitch force on $[Na^+]_i$ (145,227a) (cf. ref. 71). This discrepancy may have arisen from the fact that Lee et al. (144) allowed $[Na^+]_i$ to reach a steady state with the preparation quiescent,

then stimulated to determine force, whereas the subsequent studies have either stimulated continuously and filtered the reference-electrode signal (145) or paused briefly (227a) to measure $[Na^+]_i$. The greater steepness of the Na_i–force relation when Na_i is measured during frequent stimulation may reflect recruitment of an amplifying mechanism that comes into play only during systole (4,153).

Although rhythmic stimulation mimics the physiologic state more closely than quiescence, two types of uncertainty plague ion-sensitive microelectrode measurements during stimulation. When stimulation is continuous and a smooth difference record is obtained by filtering the reference-electrode signal, the result is indeterminate because of the phasic changes in the underlying ion concentration as filtered by the time response and nonlinearity of the individual electrode. The errors that could be introduced in this manner are likely to be much more severe for $[Ca^{2+}]_i$ [e.g., Lee and Dagostino (145), Fig. 11] than for $[Na^+]_i$ measurements, because the phasic change in $[Ca^{2+}]_i$ relative to the baseline level is likely to be much higher than the relative change in $[Na^+]_i$ during each action potential.

Optical Indicators

Such indicators for Na^+ are not available; so this review will be limited to the Ca^{2+} indicators aequorin and quin2. Metallochromic indicators have been used to measure extracellular Ca^{2+} depletion signals (50) but have not proved useful for intracellular measurements in heart cells. A detailed recent review of Ca^{2+} indicators is available (32).

Aequorin has been the most useful indicator of $[Ca^{2+}]_i$ to be applied to heart tissue. The experimental findings with regard to digitalis action were reviewed earlier. This indicator has proved useful because its time response and its minimal Ca-buffering properties do not attenuate the cardiac $[Ca^{2+}]_i$ transient during twitches. The main limitations with aequorin arise from possible spatial and temporal inhomogeneity of $[Ca^{2+}]_i$. The presence of such inhomogeneities will mean that estimates of $[Ca^{2+}]_i$ from aequorin luminescence can serve only as upper limits for spatial average $[Ca^{2+}]_i$.

Quin2 is the first widely used Ca^{2+} indicator of the family of EGTA analogues designed by Tsien and colleagues for this purpose. The fluorescence characteristics of these indicators change when they bind Ca. Esterified derivatives of the parent dye diffuse freely into cells, and once inside, the dye is liberated by the actions of intracellular esterases. This eliminates the need for disruptive loading procedures such as microinjection. Quin2 has been used extensively, particularly in suspensions of small cells (e.g., platelets) for which other Ca^{2+} indicators are ill-suited. Although quin2 has also been applied to suspensions of cardiac ventricular myocytes

(186a,205a), those measurements are of limited usefulness for two reasons: (a) The intracellular dye concentrations required are high (0.1–1 mM) and produce
considerable Ca buffering; (b) suspensions of enzymatically dissociated cells are not a homogeneous population,
at least partly because of a significant percentage of
damaged cells (35%, see ref. 205a) that may distort the
$[Ca^{2+}]_i$ determinations. Newly available indicators in
this family (particularly fura2) (102a) appear to have
overcome the major deficiencies of quin2 and have
already been applied for imaging of $[Ca^{2+}]_i$ in single
isolated smooth-muscle cells (233a).

Radioisotope Methods

Radioisotope methods have the unique capacity to
report unidirectional as well as net transmembrane ion
fluxes, but they must be used and interpreted with care
to avoid a variety of pitfalls. Of particular importance
is the need to work with homogeneous preparations that
avoid diffusion limitations as much as possible, as well
as to consider and control for backflux problems (14).

Monolayer preparations of cultured heart cells most
nearly meet these requirements, while at the same time
allowing continuous measurements of contractile behavior in response to interventions such as cardiac glycoside
exposure and also sufficient quantities of tissue for
measurements of receptors and intracellular mediators.
Use of these techniques to determine $[Ca^{2+}]_i$ kinetics
(18) and $[Na^+]_i$ and $[Ca^{2+}]_i$ responses to cardiac glycoside
exposure (16,19,28) has been considered previously.

Langer and colleagues have used radioisotope methods
to elucidate basic mechanisms of cardiac glycoside action,
first in the isolated perfused rabbit septal preparation
(139). More recent studies using neonatal rat myocardial
cells and a novel scintillation disc technique (39) support
the view that inhibition of the Na pump with ouabain
or low $[K^+]_o$ augments the cell-associated Ca pool via
Na-Ca exchange. ^{45}Ca binding to isolated sarcolemma
was not altered by ouabain or low $[K^+]_o$. Because the
majority of the 11 to 15% increase observed in cell-
associated Ca was La^{3+}-displaceable under the conditions
used, Burt and Langer (39) argued that this Ca increment
was localized to the sarcolemma-glycocalyx complex.

Nayler and Noack (172) reviewed much of the earlier
literature on studies of the influence of cardiac glycosides
on electrolyte exchange and content in cardiac muscle
cells using radioisotope as well as chemical techniques.

Recent experiments to examine changes in transsarcolemmal Ca^{2+} fluxes in response to catecholamines (131)
have been instructive with respect to the limitations of
such measurements as conventionally made. Brief incubation of cultured chick heart cells in Ca^{2+}-free medium improved the resolution of ^{45}Ca-influx measurements, permitting demonstration of at least 30%
enhancement of the ^{45}Ca-influx rate by 1 μM isoproter-

enol. This was fully inhibitable by nifedipine or by
propranolol. Among several possible explanations, experimental evidence favored increased ^{45}Ca specific activity near the sarcolemmal boundary at the time of
initial uptake measurements as the basis for improvement
by brief zero-$[Ca^{2+}]_o$ preincubation of the sensitivity of
the ^{45}Ca-uptake response to isoproterenol.

CONCLUSIONS

Evidence from electrophysiologic studies, including
those using ion-sensitive microelectrodes, together with
improved cation flux and content measurements, now
provides a reasonably cohesive picture of the sequence
of events leading from digitalis-induced inhibition of the
Na pump to enhancement of contractile force generation
by isolated cardiac muscle. The commonality of Na-
pump inhibition producing elevated $[Na^+]_i$ and $[Ca^{2+}]_i$
in the generation of both therapeutic (positive inotropic)
and toxic (arrhythmic) responses of the heart accounts
for the long-recognized difficulty in separating therapeutic
and toxic clinical effects of cardiac glycosides. Responses
of intact patients or experimental animals to digitalis
glycosides, however, are also conditioned by neurally
mediated mechanisms that can exert important influences on the integrated effect of digitalis administration.
This review has emphasized the basic cellular mechanisms that underlie the direct effects of digitalis on the
heart, with the expectation that enhanced understanding
of these mechanisms will ultimately lead to improved
ability to reap the clinical benefits of digitalis glycosides
and other positively inotropic agents while limiting the
risk of untoward responses.

REFERENCES

1. Akera, T. (1977): Membrane adenosine triphosphatase: A digitalis receptor? *Science,* 198:569.
2. Akera, T., Larson, F. S., and Brody, T. M. (1970): Correlation of cardiac sodium- and potassium-activated adenosine triphosphatase activity with ouabain-induced inotropic stimulation. *J. Pharmacol. Exp. Ther.,* 173:145.
3. Akera, T., Baskin, S. I., Tobin, T., and Brody, T. M. (1973): Ouabain: Temporal relationship between the inotropic effect and the in vitro binding to, and dissociation from, (Na^+,K^+)-activated ATPase. *Naunyn Schmiedebergs Arch. Pharmacol.,* 277:151.
4. Akera, T., and Brody, T. M. (1977): The role of Na,K-ATPase in the inotropic action of digitalis. *Pharmacol. Rev.,* 29:187–210.
5. Akera, T., Olgaard, M. K., Temma, K., and Brody, T. M. (1977): Development of the positive inotropic action of ouabain: Effects of transmembrane sodium movement. *J. Pharmacol. Exp. Ther.,* 203:675.
6. Alaghband-Zadeh, J., Fenton, S., Hancock, K., Millett, J., and de Wardener, H. E. (1983): Evidence that the hypothalamus may be a source of a circulating Na^+-K^+-ATPase inhibitor. *J. Endocrinol.,* 98:221–226.
7. Albers, R. W. (1967): Biochemical aspects of active transport. *Annu. Rev. Biochem.,* 36:727–756.
8. Allen, D. G., and Blinks, J. F. (1978): Calcium transients in aequorin injected cardiac muscle. *Nature,* 273:509–513.
9. Allen, D. G., and Kurihara, S. (1980): Calcium transients in

mammalian ventricular muscle. *Eur. Heart J.* [*Suppl. A*], 1:5–15.

10. Allen, D. G., and Kurihara, S. (1982): The effect of muscle length on intracellular calcium transients in mammalian cardiac muscle. *J. Physiol. (Lond.)*, 327:79–94.

11. Allen, J. C., and Schwartz, A. (1969): A possible biochemical explanation for the sensitivity of the rat to cardiac glycosides. *J. Pharmacol. Ther.*, 168:42.

12. Arlock, P., and Katzung, B. G. (1985): Effects of sodium substitutes on transient inward current and tension in guinea pig and ferret papillary muscle. *J. Physiol. (Lond.), (in press).*

13. Arnold, S. B., Byrd, R. C., Meister, W., Melmon, K., Cheitlin, M. D., Bristow, J. D., Parmley, W. W., and Chatterjee, K. (1980): Long-term digitalis therapy improves left ventricular function in heart failure. *N. Engl. J. Med.*, 303:1443–1448.

14. Attwell, D., Eisner, D., and Cohen, I. (1979): Voltage clamp and tracer flux data: Effects of a restricted extracellular space. *Q. Rev. Biophys.*, 12:213–261.

15. Baker, P. F., Blaustein, M. P., Hodgkin, A. L., and Steinhardt, R. A. (1969): The influence of calcium on sodium efflux in squid axions. *J. Physiol. (Lond.)*, 200:431.

16. Barry, W. H., Biedert, S., Miura, D. S., and Smith, T. W. (1981): Changes in cellular Na^+, K^+, and Ca^{++} contents, monovalent cation transport rate, and contractile state during washout of cardiac glycosides from cultured chick heart cells. *Circ. Res.*, 49:141–149.

17. Barry, W. H., and Smith, T. W. (1982): Mechanisms of transmembrane calcium movement in cultured chick embryo ventricular cells. *J. Physiol. (Lond.)*, 325:243–260.

18. Barry, W. H., and Smith, T. W. (1984): Movement of Ca^{2+} across the sarcolemma: Effects of abrupt exposure to zero external Na concentration. *J. Mol. Cell. Cardiol.*, 16:155–164.

19. Barry, W. H., Hasin, Y., and Smith, T. W. (1985): Sodium pump inhibition, enhanced Ca-influx via Na-Ca exchange, and positive inotropic response in cultured heart cells. *Circ. Res.*, 56:231–241.

20. Bealer, S. L., Haywood, J. R., Gruber, K. A., Buckalew, V. M., Fink, G. D., Brody, M. J., and Johnson, A. K. (1983): Preoptic hypothalamic periventricular lesions reduce natriuresis to volume expansion. *Am. J. Physiol.*, 244:R51–R57.

21. Bean, B. P. (1984): Nitrendipine block of cardiac calcium channels: High-affinity binding to the inactivated state. *Proc. Natl. Acad. Sci. USA*, 81:6388–6392.

22. Bean, B. P. (1985): Two kinds of calcium channels in atrial cells from dog and frog hearts. *Biophys. J.*, 47:497a.

23. Bean, B. P., Cohen, C. J., and Tsien, R. W. (1983): Lidocaine block of cardiac sodium channels. *J. Gen. Physiol.*, 81:613–642.

24. Bean, B. P., Nowycky, M. D., and Tsien, R. W. (1984): Beta-adrenergic modulation of Ca channels in frog ventricular heart cells. *Nature*, 307:371–375.

25. Bentfeld, M., Lüllmann, H., Peters, T., and Proppe, D. (1977): Interdependence of ion transport and the action of ouabain in heart muscle. *Br. J. Pharmacol.*, 61:19–27.

26. Beresewicz, A., Isenberg, G., and Klöckner, U. (1984): Inhibition of the Na-pump increases the release component of I_{Ca}. *Pfluegers Arch.*, 400:R5.

27. Bers, D. M., and Ellis, D. (1982): Intracellular calcium and sodium activity in sheep heart Purkinje fibers. Effects of changes of external sodium and intracellular pH. *Pfluegers Arch.*, 393:171–178.

28. Biedert, S., Barry, W. H., and Smith, T. W. (1979): Inotropic effects and changes in sodium and calcium contents associated with inhibition of monovalent cation active transport by ouabain in cultured myocardial cells. *J. Gen. Physiol.*, 74:479–494.

29. Blaustein, M. P. (1977): Sodium ions, calcium ions, blood pressure regulation, and hypertension: a reassessment and a hypothesis. *Am. J. Physiol.*, 232:C165–C173.

30. Blaustein, M. P., and Russell, J. M. (1975): Sodium-calcium exchange and calcium-calcium exchange in internally dialyzed squid giant axons. *J. Membr. Biol.*, 22:285–312.

31. Blaustein, M. P., and Nelson, M. T. (1982): Sodium-calcium exchange: Its role in the regulation of cell calcium. In: *Membrane Transport of Calcium*, edited by E. Carafoli, pp. 217–236. Academic Press, London.

32. Blinks, J. R., Wier, W. G., Hess, P., and Prendergast, F. G.

(1982): Measurement of Ca^{2+} concentrations in living cells. *Prog. Biophys. Mol. Biol.*, 40:1–114.

33. Bonting, S. L., Hawkins, N. M., and Canady, M. R. (1964): Studies of sodium-potassium activated adenosine triphosphatase. VII. Inhibition by erythrophleum alkaloids. *Biochem. Pharmacol.*, 13:13.

34. Bridge, J. H. B., and Bassingthwaighte, J. B. (1983): Uphill sodium transport driven by an inward calcium gradient in heart muscle. *Science*, 219:178–180.

35. Brody, T. M., and Akera, T. (1977): Relations among Na,K-ATPase activity, sodium pump activity, transmembrane sodium movement, and cardiac contractility. *Fed. Proc.*, 36:2219–2224.

36. Brum, G., Osterrieder, W., and Tautwein, W. (1984): Beta-adrenergic increase in the calcium conductance of cardiac myocytes studied with the patch clamp. *Pfluegers Arch.*, 401:111–118.

37. Buckalew, V. M., Martinez, F. J., and Green, W. (1970): The effect of dialysates and ultrafiltrates of plasma from saline loaded dogs on toad bladder sodium transport. *Eur. J. Clin. Invest.*, 49:926–935.

38. Buggy, J., Huot, S., Pamnani, M., and Haddy, F. (1984): Periventricular forebrain mechanisms for blood pressure regulation. *Fed. Proc.*, 43:25–31.

39. Burt, J. M., and Larger, G. A. (1982): Ca^{++} distribution after Na^+ pump inhibition in cultured neonatal rat myocardial cells. *Circ. Res.*, 51:543–550.

40. Cachelin, A. B., DePyer, J. E., Kokubun, S., and Reuter, H. (1983): Ca channel modulation by 8-bromocyclic AMP in cultured heart cells. *Nature*, 304:462–464.

41. Calhoun, J. A., and Harrison, T. R. (1931): Studies in congestive heart failure. IX. The effect of digitalis on the potassium content of the cardiac muscle of dogs. *J. Clin. Invest.*, 10:139.

42. Caroni, P., and Carafoli, E. (1980): An ATP-dependent Ca^{2+}-pumping system in dog heart sarcolemma. *Nature*, 283:765–767.

43. Caroni, P., and Carafoli, E. (1981): The Ca^{2+}-pumping ATPase of heart sarcolemma. *J. Biol. Chem.*, 256:3263–3270.

44. Caroni, P., and Carafoli, E. (1981): Regulation of Ca-pumping ATPase of heart sarcolemma by a phosphorylatio-dephosphorylation process. *J. Biol. Chem.*, 256:9371–9373.

45. Caroni, P., Zurini, M., Clark, A., and Carafoli, E. (1983): Further characterization and reconstitution of the purified Ca^{2+}-pumping ATPase of heart sarcolemma. *J. Biol. Chem.*, 258:7305–7310.

46. Cattell, M., and Gold, H. (1938): The influence of digitalis on the force of contraction of mammalian cardiac muscle. *J. Pharmacol. Exp. Ther.*, 62:116.

47. Chapman, R. A. (1979): Excitation-contraction coupling in cardiac muscle. *Prog. Biophys. Mol. Biol.*, 35:1–52.

48. Chapman, R. A. (1983): Control of cardiac contractility at the cellular level. *Am. J. Physiol. (Heart Circ. Physiol., 14)*, 245:H535–H552.

49. Charnock, J. S., and Post, R. L. (1963): Evidence of the mechanism of ouabain inhibition of cation activated adenosine triphosphatase. *Nature (Lond.)*, 199:910–911.

50. Cleemann, L., Pizarro, G., and Morad, M. (1984): Optical measurements of extracellular calcium depletion during a single heartbeat. *Science*, 266:173–176.

51. Cloix, J.-F., Miller, E. D., Pernollet, M. G., Devynck, M. A., and Meyer, P. (1983): Purification d'un inhibiteur endogene de la sodium-potassium-ATPase. *C. R. Acad. Sci. Paris*, 296:213–216.

52. Cohen, C. J., Fozzard, H. A., and Sheu, S.-S. (1982): Increase in intracellular sodium ion activity during stimulation in mammalian cardiac muscle. *Circ. Res.*, 50:651–662.

53. Cohen, C. J., Bean, B. P., and Tsien, R. W. (1984): Maximal upstroke velocity as an index of available sodium conductance. Comparison of maximal upstroke velocity and voltage clamp measurements of sodium current in rabbit Purkinje fibers. *Circ. Res.*, 54:636–651.

54. Cohen, I., Daut, J., and Noble, D. (1976): An analysis of the actions of low concentrations of ouabain on membrane currents in Purkinje fibers. *J. Physiol. (Lond.)*, 260:75–103.

55. Colquhoun, D., Neher, E., Reuter, H., and Stevens, C. F. (1981): Inward current channels activated by intracellular Ca in cultured cardiac cells. *Nature*, 294:752–754.

56. Coraboeuf, E., Gautier, P., and Guiraudou, P. (1981): Potential and tension changes induced by sodium removal in dog Purkinje

fibers: Role of an electrogenic sodium-calcium exchange. *J. Physiol. (Lond.)*, 311:605–622.

57. Curfman, G. D., Crowley, T. J., and Smith, T. W. (1977): Thyroid-induced alterations in myocardial sodium and potassium-activated adenosine triphosphatase, monovalent cation active transport, and cardiac glycoside binding. *J. Clin. Invest.*, 59:586–590.

58. Dagostino, M., and Lee, C. O. (1982): Neutral carrier Na$^+$- and Ca^{2+}-selective microelectrodes for intracellular application. *Biophys. J.*, 40:199–207.

59. Deitmer, J. W., and Ellis, D. (1978): The intracellular sodium activity of cardiac Purkinje fibers during inhibition and reactivation of the Na-K pump. *J. Physiol. (Lond.)*, 284:241–259.

60. Deitmer, J. W., and Ellis, D. (1980): Interactions between the regulation of the intracellular pH and Na activity of sheep cardiac Purkinje fibers. *J. Physiol. (Lond.)*, 304:471–488.

61. de Wardener, H. E., and MacGregor, G. H. (1983): The relation of a circulating sodium transport inhibitor (the natriuretic hormone?) to hypertension. *Medicine (Baltimore)*, 62:310–326.

62. DiFrancesco, D. (1981): A new interpretation of the pace-maker current in calf Purkinje fibers. *J. Physiol. (Lond.)*, 314:359–376.

63. DiFrancesco, D. (1984): Characterization of the pace-maker current kinetics in calf Purkinje fibers. *J. Physiol. (Lond.)*, 348: 341–367.

64. DiFrancesco, D., and Noble, D. (1980): Reconstruction of Purkinje fiber currents in sodium-free solution. *J. Physiol. (Lond.)*, 308: 35P.

65. Eckert, R., and Chad, J. (1984): Inactivation of Ca channels. *Prog. Biophys. Mol. Biol.*, 44:215–267.

66. Edelman, I. S. (1974): Thyroid thermogenesis. *N. Engl. J. Med.*, 290:1303–1308.

67. Eisner, D. A., and Lederer, W. J. (1979): Does sodium pump inhibition produce the positive inotropic effects of strophanthidin in mammalian cardiac muscle? *J. Physiol. (Lond.)*, 296:75P–76P.

68. Eisner, D. A., and Lederer, W. J. (1985): Na-Ca exchange: Stoichiometry and electrogenicity. *Am. J. Physiology (Cell)*, (in press).

69. Eisner, D. A., and Lederer, W. J. (1980): Characterization of the electrogenic sodium pump in cardiac Purkinje fibers. *J. Physiol. (Lond.)*, 303:441–474.

70. Eisner, D. A., and Lederer, W. J. (1980): The relationship between sodium pump activity and twitch tension in cardiac Purkinje fibers. *J. Physiol. (Lond.)*, 303:475–494.

71. Eisner, D. A., Lederer, W. J., and Vaughan-Jones, R. D. (1981): The dependence of sodium pumping and tension on intracellular sodium activity in voltage-clamped sheep Purkinje fibers. *J. Physiol. (Lond.)*, 317:163–187.

72. Eisner, D. A., Lederer, W. J., and Vaughan-Jones, R. D. (1983): The control of tonic tension by membrane potential and intracellular sodium activity in the sheep cardiac Purkinje fiber. *J. Physiol. (Lond.)*, 335:723–743.

73. Eisner, D. A., Lederer, W. J., and Sheu, S. S. (1983): The role of intracellular sodium activity in the antiarrhythmic action of local anesthetics in sheep Purkinje fibers. *J. Physiol. (Lond.)*, 340:239–257.

74. Eisner, D. A., Lederer, W. J., and Vaughan-Jones, R. D. (1984): The quantitative relationship between twitch tension and intracellular sodium activity in sheep cardiac Purkinje fibers. *J. Physiol. (Lond.)*, 355:251–266.

75. Ellis, D. (1977): The effects of external cations and ouabain on the intracellular sodium activity of sheep heart Purkinje fibers. *J. Physiol. (Lond.)*, 273:211–240.

76. Endo, M. (1975): Conditions required for calcium-induced release of calcium from the sarcoplasmic reticulum. *Proc. Japan. Acad.*, 51:467–472.

77. Fabiato, A. (1981): Myoplasmic free calcium concentration reached during the twitch of an intact isolated cardiac cell and during calcium-induced release of calcium from the sarcoplasmic reticulum of a skinned cardiac cell from the adult rat or rabbit ventricle. *J. Gen. Physiol.*, 78:457–497.

78. Fabiato, A. (1983): Calcium-induced release of calcium from the cardiac sarcoplasmic reticulum. *Am. J. Physiol.*, 245:C1–C14.

79. Fabiato, A., and Fabiato, F. (1973): Activation of skinned cardiac

80. Fabiato, A., and Fabiato, F. (1978): Effects of pH on the myofilaments and the sarcoplasmic reticulum of skinned cells from cardiac and skeletal muscles. *J. Physiol. (Lond.)*, 276:233–255.

81. Ferrier, G. R., Saunders, J. H., and Mendez, C. (1973): A cellular mechanism for the generation of ventricular arrhythmias by acetylstrophanthidin. *Circ. Res.*, 32:600–609.

82. Fischmeister, R., Argibay, J. A., and Vassort, G. (1985): The effects of cardiotonic steroids on Ca current in frog ventricular myocytes. *Biophys. J.*, 47:498a.

83. Flasch, H., and Heinz, N. (1978): Correlation between inhibition of NaK-membrane-ATPase and positive inotropic activity of cardenolides in isolated papillary muscles of guinea pig. *Naunyn Schmiedebergs Arch. Pharmacol.*, 304:37–44.

84. Forbush, B., III, Kaplan, J. H., and Hoffman, J. F. (1978): Characterization of a new photoaffinity derivative of ouabain: Labelling of the large polypeptide and of a proteolipid component of the Na,K-ATPase. *Biochemistry*, 17:3667.

85. Fossel, E. T., Post, R. L., O'Hara, D. S., and Smith, T. W. (1981): ^{31}P nuclear magnetic resonance observation of the phosphoenzymes of sodium and potassium-activated and of calcium-activated adenosine triphosphatase. *Biochemistry*, 20:7215–7218.

86. Fozzard, H. A. (1973): Excitation-contraction coupling and digitalis. *Circulation*, 47:5–7.

87. Fozzard, H. A., and Beeler, G. W. (1975): The voltage clamp and cardiac electrophysiology. *Circ. Res.*, 37:403–413.

88. From, A. H. L., Fullerton, D. S., Deffo, T., Kitatsuji, E., Rohrer, D. C., and Ahmed, K. (1984): The inotropic activity of digitalis genins is dependent upon C(17) side-group carbonyl oxygen position. *J. Mol. Cell. Cardiol.*, 16:835–842.

89. Gadsby, D. C. (1980): Activation of electrogenic Na$^+$/K$^+$ exchange by extracellular K$^+$ in canine cardiac Purkinje fibers. *Proc. Natl. Acad. Sci. USA*, 77:4035–4039.

90. Gadsby, D. C., and Cranefield, P. F. (1979): Electrogenic sodium extrusion in cardiac Purkinje fibers. *J. Gen. Physiol.*, 73:819–837.

91. Gadsby, D. C., and Cranefield, P. F. (1979): Direct measurement of changes in sodium pump current in canine cardiac Purkinje fibers. *Proc. Natl. Acad. Sci. USA*, 76:1783–1787.

92. Gadsby, D. C., Kimura, J., and Noma, A. (1985): Voltage dependence of Na/K pump current in isolated heart cells. *Nature*, 315:63–65.

93. Gervais, A., Lane, L. K., Anner, B. M., Lindenmayer, G. E., and Schwartz, A. (1977): A positive molecular mechanism of the action of digitalis: Ouabain action on calcium binding to sites associated with a purified sodium-potassium-activated adenosine triphosphatase. *Circ. Res.*, 40:8.

94. Glitsch, H. G. (1973): An effect of the electrogenic sodium pump on the membrane potential in beating guinea-pig atria. *Pfluegers Arch.*, 344:169–180.

95. Glitsch, H. G. (1979): Characteristics of active Na transport in intact cardiac cells. *Am. J. Physiol.*, 236:H189–H199.

96. Glitsch, H. G., Reuter, H., and Scholz, H. (1970): The effect of the internal sodium concentration on calcium fluxes in isolated guinea pig auricles. *J. Physiol. (Lond.)*, 209:25–43.

97. Glynn, I. (editor) (1985): *The Sodium Pump. Proceedings of the 4th International Symposium on Na$^+$,K$^+$-ATPase*. The Company of Biologists, Ltd., Cambridge, U.K.

98. Gonick, H. C., Kramer, H. J., Paul, W., and Lu, E. (1977): Circulating inhibitor of sodium-potassium-activated adenosine triphosphatase after expansion of extracellular fluid volume in rats. *Clin. Sci. Mol. Med.*, 53:329–334.

99. Graves, S. W., Valdes, R., Brown, B. A., Knight, A. B., and Craig, H. R. (1984): Endogenous digoxin-immunoreactive substance in human pregnancies. *J. Clin. Endocrinol. Metab.*, 59: 748–751.

100. Greenspan, A. M., and Morad, M. (1975): Electromechanical studies on the inotropic effects of acetylstrophanthidin in ventricular muscle. *J. Physiol. (Lond.)*, 253:357–384.

101. Gruber, K. A., Whitaker, J. M., and Buckalew, V. M. (1980):

Endogenous digitalis-like substance in plasm of volume-expanded dogs. *Nature*, 287:743–745.

102. Gruber, K. A., Rudel, L. L., and Bullock, D. V. M. (1982): Increased circulating levels of an endogenous digoxin-like factor in hypertensive monkeys. *Hypertension*, 4:348–354.

102a. Grynkiewicz, G., Poenie, M., and Tsien, R. Y. (1985): A new generation of Ca^{2+} indicators with greatly improved fluorescence properties. *J. Biol. Chem.*, 260:3440.

103. Güntert, T. W., and Linde, H. H. A. (1981): Chemistry and structure-activity relationships of cardioactive steroids. In: *Handbook of Experimental Pharmacology, Vol. 56/I, Cardiac Glycosides*, edited by K. Greeff, pp. 13–24. Springer-Verlag, Berlin.

104. Gusdon, J. P., Buckalew, V. M., and Hennessy, J. F. (1984): A digoxin-like immunosubstance in pre-eclampsia. *Am. J. Obstet. Gynecol.*, 150:83–85.

105. Haddy, F. J., and Pamnani, M. B. (1983): The role of a hormonal sodium-potassium pump inhibitor in low-renin hypertension. *Fed. Proc.*, 42:2673–2680.

106. Hamill, O. P., Marty, A., Neher, E., Sakmann, B., and Sigworth, F. J. (1981): Improved patch-clamp techniques for high-resolution current recording from cells and cell-free membrane patches. *Pfluegers Arch.*, 391:85–100.

107. Hamlyn, J. M., Ringel, R., Schaeffer, J., Levinson, P. D., Hamilton, B. P., Kowarski, A. A., and Blaustein, M. P. (1982): A circulating inhibitor of $(Na^+ + K^+)$ATPase associated with essential hypertension. *Nature*, 300:650–652.

108. Hansen, O. (1984): Interaction of cardiac glycosides with $(Na^+ + K^+)$-activated ATPase. A biochemical link to digitalis-induced inotropy. *Pharmacol. Rev.*, 36:143–163.

109. Hart, G., Noble, D., and Shimoni, Y. (1983): The effects of low concentrations of cardiotonic steroids on membrane currents and tension in sheep Purkinje fibers. *J. Physiol. (Lond.)*, 334:103–131.

110. Haupert, G. T., and Sancho, J. M. (1979): Sodium transport inhibitor from bovine hypothalamus. *Proc. Natl. Acad. Sci. USA*, 76:4658–4660.

111. Hess, P., and Müller, P. (1982): Extracellular versus intracellular digoxin action on bovine myocardium, using digoxin antibody and intracellular glycoside application. *J. Physiol. (Lond.)*, 322:197–210.

112. Hess, P., Metzger, P., and Weingart, R. (1982): Free magnesium in sheep, ferret and frog striated muscle at rest measured with ion-selective micro-electrodes. *J. Physiol. (Lond.)*, 333:173–188.

113. Hibberd, M. D., and Jewell, B. R. (1982): Calcium- and length-dependent force production in rat ventricular muscle. *J. Physiol. (Lond.)*, 329:527–540.

114. Hougen, T. J., Spicer, N., and Smith, T. W. (1981): Stimulation of monovalent cation active transport by low concentrations of cardiac glycosides: Role of catecholamines. *J. Clin. Invest.*, 68:1207–1214.

115. Isenberg, G. (1982): Ca entry and contraction as studied in isolated bovine ventricular myocytes. *Z. Naturforsch.*, 37:502–512.

116. Isenberg, G. (1984): Contractility of isolated bovine ventricular myocytes is enhanced by intracellular injection of cardioactive glycosides. Evidence for an intracellular mode of action. *Basic Res. Cardiol. [Suppl.]*, 79:56–71.

117. Isenberg, G., and Klockner, U. (1982): Calcium currents of isolated bovine ventricular myocytes are fast and of large amplitude. *Pfluegers Arch.*, 395:30–41.

118. January, C., and Fozzard, H. A. (1984): The effects of membrane potential, extracellular potassium, and tetrodotoxin on the intracellular sodium ion activity of sheep cardiac muscle. *Circ. Res.*, 54:652–665.

119. Jensen, J., Norby, J. G., and Ottolenghi, P. (1984): Sodium and potassium binding to the sodium pump: Stoichiometry and affinities evaluated from nucleotide-binding behaviour. *J. Physiol. (Lond.)*, 346:219–241.

120. Jorgensen, P. L. (1982): Mechanism of the Na^+,K^+ pump. Protein structure and conformations of the pure $(Na^+ + K^+)$-ATPase. *Biochem. Acta*, 694:27–68.

121. Kass, R. S., and Tsien, R. W. (1975): Multiple effects of calcium antagonists on plateau currents in cardiac Purkinje fibers. *J. Gen. Physiol.*, 66:169–192.

122. Kass, R. S., and Tsien, R. W. (1976): Control of action potential duration by calcium ions in cardiac Purkinje fibers. *J. Gen. Physiol.*, 67:599–617.

123. Kass, R. S., Lederer, W. J., Tsien, R. W., and Weingart, R. (1978): Role of calcium ions in transient inward currents and aftercontractions induced by strophanthidin in cardiac Purkinje fibers. *J. Physiol. (Lond.)*, 281:187–208.

124. Kass, R. S., and Tsien, R. W. (1982): Fluctuations in membrane current driven by intracellular calcium in cardiac Purkinje fibers. *Biophys. J.*, 38:259–269.

125. Katz, A. M. (1972): Increased Ca entry during the plateau of the action potential: A possible mechanism of cardiac glycoside action. *J. Mol. Cell. Cardiol.*, 4:87–89.

126. Katz, A. M., and Hecht, H. H. (1969): The early "pump" failure of the ischemic heart. *Am. J. Med.*, 47:497–502.

127. Katz, A. M., Tada, M., and Kirchberger, M. A. (1975): Control of calcium transport in the myocardium by the cyclic AMP-protein kinase system. *Adv. Cyclic Nucleotide Res.*, 5:453–472.

128. Kelly, R. A., O'Hara, D. S., Mitch, W. E., and Smith, T. W. (1985): Characterization of digitalis-like factors in human plasma: Interactions with NaK-ATPase and crossreactivity with cardiac glycoside-specific antibodies. *J. Biol. Chem., (in press)*.

129. Kim, D., and Smith, T. W. (1984): Effects of thyroid hormone on sodium pump sites, sodium content, and contractile response to cardiac glycosides in cultured chick ventricular cells. *J. Clin. Invest.*, 74:1481–1488.

130. Kim, D., Barry, W. H., and Smith, T. W. (1984): Kinetics of ouabain binding and changes in cellular sodium content, ^{42}K transport and contractile state during ouabain exposure in cultured chick heart cells. *J. Pharmacol. Exp. Ther.*, 231:326–333.

131. Kim, D., Marsh, J. D., Barry, W. H., and Smith, T. W. (1984): Effects of growth in low potassium medium or ouabain on membrane NaK-ATPase, cation transport and contractility in cultured chick heart cells. *Circ. Res.*, 55:39–48.

132. Kim, R. S., and Labella, F. S. (1981): Endogenous ligands and modulators of the digitalis receptor: Some candidates. *Pharmacol. Ther.*, 14:391–409.

133. Koch-Weser, J. (1971): Beta receptor blockade and myocardial effects of cardiac glycosides. *Circ. Res.*, 28:109–118.

134. Koch-Weser, J., and Blinks, J. R. (1962): Analysis of the relation of the positive inotropic action of cardiac glycosides to the frequency of contraction of heart muscle. *J. Pharmacol. Exp. Ther.*, 136:305–317.

135. Koch-Weser, J., and Blinks, J. R. (1963): The influence of the interval between beats on myocardial contractility. *Pharmacol. Rev.*, 15:601–652.

136. Kojima, I. (1984): Circulating digitalis-like substance is increased in DOCA-salt hypertension. *Biochem. Biophys. Res. Commun.*, 122:129–136.

137. Kort, A. A., Lakatta, E. G., Marban, E., Stern, M. D., and Wier, W. G. (1985): Fluctuations in intracellular Ca^{2+} and their effect on tonic tension in canine cardiac Purkinje fibres. *J. Physiol. (Lond.), (in press)*.

138. Kronenberg, G., Meyer, K. H., Schraufstaater, E., Schutz, S., and Stoepel, K. (1964): Synthetische Verbindungen mit Digitaliswirkung. *Naturwissenschaften*, 51:192–193.

139. Langer, G. A., and Serena, S. D. (1970): Effects of strophanthidin upon contraction and ionic exchanges in rabbit ventricular myocardium: Relation to control of active state. *J. Mol. Cell. Cardiol.*, 1:65–90.

140. Lechat, P., Malloy, C. R., and Smith, T. W. (1983): Active transport and inotropic state in guinea pig left atrium. *Circ. Res.*, 52:411–422.

141. Lederer, W. J., and Eisner, D. A. (1982): The effects of sodium pump activity on the slow inward current in sheep cardiac Purkinje fibers. *Proc. R. Soc. Lond.*, B214:249–262.

142. Lederer, W. J., and Nelson, M. T. (1983): Effects of extracellular sodium on calcium efflux and membrane current in single muscle cells from the barnacle. *J. Physiol. (Lond.)*, 341:325–339.

143. Lederer, W. J., Sheu, S.-S., Vaughan-Jones, R. D., and Eisner, D. A. (1984): The effects of Na-Ca exchange on membrane

currents in sheep cardiac Purkinje fibers. In: *Electrogenic Transport: Fundamental Principles and Physiological Implications,* edited by M. P. Blaustein and M. Lieberman, pp. 373–380. Raven Press, New York.

144. Lee, C. O., Kang, D. H., Sokol, J. H., and Lee, K. S. (1980): Relation between intracellular Na ion activity and tension of sheep cardiac Purkinje fibers exposed to dihydro-ouabain. *Biophys. J.,* 29:315–330.

145. Lee, C. O., and Dagostino, M. (1982): Effect of strophanthidin on intracellular Na ion activity and twitch tension of constantly drive canine cardiac Purkinje fibers. *Biophys. J.,* 40:185–198.

146. Lee, D. C.-S., Johnson, R. A., Bingham, J. B., Leahy, M., Dinsmore, R. E., Goroll, A. H., Newell, J. B., Strauss, H. W., and Haber, E. (1982): Heart failure in outpatients. A randomized trial of digoxin versus placebo. *N. Engl. J. Med.,* 306:699–705.

147. Lee, K. S., and Klaus, W. (1971): The subcellular basis for the mechanism of inotropic action of cardiac glycosides. *Pharmacol. Rev.,* 23:193.

148. Lee, K. S., Marban, E., and Tsien, R. W. (1985): Inactivation of calcium channels in mammalian heart cells. Joint dependence on membrane potential and intracellular calcium. *J. Physiol. (Lond.),* 364:395–441.

149. LePeuch, C. J., Haiech, J., and Demaille, J. G. (1979): Concerted regulation of cardiac sarcoplasmic reticulum calcium transport by cyclic AMP-dependent and Ca-calmodulin-dependent phosphrylations. *Biochemistry,* 18:5150–5157.

150. Lüllmann, H., and Peters, T. (1979): Action of cardiac glycosides on the excitation-contraction coupling in heart muscle. *Prog. Pharmacol.,* 2:1.

151. Marban, E., Rink, T. J., Tsien, R. W., and Tsien, R. Y. (1980): Free calcium in heart muscle at rest and during contraction measured with Ca^{2+}-sensitive microelectrodes. *Nature,* 286:845–850.

152. Marban, E., and Tsien, R. W. (1982): Effects of nystatin-mediated intracellular ion substitution on membrane currents in calf Purkinje fibers. *J. Physiol. (Lond.),* 329:569–587.

153. Marban, E., and Tsien, R. W. (1982): Enhancement of calcium current during digitalis inotropy in mammalian heart: Positive feedback regulation by intracellular calcium. *J. Physiol. (Lond.),* 329:589–614.

154. Marban, E., and Wier, G. (1985): Ryanodine as a tool to determine the contributions of calcium entry and calcium release to the calcium transient and contraction of cardiac Purkinje fibers. *Circ. Res.,* 56:133–138.

154a.Marsh, J. D., Loh, E., Lachance, D., Barry, W. H., and Smith, T. W. (1983): Relationship of binding of a calcium channel blocker to inhibition of contraction in intact cultured ambryonic chick ventricular cells. *Circ. Res.,* 53:539–543.

155. Marshall, P. G. (1970): Steroids: Cardiotonic glycosides and aglycons; toad poisons. In: *Rodd's Chemistry of Carbon Compounds, Vol. 2D, Steroids,* 2nd ed., edited by S. Coffy, p. 360. Elsevier, Amsterdam.

156. Mary-Rabine, L., Hoffman, B. F., and Rosen, M. R. (1979): Participation of slow inward current in the Purkinje fiber action potential overshoot. *Am. J. Physiol.,* 237:H204–H212.

157. Matsuda, H., Noma, A., Kurachi, Y., and Irisawa, H. (1982): Transient depolarization and spontaneous voltage fluctuations in isolated single cells from guinea pig ventricles. *Circ. Res.,* 51:142–151.

158. Matsui, H., and Schwartz, A. (1968): Mechanism of cardiac glycoside inhibition of the $(Na^+ + K^+)$-dependent ATPase from cardiac tissue. *Biochim. Biophys. Acta,* 151:655–663.

159. McCans, J. L., Lindenmayer, G. E., Pitts, B. J. R., Ray, M. V., Raynor, B. D., Butler, V. P., Jr., and Schwartz, A. (1975): Antigenic differences in (Na^+,K^+)-ATPase preparations isolated from various organs and species. *J. Biol. Chem.,* 250:7257–7265.

160. McClellan, G., and Winegrad, S. (1980): Cyclic nucleotide regulation of the contractile proteins in mammalian cardiac muscle. *J. Gen. Physiol.,* 72:737–764.

161. Mentrard, D., Vassort G., and Fischmeister, R. (1984): Changes in external Na induce a membrane current related to the Na-Ca exchange in cesium-loaded frog heart cells. *J. Gen. Physiol.,* 84:201–220.

162. Mitchell, M. R., Powell, T., Terrar, D. A., and Twist, V. W.

(1984): Ryanodine prolongs Ca-currents while suppressing contraction in rate ventricular muscle cells. *Br. J. Pharmacol.,* 81:13–15.

163. Morad, M., and Rolett, E. L. (1972): Relaxing effects of catecholamines on mammalian heart. *J. Physiol. (Lond.),* 224:537–558.

164. Morad, M., and Goldman, Y. (1973): Excitation-contraction coupling in heart muscle: Membrane control of development of tension. *Prog. Biophys. Mol. Biol.,* 27:257–312.

165. Morcos, N. S., and Drummond, G. I. (1980): $(Ca^{2+} + Mg^{2+})$-ATPase in enriched sarcolemma from dog heart. *Biochim. Biophys. Acta,* 598:29–39.

166. Morgan, J. P., and Blinks, J. R. (1982): Intracellular Ca^{2+} transients in the cat papillary muscle. *Can. J. Physiol. Pharmacol.,* 60:520–528.

167. Movsesian, M. A., Nishikawa, M., and Adelstein, R. S. (1984): Phosphorylation of phospholamban by calcium-activated phospholipid-dependent protein kinase. *J. Biol. Chem.,* 259:8029–8032.

168. Mudge, G. H., Jr., Lloyd, B. L., Greenblatt, D. J., and Smith, T. W. (1978): Inotropic and toxic effects of a polar cardiac glycoside derivative in the dog. *Circ. Res.,* 43:847–854.

169. Mullins, L. J. (1979): The generation of electric currents in cardiac fibers by Na/Ca exchange. *Am. J. Physiol.,* 263:C103–C110.

170. Mullins, L. J. (1984): An electrogenic saga: Consequences of sodium-calcium exchange in cardiac muscle. In: *Electrogenic Transport: Fundamental Principles and Physiological Implications,* edited by M. P. Blaustein and M. Lieberman, pp. 161–179. Raven Press, New York.

171. Mulvany, M. J. (1984): Effect of electrolyte transport on the response of arteriolar smooth muscle. *J. Cardiovasc. Pharmacol.,* 6:582–587.

172. Nayler, W., and Noack, E. A. (1981): Influence of cardiac glycosides on electrolyte exchange and content in cardiac muscle cells. In: *Handbook of Experimental Pharmacology, Vol. 56/I, Cardiac Glycosides,* edited by K. Greeff, pp. 405–436. Springer-Verlag, Berlin.

173. Nizet, A., Tost, H., and Foidant-Willems, J. (1974): The control of sodium excretion following saline infusion in the dog. *Pfluegers Arch.,* 350:287–298.

174. Noble, D. (1980): Mechanism of action of therapeutic levels of cardiac glycosides. Review. *Cardiovasc. Res.,* 14:495–514.

175. Noble, D. (1984): The surprising heart: A review of recent progress in cardiac electrophysiology. *J. Physiol. (Lond.),* 353:1–50.

176. Noda, M., Shimizu, S., Tanage, T., et al. (1984): Primary structure of *Electrophorus electricus* sodium channel deduced from cDNA sequence. *Nature,* 312:121–127.

177. Norby, J. G. (1983): Ligand interactions with the substrate site of Na,K-ATPase: Nucleotids, vanadate, and phosphorylation. In: *Current Topics in Membranes and Transport, Vol. 19,* edited by J. F. Hoffman and B. Forbuss III, pp. 281–314. Academic Press, New York.

178. Okada, M., and Saito, Y. (1968): Synthesis of 3-hydroxy-5-card-20(22)-enolide(14-deoxy-14-uzarigenin). *Chem. Pharm. Bull. (Tokyo),* 16:2223–2227.

179. Orchard, C. H., Eisner, D. A., and Allen, D. G. (1983): Oscillations of intracellular Ca^{2+} in mammalian cardiac muscle. *Nature,* 304:735–738.

180. Ottolenghi, P., and Ellory, J. C. (1983): Radiation inactivation of (Na,K)-ATPase, an enzyme showing multiple radiation-sensitive domains. *J. Biol. Chem.,* 258:14895–14907.

181. Patnaik, G. K., and Dhawan, B. N. (1978): Pharmacological investigations on asclepin—a new cardenolid from *Asclepius curassavica. Arzneim. Forsch.,* 28:1095–1099.

182. Penniston, J. T. (1983): Plasma membrane Ca^{2+}-ATPases as active Ca^{2+} pumps. In: *Calcium and Cell Function, Vol. IV,* pp. 99–149. Academic Press, New York.

183. Pike, M. M., Frazer, J. C., Dedrick, D. F., Ingwall, J. S., Allen, P. D., Springer, C. B., Jr., and Smith, T. W. (1985): ^{23}Na and ^{39}K NMR studies of perfused rat hearts: Discrimination of intra- and extracellular ions using a shift reagent. *Biophys. J., (in press).*

184. Pitts, B. J. R. (1979): Stoichiometry of sodium-calcium exchange in cardiac sarcolemmal vesicles. *J. Biol. Chem.*, 254:6232–6235.

185. Plesner, I. W., Plesner, L., Norby, J. G., and Klodos, I. (1981): The steady-state kinetic mechanism of ATP hydrolysis catalyzed by membrane-bound ($Na^+ + K^+$)-ATPase from ox brain. III. A minimal model. *Biochim. Biophys. Acta*, 643:483–494.

186. Post, R. L., Kume, S., Tobin, T., Orcutt, B., and Sen, A. K. (1969): Flexibility of an active center in sodium-plus-potassium adenosine triphosphatase. *J. Gen. Physiol.*, 54:306s–326s.

186a. Powell, T., Trentham, P. E. R., and Twist, V. W. (1984): Cytoplasmic free calcium measured by quin 2 fluorescence in isolated ventricular myocytes at rest and during potassium-depolarization. *Biochem. Biophys. Res. Commun.*, 122:1012–1020.

187. Prindle, K. H., Jr., Skelton, C. L., Epstein, S. E., and Marcus, F. I. (1971): Influence of extracellular potassium concentration on myocardial uptake and inotropic effect of tritiated digoxin. *Circ. Res.*, 28:337.

188. Reiter, M. (1981): The positive inotropic action of cardiac glycosides on cardiac ventricular muscle. In: *Handbook of Experimental Pharmacology, Vol. 56/I, Cardiac Glycosides*, edited by K. Greeff, pp. 187–219. Springer-Verlag, Berlin.

189. Repke, K. R. H. (1964): Uber den biochemischen Wirkungsmodus von Digitalis. *Klin. Wochenschr.*, 42:157–165.

190. Repke, K. R. H., and Schönfeld, W. (1984): Na^+/K^+-ATPase as the digitalis receptor. *Trends Pharmacol. Sci.*, 5:393–397.

191. Reuter, H. (1974): Exchange of calcium ions in the mammalian myocardium. *Circ. Res.*, 34:599–605.

192. Reuter, H. (1983): Calcium channel modulation by neurotransmitters, enzymes and drugs. *Nature*, 301:569–574.

193. Reuter, H., and Seitz, N. (1968): The dependence of calcium efflux from cardiac muscle on temperature and external ion composition. *J. Physiol. (Lond.)*, 195:451–470.

194. Reuter, H., Stevens, C. F., Tsien, R. W., and Yellen, G. (1982): Properties of single calcium channels in cardiac cell culture. *Nature*, 297:501–504.

195. Roelofson, B. (1981): The nonspecificity in the lipid requirement of calcium- and (sodium plus potassium)-transporting adenosine triphosphatases. *Life Sci.*, 29:2235–2247.

196. Rosen, M. R., Gelband, H., and Hoffman, B. F. (1973): Correlation between effects of ouabain on the canine electrocardiogram and transmembrane potentials in isolated Purkinje fibers. *Circulation*, 47:65–72.

197. Rosen, M. R., and Danilo, P., Jr. (1980): Effects of tetrodotoxin, lidocaine, verapamil, and AHR-2666 on ouabain-induced delayed afterdepolarizations in canine Purkinje fibers. *Circ. Res.*, 46:117–124.

198. Saito, Y., Kanemasa, Y., and Okada, M. (1970): Preparation of 3-deoxy and 17-hydroxy cardenolide. *Chem. Pharm. Bull. (Tokyo)*, 18:629–631.

199. Schmalzing, G., and Katschberg, P. (1982): Modulation of ATPase activities of human erythrocyte membranes by free fatty acids or phospholipase A_2. *J. Membr. Biol.*, 69:65–76.

200. Schneider, M. F., and Chandler, W. K. (1973): Voltage-dependent charge movement in skeletal muscle: A possible stop in excitation-contraction coupling. *Nature*, 242:244–246.

201. Schramm, M., Thomas, G., Toward, R., and Franckowiak, G. (1983): Novel dihydropyridines with positive inotropic action through activation of Ca^{2+} channels. *Nature*, 303:535–537.

202. Schwartz, A., Lindemayer, G. E., and Allen, J. C. (1075): The sodium-potassium adenosine triphosphatase: Pharmacological, physiological and biochemical aspects. *Pharmacol. Rev.*, 27:1.

203. Seifen, E. (1974): Evidence for preparation of catecholamines in cardiac action of ouabain. *Eur. J. Pharmacol.*, 26:115–118.

204. Sen, A. K., Tobin, T., and Post, R. L. (1969): A cycle for ouabain inhibition of sodium- and potassium-dependent adenosine triphosphatase. *J. Biol. Chem.*, 244:6596–6604.

205. Sheu, S.-S., and Fozzard, H. A. (1982): Transmembrane Na^+ and Ca^{2+} electromechanical gradients in cardiac muscle and their relationship to force development. *J. Gen. Physiol.*, 80:325–351.

205a. Sheu, S.-S., Sharma, V. K., and Banerjee, S. P. (1984): Measurement of cytosolic free calcium concentration in isolated rat ventricular myocytes with quin 2. *Circ. Res.*, 55:830–834.

206. Siegl, P. K. S., Cragoe, E. J., Jr., Trumble, M. J., and Kaczorowski, G. J. (1984): Inhibition of Na^+/Ca^{++} exchange in membrane vesicle and papillary muscle preparations from guinea pig heart by analogs of amiloride. *Proc. Natl. Acad. Sci. USA*, 81:3238–3242.

207. Smith, P., Brown, L., Boutagy, J., and Thomas, R. (1984): Cardenolid analogues. 14. Synthesis and biological activity of glycosides of C17 β-modified derivatives of digitoxigenin. (*in press*).

208. Smith, T. W. (1982): Medical treatment of advanced congestive heart failure: Digitalis and diuretics. In: *Congestive Heart Failure*, edited by E. Braunwald, M. B. Mock, and J. Watson, pp. 261–278. Grune & Stratton, New York.

209. Smith, T. W., and Wagner, H., Jr. (1975): Effects of ($Na^+ + K^+$)-ATPase-specific antibodies on enzymatic activity and monovalent cation transport. *J. Membr. Biol.*, 25:341–360.

210. Smith, T. W., and Barry, W. H. (1983): Monovalent cation transport and mechanisms of digitalis-induced inotropy. In: *Current Topics in Membranes and Transport: Structure, Mechanisms, and Function of the Na/K Pump*, edited by J. F. Hoffman and B. Forbush, pp. 843–856. Academic Press, Orlando.

211. Smith, T. W., Antman, E. A., Friedman, P. L., Blatt, C. M., and Marsh, J. D. (1984): Digitalis glycosides: Mechanisms and manifestations of toxicity. *Prog. Cardiovasc. Dis.*, 26:413–441, 495–523; 27:21–56.

212. Somberg, J. C., and Smith, T. W. (1979): Localization of the neurally mediated arrhythmogenic properties of digitalis. *Science*, 204:321–323.

213. Somberg, J. C., Mudge, G. H., Jr., Risler, T., and Smith, T. W. (1980): Neurally mediated augmentation of the arrhythmogenic properties of highly polar cardiac glycosides. *Am. J. Physiol.*, 238:H202–H208.

214. Songu-Nize, E., Bealer, S. L., and Caldwell, R. W. (1982): Effect of AV3V lesions on the development of DOCA-salt hypertension and vascular Na^+ pump activity. *Hypertension*, 4:575–580.

215. Sonnenblick, E. H., Williams, J. F., Jr., Glick, G., Mason, D. T., and Braunwald, E. (1966): Studies on digitalis. XV. Effects of cardiac glycosides on myocardial force-velocity relations in the nonfailing human heart. *Circulation*, 34:532.

216. Stern, M. D., Kort, A. A., Bhatnagar, G. M., and Lakatta, E. G. (1983): Scattered light intensity fluctuations in diastolic rat cardiac muscle caused by spontaneous Ca^{++}-dependent cellular mechanical oscillations. *J. Gen. Physiol.*, 82:119–153.

217. Sweadner, K. J. (1979): Two molecular forms of ($Na^+ + K^+$)-stimulated ATPase in brain. Separation, and difference in affinity for strophanthidin. *J. Biol. Chem.*, 254:6060–6087.

218. Tamm, C. (1963): In: *Proceedings of the 1st International Pharmacology Meeting, Vol. 3*, edited by W. Wilbrandt and P. Lindgren, pp. 11–26. Pergamon Press, Oxford.

219. Thomas, R., Boutagy, J., and Gelbart, A. (1974): Synthesis and biological activity of semisynthetic digitalis analogs. *J. Pharm. Sci.*, 63:1649–1683.

220. Trautwein, W., Taniguchi, J., and Noma, A. (1982): The effect of intracellular cyclic nucleotides and calcium on the action potential and acetylcholine response of isolated cardiac cells. *Pfluegers Arch.*, 392:307–314.

221. Tsien, R. W. (1983): Ca channels in excitable cell membranes. *Annu. Rev. Physiol.*, 45:341–358.

222. Tsien, R. W., Kass, R. S., and Weingart, R. S. (1979): Cellular and subcellular mechanisms of cardiac pacemaker oscillations. *J. Exp. Biol.*, 81:205–215.

223. Tsien, R. Y. (1980): New calcium indicators and buffers with high selectivity against magnesium and protons: Design, synthesis, and properties of prototype structures. *Biochemistry*, 19:2396–2404.

224. Tsien, R. Y. (1981): A nondisruptive technique for loading calcium buffers and indicators into cells. *Nature*, 290:527–528.

225. Vassalle, M., and Lin, C. I. (1979): Effect of calcium on strophanthidin-induced electrical and mechanical toxicity in cardiac Purkinje fibers. *Am. J. Physiol.*, 236:H689–H697.

226. Wakabayashi, S., and Goshima, K. (1981): Kinetic studies on sodium-dependent calcium uptake by myocardial cells and neuroblastoma cells in culture. *Biochim. Biophys. Acta*, 642:158–172.

227. Wasserman, O., and Holland, W. C. (1969): Effects of tetrodotoxin

and ouabain on atrial contractions. *Pharmacol. Res. Commun.,* 1:236.

227a. Wasserstrom, J. A., Schwartz, D. J., and Fozzard, H. A. (1982): Catecholamine effects on intracellular sodium activity and tension in dog heart. *Am. J. Physiol.,* 243:H670–H675.

228. Weingart, R., Kass, R. S., and Tsien, R. W. (1978): Is digitalis inotropy associated with enhanced slow inward calcium current? *Nature,* 273:389–392.

229. Wendt-Gallitelli, M. F., and Jacob, R. (1984): Effects of nontoxic doses of ouabain on sodium, potassium, calcium distribution in guinea pig papillary muscles. Electronprobe microanalysis. *Basic Res. Cardiol. [Suppl.],* 79:79–86.

230. Whitmer, K. R., Wallick, E. T., Epps, P. E., Lane, L. K., Collins, J. H., and Schwarts, A. (1982): Effects of extracts on rat brain on the digitalis receptor. *Life Sci.,* 30:2261–2275.

230a. Weidmann, S. (1955): The effects of calcium ions and local anesthetics on electrical properties of Purkinje fibers. *J. Physiol. (Lond.),* 129:568–582.

231. Wier, W. G., Kort, A. A., Stern, M. D., Lakatta, E. G., and Marban, E. (1983): Cellular calcium fluctuations in mammalian heart: Direct evidence from noise analysis of aequorin signals in Purkinje fibers. *Proc. Natl. Acad. Sci. USA,* 80:7367–7371.

232. Wier, W. G., and Hess, P. (1984): Excitation-contraction coupling in cardiac Purkinje fibers. Effects of cardiotonic steroids on the intracellular [Ca^{2+}] transient, membrane potential, and contraction. *J. Gen. Physiol.,* 83:395–415.

233. Wiggers, C. J., and Stimson, B. (1927): Studies on cardiodynamic action of drugs. III. The mechanism of cardiac stimulation by digitalis and g-strophanthin. *J. Pharmacol. Exp. Ther.,* 30:251.

233a. Williams, D. A., Tsien, R. Y., and Fay, F. S. (1985): Ca^{++} measured in a single muscle cell using a new powerfully fluorescent dye (Fura2) and the digital image microscope. *Biophys. J. (Abstr.),* 47:131a.

234. Winegrad, S. (1984): Regulation of cardiac contractile proteins. Correlations between physiology and biochemistry. *Circ. Res.,* 55:565–574.

235. Yue, D. T., Marban, E., and Wier, W. G. (1985): Relationship between force and [Ca^{2+}] in tetanized ventricular myocardium. *Biophys. J.,* 47:353a.

The Heart and Cardiovascular System,
edited by H. A. Fozzard et al.
Raven Press, New York © 1986.

CHAPTER 67

Calcium-Channel-Blocking Drugs

Arnold M. Katz, Achilles J. Pappano, Frank C. Messineo,
Henry Smilowitz, and Priscilla Nash-Adler

Calcium-channel-blocking drugs include a diverse group of chemical structures that block calcium-selective ion channels in the plasma membranes of a variety of excitable cells. The ionized calcium (Ca^{2+}) carried by these channels to the interior of these cells generally serves as an activator messenger, so that calcium-channel blockers can inhibit a variety of key cell functions by preventing Ca^{2+} from gaining access to its intracellular receptors. The calcium-channel blockers also inhibit excitatory processes that depend on the depolarizing ionic currents that are generated when Ca^{2+} crosses the plasma membrane. Most of the effects of calcium-channel blockers on the cardiovascular system can be understood, therefore, in terms of their ability to reduce both the chemical and electrical signals that are generated when Ca^{2+} enters the cells of the heart and vascular smooth muscle.

Calcium-channel blockers cause vasodilatation and exert a negative inotropic action on the heart by inhibiting contractile function in both vascular smooth muscle and the working myocardial cells of the atria and ventricles. These drugs also reduce Ca^{2+}-dependent depolarizing currents in the sinoatrial and atrioventricular nodes and thereby slow heart rate and prolong atrioventricular conduction. In addition to these well-established effects on the heart and blood vessels, calcium-channel blockers can have many effects on tissues other than those of the cardiovascular system. These include inhibition of contraction in nonvascular smooth muscle and inhibition of stimulus-secretion coupling in a variety of

nonmotile tissues. As is true in the heart and vascular smooth muscle, these actions of the calcium-channel blockers arise from inhibition of activation signals initiated when Ca^{2+} enters a variety of cell types.

The mechanisms by which these drugs influence calcium-channel functions remain to be resolved. Rapid progress now being made in this field indicates that the different chemical structures that block these ion channels most likely act by first dissolving in the plasma membrane bilayer and then binding to sites on the proteins that compose and control these channels.

The calcium-channel blockers represent a diverse group of organic structures that inhibit the flux of calcium ions (Ca^{2+}) through calcium-selective channels in the plasma membranes of a large number of different cell types. The functional effects of these drugs generally involve inhibition of cellular function as the calcium-channel blockers interfere with the ability of Ca^{2+} to play its important biological role as a second messenger. This ion, which is the most important of the *chemical messengers,* generally activates one or another cellular function by binding to members of a class of high-affinity Ca^{2+}-binding proteins within a number of eukaryotic cells (72). Because Ca^{2+} also serves as an *electrical messenger* that carries electric charges across membranes, the calcium-channel blockers can also attenuate a number of important depolarizing inward currents carried by Ca^{2+}.

The ability of the calcium-channel blockers to inhibit Ca^{2+} entry through calcium-selective plasma membrane "channels" allows these drugs to modify a number of Ca²⁺-dependent processes in the cardiovascular system, notably excitation and excitation-contraction coupling in both cardiac and vascular smooth muscle (Table 1). In the working myocardium of the atria and ventricles, these drugs inhibit Ca²⁺ entry during the plateau phase of the action potential and thereby reduce myocardial contractility. In addition, by reducing the entry of positively charged Ca²⁺ into the cells of the sinoatrial and atrioventricular nodes, these drugs slow pacemaker activity and inhibit atrioventricular conduction in the heart (Table 1).

The general view of the calcium-channel blockers as being cardiovascular drugs reflects the initial discovery of calcium channels in cardiac muscle and the fact that most of the pioneering work on these drugs was carried out using cardiac and vascular smooth muscle. Whereas their cardiovascular effects represent the best understood of the actions of these drugs, the central role of Ca²⁺ in both depolarizing and activating a variety of excitable cells allows some of these calcium-channel-blocking drugs to inhibit excitation-contraction coupling in non-vascular smooth muscle and stimulus-secretion coupling in a number of nonmotile cells (Table 1).

The most appropriate name for this class of drugs

remains controversial. Fleckenstein (36) favors his initial term "calcium antagonist," rather than "blocker," because complete blockade of calcium influx via the slow inward current would be incompatible with cell function. Godfraind and Kaba (45), however, introduced the term "blockade" to describe the actions of this class of drugs. We believe the designation *calcium antagonist* is misleading, because these drugs are not calcium analogues that directly antagonize the effects of Ca²⁺ on cellular processes; indeed, their important biological effects do not arise from actions on such Ca²⁺-binding structures as the contractile proteins (81) and sarcoplasmic reticulum (21). Furthermore, the designation calcium antagonist has engendered some confusion, because drugs that interfere with the activation of calmodulin by Ca²⁺ can also be viewed as calcium "antagonists" even though their effects involve actions quite different from those produced by blockade of calcium influx across the plasma membrane (88,115). Because these drugs act primarily by inhibiting calcium entry into cells, the term "calcium entry blockers" has been proposed (108); however, these drugs do not interfere with all of the mechanisms by which calcium enters the cell, notably Na-Ca exchange (80,85) and the background calcium current. Instead, they act mainly to inhibit the flux of

TABLE 1. *Some important calcium-regulated processes in the heart, smooth muscle, and nonmotile tissues and functional effects of calcium-channel blockers*

Tissue	Process	Functional effect
Heart		
SA node	Depolarization	Inhibit pacemaker activity
AV node	Depolarization	Inhibit A-V conduction
Working myocardium	Contraction	Reduce myocardial contractility
	Depolarization	Inhibit action-potential plateau
Vascular smooth muscle		
Arteriolar		
Systemic	Contraction	Decrease peripheral resistance
Pulmonary	Contraction	Decrease pulmonary resistance
Coronary	Contraction	Inhibit coronary vasospasm
Venous	Contraction	Decrease venous return
Nonvascular smooth muscle		
Bronchial	Contraction	Decrease bronchomotor tone
Gastrointestinal	Contraction	Decrease esophageal spasm and GI motility
Genitourinary	Contraction	Inhibit ureteric spasm and bladder contraction
Uterine	Contraction	Inhibit dysmenorrhea, labor
Nonmotile tissues		
Pancreas	Glucose-induced insulin release	Decrease insulin secretion
Pituitary	Hormone release	Decrease hormone secretion
Adrenal medulla	Catecholamine release	Decrease catecholamine secretion
Salivary glands	Saliva formation	Decrease salivation
Lacrimal glands	Tear formation	Decrease tearing
Gastric mucosa	Gastrin secretion	Decrease gastrin secretion
Mast cells	Exocytosis, histamine release	Inhibit degranulation
Polymorphonuclear leukocytes	Lysosomal enzyme release, locomotion	Inhibit neutrophil activation
Platelets	Exocytosis, aggregation, contraction	Inhibit platelet activation

calcium through calcium-selective channels in the plasma membrane in cardiac-muscle, smooth-muscle, and other cells. For this reason we believe that the most accurate phrase to describe these drugs is "blockers of calcium entry through a diverse group of calcium-selective plasma membrane ion channels," recognizing that the extent of this inhibition need not be complete. We choose to abbreviate this description to *calcium-channel blockers.*

INTERACTION OF CALCIUM-CHANNEL BLOCKERS WITH PLASMA MEMBRANE

The plasma membrane (in muscle, often referred to as the sarcolemmal membrane) controls Ca^{2+} fluxes into and out of the cytosol of the heart and vascular smooth muscle. This membrane can be viewed primarily as a barrier that impedes the movement of this ion between the two aqueous compartments on either side: the cytosol within the cell, where Ca^{2+} concentration is in the micromolar range, and the extracellular space, where Ca^{2+} concentration is in the millimolar range. As discussed in *Chapter* 5, the basic structure of the plasma membrane is a lipid bilayer that is composed of two sheets of phospholipid molecules. The central core of the membrane bilayer is a lipid barrier that is composed of the hydrocarbon chains of the fatty acid moieties of the membrane phospholipids, whereas the two surfaces of the bilayer are lined by charged groups that interact with the ionic environments of the aqueous spaces on the two sides of the membrane. The barrier to Ca^{2+} fluxes across the membrane thus resides in the hydrophobic region at the center of the bilayer.

The ion channels that allow Ca^{2+} to move across membranes, whether passively as in the case of the voltage-sensitive sarcolemmal Ca^{2+} channels (*Chapter* 31) or actively as in the case of the Ca^{2+} pump of the sarcoplasmic reticulum (*Chapter* 36) are composed of intrinsic membrane proteins. These proteins, which are embedded within and span one or both leaflets of the bilayer membrane, are amphiphilic in that they contain both hydrophobic and hydrophilic regions. The hydrophobic regions of these intrinsic membrane proteins are found within the core of the membrane bilayer, where they interact with the hydrophobic fatty acyl chains at the center of the bilayer. Their hydophilic surfaces project toward both membrane surfaces, where they interact with the aqueous environments on either side of the membrane. It is likely that the calcium channel itself is a water-filled "pore" that is surrounded by hydrophilic surfaces of one or more of the channel proteins; it is within this pore that Ca^{2+} is able to cross the membrane in a highly regulated fashion.

In general terms, there are two types of calcium channels: those that open in response to membrane depolarization (voltage-dependent calcium channels), and those whose opening is controlled by hormones, humoral

agents, and neurotransmitters that bind to specific receptor sites within or related to these channels (receptor-operated calcium channels). Both types of Ca^{2+} channels are commonly found in a given cell type (10). It is now apparent that differences in calcium-channel regulation reflect the presence of separate pathways through which Ca^{2+} crosses the plasma membrane (77).

Calcium channels differ not only in the nature of the stimulus that causes them to open but also in their responses to calcium-channel blockers. The voltage-dependent calcium channels are more readily blocked by these drugs than are receptor-operated channels (10), but this rule is not inviolate, because some calcium-channel blockers inhibit contraction in smooth muscle in which activator Ca^{2+} appears to enter the cell by way of receptor-operated calcium channels (102). The complexity of the interactions between calcium-channel-blocking drugs and their receptors within these ion channels is highlighted by marked differences in the responses to a given calcium-channel blocker of the calcium channels in different tissues, and even different regions of the same tissue (6,43). These differences are of considerable theoretical importance, because they offer a rationale for efforts to develop new and more selective calcium-channel-blocking drugs for clinical use.

PHARMACOLOGY OF CALCIUM-CHANNEL BLOCKERS

A variety of organic compounds (and some inorganic ions like Mn^{2+}) can block calcium channels with variable degrees of specificity. In general, the organic calcium-channel blockers are amphiphiles that contain a large hydrophobic region, usually one or more ring structures, and a hydrophilic portion such as an amine or other charged group. The chemical structures of a number of these drugs are shown in Figs. 1 through 4. Most of the calcium-channel-blocking drugs now being studied fall into three structural groups: the phenylalkylamines (e.g., verapamil, methoxyverapamil [D-600 or gallopamil], desmethoxyverapamil [D-888], tiapamil, and bepridil) (Figs. 1 and 2), the benzothiazepines (e.g., diltiazem) (Fig. 1), and the 1,4-dihydropyridines (e.g., nifedipine, nitrendipine, nimodipine) (Figs. 1, 3, and 4). The so-called calcium agonists, Bay K-8644 and CGP 28-392, are dihydropyridines that increase rather than inhibit calcium entry via sarcolemmal calcium channels.

Verapamil, nifedipine, and diltiazem have been approved for use in the United States, and a number of dihydropyridines that are closely related to nifedipine are being examined in both animal and clinical studies. Many of these drugs (e.g., nimodipine, nitrendipine, nisoldipine, and felodipine) (105) (Fig. 4) appear to have relatively high selectivities for calcium channels in certain smooth muscles (102). Methoxyverapamil (D-600), which has actions generally similar to those of verapamil, has

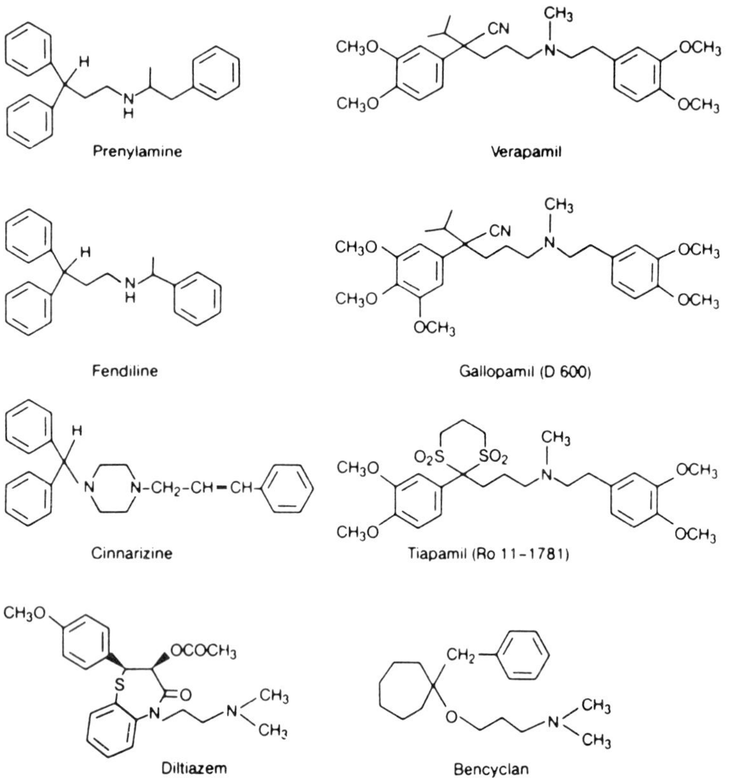

FIG. 1. Chemical structures of a number of different organic calcium-channel blockers. (From ref. 79, with permission.)

Prenylamine

Verapamil

Fendiline

Gallopamil (D 600)

Cinnarizine

Tiapamil (Ro 11-1781)

Diltiazem

Bencyclan

been used extensively in animal studies, and several related phenylalkylamines are under study. A number of additional drugs, including bepridil, a phenylalkyl-amine with significant nonspecific "quinidine-like" activity, are now undergoing extensive clinical testing. Other calcium-channel-blocking drugs that are now mainly of historical interest include prenylamine, cinnarizine, flunarizine, and lidoflazine, which have been studied and used clinically outside the United States but appear unlikely to be introduced in this country. Perhexiline has been tested clinically but has toxic side effects that preclude its routine clinical use.

Calcium-channel blockers often exert their actions at nanomolar concentrations, and the effects of these drugs are stereospecific (63). As expected, these drugs bind tightly to purified plasma membrane preparations, presumably to receptor sites on structures that are involved in calcium-channel function (9,25,28,40,95,116). It is now generally agreed that members of the three classes of calcium-channel-blocking drugs do not bind to the same site in these isolated membranes (8,43,49,50). Instead, the interactions involved in the bindings of the three types of calcium-channel blockers are quite complex (Fig. 7), probably because of allosteric interactions that occur when the dihydropyridine, phenylalkylamine, and benzothiazepine calcium-channel-blocking drugs bind to their specific sites on proteins related to the calcium channel. However, certain interactions appear to be constant; for example, phenylalkylamines inhibited, but diltiazem enhanced, dihydropyridine binding in virtually all reported studies. The degrees of these interactions depended on temperature and duration of drug exposure

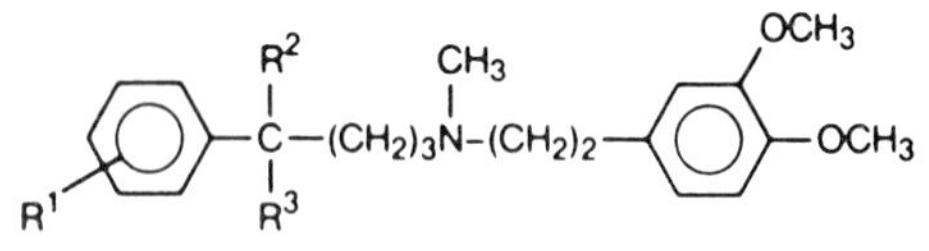

Verapamil	$R^1 = 3,4-(OCH_3)_2$	$R^2 = CH(CH_3)_2$	$R^3 = CN$
Gallopamil	$R^1 = 3,4,5-(OCH_3)_3$	$R^2 = CH(CH_3)_2$	$R^3 = CN$
Tiapamil	$R^1 = 3,4-(OCH_3)_2$	$R^2, R^3 = SO_2(CH_2)_3SO_2$	

FIG. 2. Chemical structures of some phenylalkylamine calcium-channel blockers. (From ref. 79, with permission.)

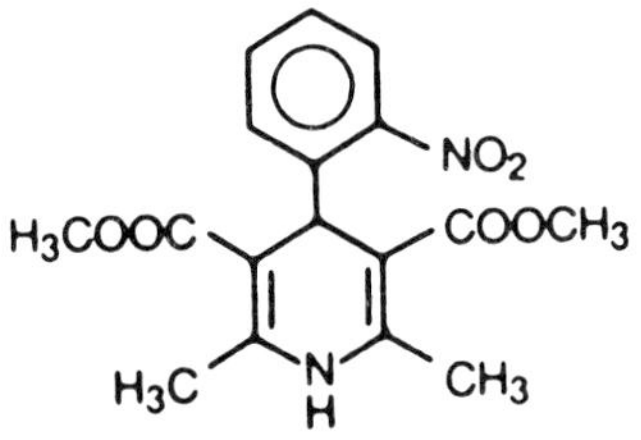

FIG. 3. Chemical structure of nifedipine. (From ref. 79, with permission.)

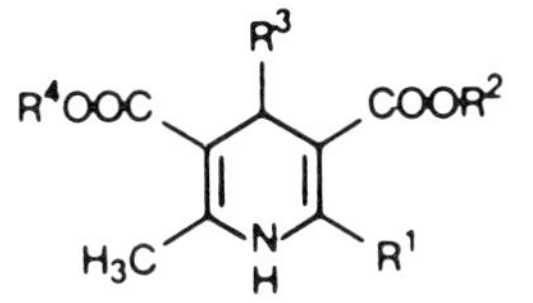

	R¹	R²	R³	R⁴
Nifedipine	CH_3	CH_3	$2\text{-}NO_2\text{-}C_6H_4$	CH_3
Nicardipine	CH_3	$CH_2CH_2N\begin{smallmatrix}CH_2C_6H_5\\CH_3\end{smallmatrix}$	$3\text{-}NO_2\text{-}C_6H_4$	CH_3
Nitrendipine	CH_3	C_2H_5	$3\text{-}NO_2\text{-}C_6H_4$	CH_3
Nimodipine	CH_3	$CH_2CH_2OCH_3$	$3\text{-}NO_2\text{-}C_6H_4$	$CH(CH_3)_2$
Nisoldipine	CH_3	CH_3	$2\text{-}NO_2\text{-}C_6H_4$	$CH_2CH(CH_3)_2$
Felodipine	CH_3	C_2H_5	$2,3\text{-}Cl_2\text{-}C_6H_3$	CH_3
FR 34235	CN	CH_3	$3\text{-}NO_2\text{-}C_6H_4$	$CH(CH_3)_2$
PN 200–110	CH_3	CH_3	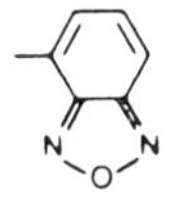	$CH(CH_3)_2$

FIG. 4. Chemical structures of some dihydro-pyridine calcium-channel blockers. (From ref. 79, with permission.)

to the membrane. Additional studies have shown that diltiazem can attenuate the inhibitory effect of verapamil on dihydropyridine binding in heart and brain membranes (8,62,63). Dihydropyridines have also been reported to enhance diltiazem binding to skeletal muscle membranes at 30°C and to inhibit at 2°C (42).

Divalent cations, especially Ca^{2+} and Mg^{2+}, have been found to alter the binding of organic calcium-channel-blocking drugs to brain, skeletal muscle, and cardiac muscle plasma membranes. In brain and skeletal muscle, Ca^{2+} and Mg^{2+} have been reported to inhibit the binding of verapamil (39) and to stimulate nifedipine binding (51,89). In cardiac membranes, on the other hand, these cations may convert nitrendipine and desmethoxyvera-pamil binding sites from low affinity to high affinity (87).

There is an important and incompletely explained discrepancy between the binding of calcium-channel-blocking drugs to isolated membranes and their actions on living cells. This discrepancy lies in differences between the affinities of the dihydropyridines for binding to cardiac membranes, involving concentrations several

orders of magnitude greater than the concentrations necessary for their actions to inhibit the contractile response in living cells (Fig. 6B). In spite of these differences in absolute potencies, the relative potencies of a number of these drugs for both binding and cellular actions in the heart are the same (96,104). Interestingly, no discrepancies are found in the binding and inhibitory actions of these drugs in smooth muscle (Fig. 6A) (96,104). There are at least two plausible explanations for the greater potencies of the dihydropyridines to bind to isolated membranes than to inhibit calcium channels in the living cells of the heart. The first is that the high-affinity binding of the dihydropyridines seen in isolated membrane preparations does not mediate their inhibitory effects in intact cells (74), but that there is a low-affinity binding site (43) that is responsible for the actions of the dihydropyridine calcium-channel blockers. The second possible explanation for the discrepancy between the high binding affinity to cardiac membranes *in vitro* and the much lower inhibitory potency of the dihydro-pyridines in cardiac muscle *in vivo* is that the ability of these drugs to bind to specific sites is potentiated in membrane fragments because of increases in the affinities of these drugs for their binding sites when, as occurs during preparation of the isolated membranes, these membranes become depolarized (*vide infra*).

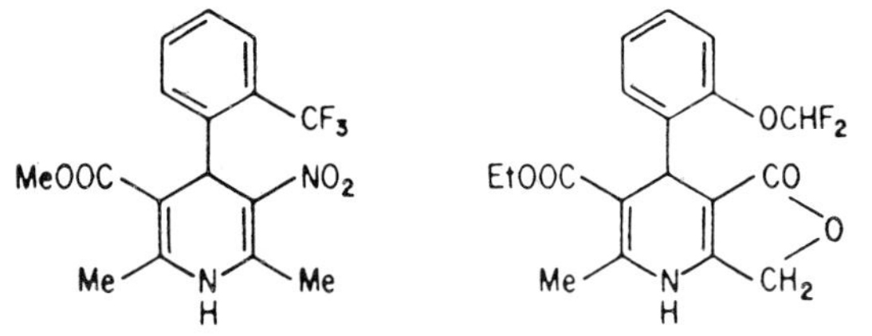

The newly developed dihydropyridine calcium agonists, which promote calcium entry into heart and vascular smooth muscle, are structurally similar to the dihydropyridine calcium-channel blockers (Fig. 5). These agents have effects opposite to those of the calcium-channel blockers; in the cardiovascular system they are vasoconstrictors and have a positive inotropic action on the heart (86). The effects of the agonists are competitively antagonized by the dihydropyridine calcium-chan-

FIG. 5. Chemical structures of two dihydropyridine calcium-channel agonists. The structure on the left is Bay K-8644; that on the right is CGP 28-392. (From ref. 62, with permission.)

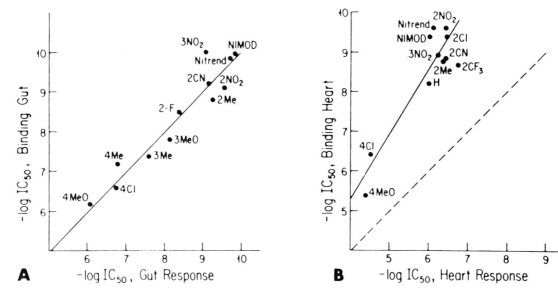

FIG. 6. Relationships between binding affinities (ordinate) and tissue responses (abscissa) to a series of dihydropyridine calcium-channel blockers containing substitutions at the 2 and 4 groups on the dihydropyridine ring, as indicated on the figures. NIMOD, nimodipine; Nitrend, nitrendipine. The dashed line is the line of identity. (From ref. 104, with permission.)

nel blockers and noncompetitively inhibited by diltiazem and verapamil, and the binding of dihydropyridine calcium-channel blockers can be displaced competitively by the dihydropyridine calcium-channel agonists (62). These findings suggest that the dihydropyridine calcium-channel blockers and agonists both bind to the same site on the calcium channel and that the opposing effects on channel function arise from subtle differences in the way in which these drug molecules act on the receptor. This interpretation is supported by studies of the mechanisms by which their opposing effects on channel function are brought about.

The effects of the "calcium agonists" have been explained by their ability to enhance calcium entry through sarcolemmal calcium channels (14,59,71) (see *Chapter* 31). The ability of the agonists to promote calcium entry is accompanied by an increased likelihood of finding the channel in a prolonged open state, which can be explained if these drugs stabilize a newly described long-lasting open state of the calcium channel. Of considerable importance to our understanding of the mechanism by which these drugs interact with the sarcolemmal proteins that control calcium-channel function is the finding that both nifedipine and nitrendipine, which are

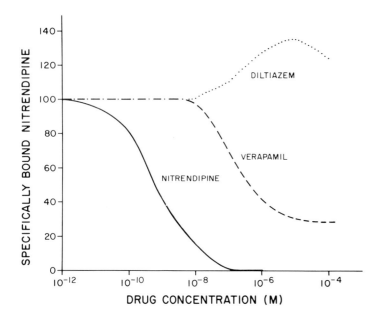

FIG. 7. Schematic diagram showing the effects of members of three classes of calcium-channel blockers on the binding of ^{3}H-nitrendipine to specific sites in the plasma membrane. (From ref. 8, with permission.)

calcium-channel blockers, also promote the appearance of this long-lived open state of the channel (59). In the case of the blockers, however, this "agonist" effect is overcome by a more pronounced action to decrease the likelihood that the channel will assume a short-lived open state in response to membrane depolarization. Thus, whereas the dihydropyridine calcium-channel blockers exhibit a weak agonist effect, their major action is to block the ability of these channels to assume their physiologically important open state. Conversely, it has been reported that the effects of Bay K-8644, one of the calcium agonists, are voltage-dependent such that at a potential of -60 mV the drug increases calcium currents, whereas at -45 mV it inhibits calcium conductance (94).

STRUCTURE OF THE CALCIUM CHANNEL

Whereas a large body of information regarding the physiological and pharmacological properties of calcium channels now exists, much less is known of the molecular structures of the membrane proteins that make up these ion channels and the manner in which the calcium-channel blockers modify their functions. The complex interactions seen between the different chemical structures that block calcium channels argue strongly against the view that these drugs compete for binding to a single class of "receptors" (vide supra). Purification and characterization of the calcium channels have recently been accomplished in studies that have used the dihydropyridines to label membrane proteins that are presumed to represent components of the calcium channels.

Because the binding of a large number of substances to the calcium channel can produce such diverse effects as prolonged channel opening, inhibition of channel opening, increased number of dihydropyridine antagonist binding sites, etc., it is not surprising that the structure of the calcium channel is complicated. At this time, our understanding of this important structure can be viewed as only in its infancy. Several features of this structure are, however, now coming into focus, notably that the channel is an oligomeric structure containing at least one integral membrane glycoprotein.

The main evidence that the calcium channel is a glycoprotein is that it binds several lectins that can be displaced from it by specific sugars. There is agreement that the dihydropyridine receptor will bind wheat germ agglutinin, which can be released by N-acetylglucosamine (11,23,42,89). This property has been found to be useful in purification of the channel by these investigators.

The main evidence that the dihydropyridine receptor is an integral membrane protein is that it can be extracted by detergents such as digitonin and CHAPS. However, recovery on extraction is usually no better than 50% and often less. Most investigators find that the calcium channel is unstable after extraction, and so quantitation by ligand binding is unreliable. Hence, 25 to 50% recovery is a minimum amount, and recovery of inactive material might be greater.

Two methods used to define the size of the dihydropyridine receptor, radiation inactivation and sucrose velocity-gradient centrifugation, both suggest that the native dihydropyridine receptor is a large macromolecular structure having a molecular weight of 150,000 to 300,000. Venter et al. (113), using guinea pig ileum, also found the molecule to be large, having a molecular weight of 278,000, whereas Ferry et al. (33), using guinea pig brain membranes and radiation inactivation, determined a molecular weight of 153,000 to 173,000. In guinea pig skeletal muscle membranes, Ferry et al. (34) found a molecular weight of 180,000. Interestingly, the molecular weight was found to decrease from 178,000 to 111,500 in the presence of D-cis-diltiazem, which suggests that the dihydropyridine receptor is oligomeric. Similarly, Goll et al. (48), using ^{3}H-PN-200-110 and target size analysis, showed the molecular weight in $(-)$diltiazem to be 136,000, and in $(+)$diltiazem 75,000. Unfortunately, some of these molecular weights do not correspond to any of the components found in the most highly purified preparations of calcium channel.

Sucrose-gradient centrifugation also suggests that the dihydropyridine receptor is large. Glossman and Ferry (42), who centrifuged membranes solubilized with CHAPS at high speed and labeled fractions with ^{3}H-nimodipine prior to filtration, found a sedimentation coefficient of 12.9 S; this value is greater than that of the Na$^+$ channel studied under the same conditions. Curtis and Catterall (23) used a 5-20 percent sucrose gradient as part of their purification scheme. Using similar sucrose gradients, Borsotto et al. (12) found several bands of dihydropyridine reactive material at 11.4 S, 14.4 S, and 21 S, with the 14.4-S band being the major species. It is possible that these different forms correspond to different oligomeric structures of the dihydropyridine receptor.

In skeletal muscle, purified T tubules contain the highest concentrations of dihydropyridine receptor (37), which suggests that the calcium channels are located in this structure. The most highly purified preparations of T tubules approach 100 pmoles dihydropyridine receptor per milligram protein, which, assuming a molecular weight of about 200,000 for the receptor, corresponds to a content of ~2.5% calcium-channel protein. Functional calcium channels have also been found when cultured skeletal muscle cells have been examined by patch-clamp methods (3). Similarly, calcium channels are found on the surface membrane in cardiac myocytes (4,58). When autoradiographic techniques were used to analyze ^{3}H-nitrendipine labeling of rat brain tissue, silver grains were found to be concentrated in regions of the brain that contained the highest concentrations of synapses (51,52).

The most successful attempts at purification of the calcium channel used relatively impure membrane preparations as starting material. This was due in part to the fact that a large fraction of the calcium channels is found in the denser membrane fractions, which contain sarcoplasmic reticulum. The finding that dihydropyridine receptors are most enriched in T-tubule-enriched fractions suggests that calcium channels may be present in the regions of membrane that bridge the T tubule to the sarcoplasmic reticulum, but there is no direct support for this hypothesis.

Purification of the calcium channels, which are present in very low concentrations on the cell surface (20), requires a great deal of starting material; for example, with skeletal muscle, most investigators have started with 40 to 400 mg of membrane material containing 6 to 10 pmoles per milligram protein dihydropyridine receptor. Curtis and Catterall (23) have emphasized the need for speed in their purification scheme, and the entire procedure is completed in about 12 hr. They achieved a 330-fold purification using digitonin solubilization of crude skeletal membranes, wheat-germ-agglutinin and DEAE Sephadex chromatography, and sucrose-gradient centrifugation. Under nonreducing conditions, three bands appeared on SDS gels that corresponded to molecular weights of 160,000 (alpha), 53,000 (beta), and 32,000 (gamma). The amount of the 53,000-dalton subunit varied in different preparations and appeared to be protease-sensitive. The apparent molecular weights of these subunits changed under reducing conditions (Table 2), which can be explained if the alpha subunit contains an interchain disulfide bond that, when reduced, increases SDS binding and hence increases mobility on SDS polyacrylamide-gel electrophoresis.

Borsotto et al. (11) also used crude skeletal microsomes as starting material, CHAPS solubilization, ion-exchange chromatography (DEAE Tris acryl gel), wheat-germ-agglutinin affinity chromatography, and gel filtration to achieve an 80-fold purification (800 pmol/mg protein) (this is probably an underestimate due to channel degradation). The subunit composition that these investigators observed is shown in Table 3. The component of 135,000 to 142,000 daltons was present in rabbit, chick, and frog preparations, whereas the low-molecular-weight polypeptide was absent in their frog preparation. As

TABLE 3. *Apparent molecular weights of calcium-channel subunits*

4–14% gel	5–12% gel
142,000	137,000
33,000	30,500
32,000	30,000

Data from Borsotto et al. (11).

with the data of Curtis and Catterall (23), it cannot be ascertained if the lower-molecular-weight polypeptides are distinct components of the calcium channel or if they are breakdown products of larger proteins.

Rengasamy et al. (89) used newborn chicken hearts as a starting material because the number of dihydropyridine binding sites in these hearts is 10-fold greater than in dog hearts. In 6 hr, these investigators were able to obtain 20 mg of membrane from 10 g of tissue containing 2 to 3 pmoles dihydropyridine receptor per milligram of membrane protein dihydropyridine receptor. Membranes extracted with digitonin and purified using DEAE Sephadex, hexylamine agarose, wheat-germ-agglutinin Sepharose columns, and sucrose-gradient centrifugation yielded 3 μg of protein containing 1,600 pmoles of receptors per milligram of protein. SDS gels showed polypeptides of 60,000, 54,000, and 34,000 daltons, but no 130,000- to 150,000-dalton polypeptide.

These early data on purification of the dihydropyridine receptor from skeletal muscle show partial agreement in that two groups found a 130,000- to 140,000-dalton subunit and a 30,000-dalton subunit; however, the status of the 50,000 subunit remains uncertain. The data for the heart dihydropyridine receptor suggest that its structure is very different from that of skeletal muscle, lacking the 130,000- to 150,000-dalton subunit. This view is strengthened by analyses of single calcium channels in membranes purified from skeletal and cardiac tissues that, when reconstituted into artificial planar lipid bilayers, exhibited significant differences in conductance and gating (92).

A number of photoaffinity labeling studies of the dihydropyridine receptor are summarized in Table 4. Most reports suggest that the dihydropyridine calcium-channel blockers label the 32,000- to 36,000-dalton subunit of the dihydropyridine receptor and a 43,000- to 45,000-dalton polypeptide. However, this conclusion must be viewed cautiously, because rather harsh conditions are used to effect the ligand-protein coupling, and the question of specificity of binding is not fully resolved.

Phosphorylation of the dihydropyridine receptor by cyclic-AMP-dependent protein kinase has been described by Curtis and Catterall (24). Both the alpha and beta subunits of the purified dihydropyridine receptor were found to be phosphorylated, the rate of phosphorylation being about 70% of that of the rate of the phosphorylation

TABLE 2. *Effects of reducing conditions*

Subunit	Nonreducing conditions	Reducing conditions	Partial reduction conditions
Alpha	160,000	130,000	130/160 doublet
Beta	53,000	50,000	
Gamma	32,000	33,000	

Data from Curtis and Catterall (23).

TABLE 4. *Dihydropyridine-binding sites determined by photoaffinity labeling studies*

Reference	Label used	Tissue	Subunits labeled
Ferry et al. (35)	^{3}H-azidopine	Skeletal muscle	145,000
Venter et al. (113)	^{3}H-isothiocyanate-dihydropyridine	Ileum	45,000
Horne et al. (61)	^{3}H-isothiocyanate-dihydropyridine	Cardiac muscle	45,000 43,000 33,000
Kirley & Schwartz (69)	^{3}H-isothiocyanate-dihydropyridine	Skeletal muscle	36,000
Campbell et al. (15)	^{3}H-nitrendipine	Cardiac muscle	32,000
Sarmiento et al. (97)	^{125}I-Bay-P	Skeletal, cardiac, and smooth muscle	33,000

of the sodium channel, which is very rapid under physiological conditions. The catalytic subunit of cyclic-AMP-dependent protein kinase selectively phosphorylates polypeptides of 145,000 and 54,000 daltons in intact T-tubule membranes. However, the phosphorylated 145,000-dalton polypeptide appears not to be the 145,000-dalton subunit of the dihydropyridine receptor, although the phosphorylated 50,000-dalton polypeptide does correspond to the 50,000-dalton subunit of the dihydropyridine receptor. Thus, the beta subunit appears to be the preferred substrate for cyclic-AMP-dependent protein kinase in intact T-tubule membranes and presumably in the intact cell. Because solubilization of the membranes appears to expose an additional site on the beta subunit that is not accessible in the membrane, this subunit of the dihydropyridine receptor is a likely site for regulation of calcium-channel function by cyclic-AMP-dependent phosphorylation. It remains to be determined if the beta subunit is a component of the calcium channel itself or if it is an extrinsic regulatory protein.

Several toxins that have recently been reported to interact with calcium channels and may serve as useful probes of the structure of the calcium channel include omega toxin, atrotoxin, and maitotoxin.

A small polypeptide toxin from the marine mollusc *Conus geographus,* called omega CgTx or omega toxin, irreversibly blocks nerve stimulus-evoked release of transmitter at the frog skeletal neuromuscular junction. Experimental evidence (68) indicates that the toxin acts presynaptically by preventing Ca^{2+} entry into the nerve terminal. The prevailing view is that omega toxin acts at the calcium channel of invertebrate neurons, as well as those of frog, chicken, and probably mammals. Another toxin, atrotoxin, has been obtained from rattlesnake venom and partially fractionated to yield a fraction that is reported to inhibit competitively the binding of dihydropyridines to cardiac tissue membranes and to serve as a calcium agonist (54a,117). Maitotoxin is a water-soluble toxin of unknown structure isolated from the poisonous dinoflagellate *Gambierdiscus toxicus.* The

purified toxin has a positive inotropic effect, causes smooth muscle to contract, stimulates transmitter release from sympathetic neurons and other cells, and releases prolactin from primary pituitary cultures. To explain these phenomena, it has been suggested that maitotoxin activates voltage-sensitive calcium channels (84), possibly by altering the voltage dependence of calcium-channel activation (38). Purification and labeling of these toxins, as well as preparation of antibodies to these potentially antigenic substances, hold promise for facilitating analysis of the structure of the calcium channel.

A powerful approach to defining the structure of the calcium channel will be the use of monoclonal antibodies prepared against components of the channel. Chin et al. (19) made polyclonal antibodies to the proposed subunits of the skeletal muscle dihydropyridine receptor, and Campbell et al. (16), who used nifedipine-protein conjugates to immunize rabbits, were able to demonstrate antibodies in post-immune sera that bound ^{3}H-dihydropyridines specifically, with dissociation constants that ranged from 0.01 nM to 0.66 nM.

MECHANISM OF CALCIUM-CHANNEL BLOCKADE

The mechanism by which channel-blocking drugs inhibit Ca^{2+} fluxes through plasma membrane channels is not yet known. In the case of the phenylalkylamines, the drugs appear to bind preferentially at the inner, or cytosolic, opening of the calcium channel (57). The view that these drugs act by insertion into the mouth of the channel (99) now seems unlikely in view of recent evidence indicating that these drugs reach the sites at which they modify channel function by first dissolving in the phospholipid bilayer, after which they inhibit channel opening by an effect on the hydrophobic portion of the calcium channel itself (14,71). Exposure to phospholipase A_2 has been reported to inhibit nitrendipine binding to brain, heart, and smooth-muscle membranes (46), indicating that membrane phospholipids play a role in the interaction between the calcium-channel blockers and the calcium channels. This interpretation is consistent with a recent kinetic analysis of the rates at which these drugs approach and come to occupy their membrane receptors (90) indicating that the approach of these lipid-soluble drugs to their receptors via the membrane is, in fact, several orders of magnitude more rapid than an approach via the bulk aqueous medium at the outside of the membrane bilayer (see *Chapter* 16).

The ability of most calcium-channel blockers to inhibit myocardial calcium-channel function is potentiated at rapid heart rates; this property is seen with the dihydropyridines and is especially marked for verapamil and diltiazem (2,27,54,70,73,103). This potentiation of the effects of these drugs when calcium channels have been activated is called "use dependence," because the ability of the drug to block the channels is enhanced when the channels have been opened, or "used."

The traditional explanation for use dependence, that the drugs enter the "mouth" of the channel when the latter is in its open state, is not in accord with recent evidence that these drugs approach their receptors via the membrane bilayer (*vide supra*). Instead, it is more likely that the receptor sites for these drugs are surfaces of the membrane proteins located at least in part near the hydrophobic region of the membrane bilayer. If this is the case, then use dependence can be explained by the ability of the drugs to bind preferentially to the calcium channels when they are in specific states that are determined by membrane voltage. According to this hypothesis, calcium-channel blockers interact preferentially with a special conformation of the hydrophobic surface of the protein; thus, the altered sensitivity of the calcium channel that occurs when the channel changes its state can be explained by a preference of the drug for binding to the specific conformation assumed by the channel during its open state. Reports that the inhibitory effects of calcium-channel blockers are potentiated by partial membrane depolarization (4,93) and removed by membrane hyperpolarization (75) are in accord with this hypothesis (see ref. 60 for review). Whereas these observations suggest an explanation for the higher affinity of the dihydropyridine calcium-channel blockers for isolated (and thus depolarized) membranes than for calcium-channel inhibition in intact tissue (*vide supra*), Green et al. (53) were not able to show that these drugs bind to isolated cardiac myocytes with greater affinity when the cells are depolarized.

DETERMINANTS OF SENSITIVITY OF TISSUE OR ORGAN TO CALCIUM-CHANNEL BLOCKERS

Source of Activator Ca^{2+}

One of the most important determinants of the sensitivity of a given organ or tissue to the inhibitory effects of the calcium-channel blockers is the source of activator Ca^{2+}. There are two general sources for this activator Ca^{2+}, and they differ markedly in their sensitivities to this class of drugs. The complexity and interplay of these mechanisms in different types of excitable cells are shown schematically in Fig. 8.

Where activator Ca^{2+} is derived from the extracellular space, and thus enters the cytosol through calcium channels in the sarcolemma, activation is generally susceptible to the calcium-channel blockers. In other cells, notably those of skeletal muscle, almost all of the activator Ca^{2+} is derived from internal stores that are separated from the cytosol by internal membranes, in which calcium-channel opening is not inhibited by the specific actions of the calcium-channel blockers. In muscle cells, for example, activation depends on the release of Ca^{2+} from internal stores that are contained within the sarcoplasmic reticulum, an internal membrane system whose calcium channels are insensitive to the calcium-channel blockers. Thus, the ability of the calcium blockers as a class to inhibit cell function will depend to a large extent on the source of the Ca^{2+} that activates cell function.

The relative contributions of extracellular and intracellular sources in providing activator Ca^{2+} for binding to the contractile proteins differ between cardiac muscle from various species. The myocardium in many amphibian species and mammalian neonates contains only a small internal calcium store, so that activation of the contractile proteins in these hearts depends primarily on calcium entry across the sarcolemma from the extracellular space. In most adult mammalian hearts, including humans, activator Ca^{2+} is derived largely from intracellular stores within the sarcoplasmic reticulum. Similar differences are seen in vascular smooth muscle; for example, in the rabbit, Ca^{2+} release from internal stores contributes differently to norepinephrine-induced contractions in different arteries (17).

One of the most important of the activator roles served by the Ca^{2+} that enters the cell from the extracellular space is to cause release of Ca^{2+} from internal stores (30,31). This "Ca^{2+}-triggered calcium release" can be viewed as an amplification mechanism that allows the entry of a small amount of Ca^{2+} into the cell interior to induce the release of a much larger internal store of this activation messenger. Thus, even in cells in which activator Ca^{2+} is derived largely from internal stores, drugs that block Ca^{2+} entry can inhibit cell activation almost completely.

Mechanism of Calcium-Channel Activation

Calcium channels in the plasma membranes of most smooth-muscle and nonmotile cells can open either in response to membrane depolarization or when a neurotransmitter or hormone binds to a receptor on the extracellular surface of the membrane. In those cells in

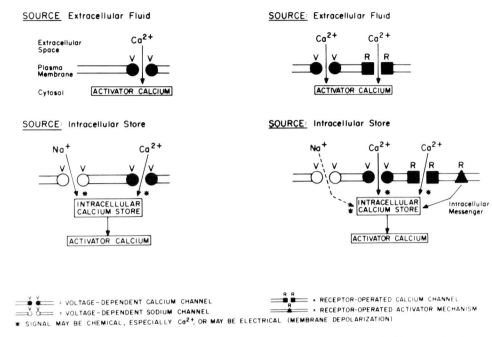

FIG. 8. Schematic diagram showing mechanisms that can provide for delivery of activator Ca²⁺ for excitation-contraction and stimulus-secretion coupling. **A:** Striated muscle. In some amphibian and embryonic mammalian hearts, activator Ca²⁺ is derived mainly from the extracellular fluid when this ion crosses the plasma membrane through voltage-sensitive calcium channels (*top*). In the adult mammalian heart (*bottom*), most of the activator Ca²⁺ is derived from intracellular stores in the sarcoplasmic reticulum. Ca²⁺ release can be initiated when a small amount of this ion crosses the plasma membrane or as the result of membrane depolarization. **B:** Smooth-muscle and nonmotile tissue. Activator Ca²⁺ derived from the extracellular fluid (*top*) can enter the cell through voltage-dependent calcium channels, one or more types of receptor-operated calcium channels, or both. In many of these cell types, all or a portion of the activator Ca²⁺ is derived from intracellular stores (*bottom*). Release of activator Ca²⁺ from these stores can be induced by Ca²⁺ entry through voltage-dependent or receptor-operated calcium channels, by membrane depolarization (which itself can be due to a calcium current), by other intracellular messengers released by the plasma membrane, or by any combination of these mechanisms. (Adapted from *Am. J. Cardiol.,* 55:2B–9B, 1985.)

which activator Ca²⁺ is derived from the extracellular fluid, calcium can enter the cytosol when membrane depolarization causes opening of voltage-dependent channels. However, the depolarizing calcium currents that result from the opening of voltage-dependent calcium channels often fail to produce propagated action potentials in many types of smooth muscle. Calcium can also enter smooth-muscle and nonmotile cells through receptor-operated channels. In many of these tissues, more than one mechanism controlling calcium-channel function can coexist, so that in a single tissue excitation-contraction or stimulus-secretion coupling can be controlled by both voltage-dependent and receptor-operated calcium channels.

Activator Ca²⁺ in smooth-muscle and nonmotile cells, as in the heart, can also be derived from internal stores (100), so that the number of possible activation mechanisms in these tissues becomes quite complex. Although the relative contributions of extracellular and intracellular sources in providing activator Ca²⁺ in most smooth muscles are not known, Bolton (10) has estimated that measured calcium currents can account for approximately 5 to 10% of this activator Ca²⁺ in a number of smooth-muscle types.

Responses to Different Transmitters

Several mechanisms may participate in the initiation of contraction in a given type of smooth muscle, and different smooth muscles may respond differently to a given transmitter or stimulus (47,105,109). In general, contraction of vascular smooth muscle initiated by membrane depolarization depends more on calcium influx across the sarcolemma than do contractions that are induced by norepinephrine, a physiological stimulus to contraction in a number of smooth muscles (10). Norepinephrine is able to open receptor-operated calcium channels in the plasma membrane and in some muscles initiate release of activator Ca²⁺ from intracellular stores, but rabbit aorta and canine coronary artery differ in their responses to norepinephrine (26,107). Whereas the major effect of norepinephrine in the aorta is to release calcium from an intracellular pool (107), in the coronary artery this neurotransmitter causes calcium to enter the cytosol from the extracellular space (26). Because the major pharmacological effect of the calcium-channel blockers is to inhibit calcium entry via plasma membrane channels, these drugs are most effective in vascular smooth muscles like the coronary artery that utilize receptor-operated calcium entry as the major mechanism to initiate contraction (6,26,107,109). In some smooth muscles, the source and pharmacological sensitivity of activator Ca^{2+} release can change during a single contraction (47), and different concentrations of a given transmitter can initiate contraction preferentially by receptor-operated or voltage-dependent channel mechanisms (10). Furthermore, there is evidence that calcium channels in vascular smooth muscle that are regulated by alpha$_1$- or alpha$_2$-receptors may have different sensitivities to various calcium-channel-blocking drugs. Thus, the different sensitivities of particular vascular beds may reflect differences in the relative distributions of alpha$_1$- or alpha$_2$-receptors in these beds (110,112).

NONSPECIFIC EFFECTS OF CALCIUM-CHANNEL BLOCKERS

The organic calcium-channel blockers are not absolutely specific in their ability to block calcium channels, and the ability of high concentrations of some of these drugs, notably bepridil, verapamil, and D-600, to exert potent nonspecific actions on membranes can be important both for their clinical use and in experimental studies. By definition, these nonspecific effects (sometimes called local anesthetic effects or quinidine-like actions) arise not from interactions of the drug with a specific site or "receptor" but by a nonspecific effect induced when the drug inserts into the membrane lipid bilayer (56). In the case of verapamil, for example, the threshold concentration that inhibits transmission through the rat phrenic nerve is almost 10 times less than that for lidocaine (55). These nonspecific effects can complicate interpretation of experimental studies of these drugs and may explain many findings in which these drugs are studied at concentrations greater than approximately 1 to 10 μM. Although of theoretical interest, effects that arise from nonspecific membrane actions are unrelated to their selective calcium-channel-blocking properties and so represent "side effects."

Other Actions of Calcium-Channel Blockers

Verapamil, nimodipine, and nifedipine have been reported to inhibit calmodulin-sensitive and calmodulin-insensitive phosphodiesterases, an effect that appears to be independent of their ability to block calcium channels (29). Felodipine, a dihydropyridine drug, has been reported to bind to calmodulin (13) but does not inhibit calcium uptake into rat heart. Although the potent smooth-muscle-relaxant effects of felodipine may arise in part from direct effects on calmodulin, this mechanism of action is quite different from those of most other calcium-channel-blocking drugs.

Interactions with Specific Plasma Membrane Receptors

Some of the calcium-channel blockers have been found to bind to neurotransmitter receptor sites. Verapamil and D-600 at high concentrations have been reported to displace some muscarinic antagonists from cardiac membranes (18,114), but these effects occurred at high drug concentrations, where nonspecific effects become significant. High concentrations of verapamil and D-600 have also been found to inhibit the uptake of serotonin, dopamine, norepinephrine, and choline by rat brain synaptosomes (76); however, this effect may be due to interference with a Na^+-channel-dependent process through nonspecific effects of these drugs. High concentrations of verapamil have also been reported to block alpha-adrenergic receptors (5,44,111), but the high concentrations of these drugs needed to inhibit agonist binding suggest that these blocking effects are also due to nonspecific effects of the calcium-channel blockers. The ability of high concentrations of verapamil and D-600 to inhibit the binding of dopaminergic agonists to dopamine receptors in the anterior pituitary (22) and agonist and antagonist binding to alpha$_1$-adrenergic and muscarinic, but not beta-adrenergic, receptors in myocardial membranes (66) can also be explained as being due in large part to nonspecific effects of these lipid-soluble drugs. High concentrations of D-600 have also been reported to interfere with the binding of several ligands to their receptors, including agonist binding to opiate receptors in rat brain homogenates (32).

It has been suggested that the site at which competition occurs between alpha-adrenergic receptor antagonists and calcium-channel blockers represents the calcium channel itself (1); however, the high drug concentrations used in many of these studies are consistent with the view that the observed effects of these drugs on muscarinic, dopaminergic, and alpha-adrenergic receptors were results of nonspecific effects of these drugs. This interpretation is supported by the finding of stereospecificity for the interactions of verapamil and D-600 with most calcium channels, but not with most other receptors. Thus, the (−) enantiomers of these drugs are more potent calcium blockers than the (+) enantiomers, whereas stereospecificity is minimal or absent for the interactions of these drugs with muscarinic and alpha-adrenergic receptors, respectively (41,64,82). Furthermore, nifedipine (which has little or no nonspecific membrane effect) displaces neither alpha$_1$- nor alpha$_2$-adrenergic agonists from cardiac membranes (82), and we have found evidence for an interaction of verapamil with muscarinic but not cardiac-glycoside-binding sites in purified cardiac sarcolemmal membranes (1a). The competitive kinetics of the interactions between verapamil and several types of membrane receptors, which are seen even at high concentrations of the drug, and the finding that these interactions exhibit some stereospecificity underscore our incomplete understanding of the nature of these "nonspecific" effects of the calcium-channel blockers.

CONCLUSION

The first descriptions of the calcium-channel blockers almost a quarter of a century ago, which were followed within a decade by the initial characterization of the calcium channels in heart muscle, led almost immediately to the introduction of this class of drugs into clinical medicine. The value of the calcium-channel blockers in therapy for several cardiovascular conditions, notably vasospastic angina, supraventricular tachycardias, and hypertension, is now established, and members of this class of drugs are finding increasing application in therapy for noncardiovascular diseases. The new information about these drugs and the structures whose functions they modify that has been presented in this chapter offers promise for important new advances in clinical therapy.

ACKNOWLEDGMENTS

The work of the authors described in this chapter was supported by Program Project Grant HL-33026 from the National Heart, Lung, and Blood Institute of the National Institutes of Health. F.C.M. is a Clinical Investigator (HL-00911) of the National Heart, Lung, and Blood Institute of the National Institutes of Health.

REFERENCES

1. Atlas, D., and Adler, M. (1981): Alpha-adrenergic antagonists as possible calcium channel inhibitors. *Proc. Natl. Acad. Sci. (USA),* 78:1237–1241.

1a. Ashavaid, T. F., Messineo, F. C., Colvin, R. A., Sarmiento, J. G., and Katz, A. M. (1984): The effect of verapamil on muscarinic, β-adrenergic, ouabain, digoxin and nitrendipine binding by purified cardiac sarcolemmal membranes. *Clin. Res.,* 32:149A.

2. Bayer, R., and Ehara, T. (1978): Comparative studies on calcium antagonsists. *Prog. Pharmacol.,* 2:31–37.

3. Beam, K. G., Knudson, C. M., and Powell, J. A. (1986): A lethal mutation in mice eliminate one slow calcium current in skeletal muscle cells. *Nature* 320:168–170.

4. Bean, B. P. (1984): Nitrendipine block of cardiac calcium channels: High affinity binding to the inactivated state. *Proc. Natl. Acad. Sci. (USA),* 81:6388–6392.

5. Blackmore, P. F., El-Refai, M. F., and Exton, J. H. (1979): Alpha-adrenergic blockade and inhibition of A23187-mediated Ca^{2+} uptake by the calcium antagonist verapamil in rat liver cells. *Mol. Pharmacol.,* 15:598–606.

6. Blakeley, A. G. H., Brown, D. A., Cunnane, T. C., French, A. M., McGrath, J. C., and Scott, N. C. (1981): Effects of nifedipine on electrical and mechanical responses of rat and guinea pig vas deferens. *Nature,* 294:759–761.

7. Blosser, J. C. (1983): β-adrenergic receptor activation increases acetylcholine receptor number in cultured skeletal muscle myotubes. *J. Neurochem.,* 40:1144–1149.

8. Boles, R. G., Yamamura, H. I., Schoemaker, H., and Roeske, W. R. (1984): Temperature-dependent modulation of [³H]nitrendipine binding by the calcium channel antagonists verapamil and diltiazem in rat brain synaptosomes. *J. Pharmacol. Exp. Ther.,* 229:333–339.

9. Bolger, G. T., Gengo, P. T., Luchowski, E. M., Siegel, H., Triggle, D. J., and Janis, R. A. (1982): High affinity binding of a calcium channel antagonist to smooth and cardiac muscle. *Biochem. Biophys. Res. Commun.,* 104:1604–1609.

10. Bolton, T. B. (1979): Mechanism of action of transmitters and other substances on smooth muscle. *Physiol. Rev.,* 59:606–718.

11. Borsotto, M., Barhanin, J., Fosset, M., and Lazdunski, M. (1985): The 1,4-dihydropyridine receptor associated with the skeletal muscle voltage-dependent Ca^{2+} channel. Purification and subunit composition. *J. Biol. Chem.,* 260:14255–14263.

12. Borsotto, M., Norman, R. I., Fosset, M., and Lazdunski, M. (1984): Solubilization of the nitrendipine receptor from skeletal muscle transverse tubule membranes. *Eur. J. Biochem.,* 142:449–455.

13. Bostrom, S.-L., Ljung, B., Mardh, S., Forser, S., and Thalin, E. (1981): Interaction of the antihypertensive drug felodipine with calmodulin. *Nature,* 292:777–778.

14. Brown, A. M., Kunze, D. L., and Yatani, A. (1984): The agonist effect of dihydropyridine on Ca channels. *Nature,* 311:570–572.

15. Campbell, K. P., Lipshutz, G. M., and Denney, G. H. (1984): Direct photoaffinity labelling of the high affinity nitrendipine binding site in subcellular membrane fractions isolated from canine myocardium. *J. Biol. Chem.,* 259:5384–5387.

16. Campbell, K. P., Sharp, A. H., Strom, M., and Kahl, S. D. (1986): High affinity antibodies to the 1,4-dihydropyridine Ca^{2+} channel blockers. *J. Biol. Chem. (in press).*

17. Cauvin, C., Saida, K., and Van Breeman, C. (1984): Extracellular Ca^{2+} dependence and diltiazem inhibition of contraction in rabbit conduit arteries and mesenteric resistance vessels. *Blood Vessels,* 21:23–31.

18. Cavey, D., Vincent, J. P., Lazdunski, M. (1977): The muscarinic receptor of heart cell membranes. Association with agonists, antagonists and antiarrhythmic agents. *FEBS Lett.,* 84:110–114.

19. Chin, H., Krueger, K., Beeler, T., and Nirenberg, M. (1985): Polyclonal antibodies with specificity for voltage-sensitive calcium channel proteins. Society for Neuroscience, abstract no. 15811.

20. Colvin, R. A., Ashavaid, T. F., and Herbette, L. G. (1985): Structure-function studies of canine cardiac sarcolemmal membranes. I. Estimation of receptor site densities. *Biochim. Biophys. Acta,* 812:609–623.

21. Colvin, R. A., Pearson, N., Messineo, F. C., and Katz, A. M. (1982): Effects of Ca channel blockers on Ca transport and Ca ATPase in skeletal and cardiac sarcoplasmic reticulum vesicles. *J. Cardiovasc. Pharmacol.,* 4:935–941.

22. Cronin, M. J. (1982): Some calcium and lysosome antagonists inhibit ³H-spiperone binding to porcine anterior pituitary. *Life Sci.,* 30:1385–1389.

23. Curtis, B. M., and Catterall, W. A. (1984): Purification of the calcium antagonist receptor of the voltage-sensitive calcium channel from skeletal muscle transverse tubules. *Biochemistry,* 23:2113–2118.

24. Curtis, B. M., and Catterall, W. A. (1985): Phosphorylation of the calcium antagonist receptor of the voltage-sensitive calcium channel by cAMP-dependent protein kinase. *Proc. Natl. Acad. Sci. (USA),* 82:2528–2532.

25. DePover, A., Matlib, M. A., Lee, S. W., Dube, G. P., Grupp, I. L., Grupp, G., and Schwartz, A. (1982): Specific binding of [³H]nitrendipine to membranes from coronary arteries and heart in relation to pharmacological effects. Paradoxical stimulation by diltiazem. *Biochem. Biophys. Res. Commun.,* 108:110–117.

26. Deth, R., and Van Breemen, C. (1977): Agonist-induced release of intracellular Ca^{2+} in rabbit aorta. *J. Membr. Biol.,* 30:363–380.

27. Ehara, T., and Kaufman, R. (1978): The voltage and time-dependent effects of (−)verapamil on the slow inward current in isolated cat ventricular myocardium. *J. Pharmacol. Exp. Ther.,* 207:49–55.

28. Ehlert, F. J., Itoga, E., Roeske, W. R., and Yamamura, H. I. (1982): The interaction of [³H]nitrendipine with receptors for calcium antagonists in the cerebral cortex and heart of rats. *Biochem. Biophys. Res. Commun.,* 104:937–943.

29. Epstein, P. M., Fiss, K., Hachisu, R., and Andrenyak, D. M. (1982): Interaction of calcium antagonists with cyclic AMP phosphodiesterases and calmodulin. *Biochem. Biophys. Res. Commun.,* 105:1142–1149.

30. Fabiato, A. (1985): Calcium-induced calcium release from the sarcoplasmic reticulum. *J. Gen. Physiol.,* 85:189–320.

31. Fabiato, A., and Fabiato, F. (1977): Calcium release from the sarcoplasmic reticulum. *Circ. Res.,* 40:119–129.

32. Fairhurst, A. S., Whittaker, M. L., and Ehlert, F. J. (1980): Interactions of D-600 (methoxyverapamil) and local anesthetics with rat brain alpha-adrenergic and muscarinic receptors. *Biochem. Pharmacol.,* 29:155–162.

33. Ferry, D. R., Goll, A., and Glossman, H. (1983): Putative calcium channel molecular weight determination by target size analysis. *Naunyn Schmiedebergs Arch. Pharmacol.,* 323:292–297.

34. Ferry, D. R., Goll, A., and Glossman, H. (1983): Calcium

channels: Evidence for oligomeric nature by target size analysis. *EMBO Journal,* 2:1729–1732.

35. Ferry, D. R., Rombusch, M., Gull, A., and Glossman, H. (1984): Photoaffinity labelling of Ca²⁺ channels with ³(H)azidopine. *FEBS Lett.,* 169:112–118.

36. Fleckenstein, A. (1983): *Calcium Antagonism in Heart and Smooth Muscle.* Wiley, New York.

37. Fosset, M., Jaimovich, E., Delpont, E., and Lazdunski, M. (1983): ³H-nitrendipine labelling of the Ca⁺⁺ channel in skeletal muscle. *Eur. J. Pharmacol.,* 86:141–142.

38. Freedman, S. B., Miller, R. J., Miller, D. M., and Tindall, D. R. (1984): Interactions of maitotoxin with voltage-sensitive calcium channels in cultured neuronal cells. *Proc. Natl. Acad. Sci. (USA),* 81:4582–4585.

39. Galizzi, J.-P., Fosset, M., and Lazdunski, M. (1984): Properties of receptors for the Ca²⁺-channel blocker verapamil in transverse tubule membranes of skeletal muscle. Stereospecificity, effect of Ca²⁺ and other inorganic cations, evidence for two categories of sites and effect of nucleotide triphosphates. *Eur. J. Biochem.,* 144:211–215.

40. Garcia, M. L., Trumble, M. J., Reuben, J. P., and Kaczorowski, G. J. (1984): Characterization of verapamil binding sites in cardiac membrane vesicles. *J. Biol. Chem.,* 259:15013–15016.

41. Gerry, R., Rauch, B., Colvin, R. A., Katz, A. M., and Messineo, F. C. (1985): Verapamil interaction with the muscarininc receptor demonstrates stereoselectivity at two sites. *Circulation [Suppl. III],* 72:330.

42. Glossman, H., and Ferry, D. R. (1983): Solubilization and partial purification of putative calcium channels labelled with ³H-nimodipine. *Naunyn Schmiedebergs Arch. Pharmacol.,* 323:279–291.

43. Glossman, H., Ferry, D. R., Goll, A., and Rombusch, M. (1985): Molecular pharmacology of the calcium channel: Evidence for subtypes, multiple drug-receptor sites, channel subtypes, and the development of a radioiodinated 1,4-dihydropyridine calcium channel label, [¹²⁵I]iodipine. *J. Cardiovasc. Pharmacol.,* 6:S608–S621.

44. Glossman, H., and Hornung, R. (1980): Calcium- and potassium-channel blockers interact with alpha-adrenoceptors. *Mol. Cell. Endocrinol.,* 19:243–251.

45. Godfraind, T., and Kaba, A. (1969): Blockade or reversal of the contraction induced by calcium and adrenaline in depolarized arterial smooth muscle. *Br. J. Pharmacol.,* 36:549–560.

46. Goldman, M. E., and Pisano, J. J. (1985): Inhibition of [³H]nitrendipine binding by phospholipase A₂. *Life Sci.,* 37:1301–1308.

47. Golenhofen, K. (1981): Differentiation of calcium activation processes in smooth muscle using selective antagonists. In: *Smooth Muscle: An Assessment of Current Knowledge,* edited by E. Bulbring, A. F. Brading, A. W. Jones, and T. Tomita, pp. 157–170. Edward Arnold, London.

48. Goll, A., Ferry, D. R., and Glossman, H. (1983): Target size analysis of skeletal muscle Ca²⁺ channels. *FEBS Lett.,* 157:63–69.

49. Goll, A., Ferry, D. R., and Glossman, H. (1984): Target-size analysis and molecular properties of Ca²⁺ channels labelled with [³H]-verapamil. *Eur. J. Biochem.,* 141:177–186.

50. Goll, A., Ferry, D. R., Streissnig, J., Schober, M., and Glossman, H. (1984): (−)-[³H]-desmethoxyverapamil, a novel Ca²⁺ channel probe. Binding characteristics and target size analysis of its receptor in skeletal muscle. *FEBS Lett.,* 176:371–377.

51. Gould, R. J., Murphy, K. M. M., and Snyder, S. H. (1982): ³H-nitrendipine labeled calcium channels discriminate in organic calcium agonists and antagonists. *Proc. Natl. Acad. Sci. (USA),* 79:3656.

52. Gould, R. J., Murphy, K. M. M., and Synder, S. H. (1985): In vitro autoradiography of ³H-nitrendipine localizes calcium channels to synaptic rich zones. *Brain Res.,* 330:217–223.

53. Green, F. J., Farmer, B. B., Wiseman, G. L., Jose, M. J. L., and Watanabe, A. M. (1985): Effect of membrane depolarization on binding of [³H]nitrendipine to rat cardiac myocytes. *Circ. Res.,* 56:576–585.

54. Hachisu, M., and Pappano, A. J. (1983): A comparative study of the blockade of calcium-dependent action potentials by verapamil, nifedipine and nimodipine in ventricular muscle. *J. Pharmacol. Exp. Ther.,* 225:112–120.

54a. Hamilton, S. L., Yatani, A., Hawkes, M. J., Redding, K., and Brown, A. M. (1985): Atrotoxin: a specific agonist for calcium currents in the heart. *Science,* 229:182–184.

55. Hay, D. W., and Wadsworth, R. M. (1981): The effects on contractions of the vas deferens of nifedipine and verapamil in relation to their local anesthetic activity. *Br. J. Pharmacol.,* 74:296P–297P.

56. Helenius, A., and Simons, K. (1975): Solubilization of membranes by detergents. *Biochim. Biophys. Acta,* 415:29–79.

57. Hescheler, J., Pelzer, D., Trube, G., and Trautwein, W. (1982): Does the organic calcium channel blocker D-600 act from inside or outside on the cardiac cell membrane? *Pfluegers Arch.,* 393:287–291.

58. Hess, P., Lansman, J. B., and Tsien, R. W. (1984): Different modes of Ca channel gating behaviour favored by dihydropyridine Ca agonists and antagonists. *Nature,* 311:538–544.

59. Hess, P., Lansman, J. B., and Tsien, R. W. (1985): Mechanism of calcium channel modulation by dihydropyridine agonists and antagonists. In: *Control and Manipulation of Calcium Movement,* edited by J. R. Parratt, pp. 189–212. Raven Press, New York.

60. Hondeghem, L. M., and Katzung, B. G. (1984): Antiarrhythmic agents: The modulated receptor mechanism of action of sodium and calcium-channel-blocking drugs. *Annu. Rev. Pharmacol. Toxicol.,* 24:387–423.

61. Horne, P., Triggle, D. J., and Venter, J. C. (1984): Nitrendipine and isoproterenol induce phosphorylation of a 42,000 dalton protein that co-migrates with the affinity labeled calcium channel regulatory subunit. *Biochem. Biophys. Res. Commun.,* 121:890–898.

62. Janis, R. A., Rampe, D., Su, C. M., and Triggle, D. J. (1985): Ca²⁺ channel: Ligand-induced antagonism and activation. In: *Calcium Entry Blockers and Tissue Protection,* edited by T. Godfraind et al., pp. 21–30. Raven Press, New York.

63. Janis, R. A., and Triggle, D. J. (1983): New developments in Ca²⁺ channel antagonists. *Med. Chem.,* 26:775–785.

64. Jim, K., Harris, A., Rosenberger, L. B., and Triggle, D. J. (1981): Stereoselective and non-stereoselective effects of D-600 (methoxyverapamil) in smooth muscle preparations. *Eur. J. Pharmacol.,* 76:67–72.

65. Kaczmarek, L. K., Jennings, K. R., Strumwasser, F., Nairn, A. C., Walter, U., Wilson, F. D., and Greengard, P. (1980): Microinjection of catalytic subunit of cyclic AMP-dependent protein kinase enhances calcium action potentials of bag cell neurons in cell culture. *Proc. Natl. Acad. Sci. (USA),* 77:7487–7491.

66. Karliner, J. S., Motulsky, J. H., Dunlap, J., Brown, J. H., and Insel, P. A. (1982): Verapamil competitively inhibits alpha₁-adrenergic and muscarinic but not beta-adrenergic receptors in rat myocardium. *J. Cardiovasc. Pharmacol.,* 4:515–520.

67. Katz, A. M., Hager, W. D., Messineo, F. C., and Pappano, A. J. (1984): Cellular actions and pharmacology of the calcium channel blocking drugs. *Am. J. Med.,* 77:2–10.

68. Kerr, L. M., and Yoshikami, D. (1984): A venom peptide with a novel presynaptic blocking action. *Nature,* 308:282–284.

69. Kirley, T. L., and Schwartz, A. (1984): Solubilization and affinity labelling of a dihydropyridine binding site from skeletal muscle: Effects of temperature and diltiazem on ³H-dihydropyridine binding to transverse tubules. *Biochem. Biophys. Res. Commun.,* 123:41–49.

70. Kohlhardt, M., and Mnich, Z. (1978): Studies on the inhibitory effect of verapamil on the slow inward current in mammalian ventricular myocardium. *J. Mol. Cell. Cardiol.,* 10:1037–1052.

71. Kokubun, S., and Reuter, H. (1984): Dihydropyridine derivatives prolong the open state of Ca channels in cultured cardiac cells. *Proc. Natl. Acad. Sci. (USA),* 81:4824–4827.

72. Kretsinger, R. H. (1979): The informational role of calcium in the cytosol. *Adv. Cyclic Nucleotide Res.,* 11:1–26.

73. Lee, K. S., and Tsien, R. W. (1983): Mechanism of calcium channel blockade by verapamil, D-600, diltiazem and nitrendipine in single dialyzed heart cells. *Nature,* 278:269–271.

74. Marsh, J. D., Loh, E., Lachance, D., Barry, W. H., and Smith, T. W. (1983): Relationship of binding of a calcium channel blocker to inhibition of contraction in intact cultured embryonic chicken ventricular cells. *Circ. Res.,* 53:539–543.

75. McDonald, T. F., Pelzer, D., and Trautwein, W. (1984): Cat

ventricular muscle treated with D600: Characteristics of calcium channel block and unblock. *J. Physiol. (Lond.)*, 352:217–241.

76. McGee, R., Jr., and Schneider, J. E. (1979): Inhibition of high affinity synaptosomal uptake systems by verapamil. *Mol. Pharmacol.*, 16:877–885.

77. Meisheri, K. D., Hwang, O., and Van Breemen, C. (1981): Evidence for two separate Ca²⁺ pathways in smooth muscle plasmalemma. *J. Membr. Biol.*, 59:19–25.

78. Messineo, F. C., Ashavaid, T., Colvin, R. A., Sarmiento, J. G., and Katz, A. M. (1984): The effect of verapamil on muscarinic, β-adrenergic, ouabain, digoxin and nitrendipine binding by purified cardiac sarcolemmal membranes. *Clin. Res.*, 32:149A.

79. Meyer, H. (1984): Structural/activity relationships in calcium antagonists. In: *Calcium Antagonists and Cardiovascular Disease*, edited by L. H. Opie, pp. 165–173. Raven Press, New York.

80. Morad, M., Tung, L., and Greenspan, A. M. (1982): Effect of diltiazem on calcium transport and development of tension in heart muscle. *Am. J. Cardiol.*, 49:595–601.

81. Nayler, W. G., and Grinwald, P. (1981): Calcium entry blockers and myocardial function. *Fed. Proc.*, 40:2855–2861.

82. Nayler, W. G., Thompson, J. E., and Jarrott, B. (1982): The interaction of calcium antagonists (slow channel blockers) with myocardial alpha-adrenoreceptors. *J. Mol. Cell. Cardiol.*, 14:185–188.

83. Norman, R. I., Borsotto, M., Fosset, M., Lazdunski, M., and Ellory, J. C. (1983): Determination of the molecular size of the nitrendipine sensitive Ca²⁺ channel by radiation inactivation. *Biochem. Biophys. Res. Commun.*, 111:878–883.

84. Ohizumi, Y., and Yasumoto, T. (1983): Contractile response of the rabbit aorta to maitotoxin, a most potent marine toxin. *J. Physiol. (Lond.)*, 337:711–721.

85. Ozaki, H., and Urakowa, N. (1979): Na-Ca exchange and tension development in guinea pig aorta. *Naunyn Schmiedebergs Arch. Pharmacol.*, 309:171–178.

86. Preuss, K. C., Gross, G. J., Brooks, H. L., and Warltier, D. C. (1985): Slow channel calcium activators, a new group of pharmacological agents. *Life Sci.*, 37:1271–1278.

87. Ptasienski, J., McMahon, K. K., and Hosey, M. M. (1985): High and low affinity states of the dihydropyridine and phenylalkylamine receptors on the cardiac calcium channel and their interconversion by divalent cations. *Biochem. Biophys. Res. Commun.*, 129:910–917.

88. Rahwan, R. G. (1985): Commentary. The methylenedioxyindene calcium antagonists. *Life Sci.*, 37:687–692.

89. Rengasamy, A., Ptasienki, J., and Hosey, M. (1985): Purification of the cardiac 1,4-dihydropyridine receptor/calcium channel complex. *Biochem. Biophys. Res. Commun.*, 126:1–7.

89a. Reynolds, I. J., Gould, R. J., and Snyder, S. H. (1983): [³H]-verapamil binding sites in brain and skeletal muscle: regulation by calcium. *Eur. J. Pharmacol.*, 95:319–321.

90. Rhodes, D. G., Sarmiento, J. G., and Herbette, L. G. (1985): Kinetics of binding of membrane-active drugs to receptor sites. Diffusion-limited rates for a membrane bilayer approach of 1,4-dihydropyridine calcium channel antagonists to their active site. *Mol. Pharmacol.*, 27:612–623.

91. Roeske, W. R., Ehlert, F. J., Itoga, E., and Yamamura, H. I. (1982): Cardiac calcium antagonist channels labelled by [³H]nitrendipine: Characterization, drug and ionic specificity. *Clin. Res.*, 30:216A.

92. Rosenberg, P. L., Hess, P., Tsien, R. W., Smilowitz, H., and Reeves, J. P. (1986): Calcium channels in planar lipid bilayers: Insights into mechanisms of ion permeation and gating. *Science*, 231:1564–1566.

93. Sanguinetti, M. C., and Kass, R. S. (1984): Voltage-dependent block of calcium channel current in the calf cardiac Purkinje fiber by dihydropyridine calcium channel antagonists. *Circ. Res.*, 55:336–348.

94. Sanguinetti, M. C., and Kass, R. S. (1984): Regulation of cardiac calcium channel current and contractile activity by the dihydropyridine Bay K8644 is voltage-dependent. *J. Mol. Cell. Cardiol.*, 16:667–670.

95. Sarmiento, J. G., Janis, R. A., Colvin, R. A., Triggle, D. J., and Katz, A. M. (1983): Binding of the calcium channel blocker

96. Sarmiento, J. G., Janis, R. A., Katz, A. M., and Triggle, D. J. (1984): Comparison of high affinity binding of calcium channel blocking drugs to vascular smooth muscle and cardiac sarcolemmal membranes. *Biochem. Pharmacol.*, 33:3119–3123.

97. Sarmiento, J. G., Epstein, P. M., Rowe, W. A., Smilowitz, H., Wehinger, E., and Janis, R. A. (1986): Photoaffinity labelling of a 35,000 dalton protein in cardiac skeletal and smooth muscle membranes using a new I¹²⁵-labelled 1,4-dihydropyridine calcium channel antagonist. *(submitted)*.

98. Schmid, A., Renaud, J. F., and Lazdunski, M. (1985): Short term and long term effects of β-adrenergic effectors and cyclic AMP on nitrendipine-sensitive voltage-dependent Ca²⁺ channels of skeletal muscle. *J. Biol. Chem.*, 260:13041–13046.

99. Schramm, M., and Towart, R. (1985): Modulation of calcium channel function by drugs. *Life Sci.*, 37:1843–1860.

100. Somlyo, A. P., Somlyo, A. V., Shuman, H., and Endo, M. (1982): Calcium and monovalent ions in smooth muscle. *Fed. Proc.*, 41:2683–2690.

101. Tada, M., Yamamoto, T., and Tonomura, Y. (1977): Molecular mechanism of active calcium transport by sarcoplasmic reticulum. *Physiol. Rev.*, 58:1–79.

102. Towart, R. (1981): The selective inhibition of serotonin-induced contractions of rabbit cerebral vascular smooth muscle by calcium-antagonistic dihydropyridines. An investigation of the mechanism of action of nimodipine. *Circ. Res.*, 48:650–657.

103. Trautwein, W., and Cavalie, A. (1985): Cardiac calcium channels and their control by neurotransmitters. *J. Am. Coll. Cardiol.*, 6:1409–1416.

104. Triggle, D. J., and Janis, R. A. (1984): The 1,4-dihydropyridine receptor: A regulatory component of the Ca²⁺ channel. *J. Cardiovasc. Pharmacol.*, 6:S949–S955.

105. Triggle, D. J. (1981): Calcium antagonists: Basic chemical and pharmacological aspects. In: *New Perspectives on Calcium Antagonists*, edited by G. B. Weiss, pp. 1–18. American Physiological Society, Bethesda.

106. Tsien, R. W. (1983): Calcium channels in excitable cell membranes. *Annu. Rev. Physiol.*, 45:341–358.

107. Van Breeman, C., and Siegel, B. (1980): The mechanism of alpha-adrenergic activation of the dog coronary artery. *Circ. Res.*, 46:426–429.

108. Vanhoutte, P. M. (1981): Calcium entry blockers and the cardiovascular system. Introduction: Why calcium blockers. *Fed. Proc.*, 40:2851.

109. Vanhoutte, P. M. (1982): Calcium-entry blockers and vascular smooth muscle. *Circulation* [Suppl. I], 65:11–19.

110. Vanhoutte, P. M. (1985): Calcium entry blockers, vascular smooth muscle and hypertension. *Am. J. Cardiol.*, 55:17–23.

111. Van Meel, J. C. A., de Jonge, A., Kalkman, H. O., Wilffert, B., Timmermans, P. B. M. W. M., and Van Zweiten, P. A. (1981): Organic and inorganic calcium antagonists reduce vasoconstriction *in vivo* mediated by postsynaptic alpha₂-adrenoceptors. *Naunyn Schmiedebergs Arch. Pharmacol.*, 316:288–293.

112. Van Zweiten, P. P., Van Meel, J., and Timmerans, P. (1983): Pharmacology of calcium entry blockers: Interactions with vascular alpha adrenoreceptors. *Hypertension* [Suppl. II], 5:8–17.

113. Venter, J. C., Fraser, C. M., Schaber, J. S., Jung, C. Y., Bolger, G., and Triggle, D. J. (1983): Molecular properties of the slow inward calcium channel. *J. Biol. Chem.*, 258:9344–9348.

114. Waelbroeck, M., Robberecht, P., deNeef, P., and Christophe, J. (1984): Effects of verapamil on the binding properties of rat heart muscarinic receptors: Evidence for an allosteric site. *Biochem. Biophys. Res. Commun.*, 121:340–345.

115. Weishaar, R. E. (1984): "Calcium antagonists" and "calcium agonists": Is there a place in pharmacology for these two misnomers? *Life Sci.*, 35:455–462.

116. Williams, L., and Tremble, P. (1982): A calcium channel antagonist, [³H]nitrendipine, binds to specific high affinity sites in vascular smooth muscle and cardiac membranes. *Clin. Res.*, 30:485A.

117. Yatani, A., Hamilton, S. L., and Brown, A. M. (1986): A component isolated from rattlesnake venom (*Crotalus atrox*) specifically activates Ca channel in mammalian heart. *Biophys J.* 47:65a.

The Heart and Cardiovascular System,
edited by H. A. Fozzard et al.
Raven Press, New York © 1986.

CHAPTER 68

Eicosanoids: Prostaglandins, Thromboxane, and Prostacyclin

Randall M. Zusman

When prostaglandins E_2 and $F_{2\alpha}$ were first identified as the vasoactive and uterine-smooth-muscle-contracting substances within seminal fluid by von Euler and associates some 50 years ago, the implications for the metabolites of arachidonic acid in human biology and physiology were unknown (1). Since the time of those original studies, four distinct classes of arachidonic acid metabolites have been identified; these compounds, prostaglandins, thromboxane, prostacyclin, and leukotrienes, are now collectively known as the eicosanoids (2). Their discovery and structural confirmation, as well as the understanding of the universality of their formation by virtually every cell type of the body, have led to intense investigations of the roles of these compounds in virtually every aspect of physiologic function (3). The common precursor for eicosanoid formation is arachidonic acid. Arachidonic acid, a polyunsaturated 20-carbon molecule, is a major component of all classes of lipids. In particular, arachidonic acid forms an important structural component of the cell membrane. In the cellular membrane, arachidonic acid is esterified within phospholipids, triglycerides, and cholesterol esters, from which it must be released for subsequent synthesis of eicosanoid material (4).

GENERAL PROPERTIES OF THE EICOSANOIDS

The individual characteristics of the various eicosanoids and their effects in human biology have been extensively reviewed, and the reader is referred to a recent article that describes the individual characteristics of these moieties in detail (5). In brief, however, the prostaglandins, thromboxane, and prostacyclin can be separated first into those agents that have vasodilating or vasoconstricting activity and those agents that are proaggregatory or antiaggregatory or inhibitory in terms of their effects on platelet aggregation (Fig. 1). Finally, the leukotrienes, which have unique chemical structures ("linear" metabolites of arachidonic acid), are predominantly thought to be mediators of immunologic reactions and processes of inflammation through their effects on vascular permeability, leukocyte adhesion, and leukocyte accumulation (6).

With regard to the "classic" prostaglandins, prostaglandin E_2 is a potent vasodilating agent that when infused into the arterial circulation results in a reduction in blood pressure, an increase in renal blood flow, and an increase in urinary sodium excretion as a result of enhanced glomerular filtration rate (7). Prostaglandin E_2, however, is rapidly metabolized by the pulmonary circulation and is not found under normal circumstances in sufficient quantity in the arterial blood supply to play an important role as the circulating vasodilating substance (8). In contrast, prostaglandin $F_{2\alpha}$ is a potent vasoconstrictor; it causes an increase in blood pressure in response to intraarterial infusion. However, like prostaglandin E_2, it is rapidly metabolized by the pulmonary circulation and plays no role as a circulating modulator

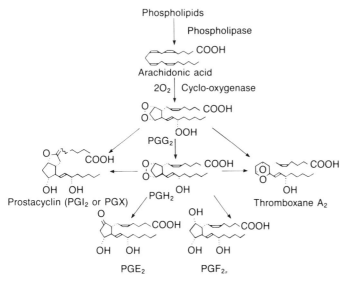

FIG. 1. Metabolic pathways of arachidonic acid leading to prostaglandins, thromboxane, and prostacyclin.

of vascular tone (9). Because of its potent effects on uterine smooth-muscle contraction and because it is released by uterine tissue, prostaglandin $F_{2\alpha}$ is thought to play an important role in the regulation of uterine contraction and the processes of fetal delivery (10).

ARTERIOSCLEROTIC VASCULAR DISEASE

With regard to the cardiovascular system, however, thromboxane A_2 and prostacyclin are thought to play much more important and potentially critical roles in both normal physiology and pathologic disease states than the prostaglandins. Thromboxane A_2, predominantly synthesized by the platelet, is a potent vasoconstrictor and stimulant of platelet aggregation (11). The activation of platelet aggregation by exposure to the collagen matrix of the vascular wall or because of activation of platelet aggregation by atherosclerotic arterial tissue has focused a great deal of attention on the potential role of thromboxane A_2 in the processes of myocardial ischemia. Similarly, prostacyclin, produced predominantly by the vascular endothelium, has characteristics that make it an important candidate to serve as an endogenous vasodilator, inhibitor of platelet aggregation, and protective agent against spontaneous platelet aggregation and thrombosis within the coronary vasculature (12). In addition, because of the vasomotor activities of all of the prostaglandins, thromboxane A_2, and prostacyclin, a potential role for these agents in the pathogenesis of hypertension has been suggested (13).

A common problem in assessing the roles of eicosanoids in human disease is inability to directly measure the rates of synthesis and function of the prostaglandins at the relevant sites of action. This inability prevents any meaningful assessment of the true importance of these substances in normal and abnormal physiology. Scientific investigation in this area is also hindered by the lack of specific inhibitors of individual synthetic pathways that might allow studies of the alterations in biological processes in the absence of a specific eicosanoid molecule.

HYPERTENSION

In the area of hypertension, the principal approach to the roles of prostaglandins in abnormal blood pressure regulation has been to measure the excretion of prostaglandin E_2 in the urine of hypertensive and normotensive subjects. Although a number of clinical studies have reported decreases in urinary prostaglandin E_2 excretion in hypertensive subjects, these data must be considered in the light of other clinical trials showing no abnormalities in urinary prostaglandin excretion (14–20). However, the use of measurements of prostaglandin moieties in the urine of patients with hypertension must be questioned as a valid technique for assessment of the roles of these substances in blood pressure control. Excretion of prostaglandins into the urine principally reflects synthesis of the molecule by the kidney, because infusion of prostaglandin E_2 into the renal artery does not result in an increase in the rate of appearance of this substance into fluid elaborated within the tubule and released into the urinary stream (21). The release of prostaglandins themselves into the urine can be dramatically affected by such factors as urinary flow rate, because these lipophilic materials are reabsorbed along the renal tubule, and the rate of reabsorption appears to be flow-dependent (22). As such, the urine flow rate, which was not considered in these clinical trials, may indicate abnormal urinary prostaglandin excretion, when in fact there is none.

An alternative approach to investigation of the roles of prostaglandins in the regulation of blood pressure has been to assess the effects of nonsteroidal antiinflammatory drugs, inhibitors of prostaglandin biosynthesis, on the control of blood pressure. Acute administration of prostaglandin synthesis inhibitors has been associated with an increase in blood pressure due to an increase in peripheral resistance. This might reflect the effects of inhibition of synthesis of vasodilating prostaglandin materials. However, chronic administration of such compounds has little effect on blood pressure in normotensives (23). The inability of such an approach to discern an etiologic role of the prostaglandins in the hypertensive process probably reflects the fact that many nonsteroidal antiinflammatory drugs have actions beyond those on the prostaglandin system. These additional effects are most notably exemplified by the effects of indomethacin, an agent often used in such trials, on cyclic AMP metabolism (25), which may result in alterations in blood pressure control unrelated to prostaglandin synthesis inhibition. In addition, inhibition of prostaglandin biosynthesis may have contradictory physiologic effects, because inhibition of thromboxane biosynthesis would be expected to result in vasodilation, but inhibition of prostacyclin biosynthesis in vasoconstriction. Alternatively, the hemodynamic effects of other vasoactive substances may be potentiated by prostaglandins, as evidenced by the vasodilatory effect of bradykinin (24), or attenuated by prostaglandins, as evidenced by the effects of angiotensin II (25). Once again, a clear determination of the roles of prostaglandins in hypertension cannot be made using these inhibitors. A third approach has been to assess the effects of nonsteroidal antiinflammatory drugs on antihypertensive therapy. Nonsteroidal antiinflammatory agents have uniformly produced inhibition of the antihypertensive activities of agents that lower blood pressure of hypertensive subjects, irrespective of their mechanisms of action. Such diverse antihypertensive agents as diuretics, beta-adrenergic blocking agents, alpha-adrenergic blocking agents, and vasodilators are all attenuated by administration of nonsteroidal antiinflammatory drugs. It is unlikely that all of these agents stimulate prostaglandin biosynthesis and thus are antagonized by the inhibition of arachidonic acid metabolism (26–29), although considerable evidence to be discussed later in this chapter would suggest that the prostaglandins do play important roles in the mechanisms of action of the converting-enzyme inhibitors.

Similarly, considerable investigation has been undertaken to assess the roles of prostaglandins and prostaglandin synthesis inhibitors in ischemic heart disease. The focus in this area has been the relationship between thromboxane A_2, the platelet aggregating and vasoconstricting agent, and prostacyclin, which inhibits platelet aggregation and promotes vasodilation. The pathologic findings of platelet thrombi within the vessels of patients with acute myocardial infarction, followed by sudden death, point to an important role for the platelet in the ischemic process and in the reduction in coronary artery blood flow in patients with ischemic heart disease (30). The potential role of platelets in regulation of coronary artery blood flow was emphasized by assessment of the role of platelets in cyclical changes in myocardial perfusion in experimental models of myocardial ischemia. Folts and associates have demonstrated that in constricted coronary arteries in the dog, spontaneous phasic reductions in coronary blood flow reflect the formation of platelet aggregates at the site of coronary constriction (31). This process was not due to spasm at the site of the coronary stenosis, but rather was due to spontaneous activation of platelets and occlusion of the vessel. Most strikingly, the observation that administration of aspirin, which selectively acetylates the enzyme responsible for initiation of the synthetic process leading to thromboxane A_2, prevented this process led to the suggestion that

platelet thromboxane biosynthesis must play an important role in the pathogenesis of myocardial ischemia (31,32). As a result of these studies, as well as the theoretical considerations suggesting that prostacyclin and thromboxane A_2 may play important roles in regulation of coronary artery tone, numerous clinical trials have been undertaken to try to identify abnormalities of eicosanoid metabolism in patients with myocardial disease. As with the studies of prostaglandin metabolism in hypertensive disorders, the results of these trials have been contradictory (33–38).

The synthesis of prostacyclin has variously been measured as being depressed and as being increased in patients with arteriosclerotic coronary vascular disease. Platelet aggregability has variously been found to be enhanced or normal in patients with coronary vascular disease. Indeed, recent developments in techniques for more accurate measurement of eicosanoids within the circulation, as well as assessment of the metabolic turnover rates of these materials, suggest that plasma concentrations of prostacyclin are 100 to 1,000 times lower than those previously reported in studies attempting to suggest a relationship between these materials and the arteriosclerotic process (39–41). The differences between results from these newly developed techniques and previous reports probably reflect the striking sensitivity of these analytical methods to sample handling and preparation prior to measurement of these labile substances.

Because of the contradictory evidence with regard to the pathophysiologic roles of eicosanoids in the pathogenesis of cardiovascular disorders, it is impossible to make any conclusive statements regarding the beneficial effects of pharmacologic intervention on the rates of synthesis of these moieties. Furthermore, because of the lack of specificity of the currently available inhibitors of prostaglandin biosynthesis, a more productive approach to modification of the eicosanoid system in clinical disorders of cardiovascular function would be to modify endogenous prostaglandin formation in the direction of a more beneficial balance of vasodilating antiaggregatory substances in comparison with the vasoconstricting agents that promote platelet aggregation. The principal focus of this discussion will therefore be to outline theoretical approaches that might result in such a beneficial balance of eicosanoid formation.

REGULATION OF EICOSANOID BIOSYNTHESIS

Modification of endogenous eicosanoid biosynthesis will be dependent on development of selective inhibitors of the synthesis of the deleterious substances or stimulants of the formation of the eicosanoid moieties with beneficial activities. Detailed knowledge of the processes leading to arachidonic acid release and subsequent formation of the eicosanoids will be critical to such a therapeutic approach.

Phospholipase-Mediated Arachidonic Acid Release

Although most mammalian cells generate arachidonic acid metabolites in response to a wide variety of physiologic, pharmacologic, or pathologic stimuli, these compounds are not stored within cells, but are released promptly following biosynthesis. The substrate for formation of such materials, arachidonic acid, must be released in a nonesterified form in order to make it accessible to the synthetic pathways within any individual cell. Under normal conditions, the intracellular level of the precursor fatty acid is extremely low, and the first step in stimulation of eicosanoid biosynthesis must be release of arachidonic acid from the intracellular lipid pool (cholesterol esters, phospholipids, and triglycerides). The principal source of arachidonic acid for cellular prostaglandin biosynthesis is from the phospholipids, in which arachidonic acid is most commonly found as the beta substitution of phosphatidylcholine and/or phosphatidylethanolamine (42). Thus, the principal regulatory enzyme for the entire eicosanoid cascade is phospholipase A_2, which hydrolyzes the beta fatty acid from these phosphatides (43).

A second potential mechanism for arachidonic acid release is activation of phospholipase C, which hydrolyzes the phosphate bond to liberate the phosphate-free diglyceride. The subsequent action of diglyceride lipase results in release of arachidonic acid. Both of these enzyme systems have been identified in prostaglandin-producing cells, and, in particular, the phospholipase-C-diglyceride pathway may be important in platelet arachidonic acid release (44,45). The phospholipase enzymes are membrane-bound proteins and are distributed ubiquitously among most cellular systems. They are calcium-dependent enzymes, and their activation by polypeptide substances is dependent on calcium translocation and formation of calcium-calmodulin complexes leading to enhanced phospholipase activity. In addition, there is a specific phospholipase enzyme pool found in the plasma membrane itself that can be activated when cell surface receptors are occupied. Bradykinin, angiotensin II, vasopressin, and antigen-antibody complexes can thus cause considerable enhancement of prostaglandin biosynthesis by cells possessing such cell surface receptors linked to phospholipase (46).

An initial approach to inhibition of eicosanoid biosynthesis is therefore presented by the possibility of inhibiting phospholipase activity. Three types of compounds have been identified with such inhibitory activity. They decrease phospholipolysis and arachidonic acid release by interacting directly with the enzyme, by interfering with binding of the phospholipid substrate, or by interfering with binding of calcium and/or the calcium-calmodulin complex. An example of an inhibitor that binds directly to the enzyme is the phospholipase inhibitory protein induced by glucocorticoids. Although the glucocorticoids have no direct action on the eicosanoid synthetic pathway, these drugs inhibit phospholipase-mediated arachidonic acid release because of their stimulation of a specific protein that interacts with the enzyme, resulting in inactivation (47,48). The second class of compounds that inhibit phospholipase activity encompasses cationic, amphiphilic substances such as mepacrine and chlorpromazine. These agents form complexes with phospholipids and prevent enzymatic attack (49). The third mechanism by which phospholipase might be inhibited is by deprivation of access to calcium; this mechanism of inhibition is exhibited by the local anesthetics. A specific antagonist of the calcium-calmodulin complex might also be a mechanism for inhibition of prostaglandin biosynthesis. However, many of the agents that are reported to be calcium-calmodulin antagonists, such as the local anesthetics and phenothiazines, are also inhibitors of purified phospholipase activity independent of calcium activity (50). Although it seems possible that agents that inhibit phospholipase activity *in vivo* might be developed by taking advantage of our knowledge of the structure and activity of phospholipase A_2 from purified preparations, the potential for inhibiting the entire eicosanoid cascade at this point with clinically beneficial effects would be limited. Inhibition of phospholipase activity would not shift eicosanoid biosynthesis toward a more beneficial therapeutic ratio, but would simply decrease arachidonic acid metabolism generally throughout the body.

Cyclooxygenase

The next step in the biosynthetic pathway of prostaglandins is the cyclooxygenase enzyme. Cyclooxygenase adds oxygen to arachidonic acid, producing prostaglandin G_2, the endoperoxide precursor for biosynthesis of prostaglandins, thromboxane A_2, and prostacyclin (51). The most specific of the cyclooxygenase inhibitors is aspirin (acetylsalicylic acid), which selectively transfers the acetyl group to a serine residue at the active site of the enzyme (52). Selective acetylation of the enzyme, rendering it permanently incapable of catalyzing this reaction, has been the basis of therapeutic attempts to selectively inhibit platelet thromboxane biosynthesis without modifying endothelial cell prostacyclin formation. The lack of a nucleus within the platelet prevents it from regenerating the cyclooxygenase enzyme after acetylation; thus, permanent inhibition of platelet thromboxane formation results from administration of even low doses of acetylsalicylic acid (53). In contrast, the ability of the endothelial cell to resynthesize cyclooxygenase results in rapid recovery of prostacyclin synthetic capabilities (54).

Thus, aspirin is an example of an irreversible inhibitor of cyclooxygenase activity. Alternatively, reversible competitive inhibitors of cyclooxygenase are fatty acid moieties closely related to arachidonic acid in structure that have comparable affinities for the enzyme but are not converted to endoperoxide metabolites. An example of this type of reversible competitive inhibitor is ibuprofen, which has a binding affinity for the enzyme similar to that of arachidonic acid. Indomethacin and naproxen, though nonsteroidal antiinflammatory drugs, do not covalently acetylate the enzyme as does aspirin; they represent time-dependent competitive inactivators of cyclooxygenase, with critical chemical dependence on carboxylic acid groups and aryl-hydrogen portions of the molecule (55). Finally, reversible noncompetitive inhibitors are the antioxidant or radical-trapping agents. Because cyclooxygenase activity is dependent on the presence of lipid peroxides, resulting in free radical chain reactions, the presence of radical scavengers or antioxidants such as paracetamol prevents ongoing cyclooxygenase activity (56). Selective inhibitors of lipoxygenase activity *in vivo* have not yet been developed. In view of the limited importance of lipoxygenase molecules in cardiovascular function, other than that associated with immunologic or inflammatory processes, the need for selective lipoxygenase inhibitors for modification of cardiovascular function is questionable.

Thromboxane Synthase

If modification of thromboxane biosynthesis should have beneficial therapeutic effects in cardiovascular disease, then development of a selective thromboxane synthase inhibitor would be an important step in pharmacologic intervention in the eicosanoid pathways. Imidazole and its analogues were the first agents to be identified that selectively inhibit thromboxane synthase at dosages that have no effect on cyclooxygenase activity (57). Indeed, a number of thromboxane synthase inhibitors have been developed, and an orally active agent, dazoxiben, with potential utility in clinical trials, has been identified (58). Unfortunately, although of some theoretical advantage, thromboxane synthase inhibitors have no effect on the generation of prostaglandin endoperoxides following platelet activation (59). Prostaglandin G_2 and its endoperoxide analogue prostaglandin H_2 are potent stimulants of platelet aggregation. Thus, although thromboxane A_2 is a more potent stimulant of platelet aggregation than are the prostaglandin endoperoxides, whether or not thromboxane A_2 is the only mediator of arachidonic-acid-induced aggregation is uncertain (60). Subsequent investigations have demonstrated that although conversion of prostaglandin endoperoxides into the more potent thromboxane A_2 usually occurs in the platelet in response to platelet activation when thromboxane synthase is inhibited and

further metabolism is blocked, prostaglandins G_2 and H_2 exert direct activity on platelets, perhaps through the thromboxane A_2 receptor, resulting in platelet aggregation (61,62). Thus, selective inhibition of thromboxane A_2 synthesis without inhibition of prostaglandin endoperoxide formation may have little or no beneficial therapeutic effect on pathophysiologic processes.

In one study, a familial bleeding tendency was identified in a patient population with partial deficiency of platelet thromboxane synthase. When platelets from this patient population were incubated with arachidonic acid, aggregation did not occur, thromboxane A_2 formation was low, and formation of other prostaglandin (PG) substances such a PGE_2 and $PGF_{2\alpha}$ was enhanced (63). The prolonged bleeding time in such patients may result from enhanced endogenous formation of platelet inhibitors such as prostacyclin by the shunting of prostaglandin endoperoxides from platelets to the endothelium. Thus, this experiment of nature suggests a potential for inhibition of *in vivo* aggregation if a favorable shift in the formation of prostacyclin, as opposed to thromboxane A_2, is produced without specific inhibition of platelet endoperoxide formation.

Prostacyclin Synthase

There are no circumstances under which prostacyclin synthase inhibition would be of theoretical advantage. Inhibition of prostacyclin synthase by lipid peroxides, however, has been demonstrated biochemically (64). Lipid peroxide inhibition of prostacyclin synthase may be important in understanding the abnormalities of endogenous prostacyclin formation in atheromatous tissue (65). The presence of lipid peroxides in atheromatous plaques could predispose to thrombus formation by inhibiting generation of prostacyclin. This possibility is supported by observations by Weksler et al. (66), who found that hypercholesterolemic animals had reduced capability for generating prostacyclin in response to vascular damage, as compared with normocholesterolemic control animals.

Substrate Modification: Eicosapentaenoic Acid Substitution

The final mechanism by which eicosanoid biosynthesis might be modified would be through dietary manipulation of the thromboxane A_2/prostacyclin ratio. Eicosapentaenoic acid is a polyunsaturated fatty acid with structural characteristics similar to those of arachidonic acid, but with a higher degree of unsaturation. It gives rise to prostaglandins of the "three" series; when incubated with vascular tissue, it serves as the substrate for formation of the prostacyclin analogue PGI_3. This compound is as potent an antiaggregatory agent as prostacyclin itself; however, thromboxane A_3, the platelet metabolite of eicosapentaenoic acid, has weaker proaggregatory activity than does thromboxane A_2, the naturally occurring arachidonic acid metabolite (67). The increased concentrations of eicosapentaenoic acid in the phospholipid fractions of cell membranes from particular populations, especially the Eskimos, have been suggested as an explanation for the low incidence of acute myocardial infarction and the increased tendency to bleeding in these patient populations (68). The prolonged bleeding time has been demonstrated to be due to a reduction in platelet aggregability, and these subjects have low concentrations of plasma cholesterol, triglyceride, and low- and very-low-density lipoproteins, whereas their concentrations of high-density lipoproteins are high (69). Eicosapentaenoic acid has inherent platelet inhibitory properties independent of its effects on thromboxane and prostacyclin formation, because it inhibits aggregation of aspirin-treated platelets (70). Eicosapentaenoic acid is incorporated into platelet phospholipids, probably replacing arachidonic acid and exerting its antithrombotic effect by decreasing the formation of arachidonic acid metabolites at the expense of formation of the less proaggregatory prostaglandin H_3 and thromboxane A_3. In addition, incubation of platelet-rich plasma with eicosapentaenoic acid prevents formation of thromboxane A_2 following exposure to arachidonate, whereas it enhances conversion of arachidonic acid to prostacyclin by vascular tissue (71). Theoretical manipulation of the formation of thromboxane and prostacyclin through such dietary manipulation is the basis of the recently reported clinical trials of fish oil substitution for patients with cardiovascular disorders.

STIMULATION OF ENDOGENOUS EICOSANOID BIOSYNTHESIS

In view of the multiple steps in the biosynthesis of the eicosanoids, the conflicting therapeutic effects of inhibition of the cyclooxygenase, thromboxane synthase, and prostacyclin synthase enzymes, and the diffuse distribution of the eicosanoids and their possible importance in multiple physiologic processes, the development of a cell- or organ-specific inhibitor of eicosanoid activity that would have a beneficial therapeutic effect is unlikely. Thus, in contrast to prior approaches to inhibition of the arachidonic acid cascade, a potentially more valuable and more effective mechanism to modify this system would be to stimulate endogenous formation of arachidonic acid metabolites in such a way as to favorably affect the prostacyclin-thromboxane relationship and thus beneficially modify those pathophysiologic processes affected by these substances.

Plasma Lipoproteins

A potentially critical but only recently identified regulatory pathway for prostacyclin formation involves the effects of plasma high- and low-density lipoproteins on cellular arachidonic acid metabolism. Incubation of vascular endothelial cells (72) or smooth-muscle cells (73) in tissue culture in the presence of high- and low-density lipoproteins has revealed that high-density lipoproteins (HDL) markedly stimulate formation of prostacyclin and prostaglandin E_2 by the cell systems. In vascular smooth-muscle cells, stimulation of prostacyclin synthesis is directly related to the amount of cholesterol-arachidonate found within the lipoprotein fraction and is not the result of interaction of the apolipoprotein with the cell in tissue culture. Low-density lipoproteins (LDL) also stimulated prostacyclin and prostaglandin E_2 formation; however, at comparable cholesterol concentrations, their ability to stimulate prostaglandin formation was greatly decreased as compared with the efficacy of the high-density lipoprotein fraction. In smooth-muscle cells, stimulation of cellular prostacyclin formation was secondary to utilization of HDL cholesterol-arachidonate and was not due to stimulation of release of endogenous arachidonic acid from the cellular storage pool.

Of additional significance from these studies was identification of a synergistic relationship between HDL-stimulated prostacyclin formation and stimulation of prostacyclin formation by agents such as bradykinin and angiotensin II, which activate phospholipase activity, thus resulting in an increase in arachidonic acid release from endogenous phospholipid stores. Bradykinin produced synergistic stimulation of prostacyclin formation, whereas angiotensin II produced an additive effect with HDL incubation.

In endothelial cells, HDL supplied exogenous arachidonate to the cells but also stimulated endogenous arachidonic acid release, indicating a dual mechanism of action leading to enhanced prostacyclin formation. Thus, there are multiple sources of arachidonate for prostacyclin formation in endothelial and vascular smooth-muscle cells. Endogenous arachidonate probably is the principal source of substrate in response to vasoactive substances such as bradykinin or angiotensin II. Lipoprotein arachidonate may also serve as a source for prostacyclin formation. The synergistic effect of HDL and bradykinin may reflect an important mechanism for endogenous regulation of prostacyclin formation. Although the molecular mechanism of this synergism is totally unknown, these data with regard to HDL effects on prostacyclin formation are of great interest when considered in light of the known epidemiologic relationships between HDL and clinical cardiovascular disease. In addition, stimulation of smooth-muscle prostacyclin formation by plasma lipoproteins may be of particular importance in view of the critical role of these cells in the formation of a neointima after vascular endothelial injury (74).

The concentration of LDL cholesterol in plasma is positively correlated with the risk of coronary artery disease, whereas as the concentration of plasma HDL cholesterol is negatively correlated. The mechanism of the protective effect of HDL has been postulated to result from the effects of HDL in mobilization of cholesterol from peripheral tissue (75,76), but these data with regard to prostacyclin formation would suggest that a second potential mechanism is reduction in thrombotic complications of atherosclerotic disease through enhanced prostacyclin formation. Mobilization of cholesterol esters from lipid-laden smooth-muscle cells by HDL may also result in lowered inhibition of endogenous prostacyclin synthase activity by cholesterol esters, and enhanced formation of prostacyclin has been implicated in further acceleration in cholesterol removal from smooth-muscle cells (77). As is apparent, a complex relationship among the vascular endothelium, the vascular smooth-muscle cell, plasma HDL and LDL, and cholesterol storage processes exists that is not subject to easy interpretation; nonetheless, enhanced prostacyclin formation seems to be universally linked with those processes leading to decreased cardiovascular morbidity.

Nitroglycerin

A second potential mechanism for modification of endogenous prostacyclin formation is to take advantage of the effects of pharmacologic agents used for treatment of cardiovascular disease. Nitroglycerin stimulates prostacyclin formation by vascular endothelial cells in tissue culture (78). Using this cell system, it has been shown that vascular endothelial cells recover their ability to synthesize prostacyclin promptly after short-term exposure to acetylsalicylic acid, and it is on these observations that aspirin therapy for treatment of patients with cardiovascular disease has been based. The major advantage of stimulation of endogenous prostacyclin formation, as opposed to its intravenous infusion in patients with myocardial ischemia (79), is that the former approach would result in release of prostacyclin at the site of greatest relevance, that being at the vascular wall, where inhibition of platelet aggregation and stimulation of vasodilation would be of greatest clinical importance. Incubation of isolated vascular endothelial cells in tissue culture in the presence of nitroglycerin results in stimulation of arachidonic acid release and formation of prostacyclin. Stimulation of prostacyclin formation by nitroglycerin results in inhibition of platelet aggregation by platelets incubated in the presence of endothelial cells and nitroglycerin, ex vivo (78). These findings have resulted in the suggestion that the biologically beneficial effects of nitroglycerin in treatment of patients with angina pectoris result from its ability to stimulate endogenous prostacyclin formation, thereby decreasing spontaneous platelet aggregation within the damaged vessels of the heart (80).

Experimental studies of the role of nitroglycerin in coronary artery blood flow have led to conflicting results with regard to the importance of nitroglycerin-stimulated arachidonic acid metabolites in the regulation of coronary artery blood flow (81). The negative studies have focused primarily on the maximal vasodilating activity of nitroglycerin, in which prior treatment with prostaglandin synthase inhibitors has not resulted in a blunting of the chemical response (82–84). A recent study, however, has reported not only on the maximal vasodilating effect but also on the duration of vasodilation in the response to nitroglycerin administration and/or prostaglandin synthesis inhibition. This study suggests that although maximal vasodilation if not affected, the duration of the effect of nitroglycerin is greatly diminished by a nonsteroidal antiinflammatory drug. As such, the importance of nitroglycerin-stimulated prostacyclin biosynthesis probably reflects the ability of prostacyclin to prolong the duration of action of nitroglycerin, thereby extending its beneficial effects on myocardial ischemia (85).

Angiotensin-Converting-Enzyme Inhibitors

The third potential mechanism for stimulation of endogenous eicosanoid biosynthesis is use of the angiotensin-converting-enzyme inhibitors.

The importance of angiotensin-converting enzyme was first documented by Skeggs and colleagues, who recognized that the vasopressor substance formed by the reaction between crudely purified porcine renin and equine angiotensinogen was the product of a reaction catalyzed by a carboxypeptidase acting on angiotensin I (86,87). Ng and Vane demonstrated that angiotensin I was converted to angiotensin II during passage through the pulmonary circulation (88,89), and subsequent studies have shown the converting enzyme to be a component of the vascular endothelium. Because the enzyme is located on the luminal surface of the plasma membrane in close contact with the vascular space, it is ideally located for catalyzing angiotensin I to angiotensin II (90). Recognizing the similarity between the disappearance of bradykinin as it passes through the pulmonary circulation and the bioactivation of angiotensin I, Ferreira and Vane suggested that the so-called angiotensin-converting enzyme also might be responsible for the metabolism of bradykinin in the pulmonary circulation (91). In 1968, Bakhle reported that a peptide substance isolated from the venom of the snake Bothrops jararaca inhibited conversion of angiotensin I to angiotensin II by canine pulmonary tissue (92). Further studies by Ferreira and colleagues confirmed that these peptides also inhibited bradykininase activity in pulmonary homogenates (93–95).

The first angiotensin-converting-enzyme inhibitor studied in humans was a synthetic nonapeptide originally known as SQ 20881 and later named teprotide (96). Teprotide blocked the vasopressor response to intravenous infusion of angiotensin I and effectively reduced blood pressure in patients with elevated plasma renin activity (97). Through careful chemical analysis of the characteristics of angiotensin-converting enzyme and its presumed similarity to other carboxypeptidase enzymes, particularly pancreatic carboxypeptidase A, an analogue of proline (D-3-mercapto-2-methylpropanoyl-1-proline) was developed and identified as a highly specific inhibitor of the converting enzyme *in vitro* (98–102).

Laboratory studies confirmed that this compound, originally known as SQ 14225 and later named captopril, was a potent competitive inhibitor of converting-enzyme activity (103). It prevented the formation of angiotensin II from angiotensin I and inhibited the metabolism of bradykinin to inactive polypeptides. Early laboratory studies led to the assumption that the hemodynamic response to captopril administration in experimental animals and humans could be explained by changes in the plasma concentrations of angiotensin II and brady-kinin. Decreases in plasma angiotensin II concentrations and the consequent decrease in aldosterone biosynthesis would diminish the mechanisms that tend to raise blood pressure. Specifically, decreased angiotensin II and al-dosterone productions decrease vascular smooth-muscle contraction, lessen sodium retention, and contract intra-vascular volume. The anticipated increases in plasma bradykinin concentrations would be expected to lead to vasodilation and thus to a decrease in blood pressure because of diminished systemic vascular resistance.

In vivo, plasma renin activity is regulated by a negative-feedback mechanism that inhibits further release of renin in response to an elevation in blood pressure or to an increase in plasma angiotensin II concentration (104). Plasma renin activity thus would be expected to increase in response to agents that decrease plasma angiotensin II concentrations and that lower blood pres-sure. But inhibition of angiotensin-converting enzyme with captopril or other converting-enzyme inhibitors would prevent the increased concentration of angiotensin I, which results when plasma renin activity rises, from being converted to angiotensin II. Indeed, many clinical trials have demonstrated that oral captopril administra-tion produces a decrease in blood pressure that is associated with decreases in plasma angiotensin II con-centration and plasma aldosterone concentration. Fur-ther, captopril-induced changes were associated with the expected elevations of plasma renin activity and angio-tensin I levels (105).

A consistent pattern of effect on the renin-angiotensin-aldosterone system has led investigators to conclude that the theoretical mechanism of action of captopril on this system is indeed observed following its administration to normal or hypertensive humans. In contrast, varying effects on the bradykinin system have been observed. Although occasional studies have reported an elevation in plasma kinin concentration, most investigators have failed to demonstrate a significant increase (106–113). Kinins are generally accepted to be local mediators of

the inflammatory response, rather than circulating sub-stances important in the control of blood pressure. Presumably, a number of proteolytic enzymes other than angiotensin-converting enzyme can inactivate bra-dykinin; therefore, failure to demonstrate an increase in circulating kinin concentration is not totally unexpected. Carretero and colleagues examined the roles of kinins in the acute and chronic hypotensive effects of captopril using specific antikinin antibodies to block the depressor effect of bradykinin. Because administration of antikinin antibodies had no effect on the hypotensive response to captopril in sodium-depleted rats, these authors con-cluded that the antihypertensive activity of captopril in this model could be attributed solely to its inhibition of the renin-angiotensin cascade (113). Although consistent changes in plasma kinin levels have not been docu-mented, the possibility cannot be excluded that tissue kinins may increase and that local mediation of hemo-dynamic parameters might contribute to the vasode-pressor response to captopril.

Although significant evidence points to a renin-depen-dent antihypertensive activity of captopril, additional studies in experimental animals and in humans suggest that a non-renin-dependent antihypertensive activity of captopril must exist. Marks and associates reported that captopril decreased blood pressure by approximately 15% in normal rats (114). Following nephrectomy, the blood pressure in these animals fell by nearly 30%. Captopril administration produced a further 10% drop in blood pressure, however, despite the absence of renin in the peripheral circulation in these anephric animals. In animals with early two-kidney one-clip hypertension, a model of hypertension known to be renin-dependent, captopril markedly decreased blood pressure. However, in animals with late two-kidney one-clip hypertension, a model of hypertension thought to be independent of the renin-angiotensin system, captopril surprisingly also produced a substantial drop in blood pressure. In addi-tion, in animals made hypertensive by chronic admin-istration of deoxycorticosterone, a potent salt-retaining steroid, and a high-salt diet, captopril reduced blood pressure significantly. These rats show markedly sup-pressed plasma renin activity and represent an experi-mental model of low-renin-volume-expansion angioten-sin-II-independent hypertension (114). Moreover, in salt-depleted rats in which the endogenous renin-angio-tensin system has been blocked by infusion of the competitive antagonist saralasin, the angiotensin II re-ceptor blocker captopril further reduced the blood pres-sure. These results all are consistent with a non-renin-dependent mechanism of action for captopril (115). Muirhead and colleagues reported that administration of captopril to rats receiving exogenous angiotensin II and a high-salt diet significantly decreased the blood pressure in these animals (116). The reduction in blood pressure in this experimental model cannot be explained on the basis of reduction in plasma angiotension II concentration, because the angiotensin II was chronically infused via a drug-infusion pump, and thus the angiotensin II concentration in the peripheral circulation was maintained constant and independent of the effects of the converting enzyme. This study, in particular, indicated the need to identify a non-renin-dependent antihypertensive activity of captopril to account for its diverse hemodynamic effects.

If captopril's antihypertensive activity were due solely to the antagonism in the generation of angiotensin II by renin in the peripheral circulation, bilateral nephrectomy would be expected to eliminate totally any hemodynamic response to administration of this converting-enzyme inhibitor. Yet Man In't Veld and associates reported that the volume status of anephric patients dramatically affects the hemodynamic response to captopril. Salt- and water-replete patients showed no response to captopril; however, following hemodialysis and relative salt and water depletion, captopril significantly reduced blood pressure (117). Finally, in a study of 26 hypertensive patients, Fagard and colleagues found that captopril had a greater antihypertensive effect than saralasin. These findings once again suggested non-renin-mediated antihypertensive activity for this orally active converting-enzyme inhibitor (118).

The importance of the prostaglandin system in the antihypertensive response to captopril was first reported by Vinci and associates, who administered teprotide, a peptidyl converting-enzyme inhibitor, at rates sufficient to lower blood pressure by 10 mm Hg in subjects with mild essential hypertension (119). The arterial concentration of PGE increased threefold during teprotide administration. These authors observed the anticipated rise in plasma renin activity and angiotensin I concentration, as well as decreases in plasma angiotensin II and aldosterone concentrations. The plasma arterial bradykinin concentration remained unchanged during converting-enzyme inhibition (119). Swartz and associates subsequently reported the effect of captopril on the prostaglandin system in normal subjects ingesting both high- and low-sodium diets. Captopril significantly increased the plasma concentration of 13,14-dihydro-15-ketoprostaglandin E_2, the major metabolite of PGE_2. The depressor response to captopril correlated closely with the increases in plasma PGE_2 metabolite concentrations but not with changes in plasma angiotensin II or bradykinin levels (120). Moore and colleagues reported increases in the plasma concentrations of PGE_2 metabolites following captopril administration in patients with essential hypertension. In these patients, administration of prostaglandin synthesis inhibitors was associated with decreased PGE_2 excretion and a significant blunting of the vasodepressor response to captopril (121). Subsequently, many investigators have reported that administration of a prostaglandin synthesis inhibitor blunts

the hemodynamic response to captopril in hypertensive and normal subjects as well as in experimental animals (122–126).

Study of the regulation of cellular prostaglandin biosynthesis became possible with the development of a technique for isolation of renomedullary interstitial cells in tissue culture (127). Previous studies have shown that this cell line synthesizes PGE_2 and $PGF_{2\alpha}$ in tissue culture. Addition of a vasoactive peptide, such as angiotensin II, vasopressin, and, importantly, bradykinin, causes an increase in prostaglandin biosynthesis (128). Incubation of these cells with radioactively labeled arachidonic acid allows identification of the endogenous arachidonic acid storage pool. Subsequent stimulation by vasoactive peptides activates the phospholipase and releases arachidonic acid from the phospholipid fraction. The arachidonic acid so released is subsequently converted to prostaglandins (129). Polypeptide-stimulated prostaglandin biosynthesis by these cells in tissue culture depends in part on translocation of calcium from the extracellular environment to the intracellular medium and can be blocked by incubation of the cells in the presence of a calcium-channel antagonist and can be stimulated through the use of a calcium-channel ionophore such as A23187 (130).

The effect of captopril on cellular regulation of prostaglandin synthesis has been assessed using renomedullary interstitial cells in tissue culture. Captopril induced up to a 30-fold stimulation of prostaglandin biosynthesis. Half-maximal stimulation of prostaglandin biosynthesis occurred at a captopril concentration of approximately 8 μM, a concentration similar to the plasma level of the drug achieved after administration of captopril to normotensive or hypertensive subjects (131).

An important consideration in the study of captopril-stimulated prostaglandin biosynthesis concerns what structural characteristics of the molecule result in its ability to promote phospholipase activation, arachidonic acid release, and subsequent formation of vasodilating prostaglandins. To address this question, the effects of captopril and three of its chemical analogues, as well as the effects of enalapril and its biologically active metabolite, enalaprilic acid, on prostaglandin biosynthesis were studied (Fig. 2). Although it is a simple chemical molecule and an analogue of proline, captopril has an optically active center at the beta carbon that allows for chemical modification. Formation of the optical enantiomer of captopril (SQ 14534) produces a molecule with less converting-enzyme inhibitory activity but does not diminish its ability to stimulate prostaglandin biosynthesis. As Fig. 2 illustrates, the increase in prostaglandin concentration evoked by this captopril analogue at a concentration of 7.5 μM was approximately eightfold. In addition, a doubling of prostaglandin biosynthesis was achieved at a concentration of approximately 2 μM; these values are identical with those for captopril. Indeed,

COMPOUND	STRUCTURE	INHIBITION OF ANGIOTENSIN CONVERTING ENZYME (IC_{50}), μm	STIMULATION OF PROSTAGLANDIN E_2 BIOSYNTHESIS	
			AT 7.5 μm	ED_{2x} (μm)
SQ 14225 (Captopril)	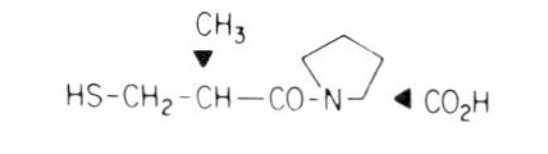 CH_3 $HS-CH_2-CH-CO-N$ ◀ CO_2H	0.023	8X	2.1
SQ 14534	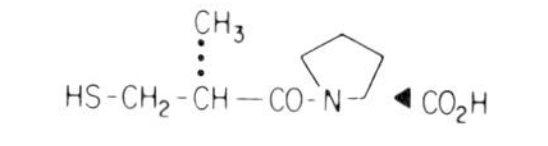 CH_3 $HS-CH_2-CH-CO-N$ ◀ CO_2H	2.4	7.8X	2.4
SQ 13863	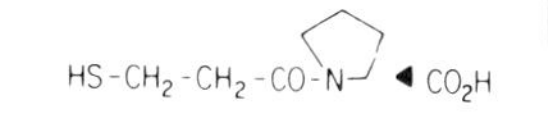 $HS-CH_2-CH_2-CO-N$ ◀ CO_2H	0.20	7.6X	2.2
SQ 13297	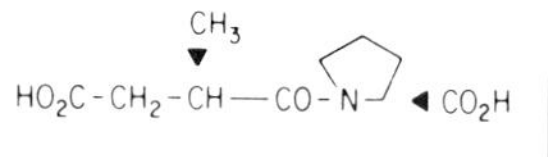 CH_3 $HO_2C-CH_2-CH-CO-N$ ◀ CO_2H	22.0	0	>1000
MK-421 (Enalapril)	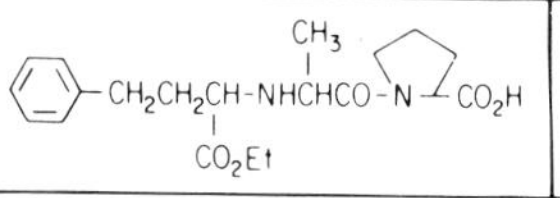 CH_3 $-CH_2CH_2CH-NHCHCO-N-CO_2H$ CO_2Et	1.2	0	>1000
MK-422	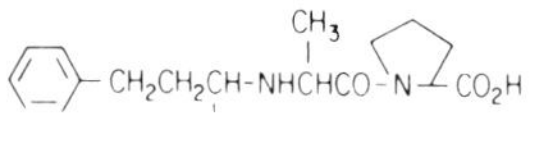 CH_3 $-CH_2CH_2CH-NHCHCO-N-CO_2H$	0.0012	0	>1000

FIG. 2. Effects of angiotensin-converting-enzyme inhibitors on converting-enzyme activity and on prostaglandin E_2 biosynthesis by rabbit renomedullary interstitial cells in tissue culture.

even removal of the methyl group at the optically active center, which produces an optically inactive molecule (SQ 13863) and affects its ability to serve as converting-enzyme inhibitor, has absolutely no effect on prostaglandin biosynthesis *in vitro*. However, substitution for the sulfhydryl group by a carboxyl group (SQ 13297) totally eliminates the ability of the compound to stimulate prostaglandin biosynthesis, even at levels 1,000-fold greater than those at which an effect is observed for the parent molecule.

Enalapril and enalaprilic acid are converting-enzyme inhibitors recently demonstrated to have significant antihypertensive activity in the treatment of patients. These two compounds do not have sulfhydryl-group substitutions as part of the chemical structure (132). After oral administration, enalapril (MK-421), and ethyl ester of its active metabolite enalaprilic acid (MK-422), is converted via bioactivation in the liver to a very potent angiotensin-converting enzyme inhibitor. Addition of either enalapril or enalaprilic acid to the incubation medium of renomedullary interstitial cells in tissue culture has no effect on prostaglandin biosynthesis.

This sequence of studies on the relationship between chemical structure and prostaglandin stimulation indicates that stimulation of prostaglandin biosynthesis is not a general property of the converting-enzyme inhibitors, but rather depends on specific chemical characteristics of the molecule involved. The sulfhydryl component of captopril is the critical chemical characteristic of this molecule. This group confers on the molecule

the ability to stimulate prostaglandin production. L. Levine (*personal communication*) and Galler et al. (133) have confirmed the ability of captopril to stimulate prostaglandin biosynthesis by aortic endothelial cells in tissue culture and in isolated renal glomeruli, respectively. In the latter study, it is of interest to note that although glomeruli synthesize PGE_2, $PGF_{2\alpha}$, thromboxane A_2, and prostacyclin, only PGE_2 and prostacyclin syntheses were increased. This observation suggests the presence of compartmentalization of the enzymes leading to the synthesis of these vasodilating substances.

A second important effect of captopril on the prostaglandin system is the synergistic activity of bradykinin and captopril in stimulating prostaglandin biosynthesis by renomedullary interstitial cells in tissue culture. Although captopril has no significant effect on plasma bradykinin concentrations, Vinci and associates noted a significant increase in urinary kinin excretion in those patients experiencing a drop in blood pressure (119). Thus, although bradykinin concentrations were unaffected in plasma, those authors did observe an increase in bradykinin in tissue, where kinins can potentially stimulate endogenous prostaglandin biosynthesis. Bradykinin is a potent stimulant of prostaglandin biosynthesis by renomedullary interstitial cells in tissue culture. The combination of captopril and bradykinin, however, increases the rates of arachidonic acid release and prostaglandin synthesis above and beyond those to be expected by the simple additive effects of the two compounds. This observation points to the possibility of synergistic prostaglandin-stimulating activity of captopril and bradykinin leading to enhanced prostaglandin synthesis *in vivo*. This synergism is similar to that seen in the effects of bradykinin and high-density lipoproteins on prostacyclin synthesis in vascular endothelial and smooth-muscle cells *in vitro*.

The significance of captopril-stimulated prostaglandin biosynthesis as an important aspect of its mechanism of antihypertensive activity is indicated by a number of clinical and experimental studies. Captopril administration to experimental animals made hypertensive by administration of deoxycorticosterone and sodium chloride resulted in a 23-mm-Hg drop in blood pressure (134). Pretreatment of these animals with indomethacin resulted in complete attenuation of the antihypertensive response to captopril. Thus, in this model of low-renin hypertension, the sole mechanism of the antihypertensive activity of captopril was increased prostaglandin biosynthesis; this finding explains the antihypertensive response to converting-enzyme inhibition in a model thought to be independent of the renin-angiotensin cascade. Goldstone and associates assessed the importance of the prostaglandin system and the renin-angiotensin system on captopril's antihypertensive activity in normal volunteers on low- and high-salt diets (135). Plasma renin activity was elevated in patients placed on a sodium-restricted diet. Administration of captopril to these subjects resulted in an approximately 12-mm-Hg drop in blood pressure. In these individuals, administration of a prostaglandin synthesis inhibitor prior to captopril administration did not attenuate the antihypertensive response. In contrast, in individuals on a high-salt diet with low plasma renin activity, captopril produced a similar 12-mm-Hg drop in blood pressure. However, prior administration of a prostaglandin synthesis inhibitor totally attenuated the antihypertensive response (135). These studies point to the importance of prostaglandin-

mediated antihypertensive activity in individuals with low plasma renin activity.

The contrasting effects of captopril and enalapril on prostaglandin stimulation also explain the difference in the responses to these molecules in experimental models of hypertension. Whereas captopril administration reduces blood pressure in animals made hypertensive by administration of deoxycorticosterone and sodium chloride through its ability to stimulate prostaglandin formation and produce peripheral vasodilation, enalapril has no significant antihypertensive activity in this model of hypertension (136). In addition, whereas captopril reduces blood pressure in animals made hypertensive by chronic infusion of angiotension II, enalapril has no antihypertensive activity when employed in this experimental model (137). In contrast, both captopril and enalapril are effective antihypertensive agents when administered in experimental models of hypertension known to be dependent on the renin-angiotensin cascade (138). Finally, the contrast between these two converting-enzyme inhibitors has been demonstrated by Shoback and associates, who administered both captopril and enalapril to human subjects and measured the plasma concentrations of PGE metabolites. Whereas captopril is a potent stimulant of PGE_2 synthesis, enalapril did not affect plasma PGE_2 metabolite concentrations (139).

A proposed summary of captopril's mechanism of action is shown in Fig. 3 (140). Inhibition of angiotensin-converting enzyme in the pulmonary circulation reduces the rate of conversion of angiotensin I to angiotensin II. The falling angiotensin II concentration and the concomitant decrease in plasma aldosterone concentration cause a decrease in peripheral vascular resistance and a decrease in sodium retention that lead to a drop in blood pressure. This effect is the predominant mechanism of action of captopril in patients with high plasma renin activity, such as those in a sodium-depleted state and in

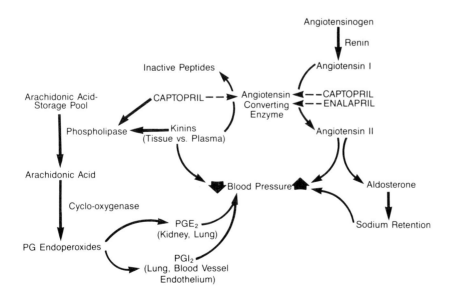

FIG. 3. Effects of captopril and enalapril on the prostaglandin, kinin, and renin-angiotensin-aldosterone systems.

patients with high-renin hypertension. Although angio-tensin-converting enzyme can metabolize bradykinin to inactive metabolites, no consistent and significant change in plasma bradykinin concentration has been documented, probably because of the multiple other enzymes capable of metabolizing bradykinin that are not affected by captopril. Despite the absence of significant changes in plasma kinin concentrations, however, increases in tissue levels of this potent polypeptide (in particular, augmented kinin formation by the kidney) may result in increased vasodilation within those tissues and heightened stimulation of prostaglandin biosynthesis. Finally, captopril directly stimulates prostaglandin biosynthesis and thus raises the arterial concentration of PGE_2, produced predominantly by the kidney and the lung, and prostacyclin (PGI_2), produced by the lung, the kidney, and the blood vessel endothelium. Increases in prostaglandin biosynthesis might result from the direct effects of captopril on cellular arachidonic acid release or from accentuation and possible acceleration of stimulation of prostaglandin biosynthesis by bradykinin, both within the peripheral circulation and at the tissue level. The vasodilation that occurs because of increased arterial prostaglandin concentrations is the major mechanism for the antihypertensive activity of captopril in the sodium-replete state and in patients with low-renin hypertension. Enalapril's mechanism of action is limited to its effect on the renin-angiotensin-aldosterone cascade.

The mechanism of the synergistic effect of captopril and bradykinin on cellular prostaglandin biosynthesis remains unknown. Indeed, the mechanism of captopril-stimulated arachidonic acid release has yet to be elucidated. Although peptide-hormone-stimulated prostaglandin biosynthesis depends on increased calcium influx following receptor activation, captopril-stimulated prostaglandin biosynthesis does not appear to be a calcium-dependent process. Additional evidence for an important role of captopril-stimulated prostaglandin/prostacyclin biosynthesis in vivo is provided by studies of platelet function in patients receiving captopril for treatment of hypertension. Platelet aggregation is diminished in patients following captopril therapy, as compared with pretreatment values (141). Ex vivo incubation of platelets with captopril does not affect aggregation parameters, and thus the decrease in aggregability must result from an in vivo response to drug therapy. This effect may be secondary to the decreased angiotensin II levels in these patients or to the antiplatelet effects of captopril-stimulated prostacyclin biosynthesis and release. Indeed, it might be speculated that the decreased mortality observed in experimental models of myocardial infarction after captopril therapy (142) or observed in patients receiving captopril for treatment of congestive heart failure (143) might reflect the beneficial effects of increases in synthesis of PGE_2 and prostacyclin by vascular endothelium, myocardium, and other arachidonic-acid-metabolizing

tissues. If, in fact, this hypothesis is true, a difference in platelet function should be observed in patients during captopril treatment versus enalapril treatment, because the former, but not the latter, directly stimulates prostaglandin formation.

CONCLUSION

It is apparent from the foregoing discussion that a simple modification of the arachidonic acid cascade in order to beneficially affect cardiovascular disease and cardiovascular performance will be impossible. In addition to those parameters already discussed, other vascular influences, including pulsatility of blood flow, shear stress, and hypoxia (144), may stimulate endogenous prostacyclin formation. Although the leukotrienes are thought principally to play a role in inflammatory or autoimmune processes, it has recently been demonstrated that leukotriene C_4, a leukocyte lipoxygenase product, stimulates prostacyclin formation by cultured endothelial cells (145). It is interesting to note that, like captopril, leukotriene C_4 is a sulfur-containing molecule and may stimulate prostaglandin biosynthesis via a sulfur-dependent pathway. The importance of this process in vivo remains unknown.

The complex relationship between arachidonic acid metabolites (particularly thromboxane A_2 and prostacyclin) and protection of patients with myocardial ischemia is indicated by a study of aspirin and sulfinpyrazone in the treatment of patients with unstable angina (146). In this large-scale double-blind placebo-controlled trial, patients with unstable angina were treated with aspirin (325 mg four times per day), or sulfinpyrazone (200 mg four times per day), or both drugs, or neither. Sulfinpyrazone had no effect on cardiovascular mortality. The patients were entered into the trial within 8 days of hospitalization and treated for up to 2 years. Significant reductions in "cardiac death" and nonfatal myocardial infarction were observed in the group receiving aspirin, as opposed to placebo. A 71% reduction in cardiac death or death from any cause was observed in the aspirin-treated patients. However, the beneficial effect from aspirin at a dosage of 325 mg four times per day contrasts with the known effects of aspirin on endothelial cell function, prostacyclin formation, thromboxane release, and platelet aggregation. Because as little as 80 mg of aspirin administered daily will completely inhibit platelet cyclooxygenase activity and prevent thromboxane formation (147), administration of aspirin on a schedule of four times per day can be expected to result in only progressive inhibition of prostacyclin formation, because the attempted regeneration of cyclooxygenase activity by these nucleus-containing cells will be continuously thwarted by the four-times-daily administration of an irreversible cyclooxygenase inhibitor. Yet these patients were observed to improve clinically following such a regimen, a regimen that cannot be rationally supported on the basis of our knowledge of the arachidonic acid cascade. Previous trials of large doses of aspirin have similarly suggested a beneficial effect of aspirin therapy in patients with coronary artery disease (148). Although individually those studies were less conclusive than the aforementioned study, when all studies are viewed together a beneficial effect of large-dosage aspirin therapy can be discerned. Beneficial effects in the recently reported study (146) must therefore be concluded to result from effects independent of those on the arachidonic acid cascade. This study, therefore, once again leaves unresolved the question of the beneficial effects of cyclooxygenase inhibition in patients with cardiovascular disease.

Despite the lack of clear-cut evidence for beneficial effects from modification of the prostacyclin-thromboxane relationship, some theoretical approaches for future investigation can be identified. The following points should be considered in such future investigation:

Plasma lipoproteins. It is apparent from epidemiologic and laboratory studies that HDL have an epidemiologic relationship to a decrease in cardiovascular mortality and also stimulate prostacyclin formation by endothelial and vascular smooth-muscle cells. Whether or not there is a direct relationship between these two observations cannot be determined except in studies that might involve a genetically deficient prostacyclin population, and no such population is currently known to exist. Nonetheless, as a mechanism for stimulating endogenous vasodilating antiaggregatory substances, efforts to enhance HDL-mediated arachidonate delivery to the vasculature would be expected to result in a therapeutically beneficial response.

Dietary supplementation of eicosapentaenoic acid. Dietary fish oil administration to replace arachidonate with eicosapentaenoic acid may have a beneficial effect if the overall response is to increase formation of vasodilating, antiaggregatory PGI_3 at the expense of formation of thromboxane A_2. Like the effect of increased HDL levels, such dietary manipulations are likely to result in changes in prostacyclin formation and formation of its potent antiaggregatory analogue PGI_3 locally at the site of greatest benefit and would not be associated with overall inhibition of the arachidonic acid cascade.

Pharmacologic agents that stimulate endogenous prostaglandin formation. As outlined previously in the discussion of the mechanisms of action of the converting-enzyme inhibitors, it is apparent that the sulfhydryl-containing angiotensin-converting-enzyme inhibitor captopril, originally designed as an antihypertensive agent, may have some protective cardiovascular effects. Evidence for endogenous inhibition of platelet aggregation, decreased cardiovascular mortality among patients with congestive heart failure, and changes in ventricular function in animals with myocardial infarctions suggests

that endogenous prostaglandin formation, either PGE_2 or prostacyclin, accounts for some of the beneficial responses to this drug. The importance of the sulfhydryl group of this compound raises the possibility that a sulfhydryl-containing molecule might be identified that dramatically stimulates endogenous prostacyclin formation. It is interesting to note the similarity of the HDL- and captopril-stimulated synergism of prostaglandin formation with bradykinin. Whether the synergistic activity of these two apparently dissimilar substances represents unique mechanisms of action of the two agents or an important and physiologically relevant regulatory mechanism remains for future investigation.

It might also be possible to design a nitroglycerin analogue with enhanced prostacyclin-stimulating activity for patients with angina pectoris. To date, the "long-acting" nitrates used in this patient population have not been associated with significant changes in arachidonic acid metabolism.

Thromboxane-endoperoxide antagonist. Recent studies have demonstrated that arachidonic acid endoperoxides formed by platelets can be effectively and efficiently converted to prostacyclin by endothelial cells, whereas utilization of endothelial-cell-derived endoperoxides by platelets does not occur (149). The extreme efficiency of conversion of platelet endoperoxides to prostacyclin by endothelial cells suggests that platelet endoperoxide formation should be maintained. However, the proaggregatory effects of PGG_2 and PGH_2 may have adverse effects, despite not being converted to thromboxane A_2. Thus, rather than inhibiting platelet endoperoxide formation, one might consider strategies to enhance endoperoxide formation, but to also inhibit thromboxane synthase, while also preventing endoperoxide receptor interactions. This strategy would decrease platelet aggregation while enhancing endothelial cell prostacyclin formation.

These speculations with regard to beneficial manipulations of the prostaglandin system await a better understanding of the mechanisms modifying endogenous eicosanoid formation and the clinical responses to modification of eicosanoid formation by therapeutic agents and/or dietary manipulation. Simple inhibition of endogenous prostaglandin formation is not likely to result in important effects on the course of cardiovascular disease; a more complex and perhaps more rational approach must be developed to deal with the multiple theoretical and actual interactions discussed earlier.

REFERENCES

1. von Euler, V. S. (1934): Zur Kenntnis der pharmakologischen Wirkungen von Natiusekreten und Extrakten mannlicher accessorischer Geschlechtsdrussen. *Arch. Exp. Pathol. Pharmakol.*, 175:78–84.
2. Crawford, M. A. (1983): Background to essential fatty acids and their prostanoid derivatives. *Br. Med. Bull.*, 39:210–213.

3. Samuelsson, B., and Paoletti, R. (editors): *Advances in Prostaglandin, Thomboxane, and Leukotriene Research, Vols. 1–14.* Raven Press, New York.
4. Flower, R. J. (1974): Drugs which inhibit prostaglandin biosynthesis. *Pharmacol. Rev.,* 26:33–67.
5. Whittle, B. J. R., and Moncada, S. (1983): Pharmacological interactions between prostacyclin and thromboxanes. *Br. Med. Bull.,* 39:232–238.
6. Piper, P. J. (1983): Pharmacology of leukotrienes. *Br. Med. Bull.,* 39:255–259.
7. Dunn, M. J., and Hood, V. J. (1977): Prostaglandins and the kidney. *Am. J. Physiol.,* 233:F169–F184.
8. Samuelsson, B., Granstrom, E., Green, K., and Hamberg, M. (1971): Metabolism of prostaglandins. *Ann. N.Y. Acad. Sci.,* 180:138–163.
9. Bakhle, Y. S., and Vane, J. R. (editors) (1977): *Metabolic Functions of the Lung.* Marcel Dekker, New York.
10. Karim, S. M. M., and Hillier, K. (1973): Pharmacology and therapeutic applications of prostaglandins in the human reproductive system. In: *The Prostaglandins: Pharmacological and Therapeutic Advances,* edited by M. F. Cuthbert, pp. 167–200. J. B. Lippincott, Philadelphia.
11. Hamberg, M., Svensson, J., and Samuelsson, B. (1975): Thrombroxanes: A new group of biologically active compounds derived from prostaglandin endoperoxides. *Proc. Natl. Acad. Sci. USA,* 72:2994–2998.
12. Vane, J. R., and Bergstrom, S. (editors) (1979): *Prostacyclin.* Raven Press, New York.
13. Vane, J. R., and McGiff, J. C. (1975): Possible contributions of endogenous prostaglandins to the control of blood pressure. *Circ. Res. [Suppl. I],* 36:68–75.
14. Dunn, M. J., and Grome, H. J. (1985): The relevance of prostaglandins in human hypertension. *Adv. Prostaglandin Thromboxane Leukotriene Res.,* 13:179–187.
15. Campbell, W. B., Holland, O. B., and Adams, B. V. (1982): Urinary excretion of prostaglandin E_2, prostaglandin $F_{2\alpha}$, and thromboxane B_2 in normotensive and hypertensive subjects on varying sodium intake. *Hypertension,* 4:735–741.
16. Lebel, M., and Grose, J. H. (1982): Renal prostaglandins in borderline and sustained essential hypertension. *Prostaglandins Leukotrienes Med.,* 8:409–418.
17. Rathaus, M., Korzets, Z., and Bernheim, J. (1983): The urinary excretion of prostaglandin E_2 and $F_{2\alpha}$ in essential hypertension. *Eur. J. Clin. Invest.,* 13:13–17.
18. Tau, S. Y., Bravo, E., and Mulrow, P. J. (1978): Impaired renal prostaglandin E_2 biosynthesis in human hypertension states. *Prostaglandins Med.,* 1:76–85.
19. Weber, P. C., Scherer, B., Held, E., Siess, W., and Stoffel, H. (1979): Urinary prostaglandins and kallikrein in essential hypertension. *Clin. Sci.,* 57:259s–261s.
20. Abe, K. (1981): The kinins and prostaglandins in hypertension. *Clin. Endocrinol. Metab.,* 10:577–605.
21. Zins, G. R. (1975): Renal prostaglandins. *Am. J. Med.,* 58:14–24.
22. Jackson, E. K., Branch, R. A., Margolius, H. S., and Oates, J. A. (1985): Physiological functions of the renal prostaglandin, renin and kallikrein systems. In: *The Kidney: Physiology and Pathophysiology,* edited by D. W. Selden and G. Giebisch, pp. 613–644. Raven Press, New York.
23. Dusting, G. J., Moncada, S., and Vane, J. R. (1979): Prostaglandins, their intermediates and precursors, their cardiovascular actions and regulatory roles in normal and abnormal circulatory systems. *Prog. Cardiovasc. Dis.,* 21:405–430.
24. Nasjletti, A., and Malik, K. U. (1981): Renal kinin-prostaglandin relationship: Implications for renal function. *Kidney Int.,* 19:860–868.
25. Aiken, J. W., and Vane, J. R. (1973): Intrarenal prostaglandin release attenuates the renal vasoconstrictor activity of angiotensin. *J. Pharmacol. Exp. Ther.,* 184:678–687.
26. Patak, R. V., Mookerjec, B. K., Bentzel, C. J., Hysert, P. E., Babej, M., and Lee, J. B. (1975): Antagonism of the effects of furosemide by indomethacin in normal and hypertensive man. *Prostaglandins,* 10:649–659.
27. Durao, B., Martins Prata, M., and Pires Goncalves, L. M. (1977):

28. Lopez-Ovejero, J. A., Weber, M. A., Drayer, J. I. M., Sealey, J. E., and Laragh, J. H. (1978): Effects of indomethacin alone and during diuretic or beta-adrenoreceptor-blockade therapy on blood pressure and the renin system in essential hypertension. *Clin. Sci. Mol. Med.,* 55:203s–205s.
29. Wing, L. M. H., Bune, A. J. C., Chalmers, J. P., Graham, J. R., and West, M. J. (1981): The effects of indomethacin in treated hypertensive patients. *Clin. Exp. Pharmacol. Physiol.,* 8:537–541.
30. Lown, B. (1984): Cardiovascular collapse and sudden cardiac death. In: *Heart Disease: A Textbook of Cardiovascular Medicine,* edited by E. Braunwald, pp. 774–806. W. B. Saunders, Philadelphia.
31. Folts, J. D., Crowell, E. B., and Rowe, G. G. (1976): Platelet aggregation in partially obstructed vessels and their elimination with aspirin. *Circulation,* 54:365–370.
32. Folts, J. D., Gallagher, K., and Rowe, G. G. (1982): Blood flow reductions in stenosed canine coronary arteries: Vasospasm or platelet aggregation. *Circulation,* 65:248–255.
33. Hirsh, P. D., Campbell, W. B., Willerson, J. T., and Hillis, L. D. (1981): Prostaglandins and ischemic heart disease. *Am. J. Med.,* 71:1009–1026.
34. Karmazyn, M., and Dhalla, N. S. (1983): Physiological and pathophysiological aspects of cardiac prostaglandins. *Can. J. Physiol. Pharmacol.,* 61:1207–1225.
35. Majerus, P. W. (1983): Arachidonate metabolism in vascular disorders. *J. Clin. Invest.,* 72:1521–1525.
36. Neri Serneri, G. G., Masotti, G., Pogessi, L., Galanti, G., Morettini, A., and Scarti, L. (1982): Reduced prostacyclin production in patients with different manifestations of ischemic heart disease. *Am. J. Cardiol.,* 49:1146–1151.
37. Pitt, B., Shea, M. J., Romson, J. L., and Lucchesi, B. R. (1983): Prostaglandins and prostaglandin inhibitors in ischemic heart disease. *Ann. Intern. Med.,* 99:83–92.
38. Weksler, B. B. (1984): Prostaglandins and vascular function. *Circulation [Suppl. III],* 70:63–71.
39. Haslam, R. J., and Mcclenaghan, M. D. (1981): Measurement of circulating prostacyclin. *Nature,* 292:364–366.
40. Siess, W., and Dray, F. (1982): Very low levels of 6-ketoprostaglandin $F_{1\alpha}$ in human plasma. *J. Lab. Clin. Med.,* 99:388–398.
41. Fitzgerald, G. A., Brash, A. R., Falardeau, P., and Oates, J. A. (1981): Estimated rate of prostacyclin synthesis in normal man. *J. Clin. Invest.,* 68:1272–1275.
42. Moncada, S., and Vane, J. R. (1979): Arachidonic acid metabolites and the interactions between platelets and blood vessel walls. *N. Engl. J. Med.,* 300:1142–1147.
43. Van den Bosch, H. (1980): Intracellular phospholipases A. *Biochim. Biophys. Acta,* 604:191–246.
44. Hofmann, S. L., and Majerus, P. W. (1982): Identification and properties of two distinct phosphatidylinositol-specific phospholipase C enzymes from sheep seminal vesicular glands. *J. Biol. Chem.,* 257:6461–6469.
45. Prescott, S. M., and Majerus, P. W. (1983): Characterization of 1,2-diacylglycerol hydrolysis in human platelets. *J. Biol. Chem.,* 258:764–769.
46. Humes, J. L., Sadowski, S., Galavage, M., Goldenberg, M., Subers, E., Bonney, R. J., and Kuehl, F. A. (1982): Evidence for two sources of arachidonic acid for oxidative metabolism by mouse peritoneal macrophages. *J. Biol. Chem.,* 257:1591–1594.
47. Flower, R. J., and Blackwell, G. J. (1976): The importance of phospholipase-A_2 in prostaglandin biosynthesis. *Biochem. Pharmacol.,* 25:285–291.
48. Hirata, F., Schiffman, E., Venkatasubramanian, K., Salomon, D., and Axelrod, J. (1980): A phospholipase A_2 inhibitory protein in rabbit neutrophils induced by glucocorticoids. *Proc. Natl. Acad. Sci. USA,* 77:2535–2536.
49. Lullmann, H., and Wehling, M. (1979): The binding of drugs to different polar lipids in vitro. *Biochem. Pharmacol.,* 28:3409–3415.
50. Levin, R. M., and Weiss, B. (1979): Selective binding of antipsychotics and other psychoactive agents to the calcium-dependent

activator of cyclic nucleotide phosphodiestrase. *J. Pharmacol. Exp. Ther.*, 208:454–459.

51. Lands, W. E. M. (1979): The biosynthesis and metabolism of prostaglandins. *Annu. Rev. Physiol.*, 41:633–652.

52. Roth, G. J., and Majerus, P. W. (1975): The mechanism of the effect of aspirin on human platelets: Acetylation of a particulate fraction protein. *J. Clin. Invest.*, 56:624–632.

53. Patrignani, P., Filabozzi, P., and Patrono, C. (1982): Selective cumulative inhibition of platelet thromboxane production by low-dose aspirin in healthy subjects. *J. Clin. Invest.*, 69:1366–1372.

54. Jaffe, E., and Weksler, B. B. (1979): Recovery of endothelial cell prostacyclin after inhibition by low doses of aspirin. *J. Clin. Invest.*, 63:532–535.

55. Rome, L. H., and Lands, W. E. M. (1975): Structural requirements for time-dependent inhibition of prostaglandin biosynthesis by anti-inflammatory drugs. *Proc. Natl. Acad. Sci. USA*, 72:4863–4865.

56. Lands, W. E. M., Cook, H. W., and Rome, L. H. (1976): Prostaglandin biosynthesis: Consequences of oxygenase mechanism upon *in vitro* assays of drug effectiveness. *Adv. Prostaglandin Thromboxane Res.*, 1:7–17.

57. Samuelsson, B., Goldyne, M., Granstrom, E., Hamberg, M., Hammarstrom, S., and Malmsten, C. (1978): Prostaglandins and thromboxanes. *Annu. Rev. Biochem.*, 47:997–1029.

58. Patrignani, P., Filabozzi, P., Catella, F., Pugliese, F., and Patrono, C. (1984): Differential effects of dazoxiben, a selective thromboxane-synthase inhibitor, on platelet and renal prostaglandin-endoperoxide metabolism. *J. Pharmacol. Exp. Ther.*, 228:472–477.

59. Hamberg, M., and Samuelsson, B. (1974): Prostaglandin endoperoxides: Novel transformations of arachidonic acid in human platelets. *Proc. Natl. Acad. Sci. USA*, 71:3400–3404.

60. Gorman, R. R., Fitzpatrick, F. A., and Miller, O. V. (1978): Reciprocal regulation of human cyclic AMP levels by thromboxane A_2 and prostacyclin. *Adv. Cyclic Nucleotide Res.*, 9:597–609.

61. Gorman, R. R., Bundy, G. L., Peterson, D. C., Sun, F. F., Miller, O. V., and Fitzpatrick, F. A. (1977): Inhibition of human platelet thromboxane synthetase by 9,11-azoprosta-5,13-dienoic acid. *Proc. Natl. Acad. Sci. USA*, 74:4007–4011.

62. Blackwell, G. J., Flower, R. J., Russell-Smith, N., Salmon, J. A., Thorogood, P. B., and Vane, J. R. (1978): Prostacyclin is produced in whole blood. *Br. J. Pharmacol.*, 64:436P.

63. Defreyn, G., Machin, S. J., Carreras, L. O., Vergara Dayden, M., Chamone, D. A. F., and Vermylen, J. (1981): Familial bleeding tendency with partial platelet thromboxane synthetase deficiency: Reorientation of cyclic endoperoxide metabolism. *Br. J. Haematol.*, 49:29–41.

64. Moncada, S., Gryglewski, R. J., Bunting, S., and Vane, J. R. (1976): An enzyme isolated from arteries transforms prostaglandin endoperoxides to an unstable substance that inhibits platelet aggregation. *Nature (London)*, 263:663–665.

65. Warso, M. A., and Lands, W. E. M. (1983): Lipid peroxidation in relation to prostacyclin and thromboxane physiology and pathophysiology. *Br. Med. Bull.*, 39:277–280.

66. Weksler, B. B., Eldor, A., Falcone, D., Levin, R. I., Jaffe, E. A., and Minick, C. R. (1982): In: *Cardiovascular Pharmacology of the Prostaglandins*, edited by A. G. Herman, P. M. Vanhoutte, H. Denolin, and A. Goosseus, pp. 137–148. Raven Press, New York.

67. Needleman, P., Raz, A., Minkes, M. S., Ferrendelli, A., and Sprecher, H. (1979): Triene prostaglandins: Prostacyclin and thromboxane biosynthesis and unique biological properties. *Proc. Natl. Acad. Sci. USA*, 76:944–948.

68. Kromhout, D., Bosschieter, E. B., and Coulander, C. de L. (1985): The inverse relation between fish consumption and 20-year mortality from coronary heart disease. *N. Engl. J. Med.*, 312:1205–1209.

69. Phillipson, B. E., Rothrock, D. W., Connor, W. E., Harris, W. S., and Illingworth, D. R. (1985): Reduction of plasma lipids, lipoproteins, and apoproteins by dietary fish oils in patients with hypertriglyceridemia. *N. Engl. J. Med.*, 312:1210–1216.

70. Lorenz, R., Spengler, V., Fischer, S., Duhm, J., and Weber, P. C. (1983): Platelet function, thromboxane formation and blood pressure control during supplementation of the western diet with cod liver oil. *Circulation*, 67:504–511.

71. Dyerberg, J., Bang, H. O., Stoffersen, E., Moncada, S., and Vane, J. R. (1978): Eisosapentaenoic acid and prevention of thrombosis and atherosclerosis. *Lancet*, 2:117–119.

72. Fleisher, L. N., Tall, A. R., Witte, L. D., Miller, R. W., and Cannon, P. J. (1982): Stimulation of arterial endothelial cell prostacyclin synthesis by high density lipoproteins. *J. Biol. Chem.*, 257:6653–6655.

73. Pomerantz, F. B., Tall, A. R., Feinmark, S. J., and Cannon, P. J. (1984): Stimulation of vascular smooth muscle cell prostacyclin and prostaglandin E_2 synthesis by plasma high and low density lipoproteins. *Circ. Res.*, 54:554–565.

74. Eldor, A., Falcone, D. J., Hajjar, D. P., Minick, R., and Weksler, B. B. (1981): Recovery of prostacyclin production by de-endothelialized rabbit aorta: Critical role of neointimal smooth muscle cells. *J. Clin. Invest.*, 67:735–741.

75. Lipid Research Clinics Program (1984): The lipid research clinics coronary primary prevention trial results. I. Reduction in incidence of coronary heart disease. *J.A.M.A.*, 251:351–364.

76. Lipid Research Clinics Program (1984): The lipid research clinics coronary primary prevention trial results. II. The relationship of reduction in incidence of coronary heart disease to cholesterol lowering. *J.A.M.A.*, 251:365–374.

77. Stein, O., Coetzee, G., and Stein, Y. (1980): Modulation of cytoplasmic cholesterol ester of smooth muscle cells in culture derived from rat, rabbit, and bovine aorta. *Biochim. Biophys. Acta*, 620:539–549.

78. Levin, R. I., Jaffe, E. A., Weksler, B. B., and Tack-Goldman, K. (1981): Nitroglycerin stimulates synthesis of prostacyclin by cultured by cultured human endothelial cells. *J. Clin. Invest.*, 67:762–769.

79. Chierchia, S., Patrono, C., Crea, F., Ciabattoni, G., DeCaterina, R., Cinotti, G. A., Distante, A., and Maseii, A. (1982): Effects of intravenous prostacyclin in variant angina. *Circulation*, 65:470–477.

80. Levin, R., Weksler, B. B., and Jaffe, E. A. (1982): The interaction of sodium nitroprusside with human endothelial cells and platelets: Nitroprusside and prostacyclin synergistically inhibit platelet function. *Circulation*, 66:1299–1307.

81. Masotti, G. (1985): Role of prostaglandins in the activity of some cardiovascular drugs. *Adv. Prostaglandin Thromboxane Leukotriene Res.*, 13:319–326.

82. Marcillio, E., Reid, P. R., Dubin, N., Ghodgaonkar, R., and Pitt, B. (1980): Myocardial prostaglandins release by nitroglycerin and modification by indomethacin. *Am. J. Cardiol.*, 45:53–57.

83. Panzenback, M. J., Baez, A., and Kaley, G. (1984): Nitroglycerin and nitroprusside increase coronary blood flow in dogs by a mechanism independent of prostaglandin release. *Am. J. Cardiol.*, 53:936–940.

84. Capurro, N. L., Borrow, R. O., Lipson, L. C., Goldstein, R. E., Shulman, N. R., and Epstein, S. E. (1980): Relative effects of aspirin on prostaglandin modulation of coronary blood flow and platelet aggregation. *Circulation*, 62:1221–1227.

85. Trimarro, B., Patrono, C., Ricciardelli, B., Volpe, M., Cuocolo, A., DeSimone, A., and Condorelli, M. (1985): Indomethacin blunts the late phase of nitroglycerin-induced coronary vasodilatation in dogs. *Adv. Prostaglandin Thromboxane Leukotriene Res.*, 13:333–340.

86. Skeggs, L. T., Marsh, W. M., and Kahn, J. R. (1954): Existence of two forms of hypertension. *J. Exp. Med.*, 99:275–282.

87. Lentz, K. E., Skeggs, L. T., and Wood, K. R. (1956): The amino acid composition of hypertension II and its biochemical relationship to hypertension I. *J. Exp. Med.*, 104:183–191.

88. Ng, K. K. F., and Vane, J. R. (1967): Conversion of angiotensin I to angiotensin II. *Nature*, 215:762–766.

89. Ng, K. K. F., and Vane, J. R. (1968): Fate of angiotensin I in the circulation. *Nature*, 218:144–150.

90. Soffer, R. L. (1976): Angiotensin-converting enzyme and the regulation of vasoactive peptides. *Annu. Rev. Biochem.*, 45:73–94.

91. Ferreira, S. H., and Vane, J. R. (1967): The disappearance of bradykinin and eledoisin the circulation and vascular beds of the cat. *Br. J. Pharmacol. Chemother.*, 30:417–424.

92. Bakhle, Y. S. (1968): Conversion of angiotensin I to angiotensin II by cell free extracts of dog lung. *Nature,* 220:919–921.

93. Ferreira, S. H. (1965): A bradykinin-potentiating factor (BPF) present in venom of *Bothrops jararaca. Br. J. Pharmacol.,* 24: 163–169.

94. Ferreira, S. H., Greene, L. J., Alabaster, V. A., Bakhle, Y. S., and Vane, J. R. (1970): Activity of various fractions of bradykinin potentiating factor against angiotensin I converting enzyme. *Nature,* 225:379–380.

95. Ferreira, S. H., Bartlet, D. C., and Greene, L. J. (1970): Isolation of bradykinin-potentiating peptides from *Bothrops jararaca* venom. *Biochemistry,* 9:2583–2593.

96. Antonaccio, M. J. (1982): Angiotensin converting (ACE) inhibitors. *Annu. Rev. Pharmacol. Toxicol.,* 22:57–87.

97. Horovitz, Z. P. (editor) (1981): *Angiotensin Converting Enzyme Inhibitors: Mechanisms of Action and Clinical Implications,* Urban and Schwarzenberg, Baltimore.

98. Hartsuck, J. A., and Lipscomb, W. N. (1971): Carboxypeptidase A. In: *The Enzyme, Vol. 3,* edited by P. D. Boyer, pp. 1–56. Academic Press, New York.

99. Das, M., and Soffer, R. L. (1975): Pulmonary angiotensin-converting enzyme: Structural and catalytic properties. *J. Biol. Chem.,* 250:6762–6768.

100. Cushman, D. W., Cheung, H. S., Sabo, E. F., and Ondetti, M. A. (1978): Design of new antihypertensive drugs: Potent and specific inhibitors of angiotensin-converting enzyme. *Prog. Cardiovasc. Dis.,* 21:176–182.

101. Byers, L. D., and Wolfenden, P. (1973): Binding of the bi-product analog benzylsuccinic acid by carboxypeptidase A. *Biochemistry,* 12:2070–2072.

102. Cushman, D. W., Cheung, H. S., Sabo, E. F., and Ondetti, A. (1977): Design of potent competitive inhibitors of angiotensin-converting enzyme. *Biochemistry,* 16:5484–5491.

103. Cushman, D. W., and Ondetti, M. A. (1980): Inhibitors of angiotensin-converting enzyme. *Prog. Med. Chem.,* 174:41–104.

104. Haber, E. (1979): The renin-angiotensin system and hypertension. *Kidney Int.,* 15:427–444.

105. Atkinson, A. B., Morton, J. J., Brown, J. J., Davies, D. L., Frazier, R., Kelly, P., Leckie, B., Lever, A. F., and Robertson, J. I. (1980): Captopril in clinical hypertension changes in components of renin-angiotensin system and in body composition in relation to fall in blood pressure with a note on measurement of angiotensin II during converting enzyme inhibition. *Br. Heart J.,* 44:290–296.

106. McCaa, R. E., Hall, J. E., and McCaa, C. S. (1978): The effects of angiotensin I-converting enzyme inhibitors on arterial blood pressure and urinary sodium excretion: Role of the renal renin-angiotensin and kallikrein-kinin systems. *Circulation [Suppl. I],* 43:32–39.

107. Johnston, C. I., Yasujima, M., and Clappison, B. H. (1981): The kallikrein-kinin system and angiotensin converting enzyme inhibition in hypertension. In: *Angiotensin Converting Enzyme Inhibitors,* edited by Z. P. Horovitz, pp. 1257–1264. Urban and Schwarzenberg, Baltimore.

108. Swartz, S. L., Williams, G. H., Hollenberg, N. K., Levine, L., Dluhy, R. G., and Moore, T. J. (1980): Captopril-induced changes in prostaglandin production: Relationship to vascular responses in normal man. *J. Clin. Invest.,* 65:1257–1264.

109. Swartz, S. L., Williams, G. H., Hollenberg, N. K., Moore, T. J., and Dluhy, R. G. (1979): Converting enzyme inhibition in essential hypertension: The hypotensive response does not reflect only reduced angiotensin II formation. *Hypertension,* 1:106–111.

110. Millar, J. A., and Johnston, C. I. (1979): Sequential changes in circulating levels of angiotensin I and II, renin, and bradykinin after captopril. *Med. J. Aust. [Suppl. 2],* 2:R15–R17.

111. Matthews, P. G., and Johnston, C. I. (1979): Responses of the renin-angiotensin system and kallikrein-kinin system to sodium and converting enzyme inhibitor (SQ 14,225). *Adv. Exp. Med. Biol.,* 120B:447–457.

112. Swartz, S. L., Williams, G. H., Hollenberg, N. K., Crantz, F. R., Moore, T. J., Levin, L., Sasahara, A. A., and Dluhy, R. G. (1980): Endocrine profile in the long-term phase of converting-enzyme inhibition. *Clin. Pharmacol. Ther.,* 28:499–508.

113. Carretero, O. A., Scicli, A. G., and Maitra, S. R. (1981): Role of kinins in the pharmacological effects of converting enzyme inhibitors. In: *Angiotensin Converting Enzyme Inhibitors: Mechanisms of Action and Clinical Implications,* edited by Z. P. Horovitz, pp. 105–122. Urban and Schwarzenberg, Baltimore.

114. Marks, E. S., Bing, R. F., Thurston, H., and Swales, J. D. (1980): Vasodepressor property of the converting enzyme inhibitor captopril (SQ 14,225): The role of factors other than renin-angiotensin blockade in the rat. *Clin. Sci.,* 58:1–6.

115. Thurston, H., and Swales, J. D. (1978): Converting enzyme inhibitor and saralasin infusion in rats: Evidence for an additional vasodepressor property of converting enzyme inhibitor. *Circ. Res.,* 42:588–592.

116. Muirhead, E. E., Brooks, B., and Brosius, W. L. (1980): Antihypertensive action of captopril in angiotensin-salt hypertension. *Arch. Pathol. Lab. Med.,* 104:631–634.

117. Man In't Veld, A. J., Schicht, I. M., Derkx, F. H. M., de Bruyn, J. H. B., and Schalekamp, M. A. D. H. (1980): Effects of an angiotensin-converting enzyme inhibitor (captopril) on blood pressure in anephric subjects. *Br. Med. J.,* 1:288–290.

118. Fagard, F., Amery, A., Lijnen, P., and Reybrouck, T. (1979): Haemodynamic effects of captopril in hypertensive patients: Comparison with saralasin. *Clin. Sci.,* 57:131s–134s.

119. Vinci, J. M., Horowitz, D., Zusman, R. M., Pisano, J. J., Catt, K. J., and Keiser, H. R. (1979): The effect of converting enzyme inhibition with SQ 20881 on plasma and urinary kinins, prostaglandin E and angiotensin II in hypertensive man. *Hypertension,* 1:416–426.

120. Swartz, S. L., Williams, G. H., Hollenberg, N. K., Crantz, F. R., Levine, L., Moore, T. J., and Dluhy, R. G. (1980): Increase in prostaglandins during converting enzyme inhibition. *Clin. Sci.,* 59:133s–135s.

121. Moore, T. J., Crantz, F. R., Hollenberg, N. K., Koletsky, R. J., Leboff, M. S., Swartz, S. L., Levine, L., Podolsky, S., Dluhy, R. G., and Williams, G. H. (1981): Contribution of prostaglandins to the antihypertensive action of captopril in essential hypertension. *Hypertension,* 3:168–173.

122. Silberbauer, K., Stanek, B., and Templ, H. (1982): Acute hypotensive effect of captopril in man modified by prostaglandin synthesis inhibition. *Br. J. Clin. Pharmacol.,* 14:87S–93s.

123. Ogihara, T., Maruyama, A., Hata, T., Mikami, H., Nakamaru, M., Naka, T., Ohde, H., and Kumahara, Y. (1981): Hormonal responses to long-term converting enzyme inhibition in hypertensive patients. *Clin. Pharmacol. Ther.,* 30:328–335.

124. Witzgall, H., Hirsch, B., Scherer, B., and Weber, P. C. (1982): Acute haemodynamic and hormonal effects of captopril are diminished by indomethacin. *Clin. Sci.,* 62:611–615.

125. Goldstone, R. M., Martin, K., Zipser, R., and Horton, R. (1981): Evidence for a dual action of converting enzyme inhibitor on blood pressure in normal man. *Prostaglandins,* 22:587–598.

126. Provoost, A. (1980): The effect of prostaglandin synthesis inhibition of the acute blood pressure reduction by captopril in pentobarbitol-anaesthetized rats. *Eur. J. Pharmacol.,* 65:425–428.

127. Muirhead, E. E., Germain, G. S., Armstrong, F. B., Brooks, B., Leach, B. E., Byers, L. W., Pitcock, J. A., and Brown, P. B. (1975): Endocrine-type antihypertensive function of renomedullary interstitial cells. *Kidney Int.,* 8:S271–S282.

128. Zusman, R. M., and Keiser, H. R. (1977): Prostaglandin biosynthesis by rabbit renomedullary interstitial cells in tissue culture: Stimulation by angiotensin II, bradykinin and arginine vasopressin. *J. Clin. Invest.,* 60:215–223.

129. Zusman, R. M., and Keiser, H. R. (1977): Prostaglandin E_2 biosynthesis by rabbit renomedullary interstitial cells in culture: Mechanisms of stimulation by angiotensin II, bradykinin and arginine vasopressin. *J. Biol. Chem.,* 252:2069–2071.

130. Ausiello, D. A., and Zusman, R. M. (1984): The role of calcium in the stimulation of prostaglandin biosynthesis in rabbit renomedullary interstitial cells. *Biochem. J.,* 220:139–145.

131. Zusman, R. M. (1983): Regulation of the prostaglandin biosynthesis in cultured renal medullary interstitial cells. In: *Prostaglandins and the Kidney,* edited by M. J. Dunn, C. Patrono, and G. A. Cinotti, pp. 17–25. Plenum, New York.

132. Abrams, W. B., Davies, J. O., and Gomez, H. J. (1984): Clinical pharmacology of enalapril. *J. Hypertens. [Suppl. 2],* 2:31–36.

133. Galler, M., Folkert, V. W., and Schlondorff, D. (1981): Effect of converting enzyme inhibitor on prostaglandin synthesis by isolated rat glomeruli. *Clin. Res.*, 29:271A (abstract).

134. Dollery, C. T., and Miyamori, I. (1979): Indomethacin and the hypotensive action of captopril in DOCA salt hypertensive rats. *Br. J. Pharmacol.*, 68:117P–118P.

135. Goldstone, R. M., Martin, K., Zipser, R., and Horton, R. (1981): Evidence for a dual action of converting enzyme inhibitor on blood pressure in normal man. *Prostaglandins*, 22:587–598.

136. Sweet, C. S., and Ulm, E. H. (1984): Enalapril. *New Drugs Annual: Cardiovascular Drugs*, 2:1–17.

137. Sweet, C. S., Gaul, S. L., Reitz, P. M., Blaine, E. H., and Ribeiro, L. T. (1983): Mechanism of action of enalapril in experimental hypertension and acute left ventricular failure. *J. Hypertens.*, 1:53–63.

138. Sweet, C. S., Gross, D. M., Arbegast, P. T., Gaul, S. L., Britt, P. M., Ludden, C. T., Weitz, D., and Stone, C. A. (1981): Antihypertensive activity of *N*-[(*S*)-1-(ethoxycarboxyl)-3-phenyl-propyl]-L-Ala-L-Pro (MK 421) on orally active converting enzyme inhibitor. *J. Pharmacol. Exp. Ther.*, 216:556–558.

139. Shoback, D. M., Williams, G. H., Swartz, S. L., Davies, R. O., and Hollenberg, N. K. (1983): Time course and effect of sodium intake on vascular and hormonal responses to enalapril (MK 421) in normal subjects. *J. Cardiovasc. Pharmacol.*, 5:1010–1018.

140. Zusman, R. M. (1984): Nephrology forum: Renin- and non-renin-mediated antihypertensive actions of converting enzyme inhibitors. *Kidney Int.*, 25:969–983.

141. Someya, N., Morotomi, Y., Kodama, K., Kida, O., Higa, T., and Tanaka, K. (1984): Suppressive effect of captopril on platelet aggregation in essential hypertension. *J. Cardiovasc. Pharmacol.*, 6:840–843.

142. Pfeffer, J. M., Pfeffer, M. A., and Bramdwald, E. (1985): Influence of chronic captopril therapy on the infarcted left ventricle of the rat. *Circ. Res.*, 57:84–95.

143. Lilly, L., Dzau, V. J., Williams, G. H., and Hollenberg, N. K. (1985): Captopril vs. hydralazine in advanced congestive heart failure: Comparison of one year survival. *Circulation* [*Suppl. IV*], 72:408.

144. Kirstein, A. (1979): Cardiac prostacyclin release: Stimulation by hypoxia, and various agents. *Scand. J. Haematol.*, 34:105–111.

145. Cramer, E. B., Pologe, L., Pawlowski, N. A., Cohn, Z. A., and Scott, W. A. (1983): Leukotriene C promotes prostacyclin synthesis by human endothelial cells. *Proc. Natl. Acad. Sci. USA*, 80:4109–4113.

146. Cairns, J. A., Gent, M., Singer, J., Finnie, K. J., Fraggatt, G. M., Holder, D. A., Jablonsky, G., Kostuk, W. J., Melendez, L. J., Myers, M. G., Sackett, D. L., Sealey, B. J., and Tauser, P. H. (1985): Aspirin, sulfinpyrazone, or both in unstable angina. *N. Engl. J. Med.*, 313:1369–1375.

147. Weksler, B. B., Tack-Goldmann, K., Subramanian, V. A., and Gay, W. A., Jr. (1985): Cumulative inhibitory effect of low-dose aspirin on vascular prostacyclin and platelet thromboxane production in patients with atherosclerosis. *Circulation*, 71:332–340.

148. May, G. S., Eberlein, K. A., Furberg, C. D., Passamani, E. R., and DeMets, D. L. (1982): Secondary prevention after myocardial infarction: A review of long-term trials. *Prog. Cardiovasc. Dis.*, 24:331–352.

149. Schafer, A. I., Crawford, D. D., and Gimbrone, M. A., Jr. (1984): Indirectional transfer of prostaglandin endoperoxides between platelets and endothelial cells. *J. Clin. Invest.*, 73:1105–1112.

The Heart and Cardiovascular System,
edited by H. A. Fozzard et al.
Raven Press, New York © 1986.

CHAPTER **69**

Renin-Angiotensin System: Biology, Physiology, and Pharmacology

Victor J. Dzau and Richard E. Pratt

The renin-angiotensin system (RAS) is a blood-borne biochemical cascade whose final product, angiotensin II, is a potent vasoconstrictor and a primary stimulus for aldosterone secretion (Fig. 1A). Numerous studies have demonstrated an important role for this circulating system in blood pressure and electrolyte and fluid homeostasis. Our understanding of the contribution of the RAS to cardiovascular and renal physiology has been made possible through the development of radioimmunoassay, techniques for protein isolation and sequencing, and the availability of synthetic peptides and pharmacologic inhibitors. More recently, molecular cloning of renin cDNA and genes was accomplished using recombinant DNA technology. Using standard biochemical methods and modern molecular biologic techniques, a number of investigators have recently demonstrated the expression of renin and angiotensinogen genes in a variety of tissues. As a result, the concept of the RAS as a hormonal system alone is in question. Locally expressed RASs may be involved in the regulation of individual tissue function, independent of the circulating counterpart. This new concept may be important in further understanding the RAS's role in physiology and the responses to pharmacologic inhibitors.

This chapter will attempt to review the biology, physiology, and pharmacology of the RAS, with emphasis on new developments and techniques. A section of this chapter is dedicated to the principles and details of the methods used in the study of this system. It is our goal to provide a comprehensive review of the subject as well as a resource on methods for students, trainees, and investigators in this field.

BIOLOGY OF THE RENIN-ANGIOTENSIN CASCADE

Renin

Characteristics and Chemistry

Renin is the first enzyme in the biochemical cascade of the RAS. It cleaves its substrate, angiotensinogen, to generate the decapeptide angiotensin I (AI) (Fig. 1B). Renin is synthesized and stored in the juxtaglomerular (JG) cells of the afferent arteriole of the kidney and is released into the circulation in response to a variety of stimuli. Renin is an aspartyl proteinase. Like the other aspartyl proteinases, renin contains two carboxyl groups contributed by aspartic acid residues in the active site

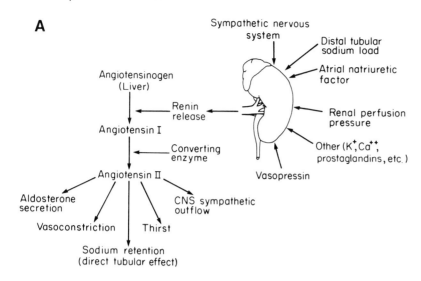

FIG. 1. A: Schematic representation of the renin angiotensin system showing major regulators of renin release, the biochemical cascade leading to AII, and the major effects of AII. **B:** Angiotensin biochemical cascade. Pathway of angiotensin production and catabolism.

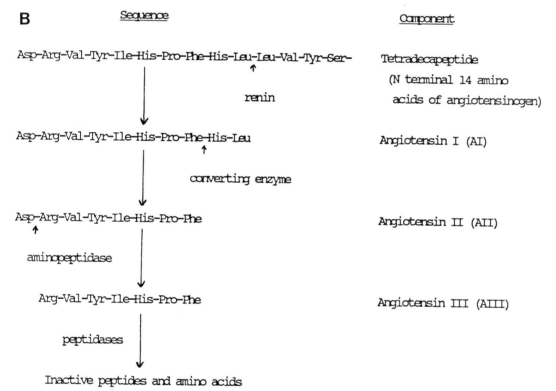

that are essential for catalytic function (150). Even though renin's primary amino acid sequence resembles, to a large extent, those of other aspartyl proteinases (Fig. 2), renin differs from these proteinases in several respects. It is active at neutral pH, has free sulfhydryl groups, and is highly selective for its substrate (149). Aspartyl proteinases, in general, are nonspecific enzymes, whereas renin's substrate specificity is stringently limited to one particular peptide bond of angiotensinogen.

Structure and Synthesis

Renin has been completely purified from various species (39,69,88,121,124). Renal renin is a glycoprotein

with a molecular weight of 37,000 to 40,000. Its isoelectric point is between 5.2 and 5.8, and the pH optimum for reaction with angiotensinogen is 5.5 to 5.6. Recent studies of the structure of mouse submandibular gland (SMG) renin indicate that renin is composed of a heavy chain (MW 31,000) and a light chain (MW 5,500) linked by a single disulfide bond (149). The active site is located in the heavy chain; the exact function of the light chain has not yet been elucidated. It is not yet clear whether human renin is a single-chain polypeptide or is composed of two polypeptide chains like mouse renin. The available evidence tends to suggest that mature human renin is a single-chain polypeptide. However, dibasic amino acid residues are located in a similar position in human

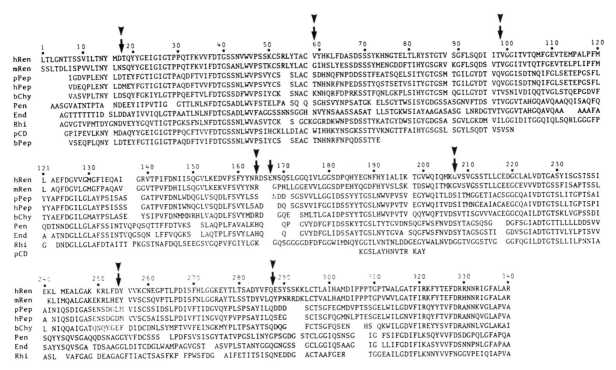

FIG. 2. Comparison of the sequences of the aspartyl proteinases. Arrows indicate locations of splice junctions in the human renin gene, and arrowheads indicate splice junctions in human pepsin gene. The alignment is based on the primary structural homologies among human renin (hRen), mouse (mRen), pig pepsin (pPep), human pepsin (hPep), bovine chymosin (bChy), penicillopepsin (Pen), endothiapepsin (End), rhizopuspepsin (Rhi), pig cathepsin D (pCD), and bovine pepsin (bPep). Note the similarities in splice junctions and amino acid sequences. (From ref. 151, with permission.)

renin, which might represent the cleavage site to generate two-chain human renin (106,109,119).

Based on the known amino acid sequence of mouse SMG and human renal renin, three-dimensional structural models have been proposed using computer graphics (5,18,33). Like other aspartyl proteinases, the catalytic site of renin is formed as a cleft between two lobes of the enzyme molecule. There are also some remarkable differences between renin and other aspartyl proteinases at the edges of the active-site cleft. Here, renin appears to contain highly basic residues. In addition, renin has a unique "flap" not present in other aspartyl residues. This flap may be important in determining the substrate specificity. Human renin contains two presumptive N-glycosylation sites at Asn-Thr-Thr (position 5–7) and Asn-Gly-Thr (position 75–77) (106,109,119). Similar sites are found in mouse kidney renin (79), but are not present in mouse SMG renin (173). Indeed, SMG renin is not glycosylated, whereas renal renins of various species are glycoproteins.

Renin is synthesized from its messenger RNA as a preproenzyme (37,65,181,182) that is rapidly translocated into the lumen of the endoplasmic reticulum and converted to prorenin. Prorenin is processed in the lumen of the rough endoplasmic reticulum and Golgi apparatus to the mature active enzyme that is finally packaged and stored in secretory granules. For mouse renin, two

proteolytic cleavages are necessary in the processing and maturation of prorenin to renin (Fig. 3A). The first cleavage occurs at the peptide bond between arginine-63-serine-64 and converts prorenin to a single-chain polypeptide. The second cleavage removes the dipeptide arginine-352-arginine-353, resulting in two chains that are held together by a disulfide bond (149,173). The biosynthetic pathway of human renin has not been fully characterized. A study of renin synthesis in a renin-producing tumor has offered useful insight. It appears that human prorenin is processed to a single-chain polypeptide that is glycosylated and stored in granules (89).

In addition to the active enzyme, heavier forms of renin, ranging from 50,000 to 140,000 MW, have been reported (121,194,195). Most of these forms have not been purified, and virtually nothing is known about their structures. Their demonstration has been dependent on the fractionation of renal extracts by gel filtration or affinity chromatography. Considerable debate exists over which of these forms are authentic renin precursors (zymogens), renin-plus-inhibitor-protein complexes, or artifacts of extraction (resulting in a nonspecific protein-protein association).

The high-MW forms of renin can be broadly divided into two groups based on the presence or absence of enzymatic activity. The first group includes inactive

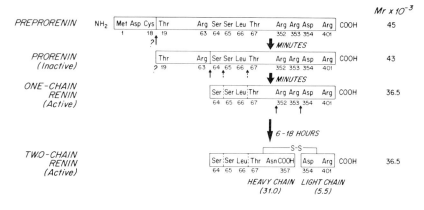

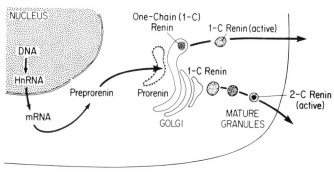

FIG. 3. Models of renin biosynthesis and secretion. **Top:** Proposed sites (*solid arrow*) and alternative sites (*broken arrow*) of processing of renin with the relative kinetics of each step shown. The molecular weights were deduced from the amino acid sequences. The question mark at the Cys-Thr cleavage site at positions 18–19 indicates the proposed but unconfirmed cleavage location of preprorenin to prorenin. **Bottom:** Proposed intracellular localizations of the various forms of renin during biosynthesis and secretion. (From ref. 182, with permission.)

enzyme, which may be activated by limited proteolysis using trypsin, pepsin, or kallikrein, or by acidification or prolonged cold exposure. These "inactive renins" have been demonstrated in plasma and kidneys of humans and hogs and possibly dogs, mice, and rats, as well as in human amniotic fluid (121,122,194,195). Plasma inactive renin appears to originate primarily from the kidney (117). Recent purification of hog renal inactive renin indicates that it has a MW of 50,000 and is probably a single-chain polypeptide (205,206). Using antibodies raised to a pentapeptide of the prosegment of prorenin, recent data suggest that inactive renin and prorenin are immunologically homologous and may be the same molecule (22,127). Based on these observations, inactive renin appears to be a zymogen (biological precursor) of the active, mature enzyme. For this reason, inactive renin has also been named "prorenin" by many investigators (121,194,195).

The second group of high-MW forms do have intrinsic enzymatic activity. They tend to be larger than inactive renin (i.e., MW approximately 60,000) and can be isolated from renal extracts in the presence of sulfhydryl-oxidizing agents such as sodium tetrathionate or *N*-ethylmaleimide (87). The available evidence suggests that these forms represent renin complexed with protein; i.e., postsynthetic modification of the enzyme has occurred (124). Although it has been postulated that these forms are renin-inhibitor complexes, *in vitro* artifacts of the extraction process cannot be ruled out.

Factors Controlling Renin Release

The release of renin (94,125) is influenced by a number of factors (Fig. 1A). The major signals controlling renin secretion are (a) renal perfusion pressure (intrarenal baroreceptor), (b) the adrenergic nervous system (via renal sympathetic nerves or circulating catecholamines), (c) distal tubular sodium concentration (macula densa), and (d) other humoral signals (potassium, angiotensin II, prostaglandins, and possibly kinins).

Effects of renal perfusion pressure.

Elevated renal perfusion pressure suppresses renin secretion, whereas reduction in renal perfusion pressure increases renin release by activating an intrarenal baroreceptor. The stimulus–response curve of pressure and renin secretion has been defined (76). Renin release is relatively unresponsive to the initial 10- to 20-mm-Hg reduction from a normal basal blood pressure. The threshold pressure is 80 to 90 mm Hg; below the threshold, renin secretion is a steep and linear function of renal perfusion pressure.

Influence of sodium on renin release.

Sodium also exerts a major influence on renin release. Both intrarenal infusion of sodium chloride and an increase in dietary sodium intake are capable of inhibiting renin release. Dietary sodium restriction is associated with increased renin secretion. There are at least two possible mechanisms by which sodium may influence renin release. Sodium may have an indirect effect by changing extracellular sodium content and fluid volume (leading to an altered volume or neural signal); there may be, potentially, a direct effect of sodium on the JG apparatus (either on the JG cells or on the macula densa sensor). There is probably little or no direct effect of changes in plasma sodium concentration within the physiologic range on renin release by JG cells. In fact, Kotchen and associates have suggested that chloride rather than sodium is responsible for the control of renin release via the macula densa (129). However, the precise effect of the sodium concentration in the distal nephron on renin release is unresolved.

Effects of adrenergic receptor stimulus.

Beta-adrenergic receptors on the JG cells are responsive to both neurally released and circulating catecholamines (125). Electrical stimulation of renal sympathetic nerves or selective areas of the vasomotor center or hypothalamus results in renin release that is blocked by propranolol. Epinephrine and isoproterenol stimulate renin release both *in vivo* and *in vitro*. Recently, specific dopaminergic nerve endings and receptors have been demonstrated in the kidney. Stimulation of receptors also results in renin release (151).

The role of alpha-adrenergic receptors in regulation of renin secretion is less clear. Since presynaptic and postsynaptic alpha receptors are present in the intact, innervated kidney, the response to non-subtype-selective adrenergic agonists or antagonists may vary depending on the dose of the agent and the physiological conditions of the study. To date, the data appear to favor an inhibitory effect of the alpha-adrenergic receptor on renin release (125).

Other influences on renin release.

Several other humoral factors also influence the secretion of renin (125). Hypokalemia stimulates renin release. Vasopressin inhibits renin secretion, but its effect on renin release is probably mediated by systemic or renal hemodynamic changes. Vasodilator prostaglandins (PGs), PGE_2 and PGI_2, appear to stimulate renin release, as does arachidonic acid. The precise contribution of endogenous PGs to the control of renin release in the intact subject is less clear. It appears that in the basal state in the sodium-replete dog, the PG synthetase inhibitor, indomethacin, has no effect on renin release (48). On the other hand, indomethacin reduces basal renin release in the sodium-depleted dog. Similarly, decreased cardiac output by vena caval constriction and hemorrhage evokes secretion of renin that can be atten-

uated by indomethacin (70). In addition, endogenous PGs may mediate many stimulatory signals, such as the renal baroreceptor signals (13).

Studies on the effect of calcium on the secretion of renin have yielded conflicting results. Several investigators have demonstrated that intrarenal infusion of calcium chloride reduces renin secretion. However, a few others have reported an increase (216,222). Moreover, removal of calcium from the perfusate of isolated kidneys increases basal renin release (83,178); but Viskoper et al. (213) reported that chelation of calcium with EGTA had no effect on renin release in the blood-perfused isolated kidney. The addition of lanthanum, a cation that "locks" calcium channels and blocks calcium efflux, to isolated perfused kidneys (139) or glomeruli (9) decreased renin release.

These experiments, using intact preparations, have several limitations. Calcium infusion may lead to changes in sodium excretion and/or alterations in renal hemodynamics that may indirectly influence renin release. Removal of calcium from perfusate or use of chelating agents can produce nonspecific effects on cell volume or membrane permeability. Furthermore, increasing calcium concentration may lead to increased calcium influx into nerve terminals or endothelial cell membranes, evoking catecholamine release in the first instance, resulting in PG release from the endothelial cells; both catecholamine and PG secretions can secondarily stimulate renin secretion from JG cells. Overall, the data favor an inhibitory effect of calcium on renin secretion; such a inhibition is in contrast to the effect of calcium on the secretion of most other hormones. In addition, calcium might play an important role as a cellular messenger for other elements that affect renin release (*vide infra*).

Feedback regulation of renin release.

Renin release is subject to feedback regulation. For example, within minutes after renal artery constriction in the experimental animal, pressure distal to constriction begins to rise toward base-line pressure as systemic pressure rises. This rise in distal pressure is also associated with rising intrarenal resistance, after the initial autoregulatory vasodilation, partly because of angiotensin-mediated renal vasoconstriction (6,68). This increase in distal pressure is, at least in part, responsible for the subsequent inhibition of renin release.

Angiotensin II also has a direct inhibitory effect on renin release by the JG cells, known as the "short feedback loop." A third mechanism of feedback inhibition involves sodium retention and extracellular fluid (ECF) volume expansion, induced by elevated plasma aldosterone or by other factors; it is known as the "long feedback loop."

Cellular Mechanisms and Pathways of Renin Release

Cellular mechanisms.

Despite extensive studies identifying the factors that influence renin release, the cellular messengers of these signals are poorly understood. The best candidates for second messengers are calcium, endogenous PGs, and cAMP.

Manipulations that increase intracellular calcium concentration, such as increased extracellular calcium, lanthanum, and calcium ionophores, tend to depress renin secretion. An increase in intracellular calcium concentration may be the mechanism by which angiotensin II (AII), norepinephrine, vasopressin, and other vasoconstrictors inhibit renin secretion. Conversely, when calcium influx is reduced by the addition of verapamil, the inhibitory action of these agents on renin release is attenuated (162,175). Increased extracellular potassium and increased intraluminal pressure in renal arterioles may exert inhibitory effects by a similar mechanism. Recently, Harada and Rubin (105) have shown that renin release mediated by the beta-adrenergic receptor is associated with a dose-related and temporally associated calcium efflux, providing indirect evidence that a decrease in intracellular calcium may be the stimulatory signal to renin release.

Since many cellular events controlled by intracellular calcium are mediated by calmodulin, the cellular calcium-binding protein, Churchill and Churchill (38) studied the effect of trifluorperazine, a putative calmodulin inhibitor, on renin release. Trifluorperazine produced a dose-dependent increase in renin release and blocked the inhibitory effect of a high extracellular potassium concentration. These investigators postulate that changes in the calmodulin-calcium complex mediate the influence of calcium on renin release.

Endogenous PGs may also act as a second messenger mediating the response to several stimuli that promote renin release; these include sodium depletion, beta-adrenergic stimulation, and reduction of renal perfusion pressure in the autoregulatory range. However, the role of PGs on renin release in response to reduction in pressure below the autoregulatory range, 60 mm Hg, is less clear.

Other cellular mechanisms, e.g., adenylate cyclase activity, may also be second messengers in response to certain stimuli of renin release (44).

Cellular pathways.

Recent studies have examined the cellular pathways of renin secretion that may be potential sites of regulation. Studies on mouse kidney and SMG show that renin may be secreted by two cellular pathways (Fig. 3B) (182,183). Renin is released by the storage granules in response to acute stimuli. This pathway is regulated by many secretagogues (e.g., isoproterenol) and releases principally the two-chain renin and is termed the "regulated" pathway. An alternative route, directly from the Golgi apparatus, secretes the one-chain renin. This "constitutive" pathway is not immediately influenced by secretagogues but appears to be dependent on the rate of renin synthesis. In the mouse kidney, the constitutive pathway also releases prorenin.

Less is known about the cellular pathways of renin secretion in humans. Studies on renin-producing tumors and cultured chorionic cells suggest that a constitutive pathway that releases prorenin is also present (1,89). In the kidney, our preliminary data demonstrated that mature renin is a glycosylated one-chain form and is released principally from the storage granules. Further studies in elucidating these secretory pathways and their regulation will provide insight into control of renin secretion.

Extrarenal Renin

Several investigators have demonstrated that reninlike enzymes exist in many tissues besides the kidney (Table 1). While some of the enzyme activity may be due to cathepsin D, immunoreactive renin has clearly been identified in brain, anterior pituitary, uterus, arterial tissue, and adrenal cortex (for reviews, see refs. 46,52,91). In addition, renin and angiotensinogen messenger RNAs have been demonstrated in many of these tissues (Table 1), indicating local expression of these genes. In most of these tissues, other components of the RAS (converting enzyme, angiotensin and its receptors) have also been identified, suggesting that the entire RAS exists locally in these sites. The role of local RAS is unclear. The brain RAS may play a role in control of blood pressure, release of antidiuretic hormone and catecholamine, and regulation of thirst (184). The vascular RAS may contribute to the regulation of flow and vascular resistance. We believe that tissue RASs are involved in the regulation of local tissue function, possibly through intracellular synthesis of AII (which would act either intracellularly or on cell surface receptors) (46,52).

Genetics of Renin

Mouse and human renin complementary DNAs have been cloned (119,173,179,189). Based on its nucleotide sequence, one can deduce that renin mRNA encodes for a preproenzyme similar to the other secretory proteins. The human and mouse renin genes have also been cloned (106,109,151,159,173). The mouse renin gene is 10 kilobases long and contains 8 introns and 9 exons. The human renin gene also spans approximately 12 kilobases and has 10 exons interrupted by 9 introns (Fig. 4). The presumptive promoter element, TATAA, termed a Hogness box, is located 73 bases 5' to the start

TABLE 1. *Presence of renin and renin mRNA in various tissues*

Tissue	Renin activity (species)[a]	Renin mRNA (species)
Kidney	+ (all)	+ (M,R,H)
SMG	+ (M)	+ (M)
Uterus	+ (Rb,M)	ND
Chorion	+ (H)	+ (cultured cells) (H)
Blood vessel	+ (Rb,S,B,M,R,D,H,Ho)	+ (cultured cells) (H)
Brain	+ (H,Ho,M,R,D)	+ (M,R)
Pituitary	+ (B,R,Ho,Rb,H)	ND
Adrenal	+ (Rb,B,M,R,H)	+ (M)
Testis	+ (M,R)	+ (M)
Heart	+ (M,R)	+ (M)

[a] Plus signal = present; ND = not determined. Parentheses contain species in which renin has been documented: M, mouse; R, rat; Rb, rabbit; H, human; S, sheep; B, bovine; Ho, hog; D, dog.
Data from various sources (46,58,79,91) and our unpublished observations.

of transcription. Interestingly, a second Hogness box was found in the first intron, 110 bases 5' to the start of exon 2 (109). The human gene also contains an extra exon (#6 or 5A) that encodes three amino acids that are not present in the mouse gene (106,151).

Finally, some insight into the genetic regulation of renin has been provided by studies on mouse SMG renin. Several investigators have obtained evidence that inbred strains of mice with low levels of SMG renin have a single renin gene (Ren-1), whereas strains that have high SMG renin levels carry duplicated renin genes (Ren-1, Ren-2) (174,179). Both genes have been mapped to the same region of mouse chromosome one. The regulation of the expression of these two genes and the tissue specificity of their expression are under active investigation.

Angiotensinogen

Chemistry and Characteristics

The renin substrate angiotensinogen, an α_2-globulin synthesized and released by the liver, has been purified from plasma of several species (20,208). Angiotensinogen is a glycoprotein that exists in two forms: MW 62,000 and MW 65,000. The 14-NH_2-terminal amino acid residue of angiotensinogen, the tetradecapeptide, is functional as renin substrate *in vitro* (Fig. 1B). Renin cleaves angiotensinogen specifically at the leucine[10]leucine[11] bond to release the physiologically inactive peptide, AI (20). The human NH_2-terminal sequence differs from those in equine and rat angiotensinogens; the cleavage site is a leucine-valine bond (208). Human angiotensinogen is not hydrolyzed by nonprimate renins. However, human renin is capable of hydrolyzing nonprimate angiotensinogen. This species specificity may be due to structural differences in renins and angiotensinogens of different species.

Angiotensinogen Secretion

Angiotensinogen is stored in low quantity in the liver. In response to an appropriate stimulus, angiotensinogen is rapidly synthesized and released. Hepatic angiotensinogen production is subject to feedback regulation by the components of the RAS (Fig. 5). It is stimulated by AII and inhibited directly or indirectly by renin or des(AI)-angiotensinogen, a product of the reaction of renin and angiotensinogen (107). This may explain, in part, the decrease in plasma angiotensinogen concentration observed with captopril therapy. Hepatic angiotensinogen production is also stimulated by several hormones, including glucocorticoids, estrogens (including the oral contraceptives), and thyroxine (19,21,60). Hypophysectomy results in marked decreases in the rate of angiotensinogen production and plasma substrate concentration that can be normalized with replacement of these hormones (67). Although plasma angiotensinogen concentration usually reflects the rate of hepatic angiotensinogen production, changes in degradation due to alterations in plasma renin concentration can also affect plasma substrate levels. The influence of these hormones on hepatic angiotensinogen release may explain the elevated plasma substrate levels observed in patients with Cushing's disease or hyperthyroidism and in women on oral contraceptives and during pregnancy (60). Other clinical conditions that affect plasma angiotensinogen levels include bilateral nephrectomy, which increases the plasma concentration, and hepatic cirrhosis, which decreases it.

Plasma angiotensinogen may be rate-limiting in the generation of AI and thus important in the regulation of blood pressure. The importance of plasma angiotensinogen in blood pressure control has been demonstrated by *in vivo* experiments in which angiotensinogen antibody was administered to rats. Under normal conditions, plasma angiotensinogen concentration is significantly

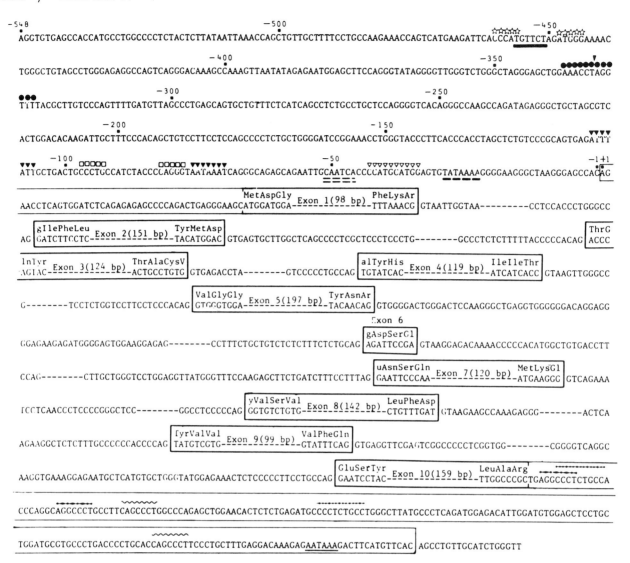

FIG. 4. Sequence and structure of the human renin gene. Position 1 corresponds to the presumptive transcription initiation site. Exons are numbered 1–10 and are indicated by boxes. In the region 5' to the start of initiation, note the presence of the presumptive promoter sequences TATA, TATAA, and CAATCA. In addition, note the many palindromic sequences (*dots, stars, triangles, squares*) found in this region, as well as a presumptive glucocorticoid-receptor-binding sequence (*bold line*). All three classes of sequences might be important in regulation of transcription of the human renin gene. (From ref. 151, with permission.)

lower than the K_m of the renin and angiotensinogen reaction (60). In conditions where plasma angiotensinogen concentration is primarily increased, the rate of AII production also increases. Substrate excess may contribute to the hypertension in Cushing's syndrome and to that associated with the use of oral contraceptives (60).

Angiotensin-Converting Enzyme

Angiotensin-converting enzyme (ACE) is a dipeptidyl peptidase that cleaves the carboxy-terminal dipeptide of AI, releasing AII (Fig. 1B). It is present in high concentrations on the luminal membrane surfaces of endothelial cells of pulmonary capillaries. Although it is found in the plasma, the plasma concentration is only a small fraction of that in the lung. Thus, the majority of plasma AI is converted to AII in a single pass through the pulmonary circulation (191). ACE and its isoenzyme(s) are also found in the kidney, brain, liver, epididymis, and most vascular beds (30). Because ACE is present in great excess in the pulmonary circulation, it is not rate-limiting in the generation of AII. ACE is a glycoprotein of MW 150,000, including an anchor peptide of MW approximately 4,000 that is submerged in the lipid bilayer of the plasma membrane; the anchor peptide is clipped after solubilization with trypsin (214). ACE is a metalloprotease that is inhibited by EDTA and other chelating agents. The enzyme is activated by chloride and other monovalent anions. The active site of ACE

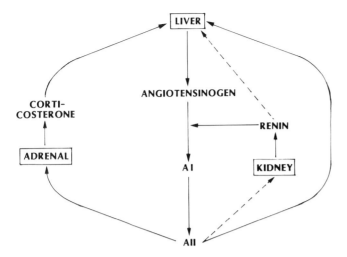

FIG. 5. Feedback regulation of angiotensinogen production by components of the renin angiotensin system. *Solid arrow* implies stimulation; *broken arrows* represent inhibition. (From ref. 107, with permission.)

contains three stereospecific groups (resembling carboxypeptidase A in this respect). A catalytically essential zinc atom in the active site appears to be directly involved in the hydrolysis of the sessile bond. Further components of the active site are both the carboxyl group of an aspartyl or glutamyl residue and tyrosyl, arginyl, and lysyl residues. The last two are probably involved in mediating the anion activation. ACE is also capable of cleaving COOH-terminal dipeptides of bradykinin ("kinase II") and enkephalins, as well as a variety of protected tripeptides (72).

The regulation of endothelial or plasma ACE has not been well characterized. The plasma ACE appear to originate from the endothelial cells. The factors that control its release are not known. Endothelial ACE synthesis is stimulated by dexamethasone and captopril and inhibited by low oxygen tension (86). In active sarcoidosis or other granulomatous diseases involving the lung, the plasma ACE concentration is elevated; changes in plasma ACE levels may be useful as an index of the activity of these diseases (49). Plasma ACE concentrations have been shown to be decreased in patients with a variety of diseases of pulmonary parenchyma, including chronic obstructive lung disease, carcinoma, and cystic fibrosis. It is also elevated, for unknown reasons, in Gaucher's disease, hyperthyroidism, and diabetes mellitus (136,137,225).

Angiotensins

AII, the physiologically active octapeptide, has multiple sites of action (Fig. 1A). It is one of the most potent vasoconstrictors found in the mammalian body. The renal and splanchnic circulations are particularly sensitive to the vasoconstrictor action of AII. AII can cause contraction of isolated glomeruli and may alter glomer-

ular dynamics and the filtration coefficient (15,28). *In vitro* experiments have suggested that AII can modify tubular sodium handling (135). The octapeptide is a potent stimulus for aldosterone release from the adrenal cortex. It has also been shown to stimulate release of catecholamine from the adrenal medulla and from peripheral sympathetic nerve endings (126,145). Injection of AII into the central nervous system can stimulate thirst, increase systemic blood pressure, and evoke secretion of antidiuretic hormone and catecholamines (184).

AI is probably physiologically inactive, although some observations suggest that it is capable of stimulating catecholamine release from adrenal medulla and inducing thirst when injected into the CNS (80,177). AII can be cleaved by aminopeptidases to yield des(aspartyl[1])angiotensin II or "angiotensin III" (Fig. 1B). This heptapeptide is a potent stimulator of aldosterone release *in situ* and *in vitro*; it induces renal vasoconstriction, stimulates PG release from perfused vessels *in vitro,* and is a potent inhibitor of renin release (17,96). However, the exact physiologic importance of AIII remains unclear. It is also unclear whether AIII interacts with a separate specific receptor or cross-reacts with AII receptors. AII and AIII can be cleaved by other peptidases to generate inactive angiotensin peptides and amino acids (Fig. 1B).

Angiotensin Receptors

AII receptors have been identified and characterized biochemically in adrenal zona glomerulosa, vascular smooth muscle, uterus, bladder, isolated glomeruli, platelets, pituitary, and brain (12,31,81,97,155). The binding of angiotensin to these receptors is sterospecific and saturable. Angiotension can be displaced from receptors by structurally related agonists and antagonists. The dissociation constant K_d is approximately 10^{-9} M.

Angiotensin receptors on smooth muscle and adrenal cortex are regulated by sodium intake. *In vivo* studies have shown that the sensitivity of adrenals to AII increases during sodium depletion, whereas vascular sensitivity decreases (4,112). The converse occurs during sodium loading. The effects of a low-sodium diet on vascular receptors can be reproduced by infusion of AII and blocked by captopril, indicating that changes in circulating AII are responsible for the regulation of AII receptors (97). Recent studies indicate that changes in glomerular AII receptors resemble those of vascular smooth muscle receptors with respect to sodium intake. The change in number of glomerular AII receptors parallels the changes in glomerular contractility and dynamics and thus may be important in the regulation of glomerular filtration (81). Sodium's influence on adrenal angiotensin receptors is converse of that on smooth muscle angiotensin receptors. Regulatory influences on brain and pituitary AII receptors have not yet been characterized.

PHYSIOLOGY OF THE RAS

The renin-angiotensin-aldosterone system plays a major role in the control of arterial blood pressure, regional blood flow, and sodium balance (Fig. 1A). AII is a potent vasoconstrictor as well as a primary stimulus for aldosterone secretion. The development of radioimmunoassays for components of the renin-angiotensin-aldosterone system and the availability of pharmacological inhibitors of this system have made it possible to address certain critical questions concerning the roles of AII and aldosterone in physiological homeostasis and in a number of pathological states.

Regulation of Blood Pressure and ECF Volume

It is now clear that the renin-angiotensin-aldosterone system is activated during sodium depletion and volume contraction. Under these conditions, the elevated plasma concentration of AII contributes to the maintenance of arterial pressure (57,100,192). The increased secretion of aldosterone promotes renal sodium and water retention and aids in the restoration of sodium and volume balance. Furthermore, AII, acting on renal tubules, also possesses a potent antinatriuretic effect. Blockade of this system in sodium-depleted animals and humans results in hypotension and prevents sodium retention.

During sodium loading, plasma renin activity is suppressed. Under this circumstance, inhibition of the renin-angiotensin-aldosterone system has no effect on blood pressure or electrolyte balance (57,100,192). In humans on a normal-sodium intake, upright posture induces a modest activation of the RAS. Pharmacological inhibition of this system under this circumstance produces minimal to mild depressor effects. This inverse relationship between sodium and renin activity is an important concept in understanding the response to pharamacological inhibitors.

The vascular response to AII is also influenced by the state of sodium balance. The pressor response to AII is blunted during sodium restriction and enhanced on a high-sodium intake in humans and in animals (112). This effect was specific for AII; norepinephrine showed no such shift in vascular responsiveness. The sensitivity to AII is particularly marked in the renal circulation. As discussed in the section on angiotensin receptors, the physiological basis for the changes in vascular responsiveness is the number of receptors in the blood vessel wall, which varies according to circulating angiotensin levels (97). With high-sodium diets, the plasma AII concentration is low, and the receptors are "up-regulated." The converse is true during sodium depletion.

Influence on the Kidney and Other Regional Circulations

Because of the differential sensitivity of various vascular beds to AII, changes in regional circulation during activation of the RAS is not uniform. When sodium intake was restricted, the kidney and skin exhibited the greatest decreases in blood flow. The skeletal muscle and splanchnic circulation flows also decreased, whereas cerebral and coronary flows remained relatively unchanged (93). Blockade of the RAS resulted in a relatively greater increase in renal blood flow and may be associated with a brisk natriuresis. This rapid response suggested that a local action of angiotensin, independent of aldosterone, had contributed to renal sodium handling (128).

AII reduces renal blood flow but maintains glomerular filtration rate, resulting in an increased filtration fraction. This is because of a preferential efferent (postglomerular) arteriolar constriction in response to angiotensin. In high doses, AII will also constrict afferent (preglomerular) as well as efferent (postglomerular) arterioles, resulting in decreases in both glomerular filtration rate and renal blood flow. In addition, glomerular mesangial cells also contain AII receptors. Activation of these receptors results in glomerular contraction, a reduction in glomerular capillary surface area, and a decrease in filtration (15,29). Indeed, evidence from experimental studies indicates that the RAS plays an important part in the autoregulation of renal blood flow and glomerular filtration rate when renal artery perfusion pressure is substantially reduced. Since glomerular capillary hydraulic pressure is determined by the balance between afferent and efferent vascular tone, efferent arteriolar vasoconstriction serves to maintain an effective filtration pressure and glomerular filtration rate when renal arterial pressure is substantially diminished. The critical role of the RAS in mediating this efferent arteriolar constriction is suggested by studies in animals in which glomerular filtration rate was impaired during infusion of an angiotensin antagonist, (Sar[1]Ile[8])AII, or of teprotide, an intravenously administered converting enzyme inhibitor (103,104). Failure to autoregulate the rate of filtration because of pharmacological blockade of the RAS was exaggerated by prior sodium depletion. Extrapolating from the foregoing experimental data, one may clinically anticipate generation of a functional form of acute renal failure when the RAS is blocked and the prevailing renal parenchyema is perfused at a sufficiently low pressure. This set of conditions appears to be satisfied when captopril is administered to patients with hemodynamically severe renal artery stenosis involving either both renal arteries or the renal artery of a solitary kidney whether native or transplanted. Severe unilateral renal artery stenosis in the presence of a contracted, atrophic contralateral kidney would also be expected to result in this functional decrement in glomerular filtration rate.

Indeed, such deterioration in glomerular filtration rate has been described in patients who fit this condition (40,116,221).

Angiotensin Effect on the CNS

Direct administration of AII to the CNS can lead to increased plasma catecholamine levels and systemic hypertension (184). These effects can be blocked by central administration of angiotensin antagonist, (Sar^{1}Ala^8)AII. AII, when administered centrally, also activates receptors in the area postrema and induces thirst (184). This dipsogenic effect can also be induced by infusion of AII into carotid arteries and can be blocked with centrally administered AII and antagonists. In certain pathological states, e.g., experimental renovascular hypertension and heart failure, this dipsogenic effect can also be observed (215). The contribution of this behavior to the development of hyponatremia in clinical conditions such as congestive heart failure is unclear.

Interaction with Sympathetic Nervous System and Other Vasoactive Hormones

The RAS interacts with the sympathetic nervous system in a number of ways. AII facilitates the release of norepinephrine and blocks the reuptake of this neurotransmitter in the peripheral nerve endings (126,145). Evidence is also accumulating that centrally produced AII can cause selective changes in catecholamine turnover in the CNS (for review, see ref. 90). In the hypothalamus, increased dopamine turnover in the media eminence and increased norepinephrine turnover in the supraoptic nuclei in the preoptic area have been described. AII also augments the sensitivity of the baroreceptor reflex. Inhibition of the RAS reduces the sensitivity of the baroreceptor reflex. This may explain the absence of plasma catecholamine release and tachycardia despite hypotension due to pharmacological inhibition of this system.

Angiotensin interacts with a number of vasoactive substances in the regulation of vascular tone. AII stimulates the biosynthesis of vasodilator PGs by blood vessel wall and kidney (146,197,228). Then endogenous PGI$_2$ and PGE$_2$ counteract angiotensin vasoconstriction. Indeed, inhibition of PG synthesis frequently unmasks and enhances the vasoconstrictive response to AII (66). In addition, PGE$_2$ modulates renal sodium excretion via hemodynamic changes or a direct tubular effect. Inhibition of its synthesis can result in sodium retention and may precipitate acute renal failure (214).

Another area of interaction between the RAS and tissue vasoactive substances is via angiotensin-converting enzyme or kininase II. This peptidyl dipeptidase degrades AI as well as bradykinin (72). Blockade of this enzyme not only prevents the production of AII but also results in accumulation of the local vasodilator bradykinin (34). It has been suggested, although not proved, that this accumulation of tissue bradykinin may contribute to the vasodilatory action of converting enzyme inhibitors.

Role of the RAS in the Pathophysiology of Hypertension and Heart Failure

Hypertension

Renovascular hypertension.

The RAS plays an important role in the initiation of experimental renovascular hypertension (59,161). In experimental models of renovascular hypertension (two-kidney one-clip, 2K-1C; one-kidney one-clip, 1K-1C), plasma renin activity and angiotensin levels increase during the acute phase immediately after renal artery constriction. These hormonal changes are associated with a rapid increase in blood pressure in both models. The causal relationship between the increase in hormonal levels and the increased blood pressure has been demonstrated by normalization of blood pressure by administration of AII antagonist, ACE inhibitor, or renin-specific antibody in this phase. Moreover, the acute hypertension can be prevented by pretreatment with pharmacological blockade of the RAS (8,63). During this phase, angiotensin also induces changes in intrarenal hemodynamics (decreases glomerular filtration rate and blood flow) and stimulates aldosterone secretion. The combination of hemodynamic and direct hormone effects on tubular function results in increased sodium reabsorption. This intrarenal action of angiotensin is probably important in the transition to the chronic phase of hypertension.

The second phase of experimental renal hypertension is characterized by a decline in hormonal levels toward normal and sodium retention, with ECF volume expansion. Acute administration of AII antagonist or converting enzyme inhibitor does not significantly affect blood pressure or renal blood flow at this stage (8,68). The time course for the development of the chronic phase varies between species and models. The 1K-1C dog can develop this non-angiotensin-dependent phase in 3 to 5 days (68). In the 1K-1C rat, several weeks are necessary, whereas the 2K-1C rat may require 2 to 4 months to reach this phase (153).

It appears that the time taken for the development of this phase may be directly related to the ability of the contralateral kidney to excrete the increased sodium and water load. Indeed, Rostand et al. (188) have demonstrated that the expected pressure natriuresis by the contralateral kidney is attenuated in the chronic phase as a result of functional changes in intrarenal hemodynamics as well as structural changes in the renal vasculature induced by hypertension. Thus, the shorter time required for the development of this phase in the 1K-1C model is explained by the reduction in excretory capacity resulting from nephrectomy. In other words, the 1K-1C model is probably analogous to the 2K-1C model at the stage in which the function of the contralateral kidney is markedly impaired.

To address the pathogenetic role of sodium and water retention in Goldblatt hypertensive rats during this nonangiotensin-dependent phase, Gavras et al. (92) induced sodium depletion and observed that blood pressure once again became sensitive to angiotensin antagonists. It has also been demonstrated that the changes in intrarenal resistance revert to angiotensin dependence upon sodium depletion (7). Furthermore, Barger and associates have shown that renovascular hypertension can be induced without volume expansion in 1K-1C dogs maintained continuously on a low sodium intake. In this preparation, the RAS remained activated in the chronic phase and was pathogenic in all phases of the hypertension (8).

Experimental data suggest that increased vascular reactivity (3,10,82,187), sympathetic nervous system activity (27,28,123), and structural changes in systemic vascular walls contribute in various degrees to the maintenance of chronic hypertension. Furthermore, recent data indicate that increased brain or vascular renin activity (187), circulating ouabain-like substance(s) (172), and vasopressin release (185) may also participate in its pathogenesis. Guyton et al. (99) also proposed the concept of "whole-body autoregulation," i.e., increased peripheral vascular resistance initiated by an early transient rise in cardiac output. However, this view is not shared by all investigators.

In summary, there are two basic models of Goldblatt renovascular hypertension. The pathogenesis of both models produces a spectrum of plasma renin and angiotensin levels from high to normal that is inversely related to sodium balance. The models are characterized by an acute hypertensive phase with elevated hormone levels in which blood pressure is normalized by renin-angiotensin blockers or nephrectomy. Although the time course varies, both models eventually reach a chronic hypertensive phase in which hormone levels have declined toward normal and ECF volume has expanded. During this stage, neither acute pharmacological blockade nor nephrectomy reduces blood pressure to normal. Removal of the stenosis during the chronic volume-expanded stage results in a natriuresis and a return of blood pressure to normal. Sodium depletion during the chronic phase can revert the hypertensive state to the angiotensin-dependent phase and restore responsiveness to pharmacological blockade and nephrectomy.

Essential hypertension.

The role of the RAS in the pathogenesis of human essential hypertension is less clear. Several investigators have demonstrated that 15 to 30% of essential hypertensives have high plasma renin activities and 30% or more have normal plasma renin levels that are inappropriate for the elevated blood pressure (26). Thus, approximately 60% of human essential hypertension potentially is renin-dependent. Indeed, converting enzyme inhibitors alone reduce the blood pressure in more than 60% of all essential hypertension patients (51). With dietary sodium restriction, over 80% of the patients respond to converting enzyme inhibition. The responses to pharmacological inhibition of the RAS in these patients include systemic blood pressure reduction, renal blood flow increase, net sodium excretion (associated with suppression of angiotension and aldosterone production), and increased plasma PG levels (24,114,201).

Primary aldosteronism.

Hypertension results from excessive adrenal output of aldosterone. This increased autonomous aldosterone production due to adrenal cortical hyperplasia or adenoma is associated with secondary suppression of plasma renin activity. Because this chapter is focused on renin-angiotensin, the authors refer the reader to an endocrine textbook for further information on this subject.

Congestive Heart Failure

Elevation of peripheral vascular resistance and expansion of the ECF volume are two prominent homeostatic mechanisms that are activated when heart failure occurs (62). Studies in conscious animals with cardiac failure have suggested that the RAS is activated early in the development of heart failure, following the acute lowering of the cardiac output (215). During the chronic compensated state of experimental heart failure, plasma renin activity and plasma aldosterone concentration decline toward normal as the ECF volume expands. These observations have been confirmed by clinical studies: Plasma renin activity and plasma aldosterone concentrations were found to be markedly elevated in patients with recent cardiac decompensation but were normal in those with chronic compensated congestive heart failure and peripheral edema (56). When sequential measurements were made in patients who were followed from the acutely decompensated state, the elevated plasma renin activity and AII concentration returned to normal as congestive heart failure stabilized and circulatory compensation occurred.

The state of the RAS also appears to be related to the severity of cardiac dysfunction. This observation has raised the possibility that angiotensin may play a role in the increased systemic vascular resistance occurring in patients with severe heart failure. The resulting increased impedance to left ventricular outflow can depress cardiac output further. Similarly, the potent antinatriuretic renal tubular effects of AII and aldosterone may be a key factor in the salt and water retention that accompanies heart failure. A third possible contribution of the RAS to the pathophysiology of cardiac failure is via redistribution of cardiac output to various organs. The renal circulation is particularly sensitive to the actions of AII and the sympathetic nervous system. In fact, the azotemia accompanying cardiac failure is the result of reductions in renal blood flow and in glomerular filtration rate, which are due to renal arteriolar vasoconstriction, mediated, in part, by AII. Indeed, close correlations between serum creatinine, blood urea nitrogen, and renal plasma flow and plasma renin activity have been observed in patients with severe congestive heart failure (23,56).

The major stimulus to renin release in patients with congestive heart failure appears to be a decrease in renal perfusion and/or arterial pressure, secondary to the reduced cardiac output. An inverse correlation between mean arterial pressure and plasma renin activity has been observed in these patients. Other possible mechanisms include activation of cardiopulmonary receptors and reductions in sodium concentrations in the macula densa. Indeed, a significant inverse relationship between serum sodium concentration and plasma renin activity has been reported (66,134,171).

In addition to the release of vasoconstrictor hormones,

vasodilator systems are activated in experimental heart failure (66,169). PGE_2 and PGI_2 are released during tissue ischemia, which results in lower vascular resistance and improved local blood flow (164). A number of vasoactive substances, including AII, norepinephrine, and bradykinin, directly stimulate the synthesis and release of PGs, which in turn modulate their actions (16,141,163). AII-induced vasoconstriction in the renal, coronary, and mesenteric vasculature, for example, is associated with enhanced PGE_2 and PGI_2 synthesis. Administration of inhibitors of PG synthesis under these conditions resulted in magnification of the vasoconstrictor response to AII (Fig. 6). Similar interactions have been reported between vasodilator PGs and norepinephrine during infusions of these agents or during sympathetic nerve stimulation (147). In addition, PGE_2 has nonvascular renal effects and enhances urinary sodium excretion and modulates the action of vasopressin on water permeability (226).

Experimental studies suggested that during activation of the RAS and/or sympathetic nervous system, maintenance of renal flow and function was critically dependent on the interplay between endogenous PGs and these vasoconstrictor hormones (163). This interaction is probably also true for many other vascular beds. Thus, during cardiac decompensation when the vasoconstrictor

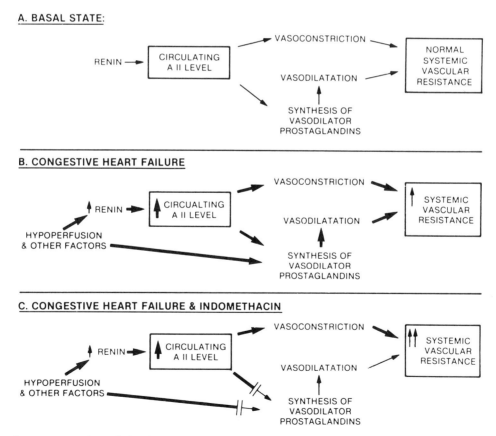

FIG. 6. Schematic representation of the interaction of vasoconstrictor angiotensin and vasodilator PGs in the control of systemic vascular resistance in CHF. (Modified from Levenson, D. J., Simmons, C. E., and Brenner, B. M., *Am. J. Med.,* 72: 354–374, 1982.)

hormonal systems are markedly activated, compensatory activation of the vasodilator PG system can play a modulating role in the regulation of organ perfusion and function. Oliver et al. (169) demonstrated that during acute reduction of cardiac output in anesthetized dogs, plasma PGE_2 concentration in renal venous blood increased fourfold, associated with the increases in plasma renin activity (PRA) and plasma norepinephrine concentration. We have documented marked elevations of plasma PGE_2 metabolite levels and 6-keto-PGF_1 (metabolite of prostacyclin) in patients with acute severe decompensated congestive heart failure (CHF) (62,68). In these patients, the RAS was also activated, and significant correlations between PGE_2 metabolite and PRA as well as AII were observed (Fig. 7A). Greater degrees of azotemia and hyponatremia were seen in these patients as compared with those with chronic stable CHF. In fact, we observed that the serum sodium concentration was inversely correlated with PRA and plasma PG concentrations (Fig. 7B). The close correlation between plasma PG levels and renin-angiotensin levels reflects

either the stimulation of PG synthesis by AII or increased renin release induced by PGI_2 (219).

The identification of patients with heart failure who have compensatory activation of the PG system may be important. It has been known for a long time that nonsteroidal antiinflammatory drugs, which block PG synthetase, such as indomethacin, can result in sodium and water retention or even precipitate renal failure in CHF. Blockade of the synthesis of renal PGE_2 and PGI_2 can result in unopposed intense systemic and renal vasoconstriction. Indeed, Walshe and Venutto (214) reported the development of acute oliguric renal failure in a patient with severe CHF as a result of indomethacin administration. Recently, we demonstrated that indomethacin resulted in determination of cardiac hemodynamics in hyponatremic CHF patients who had elevated plasma PG levels (66). Also of relevance are the recent observations that captopril increases plasma PGE_2 metabolite concentrations (201) and that indomethacin and aspirin attenuates the vasodilator and renal responses to captopril in normal and hypertensive subjects (154). We

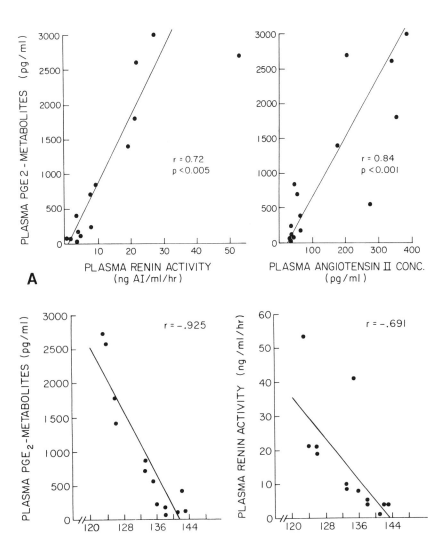

FIG. 7. A: Relationships of plasma PGE_2 metabolite concentrations to PRAs and plasma angiotensin concentrations in patients with CHF. **B:** Inverse relationship of serum sodium concentration to PRAs and PGE_2 metabolite levels in patients with CHF. (From refs. 62 and 66 with permission.)

demonstrated that indomethacin impaired the cardiac hemodynamic response to captopril in CHF patients. Recognition of this drug interaction is particularly critical for patients with decompensated cardiac failure, because captopril appears to be an effective drug in their management.

Based on our knowledge of the contribution of vasoconstrictor hormones to increased systemic vascular resistance in CHF, inhibitors of the RAS have been studied and widely employed as vasodilators in the treatment of CHF (see the later section on pharmacology). In summary, the RAS plays an important role in blood pressure and ECF volume homeostasis. In hypertension and CHF, the RAS is activated and contributes to the pathogenesis of these pathological states.

METHODS IN RENIN-ANGIOTENSIN MEASUREMENTS AND RESEARCH

Early methods for detection and quantification of the components of the RAS were based on the ability of the component to generate AII either directly or indirectly. The resultant AII would then be quantified with a bioassay, either *in vivo* or *in vitro* by measuring the contraction of aortic, intestinal, or uterine strips. Such methods were time-consuming and lacking in sensitivity and reproducibility. Because of these drawbacks, measurements of these components were restricted to the research laboratory and therefore were of limited usefulness to clinicians.

Today, radioimmunoassays are used for measurements of many of the components of the RAS. Because other chapters have dealt with the theoretical aspects of these assays, we shall concentrate on the specific assays for each component.

Assays for Components of the RAS

Angiotensins

The radioimmunoassay (RIA) for angiotensins involves the competition for antibody binding between angioten-

sin in a sample and radiolabeled angiotensin (Table 2). The radiolabeled antigen (AI or AII) can be readily prepared by iodination using described methods (84). In our experience, the cost of commercially available ^{125}I-labeled AI and AII is more than offset by the convenience and safety aspects. Most suppliers of radiochemicals will provide iodinated angiotensins with sufficiently high specific activity for a modest price.

AI assay.

The procedure used in most laboratories is based on that of Haber et al. (102). The radiolabeled tracer is diluted in 0.1-M Tris-HCl, pH 7.4, plus BSA at 1 mg/ml, to give 5,000 to 10,000 cpm/0.5 ml. The antibody is diluted in the same buffer such that 0.5 ml contains sufficient antisera to bind 45 to 55% of the ^{125}I-AI. A standard curve is constructed containing AI (0.1–1.2 ng) in 100 μl of the same buffer and incubated with radiolabeled AI and antibody at 4°C for >12 hr. To separate the free AI from the antibody-bound AI, dextran-coated charcoal (0.5% charcoal, dextran T-70) is added, and the samples are immediately centrifuged at 2,000 rpm for 10 min. The supernatant is decanted and counted. The amount of angiotensin in the sample is determined by comparison with the standards.

AII assay.

The buffer used for this assay (84) is 0.01-M potassium phosphate (pH 7.4) containing 3 mM Na$_2$-EDTA, 0.15 mM 8-hydroxyquinoline sulfate, 0.02% neomycin, and BSA at 2.5 mg/ml. Prior to use, the buffer is heated to 56°C for 30 min and stored at 4°C. ^{125}I-AII tracer (10,000 cpm/0.1 ml) is added to the sample or standards (0.3–80 pg AII). As in the preceding assay, sufficient antibody to bind 50% of the ^{125}I-AII is added (0.1 ml), and the sample is incubated at 4°C for 24 hr. Dextran-coated charcoal is added, the sample is spun and decanted, and the supernatant is counted.

Although the foregoing assay is straightforward, sen-

TABLE 2. *Summary of techniques employed in study of the RAS*

Component	Method of analysis	Refs.
Renin mRNA	Northern-blot analysis	58,79,209
Prorenin (inactive renin)	Trypsin activation	194,195
	Acid activation	117,118
	Direct radioimmunoassay	98,108,110,142,148
Renin	AI generation	102,196,198
	Direct radioimmunoassay	98,108,110,142,148
Angiotensinogen	Exhaustive digestion with renin; AI RIA	60,67,107
	Direct RIA	19
AI, AII, AIII	RIA	84,102
	HPLC, RIA	167
Converting enzyme	Conversion of AI to AII, HPLC, RIA	130
	Cleavage of tripeptid Hip-Gly-Gly, Hip-His-Leu	41,42,85,193

* Direct radioimmunoassay measures total immunoreactive renin (active plus prorenin).

sitive, and reproducible, there are certain limitations. The low levels of AI and AII in plasma require concentration and extraction to remove interfering substances. Whereas it is possible to obtain antisera specific for AI that show low cross-reactivity with the other angiotensins, it has been more difficult to obtain a highly specific antiserum to AII. All currently available antisera show considerable cross-reactivity with the smaller angiotensin fragments, especially AIII (50,157,166–168).

A recent approach to circumvent these problems has been to perform reverse-phase high-performance liquid chromatography (HPLC) prior to RIA analysis of the angiotensins, particularly for AII (167). Because of the time and expense involved, this procedure is not likely to be routinely available for clinical use; however, it has gained rapid acceptance in clinical and laboratory research. Using these procedures, the presence and quantities of the various angiotensins have been determined not only in plasma but also in other biological fluids (i.e., CSF), as well as various tissues and cells.

In this procedure (167), 10 ml of blood is collected into tubes containing 0.5 ml of inhibitor solution (2% ethanol, 0.025 M phenanthroline, 0.125 M Na$_2$-EDTA, neomycin at 2 g/liter), chilled, and centrifuged. The plasma (2 ml) is rapidly chromatographed on a phenylsilyl silica cartridge (100 mg) previously washed with methanol followed by water. Following a water wash, the absorbed angiotensins are eluted in 0.5 ml methanol and collected into polypropylene tubes previously washed with 0.5% BSA in Tris-HCl (pH 7.5). The eluate is dried, dissolved in 0.1-M acetic acid, and chromatographed by isocratic reverse-phase HPLC using a 10-μ C-18 silica column with methanol/0.085% phosphoric acid (33.5:66.5) as the mobile phase. Because the retention time for AII is consistent, only the region of the elution previously shown to contain AII is collected and assayed. The limit of detection for this assay was determined to be 0.45 fmol/ml plasma.

Renin Assay

The standard renin assay, which is commercially available, depends on measuring the amount of AI formed during a given *in vitro* incubation period. The results are expressed as quantity of AI generated in a volume of sample per unit time (e.g., ng AI/ml/hr, as in plasma, or ng AI generated per mg protein per unit time, as in tissue homogenate).

Plasma renin level.

Renin levels in plasma are assayed by two separate protocols. PRA measures the intrinsic ability of the plasma sample to generate AI. It involves no manipulations of the sample other than addition of buffer and

protease inhibitors. The value obtained is dependent on the renin levels and the amount of endogenous substrate, which usually is not present at saturating levels. Plasma renin concentration (PRC), on the other hand, measures renin activity in the presence of excess endogenously added substrate. In this case, the plasma sample is supplemented with substrate, ideally in saturating amounts such that the rate of AI generation is dependent only on the levels of renin. The term PRC is probably a misnomer, because the concentration of renin is not truly being measured.

In these assays, addition of protease inhibitors to the samples is important, because plasma (as well as tissue extracts) contains numerous angiotensinases as well as other nonspecific proteases that will degrade not only the generated AI but also the renin itself. For this reason, EDTA, phenylmethylsulfonyl fluoride (PMSF), 8-hydroxyquinoline sulfate, and dimercaprol are present in the reaction mixture (11,170). Because the inhibition of these proteases is of such importance, it is recommended that the stability of exogenously added AI be measured routinely as a control to document complete inhibition of these proteases.

The pH chosen for the assay is also of importance (11,84,102,170,196). Renin's pH optimum is between 5 and 6, depending on the sources of substrate and renin. However, because the plasma pH is 7.4, some investigators argue that PRA or PRC should be performed at the physiological pH. This also provides an added advantage of inhibiting certain acid proteases (other than renin) whose pH optimum is much lower. A drawback is that the amount of AI generated will be twofold to fourfold less than that obtained at the pH optimum. In fact, some investigators feel that it is preferable to generate at the lower pH, especially for low-renin samples. However, the comparisons of data obtained at different pHs are questionable at best.

The duration of incubation for AI generation will, of course, depend on the levels of renin in the sample as well as the avidity of the AI antisera. Periods of incubation as long as 24 hr can be used, but other factors become important, such as the stability of the protease inhibitors as well as the stability of both renin and substrate. Whenever possible, multiple time points should be used to assure that the rate of generation is linear. The details of the assays are described next.

PRA. Blood is collected into chilled tubes containing NA$_2$-EDTA to give a final concentration of 4 mM, then chilled and centrifuged (102,196). Plasma (250 μl) is mixed with 0.34 M 8-hydroxyquinoline sulfate (5 μl) and is then diluted with 250 μl of 0.6-M Tris-HCl (pH 7.4) containing 0.2 mM PMSF, 3.2 mM dimercaprol, and 0.02% neomycin. The sample is divided in two, one incubated at 4°C (control sample) and the other at 37°C for 3 to 24 hr. The samples are then assayed in duplicate for AI. For assays employing a lower pH, the Tris-HCl is replaced with 0.6 M potassium phosphate or maleate (pH 5.7) (196).

PRC. Plasma (100 μl) collected as described earlier (198) is mixed with 250 μl of substrate mix [plasma from anephric sheep diluted 1:3 in 0.1 M Tris-HCl (pH 7.4) or 0.6 M potassium phosphate or maleate (pH 5.7) containing 3.4 mM 8-hydroxyquinoline sulfate, 0.25 mM EDTA, 0.1 mM PMSF, and 1.6 mM dimercaprol]. The sample is incubated at 37°C for 1 to 3 hr and then assayed in duplicate for AI.

Source of substrate. Sheep angiotensinogen is the preferred substrate for the foregoing assay (84,117,199). However, plasma from nephrectomized dog, hog, or rat is also used. The animal is nephrectomized 48 hr prior to collecting plasma. For the large animals, the blood is collected into 600-ml blood bags (on ice) containing 10 ml of 9% Na_2-EDTA in saline. During the collection, the bags are gently mixed. After collection, the blood is transferred to centrifuge bottles and centrifuged at 3,000 rpm for 20 min at 4°C. The decanted plasma is stored at −70°C. Prior to use, the plasma is assayed for residual renin activity (PRA) as described earlier. In addition, the substrate concentration is determined by exhaustive digestion with renin (*vide infra*). Usually the concentration of angiotensinogen in plasma from nephrectomized animals is greater than 1,000 ng equivalent AI/nl.

Tissue renin.

Tissue is removed from the animal and processed as quickly as possible. For storage and subsequent analysis, the tissue should be snap-frozen in liquid nitrogen or on dry ice and stored at −20°C. The tissue is homogenized in 0.1-M Tris-HCl, pH 7.4, containing 0.1% Triton X-100, 0.25 mM Na_2-EDTA, 0.1 mM PMSF, 0.25 mM sodium tetrathionate (NaTT). In addition, SBTI or aprotinin at 0.1 mg/ml is occasionally used. To lyse cultured cells, addition of the foregoing buffer is usually sufficient, with mild agitation of the sample, to solubilize both external and internal membranes. However, with tissue, additional mechanical disruption is usually necessary. In the past, we have used a close-fitting Teflon or ground-glass hand homogenizer, a polytron, or a sonicator with equal success. Our preference is to use a polytron or sonicator; however, care must be taken to keep the sample as cold as possible and to minimize foaming. After extraction, the solution is centrifuged (15,000 rpm, 10 min, 4°C) to remove cell debris, and the supernatant is assayed for renin concentration as described earlier. If necessary, the sample is first diluted in Tris-HCl (0.1 M, pH 7.4) containing BSA at 1 mg/ml and the same inhibitors.

The same controls that were discussed for plasma are performed for tissue. Documentation of the stability of AI is of critical importance, especially if the tissue is rich in nonspecific proteases or, as in the case of

endothelial cells (138), rich in converting enzyme and angiotensinases. If the tissue has low activity, it is conceivable that some or all of the activity is due to contamination with plasma. For this reason, the tissue should be cleared of blood prior to extraction either by washing or, if possible, by perfusion with an isotonic solution. However, even with washed tissue, the only method to assure that the renin activity represents local synthesis is to demonstrate the presence of renin mRNA in the tissue (*vide infra*).

Because of the presence of other intracellular nonspecific proteases (cathepsin D) that can liberate AI from substrate, it is often necessary to document that the AI-generating activity is, in fact, renin. This has been accomplished either by demonstrating inhibition of activity with renin-specific antisera or by inhibition with synthetic peptide inhibitors (53,138). Comparison of the inhibitory kinetics of the tissue renin with those of authentic renin (usually kidney or plasma renin) from the same species is usually required. For this assay, the sample at the proper dilution (50 μl) is incubated with the antibody or inhibitor (100 μl) at 37°C for 1 hr. For exact comparisons, the inhibitor or antibody is used in multiple concentrations in order to compare the IC_{50} values. After the incubation, the residual renin activity is assayed by addition of renin substrate as described earlier. Differences in inhibitory curves and IC_{50} values as compared with those for authentic renin are indications that other nonrenin proteases are contributing to the AI generation.

Inactive renin.

As described earlier, there exists an inactive form of renin, termed prorenin, that can be activated by a number of manipulations. The evidence that inactive renin may be the biosynthetic precursor was discussed earlier. Treatment of inactive renin with brief exposure to trypsin or other proteases, dialysis to acidic pH, or cryoactivation results in an increase in activity. Unfortunately, it seems that the procedure details vary between laboratories. Moreover, sources of inactive renin frequently vary in other constituents that influence the condition of activation, i.e., variations in total protein concentrations, endogenous proteases and endogenous serine protease inhibitors, etc. Therefore, the methods may have to be modified and adapted for different tissues and fluids. The following are some basic principles.

Trypsin activation. Plasma samples are prepared without serine protease inhibitors (PMSF, DFP, SBTI, aprotinin) and aliquoted in 100-μl samples to which 10 μl of trypsin [10 × final concentration dissolved in 10 mg/ml BSA in 0.1-M Tris-HCl (pH 7.4)] is added (194,195). The final concentration of trypsin usually used is 5 mg/ml to 10^{-3} mg/ml, depending on the level of endogenous protease inhibitors and total protein concentration of the sample. Following incubation at 25°C for 60 min, the reaction is brought to 1.0 mg/ml soybean trypsin inhibitor (SBTI) and 1.0 mM DFP or PMSF to inhibit the trypsin. Renin substrate is then added, and the renin concentration is determined as before. These conditions (time, temperature) were developed for plasma. Tissue inactive renin is activated in a similar procedure at 25°C for 30 min. As a positive control in these experiments, we use human amniotic fluid, which contains high levels of inactive renin.

Other proteases have also been used to activate pro-renin. Treatment with pepsin (156) at pH 4.5 will lead to activation with little or no further degradation of the renin molecule. Kallikrein (121,224) (pancreatic, urinary, and plasma) will activate prorenin only after prior exposure to pH 3.3. The lysosomal proteases cathepsin D, H, and B have also been shown to activate inactive renin (140). Because cathepsin B has been implicated in the intracellular processing of proinsulin to insulin and proalbumin to albumin, it has been speculated that this protease might play a role in the intracellular processing of prorenin in the kidney.

Acid activation. Dialysis of a sample containing inactive renin to pH 3.3, followed by dialysis back to 7.4, leads to irreversible activation (117,118). However, if the acidic sample is immediately titrated to 7.4 without dialysis, the activation is reversible within 2 hr. It has been suggested that the activation occurs in two stages: an acidic-pH-induced conformational change that is reversible, followed by a proteolytic cleavage at neutral pH that is irreversible. Thus, samples are dialyzed for 24 hr at 4°C against 0.05 M glycine, pH 3.3, containing 0.1 N NaCl and 5 mM EDTA. The samples are immediately titrated by addition of $\frac{1}{3}$ vol. 1 M phosphate, pH 8.0, and then assayed for renin activity as before. Multiple time points of generation (maximum time 1 hr) are obtained, and the initial velocity is obtained. If the samples contain low renin activity such that longer generation time is necessary, the acidic sample must be dialyzed to pH 7.4 prior to assay.

Inactive renin concentration is calculated as the difference between total renin concentration (as a result of activation) and active renin as measured prior to activation treatment. The data can also be expressed as percentage increase in renin activity of the sample prior to treatment.

Direct assay for renin.

Many of the problems discussed earlier concerning the renin assay (stability of AI, inexact measurements of inactive renin, etc.) will be eliminated if a direct assay for renin can be developed. However, this necessitates the development of antibodies with very high avidities, as well as purification of reagent amounts of renin to

use as labeled tracer. In the past 15 years, these developments have been the goal of many research laboratories.

One of the first reported RIAs for renin was developed for the mouse (142,148). Certain strains of mice have extremely high renin levels in the SMG, constituting 2 to 5% of total protein. The tissue yields large quantities of highly purified renin that can be used as an antigen as well as for radiolabeling. This has enabled several investigators to successfully develop a direct RIA. However, this RIA was limited to studies in the mouse and has not gained widespread use. Other direct RIAs have been reported for hog and rat renins (108,205). Development of RIA for human renin has been hindered because of lack of sufficient quantities of highly purified antigen. However, one research group obtained a renin-producing tumor that yielded sufficient amounts of pure human renin and led to the development of a direct RIA (98). Unfortunately, the sensitivity of this assay was low, and its use was limited because of the need for a continuous source of radiolabeled pure renin.

Many of the problems associated with establishment of a direct assay for renin may have been resolved using the techniques for monoclonal antibodies. In the development of a polyclonal antisera, the specificity of the antisera is directly related to the purity of antigen. However, because the development of monoclonal antibodies involves cloning the antibody-producing cell, the use of impure antigen may still result in isolation of a pure, highly specific antibody. This antibody can then be used in the development of a radioimmunoreactive assay. In addition, these specific antibodies, when bound to Sepharose, provide specific immunoaffinity columns for purification of the antigen necessary as a standard in the assay.

Recently, a solid-phase ELISA for human renin has been described (110). Microtiter plates are first coated with a monoclonal antirenin antibody by incubation at 37°C for 2 hr. This solution is removed, and the plates are washed extensively and then incubated with PBS containing 1% BSA to block any remaining protein-binding sites. The plates are then incubated sequentially (1 hr at 37°C each) with the renin sample or standards, a rabbit antihuman renin antisera, and alkaline-phosphatase-conjugated goat antirabbit IgG, with extensive washing between steps. Following addition of the substrate, *p*-nitrophenyl phosphate, the plates are again incubated at 37°C for 30 min, at which time the optimal density at 405 nm is determined. The sensitivity of this method has been reported to be in the attomole range for both human renin and renin from other primate plasma. However, the antibodies do not react with renin from the nonprimates, such as rat or mouse.

This assay has been further modified and improved (C. Heusser and K. G. Hofbauer, *personal communication*) by the substitution of phosphatase-conjugated second monoclonal antibody for the two-step method employing rabbit antihuman renin antisera and phosphate-conjugated goat antirabbit IgG. The two monoclonal antibodies that are used recognize different epitopes on the renin molecule and as such do not compete for the same binding site. Using two different monoclonal antibodies theoretically should increase the specificity of the assay. In addition, this assay can be performed using a ^{125}I-labeled second monoclonal antibody substituted for the alkaline-phosphatase-conjugated monoclonal antibody. This has resulted in a slightly more reliable and reproducible RIA (C. Heusser and K. G. Hofbauer, *personal communication*).

Western blot analysis of renin.

Antibodies can be used to determine the molecular size of renin using a technique known as "Western" blotting (210) (Table 3). An impure renin sample is analyzed by SDS–PAGE (131) to separate the proteins by molecular weight. The protein is then electrophoretically transferred from the gel to a nitrocellulose sheet. The sheets are incubated in 20-mM Tris-HCl (pH 7.4), 0.15 M NaCl (TBS), containing 3% gelatin to block the remaining protein-binding sites, and then reacted sequentially with a renin-specific rabbit antisera diluted in PBS plus 1% gelatin, followed by a second antibody (goat antirabbit IgG) that is conjugated with horseradish peroxidase. The blot is then developed by the addition of peroxidase substrate (4-chloronaphthol plus H_2O_2). Alternatively, the second antibody can be labeled with ^{125}I and the blot analyzed by autoradiography.

Unfortunately, the Western technique is not at the present time very sensitive, requiring renin activities of approximately 2,000 to 3,000 ng AI per hour per sample for detection. This technique has been used successfully in characterization of the renins in the SMG of immature and adult mice (122) and in the subcellular fractions of SMG (182). In addition, this technique has been used to analyze the forms of renin secreted from SMG; moreover, it has been used to compare the molecular forms of SMG and kidney renin (R. E. Pratt, T. P. Roth, and V. J. Dzau, *unpublished data*). In order to study lower quantities of renin, e.g., renin secreted into culture medium from minced kidney, it is first necessary to perform a partial purification and concentration of the renin. This involves ammonium sulfate precipitation, followed by affinity chromatography using pepstatin-Sepharose or antibody-Sepharose. This technique has also been employed recently in characterization of partially purified inactive renin from rat kidney (205).

Angiotensinogen

There are two assays for angiotensinogen currently in use. The first assay involves exhaustive digestion of the substrate with excess renin, followed by quantification of the released AI (60,67,107). The second assay is a direct RIA for angiotensin (19).

The exhaustion assay, originally described for plasma angiotensinogen, can be used to determine substrate levels in cultured cells or tissue as well as culture medium. Briefly, plasma or sample (50 μl) is mixed with 50 mM NaAc (pH 5.4) containing the protease inhibitors EDTA (15 mM), NaTT (15 mM), PMSF (0.3 mM), dimercaprol (1.6 mM), and 8-hydroxyquinoline (0.6 mM) to give a final volume of 600 μl. Partially purified renin is added and the reaction incubated at 37°C. At various times (30 min to 3 hr), aliquots are removed, diluted with two volumes of water, and boiled for 2 min, and 20- to 100-μl aliquots are assayed for AI. Incubation up to 3 hr is performed to assure complete digestion of the angiotensinogen. As with the renin assay, it is important to document that the AI released is stable during the procedure. The result is expressed as ng AI equivalent/hr/unit volume or mg protein. Alternatively, an estimation of concentration of angiotensinogen based on AI generated can be made assuming that 1 mole of AI represents 1 molecule of angiotensinogen.

ACE

The enzymatic activity of ACE is based on the action of ACE on the tripeptide benzoyl-Gly-Gly-Gly (Hip-Gly-Gly) or benzoyl-Gly-His-Leu (Hip-His-Leu). The most widely used assay is a radiometric assay using ^{3}H-Hip-Gly-Gly as substrate (41). Converting enzyme cleaves this, forming ^{3}H-hippuric acid plus the dipeptide Gly-Gly. Following acidification, the ^{3}H-hippuric acid is extracted into ethylacetate and quantitated by liquid scintillation spectroscopy (under these conditions the substrate remains in the aqueous phase and is not extracted in the ethylacetate). Variations of this assay have been proposed. The released hippuric acid can be quantified spectrophotometrically after extraction by ethylacetate, evaporated to dryness, and solubilization of the hippuric acid in aqueous solution (42). A more sensitive assay is to measure the released dipeptide fluorometrically (85,193). Serum (1–10 μl) is added to 490 μl of 0.4-M sodium borate (pH 8.3), 0.9 M NaCl, containing 5 mM Hip-His-Leu, and incubated for 15 min at 37°C. Following addition of 1.2 ml of 0.34 M NaOH to stop the reaction, o-phthaldialdehyde is added (100 μl, 20 mg/nl, in methanol). After a 10-min reaction, the sample is acidified with 200 μl 3-N HCl and centrifuged at 800 g for 5 min, and the fluorescence of the supernatant is measured (365 nm excitation/495 emission). Care must be exercised in this assay, because the dipeptide, His-Leu, might not be stable because of dipeptidases present in serum. However, choice of the buffer (borate–sodium chloride) was made specifically to inhibit this enzyme.

Recently, another very sensitive assay for ACE based on the cleavage of an enkephalin-containing octapeptide (Tyr-Gly-Gly-Phe-Met-Arg-Gly-Leu, YGGFMRGL) was reported (165). ACE cleaves at the carboxy side of Arg-6, releasing the dipeptide Gly-Leu. The products are derivatized and separated by HPLC and quantitated by UV absorption. Smaller peptides Tyr^1-Arg^6 and Tyr^1-Met^5 can also be used for substrate. This new technique has not yet been fully explored. However, it is claimed to be a very successful and sensitive procedure.

In addition to the foregoing assays using synthetic substrates, ACE can also be assayed using its natural substrate, AI. The product AII is separated from AI by reverse-phase HPLC and quantitated either by UV absorption (130) or by the RIA described earlier. Care must be taken, however, to assure that the AII is stable and that the AII is being digested only by ACE, because there are many other plasma and tissue proteases that will cleave these two peptides.

Angiotensin Receptors

The sample (cells or isolated membranes) to be assayed (3,4,97,155,200) is incubated with ^{125}I-AII (10–20 pM) and increasing amounts of AII (0.01–1,000 nM) in sodium phosphate (pH 2.4) containing 120 mM NaCl, 5 mM EDTA, 5 mM MgCl$_2$, 10 mM glucose, and 2% BSA at 22°C for 30 to 90 min. Following this, bound AII is separated from free AII by dilution of the sample with ice-cold phosphate buffer, followed by rapid filtration through glass-fiber filters. The filters are then counted to determine the quantity of bound AII.

An alternative method for separation of free and bound AII is by centrifugation. After incubation, the reaction is layered on dibutyl phthalate oil and centrifuged in a microcentrifuge (15,000 rpm), which performs the separation within 15 sec. The tube is then cut, and the cell pellet is counted for bound AII. The data are analyzed by Scatchard plots or by computer program to determine the number of binding sites as well as the affinity of binding.

Molecular Biological Techniques

In the last 5 years, the molecular genetics of renin has become an area of great interest. It is beyond the scope of this chapter to review the molecular biological techniques, which are discussed in detail in another chapter. In this section we shall briefly discuss the advances that have been obtained using these procedures.

cDNA Cloning

Using established techniques (119,179,189), poly(A)-mRNA was isolated from mouse SMG and used as a template for cDNA synthesis. The cDNA was made double-stranded, inserted into pBR322 (pst site), and introduced into *E. coli*. The transformed colonies of *E. coli* were then screened for the presence of renin cDNA. The screening rationale was based on the fact that renin is among a few proteins that are abundant in the male gland but not in the female gland. Thus, the transformed bacterial colonies were grown on bacterial plates, transferred to nitrocellulose sheets, lysed, and exposed to labeled cDNA transcribed from mRNA from male or female glands. Those colonies that contained DNA that would hybridize to cDNA transcribed from the male-gland mRNA but not that from the female gland would contain cDNA to the "male-specific" mRNA. These colonies were then further screened for the presence of renin cDNA by a technique called hybrid selection of mRNA. The plasmid containing the male-specific cDNA was bound to nitrocellulose and incubated with total RNA from the SMG of male mice. The RNA that was specifically bound to the cDNA was eluted and translated in a cell-free system, and the translation products were analyzed for the presence of preprorenin by SDS–PAGE and fluorography. Only the clones that contained the renin cDNA would have specifically bound the renin mRNA.

Mouse renin cDNA has been sequenced (173). It was also utilized to isolate mouse as well as human renin genes (109,159,173). In addition, it was employed as a probe to detect the presence and regulation of renin mRNA in different tissues (58,79,179) using the Northern-blot hybridization method (Table 3). In the following discussion, the numbering system for the human renin mRNA and gene is used (109).

TABLE 3. *Solid-phase analysis of renin and renin mRNA*

Renin mRNA: Northern-blot analysis	Renin: Western-blot analysis
1 RNA isolation	1 Protein isolation
2 Size separation by agarose-gel electrophoresis	2 Size separation by NaDod SO$_4$/polyacrylamide-gel electrophoresis
3 Capillary blotting of RNA from agarose to nitrocellulose	3 Electroblotting of protein from acrylamide gel to nitrocellulose
4 Hybrid formation between ^{32}P-labeled cDNA probe and bound renin mRNA	4 Antigen-antibody complex between renin antibody and bound renin; second antibody (horseradish peroxidase conjugated or ^{125}I labeled) specific for first antibody
5 Detection by autoradiography	5 Detection by colorimetry or autoradiography

mRNA Structure

Sequencing of the cloned DNA complementary to renin mRNA yielded the primary sequence of renin (106,109,151). As with many mRNAs for secretory proteins, human renin mRNA codes for a protein with a pre or signal peptide approximately 23 amino acids in length that contains the characteristic hydrophobic leucine-rich region. Because the cleavage site between the pre and pro is not known, the length of the pre region can be determined only by comparison to other signal peptides. Removal of the pro sequence probably occurs at position lysine(−2)/lysine(−1), because this sequence coincides with the mature mouse renin. However, there are other dibasic residues, (−35/−34), (−30/−29), where cleavage could occur, suggesting alternative processing sites. Mouse SMG renin is nonglycosylated, whereas mouse and human kidney renins are glycoproteins. Consistent with this fact, human renin contains two presumptive N-glycosylation sites at Asn-Thr-Thr (position 5–7) and Asn-Gly-Thr (position 75–77). Similar sites are found in mouse kidney renin but are not present in mouse SMG renin.

Gene Structure

The mouse gene is 10 kilobases long and contains 8 introns and 9 exons (106,109,151). The human renin gene spans approximately 12 kilobases and is interrupted by nine introns (Fig. 4). The presumptive promotor element, TATAAA, termed a Hogness box, is located 73 bases 5′ to the start of translation. Interestingly, a second Hogness box was found in the first intron, 110 bases 5′ to the start of exon 2 (109). If this promoter was utilized, a mRNA would be transcribed that would encode only prorenin, not preprorenin, because the pre region is located in exon 1. This foreshortened renin might be a nonsecreted protein. Because extrarenal renin (other than SMG renin) does not appear to be secreted, this alternative promoter might be functional in these tissues.

As mentioned, the sequence of the human renin gene showed extensive homology with the mouse renin sequence and the sequences of the other acid proteases (Fig. 2). However, one novel sequence was found in human renin that was absent from mouse SMG renin and the other acid proteases. The human renin gene contains an extra exon (#6 or 5A) that encodes three amino acids (Asp-165, Ser-166, Glu-167). The significance of these extra amino acids is at this time unclear (106,151).

Renin mRNA Determination

The technique for quantitation of renin mRNA (Table 3) is based on hybridization of a radiolabeled probe, usually nick-translated cDNA, with the renin mRNA, immobilized on nitrocellulose. The most stringent analysis involves denaturation of the RNA with methyl mercury, formaldehyde, or glyoxal (209), followed by size separation of the RNA on agarose gels. The RNA is then transferred either electrophoretically or by capillary action to nitrocellulose, and the renin mRNA is detected by hybridization with [35]P-labeled cDNA, followed by autoradiography. This technique is termed Northern-blot analysis.

A simpler method is to apply the RNA directly to the nitrocellulose sheets without prior separation on agarose gels. This procedure, termed dot-blot analysis, while being less time-consuming, is not as stringent as Northern blot. Size separation of the RNA prior to blotting allows one to inspect visually the integrating of the RNA to determine the extent of degradation during isolation. Moreover, Northern-blot analysis will eliminate signals due to hybridization with mRNA fragments and to nonspecific hybridization, which may be a problem using the dot-blot analysis.

Extrarenal Renin

As discussed earlier, renin has been found in many tissues other than the kidney and SMG. Because these tissues contain relatively low levels of activity (10–100-fold lower than kidney), the possibility existed that this activity resulted from nonspecific plasma contamination or specific uptake from the plasma, as opposed to synthesis in these tissues. Definitive proof for the local synthesis of renin in certain cells in culture was provided by pulse-labeling studies, which documented *de novo* synthesis of renin (138). However, the low level of renin in most tissues and cells makes this approach technically difficult. A more sensitive method is to determine the presence or absence of renin mRNA by Northern-blot analysis. Using this approach, the presence of renin mRNA in mouse adrenal glands, testis, heart, and brain has been determined (58,79). In addition, cultured human chorionic cells and vascular endothelial cells both contain renin mRNA. Thus, expression of the renin gene in these extrarenal sites has been documented.

Analysis of Renin Biosynthesis

An understanding of renin biosynthesis has added greatly to our understanding of renin biochemistry and physiology (*vide supra*). Initial experiments were performed on mouse SMG *in vivo* or *in vitro* (182; R. E. Pratt, T. P. Roth, and V. J. Dzau, *unpublished data*) using the technique to be described later. However, these techniques have also been used to study mouse kidney, human kidney and tumors, and various cell types in culture. This technique can be used to investigate the effects of various *in vivo* or *in vitro* perturbations on the biosynthesis and secretion of renin.

Following surgical removal, the glands are minced, washed four times, and preincubated for 15 min at 37°C in methionine-free Dulbecco's modified Eagle medium (DMEM) saturated with 95% O_2/5% CO_2. At this time, the medium is removed, replaced with fresh medium containing ^{35}S-methionine (>1,000 Ci/mmol, 250 µCi/ml, 1.0 ml/gland), and incubated at 37°C. Usually the incubation is performed in 20-ml glass scintillation vials that are flushed with O_2/CO_2 and tightly sealed. At various times, tissue representing one-half pair of glands is separated from medium by centrifugation and is sonicated in 2 ml of PBS (pH 7.4) containing 0.1% Triton X-100 and the following protease inhibitors: 0.1 mM EDTA, 0.1 mM NaTT, 1 mM PMSF, 0.1 mg/ml SBTI, and 0.1 mg/ml aprotinin. The levels of ^{35}S-radiolabeled proteins in medium and tissue homogenate were determined by trichloroacetic acid precipitation. Prior to immunoprecipitation, the medium and tissue were brought to 0.01% SDS and 1.0% Triton X-100. Renin-specific antiserum or control serum is added, and the reaction is incubated overnight at 4°C. The immune complex is isolated by absorption to protein-A-Sepharose and analyzed by SDS-PAGE under reducing conditions with 2-mercaptoethanol, followed by fluorography using Enhance. Reduction with 2-mercaptoethanol allows separation of one-chain renin (M_r 37 kd) from two-chain renin in SDS-PAGE, because the latter will migrate as the heavy chain (M_r 32 kd).

Procedures similar to the foregoing techniques have also been used to study the synthesis and secretion of angiotensinogen from the liver as well as hepatocytes and hepatoma cells (21,60,67,107).

PHARMACOLOGIC INTERVENTION

Specific inhibition of the RAS is an important strategy in the treatment of hypertension and CHF. The renin-angiotensin cascade offers a series of sites for selective inhibition (Table 4).

Angiotensin Antagonists

The angiotensin receptor is a primary site that can be pharmacologically inhibited by analogues of AII (14,81,104,113). The octapeptide analogues [(Sar^{1}Ala^9)-AII, (Sar^1-Ile^8)AII, (Sar^{1}Thr^8)AII, etc.] act as antagonists by competing with angiotensin at its receptor site in vascular smooth muscle, the adrenal cortex, and the nervous system. These peptide analogues produce a depressor response in humans during sodium depletion comparable to those induced by renin or ACE inhibition. Interestingly, in sodium-replete humans, angiotensin analogues produce a pressor response. Under these conditions, vascular angiotensin receptors are up-regu-

TABLE 4. *Pharmacological interruption of the RAS*

Site of inhibition	Pharmacological agent
Renin release	1. β-adrenergic blockers (e.g., propranolol) 2. α-adrenergic agonist (e.g., clonidine)
Renin-substrate interaction	1. Peptide analogues of angiotensinogen 2. Pepstatin 3. Antirenin antibody
Angiotensin-converting enzyme	1. Peptide analogues of AI (e.g., teprotide)
AII receptor	1. Peptide analogues of AII (e.g., saralasin)

lated, and these analogues behave as weak agonists. This partial agonist response is particularly evident with high doses of these analogues (115,207). Infusion of (Sar^{1}Ala^8)AII lowered blood pressure in AII-induced hypertension, experimental renovascular hypertension (during the renin-dependent phase), and spontaneous hypertension in rats. (Sar^{1}Ala^8)AII produced a decrease in blood pressure in patients with essential, renovascular, or renal hypertension. The magnitude of blood pressure decline correlated with pretreatment PRA. Unfortunately, no orally active angiotensin antagonist has been developed to date for investigative or clinical use.

Renin Inhibition

Renin is the first and rate-limiting step in plasma angiotensin production. This enzyme is specific for its substrate, angiotensinogen. To date, no other substrate has been reported. Therefore, renin provides an ideal target for the blockade of this system. The most promising inhibitors of renin include four classes of compounds (Table 5A).

Specific blockade of renin using antibodies raised against purified renin is now possible. Antirenin antisera, purified IgG, and Fab have been administered to conscious animals. Complete renin inhibition was accompanied by a hypotensive response in the sodium-deplete but not sodium-replete animals. Antirenin antibodies normalized the blood pressure of animals with acute renovascular hypertension (57,63). Recently, monoclonal antibodies to dog and human renal renin have been obtained (64,220). The antihuman antibodies selectively inhibited human and monkey renin activities. Monoclonal antirenin antibodies lowered blood pressure in sodium-deplete monkeys as well as those with renin-dependent hypertension. The overall blood pressure responses to polyclonal or monoclonal antibodies were comparable to those of ACE inhibitors (47,57,220). This immunological approach provides a highly specific method of renin blockade *in vivo,* but its therapeutic potential is limited by the potential immunogenicity of these foreign proteins and by the lack of activity when orally administered.

Chemical renin inhibitors include peptides from the pro segment of prorenin, general inhibitors of aspartyl proteinases, or angiotensinogen analogues: (a) Evin et al. (74) synthesized peptide 11–19 of mouse SMG prorenin and demonstrated its inhibitory activity on the enzyme. More recently, human pro-segment peptide has also been synthesized. This peptide has a relatively weak inhibitory activity (IC$_{50}$ 10^{-4} M) on human plasma renin (73). However, one may anticipate that further manipulation of the amino acid sequences of these peptides may result in the development of more potent inhibitors of renin in the future. (b) Pepstatin inhibits many aspartyl proteinases. Its application has been limited by its relative insolubility and nonselectivity. The addition of charged amino acids at its carboxy terminus has rendered it more useful (71). (c) The most promising approach in the development of chemical renin inhibitors appears to be the synthesis of angiotensinogen analogues (Table 5B).

Analogues of the minimal octapeptide sequence of angiotensinogen have yielded highly specific competitive inhibitors (101). The first modifications made in the octapeptide sequences were aimed at producing peptides that bind to and are not cleaved by renin. Replacement of leucyl residue (position 10 or 11) with D-stereoisomer resulted in an effective renin inhibitor. Replacement of leucyl residues with phenylalanine yielded an even more potent inhibitor. Addition of a prolyl residue to the amino terminus and a lysyl residue to the carboxy

terminus increased solubility. This renin inhibitory peptide (RIP) has a K_i of 1 μM for human renin (101). Recently, several laboratories have synthesized transition-state analogues of renin substrate, based on the theory that enzymes have a greater binding affinity for the transition state than the ground state of the substrate. These consist of two classes of compounds: (a) those that contain a statine substitution for residues at the scissile bond (e.g., SCRIP) (14) and (b) those that incorporate transition-state isotere into the octapeptide (202,203). In place of the scissile Leu-Leu peptide bond, the secondary amine —CH$_2$—NH— (i.e., Leu^{R}Leu) or the hydroxyethylene moiety —CH(OH)—CH$_2$— (i.e., Leu^{OH}Leu) was incorporated (Table 5B). These transition-state analogues are highly potent inhibitors (IC$_{50}$ 10^{-9} to 10^{-10} M) with increased *in vivo* stability. However, all these compounds are limited by the relatively short duration of action and susceptibility to digestive enzymes.

In vivo experimental studies employing different renin inhibitors have yielded similar overall results (14,202–204,211). All renin inhibitors effectively inhibited PRAs *in vivo* and lowered blood pressure in sodium-deplete animals as well as in those with renin-dependent hypertension. The acute depressor responses were comparable to those of teprotide or captopril in all cases. However, an additional interesting observation was made with the statine-containing renin inhibitor SCRIP (14). Although a dose-dependent decrease in blood pressure was observed with SCRIP, its effects on blood pressure and PRA appeared to be dissociated. At lower infusion rates (up to 20 μg/kg/min), the slope for inhibition of PRA was steeper than that for the decline in blood pressure. At doses greater than 20 μg/kg/min, when PRA was completely suppressed, blood pressure continued to fall in a dose-dependent fashion, independent of PRA.

To date, only two clinical trials with renin inhibitors have been reported (218,227). Infusion of H-142 (1 and 2.5 mg/kg/hr) reduced diastolic blood pressure in sodium-deplete normal human subjects, accompanied by large reductions in circulating AI and AII (227). In a separate study, infusion of RIP in doses effective in monkeys (0.2 mg/kg/min) had little effect in sodium-deplete or sodium-replete humans. In higher doses (1

TABLE 5B. *Substrate analogues as renin inhibitors*

Compound	Amino acid sequence[a]	IC$_{50}$ (M)[b]
Minimal substrate	His-Pro-Phe-His-Leu-Leu- Val-Tyr (Val-Ile-His)	
RIP	Pro-His-Pro-Phe-His-Phe-Phe- Val-Tyr-Lys	7 × 10^{-6}
H-77	D His-Pro-Phe-His-Leu^{R}Leu- Val-Tyr	1 × 10^{-6}
H-142	Pro-His-Pro-Phe-His-Leu^{R}Val- Ile-His	1 × 10^{-8}
H-261	His-Pro-Phe-His-Leu^{OH}Val-Ile-His	6.9 × 10^{-10}
SCRIP	His-Pro-Phe-His----Sta----Ile-His	2 × 10^{-9}

[a] R = —CH$_2$—NH—; OH = —CH(OH)—CH$_2$—.
[b] Human renin.

mg/kg/min), RIP resulted in large reductions of systolic and diastolic blood pressure in the supine position and induced syncope when the subject was tilted upright. This response was significantly greater than that seen with captopril in the same subject. Similar responses were also seen in sodium-replete subjects and in a patient with low-renin hypertension (218).

Although the overall acute blood pressure response to renin inhibitors appeared to be comparable to that for ACE inhibitors, the responses to RIP in humans and SCRIP in animals raise the possibility that the mechanisms of action of renin and ACE inhibitors may differ to some extent. Are renin inhibitors acting at another site(s) of renin action other than plasma, e.g., brain, vascular, or intracardiac renin? Is the additional blood pressure response to some of the renin inhibitors due to nonrenin effects? It should be pointed out that all studies with renin inhibitors to date employed short-term administration of these compounds. Comparison of chronic effects of renin and ACE inhibitors will provide further information on the differences and similarities of these compounds and their relative therapeutic potentials in hypertension.

ACE Inhibition

Inhibition of ACE (peptidyl dipeptidase) was first made possible by the discovery of the nonapeptide inhibitor (teprotide) in the snake venom of *Bothrops jararaca* (51). Subsequently, an orally active ACE inhibitor, D-3-mercapto-2-methylpropanoyl-L-proline (captopril), was synthesized based on a hypothetical model of ACE extrapolated from the known properties of the active site of carboxypeptidase A (51). Captopril has been approved for clinical use. Recently, a series of substituted N-carboxymethyl dipeptides has been synthesized (176). One of these compounds, enalapril (MK-421) has been employed for animal and clinical studies. Several other ACE inhibitors are also under active study.

Mechanism of Action of Converting Enzyme Inhibitors

Inhibition of ACE (51,190) blocks the conversion of AI to AII, both *in vivo* and *in vitro* (51). As a consequence, plasma AII and aldosterone concentrations are suppressed by ACE inhibitors, both in animals and in humans. This is probably the primary mechanism by which ACE inhibitors exert their effect. However, ACE inhibitors may also have actions that are mediated outside the RAS. One likely such action is to increase the concentration of circulating bradykinin, a potent vasodilator (34). Indeed, ACE is also a kininase that cleaves bradykinin to inactive products, and both teprotide and captopril have been shown to potentiate vasodepressor responses to infused bradykinin in the rat. However, in human plasma, kinin levels have shown variable responses to teprotide and captopril. The action of converting enzyme inhibitor may also be mediated, in part, by PG activation. Captopril has been shown to increase plasma concentrations of the metabolites PGE_2 and PGF_2 in patients with hypertension. The increase in the PGE_2 metabolite correlated with the reduction in arterial pressure in response to captopril. Furthermore, indomethacin attenuates the fall in diastolic pressure produced by captopril (154,201). Enalapril, a nonsulfhydryl ACE inhibitor, appears not to have an effect on plasma PG levels (95).

An additional action of AII is facilitation of the release of norepinephrine and an increase in reuptake at nerve endings (126,145). When administered directly into the CNS, AII increases arterial pressure and plasma catecholamine levels (184). Conversely, interference with AII production appears to interfere with sympathetic reflexes. Therefore, inhibition of AII production also affects the sympathetic nervous system. Reflex tachycardia is not observed with converting-enzyme-inhibitor-induced hypotension, and plasma catecholamine levels remain unchanged during converting enzyme inhibitor administration to dogs subjected to hemorrhage or to patients with CHF. Captopril elicits selective prejunctional and postjunctional inhibitory effects on vascular responses to sympathetic nerve stimulation (190). It is therefore possible that part of the non-angiotensin-mediated action of captopril is through inhibition of sympathetic activity. This unique dual inhibitory effect on cardiovascular compensatory mechanisms (the RAS and the sympathetic nervous system) may account for the sustained effectiveness of ACE inhibition in long-term treatment of hypertension and CHF.

ACE Inhibitors in Clinical Medicine

In patients with hypertension, ACE inhibitors reduce systemic vascular resistance and pulmonary capillary wedge pressure, while the heart remains largely unchanged and cardiac output tends to rise; these changes are sustained with long-term therapy. Captopril and enalapril have been reported to be efficacious in the treatment of various forms of hypertension. In most human subjects, as in experimental animals, the acute response to ACE inhibitors correlated with pretreatment PRA. The correlation between the long-term response to treatment and PRA is less clear. Indeed, an antihypertensive response has been reported even in patients with low renin activity. Some authors have reported an increased responsiveness of arterial pressures to ACE inhibitors over several days, whereas others have found a progressive loss of response. Laragh and associates reported a triphasic pressure response during short-term therapy in some patients: an initial drop in blood pressure, followed by a plateau phase or gradual increase, and then a further reduction (132).

Hypertension.

Clinical trials have demonstrated that captopril results in significant decreases in arterial pressure in many patients with essential hypertension. In patients with mild to moderate essential hypertension, ACE inhibitors alone produced a 20% reduction in supine diastolic pressure. Generally, about 70% of patients were adequately controlled on ACE inhibitors alone, compared with 60% of patients treated only with hydrochlorothiazide (75,212). Addition of a diuretic to captopril resulted in control of arterial pressure in over 95% of hypertensive patients (75,111,212). ACE inhibitors and propranolol were similar in effectiveness as antihypertensive agents, and the addition of propranolol to captopril resulted in an additive effect.

Captopril and enalapril has been employed successfully in the management of several different forms of treatment-resistant hypertension. Therapy with captopril or enalapril alone has resulted in responses similar to those produced by standard triple-drug therapy (diuretic, propranolol, and hydralazine) in many refractory hypertensive patients (36). However, when used alone, the doses of ACE inhibitors needed to control treatment-resistant hypertension are often high. Lower doses can be used when it is given in combination with a diuretic or with sodium restriction. Moreover, a beta-adrenergic antagonist may normalize blood pressure in patients in whom the combination of ACE inhibitors and a diuretic has failed.

The salutary effect of captopril on arterial pressure is sustained during long-term administration of the drug. ACE inhibitors increase renal blood flow in experimental animals and humans with hypertension, especially in states of sodium depletion. Their effect on the glomerular filtration rate varies. Hollenberg and Dzau (113) observed that teprotide produced a modest improvement in the glomerular filtration rate in patients with essential hypertension and impaired creatinine clearance. An increase in sodium excretion has been reported with both agents, an effect that may be related to decreased AII and aldosterone levels. These renal responses have also been observed in patients treated with captopril and may account in part for the long-term effectiveness of this drug in the treatment of hypertension.

ACE inhibition is particularly effective in controlling arterial pressure in patients with renovascular hypertension and elevated PRA (24,35,36). The blood pressure response correlates closely with the base-line PRA in these patients. The dose required to control pressure is often small. In our experience, long-term treatment with ACE inhibitors resulted in good control of hypertensives with renovascular hypertension. However, patients with severe bilateral or unilateral renal arterial stenosis and impaired renal function prior to captopril or enalapril administration showed acute deterioration of renal func-

tion with the drug (40,116,221). The relative roles of ACE inhibition and of surgery in the treatment of renovascular hypertension require further clarification.

CHF.

Captopril and enalapril appear to be effective dilators of the arteriolar and venous beds. Acutely, they lowered left ventricular filling pressure and elevated cardiac output, stroke volume, and stroke work (2,32,134,144). In patients with severe heart failure, the average increases in cardiac output are 10 to 25%, whereas reductions in left ventricular filling pressure of 30 to 50%, systemic and pulmonary vascular resistance of 30 to 40%, and mean arterial pressure of 20 to 25% have been reported. Heart rate shows little change.

The magnitudes of acute decline in systemic vascular resistance and blood pressure with converting enzyme inhibitor appear to depend on the pretreatment PRA. However, even patients with heart failure who have normal or low PRA often respond to ACE inhibition, and the beneficial hemodynamic effect is sustained during long-term therapy (32,45).

There has been considerable debate on the renal effects of captopril and enalapril therapy in patients with heart failure. Pierpont et al. (180) reported increases in blood urea nitrogen and creatinine in 3 of 9 patients after 3 days of captopril therapy. Faxon et al. (77) saw an improvement in renal plasma flow without affecting the glomerular filtration rate after a single dose of captopril, whereas Mujais et al. (158) reported that captopril reduced both renal plasma flow and glomerular filtration rate. In contrast, studies with prolonged captopril administration have shown sustained improvement in both renal plasma flow and glomerular filtration rate (53,158).

The apparent discrepancies may have been due to differences in study design. For example, in studies of its short-term effects, a single captopril dose was not titrated to blood pressure or the hemodynamic response; furthermore, diuretic agents were withheld in these studies. On the other hand, in studies in which captopril doses were titrated and the glomerular filtration rate and renal plasma flow were studied during chronic therapy, sustained improvements in renal plasma flow and glomerular filtration rate were reported (55,61,158). As shown by the work of Pierpont et al. (180), the initial deterioration of renal function with acute captopril administration may be related to an excessive decrease in renal perfusion pressure, complicated by blockade of angiotensin-mediated autoregulation of glomerular filtration rate. The mean blood pressure of these patients with severe CHF is often very near the autoregulatory break. Thus, a further fall in blood pressure can result in a substantial decrease in renal plasma flow and glomerular filtration rate.

Chronic therapy with dosage adjustments, as done in our studies, can avoid excessive and precipitous reduction in renal pressure and optimize renal hemodynamic changes. Indeed, in our study, effective renal plasma flow and glomerular filtration rate have been found to be increased 5 to 7 days after the start of therapy (55,61). Blood urea nitrogen and serum creatinine decline, and these favorable changes are sustained with continued therapy. We have also observed that captopril enhances the diuretic effect of furosemide (61). Indeed, in some patients with severe heart failure, attempts at initiating diuresis to reverse pulmonary and systemic edema result in progressive azotemia, which is reversed after initiation of captopril therapy, despite prompt diuresis with clearance of edema and reduction of body weight. In addition, captopril plus furosemide corrected hyponatremia in these patients (61). Thus, a major renal action of ACE inhibitors may be to enhance the effectiveness of furosemide or other diuretics (Fig. 8). Hyperkalemia may develop in patients on long-term captopril therapy, especially if overall KCl supplements are continued. This may be due to the effect of captopril-induced deficiency of aldosterone. The salutary effect of captopril as vasodilator therapy in CHF has been documented by the controlled prospective multicenter trial (160). Patients treated with captopril showed objective and subjective improvement that was sustained over time.

In summary, ACE inhibitors appear to be effective vasodilators for treatment of patients with advanced CHF. They are especially useful in patients in whom other vasodilators have failed, because tolerance to these

drugs may be due to secondary activation of the RAS. Captopril dilates both resistance and capacitance vessels, and this dilation leads to a reduction in left ventricular filling pressure and improved cardiac performance. These effects appear to be sustained with continued administration of the drug. Particularly striking is the prolonged improvement in renal function and in clinical well-being.

FUTURE DIRECTIONS IN RENIN-ANGIOTENSIN RESEARCH

Structure and Drug Design

The RAS has become a major therapeutic target in cardiovascular pharmacology. It has been possible to develop inhibitors to every component of the RAS. At present, with the exception of ACE inhibitors, antagonists of renin and angiotensin are not orally active. In addition, the specificity of action of these inhibitors continues to be a subject of concern. The future in drug design lies in a better understanding of the structures of the various components. Isolation of all these components has been accomplished. Determination of three-dimensional structures by X-ray crystallography or computer graphics should aid in the development of specific inhibitors.

Tissue RAS

An understanding of the regulation and role of the tissue RAS is an important area of current and future research. The availability of a number of molecular probes makes investigation in this area feasible. What controls the expression of renin and angiotensinogen genes in various tissues? What is the role of the local RAS? How do pharmacological inhibitors of this system influence the tissue renin-angiotensin cascade and local function? These questions are important for understanding of the physiology of the RAS and the influence of pharmacological inhibitors.

Genetic Control and DNA Polymorphism in Hypertension

Although human essential hypertension has a multifactorial pathogenesis, aberrant renin-angiotensin expression may play a role in elevating blood pressure. Structural mutations in or near human renin genes could result in aberrant expression of human renin and may correlate with hypertension. Future research should investigate this possibility by undertaking close analysis of the structure of the renin gene in hypertensives relative to that found in normotensives. Restriction-fragment length polymorphisms may provide markers for the inheritance of an aberrantly expressed gene. Genetic anal-

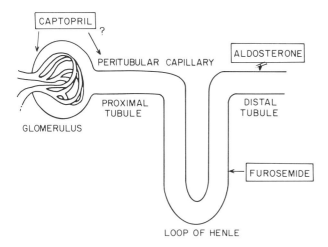

FIG. 8. Effect of converting enzyme inhibition (CEI) (captopril) on renal function: CEI increases glomerular filtration rate and renal plasma flow, which probably increases peritubular capillary hydraulic pressure and reduces proximal tubular sodium reabsorption. CEI also increases delivery of furosemide to its locus of action (*ascending loop*) by increasing renal plasma flow. In addition, plasma aldosterone levels decreases with CEI therapy. These actions of CEI enhance the renal effects of furosemide and other diuretics.

ysis, testing the linkage between specific renin haplotypes in hypertension, will be an exciting area of research.

ACKNOWLEDGMENTS

We wish to acknowledge the assistance of Dr. Julie Ingelfinger and Mr. Thomas Brody in the preparation of this manuscript. We also wish to thank Ms. Sarah Curwood and Ms. A. Ines Nolasco for their excellent secretarial assistance. This work was partly supported by a grant from the NIH (HL-19259) and by a gift from the R. J. Reynolds industry.

REFERENCES

1. Acker, G. M., Galen, F. X., Devaux, C., Foote, S., Papernik, E., Pesty, A., Menard, J., and Corvol, P. (1982): Human chorionic cells in primary culture: A model for renin biosynthesis. *J. Clin. Endocrinol. Metab.*, 55:902–909.
2. Adler, R., Cahatterjee, K., Ports, T., Brundage, B., Hirmatzu, B., and Parmsley, W. (1980): Immediate and sustained hemodynamic and clinical improvement in chronic heart failure by an oral angiotensin-converting enzyme inhibitor. *Circulation*, 61:931–937.
3. Aguilera, G., and Catt, K. (1981): Regulation of vascular angiotensin II receptors in the rat during altered sodium intake. *Circ. Res.*, 49:751–758.
4. Aquilera, G., Schirar, A., Baukal, A., and Catt, K. J. (1980): Angiotensin II receptors. Properties and regulation in adrenal glomerulosa cells. *Circ. Res. [Suppl. I]*, 46:118–127.
5. Akahane, K., Umeyama, H., Nakagawa, S., Moriguchi, I., Hirose, S., Iizuka, K., and Murakami, K. (1985): Three-dimensional structure of human renin. *Hypertension*, 4:3–12.
6. Ayers, C. R., Darracott, E., Yancey, M. R., Bing, K. T., Johnson, C. C. J., and Morton, C. (1974): Effect of 1-sarcosine-8-alanine angiotensin II in dog acute renovascular hypertension. *Circ. Res. [Suppl. I]*, 34/35:27–34.
7. Ayers, C. R., Katholi, R. E., Vaughan, E. D., Carey, R. M., Kimbrough, H. M., Yancey, M. R., and Morton, C. L. (1977): Intrarenal renin angiotensin-sodium interdependent mechanism controlling post clamp renal artery pressure and renin release in the conscious dog with chronic one-kidney Goldblatt hypertension. *Circ. Res.*, 40:238–242.
8. Barger, A. C. (1979): The Goldblatt memorial lecture. Part I: Experimental renovascular hypertension. *Hypertension*, 1:447–455.
9. Baumbach, L., and Leyssacc, P. P. (1977): Studies on the mechanism of renin release from isolated superfused rat glomeruli: Effects of calcium, calcium ionophore and lanthanum. *J. Physiol. (Lond.)*, 273:745–764.
10. Bean, B. L., Brown, J. J., Casals-Stenzel, J., Frazier, R., Lever, A. F., Millar, J. A., Morton, J. J., Petch, B., Riegger, A. J. G., Robertson, J. I. S., and Tree, M. (1979): The relation of arterial pressure and plasma angiotensin II concentration: A change produced by prolonged infusion of angiotensin II in the conscious dog. *Circ. Res.*, 44:452–458.
11. Beckerhoff, R., Uhlschmid, G., Furrer, J., Nussberger, J., Schmied, U., Vetter, W., and Siegenthaler, W. (1975): In vivo effects of angiotensin antagonists on plasma aldosterone in the dog. *Eur. J. Pharmacol.*, 34:363–367.
12. Bennett, J. P., and Snyder, S. H. (1976): Angiotensin II binding to mammalian brain membranes. *J. Biol. Chem.*, 251:7423.
13. Berl, T., Henrich, W. L., Erickson, A. L., and Schrier, R. W. (1979): Prostaglandins in the beta-adrenergic and baroreceptor-mediated secretion of renin. *Am. J. Physiol.*, 236:F472–477.
14. Blaine, E. H., Schorn, T. W., and Boger, J. (1984): Statin-containing renin inhibitor. Dissociation of blood pressure lowering and renin inhibition in sodium-deficient dogs. *Hypertension [Suppl. I]*, 6:11–118.
15. Blantz, R. C., Konnen, K. S., and Tucker, B. J. (1976): Angiotensin II effects upon the glomerular microcirculation and ultrafiltration coefficient of the rat. *J. Clin. Invest.*, 57:419–434.
16. Blumberg, A., Denny, S. E., Marshall, G. R., and Needleman, P. (1977): Blood vessel–hormone interactions: Angiotensin, bradykinin and prostaglandins. *Am. J. Physiol.*, 232:H305–H310.
17. Blumberg, A. S., Denny, S., Nishikawa, K., Pure, E., and Needleman, P. (1976): Angiotensin II induced prostaglandin release. *Prostaglandins*, 11:195–197.
18. Blundell, T., Sibanda, B. L., and Pearl, L. (1983): Three-dimensional structure, specificity and catalytic mechanism of renin. *Nature*, 304:273–275.
19. Bouhnik, J., Clauser, E., Gardes, J., Corvol, P., and Menard, J. (1982): Direct radioimmunoassay of rat angiotensinogen and its application to rats in various endocrine states. *Clin. Sci.*, 62:355–360.
20. Bouhnik, J., Clauser, E., Strosberg, D., Frenoy, J. P., Menard, J., and Corvol, P. (1981): Rat angiotensinogen and des (angiotensin I) angiotensinogen: Purification, characterization and partial sequencing. *Biochemistry*, 20:7010–7015.
21. Bouhnik, J., Galen, F. X., Clauser, E., Menard, J., and Corvol, P. (1981): The renin angiotensin system in thyroidectomized rats. *Endocrinology*, 108:647–650.
22. Bouhnik, J., Fehrentz, J. A., Galen, F. X., Seyer, R., Evin, G., Castro, B., Menard, J., and Corvol, P. (1985): Immunologic identification of both plasma and human renal inactive renin as prorenin. *J. Clin. Endocrinol. Metab.*, 60:399–401.
23. Brown, J. J., Davis, D. L., Lever, A. F., and Robertson, J. I. S. (1965): Plasma renin concentration in human heart failure. I: Relationship between renin, sodium, potassium. *Br. Med. J.*, 2:144–148.
24. Brunner, H. R., Gavras, J., Waeber, B., Kershaw, G. R., Turini, G. A., Vokovich, R. A., McKinstry, D. N., and Gavras, I. (1979): Oral angiotensin-converting enzyme inhibitor in long-term treatment of hypertensive patients. *Ann. Intern. Med.*, 90:19–23.
25. Brunner, H. R., Gavras, H., Waeber, B., Textor, S. C., Turini, G. A., and Wauters, J. P. (1980): Clinical use of an orally active converting enzyme inhibitor: Captopril. *Hypertension*, 2:558–566.
26. Brunner, H. R., Laragh, J. M., Baer, L., Newton, M. A., Goodwin, F. T., Krakoff, L. R., Bard, R. H., and Buhler, F. R. (1972): Essential hypertension: Renin and aldosterone, heart attack and stroke. *N. Engl. J. Med.*, 286:441–449.
27. Buggy, J., Fink, G. D., Johnson, A. K., and Brody, M. J. (1977): The effect of anteroventral third ventricle tissue lesions on the development of renal hypertension in rats. *Circ. Res. [Suppl. I]*, 40:110–117.
28. Bumpus, F. M. (1977): Intrarenal effects of angiotensin. In: *Hypertension: Mechanisms, Diagnosis and Management*, edited by J. O. Davis et al., p. 254. HP Publishing, New York.
29. Caldicott, W. J. H., Taub, K. J., Margulies, S. S., and Hollenberg, N. K. (1981): Angiotensin receptors in glomeruli differ from those in renal arterioles. *Kidney Int.*, 19:687–693.
30. Caldwell, P. R. B., Seegal, B. C., Hsu, K. C., Das, M., and Softer, R. L. (1976): Angiotensin converting enzyme: Vascular endothelial localization. *Science*, 191:1050–1051.
31. Capponi, A. M., and Catt, K. J. (1979): Angiotensin II receptors in adrenal cortex and uterus. *J. Biol. Chem.*, 254:5120–5127.
32. Captopril Multicenter Research Group (1985): A cooperative multicenter study of captopril in congestive heart failure: Hemodynamic effects and long-term response. *Am. Heart J.*, 110:439–447.
33. Carlson, W., Karplus, M., and Haber, E. (1985): Construction of a model for the three-dimensional structure of human renal renin. *Hypertension*, 7:13–26.
34. Carretero, O. A., Scicli, A. G., and Mitra, S. R. (1981): Role of kinins in the pharmacologic effects of converting enzyme inhibitors. In: *Angiotensin Converting Enzyme Inhibitors*, edited by Z. P. Horovitz, pp. 105–121. Urban & Schwarzenberg, Baltimore.
35. Case, D. B., Atlas, S. A., Laragh, J. H., Sealey, J. E., Sullivan, D. A., and McKinstry, D. N. (1978): Clinical experience with blockade of the renin-angiotensin-aldosterone system by an oral converting enzyme inhibitor (SQ 14,225, captopril) in hypertensive patients. *Prog. Cardiovasc. Dis.*, 21:195–206.

36. Case, D. B., Atlas, S. A., Sullivan, P. A., and Laragh, J. M. (1981): Acute and chronic treatment of severe and malignant hypertension in the oral angiotensin converting enzyme inhibitor captopril. *Circulation,* 64:765–771.
37. Catanzaro, D. F., Mullins, J. J., and Morris, B. U. (1982): The biosynthetic pathway of renin in mouse submandibular gland. *J. Biol. Chem.,* 258:7364–7368.
38. Churchill, P. C., and Churchill, M. C. (1983): Effects of trifluoperazine on renin secretion of rat kidney slices. *J. Pharmacol. Exp. Ther.,* 224:68–72.
39. Cohen, S., Taylor, J. M., Murakami, K. Michelakis, A. M., and Inagami, T. (1972): Isolation and characterization of renin-like enzymes from mouse submandibular glands. *Biochemistry,* 11: 4286–4293.
40. Curtis, J. J., Luke, R. G., Whelchel, J. D., Dietehlm, A. G., Jones, P., and Dustan, H. P. (1983): Inhibition of angiotensin-converting enzyme in renal transplant recipients with hypertension. *N. Engl. J. Med.,* 308:377–381.
41. Cushman, D. W., and Cheung, H. S. (1969): A simple substrate for assay of dog lung angiotensin converting enzyme. *Fed. Proc.,* 28:799.
42. Cushman, D. W., and Cheung, H. S. (1971): Spectrophotometric assay and properties of the angiotensin converting enzyme of rabbit lung. *Biochem. Pharmacol.,* 20:1637–1648.
43. Cushman, D. W., Cheung, H. S., Sabo, E. F., and Ordetti, M. A. (1977): Design of potent competitive inhibitors of angiotensin-converting enzyme. Carboxylalkanoyl and mercapotoalkanoyl amino acids. *Biochemistry,* 16:5484–5491.
44. Davis, J. O., and Freeman, R. H. (1976): Mechanisms regulating renin release. *Physiol. Rev.,* 56:1–56.
45. Davis, R., Ribner, H. S., Keung, E., Sonnenblick, E., and LeJemiel, T. (1979): Treatment of chronic congestive heart failure with captopril, an oral inhibitor angiotensin-converting enzyme. *N. Engl. J. Med.,* 301:117–121.
46. Deboben, A., Inagami, T., and Ganten, G. (1983): Tissue renin. In: *Hypertension,* ed. 2, edited by J. Genest, O. Kuchel, P. Hamet, and M. Cantin, pp. 194–209. McGraw-Hill, New York.
47. de Claviere, M., Lacour, C., Gayraud, R., Roccon, A., Cazaubon, C., Carlet, C., Pau, B., and Gagnol, J. P. (1984): Effects of a human renin monoclonal antibody on blood pressure and hormonal parameters in conscious monkeys under various sodium conditions. In: *Proceedings of the Tenth Scientific Meeting of the International Society of Hypertension* (abstract 279), p. 139.
48. Deforrest, J. M., Davis, J. O., Freeman, R. H., Seymour, A. A., Rowe, B. P., Williams, G. M., and Davis, T. P. (1980): Effects of indomethacin and meclofenamate on renin release and renal hemodynamic function during chronic sodium depletion in conscious dogs. *Circ. Res.,* 47:99–107.
49. DeRemee, R. A., and Rohrbach, J. (1980): Serum angiotensin converting enzyme activity in evaluating the clinical course of sarcoidosis. *Ann. Intern. Med.,* 92:361–365.
50. Duesterdieck, G., and McElwee, G. (1971): Estimation of angiotensin II concentration in human plasma by radioimmunoassay: Some applications to physiological and clinical states. *Eur. J. Clin. Invest.,* 2:32–38.
51. Dzau, V. J. (1983): Angiotensin converting enzyme inhibition in treatment of congestive heart failure and hypertension: In: *Harrison's Principles of Internal Medicine,* updates IV, edited by K. Isselbacher, R. D. Adams, E. Braunwald, J. B. Martin, R. G. Pedersdorf, and J. D. Wlson, pp. 137–146. McGraw-Hill, New York.
52. Dzau, V. J. (1984): Vascular wall renin-angiotensin pathway in control of the circulation: A hypothesis. *Am. J. Med.,* 77:31–36.
53. Dzau, V. J., Brenner, A., and Emmett, N. L. (1982): Evidence for renin in rat brain. Characterization and differentiation from other renin like enzymes. *Am. J. Physiol.,* 242:E292–E297.
54. Dzau, V. J., Brenner, A., Kapler, J., Churchill, S., and Emmett, N. (1980): Characterization of renin-like enzymes in the rabbit uterus by renin specific antibody. *Circulation,* 62:111–238.
55. Dzau, V. J., Colucci, W. S., Williams, G. H., Curfman, G., Meggs, L., and Hollenberg, N. K. (1980): Sustained effectiveness of converting-enzyme inhibition in patients with severe congestive heart failure. *N. Engl. J. Med.,* 302:1371–1379.
56. Dzau, V. J., Colucci, W. S., Williams, G. H., and Hollenberg,

N. K. (1981): Relation of renin-angiotensin-aldosterone to clinical state in congestive heart failure. *Circulation,* 63:645–651.
57. Dzau, V. J., Devine, D., Mudgett-Hunter, M., Kopelman, R. E., Barger, A. C., and Haber, E. (1983): Antibodies as specific renin inhibitors: Studies with polyclonal and monoclonal antibodies and Fab fragments. *Clin. Exp. Hypert.,* 7/8:1207–1220.
58. Dzau, V. J., Ellison, K., McGowan, D., Gross, K. W., and Ouellette, A. (1984): Hybridization studies with a renin cDNA probe: Evidence for widespread expression of renin in the mouse. *J. Hyper.,* 2:235–237.
59. Dzau, V. J., Gibbons, G., and Levin, D. (1983): Renovascular hypertension. An update on pathophysiology, diagnosis and management. *Am. J. Nephrol.,* 3:172–184.
60. Dzau, V. J., and Hermann, H. C. (1982): Hormonal regulation of angiotensinogen synthesis. *Life Sci.,* 30:577–584.
61. Dzau, V. J., and Hollenberg, N. K. (1984): Renal response to captopril in severe heart failure: Role of furosemide in natriuresis and reversal of hyponatremia. *Ann. Intern. Med.,* 100:777–782.
62. Dzau, V. J., Hollenberg, N. K., and Williams, G. H. (1983): Neurohormonal mechanism in heart failure. Role in pathogenesis, therapy and drug tolerance. *Fed. Proc.,* 41:3162–3169.
63. Dzau, V. J., Kopelman, R. I., Barger, A. C., and Haber, E. (1980): Renin-specific antibody for study of cardiovascular homeostasis. *Science,* 297:1091–1093.
64. Dzau, V. J., Mudgett-Hunter, M., Kapler, G., and Haber, E. (1981): Monoclonal antibodies binding renal renin. *Hypertension,* 3:4–8.
65. Dzau, V. J., Ouellette, A. J., and Pratt, R. (1981): Studies of the biosynthesis of renin using a cell-free translation system. *Clin. Sci.,* 61:241s–243s.
66. Dzau, V. J., Packer, M., Swartz, S. L., Lilly, L. S., Hollenberg, N. K., and Williams, G. H. (1984): Prostaglandins in heart failure: Relationship to renin angiotensin system and hyponatremia. *N. Engl. J. Med.,* 310:347–352.
67. Dzau, V. J., and Sands, K. (1982): Role of pituitary gland in regulation of angiotensinogen production. *Fed. Proc.,* 41:6265.
68. Dzau, V. J., Siwek, L. G., Rosen, S., Farhi, E. R., Mizoguchi, H., and Barger, A. C. (1981): Sequential renal hemodynamics in experimental benign and malignant hypertension. *Hypertension [Suppl. I],* 3:63–68.
69. Dzau, V. J., Slater, E. E., and Haber, E. (1979): Complete purification of dog renal renin. *Biochemistry,* 18:5224–5228.
70. Echtenkamp, S. F., Davis, J. D., DeForrest, J. M., Rowe, B. P., Freeman, R. H., Seymour, A. A., and Dietz, J. R. (1981): Effects of indomethacin, renal denervation and propranolol on plasma renin activity in conscious dogs with chronic thoracic caval constriction. *Circ. Res.,* 49:492–500.
71. Eid, M., Evin, G., Castro, B., Menard, J., and Corvol, P. (1981): New renin inhibitors homologous with pepstatin. *Biochem. J.,* 197:465–471.
72. Erdos, E. F., Johnson, A., and Boyden, N. T. (1978): Hydrolysis of enkephalin by cultured endothelial cells and purified dipeptidyl peptidase. *Biochem. Pharmacol.,* 27:843–848.
73. Evin, G., Cumin, F., Menard, J., and Corvol, P. (1984): Renin inhibition by synthetic peptides related to mouse and human renin prosegments. In: *Proceedings of the Tenth Scientific Meeting of the International Society of Hypertension* (abstract 44), p. 22.
74. Evin, G., Devin, J., Castro, B., Menard, J., and Corvol, P. (1984): Synthesis of peptides related to the prosegment of mouse submaxillary gland renin precursors: An approach to renin inhibitors. *Proc. Natl. Acad. Sci. USA,* 81:48–52.
75. Fagard, R., Bolpett, C., Lijneva, P., and Avery, A. (1982): Response of the systemic and pulmonary circulation to converting-enzyme inhibition (captopril) at rest and during exercise in hypertensive patients. *Circulation,* 65:33–39.
76. Farhi, E. R., Cant, J. R., and Barger, A. C. (1982): Interactions between intrarenal epinephrine receptors and the renal baroreceptor in the control of PRA in conscious dogs. *Circ. Res.,* 50: 477–485.
77. Faxon, D. P., Halperin, J. L., Creager, M. A., Gavras, H., Schick, E. C., and Ryan, T. J. (1981): Angiotensin inhibition in severe heart failure, acute central and limb hemodynamic effects of captopril, with observations on sustained oral therapy. *Am. Heart J.,* 101:548–556.

78. Ferrario, C. M., Gildenberg, P. L., and McCubbin, J. W. (1972): Cardiovascular effects of angiotensin mediated by the central nervous system. *Circ. Res.*, 30:257–262.
79. Field, L. J., McGowan, R. A., Dickinson, D. P., and Gross, K. W. (1984): Tissue and gene specificity of mouse renin expression. *Hypertension*, 6:597–603.
80. Fitzsimmons, J. T. (1971): The effect on drinking of peptide precursors and short chain peptide fragments of angiotensin II injected into the rat's diencephalon. *J. Physiol. (Lond.)*, 214:295–301.
81. Foidart, J., Sraer, J., Delarue, F., Mahieu, P., and Ardaillou, R. (1980): Evidence for mesangial glomerular receptors for angiotensin II linked to mesangial cell contractility. *FEBS Lett.*, 121:333–339.
82. Folkow, B. (1971): The hemodynamic consequences of adaptive structural changes of the resistance vessels in hypertension. *Clin. Sci.* 41:1–12.
83. Fray, J. C. S. (1977): Stimulation of renin release in perfused kidney by low calcium and high magnesium. *Am. J. Physiol.*, 232:F377–382.
84. Freedlender, A. E., and Goodfriend, T. L. (1979): Renin and the angiotensins. In: *Methods of Hormone Radioimmunoassays*, edited by B. M. Jaffe and H. R. Berman, pp. 889–907. Academic Press, New York.
85. Friedland, J., and Silverstein, E. (1976): A sensitive fluorimetric assay for serum angiotensin-converting enzyme. *Am. J. Clin. Pathol.*, 66:416–424.
86. Friedland, J. C., Setton, C., and Silverstein, E. (1977): Angiotensin converting enzyme: Induction by steroids in rabbit alveolar macrophages in culture. *Science*, 197:64–65.
87. Funakawa, S., Dunae, Y., and Yamamoto, K. (1978): Conversion between renin and high molecular weight renin in the dog. *Biochem. J.*, 176:977–981.
88. Galen, F. X., Devaux, C., Guyenne, T., Menard, J., and Corvol, P. (1979): Multiple forms of human renin: Purification and characterization. *J. Biol. Chem.*, 254:4848–4855.
89. Galen, F. X., Devaux, C., Hovot, A. M., Menard, J., Corvol, P., Corvol, M. T., Gubler, M. C., Mounier, F., and Cammilleri, J. P. (1984): Renin biosynthesis of human tumoral juxtaglomerular cells. *J. Clin. Invest.*, 73:1144–1155.
90. Ganong, W. F. (1984): The brain renin angiotensin system. In: *Annual Review of Physiology, Vol. 46*, edited by R. M. Berne and J. F. Hoffman, pp. 17–32. Annual Reviews, Palo Alto.
91. Ganten, D., Schelling, P., Vecsei, P., and Ganten, U. (1976): Isorenin of extrerenal origin. "The tissue angiotensinogenase systems." *Am. J. Med.*, 60:760–772.
92. Gavras, H., Brunner, H. R., Vaugham, E. D., and Laragh, J. H. (1973): Angiotensin-sodium interaction in blood pressure maintenance of renal hypertensive and normotensive rats. *Science*, 180:1369–1372.
93. Gavras, H., Liang, C.-S., and Brunner, H. R. (1978): Redistribution of regional blood flow after inhibition of the angiotensin converting enzyme. *Circ. Res. [Suppl. 1]*, 43:159–163.
94. Gibbons, G., Dzau, V. J., Farhi, E., and Barger, A. C. (1984): Interactions of signals influencing renin release. *Annu. Rev. Physiol.*, 46:291–308.
95. Given, B. D., Taylor, T., Hollenberg, N. K., and Williams, G. H. (1984): Duration of action and short term hormonal responses to Enalapril (MK421) in normal subjects. *J. Cardiovasc. Pharmacol.*, 6:436–441.
96. Goodfriend, T. L., and Peach, M. J. (1975): Angiotensin III: Evidence and speculation for its role as an important agonist in the renin-angiotensin system. *Circ. Res. [Suppl. I]* 36/37:38–40.
97. Gunther, S., Gimbrone, M. A., Jr., and Alexander, R. W. (1980): Regulation by angiotensin II of its receptors in resistance blood vessels. *Nature*, 287:230–232.
98. Guyene, T. T., Galen, F. X., Devaux, C., Corvol, P., and Menard, J. (1980): Direct radioimmunoassay of human renin. *Hypertension*, 2:465–470.
99. Guyton, A. C., Coleman, T. G., Cowley, A. W., Scheel, K. W., Manning, R. D., and Normal, R. A. (1972): Arterial pressure regulation. *Am. J. Med.*, 52:485–594.
100. Haber, E. (1976): The role of renin in normal and pathological cardiovascular homeostasis. *Circulation*, 54:849–861.
101. Haber, E. (1983): Inhibitors of renin: Present and future. *Clin. Exp. Hyper.*, 7/8:1193–1205.
102. Haber, E., Koerner, T., Page, L. B., Kliman, B., and Purnode, A. (1969): Application of a radioimmunoassay for angiotensin I to the physiologic measurement of plasma renin activity in normal human subjects. *J. Clin. Endocrinol. Metab.*, 29:1349–1355.
103. Hall, J. E., Guyton, A. C., and Cowley, A. W., Jr. (1977): Dissociation of renal blood flow and filtration rate autoregulation by renin depletion. *Am. J. Physiol.*, 236:F252–F259.
104. Hall, J. E., Guyton, A. C., Jackson, T. E., Coleman, T. G., Lohmeier, T. E., and Trippodo, N. C. (1977): Control of glomerular filtration rate by renin-angiotensin system. *Am. J. Physiol.*, 233:F366–F372.
105. Harada, E., and Rubin, R. P. (1978): Stimulation of renin secretion and calcium efflux from the isolated perfused cat kidney by noradrenaline after prolonged calcium deprivation. *J. Physiol. (Lond.)*, 274:367–379.
106. Hardman, J. A., Hart, Y. J., Catazanio, D. F., Tellam, J. T., Baxter, J. D., Morris, B. J., and Shine, J. (1984): Primary structure of the human renin gene. *DNA*, 3:457–468.
107. Herrmann, H. C., and Dzau, V. J. (1983): Feedback regulation of angiotensinogen produced by components of the renin-angiotensin system. *Circ. Res.*, 52:328–334.
108. Hirose, S., Workman, R. J., and Inagami, T. (1979): Specific antibody to hog renal renin and its application to the direct radioimmunoassay of renin in various organs. *Circ. Res.*, 45:275–281.
109. Hobart, P. M., Fogliano, M., O'Connor, B. A., Schaefer, I. M., and Chirgwin, J. M. (1984): Human renin gene: Structure and sequence analysis. *Proc. Natl. Acad. Sci. USA*, 81:5026–5030.
110. Hofbauer, K. G., Wood, J. M., Gulati, N., Heusser, C., and Menard, J. (1985): Increased plasma renin during renin inhibition. *Hypertension [Suppl. 1]*, 7:61–65.
111. Holland, O. B., Ruhnert, L. V., Campbell, W. B., and Anderson, R. J. (1983): Synergistic effect of captopril with hydrochlorothiazide for the treatment of low-renin hypertensive black patients. *Hypertension*, 5:235–239.
112. Hollenberg, N. K., Chenitz, W. R., Adams, D. F., and Williams, G. H. (1974): Reciprocal influence of salt intake on adrenal glomerulosa and renal vascular responses to angiotensin II in normal man. *J. Clin. Invest.*, 54:34–42.
113. Hollenberg, N. K., and Dzau, V. J. (1986): The renin angiotensin system. In: *Clinical Disorders in Fluid and Electrolyte Metabolism*, edited by M. H. Maxwell, C. R. Kleeman, and R. J. Narins. McGraw-Hill, New York.
114. Hollenberg, N. K., Swartz, S. L., Passan, D. R., and Williams, G. H. (1979): Increased glomerular filtration rate after converting enzyme inhibition in essential hypertension. *N. Engl. J. Med.*, 301:9–12.
115. Hollenberg, N. K. Williams, G. H., Brown, C., Taub, K. J., Adams, D. F., and Ishikawa, I. (1977): Renal vascular response to interruption of the renin-angiotensin system in normal man. *Kidney Int.*, 12:285–293.
116. Hricik, D. E., Browning, R. J., Kopelman, R. I., Goorno, W. E., Medias, N. E., and Dzau, V. J. (1983): Captopril induced functional renal insufficiency in patients with bilateral renal-artery stenosis or renal artery stenosis in the solitary kidney. *N. Engl. J. Med.*, 308:373–376.
117. Hseuh, W. A., Carlson, E. J., and Dzau, V. J. (1983): Characterization of inactive renin from human kidney and plasma. *J. Clin. Invest.*, 71:506–517.
118. Hseuh, W. A., Carlson, E. J., and Israel-Hagman, M. (1981): Mechanism of acid activation of renin: Role of kallikrein in renin activation. *Hypertension [Suppl. 1]*, 3:22–29.
119. Imai, T., Miyazaki, H., Hirose, S., Hori, H., Hayashi, T., Kageyama, R., Ohkubo, H., Nakanishi, S., and Murakami, K. (1983): Cloning and sequence analysis of cDNA for human renin precursor. *Proc. Natl. Acad. Sci. USA*, 80:7405–7409.
120. Inagami, T., and Murakami, K. (1977): Pure renin isolation from hog kidney and characterization. *J. Biol. Chem.*, 252:2978–2983.
121. Inagami, T., and Murakami, K. (1980): Prorenin. *Biomed. Res.*, 1:456–475.
122. Inglefinger, J. R., Pratt, R. E., Ellison, K. E., and Dzau, V. J.

(1985): Regulation of mouse renin expression during ontogeny. *Clin. Res.*, 33:362A.

123. Katholi, R. E., Winternitz, S. R., and Oparil, S. (1982): Decrease in peripheral sympathetic nervous system activity following renal denervation or unclipping in the one-kidney one-clip Goldblatt hypertensive rat. *J. Clin. Invest.*, 69:55–62.

124. Kawamura, M., Ikemoto, F., Funakawa, S., and Yamamoto, K. (1979): Characteristics of a renin-binding substance for the conversion of renin into a higher molecular-weight form in the dog. *Clin. Sci.*, 57:345–350.

125. Keeton, T. K., and Campbell, W. B. (1980): The pharmacologic alteration of renin release. *Pharmacol. Rev.*, 32:81–227.

126. Khairallah, P. A. (1972): Action of angiotensin on adrenergic nerve endings: Inhibition of norepinephrine uptake. *Fed. Proc.*, 31:1351–1357.

127. Kim, S. J., Hirose, S., Miyazaki, H., Ueno, N., Higashimori, K., Morinaga, S., Kimura, T., Sakakibara, S., and Murakami, K. (1985): Identification of plasma inactive renin as prorenin with a site-directed antibody. *Biochem. Biophys. Res. Commun.*, 126:641–645.

128. Kimbrough, H. R., Jr., Vaughan, D. E., Carey, R. M., and Ayers, C. R. (1977): Effect of intrarenal AII blockade on renal function in conscious dogs. *Circ. Res.*, 40:174–178.

129. Kirchner, K. A., Kotchen, T. A., Galla, J. H., and Luke, R. G. (1978): Importance of chloride for acute inhibition of renin by sodium chloride. *Am. J. Physiol.*, 235:F444–450.

130. Klickstein, L. B., and Wintroub, B. U. (1982): Separation of angiotensins and assay of angiotensin generating enzymes by HPLC. *Anal. Biochem.*, 120:146–150.

131. Laemmli, U. K. (1970): Cleavage of structural proteins during the assembly of the head of bacteriophage T4. *Nature*, 227:580–685.

132. Laragh, J. H., Case, D. B., Atlas, S. A., and Sealey, J. E. (1980): Captopril compared with other antirenin system agents in hypertensive patients: Its triphasic effects on blood pressure and its use to identify and treat the renin factor. *Hypertension*, 2:586–593.

133. Levine, T. B., Franciosa, J. A., and Cohn, J. N. (1980): Acute and long-term response to an oral converting-enzyme inhibition in patients with severe congestive heart failure. *Circulation*, 62:35–41.

134. Levine, T. B., Franciosa, J. A., Vrobel, T., and Cohn, J. N. (1982): Hyponatremia as a marker for high renin heart failure. *Br. Heart J.*, 47:161–166.

135. Leyssac, P. P. (1967): Intrarenal function of angiotensin. *Fed. Proc.*, 26:55.

136. Lieberman, J., and Buetler, E. (1976): Elevation of serum angiotensin-converting enzyme in Gaucher's disease. *N. Engl. J. Med.*, 294:1442–1444.

137. Lieberman, J., and Sastre, A. (1980): Serum angiotensin converting enzyme: Elevation in diabetes mellitus. *Ann. Intern. Med.*, 93:825–826.

138. Lilly, L., Pratt, R. E., Alexander, R. W., Larson, D. M., Ellison, K. E., Gimbrone, M. A., and Dzau, V. J. (1985): Renin expression by vascular endothelial cells in culture. *Circ. Res.*, 57:312–318.

139. Logan, A. G., Tenyi, I., Peart, W. S., Breathnach, A. S., and Martin, B. G. H. (1977): The effect of lanthanum on renin secretion and renal vasoconstriction. *Proc. R. Soc. Lond.*, 195:327–342.

140. Luetscher, J. A., Bialek, J. W., and Gris, I. S. (1982): Human kidney cathepsin B and H activate and lower the molecular weight of human inactive renin. *Clin. Exp. Hyper.*, A4:2149–2158.

141. Malik, K. U., Ryan, P., and McGiff, J. C. (1976): Modification by prostaglandins E_1 and E_2 indomethacin and arachidonic acid of the vasoconstrictor responses of the isolated perfused rabbit and rat mesenteric arteries to adrenergic stimuli. *Cir. Res.*, 39:163–168.

142. Malling, C., and Poulsen, K. (1977): A direct radioimmunoassay for plasma renin in mice and its evaluation. *Biochim. Biophys. Acta*, 491:532–541.

143. Marshall, G. R. (1976): Structure–activity relations of antagonist of the renin-angiotensin system. *Fed. Proc.*, 35:2494–2501.

144. Massie, B. M., Kramer, B. L., Topic, N., and Henderson, S. G. (1982): Hemodynamic and radionuclide effects of acute captopril therapy for heart failure: Changes in left and right ventricular volumes and function at rest and during exercise. *Circulation*, 65:1374–1381.

145. McCubbin, J. W. (1974): Peripheral effects of angiotensin on the autonomic nervous system. In: *Angiotensin*, edited by I. H. Page and F. M. Bumpus, pp. 417–422. Springer-Verlag, New York.

146. McGiff, J. C., Croshaw, K., Terragno, N. A., and Lonigro, A. J. (1970): Release of a prostaglandin-like substance in renal venous blood in response to angiotensin II. *Circ. Res. [Suppl. 1]*, 27:121–130.

147. Messina, E. J., Weinger, R., and Keley, G. (1975): Inhibition of bradykinin vasodilation and potentiation of norepinephrine and angiotensin vasoconstriction by inhibitors of prostaglandin synthesis in skeletal muscle in the rat. *Circ. Res.*, 37:430–437.

148. Michelakis, A. M., Yoshida, H., Menzie, J., Murakami, K., and Inagami, T. (1974): A radioimmunoassay for the direct measurement of renin in mice and its application to submaxillary gland and kidney studies. *Endocrinology*, 94:1101–1105.

149. Misono, K. S., Chang, J.-J., and Inagami, T. (1982): Amino acid sequence of mouse submaxillary gland. *Proc. Natl. Acad. Sci. USA*, 78:4858–4862.

150. Misono, K. S., and Inagami, T. T. (1980): Characterization of the active site of mouse submandibular gland renin. *Biochemistry*, 19:2616–2622.

151. Miyazaki, H., Fukamizu, A., Hirose, S., Hayasji, T., Hori, H., Ohkubo, H., Nakanishi, S., and Murakami, K. (1984): Structure of the human renin gene. *Proc. Natl. Acad. Sci. USA*, 81:5999–6003.

152. Mizoguchi, J., Dzau, V. J., Siwek, L., and Barger, A. C. (1983): Effect of intrarenal administration of dopamine on renin release in conscious dogs. *Am. J. Physiol.*, 224:H39–H45.

153. Mohring, J., Mohring, B., Naumann, H., Philippi, A., Homsey E., Orth, H., Dauda, G., Kazda, S., and Gross, F. (1975): Salt and water balance and renin activity in renal hypertension of rats. *Am. J. Physiol.*, 228:1847–1855.

154. Moore, T. J., Crantz, F. R., Hollenberg, N. K., Koletsky, R. J., Leboff, M. S., Swatz, S. L., Levine, L., Podolsky, S., Dluhy, R. G., and Williams, G. H. (1981): Contribution of prostaglandins to the antihypertensive action of captopril in essential hypertension. *Hypertension*, 3:168–173.

155. Moore, T. J., and Williams, G. H. (1981): Angiotensin II receptors in human platelets. *Circ. Res.*, 51:314–320.

156. Morris, B. J. (1978): Properties of the activation of pepsin of inactive renin in human amniotic fluid. *Biochim. Biophys. Acta*, 572:86–97.

157. Morton, J. J., Tree, M., and Casals-Stenzel, J. (1980): The effect of captopril on blood pressure and angiotensin I, II and III in sodium-depleted dogs. Problems associated with the measurement of angiotensin II after inhibition of converting enzyme. *Clin. Sci.*, 58:445–450.

158. Mujais, S. K., Fouad, F. M., Textor, S. C., Tarazi, R. C., and Bravo, E. L. (1981): Contrast between acute and chronic effects of converting enzyme inhibition on renal function in heart failure. *Clin. Res.*, 29:472 (abstract).

159. Mullins, J. J., Burt, D. W., Windass, J. D., McTurk, P., and Brammer, W. J. (1982): Molecular cloning og two distinct renin genes from the DBA/2 mouse. *EMBO J.*, 1:1461–1466.

160. Multicenter Heart Failure Group (1983): A placebo-controlled trial of captopril in refractory chronic congestion heart failure. *J. Am. Coll. Cardiol.*, 2:755–763.

161. Nabel, E., Gibbons, G., and Dzau, V. J. (1985): Pathophysiology of experimental renovascular hypertension. *Am. J. Kidney Disease*, 5:A111–A119.

162. Naftilan, A., and Oparil, S. (1982): The role of calcium in the control of renin release. *Hypertension*, 4:670–675.

163. Nasjletti, A., and Malik, K. U. (1981): Interrelationship among prostaglandins and vasoactive substances. *Med. Clin. North Am.*, 65:881–889.

164. Needleman, P., Bronson, S. D., Wyche, A., and Sivakoff, M. (1978): Cardiac and renal prostaglandin I_2. Biosynthesis and biological effects in isolated perfused rabbit tissue. *J. Clin. Invest.*, 61:839–849.

165. Norman, J. A., and Chang, J. Y. (1985): Protelytic conversion of [Met]enkephalin-Arg⁶-Gly⁷-Leu⁸ by Braun synaptic membranes. *J. Biol. Chem.*, 260:2653–2656.
166. Nussberger, J., Brunner, D. B., Waeber, B., and Brunner, H. R. (1984): Measurement of low angiotensin concentrations after ethanol and Dowex extraction process. *J. Lab. Clin. Med.*, 103:304–312.
167. Nussberger, J., Brunner, D. B., Waeber, B., and Brunner, H. R. (1985): True verus immunoreactive angiotensin II in human plasma. *Hypertension [Suppl I]*, 7:1–7.
168. Nussberger, J., Matsueda, G. R., Re, R. N., and Haber, E. (1983): Selectivity of angiotensin II antisera. *J. Immunol. Methods*, 56:85–96.
169. Oliver, J. A., Sciacca, R. R., Pinto, J., and Cannon, P. J. (1981): Participation of the prostaglandins in the control of renal blood flow during acute reduction of cardiac output in the dog. *J. Clin. Invest.*, 67:229–237.
170. Oparil, S., Koerner, T. J., and Haber, E. (1974): Effects of pH and enzyme inhibitors on apparent generation of angiotensin I in human plasma. *J. Clin. Endocrinol. Metab.*, 39:965–968.
171. Packer, M., Medina, N., and Yushak, M. (1984): Relationship between serum sodium concentration and the hemodynamic and clinical responses to converting-enzyme inhibition in severe heart failure. *J. Am. Coll. Cardiol.*, 3:1035–1043.
172. Pamnani, M., Huot, S., Buggy, J. B., Clough, D., and Haddy, F. (1981): Demonstration of a humoral inhibitor of the Na⁺-K⁺ pump in some models of experimental hypertension. *Hypertension [Suppl. II]*, 3:96–101.
173. Panthier, J. J., Foote, S., Chambraud, B., Strosberg, A. D., Corvol, P., and Rougeon, F. (1982): Complete amino acid sequence and maturation of the mouse submaxillary gland renin precursor. *Nature*, 298:90–92.
174. Panthier, J. J., Holm, I., and Rougeon, F. (1982): The mouse RN locus: S allele of the renin regulator gene results form a single structural gene duplication. *EMBO J.*, 1:1417–1421.
175. Park, C. S., Han, D. S., and Fray, J. C. S. (1980): Calcium in the control of renin secretion: Ca²⁺ influx as an inhibitory signal. *Am. J. Physiol.*, 240:F70–F74.
176. Patchett, A. A., Harris, E., Tristram, E. W., and Wgvratt, M. J. (1980): A new class of antigiotensin-converting enzyme inhibitor. *Nature*, 288:280–283.
177. Peach, M. J. (1974): Adrenal medulla. In: *Angiotensin*, edited by I. M. Page and F. M. Bumpus, pp. 400–407. Springer-Verlag, New York.
178. Peart, W. S., Quesada, T., and Tenyi, I. (1977): The effects of EDTA and EGTA on renin secretion. *Br. J. Pharmacol.*, 59:247–252.
179. Piccini, N., Knopf, J. L., and Gross, K. W. (1982): A DNA polymorphism, consistent with gene duplication correlates with high renin levels in mouse submaxillary gland. *Cell*, 30:205–213.
180. Pierpont, G. L., Francis, G. S., and Cohn, J. N. (1981): Effect of captopril on renal function in patients with congestive heart failure. *Br. Heart J.*, 46:522–527.
181. Poulsen, K., Vuust, J., Lykkegaard, S., Nielsen, A., and Lunt, T. (1979): Renin is synthesized as a 50,000-dalton single-chain polypeptide in cell-free translation systems. *FEBS Lett.*, 98:135.
182. Pratt, R. E., Ouellette, A. J., and Dzau, V. J. (1983): Renin biosynthesis: Multiplicity of active and intermediate forms. *Proc. Natl. Acad. Sci. USA*, 80:6809–6813.
183. Pratt, R. E., Roth, T. P., and Dzau, V. J. (1984): Evidence for two pathways of renin secretion. *Circulation [Suppl. II]*, 70:315.
184. Printz, M., Phillips, M., and Ganten, D. (1982): The brain renin angiotensin system (minireview). In: *The Renin-Angiotensin System in the Brain*, edited by D. Ganten, M. Printiz, and M. I. Phillips, p. 3. Springer-Verlag, New York.
185. Rabito, S. F., Carretero, O. A., and Scicli, A. G. (1981): Evidence against a role of vasopressin in the maintenance of high blood pressure in mineralocorticoid and renovascular hypertension. *J.A.M.A.*, 220:1209–1218.
186. Regoli, D., Park, W. K., and Rioux, F. (1974): Pharmacology of angiotensin. *Pharmacol. Rev.*, 26:69–123.
187. Riegger, A. J. G., Lever, A. F., Millar, J. A., Morton, J. J., and Slack, B. (1977): Correction of renal hypertension in the rat by prolonged infusion of angiotensin inhibitors. *Lancet*, 2:1317–1319.
188. Rostand, S. G., Lewis, D., Watkins, J. B., Huang, W., and Navar, L. G. (1982): Attenuated pressure natriuresis in hypertensive rats. *Kidney Int.*, 21:330–338.
189. Rougeon, F., Chambraud, D., Foote, S., Panthier, J.-J., Nageotte, R., and Corvol, P. (1981): Molecular cloning of a mouse submaxillary gland renin cDNA fragment. *Proc. Natl. Acad. Sci. USA*, 78:6367–6371.
190. Rubin, B., Antonaccio, M. J., and Horovitz, Z. P. (1981): The antihypertensive effects of captopril in hypertensive animal models. In: *Angiotensin Converting Enzyme Inhibitors*, edited by A. P. Horovitz, pp. 27–54. Urban & Schwarzenberg, Baltimore.
191. Ryan, J. W., Stewart, J. M., Leary, W. P., and Ledingham, J. G. (1970): Metabolism of angiotensin I in the pulmonary circulation. *Biochem. J.*, 120:221–223.
192. Sancho, J., Re, R., Burton, J., Barberg, A. C., and Haber, E. (1976): The role of the renin-angiotensin aldosterone system in cardiovascular homeostasis in normal human subjects. *Circulation*, 53:400–405.
193. Santos, R. A. S., Krieger, E. M., and Greene, L. J. (1985): An improved fluorometric assay of rat serum and plasma converting enzyme. *Hypertension*, 7:244–252.
194. Sealey, J. E., Atlas, S. A., and Laragh, J. H. (1980): Prorenin and other large molecular weigh forms of renin. *Endocrinol. Rev.*, 1:365–391.
195. Sealey, J. E., Atlas, S. A., Laragh, J. H., Oza, N. B., and Ryan, J. W. (1979): Activation or prorenin-like substance in human plasma by trypsin and by urinary kallikrein. *Hypertension*, 1:179–189.
196. Sealey, J. E., and Laragh, J. H. (1975): Radioimmunoassay of plasma renin activity. *Semin. Nucl. Med.*, 5:189–192.
197. Shebuski, R. J., and Aiken, J. W. (1980): Angiotensin II stimulation of renal prostaglandin synthesis elevates circulating prostacylcin in the dog. *J. Cardiovasc. Pharmacol.*, 2:667–677.
198. Skinner, S. L. (1967): Improved assay methods for renin "concentration" and "activity" in human plasma. *Circ. Res.*, 20:391–402.
199. Skinner, S. L., Dunn, J. R., Mazzett, J., Campbell, D. J., and Fidge, N. H. (1975): Purification properties and kinetics of sheep and human renin substrates. *Aust. J. Exp. Biol.*, 53:77–87.
200. Skorecki, K. L., Bellermann, B. J., Rennke, H. G., and Brenner, B. M. (1983): Angiotensin II receptor regulation in isolated renal glomeruli. *Fed. Proc.*, 42:3064–3070.
201. Swartz, S. L., Williams, G. H., Hollenberg, N. K., Levine, L., Dluhy, R. G., and Moore, T. J. (1980): Captopril-induced changes in prostaglandin production. *J. Clin. Invest.*, 65:1257–1264.
202. Szelke, M., Jones, D. M., Atrash, B., Hallet, A., and Leckie, B. J. (1983): Novel transition-state analogue inhibitors of renin. In: *Peptides: Structure and Function*, edited by V. J. Hruby and D. H. Rich, pp. 579–583. Proceedings of the 8th American Peptide Symposium.
203. Szelke, M., Leckie, B., Hallet, A., Jones, D. M., Sveiras, J., Atrash, B., and Lever, A. F. (1982): Potent new inhibitors of human renin. *Nature*, 299:555–557.
204. Szelke, M., Leckie, B. J., Tree, M., Brown, A., Grant, J., Hallet, A., Hughes, M., Jones, D. M., and Lever, A. F. (1982): H-77 a potent new renin inhibitor—in vitro and in vivo studies. *Hypertension [Suppl. II]*, 4:59–69.
205. Takii, Y., Figueiredo, A. F. S., and Inagami, T. (1985): Application of immunochemical methods to the identification of rat kidney inactive renin. *Hypertension*, 7:236–243.
206. Takii, Y., and Inagami, T. (1982): Purification of a completely inactive renin from hog kidney and identification of renin zymogen. *Biochem. Biophys. Res. Commun.*, 104:133–140.
207. Taub, K. J. (1977): Angiotensin antagonists with increased specificity for the renal vasculature. *J. Clin. Invest.*, 59:528–535.
208. Tewksbury, D. A., Dart, R. A., and Travis, J. (1981): The amino terminal amino acid sequence of human angiotensinogen. *Biochem. Biophys. Res. Commun.*, 99:1311–1315.
209. Thomas, P. S. (1983): Hybridization of denatured RNA transferred or dotted to nitrocellulose paper. *Methods Enzymol.*, 100:255–266.

210. Towbin, H., Staehelin, T., and Gordon, J. (1979): Electrophoretic transfer of proteins from polyacrylamide gels to nitrocellulose sheets: Procedure and some application. *Proc. Natl. Acad. Sci. USA,* 76:4350–4354.

211. Tree, M., Atrash, B., Donovan, B., Gamble, J., Hallett, A., Highes, M., Jones, D. M., Leckie, B., Lever, A. F., Morton, J. J., and Szelke, M. (1983): New inhibitors of human renin tested in the anaesthetised baboon. *J. Hyper.,* 1:399–403.

212. Veterans Administration Cooperative Study Group on Antihypertensive Agents (1982): Captopril: Evaluation of low doses, twice daily doses and the addition of diuretic for the treatment of mild to moderate hypertension. *Clin. Sci.,* 63:443S–445S.

213. Viskoper, R. J., Rosenfeld, S., Maxwell, M. H., DeLima, J., Lupo, A. N., and Rosenfed, J. B. (1976): Effect of Ca^{2+} binding by EGTA on renin release in the isolated perfused rabbit kidney. *Proc. Soc. Exp. Biol. Med.,* 142:415–418.

214. Walshe, J. J., and Venutto, R. C. (1979): Acute oliguric renal failure induced by indomethacin: Possible mechanisms. *Ann. Intern. Med.,* 91:47–49.

215. Watkins, L., Jr., Burtin, J. A., Haber, E., Cant, J. R., Smith, F. W., and Barger, A. C. (1976): The renin-angiotensin-aldosterone system in congestive failure in conscious dogs. *J. Clin. Invest.,* 517:1606–1617.

216. Watkins, B. E., et al. (1976): Intrarenal site of action of calcium on renin secretion in dogs. *Circ. Res.,* 39:847–853.

217. Weare, J. A., Gafford, J. T., Lu, H. S., and Erdos, E. G. (1982): Purification of human angiotensin converting enzyme using reverse immunoadsorption chromatography. *Anal. Biochem.,* 123: 310–319.

218. Webb, D. J., Cumming, A. M., Leckie, B. J., Lever, A. F., Morton, J. J., Robertson, J. I. S., Szelke, M., and Donovan, B. (1983): Reduction of blood pressure in man with H-142, a potent new renin inhibitor. *Lancet,* 2:1486–1487.

219. Whorton, A. R., Nisono, K., Hollifield, J., Frolich, J. C., Inagami, T., and Oates, J. A. (1977): Prostaglandin and renin release. I. Stimulation of renin release from rabbit renal cortical slices by PGI_2. *Prostaglandins,* 14:1095–1099.

220. Wood, J. M., Heusser, C., Alkan, S., Dietrich, F. M., and Gulati, N. (1984): In vivo studies with a monoclonal antibody against human renin. In: *Proceedings of the Tenth Scientific Meeting of the International Society of Hypertension* (abstract 941), p. 470.

221. Woodhouse, K., Farrow, P. R., and Wilkinson, R. (1979): Reversible renal failure during treatment with captopril. *Br. Med. J.,* 2:1146–1147.

222. Yamamoto, K., Iwao, H., Abe, Y., and Morimoto, S. (1974): Effect of Ca^{2+} on renin release in vitro and in vivo. *Jpn. Circ.,* 38:1127–1131.

223. Yokosawa, J., Holladay, L. A., Inagami, T., Haas, E., and Murakami, K. (1980): Human renal renin: Complete purification and characterization. *J. Biol. Chem.,* 255:3498–3502.

224. Yokosawa, N., Takahashi, N., Inagami, T., and Page, D. L. (1979): Isolation of completely inactive plasma prorenin and its activation by kallikreins. *Biochim. Biophys. Acta,* 569:211–219.

225. Yotsumoto, H., Imai, Y., Kuzuya, N., and Uchimura, H. (1982): Increased levels of serum angiotensin converting enzyme activity in hyperthyroidism. *Ann. Intern. Med.,* 96:326–328.

226. Zusman, R. M. (1981): Prostaglandins, vasopressin and renal water reabsorption. *Med. Clin. North Am.,* 65:915–925.

227. Zusman, R. M., Burton, J., Christianson, D., Nussberger, J., Dodds, A., and Haber, E. (1983): Hemodynamic aspects of a competitive renin inhibitory peptide in man: Evidence for multiple mechanisms of action. *Trans. Am. Assoc. Phys.,* 96:365–374.

228. Zusman, R. M., and Keiser, H. R. (1977): Prostaglandin biosynthesis by rabbit renomedullary interstitial cells in tissue culture: stimulation by angiotensin II, bradykinin and arginine vasopressin. *J. Clin. Invest.,* 60:215–223.

The Heart and Cardiovascular System,
edited by H. A. Fozzard et al.
Raven Press, New York © 1986.

CHAPTER 70

Kinins

O. A. Carretero, A. G. Scicli, S. F. Rabito, and A. Nasjletti

There are many mechanisms by which blood pressure can be regulated. These mechanisms interact in a complex fashion with each other to maintain blood pressure homeostasis.

Vasopressor systems such as the renal renin-angiotensin system have been clearly shown to have major roles in the control of blood pressure and in the pathogenesis of certain types of hypertension (120). The roles of vasodepressor systems in the control of blood pressure and in the pathogenesis of hypertension are less well defined. However, the hypothesis that a balance among vasopressor and vasodepressor systems contributes to maintenance of normal blood pressure and that an alteration in this balance can cause hypertension or hypotension is reasonable (Fig. 1). Kinins are among the most potent vasodilator substances known. These peptides are released from precursor proteins called kininogens (substrate) by a group of enzymes named kininogenases. The best known and most potent kininogenases are plasma and glandular kallikreins. Plasma kallikrein (EC 3.4.21.33) circulates as a proenzyme complexed to its substrate, high-molecular-weight kininogen (HMWK). Plasma prekallikrein is activated by and in turn activates Hageman factor (coagulation factor XII). This system, in addition to its kinin-generating and procoagulant activities, has fibrinolytic activity (through activation of plasminogen to plasmin) and complement-activating capability (36). Glandular kallikreins (EC 3.4.21.34) are serine proteases with 60 to

75% homology with tonin, the γ subunit of nerve growth factor, and epidermal-growth-factor-binding protein (9,45,72,76) and 35 to 50% homology with trypsin, chymotrypsin, and elastase (13,38,76,123). Kallikreins appear to originate from expression of 25 to 30 different genes located in chromosome 7 (76). Kallikreins are found in the salivary and sweat glands, pancreas, intestines, kidney, prostate, spleen, arteries and veins, and brain (Fig. 2). The ubiquity in location and presence of multiple kallikrein genes suggests multiple functions for these enzymes.

Although glandular kallikrein has a much narrower range of substrate specificity than trypsin, it can hydrolyze many other substrates. In addition to its kininogenase activity (kinin-generating capacity), glandular kallikrein has the capability to process prohormone to hormone [proinsulin (92), prorenin (42,114), proatrial natriuretic factor (39)], to activate growth factors (18,22,53), to generate angiotensin from plasma (78), to break down apoprotein B from low-density lipoproteins (LDL) (25), to stimulate release of renin and PGI_2 (14,27,83,122,126), and to produce contraction of the uterus (15,16,31) and ureter (74) (Fig. 3). These *in vitro* and pharmacological effects of the enzyme are not mediated by the release of kinins. Although at the present time it is not known if these events also occur in physiologic and pathologic situations, they open the possibility that kallikrein participates in multiple biological regulatory functions.

The kininogenase activity of kallikrein is an important

VASODEPRESSOR

KININS (?)
KALLIKREIN (?)
ICOSANOIDS
A.N.F. (?)
ADENOSINE (?)
ATP, ADP (?)
P.A.F. (?)
THROMBIN (?)
SUBSTANCE P, V.I.P. (?)
E.D.R.F. (?)
HISTAMINE (?)
RENOMEDULLARY LIPIDS (?)
ACETYLCHOLINE (?)
CATECHOLAMINES (?)

$\downarrow$ C.O. $\uparrow$
T.P.R.

VASOPRESSOR

RENIN(S)
TONIN (?)
VASOPRESSIN
CATECHOLAMINES
ICOSANOIDS (?)
STEROIDS
RENOPRESSIN (?)
SEROTONIN (?)
NEUROPEPTIDE Y (?)

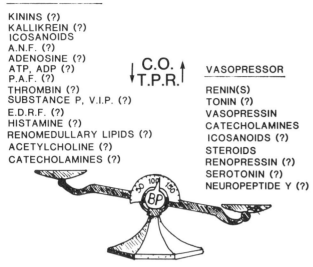

FIG. 1. Hypothetical roles of vasoactive substances in hypertension.

one, although kininogen is not the exclusive substrate for this enzyme. Glandular kallikrein can release kinins from both HMWK and low-molecular-weight kininogen (LMWK). When released into the circulation, glandular kallikrein is rapidly inactivated by plasma inhibitors, while generated kinins are destroyed by a group of peptidases known as kininases. Thus, both the rapid inactivation of glandular kallikrein and the rapid degradation of kinins in normal circumstances suggest that

if this vasodepressor system plays a role in the regulation of blood pressure, it is not as a systemic, but as a local, hormone (autacoid).

In our laboratory, Salgado et al. (107) showed that during infusion of bradykinin, the arterial blood kinin concentration required to decrease blood pressure in normotensive and hypertensive rats was 40 to 100 times higher than that in noninfused rats. This finding makes it unlikely that circulating kinins play a role in the regulation of blood pressure. As autacoids, the glandular kallikrein-kinin system could regulate vascular resistance, particularly in tissues rich in glandular kallikrein. Furthermore, in the kidney, the renal kallikrein-kinin system could participate in control of sodium and water excretion and consequently in regulation of blood pressure (30).

KININ ASSAYS

Free kinins are found in blood and urine and, under pathologic conditions, have been identified in spinal, synovial, and ascitic fluids. Measurement of free kinins in biological fluids is necessary for better knowledge of their roles in physiologic and pathologic conditions. Several studies have been reported concerning methods to measure kinins in blood and other biological fluids (20,64,75,84,112,115,125,133,136). Basically, these methods involve two parts: (a) collection of fluid and extraction of kinins and (b) bioassay or radioimmunoassay of the purified kinins.

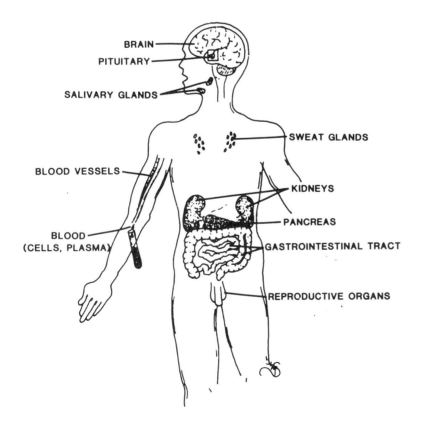

FIG. 2. Localization of kallikrein.

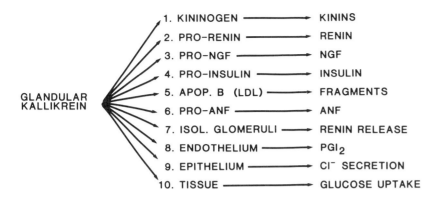

FIG. 3. Proposed functions of glandular kallikrein.

Collection and Extraction of Samples

Table 1 shows some of the methods used for harvesting blood and extracting kinins. The concentration of kinins found in blood or plasma is also shown. The manner in which the biological fluids are collected is very important, and if true endogenous free kinins are to be measured, formation and destruction of kinins during the fluid harvest must be avoided. For this purpose, two basically different methods have been used.

In one of these procedures, the blood is collected directly in ethanol, thereby instantly stopping all enzymatic reactions (20). After the proteins are separated and the alcohol is evaporated, the lipids are extracted with ether or dichloromethane. This is important, because lipids interfere with both bioassay and radioimmunoassay (RIA) (89). Further, purification of kinins can be accomplished with butanol extraction followed by extraction into aqueous solvents (20).

The other procedure consists of collecting blood in a plastic syringe containing inhibitors such as hexadimethyl bromide, to inhibit Hageman-factor activation, and EDTA or 1,10-phenanthroline, to inhibit kininases. This is usually followed by separation of the plasma and precipitation of the proteins by trichloroacetic acid (TCA). This method has been applied to other biological fluids such as spinal, synovial, and ascitic fluids, and urine (125).

The recoveries of kinins using these two methods of collection are similar. However, if the studies in which kinins were measured by bioassay are excluded, the methods that use enzyme inhibitors, plasma, and precipitation with TCA give higher normal blood levels of kinins than methods in which the blood is collected

TABLE 1. *Concentrations of kinins in human blood*

Collection method	Processing steps	Kinins[a] (ng ml^{-1})	Refs.
50 ml blood, directly in ethanol[b]	Ethanol supernat., evap.; ether and butanol ext.; water ext.	1–3	20
5 ml blood plastic syringe, 1,10-phenanthroline, ethanol	Ethanol evap.; ether ext.	0.07 ± 0.01	75
Plastic syringe, hexadimethrine bromide, EDTA	2 ml plasma, TCA precip., Amberlite IRC-50	<3.0 <1.5	125
Plastic syringe, hexadimethrine bromide, EDTA	2 ml plasma, TCA precip., QAE-Sephadex, IRC-50	5.00 ± 2.00 2.95 ± 1.75	136 134
6 ml blood, plastic syringe, 1,10-phenanthroline, ethanol	Ethanol supernat., evap.; dichloromethane evap.	0.22 ± 0.03	64
5 ml blood, directly in ethanol	Ethanol, boiled, evap.; ether ext.; QAE-Sephadex, IRC-50	0.025 ± 0.003	112
6 ml blood in acetone, EDTA, 1,10-phenanthroline, Polybrene	Ether ext., evap.; QAE-Sephadex	<0.003	84
Plastic syringe, HCl	Butanol, ether, H$_2$O, evap.	0.005 ± 0.001	115
2.5 ml blood, plastic syringe, 1,10-phenanthroline, ethanol	Ethanol supernat.; ether ext.; CM-Sephadex C-25	0.46 ± 0.04	133

[a] Mean ± SEM.
[b] Measured by bioassay.

directly into alcohol or acetone. These higher values probably do not reflect the true concentration of endogenous kinins but rather reflect inability to completely control kinin generation during the collection of blood, separation of the plasma, and precipitation with TCA. Another drawback to the use of enzyme inhibitors such as 1,10-phenanthroline, EDTA, and hexadimethrine bromide (Polybrene) is that they interfere with the RIA (89). Furthermore, we and others have found that antibodies against kinins cross-react with kininogen (28,89). Samples of plasma are still contaminated with kininogen after precipitation with ethanol or TCA and after chromatography with Amberlite IRC-50 (28). These two findings have led to the introduction of a column of QAE-A25-Sephadex in the processing of plasma or blood samples prior to RIA (28,136). This step is extremely important, because plasma has a high concentration of kininogen, and a small contamination could cause spuriously high estimates of kinins. The QAE-A25-Sephadex equilibrated with 3.5 mM phosphate buffer, pH 8.0, binds the kininogens while the kinins are recovered in the effluent. However, because the kinins are now diluted in a high volume of buffer, it is necessary to pass the samples through an Amberlite IRC-50 column. This step has the advantage of concentrating and desalting the samples, which is important, because a high concentration of salt may also interfere with the RIA. Once the kinins are extracted, they are subject to either bioassay or RIA. The latter is preferred, because it is more specific and sensitive than the bioassay. Kinins can be measured in urine for an indication of the intrarenal activity of the kallikrein-kinin system. However, because urine also contains kininogen and kininases in addition to kallikrein, special precautions must be taken to avoid formation and/or destruction of kinins while the urine is in the bladder and also while it is in the collecting vessel. The ideal method would be to collect the urine from the ureters directly into a vessel containing alcohol. However, except for experiments utilizing animals, this method is not usually feasible. An alternative method is to limit the time of incubation of the urine outside the kidneys by frequent voiding of the bladder. This can be accomplished without difficulty if the experiments last no more than a few hours. The voided urine should be collected directly in alcohol (final concentration of alcohol 70–80%) or some other suitable deproteinizing agent. After evaporation of the alcohol, usually no further purification of the urinary kinins is necessary for the RIA method. However, if the kinins are to be measured using a bioassay, butanol extraction seems to give a reasonable recovery while eliminating interference from other bioactive compounds (24). Table 2 summarizes some of the values found for the rate of secretion of kinins in urine.

Bioassay

Bioassay procedures to measure kinins are many and diverse, reflecting the wide spectrum of pharmacologic activities of kinin peptides. Any biological structure that reacts to a kinin with a reproducible and dose-related response can serve to quantitate the peptide. Most biological procedures to assay kinins rest on the ability of this class of peptides to produce contraction of nonvascular smooth muscle *in vitro* and to produce vasodilation *in vivo*. The bioassay of kinins, like all biological methods of assay, involves determining the potency of a sample of unknown kinin content relative to that of an appropriate reference standard (55). The major kinins in mammals (bradykinin, lysyl-bradykinin, and methionyl-lysyl-bradykinin) bring about the same qualitative response in the bioassay preparations. However, the three related kinins differ in pharmacologic potency (104). This is a drawback when assaying samples that contain a mixture of two or more kinin peptides, because a mere change in the concentration ratio of the peptides affects the results of the assay. Additional drawbacks of the biological methods to assay kinins may include lack of specificity and insufficient sensitivity. One can increase the specificity of the assay by separating

TABLE 2. *Urinary excretion of kinins (bradykinin and Lys-bradykinin)*

Method	Species	Kinins[a] (ng hr^{-1})	Refs.
Bioassay	Human males, 24-hr collection	458 ± 71	63
RIA	Human, 24-hr collection	554 ± 363	134
RIA	Human, nonretained urine	1,200	113
	Same urine after 3-hr incubation (37°C)	685 ± 437	
RIA	Human, 1-hr collection	690 ± 108	2
RIA	Dog, by ureterotomy, collected in alcohol	84 ± 15	Scicli et al. (*unpublished data*)
RIA	Rat, by ureterotomy, collected in alcohol	1.2–3	111

[a] Values are expressed as means ± SEM.

the kinins from other substances, e.g., catecholamines, acetylcholine, histamine, serotonin, substance P, and prostaglandins, that also affect the assay preparation and consequently obscure the interpretation of the kinin bioassay (41). Also, in many instances it is possible to render the assay structure insensitive to such interfering substances by the use of specific receptor blockers.

Assay of Kinins in Isolated
Smooth-Muscle Preparations

Trautschold has extensively reviewed the procedures that utilize isolated nonvascular smooth muscle to assay kinins (128). Bradykinin and related kinins bring about relaxation of the duodenum of the rat and the rectal cecum of the hen, but cause contraction of most other smooth-muscle preparations, including the ileum of the guinea pig, the uterus and the stomach of the rat, and the jejunum and the terminal ileum of the cat (104). Generally, these tissues are suspended in a small organ bath (5–10 ml) containing an appropriate nutrient fluid oxygenated with a gas mixture containing 95% O_2 and 5% CO_2 (136). Alternatively, the isolated tissues may be suspended and superfused by a stream of nutrient solution delivered continuously over the tissues (54). Changes in the tone of the smooth muscle are sensed by either mechanical or electrical (transducer) devices and are recorded. The superfusion technique permits arranging several strips from the same or from different organs in a cascade system superfused by the same stream of fluid. This, in turn, permits assay of an unknown sample simultaneously on several different assay organs (132).

The threshold concentration of bradykinin that contracts the isolated guinea pig ileum is in the range of 1 to 10 ng ml^{-1} (104). The responses are quite reproducible. However, the tissue is also contracted by several substances other than kinins, including prostaglandins, substance P, angiotensins, histamine, acetylcholine, and serotonin (64). Interference in the kinin assay by any of these agents can be prevented by adding the appropriate antagonist to the nutrient solution or by prior purification of the kinins.

The uterine horn taken from a rat pretreated with stilbestrol 18 hr before experimentation, suspended and bathed by either Tyrode or de Jalon solution at 29 to 31°C, is contracted by bradykinin and related kinins at a concentration as low as 0.1 ng ml^{-1} (104,128). A drawback to this preparation, however, is that the tissue is also sensitive to angiotensin II and to oxytocin. In addition, it exhibits marked seasonal variations in spontaneous contractility; excessive motility during spring contributes to make kinin assay a laborious task. Interestingly, the rat uterus can also be used to assay rat glandular kallikrein directly (17). The assay rests on the ability of kallikrein to evoke dose-related contraction of the uterine horn.

The duodenum of the rat is relaxed by bradykinin and related kinins in concentrations of 1 to 10 ng ml^{-1} (6). Epinephrine and norepinephrine also produce relaxation. In contrast, several other agents, including angiotensins, substance P, acetylcholine, and serotonin, bring about contraction of the tissue. It would appear, then, that the isolated duodenum of the rat, particularly when bathed or superfused with a nutrient solution containing α- and β-adrenoreceptor-blocking agents, is an adequate preparation for identification and assay of kinins in biological samples. A major drawback is the poor reproducibility of the kinin-evoked responses (11).

Longitudinal strips of cat jejunum, bathed or superfused with Krebs solution, respond to bradykinin and related kinins by contraction; the response is reproducible, and the threshold sensitivity is about 0.5 ng ml^{-1}. The sensitivity toward bradykinin of the cat jejunum bathed in Krebs solution increases with storage (18–48 hr) at 4°C. Acetylcholine also contracts the cat jejunum; but the smooth-muscle preparation is almost insensitive to other substances, including angiotensins, prostaglandins, histamine, serotonin, oxytocin, and substance P. Catecholamines cause relaxation of the cat jejunum; they also reduce the tissue's sensitivity to bradykinin (50).

The sensitivity of smooth-muscle preparations, including guinea pig ileum, rat uterus, and cat jejunum, toward bradykinin, but not toward other agonists, is greatly increased by transient exposure of the isolated tissues to chymotrypsin or to other proteolytic enzymes. The action of chymotrypsin in sensitizing the smooth muscle to bradykinin has been attributed to the uncovering of kinin receptors (44).

Because of its sensitivity and relative specificity toward bradykinin and related peptides, cat jejunum superfused with Krebs solution appears to be the most appropriate smooth-muscle preparation for assay of kinins in biological samples. The specificity of the bioassay can be further increased by the use of appropriate antagonists and by adding another assay organ, e.g., rat duodenum, to the superfusion cascade. Ferreira and Vane (50) successfully utilized strips of cat jejunum superfused with blood to monitor changes in blood kinin levels in the cat and dog. The blood was taken from a cannulated blood vessel, pumped at about 15 ml min^{-1} over the assay organs arranged in a cascade, collected in a reservoir, and then infused back into the animal. The cat jejunum superfused by blood contracted when the concentration of bradykinin in the blood increased by as little as 0.1 to 0.5 ng ml^{-1}.

Assay of Kinins by Their Effects on Blood
Pressure and Vascular Tone

When injected into the systemic circulation, the most conspicuous effects of kinins are lowering of arterial pressure and dilation of peripheral arterioles. These actions are the basis of several bioassay procedures that have been reviewed by Trautschold (128). In the rat pretreated with phenoxybenzamine and 2-mercaptoethanol, a bolus injection of bradykinin (10–100 ng) into the ascending aorta causes a dose-related fall in blood pressure. However, this procedure's usefulness in assaying kinins in biological samples appears to be limited, because the dose–response curve is quite flat, and the sensitivity is inadequate for assay of the small amounts of kinins present in biological fluids (103).

Kinins injected arterially are capable of reducing hindlimb vascular resistance (1,20,82). Assays that utilize this property are more sensitive than those mentioned earlier. Bradykinin injected as a bolus produces a dose-related reduction in perfusion pressure in dog and rabbit hindquarters perfused with their own blood by a pump (1,20). A modification of this preparation results in an easier bioassay procedure of improved simplicity, reliability, and sensitivity that permits assay of a large number of samples in a single preparation (82). Injected as a bolus into the femoral artery of a dog anesthetized with pentobarbital sodium, both bradykinin and lysyl-bradykinin bring about an increase in femoral blood flow, measured by an electromagnetic flowmeter. This increase subsides in about 80 sec. Increases in femoral blood flow produced by kinins are related to dosage (0.5–10 ng), and the steepest segment of the log dose–response curve is between 2.5 and 10 ng. Inhibition of kininase II by intravenous administration of the nonapeptide inhibitor SQ 20,881 enhances the sensitivity of the preparation and permits detection of as little as 0.10 ng of either bradykinin or lysyl-bradykinin.

The major drawback of these procedures is their lack of specificity. For example, several substances other than kinins, e.g., prostaglandins, histamine, substance P, and acetylcholine, also increase femoral blood flow in the dog. As previously indicated, these drawbacks can be overcome by appropriate extraction and purification of the sample prior to bioassay.

Radioimmunoassay

Induction of kinin antibodies is difficult because they have weak immunogenicity. Also, when kinins are injected, they are rapidly destroyed by kininases. In 1964, Goodfriend et al. (59) were the first to induce kinin antibodies by using bradykinin conjugated to albumin. They also reported an immunoassay for bradykinin employing inhibition of complement fixation; the sensitivity of this assay was only in the microgram range. In 1966, Spraag et al. (121) reported the first kinin RIA. Because labeled antigen ([³H]bradykinin) of relatively low specific activity was used, the sensitivity of this RIA was still low, on the order of nanograms. With the introduction of ^{125}I-labeled bradykinin analogs with high

specific activity, the sensitivity of the assay was increased to the level of picograms, thus allowing measurement of kinins in physiologic situations (49,58). The absence of a tyrosine ring in the native bradykinin required the use of tyrosine-bradykinin analogs for iodination of this peptide.

Because the various kinin RIAs reported are quite similar, we shall briefly describe one of them as well as some of the general principles it employs. For more details, the reader may refer to the report of Odya et al. (89).

Antisera

Antibodies against kinins have been produced by injecting rabbits with bradykinin or kallidin coupled with plasma albumin, ovalbumin, and thyroglobulin. Further, antibodies against kininogen have cross-reactivity with kinins, and some investigators have used these antibodies for RIA of kinins (30). In our own experience, immunization of rabbits with kallidin coupled with ovalbumin has produced a serum with a high antikinin titer (28). We had a rabbit that was injected with this complex for 16 months and produced antiserum that could be used in a final dilution of 1 : 360,000 to obtain 40 to 50% binding of approximately 10 pg of ^{125}I-Tyr-8-bradykinin. All antibodies against one of the kinins exhibited cross-reactivity with one of the other kinin analogs (bradykinin, kallidin, and Met-Lys-bradykinin) and with kininogen. The cross-reactivity with the kinin analog was not 1:1.

The antisera should be treated at 56 to 60°C for at least 30 min. This reduces the possibility of activation of plasma prekallikrein, which could generate kinins and interfere with the RIA.

Labeled Antigen

^{125}I-Tyr-8-bradykinin is the labeled antigen used most frequently; however, it has been shown that some antibodies have a higher affinity for either ^{125}I-Tyr-8-bradykinin or ^{125}I-Tyr-1-kallidin (89). Usually, the labeled antigen that gives 50% binding at the highest dilution of a particular antiserum is also the antigen that gives an RIA with the highest sensitivity. Tyrosine derivatives of bradykinin are iodinated using standard techniques such as the chloramine-T method (60). Purification of the iodinated kinin can be done by column chromatography with either CM-Sephadex C-25 or SP-Sephadex C-25 (108). In our experience, SP-Sephadex C-25 gives a better and faster separation.

Standard Plot

Care should be taken to avoid adsorption of labeled or unlabeled kinins to the test tube. To prevent adsorption, we performed the RIA in polystyrene tubes and used 0.1-M Tris–HCl buffer, pH 7.4, in which 0.2% gelatin and 0.1% neomycin had been added. In addition to the buffer, the incubation mixture contained ^{125}I-Tyr-8-bradykinin (approximately 3,000–5,000 cpm), antiserum in appropriate dilution, and kinin standard (10–500 pg or 2–100 μl) of the unknown sample in a final volume of 0.6 ml. However, the higher the amount of unknown sample, the greater the possibility of having substances that interfere with the antigen-antibody reaction. Usually, the samples are incubated at 4°C for 24 hr.

To separate bound and free labeled bradykinins, different procedures have been used, such as (a) precipitation of the antibody using ammonium sulfate, polyethylene glycol, double antibodies, and so on, (b) adsorption of antibody on solid-phase supports, or (c) adsorption of the free antigen in coated-charcoal suspension. In our experience, dextran-coated charcoal works well if the appropriate dilution of charcoal and time of adsorption are used (28). However, if antisera of low affinity are used, charcoal should not be used as a method of separation, because it could result in partial dissociation of the bound labeled hormone. Double antibody or polyethylene glycol would be the method of choice in this case. In our laboratory, this RIA can measure as little as 2 pg of kallidin or bradykinin in 100 μl of sample.

KALLIKREIN ASSAYS

Kininogenase Assay

Through this method, kallikrein is measured by its capacity to generate kinins when incubated with kininogen (kallikrein substrate) in vitro. The kinins generated are measured either by bioassay or RIA (the bioassay and RIA for kinins were described earlier). The method is not difficult, but requires the following precautions:

1. The kininase activity of the substrate and of the fluid containing the enzyme should be inhibited. This is accomplished by the use of 1,10-phenanthroline and EDTA.
2. In the collection of blood for substrate preparation, activation of the plasma prekallikrein should be prevented by using siliconized or plastic material and by avoiding cooling or dilution of the blood. Because it has been demonstrated that heparin is an inhibitor of kallikrein (10), it is not advisable to use it as an anticoagulant unless the kininogen of the plasma is to be further purified, thus removing the heparin from the preparation. If the plasma substrate is used without extensive purification, it should be treated at 58°C for 2 to 3 hr. This procedure inactivates not only part of the plasma kininases but also the kallikrein inhibitors and the plasma prekallikrein.

3. To measure the activity of any enzyme, it is very important to use initial velocity, and kallikrein is not an exception. If enough substrate is used, the reaction is usually linear for 60 min. Kininogen should be used in a concentration sufficient to produce zero-order reaction or at least high enough that the velocity of the reaction does not change during the incubation time. Further, it is important to carry out the reaction close to the optimum pH of the enzyme (pH 8.5), because the velocity of the reaction decreases significantly at a lower pH (135). Kininogen blanks should be run simultaneously, because the kininogen interferes with the kinin RIA, and also, because of contamination with plasma kallikrein and/or other kininogenases, the preparations of kininogen alone sometimes generate kinins.
4. Siliconized glassware should be used, because the kinins generated are easily adsorbed to glass and also to some types of plastic. If kallikrein is being measured in renal tissue, it is important that the homogenized tissues be frozen and thawed repeatedly or treated with detergents such as deoxycholic acid to release the kallikrein bound to the membranes (85). The latter method, in our experience, has yielded satisfactory results (29,110).

The kininogenase methods are very sensitive; only 1 to 100 μl of urine, depending on the species, or 1 to 100 mg of renal tissue is necessary for incubation with the substrate to generate sufficient amounts of kinin for measurement by RIA or bioassay. However, it should be remembered that other enzymes generate kinins at alkaline pH, such as plasma kallikrein, plasmin, and trypsin. Further, the specificity of the kininogenase assay to measure kallikrein depends greatly on the method used to measure the kinins generated, the RIA being more specific than the bioassays (vide supra).

Direct RIA for Enzymic Protein

Several RIAs for direct measurement of urinary kallikrein have been reported (26,51,71,73,86,95,116,117). In these RIAs, rabbit or sheep antiserum against purified urinary kallikrein and ^{125}I-kallikrein is used. The purification of the enzyme is done by using ion-exchange (DEAE cellulose), affinity (Trasylol-Sepharose), and Sephadex G-100 chromatography (96). The iodination of the kallikrein is done with chloramine-T. Sheep antirabbit gamma globulin or polyethylene glycol is used to separate the free from bound ^{125}I-kallikrein. These RIAs are sensitive to 8 to 50 pg of pure kallikrein, and they are highly specific for glandular kallikrein. This assay is not devoid of problems, and inhibitors of kallikrein interfere with it. For example, if Trasylol (aprotinin) is added to urine, the values obtained by direct RIA are three times higher than those for urine to which the inhibitors have not been added (99,100). Blood added to urine also interferes with the direct RIA. These findings suggest that plasma and tissue inhibitors of kallikrein interfere with the binding of antigen to the antibody. Benzamidine, a low-molecular-weight inhibitor (MW 157), does not interfere, suggesting that the antigenic site is not the same as the active site of the enzyme. When urinary kallikrein was measured by the direct RIA and by the kininogenase method in 11 different dilutions of pure kallikrein ranging from 100 ng to 100 μg ml^{-1}, the correlation coefficient between the results obtained by these methods was $r = 0.98$. Similarly, strong correlation was observed between the results obtained by the direct RIA and the kininogenase method in urine of rats in different experimental situations ($r = 0.90$). However, when urinary kallikrein was measured in rats bred to be susceptible to the hypertensive effect of salt (Dahl rats) by the direct RIA and by the kininogenase method, the correlation coefficient was only $r = 0.53$. Further, the ratios (direct RIA/kininogenase) obtained when kallikrein was measured by these two methods were 1.0 with pure kallikrein, 0.8 to 1.3 with urine of normal rats, and 6.0 with urine of S rats. This, in addition to the fact that S rats have significant proteinuria (plasma inhibitors?), suggests that inhibitors of kallikrein could affect the results obtained with these two methods in an opposite manner in certain experimental situations. Furthermore, the kininogenase assay measures only active kallikrein, whereas the direct assay can measure both active and inactive kallikrein (prekallikrein and/or kallikrein bound to an inhibitor) (26,100).

RIAs that directly measure immunoreactive glandular kallikrein have been applied to measure the antigen in plasma or serum. In some of these assays the displacement of the tracer produced by different aliquots of plasma did not parallel the displacement produced by kallikrein standards (51,71,86), whereas in others, parallelism to standard displacement was always seen (118,127). The lack of parallelism between the plasma dilution curves and the standard curve may be due to kallikrein inhibitors present in plasma, and it can be corrected by inactivating the tracer with phenylmethyl-sulfonyl fluoride (101).

Immunoradiometric Assay

This excess-antibody assay is based on coupling an antikallikrein antibody to a solid phase. Kallikrein in the sample or standard is bound to the immobilized antibody. In a second incubation step, kallikrein is determined immunologically by adding iodinated antikallikrein antibody or enzymatically by adding a kallikrein substrate (65,66). Because the specificity of this assay depends on the specificity of the antibody, interference of cross-reacting antigens can be overcome by preadsorption of the antibody. In addition, because this assay allows for measurement of the enzymatic activity of kallikrein bound to the immobilized antikallikrein

antibody, the specificity of the method is highly enhanced. The sensitivity of this assay ranges from 0.3 to 1.7 ng/ml, the sample dilution curves are parallel to the standard curve, and the recovery of added kallikrein is 100%. All these assay characteristics make this method one of the best for measurement of kallikrein.

Esterolytic and Amidolytic Assays

Esterolytic Assays

Of the methods described for measuring kallikrein activity, the most widely used because of their simplicity are the esterolytic assays. Esters having the general formula R-Arg-O-X are used as substrates; R is an acyl group such as benzoyl or tosyl, and X consists of methyl or ethyl groups. When proteases such as kallikrein cleave one of these esters, the alcohol is released and an acid is formed. Therefore, the hydrolysis of the ester can be followed by measuring (a) the change in optical density when the molar extinction coefficient of the liberated acid is higher than that of the ester, as is the case for benzoyl arginine ethyl ester (BAEE, spectrophotometric method), (b) the liberated alcohol, (c) the liberated acid, and (d) the unhydrolyzed ester.

Spectrophotometric method. The optimum hydrolysis of BAEE by kallikrein occurs at pH 8.5. At 253 nm, the molar extinction coefficients for BAEE and benzoyl arginine are 2.3×10^{-3} and 3.45×10^{-3}, respectively. Detailed descriptions of this method can be found in previous publications (109,129,137).

Measurement of esterase activity by liberated alcohol. Basically, three methods are being used to measure the liberated alcohol. Trautschold et al. (129) have used alcohol dehydrogenase to reduce the ethanol liberated from BAEE with NAD (nicotinamide adenine dinucleotide) as a proton acceptor. The reduced NAD shows increased absorbance at 366 nm. Colman et al. (37) have developed a colorimetric assay for determination of kallikrein activity. In this method, methanol released from α-N-tosyl-L-arginine methyl ester (TAME) is quantitated by a modification of the method of Siegelman et al. (119). A third method employs [^{3}H]TAME labeled in the methyl group of the alcohol moiety (12). This sensitive method is similar to that developed by Roffman et al. (105) for measuring trypsin esterase activity. The isotopic method depends on the partitioning of liberated [^{3}H]methanol and the substrate TAME by their differential solubilities in the aqueous and toluene phases of a scintillation-counting solution. TAME is insoluble in toluene, and in the absence of an agent that will enhance its solubility, it will not be counted, because it will remain in the aqueous phase. This method is fairly simple and, after careful standardization, reproducible. Because of its high sensitivity, human urine can be tested without prior concentration.

Titrimetric assay of liberated acid. Titration of the liberated acid is an accurate technique for measuring esterase activity. Nustad et al. (87) selected a pH of 8 and a temperature of 25°C to conduct their titrimetric analysis, probably because optimum substrate concentration can be maintained under these conditions. Nustad and Pierce (88) used 0.01-M NaOH in an automatic titrator to determine the acid released by the esterase. The low sensitivity and the need for an automatic titrator are this method's drawback.

Determination of unhydrolyzed ester. The colorimetric means of detecting organic esters was first introduced by Feigl as a spot test (48) and later as a quantitative test by Hestrin (62). The test involves measurement of the amount of ester remaining after incubation with a test sample. The unhydrolyzed ester, after treatment with alkaline hydroxylamine, is treated with ferric chloride. The arginine iron hydroxamate formed absorbs at 525 nm.

Roberts (102) introduced TCA to precipitate proteins and terminate the reaction. He also changed the relative composition of the reactant, thus optimizing the conditions for reading the color developed. Nustad and Pierce (88) have standardized this method and given very precise concentrations and times for each step in measurement of rat urinary kallikrein. The esterase activity in human urine is relatively low, and this method is not sensitive enough to detect it, although this can be overcome by concentrating the urine prior to assay.

Amidolytic Assays

With partial or complete elucidation of the primary structures of many serine proteases and identification of proteolytic cleavage sites, a number of synthetic peptide substrates mimicking the amino acid sequences adjacent to proteolytic activation cleavage have been developed in recent years. One example is the peptide N-α-benzoyl-L-proline-L-phenylalanine-L-arginine-p-nitroanilide, in which the chromophore p-nitroanilide (PNA) is attached to the peptide in amide linkage. This peptide represents the amino acid sequence at the carboxyl end of bradykinin. Kallikrein will cleave the amido bond and release PNA, which has a yellow color, in contrast to the colorless substrate. Thus, reaction rates can be obtained using a recording spectrophotometer at 405 nm. Working with 1 mM substrate, Amundsen et al. (7) were able to detect as little as 10 ng of plasma kallikrein with 30 min of incubation. Mattler and Bang (77) determined that other proteases that are kininogenases, such as trypsin and plasmin, also showed amidolytic activity toward the tripeptide, whereas nonkininogenases such as thrombin and factor X had poor catalytic capacity. Amundsen et al. (7) claimed that bovine pancreatic kallikrein, a glandular kallikrein that is a powerful esterase, was virtually devoid of amidolytic activity against the peptide. In contrast, Halabi and Baek (61), using β-Phe-Val-Arg-PNA, found that hog pancreatic kallikrein has good amidolytic properties with a calculated K_m of 2.2×10^{-4} M. The best substrate for glandular kallikrein appears to be H-D-Val-Leu-Arg-PNA (S-2266, Kabi).

The amidolytic assays are relatively specific because the amino acid residues preceding the scissile bond (P_2 and P_3 sites) are of importance in the interaction of enzymes and substrates (21). Zimmerman (138) used peptide amides of 7-amino-4-methyl coumarin (MCA) as a sensitive substrate for assay of chymotrypsin. This assay method is more sensitive than the chromogenic assay because the 7-amino-4-MCA group is highly fluorescent (138). Based on the same premise, a peptidyl-MCA substrate used to measure kallikrein has been synthesized by Morita et al. (81). These authors have shown that glandular kallikrein readily releases MCA from Pro-Phe-Arg-MCA. This is a better substrate for glandular than for plasma kallikrein, as evidenced by the 10-fold higher V_{max}/K_m for urinary kallikrein (81). The substrate is first dissolved in dimethyl sulfoxide (DMSO) and then diluted to give a final concentration of 0.1 mM, using 0.05 M Tris–HCl buffer, pH 8.0, containing 0.1 M NaCl and 0.01 M CaCl$_2$. The enzyme activity can be measured by either the initial-rate method or the end-point method. The amount of MCA liberated is measured with excitation at 380 mm and emission at 460 nm. The fluorescence spectrophotometer is standardized so that a 0.01-mM solution of MCA in 0.1% DMSO gives 1.0 relative fluorescence unit.

Another very sensitive substrate to measure glandular kallikrein has been shown to be the dipeptide ester Ac-Phe-Arg-O ethanol, which is 40 times more sensitive than H-D-Val-Leu-Arg-PNA (S-2266, Kabi). The drawback in using this substrate is the need for a coupled enzymatic determination of the ethyl alcohol (47). Chung et al. (33) have developed an extremely sensitive assay for urinary kallikrein using H-Pro-Phe-Arg-[³H]anilide or H-Pro-Phe-Arg-[³H-benzylamide]. For comparative purposes, using human urinary kallikrein, Claeson and Aurell (35) reported that K_{cat}/K_m for H-Pro-Phe-Arg-[³H]anilide was $3,700 \times 10^5$, and for H-Pro-Phe-Arg-MCA, 1×10^5.

Comments

With the introduction of synthetic esters such as BAEE and TAME, purified preparations of serine proteases can be rapidly characterized without performance of tedious assays. However, the lack of specificity seen with esterolytic assays is a major disadvantage when glandular kallikrein activities are being measured in biological fluids or tissues. This lack of specificity should be carefully evaluated when renal and/or urinary kallikreins are estimated through any of the esterase methods.

Esterase assays should not be used to measure glandular kallikrein in tissues, because tissue esterase activity does not always correlate with kininogenase activity (8,23). Furthermore, because alkaline esterases other than kallikrein have been reported in rat (88,96) and dog urine (79), these assays are not convenient for accurate determination of urinary kallikrein excretion in these species.

Data on the existence of more than one alkaline esterase in human urine conflict. Moriya et al. (80) reported the presence of only one esterase in human urine. However, Geiger et al. (57) noted a sharp fall in the ratio of esterase to kinin-generated activity during purification, implying the presence of esterase with nonkininogenase activity, and Ole-Moi Yoi et al. (91) found that almost 40% of the esterase activity in human urine was due to enzymes other than kallikrein. Thus, regardless of which esterolytic method is used, alkaline esterase activity in human urine may not be synonymous with kallikrein activity.

There are available a number of very sensitive assays using peptide-derived substrates that can be used to measure glandular kallikreins. These substrates resemble short amino acid sequences in the natural enzyme's substrate. However, when one goes from the large natural substrate to the small synthetic peptide, one loses many interaction sites that have roles in determining specificity. Thus, small synthetic substrates may be preferentially cleaved by a particular enzyme, such as glandular kallikrein, but other proteases able to cleave arginine peptide bonds could also release the chromophore group from the short peptide chain. It is because of this potential interference that the use of peptide amides or peptide esters to measure glandular kallikrein in biological fluids (which may contain other proteases, such as urine, saliva, or tissue homogenates) should always be preceded by validation of the specificity of the assay.

It is possible that further development of the PNA derivatives or the fluorogenic substrates (81) will provide an artificial substrate specific for glandular kallikrein. In the meantime, in order to avoid acquisition of data that may be misleading, more accurate and more specific methods than esterase or amidolytic assays alone should be used to measure kallikrein in biological samples.

KININOGEN ASSAYS

Total Kininogen Assays

Total kininogen in plasma has been indirectly determined by fully releasing the bradykinin moiety with a kininogenase such as trypsin, pancreatic kallikrein, or snake venom and then measuring the free peptide. For accurate results when using this method, the following are important: (a) Inhibitors of kininogenases should be eliminated from the plasma, because they will impair the action of enzyme. (b) Kininase activity should be absent. (c) Precautions should be taken to avoid activation of plasma kallikrein. (d) The kininogenase should be capable of releasing all available kinins from the kininogens.

The most commonly used method to determine kininogen in plasma was published by Dinitz and Carvalho (43). Through this method, plasma inhibitors of kininogenase, plasma prekallikrein, and kininases are destroyed by acidification (pH 3.8) and 30 min of boiling. All the kinins present in 0.2 ml of plasma are released from kininogen by incubation with 200 μg of trypsin for 30 min. Trypsin activity is then destroyed by adding hot alcohol and heating the mixture for 10 min at 70°C. The extract is dried and reconstituted, and bradykinin is assayed.

A slightly different method was published by Fasciolo et al. (46), who accomplished the destruction of plasmatic trypsin inhibitors, prekallikrein, and kininases by diluting the plasma 35-fold and placing it in a boiling-water bath for 3 min. All the kinins from plasmatic kininogen are released by incubation for 30 min with 0.5 mg of trypsin. The trypsin is then destroyed by boiling, and the free kinins are measured without further extraction. In our experience, this method has proved to be both fast and accurate.

Because incubation of plasma with trypsin induces the generation of potentiating peptides, these assays may overestimate kininogen when kinins are measured by bioassay.

Low- and High-Molecular-Weight Kininogen Assay

Whereas the methods previously described measure only total kininogen, Uchida et al. (130) have described a method by which both low- and high-molecular-weight kininogens can be determined. They base their method on the fact that plasma kallikrein releases bradykinin only from high-molecular-weight kininogen. Plasma kallikrein is activated with glass beads in the absence of peptidase inhibitors; so the plasmatic peptidases will destroy all the released kinins. After destroying peptidases by acidification at pH 2, further incubation with trypsin or a glandular kallikrein will release kinins only from the remnant low-molecular-weight kininogen. Simultaneously, total kininogen is also measured in another sample following Dinitz and Carvalho. Subtracting low-molecular-weight kininogen values from total kininogen will give the concentration of high-molecular-weight kininogen. These results can be confirmed by incubating plasma with glass beads in the presence of the peptidase inhibitor 1,10-phenanthroline. The disadvantage is that this method depends on normal levels of Hageman factor and prekallikrein.

RIA

RIAs for high- and low-molecular-weight kininogens have been developed using antibodies raised against highly purified kininogens of high and low molecular masses (3,69,98,124). These assays are sensitive, accurate, and reproducible and allow for measurement of several samples simultaneously. However, if part of the antibodies to high- or low-molecular-weight kininogens are directed to antigenic determinants on the heavy chain of the kininogen molecule, they will react with both high- and low-molecular-weight kininogens. In this case the antiserum needs to be adsorbed with low-molecular-weight kininogen to become specific for high-molecular-weight kininogen or with high-molecular-weight kininogen to recognize only low-molecular-weight kininogen. In addition, because the antibody may recognize kinin-free kininogen and antigenic fragments, these RIAs may overestimate kininogen.

KININASE ASSAYS

Assay of Total Kininase Activity

Because cleavage at any of the peptide bonds of the bradykinin molecule inactivates the peptide, an assay has been devised in which a given amount of bradykinin is incubated with a test solution for a known period of time. The reaction is then stopped by heating, acidification, or denaturation with alcohol, and the residual kinins are measured (34,67).

Assay of Kininase I

Kininase I is a carboxypeptidase called carboxypeptidase N or arginin carboxypeptidase. It has also been identified as an anaphylotoxin inactivator, because it cleaves the C-terminal Ala-Arg sequence of C3a anaphylotoxin. This enzyme hydrolyzes hippuryl-L-argininic acid, allowing its activity to be measured using the method of Folk et al. (52), which is based on the difference in absorbance of hippuric acid and hippuryl-L-arginine or lysine at 254 μm. Oshima et al. (94) reported that the reaction follows zero-order kinetics until 40% of the substrate is destroyed.

Assay of Kininase II

Several methods have been developed for measuring kininase II, otherwise known as converting enzyme. The most commonly used assay method was described by Cushman and Cheung (40), who measured the amount of p-hippuric acid released from hippuryl-histidyl-leucine by an increase in absorbance at 228 nm. This assay is not affected by chymotrypsin or aminopeptidases and is reproducible with careful timing of the various steps. The sensitivity of the method can be improved by working with [³H]hippuryl-glycyl-glycine, as described by Ryan et al. (106). Other methods described to

measure kininase II include (a) measuring the conversion rate of angiotensin I to angiotensin II with a specific RIA (19), (b) measuring ¹²⁵I-Tyr-8-bradykinin (32), and (c) fluorimetrically measuring the histidyl-leucine released from a phenyl-histidyl-leucyl substrate (97). All these methods have been proved adequate for measurement of kininase II in plasma or biological fluids.

Odya et al. (90) and Alhenc-Gelas et al. (4) have reported direct RIAs for hog and human converting enzyme, and Lanzillo and Fanburg (70) have developed a competitive enzyme-linked immunoassay (CELIA) for human serum-converting enzyme. One major advantage of these methods is that they can be used to measure the enzyme level in the presence of endogenous or therapeutically administered inhibitors.

Assay of Neutral Metalloendopeptidase

A neutral metalloendopeptidase (NEP) recently purified from human kidney cleaves bradykinin by releasing the C-terminal dipeptide (4,56). Although the K_m of bradykinin is lower with kininase II than with NEP, NEP has a 10-fold higher turnover number (56). The importance of this NEP for in vivo degradation of kinins is now being investigated. Ura et al. (131) in our laboratory have studied the participation of NEP in the metabolism of urinary kinins in vitro and in vivo. NEP was responsible for 68% of the total kininase activity of urine, and kininase I and II contributed 9% and 23%. When NEP was inhibited in vivo by infusing phosphoramidon, total kininase activity of urine decreased 77%, and urinary kinin excretion increased 73%. NEP activity could be determined either with Hip-Arg-Arg-Leu-2-naphthylamide or Glu-Ala-Ala-Phe-4-methoxy-2-naphthylamide in a two-step procedure (93). With Glu-Ala-Ala-Phe-4-methoxy-2-naphthylamide as substrate, the reaction involves cleavage of the substrate at the Ala-Phe bond to release 4-methoxy-2-naphthylamide (Phe-MNA). This product is then hydrolyzed by addition of an excess of aminopeptidase M to release the fluorescent product MNA. NEP activity in tissue homogenates is measured in a reaction mixture of 0.1-M 2-(N-morpholino)ethanesulfonic acid buffer with 0.1% Triton X-100, pH 6.5. Free MNA is measured fluorometrically at an excitation wavelength of 340 nm and an emission wavelength of 425 nm (68). The specificity of the reaction is determined by adding phosphoramidon, an inhibitor of NEP, to the reaction mixture (68).

ACKNOWLEDGMENTS

Supported in part by NIH grants HL-28982, HL-15839, and HL-18579.

Published in part in *Modern Pharmacology-Toxicology,* Vol. 19, Marcel Dekker, 1982, and in *Primary Hypertension,* Springer-Verlag, 1986. Reproduced with permission from the publishers.

REFERENCES

1. Abe, K., Mouri, T., Seki, T., Suzuki, M., Takano, T., and Yoshinaga, K., (1968): An improved bioassay method for kinins. *Experientia,* 24:455–457.
2. Abe, K., Irokawa, H., Yasujima, M., Seino, M., Chiba, S., Sakurai, Y., Yoshinaga, K., and Saito, K. T. (1978): The kallikrein-kinin system and prostaglandins in the kidney: Their relation to furosemide-induced diuresis and to the renin-angiotensin-aldosterone system in man. *Circ. Res.,* 43:254–260.
3. Adam, A., Albert, A., Calay, G., Closset, J., Damas, J., and Franchimont, P. (1985): Human kininogens of low and high molecular mass: Quantification by radioimmunoassay and determination of reference values. *Clin. Chem.,* 31:423–426.
4. Alhenc-Gelas, F., Weare, J. A., Johnson, R. L., and Erdos, E. G. (1983): Measurement of human converting enzyme level by direct radioimmunoassay. *J. Lab. Clin. Med.,* 101:83–96.
5. Almenoff, J., and Orlowski, M. (1983): Membrane-bound kidney metalloendopeptidase: Interaction with synthetic substrates, neutral peptides, and inhibitors. *Biochemistry,* 22:590–599.
6. Antonio, A. (1968): The relaxing effect of bradykinin on intestinal smooth muscle. *Br. J. Pharmacol.,* 32:78–86.
7. Amundsen, E., Svenosen, L., Vennerod, A. M., and Laake, K. (1974): Determination of plasma kallikrein with a new chromogenic tripeptide derivative. In: *Chemistry and Biology of the Kallikrein-Kinin System in Health and Disease,* edited by J. J. Pisano and K. F. Austen, pp. 215–270. U.S. Government Printing Office, Washington, D.C.
8. Arens, S. A., and Haberland, G. L. (1977): Determination of kallikrein activity in animal tissues, using biochemical methods. In: *Kininogenases,* edited by G. L. Haberland, J. W. Rohen, and T. Suzuki, pp. 43–53. Schattauer-Verlag, Stuttgart.
9. Ashley, P. L., and MacDonald, R. J. (1985): Kallikrein-related mRNAs of the rat submaxillary gland: Nucleotide sequences of four distinct types including tonin. *Biochemistry,* 24:4512–4520.
10. Back, H., and Steger, R. (1970): Effect of heparin on the kinin-forming activity of trypsin, plasmin, and various kallikreins. *Proc. Soc. Exp. Biol. Med.,* 133:740–743.
11. Barabe, J., Park, W. K., and Regoli, D. (1975): Application of drug receptor theories to the analysis of the myotropic effects of bradykinin. *Can. J. Physiol. Pharmacol.,* 53:345–353.
12. Beaven, V. N., Pierce, J. V., and Pisano, J. J. (1971): A sensitive isotopic procedure for the assay of esterase activity: Measurement of human urinary kallikrein. *Clin. Chim. Acta,* 32:67–73.
13. Bell, G. I., Quinto, C., Quiroga, M., Valenzuela, P., Craik, C. S., and Rutter, W. J. (1984): Isolation and sequence of a rat chymotrypsin B gene. *J. Biol. Chem.,* 259:14265–14270.
14. Beierwaltes, W. H., Prada, J., and Carretero, O. A. (1985): Effect of glandular kallikrein on renin release in isolated rat glomeruli. *Hypertension,* 7:27–31.
15. Beraldo, W. T., Araujo, R. L., and Mares-Guia, M. (1966): Oxytocic esterase in rat urine. *Am. J. Physiol.,* 211:975–980.
16. Beraldo, W. T., Lauar, N. S., Siqueira, G., Heneine, I. F., and Catanzaro, O. L. (1976): Peculiarities of the oxytocic action of rat urinary kallikrein. In: *Chemistry and Biology of the Kallikrein-Kinin System in Health and Disease,* edited by J. J. Pisano and K. F. Austen, pp. 375–378. Fogarty International Center Proceedings, Washington, D.C.
17. Beraldo, W. T., Siqueira, G., Rodriguez, J. A., and Machado, C. R. S. (1972): Changes in kallikrein activity of rat submandibular gland during post-natal development. In: *Advances in Experimental Medicine and Biology, Vol. 21,* edited by F. Sicuteri and N. Back, pp. 239–250. Plenum, New York.
18. Berger, E. A., and Shooter, E. M. (1977): Evidence for pro-β-nerve growth factor, a biosynthetic precursor to β-nerve growth factor. *Proc. Natl. Acad. Sci. (USA),* 74:3647–3651.
19. Bing, J., Poulson, K., and Markussen, J. (1974): The ability of various insulins and insulin fragments to inhibit the angiotensin I converting enzyme. *Acta Pathol. Microbiol. Scand.,* 82:777–782.
20. Binia, A., Fasciolo, J. C., and Carretero, O. A. (1963): A method for the estimation of bradykinin in blood. *Acta Physiol. Lat. Am.,* 13:101–109.
21. Blomback, B. (1970): Selectional trends in the structure of fibrinogen of different species. In: *The Hemostatic Mechanism in Man and Other Animals,* edited by R. G. MacFarlane, pp. 167–187. Academic Press, New York.
22. Bothwell, M. A., Wilson, W. H., and Shooter, E. M. (1979): The relationship between glandular kallikrein and growth factor-processing proteases of mouse submaxillary gland. *J. Biol. Chem.,* 254:7287–7294.
23. Brandtzaeg, P., Gautvik, K. M., Hustad, K., and Pierce, J. V. (1976): Rat submandibular gland kallikreins: Purification and cellular localization. *Br. J. Pharmacol.,* 56:155–167.
24. Brocklehurst, W. E., and Zeitlin, I. J. (1967): Determination of plasma kinin and kininogen levels in man. *J. Physiol. (Lond.),* 191:417–426.
25. Cardin, A. D., Witt, K. R., Chao, J., Margolius, H. S., Donaldson, V. H., and Jackson, R. L. (1984): Degradation of apolipoprotein B-100 of human plasma low density lipoproteins by tissue and plasma kallikreins. *J. Biol. Chem.,* 259:8522–8528.
26. Carretero, O. A., Amin, V. M., Ocholik, T., Scicli, A. G., and Koch, J. (1978): Urinary kallikrein in rats bred for their susceptibility and resistance to the hypertensive effect of salt: A new radioimmunoassay for its direct determination. *Circ. Res.,* 42: 727–731.
27. Carretero, O. A., and Beierwaltes, W. H. (1984): Effect of glandular kallikrein, kinins and aprotinin (a serine protease inhibitor) on renin release. *J. Hypert. [Suppl. 1],* 2:125–130.
28. Carretero, O. A., Oza, N. V., Piwonska, A., Ocholik, T., and Scicli, A. G. (1976): Measurement of urinary kallikrein activity by kinin radioimmunoassay. *Biochem. Pharmacol.,* 25:2265–2270.
29. Carretero, O. A., Oza, N. B., Scicli, A. G., and Schork, A. (1974): Renal tissue kallikrein, plasma renin and plasma aldosterone in renal hypertension. *Acta Physiol. Lat. Am.,* 24:448–452.
30. Carretero, O. A., and Scicli, A. G. (1978): The renal kallikrein-kinin system in human and in experimental hypertension. *Klin. Wochenschr. [Suppl. 1],* 56:113–125.
31. Chao, J., Shimamoto, K., and Margolius, H. S. (1981): Kallikrein-induced uterine contaction independent of kinin formation. *Proc. Natl. Acad. Sci. (USA),* 78:6154–6157.
32. Chiu, A. T., Ryan, J. W., and Ryan, V. (1975): A sensitive radiochemical assay for angiotensin converting enzyme (kininase II). *Biochem. J.,* 149:297–300.
33. Chung, A., Ryan, S. W., Pena, G., and Oza, N. B. (1978): A simple radioassay for human urinary kallikrein. In: *Kinins II: Biochemistry, Pathophysiology, and Clinical Aspects,* edited by S. Fuji, H. Moriya, and T. Suzuki, pp. 115–125. Plenum Press, New York.
34. Cicilini, M. A., Caldo, H., Berti, J. D., and Camargo, A. (1977): Rabbit tissue peptidases that hydrolyze the peptide hormone bradykinin. *Biochem. J.,* 163:433–439.
35. Claeson, G., and Aurell, L. (1981): Small synthetic peptides with affinity for proteases in coagulation and fibrino lysis: An overview. *Ann. N.Y. Acad. Sci.,* 370:798–811.
36. Colman, R. W. (1980): Patho-physiology of the kallikrein system. *Ann. Clin. Lab. Sci.,* 10:220–226.
37. Colman, R. W., Mason, J. W., and Sherry, S. (1969): The kallikreinogen-kallikrein enzyme system of human plasma. Assay of components and observations in disease states. *Ann. Intern. Med.,* 71:763–773.
38. Craik, C. S., Choo, Q. L., Swift, G. H., Quinto, C., MacDonald, R. J., and Rutter, W. J. (1984): Structure of two related rat pancreatic trypsin genes. *J. Biol. Chem.,* 259:14255–14264.
39. Currie, M. G., Geller, D. M., Chao, J., Margolius, H. S., and Needleman, P. (1984): Kallikrein activation of a high molecular weight atrial peptide. *Biochem. Biophys. Res. Commun.,* 120: 461–466.
40. Cushman, D. W., and Cheung, H. S. (1971): Spectrophotometric assay and properties of the angiotensin-converting enzyme of rabbit lung. *Biochem. Pharmacol.,* 20:1637–1648.
41. Dale, H. H. (1912): The anaphylactic reaction of plain muscle in the guinea pig. *J. Pharmacol. Exp. Ther.,* 4:167–223.
42. Derkx, F. H. M., Tan-Tjiong, H. L., Man In't Veld, A. J., Schalekamp, M. P. A., and Schalekamp, M. A. H. (1979): Activation of inactive plasma renin by tissue kallikreins. *J. Clin. Endocrinol. Metab.,* 49:765–769.

43. Dinitz, C. R., and Carvalho, I. F. (1963): A micromethod for determination of bradykininogen under several conditions. *Ann. N.Y. Acad. Sci.,* 104:77–89.

44. Edery, H., and Abraham, Z. (1976): An improved preparation for determination of bradykinin. In: *Advances in Experimental Medicine and Biology, Vol. 70,* edited by F. Sicuteri, N. Back, and G. L. Haberland, pp. 103–107. Plenum, New York.

45. Evans, B. A., and Richards, R. I. (1985): Genes for the α and γ subunits of mouse nerve growth factor are contiguous. *EMBO Journal,* 4:133–138.

46. Fasciolo, J. C., Espada, J., and Carretero, O. A. (1963): The estimation of bradykininogen content of the plasma. *Acta Physiol. Lat. Am.,* 13:215–220.

47. Fiedler, F., Geiger, C., Hirschauer, C. and Leysath, G. (1978): Peptide esters and nitroanilides as substrates for the assay of human urinary kallikrein. *Hoppe Seylers Z. Physiol. Chem.,* 259: 1667–1673.

48. Feigl, F., Anger, V., and Frehden, O. (1934): Ueber die Verwendung von tupfel Reaktionen zum Nachweiss von organischen Verbildungen. *Mikrochemie,* 15:9.

49. Fejes-Toth, G., Naray Fejes-Toth, A., and Frölich, J. C. (1984): Measurements of urinary kinins by HPLC-radioimmunoassay. *Clin. Chim. Acta,* 140:21–29.

50. Ferreira, S. H., and Vane, J. R. (1967): The detection and estimation of bradykinin in the circulating blood. *Br. J. Pharmacol.,* 29:267–277.

51. Fink, E., Seifert, J., and Güttel, C. (1978): Development of a radioimmunoassay for pig pancreatic kallikrein and its application in physiological studies. *Fresenius Z. Anal. Chem.,* 240:183.

52. Folk, J. E., Piez, K. E., Carroll, W., and Gladner, S. A. (1960): Carboxypeptidase B. Purification and characterization of the porcine enzyme. *J. Biol. Chem.,* 235:2272–2277.

53. Frey, P., Forand, R., Maciag, T., and Shooter, E. M. (1979): The biosynthetic precursor of epidermal growth factor and the mechanism of its processing. *Proc. Natl. Acad. Sci. (USA),* 76:6294–6298.

54. Gaddum, J. H. (1953): The technique of superfusion. *Br. J. Pharmacol. Chemother.,* 8:321–326.

55. Gaddum, J. H. (1959): Measurement of epinephrine, norepinephrine, and related compounds: Bioassay procedures. *Pharmacol. Rev.,* 11:241–249.

56. Gafford, J. T., Skidgel, R. A., Erdös, E. G., and Hersh, L. B. (1983): Human kidney "enkephalinase." A neutral metalloendopeptidase that cleaves active peptides. *Biochemistry,* 22:3265–3271.

57. Geiger, R., Mann, K., and Bettels, T. (1977): Isolation of human urinary kallikrein by affininty chromatography. Determination of human urinary kallikrein. *J. Clin. Chem. Clin. Biochem.,* 15: 479–483.

58. Goodfriend, T. L., and Ball, D. L. (1969): Radioimmunoassay of bradykinin chemical modification to enable use of radioactive iodine. *J. Lab. Clin. Med.,* 73:501–511.

59. Goodfriend, T. L., Levine, L., and Fasman, G. (1964): Antibodies to bradykinin and angiotensin: A use of carbodiimides in immunology. *Science,* 144:1344–1346.

60. Greenwood, D. L., and Hunter, W. M. (1963): The preparation of [131I]labeled growth hormone of high specific activity. *Biochem. J.,* 89:114–118.

61. Halabi, M., and Baek, N. (1977): Kinetic studies with serine proteases and protease inhibitors utilizing a synthetic nitro amilide chromogenic substrate. In: *Kininogenases,* edited by G. L. Haberland, J. W. Rohen, and T. Suzuki, pp. 35–46. Schattauer-Verlag, Stuttgart.

62. Hestrin, S. (1949): The reaction of acetylcholine and other carboxylic acid derivatives with hydroxylamine and its analytical application. *J. Biol. Chem.,* 180:240–255.

63. Hial, V., Keiser, H. R., and Pisano, J. J. (1976): Origin and content of methyonil-lysil-bradykinin, lysil-bradykinin and bradykinin in human urine. *Biochem. Pharmacol.,* 25:2499–2503.

64. Hulthen, U. L., and Borge, T. (1976): Determination of bradykinin by a sensitive radioimmunoassay. *Scand. J. Clin. Lab. Invest.,* 36:833–839.

65. Johansen, L., Nustad, K., Orstavik, T. B., Ugelstad, J., Berge, A., and Ellingsen, T. (1983): Excess antibody immunoassay for rat glandular kallikrein. Monosized polymer particles as the preferred solid phase material. *J. Immunol. Methods,* 59:255–264.

66. Johansen, L., Orstavik, T. B., Nustad, K., and Holck, M. (1983): Excess antibody immunoassays for rat glandular kallikreins. Measurement of kallikrein from different organs in the presence of cross-reacting antigens. *J. Immunol. Methods,* 59:315–326.

67. Johnson, A. R., and Erdös, E. G. (1977): Metabolism of vasoactive peptides by human endothelial cells in culture. Angiotensin I converting enzyme (kininase II) and angiotensinase. *J. Clin. Invest.,* 59:684–695.

68. Johnson, A. R., Skidgel, R. A., Gafford, J. T., and Erdös, E. G. (1984): Enzymes in placenta microvilli: Angiotensin I converting enzyme, angiotensinase A, carboxypeptidase, and neutral endopeptidase ("enkephalinase"). *Peptides,* 5:789–796.

69. Kerbiriou-Nabias, D. M., Garcia, F. O., and Larrieu, M. J. (1984): Radioimmunoassays of human high and low molecular weight kininogens in plasmas and platelets. *Br. J. Haematol.,* 56: 273–286.

70. Lanzillo, J. J., and Fanburg, B. L. (1982): Development of competitive enzyme immunoassays for human serum angiotensin-1-converting enzyme: A comparison of four assay configurations. *Anal. Biochem.,* 126:156–164.

71. Lawton, W., Proud, D., Frech, M. E., Pierce, J. V., Keiser, H. R., and Pisano, J. J. (1981): Characterization and origin of immunoreactive glandular kallikrein in rat plasma. *Biochem. Pharmacol.,* 30:1731–1737.

72. Lazure, C., Leduc, R., Seidah, N. G., Thibault, G., Genest, J., and Chretien, M. (1984): Amino acid sequence of rat submaxillary tonin reveals similarities to serine proteases. *Nature,* 309:555–558.

73. Mann, K., Lipp, B., Grunst, J., Geiger, R., and Karl, H. J. (1980): Determination of kallikrein by radioimmunoassay in human body fluids. *Agents Actions,* 1074:329–334.

74. Marin-Grez, M., Bonner, G., and Gross, F. (1980): Ureteral contractions induced by rat urine in vitro: Probable involvement of renal kallikrein. *Experientia,* 36:865–866.

75. Mashford, M. L., and Roberts, M. L. (1972): Determination of blood kinin levels by radioimmunoassay. *Biochem. Pharmacol.,* 21:2727–2735.

76. Mason, A. J., Evans, B. A., Cox, D. R., Shine, J., and Richards, R. I. (1983): Structures of mouse kallikrein gene family suggest a role in specific processing of biologically active peptides. *Nature,* 303:300–307.

77. Mattler, L. E., and Bang, N. V. (1978): Serine protease specificity for peptide chromogenic substrate. *Thromb. Haemost.,* 38:776–792.

78. Mills, I. H. (1979): Kallikrein, kininogen and kinins in control of blood pressure. *Nephron,* 23:61–71.

79. Moriya, H., Mazsuda, Y., Miyazaki, K., Moriwaki, C, and Hojima, Y. (1977): Some aspects of urinary and renal kallikrein. In: *Kininogenases,* edited by G. L. Haberland, S. W. Rohen, and T. Suzuki, pp. 29–34. Schattauer-Verlag, Stuttgart.

80. Moriya, H., Webster, M. E., and Pierce, J. V. (1963): Purification and some properties of three kallikreins. *Ann. N.Y. Acad. Sci.,* 104:172.

81. Morita, T., Kato, H., Iwanaga, S., Takada, K., Kimura, T., and Sahakibara, S. (1977): New fluorogenic substrates for thrombin, factor x, kallikreins and urokinase. *J. Biochem.,* 82:1495.

82. Nasjletti, A., Colina-Chourio, J., and McGiff, J. C. (1975): Assay of kinins by their effects on canine femoral blood flow. *Proc. Soc. Exp. Biol. Med.,* 150:493–497.

83. Nasjletti, A., and Malik, K. U. (1979): Relationships between the kallikrein-kinin and prostaglandin system. *Life Sci.,* 25:99–110.

84. Neilsen, M. D., Nielsen, F., Kappelgaard, A. M., and Giese, J. (1982): Double-antibody solid-phase radioimmunoassay for blood bradykinin. *Clin. Chim. Acta,* 125:145–156.

85. Nustad, K. (1970): The relationship between kidney and urinary kininogenases. *Br. J. Pharmacol. Chemother.,* 39:73–86.

86. Nustad, K., Gautvik, K., and Orstavik, T. (1979): Radioimmunoassay of rat submandibular gland kallikrein and the detection of immunoreactive antigen in blood. *Adv. Exp. Med. Biol.,* 120: 225–234.

87. Nustad, K., Gautvik, K. M., and Pierce, J. V. (1974): Glandular kallikreins: Purification, characterization and biosynthesis. In:

Chemistry and Biology of the Kallikrein-Kinin System in Health and Disease, edited by J. J. Pisano and F. Austen, pp. 77–92. U.S. Government Printing Office, Washington, D.C.

88. Nustad, K., and Pierce, J. V. (1974): Purification of rat urinary kallikrein and their specific antibody. *Biochemistry,* 13:2312–2319.

89. Odya, C. E., Goodfriend, J. M., Stewart, J. M., and Pena, C. (1978): Aspects of bradykinin radioimmunoassay. *J. Immunol. Methods,* 19:243–257.

90. Odya, C. E., Hall, E. R., and Robinson, C. J. G. (1979): Radioimmunoassay for pig angiotensin 1 converting enzyme: A comparison of immunologic with enzymatic activity. *Biochem. Biophys. Res. Commun.,* 86:508–513.

91. Ole-Moi Yoi, O., Austen, F., and Spraag, J. (1977): Kinin generating and esterolytic activity of purified human urinary kallikrein. *Biochem. Pharmacol.,* 26:1893–1900.

92. Ole-Moi Yoi, O., Seldin, D. C., Spragg, J., Pinkus, G. S., and Austen, F. K. (1979): Sequential cleavage of proinsulin by human pancreatic kallikrein and a human pancreatic kininase. *Proc. Natl. Acad. Sci. (USA),* 76:3612–3616.

93. Orlowski, M., and Wilk, S. (1981): Purification and specificity of a membrane-bound metalloendopeptidase from bovine pituitaries. *Biochemistry,* 20:4942–4950.

94. Oshima, G., Kato, J., and Edrös, E. G. (1975): Plasma carboxypeptidase N. Subunits and characteristics. *Arch. Biochem. Biophys.,* 170:132–138.

95. Oza, N. B. (1981): Development of a rat urinary kallikrein-binding radioimmunoassay and identification of homologous enzyme in plasma. *J. Clin. Chem. Clin. Biochem.,* 19:1033–1038.

96. Oza, N. B., Amin, V. M., McGregor, R., Scicli, A. G., and Carretero, O. A. (1976): Isolation of rat urinary kallikrein and properties of its antibodies. *Biochem. Pharmacol.,* 25:1607–1612.

97. Piquilloud, Y., Reinharz, A., and Roth, M. (1970): Studies on the angiotensin converting enzyme with different substrates. *Biochem. Biophys. Acta,* 206:136–142.

98. Proud, D., Pierce, J. U., and Pisano, J. J. (1980): Radioimmunoassay of human high molecular weight kininogen in normal and deficient plasmas. *J. Lab. Clin. Med.,* 95:563–574.

99. Rabito, S. F., Amin, V., Scicli, A. G., and Carretero, O. A. (1979): Glandular kallikrein in plasma and urine: Evaluation of a direct RIA for its determination. *Adv. Exp. Med. Biol.,* 120:127–142.

100. Rabito, S. F., Scicli, A. G., and Carretero, O. A. (1979): Glandular kallikrein in plasma and urine: Evaluation of a direct RIA for its determination. In: *Kinins II: Biochemistry, Pathophysiology, and Clinical Aspects,* edited by S. Fuji, H. Moriya, and T. Suzuki, pp. 127–142. Plenum, New York.

101. Rabito, S. F., Scicli, A. G., Kher, V., and Carretero, O. A. (1982): Immunoreactive glandular kallikrein in rat plasma: A radioimmunoassay for its determination. *Am. J. Physiol.,* 242:H602–H610.

102. Roberts, P. S. (1958): Measurement of the rate of plasmin action on synthetic substrates. *J. Biol. Chem.,* 232:285–291.

103. Roblero, J., Ryan, J. W., and Stewart, J. M. (1973): Assay of kinins by their effects on blood pressure. *Res. Commun. Chem. Pathol. Pharmacol.,* 6:206–212.

104. Rocha e Silva, M. (1970): Isolation of bradykinin: Biological assay and occurrence in nature. In: *Kinin Hormones,* edited by I. N. Kugelmass, pp. 28–58. Thomas, Springfield, Ill.

105. Roffman, S. V., Sanock, A., and Troll, W. (1970): Sensitive proteolytic enzyme assay using differential solubilities of radioactive substrate and products in biphasic systems. *Anal. Biochem.,* 36:11–17.

106. Ryan, J. W., Chung, A., Ammons, C., and Carlton, M. L. (1977): A simple radioassay for angiotensin-converting enzyme. *Biochem. J.,* 167:501–504.

107. Salgado, M. C. O., Rabito, S. F., and Carretero, O. A. (1985): Blood kinin in one-kidney, one-clip hypertensive rats. *Hypertension,* 8:I110–I113, 1986.

108. Sampaio, M. V., Reis, M. L., Fink, E., Camargo, A. C., and Greene, L. J. (1977): SP-Sephadex equilibrium chromatography of bradykinin and related peptides: Application to trypsin-treated human plasma. *Anal. Biochem.,* 81:369–383.

109. Schwert, G., and Takehaka, Y. (1955): A spectrophotometric determination of trypsin and chymotrypsin. *Biochim. Biophys. Acta,* 16:570–575.

110. Scicli, A. G., Carretero, O. A., Oza, N. B., and Schork, A. (1976): Distribution of kidney kininogenases. *Proc. Soc. Exp. Biol. Med.,* 151:57–60.

111. Scicli, A. G., Diaz, M. A., and Carretero, O. A. (1983): Effect of pH and amiloride on the intrarenal formation of kinins. *Am. J. Physiol.,* 245:F198–F203.

112. Scicli, A. G., Mindroiu, T., Scicli, G., and Carretero, O. A. (1982): Blood kinins, their concentration in normal subjects and in patients with congenital deficiency in plasma pre-kallikrein and kininogen. *J. Lab. Clin. Med.,* 100:81–93.

113. Scicli, A. G., Rabito, S. F., and Carretero, O. A. (1983): Blood and urinary kinins in human subjects during normal and low sodium intake. *Adv. Exp. Med. Biol.,* 156:877–882.

114. Sealey, J. E., Atlas, S. A., Laragh, J. H., Oza, N. B., and Ryan, J. W. (1978): Human urinary kallikrein converts inactive renin to active renin and is a possible physiological activator of renin. *Nature,* 275:144–145.

115. Shimamoto, K., Ando, T., Tanaka, S., Nakahashi, Y., Nishitani, T., Hosoda, S., Ishida, H., and Iimura, O. (1982): An improved method for the determination of human blood kinin levels by sensitive kinin radioimmunoassay. *Endocrinol. Jpn.,* 29:487–494.

116. Shimamoto, K., Chao, J., and Margolius, H. S. (1980): The radioimmunoassay of human urinary kallikrein and comparisons with kallikrein activity measurements. *J. Clin. Endocrinol. Metab.,* 51:840–848.

117. Shimamoto, K., Margolius, H. S., Chao, J., and Crosswell, A. R. (1979): A direct radioimmunoassay of rat urinary kallikrein and comparison with other measures of urinary kallikrein activity. *J. Lab. Clin. Med.,* 94:172–179.

118. Shimamoto, K., Mayfield, R. K., Margolius, H. S., Chao, J., Stroud, W., and Kaplan, A. P. (1984): Immunoreactive tissue kallikrein in human serum. *J. Lab. Clin. Med.,* 103:731–738.

119. Siegelman, A. M., Carlsen, A. S., and Robertson, T. (1962): Investigation of serum trypsin and related substances. The quantitative demonstration of trypsin-like activity in human blood serum by a micromethod. *Arch. Biochem. Biophys.,* 97:159–164.

120. Skeggs, L. T., Dorer, F. E., Kahn, J. R., Lentz, K. E., and Levine, M. (1976): The biochemistry of the renin-angiotensin system and its role in hypertension. *Am. J. Med.,* 60:737–748.

121. Spraag, J., Austen, K. F., and Haber, E. (1966): Production of antibody against bradykinin: Demonstration of specificity by complement fixation and radioimmunoassay. *J. Immunol.,* 96:865–872.

122. Suzuki, S., Franco-Saenz, R., Tan, S. Y., and Mulrow, P. J. (1980): Direct action of rat urinary kallikrein on rat kidney to release renin. *J. Clin. Invest.,* 66:757–762.

123. Swift, G. H., Craik, C. S., Stary, S. J., Qunito, C., Lahaie, R. G., Rutter, W. J., and MacDonald, R. J. (1984): Structure of the two related elastase genes expressed in the rat pancreas. *J. Biol. Chem.,* 259:14271–14278.

124. Syvanen, A. C., Turpeinen, U., Siimesmaa, S., and Hamberg, U. (1981): A radioimmunoassay for the detection of molecular forms of human plasma kininogen. *FEBS Lett.,* 129:241–245.

125. Talamo, R. C., Haber, E., and Austen, K. F. (1969): A radioimmunoassay for bradykinin in plasma and synovial fluid. *J. Lab. Clin. Med.,* 74:816–927.

126. Terragno, N. A., Lonigro, A. J., Malik, K. U., and McGiff, J. C. (1972): The relationship of the renal vasodilator action of bradykinin to the release of prostaglandin E-like substances. *Experientia,* 28:437–439.

127. Tanaka, S., Chao, J., and Margolius, H. S. (1982): A direct radioimmunoassay for immunoreactive glandular kallikrein in rat serum. *Fed. Proc.,* 41:1473.

128. Trautschold, I. (1970): Assay mathods in the kinin system. In: *Handbook of Experimental Pharmacology, Vol. 25,* edited by E. G. Erdös, pp. 52–81. Springer-Verlag, Berlin.

129. Trautschold, I. P., Werle, E., and Schweitzer, G. (1970): Kallikrein. In: *Methoden der enzymatischen Analyse,* edited by N. Bergmayer, p. 1011. Verlag-Chemie, Weinheim.

130. Uchida, Y., Oh-Ishi, S., and Katori, M. (1977): A determination method for plasma kininogen and its application. In: *Kininogen-*

ases, edited by G. L. Haberland, J. W. Rohen, and T. Suzuki, pp. 99–105. Schattauer-Verlag, Stuttgart.

131. Ura, N., Carretero, O. A., and Erdös, E. G. (1986): Participation of neutral endopeptidase 24.11 (NEP; enkephalinase A) in kinin metabolism *in vitro* and *in vivo. Fed. Proc.,* 45:790 (abstract).

132. Vane, J. R. (1969): The release and fate of vasoactive hormones in the circulation. *Br. J. Pharmacol.,* 35:209–242.

133. Van Leeuwen, B. H., Millar, J. A., Hammat, M. T., and Johnston, C. I. (1983): Radioimmunoassay of blood bradykinin: Purification of blood extracts to prevent cross-reaction with endogenous kininogen. *Clin. Chim. Acta,* 127:343–351.

134. Vinci, J. M., Gill, J. R., Bowden, R. E., Pisano, J. J., Izzo, J. L., Radfar, N., Taylor, A. A., Bartter, F. C., and Keiser, H. R. (1978): The kallikrein-kinin system in Bartter syndrome and its response to prostaglandin synthetase inhibition. *J. Clin. Invest.,* 61:1671–1682.

135. Webster, M. E. (1970): Kallikreins in glandular tissue. In: *Handbook of Experimental Pharmacology,* edited by E. G. Erdös, pp. 131–156. Springer-Verlag, Berlin.

136. Wintroub, B. A., Spraag, S., Stechschulte, D. J., and Austen, K. F. (1973): Characterization and immunoassay for components of the kinin generating system. In: *Mechanisms in Allergy Mediated Hypersensitivity,* edited by T. L. Goodfriend, A. Sehan, and R. Orange, pp. 495–512. Dekker, New York.

137. Worthington, K., and Cuscheri, A. (1974): A study on the kinetics of pancreatic kallikrein with the substrate benzoyl arginine ethyl ester using a spectrophotometric assay. *Clin. Chim. Acta,* 52:129–136.

138. Zimmerman, M., Yurewicz, E. C., and Patel, G. (1970): A new fluorogenic substrate for chymotrypsin. *Anal. Biochem.,* 70:258–262.

The Heart and Cardiovascular System,
edited by H. A. Fozzard et al.
Raven Press, New York © 1986.

CHAPTER 71

Biochemical Mechanisms of Parasympathetic Regulation of Cardiac Function

John W. Fleming and August M. Watanabe

DUAL REGULATION OF CARDIAC FUNCTION

The major system extrinsic to the heart that regulates its function is the autonomic nervous system. This system is divided on the basis of anatomical differences, differences in physiological effects, differences in neurotransmitters, and differences in receptors into the sympathetic and parasympathetic nervous systems. In general, activation of the sympathetic nervous system is excitatory, whereas activation of the parasympathetic nervous system is inhibitory to cardiac function. The net physiological effect of the influences of these two limbs of the autonomic nervous system on cardiac function is not simply the algebraic sum of their individual levels of activity (24). Rather, the two limbs interact in a complex manner such that the parasympathetic nervous system can modulate the effects of the sympathetic nervous system. This parasympathetic modulation of sympathetic effects on the heart occurs at both the prejunctional level (i.e., between nerve endings) and the postjunctional level (for reviews, see refs. 24, 44). In the prejunctional interaction, activation of the parasympathetic nervous system can inhibit the release of norepinephrine from sympathetic nerve terminals. In the postjunctional interaction, activation of muscarinic receptors can inhibit the response of cardiac myocytes to β-adrenergic receptor stimulation. This phenomenon of parasympathetic modulation of sym-

pathetic effects is magnified when sympathetic tone to the heart is high. In ventricular myocardium, parasympathetic effects on most physiological properties of the tissue are apparent only in the presence of sympathetic activity. In other words, in ventricular muscle the predominant mode by which the physiological effects of the parasympathetic nervous system become manifest is by modulation of sympathetic effects. This phenomenon of increased parasympathetic efficacy in the presence of sympathetic activity was originally observed in physiological experiments in whole animals and was termed accentuated antagonism by Levy and Martin (24). Subsequent studies have demonstrated the phenomenon of accentuated antagonism when certain biochemical effects of catecholamines and acetylcholine on the isolated heart are examined.

The proximal mediator of the effects of acetylcholine, released from parasympathetic nerve terminals, on cardiac myocytes is the muscarinic cholinergic receptor. The advances of the past decade in biochemical approaches to the study of receptors have been applied as well to muscarinic receptors. These approaches, based primarily on the use of radiolabeled ligands that possess high affinity for muscarinic receptors, have facilitated characterization of muscarinic receptors in cardiac membranes. However, the biochemical mechanisms by which activation of muscarinic receptors alters cell function have been relatively less well-understood. Several processes have been implicated as mediating the cellular effects of muscarinic receptor stimulation, including opening of potassium channels, stimulation of guanylate cyclase, stimulation of phosphatidylinositol turnover, inhibition of protein phosphorylation, and inhibition of adenylate cyclase activity (44). The latter effect could reasonably be hypothesized as a biochemical mechanism for muscarinic modulation of β-adrenergic effects on cardiac myocytes.

Early descriptions of the biochemistry of adenylate cyclase included studies showing muscarinic inhibition of activity (27). However, these types of studies were not followed up for a number of years, even though experiments with intact cardiac tissues showed muscarinic inhibition of cyclic AMP accumulation in response to β-adrenergic receptor stimulation. Muscarinic inhibition of cardiac adenylate cyclase activity was "rediscovered" in 1978 (45), and simultaneously it was observed for the first time that this was a GTP-dependent phenomenon. These observations were shortly thereafter confirmed in another laboratory (16). Subsequently, molecular understanding of inhibitory regulation of the adenylate cyclase system has developed at an explosive rate, and it is now generally accepted that the enzyme is dually regulated. E. Neer (see *Chapter 62*) has given a detailed molecular description of the hormonally regulated adenylate-cyclase/cyclic-AMP system as characterized in several tissues. The focus of this chapter will be our current understanding of the mechanism of muscarinic inhibition of adenylate cyclase activity in cardiac sarcolemma.

COMPONENTS OF THE HORMONE-SENSITIVE ADENYLATE CYCLASE SYSTEM

Hormonal regulation of cyclic AMP synthesis by the catalytic subunit (C) requires the presence of two additional proteins: a hormone receptor (R) and regulatory protein (N) (for reviews, see refs. 14,25,34,35,37,40) (also see *Chapter 62*). Our biochemical understanding of adenylate cyclase systems has been greatly facilitated by the discovery and purification of unique guanine-nucleotide-binding regulatory proteins that mediate stimulation (N_s) and inhibition (N_i) of adenylate cyclase activity (3,4,10,21,29–34,41,43). These regulatory proteins appear to have a large degree of structural and functional analogy. Both are activated when bound with GTP; both hydrolyze GTP; and both have similar subunit compositions composed of α and β peptides,[1] the 35-kilodalton (35-kd) β subunits being apparently

identical (14,40). A schematic model of stimulation and inhibition of adenylate cyclase is shown in Fig. 1.

Hormonal Stimulation of Adenylate Cyclase Activity

The proximal activator of C is the 45-kd α subunit of N_s bound with GTP ($\alpha_s \cdot$ GTP). Catalytic activity is "turned off" or reduced to a basal level by the hydrolysis of GTP to GDP by GTP hydrolytic (GTPase) activity at N_s (2,5,9,36). It appears that GTPase activity requires the presence of both α and β subunits of N_s (20). Stimulatory hormone receptors bound with agonist facilitate the exchange of GTP for GDP at N_s, resulting in subunit dissociation and regeneration of the active complex.

Inhibition of Adenylate Cyclase Activity

Inhibitory regulation of adenylate cyclase activity is mediated by N_i (21,43), whose inhibitory activity is apparently determined by a GTP regulatory cycle similar to that for N_s. Analogous to activation of N_s by stimulatory hormones, inhibitory hormones may activate N_i by facilitating the activation of N_i by GTP (10,17,40). After GTP-induced dissociation of N_i into its 41-kd α_i and 35-kd β subunits, two general mechanisms have been described for the inhibition of adenylate cyclase activity by the dissociated N_i subunits: (a) direct inhibition of C by $\alpha_i \cdot$ GTP and (b) indirect inhibition of C mediated by N_i inhibition of $\alpha_s \cdot$ GTP. Seamon and Daly (39) first suggested that inhibition of C by the nonhydrolyzable GTP analog Gpp(NH)p represented direct inhibition of C by $N_i \cdot$ Gpp(NH)p. Gpp(NH)p inhibition of enzymatic activity is seen only in various dually regulated adenylate cyclase systems, including cardiac, but this appears to be true only in the presence of the plant diterpene activator of C, forskolin. Gilman and associates have demonstrated that purified β subunit is inhibitory to activated α_s and have therefore suggested that one mechanism of inhibitory hormone attenuation of adenylate cyclase activity may involve an inhibitory-receptor-induced increase in the pool of β subunits (40). Because the stoichiometric ratio of N_i to N_s has been found to be 10 to 20 in those tissues studied, inhibitory receptor facilitation of GTP-induced N_i subunit dissociation could increase the pool of β subunits significantly. Increasing the pool of β subunits could lead to the formation of $\beta\alpha_s \cdot$ GTP and, subsequently, $\beta\alpha_s \cdot$ GDP, resulting in attenuation of adenylate cyclase activity. This latter mechanism appears to be the most physiologically relevant at this time. The role of GTPase activity in the inhibition of GTP-activated N_s by N_i has not been determined unequivocally. Sunyer et al. (42) have demonstrated GTPase activity by purified N_i, and

---

[1] Most preparations of N_s and N_i contain a less well characterized 10-kd peptide that is probably a third (γ) subunit of the N proteins (14). We have limited the present discussion to the α and β subunits, but note that activities attributed to the β subunit probably reflect the activity of the $\beta\gamma$ complex.

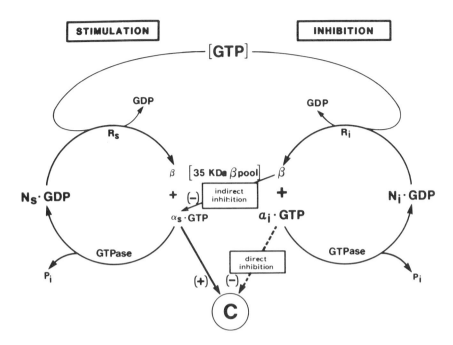

FIG. 1. Hypothetical GTP regulatory cycle for dually regulated adenylate cyclase activity.

Kanaho et al. (20) recently demonstrated that GTPase activity is not intrinsic to isolated α or β, but is observed only in the presence of both subunits. It seems reasonable to speculate that inhibitory-hormone-induced increases in the β subunit pool may inhibit $\alpha_s \cdot$ GTP and therefore adenylate cyclase activity by formation of $\beta\alpha_s \cdot$ GTP, with subsequent hydrolysis of GTP to GDP.

MUSCARINIC INHIBITION OF CARDIAC ADENYLATE CYCLASE ACTIVITY

Our biochemical investigations of inhibitory mechanisms of cardiac adenylate activity have been greatly facilitated by the availability of highly purified and characterized preparations of canine sarcolemma, as described by L. Jones (see *Chapter 19*). The use of cholera and pertussis toxins has proved to be indispensable for the study and purification of N_s and N_i. The use of these bacterial toxins has allowed selective identification and functional modification of N_s and N_i because of the ability of these toxins to selectively catalyze the covalent modification of the α subunit of each regulatory protein. After intoxication of a membrane preparation, the membranes can be solubilized and electrophoresed on SDS polyacrylamide gels. After electrophoresis, an autoradiogram can be made from the resulting slab gel, allowing identification and quantitation of the covalently labeled α subunit of N_s or N_i.

Identification of N_s and N_i in Cardiac Sarcolemma

Using [^{32}P]NAD as substrate, we have used cholera toxin to catalyze [^{32}P]ADP-ribosylation of the 45-kd α

subunit of N_s (Fig. 2). Because of GTP hydrolysis, the GTP-stimulated adenylate cyclase activity of cardiac sarcolemma is only a fraction of the activity obtained in the presence of the nonhydrolyzable GTP analog Gpp(NH)p. ADP-ribosylation functionally modifies N_s, inhibiting its ability to hydrolyze GTP (8,26), and therefore allows GTP to activate adenylate cyclase activity to a level near that obtained with Gpp(NH)p (Table 1).

Ui and associates first demonstrated that pertussis

cholera toxin	–	+	–	–
IAP	–	–	–	+
ARF	+	+	–	–

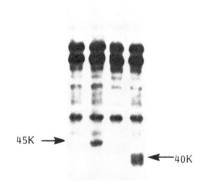

45K →

←40K

FIG. 2. Identification of the α subunits of N_s and N_i in cardiac sarcolemma. Sarcolemmal membranes were incubated with [^{32}P]NAD in the absence and presence of cholera toxin or IAP, as indicated. In cardiac sarcolemma, cholera-toxin-catalyzed [^{32}P]ADP ribosylation of α_s requires the presence of an additional protein (12), "ADP ribosylation factor" (ARF). ARF is not necessary for IAP-catalyzed [^{32}P]ADP ribosylation of α_i.

TABLE 1. *Effects of IAP and cholera toxin on the ratio of cardiac adenylate cyclase activity in the presence of isoproterenol (ISO) and GTP to that in the presence of ISO and Gpp(NH)p*

Pretreatment	Adenylate cyclase activity: ISO + GTP/ISO + Gpp(NH)p
None	0.34
IAP	0.34
Cholera toxin	0.83

Sarcolemmal membranes were intoxicated in a preincubation with IAP or cholera toxin, as indicated. The membranes were then diluted, pelleted, and resuspended for adenylate cyclase assay in the presence of 10 μM ISO and 10 μM GTP or Gpp(NH)p.

toxin (islet-activating protein, IAP) treatment of rat myocytes attenuated the ability of inhibitory hormones to decrease cyclic AMP accumulation in response to stimulatory hormones (15). It was subsequently shown that IAP catalyzes the incorporation of ADP ribose into the 41-kd α subunit of N_i and that this modification correlates with attenuation of the response to inhibitory receptor agonists (28). We have recently used IAP to identify the α subunit of N_i in canine cardiac sarcolemma (Fig. 2). In contrast to the intoxication of cardiac sarcolemma with cholera toxin, treatment of sarcolemma with IAP has no effect on the ability of GTP to activate adenylate cyclase activity (Table 1). However, the ability of the muscarinic agonist oxotremorine to inhibit GTP-stimulated adenylate cyclase activity was reduced following ADP ribosylation of N_i (13). These studies demonstrate (a) the presence of N_s and N_i in cardiac sarcolemma, (b) that ADP-ribosylation of N_i has no effect on $\alpha_s \cdot$ GTP in the absence of inhibitory hormones, and (c) that ADP-ribosylation of N_i attenuates the ability of muscarinic agonists to inhibit GTP-stimulated adenylate cyclase activity.

Studies with Forskolin

In our previous studies, muscarinic agonists had no effect on basal adenylate cyclase activity, suggesting that these agents and their receptors do not directly inhibit the catalyst in cardiac sarcolemma (45). However, possible direct inhibition of C was further evaluated by use of forskolin, which is thought to stimulate C directly (38). In those tissues that are characterized by having GDP tightly bound to N_s and therefore very low basal adenylate cyclase activity, other investigators have added forskolin to their assays to stimulate C so that possible effects of inhibitory hormones can be measured (40). Although purified cardiac sarcolemma displays relatively high basal adenylate cyclase activity, we have included forskolin in certain assays to stimulate enzymatic activity

further, possibly magnifying or unmasking direct inhibitory effects of muscarinic agonists on the catalyst. As in membranes from other tissues, forskolin is a powerful stimulator of canine cardiac adenylate cyclase activity. Although basal Mg^{2+}-dependent adenylate cyclase activity was stimulated approximately sixfold by 50 μM forskolin, 10 μM methacholine had no effect on catalytic activity at any concentration of forskolin tested (0.1–100 μM, data not shown). These experiments suggested that muscarinic receptors do not directly inhibit C, and that forskolin alone was insufficient to permit muscarinic inhibition of the enzyme. However, the data did not address the possibility of N_i-mediated mechanisms due to the absence of guanine nucleotides.

In dually regulated adenylate cyclase systems, forskolin activation of C unmasks a special type of adenylate cyclase inhibition, i.e., inhibition of forskolin-activated C by Gpp(NH)p in the absence of inhibitory hormones (39). Inhibition of forskolin-stimulated adenylate cyclase activity by Gpp(NH)p may represent direct inhibition of the catalyst by a complex of the 41-kd α subunit of N_i and the guanine nucleotide [$\alpha_i \cdot$ Gpp(NH)p] (21). However, Gpp(NH)p did not inhibit forskolin-stimulated adenylate cyclase activity in cardiac sarcolemma under "normal" incubation conditions, which included 1 mM ATP and 9.75 mM $MgCl_2$. As seen in other tissues (e.g., ref. 22), Gpp(NH)p inhibition of forskolin-stimulated adenylate cyclase activity was dependent on the concentration of $MgCl_2$ present, the maximal inhibition being 30% at $MgCl_2$ concentrations below 1 mM. The ability of forskolin to convert Gpp(NH)p modification of cardiac adenylate cyclase activity from stimulatory to inhibitory and the dependence of this conversion on the concentration of $MgCl_2$ are shown in Fig. 3. In the presence of 10 mM $MgCl_2$ (excess [Mg^{2+}]), 10 μM Gpp(NH)p characteristically stimulated basal adenylate cyclase activity (Fig. 3, right panel), and 10 μM methacholine had no effect on either basal or Gpp(NH)p-stimulated activity (data not shown). In the presence of excess [Mg^{2+}] and forskolin, Gpp(NH)p had no effect on the forskolin-stimulated enzyme (Fig. 3, right panel). Although control adenylate cyclase activity was considerably lower in the presence of 1 mM $MgCl_2$, the effect of Gpp(NH)p on the enzyme was also stimulatory under these conditions of limiting [Mg^{2+}] (Fig. 3, left panel). However, Gpp(NH)p activation of adenylate cyclase activity was converted to an inhibition of the enzyme in the presence of forskolin and limiting [Mg^{2+}] (Fig. 3, left panel). Forskolin-stimulated adenylate cyclase activity was inhibited 22% by 0.1 μM Gpp(NH)p, and methacholine had no effect on control or Gpp(NH)p-inhibited activity (data not shown). Therefore, Gpp(NH)p produced small, but characteristic, adenylate cyclase inhibition under special conditions (limiting [Mg^{2+}] in excess of ATP, in the presence of forskolin), but stimulated enzymatic

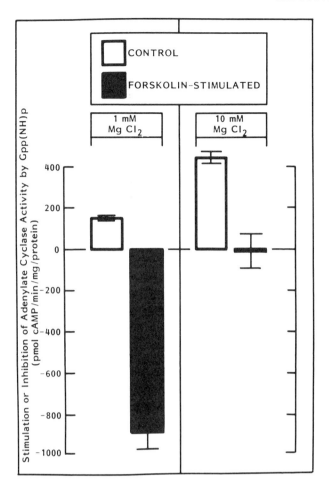

FIG. 3. Conversion of Gpp(NH)p modulation of adenylate cyclase activity from stimulatory to inhibitory by forskolin and limiting [MgCl₂]. Sarcolemmal membranes were incubated in adenylate cyclase assays containing 1 mM [³²P]ATP and the indicated concentrations of MgCl₂, in the absence and presence of 10 μM forskolin. (The IAP substrate was later resolved into two distinct proteins with M_r = 40,000 and 42,000).

activity under more physiological assay conditions (higher [Mg²⁺] in excess of ATP, in the absence of forskolin).

As mentioned earlier, it has recently been suggested that activation of N_i by inhibitory hormones may be analogous to activation of N_s by stimulatory hormones. Similar to the stimulatory hormone-catalyzed activation of the α subunit of N_s, inhibitory hormones may lead to activation of the α subunit of N_i, with subsequent direct inhibition of C by $\alpha_i \cdot$ GTP. Schultz and associates have proposed that the mechanism of direct inhibition of the catalyst by activated N_i involves a change in affinity for Mg²⁺ of an allosteric site on C (18). These investigators found that activated N_s decreases the K_{act} for Mg²⁺ stimulation of adenylate cyclase activity and that activation of N_i with nonhydrolyzable GTP analogs results in an increase in the K_{act} for Mg²⁺. Two predictions result from the assumption that direct inhibition

of the catalyst by this mechanism is significant in cardiac sarcolemma: (a) direct inhibition of the catalyst [as measured by Gpp(NH)p inhibition of forskolin-stimulated adenylate cyclase activity] should be observed only at limiting concentrations of Mg²⁺, and (b) muscarinic agonists should increase inhibition of forskolin-stimulated adenylate cyclase activity by Gpp(NH)p if the Gpp(NH)p effect is not maximally attained [Gpp(NH)p concentration is not excessively high (near its apparent K_{act})]. If N_i inhibits C directly, it follows that concentrations of Gpp(NH)p might be found that would inhibit basal adenylate cyclase activity, especially since the K_{act} for guanine nucleotide activation of N_i has been found to be lower than that for N_s (17,22). Inhibition of basal adenylate cyclase activity by submaximal concentrations of Gpp(NH)p should be increased by the addition of muscarinic agonists. Several experiments designed to test these hypotheses were performed using various low concentrations of MgCl₂ and Gpp(NH)p.

In the presence of 0.25 mM ATP and 1 mM MgCl₂, one-half maximal inhibition of forskolin-stimulated adenylate cyclase activity occurred at approximately 20 nM Gpp(NH)p, with the maximal inhibition being 31%. Methacholine had no effect on Gpp(NH)p inhibition of forskolin-stimulated adenylate cyclase activity at any concentration of Gpp(NH)p tested (0.1 μM to 1 μM, data not shown). The effects of various concentrations of MgCl₂ on the ability of methacholine to inhibit basal or isoproterenol- plus Gpp(NH)p-stimulated adenylate cyclase activity were examined at 0.25 mM ATP. The apparent K_{act} for MgCl₂ activation of basal adenylate cyclase activity was 7.9 mM. Although methacholine had little effect on the activation of basal adenylate cyclase activity by MgCl₂, 33 nM Gpp(NH)p plus 10 μM isoproterenol decreased the K_{act} for MgCl₂ by 70% to 2.4 mM. Methacholine had no effect on basal adenylate cyclase activity at any concentration of MgCl₂ tested (0.25–10 mM, data not shown). Isoproterenol plus 33 nM Gpp(NH)p stimulated adenylate cyclase activity 100 to 200% at all concentrations of MgCl₂ tested. Methacholine had no effect on adenylate cyclase activity in the presence of isoproterenol and Gpp(NH)p at any concentration of MgCl₂ (K_{act} = 2.5 mM), even at limiting concentrations near that of the ATP. Table 2 summarizes the effects of methacholine and Gpp(NH)p on control and forskolin-stimulated adenylate cyclase activities in the presence of 0.05 mM ATP, in the presence of limiting (0.05 mM) and excess (0.5 mM) MgCl₂. In the presence of forskolin, both 33 nM and 10 μM Gpp(NH)p characteristically inhibited adenylate cyclase activity 30 to 50%. Gpp(NH)p inhibition of forskolin-stimulated activity was not further increased by addition of methacholine at either 33 nM or 10 μM Gpp(NH)p, whether in the presence of limiting (0.05 mM) MgCl₂ or excess MgCl₂. In the absence of forskolin, 33 nM Gpp(NH)p

TABLE 2. *Effects of MgCl₂ concentration and forskolin on Gpp(NH)p modulation of cardiac adenylate cyclase activity*

Additions	[MgCl₂]	Adenylate cyclase activity (relative to control)	
		No forskolin	10 μM forskolin
33 nM Gpp(NH)p	Limiting	0	− −
	Excess	0	−
33 nM Gpp(NH)p + 10 μM METH	Limiting	0	− −
	Excess	0	−
10 μM Gpp(NH)p	Limiting	+ +	− − −
	Excess	+ + +	− −
10 μM Gpp(NH)p + 10 μM METH	Limiting	+ +	− − −
	Excess	+ + +	− −

Sarcolemmal membranes were incubated in the presence of the indicated concentrations of Gpp(NH)p and methacholine (METH), in the absence and presence of forskolin. A plus sign indicates stimulation relative to control adenylate cyclase activity [no Gpp(NH)p or METH]; minus indicates inhibition relative to control; zero indicates no change. [ATP] = 0.05 mM; limiting [MgCl₂] = 0.05 mM; excess [MgCl₂] = 0.5 mM.

had no effect on adenylate cyclase activity in the absence or presence of methacholine, at either limiting or excess MgCl₂. In the absence of forskolin, 10 μM Gpp(NH)p was stimulatory, and the Gpp(NH)p-stimulated adenylate cyclase activity was not significantly inhibited by methacholine at either concentration of MgCl₂. In summary, although Gpp(NH)p was found to inhibit the forskolin-stimulated enzyme under certain conditions, this inhibition was not enhanced by methacholine under any conditions tested, including limiting concentrations of MgCl₂ and Gpp(NH)p. In addition, in the absence of forskolin, methacholine did not inhibit adenylate cyclase activity in the absence (basal) or presence of low concentrations (33 mM) of Gpp(NH)p at any concentration of MgCl₂.

Muscarinic Inhibition of GTP-Stimulated Adenylate Cyclase Activity

Substantial experimental findings in cardiac sarcolemma have indicated that muscarinic inhibition of β-adrenergic stimulation of adenylate cyclase activity occurs at the level of the guanine nucleotide regulatory proteins. We have shown that muscarinic agonists oppose the regulatory effect of GTP on β-adrenergic receptor affinity for catecholamines (45). Guanine nucleotide triphosphates are now known to regulate agonist binding to both β-adrenergic and muscarinic cholinergic receptors, and this regulation is mediated by N_s and N_i, respectively. Our previous data indicate that adenylate cyclase activity in canine cardiac sarcolemma is subject to dual regulation by muscarinic cholinergic and β-adrenergic receptors. The muscarinic agonist methacholine inhibited GTP- but not Gpp(NH)p-activated adenylate cyclase activity

(45). These observations and others prompted us to suggest a role for GTP hydrolytic activity in the mechanism by which muscarinic agonists inhibit GTP-activated adenylate cyclase.

Studies of Guanine Nucleotide Activation and Inactivation Rates of Adenylate Cyclase Activity

Activation of adenylate cyclase activity by guanine nucleotides proceeds with a certain lag of time due to slow activation of N_s. β-adrenergic agonists stimulate adenylate cyclase activity by increasing the rate of N_s activation by guanine nucleotides. In cardiac sarcolemma, the lag time for Gpp(NH)p activation of adenylate cyclase activity is shortened 60% by isoproterenol (data not shown). In contrast, methacholine has no effect on the rate of activation of adenylate cyclase activity by Gpp(NH)p. As mentioned above, inhibition of GTP- but not Gpp(NH)p-activated adenylate cyclase activity by methacholine suggested that a specific GTPase activity might be involved in the inhibitory mechanism.

TABLE 3. *Effects of methacholine on the inactivation rate constant (k_{off}) for cardiac adenylate cyclase activity*

Additions	k_{off}
None	0.9 min^{-1}
10 μM methacholine	13.3 min^{-1}
10 μM methacholine + 1 μM atropine	1.7 min^{-1}

Effects of methacholine and methacholine plus atropine on the inactivation rate constant for adenylate cyclase activity were determined as described in the text.

As $\alpha_s \cdot$ GTP is hydrolyzed to $\alpha_s \cdot$ GDP, adenylate cyclase activity is returned to a basal level. Kinetic determination of the inactivation rate constant (k_{off}) for this turn-off reaction provides a measure of GTPase activity at N_s (6,7). To determine k_{off}, cardiac sarcolemma was first preincubated with GTP in the presence of isoproterenol. After preactivation, a solution was added containing [^{32}P]ATP, GDPβS, propranolol, and, where indicated, muscarinic ligands, and adenylate cyclase activity was measured for 210 sec. The propranolol and GDPβS added at time zero prevented regeneration of activated adenylate cyclase (GTP$\cdot\alpha_s\cdot$C), and thereby permitted measurement of decreasing enzymatic activity as GTP was hydrolyzed to GDP at N_s. Basal adenylate cyclase activity was linear for the duration of the time course and was increased 4.3-fold by preactivation of the sarcolemma with GTP plus isoproterenol. When propranolol and GDPβS were added at time zero, the rate of cyclic AMP synthesis slowed to a rate similar to the basal rate (74% inhibited), and k_{off} was calculated to be 2.14 min^{-1} (data not shown). The turn-off reaction rate was substantially increased in the presence of a muscarinic agonist (Table 3). Methacholine stimulated the rate constant nearly 15-fold, from 0.9 min^{-1} to 13.3 min^{-1}; inclusion of atropine at time zero essentially abolished the methacholine-induced increase in k_{off} (k_{off} = 1.7 min^{-1}). These data suggest that methacholine stimulated a specific GTPase activity that was intimately related to adenylate cyclase activity, and that this stimulation was mediated by muscarinic receptors.

TABLE 4. *Muscarinic stimulation of a specific, low-K_m GTPase activity in cardiac sarcolemma*

Additions	V_{max}: P_i released (pmol/min/mg)	K_m (μM)
None	22.8 (21.0–24.8)	0.18 (0.14–0.23)
10 μM oxotremorine	51.0 (47.3–54.9)	0.26 (0.20–0.32)

Sarcolemmal membranes were incubated with [γ-^{32}P]GTP in the absence and presence of oxotremorine. Specific GTPase activity was determined by subtracting nonspecific P_i release (in assays containing 100 μM unlabeled GTP) from the total P_i release in the presence of varying concentrations of GTP (0.1–5.1 μM). The values in parentheses are the asymmetric confidence intervals of the constants calculated as described by Johnson and Frasier (19).

Identification of a Specific, Muscarinic-Stimulated GTPase Activity in Cardiac Sarcolemma

The foregoing experiments indirectly indicated the presence of a muscarinic-sensitive GTPase activity closely associated with adenylate cyclase activity. Several investigators have described specific GTPases in dually regulated noncardiac adenylate cyclase systems using direct assessment of GTP hydrolysis by measuring the release of ^{32}P$_i$ from [γ-^{32}P]GTP (1,9,23). Using this technique, we have identified a specific, low-K_m GTPase activity in

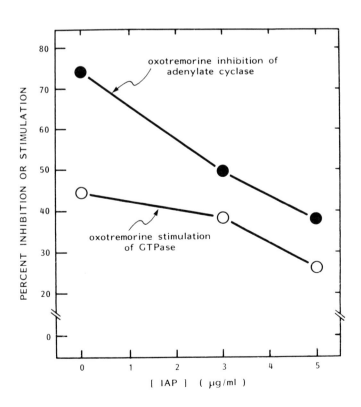

FIG. 4. Effects of pretreatment of sarcolemma with IAP on muscarinic inhibition of GTP-stimulated adenylate cyclase activity and on muscarinic-stimulated GTPase activity. Sarcolemmal membranes were pretreated with the indicated concentrations of IAP; the membranes were then diluted, pelleted, and resuspended for subsequent assays. GTP-stimulated adenylate cyclase and GTPase activities were determined in the absence and presence of 10 μM oxotremorine. The percentage change in enzymatic activity due to oxotremorine is indicated.

canine cardiac sarcolemma that is stimulated by muscarinic agonists (11). The V_{max} of the unstimulated GTPase activity was 22.8 pmol P_i released per minute per milligram protein, and the K_m for GTP was 0.18 μM (Table 4). The muscarinic agonist oxotremorine stimulated the V_{max} of the GTPase 124% and had no effect on the affinity of the enzyme for GTP (Table 4). The K_{act} for oxotremorine stimulation of this GTPase activity was 140 nM, in good agreement with the K_d for oxotremorine binding to sarcolemmal muscarinic receptors (64.9 nM). Atropine competitively antagonized oxotremorine stimulation of GTPase activity, decreasing the K_{act} for the muscarinic agonist approximately 1,000-fold (data not shown). In other experiments we have shown that the K_i for oxotremorine inhibition of specific [^{3}H]QNB binding to muscarinic receptors, the apparent K_i for oxotremorine inhibition of GTP-stimulated adenylate cyclase activity, and the K_{act} for oxotremorine stimulation of the specific GTPase activity are nearly identical. We have also shown that ADP-ribosylation of N_s using cholera toxin has no effect on the muscarinic-stimulated GTPase activity (12). In contrast, ADP-ribosylation of N_i using IAP reduced oxotremorine inhibition of GTP-stimulated adenylate cyclase activity from 72% to 38% (Fig. 4). In parallel, IAP treatment of the sarcolemma attenuated oxotremorine stimulation of the muscarinic-stimulated GTPase activity (Fig. 4). In summary, these experiments indicate (a) that muscarinic agonists stimulate a specific GTPase activity in cardiac sarcolemma, (b) that the muscarinic GTPase activity is not identical with the GTPase inhibited by cholera toxin, and (c) that muscarinic stimulation of this GTPase is reduced when N_i is ADP-ribosylated using IAP.

SUMMARY AND CONCLUSIONS

Many studies have suggested the general model for dually regulated adenylate cyclase systems shown in Fig. 1. Although many details are lacking even in the best-characterized systems, certain general themes emerge, greatly organizing our thinking and stimulating further thought. It appears clear that active adenylate cyclase consists of $GTP \cdot \alpha_s \cdot C$. Enzymatic activity is turned off by hydrolysis of GTP to GDP, apparently requiring the presence of both the α_s and β subunits. Muscarinic inhibition of GTP-stimulated adenylate cyclase activity appears to be mediated by N_i, although the exact role of the muscarinic-stimulated GTPase activity in this process is not unequivocally known at present. Analogous to descriptions of catecholamine-stimulated GTPase activities, the scheme depicted in Fig. 1 indicates that muscarinic agonists could appear to stimulate GTP hydrolysis by increasing substrate availability at α_i. Thus, as [γ-^{32}P]GTP exchange for GDP at N_i is stimulated by agonist-occupied muscarinic receptors, an ap-

parent muscarinic stimulation of P_i release would be observed. The distinction between muscarinic effects on guanine nucleotide exchange and/or activation of N_i and direct muscarinic stimulation of GTPase activity is important. Some investigators have suggested that the role of GTPase is simply to turn off the "activated" regulatory proteins ($\alpha_s \cdot GTP$ or $\alpha_i \cdot GTP$). In elegant reconstitution experiments, Gilman's laboratory demonstrated that the purified β subunit stimulated the rate of inactivation of $\alpha_s \cdot GTP\gamma S$. Because $GTP\gamma S$ is a relatively nonhydrolyzable GTP analog, these data might suggest that GTP hydrolysis per se is not the mechanism responsible for hormonal inhibition of adenylate cyclase. However, those investigators point out that although it is demonstrable, inhibition of the $GTP\gamma S$-activated protein by β subunits is not particularly rapid, suggesting that the affinity of $\alpha_s \cdot GTP\gamma S$ for the β subunit may be low (29).

All of our data suggest that an IAP-sensitive GTPase activity is intimately related to muscarinic inhibition of adenylate cyclase activity in canine cardiac sarcolemma. We have never observed muscarinic inhibition of basal or Gpp(NH)p-stimulated adenylate cyclase activity under any assay conditions, including low concentrations of guanine nucleotides and Mg^{2+}. The possible role of direct inhibition of the catalyst by $\alpha_i \cdot GTP$ in cardiac sarcolemma cannot be unequivocally ruled out at present because of our observation of Gpp(NH)p inhibition of the forskolin-stimulated enzyme. However, this phenomenon has generally been noted by others only in the presence of forskolin, and we have not been able to observe any effect of muscarinic agonists on Gpp(NH)p inhibition of the forskolin-stimulated enzyme. These data and those from other laboratories suggest that the physiologically significant mechanism of adenylate cyclase inhibition is an inhibitory-hormone-induced increase in the pool of β subunits (presumably released from α_i). The question remains as to the role of GTP hydrolytic activity in the inhibitory effect of these β subunits on activated α_s.

While dispelling certain apparent paradoxes presented by older studies, recent insights into the molecular details of dual hormonal regulation of adenylate cyclase activity at the same time raise exciting new questions regarding regulation of cardiac adenylate cyclase activity. What, exactly, comprises the muscarinic-stimulated GTPase activity? Is the GTP regulatory cycle for N_i significantly different in cardiac tissue than that for N_s? Are certain muscarinic effects mediated by N_i by mechanisms in addition to those related to adenylate cyclase activity? Are other GTP-binding proteins present in sarcolemma that mediate cardiac responses to muscarinic and other inhibitory receptors? It appears that GTP-binding proteins play significant pivotal roles in cardiac regulation by the autonomic nervous system. Characterization of the mechanisms underlying the functions of these GTP-binding proteins will undoubtedly add significantly to our understanding of autonomic control of cardiac performance.

ACKNOWLEDGMENTS

The authors thank Paul Cantrell and Elizabeth Price for excellent technical assistance, Terri Young for her help with the preparation and use of IAP, Dr. Erik Hewlett and Gwendolyn Meyers of the University of Virginia for their gift of *Bordetella pertussis* and suggestions for the purification of IAP, and Phil and Becky Wilson for preparing the illustrations. Studies performed in the authors' laboratories were supported by USPHS grant R01-HL-29208 and by a grant-in-aid from the American Heart Association, Indiana Affiliate (to J.W.F.).

REFERENCES

1. Aktories, K., Schultz, G., and Jacobs, K. H. (1982): Stimulation of a low K_m GTPase by inhibitors of adipocyte adenylate cyclase. *Mol. Pharmacol.*, 21:336–342.
2. Blume, A. J., and Foster, C. J. (1976): Neuroblastoma adenylate cyclase. Role of 2-chloroadenosine, prostaglandin E₁, and guanine nucleotides in regulation of activity. *J. Biol. Chem.*, 251:3399–3404.
3. Bokoch, G. M., Katada, T., Northup, J. K., Hewlett, E. L., and Gilman, A. G. (1983): Identification of the predominant substrate for ADP-ribosylation by islet activating protein. *J. Biol. Chem.*, 258:2072–2075.
4. Bokoch, G. M., Katada, T., Northup, J. K., Ui, M., and Gilman, A. G. (1984): Purification and properties of the inhibitory guanine nucleotide-binding regulatory component of adenylate cyclase. *J. Biol. Chem.*, 259:3560–3567.
5. Brandt, D. R., Pedersen, S. E., and Ross, E. M. (1983): Reconstitution of catecholamine-stimulated guanosinetriphosphatase activity. *Biochemistry*, 22:4357–4362.
6. Cassel, D., Eckstein, F., Lowe, M., and Selinger, Z. (1979): Determination of the turn-off reaction for the hormone-activated adenylate cyclase. *J. Biol. Chem.*, 254:9835–9838.
7. Cassel, D., Levkovitz, H., and Selinger, Z. (1977): The regulatory GTPase cycle of turkey erythrocyte adenylate cyclase. *J. Cyclic Nucleotide Res.*, 3:393–406.
8. Cassel, D., and Pfeuffer, T. (1978): Mechanism of cholera toxin action: Covalent modification of the guanyl nucleotide-binding protein of the adenylate cyclase system. *Proc. Natl. Acad. Sci. U.S.A.*, 75:2669–2673.
9. Cassel, D., and Selinger, D. (1976): Catecholamine-stimulated GTPase activity in turkey erythrocyte membranes. *Biochim. Biophys. Acta*, 452:538–551.
10. Codina, J., Hildebrandt, J., Sunyer, T., Sekura, R. D., Manclark, C. R., Iyengar, R., and Birnbaumer, L. (1984): Mechanisms in the vectorial receptor-adenylate cyclase signal transduction. *Adv. Cyclic Nucleotide Phosphorylation Res.*, 17:111–125.
11. Fleming, J. W., and Watanabe, A. M. (1983): Muscarinic agonists stimulate GTPase activity and inhibit adenylate cyclase activity in cardiac membranes. *Fed. Proc.*, 42:1149.
12. Fleming, J. W., and Watanabe, A. M. (1984): Requirement of a soluble factor for the [³²P]ADP-ribosylation of the cholera toxin substrate of cardiac sarcolemmal adenylate cyclase. *Fed. Proc.*, 43:1584.
13. Fleming, J. W., Young, T. L., and Watanabe, A. M. (1984): Identification of the inhibitory guanine nucleotide regulatory protein of cardiac adenylate cyclase. *Pharmacologist*, 26:164.
14. Gilman, A. G. (1984): G proteins and dual control of adenylate cyclase. *Cell*, 36:577–579.
15. Hazeki, O., and Ui, M. (1981): Modification by islet-activating protein of receptor-mediated regulation of cyclic AMP accumulation in isolated rat heart cells. *J. Biol. Chem.*, 256:2856–2862.
16. Jacobs, K. H., Aktories, K., and Schultz, G. (1979): GTP-dependent inhibition of cardiac adenylate cyclase by muscarinic cholinergic agonists. *Naunyn Schmiedebergs Arch. Pharmacol.*, 310:113–119.
17. Jacobs, K. H., Aktories, K., and Schultz, G. (1984): Mechanisms and components involved in adenylate cyclase inhibition by hormones. *Adv. Cyclic Nucleotide Phosphorylation Res.*, 17:135–143.
18. Jacobs, K. H., Schultz, G., Gaugler, B., and Pfeuffer, T. (1983): Inhibition of Nₛ-protein-stimulated human-platelet adenylate cyclase by epinephrine and stable GTP analogs. *Eur. J. Biochem.*, 134:351–354.
19. Johnson, M. L., and Frasier, S. G. (1984): Analysis of hormone binding data. In: *Methods in Diabetes Research*, edited by J. Larner and S. Pohl, Vol. I, pp. 45–61. John Wiley & Sons, New York.
20. Kanaho, Y., Tsai, S.-C., Adamik, R., Hewlett, E. L., Moss, J., and Vaughan, M. (1984): Rhodopsin-enhanced GTPase activity of the inhibitory GTP-binding protein of adenylate cyclase. *J. Biol. Chem.*, 259:7378–7381.
21. Katada, T., Bokoch, G. M., Northup, J. K., Ui, M., and Gilman, A. G. (1984): The inhibitory guanine nucleotide-binding regulatory component of adenylate cyclase. Properties and function of the purified protein. *J. Biol. Chem.*, 259:3568–3577.
22. Katada, T., Northup, J. K., Bokoch, G. M., Ui, M., and Gilman, A. G. (1984): The inhibitory guanine nucleotide-binding regulatory component of adenylate cyclase. Subunit dissociation and guanine nucleotide-dependent hormonal inhibition. *J. Biol. Chem.*, 259:3578–3585.
23. Koski, G., and Klee, W. A. (1981): Opiates inhibit adenylate cyclase by stimulating GTP hydrolysis. *Proc. Natl. Acad. Sci. U.S.A.*, 78:4185–4189.
24. Levy, M. N., and Martin, P. J. (1979): Neural control of the heart. In: *Handbook of Physiology, Section 2: The Cardiovascular System*, edited by R. M. Berne, Vol. 1, pp. 581–620. American Physiological Society, Bethesda, Md.
25. Limbird, L. E. (1981): Activation and attenuation of adenylate cyclase. The role of GTP-binding proteins as macromolecular messengers in receptor-cyclase coupling. *Biochem. J.*, 195:1–13.
26. Moss, J., and Vaughan, M. (1979): Activation of adenylate cyclase by choleragen. *Annu. Rev. Biochem.*, 48:581–600.
27. Murad, F., Chi, Y.-M., Rall, T. W., and Sutherland, E. M. (1962): Adenyl cyclase. III. The effect of catecholamines and choline esters on the formation of adenosine 3′,5′-phosphate by preparations from cardiac muscle and liver. *J. Biol. Chem.*, 237:1233–1238.
28. Murayama, T., and Ui, M. (1983): Loss of the inhibitory function of the guanine nucleotide regulatory component of adenylate cyclase due to its ADP ribosylation by islet-activating protein, pertussis toxin, in adipocyte membranes. *J. Biol. Chem.*, 258:3319–3326.
29. Northup, J. K., Smigel, M. D., Sternweis, P. C., and Gilman, A. G. (1983): The subunits of the stimulatory regulatory component of adenylate cyclase. Resolution of the activated 45,000-dalton (α) subunit. *J. Biol. Chem.*, 258:11369–11376.
30. Northup, J. K., Sternweis, P. C., and Gilman, A. G. (1983): The subunits of the stimulatory regulatory component of adenylate cyclase. Resolution, activity, and properties of the 35,000-dalton (β) subunit. *J. Biol. Chem.*, 258:11361–11368.
31. Northup, J. K., Sternweis, P. C., Smigel, M. D., Schleifer, L. S., Ross, E. M., and Gilman, A. G. (1980): Purification of the regulatory component of adenylate cyclase. *Proc. Natl. Acad. Sci. U.S.A.*, 77:6516–6520.
32. Pfeuffer, T. (1977): GTP-binding proteins in membranes and the control of adenylate cyclase activity. *J. Biol. Chem.*, 252:7224–7234.
33. Pfeuffer, T., and Helmreich, E. J. M. (1975): Activation of pigeon erythrocyte membrane adenylate cyclase by guanylnucleotide analogues and separation of a nucleotide binding protein. *J. Biol. Chem.*, 250:867–876.
34. Rodbell, M. (1980): The role of hormone receptors and GTP-

regulatory proteins in membrane transduction. *Nature,* 284:17–22.

35. Ross, E. M., and Gilman, A. G. (1980): Biochemical properties of hormone-sensitive adenylate cyclase. *Annu. Rev. Biochem.,* 49:533–564.

36. Ross, E. M., Maguire, M. E., Sturgill, T. W., Biltonen, R. L., and Gilman, A. G. (1977): Relationship between the β-adrenergic receptor and adenylate cyclase. Studies of ligand binding and enzyme activity in purified membranes of S49 lymphoma cells. *J. Biol. Chem.,* 252:5761–5775.

37. Schramm, M., and Selinger, Z. (1984): Message transmission: Receptor controlled adenylate cyclase system. *Science,* 225:1350–1356.

38. Seamon, K., and Daly, J. W. (1981): Activation of adenylate cyclase by the diterpene forskolin does not require the guanine nucleotide regulatory protein. *J. Biol. Chem.,* 256:9799–9801.

39. Seamon, K. B., and Daly, J. W. (1982): Guanosine 5′-(β,γ-imido)triphosphate inhibition of forskolin-activated adenylate cyclase is mediated by the putative inhibitory guanine nucleotide regulatory protein. *J. Biol. Chem.,* 257:11591–11596.

40. Smigel, M., Katada, T., Northup, J. K., Bokoch, G. M., Ui, M., and Gilman, A. G. (1984): Mechanisms of guanine nucleotide-mediated regulation of adenylate cyclase activity. *Adv. Cyclic Nucleotide Protein Phosphorylation Res.,* 17:1–18.

41. Sternweis, P. C., Northup, J. K., Hanski, E., Schleifer, L. S., Smigel, M. D., and Gilman, A. G. (1981): Purification and properties of the regulatory component (G/F) of adenylate cyclase. *Adv. Cyclic Nucleotide Res.,* 14:23–36.

42. Sunyer, T., Codina, J., and Birnbaumer, L. (1984): GTP hydrolysis by pure N_i, the inhibitory regulatory component of adenylyl cyclases. *J. Biol. Chem.,* 259:15447–15451.

43. Ui, M., Katada, T., Murayama, T., Kurose, H., Yajima, M., Tamura, M., Nakamura, T., and Nogimori, K. (1984): Islet-activating protein, pertussis toxin: A specific uncoupler of receptor-mediated inhibition of adenylate cyclase. *Adv. Cyclic Nucleotide Protein Phosphorylation Res.,* 17:145–151.

44. Watanabe, A. M. (1984): Cellular mechanisms of muscarinic regulation of cardiac function. *In: Nervous Control of Cardiac Function,* edited by W. Randall, pp. 130–164. Oxford University Press, New York.

45. Watanabe, A. M., McConnaughey, M. M., Strawbridge, R. A., Fleming, J. W., Jones, L. R., and Besch, H. R., Jr. (1978): Muscarinic cholinergic receptor modulation of β-adrenergic receptor affinity for catecholamines. *J. Biol. Chem.,* 253:4833–4836.

The Heart and Cardiovascular System,
edited by H. A. Fozzard et al.
Raven Press, New York © 1986.

CHAPTER 72

Cardiovascular Growth Factors

Lewis T. Williams and Shaun R. Coughlin

Local stimulation of cell proliferation is fundamental to processes such as wound healing, neovascularization, tissue regeneration, fibrosis, atherosclerosis, and tumor formation. During the last decade, many new data have suggested that an important mechanistic feature shared by these local perturbations in cell growth is local release and action of growth-promoting compounds.

In the cardiovascular system, growth factors mediate several clinically important phenomena. The development of atherosclerotic plaques involves proliferation of smooth muscle cells in the blood vessel wall, a process that is stimulated by platelet-derived growth factor (PDGF). This factor is also likely to be important in the intense intimal thickening seen almost universally in vein bypass grafts placed into the arterial circulation. When proliferation of smooth muscle cells is especially intense, the vein lumen can be narrowed to a clinically significant extent. Another cell type, the vascular endothelial cell, is maintained by a distinct set of growth-promoting substances and may play a protective role by providing a nonthrombogenic surface for platelets. Thus, restoration of the integrity of the endothelial lining of a blood vessel may be important in preventing the development of smooth muscle proliferation in regions of endothelial damage caused by hemodynamic, metabolic, or mechanical insults. A recently described property of endothelial cells, the production of a PDGF-like growth factor, may also be involved in the interaction between endothelial cells and smooth muscle cells (3,16). Finally, hypertrophy of myocardial cells is also likely to be mediated by polypeptide factors and catecholamines (27,46). Although these cells do not divide, their hyper-

trophic responses to growth-promoting substances may be mechanistically similar to the proliferative responses of vascular tissue.

The purpose of this chapter is to review some pathological processes in the cardiovascular system that appear to involve growth factors and their receptors. Special emphasis will be placed on the specific growth factors known to be important in proliferation of cardiovascular tissues. Included in the discussion is speculation on future directions in growth factor research and on how these studies might be useful in understanding cardiovascular disease.

BLOOD VESSELS: ATHEROGENESIS AND INTIMAL PROLIFERATION

Normal blood vessels consist of an endothelial cell layer, an internal elastic lamina, and the vascular media composed of connective tissue and vascular smooth muscle cells. In the localized lesions of atherosclerosis there is intense proliferation of smooth muscle cells and migration of these cells through the internal elastic lamina to the intimal region. This proliferation is especially prominent in fibrous plaques and even in advanced atherosclerotic lesions. Although the relative roles of the proliferative response and the deposition of lipid have been debated, it is likely that both processes are important in the progression of atherosclerotic lesions. In experimental models a similar proliferation of smooth muscle cells is seen following chemical or mechanical injury to the endothelium. By analogy, atherosclerotic lesions may be initiated following subtle injury to the endothelium, caused, for example, by hypercholesterolemia or hypertension, and consequent activation of platelets, with release of their granule contents into the vessel wall and stimulation of cell proliferation by PDGF. The evidence that platelet factors are involved in this process came from studies in which thrombocytopenic animals developed less extensive plaques than control animals following endothelial injury (37). Other studies have found that antiplatelet drugs ameliorate atherosclerosis in rabbits (7) and that pigs with von Willebrand's disease develop less atherosclerosis than their normal counterparts (6). In 1976, Ross and associates provided further support for the proposed role of platelets in atherogenesis when they described a material released from platelets that induces proliferation of cultured vascular smooth muscle cells (42,43). This material was termed PDGF and was subsequently purified by several groups of investigators. It is likely that PDGF is involved not only in atherosclerotic lesions but also in the smooth muscle cell proliferation observed in coronary artery bypass grafts (48) and perhaps in the recurrence of atherosclerosis following angioplasty procedures.

PDGF

PDGF is a potent mitogen for fibroblasts, vascular smooth muscle cells, and glial cells in culture (1). It is normally not present in substantial amounts in plasma, but is released when platelets are activated by chemical or physical stimuli. Vascular smooth muscle cells are highly responsive to the mitogenic effects of PDGF, but endothelial cells apparently are not responsive (22). PDGF has been purified by several groups of investigators by following its activity as a mitogen for cultured fibroblasts (1,15). Although it can be isolated from whole serum or from supernatants of activated platelet preparations, it is most easily purified from lysates of intact human outdated platelets. The purification relies heavily on the cationic nature of PDGF (PI = 10) and the avidity of PDGF for hydrophobic resins such as blue Sepharose. The purified protein is a glycoprotein with a molecular mass in the range of 32 to 35 kd. PDGF binds tenaciously to tissues and to plastic and glass substrates. It is stable to heating and to both acid and base treatment, but its activity is rapidly lost following reduction and alkylation. The 32-kd PDGF molecule consists of at least two polypeptides (A and B) that are linked through disulfide bonds. Its primary structure is not related to those of other known growth factors. However, the N-terminal 109 amino acids of the B polypeptide chain of PDGF are virtually identical with the predicted sequence of the transforming protein p28^{sis} of simian sarcoma virus (SSV) (17,50). Tumor cells transformed by SSV produce and release large amounts of a protein that is functionally indistinguishable from

PDGF and is encoded by the v-*sis* sequence of the viral genome (23,29,39). The released PDGF-like protein acts on cell surface PDGF receptors to cause a continuous mitogenic response by an "autocrine" mechanism, thus making the cells independent of exogenously added growth factors. The growth properties of these transformed cells can be altered by blocking the interaction of the released PDGF-like peptides with the cell surface receptors (23,29). This area of research is of potential clinical importance in oncology, because several lines of human tumor cells are known to express high levels of PDGF-like peptides. In addition, vascular smooth muscle cells have recently been found to be capable of producing a PDGF-like growth factor. Thus, a similar autocrine mechanism could contribute to the intimal proliferation of atherogenesis.

Chromosome 22 of the human genome contains the proto-oncogene c-*sis* that encodes the B chain of PDGF (33). From the standpoint of the cardiovascular system, it is intriguing that vascular endothelial cells have relatively high levels of c-*sis* RNA and produce a molecule that has PDGF-like functional properties, even though these cells lack PDGF receptors. The role of endothelial-derived *sis*-encoded protein in atherosclerosis and endothelial injury is not yet clear, but it suggests the potential for paracrine stimulation of smooth muscle cell proliferation.

The action of PDGF in stimulating mitogenesis of cultured cells is especially prominent early in the cell cycle (1). In one specific cell type, the BALB/c 3T3 cell, PDGF induces a state of "competence" that confers on the cell the ability to respond to subsequent addition of other growth factors termed "progression" factors. For most cultured cells, PDGF alone does not give a maximal mitogenic response; other supporting growth factors are usually required. However, for a few cell types, such as glial cells, PDGF can support growth in almost total absence of other growth-promoting substances. Because PDGF is not normally found in plasma, its effects are often measured on cells in the presence of plasma. The circulating levels of PDGF in plasma are extraordinarily low and are below the level required to activate PDGF receptors. However, the level of PDGF present in serum is high enough to provide at least half occupancy of PDGF receptors.

PDGF RECEPTORS

PDGF triggers the sequence of intracellular events leading to DNA replication by first binding to specific cell surface receptors. The PDGF receptor has been characterized by radioligand binding and cross-linking studies as a 180-kd plasma membrane glycoprotein with high affinity and specificity for PDGF (4,28,51). Like the receptors for epidermal growth factor (EGF), insulin, and somatomedin C, the PDGF receptor is closely coupled to tyrosine kinase activity, which is maximally stimulated when the receptor is occupied. PDGF receptors are found on 3T3 cells, diploid human fibroblasts, arterial smooth muscle cells, and other connective tissue cells from several species. Lymphoid cells (peripheral blood lymphocytes), epithelial cells, endothelial cells, and some transformed cells do not have binding sites for ^{125}I-PDGF (4,9). The number of receptors in responsive cells is approximately 100,000 sites per cell. These receptors have an equilibrium dissociation constant of approximately 0.1 nM (ranging from 0.01 nM to 1 nM in studies by various authors) (4,28).

The mechanism by which PDGF receptors initiate the intracellular events leading to DNA replication is not known. It is clear that the PDGF response is one of the earliest hormone responses in the cell cycle (49). An exposure of cells to PDGF for only an hour, or less, is sufficient to commit the cells to progression to DNA replication, assuming the culture medium contains other factors such as EGF and somatomedin C that act at later phases in the cell cycle. Like other polypeptide hormone receptors, the PDGF receptor internalizes during its activation (28). Early responses to receptor occupation include rapid stimulation of the turnover of phosphatidylinositol in the membrane (26), alterations in cellular pH (9), and stimulation of transcription of the fos and myc proto-oncogenes and several other RNA species that are as yet undefined (10,35). Because the fos and myc gene inductions are associated with a number of mitogenic stimuli, their importance has recently been emphasized.

Much attention has also focused on the activation of tyrosine kinase that occurs when PDGF binds to its receptor. The possible role of tyrosine-specific protein kinase in PDGF action has been supported by observations that other mitogenic hormones such as EGF (8), insulin (34), somatomedin C (30), and the tumor growth factors (40) are potent activators of receptor-associated tyrosine kinases. Additional evidence implicating phosphotyrosine in growth control has come from studies of oncogenic retroviruses, where it was found that the ability of the viruses to transform cells was critically dependent on the presence of active, virally encoded tyrosine kinases (45). The relationships among the cellular activities associated with PDGF action are not clear, and their relative importances in mediating mitogenic responses remain to be determined.

RELATIONSHIP OF THE PDGF RECEPTOR TO OTHER GROWTH FACTOR RECEPTORS

The PDGF receptor shares with the receptors for EGF, insulin, and somatomedin C the ability to stimulate tyrosine kinase activity. However, the PDGF receptor is clearly a distinct molecular entity, because its ligand

binding characteristics, molecular size, isoelectric point, and tissue distribution are different from those for the other receptors. In addition, its mechanism of action appears to be different, at least in part, because it is more effective earlier in the cell cycle than the other known growth factors, with the possible exception of fibroblast growth factor.

The recent finding that the EGF receptor is encoded by c-erb, the proto-oncogene of the v-erb gene of avian erythroblastosis virus (18), has raised the question whether or not the PDGF receptor is also encoded by a cellular counterpart of an oncogene. At the time of this writing, no such relationship is known for the PDGF receptor. Receptor sequence information should provide insight into this issue in the near future.

UNRESOLVED ISSUES

There have been numerous major advances and unexpected findings in the field of growth factor research in the last 3 years. Most of the mitogenic responses to PDGF and other platelet growth factors have been studied in cultured cell systems. However, there has never been a convincing demonstration that these growth factors are operative in vivo. This lack of documentation is more related to the difficulty in performing appropriate experiments than to negative findings. For example, because these growth factors act locally at sites of platelet activation, their in vivo action is normally restricted to a very localized area where the growth factor is deposited. Experimentally it is very difficult to mimic this situation in vivo. For this reason, documentation of the roles of growth factors in vascular repair and in atherosclerosis has become an important issue. When specific blockers for these factors are available, this issue will be easier to address. Other unresolved issues in this field include the following:

1. What is the structure of the PDGF receptor? Is it related to one of the oncogenes? What are the functional domains of the receptor? How is the expression of the receptor regulated?
2. What is the mechanism by which the receptor transmits a mitogenic signal to the nucleus?
3. What are the roles of the PDGF system in atherogenesis, in the proliferative response seen after endothelial denudation, and in coronary artery bypass grafts? Are other growth factors involved? Will receptor antagonists prevent these responses?
4. How are PDGF receptors involved in normal growth and differentiation, in carcinogenesis, and in disease in which there is local abnormal proliferation of mesenchymal cells (e.g., scleroderma, keloid formation, glomerulonephritis, pulmonary fibrosis).
5. What is the role of the PDGF-like peptides produced by endothelial cells? Are these peptides involved in

the smooth muscle proliferation in response to endothelial injury? Are they important in new blood vessel formation?

6. Do some patients have abnormal levels of PDGF or hyperresponsive PDGF receptors?

OTHER GROWTH FACTORS FROM PLATELETS

Ross and associates clearly demonstrated that platelets contain mitogenic activity for fibroblasts and smooth muscle cells. Purification of this mitogenic activity led to the discovery of PDGF. However, for several years it was not recognized that platelets contain more than one mitogenic compound. Within the last few years, two additional mitogens have been isolated from human platelets. These include a growth factor that binds to epidermal growth factor receptors and mimics the action of epidermal growth factor *in vitro* (2). The third factor isolated from platelets is a factor termed transforming growth factor beta (2). This growth factor was first discovered by its ability to potentiate the growth of cells in soft agar, a characteristic of transformed cells. The growth responses of cells to this mitogen are extremely complex and are currently under investigation in several laboratories. The finding of these three growth factors in platelets shows that platelets contain all the factors necessary to support proliferation of fibroblasts and vascular smooth muscle cells.

Monocyte-Derived Growth Factors

One of the first observable changes early in atherosclerotic lesions is infiltration of the plaque by mononuclear cells that presumably are derived from the circulation. Several investigators have demonstrated the presence of growth factor activity in cultured mononuclear cells and have shown that this activity stimulates the growth of 3T3 cells and mesenchymal cells (36,41). Thus, circulating mononuclear cells may provide a source of mitogens in early atherosclerotic lesions and in neovascularization. Whether mononuclear cells contain a single polypeptide growth factor or multiple factors has not been conclusively determined. Several of these factors, including interleukin I, endogenous pyrogen, and monocyte-derived growth factor, are likely to be closely related or identical molecules.

Other Growth-Promoting Substances for Smooth Muscle Cells

It is likely that other plasma peptides such as insulin, somatomedin C, and epidermal growth factor may be involved in proliferative responses of smooth muscle cells. In addition, certain lipoproteins, cell-cell interac-tions, cell-matrix interactions, and platelet-released serotonin may play important roles in supporting the complex process of cell growth (12,24,25).

ENDOTHELIAL CELL GROWTH

Human vascular epithelial cells serve a number of important physiological functions. Normally the endothelial lining of blood vessels is relatively quiescent, and the low level of cell proliferation is probably a method for slow cell replacement. However, this slow pattern of growth can be increased dramatically by a number of stimuli, including damage of the blood vessel. Following endothelial damage, the subendothelial region of the blood vessel is exposed, and platelet aggregation and adhesion occur rapidly, leading to release of growth factors that act on the underlying smooth muscle cells. Thus, the endothelium serves a protective function in that it provides a nonthrombogenic surface and a barrier against mitogenic platelet products. In addition, recent studies have demonstrated that endothelial cells produce and release a number of PDGF-like materials that may also stimulate vascular smooth muscle proliferation (3,16). Regulation of the release of these peptides from endothelial cells has not been studied, and the roles of these compounds in atherogenesis and vascular injury are unknown.

Until the 1970s it was difficult to study endothelial cells directly, because they represent only a small percentage of the total cell population of the blood vessel. The significant advances in this field were based on the ability to grow endothelial cells in culture and to study these cells as a distinct tissue type. Endothelial cells have been cultured from human umbilical vein (31) and lung (32), bovine capillaries (20), rat brain capillaries (14), bovine aorta (47), rabbit aorta, and swine aorta (47). For each of these cell types there is a specific set of conditions, including the presence of exogenous growth factors, for optimal growth in culture. Despite differences among these specific cell types, there are some generalizations that can be made with respect to growth factor requirements. For most endothelial cells, PDGF does not seem to play a significant role in cell proliferation. However, fibroblast growth factor, a polypeptide isolated from brain or pituitary (24), stimulates the growth of most endothelial cells and is required for optimal growth and passaging of some endothelial cells. Another effective mitogen for most endothelial cells is macrophage-derived growth factor, a polypeptide released by activated monocytes or macrophages. Another polypeptide extracted from brain, endothelial cell growth factor, has been reported to enhance proliferation of human umbilical vein endothelial cells plated at low densities. This material has been purified by several groups of investigators. Finally, endothelial cells appear to have the ability to "self-condition" their media. That is, material produced and released by endothelial cells appears to stimulate the growth of other endothelial cells. The significance of this finding *in vivo* has not been determined. Thus, the area of growth factor research for endothelial cells is a complex field. During the next few years it will be important to determine if findings *in vitro* can be extrapolated to *in vivo* systems and whether or not certain growth factors are specific for the endothelial cells in specific vascular beds.

MYOCARDIAL HYPERTROPHY

Myocardial hypertrophy is a common occurrence *in vivo*. This response of cardiac cells appears to be cell hypertrophy in the classic sense, because adult myocardial cells do not proliferate. In recent years there have been several attempts to identify substances that mediate myocardial hypertrophy. Hammond et al. (27) demonstrated that extracts from hypertrophying dog hearts initiate synthesis of messenger RNA and stimulate hypertrophy when perfused through isolated rat hearts. Precise identification of the factor(s) responsible for this activity has not been reported. Simpson (46) has taken a more defined approach by demonstrating that non-epinephrine stimulates hypertrophy of cultured rat myocardial cells through an α_1-adrenergic mechanism. These studies were the first to demonstrate a clear direct effect of a growth-promoting substance on cardiac cells *in vitro*. This area of research should provide insight on the complex phenomenon of hypertrophy *in vivo*, as well as provide model systems for studying the molecular mechanism of the hypertrophic response.

REFERENCES

1. Antoniades, H. N., Scher, C. D., and Stiles, C. D. (1979): Purification of platelet-derived growth factor. *Proc. Natl. Acad. Sci. U.S.A.,* 76:1809–1813.
2. Assoian, R. K., Grotendorst, G. R., Miller, D. M., and Sporn, M. D. (1984): Cellular transformation by coordinated action of those peptide growth factors from human platelets. *Nature,* 309:804–806.
3. Barrett, T. B., Gajdusek, C. M., Schwartz, S. M., McDougall, J. K., and Benditt, E. P. (1984): Expression of the sis gene by endothelial cells in culture and *in vivo. Proc. Natl. Acad. Sci. U.S.A.,* 81:6772–6774.
4. Bowen-Pope, D. F., and Ross, R. (1982): Platelet-derived growth factor-specific binding to cultured cells. *J. Biol. Chem.,* 257:5161–5166.
5. Bowen-Pope, D. F., Vogel, A., and Ross, R. (1984): Production of PDGF-like molecules and reduced expression of PDGF receptors accompany transformation by a wide spectrum of agent. *Proc. Natl. Acad. Sci. U.S.A.,* 81:2396–2400.
6. Bowie, E., Fuster, V., Owen, C. A., and Brown, A. L. (1975): Resistance to the development of spontaneous atherosclerosis in pigs with von Willebrand's disease. *Thromb. Diath. Haemorrh.,* 34:599.
7. Burns, E. R., Friedman, R., Puszkin, E. G., et al. (1976): The effects of dipyridamole and aspirin on arterial sclerotic plaque formation in rabbits. *Circulation,* 54:138A.
8. Carpenter, G. (1984): Properties of the receptor for epidermal growth factor. *Cell,* 37:3573–3578.
9. Cassel, D., et al. (1983): Platelet-derived growth factor stimulates

10. Na/H exchange and induces cytoplasmic alkalinization in NR6 cells. *Proc. Natl. Acad. Sci. U.S.A.,* 80:6224–6228.
10. Cochran, B. H., Zullo, J., Verma, I. M., and Stiles, C. D. (1984): Expression of the c-fos gene and of an fos-related gene is stimulated by PDGF. *Science,* 226:1080–1082.
11. Cooper, J. A., Bowen-Pope, D. F., Raines, E., Ross, R., and Hunter, T. (1982): Similar effects of platelet-derived growth factor and epidermal growth factor on the phosphorylation of tyrosine in cellular proteins. *Cell,* 31:263–268.
12. Coughlin, S. R., and Moskowitz, M. (1981): Serotonin stimulates mitogenesis of vascular smooth muscle cells. *Circulation [Suppl.],* 54:1100 (abstract).
13. Daniel, T. O., Frackelton, A. R., Jr., Tremble, P. M., and Williams, L. T. (1985): Purification of the platelet-derived growth factor receptor using an antiphosphotyrosine antibody. *Proc. Natl. Acad. Sci. USA,* 82:2684–2687.
14. Debault, L. E., Kahn, L. E., Frommes, S. P., and Cancilla, P. A. (1979): Cerebral micro vessels in derived cells in tissue culture: Isolation and preliminary characterization. *In Vitro,* 15:473–487.
15. Deuel, T. F., Huang, J. S., Proffitt, R. T., et al. (1981): Human platelet-derived growth factor: Purification and resolution into two active protein fractions. *J. Biol. Chem.,* 256:8896–8899.
16. Corleto, D., and Bowen-Pope, D. F. (1983): Cultured endothelial cells produce a platelet-derived growth factor-like protein. *Proc. Natl. Acad. Sci. U.S.A.,* 80:1919–1923.
17. Doolittle, R. F., Hunkapiller, M. W., Hood, L. E., et al. (1983): Simian sarcoma virus oncogene v-sis is derived from the gene encoding a platelet-derived growth factor. *Science,* 221:275–277.
18. Downward, J., Yarden, Y., Mayes, E., et al. (1984): Close similarity of epidermal growth factor receptor and v-erb-B oncogene protein sequences. *Nature,* 307:521–526.
19. Ek, B., and Heldin, C.-H. (1982): Characterization of a tyrosine specific kinase activity in human fibroblast membranes stimulated by platelet-derived growth factor. *J. Biol. Chem.,* 257:10486–10491.
20. Folkman, J., Haudenschield, C. C., and Zetter, B. R. (1979): Long term culture of capillary endothelial cells. *Proc. Natl. Acad. Sci. U.S.A.,* 76:5217–5221.
21. Frackelton, A. R., Jr., Tremble, P. M., and Williams, L. T. (1984): Evidence for the platelet-derived growth factor stimulated tyrosine phosphorylation of the platelet-derived growth factor receptor *in vivo. J. Biol. Chem.,* 259:7907–7915.
22. Gajdusek, C. M., and Schwartz, S. M. (1984): Growth requirements for bovine aortic endothelium *in vitro.* In: *Endothelial Cells,* edited by E. A. Jaffe, pp. 59–63. Martinus Nijhoff, Boston.
23. Garrett, J. S., Coughlin, S. R., Niman, H. L., Tremble, P. M., Giels, G. M., and Williams, L. T. (1984): Blockade of autocrine stimulation in simian sarcoma virus transformed cells. *Science,* 221:1348–1350.
24. Gospodarowicz, D., Moran, J., Braun, D., and Birdwell, C. (1976): Clonal growth of bovine vascular endothelial cells: Fibroblast growth factor as a survival agent. *Proc. Natl. Acad. Sci. U.S.A.,* 73:4120–4124.
25. Gospodarowicz, D., and Dill, C. (1980): Extracellular matrix and control of proliferation of vascular endothelial cells. *J. Clin. Invest.,* 65:1351–1364.
26. Habenicht, A. J. R., Glomset, J. A., King, W., et al. (1981): Early changes in phosphatidylinositol and arachidonic acid metabolism in quiescent Swiss 3T3 cells stimulated to divide by PDGF. *J. Biol. Chem.,* 256:12329–12335.
27. Hammond, G. L., Lai, Y.-K., and Markert, C. L. (1982): Molecules that initiate cardiac hypertrophy are species specific. *Science,* 216:529–531.
28. Heldin, C.-H., Ek, B., and Ronnstrand, L. (1983): Characterization of the receptor for platelet-derived growth factor on human fibroblast. *J. Biol. Chem.,* 258:10054–10059.
29. Huang, J. S., Huang, S. S., and Deuel, T. F. (1984): Transforming protein of simian sarcoma virus stimulates autocrine growth of SSV-transformed cells through PDGF cell surface receptors. *Cell,* 39:79–87.
30. Jacobs, S., Kull, F. C., and Earp, H. S. (1983): Somatomedin-C stimulates the phosphorylation of the beta-subunit of its own receptor. *J. Biol. Chem.,* 258:9581–9584.
31. Jaffe, E. A., Nachman, R. L., Becker, C. G., and Minick, C. R. (1973): Culture of human endothelial cells derived from umbilical

veins. Identification by morphological and immunologic bacteria. *J. Clin. Invest.,* 52:2745–2756.

32. Johnson, A. R., and Erdos, E. G. (1977): Metabolism of vasoactive peptides by human endothelial cells in culture: Angiotensin I converting enzyme and angiotensinase. *J. Clin. Invest.,* 59:684–695.

33. Josephs, S. F., Gallo, C., Ratner, L., and Wong-Staal, F. (1984): Human proto-oncogene nucleotide sequences corresponding to the transforming region of simian sarcoma virus. *Science,* 23:487–491.

34. Kasuga, M., Fujita-Yamaguchi, Y., Blithe, D. L., and Kahn, C. R. (1983): Tyrosine specific protein kinase activity is associated with the purified insulin receptor. *Proc. Natl. Acad. Sci. U.S.A.,* 80:2137–2141.

35. Kelly, K., Cochran, B. H., Stiles, C. D., and Leder, P. (1983): Cells specific regulation of the c-*myc* gene by lymphocyte mitogens and PDGF. *Cell,* 35:603–610.

36. Martin, B. M., Gimbrone, M. A., Jr., Unanue, E. R., and Coltrain, R. S. (1981): Stimulation of nonlymphoid mesenchymal cell proliferation by a macrophage-derived growth factor. *J. Immunol.,* 126:1510–1515.

37. Moore, S., Friedman, R., Singal, D., et al. (1976): Inhibition of injury induced thromboatherosclerotic lesions by anti-platelet serum in rabbits. *Thromb. Diath. Haemorrh.,* 35:70–81.

38. Nishimura, J., Huang, J. S., and Deuel, T. F. (1982): Platelet-derived growth factor stimulates tyrosine specific protein kinase activity in Swiss mouse 3T3 cell membranes. *J. Biol. Chem.,* 258:9383–9388.

39. Owen, A. J., Pantazis, P., and Antoniades, H. N. (1984): Simian sarcoma virus-transformed cells secrete a mitogen identical to platelet-derived growth factor. *Science,* 225:54–56.

40. Pike, L. J., Marquart, H., Todaro, G. J., et al. (1982): Transforming growth factor and epidermal growth factor stimulate the phos-

41. Polverini, P. J., Coltrain, R. S., Gimbrone, M. A., Jr., and Unanue, E. R. (1977): Activated macrophages induce vascular proliferation. *Nature,* 269:804–806.

42. Ross, R., and Glomset, J. A. (1973): Atherosclerosis and the arterial smooth muscle cell. *Science,* 180:1332–1339.

43. Ross, R., and Glomset, J. A. (1976): The pathogenesis of atherosclerosis. *N. Engl. J. Med.,* 295:369–377.

44. Schwartz, S. M. (1978): Selection and characterization of bovine aortic endothelial cells. *In Vitro,* 14:966–980.

45. Sefton, B., et al. (1980): Evidence that the phosphorylation of tyrosine is essential for cellular transformation by Rous sarcoma virus. *Cell,* 20:807–816.

46. Simpson, P. (1983): Norepinephrine-stimulated hypertrophy of cultured myocardial cells is in alpha$_1$ adernergic response. *J. Clin. Invest.,* 72:732–738.

47. Slater, D. N., and Sloan, J. M. (1975): The porcine endothelial cell in tissue culture. *Atherosclerosis,* 21:259–272.

48. Spray, T. L., and Roberts, W. C. (1977): Changes in saphenous veins used as aorta coronary bypass grafts. *Am. Heart J.,* 94:500–516.

49. Stiles, C. D. (1983): The molecular biology of platelet-derived growth factor. *Cell,* 33:653–655.

50. Waterfield, M. D., Scrace, T., Whittle, N., et al. (1983): Platelet-derived growth factor is structurally related to the putitive transforming protein p28^{sis} of simian sarcoma virus. *Nature,* 304:35–39.

51. Williams, L. T., Tremble, P. M., Lavin, M., and Sunday, M. E. (1984): Platelet-derived growth factor receptors in membrane preparations: Kinetics and affinity cross-linking studies. *J. Biol. Chem.,* 259:5287–5292.

phorylation of a synthetic tyrosine-containing peptide in a similar manner. *J. Biol. Chem.,* 257:14628–14631.

Subject Index

Subject Index